Obstetrics and Gynecology

Principles for Practice

To my wife, Janis, who has modeled the faith-filled life,
who has dedicated herself to serving others, and
who has patiently taught me the importance of priorities.
Thank you for the constant joy and love
that you send to Mandy, Trevor, and me.
"For 80 years."

—*Frank W. Ling, M.D.*

I dedicate this book to my wife of 32 years, Judy.
Thank you for enriching beyond measure my life and the lives of our four children.
Thank you also for teaching me so much about the importance
of having compassion, sensitivity, and a kind, gentle heart.

—*Patrick Duff, M.D.*

Contents

Contributors

Patricia Adams-Graves, M.D.
Department of Medicine
Division of Hematology
University of Tennessee
Memphis, Tennessee

Melissa Appleton, M.D.
Assistant Professor of Medicine
Director of Adult Special Care Clinic
University of Tennessee
Memphis, Tennessee

Charles R.B. Beckmann, M.D.
Chief
Women's Health/Obstetrics & Gynecology
Samuel U. Rodgers Community Health Center
and
Clinical Professor
Department of Obstetrics & Gynecology
University of Missouri at Kansas City School of Medicine
Kansas City, Missouri

Amy Boardman, M.D.
Assistant Professor
Division of General Obstetrics & Gynecology
Department of Obstetrics & Gynecology
University of South Florida College of Medicine
Tampa, Florida

Candace S. Brown, Pharm.D., CFNP
Professor
Departments of Pharmacy Practice & Pharmacoeconomics,
    Obstetrics & Gynecology, and Medicine
Colleges of Medicine and Pharmacy
University of Tennessee, Memphis
Memphis, Tennessee

Cynthia G. Brumfield, M.D.
Professor of Obstetrics & Gynecology
Division of Maternal–Fetal Medicine
Medical Director of University Obstetrical Service
The University of Alabama at Birmingham
Birmingham, Alabama

Michael Bryer-Ash, M.D.
Associate Professor of Medicine and Biochemistry
Department of Medicine
University of Tennessee
and
Associate Director
General Clinical Research Center
Medical Staff Endocrinologist
Veterans Administration Medical Center
    and University Medical Center
Memphis, Tennessee

David J. Burchfield, M.D.
Professor of Pediatrics & Physiology
Department of Pediatrics
Sharrds Children's Hospital at the University of Florida
Gainesville, Florida

Eleanor Capeless, M.D.
Professor and Vice Chairman
Division of Maternal–Fetal Medicine
Department of Obstetrics & Gynecology
University of Vermont
and
Vice Chairman and Director of Obstetrics
Division of Maternal–Fetal Medicine
Department of Obstetrics & Gynecology
Fletcher Allen Health Care
Burlington, Vermont

Laura Carbone, M.D.
Associate Professor
Department of Medicine
University of Tennessee
Memphis, Tennessee

Robert C. Cefalo, M.D., Ph.D.
Professor of Obstetrics & Gynecology
Director of Maternal–Fetal Medicine
University of North Carolina School of Medicine
Chapel Hill, North Carolina

Beth Choby, M.D.
Resident
Department of Family Medicine
University of Tennessee
Memphis, Tennessee

Gregory E. Chow, M.D.
Associate Program Director
Department of Obstetrics & Gynecology
Madigan Army Medical Center
Fort Lewis, Washington

Mary D'Alton, M.D.
Professor of Clinical Obstetrics & Gynecology
Columbia University College of Physicians & Surgeons
Director, Division of Maternal–Fetal Medicine
Department of Obstetrics & Gynecology
New York Presbyterian Hospital
New York, New York

Jed Delmore, M.D.
Professor
Director, Division of Gynecologic Oncology
Department of Obstetrics & Gynecology
University of Kansas School of Medicine—Wichita
Wichita, Kansas

Patrick Duff, M.D.
Professor and Residency Program Director
Department of Obstetrics & Gynecology
University of Florida College of Medicine
Gainesville, Florida

Robert S. Egerman, M.D.
Associate Professor
Division of Maternal–Fetal Medicine
Department of Obstetrics & Gynecology
University of Tennessee
Memphis, Tennessee

Joseph N. Fisher, M.D.
Professor of Medicine & Pediatrics
Department of Medicine
University of Tennessee Health Science Center
and
Chief of Medicine
University of Tennessee Bowld Hospital
Memphis, Tennessee

James Franks, M.D.
Resident
Department of Family Medicine
University of Tennessee
Memphis, Tennessee

A. Gordon Fry III, M.D.
Assistant Professor
Division of Maternal–Fetal Medicine
Department of Obstetrics & Gynecology
University of Rochester
Rochester, New York

Nancy S. Fuller, M.D.
Assistant Professor of Medicine
Division of General Internal Medicine
Department of Medicine
University of Tennessee
Memphis, Tennessee

Randall K. Gibb, M.D.
Assistant Professor
Department of Obstetrics & Gynecology
Division of Gynecologic Oncology
Washington University School of Medicine
St. Louis, Missouri

Carol A. Glowacki, M.D.
Department of Obstetrics & Gynecology
Stanford University School of Medicine
Stanford, California

Alice R. Goepfert, M.D.
Assistant Professor
Department of Obstetrics & Gynecology
University of Alabama at Birmingham
Birmingham, Alabama

Laura Goetzl, M.D.
Maternal–Fetal Medicine Fellow
Division of Maternal–Fetal Medicine
Department of Obstetrics & Gynecology
New England Medical Center
Boston, Massachusetts

Michael F. Greene, M.D.
Associate Professor
Department of Obstetrics, Gynecology,
    and Reproductive Biology
Harvard Medical School
and
Director of Maternal–Fetal Medicine
Department of Obstetrics & Gynecology
Massachusetts General Hospital
Boston, Massachusetts

Jennifer Gunter, M.D.
Assistant Professor
Department of Obstetrics & Gynecology
The University of Kansas
Kansas City, Kansas

James A. Hall, M.D.
Clinical Associate Professor
Department of Obstetrics & Gynecology
Indiana University
Indianapolis, Indiana
and
Private Practice
Women's Health Center of Logansport
Logansport, Indiana

Terri H. Henson, M.D.
Dermatology Clinic of North Mississippi
Southaven, Mississippi

Douglas Horbelt, M.D.
Professor and Chairman
Department of Obstetrics & Gynecology
University of Kansas School of Medicine—Wichita
Wichita, Kansas

Lynda Hudon, M.D.
Assistant Professor
Division of Maternal–Fetal Medicine
Department of Obstetrics & Gynecology
University of Montreal
Ste-Justine Hospital
Montreal, Quebec, Canada

Thomas A. Hughes, M.D.
Professor of Medicine
Division of Endocrinology
Department of Medicine
University of Tennessee
Memphis, Tennessee

Christopher F. James, M.D.
Assistant Professor of Anesthesiology
Mayo Graduate School
Courtesy Visiting Associate Professor of Anesthesiology
University of Florida
Director, Obstetric Anesthesia
Consultant
Department of Anesthesiology
Mayo Clinic–Jacksonville
Jacksonville, Florida

Christine W. Jordan, M.D.
Instructor
Department of Obstetrics & Gynecology
University of Florida Health Sciences Center—Jacksonville
Jacksonville, Florida

Gurjit Kaeley, M.D.
Department of Medicine
University of Tennessee
Memphis, Tennessee

Ward A. Katsanis, M.D.
Assistant Professor
Division of Gynecologic Oncology
Department of Obstetrics & Gynecology
University of Tennessee
Memphis, Tennessee

Andrew Kaunitz, M.D.
Professor and Assistant Chair
Department of Obstetrics & Gynecology
University of Florida Health Sciences Center
Jacksonville, Florida

Raymond W. Ke, M.D.
Associate Professor
Division of Reproductive Endocrinology
Department of Obstetrics & Gynecology
University of Tennessee
Memphis, Tennessee

Melanie Kennedy

Abbas E. Kitabchi, Ph.D., M.D.
Professor of Medicine & Biochemistry
Department of Medicine
University of Tennessee, Memphis
Director
Division of Endocrinology, Diabetes, and Metabolism
University of Tennessee Bowld Hospital
Memphis, Tennessee

Jeffrey A. Kuller, M.D.
Assistant Professor
Division of Maternal–Fetal Medicine
Department of Obstetrics & Gynecology
University of North Carolina School of Medicine
Chapel Hill, North Carolina

William H. Kutteh, M.D., Ph.D.
Associate Professor
Director, Division of Reproductive Endocrinology
Director of Reproductive Immunology
University of Tennessee
Memphis, Tennessee

Mark Landon, M.D.
Professor and Vice Chair
Department of Obstetrics & Gynecology
Ohio State University College of Medicine
Columbus, Ohio

Hal C. Lawrence, M.D.

James B. Lewis, Jr., M.D.
Associate Professor and Program Director
Department of Medicine
University of Tennessee
Memphis, Tennessee

Rani Lewis, M.D.
Assistant Professor
Department of Obstetrics & Gynecology
University of Tennessee College of Medicine
Memphis, Tennessee

Stephen R. Lincoln, M.D.
Division of Reproductive Endocrinology
Department of Obstetrics & Gynecology
University of Tennessee College of Medicine
Memphis, Tennessee

Frank W. Ling, M.D.
Faculty Professor and Chair
Department of Obstetrics & Gynecology
University of Tennessee College of Medicine
Memphis, Tennessee

Gary H. Lipscomb, M.D.
Professor and Director
Division of Gynecology
Department of Obstetrics & Gynecology
University of Tennessee, Memphis
Chief
Division of Gynecology
Regional Medical Center at Memphis
Memphis, Tennessee

Gregory J. Locksmith, M.D.
Assistant Professor
Division of Maternal–Fetal Medicine
Department of Obstetrics & Gynecology
The University of Texas Medical Branch
Galveston, Texas

Geeta Malik, M.D.

J. Sloan Manning, M.D.
Associate Professor
Department of Family Medicine
University of Tennessee
Memphis, Tennessee

Charles Masbach II, M.D.
Professor of Medicine and Physiology
Chief, Division of Gastroenterology
Department of Medicine
University of Tennessee
Memphis, Tennessee

Susan F. Meade, M.D., FPNP

Brigitte E. Miller, M.D.
Associate Professor
Section of Gynecologic Oncology
Department of Obstetrics & Gynecology
Wake Forest University School of Medicine
Winston-Salem, North Carolina

Debra A. Minjarez, M.D.
Instructor
Department of Obstetrics & Gynecology
University of Texas Southwestern Medical Center
Dallas, Texas

Robert E. Morrison, M.D.
Professor of Medicine
Division of General Internal Medicine
Department of Medicine
University of Tennessee
Memphis, Tennessee

Michael Murphy, M.D.
Associate Professor
Department of Family Medicine
University of Tennessee
Memphis, Tennessee

Thomas E. Nolan, M.D.
Professor of Obstetrics & Gynecology and Medicine
Louisiana State University Health Sciences Center
and
Hospital Center Director of Women's and Newborn Services
Medical Center of Louisiana
New Orleans, Louisiana

Richard O'Shaughnessy, M.D.
Professor
Department of Obstetrics & Gynecology
Ohio State University College of Medicine
Columbus, Ohio

Linn H. Parsons, M.D.
Associate Professor
Department of Obstetrics & Gynecology
Wake Forest University
Winston-Salem, North Carolina

Mark D. Pearlman, M.D.
Associate Professor and Vice Chair
Department of Obstetrics & Gynecology
and
Associate Professor
Department of Surgery
University of Michigan Health System
Ann Arbor, Michigan

B. Denise Raynor, M.D.
Assistant Professor
Division of Maternal–Fetal Medicine
Department of Obstetrics & Gynecology
Emory University School of Medicine
Atlanta, Georgia

John A. Read, M.D.
Professor and Director of Medical Student Education
   in Obstetrics & Gynecology
Department of Obstetrics & Gynecology
University of Kentucky College of Medicine
Lexington, Kentucky

Cesar Rosa, M.D.
Associate Professor
Department of Obstetrics & Gynecology
Uniformed Services University of the Health Sciences
Bethesda, Maryland

Renate H. Rosenthal, Ph.D.
Professor
Department of Psychiatry
Director
Medical Student Education
University of Tennessee
Memphis, Tennessee

R. James St. Hilaire, M.D.
Assistant Professor of Medicine
University of Tennessee Health Science Center
Section Chief, Gastroenterology Service
Director, Outpatient Gastroenterology Clinic
Chief, Endoscopy Laboratory
Regional Medical Center at Memphis
Memphis, Tennessee

Philip Samuels, M.D.
Associate Professor
Division of Maternal–Fetal Medicine
Department of Obstetric & Gynecology
Ohio State University College of Medicine
Columbus, Ohio

Joshua Sepesi, M.D.
Department of Obstetrics & Gynecology
University of Tennessee
Memphis, Tennessee

Claudette Jones Shephard, M.D.
Assistant Professor
Chief, Section of Pediatric and Adolescent Gynecology
Department of Obstetrics & Gynecology
University of Tennessee
Memphis, Tennessee

Robert A. Skinner, Jr., M.D.
Division of Dermatology
Department of Medicine
University of Tennessee
Memphis, Tennessee

Roger P. Smith, M.D.
Professor and Vice Chairman
Department of Obstetrics & Gynecology
Program (Residency) Director
Director of Ambulatory Care
University of Kansas Truman Medical Center
Kansas City, Missouri

Thomas E. Snyder, M.D.
Associate Professor
Department of Obstetrics & Gynecology
Wake Forest University School of Medicine
Baptist Medical Center
Winston-Salem, North Carolina

Edward J. Stanford, M.D.
Clinical Assistant Professor
Departments of Obstetrics & Gynecology and Family
    Medicine
University of Illinois
and
Director
Rockford Uro-Gynecology
Rockford, Illinois

Thomas G. Stovall, M.D.
Professor
Department of Obstetrics & Gynecology
University of Tennessee
Memphis, Tennessee

Robert A. Strauss, M.D.
Fellow
Division of Maternal–Fetal Medicine
Department of Obstetrics & Gynecology
University of North Carolina
Chapel Hill, North Carolina

Robert L. Summitt, Jr., M.D.
Professor and Chief
Section of Urogynecology
Director, Residency Training Program
University of Tennessee
Memphis, Tennessee

Dean T. Theophilopoulos, M.D.
Clinical Fellow
Division of Neonatology
Department of Pediatrics
University of Florida
Gainesville, Florida

Val Y. Vogt, M.D.
Assistant Professor
Department of Obstetrics & Gynecology
University of Tennessee
Memphis, Tennessee

Ray Walker, M.D.
Assistant Professor and Director of Clinical Affairs
Department of Family Medicine
University of Tennessee
Memphis, Tennessee

Virginia W. Ward, M.D.

Isabelle Wilkins, M.D.
Associate Professor
Director, Division of Maternal–Fetal Medicine
Department of Obstetrics & Gynecology
Baylor College of Medicine
Houston, Texas

Verneeta L. Williams, M.D.
Resident
Department of Family Medicine
University of Tennessee
Memphis, Tennessee

Michael K. Yancey, M.D.
Associate Professor
Department of Obstetrics & Gynecology
F. Edward Hebert School of Medicine
Uniformed Services University of Health Sciences Center
Honolulu, Hawaii

Khaled Zeitoun, M.D.
Division of Reproductive Endocrinology
Department of Obstetrics & Gynecology
University of Tennessee
Memphis, Tennessee

Preface

The discipline of obstetrics and gynecology has changed dramatically in recent years. We are witnessing a literal explosion in our knowledge of human reproduction and a corresponding refinement in our technical ability to diagnose and treat complicated disease processes. We now can fertilize human eggs in the laboratory and reimplant the conceptus in the womb. We can test the early embryo for selected genetic disorders. Through ultrasound, amniocentesis, chorionic villus sampling, and fetal blood sampling we can identify karyotype abnormalities, congenital anomalies, and congenital infections and, in selected instances, offer life-saving medical and surgical treatments. Through electronic fetal monitoring, Doppler velocimetry, and biophysical assessment, we can evaluate fetal well-being and determine the optimal timing of delivery. Because of improvements in supportive care, we now can offer pregnant women with severe medical illnesses such as diabetes and heart disease an excellent prognosis for perinatal outcome.

In the realm of gynecology, we now have available new and potent antibiotics for the treatment of genital tract infections. We have developed several new and exciting therapies for prevention of osteoporosis. Medical management has largely replaced surgical treatment for abnormal uterine bleeding and ectopic pregnancy. In situations where open abdominal surgery used to be the norm, sophisticated laparoscopic approaches now are possible. Treatments for gynecologic malignancies continue to improve, and many patients now can have a remarkably good prognosis for complete cure.

Even as requirements for expertise in the traditional disciplines of obstetrics and gynecology have intensified, our specialty has broadened its perspective to include the responsibility for primary care. In essence, we have clearly identified obstetrician–gynecologists as the key resource for provision of *comprehensive women's health care*. Accordingly, we have had to broaden our knowledge base to include a secure understanding of common medical illnesses. We also have had to learn to administer preventive services, such as immunizations, and to correctly orchestrate periodic screening for serious disorders such as breast and colon cancer, hyperlipidemia, and coronary artery disease.

This textbook is intended to provide a comprehensive review of women's health care. It is targeted primarily at obstetrician–gynecologists, nurse midwives, and obstetrics and gynecology nurse–practitioners. However, it also should be of value to internal medicine specialists who provide gynecologic care to their patients and to family practitioners who serve both the gynecologic and obstetric needs of women. The pocketbook edition of this text, soon to be published, should be of particular interest to those providers seeking a convenient single text as they address the health care needs of women.

Our text was written by many different authors, each with unique expertise in a special area of study. It seeks to provide straightforward, practical information that is immediately applicable to clinical practice. The text is complemented by summary tables, pertinent illustrations and graphics, and a succinct "five key points" summary for each chapter. We sincerely hope that you find this new textbook informative and helpful as you pursue the exciting, fulfilling challenge of providing comprehensive health care to women.

PART I

Obstetrics

Chapter 1
Maternal Physiology

Eleanor Capeless
A. Gordon Fry, III

Five Key Points

- Cardiac output increases 30 to 50% during pregnancy. This change begins early in gestation and persists longer than the traditional six weeks "postpartum" time period. Positioning influences cardiac output. Both the standing and supine position cause cardiac output to fall.

- Both systolic and diastolic blood pressure drop early in pregnancy, followed by a nadir at 20 to 28 weeks, and a return to nonpregnant values by term.

- Minute ventilation increases in pregnancy because of increased tidal volume. The respiratory rate remains unchanged. These changes result in higher PO_2 values and lower PCO_2 values in pregnancy.

- Both ureters and calices are normally dilated in pregnancy. Although usually the right is more dilated, the left is also markedly expanded as compared with its nonpregnant state.

- Plasma volume and red-cell mass both increase in pregnancy. A proportionately larger increase in plasma volume (50% vs. 30%) produces the "physiologic" anemia seen in pregnancy.

Pregnancy initiates profound physiologic changes in almost all organ systems. In general, there is an improvement in function, especially in the cardiovascular and renal systems. However, endocrine changes may reflect a less sensitive system during pregnancy. It is as important to recognize failure of the "normal" changes as to recognize a deterioration in function. Thus, a firm understanding of physiologic changes in pregnancy is necessary for the optimal care of the pregnant woman.

CARDIOVASCULAR PHYSIOLOGY

Adaptations within the cardiovascular system during pregnancy are among the most difficult to characterize. Nevertheless, it is vital to understand the currently available data in this area in order to distinguish pathologic changes from normal ones in the gravid patient.

Anatomic Considerations

The heart itself is displaced upward by elevation of the diaphragm. This process also causes a forward rotation and lateral displacement of the apex and left heart border, which gives an exaggerated impression of cardiac enlargement.[1] In addition, this shift causes the left heart border to straighten, which can be detected radiographically. Overall, cardiac size does appear to enlarge modestly.[2-4]

Heart Sounds

A change in the character of heart sounds during pregnancy often can be appreciated. The **first heart sound** (atrioventricular [AV] valve closure) becomes louder, and splitting may be enhanced. The **second heart sound** (closure of the valves of the great vessels) does not change appreciably in quality; however, the splitting interval may be less affected by respiration than in nonpregnant individuals. The **third heart sound** (rapid ventricular filling) can be heard in most pregnant subjects when auscultation is performed after midgestation. It usually persists and then disappears in the early postpartum period. A **fourth heart sound** (atrial contraction) is rarely auscultated in pregnancy but can be detected by phonocardiography in approximately 16% of gravid patients. It usually disappears by the time of delivery.[5]

Murmurs

Systolic murmurs caused by increased flow across normal valves are almost universal in pregnancy. These ejection murmurs most commonly are early systolic, but some are midsystolic; and they are usually most easily detected along the left sternal border. Another type of systolic murmur arising from the increased blood flow through the mammary vessels can sometimes be heard (the so-called mammary souffle). This sound generally manifests itself in late pregnancy and early puerperium and is heard in the precordium bilaterally in the second, third, or fourth intercostal space.[6] Although a transient diastolic murmur detected along the left sternal border may be normal, most diastolic murmurs require further evaluation.[5]

Electrocardiography

ECG changes in pregnancy result from the previously described changes in cardiac positioning. Left-axis deviation may range from 15 to 28 degrees.[7] Flattened T waves in lead III and ST-segment depression in both the precordial and limb leads are also normal findings occasionally seen during gestation.[2,7-11] AV conduction and conduction within the ventricles is not altered, but premature atrial and ventricular contractions have been reported,[12] as well as a higher propensity for the development of supraventricular tachycardia, especially in the third trimester, presumably due to the increased hemodynamic burden.[13]

TABLE 1-1
NORMAL CARDIOVASCULAR ADAPTATIONS TO PREGNANCY THAT MAY BE MISTAKEN FOR PATHOLOGIC PROCESSES

Altered heart borders
   Left lateral displacement of apex
   Straightening of left heart border
Changes in heart sounds
   S3 gallop
   S4 gallop
   Systolic ejection murmur
   Continuous murmur
   Enhanced splitting of S1
ECG
   Left-axis deviation
   Flattened T waves in lead III
   ST depression in limb and chest leads
Symptoms
   Decreased exercise tolerance
   Increased fatigue
   Dyspnea

Table 1-1 summarizes the normal cardiovascular features of pregnant women that are commonly mistaken as signs of pathologic processes. In addition, lower-extremity edema results from decreased venous return from this region as well as reduced plasma oncotic pressure. Jugular venous distention and pulsations are often readily observed in the latter half of pregnancy due to the increase in venous cardiac filling.

Cardiac Output

Cardiac output is the product of stroke volume and heart rate and is influenced by other factors such as peripheral resistance and arterial and venous blood pressure. Since all these factors undergo profound adaptations in pregnancy, it follows that cardiac output will likewise be similarly affected.

Early catheterization and dye-dilution studies suggested a slow rise of cardiac output to a peak value in the late second trimester, after which values gradually returned to approach their prepregnant values. Unfortunately, these techniques had large degrees of variability, and the impact of maternal positioning was not recognized. In pregnancy, the supine position can lead to compression of the inferior vena cava by the gravid uterus. Impaired venous return can lead to a reduction in cardiac output of up to 14% at 28 to 32 weeks[14] and up to 25 to 30% at term.[15] Such changes associated with positioning were not accounted for in many early studies.[16] Recent studies

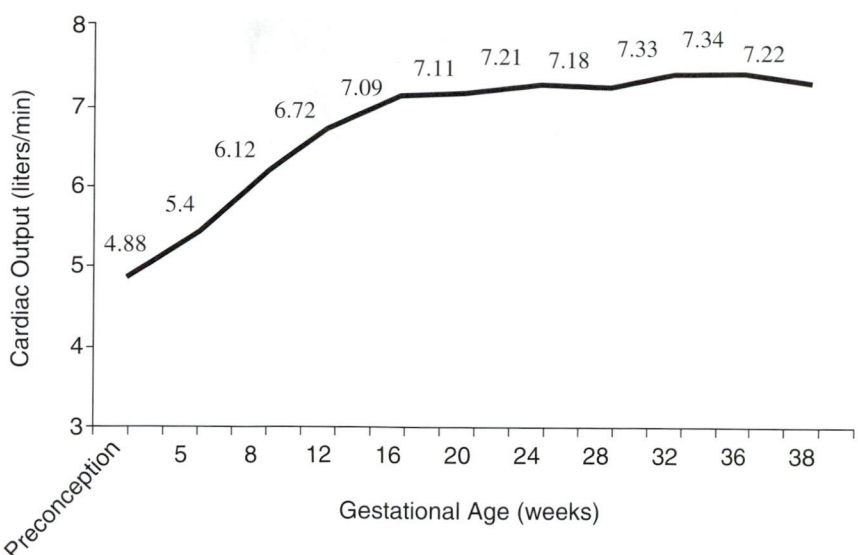

Figure 1-1 Longitudinal changes in cardiac output during pregnancy. *Derived from Robson et al.*[20]

have demonstrated that the previously perceived decrease in cardiac output in late pregnancy seems to be a spurious result of testing in the supine position.

More recent studies of cardiac output have used noninvasive techniques such as Doppler and M-mode echocardiography. Cardiac output has been demonstrated to increase by 30 to 50% over the course of pregnancy.[4,17–20] When studied prior to conception and throughout pregnancy, the rise in cardiac output occurs rapidly and early, with more than 50% of the total increase present at 8 weeks of gestation.[21] Cardiac output continues to increase, albeit at a slower rate, and reaches a peak between 24 and 32 weeks, which is maintained until term (Fig. 1-1).[20]

While it is commonly believed that most hemodynamic parameters have returned to preconception values by 6 weeks postpartum, these assumptions were based on observations during pregnancy, when significant increases in cardiac output have already taken place. When Capeless and Clapp compared cardiovascular parameters after pregnancy to measurements obtained prior to conception, they found that cardiac output remained elevated at 12 weeks postpartum.[22]

The changes responsible for increased cardiac output are stroke volume and heart rate. At early gestational ages, coinciding with the early increase in ventricular muscle mass, stroke volume seems to be the larger contributor to an increase in cardiac output.[20,21] The actual increment has been calculated to be approximately 7 ml (rising from 64 ml to 71 ml).[5] However, as stroke volume remains stable, the continued elevation in cardiac output is maintained by an increase in maternal heart rate. From about 5 weeks of

gestation on, the maternal heart rate begins to rise to a maximal gain of 15 to 20 bpm by 32 weeks, where it remains until term.[15,19,23]

As the total amount of blood distributed by the heart changes in pregnancy, so too does the relative distribution of blood flow. Uterine blood flow shows the most dramatic change. Although technically difficult to measure, reasonable values of longitudinal changes in uterine blood flow have been achieved by Asali and Romney and their colleagues.[24,25] In the nonpregnant state and during the first trimester, the uterus receives about 2 to 3% (90 to 100 ml/min) of total cardiac output. A steady and more or less linear increase in uterine blood flow continues to about 24 weeks. After this, the increase becomes more accelerated, until at term the uterus is receiving a blood supply on the order of 500 ml/min, and possibly as high as 800 ml/min (10 to 15% of cardiac output). The supply to the breasts also increases from less than 1% to 2%. Although total flow to other areas increases as a result of the overall rise in cardiac output, the fractions supplying the brain (10%), kidneys (20%), and skin (10%) remain relatively stable as compared with nonpregnant values (Fig. 1-2).

Blood Pressure

Arterial Pressure

Attempts to characterize normal blood pressure in pregnancy are complicated by methodological problems and lack of agreement on a "gold" standard. Intraarterial determinations may be significantly lower than manual cuff measurements but higher than

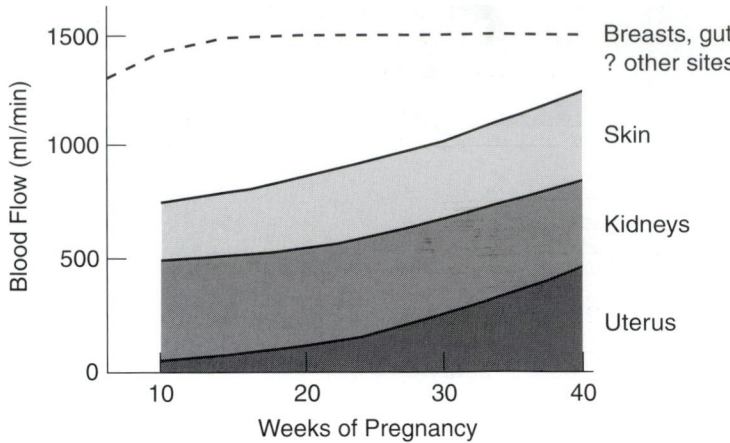

Figure 1-2 Distribution of increased cardiac output in pregnancy. *Reproduced with permission from de Swiet M. The cardiovascular system. In: Hytten FE and Chamberlain G, eds. Clinical physiology in obstetrics. 2nd ed. Oxford: Blackwell Scientific, 1991:25.*

automated cuff values.[26–28] Also, values are influenced by maternal positioning. Most investigators have found that measurements of systolic blood pressure recorded when a woman is standing or sitting is higher than when she is lying supine; in turn it is higher than when recorded in the left lateral decubitus position. Diastolic pressure also follows a similar response to positioning (Fig. 1-3).[29,30] Finally, defining diastolic pressure in pregnancy has been debated. Measurement of Korotkoff phase 4 (muffling of sound) results in an average increase in diastolic pressures of 13 mm Hg as compared with measurement of phase 5 (disappearance of sound).[31] The National High Blood Pressure Education Program Working Group Report on High Blood Pressure in Pregnancy recommends use of the fifth Korotkoff sound for designation of the diastolic value.[32]

The above problems notwithstanding, the general pattern of blood pressure can be summarized as an early drop in mean arterial pressure at 7 weeks,[21] with a relatively greater drop in diastolic levels and a concomitant widening of pulse pressure. Systolic pressure throughout pregnancy remains fairly stable when measured in the standing or sitting position. A more marked drop in diastolic pressure occurs, falling to a nadir at midgestation (20 to 28 weeks). This represents an incremental decrease of up to 10 to 15 mm Hg below nonpregnant values. Thereafter, a steady increase follows, eventually reaching nonpregnant values at term. A similar but less dramatic fall in systolic pressure (5 to 10 mm Hg) has also been reported when measurements are taken in the left lateral decubitus position.[29,30,33]

Peripheral resistance is mean arterial pressure divided by cardiac output. Because pregnancy is associated with an elevated cardiac output but not arterial pressure, peripheral resistance must necessarily be decreased. The pattern of change parallels that described

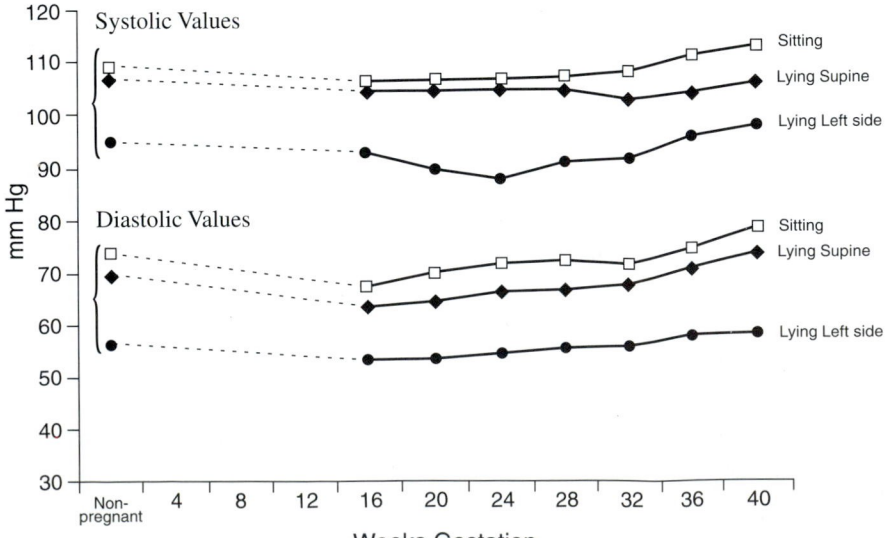

Figure 1-3 Longitudinal changes in blood pressure related to posture during pregnancy. *Derived from Schwarz,[29] with permission.*

TABLE 1-2 CENTRAL HEMODYNAMIC CHANGES		
	Nonpregnant	Pregnant
Cardiac output (liters/min)	4.3±0.9	6.2±1.0
Heart rate (beats/min)	71±10.0	83±10.0
Systemic vascular resistance (dyne · cm · sec^{-5})	1530±520	1210±266
Pulmonary vascular resistance (dyne · cm · sec^{-5})	119±47.0	78±22
Colloid oncotic pressure (mm Hg)	20.8±1.0	18.0±1.5
Colloid oncotic pressure– pulmonary capillary wedge pressure (mm Hg)	14.5±2.5	10:5±2.7
Mean arterial pressure (mm Hg)	86.4±7.5	90.3±5.8
Pulmonary capillary wedge pressure (mm Hg)	6.3±2.1	7.5±1.8
Central venous pressure (mm Hg)	3.7±2.6	3.6±2.5
Left ventricular stroke work index (g · m · m^{-2})	41±8	48±6

Reproduced, with permission, from Clark et al.[19]

for blood pressure, namely a decrease beginning early with a nadir at 14 to 24 weeks, followed by a progressive rise toward term.[17,34] Absolute values are given in Table 1-2. Explanations for this phenomenon include a vasodilatory response to progesterone or prostaglandins and the presence of the uteroplacental circulation that may function as a physiologic low-resistance shunt.

Venous Pressure

Central venous (Table 1-2) and upper extremity venous pressure do not change significantly in pregnancy.[35-37] However, pressure in the veins of the lower extremities seem to undergo progressive and significant increases throughout pregnancy, from approximately 10 mm Hg at 10 weeks to 25 mm Hg at term.[38]

Central Hemodynamics

Clark et al.[19] obtained information regarding changes in cardiovascular parameters during pregnancy using invasive methods in 10 carefully selected patients at 25 to 28 weeks of gestation and again at 11 to 13 weeks postpartum (Table 1-2). In addition to changes already discussed, these investigators found significant decreases in pulmonary vascular resistance and colloid oncotic pressure. No change was observed in the pulmonary capillary wedge pressure, despite increases in blood volume and cardiac output, perhaps because of

the fall in pulmonary vascular resistance. Nevertheless, the colloid oncotic pressure–pulmonary capillary wedge pressure gradient was lower, which may explain the increased susceptibility to the development of pulmonary edema seen during pregnancy.

Intrapartum Changes

Hemodynamic parameters undergo further alterations during labor. Cardiac output increases in early labor by 15%, largely reflecting an increase in stroke volume. This translates to a rise of 2 ml/min when a uterine contraction occurs, partly due to augmented venous return to the heart when 300 to 500 ml of venous blood is forced from the uterus.[39,40] Further elevation occurs as labor progresses, with a mean increase of 34% by the onset of the second stage.[41] Mean arterial pressure also increases by 10 mm Hg during contractions. It is important to keep in mind that some of the observed hemodynamic changes during labor and delivery are diminished by regional anesthesia.[40]

Postpartum Changes

In the immediate postpartum period, release of uterine caval compression and autotransfusion of the uteroplacental circulation cause a dramatic increase in cardiac output. The magnitude of the rise following vaginal delivery varies from 60%, when regional anesthesia is used, to 80%, with local anesthesia.[40,42] A large increase also follows cesarean delivery; however, the shift is not as great (in the range of 25%) when measured in the presence of regional anesthesia.[43]

PULMONARY PHYSIOLOGY

Physiologic adaptation of the respiratory system during pregnancy results in profound changes that must be recognized and understood in order to effectively diagnose and treat pulmonary disease complicating pregnancy. Although cardiac output and minute ventilation (the respiratory equivalent of cardiac output) both increase by similar proportions during pregnancy, the added cardiac output represents a much greater fraction of normal cardiac reserve than does the parallel rise in minute ventilation to pulmonary reserve. Consequently, individuals with lung disease tend to tolerate pregnancy better than their counterparts with cardiac disease.

Anatomic Changes

Structural changes in the shape of the chest have been well described for some time. Over the course of pregnancy, the configuration of the thoracic cavity becomes more barrel-shaped as a result of a flaring of the subcostal angle, an increase in the transverse diameter of the rib cage, and an elevation of the diaphragm. Radiographic observations by early investigators documented an increase in the subcostal angle from 68 degrees to 103 degrees and an elevation of the diaphragm of about 4 cm. These changes are also accompanied by an increase in the transthoracic diameter of about 2 cm.[44,45] Although many clinicians assume that movement of the diaphragm is impeded by the expanding pregnancy, it has been well demonstrated that diaphragmatic excursion is actually greater in pregnancy, whether measured sitting, standing, or supine. This pattern occurs as breathing in pregnancy becomes more diaphragmatic than costal.[46]

Radiographically, lung markings are enhanced due to an increase in the volume of the pulmonary vessels and a more collapsed state of the lungs,[47] which will be discussed further below.

Respiratory Function

Pulmonary function is described by four, nonoverlapping volumes and four capacities, each consisting of two or more of these volumes (Fig. 1-4).

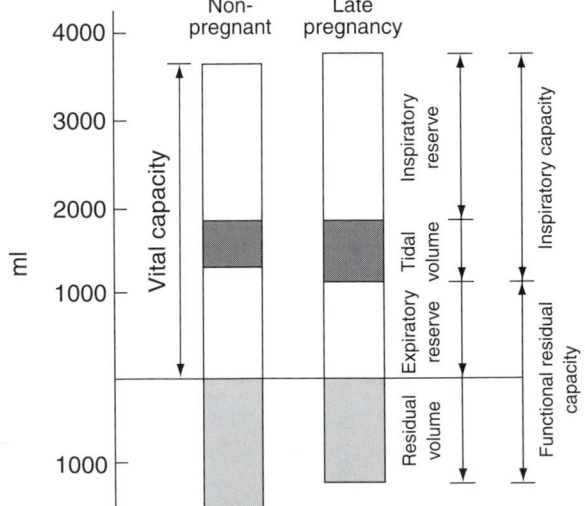

Figure 1-4 Division of lung volumes and capacities and their changes in pregnancy. *Reproduced with permission from de Swiet M. The respiratory system. In: Hytten FE, Chamberlain G, eds. Clinical physiology in obstetrics. 2nd ed. Oxford: Blackwell Scientific, 1991:84.*

Tidal volume, the volume of gas that enters and exits the lung during each respiratory cycle, is measured during normal respiration. Tidal volume increases during pregnancy, from about 500 cc to 700 cc, or approximately 40%.[44,49]

Expiratory reserve volume (ERV) is the volume of gas that can be forcibly expired from the lungs at the end of a normal respiration. Changes in ERV account for the majority of the adaptation that allows tidal volume to expand. A progressive decline of about 200 cc occurs throughout pregnancy, from about 1300 cc to 1100 cc, and likely begins to drop early in gestation.[50,51]

Inspiratory reserve volume is the maximal amount of gas that can be inspired beyond the limits of a normal tidal breath at end inspiration. This volume does not change in pregnancy.

Residual volume is the amount of gas remaining in the lungs after maximal, forced expiration. This value does not include anatomic dead space. Although results have varied with different measuring techniques, investigators agree that this volume is significantly reduced in pregnancy. The modern studies describe a fall of about 20%, from 1500 cc to 1200 cc.[50-52] Decreased lung volume in the resting state, alluded to earlier, brought about by elevation of the diaphragm, accounts for this decrease.

Total lung capacity (TLC) is the sum of all the previously described volumes. The decrease in expiratory reserve volume and residual volume results in approximately a 5% decrease in TLC.

Vital capacity includes all lung volumes except the residual volume. It is measured as the amount of gas that can be expired following maximum inspiration. Given the conflicting data available,[48,50,51,53,54] it appears that it may be normal for vital capacity to increase in some but not all women by 100 cc to 200 cc as gestation proceeds. This finding may very well be related to body habitus since vital capacity has been shown to be reduced in obese pregnant women.[52]

Inspiratory capacity, calculated as tidal volume plus inspiratory reserve volume, has been shown to consistently increase in pregnancy. The absolute increase is approximately 5%, which represents a volume of about 300 cc.[52,53] The rise in inspiratory capacity occurs progressively over the course of pregnancy.

Functional residual capacity (FRC) is the sum of ERV and residual volume. It represents the total amount of gas remaining in the lung at the end of a normal tidal breath. Since both ERV and residual volume fall during pregnancy, it follows that FRC concomitantly decreases. The magnitude of the volume loss is approximately 20%, or an absolute decrease of 500 cc.[52,53] This change further reflects the relatively collapsed state of the resting lung seen during pregnancy.

Pulmonary Function Testing

Adequacy of ventilation is assessed by standardized pulmonary function testing. The **forced expiratory volume in one second (FEV₁)** and **peak flow rate (PFR)** are tests designed to assess large airway function.

FEV_1 is the volume of gas that can be forcibly expelled from the lungs in one second. It is usually expressed as either an absolute volume or as a fraction of vital capacity. Typically, it is the procedure of first choice given its ease of performance, its high degree of reproducibility, and its independence of patient effort. Most investigators agree that pregnancy does not affect FEV_1 and that it should remain at 80 to 85% of vital capacity. PFR indicates the maximal velocity of gas flow during a forced expiration. As might be expected in light of the stability of FEV_1, PFR is not altered in pregnancy.[48,50–53,55–58]

Gas Exchange

Minute ventilation is the amount of air inspired in one minute. Thus, it is the product of respiratory rate and tidal volume. Pregnancy is characterized by an increase in minute ventilation volume of 10 to 40%.[49,51,59] Because respiratory rate is unchanged, remaining at 14 to 15 breaths per minute, the augmented minute volume is explained by the increase in tidal volume. By augmenting minute ventilation through breathing more deeply rather than more frequently, the gravid patient is able to increase alveolar ventilation even more so than overall ventilation.

Gas transfer across the alveolar–endothelial membrane appears to be impaired in pregnancy. This mild effect (a decrease from 26.5 ml/min to 22.5 ml/min)[49] is possibly explained by the normal, pregnancy-associated drop in hemoglobin concentration or even through an estrogen-induced change in alveolar mucopolysaccharide consistency.[50] Whatever the cause, this diffusion impairment results in an expected

increase in the alveolar–arterial oxygen (A-a) gradient[60] which is well compensated by the increased alveolar partial pressure of oxygen (PO_2) ventilation achieved through greater ventilation. Shunting values of up to three times those seen in nonpregnant patients have been observed in healthy pregnant women.[61]

Oxygen consumption in pregnancy increases by 30 to 40 ml/min, representing an increase of 15 to 30% over nonpregnant conditions. Since this is of a smaller magnitude than the associated increase in ventilation, PO_2, and consequently arterial O_2 pressures (PaO_2), rise. A change in PaO_2 from normal nonpregnant values (85 to 90 mm Hg) to 101 to 104 mm Hg at term has been described.[61] Importantly, maternal positioning has been reported to influence the values of arterial blood gases in pregnancy with an increase in the A-a gradient when measured in the supine position.[62]

With increased ventilation, the **arterial carbon dioxide partial pressure ($PaCO_2$)** falls. In normal pregnancies, PCO_2 levels range from 27 to 32 mm Hg, as compared with 35 to 40 mm Hg in nonpregnant subjects.[63–65] This reduction in maternal $PaCO_2$ levels benefits the fetus by facilitating CO_2 exchange through the generation of a larger transplacental CO_2 gradient than would otherwise exist at nonpregnant CO_2 concentrations.

Pregnant women maintain a normal arterial pH of 7.4 to 7.45; therefore, a means of compensating for this respiratory alkalosis must exist. This compensation is achieved through a fall in serum bicarbonate through renal excretion, so that pregnancy is associated with normal serum bicarbonate concentrations of 18 to 31 mEq/liter.[64] Normal blood gas values in pregnancy are summarized in Table 1-3.

The stimulus responsible for the increase in ventilation and thus reduced CO_2 levels appears to be progesterone.[66] Although the mechanism behind this observation is undetermined, various proposals include a direct effect on the central respiratory center,[67] an

TABLE 1-3 NORMAL ARTERIAL BLOOD GAS VALUES IN PREGNANCY	
PH	7.40–7.45
$PaCO_2$	27–32 mm Hg
PaO_2	101–104 mm Hg
HCO_3	18–31 mEq/liter

increase in the sensitivity of the respiratory center to CO_2, and an increase in the activity of carbonic anhydrase in red blood cells.[68]

Dyspnea

Defined as an uncomfortable, conscious awareness of the normal process of breathing, dyspnea is commonly reported in pregnancy. Present even early in the first trimester, it has been reported in up to 50% of women by 20 weeks, and 75% by 31 weeks.[69] The etiology of this symptom is not understood, but may be related to the low CO_2 tensions or an awareness of the increase in minute ventilation.

URINARY SYSTEM AND VOLUME HOMEOSTASIS

Anatomic Adaptations

During pregnancy, the kidneys enlarge due an increase in both their interstitial space and the intravascular volume.[70] The right kidney appears to expand slightly more than the left. Radiologic evidence[71] suggests that normal kidney size is approximately 1 cm longer in pregnant as compared with nonpregnant women. Ultrasound evidence suggests an increase in renal parenchyma volume of about 70% by the third trimester.[70,72]

Dilation of the ureters and calices also seems to be a normal finding in pregnancy. Normal ureteral diameter in pregnancy can be up to 2 cm and persists at this level up to 16 weeks postpartum.[73] The clinical implications of this adaptation include an increased risk of the development of pyelonephritis and difficulty in the interpretation of radiologic studies of the urinary collecting system of pregnant women. Normal findings from excretory urograms obtained in pregnancy include proximal ureteral dilation, an apparent filling defect at the pelvic brim, and lateral displacement.[71] The right-sided collecting system tends to undergo a greater change than the left. The pelvicaliceal dilation on the right side is about 15 mm and 5 mm on the left.[74] The cause of this dilation may be hormonal and/or mechanical. Mechanical obstruction results from compression of the collecting system from the gravid uterus. Furthermore, on excretory urograms, the ureteric dilation often ends at the pelvic brim, where the pregnant uterus may be resting on the ureters.[75] However, this mechanism does not explain why such dilation is seen in the first trimester,

when such mechanical obstruction should be minimal. Thus, hormonal mechanisms such as the smooth-muscle relaxant effects of progesterone are often offered as an explanation. Interestingly, tonometric studies have revealed an actual increase in ureteral tone during pregnancy.[76]

Renal Hemodynamics

Because an immediate reduction in urine flow, sodium excretion, **effective renal plasma flow (ERPF),** and **glomerular filtration rate (GFR)** occurs when a pregnant women changes from the lateral decubitus position to the supine or standing position, it is important to consider the influence of positioning when designing and interpreting studies of renal function in pregnancy.

ERPF increases by 70 to 80% to reach a level of 840 ml/min at 16 weeks.[77,78] Near term, a small but significant decrease in ERPF occurs. Since this effect is present in both the seated and left lateral recumbent positions,[79] it seems to represent a true physiologic change rather than a postural artifact.

GFR, as estimated by inulin clearance, increases by about 50%, beginning quite early in pregnancy and reaching a maximum in the late first to early second trimester. This elevated level is maintained until term.[80–82] In clinical practice, creatinine clearance rather than inulin clearance is used to determine GFR, although the values obtained are higher than those with inulin clearance. In a pattern similar to inulin clearance, creatinine clearance increases early in pregnancy and is 45% higher than that in nonpregnant women by 9 weeks.[83] Normal values for creatinine clearance in pregnancy generally lie between 150 and 200 ml/min, and these levels are usually sustained until delivery and beyond in normal pregnancies. Filtration fraction is the ratio of GFR to ERPF. Because the ERPF increase is of a greater magnitude than the increase in GFR, the filtration fraction in pregnancy decreases. Near delivery, when ERPF drops but GFR does not, filtration fraction consequently falls, returning to normal nonpregnant levels of 20 to 21% (Fig. 1-5).[84]

Volume Regulation

Total body water in pregnancy increases by 6 to 8 liters, 4 to 6 of which are extracellular.[85] Shortly after conception, plasma osmolality begins to decline,

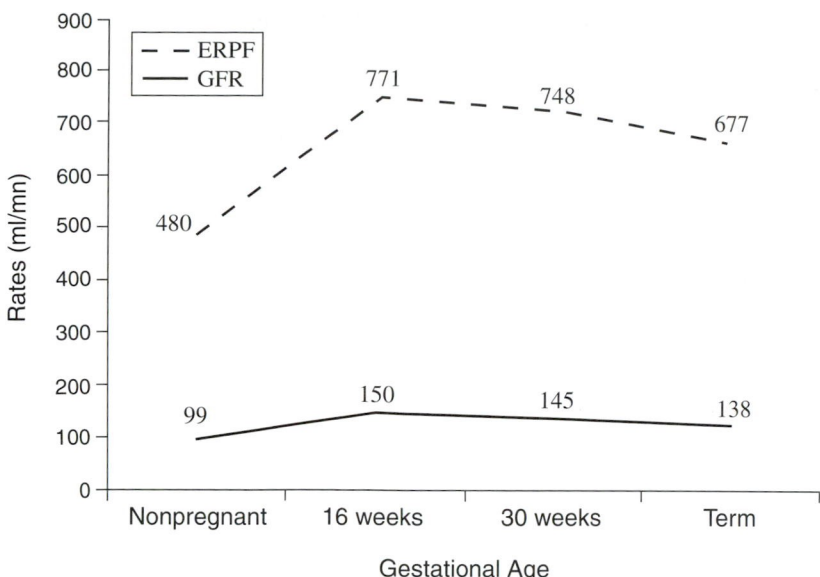

Figure 1-5 Longitudinal changes in renal hemodynamics and filtration during pregnancy. *From data in Equimokhai et al.*[79] *and Davison and Dunlop.*[80]

falling by about 10 mOsm/kg H_2O from normal nonpregnant values of 280 to 290 mOsm/kg H_2O to levels of 270 to 280 mOsm/kg H_2O by 5 weeks of gestation.[86,87] The pregnant women are able to maintain this lowered plasma osmolality through a resetting of the osmoreceptor system to a lower level, thus decreasing the osmotic threshold for antidiuretic hormone (ADH) release.

Sodium regulation is the primary determinant of volume status. Pregnancy is associated with an increase in the filtered load of sodium from 20,000 to 30,000 mmol/day. Tubular sodium resorption during pregnancy not only meets this additional requirement but also allows an additional 2 to 6 mmol of sodium to be resorbed per day. This change results in a net sodium accumulation of 900 to 1000 mEq of sodium, which is partitioned between the fetus, placenta, and maternal intravascular and interstitial fluids. Given that this takes place against the background of a 50% increase in GFR and in the presence of the natriuretic properties of progesterone, it is clear that the adjustment of renal tubular function to promote increased sodium resorption is among the most profound renal adaptations that occurs in pregnancy.[86,88,89]

Aldosterone, deoxycortisone and estrogen are hormones that enhance sodium resorption. All of these hormones circulate in greater concentrations during pregnancy. Plasma aldosterone levels range from 200 to 700 ng/liter in pregnancy as compared with 100 to 200 ng/liter in nonpregnant women.[90] Plasma deoxycortisone levels also increase in pregnancy, most

dramatically in the third trimester.[91] Although some of the additional deoxycortisone is accounted for by fetal production, the predominant source of the increment most likely is via peripheral conversion of circulating progesterone.[91,93] Estrogens not only have the endogenous ability to induce sodium retention, but it appears that the elevated plasma levels in pregnancy also enhance the conversion of progesterone to deoxycortisone through extraadrenal enhancement of 21-hydroxylase activity.[94]

Other factors influencing volume regulation in pregnancy also are altered in pregnancy. The serum concentration of atrial natriuretic peptide increases roughly twofold, from 44 pg/ml to 99 pg/ml.[95] Distention of the atrial wall from the increased plasma volume of pregnancy is the likely source of this change. Plasma renin activity increases 5- to 10-fold while angiotensin levels increase 4- to 5-fold.[96] The higher angiotensin levels exert their influence primarily through increased aldosterone production rather than hypertensive effects, which results in increased sodium retention. In fact, pregnant women show a decreased response to the pressor effects of angiotensin.[88]

Tubular Function and Excretion of Nitrogenous Metabolites

Blood urea nitrogen (BUN) and serum creatinine levels decrease early in normal pregnancies. While creatinine levels of 0.8 mg/dl and BUN levels of 10 mg/dl are normal outside of pregnancy, these levels average 0.6 mg/dl and 9 mg/dl, respectively, in pregnant women by the end of the first trimester. They remain at these levels until term. BUN values above 14 mg/dl and creatinine values above 0.9 mg/ml in pregnant women should arouse suspicion.[97]

Uric acid is the end product in the metabolic pathway of purine breakdown. Nearly all the filtered uric acid is resorbed in the proximal tubule.[98] In pregnancy, a decrease in tubular resorption causes plasma uric acid levels to fall early, reaching a nadir at 24 weeks, at which point serum levels are normally between 2.0 and 3.0 mg/dl, or about 25% of the normal nonpregnant serum concentration.[99] Because net tubular resorption of uric acid rises late in pregnancy, serum levels begin a trend toward their normal, nonpregnant levels at term. Glucose excretion is regulated by tubular resorption occurring on both the luminal and basolateral surface of the tubular membrane. The vast majority of pregnant women have a significant increase in glucose excretion during gestation.[100] Although glucose excretion is no doubt greater in pregnancy because of the increased GFR, resorption is decreased as early as 8 to 12 weeks. However, the previously widely accepted concept of a fixed, maximal glucose resorptive capacity is now known to be false.[101,102]

Renal excretion of most amino acids increases in pregnancy; however, the normal nonpregnant 24-hour urinary protein loss of 100 to 300 mg remains constant during pregnancy.[90] The most comprehensive investigation of urinary amino acids revealed different patterns of excretion for different groups of amino acids. Glycine, histidine, threonine, serine, and alanine excretion increased early in pregnancy, doubling by 16 weeks, and remained elevated up to term. Excretion of lysine, cystine, taurine, phenylalanine, valine, leucine, and tyrosine significantly increased early in pregnancy but fell thereafter. Glutamic acid, methionine, and ornithine showed minimally increased rates of excretion, while arginine excretion actually fell.[103]

Acid–base balance is also altered in pregnancy. The concentration of hydrogen ions falls by 2 to 4 mmol/l in the first trimester. Since minute ventilation normally increases in pregnant women, the decrease in arterial PCO_2 is accompanied by a fall in plasma bicarbonate to normal pregnant levels of 18 to 22 mmol/l, which is necessary in order to maintain normal blood pH values.

THE DIGESTIVE SYSTEM

Changes in Oral Intake

An increase in appetite and thirst are among the first symptoms reported by a large majority of pregnant women, beginning early in the first trimester and persisting up to delivery.[104] It is believed that most pregnant women, if they eat to satiety, will increase their energy intake by 200 kcal during the first trimester.[105]

Unusual food cravings and aversions are well recognized in both the public and medical communities. Women in the United Kingdom commonly hunger for highly seasoned foods such as pickles, kippers, and cheese, while their U.S. counterparts often crave such foods as ice cream, sweets, fruit, and fish. Aversions also occur, involving many foods.[104,106] Pica may occur commonly, although the substances consumed vary by region and culture. Southern black women have been known to consume starch and clay, while others in the U.S. report ingestion of ice, newspaper, and coffee grounds.[107] Even more prevalent than increased appetite in pregnancy is increased thirst, although the mechanism remains unclear.

Mouth and Teeth

Salivary production is unchanged during gestation, with rates of secretion from the submandibular gland of 0.1 ml/min as compared with 0.15 ml/min in nonpregnant women.[108] It is reasonable to conclude, given available evidence, that no significant change in salivary pH occurs during pregnancy.

Pregnant women often have swollen or spongy gums that bleed rather easily. Although gingivitis and periodontal disease have been reported to occur as a result of this edema, there is no evidence that pregnancy leads to an increase in the formation or progression of dental caries.[109–111]

Esophagus

Heartburn, interpreted by most clinicians as a sign of gastroesophageal reflux, is among the most common symptoms reported by pregnant women. Although a drop in tone of the lower esophageal sphincter has been demonstrated,[112,113] symptoms of heartburn may be absent in women who actually are experiencing reflux confirmed by direct esophageal pH measurement.

This discrepancy raises the question of an alternative cause for heartburn symptoms in pregnancy, such as symptomatic changes in esophageal peristalsis.[113]

Stomach

Gastric emptying times have been evaluated by many different methods, all of which are associated with potential technical and methodologic flaws. Early radiographic studies generally suggest a decrease in gastric tone and motility associated with pregnancy.[114] These findings are consistent with a 50% decrease in circulating levels of **motilin**, a hormone that stimulates gastrointestinal motility.[115] However, delayed gastric emptying has been difficult to corroborate physiologically.

With the widespread use of analgesia in labor, it is important to keep in mind that narcotics and regional anesthesia can independently prolong gastric emptying.[116] Although fentanyl-containing epidural anesthesia has been particularly implicated,[117] the delay in gastric emptying associated with its use may well be dose-dependent.[118]

There is some evidence that gastric secretion is decreased in pregnancy. Such a reduction may help explain the infrequency of peptic ulcer disease and improvement in preexisting ulcer symptoms reported in pregnancy.[119] Increased mucus production from the gastric mucosa in response to estrogen and progesterone[120] may also be involved in the improvement of peptic ulcer disease in pregnancy. Blood pepsin levels in pregnancy are also lower than nonpregnant and postpartum levels but begin to rise to nonpregnant levels in the third trimester.[121]

Small Intestine

Small intestine motility decreases in pregnancy, with a mean increased transit time from the stomach to cecum of about 6 hours in the second trimester as compared with the nonpregnant state.[122] The absorption of nutrients from the small bowel does not change appreciably with the exception of enhanced absorption of calcium and iron.[123,124]

Large Intestine

The general decrease in motility seen in other parts of the gastrointestinal tract is shared by the large intestine.

Constipation may also result from enhanced water absorption from the colon. A 59% increase in water absorption coupled with a 45% increase in sodium absorption has been demonstrated in pregnancy using colon perfusion techniques.[125] These changes contribute to the constipation encountered by many women.

Liver

Certain changes occur in normal pregnancy that would otherwise suggest liver disease. Physical findings include spider angiomata and palmar erythema, probably caused by elevated estrogen levels. Serum albumin levels fall in normal pregnancies to about 3.0 mg/dl, which represents a 30% decrease from nonpregnant values. Serum alkaline phosphatase levels undergo a significant increase, up to two to four times nonpregnant levels. The higher levels result from placental production of a heat-stable isoenzyme.[126] Levels of bilirubin, aspartate aminotransferase (AST), alanine aminotransferase (ALT), and prothrombin time remain essentially unchanged. Both unchanged and increased levels of γ-glutamyltranspeptidase (GGT) levels have been reported.[127–129]

Other proteins produced by the liver also undergo a characteristic rise during pregnancy. These include fibrinogen (50% increase), ceruloplasmin, and sex hormone, thyroid, vitamin D, and corticosteroid binding proteins.[126]

Gallbladder

Because cholesterol gallstones are more common in women than in men, a link between biliary disease and pregnancy has been widely accepted.[130] Such epidemiologic evidence has been challenged, but the number of pregnancies has been thought to increase the risk of gallstone development. Changes in bile acid composition can influence the likelihood of the occurrence of cholelithiasis. An increase in the bile acid pool, a decreased proportion of chenodeoxycholic acid, and an increased proportion of cholic acid are findings that cause increased lithogenicity of bile in pregnancy.[131,132] Decreases in gallbladder emptying can also promote biliary stasis and thus predispose pregnant women to biliary disease. At early gestational ages, fasting and residual gallbladder volumes may be 30% higher and continue to rise to levels up to twice as high as those of nonpregnant controls in the second and third trimesters. The rate of emptying of the gallbladder is also reduced.[131,132]

Despite the increased lithogenic environment of bile, a large study of the incidence of biliary sludge and gallstones in pregnancy revealed that although the incidence of biliary sludge significantly increased, the presence of true gallstones did not. Biliary colic was only firmly associated with gallstones, not sludge.[135]

HEMATOLOGICAL SYSTEM

Blood Volume

Blood volume is determined primarily by plasma volume and red-cell mass. These two components have no fixed relationship and change independently. In pregnancy both increase, but by different degrees and over different time courses.

Plasma Volume

Plasma volume is usually estimated using dilution techniques. The substances most commonly used are Evans' blue dye or radioactive tracers such as radioactive iodinated albumin. Pregnant women begin to show an increase in plasma volume at about 10 weeks and a steady increase occurs until about 32 to 34 weeks, when a plateau is reached; relatively little change takes place until after delivery.[136] Confusion as to whether a fall in plasma volume occurs near term stems from artifactual changes caused by measurement techniques and postural changes. Pregnant women undergo an average increase of about 1250 ml from a prepregnant volume of 2600 ml.[137] This change represents a 50% increase in plasma volume. However, the habit of expressing volume expansion in pregnancy as a percentage increase is misleading. Since women enter pregnancy with widely differing plasma volumes, the proportion by which it increases in pregnancy will also vary widely. Unquestionably, the degree of plasma volume expansion can be correlated with clinical pregnancy outcome and birthweight.[136,138] Because favorable outcomes have been reported with increases ranging from 20 to 100%,[139] it is likely that the absolute increase in plasma volume is more important than the fractional change.

Red-Cell Mass

Red-cell labeling studies demonstrate a significant increase in red-cell mass, beginning at around 10 weeks, with a steady rise continuing up to term. Unlike plasma volume, no plateau at 32 to 34 weeks is observed. The magnitude of this increase is influenced by iron supplementation. The red-cell volume prior to pregnancy is about 1400 ml, and it rises by approximately 400 ml (30%) in women taking iron supplements and 200 ml (18%) in the absence of iron supplementation over the course of pregnancy.[140–144] Because the red-cell mass increases by a smaller amount than the plasma value, a fall in hematocrit, so-called physiologic anemia, occurs in pregnancy. Since plasma volume does not continue to increase near term but red-cell mass does, the falling hematocrit nadirs at about 32 to 34 weeks and slowly increases until delivery.

The clinical implications of increased blood volume make sense from a teleologic viewpoint. Uncomplicated vaginal delivery is associated with an average blood loss of 500 ml, while figures for cesarean delivery are estimated at 1000 ml.[145,146] The increased blood volume thus serves to protect the mother from the dangers of significant hemorrhage at the time of delivery. The additional red-cell mass also serves to meet the additional oxygen requirements of pregnancy, as described earlier. Finally, the disproportionately elevated plasma volume results in less viscous blood and thus a decreased intravascular resistance to flow.

White Cells and Platelets

An increase in the peripheral white-cell count normally occurs in pregnancy with a mean of $9500/mm^3$ and normal range of 3000 to $15,000/mm^3$ in the first trimester. In the later trimesters, a further increase raises the normal range from 6,000 to $16,000/mm^3$, with a mean of $10,500/mm^3$. Labor is associated with an even greater increase in white-cell count, with values ranging from 20,000 to $30,000/mm^3$.[145,147] The elevated white-cell counts seen in pregnancy are the result of an increased polymorphonuclear neutrophil leukocyte (PMN, or granulocyte) fraction[148] and usually return to normal by 6 weeks postpartum.[149] Eosinophil percentage of total white cells remains stable during pregnancy, although the absolute number rises.[150] Lymphocyte counts remain stable, as do the numbers of circulating T and B cells.[151,152] The monocyte count also does not appear to change in pregnancy, but basophil counts may drop slightly.[150]

Studies addressing the changes in platelet counts have reported increasing, decreasing, and stable counts in normal pregnancies. These discrepancies resulted from widely varying measurements prior to the use of automated cell-counting devices. The current consensus is that a detectable, progressive fall in platelet count occurs in pregnancy, but the decrease is not large enough to drop the platelet count below the lower limit of normal for nonpregnant women. Mean platelet counts of 275,000/mm^3 prior to 20 weeks of gestation gradually fall to reach a mean of 260,000/mm^3 after 35 weeks.[153] The finding of a shorter platelet life span during the latter part of pregnancy suggests that the slight fall in platelet count probably results from increased peripheral platelet consumption rather than decreased production or dilutional changes.[154]

Hemostasis

Normal gestations are associated with significant changes in several clotting factors. These changes can usually be detected by the end of the first trimester. The circulating levels of factors VII through X progressively increase through pregnancy. Factor I (fibrinogen) levels show a dramatic increase from a normal nonpregnant range of 250 to 400 mg/dl to normal pregnant levels of 400 to 500 mg/dl. Factors II (prothrombin), V, and VII remain unchanged, while levels of factors XI and XIII may actually show a slight decrease.[155,156]

Pregnancy is commonly referred to as a hypercoagulable state. In fact, thromboembolism accounts for more than half of the pregnancy-related deaths caused by an embolic event, and it is the direct cause of about 10% of all pregnancy-related deaths in the United States.[157] However, parameters commonly used to assess coagulability, such as the prothrombin time, activated partial plastin time, and bleeding time are not affected by normal pregnancy. The fact that most thromboembolic events occur in the puerperium, when activity levels are typically decreased, implies that stasis and vessel-wall injury may be more significant components than elevated levels of clotting factors.

Iron Metabolism

The total iron requirement for pregnancy is estimated to range from 700 to 1400 mg.[138,158] The various components of this requirement are 500 to 600 mg from expansion of the maternal red-cell mass; 270 mg

lost daily by excretion through the urine, stool, and skin; fetal needs of 200 to 370 mg; and 100 to 250 mg through blood lost at delivery. Breast-feeding for 6 months carries an additional iron requirement of 100 to 180 mg. Fortunately, the amount of iron conserved during 15 months of amenorrhea (representing pregnancy and 6 months of breast feeding) averages between 240 and 480 mg.[159]

Because only about 5 to 10% of ingested iron is absorbed, a typical diet provides only about 1 to 2 mg of iron. However, the fraction of iron absorbed can increase under conditions of deficiency or increased needs, and dietary absorption rates in pregnancy have been reported to increase up to the 20 to 40% range.[160,161] Dietary iron comes from two sources: heme (organic) iron, which is found in hemoglobin and myoglobin from animal food sources, and inorganic iron, from vegetable food sources. Inorganic iron is in the ferric (or trivalent) form and must be converted to the organic ferrous (or divalent) form before it can be absorbed from the duodenum.[159] From the duodenal mucosa cells where it is absorbed in the gut, iron is released into the circulation, where it circulates bound to the protein transferrin and is then transported to the liver, bone marrow, and spleen. Once delivered to these sites, it is released from transferrin and either incorporated into hemoglobin or myoglobin or stored in the form of ferritin or hemosiderin. Iron is supplied to the fetus through a specialized transport mechanism, which transfers iron from the maternal circulation to the fetal circulation against a steep concentration gradient.[162]

The benefits of routine iron supplementation in healthy pregnant women have been a longstanding source of debate. It is estimated that 74 to 78% of U.S. women between the ages 20 and 40 have inadequate daily iron intake; thus, a significant percentage of women are at risk for entering pregnancy with low iron stores.[163,164] Women with normal iron stores, who are not given iron supplementation during pregnancy may require up to 2 years to restore their reserves. Pregnant women with inadequate iron stores without added iron supplementation are at especially high risk for long-term iron deficiency.

While universal iron supplementation has not been proven to prevent adverse pregnancy outcomes in large, well-designed, randomized trials, there is evidence associating iron-deficiency anemia with preterm birth and low-birth-weight infants.[165] Iron supplementation in pregnancy is not associated with significant

TABLE 1-4
MINIMUM VALUES FOR DIAGNOSING ANEMIA
BY AGE GROUP AND GESTATIONAL AGE

	Hemoglobin Concentration (g/dl)	Hematocrit (%)
Nonpregnant women and lactating women (age, in years)		
12–<15	11.8	35.7
15–<18	12.0	35.9
≥18	12.0	35.7
Pregnant women		
Weeks of gestation		
12	11.0	33.0
16	10.6	32.0
20	10.5	32.0
24	10.5	32.0
28	10.7	32.0
32	11.0	33.0
36	11.4	34.0
40	11.9	36.0
Trimester		
First	11.0	33.0
Second	10.5	32.0
Third	11.0	33.0

From Rees et al.,[167] with permission.

health risks. Because of the maternal risks of long-term iron depletion during pregnancy and possible association of poor pregnancy outcome with iron deficiency anemia, the Centers for Disease Control and Prevention (CDC) recommends both primary and secondary intervention for iron deficiency during pregnancy.[166] Primary prevention involves providing low-dose (30 mg/day) iron supplementation beginning as early in the pregnancy as possible. Secondary prevention involves screening for and treating anemia in pregnancy. Because of the known physiologic decrease in circulating red cells, anemia should be defined by pregnancy-specific standards (Table 1-4). Red-cell mass should be measured at the first prenatal visit. Anemia should be treated using 60 to 120 mg/day of supplemental iron. Iron therapy should result in an increase in hemoglobin by 1 g (3% increase in hematocrit) after 4 weeks of therapy. If this response does not occur and the woman remains anemic for her stage of pregnancy, a work-up for causes of anemia other than iron deficiency should be undertaken (i.e., acute illness, hemoglobinopathy, hemolysis, etc.). When the red-cell mass returns to normal for gestational age, the iron dose should decrease to 30 mg/day until delivery.[166]

ENDOCRINE METABOLISM

The Adrenal Gland

The adrenal glands are situated overlying the upper poles of the kidneys and are divided into an outer cortex and an inner medulla. The cortex is responsible for the production of steroid hormones, while the medulla secretes catecholamines.

Adrenal hormone release is regulated by the hypothalamic–pituitary axis. The diurnal rhythm in release of corticotropin-releasing hormone (CRH) from the hypothalamus is matched by adrenocorticotropic hormone (ACTH). ACTH, in turn, influences steroid secretion from the adrenal cortex. ACTH levels in pregnancy remain within the normal range for nonpregnant individuals.[167–169]

Glucocorticoids function in glucose homeostasis by stimulating gluconeogenesis and glycogen formation as well as promoting fatty acid synthesis. They also possess an antagonistic effect toward insulin. Cortisol, like most hormones, circulates bound to a plasma protein. About 75% is bound to corticosteroid-binding globulin (CBG) and 15% to albumin, leaving about 10% freely circulating.[170–172] The relative distribution of these binding fractions does not change appreciably in pregnancy. Since plasma CBG concentrations increase during pregnancy, plasma cortisol concentrations also rise. A two-fold increase occurs in the first trimester, and, by the third trimester, the plasma concentration is about three times its nonpregnant level.[173] Only the free fraction of the hormone is metabolically active, and since the binding affinity of cortisol for CBG remains unaltered, there is a concomitant rise in the circulating free cortisol concentration. By the end of a normal pregnancy, free hormone concentrations can reach levels seen in Cushing syndrome. However, unlike Cushing syndrome, the diurnal pattern in pregnancy is retained.[174] The increased free levels of cortisol in pregnancy may help explain the presence of cushingoid changes associated with normal pregnancies, such as striae gravidarum and carbohydrate intolerance.[175,176]

Aldosterone is a mineralocorticoid involved in salt and water regulation, causing sodium to be resorbed and potassium to be secreted from the distal tubules of the kidney. It circulates with a total plasma concentration that is 50 to 60% bound to albumin, 5 to 10% bound to CBG, and the remainder in the metabolically active free form.[172] Its release is stimulated by factors that activate the renin–angiotensin–aldosterone axis, such as low renal perfusion, decreased plasma volume, and hyponatremia. Pregnancy is associated with elevated plasma aldosterone concentrations. This occurs in response to the natriuretic effect of pregnancy caused by high progesterone levels coupled with increased glomerular filtration, as well as the loss of sodium to meet fetal requirements. These factors activate the release of renin from the kidney, which, in turn, ultimately leads to angiotensin II release. Angiotensin II then directly stimulates aldosterone secretion.[90,177–182]

Deoxycortisone is a less potent mineralocorticoid than aldosterone. It displays a greater relative increase in concentration during pregnancy than any other adrenal steroid.[183] It begins to rise at 8 weeks of gestation, which is earlier than the other corticosteroids,[184] and it is neither suppressible by dexamethasone nor responsive to changes in salt balance during pregnancy.[184,185] These unusual findings strongly indicate an alternate site of deoxycortisone secretion, most likely the fetal-placental unit.[184]

Androgens produced by the adrenals include testosterone, androstenedione, dehydroepiandrosterone (DHEA), and dehydroepiandrosterone sulfate (DHEAS). These hormones circulate bound to the plasma protein sex-hormone-binding globulin, which increases during pregnancy. Therefore, plasma concentrations of testosterone and androstenedione increase due to higher binding. In contrast, because of significant increases in metabolic clearance, DHEAS and DHEA levels are slightly lower in pregnancy.[186] Adrenal androgens, under conditions of normal pregnancy, have little physiologic impact.

The catecholamines epinephrine and norepinephrine are secreted by the adrenal medulla. Plasma levels of these are unchanged in pregnancy.

Pituitary

Pituitary imaging studies of pregnant women have shown a dramatic enlargement of the pituitary during pregnancy. By 12 weeks of gestation, pituitary volume increases by 45%, and continued growth results in an increase of 136% at term as compared with nonpregnant controls.[187] This growth occurs as a result of an increase in the number of prolactin-secreting cells, with the proportion of lactotrophs increasing from 1% to 40%.[188] This increase in prolactin-producing cells results in elevated plasma prolactin levels. Plasma concentrations of prolactin rise soon after conception and steadily increase to reach levels 10 to 20 times those of normal, nonpregnant values.[189]

The basal postpartum prolactin level depends on the frequency and quality of breast-feeding, with more frequent feeders maintaining higher basal levels. During suckling, prolactin levels increase 5- to 10-fold and remain elevated for about 30 minutes.[190,191] Elevated prolactin may play a role in the conservation of calcium. Animal studies reveal that prolactin enhances the conversion of 25-hydroxycholecalciferol to 1,25-dihydroxycholecalciferol.[192] An increased presence of this more potent vitamin D metabolite resulting from high prolactin values may be an adaptive mechanism that protects women from bone mineral loss, which could occur over long periods of breast-feeding because of the associated decrease in circulating estrogen.

Gonadotropins and growth hormone are both decreased in pregnancy because of feedback inhibition from high levels of estrogen and progesterone. Plasma levels of growth hormone return to normal within a few weeks of delivery, even in the presence of lactation. Gonadotropin release, on the other hand, remains inhibited in women who breast-feed.[193]

Thyroid

Hormones produced by the thyroid gland are central to basic cellular functions such as energy utilization and heat regulation. Pregnancy is associated with profound but reversible changes in laboratory tests used to assess thyroid function, which present a challenge to monitoring preexisting thyroid disease and detecting suspected thyroid abnormalities during pregnancy.

Thyroid Physiology

The normal thyroid gland undergoes a modest 13% increase in size during pregnancy.[194,195] The thyroid secretes the hormones thyroxine (T_4), which represents about 80% of thyroid hormone secretion, and triiodothyronine (T_3), which makes up the remaining 20% of thyroid secretion.[196]

Iodine is supplied from intestinal absorption of dietary sources and is incorporated into thyroglobulin in the thyroid. Thyroglobulin is then hydrolyzed to form individual T_3 and T_4 molecules, which are released from the gland.[197] Thionamides, drugs that are commonly used to treat hyperthyroidism in pregnancy, inhibit the enzyme that catalyzes the synthesis of iodothyronines.[198]

Thyroid-stimulating hormone (TSH), secreted from the anterior pituitary, controls the release of T_4 and T_3 from the thyroid gland by stimulating entry of iodine into the gland, thyroglobulin synthesis, and cleavage of thyroglobulin to form T_3 and T_4.[199,200] TSH secretion is, in turn, inhibited through a feedback mechanism by circulating levels of T_3 and T_4. TSH release, on the other hand, is promoted by thyrotropin-releasing hormone (TRH).

T_3 is the metabolically active form of thyroid hormone. The majority of T_3 is derived from peripheral conversion of T_4. Another form of thyroid hormone, reverse T_3 (rT_3) is produced through removal of a different iodine atom from T_4. rT_3 has no apparent metabolic activity and probably serves as a means of inactivating T_4.

Thyroid Function in Pregnancy

Iodine uptake by the thyroid in pregnancy seems to remain normally responsive to stimulation by TSH and suppression by thyroid hormones.[201] T_3 and T_4 circulate bound to thyroxine-binding globulin (TBG). Since TBG synthesis increases in pregnancy, serum levels of total T_3 and T_4 also increase. Consequently, the commonly measured total serum hormone levels will be increased in pregnancy. Total T_4 levels increase from euthyroid nonpregnant values of 5 to 12 μg/dl to 9 to 16 μg/dl in euthyroid pregnant women. Despite the increase in total hormone levels, the free fractions of T_3 and T_4, which are biologically active, remain unchanged in normal pregnancy.[202] With the advent of new assays by equilibrium dialysis techniques, free T_3 and T_4 levels can be measured directly rather than relying on the more cumbersome free T_4 index. Free T_3 and T_4 levels remain the most reliable indexes of thyroid function in pregnancy.[203]

The response of TSH to TRH also remains unchanged in pregnancy. In general, TSH is useful in screening for thyroid disease. However, it can be misleading when used alone in individuals being monitored for known thyroid disease,[204] women in the first trimester, women with hyperemesis gravidarum, or in molar pregnancies. In these situations, free T_3 or T_4 levels should also be obtained. T_3 and T_4 are able to cross the placenta but do so poorly.[205,206] TSH does not cross the placenta. The developing fetus is completely dependent on maternal transfer for its iodine supply and begins to concentrate iodine in the thyroid at about 12 weeks, when TSH and TRH are first detectable in the fetal pituitary and hypothalamus.[207]

Glucose Metabolism

An insulin-resistant condition, similar to that of Type II diabetes, accompanies normal pregnancy. Early in pregnancy, increasing estrogen and progesterone levels, which lead to pancreatic β-cell hypertrophy and insulin excretion, alters maternal carbohydrate metabolism. Meanwhile, the placental peptide hormone, human chorionic somatomammotropin (HCS, also known as human placental lactogen), has been implicated in inducing insulin resistance, as have prolactin, cortisol, estrogen, and progesterone.[208] The level of all these substances is significantly greater in pregnancy than in nonpregnant states. Euglycemic clamp techniques have been used to characterize the changes in insulin release and insulin resistance in pregnancy.[209] These methods have demonstrated a two-phase insulin response to increases in blood glucose as might occur after feeding. The first phase takes place from 0 to 5 minutes, and is proportional to the magnitude of the glucose concentration that provoked the response. The second phase takes place from 5 to 60 minutes after eating and is caused by continued secretion of insulin from β cells in the pancreas when glucose levels remain above a certain threshold following the first phase. In pregnancy, the first and second phases were significantly elevated, and peripheral insulin sensitivity decreased by 56% as pregnancy continued. This relative state of hyperinsulinemia and exaggerated glycemic response are often referred to as the diabetogenic effect of pregnancy. Despite this trend toward insulin resistance, during the overnight nonfeeding hours, glucose levels steadily fall to reach lower fasting values; maternal fasting plasma glucose levels are 10 to 15 mg/dl lower than in nonpregnant women.[210,211] The exaggerated starvation also leaves pregnant women prone to ketone formation, with elevated levels of β-hydroxybutyric acid and acetoacetic acid following overnight fasting.[212]

In contrast, the maternal response to feeding is more consistent with an insulin-resistant picture. Plasma glucose responses to similar carbohydrate loads are higher in pregnant women than nonpregnant women.[213] Although pregnancy is usually associated with relatively small glucose excursions after feeding, this requires a dramatic increase in insulin response, with mean 24-hour plasma values approximately one-third higher than those in nonpregnant women.[210,211,214]

The fetus meets nearly all its energy needs through glucose. Glucose is transferred across the placenta by **facilitated diffusion**, which is carrier-mediated but not energy-dependent. Although the fetus depends on maternal glucose for fuel, it has no requirement for maternal insulin. In fact, insulin does not cross the placenta, and the fetus produces insulin after the early part of pregnancy.

Amino acids are actively transported across the placenta against a gradient where they are used for fuel and protein synthesis. The rate of transfer depends on the amino acid structure. Branched-chained varieties are relatively rapidly transported while neutral straight chains undergo less rapid transfer.[215] Glutamate and aspartate (the acidic amino acids) are only negligibly transported across the placenta but are synthesized by the fetus.[216,217]

Although relatively impermeable to esterified lipids, the placenta permits free fatty acids to readily cross, governed by gradient-dependent diffusion, exceeding the amount needed for lipid storage needs. Free fatty acids in the fetal circulation are taken up by the fetal liver, where they undergo esterification and are then released into the circulation as very-low-density lipoproteins.[215,218]

REFERENCES

1. Swiet M. The cardiovacular system. In: Hytten FE, Chamberlain G, eds. Clinical physiology in obstetrics. 2nd ed. Oxford: Blackwell Scientific, 1991:3.
2. Gemzell CA, Robbe H, Ström G. Total amount of haemoglobin and physical working capacity in normal pregnancy and puerperium with iron medication. Acta Obstet Gynaecol Scand 1957;36:93.
3. Ihrman K. A clinical and physiological study of pregnancy in a material from Northern Sweden. III. Vital capacity and maximal breathing capacity during and after pregnancy. Acta Soc Med Ups 1960;65:147.
4. Rubler S, Damani P, Pinto ER. Cardiac size and performance during pregnancy estimated with echocardiography. Am J Cardiol 1977;40:534.
5. Cutforth R, MacDonald CB. Heart sounds and murmurs in pregnancy. Am Heart J 1966;71:741.
6. Tabatznik B, Randall TW, Hearsch C. The mammary souffle in pregnancy and lactation. Circulation 1960; 22:1069.
7. Hollander AG, Crawford JH. Roentgenologic and electrocardiographic changes in the normal heart during pregnancy. Am Heart J 1943;26:364.
8. Landt H, Benjamin JE. Cardiodynamic and electrocardiographic changes in normal pregnancy. Am Heart J 1936;12:592.
9. Zatuchni J. The electrocardiogram in pregnancy and the puerperium. Am Heart J 1951;42:11.
10. Oram S, Holt M. Innocent depression of the S–T segment and flattening of the T-wave during pregnancy. J Obstet Gynaecol Br Commonw 1961;68:765.
11. Boyle D McC, Lloyd-Jones RL. The electrocardiographic S–T segment in pregnancy. J Obstet Gynaecol Br Commonw 1966;73:986.
12. Szekely P, Snaith L. Heart disease and pregnancy. Edinburgh: Churchill Livingstone, 1974.
13. Rotmensch HH, Rotmensch S, Elkayam U. Management of cardiac arrhythmias during pregnancy: current concepts. Drugs 1987;33(6):623.
14. Kerr MG, Scott DB, Samuel E. Studies of the inferior vena cava in late pregnancy. BMJ 1964;1:532.
15. Ueland K, Novy MJ, Peterson EN, Metcalfe J. Maternal cardiovascular dynamics. IV. The influence of gestational age on the maternal cardiovascular response to posture and exercise. Am J Obstet Gynecol. 1969;104(6):856.
16. de Swiet M. The cardiovascular system. In: Hytten FE, Chamberlain G, eds. Clinical physiology in obstetrics. 2nd ed. Oxford: Blackwell Scientific, 1991:6.
17. Bader RA, Bader MG, Rose DJ, et al. Hemodynamics at rest and during exercise in normal pregnancy as studied by cardiac catheterization. J Clin Invest 1955;34:1524.
18. Walters WAW, MacGregor WG, Hills M. Cardiac output at rest during pregnancy and the puerperium. Clin Sci 1966;30:1.
19. Clark SL, Cotton DB, Lee W, et al. Central hemodynamic assessment of normal term pregnancy. Am J Obstet Gynecol 1989;161(6 Pt 1):1439.
20. Robson SC, Hunter S, Boys RJ, Dunlop W. Serial study of factors influencing changes in cardiac output during human pregnancy. Am J Physiol 1989;256(4 Pt 2):H1060.

21. Capeless EL, Clapp JF. Cardiovascular changes in early phase of pregnancy. Am J Obstet Gynecol 1989; 161(6 Pt 1):1449.

22. Capeless EL, Clapp JF. When do cardiovascular parameters return to their preconception values? Am J Obstet Gynecol 1991;165(4 Pt 1):883.

23. Clapp JF. Maternal heart rate in pregnancy. Am J Obstet Gynecol 1985;52:659.

24. Assali NS, Rauramo L, Peltonen T. Uterine and fetal blood flow and oxygen consumption in early human pregnancy. Am J Obstet Gynecol 1960;79:86.

25. Romney SL, Reid DE, Metcalfe J, Burwell CS. Oxygen utilization by the human fetus in utero. Am J Obstet Gynecol 1955;70:791.

26. Bordley J, Connor CAR, Hamilton WF, et al. Recommendations for human blood pressure determinations by sphygmomanometer. Circulation 1951;4:503.

27. Koller O. The clinical significance of hemodilution during pregnancy. Obstet Gynecol Surv 1982;37(11):649.

28. Kirshon B, Lee W, Cotton DB, Giebel R. Indirect blood pressure monitoring in the postpartum patient. Obstet Gynecol 1987;70(5):799.

29. Schwarz R. Das Verhalten des Kreislaufs in der normalen Schwangershaft. 1. Der arterielle Blutdruck. Arch Gynekol 1964;199:54.

30. Wilson M, Morganti AA, Zervoudakis I, et al. Blood pressure, the renin-aldosterone system and sex steroids throughout normal pregnancy. Am J Med 1980; 68(1):97.

31. Wichman K, Ryden G, Wichman M. The influence of different positions and Korotkoff sounds on the blood pressure measurements in pregnancy. Acta Obstet Gynecol Scand Suppl 1984;118:25.

32. National High Blood Pressure Education Program Working Group Report on High Blood Pressure in Pregnancy. Am J Obstet Gynecol 1990;163(5 Pt 1):1691.

33. MacGillivray I, Rose GA, Rowe B. Blood pressure survey in pregnancy. Clin Sci 1969;37:95.

34. Pyorala AT. Cardiovascular response to the upright position during pregnancy. Acta Obstet Gynecol Scand 966;45(Suppl. 5):1.

35. Thomson KJ, Hirsheimer A, Gibson JG, et al. Studies on the circulation in pregnancy. III. Blood volume changes in normal pregnant women. Am J Obstet Gynecol 1938; 36:48.

36. Bickers W. The placenta: a modified arteriovenous fistula. South Med J 1942;35:593.

37. McLennan CE. Antecubital and femoral venous pressure in normal and toxemic pregnancy. Am J Obstet Gynecol 1943;45:568.

38. de Swiet M. The cardiovascular system. In: Hytten FE, Chamberlain G, eds. Clinical physiology in obstetrics. 2nd ed. Oxford: Blackwell Scientific, 1991:14.

39. Ueland K, Hansen JM. Maternal cardiovascular dynamics. II. Posture and uterine contractions. Am J Obstet Gynecol 1969;103:1.

40. Ueland K, Hansen JM. Maternal cardiovascular dynamics. III. Labor and delivery under local and caudal analgesia. Am J Obstet Gynecol 1969;103:8.

41. Hunter D, Robson SC. Adaptation of the maternal heart in pregnancy. Br Heart J 1992;68:540.

42. Ueland K, Metcalfe J. Circulatory changes in pregnancy. J Clin Obstet Gynecol 1975;18(3):41.

43. Ueland K, Gills RE, Hansen JM. Maternal cardiovascular dynamics. I. Cesarean section under subarachnoid block anesthesia. Am J Obstet Gynecol 1968;100(1):42.

44. Thomson KJ, Cohen ME. Studies on the circulation in pregnancy. II. Vital capacity observations in normal pregnant women. Surg Gynecol Obstet 1938;66:591.

45. Gilroy RJ, Mangura BT, Lavietes MH. Rib cage and abdominal volume displacement during breathing in pregnancy. Am Rev Respir Dis 1988;137:668.

46. McGinty AP. The comparative effect of pregnancy and phrenic nerve interruption on the diaphragm and their relation to pulmonary tuberculosis. Am J Obstet Gynecol 1938;35:237.

47. de Swiet M. The respiratory system. In: Hytten FE, Chamberlain G, eds. Clinical physiology in obstetrics. 2nd ed. Oxford: Blackwell Scientific, 1991:88.

48. Cugell DW, Frank NR, Gaensler EA, et al. Pulmonary function in pregnancy. 1. Serial observations in normal women. Am Rev Tuberc Pulm Dis 1953;67:568.

49. Lehmann V, Fabel H. Lungen funktionsuntersuchungen an Schwangeren Teil II: Ventilation, Atemmechanik und Diffusionkapazitat. Z Geburtshilfe Perinatol 1973; 177:397.

50. Gazioglu K, Kaltreider NL, Rosen M, et al. Pulmonary function during pregnancy in normal women and in patients with cardiopulmonary disease. Thorax 1970; 25:445.

51. Knuttgen HG, Emerson K. Physiological response to pregnancy at rest and during exercise. J Appl Physiol 1974;36:549.

52. Etig M, Butler J, Bonica JJ. Respiratory function in pregnant obese women. Am J Obstet Gynecol 1975; 123:241.

53. Rubin A, Russo N, Goucher D. The effect of pregnancy upon pulmonary function in normal women. Am J Obstet Gynecol 1956;72:963.

54. Woolcock AJ, Read J. In: Shearman RP, ed. Human reproductive physiology. Oxford: Blackwell Scientific, 1972:639.

55. Sims CD, Chamberlain GVP, de Swiet M. Lung function tests in bronchial asthma during and after pregnancy. Br J Obstet Gynaecol 1976;83:434.

56. Kruniholz RA, Echt CR, Ross JC. Pulmonary diffusing capacity, capillary blood volume, lung volumes and mechanics of ventilation in early and late pregnancy. J Lab Clin Med 1964;63:648.

57. Cameron SJ, Bain HH, Grant IWB. Ventilatory function in pregnancy. Scott Med J 1970;15:243.

58. Milne JA, Mills RJ, Howie AD, et al. Large airways function during normal pregnancy. Br J Obstet Gynaecol 1977;84:448.

59. Pernoll ML, Metcalfe J, Kovach PA, et al. Ventilation during rest and exercise in pregnancy and postpartum. Respir Physiol 1975;25:295.

60. Omatsu Y. Basal metabolism in pregnancy. Kobe Med Sci 1957;27:21.

61. Templeton A, Kelman GR. Maternal blood gases (PAO_2-PaO_2) physiological shunt and VD/VT in normal pregnancy. Br J Anaesth 1976;48:1001.

62. Pecora LJ, Putnam LR, Baum GL. Effects of intravenous estrogens on pulmonary diffusing capacity. Am J Med Sci 1963;246:48.

63. Pernoll ML, Metcalfe J, Schlenker TL, et al. Oxygen consumption at rest and during exercise in pregnancy. Respir Physiol 1975;25:285.

64. Lucius H, Gahlenbeck H, Kleine HO, et al. Respiratory functions, buffer system, and electrolyte concentrations of blood during human pregnancy. Respir Physiol 1970; 9:311.

65. Kelman GR, Templeton A. Maternal blood gases during human pregnancy. J Physiol 975;244:66P.

66. Goodland RL, Reynolds JG, McCoord AB, et al. Respiratory and electrolyte effects induced by estrogen and progesterone. Fertil Steril 1953;4:300.

67. Skatrud JB, Dempsey JA, Kaiser DG. Ventilatory response to medroxyprogesterone acetate in normal subjects: time course and mechanisms. J Appl Physiol 1978;44:939.

68. Paciorek J, Spencer N. An association between plasma progesterone and erythrocyte carbonic anhydrase 1 concentration in women. Clin Sci 1980;58:161.

69. Milne JA, Howie AD, Pack Al. Dyspnoea during normal pregnancy. Br J Obstet Gynaecol 1978;85(4):260.

70. Cietak KA, Newton JR. Serial quantitative nephrosonography in pregnancy. Br J Radiol 1985;58:405.

71. Bailey RR, Rolleston GL. Kidney length and ureteric dilatation in the puerperium. J Obstet Gynaecol Br Commonw 1971;78:55.

72. Cietak KA, Rolieston GL. Serial qualitative nephrosonography in pregnancy. Br J Radiol 1985;58:399.

73. Rasmussen PE, Nielsen FR. Hydronephrosis during pregnancy: a literature survey. Eur J Obstet Gynaecol Reprod Bio 1988;27:249.

74. Fried A, Woodring JH, Thompson TJ. Hydronephrosis of pregnancy. J Ultrasound Med 1983;2:225.

75. Bayless C, Davison J. The urinary system. In: Hytten FE, Chamberlain G, eds. Clinical physiology in obstetrics. 2nd ed. Oxford: Blackwell Scientific, 1991:247.

76. Rubi RA, Sala NL. Ureteral functions in pregnant women. III. Effect of different positions and of fetal delivery upon ureteral tonus. Am J Obstet Gynecol 1968; 101:230.

77. Dunlop W. Investigations into the influence of posture on renal plasma flow and glomerular filtration rate during late pregnancy. Br J Obstet Gynaecol. 1976;83:17.

78. Dunlop W. Serial changes in renal haemodynamics during normal human pregnancy. Br J Obstet Gynaecol 1981;88:1.

79. Equlmokhai M, Davison JM, Philips PR, et al. Nonpostural serial changes in renal function during the third trimester of normal human pregnancy. Br J Obstet Gynaecol 1981;88:465.

80. Davison JM, Dunlop W. Renal haemodynamics and tubular function in normal human pregnancy. Kidney Int 1980;18:152.

81. Davison JM, Dunlop W. Changes in renal haemodynamics and tubular function induced by normal human pregnancy. Semin Nephrol 1984:198.

82. Davison JM, Hytten FE. Glomerular filtration during and after pregnancy. J Obstet Gynaecol Commonw 1975;81:583.

83. Davison JM, Noble MCB. Serial changes in 24-hour creatinine clearance during normal menstrual cycles and the first trimester of pregnancy. Br J Obstet Gynaecol 1981;88:10.

84. Whaley PJ. Bacteriuria of pregnancy. Am J Obstet Gynecol 1967;97:723.

85. Bayless C, Davison J. The urinary system. In: Hytten FE, Chamberlain G, eds. Clinical physiology in obstetrics. 2nd ed. Oxford: Blackwell Scientific, 1991:270.

86. Cruikshank DP, Wigton TR, Hays PM. Maternal physiology in pregnancy. In: Gabbe SG, Niebyl JL, Simpson JL, eds. Obstetrics: normal and problem pregnancies. 3rd ed. New York: Churchill Livingstone, 1996:97.

87. Davison JM, Vallotton MB, Lindheimer MD. Plasma osmolality and urinary concentration and dilution during and after pregnancy: evidence that lateral recumbency inhibits maximal urinary concentrating ability. Br J Obstet Gynaecol 1981;88:472.

88. Gallery EDM, Brown M. Volume homeostasis in normal and hypertensive human pregnancy. Clin Obstet Gynecol 1987;1:835.

89. Lindheimer MD, Katz AI. Normal and abnormal pregnancy. In: Arieff AI, Defronzo R, eds. Fluid, electrolyte and acid-base disorders. New York: Churchill Livingstone, 1985:1041.

90. Smeaton TC, Andersen GJ, Fulton IS. Study of aldosterone levels in plasma during pregnancy. J Clin Endocrinol Metab 1977;44(1):1.

91. Nolten WE, Lindheimer MD, Oparil S, et al. Desoxycorticosterone in normal pregnancy. II. Cortisol dependent fluctuations in free plasma desoxycorticosterone. Am J Obstet Gynecol 1979;133:644.

92. Casey ML, MacDonald PC. Metabolism of deoxycorticosterone and deoxycorticosterone sulfate in men and women. J Clin Invest 1982;70:312.

93. Nolten WE, Holt LH, Ruerckert P. Desoxycorticosterone in normal pregnancy. III. Evidence of a fetal source of desoxycorticosterone. Am J Obstet Gynecol 1980; 139:477.

94. MacDonald PC, Cutrer S, MacDonald SC, et al. Regulation of extraadrenal steroid 21-hydroxylase activity: increased conversion of plasma progesterone during estrogen treatment of women pregnant with a dead fetus. J Clin Invest 1982;69:469.

95. Miyamoto S, Shimokawa H, Stimioki H, et al. Circadian rhythm of plasma atrial natriuretic peptide, aldosterone, and blood pressure during the third trimester in normal and preeclamptic pregnancies. Am J Obstet Gynecol 1988;158:393.

96. Cruikshank DP, Wigton TR, Hays PM. Maternal physiology in pregnancy. In: Gabbe SG, Niebyl JR, Simpson JL, eds. Obstetrics: normal and problem pregnancies. 3rd ed. New York: Churchill Livingstone, 1996:97.

97. Davison JM, Lindheimer MD. Renal disorders. In: Creasey RK, Resnik R, eds. Maternal-fetal medicine: principles and practice. 3rd ed. Philadelphia: Saunders, 1994:847.

98. Rieselbach RE, Steele TH. Influence of the kidney upon urate homeostasis in health and disease. Am J Med 1974; 56:575.

99. Lind T, Godfrey KA, Otun H, et al. Changes in serum uric acid concentration during normal pregnancy. Br J Obstet Gynaecol 1984;91:128.

100. Davison JM, Hytten FE. The effect of pregnancy on the renal handling of glucose. J Obstet Gynaecol Br Commonw 1975;82:374.

101. Davison JM, Cheyne GA. Renal reabsorption of glucose. Lancet 1972;1:787.

102. Schultze RG, Burger H. The influence of GFR and saline expansion on TmG of the dog kidney. Kidney Int 1973;3:291.

103. Hytten FE, Clieyne GA. The aminoaciduria of pregnancy. J Obstet Gynaecol Br Commonw 1972;79:424.

104. Taggart N. Food habits in pregnancy. Proc Nutr Soc 1961;20:35.

105. Hytten FE, Lind T. Indices of alimentary function. In: Hytten FE, Chamberlain G, eds. Clinical physiology in obstetrics. 2nd ed. Oxford: Blackwell Scientific, 1991:13.

106. Hook EB. Dietary cravings and aversions during pregnancy. Am J Clin Nutr 1978;31:1355.

107. Cruikshank DP, Wigton TR, Hays PM. Maternal physiology in pregnancy. In: Gabbe SG, Niebyl JR, Simpson JL, eds. Obstetrics: normal and problem pregnancies. 3rd ed. New York: Churchill Livingstone, 1996:91.

108. Kallendar D, Sonesson B. Studies on saliva in menstruating, pregnant and post-menopausal women. Acta Endocrinol (Copenh) 1965;48:329.

109. James JD. Dental caries in pregnancy. J Am Dent Assoc 1941;28:1857.

110. Deakins M, Looby J. Effect of pregnancy on the mineral content of dentin in human teeth. Am J Obstet Gynecol 1943;46:265.

111. Dragiff DA, Karshan M. Effect of pregnancy on the chemical composition of human dentin. J Dent Res 1943;22:261.

112. Lind JF, Smith AM, McIver DK, et al. Heartburn in pregnancy—a manometric study. Can Med Assoc J 1968;98:571.

113. Hey VMF, Cowley DJ, Ganguli PC, et al. Gastro-oesophageal reflux in late pregnancy. Anaesthesia 1977;32:372.

114. Hytten FE. The alimentary system. In: Hytten FE, Chamberlain G, eds. Clinical physiology in obstetrics. 2nd ed. Oxford: Blackwell Scientific, 1991:141.

115. Christofides ND, Ghatei MA, Bloom SR, et al. Decreased plasma motilin concentrations in pregnancy. BMJ 1982;285:1453.

116. Nimmo WS, Wilson J, Prescott LF. Narcotic analgesics and delayed gastric emptying during labour. Lancet 1975;1:890.

117. Wright PM, Allen RW, Moore J, et al. Gastric emptying during lumbar extradural analgesia in labour: effect of fentanyl supplementation. Br J Anaesth 1992;68(3):248.

118. Porter JS, Bonnello E, Reynolds F. The influence of epidural administration of fentanyl infusion on gastric emptying in labour. Anaesthesia 1997;52(12):1151.

119. Clarke DH. Peptic ulcer in women. BMJ 1953;1:1254.

120. Parbhoo SP, Johnston IDA. Effect of oestrogens and progestogens on gastric secretion in patients with duodenal ulcer. Gut 1966;7:612.

121. Gryboski WA, Spiro HM. The effect of pregnancy on gastric secretion. N Engl J Med 1956;255:1131.

122. Parry E, Shields R, Turnbull AC. Transit time in the small intestine in pregnancy. J Obstet Gynaecol Br Commonw 1970;77:900.

123. Svanberg B. Absorption of iron in pregnancy. Acta Obstet Gynecol Scand (Suppl) 1975;48:69.

124. Haeney RP, Skillman TG. Calcium metabolism in normal human pregnancy. J Clin Endocrinol Metab 1971;33:661.

125. Parry E, Shields R, Turnbull AC. The effect of pregnancy on the colonic absorption of sodium, potassium and water. J Obstet Gynaecol Br Commonw 1970;77:616.

126. Cruikshank DP, Wigton TR, Hays PM. Maternal physiology in pregnancy. In: Gabbe SG, Niebyl JR, Simpson JL, eds. Obstetrics: normal and problem pregnancies. 3rd ed. New York: Churchill Livingstone, 1996:92.

127. Walker FB, Hobilt DL, Cunningham FG. Gamma glutamyl transpeptidase in normal pregnancies. Obstet Gynecol 1974;43:745.

128. Carter J. Liver function in normal pregnancy. Aust NZ J Obstet Gynaecol 1990;30:296.

129. Cerutti R, Ferrari S, Grella P. Behavior of serum enzymes in pregnancy. Clin Exp Obstet Gynecol 1976;3:22.

130. Bennion LJ, Grundy SM. Risk factors for the development of cholelithiasis in man. N Engl J Med 1978;299(21):1161.

131. Kern F Jr, Everson GT, DeMark B, et al. Biliary lipids, bile acids, and gallbladder function in the human female: effects of contraceptive steroids. J Lab Clin Med 1982;99(6):798.

132. Laatikainen T, Lehtonen P, Hesso A. Biliary bile acids in uncomplicated pregnancy and in cholestasis of pregnancy. Clin Chim Acta 1978;85(2):145.

133. Gerdes MM, Boyden EA. The rate of emptying of the human gall-bladder in pregnancy. Surg Gynecol Obstet 1938;66:145.

134. Bracerman DZ, Johnson ML, Kern F. Effects of pregnancy and contraceptive steroids on gallbladder function. N Engl J Med 980;302:363.

135. Maringhini A, Meddalena Ciambra MD, Baccelliere P, et al. Biliary sludge and gallstones in pregnancy: incidence, risk factors, and natural history. Ann Intern Med 1993;119(2):116.

136. Pirani BBK, Campbell DM, MacGilivray I. Plasma volume in normal first pregnancy. J Obstet Gynaecol Br Commonw 1973;80:884.

137. Letsky E. The haematological system. In: Hytten FE, Chamberlain G, eds. Clinical physiology in obstetrics. 2nd ed. Oxford: Blackwell Scientific, 1991:42.

138. Hytten FE, Leitch I. The volume and composition of the blood. In Hytten FE, Leitch I, eds. The physiology of human pregnancy. 2nd ed. Oxford: Blackwell Scientific, 1971:1.

139. Pritchard JA. Changes in blood volume during pregnancy and delivery. Anesthesiology 1965;26:393.

140. Caton WL, Roby CC, Reid DE, et al. The circulating red cell volume and body haematocrit in normal pregnancy and the puerperium. Am J Obstet Gynecol 1951;61:1207.

141. Verel D, Bury JD, Hope A. Blood volume changes in pregnancy and the puerperium. Clin Sci 1956;15:1.

142. Berlin NI, Goetsch C, Hyde GM, et al. The blood volume in pregnancy as determined with p3'-labelled red blood cells. Surg Gynecol Obstet 1953;97:173.

143. Pritchard JA, Wiggins KM, Dickey JC. Blood volume changes in pregnancy and the puerperium. 1. Does sequestratium of red blood cells accompany parturition? Am J Obstet Gynecol 1960;80:956.

144. Paintin DB. The size of the total red cell volume in pregnancy. J Obstet Gynaecol Br Commonw 1962;69:719.

145. Pritchard JA, Baldwin RM, Dickey JC, et al. Blood volume changes in pregnancy and the puerperium. II. Red blood cell loss and changes in apparent blood volume during and following vaginal delivery, cesarean section, and cesarean section plus total hysterectomy. Am J Obstet Gynecol 1962;84:1271.

146. Euland K. Maternal cardiovascular dynamics. VII. Intrapartum blood volume changes. Am J Obstet Gynecol 1976;126:671.

147. Gibson A. On leucocyte changes during labour and the puerperium. J Obstet Gynaecol Br Emp 1937;44:500.

148. Efrati P, Presentey B, Margalith M, et al. Leukocytes of normal pregnant women. Obstet Gynecol 1964;23:429.

149. Polishuk WZ, Diamant YZ, Zuckerman H, et al. Leukocyte alkaline phosphatase in pregnancy and the puerperium. Am J Obstet Gynecol 1970;107:604.

150. Andrews WC, Bonsnes RW. The leucocytes during pregnancy. Am J Obstet Gynecol 1951;61:1129.

151. Cruickshank JM. The effects of parity on the leucocyte count in pregnant and non-pregnant women. Br J Haematol 1970;18:531.

152. Brain P, Marston RH, Gordon J. Immunological responses in pregnancy. BMJ 1972;4:488.

153. Fay RA, Hughes AO, Farron NT. Platelets in pregnancy: hyperdestruction in pregnancy. Obstet Gynecol 1983; 61:238.

154. Wallenberg HCS, VanKessel PH. Platelet lifespan in normal pregnancy as determined by a nonradioisotope technique. Br J Obstet Gynaecol 1978;85:33.

155. Hytten FE, Lind T. Volume and composition of the blood. In: Hytten FE, Lind T, eds. Diagnostic indices in pregnancy. Basel: Documenta Geigy, 1973:36.

156. Laros RK, Alger LS. Thromboembolism and pregnancy. Clin Obstet Gynecol 1979;22:871.

157. Berg CJ, Atrash HK, Koonon LM, et al. Pregnancy-related mortality in the United States, 1987–1990. Obstet Gynecol 1996;88(2):161.

158. De Leeuw NKM, Lowenstein L, Hsieh YS. Iron deficiency and hydremia in normal pregnancy. Medicine (Baltimore) 1966;45:291.

159. Letsky E. The haematological system. In: Hytten FE, Chamberlain G, eds. Clinical physiology in obstetrics. 2nd ed. Oxford: Blackwell Scientific, 1991:48.

160. Apte SV, Iyenger L. Absorption of dietary iron in pregnancy. Am J Clin Nutr 1970;23:73.

161. Svanberg B. Absorption of iron in pregnancy. Acta Obstet Gynaecol Scand Suppl 1975;48:7.

162. Stacey TE. Placental transfer. In: Hytten FE, Chamberlain G, eds. Clinical physiology in obstetrics. 2nd ed. Oxford: Blackwell Scientific, 1991:431.

163. National Research Council. Recommended dietary allowances. 10th ed. Washington, DC: National Academy Press, 1989.

164. Centers for Disease Control and Prevention. Recommendations to prevent and control iron deficiency in the United States. MMWR 1998;47(RR-3):9.

165. Scholl TO, Hediger ML, Fischer RL, et al. Iron deficiency: increased risk of preterm delivery in a prospective study. Am J Clin Nutr 1992;55:985.

166. Centers for Disease Control and Prevention. Recommendations to prevent and control iron deficiency in the United States. MMWR 1998;47(RR-3):24.

167. Rees, LH, Burke CW, Chard T, et al. Possible placental origin of ACTH in normal human pregnancy. Nature 1975;254:620.

168. Genazzani AR, Fraioli F, Hurlimann I, et al. Immuno-reactive ACTH and cortisol plasma levels during pregnancy: detection and partial purification of corticotrophin-like placental hormone: the human chorionic corticotrophin (hCG). Clin Endocrinol 1975;4:1.

169. Carr BR, Parker CR, Madden JD, et al. Maternal plasma adrenocorticotrophin and cortisol relationships throughout human pregnancy. Am J Obstet Gynecol 1981; 139:416.

170. Daughaday WH. Binding of corticosteroids by plasma proteins. III. The binding of corticosteroid and related hormones by human plasma and plasma fractions as measured by equilibrium dialysis. J Clin Invest 1958;37:511.

171. Doe RP, Fernandez R, Seal US. Measurement of corticosteroid-binding globulin in man. J Clin Endocrinol Metab 1964;24:1029.

172. Burke CW. The adrenal cortex in practical medicine. London: Gray-Mills, 1973:16.

173. Rosenthal HE, Slaunwhite NVR Jr, Sandberg AA. Transcortin: a corticosteroid-binding protein of plasma, X: Cortisol and progesterone interplay and unbound levels of these steroids in pregnancy. J Clin Endocrinol Metab 1969;29:352.

174. Nolten NVE, Lindheimier MD, Rueckert PA, et al. Diurnal patterns and regulation of cortisol secretion in pregnancy. J Clin Endocrinol Metab 1980;51:466.

175. Browne FJ. Aetiology of pre-eclamptic toxaemia and eclampsia: fact and theory. Lancet 1958;1:115.

176. Sophian J. Aetiology of pre-eclamptic toxaemia and eclampsia. Lancet 1958;1:434.

177. Düsterdieck G, McElwee G. Estimation of angiotensin II concentration in human plasma by radioimmunoassay: some applications to physiological and clinical states. Eur J Clin Invest 1971;2:32.

178. Venning EH, Dyrenfurth I. Aldosterone excretion in pregnancy. J Clin Endocrinol Metab 1956;16:426.

179. Rinsier MG, Rigby B. Function of aldosterone in the metabolism of sodium and water in pregnancy. BMJ 1957;2:966.

180. Weir RI, Paintin DB, Robertson IIS, et al. Renin, angiotensin and aldosterone relationships in normal pregnancy. Proc R Soc Med 1970;63:1101.

181. Weir RJ, Paintin DB, Brown JJ, et al. A serial study in pregnancy of the plasma concentration of renin, corticosteroids, electrolytes and proteins and of haematocrit and plasma volume. J Obstet Gynaecol Br Commonw 1971;78:590.

182. Alhenc-Celas F, Tache A, Saint-Andre JP. In: Grunfeld JP, Maxwell MH, Bach JF, et al., eds. Advances in nephrology. Vol. 15. Chicago: Year Book, 1986:25.

183. Wintour EM, Coghlan JP, Oddie CJ, et al. A sequential study of adrenocorticosteroid level in human pregnancy. Clin Exp Pharmacol Physiol 1978;5:399.

184. Brown RD, Strott CA, Liddle GW. Plasma deoxycorticosterone in normal and abnormal human pregnancy. J Clin Endocrinol Metab 972;35:736.

185. Ehrlich EN, Nolten WE, Oparil S, et al. Mineralocorticoids in normal pregnancy. In: Lindheimer MD, Katz AI, Zuspan FP, eds. Hypertension in pregnancy. New York: Wiley, 1976:189.

186. Cruikshank DP, Wigton TR, Hays PM. Maternal physiology in pregnancy. In: Gabbe SG, Niebyl JR, Simpson JL, eds. Obstetrics: normal and problem pregnancies. 3rd ed. New York: Churchill Livingstone, 1996:104.

187. Gonzalez JG, Elizondo G, Saldivar D, et al. Pituitary gland growth during normal pregnancy: an in vivo study using magnetic resonance imaging. Am J Med 1988; 85:217.

188. Goluboff LG, Ezrin C. Effect of pregnancy on the somatotroph and prolactin cell of the human adenohypophysis. J Clin Endocrinol Metab 1969;29:1533.

189. Rigg LA, Lein A, Yen SSC. The pattern of increase in circulating prolactin levels during human gestation. Am J Obstet Gynecol 1977;129:454.

190. Delvoye P, Badawi M, Demaega M. Long lasting lactation is associated with hyperprolactinaemia and amenorrhoea. In: Robyn C, Harter M, eds. Progress in prolactin physiology and pathology. Amsterdam: Elsevier/North Holland, 1978:213.

191. Noel GL, Suh HK, Frantz AG. Prolactin release during nursing and breast stimulation in post partum and non post partum subjects. J Clin Endocrinol Metab 1974; 38:413.

192. Spanos E, Pike JW, Haussler MR, et al. Circulating 1α,25-dihydroxy vitamin D in the chicken: enhancement by injection of prolactin and during egg laying. Life Sci 1976;19:1751.

193. Faiman C, Ryan RJ, Zwirck SJ, et al. Serum FSH and hCG during human pregnancy and puerperium. J Clin Endocrinol Metab 1968;28:1323.

194. Nelson M, Wickus GC, Caplan RH, Beguin EA. Thyroid gland size in pregnancy: an ultrasound and clinical study. J Reprod Med 1987;32:888.

195. Seely LB, Burrow GN. Thyroid disease in pregnancy. In: Creasey RK, Resnik R, eds. Maternal-fetal medicine: principles and practice. 3rd ed. Philadelphia: Saunders, 1994:979.

196. Brent GA. The molecular basis of thyroid hormone action. N Engl J Med 1994;331:847.

197. DeGroot LJ, Niepomnizcze H. Biosynthesis of thyroid hormone: basic and clinical aspects. Metabolism 1977; 26:665.

198. Cooper DS. Antithyroid drugs. N Engl J Med 1984; 311:1353.

199. Weinberger C, Thompson CC, Ong ES, et al. The c-erb-A gene encodes a thyroid hormone receptor. Nature 1986;324:641.

200. Sap J, Munoz A, Damm K, et al. The c-erb-A protein is a high-affinity receptor for thyroid hormone. Nature 1986;324:635.

201. Pochin EE. The iodine uptake of the human thyroid throughout the menstrual cycle and in pregnancy. Clin Sci 1952;11:441.

202. Harada A, Hershman JM, Reed AW, et al. Comparison of thyroid stimulators and thyroid hormone concentrations in the sera of pregnant women. J Clin Endocrinol Metab 1979;48:793.

203. Chopra IJ, Van Herle AJ, Chua Teco GN, et al. Serum free thyroxine in thyroidal and nonthyroidal illnesses: a comparison of measurements by radioimmunoassay, equilibrium dialysis, and free thyroxine index. J Clin Endocrinol Metab 1980;51:135.

204. Ross DS, Daniels GH, Goveia D. The use and limitations of a chemiluminescent thyrotropin assay as a single thyroid function test in an out-patient endocrine clinic. J Clin Endocrinol Metab 1990;71:764.

205. Bernal J, Pekonen F. Ontogenesis of nuclear 3,5,3′ triiodothyronine receptors in human fetal brain. Endocrinology 1984;114:677.

206. Fisher DA, Lehman H, Lackey D. Placental transport of thyroxine. J Clin Endocrinol Metab 964;24:393.

207. Fisher DA, Filey BL. Early treatment of congenital hypothyroidism. Pediatrics 1989;83:785.

208. Moore TR. Diabetes in pregnancy. In: Creasey PK, Resnik R, eds. Maternal-fetal medicine: principles and practice. 3rd ed. Philadelphia: Saunders, 1994:937.

209. Catalano PM, Tyzbir ED, Roman MM, et al. Longitudinal changes in insulin release and insulin resistance in nonobese pregnant women. Am J Obstet Gynecol 1991; 165:1667.

210. Cousins L, Rigg L, Hollingsworth D, et al. The 24-hour excursion and diurnal rhythm of glucose, insulin and C peptide in normal pregnancy. Am J Obstet Gynecol 1980;136:483.

211. Phelps RL, Metzger BE, Freinkel N. Carbohydrate metabolism in pregnancy. XVII. Diurnal profiles of plasma glucose, insulin, free fatty acids, triglycerides, cholesterol and individual amino acids in late normal pregnancy. Am J Obstet Gynecol 981;140:730.

212. Felig P, Lynch V. Starvation in human pregnancy: hypoglycemia, hypoinsulinemia, and hyperketonemia. Science 1970;170:990.

213. O'Sullivan JB, Malian CNI. Criteria for the oral glucose tolerance test in pregnancy. Diabetes 1964;13:278.

214. Hollingsworth DR. Maternal metabolism in normal pregnancy and pregnancy complicated by diabetes mellitus. Clin Obstet Gynecol 1985;28:457.

215. Hollingsworth DR. Alterations of maternal metabolism in normal and diabetic pregnancies: differences in insulin-dependent, non-insulin-dependent, and gestational diabetes. Am J Obstet Gynecol 1983;146(4):417.

216. Schneider H, Mohlen JH, Dancis J. Transfer of amino acids across the in vitro perfused human placenta. Ped Res 1979;13:236.

217. Schneider H, Mohlen JH, Challier JC, Dancis J. Transfer of glutamic acid across the human placenta perfused in vitro. Br J Obstet Gynaecol 1979;86:299.

218. Moore TR. Diabetes in pregnancy. In: Creasey RK, Resnik R, eds. Maternal-fetal medicine: principles and practice. 3rd ed. Philadelphia: Saunders, 1994:939.

Chapter 2

Preconceptional and Prenatal Care

Jeffrey A. Kuller
Robert A. Strauss
Robert C. Cefalo

Five Key Points

- **Preconceptional counseling is appropriate for all women contemplating pregnancy, not just those with obvious medical illnesses.**

- **The recommended weight gain for pregnancy is 28 to 40 lb for underweight women, 25 to 35 lb for women of normal weight, and 15 to 25 lb for women who are overweight.**

- **Ideally, all women should take supplemental folic acid (0.4 mg/day) prior to conception and during pregnancy to reduce the occurrence of fetal neural-tube defects. Women with a history of an affected child should take 4.0 mg of folic acid for 4 to 6 weeks prior to conception through the first trimester. This intervention reduces the risk of recurrence by approximately 50 to 60%.**

- **In the absence of obstetric or medical complications, pregnant women who engage in a moderate level of physical activity can maintain this activity throughout pregnancy.**

- **Inactivated vaccines, such as influenza, hepatitis A and B, and tetanus/diphtheria, may be safely administered during pregnancy.**

The goal of prenatal care is to optimize maternal and neonatal outcome. This process is best realized when begun prior to pregnancy. Although the maternal mortality rate in the United States has decreased significantly in the past 50 years, preventable pregnancy-related deaths continue to occur. Data from the Centers for Disease Control and Prevention indicate that the mortality rate increased from 7.2/100,000 in 1987 to 10.0/100,000 in 1990.[1] The leading causes of pregnancy-related death were hemorrhage, embolism, and hypertensive disorders of pregnancy.[1,2]

PRECONCEPTIONAL COUNSELING AND INTERVENTION

Preconceptional counseling is appropriate not only for women with medical complications but for any woman or couple contemplating pregnancy. The goal is to improve pregnancy outcome by assessing and optimizing a patient's medical, social, and genetic issues prior to pregnancy.[3] Targeting of only those women who are actively attempting pregnancy would exclude the greater than 50% of women who become

TABLE 2-1 **LABORATORY TESTS THAT MAY BE** **ORDERED PRECONCEPTIONALLY**

Complete blood count
Screening for:
    Rubella
    Syphilis
    Toxoplasmosis
    Hepatitis B surface antigen
    Chlamydia
    Gonorrhea
    Tuberculosis
    Human immunodeficiency virus
    Varicella

pregnant unintentionally. In a population-based survey of 12,452 new mothers, women with unintended pregnancies were more likely to have an indication for preconceptional counseling than women with planned pregnancies.[4]

A preconceptional visit involves risk identification, education, and recommended interventions. A preconceptional assessment ideally should be mailed to the patient prior to the visit. The answers can be expanded during the visit (see Figure 2-1). Table 2-1 lists laboratory tests that may be ordered during a preconception visit. These tests should be tailored to the patient's answers to the questionnaire, her specific concerns, and her home and work environments.

Medical History

Diabetes Mellitus

Diabetes mellitus presents one of the most compelling arguments supporting preconceptional care. Preconceptional care of the insulin-dependent diabetic, which strives for strict plasma glucose control, has been repeatedly demonstrated to decrease the prevalence of congenital malformations, preeclampsia, macrosomia, intrauterine growth restriction, and intrauterine fetal death.[5,6] Target glucose values are a preprandial level of 70 to 100 mg/dl and postprandial levels of <140 mg/dl at 1 hour and <120 mg/dl at 2 hours and a glycosolated hemoglobin value within or near the upper limit of normal for the laboratory. Prepregnancy is an ideal time to teach the patient about use of an appropriate meal plan, including timing of snacks, planning a physical exercise program, choosing time and site of insulin injections, the importance of testing and recording capillary blood glucose

results and the use of carbohydrate and glucagon for hypoglycemia.[7] Obstetric-care provders must consider every visit with a diabetic woman in her reproductive years as a preconception visit; if the patient is not planning a pregnancy at present, contraception should be explicitly discussed.[8]

In a cost–benefit analysis of the relevant literature, a consensus panel for the Agency for Health Care Policy and Research, Department of Health and Human Services, concluded that a preconception care program of a diabetic, along with intensive medical care continued throughout pregnancy, results in cost savings through the prevention of maternal and neonatal complications as compared with prenatal care alone. Preconceptional health care of diabetic women has been shown to result in improved infant and maternal outcome and significant cost savings. Unfortunately, a high rate of unplanned pregnancies occurs among diabetics, and lack of knowledge of the potential benefts of preconceptional care exists among both health care providers and patients, indicating that dissemination of information in this area is a problem.

Phenylketonuria

Phenylketonuria is an autosomal recessive condition usually diagnosed in the neonatal period as a result of newborn screening programs. Patients should be asked if they were ever on a special restricted diet as a child or young adult. Childhood restriction to a low-phenylalanine diet may have been long forgotten by the patient. Infants who do not themselves have phenylketonuria (PKU) may be born to women with classic PKU or atypical hyperphenylalaninemia. Maternal blood phenylalanine levels greater than 20 mg/dl are associated with a high prevalence of serious abnormalities such as microcephaly, mental retardation, congenital heart disease, and fetal growth restriction.[9-11] Excessive blood levels of phenylalanine are destructive to the fetal brain; to achieve a protective effect for the fetus, preconceptional reduction of the maternal blood level of phenylalanine to the range of 4 to 10 mg/dl with maintenance throughout pregnancy is essential.[10] In order to achieve this goal, a phenylalanine-restricted diet must be instituted 3 to 4 months prior to pregnancy. In the United States, there are approximately 3000 hyperphenylalaninemic women of childbearing age who may no longer be on a low phenylalanine diet and who may be at significant risk of having children who suffer the consequences.

MR# _____

(for clinic use)

_____ /____ / ____

_____ | _____ | _____ | _____
last name | first name | mi | date of birth

_____ | _____
street | apt/unit #

_____ | _____ | _____
city | state | zip code

(____) _____ | (____) _____ | _____
home phone number | work phone number | e-mail address (optional)

In order to address your specific interests and concerns for your visit, we ask that you complete the following questionnaire. You may use the back of this form to provide additional information when necessary.

What is your main reason for seeking preconceptional counseling?

_____

_____

_____

_____

ALLERGIES

Are you allergic to any medications? If yes, list the names and types of reactions:

_____

_____

MEDICATION HISTORY

Do you routinely or occasionally take prescribed medications?

If yes, list names and dosages:

_____

_____

_____

Do you routinely or occasionally take over-the-counter medications? If yes, list names and dosages:

_____

_____

_____

MEDICAL HISTORY

Do you now have, or have you ever had:
(Place an **X** next to any item(s) that applies to you)

❏ diabetes
❏ thyroid disease
❏ phenylketonuria (PKU)
❏ asthma
❏ other, describe below:

❏ heart disease
❏ high blood pressure
❏ deep venous thrombosis (blood clots)
❏ kidney disease

❏ systemic lupus erythematosus (SLE)
❏ epilepsy
❏ sickle cell disease
❏ cancer

_____

_____

_____

SURGICAL HISTORY

Please list any surgeries you have had in the past:

_____

_____

_____

Figure 2-1 Preconceptional Health Assessment. *Modified from Cefalo RC, Moos MK. Preconceptional care: a practical guide. St. Louis: Mosby, 1995.*

(figure continues on following page)

INFECTIOUS DISEASE HISTORY

Do you or your partner have a history of:

(Place an **X** next to any item(s) that applies to you)

- ❏ herpes simplex
- ❏ *Chlamydia* infection
- ❏ human papillomavirus (genital warts)
- ❏ gonorrhea
- ❏ syphilis
- ❏ recurrent genital infections
- ❏ viral hepatitis or high-risk behavior, including use of intravenous street drugs, intimate bisexual/homosexual contact, or multiple sexual partners
- ❏ acquired immunodeficiency syndrome (AIDS) or high-risk behavior, including use of intravenous street drugs, intimate bisexual/homosexual contact, or multiple sexual partners
- ❏ occupational exposure to the blood or bodily secretions of others
- ❏ blood transfusions

REPRODUCTIVE HISTORY

Do you have a history of:

(Place an **X** next to any item(s) that applies to you)

- ❏ uterine or cervical abnormalities
- ❏ two or more pregnancies that ended in first-trimester miscarriages
- ❏ one or more pregnancies that ended between 14 and 28 weeks of gestation
- ❏ one or more fetal deaths
- ❏ one or more infants who weighed less than 5 lb at birth
- ❏ one or more infants who were admitted to a neonatal intensive care unit
- ❏ one or more infants with a birth defect

FAMILY HISTORY

Do you, your partner, or members of either of your families, including children, have:

(Place an **X** next to any item(s) that applies to you)

❏ hemophilia	❏ Tay–Sachs disease	❏ phenylketonuria (PKU)	❏ a birth defect
❏ thalassemia	❏ sickle cell disease or trait	❏ cystic fibrosis	❏ mental retardation

- ❏ Are you and your partner related outside of marriage (i.e., cousins)?
- ❏ Do you and your partner have the same ethnic or racial background, such as Ashkenazi Jew, Mediterranean, or African-American?

NUTRITION HISTORY

On the back of this sheet, list by meal everything you ate and drank yesterday, including the approximate amount; indicate snacks separately.

Do you:

(Place an **X** next to any item(s) that applies to you)

- ❏ practice vegetarianism
- ❏ eat unusual substances, such as laundry starch or clay
- ❏ have a history of bulimia or anorexia
- ❏ follow a special diet
  (if yes, describe):

_____

_____

_____

- ❏ supplement your diet with vitamins
  (if yes, list vitamins and dosages):

_____

_____

- ❏ have an intolerance for milk
- ❏ use well water

Figure 2-1 Continued

SOCIAL HISTORY

Do you:

(Place an **X** next to any item(s) that applies to you)

❑ drink beer, wine, or hard liquor
❑ smoke cigarettes or use any other tobacco products
❑ use marijuana, cocaine, or any recreational drugs
❑ use lead or chemicals at home or at work
  (if yes, list the specific chemicals, if you know what they are):

_____

_____

❑ own or work with cats
❑ work with children
❑ work with radiation
❑ participate in activities that could result in overheating (e.g., sauna, hot tub, exercise in hot, humid conditions)
❑ know the extent of your health insurance maternity benefits
❑ know your employer's policies regarding pregnancy and birth

Have you:

❑ ever been emotionally or physically abused by your partner or someone important to you

Are you:

❑ 34 years of age or older

IMMUNIZATIONS

Do you have you documented immunity to:

❑ tetanus
❑ rubella
❑ measles
❑ mumps
❑ hepatitis
❑ varicella (chickenpox)

Please feel free to express any additional concerns you may have in the space below (add additional sheets, if necessary):

_____

_____

_____

_____

_____

_____

_____

_____

_____

_____

_____

_____

_____

_____

_____

_____

Figure 2-1 Continued

that congenital defects associated with varicella occurred in 4 infants (1.2%). There were 14 patients who had varicella after 20 weeks gestation with no evidence of teratogenicity.[34] Varicella-Zoster immune globulin is a live attenuated virus and provides immunity to varicella. In the preconceptional period, if there is no history of varicella, varicella titres can be performed. If the patient is susceptible, Varicella-Zoster immune globulin should be given. Adults should avoid salicylates for 6 weeks after vaccination due to the theoretical risk of Reye syndrome. Women receiving the vaccine should not become pregnant for 3 months following the vaccination.

Toxoplasmosis

Approximately 30% of adults in the United States have antibodies to *Toxoplasma gondii*. All patients, particularly those who own outdoor cats, should be counseled about ways to minimize the risk of toxoplasmosis. Human infection occurs primarily through ingestion of toxoplasma cysts from raw or undercooked meat (frozen food is not a source of infection) and contact with sporulated oocysts from infected cat feces or through transplacental transmission. Therefore, pregnant women should wash their hands thoroughly after handling raw meat and should avoid contact with their mouths and eyes. They also should wash uncooked fruits, berries, and vegetables thorougly before consumption and wash kitchen utensils carefully after use in preparing foods. Cats should be fed well-cooked or canned food and kept indoors. Pregnant women should not handle cat litter, and should wear gloves when handling other materials potentially contaminated by cat feces.

Cytomegalovirus and Parvovirus

To allay their anxiety, day-care workers can be offered cytomegalovirus and parvovirus antibody testing. Maternal infections with primary cytomegalovirus and parvovirus potentially have severe consequences to the developing fetus. No specific recommendations for health care and day-care workers, other than universal precautions, are recommended because of the lack of evidence for efficacy of screening and/or treatment programs to prevent infection.[32,35]

Genetics

The relationship of genetics and reproductive outcome relates not only to the ethnic and racial background of the patient, but also to the family history. Individual as well as family risk may prompt carrier screening such as Tay–Sachs testing for patients of Eastern European Jewish or French Canadian descent; β-thalassemia screening for Greeks and Italians; α-thalassemia testing for Indians, Pakistanis, Southeast Asians, and Filipinos; and sickle cell anemia screening for those of African, Mediterranean, and Middle Eastern ancestry.[36] For some couples, such as those with a family history of cystic fibrosis or mental retardation suggestive of fragile X syndrome or Down syndrome, preconceptional counseling should include a discussion of both prepregnancy screening and prenatal diagnosis, including its risks and limitations. Advanced paternal age (>55) is associated with a greater prevalence of new mutations in autosomal dominant diseases such as Marfan syndrome, neurofibromatosis, and achondroplasia.[37,38]

Work and Environment

The patient and her partner should be queried about their work environment and work hours, potential stressors, and use of tobacco, alcohol, illicit drugs, and teratogenic exposure to heavy metals and organic solvents. Health care and disability insurance may be important family and economic concerns. Screening questions directly related to domestic violence should be included in the psychosocial assessment. The male partner is of potentially great help in supporting lifestyle modifications related to smoking, alcohol, drug exposures, medication, and exercise. The male's preconceptional health status may also potentially be of consequence. An ovum fertilized by an altered spermatozoon altered by paternal smoking or alcohol intake may theoretically be at increased risk of spontaneous abortion, a live birth with malformations, or a child who appears normal at birth but is at increased risk for later disease such as cancer.[39]

The patient or her partner may be exposed to organic chemicals such as tetrachloroethylene, xylene, styrene, or toluene. Overall, most studies show a fairly consistent association between maternal exposure to organic solvents and spontaneous abortion when high rates of exposure occur, but investigators have not characterized a dose response. Paternal exposure to organic solvents has not demonstrated an increased incidence of spontaneous abortion in the partners.[40,41] There is no epidemiologic evidence for an association of paternal or maternal exposure to Agent Orange and increased prevalence of offspring with congenital malformations.

The issue of video display terminals (VDTs) and spontaneous abortion has been debated. In 1988, Goldhaber and associates in a case-controlled study found that women who used VDTs more than 20 hours per week had a significantly increased rate of abortion as compared with women who used VDTs for less than 20 hours per week.[42] However, in another case-controlled study, the experiences of women employed as directory assistance operators and general operators at two companies in eight southeastern states were compared. There were 882 women who had been pregnant during a 3-year period. The difference in spontaneous abortion rates between the exposed and the nonexposed group was not significant.[43] Thus, there appears to be a lack of association in most studies between VDT exposure and spontaneous abortion, but the question has not been definitively answered, since all existing research has been retrospective in design.

To date, there is no convincing evidence to support a relationship between residential electromagnetic field exposure such as electric blankets, heated water beds, and ceiling cable heat.[44]

NUTRITION

Weight Gain

In 1990, the Institute of Medicine published guidelines for weight gain during pregnancy. It recommended weight gains of 12.5 to 18 kg (28 to 40 lb) for underweight women, 11.5 to 16 kg (25 to 35 lb) for normal weight women, and 7 to 11.5 kg (15 to 25 lb) for overweight women.[45] Their categories were based on body-mass index, which is defined as prepregnant weight in kilograms divided by the square of the height in meters. Although it was argued that the Institute had insufficient scientific data to justify specific weight-gain recommendations for pregnant patients,[46] the aforementioned guidelines were generally supported by the American College of Obstetricians and Gynecologists.[47] Parker and Abrams have shown that maternal weight gain within the Institute of Medicine guidelines reduced the risk of perinatal morbidity. In their investigation, low prenatal weight gain was associated with a more than doubled risk of small-for-gestational-age babies. Increased prenatal weight gain doubled the risk of large-for-gestational-

age infants and increased the rate of cesarean delivery by 20 to 30%, even after controlling for fetal size.[48] In subsequent investigations, a low third-trimester rate of weight gain, defined by the Institute of Medicine guidelines, was associated with an increased risk of preterm delivery.[49,50]

Diet (Including Vitamin and Mineral Supplementation)

Throughout pregnancy, a daily caloric increase of 300 kcal over base-line values is recommended by the National Research Council.[51] The recommended daily dietary allowance is increased from 2200 kcal in nonpregnant subjects to 2500 kcal in pregnant women and 2600 kcal in lactating women.

Ideally, a balanced diet that results in appropriate weight gain during pregnancy will provide the requisite vitamins for pregnancy. However, because many patients admittedly do not eat a nutritious diet, multivitamins are widely prescribed in pregnancy. Although it did not recommend routine multivitamin supplementation for all pregnant women, the Institute recommended a daily multivitamin–mineral supplement for women who do not consume an adequate diet. The Institute of Medicine concluded that iron was the only known nutrient for which requirements during pregnancy could not be met by diet alone.[45] Because of the continuous loss of iron with monthly menstruation, most women enter pregnancy with less than optimal iron stores. Prenatal vitamins typically include 25 to 65 mg of elemental iron. Iron is prescribed frequently, even without laboratory evidence of anemia or iron deficiency, because both conditions are thought to be common in pregnancy, potentially harmful to the mother and fetus, and preventable through iron supplementation.

The U.S. Preventive Service Task Force recently examined the efficacy of iron in improving perinatal outcome.[52] The task force concluded that there is currently little evidence from available published data to suggest that routine iron supplementation during pregnancy is beneficial in improving clinical outcomes for the mother, fetus, or newborn. It was felt that the evidence was insufficient to recommend for or against routine iron supplementation during pregnancy. The American College of Obstetricians and Gynecologists notes that since iron needs during pregnancy usually cannot be met with the average diet, second- and third-trimester supplementation with a daily dose of 30 mg of elemental ferrous iron (available separately or in prenatal vitamins) is recommended to prevent anemia.[47] An evaluation for anemia should be undertaken if a pregnant patient's hematocrit falls below 30%. If red-cell indexes, peripheral blood smear evaluation, and iron storage studies, including ferritin levels, are consistent with iron deficiency, iron supplementation is warranted. Severely anemic patients pose a particular problem at the time of delivery because they may have insufficient reserves to handle acute blood loss.[53]

Periconceptional folic acid is recommended on a regular basis to all American women of reproductive age as a public health measure to prevent neural-tube defects.[54,55] Women with a previous infant or fetus with a neural tube defect should take 4 mg per day of folic acid starting at the time they plan to become pregnant. This recommendation of the U.S. Preventive Service Task Force and the CDC is based on an international multicenter, double-blind, randomized trial in Europe in which over 1800 women with a previous pregnancy affected by a neural tube defect were enrolled; the group who received 4 mg of folic acid per day periconceptionally had a 72% protective effect for recurrence with no demonstrable harm from the large folate dose.[56] Women should take the supplement from at least 4 to 6 weeks before conception through the first 3 months of pregnancy. The folic acid dose should be obtained from pills containing only folic acid. In patients who require the 4-mg dose, multivitamin preparations containing folic acid should not be used to attain the 4-mg dose because harmful levels of vitamin A and D could also be reached.[57]

In addition, at least two studies have shown that periconceptional folate reduces the risk of first occurrence of neural tube defects by as much as 60%.[58,59] Because of these studies, the U.S. Preventive Service Task Force and the Centers for Disease Control and Prevention now recommend that all women of childbearing age consume 0.4 mg of folic acid on a continuous basis.[55] In addition, there are preliminary data that women who used multivitamins containing folic acid had a reduced rate of offspring with orofacial clefts and heart defects.[60] Although folate supplementation by diet has been suggested, it is difficult to achieve the recommended daily intake of 0.4 mg by diet alone. Folic acid supplementation of grains and juices is also helpful, but its potential impact is too variable to warrant a change in the above recommendations.

An association has been noted between the use of high doses of vitamin A during early pregnancy and birth defects similar to those prescribed by the vitamin A derivative, isotretinoin.[61] Data indicate that high dietary intake of vitamin A appears to be teratogenic. Among babies born to women who took more than 10,000 IU of vitamin A per day in the form of supplements, approximately 1 in 57 had a malformation attributable to the supplement.[62]

One study noted a markedly lower incidence of dental caries in children whose mothers ingested 2.2 mg/day of sodium fluoride during pregnancy as compared with mothers who used only fluorinated water.[63] Despite this report, fluoride supplementation during pregnancy has not been endorsed by the American Dental Association.[45]

Some reports have implicated zinc deficiency with poor perinatal outcome. One study found that daily zinc supplementation in women with relatively low plasma zinc concentrations in early pregnancy was associated with greater infant birth weight and head circumferences.[64] These beneficial effects were demonstrated with a daily zinc supplement of 25 mg, the typical dose in a prenatal vitamin. In contradiction, magnesium supplementation during pregnancy has not been shown to improve pregnancy outcome and did not reduce the incidence of either preeclampsia or fetal growth restriction.[65] Iodized salt will prevent maternal iodine deficiency and its risk of cretinism, the world's most common preventable cause of mental retardation.[66] Excessive iodine intake, on the other hand, can cause congenital goiter.[47]

WORK AND EXERCISE

In the absence of obstetric or medical complications, pregnant women who engage in a moderate level of physical activity can maintain this throughout pregnancy and the postpartum period.[67] For women without risk factors for adverse perinatal outcome, the following recommendations are made by the American College of Obstetricians and Gynecologists:

1. Regular exercise, at least three times per week, is preferable to intermittent activity.
2. Women should avoid exercise in the supine position after the first trimester. Prolonged periods of motionless standing should be avoided.
3. Women should be aware of the decreased oxygen available for aerobic exercise during pregnancy.

They should modify the intensity of their exercise according to their symptoms.

4. Exercise involving the potential for even mild abdominal trauma should be avoided.
5. Women who exercise during pregnancy should be careful to ensure an adequate diet.
6. Pregnant women who exercise in the first trimester should ensure adequate hydration, appropriate clothing, and optimal environmental surroundings during exercise.
7. Because physiologic and morphologic changes of pregnancy persist 4 to 6 weeks postpartum, prepregnancy exercise routines should be resumed gradually.

Contraindications to exercise during pregnancy include severe, chronic, or gestational hypertension, preterm rupture of membranes, preterm labor during the prior or current pregnancy, incompetent cervix, persistent second- and third-trimester bleeding, and intrauterine growth restriction. There is no evidence that beginning or continuing an exercise regimen during pregnancy increases the incidence of preterm labor or preterm rupture of the membranes. There are no apparent reports of an increase in fetal cord entanglement, meconium staining, fetal heart rate abnormalities during labor, low Apgar scores, or neonatal complications in exercising women.[68] Most studies report that mild exercise during pregnancy has no effect on the course and outcome of labor. However, well-conditioned recreational athletes, who continued a regular aerobic or running exercise program above maintenance level throughout pregnancy were found to have shorter labors, less need for obstetric intervention and fewer signs of fetal distress as compared with women who did not exercise regularly.[69]

The issue of work and physical activity and its impact on pregnancy is an important one. Long hours of standing appear to be associated with an increased risk of preterm delivery.[70,71] Strenuous work, in general, does not seem to predispose to preterm delivery, although women who continue employment into the third trimester have been found to have lower birth weights, especially those engaged in heavy work.[71]

COITUS

It is generally accepted in healthy pregnant women that sexual intercourse is permissible. Coitus should generally be avoided whenever spontaneous abortion or preterm labor threatens. The relationship between sexual intercourse during pregnancy and gestational age at delivery was recently examined in a multicenter study entitled the Vaginal Infection and Prematurity Study Group.[72] The investigation showed that frequent sexual intercourse by itself was not associated with an increased risk of preterm birth. However, women colonized with specific microorganisms, including *Trichomonas vaginalis* and *Mycoplasma hominis* who engaged in frequent intercourse (once per week or more), had an increased rate of preterm delivery. The relationship between sexual positions and activities and pregnancy outcome has also been analyzed, only the male superior position was significantly associated with preterm premature rupture of membranes and preterm delivery.[73] There have been several reported cases of fatal air embolism during oral sex when air was blown into the vagina.[74]

TRAVEL

Air travel in properly pressurized aircrafts offers no unusual risks. Thus, air travel does not need to be proscribed during pregnancy. Pregnant woman should be advised to walk about the cabin approximately every 2 hours and maintain good hydration with water and/or juices. Probably the greatest risk with travel is the development of a complication remote from the patient's home and her care providers. If a complication were to develop during travel, the patient could potentially require care in an area with suboptimal services.

The American College of Obstetricians and Gynecologists have formulated guidelines for automobile passenger restraints during pregnancy.[75] Pregnant women should be encouraged to wear properly positioned three-point restraints throughout pregnancy during automobile travel. The lap belt portion should be placed snugly under the abdomen and across the thighs. The shoulder belt should be positioned snugly between the breasts. Importantly, there is no evidence that safety restraints increase the chance of fetal injury.

VACCINATIONS AND INFECTIONS

Perinatal risks from vaccinations are largely theoretical. Immunization in pregnancy is generally indicated when the risk for exposure is high, infection poses a particular risk to the mother or fetus, and the vaccine is not likely to cause harm. There are four types of immunologic agents commonly used in the United States. Toxoids are preparations of chemically altered bacterial exotoxin. Inactivated vaccines contain a suspension of heat-inactivated or chemically inactivated microorganisms. Live viral and bacterial vaccines are suspensions of viral or bacterial strains selected for their reduced virulence. Although no significant illness is produced, the live viral or bacterial vaccine has sufficient antigenic properties in common with the infectious viral-type agent to stimulate protective immunity. Immune globulin preparations are protein fractions of pooled human plasma containing antibodies that can produce transient passive protection in the recipient.[76] Each vaccine must be assessed with regard to both its effectiveness in confirming immunity and the potential for causing complications in pregnancy. In the United States, the only immunologic agents that are recommended for routine administration during pregnancy are tetanus and diphtheria toxoids. The hepatitis B vaccine series can be administered to pregnant patients who are at high risk because of their behavior, work, household contact, or requirement for transfusions of clotting factors.[77]

The introduction of effective attenuated viral vaccines against measles, mumps, and rubella (MMR) in the United States in the 1960s resulted in a dramatic decrease in the incidence of these diseases.[78] MMR vaccine should be given at least 3 months prior to pregnancy or in the immediate postpartum period.[79] Rubella vaccine virus is known to cross the placenta and may theoretically infect the fetus during the early stages of development. However, there is no evidence that it causes birth defects or illness. The observed risk of congenital malformation following the rubella vaccine has been zero, although several infants have shown laboratory evidence of subclinical fetal infection.[80]

Pregnant women may be cultured for *Neisseria gonorrhoeae* and tested for *Chlamydia trachomatis* based on their history and physical examination.[81] Routine testing of pregnant women for chlamydia is not recommended by ACOG. However, in high-risk populations (age <25 years, history of other sexually transmitted diseases, a new sexual partner within the preceding 3 months, and multiple sexual partners) testing is warranted. The recommended treatment for gonorrhea in pregnancy is ceftriaxone 125 mg intramuscularly once, or cefixime, 400 mg orally in a single dose. The recommended regimen for chlamydia infection in pregnancy is erythromycin base, 500 mg orally four times daily for 7 days. Azithyromycin 1 g orally in a single dose is also approved for the treatment of chlamydia. Follow-up cervical and rectal cultures for *N. gonorrhoeae* should be obtained, although test-of-cure evaluation is not necessary for chlamydia. At least 50% of patients with either gonorrhea or chlamydia are positive for the other disease. Thus, simultaneous empiric treatment for both sexually transmitted diseases can be justified when either is diagnosed. Sexual partners should be tested and treated. Routine screening for syphilis should be performed as early in pregnancy as possible. Syphilis in pregnancy must be treated with penicillin since erythromycin, an alternative drug, does not adequately treat the fetus.[82] Patients allergic to penicillin should undergo a desensitization program.

The association between trichomoniasis and preterm birth has been debated over the years. By itself, trichomonas does not appear to be a major cause of prematurity. However, when present concomitantly with other genital tract infections such as bacterial vaginosis or chlamydia, the preterm birth rate is increased.[83] The commonly used wet preparation is considerably less sensitive than culture technique.

It is increasingly clear that bacterial vaginosis may be a preventable cause of preterm labor and preterm premature rupture of the membranes.[84] It has been shown in a double-blind randomized trial that women who were at increased risk for preterm delivery and who had bacterial vaginosis had significantly lower rates of delivery prior to 37 weeks of gestation when they were treated with metronidazole and erythromycin.[85] Although screening all pregnant women for bacterial vaginosis is not yet standard care, women at high risk for preterm delivery (prior preterm delivery, low maternal weight) should be screened for bacterial vaginosis and, if positive, treated.[86]

The U.S. Public Health Service has published recommendations for human immunodeficiency virus counseling and voluntary testing in pregnant women.[87] Health care providers should ensure that all pregnant women are counseled and encouraged to have HIV testing. Knowledge of the mother's serostatus has become of increasing importance, both with respect to her treatment and prevention of perinatal transmission. Maternal zidovudine treatment has been shown to markedly lower the perinatal transmission rate.[88] Newer protocols from the AIDS Clinical Trials Group and increasing use of protease inhibitors in pregnant patients may potentially lower the perinatal transmission rate even further. HIV testing of pregnant women and their infants should be voluntary. HIV testing should be performed according to the recommended algorithm, which includes the use of enzyme immunoassay to test for antibody to HIV and confirmatory testing with an additional more specific assay such as the Western blot.

The Centers for Disease Control and Prevention has published a new protocol on group B streptococcus (GBS) in pregnancy. GBS disease is the leading bacterial infection associated with illness and death among newborns in the United States. Many perinatal GBS infections are preventable through intrapartum antimicrobial prophylaxis. In most populations, 10 to 30% of pregnant women are colonized with GBS in the genitourinary or gastrointestinal tracts. The CDC has proposed two preventive strategies. The first uses a screening-based approach. In this strategy, all patients between 35 to 37 weeks of gestation are screened for GBS using a culturette placed into the lower third of the vagina and then swabbed posteriorly toward the rectum. The culturette should be placed in a nutrient broth rather than a nonselective solid agar in order to maximize isolation rates of GBS. Patients with positive cultures or who present with preterm labor or preterm premature rupture of the membranes are treated with intrapartum penicillin or ampicillin. The other strategy uses a risk factor approach. Intrapartum penicillin or ampicillin is used for women with the following risk factors: patients who are less than 37 weeks of gestation, duration of membrane rupture >18 hours, or maternal temperature of 100.4°F (38.0°C). Regardless of which preventive strategy is used, a woman with symptomatic or asymptomatic GBS bacteriuria detected during pregnancy should be treated at the time of diagnosis and should also receive intrapartum chemoprophylaxis. Also, women who have previously given birth to an infant with GBS disease should receive intrapartum chemoprophylaxis.[89]

SUBSTANCE ABUSE

Smoking

Tobacco smoking is associated with multiple types of cancer (e.g, lung, head and neck, esophageal, bladder) and with chronic cardiovascular and pulmonary disease. Despite this, 26% of reproductive age women smoke, and 19 to 30% of pregnant women continue to smoke.[90] Smokers have a higher rate of both infertility and spontaneous abortion. Women who smoke during pregnancy have a higher rate of placental abnormalities, including placental abruption and placenta previa.[91–93] The rate of prematurity is also increased in smoking mothers.[94] Epidemiologic studies have consistently shown that the mean birth weight of infants of women who smoke during pregnancy is 170 to 200 g less than that of infants of nonsmokers.[95] Multiple studies have shown a definite association between maternal smoking and perinatal loss.[90]

Comprehensive smoking cessation programs during pregnancy have proven efficacious.[96] Outside of pregnancy, nicotine replacement therapy (patch, gum) clearly improves the rate of smoking cessation.[97] There are only preliminary data on the safety of the nicotine patch in pregnancy.[96] Whereas pilot data in this study did not show untoward maternal or fetal effects from the nicotine patch, until further information is available, it is appropriate to inform the patient about the presumed risks and benefits of this therapy and to individualize decisions. Although most studies have not found a relationship between smoking in pregnancy and birth defects, a recent case-controlled study found that smoking during pregnancy increased the relative odds for terminal transverse limb deficiencies.[98–99]

Caffeine

Caffeine is consumed in great quantities through coffee, tea, cola, and cocoa drinks. There are conflicting data regarding caffeine consumption and adverse pregnancy outcomes, including spontaneous abortion. In 1980, mainly on the basis of animal data, the Food and Drug Administration (FDA) cautioned pregnant women to limit their caffeine intake.[100] A recent Canadian case-controlled study showed that caffeine intake before and during pregnancy was associated with an increased rate of fetal loss, supporting the FDA recommendation.[101] In contradiction, several studies have shown no association between caffeine use and adverse perinatal outcome.[102,103] Based on these studies, it is reasonable to counsel patients that caffeine use in moderation (1 to 2 cups coffee per day) is most likely safe.

Alcohol

As a general rule, alcohol use in pregnancy should be proscribed. Maternal alcohol abuse is the leading cause of mental retardation in this country.[104] Although an occasional drink during pregnancy has not been proven to be harmful, patients should be counseled that there is no level of alcohol use during pregnancy that is known to be safe. The fetal alcohol syndrome is characterized by growth restriction, facial abnormalities, and central nervous system dysfunction.[105] Even among chronic alcoholics, the incidence of fetal alcohol syndrome is variable, ranging from 6 to 50%.[106] The prevalence of alcohol consumption in pregnant women has declined steadily from 32% in 1985 to 20% in 1988. However, no decline in alcohol consumption was observed among the less educated and those under the age of 25 years. The prevalence of alcohol use among pregnant women has remained highest among smokers and the unmarried.[107]

Cocaine

Cocaine use during pregnancy is widespread, with estimates of frequency ranging from 2 to 17%. Crack cocaine, the alkaloid form of cocaine that is not destroyed by heating, is extremely addictive and results in high blood levels of the drug. Several complications of pregnancy are increased in cocaine users, including spontaneous abortion and fetal death in utero, premature rupture of the membranes, preterm labor and delivery, intrauterine growth restriction, meconium-stained amniotic fluid, and placental abruption. In utero cerebral infarction resulting in porencephaly has been reported, presumably due to fetal hypoxemia caused by decreasing placental flow resulting in impaired fetal cerebrovascular autoregulation.[108]

Whether or not cocaine is a teratogen has been debated. Several studies have noted an increased frequency of microcephaly, limb-reduction defects, and genitourinary abnormalities.[109] These malformations are thought to be due to vascular interruption during development caused by cocaine's intense vasoconstrictive effects. Neurobehavioral abnormalities in infants have been associated with maternal cocaine use.[108] Sudden infant death syndrome has been linked to cocaine exposure in utero.[111] A fetal cocaine syndrome of facial dysmorphology including large fontanels, prominent glabella, marked periorbital and eyelid edema, and short nose with a low bridge and lateral soft-tissue nasal hypertrophy, has been reported but has not been widely accepted.[112]

Others

There is no evidence that marijuana is a teratogen. However, since it is commonly used by multiple substance abusers, the presence of cannabinoid metabolites in the urine may identify patients who are at increased risk for being users of more dangerous substances.[113] Narcotic addiction during pregnancy is a serious concern for the pregnant patient and her fetus. Heroin addicts have higher rates of stillbirths, fetal growth restriction, and prematurity. The neonate is at risk for a severe and potentially fatal narcotic withdrawal syndrome.[113] There is less information available on amphetamines. A crystal intravenous methamphetamine, with the street name *ice*, is a potent stimulant. It has been associated with a pattern of abnormalities that is similar to those seen in cocaine users, including placental abruption, intrauterine growth restriction, and fetal death in utero.[114] The pathophysiologic mechanism is thought to be related to the vasoconstrictive properties of the drug. There is no convincing evidence that lysergic acid diethylamide (LSD) is a teratogen, but data are limited.

Because substance abuse is one of the most important risks encountered in pregnancy, all patients should be questioned about alcohol, tobacco, and substance abuse at their first prenatal visit. There are several screening questionnaires to assess alcohol use, referred to as CAGE and T-ACE, that are useful.[113] Many academic centers have developed multidisciplinary programs to manage the associated social and psychiatric issues that so frequently interplay in the drug-addicted patient.[115]

COMMON COMPLAINTS

Nausea and vomiting are common complaints in the first trimester, with an incidence of approximately 50%.[116] In certain instances, antiemetic pharmacologic treatment is necessary. Phenothiazines, including promethazine and prochlorperazine do not appear to be teratogenic.[117] Some practitioners recommend the use of both vitamin B_6 (pyridoxine) 25 mg and doxylamine 25 mg, a sleep agent, as an antiemetic. This drug combination constitutes the contents of the preparation, Bendectin, which was removed from the market years ago over fears of litigation, but was never proven to be a teratogen.

Heartburn is one of the most common complaints of pregnancy. It is caused by reflux of gastric contents into the lower esophagus. Relief is often found by eating more frequent, smaller meals and avoidance of bending or lying flat. Antacid preparations and H_2 blockers are recommended when dietary and positional changes have proven to be unsuccessful and do not appear to be teratogenic.

Constipation is a physiologic change of pregnancy due to decreased bowel transit time, in part due to the effects of progesterone. Iron supplementation can often exaggerate this condition. Dietary modification with increased fiber and additional water intake are generally the first lines of treatment. Stool softeners, such as docusate and/or dietary fiber agents such as psyllium hydrophilic muciloid should be used in lieu of laxatives.

Hemorrhoids, which are varicose veins of the rectum, can be exacerbated by pregnancy, related in part to the increased venous pressure within the rectal veins caused by the expanding uterus. Relief is obtainable by avoidance of constipation, use of stool softeners, topically applied anesthetics, warm soaks, and wiping agents such as Tucks, which are less abrasive than toilet paper. Hemorrhoids generally regress after delivery but usually do not entirely disappear.

Varicosities of the lower extremities and vulva often become more prominent as pregnancy advances, and maternal weight increases, and they are exacerbated by prolonged periods of standing. Treatment is generally periodic rest, leg elevation, and elastic stockings.

Urinary frequency is common, especially in the first trimester, in part due to pressure that the growing uterus places against the bladder. When there is concomitant dysuria or hematuria, however, evaluation for cystitis is important. A urine culture should be obtained in all pregnant women with their laboratory studies to assess for asymptomatic bacteriuria, a preventable cause of pyelonephritis.

Pregnant women frequently complain of increased vaginal discharge, which is often due to increased mucus formation from the cervical glands. However, other infectious causes should be considered, assessed, and treated when appropriate.

Low back pain during pregnancy is also common, with an incidence of over 50%. Back pain in previous pregnancies and obesity are thought to be risk factors. The pathogenesis of low back pain during pregnancy is attributed to direct pressure of the fetus and uterus on lumbosacral nerve roots, laxity of ligaments, and increased lumbar lordosis.[118] Other more difficult to treat concerns include pica, ptyalism (profuse salivation), and fatigue.

PRENATAL CARE

Repeat Prenatal Visits

The frequency of return visits should be determined by the individual needs of the woman and her risk assessment. The American College of Obstetricians and Gynecologists has recommended that women with uncomplicated pregnancies be seen every 4 weeks until 28 weeks of gestation, every 2 to 3 weeks until 36 weeks of gestation, and then weekly thereafter.[119,120] Some studies have suggested that low-risk pregnancies can be seen less frequently than routinely advised without jeopardizing perinatal outcome, although this may be at the expense of reduced patient satisfaction.[121,122] Women with complicated pregnancies may need to be seen more often in order to optimize pregnancy outcome.

At each visit, physical examination should include measurement of blood pressure, weight, fundal height, and fetal heart rate. Diastolic blood pressures >90 mm Hg are abnormal at any time during pregnancy, and further evaluation is warranted. Excessive weight gain or weight loss should be evaluated, as this may herald other problems (see "Weight Gain," page 33). Pretibial edema occurs in the majority of normotensive uncomplicated pregnancies. However, marked edema of the fingers and face may be one of the initial manifestations of preeclampsia.

Serial fundal height measurements through gestation are a simple and inexpensive screening technique for fetal growth abnormalities. The measurement of fundal height in centimeters, when performed between 20 and 32 weeks, approximates the gestational age.[123,124] A fundal height lag of $\geq$4 cm may represent intrauterine growth restriction, justifying further clinical investigation.[123,125] The value of these measurements in diagnosing fetal macrosomia is limited; however, measurements 2 to 3 cm greater than gestational age require evaluation for polyhydramnios or multiple gestation.[126] Although some controversy surrounds the utility of fundal height measurements in clinical practice, they appear to be a simple and valuable method of screening for abnormal fetal growth.[127-129]

Digital cervical examination at every prenatal visit has not been shown to decrease the rates of preterm delivery or premature rupture of the membranes in asymptomatic patients.[130] In general, digital cervical exams need be done only if they will influence clinical management. In patients at high risk for preterm labor, such as a twin gestation, frequent cervical exams are warranted. If a breech presentation is detected at ≥36 weeks of gestation, external cephalic version should be offered at 37 weeks.[131]

The American College of Obstetricians and Gynecologists recommends routine screening for urinary protein and glucose at each prenatal visit. The value of routine urinary dipstick screening for protein has been questioned due to the limitations of this test in diagnosing preeclampsia.[132–134] Measurable proteinuria usually occurs after the onset of hypertension and, therefore, is not useful for early detection of preeclampsia.[135] In addition, the normal fluctuations in urine protein excretion and subjective interpretation of urine dipstick determinations can result in inaccurate measurements.[132,133] Because the conventional urine dipstick test is unreliable in detecting elevations in proteinuria that can occur early in the course of preeclampsia, any suspicion for preeclampsia should prompt a definitive test for proteinuria, the 24-hour urine collection.

Glucosuria is more common in pregnancy due to the increase in glomerular filtration and impaired tubular resorptive capacity for filtering glucose that normally occur. Approximately one-sixth of all pregnant women have glucosuria at some time during their pregnancy.[136] The correlation between urine and blood glucose is poor in pregnancy.[137] When performed prior to 28 weeks, routine dipstick analysis reported as greater than "trace" glucose may identify pregnant women at increased risk for gestational diabetes; however, this test lacks sensitivity for detecting gestational diabetes mellitus.[138] The value of routine urine screening for glucose remains to be proven.[134]

Subsequent visits should include certain routine laboratory values. Repeat hemoglobin or hematocrit should be done at 26 to 28 weeks of gestation and repeated again at 36 weeks if anemia is present. If the patient is Rh-negative and unsensitized, she should have repeat antibody screening at 28 weeks. If the patient is unsensitized, Rho(D) immune globulin (RhIg) should be administered prophylactically at 28 weeks. A screening test for gestational diabetes should be performed at 24 to 28 weeks using a 50-g glucose challenge test (Chapter 27 on Diabetes). If a culture-based strategy for the prevention of group B streptococcal disease is used, vaginorectal cultures should be obtained at 35 to 37 weeks of gestation.[139,140]

For low-risk patients, assessment of fetal well-being may begin at 28 weeks of gestation using daily kick counts. Fetal movement counts appear to be an effective form of surveillance (see "Fetal Assessment," page 46). In the uncomplicated pregnancy, antepartum fetal testing should begin at 41 to 42 weeks gestation.

The Prenatal Record

The prenatal record should accurately reflect the necessary prenatal information in a clear and thorough fashion. These records commonly contain:

Demographic data

Obstetrical, medical, and surgical history

Genetic screening

Physical examination

Dating parameters (menstrual history and any clinical or ultrasound dating criteria)

Record of individual visits

Laboratory data

Problem list

Delivery and discharge information

Postpartum information

Several different records have been adopted in different parts of the United States and other countries. In 1997, the American College of Obstetricians and Gynecologists updated their version of the antepartum record (Figure 2-2).

Assessment of Gestational Age

The establishment of an accurate estimated date of confinement is one of the most important parts of prenatal care. There are several clinical implications of inaccurate dates. The rate of postterm pregnancy is reduced from about 9% to 3% for patients who receive early ultrasound.[141–143] Similarly, the rate of an incorrect diagnosis of intrauterine growth restriction may be decreased with the use of early ultrasound dating.[143] Determination of accurate dates is essential

DATE _____

NAME _____
LAST   FIRST   MIDDLE

ID # _____ HOSPITAL OF DELIVERY _____

NEWBORN'S PHYSICIAN _____ REFERRED BY _____

FINAL EDD _____   PRIMARY PROVIDER/GROUP _____

BIRTH DATE	AGE	RACE	MARITAL STATUS	ADDRESS:			
MONTH DAY YEAR			S M W D SEP				
OCCUPATION □ HOMEMAKER □ OUTSIDE WORK □ STUDENT Type of Work		EDUCATION (LAST GRADE COMPLETED)		ZIP: PHONE: (H) (O)			
				INSURANCE CARRIER/MEDICAID #			
HUSBAND/FATHER OF BABY: PHONE:				EMERGENCY CONTACT: PHONE:			

TOTAL PREG	FULL TERM	PREMATURE	AB, INDUCED	AB, SPONTANEOUS	ECTOPICS	MULTIPLE BIRTHS	LIVING

MENSTRUAL HISTORY

LMP □ DEFINITE □ APPROXIMATE (MONTH KNOWN)   MENSES MONTHLY □ YES □ NO   FREQUENCY: Q _____ DAYS   MENARCHE _____ (AGE ONSET)
□ UNKNOWN □ NORMAL AMOUNT/DURATION   PRIOR MENSES _____ DATE   ON BCP AT CONCEPT. □ YES □ NO   hCG + ____ / ____ / ____
□ FINAL _____

PAST PREGNANCIES (LAST SIX)

DATE MONTH / YEAR	GA WEEKS	LENGTH OF LABOR	BIRTH WEIGHT	SEX M/F	TYPE DELIVERY	ANES.	PLACE OF DELIVERY	PRETERM LABOR YES / NO	COMMENTS / COMPLICATIONS

PAST MEDICAL HISTORY

	O Neg + Pos.	DETAIL POSITIVE REMARKS INCLUDE DATE & TREATMENT		O Neg + Pos.	DETAIL POSITIVE REMARKS INCLUDE DATE & TREATMENT
1. DIABETES			16. D (Rh) SENSITIZED		
2. HYPERTENSION			17. PULMONARY (TB, ASTHMA)		
3. HEART DISEASE			18. ALLERGIES (DRUGS)		
4. AUTOIMMUNE DISORDER			19. BREAST		
5. KIDNEY DISEASE / UTI			20. GYN SURGERY		
6. NEUROLOGIC/EPILEPSY					
7. PSYCHIATRIC			21. OPERATIONS / HOSPITALIZATIONS (YEAR & REASON)		
8. HEPATITIS / LIVER DISEASE					
9. VARICOSITIES / PHLEBITIS					
10. THYROID DYSFUNCTION			22. ANESTHETIC COMPLICATIONS		
11. TRAUMA/DOMESTIC VIOLENCE			23. HISTORY OF ABNORMAL PAP		
12. HISTORY OF BLOOD TRANSFUS.			24. UTERINE ANOMALY/DES		
	AMT/DAY PREPREG	AMT/DAY PREG #YEARS USE	25. INFERTILITY		
13. TOBACCO			26. RELEVANT FAMILY HISTORY		
14. ALCOHOL					
15. STREET DRUGS			27. OTHER		

COMMENTS: _____

The American College of Obstetricians and Gynecologists, 409 12th Street, SW, PO Box 96920, Washington, DC 20090-6920   Copyright © 1997 (Version 4)

ACOG ANTEPARTUM RECORD (FORM A)

Figure 2-2 ACOG Prenatal Care Form (1997 version). *American College of Obstetricians and Gynecologists. Antepartum Record Washington, DC,* © ACOG, 1997.

(figure continues on following page)

in evaluating maternal serum screening for fetal open neural tube defects and aneuploidy. Dating is also important for timing of repeat cesarean delivery or in management of a pregnancy with medical complications. Finally, dating error can have important clinical consequences in the management of preterm labor. Inaccurate dating may alter management decisions for fetuses with borderline viability.

Clinical Dating

The length of pregnancy is 280 to 281 days from the first day of the last menstrual period until delivery.[141,144,145] This correlates with a 40-week gestational period, assuming that ovulation and conception occurred on day 14 of a 28-day cycle. Failure to recognize this assumption may result in inaccurate dating

SYMPTOMS SINCE LMP

GENETIC SCREENING/TERATOLOGY COUNSELING
INCLUDES PATIENT, BABY'S FATHER, OR ANYONE IN EITHER FAMILY WITH:

	YES	NO			YES	NO
1. PATIENT'S AGE ≥ 35 YEARS			12. MENTAL RETARDATION/AUTISM			
2. THALASSEMIA (ITALIAN, GREEK, MEDITERRANEAN, OR ASIAN BACKGROUND): MCV < 80			IF YES, WAS PERSON TESTED FOR FRAGILE X?			
3. NEURAL TUBE DEFECT (MENINGOMYELOCELE, SPINA BIFIDA, OR ANENCEPHALY)			13. OTHER INHERITED GENETIC OR CHROMOSOMAL DISORDER			
4. CONGENITAL HEART DEFECT			14. MATERNAL METABOLIC DISORDER (EG. INSULIN-DEPENDENT DIABETES, PKU)			
5. DOWN SYNDROME			15. PATIENT OR BABY'S FATHER HAD A CHILD WITH BIRTH DEFECTS NOT LISTED ABOVE			
6. TAY-SACHS (EG. JEWISH, CAJUN, FRENCH CANADIAN)			16. RECURRENT PREGNANCY LOSS, OR A STILLBIRTH			
7. SICKLE CELL DISEASE OR TRAIT (AFRICAN)			17. MEDICATIONS/STREET DRUGS/ALCOHOL SINCE LAST MENSTRUAL PERIOD			
8. HEMOPHILIA			IF YES, AGENT(S):			
9. MUSCULAR DYSTROPHY						
10. CYSTIC FIBROSIS						
11. HUNTINGTON CHOREA			18. ANY OTHER			

COMMENTS/COUNSELING: _____

_____

_____

INFECTION HISTORY	YES	NO		YES	NO
1. HIGH RISK HEPATITIS B/IMMUNIZED?			4. RASH OR VIRAL ILLNESS SINCE LAST MENSTRUAL PERIOD		
2. LIVE WITH SOMEONE WITH TB OR EXPOSED TO TB			5. HISTORY OF STD, GC, CHLAMYDIA, HPV, SYPHILIS		
3. PATIENT OR PARTNER HAS HISTORY OF GENITAL HERPES			6. OTHER (SEE COMMENTS)		

COMMENTS: _____

_____

_____ INTERVIEWER'S SIGNATURE _____

INITIAL PHYSICAL EXAMINATION

DATE _____ / _____ / _____   PREPREGNANCY WEIGHT _____   HEIGHT _____   BP _____

1. HEENT	☐ NORMAL	☐ ABNORMAL	12. VULVA	☐ NORMAL	☐ CONDYLOMA	☐ LESIONS	
2. FUNDI	☐ NORMAL	☐ ABNORMAL	13. VAGINA	☐ NORMAL	☐ INFLAMMATION	☐ DISCHARGE	
3. TEETH	☐ NORMAL	☐ ABNORMAL	14. CERVIX	☐ NORMAL	☐ INFLAMMATION	☐ LESIONS	
4. THYROID	☐ NORMAL	☐ ABNORMAL	15. UTERUS SIZE	_____ WEEKS		☐ FIBROIDS	
5. BREASTS	☐ NORMAL	☐ ABNORMAL	16. ADNEXA	☐ NORMAL	☐ MASS		
6. LUNGS	☐ NORMAL	☐ ABNORMAL	17. RECTUM	☐ NORMAL	☐ ABNORMAL		
7. HEART	☐ NORMAL	☐ ABNORMAL	18. DIAGONAL CONJUGATE	☐ REACHED	☐ NO	_____ CM	
8. ABDOMEN	☐ NORMAL	☐ ABNORMAL	19. SPINES	☐ AVERAGE	☐ PROMINENT	☐ BLUNT	
9. EXTREMITIES	☐ NORMAL	☐ ABNORMAL	20. SACRUM	☐ CONCAVE	☐ STRAIGHT	☐ ANTERIOR	
10. SKIN	☐ NORMAL	☐ ABNORMAL	21. SUBPUBIC ARCH	☐ NORMAL	☐ WIDE	☐ NARROW	
11. LYMPH NODES	☐ NORMAL	☐ ABNORMAL	22. GYNECOID PELVIC TYPE	☐ YES	☐ NO		

COMMENTS (Number and explain abnormals): _____

_____

_____ EXAM BY _____

ACOG ANTEPARTUM RECORD (FORM B)

Figure 2-2 Continued

in women whose menstrual cycles do not follow a 28-day cycle. Common practice is to measure menstrual age as opposed to conceptional or ovulatory age, both of which are usually 2 weeks shorter. The term gestational age should be equivalent to conceptional age; however, in practice, gestational age is used interchangeably with menstrual age.

Several clinical parameters can be used to estimate gestational age. The most reliable clinical criteria is an accurate last menstrual period (LMP). Naegele's rule, which adds 280 to 284 days to the LMP, can be used to predict the estimated date of confinement (EDC) by subtracting 3 months and adding 1 week from the first day of the LMP. A careful patient history should verify the first day of the LMP, cycle length, and use of hormonal contraceptives that might alter ovulation. "Pregnancy wheels" are commonly used to calculate the EDC based on a reliable LMP. Bracken

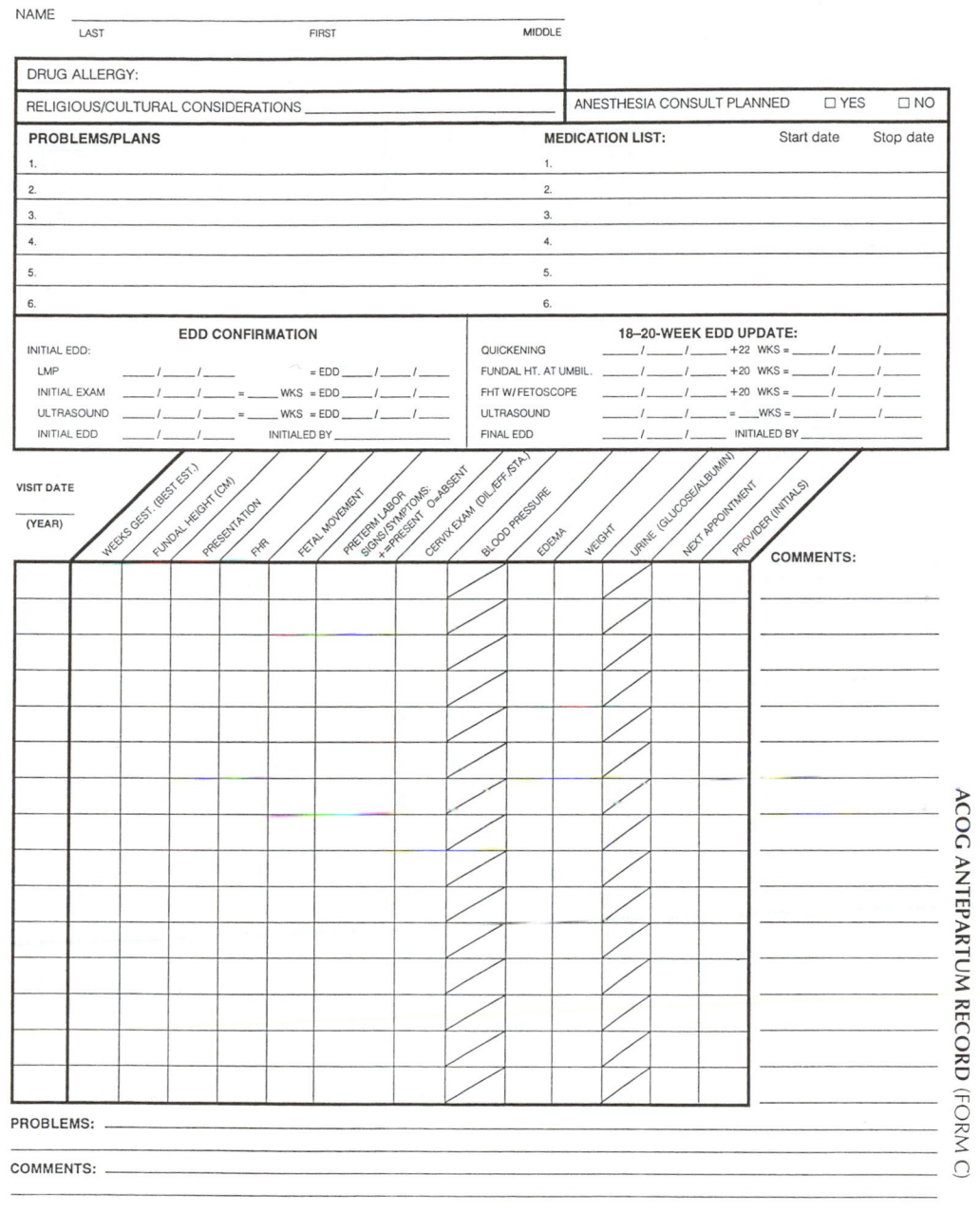

NAME _____

LAST   FIRST   MIDDLE

DRUG ALLERGY:

RELIGIOUS/CULTURAL CONSIDERATIONS _____   ANESTHESIA CONSULT PLANNED   ☐ YES   ☐ NO

PROBLEMS/PLANS	MEDICATION LIST:	Start date	Stop date
1.	1.		
2.	2.		
3.	3.		
4.	4.		
5.	5.		
6.	6.		

EDD CONFIRMATION

INITIAL EDD:

LMP ____/____/____ = EDD ____/____/____

INITIAL EXAM ____/____/____ = ____ WKS = EDD ____/____/____

ULTRASOUND ____/____/____ = ____ WKS = EDD ____/____/____

INITIAL EDD ____/____/____ INITIALED BY _____

18–20-WEEK EDD UPDATE:

QUICKENING ____/____/____ +22 WKS = ____/____/____

FUNDAL HT. AT UMBIL. ____/____/____ +20 WKS = ____/____/____

FHT W/FETOSCOPE ____/____/____ +20 WKS = ____/____/____

ULTRASOUND ____/____/____ = ____WKS = ____/____/____

FINAL EDD ____/____/____ INITIALED BY _____

VISIT DATE ____ (YEAR)

Columns: WEEKS GEST. (BEST EST.) / FUNDAL HEIGHT (CM) / PRESENTATION / FHR / FETAL MOVEMENT / PRETERM LABOR SIGNS/SYMPTOMS: + =PRESENT O=ABSENT / CERVIX EXAM (DIL/EFF/STA.) / BLOOD PRESSURE / EDEMA / WEIGHT / URINE (GLUCOSE/ALBUMIN) / NEXT APPOINTMENT / PROVIDER (INITIALS) / COMMENTS:

PROBLEMS: _____

COMMENTS: _____

ACOG ANTEPARTUM RECORD (FORM C)

Figure 2-2 Continued   *(figure continues on following page)*

found that these devices are often prone to error, with a 5-day error being typical.[146]

Other clinical measures can be used to support gestational dating. Uterine size during first-trimester pelvic examination can be assessed with reproducibility by experienced examiners. At about 20 weeks of gestation, the uterus can be palpated at the level of the umbilicus. This marker can vary depending on patient height, umbilical location, bladder size, uter-ine fibroids, presence of multiple gestation, and previous cesarean delivery, which may elevate the uterus in early pregnancy.

Fetal heart tones can also be used to estimate gestational age. An electronic Doppler device can allow detection of the fetal heart by 11 to 12 weeks. The mother's first perception of fetal movement, or quickening, occurs at predictable times in gestation. Anderson found that quickening occurred at an average

Patient Addressograph

LABORATORY AND EDUCATION

INITIAL LABS	DATE	RESULT	REVIEWED
BLOOD TYPE	/ /	A B AB O	
D (Rh) TYPE	/ /		
ANTIBODY SCREEN	/ /		
HCT/HGB	/ /	_____ % _____ g/dL	
PAP TEST	/ /	NORMAL / ABNORMAL / _____	
RUBELLA	/ /		
VDRL	/ /		
URINE CULTURE/SCREEN	/ /		
HBsAg	/ /		
HIV COUNSELING/TESTING	/ /	☐ POS. ☐ NEG. ☐ DECLINED	

OPTIONAL LABS	DATE	RESULT	
HGB ELECTROPHORESIS	/ /	AA AS SS AC SC AF ↑A$_2$	
PPD	/ /		
CHLAMYDIA	/ /		
GC	/ /		
TAY-SACHS	/ /		
OTHER			

8–18-WEEK LABS (WHEN INDICATED/ELECTED)	DATE	RESULT	
ULTRASOUND	/ /		
MSAFP/MULTIPLE MARKERS	/ /		
AMNIO/CVS	/ /		
KARYOTYPE	/ /	46, XX OR 46, XY / OTHER_____	
AMNIOTIC FLUID (AFP)	/ /	NORMAL_____ ABNORMAL_____	

24–28-WEEK LABS (WHEN INDICATED)	DATE	RESULT	
HCT/HGB	/ /	_____ % _____ g/dL	
DIABETES SCREEN	/ /	1 HOUR_____	
GTT (IF SCREEN ABNORMAL)	/ /	_____ FBS _____ 1 HOUR _____ 2 HOUR _____ 3 HOUR	
D (Rh) ANTIBODY SCREEN	/ /		
D IMMUNE GLOBULIN (RhIG) GIVEN (28 WKS)	/ /	SIGNATURE _____	

32–36-WEEK LABS (WHEN INDICATED)	DATE	RESULT	
HCT/HGB (RECOMMENDED)	/ /	_____ % _____ g/dL	
ULTRASOUND	/ /		
VDRL	/ /		
GC	/ /		
CHLAMYDIA	/ /		
GROUP B STREP (35–37 WKS)	/ /		

COMMENTS/ADDITIONAL LABS

PLANS/EDUCATION (COUNSELED ☐)

☐ ANESTHESIA PLANS _____
☐ TOXOPLASMOSIS PRECAUTIONS (CATS/RAW MEAT) _____
☐ CHILDBIRTH CLASSES _____
☐ PHYSICAL/SEXUAL ACTIVITY _____
☐ LABOR SIGNS _____
☐ NUTRITION COUNSELING _____
☐ BREAST OR BOTTLE FEEDING _____
☐ NEWBORN CAR SEAT _____
☐ POSTPARTUM BIRTH CONTROL _____
☐ ENVIRONMENTAL/WORK HAZARDS _____

☐ TUBAL STERILIZATION _____
☐ VBAC COUNSELING _____
☐ CIRCUMCISION _____
☐ TRAVEL _____
☐ LIFESTYLE, TOBACCO, ALCOHOL _____

REQUESTS _____
_____

TUBAL STERILIZATION   DATE   INITIALS
CONSENT SIGNED   ____ / ____ / ____   _____

AA128   12345/10987

PROVIDER SIGNATURE (AS REQUIRED) _____

ACOG ANTEPARTUM RECORD (FORM D)

Figure 2-2 Continued

of 18 ± 2.5 weeks of gestation.[147] Fetal movement tends to be perceived earlier after the first pregnancy, probably because of the experience of the mother.

Ultrasound Dating

Clinical parameters to estimate gestational age can be unreliable. The menstrual history can be especially misleading for several reasons. As many as 30 to 45% of women may not recall their LMP.[147,148] Even certainty of the LMP can give unreliable dating criteria. Every woman has a relatively large degree of variation in her cycle length, with fluctuations of ± 4 days (1 SD) existing in "regular" cycles.[149] In addition, cycles of 25 to 31 days have been found in only 77% of women.[149] Even in women who do recall their LMP with certainty and know their cycle length, the LMP may be unreliable because of implantation bleeding, the use of oral contraceptive pills, or ovulatory variation.

When clinical parameters of gestational age are unreliable, ultrasound determination of gestational age in the first half of pregnancy provides an accurate estimate of gestational age. The American College of Obstetrics and Gynecology does not support the routine use of ultrasound for determining gestational age in all low-risk patients; however, the ACOG states that ultrasound is indicated for patients with uncertain clinical dates or vaginal bleeding of undetermined cause.

The earliest ultrasound estimate of gestational age can be obtained by measuring the mean gestational sac diameter at 5 to 6 weeks. Although this measurement can provide a reasonable estimate of menstrual age, the mean sac diameter becomes progressively less reliable as pregnancy advances.[150] By 7 gestational weeks a fetal pole can be identified in all viable pregnancies, making it possible to measure the fetal crown-to-rump length.[151] The crown-to-rump length provides a highly accurate estimate of gestational age in the first trimester.[152,153] Beyond the 12th week, crown-to-rump length determination becomes more difficult because of the variable flexion of the fetal head. After the first trimester, other fetal parameters can be reliably measured. The accuracy of gestational age estimates by ultrasound increases by using several parameters to derive a composite gestational age. There is no consensus on which parameters to include in composite estimates; however, the basic fetal measurements used to estimate age are the biparietal diameter, head circumference, abdominal circumference, and femur length.[154] The accuracy of ultrasound estimates of fetal gestation is inversely related to fetal age. Ultrasound determination of fetal age beyond 24 weeks and 36 weeks is associated with an error of >2 weeks and >3 weeks, respectively (Table 2-2).[155]

Fetal Maturity Assessment

The assessment of fetal lung maturity is important before elective induction or repeat cesarean delivery. The risk of respiratory illness for an infant born by elective cesarean delivery decreases with each week of gestation from 37 to 39 weeks.[156] Transient tachypnea of the newborn related to elective cesarean delivery is not prevented by confirmation of fetal lung maturity because the respiratory morbidity is not caused by surfactant deficiency, but rather by excess lung fluid. The only preventive measure to decrease

TABLE 2-2 ACCURACY OF ULTRASOUND ASSESSMENT OF GESTATIONAL AGE		
Gestational Age (wk)	Parameter	Range (2 SD) (days)
5–6	Mean gestational sac diameter	±4
6	Crown-to-rump length	±3
7		±4
8–9		±5
10–11		±6
12–13		±7
12–18	Biparietal diameter	±8
	Head circumference	±9
	Abdominal circumference	±13
	Femur length	±7
24–30	Biparietal diameter	±15
	Head circumference	±16
	Abdominal circumference	±15
	Femur length	±14
36–42	Biparietal diameter	±22
	Head circumference	±24
	Abdominal circumference	±18
	Femur length	±22

SD = Standard deviation
From Hadlock.[155]

transient tachypnea of the newborn is for elective cesarean deliveries to be performed after the 39th week of gestation or after the onset of labor. ACOG states that fetal maturity may be assumed and amniocentesis need not be performed if any one of the following criteria confirms gestational age assessment on the basis of menstrual dates in a patient with regular menstrual cycles and no immediate antecedent use of oral contraceptives:

1. Fetal heart tones have been documented for 20 weeks by nonelectronic fetoscope or for 30 weeks by Doppler.
2. It has been 36 weeks since a positive serum or urine human chorionic gonadotropin pregnancy test was performed by a reliable laboratory.
3. An ultrasound measurement of the crown-to-rump length, obtained at 6 to 11 weeks, supports a gestational age of ≥39 weeks. (Ultrasound may be considered confirmatory of menstrual dates if there is gestational age agreement within 1 week by crown-to-rump length.)
4. An ultrasonography performed at 12 to 20 weeks confirms a gestational age of ≥39 weeks determined by clinical history and physical examination. (Ultrasound may be considered confirmatory of

menstrual dates if there is gestational age agreement within 10 days by the average of multiple fetal measurements.)[157]

FETAL ASSESSMENT

Perinatal Mortality

The goal of antepartum fetal assessment is to reduce perinatal mortality. There are several different definitions of perinatal death, a situation that has contributed to discrepancies in perinatal statistics between the United States and other countries.[158] The perinatal mortality rate (PMR) as defined by the National Center for Health Statistics (NCHS) is the number of fetal deaths at $\geq$28 weeks of gestation plus neonatal deaths of infants 0 to 6 days of age per 1000 live births and fetal deaths.[159] Using this definition, the PMR in the United States in 1991 was 8.7 per 1000.[160] The definition of the perinatal period recommended by the American College of Obstetricians and Gynecologists is broader, including the number of fetuses and live births from 22 weeks of gestation (or 500 g) through 28 completed days of life.[161] For purposes of comparison on an international basis, perinatal statistics should include only deaths of fetuses and infants weighing $\geq$1000 g at delivery.[161]

Antepartum fetal testing identifies fetuses at risk for asphyxia, which accounts for about 30% of antepartum fetal deaths.[162] Two large retrospective studies have concluded that fetal testing can decrease the rate of fetal death or stillbirth.[163,164] Antenatal fetal monitoring may even identify fetal asphyxia early enough to prevent brain damage. The risk of cerebral palsy is increased with low biophysical profile scores.[165]

Not all authors agree that the use of antepartum fetal surveillance has proven to be beneficial.[166] Several small randomized trials do not support the use of nonstress tests as a supplementary evaluation of fetal well-being in "high-risk" pregnancies.[167–170] Because many of the studies of antepartum fetal assessment have been limited by small sample sizes, however, one cannot assume that fetal testing is without value.[171] There are several antepartum tests of fetal well-being currently used in clinical practice.

Fetal Movement Assessment

Maternal assessment of fetal activity is a simple and inexpensive method of fetal surveillance. During the third trimester, the human fetus makes about 30 gross body movements per hour.[172] About 80% of these movements can be appreciated by the mother.[173] Fetal movement increases between 9:00 p.m. and 1:00 a.m., probably because this is a time of decreasing maternal serum glucose, which is associated with increased fetal movement.[172,174] Contrary to popular belief, fetal movements are not increased after a meal or after a sugar-based drink.[162,175]

Several studies have shown that maternal assessment of fetal movement can reduce fetal death, while others have found no benefit from this approach.[176–178] Different protocols for fetal movement or "kick counts" have been used; however, the ideal number of kicks and time period for assessment have yet to be defined.[179] The method developed by Moore and Picquadio was shown to have greater than 90% patient compliance.[176] Patients were told to monitor fetal activity in the evening. The amount of time to perceive 10 movements was recorded, which averaged 21 minutes. Patients who do not appreciate 10 movements within 2 hours were instructed to report immediately for further evaluation. By instituting a formal program of fetal movement counting, the authors found the fetal mortality rate decreased from 8.7/1000 to 3.6/1000.[180] During the study period, the number of antepartum tests required to assess patients with decreased fetal movement increased only 13%. This method appears to be a simple and effective way to perform fetal activity assessment.

The Nonstress Test

The nonstress test (NST) is the most widely applied test for antepartum fetal assessment. This test is based on the premise that the heart rate of a healthy fetus will accelerate in response to fetal movement. At term, more than 90% of fetal movements are associated with fetal heart rate accelerations.[172] A healthy, term fetus typically exhibits heart rate accelerations at least every 40 minutes; absence of accelerations for 90 minutes is frequently associated with significant perinatal pathology.[181]

The NST is performed by monitoring the fetal heart rate with an external transducer. The patient should be in either a semi-Fowler or supine position and tilted to the left to avoid maternal hypotension. The tracing is continued until fetal heart reactivity is observed. A reactive test is defined as two or more accelerations peaking at least 15 beats per minute above the baseline and lasting 15 seconds from baseline to baseline, all occurring within 20 minutes.[179,182] The test may be continued for 40 minutes to take into account fetal sleep–wake cycles.

About 85% of NSTs will be reactive on initial testing of a term fetus. This is a reassuring measure of fetal well-being, as the rate (corrected for congenital anomalies) of stillbirth occurring within 1 week of a reactive NST is only 1.4 per 1000.[183] About 15% of NSTs will be nonreactive, although 90% of these fetuses will tolerate labor well.[184] The most common cause of a nonreactive NST is a period of fetal sleep. Absence of fetal heart rate accelerations may also be due to medications (i.e., narcotics, magnesium sulfate, β-blockers, phenobarbital), smoking or fetal hypoxia.[185–187] If reactivity has not been confirmed after 40 minutes of observation, a contraction stress test (CST) or biophysical profile (BPP) should be performed, since 13% of such fetuses will be found to have a positive CST.[182]

Vibroacoustic stimulation (VAS) may be used to awaken the fetus from quiet to active sleep and shorten the testing period. Most studies have used an electronic artificial larynx to generate a stimulus of 3 seconds or less applied near the fetal head. If the fetal heart tracing remains nonreactive, acoustic stimulation is repeated at 1-minute intervals up to 3 times.[188] If the tracing remains nonreactive, further evaluation should be performed with a CST or BPP. VAS has been shown to decrease the incidence of nonreactive NSTs from 14% to 9%.[189] A reactive NST after VAS is as reassuring of fetal well-being as a spontaneously reactive NST.

Contraction Stress Test

The CST identifies the fetus at risk for uteroplacental insufficiency by examining the response of the fetal heart to the stress of uterine contractions. Uterine contractions may produce late decelerations suggestive of marginally adequate fetal oxygenation. Contractions may also produce variable decelerations indicating cord compression, which often is secondary to oligohydramnios.

To perform the CST, the patient should be in either a semi-Fowler or supine position and tilted to the left. Baseline fetal heart rate tracing and uterine activity are obtained. If three contractions of $\geq$40 seconds' duration occur within 10 minutes, no uterine stimulation is necessary. If necessary, contractions may be produced with nipple stimulation or low-dose oxytocin. Nipple stimulation has the advantage of completing the CST in about half the time and without an intravenous transfusion. The patient gently strokes the nipple of one breast through her clothes for 2 minutes and then rests for 5 minutes. This cycle is repeated until adequate contractions are achieved. About two-thirds of patients can be expected to complete the test within 40 minutes.[190] If nipple stimulation is unsuccessful, a low-dose intravenous infusion of oxytocin can be initiated and increased at the same rates as used for labor induction.

Table 2-3 summarizes the ACOG interpretation and management of the CST. A negative CST has been associated with a stillbirth rate (corrected for congenital anomalies) of only 0.4 per 1000 within 1 week of the test.[191] Although a positive CST has been associated with an increased rate of intrauterine death, this test is limited by a high rate (30%) of false positive results.[191,192] Relative contraindications to the CST include a risk factor for preterm labor, premature rupture of membranes, classical uterine incision scar, and placenta previa.

TABLE 2-3
INTERPRETATION AND MANAGEMENT OF THE CONTRACTION STRESS TEST

Interpretation	Definition	Management
Negative	No late decelerations	Repeat study in 1 week
Positive	Late decelerations following ≥50% of contractions regardless of contraction frequency	Real-time ultrasonography for fetal anomalies Delivery is warranted*
Suspicious (equivocal)	Intermittent late or variable decelerations	Assess amniotic fluid volume Repeat test within 24 hr
Unsatisfactory	Inadequate contractions (<3 contractions per 10 minutes)	Repeat test within 24 hr

*If the fetus is premature without documented pulmonary maturity but the NST is still reactive, delivery may be temporarily delayed while frequently monitoring for reactivity and administering of corticosteroids for fetal lung maturation.
From ACOG.[179]

Biophysical Profile

Real-time ultrasound evaluation of fetal movement can be used to screen for fetal asphyxia. The biophysical profile is based on the premise that changes in fetal biophysical activities accompany central nervous system hypoxemia or asphyxia or both.[193] The test combines the use of four observations made by ultrasound with an NST. Each of these five variables is assigned a score of 2 if normal and 0 if abnormal. The highest possible score is 10. The four ultrasound variables (fetal breathing, movement, tone, and amniotic fluid) are observed simultaneously until each variable meets normal criteria or 30 minutes has elapsed. The normal duration of the ultrasound is usually less than 10 minutes. The normal components and technique of the biophysical profile are as follows:

1. Fetal breathing movements: The presence of at least one episode of fetal breathing of ≥30 seconds' duration during a 30-minute observation period.
2. Gross fetal body movements: The presence of ≥3 discrete body/limb movements during a 30-minute observation period.
3. Fetal tone: ≥1 episode of active extension with return to flexion of fetal limb(s) or trunk.
4. Amniotic fluid volume: ≥1 pocket of fluid measuring ≥2 cm in its largest vertical axis.
5. Reactive nonstress test: ≥2 episodes of fetal heart rate acceleration of ≥15 bpm and of ≥15 seconds in a 20-minute period (The NST can be eliminated for patients with normal ultrasound components of the test, yielding an additional normal score category of 8 of 8).[194,195]

Management based on the biophysical profile is always considered within the overall clinical context of each case and depends on the test score and gestational age of the fetus (Table 2-4). The incidence of

---

TABLE 2-4
PREGNANCY MANAGEMENT BASED ON THE BIOPHYSICAL PROFILE SCORE (PBS)

BPS Result	Interpretation	Risk of Asphyxia (Umbilical Venous Metabolic Acidosis <7.25) (%)	Risk of Fetal Death (per 1000/week)	Management
10/10 8/10 with normal fluid 8/8 (NST not done)	Normal infant; nonasphyxiated	0	0.565	No fetal indication for intervention; repeat testing per protocol
8/10 with oligohydramnios	Chronic compensated asphyxia	5–10 (estimate)	20–30	If mature (≥37 weeks), deliver. Serial testing (twice weekly) in the immature fetus
6/10 with normal fluid	Possible acute asphyxia	10	50	If mature (≥37 weeks), deliver. Repeat test in 24 hours in immature fetus. Repeat test; if ≤6/10, deliver
6/10 with oligohydramnios	Chronic asphyxia with possible acute asphyxia	>10 (?)	>50	Consider gestational age; if ≥32 weeks, deliver. If ≤32 weeks, test daily
4/10 with normal fluid	Acute asphyxia likely	36	115	Consider gestational age; if ≥32 weeks, deliver. If ≤32 weeks, test daily
4/10 with oligohydramnios	Chronic asphyxia, acute asphyxia likely	>36	>115	If ≥26 weeks, deliver
2/10 with normal fluid	Acute asphyxia nearly certain	73	220	If ≥26 weeks, deliver
2/10 with oligohydramnios	Chronic asphyxia with superimposed acute asphyxia	>73	>220	If ≥26 weeks, deliver
0/10	Gross severe asphyxia	100	550	If ≥26 weeks, deliver

Oligohydramnios = maximal fluid pocket ≤2 cm in vertical axis

Adapted from Manning,[196] with permission.

stillbirth occurring within 1 week of a reassuring BPP is reported to be 0.6/1000.[195]

The modified biophysical profile score was developed by Clark and co-workers to shorten the testing time and decrease the labor-intensiveness required by the BPP.[197] This test combines the vibroacoustic NST and amniotic fluid volume, which are reflective of both acute and chronic asphyxia, respectively. This approach appears to be an excellent method of antepartum fetal surveillance. The incidence of stillbirth occurring within 1 week of a normal modified BPP has been reported to be 0/1000.[197]

Umbilical Artery Doppler Flow Assessment

Doppler ultrasound has been used to measure blood flow in uterine and fetal vessels. Evaluation of the umbilical artery is the most widely used approach. The peak systolic:diastolic (S:D) ratio is characterized by a progressive decline from early pregnancy until term. Abnormal umbilical artery blood flow is defined as decreased, absent, or reversed end-diastolic flow.

The appropriate use of umbilical artery flow patterns remains to be defined.[179] There is no evidence that Doppler velocimetry is beneficial in screening low-risk pregnancies. In contrast, women with high-risk pregnancies, including preeclampsia and intrauterine growth restriction, may benefit from doppler ultrasonography. A meta-analysis of Doppler ultrasonography in high-risk pregnancies found that clinical action guided by Doppler measurements reduced the odds of perinatal death by 38%.[198] According to ACOG, it appears "reasonable to consider extremely abnormal umbilical arterial flow patterns (i.e., absent or reversed umbilical flow during fetal cardiac diastole) in the context of other abnormal test results in formulating a management plan."[179]

REFERENCES

1. Centers for Disease Control. Surveillance for reproductive health. MMWR 1997;46(SS-4).
2. Berg CJ, Atrash HK, Koonin LM, et al. Pregnancy-related mortality in the United States, 1987–1990. Obstet Gynecol 1996;88:161.
3. Kuller JA, Laifer SA. Preconceptional counseling and intervention. Arch Intern Med 1994;154:2273.
4. Adams MM, Bruce FC, Shulman HB, et al. Pregnancy planning and preconception counseling. Obstet Gynecol 1993;82:955.
5. Fuhrmann K, Reiher H, Semmler K, et al. The effect of intensified conventional insulin therapy before and during pregnancy on the malformation rate in offspring of diabetic mothers. Exper Clin Endocrinol 1984;83:173.
6. Kitzmiller JL, Gavin Al, Gin GD, et al. Preconception care of diabetes: glycemic control prevents congenital anomalies. JAMA l991;265:731.
7. American Diabetes Association. Preconception care of women with diabetes. Diabetes Care 1997;20:540.
8. Janz, NK, Herman WH, Becker MP, et al. Diabetes and pregnancy. Factors associated with seeking preconception care. Diabetes Care 1995;18:157.
9. Lenke RR, Levy HL. Maternal phenylketonuria—results of dietary therapy. Am J Obstet Gynecol 1982;142:548.
10. Platt LD, Kock R, Azen C, et al. Maternal phenylketonuria collaborative study, obstetric aspects and outcome: the first 6 years. Am J Obstet Gynecol 1992;166:1150.
11. Lenke RR, Levy HL. Maternal phenylketonuria and hyperphenylalaninemia: an international survey of the outcome of untreated and treated pregnancies. N Engl J Med 1980;303:1202.
12. Koch R, Levy HL, Matalon R, et al. The North American Collaborative Study of maternal phenylketonuria: status report 1993. Am J Dis Child 1993;147:1224.
13. Hanley WB, Demshar H, Preston MA, et al. Newborn phenylketonuria (PKU) Guthrie (BIA) screening and early hospital discharge. Early Hum Dev 1997;47:87.
14. Baily CJ, Poole RW, Poskitt EM, et al. Valproic acid and fetal abnormality. BMJ 1983;286:190.
15. Hanson JW, Smith DW. The fetal hydantoin syndrome. J Pediatr 1975;87:285.
16. Meadow R. Anticonvulsants in pregnancy. Arch Dis Child 1991;60:62.
17. Jones KL, Lacro RV, Johnson KA, et al. Pattern of malformations in children of women treated with carbamazepine during pregnancy. N Engl J Med 1989;320:1661.
18. Callaghan N, Garrett A, Goggin T. Withdrawal of anticonvulsant drugs in patients free of seizures for two years: a prospective study. N Engl J Med 1988;318:942.
19. Hall JG, Pauli RM, Wilson KM. Maternal and fetal sequelae of anticoagulation during pregnancy. Am J Med 1980;68:122.
20. Surian M, Imbasciati E, Cosci P, et al. Glomerular disease and pregnancy: a study of 123 pregnancies in patients with primary and secondary glomerular diseases. Nephron 1984;36:101.
21. Jungers P, Houillier P, Forget D, et al. Influence of pregnancy on the course of primary chronic glomerulonephritis. Lancet 1995;346:1122.
22. Hemmelder MH, deZeeuw D, Fidler V, et al. Proteinuria: a risk factor for pregnancy-related renal function decline in primary glomerular disease? Am J Kidney Dis 1995;25:187.
23. Sibai BM, Abdella TY, Anderson GD. Pregnancy outcome in 211 patients with mild chronic hypertension. Obstet Gynecol 1983;61:571.
24. Barr M, Cohen MM. ACE inhibitor fetopathy and hypocalvaria: the kidney–skull connection. Teratology 1991;44:485.
25. Piper JM, Raj WA, Rosa FW. Pregnancy outcome following exposure to angiotensin-converting enzyme. Obstet Gynecol 1992;80:429.

26. Dawson J, Lind T, Uldal P. Planned pregnancy in a renal transplant recipient. Br J Obstet Gynaecol 1976;83:518.

27. El-Khatib M, Becker GJ, Kincaid-Smith. Pregnancy-related complications in women with reflux nephropathy. Clin Nephrol 1994;41:50.

28. Floyd RC, Roberts WE. Autoimmune disease in pregnancy. Obstet Gynecol Clin North Am 1992;19:719.

29. Mintz G, Nez J, Gutierrez G. Prospective study of pregnancy in systemic lupus erythematosus. J Rheumatol 1986;13:732.

30. Cheron RG, Kaplan MM, Larsen PK, et al. Neonatal thyroid function after propylthiouracil: subsequent intellectual and physical development. Am J Dis Child 1986; 116:161.

31. Leung AS, Miller LK, Kooningo PP, et al. Perinatal outcome in hypothyroid pregnancies. Obstet Gynecol 1993; 81:349.

32. Cefalo RC, Moos MK. Preconceptional health care: a practical guide. 2nd ed. St. Louis: Mosby, 1995.

33. Lee SH, Ewert DP, Frederick PD, et al. Resurgence of congenital rubella syndrome in the 1990's: report on missed opportunities and failed prevention policies among women of childbearing age. JAMA 1992; 267:2616.

34. Pastuszak AL, Levy M, Schik B, et al. Outcome after maternal varicella infection in the first 20 weeks of pregnancy. N Engl J Med 1994;330:901.

35. American College of Obstetricians and Gynecologists. Perinatal viral and perinatal infections. ACOG Tech Bull 1973;177.

36. Kuller JA, Yankowitz J. Genetics for the obstetrician-gynecologist. Primary Care Update Obstet Gynecol 1995;2:71.

37. Friedman JM. Genetic disease in the offspring of older fathers. Obstet Gynecol 1981;57:74509.

38. American College of Obstetricians and Gynecologists, Committee on Genetics. Advanced paternal age: risk to the fetus. Committee Opinion No. 189. October 1997.

39. Savitz DA, Schwingl PJ, Keels MA. Influence of paternal age, smoking and alcohol consumption on congenital anomalies. Teratology 1991;44:429.

40. Taskinen HK. The effects of parental occupation exposure on spontaneous abortion and congenital malformation. Scand J Work Environ Health 1990;16:297.

41. McDonald AD, McDonald JC, Armstrong B, et al. Occupation and pregnancy outcome. Br J Ind Med 1987;44:521.

42. Goldhaber MK, Polen MR, Hyatt RH. The risk of miscarriage or birth defects among women who use video display terminals during pregnancy. Am J Ind Med 1988; 13:695.

43. Schnorr TM, Gragewiski BA, Hornung RW, et al. Video display terminals and the risk of spontaneous abortion. N Engl J Med 1991;324:727.

44. Chernoff N, Rogers JM, Kavet R. A review of the literature on potential reproductive and developmental toxicity of electric and magnetic fields. Toxicology 1992; 774:91.

45. Institute of Medicine. Nutrition during pregnancy. 1. Weight gain; 2. Nutrient supplements. Washington, DC: National Academy Press, 1990.

46. Johnson JWC, Yancey MK. A critique of the new recommendations for weight gain in pregnancy. Am J Obstet Gynecol 1996;174:254.

47. American College of Obstetrics and Gynecologists. Nutrition during pregnancy. ACOG Technical Bulletin 1993;179.

48. Parker JD, Abrams B. Prenatal weight gain advice: An examination of the recent prenatal weight gain recommendations of the Institute of Medicine. Obstet Gynecol 1992;79:664.

49. Hickey CA, Cliver SP, McNeal SF, et al. Prenatal weight gain patterns and spontaneous preterm birth among nonobese black and white women. Obstet Gynecol 1995;85:909.

50. Seiga-Riz AM, Adair LS, Hobel CJ. Institute of Medicine maternal weight gain recommendations and pregnancy outcome in a predominantly hispanic population. Obstet Gynecol 1994;84:565.

51. National Research Council. Recommended dietary allowances. 10th ed. Washington, DC: National Academy Press, 1989:240.

52. United States Preventive Services Task Force. Routine iron supplementation during pregnancy. JAMA 1986; 270:2846.

53. United States Public Health Service. Healthy people 2000, national health promotion and disease preventing objectives. Washington, DC: Department of Health and Human Services, Public Health Service, 1992:381.

54. Milunsky A, Jick H, Jick SS, et al. Multivitamin/folic acid supplementation in early pregnancy reduces the prevalence of neural tube defects. JAMA 1989;262:2847.

55. Centers for Disease Control and Prevention. Recommendations for the use of folic acid to reduce the number of cases of spina bifida and other neural tube defects. MMWR 1992;41:1.

56. MRC Vitamin Study Research Group. Prevention of neural tube defects: results of the medical research council vitamin study. Lancet 1991;338:131.

57. Centers for Disease Control and Prevention. Use of folic acid for prevention of spina bifida and other neural tube defects. MMWR 1991;40:513.

58. Werler MM, Shapiro S, Mitchell AA. Periconceptional folic acid exposure and risk of occurrent neural tube defects. JAMA 1993;269:1257.

59. Czizel AE, Dudas I. Prevention of the first occurrence of neural-tube defects by periconceptional vitamin supplementation. N Engl J Med 1992;327:1832.

60. Shaw GM, Lammer EJ, Wasserman CR, et al. Risks of orofacial clefts in children born to women using multivitamins containing folic acid periconceptionally. Lancet 1995;346:393.

61. American College of Obstetricians and Gynecologists Committee on Obstetrics. Vitamin A supplementation during pregnancy. Committee Opinion No. 157, September 1995.

62. Rothman KJ, Moore CC, Singer JR, et al. Teratogenicity of high vitamin A intake. N Engl J Med 1995;333:1369.

63. Glenn FB, Glenn WD III, Duncan RC. Fluoride tablet supplementation during pregnancy for caries immunity: a study of the offspring produced. Am J Obstet Gynecol 1982;143:560.

64. Goldenberg RL, Ramura T, Neggers Y, et al. The effect of zinc supplementation on pregnancy outcome. JAMA 1995;274:463.

65. Sibai BM, Villar MA, Brau E. Magnesium supplementation during pregnancy: a double-blind randomized controlled clinical trial. Am J Obstet Gynecol 1989;161:115.

66. Cao XY, Jiang WM, Dou ZH, et al. Timing of vulnerability of the brain to iodine deficiency in endemic cretinism. N Engl J Med 1994;26:1739.

67. American College of Obstetricians and Gynecologists. Exercise during pregnancy and the postpartum period. ACOG Technical Bulletin No. 189, February 1994.

68. Clapp JC III, Little KD. The interaction between regular exercise and selected aspects of women's health. Am J Obstet Gynecol 1995;173:2.

69. Clapp JC. The course of labor after endurance exercise during pregnancy. Am J Obstet Gynecol 1990;163:1799.

70. Teitelman AM, Welch LS, Hellenbrand KG, et al. Effect of maternal work activity on preterm birth and low birthweight. Am J Epidemiol 1990;131:104.

71. Klebanoff MA, Shiono PH, Carey JC. The effect of physical activity during pregnancy on preterm delivery and birth weight. Am J Obstet Gynecol 1990;163:1450.

72. Read JS, Klebanof MA. Sexual intercourse during pregnancy and preterm delivery: effects of vaginal microorganisms. Am J Obstet Gynecol 1993;168:514.

73. Ekwo EE, Gosselink CA, Woolson R, et al. Coitus late in pregnancy: risk of preterm rupture of amniotic sac membranes. Am J Obstet Gynecol 1993;168:22.

74. Aronson ME, Nelson PK. Fatal air embolism in pregnancy resulting from an unusual sex act. Obstet Gynecol 1967;30:127.

75. American College of Obstetricians and Gynecologists. Automobile passenger restraints for children and pregnant women. ACOG Technical Bulletin No. 151, January 1991.

76. American College of Obstetricians and Gynecologists. Immunization during pregnancy. ACOG Technical Bulletin No. 160, October 1991.

77. American College of Obstetricians and Gynecologists. Hepatitis in pregnancy. ACOG Technical Bulletin No. 174, November 1992.

78. Garner P, Schaffner W. Immunization of adults. N Engl J Med 1993;328:1252.

79. American College of Obstetricians and Gynecologists. Rubella and pregnancy. ACOG Technical Bulletin No. 171, August 1992.

80. Centers for Disease Control and Prevention, Immunization Practices Advisory Committee. Outbreaks of rubella among the Amish—United States, 1991. MMWR 1991; 40:264.

81. American Academy of Pediatrics, American College of Obstetricians and Gynecologists. Guidelines for perinatal care. 4th ed. Washington, DC: AAP/ACOG, 1992:52, 137.

82. American College of Obstetricians and Gynecologists. Gonorrhea and chlamydial infections. ACOG Technical Bulletin No. 190, March 1994.

83. McGregor JA, French JI, Parker R, et al. Prevention of premature birth by screening and treatment for common genital tract infections: results of a prospective controlled evaluation. Am J Obstet Gynecol 1995;173:157.

84. MacDermott RJ. Bacterial vaginosis. Br J Obstet Gynaecol 1995;102:92.

85. Hauth JC, Goldenberg RL, Andrews WW, et al. Reduced incidence of preterm delivery with metronidazole and erythromycin in women with bacterial vaginosis. N Engl J Med 1995;333:1732.

86. McCoy MC, Katz VL, Kuller JA, et al. Bacterial vaginosis in pregnancy: an approach for the 1990s. Obstet Gynecol Surv 1995;50:482.

87. Centers for Disease Control and Prevention. U.S. Public Health Service recommendations for human immunodeficiency virus counseling and voluntary testing for pregnant women. MMWR 1995;44(RR-7).

88. Connor EM, Sperling RS, Gelber R, et al. Reduction of maternal–infant transmission of human immunodeficiency virus type 1 with zidovudine treatment. N Engl J Med 1994;331:1173.

89. Centers for Disease Control and Prevention. Prevention of perinatal group B streptococcal disease: a public perspective. MMWR 1996;45:1.

90. American College of Obstetricians and Gynecologists. Smoking and reproductive health. ACOG Technical Bulletin No. 180, May 1993.

91. Jauniaux E, Burton GJ. The effect of smoking in pregnancy on early placental morphology. Obstet Gynecol 1992;79:645.

92. Brown HL, Miller JM, Khawli O, et al. Premature placental calcification in maternal cigarette smokers. Obstet Gynecol 1988;71:914.

93. Naeye RL. Factors that predispose to premature rupture of the fetal membranes. Obstet Gynecol 1982; 60:93.

94. U.S. Department of Health and Human Services. The health benefits of smoking cessation: a report of the Surgeon General. Washington, DC: Department of Health and Human Services, publication no. (CDC) 90-8416, 1990:371.

95. Wen Shi Wu, Goldenberg RL, Cutter GR, et al. Smoking, maternal age, fetal growth, and gestational age at delivery. Am J Obstet Gynecol 1990;162:53.

96. Wright LN, Pahel-Short L, Hartmann K, et al. Statewide assessment of a behavioral intervention to reduce cigarette smoking by pregnant women. Am J Obstet Gynecol 1996;175:283.

97. Wright LN, Thorp JM, Kuller JA, et al. Transdermal nicotine replacement in pregnancy: maternal pharmacokinetics and fetal effects. Am J Obstet Gynecol 1997; 176:1090.

98. Sachs BP. The effect of smoking on late pregnancy outcome. Semin Reprod Endocrinol 1989;7:319.

99. Czeil AE, Kodaj I, Lenz W. Smoking during pregnancy and congenital limb deficiency. BMJ 1994;308:1473.

100. FDA Drug Bulletin, 1980;10(3):19–20.

101. Infante-Rivard C, Fernandez A, Gauthier R, et al. Fetal loss associated with caffeine intake before and during pregnancy. JAMA 1993;270:2940.

102. Mills JI, Holmes LB, Aarons JH, et al. Moderate caffeine use and the risk of spontaneous abortion and intrauterine growth retardation. JAMA 1993;269:593.

103. Kurppa K, Holmberg PC, Puosma E, et al. Coffee consumption during pregnancy and selected congenital

malformations: a nationwide case-control study. Am J Public Health 1983;73:1397.

104. Abel EL, Sokol RJ. Fetal alcohol syndrome is now leading cause of mental retardation. Lancet 1986;2:1222.

105. Jones KL, Smith DW, Ulleland CN, et al. Pattern of malformation in offspring of chronic alcoholic mothers. Lancet 1973;1:1267.

106. Abel EL, Sokol RJ. Incidence of fetal alcohol syndrome and economic impact of FAS-related anomalies. Drug Alcohol Depend 1987;19:51.

107. Serdula M, Williamson DF, Kendrick JS, et al. Trends in alcohol consumption by pregnant women. JAMA 1991; 265:876.

108. Eller KM, Kuller JA. Fetal porencephaly: a review of etiology, diagnosis, and prognosis. Obstet Gynecol Surv 1995;50:684.

109. Volpe JJ. Effect of cocaine use on the fetus. N Engl J Med 1992;327:399.

110. Chasnoff IJ, Griffith DR, MacGregor S, et al. Temporal patterns of cocaine use in pregnancy: perinatal outcome. JAMA 1989;261:1741.

111. Durand DJ, Espinoza AM, Nickerson BG. Association between prenatal cocaine exposure and sudden infant death syndrome. J Pediatr 1990;117:909.

112. Fries MH, Kuller JA, Norton ME, et al. Facial features of infants exposed prenatally to cocaine. Tetrology 1993; 48:413.

113. American College of Obstetricians and Gynecologists. Substance abuse in pregnancy. ACOG Technical Bulletin No. 195, July 1994.

114. Little BB, Snell LM, Gilstrap LC III. Methamphetamine abuse during pregnancy: outcome and fetal effects. Obstet Gynecol 1988;72:541.

115. Thorp JM. Management of drug dependency, overdose, and withdrawal in the obstetric patient. Obstet Gynecol Clin North Am 1995;22:131.

116. Soules MR, Hughes CL Jr, Garcia JA, et al. Nausea and vomiting of pregnancy: role of human chorionic gonadotropin and 17-hydroxyprogesterone. Obstet Gynecol 1980;55:696.

117. Kuller JA, McMahon MJ, Wells Sr, et al. Pharmacologic treatment of psychiatric disease in pregnancy and lactation: fetal and neonatal effects. Obstet Gynecol 1996;87:789.

118. Orvieto R, Achiron A, Ben-Rafael Z, et al. Low-back pain of pregnancy. Acta Obstet Gynecol Scand 1994; 73:209.

119. American Academy of Pediatrics/American College of Obstetricians and Gynecologists. Guidelines for Perinatal Care. 4th ed. Washington, DC: AAP/ACOG, 1992.

120. American College of Obstetricians and Gynecologists: Standard for Obstetric and Gynecologic Services. 7th Ed. ACOG, Washington, DC, 1989.

121. McDuffie RS Jr, Beck A, Bischoff K, et al. Effect of frequency of prenatal care visits on perinatal outcome among low-risk women: a randomized controlled trial. JAMA 1996;275:847.

122. Sikorski J, Wilson J, Clement S, et al. A randomized controlled trial comparing two schedules of antenatal visits: the antenatal care project. BMJ 1996;312:546.

123. Calvert JP, Crean EE, Newcombe RG, et al. Antenatal screening by measurement of symphysis-fundus height. BMJ 1982;285:846.

124. Jimenez JM, Tyson JE, Reisch JS. Clinical measures of gestational age in normal pregnancies. ObstetGynecol 1983;61:438.

125. Belizan JM, Villar J, Nardin JC, et al. Diagnosis of intrauterine growth retardation by a simple clinical method: measurement of uterine height. Am J Obstet Gynecol 1978;131:643.

126. Wikstrom I, Bergstrom R, Bakketeig L, et al. Prediction of high birthweight from maternal characteristics, symphysis fundal height and ultrasound biometry. Gynecol Obstet Invest 1993;35:27.

127. Lindhard A, Nielsen PV, Mouritsen LA, et al. The implications of introducing the symphyseal-fundal height-measurement: a prospective randomized controlled trial. Br J Obstet Gynaecol 1990;97:675.

128. Person B, Stangenberg M, Lunnell NO, et al. Prediction of size of infants at birth by measurement of symphysis fundus height. Br J Obstet Gynaecol 1986; 93:206.

129. Rosenberg K, Grant JM, Tweedi I, et al. Measurement of fundal height as a screening test for fetal growth retardation. Br J Obstet Gynaecol 1982;89:447.

130. Buekens P, Alexander S, Boutsen M, et al. Randomized controlled trial of routine cervical examinations in pregnancy. Lancet 1994;344:841.

131. American College of Obstetricians and Gynecologists. Practice patterns—external cephalic version. ACOG Technical Bulletin No. 4, July 1997.

132. Meyer NL, Mercer BM, Friedman SA, et al. Urinary dipstick protein: a poor predictor of absent or severe proteinuria. Am J Obstet Gynecol 1994;170:137.

133. Kuo VS, Lournantakis G, Gallery EDM. Proteinuria and its assessment in normal and hypertensive pregnancy. Am J Obstet Gynecol 1992;167:723.

134. Gribble RK, Meier PR, Berg RL. The value of urine screening for glucose at each prenatal visit. Obstet Gynecol 1995;86:405.

135. Chesley LC. History and epidemiology of preeclampsia-eclampsia. Clin Obstet Gynecol 1984;27:801.

136. Chesley LC. Renal function during pregnancy. In: Carey HM, ed. Modern trends in human reproductive physiology. London, Butterworth, 1963.

137. Lind T, Hytten FE. The excretion of glucose during normal pregnancy. J Obstet Gynaecol Br Commonw 1972; 79:961.

138. U.S. Preventive Services Task Force. Guide to Clinical Preventive Services. 2nd ed. Alexandria, VA: International Medical Publishing, 1996:193.

139. Centers for Disease Control. Prevention of perinatal group B streptococcal disease: a public health perspective. MMWR 1996;45(RR-7).

140. American College of Obstetricians and Gynecologists. Committee on Obstetrics. Prevention of early-onset group B streptococcal disease in newborns. Committee Opinion No. 173, June 1996.

141. Tunon K, Eik-Nes SH, Grottum P. A comparison between ultrasound and a reliable last menstrual period as predictors of the day of delivery in 15,000 examinations. Ultrasound Obstet Gynecol 1996;8:178.

142. Eik-Nes SH, Okland O, Aure JC. Ultrasound screening in pregnancy: a randomized controlled trial. Lancet 1984; 1:1347.

143. Grennert L, Persson P, Gerrser G, et al. Benefits of ultrasound screening of a pregnancy population. Acta Obstet Gynecol Scand 1978;78:5.

144. Wilcox M, Gardosi J, Mongelli M, et al. Birth weight from pregnancies dated by ultrasonography in a multicultural British population. BMJ 1993;307:588.

145. Kieler H, Axelsson O, Nilsson S, et al. The length of human pregnancy as calculated by ultrasonographic measurement of the fetal biparietal diameter. Ultrasound Obstet Gynecol 1995;6:353.

146. Bracken MB, Belanger K. Calculation of delivery dates. N Engl J Med 1989;321:1483.

147. Anderson HF, Johnson TRB, Flora JD, et al. Gestational age assessment. II. Prediction from combined clinical observations. Am J Obstet Gynecol 1981;140:770.

148. Campbell S, Warsof SL, Little D, et al. Routine ultrasound screening for the prediction of gestational age. Obstet Gynecol 1985;65:613.

149. Chiazze L, Brayer FT, Macisco JJ, et al. The length and variability of the human menstrual cycle. JAMA 1968;203:377.

150. Daya S, Woods S, Ward S, et al. Early pregnancy assessment with transvaginal ultrasound scanning. Can Med Assoc J 1991;144:441.

151. Warren WB, Timor-Tritsch I, Peisner DB, et al. Dating the early pregnancy by sequential appearance of embryonic structures. Am J Obstet Gynecol 1989;161:747.

152. Robinson HP. Sonar measurement of fetal crown-rump length as a means of assessing maturity in first trimester of pregnancy. BMJ 1973;4:28.

153. Hadlock FP, Shah YP, Kanon DJ, et al. Fetal crown-rump length: reevaluation of relation to menstrual age (5–18 weeks) with high-resolution realtime US. Radiology 1992;182:501.

154. Hadlock FP. Sonographic estimation of fetal age and weight. Radiol Clin North Am 1990;28:39.

155. Hadlock FP. Ultrasound determination of menstrual age. In: Callen PW, ed. Ultrasonography in obstetrics and gynecology. 3rd ed. Philadelphia: Saunders, 1994:86.

156. Morrison JJ, Rennie JM, Milton PJ. Neonatal respiratory morbidity and mode of delivery at term: influence of timing of elective cesarean section. Br J Obstet Gynaecol 1995;102:101.

157. American College of Obstetricians and Gynecologists Committee on Obstetrics. Fetal maturity assessment prior to elective repeat cesarean delivery. Committee Opinion No. 98, September 1991.

158. Sachs BP, Fretts RC, Gardner R, et al. The impact of extreme prematurity and congenital anomalies on the interpretation of international comparisons of infant mortality. Obstet Gynecol 1995;85:941.

159. Friede A, Rochat R. Maternal mortality and perinatal mortality: definitions, data, and epidemiology: obstetric epidemiology, Littleton, MA: PSG Publishing Company, 1985, p 35.

160. U.S. Department of Health and Human Services. Childhealth USA '94. Washington, DC: Government Printing Office, 1995.

161. American College of Obstetricians and Gynecologists, Committee on Obstetrics. Perinatal and infant mortality statistics. Committee Opinion No. 167, December 1995.

162. Druzin ML, Gabbe SG. Antepartum fetal evaluation. In: Gabbe SG, Niebyl JR, Simpson JL, eds. Obstetrics: normal and problem pregnancies. 3rd ed. New York: Churchill Livingstone, 1996:329.

163. Platt LD, Paul RH, Phelan J, et al. Fifteen years of experience with antepartum fetal testing. Am J Obstet Gynecol 1987,156:1509.

164. Schneider EP, Hutson JM, Petrie RH. An assessment of the first decade's experience with antepartum fetal heart rate testing. Am J Perinatol 1988;5:134.

165. Manning FA, Harman C, Menticoglou S. Fetal biophysical score and cerebral palsy at age 3 years. Am J Obstet Gynecol 1996;174:319.

166. Erkin M, Keirse MJNC, Renfrew M, et al. A guide to effective care in pregnancy and childbirth. 2nd ed. New York: Oxford University Press, 1995:410.

167. Flynn AM, Kelly J, Mansfield H, et al. A randomized controlled trial of non-stress antepartum cardiotocography. Br J Obstet Gynaecol 1982;89:427.

168. Brown VA, Sawers RS, Parsons S, et al. The value of antenatal cardiotocography in the management of high-risk pregnancy: a randomized controlled trial. Br J Obstet Gynaecol 1982;89:716.

169. Lumley J, Lester A, Anderson I, et al. A randomized trial of weekly cardiotocography in high-risk obstetric patients. Br J Obstet Gynaecol 1983;90:1018.

170. Kidd LC, Patel NB, Smith R. Non-stress antenatal cardiotocography—a prospective randomized clinical trial. Br J Obstet Gynaecol 1985;92:1156.

171. Neilson JP, Alfirevic Z. Biophysical profile for antepartum fetal assessment. Cochrane Pregnancy & Childbirth Database 1995;2.

172. Patrick J, Campbell K, Carmichael L, et al. Patterns of gross fetal body movements over 24-hours observation intervals during the last 10 weeks of pregnancy. Am J Obstet Gynecol 1982;142:363.

173. Rayburn WF. Clinical significance of perceptible fetal motion. Am J Obstet Gynecol 1980;138:210.

174. Holden K, Jovanovic L, Druzin M, et al. Increased fetal activity with low maternal blood glucose levels in pregnancies complicated by diabetes. Am J Perinatol 1984;1:161.

175. Phelan JP, Kester R, Labudovich ML. Nonstress test and maternal glucose determinations. Obstet Gynecol 1982;67:4.

176. Moore TR, Piacquadio K. A prospective evaluation of fetal movement screening to reduce the incidence of antepartum fetal death. Am J Obstet Gynecol 1989;160:1075.

177. Neldam S. Fetal movements as an indicator of fetal well-being. Lancet 1980;1:1222.

178. Grant A, Valentin L, Elbourne D, et al. Routine formal fetal movement counting and risk of antepartum late death in normally formed singletons. Lancet 1989;2:345.

179. American College of Obstetricians and Gynecologists. Antepartum fetal surveillance. ACOG Technical Bulletin No. 188, January 1994.

180. Moore TR, Piacquadio K. Study results vary in count-to-10 method of fetal movement screening. Am J Obstet Gynecol 1990;163:264.

181. Devoe LD, McKenzie J, Searle NS, et al. Clinical sequelae of the extended nonstress test. Am J Obstet Gynecol 1985;151:1074.

182. Evertson L, Gauthier R, Schifrin B, et al. Antepartum fetal heart rate testing. I. Evolution of the nonstress test. Am J Obstet Gynecol 1979;133:29.

183. Freeman RK, Anderson G, Dorchester W. A prospective multi-institutional study of antepartum fetal heart rate monitoring. II. Contraction stress test versus nonstress test for primary surveillance. Am J Obstet Gynecol 1982; 143:778.

184. Laxery J. Nonstress fetal heart rate testing. Clin Obstet Gynecol 1982;25:689.

185. Margulis E, Binder D, Cohen A. The effect of propranolol on the nonstress test. Am J Obstet Gynecol 1984; 148:340.

186. Keegan K, Paul R, Broussard P, et al. Antepartum fetal heart rate testing. III. The effect of phenobarbital on the nonstress test. Am J Obstet Gynecol 1979;133:579.

187. Phelan J. Diminished fetal reactivity with smoking. Am J Obstet Gynecol 1985;136:230.

188. Phelan JP. Antepartum fetal assessment—new techniques. Semin Perinatol 1988;12:57.

189. Smith CV, Phelan JP, Platt LD, et al. Fetal acoustic stimulation testing. II. A randomized clinical comparison with the nonstress test. Am J Obstet Gynecol 1986; 155:131.

190. Huddleston J, Stuliff G, Robinson D. Contraction stress test by intermittent nipple stimulation. Obstet Gynecol 1984;63:669.

191. Freeman RK, Anderson G, Dorchester W. A prospective multi-institutional study of antepartum fetal heart rate monitoring. I. Risk of perinatal mortality and morbidity according to antepartum fetal heart rate test results. Am J Obstet Gynecol 1982;143:771.

192. Collea J, Hollis W. The contraction stress test. Clin Obstet Gynecol 1982;25:707.

193. Manning FA, Platt LD. Maternal hypoxemia and fetal breathing movements. Obstet Gynecol 1979;53:758.

194. Manning FA, Morrison I, Lange IR, et al. Fetal assessment based on fetal biophysical profile scoring: experience in 12,620 referred high-risk pregnancies. I. Perinatal mortality by frequency and etiology. Am J Obstet Gynecol 1985;151:343.

195. Manning FA, Harman CR, Morrison I, et al. Fetal assessment based on fetal biophysical profile scoring. IV. An analysis of perinatal morbidity and mortality. Am J Obstet Gynecol 1990;162:703.

196. Manning FA. Fetal medicine: principles and practice. Norwalk, CT: Appleton and Lange, 1995:255.

197. Clark SL, Sabey P, Jolley K. Nonstress testing with acoustic stimulation and amniotic fluid volume assessment: 5973 tests without unexpected fetal death. Am J Obstet Gynecol 1989;160:694.

198. Alfirevic Z, Neilson JP. Doppler ultrasonography in high-risk pregnancies: Systematic review with meta-analysis. Am J Obstet Gynecol 1995;172:1379.

Chapter 3
Teratology

Michael F. Greene

Five Key Points

- Approximately 4.5% of all live births in the United States are associated with major or minor congenital malformations. Congenital malformations are one of the two most important causes of perinatal mortality.

- Several factors determine the extent to which a drug or chemical agent crosses the placenta: molecular size, lipid solubility, degree of ionization at physiologic pHs, and degree of protein binding.

- Diagnostic radiology and nuclear medicine procedures do not pose a risk of fetal teratogenicity.

- Thalidomide and isotretinoin are extremely potent teratogens. The former is associated with severe limb and craniofacial malformations. The latter is associated with defects of the central nervous system, cranium, face, and heart.

- Oral anticoagulants should not be used in pregnancy because of their teratogenic effects.

HISTORICAL PERSPECTIVE

The notion that environmental factors could have a major impact on embryonic and fetal development dates to antiquity. Over the centuries, however, our concept of what factors are dangerous and their mechanisms of action have changed. The ancient Romans believed that if a pregnant woman viewed a particularly horrifying or shocking sight, it could adversely affect her pregnancy. Median cleft lip, or hare-lip, was thought to result from staring at a rabbit for too long. This belief was known as the doctrine of maternal impressions. In early colonial times, some anomalies were thought to result from human liaisons with animals. A woman who delivered a cyclopic fetus with a single midline eye and a proboscis was thought to

have had intercourse with a pig and was in danger of being put to death for the offense. It was not until 1933, when Hale noted that intentionally depriving pigs of food and water during a specific period of gestation could produce a high incidence of anophthalmia, that the science of experimental teratology was born.[1] In 1941 Gregg recognized the association between maternal rubella infection during pregnancy and the constellation of malformations that we now know as the congenital rubella syndrome.[2] Despite Gregg's clinical work and the experimental animal studies of a small number of investigators during the 1940s and '50s, the potential impact of noxious environmental agents on human pregnancy was not fully appreciated until the thalidomide disaster.

LESSONS OF THE THALIDOMIDE EPIDEMIC

Thalidomide is a compound with antiemetic and hypnotic properties that was introduced in Europe to treat nausea, vomiting, and sleeplessness. Its introduction as a sleeping pill was hailed for its safety because intentional massive overdose was rarely, if ever, lethal. Thalidomide quickly became popular for treating the nausea and vomiting of early pregnancy. In 1961 and 1962, McBride in Australia[3] and Lenz in Germany[4] independently suggested that thalidomide was responsible for dramatic limb reduction malformations, termed *phocomelia*. A number of lessons were learned from that experience. These can be grouped into lessons in biology and epidemiology.

Biologic Lessons

The vulnerability of the developing fetus to environmental agents was reemphasized. The human placenta is neither impermeable to small xenobiotic molecules, nor is it necessarily capable of detoxifying them prior to transplacental passage.

An agent that is extremely safe and nontoxic for an adult may nonetheless be very toxic to a developing embryo at a normal adult therapeutic dose.

The fallibility of the existing reproductive toxicity testing system was obvious. Thalidomide had been tested and passed all the necessary toxicology testing of the day with no hint of its potential hazard. Much greater care was needed when extrapolating results from animal testing to humans.

Epidemiologic Lessons

The uniqueness of the malformation complex produced by thalidomide, and its very rare spontaneous occurrence, led to the relatively rapid recognition of cause and effect. If thalidomide caused a malformation that occurred relatively commonly spontaneously, it would have taken considerably longer to recognize a relatively small increase in the incidence of that malformation. It was obvious that a formal and sensitive population-based system for monitoring the incidence of congenital anomalies would be necessary to detect any introduction of such an insidious teratogen in the future.

The very high attack rate among exposed fetuses made recognition of the association between exposure and outcome relatively easy. The incidence of limb reduction defects among individuals exposed during the critical period of limb development was thought at one time to be almost 100%. It is now clear that the correlation is not that high and that the true figure is more like 50%. Nonetheless, this is quite a bit higher than the incidence for most documented teratogens. As the attack rate among the exposed individuals falls, larger numbers of exposed individuals must be studied for the association to become apparent.

The dramatic nature of the malformation and the fact that it could be readily appreciated on surface physical examination led to essentially 100% ascertainment of affected individuals at birth. Many congenital malformations (for example, congenital heart defects, or the genital tract changes associated with diethylstilbestrol exposure) are not noted until much later in life. The relationship between an exposure and its outcome will be more readily apparent when there is a short time between them.

Severe, permanent damage can be done to a fetus by a drug taken by its mother prior to the time that she realizes that she is pregnant.

MAGNITUDE OF THE MODERN PROBLEM

Approximately 4.5% of the live births in the United States are associated with major or minor congenital malformations. This incidence translates to approximately 160,000 malformed live births in the U.S. annually. Data from the Perinatal Collaborative Study of 50,000 mother–infant pairs reveals that these malformations break down by organ system as shown in Table 3-1.[5]

TABLE 3-1
CONGENITAL MALFORMATIONS OBSERVED IN THE COLLABORATIVE PERINATAL PROJECT

	Rate per 1000 Live Births
Any malformation	45.3
Major malformations	27.7
Minor malformations	17.9
Central nervous system	5.3
Cardiovascular system	8.0
Musculoskeletal system	14.3
Respiratory system	4.3
Gastrointestinal tract	6.0
Genitourinary system	9.2
Eye and ear	2.4
Syndromes	3.5
Tumors	3.3

TABLE 3-2
CAUSES OF DEVELOPMENTAL ABNORMALITIES IN HUMANS

	Wilson	Holmes
Genetic and chromosomal disorders	25%	54%
Environmental factors		
Drugs	4–5%	1.5%
Maternal conditions	1–2%	3.0%
Maternal infections	2–3%	0
Deformations	—	5.4%
Amniotic bands	—	1.1%
Ionizing radiation	<1%	0
Unknown	65–70%	35.1%

A number of attempts have been made to ascribe causes to these malformations. From a survey of the literature, Wilson estimated the causes of the developmental defects found in humans.[6] Holmes made a similar tabulation, but his figures were from an actual survey and investigation of the anomalies found among more than 18,000 consecutive live births at the Boston Lying-In Hospital from 1972 to 1975.[7] Wilson's estimates and Holmes's study findings are compared in Table 3-2. There are several important points to note when examining these figures. First, the major difference between the sets of figures is in the percentage of anomalies that Holmes was able to attribute to genetic or chromosomal causes. Second, by both accounts a major percentage of anomalies are due to unknown causes. Third, only a minor percentage of all anomalies is attributable to the sum total of all environmental factors. If such a minor fraction of anomalies is due to environmental exposures, why then is there such seemingly inordinate concern about environmental exposures such as Bendectin, Agent Orange, and nuclear power plants? The answer is twofold. First is the concern that a significant percentage of the unknown group might be attributable to some as-yet unrecognized environmental exposure. Second, if there are congenital anomalies that might be preventable, they are in this category.

Drug exposure during pregnancy in American women is virtually universal. Among the 50,282 mother–infant pairs in the drug exposure portion of the Collaborative Perinatal Project, in excess of 360 different drugs were taken during the pregnancies. Estimates of the average number of drugs taken by women during the course of pregnancy in the United States range between 4 and 9. A major percentage of these drugs are taken very early in pregnancy, often prior to the time that patients realize they are pregnant. Many are over-the-counter preparations that patients do not consider important.

GENERAL PRINCIPLES OF TERATOLOGY

Several principles of teratology pertain across species. Their appreciation is important to clinical medicine.

An environmental agent must gain access to the developing organism, and ease of access depends on the nature of the agent. Ionizing radiation reaches a fetus based on relatively simple physical considerations of the energy of the radiation and the amount of tissue to be traversed. Very-low-energy particles such as α and β particles will be attenuated in the superficial skin and never reach a mammalian fetus in utero. Very-high-energy γ-rays will pass through tissue, giving up only very small amounts of energy and, therefore, doing relatively little damage to the tissue. Lower-energy γ-rays, which are completely attenuated within the tissue (rather than passing through and through), will give up more energy within the tissue and, therefore, do more damage. Relatively few infectious agents are capable of crossing the placenta to infect fetal tissues. The factors that control fetal infection are poorly understood. Once fetal infection has been established, tissue damage may occur as a direct result of the action of the organism or from the fetal immune response.

Placental transfer of chemical agents is dependent on a complex interaction of physical and chemical factors. The characteristics of the chemical itself are paramount. Generally, any agent of molecular weight less than 600 daltons will cross the placenta relatively freely. Molecules greater than 1000 daltons will not cross the placenta to any great extent. Between 600 and 1000 daltons, the lipid solubility and degree of ionization of the compound are very important. The more highly charged the molecule, the less lipid-soluble it is and the less readily it will cross the placenta. Most drugs have molecular weights less than 600 and are able to pass the placenta relatively freely. There are a few notable exceptions, such as heparin, which is a very large molecule (~5000 daltons) with a strong negative charge. Its placental passage is insignificant, which is a clinically useful fact. Neostigmine is a quaternary ammonium compound with a strong positive charge, which does not cross the placenta to a significant degree. The degree to which a compound is protein-bound determines the amount of drug free to cross the placenta.

Other factors such as the concentration of drug on both sides of the placenta and placental blood flow will influence the rate at which a drug crosses. The placenta is capable of metabolizing many xenobiotics, and its enzyme systems can be induced by chronic exposure to a variety of foreign compounds, for example cigarette smoke. The degree to which the placenta can metabolize a drug will help to determine how much of the drug reaches the fetus.

The genetic constitution of an organism determines how an environmental insult will affect the developing organism. The response may vary on the basis of species, strain, or even individual differences. This effect can be shown very easily in experimental animals. Hydrocortisone, for example, will produce clefts of the palate in 100% of exposed AJAX mouse fetuses, only 19% of C57BL mouse fetuses, and not at all in rats. Following recognition of the human teratogenicity of thalidomide, extensive testing in a variety of animal species showed that the human species is 50 to 200 times more sensitive to thalidomide than any common test animals. Even different fetuses developing within the same uterus may have different sensitivities to a teratogen. A case has been reported in which the mother of triplets was taking phenytoin during pregnancy.[8] Each of the triplets manifested phenytoin teratogenicity differently. In another case report, a pair of twins was shown by HLA typing to have been fathered by different men.[9] One twin manifested the full fetal hydantoin syndrome while the other was entirely normal. These differences may arise from differences in drug metabolism or from intrinsic differences in morphogenesis.

The developmental stage at which an organism is insulted is critical in determining the response. During the blastocyst stage, no significant differentiation has occurred among the cells destined to become the embryo and extraembryonic structures. These cells are all still totipotent. At this stage, the embryo generally responds in an all-or-none fashion. If a sufficiently large number of cells are destroyed, no new organism will develop. A sublethal injury, however, can generally be repaired by the remaining cells, resulting in no deficit but a possible temporal delay.

The embryonic period, during which major organogenesis occurs, is most sensitive to teratogenic insult. During this period major developmental disturbances result in such classic congenital malformations as anencephaly, heart and limb defects, omphalocele, and others. Later in development, during the fetal period, environmental insults are more likely to result in poor fetal growth and more subtle developmental disturbances. With recognition of these effects, and the knowledge that certain areas of the brain (for example the external granular cell layer of the cerebellum) continue to accumulate neurons through the first year of life after birth, it has become more difficult to place a limit on the sensitive period of development.

Different agents may act through different mechanisms to produce the same malformation. There are a limited number of ways in which an embryo can respond to a developmental disturbance. A malformation as viewed in a newborn is the end stage of a distorted developmental process. Similar or identical malformations cannot be assumed to have arisen through identical or even similar mechanisms or agents.

Any one agent may produce malformations in a variety of developing structures or organ systems, depending on the dose, route of administration, or timing of exposure.

Malformation may be seen as a part of the spectrum of adverse outcomes that may result from insults during the course of development. This spectrum may be seen as:

Death

Congenital malformation

Growth restriction

Functional disorder

No effect

Where along this spectrum any given conceptus will fall depends upon the intensity and timing of the insult as well as other possible modifiers.

Agents may interact to antagonize or synergize with one another. This effect may occur through simple mutual augmentation or inhibition of their metabolism or through more complex interactions. The antimetabolite 6-amino-nicotinamide (6AN) is an analogue of nicotinamide and a potent experimental teratogen. Its teratogenic effect can be completely eliminated, however, if it is administered simultaneously with a sufficient dose of the vitamin nicotinamide. Phenytoin is teratogenic in mice, with the teratogenic potency belonging to the native drug. Hydroxylation to the first metabolite eliminates its teratogenicity. Pretreatment of mice with a competitive inhibitor of the hydroxylation enzyme enhances the teratogenic effect of phenytoin. In contrast, pretreatment with phenobarbital, which stimulates the levels of the hydroxylation enzyme, reduces the teratogenicity of phenytoin.

A special case of this principle is that many compounds are capable of inducing enzymes responsible for their own metabolic destruction. Thus, chronic administration of a drug may result in lower circulating levels of the drug than a brief exposure to the same dose. If this brief exposure should happen during a sensitive period of embryogenesis, teratogenesis might result from an apparently benign drug.

In clinical practice, the concept of a dose ratio is very important. The dose ratio is the relationship between the dose of a medication that is necessary for the desired therapeutic effect and the dose that produces undesirable toxic effects. As a general rule, the dose necessary to produce the maternal therapeutic effect is relatively low. Increasingly higher doses may be responsible for teratogenesis, fetal toxicity, and ultimately maternal toxicity. One of the factors that makes thalidomide so uniquely dangerous as a human teratogen is that the maternal therapeutic and teratogenic doses are the same. There is no margin of safety. It is also important to keep this principle in mind when evaluating experimental studies that purport to demonstrate the teratogenicity of a drug. The critical question is: Was the teratogenic dose reasonable in relation to what would be used therapeutically? If the answer is that teratogenicity is seen only at doses that are toxic to the mother and several-fold higher than therapeutic, then the teratogenic effect is not of practical concern. Virtually any agent can be shown to be teratogenic at extremely high exposure levels.

SPECIFIC EXPOSURES

Ionizing Radiation

Few, if any, exposures raise the level of concern and fear quite as high as radiation. Three potential consequences of radiation exposure must be considered: teratogenicity, mutagenicity, and carcinogenicity. Central to understanding all three of these is appreciating the issue of dose. How much is too much, and how much is encountered in the course of routine diagnostic procedures?

It is generally agreed that less than 5 rad (5000 mrad) of exposure is not capable of producing a teratogenic

TABLE 3-3 **RADIATION EXPOSURE TO FIRST-TRIMESTER GRAVID UTERUS FROM DIAGNOSTIC PROCEDURES**	
Examination	Millirad
Chest x-ray	0.1
Pelvis and hip x-ray	220
Upper gastrointestinal series	3.7
Barium enema	1080
Flat plate abdomen	140
Intravenous pyelogram	308
Bilateral venogram (lower extremities)	628
Pulmonary angiogram (femoral approach)	374
Pulmonary angiogram (brachial approach)	50

effect in a mammalian fetus. Human and animal data indicate that the threshold for a detectable increase in malformations is between 5 and 25 rad, with a 40% incidence at 50 rad.[10] Among the in utero atomic bomb blast survivors at Hiroshima and Nagasaki, the most common congenital malformation was microcephaly, with its associated mental retardation. The threshold for this effect at 10 to 17 weeks of gestation was 12 rad, reaching a 40% risk at 100 rad. That threshold rises to greater than 50 rad after 17 weeks. Given this framework, how much radiation could a pregnant woman encounter diagnostically? Table 3-3 lists the radiation exposure for a gravid uterus in the first trimester resulting from some common diagnostic procedures.[11] Note that a chest x-ray examination results in 0.1 mrad (0.0001 rad) exposure to the uterus. Even with an extensive examination such as a barium enema, the exposure is only 1100 mrad (1.1 rad). It should be obvious that an upper gastrointestinal series done to investigate nausea and vomiting during what later is recognized as the first trimester of pregnancy is no cause for panic or pregnancy termination. Computed tomographic (CT) scanning is associated with a dose of as much as 1.5 rad per slice with minimal scatter to adjacent slices. Thus, even a CT scan of the pelvis during the first trimester is unlikely to result in an exposure with significant teratogenic risk.

Note in Table 3-2 that Holmes did not find a single baby in more than 18,000 whose anomalies could be attributed to radiation exposure. Given the incidence of major congenital malformations in the general population, approximately 2.7% of the time that an x-ray examination is done on a pregnant woman, it will be one who already has, or is destined to have, a fetus with a major malformation. When this coincidence occurs, causality should not be inferred without thorough investigation of the dose and timing of the exposure. Essentially, the only way that a woman would be likely to receive a dangerously large dose of radiation from an external beam would be in the course of radiation therapy. Doses to treat malignancies are on the order of thousands of rad and would be cause for concern.

Most diagnostic studies using radioisotopes involve very low levels of radiation exposure and are not hazardous to the fetus. A typical technetium-99m scan results in a fetal dose of less than 0.5 rad, and a thallium-201 scan results in a similarly small dose. Many of these isotopes are excreted in the urine. Therefore, to further minimize their exposure, women should be advised to drink plenty of fluids and void frequently following a radionuclide study. An important exception is the therapeutic use of iodine-131 to ablate the thyroid gland to treat maternal hyperthyroidism. The fetal thyroid gland begins to accumulate iodine by the end of the first trimester. Administration of a therapeutic dose of iodine-131 after this time can result in a several-thousand-rad dose to the fetal thyroid, destroying the gland.

The subject of mutagenicity is somewhat more complex, and involves a discussion of the relative risk of a large dose single exposure versus chronic exposure at low dose. (For a full discussion of this issue, as well as the methodologic problems in measuring the adverse outcome, refer to Schull et al.[12]) Data from the atomic-bomb survivors show that the dose required for significant damage is approximately 156 rem, which is 4 times higher than prior animal estimates. (A rem is roughly equivalent to a rad in this context.) The equivalent chronically administered dose would be approximately 468 rem.

Radiation exposure in infants and young children clearly places them at greater risk for the development of leukemia. Children under 10 years of age irradiated by the atomic-bomb blasts at Hiroshima and Nagasaki had a six times greater risk of leukemia developing than nonirradiated children. Radiation therapy in children is associated with an increased risk for malignancy later in life. It is not at all clear whether radiation exposure at levels encountered in the course of diagnostic studies in children can increase the incidence of malignancy later in life. In the 1960s, a series of studies and reviews appeared (summarized by Bithell and Stewart[13]) that concluded that diagnostic radiation exposure of a fetus in utero could increase the risk of leukemia by a factor of 1.3 to 1.8. Other studies have subsequently cast considerable doubt on the conclusions of those reviews.[14] At present, it is not at all clear whether diagnostic radiation exposure in utero is capable of increasing the incidence of malignancy.[15]

DRUGS

A teratogenic exposure has been narrowly defined as a chemical, physical, or infectious exposure during pregnancy that disturbs morphogenesis and results in a structural abnormality of the embryo, fetus, or neonate. A more expanded definition would include functional or behavioral abnormalities as well as structural abnormalities. There is also a distinction between a malformation and a deformation. A malformation is a structural abnormality that results from a disturbance in morphogenesis. A deformation is a structural abnormality that results from external compression or forces acting on a structure that was normally formed during embryogenesis. This discussion will be restricted to the narrow definition of teratogens that produce malformations. Despite widespread public concern, there are only a small number of drugs that are known to be human teratogens. The list of drugs and exposures that can have an adverse impact on reproduction or the neonate, however, is longer than the list of true teratogens. Cigarette smoking, for example, is associated with an increased risk of first-trimester spontaneous abortion, but not with congenital malformations. Exposures to anticholinergic and ganglionic blocking agents during pregnancy are associated with meconium ileus and paralytic ileus in the neonate, but these are not structural abnormalities. The reader is referred to the review of Koren et al. for a discussion of some of the more controversial nonteratogens such as Agent Orange, diazepam, and Bendectin that have received considerable public attention.[16] Table 3-4 is a list of the known human teratogens.

Angiotensin-Converting–Enzyme Inhibitors

Attention was first called to angiotensin-converting–enzyme (ACE) inhibitors as potential reproductive toxins by Broughton-Pipkin, who noted that they caused spontaneous abortion among rabbits.[17] Subsequently, human case reports began to appear linking prenatal exposure to ACE inhibitors with a variety of congenital malformations and fetal and neonatal

TABLE 3-4
KNOWN HUMAN TERATOGENS

Angiotensin-converting enzyme
Anticonvulsant agents
   Trimethadione and paramethadione
   Phenytoin
   Valproic acid
   Carbamazepine
Cytotoxic agents
   Aminopterin and methotrexate
   Cyclophosphamide
Ethanol
Lithium
Methimazole
Methyl mercury
Methylene blue
Misoprostol
Sex hormones
   Androgens
   Progestins
   Diethylstilbestrol
Tetracycline
Thalidomide
Vitamin A analogues
   Isotretinoin
   Etretinate
Warfarin

functional disorders. The teratogenic effects are inadequate calcification of the calvarial plates in the skull (hypocalvaria) and renal tubular dysgenesis.[18] The renal tubular dysgenesis may be associated with oligohydramnios, pulmonary hypoplasia, and intrauterine growth restriction. Neonatal complications may include hypotension, oliguria, or anuria and be of severe or fatal degree. Many of these complications are thought to result from fetal hypotension during the second and third trimester as the direct effect of fetal drug exposure. First trimester exposure to ACE inhibitors does not appear to be teratogenic, which is contrary to the general rule that earlier pregnancy exposures result in more serious consequences.[19]

Anticonvulsants in Pregnancy

There are reports in the literature suggesting that the increased incidence of congenital anomalies among infants of epileptic mothers is due to some cause other than the antiseizure medications. Speculation has included a genetic predisposition to anomalies associated with a genetic predisposition to seizures and an effect on development due to repeated seizures during pregnancy. Evidence has accumulated along two lines to indicate that this is not true and that some anticonvulsants are indeed teratogenic. (1) The incidence of anomalies among infants of epileptic mothers on therapy is higher than that for epileptic mothers not on therapy. (2) The incidence of anomalies in infants born to epileptic fathers is no higher than that of the general population.

Trimethadione and Paramethadione

Trimethadione and paramethadione are oxazolidene derivatives that have been used extensively, especially for petit mal epilepsy. They seem to be strongly associated with a syndrome of mental retardation, speech difficulty, V-shaped eyebrows, which virtually meet in the midline, backward-sloped ears, cleft or high arched palate, dental abnormalities, intra- and extrauterine growth restriction, inguinal hernias, myopia, and strabismus.[20] Estimates of fetal risk following exposure are difficult due to the small number of cases, but the risks seem high, and the syndrome can be very severe. These compounds are best avoided during pregnancy, and, in fact, they have been replaced by newer drugs.

Phenytoin

Phenytoin is commonly used for grand mal epilepsy and is frequently used in combination with phenobarbital and other agents. Several factors relating to its pharmacology should be emphasized. Changes occur during pregnancy that result in a dramatic fall in serum phenytoin levels from the nongravid state. A patient who has done well with therapeutic serum levels of phenytoin on 300 mg per day may, when pregnant, requires 500 to 600 mg per day to maintain the same serum levels. Dosage requirements do not revert back to the nongravid condition until approximately 6 weeks postpartum. Between 35 and 65% of the ingested phenytoin is excreted as the single hydroxylated metabolite, parahydroxyphenylhydantoin. Animal studies have shown that this metabolite is not teratogenic but that native phenytoin or more proximate metabolites are teratogenic. At therapeutic serum levels in humans, the metabolism of phenytoin operates essentially at saturation. Therefore, excesses in phenytoin dose quickly raise serum levels of the apparent proximate teratogen(s).

Individual differences in response to the teratogenic stimulus of phenytoin exposure may well be due to genetic differences in drug metabolism. If the fetal hydantoin syndrome is due to excessive phenytoin levels, and substantial adjustments in dosage are necessary in pregnancy to maintain therapeutic levels, then it would seem prudent to monitor serum phenytoin levels carefully during pregnancy.

The fetal hydantoin syndrome has been characterized as: (1) dysmorphic facies with a broad, low nasal bridge, epicanthal folds, short up-turned nose, hypertelorism, ptosis, strabismus, prominent and slightly malformed ears, wide mouth, and long philtrum; (2) hypoplasia of the distal phalanges and nails; and (3) prenatal and postnatal growth deficiency with microcephaly and motor or mental deficiency.[21,22] Risk estimates for the incidence of the fetal hydantoin syndrome among exposed fetuses vary widely in the literature. The highest estimates for major manifestations are approximately 10%. Most studies have found risks considerably less than that, although not zero. A reasonable estimate is a risk of major malformation of approximately 6%, or about double the risk for the general population.[23]

A coagulation defect in the newborn characterized by deficiency of factors II, VII, IX, and X (the vitamin K–dependent factors) has been well described. This is demonstrable in the laboratory in most neonates born to mothers on therapeutic doses of phenytoin, but it is only clinically significant in approximately 10% of them. It can be reversed by administration of vitamin K and/or fresh frozen plasma to the newborn.

Valproic Acid

Valproic acid is also used to treat grand mal seizures. A birth defects surveillance program in Lyon, France, noted a dramatic increase in the incidence of spina bifida in southern France. Investigation of the epidemic revealed that many of the cases were associated with intrauterine exposure to valproic acid.[24] Many of the neurologists in that area had turned to valproic acid as an alternative to phenytoin to avoid its known teratogenicity. Subsequent studies have confirmed that there is a 10- to 20-fold greater risk of open neural-tube defects following valproic acid treatment during pregnancy.[25-28] Most of this risk is due to myelomeningocele relatively low on the spine, but the incidence of anencephaly may also be increased. The risk of open neural-tube defect in the general population in the United States is approximately 1/1000, but it rises to 1/100 among fetuses exposed to valproic acid.

Carbamazepine

Carbamazepine is a tricyclic anticonvulsant that is also used to treat grand mal epilepsy. Like valproic acid, it was initially seen as a potentially safer alternative to phenytoin. It has proven, however, to cause a spectrum and incidence of malformations comparable to both phenytoin and valproic acid. Jones et al. reported a syndrome of craniofacial defects, fingernail hypoplasia, and developmental delay among 35 exposed children that was comparable to the fetal hydantoin syndrome.[29] Subsequently, Rosa studied data from pregnant Medicaid recipients in Michigan and summarized prior reports to conclude that carbamazepine exposure was associated with a 1% risk of neural-tube defects, very similar to valproic acid.[30]

Combined Therapy

Anticonvulsants have frequently been used in combination with one another to achieve optimal seizure control. Studies of the congenital malformations and developmental delay resulting from these exposures during pregnancy have consistently found a greater risk from multidrug therapy than from single-agent treatment. For this reason, it is advisable to attempt to achieve acceptable seizure control during pregnancy by optimizing therapy with a single agent whenever possible.

Cytotoxic Agents

Embryos, fetuses, and malignancies share the fact that they are all composed of rapidly multiplying cells. Therefore, it should not be surprising that agents designed to destroy one type of rapidly growing cell would also damage others. Indeed, in experimental animal models virtually all antitumor agents can be shown to be teratogenic when administered in the right dose at the right gestational age.

Aminopterin is an antineoplastic folic acid antagonist closely related to methotrexate. It was used as a black-market abortifacient in the 1950s. At doses inadequate to result in abortion, first-trimester exposure frequently resulted in fetuses with a constellation of severe congenital malformations, including hydrocephaly, mental retardation, facial malformations, and a variety of limb abnormalities. Methotrexate is now used in place of aminopterin as an antineoplastic agent. Inadvertent first-trimester fetal exposures to methotrexate seem to be rare but have resulted in congenital malformations very similar to those seen with aminopterin exposure.[31]

Cyclophosphamide exposure in the first trimester has resulted in a variety of congenital malformations, including facial malformations, digital abnormalities, and umbilical and inguinal hernias. Exposure later in pregnancy has been associated with intrauterine growth restriction, premature delivery, and transient neonatal marrow suppression. Many of these reported patients have been systemically ill and have received other chemotherapeutic agents and radiation.[32] The degree to which some of these complications are due to the cyclophosphamide per se is conjectural.

Obviously, the use of chemotherapeutic agents should be avoided during pregnancy and especially the first trimester whenever possible. When it is necessary to use them during pregnancy, the patient must be apprised of the potential fetal risks.

Ethanol

Descriptions of the human teratogenic effect of alcohol are as old as antiquity, and resulted in proscriptions in ancient Greece against drinking on a bridal couple's wedding night. Within the past 25 years, interest in this teratogen has been rekindled, and the term *fetal alcohol syndrome* (FAS) has been coined. The most striking and consistent feature of FAS is intra- and extrauterine growth retardation. Microcephaly and mental deficiency are seen but are highly variable in degree. Facial features are distinctive, and in the more severely affected cases include a broad flat midface, broad low nasal bridge, epicanthal folds, narrow palpebral fissures, and facial hirsutism. A tendency toward an increased incidence of anomalies in other organ systems, including the heart and kidneys, has also been noted.[33] There is no question that heavy drinking during pregnancy by chronic alcoholics confers a risk of fetal alcohol syndrome. It is not possible to quantitate that risk with any precision. Much more controversial are the possible risks of low or moderate alcohol consumption and the risks of binge drinking. If consumption of a large amount of alcohol during pregnancy is clearly very bad, is a small amount of alcohol still bad but to a lesser degree? Is there any level of alcohol consumption during pregnancy that is safe? These are much more difficult questions to answer and remain controversial.

Lithium

Lithium ion is used to treat the mania associated with manic–depressive disorder and is available as either the carbonate or citrate salt. Manic–depressive disorder

may affect as much as 1% of the population, and, among women, is most common during the reproductive years. As many as 1/1000 pregnant women may be taking lithium. Registries to record pregnancy outcomes among women taking lithium were established in North America and Europe during the 1960s. Registries of this nature undoubtedly result in selective reporting of adverse events and underreporting of uncomplicated pregnancies. The initial report of data from the Danish registry through 1973 found 9 congenital malformations among 118 exposed fetuses.[34] Six babies had congenital heart disease and two of these were the very rare Ebstein anomaly. Ebstein anomaly is a downward displacement of the tricuspid valve into the right ventricle with atrialization of the ventricle above the valve. The degree of severity is variable, ranging from mild and noted only on echocardiography, to severe and resulting in fatal congestive heart failure. It occurs in only 0.5% of fetuses with congenital heart disease. This early report undoubtedly further encouraged selective reporting of malformed cases, especially of heart disease.

Kallen reported a cohort study of women hospitalized for manic-depressive illness, 59 of whom were lithium-exposed cases, and compared them with 228 controls unexposed to lithium.[35] There were four cases of congenital heart disease among the exposed infants and two cases among the unexposed, which was a statistically significant difference, but there were no cases of Ebstein anomaly. Subsequently, four case-controlled studies did not find lithium exposure in any of 207 cases of Ebstein anomaly. Jacobson et al. reported 3 congenitally malformed infants among 108 lithium-exposed live births, which was not significantly different from the 3 cases among 126-live born controls.[36] Interestingly, one of the lithium-exposed cases did have a severe Ebstein anomaly. A published review of the available data concluded that the risk of malformation due to lithium exposure is probably 4 to 12%, which is higher than the 2 to 4% found among controls.[37] Although this is not as high as initially thought, it is greater than the risk for the unexposed population, and treated patients should be informed of the risks involved.

Methimazole

Methimazole and carbimazole (which is metabolized to methimazole) are thioureylenes structurally related to propylthiouracil and used to treat hyperthyroidism. Several cases of aplasia cutis of the scalp have been reported after methimazole or carbimazole treatment during pregnancy. This is a very rare lesion that appears as a punched-out area of the scalp, leaving the underlying skull exposed.[38] The very rare occurrence of this lesion in the general population lent credibility to a causal relationship with methimazole exposure. Establishing causality with methimazole has been difficult, however, because hyperthyroidism itself probably leads to a greater risk of congenital malformations, small cohort studies have failed to confirm the association, and several drugs have frequently been used in combination. It is noteworthy, though, that aplasia cutis has not been described after propylthiouracil exposure. Whenever possible, propylthiouracil should be used during pregnancy rather than methimazole.

Methyl Mercury

There are no therapeutic uses for methyl mercury, which is used as an industrial fungicide, but it is mentioned here because it is a potent human teratogen. The initial report of its teratogenicity came from Japan, where its discharge from paper mills contaminated the fish in Minamata Bay. Pregnant women who ate the fish delivered babies with severe cerebral palsy and microcephaly that became known as Minamata disease.[39] Another outbreak occurred in Iraq when bread was made from methyl-mercury-treated wheat that was intended for use as crop seed.

Methylene Blue

Although methylene blue has some weak activity as a urinary antiseptic when taken by mouth, it is more commonly used as a diagnostic dye. It was frequently used as a marker for the first sac during second-trimester diagnostic amniocentesis in twins. Numerous case reports and small series have confirmed that intraamniotic instillation of methylene blue at 15 to 17 weeks of gestation is associated with both jejunal and ileal atresia. Depending on the dose used, up to 20% of the exposed fetuses may be affected with small intestinal atresia.[40,41] Intraamniotic injection later in pregnancy to diagnose rupture of the membranes has been associated with fetal hemolysis, methemoglobinemia, and hyperbilirubinemia. Intraamniotic injection of methylene blue should be avoided. Other

dyes such as indigo carmine are available for these purposes and seem to be safer.

Misoprostol

Misoprostol is a synthetic analogue of prostaglandin E_1 that was developed to protect the gastric mucosa during treatment with nonsteroidal antiinflammatory agents. It has oxytocic activity and has found use in obstetrics to prepare the cervix prior to induction of labor or dilatation and evacuation. It has also been used with mifepristone (RU 486) or methotrexate to induce abortion in the first trimester. In Brazil, where the drug has been available over the counter and abortion is illegal, it has found its way into use as a black-market abortifacient. Used alone it is not very efficacious in producing abortion, and a variety of congenital malformations have been described among nonaborted survivors. In a series of 42 Brazilian infants and children with congenital malformations associated with first-trimester misoprostol exposure, the most common malformations were equinovarus and cranial-nerve abnormalities especially of nerves V, VI, and VII.[42] In a case-control study from Brazil, 96 infants with Mobius syndrome (facial nerve paralysis) were compared to 96 infants with neural-tube defects.[43] A history of first-trimester misoprostol exposure was obtained in 47 (49%) of the Mobius cases but only 3 (3%) of the neural-tube defect cases, for a statistically significant odds ratio of 29.7. These studies make a convincing argument for the teratogenicity of misoprostol and provide a clear description of the phenotype but they do not provide any estimate of the risk for the syndrome among the exposed.

Sex Hormones

Sex hormones have clearly been teratogenic to the developing genital system in humans. The only serious controversy has been related to their ability to cause extragenital malformations.

In the 1950s and 1960s a number of androgens, including testosterone, methyltestosterone, methandriol, and normethandrone were used for a variety of indications, including the treatment of breast cancer. There was a series of reports of masculinized female fetuses resulting from exposures to these potent androgens. The most common manifestation of masculinization is phallic enlargement (clitoromegaly), which can be stimulated at any time during pregnancy.

Less commonly, labioscrotal fusion can be seen if sufficiently high doses are given between 8 and 13 weeks of gestation.[44]

Danazol is a synthetic steroid with androgenic activity that is used most commonly to treat endometriosis. It usually produces anovulatory amenorrhea, thus preventing pregnancy. On occasion, however, treated patients may ovulate and become pregnant, resulting in inadvertent danazol administration for considerable lengths of time during early pregnancy. Exposure to this drug has resulted in masculinized female infants with both clitoromegaly and labioscrotal fusion. Most cases have involved relatively high doses (800 mg per day), but some have been reported with as little as 400 mg per day.[45]

Many of the synthetic progestins, especially the 19-nortestosterone derivatives ethisterone and norethindrone, possess a substantial degree of androgenic activity. Treatment of threatened abortion in the first trimester with these hormones has produced masculinized female fetuses. It has been estimated that only approximately 0.3% of exposed pregnancies actually manifest hormonally induced masculinization. Dosage and timing of the exposure together with genetic susceptibility probably determine which individuals will be affected.

Diethylstilbestrol (DES) is a potent synthetic estrogen that was used from the 1940s through 1971 to attempt to prevent first-trimester spontaneous abortion. It became infamous because it was ineffective, and because it caused an epidemic of abnormalities in the reproductive tracts of exposed female fetuses that was not recognized until decades later. These abnormalities included vaginal adenosis, a characteristic hood (or cock's comb) on the cervix, a hypoplastic cervix, a small T-shaped uterine cavity, and tubal abnormalities.[46] The consequence of these exposures that received the greatest attention was the occurrence of an otherwise very rare cancer, clear-cell adenocarcinoma of the vagina, in 1 to 2/1000 exposed individuals.[47] Although DES has been termed a transplacental carcinogen, it should truly be considered a teratogen that caused columnar epithelium to be present inappropriately in the vagina. There the columnar epithelium was probably subject to an environment that proved carcinogenic in a small percentage of cases. The reproductive consequences of these anomalies included increased incidences of pregnancy loss, premature delivery, and tubal ectopic gestation.

Combined estrogen/progestin oral contraceptives were suspected for several years of teratogenicity in extragenital sites. Janerich et al. first suggested, in a study of 108 cases, that exposure to oral contraceptives in the first trimester could produce limb-reduction defects.[48] They were unable to confirm their own findings in a subsequent larger study of 715 cases.[49] Oral contraceptives were also suspected of causing congenital heart disease. The incidence of all types of congenital heart disease among the 50,000 infants in the Collaborative Perinatal Project was 7.8/1000 live births. Among the 278 women known to have taken oral contraceptives during the first 4 months of pregnancy, there were 6 children with congenital heart defects, for a rate of 21/1000. Although this difference (7.8/1000 vs. 21/1000) did not reach statistical significance when formally tested, it seemed worrisome.[5] Subsequent epidemiologic studies employing both cohort and case control designs yielded conflicting results. Critics who doubted the association of oral contraceptives with congenital heart disease cited the conflicting epidemiologic data and the facts that there was no reasonable biologic explanation for such an effect and no good animal model that duplicated the proposed human effect. Subsequent studies and meta-analyses have resolved these concerns.[50]

Tetracycline

Members of the tetracycline family bind avidly to divalent cations, including calcium. As a result, they are deposited in both bone and teeth in a complex with calcium orthophosphate. This compound will discolor deciduous teeth, which begin to calcify after 20 weeks of gestation. This problem is of minimal concern because these teeth are lost during childhood and the permanent teeth do not begin to calcify in utero. It has been suggested that a variety of true congenital malformations might be associated with intrauterine tetracycline exposure but these have not been consistently supported by the data. Of greater practical importance in the care of pregnant women is the association of tetracycline treatment with a toxicity syndrome very similar to acute fatty liver of pregnancy. Generally, tetracycline treatment should be avoided during pregnancy.

Thalidomide

The introduction of thalidomide and the epidemic of malformations that it caused is discussed above as a sentinel event in modern medicine. U.S. citizens were largely spared from the epidemic in Europe and Australia because the Food and Drug Administration refused to license the drug in this country. Awareness of the potent teratogenicity of this drug is of practical importance and not just of historic interest because the FDA has recently licensed thalidomide for sale in the United States to treat leprosy. Reports of its efficacy in treating recalcitrant oral aphthous ulcers in patients with human immunodeficiency virus infection will undoubtedly further expand the indications for its use.[51] The manufacturer has recommended very strict rules for its use to avoid exposures of pregnant women and resultant congenital malformations, but as with isotretinoin, it is fair to anticipate that exposures and malformations will occur.

The thalidomide embryopathy consists of malformations of both the upper and lower extremities, craniofacial malformations, and malformations of internal organs. The limb malformations range from complete absence of one or more limbs (amelia) to varying degrees of reduction defects, particularly of the radial side of the upper extremity. Craniofacial malformations include anotia, microtia, anophthalmos, microphthalmos, coloboma, facial palsy, and external ophthalmoplegia. Other manifestations include congenital heart disease, renal anomalies, anomalies of the alimentary tract, and choanal atresia.[52]

Vitamin A Analogues

Isotretinoin

Isotretinoin is 13-*cis*-retinoic acid, a potent synthetic isomer of vitamin A. It was introduced in 1982 for the oral treatment of recalcitrant acne. Hypervitaminosis A was one of the earliest experimental teratogenic agents to be studied in animals. On the basis of those data, and a few case reports of vitamin A overdose in humans, it was assumed that isotretinoin would be teratogenic if taken by pregnant women. The age group at greatest risk for acne is also the age group at greatest risk for pregnancy. Accordingly, strong warnings against administration to pregnant women or women who could become pregnant were included with the drug. In spite of this, there have been a relatively large number of women who have taken isotretinoin during pregnancy. Approximately one-quarter of the pregnancies exposed in the first

trimester spontaneously abort. One-fifth of those that continue are affected with major congenital malformations. Almost half of the malformed infants die from their malformations before 1 year of age.

The most prominent features of the malformation syndrome are defects of the central nervous system (CNS), cranium, face, and heart.[53] The CNS defects include hydrocephaly, microcephaly, cortical blindness, microphthalmia, optic-nerve hypoplasia, and facial-nerve palsy. Craniofacial malformations include microtia, anotia, agenesis or severe stenosis of the external auditory canals, cleft palate, micrognathia, and hypertelorism. Cardiac defects include transposition of the great vessels, tetralogy of Fallot, double-outlet right ventricle, truncus arteriosus, and interrupted aortic arch. The critical period for exposure seems to be 28 to 70 days following the last menstrual period.

The package insert warnings have been strengthened and include recommendations that women use two forms of reliable contraception while taking the drug and that the drug be stopped at least 1 month prior to conception. The drug manufacturer will pay most of the cost of an initial visit to a gynecologist to rule out pregnancy and provide contraception prior to beginning the drug. Blood banks will not accept donors who are taking isotretinoin to avoid inadvertent administration to pregnant women who may require a transfusion. Despite these precautions, occasional accidents will undoubtedly continue to occur as long as the drug is available.

Etretinate

Etretinate is another potent synthetic vitamin A analogue that is used to treat severe psoriasis. It is highly lipid-soluble and accumulates in fat tissue. After discontinuing long-term therapy, etretinate is released from fat stores, resulting in detectable serum levels literally for years. Lammer reported the case of a woman who took etretinate for 5 months and conceived 51 weeks after discontinuing the medication.[54] That baby was born with multiple congenital malformations, including tetralogy of Fallot, malformed ears, and microcephaly strikingly similar to the pattern seen with isotretinoin exposure. More than 3 months after the baby's birth, the mother still had etretinate detectable in her serum. Because of the documented persistence of etretinate and reports of cases of malformations like this one, it is not clear how long after discontinuing therapy it is safe to become pregnant.

Warfarin

Warfarin is an anticoagulant that works by antagonizing the action of vitamin K. Fetuses exposed to warfarin are characterized by a syndrome including dysmorphic facies with a broad, flat bridge of the nose, and an unusual bony defect called chondrodysplasia punctata.[55] On x-ray examination, the ends of the long bones demonstrate numerous small punctate areas of calcification, rather than the typical single organized epiphyseal growth plate. Even second-trimester exposure can be harmful, resulting in hydrocephalus due to periventricular intracranial hemorrhage and optic-nerve atrophy. The incidence of these anomalies among exposed individuals is not known. The problem can be completely avoided if heparin is used for the duration of any pregnancy that requires anticoagulation.

CONCLUSION

Congenital malformations and prematurity are the two most important causes of perinatal mortality in the United States. The Centers for Disease Control and Prevention list congenital malformations as the fifth leading cause of years of potential life lost. Although only a minor fraction of all congenital malformations are known to result from environmental exposures, health care professionals have an obligation to help minimize these exposures and reduce the burden of morbidity and mortality they can impose. Consciousness of the possibility of pregnancy in young women in their child-bearing years, understanding the timing of periods of vulnerability during human gestation, and knowledge of the relatively few human teratogens should keep potentially harmful exposures to a minimum.

REFERENCES

1. Hale F. Pigs born without eyeballs. J Hered 1933;24:105.
2. Gregg NM. Congenital cataract following German measles in the mother. Trans Ophthalmol Soc Aust 1941; 3:34.
3. McBride WG. Thalidomide and congenital abnormalities. Lancet 1961;2:1358.
4. Lenz W. Thalidomide and congenital abnormalities. Lancet 1962;1:45.
5. Heinonen OP, Slone D, Shapiro S. Birth defects and drugs in pregnancy. Littleton, MA: Publishing Science Group, 1977:65.
6. Wilson JG. Embryotoxicity of drugs in man. In: Wilson JG, Fraser FC, eds. Handbook of teratology. New York: Plenum, 1977:310.
7. Holmes LB. Congenital malformations: incidence, racial differences and recognized etiologies in biologic and clinical aspects of malformations. Mead Johnson Symposium, June 8–12, 1975;7:3.
8. Bustamante SA, Stumpff LC. Fetal hydantoin syndrome in triplets. Am J Dis Child 1978;132:978.
9. Phelan MC, Pellock JM, Nance WE. Discordant expression of fetal hydantoin syndrome in heteropaternal dizygotic twins. N Engl J Med 1982;307:99.
10. Stovall M, Blackwell CR, Cundiff J, et al. Fetal dose from radiotherapy with photon beams: report of AAPM Radiation Therapy Committee Task Group No. 36. Med Phys 1995;22:63.
11. Ginsberg JS, Hirsh J, Rainbow AJ, Coates G. Risks to the fetus of radiologic procedures used in the diagnosis of maternal venous thromboembolic disease. Thromb Haemost 1989;61:189.
12. Schull WJ, Otake M, Neel J. Genetic effects of the atomic bombs: a reappraisal. Science 1981;213:1220.
13. Bithell JF, Stewart AM. Prenatal irradiation and childhood malignancy: a review of British data from the Oxford survey. Br J Cancer 1975;31:271.
14. Harvey E, Boice JD, Honeyman M, Flannery JT. Prenatal x-ray exposure and childhood cancer in twins. N Engl J Med 1985;312:541.
15. MacMahon B. Prenatal x-ray exposure and twins. N Engl J Med 1985;312:576.
16. Koren G, Pastuszak A, Ito S. Drugs in pregnancy. N Engl J Med 1998;338:1128.
17. Broughton-Pipkin F, Symonds EM, Turner SR. The effect of captopril (SQ14, 225) upon mother and fetus in the chronically cannulated ewe and in the pregnant rabbit. J Physiol (Lond) 1982;323:415.
18. Barr M Jr, Cohen M Jr. ACE inhibitor fetopathy and hypocalvaria: the kidney–skull connection. Teratology 1991;44:485.
19. Barr M Jr. Teratogen update: angiotensin-converting enzyme inhibitors. Teratology 1994;50:399.
20. Rosen R, Lightner E. Phenotypic malformations in association with maternal trimethadione therapy. J Pediatr 1978;92:240.
21. Hanson JW, Smith DW. The fetal hydantoin syndrome. J Pediatr 1975;87:285.
22. Scolnik D, Nulman I, Rovet J, et al. Neurodevelopment of children exposed in utero to phenytoin and carbamazepine monotherapy. JAMA 1994;271:767.
23. Kaneko S. Antiepileptic drug therapy and reproductive consequences: functional and morphologic effects. Reprod Toxicol 1991;5:179.
24. Robert E, Guibaud P. Maternal valproic acid and congenital neural tube defects. Lancet 1982;2:937.
25. Bjerkedal T, Czeizel A, Goujard J, et al. Valproic acid and spina bifida. Lancet 1982;2:1096.
26. Lindhout D, Meinardi H. Spina bifida and in-utero exposure to valproate. Lancet 1984;2:396.
27. Robert E, Lofkvist E, Mauguiere F. Valproate and spina bifida. Lancet 1984;2:1392.

28. Ardinger HH, Atkin JF, Dwain-Blackston R, et al. Verification of the fetal valproate syndrome phenotype. Am J Med Genet 1988;29:171.

29. Jones KL, Lacro RV, Johnson KA, et al. Pattern of malformations in the children of women treated with carbamazepine during pregnancy. N Engl J Med 1989; 320:1661.

30. Rosa FW. Spina bifida in infants of women treated with carbamazepine during pregnancy. N Engl J Med 1991; 324:674.

31. Milunsky A, Graef JW, Gaynor MF Jr. Methotrexate-induced congenital malformations. J Pediatr 1968;72:790.

32. Gilland J, Weinstein L. The effects of cancer chemotherapeutic agents on the developing fetus. Obstet Gynecol Surv 1983;38:6.

33. Pytkowicz Streissguth A, Clarren SK, Jones KL. Natural history of the fetal alcohol syndrome: a 10-year follow-up of eleven patients. Lancet 1985;2:85.

34. Schou M, Goldfield MD, Weinstein MR, et al. Lithium and pregnancy. I. Report from the register of lithium babies. BMJ 1973;2:135.

35. Kallen B, Tandberg A. Lithium and pregnancy. Acta Psychiatr Scand 1983;68:134.

36. Jacobson SJ, Jones K, Johnson K, et al. Prospective multicentre study of pregnancy outcome after lithium exposure during first trimester. Lancet 1992;339:530.

37. Cohen LS, Friedman JM, Jefferson JW, Johnson M, Weiner ML. A reevaluation of risk of in utero exposure to lithium. JAMA 1994;271:146.

38. Milham S Jr. Scalp defects in infants of mothers treated for hyperthyroidism with methimazole or carbimazole during pregnancy. Teratology 1985;32:321.

39. Koos BJ, Longo L. Mercury toxicity in the pregnant woman, fetus, and newborn infant. Am J Obstet Gynecol 1976;126:390.

40. Nicolini U, Monni G. Intestinal obstruction in babies exposed in utero to methylene blue. Lancet 1990;336:1258.

41. Cragan JD, Martin ML, Khoury MJ, Fernhoff PM. Dye use during amniocentesis and birth defects. Lancet 1993;341:1352.

42. Hajaj Gonzalez C, Marques-Dias J, Kim CA, et al. Congenital abnormalities in Brazilian children associated with misoprostol misuse in first trimester of pregnancy. Lancet 1998;351:1624.

43. Pastuszak AL, Schuler L, Speck-Martins CE, et al. Use of misoprostol during pregnancy and Mobius' syndrome in infants. N Engl J Med 1998;338:1881.

44. Schardein JL. Congenital abnormalities and hormones during pregnancy: a clinical review. Teratology 1980; 22:251.

45. Rosa FW. Virilization of the female fetus with maternal danazol exposure. Am J Obstet Gynecol 1984;149:99.

46. Kaufman RH, Adam E, Noller K, et al. Upper genital tract changes and infertility in diethylstilbestrol-exposed women. Am J Obstet Gynecol 1986;154:1312.

47. Melnick S, Cole P, Anderson D, et al. Rates and risks of diethylstilbestrol-related clear-cell adenocarcinoma of the vagina and cervix. N Engl J Med 1987;316:514.

48. Janerich DT, Piper MS, Glebatis DM. Oral contraceptives and congenital limb-reduction defects. N Engl J Med 1974;291:697.

49. Janerich DT, Piper JM, Glebatis DM. Oral contraceptives and birth defects. Am J Epidemiol 1980;112:73.

50. Martinez-Frias M, Rodriguez-Pinella E, Bermejo E, Prieto L. Prenatal exposure to sex hormones: a case control study. Teratology 1998;57:8.

51. Jacobson JM, Greenspan JS, Spritzler J, et al. Thalidomide for the treatment of oral aphthous ulcers in patients with human immunodeficiency virus infection. N Engl J Med 1997;336:1487.

52. McBride WG. Thalidomide embryopathy. Teratology 1977; 16:79.

53. Lammer EJ, Chen DT, Hoar RM, et al. Retinoic acid embryopathy. N Engl J Med 1985;313:837.

54. Lammer EJ. Embryopathy in infant conceived one year after termination of maternal etretinate. Lancet 1988; 2:1080.

55. Hall JG, Pauli RM, Wilson KM. Maternal and fetal sequelae of anticoagulation during pregnancy. Am J Med 1980; 68:122.

Chapter 4
Prenatal Diagnosis

Laura Goetzl
Mary D'Alton

Five Key Points

- Maternal serum α-fetoprotein testing can identify approximately 80% of fetuses with spina bifida.

- The triple screen or triscreen test can identify approximately 60 to 65% of fetuses with Down syndrome.

- Ultrasound findings associated with Down syndrome include thickened nuchal fold, shortened humerus and femur, cardiac anomalies, duodenal atresia, and echogenic bowel.

- The procedure-related loss rate from amniocentesis at 15 to 16 weeks of gestation is approximately 1/200.

- Compared to amniocentesis at ≥ 15 weeks of gestation, early amniocentesis is associated with an increased risk of fetal talipes equinus, procedure-related pregnancy loss, and amniotic fluid leakage.

GOALS OF PRENATAL DIAGNOSIS

There are two main goals of prenatal diagnosis: first, to identify pregnancies at high risk for abnormalities so they can be targeted for specific antenatal testing, and second, to effectively screen low-risk pregnancies for potential problems. Ultimately, the goal of prenatal diagnosis is to identify fetal abnormalities early enough in gestation to be able to treat them and perhaps reverse their consequences (Table 4-1). In situations where treatment is not possible, antenatal diagnosis of an abnormal fetus allows women to exercise their full reproductive choices. Many women decide to continue a pregnancy in the face of an abnormality; in these cases prenatal diagnosis can influence antepartum and intrapartum management, permit planning regarding delivery timing and site, and prepare the intensive care nursery for the arrival of a potentially compromised neonate, thus ensuring optimal care of the newborn.

TABLE 4-1
ANTENATAL FETAL TREATMENT

Administration of medication to mother to treat fetal conditions
  Corticosteroids for females with congenital adrenal hyperplasia
  Digoxin for fetal arrhythmias and congestive heart failure
  Vitamin B_{12} in B_{12}-responsive methylmalonic acidemia
Fetal medical treatment
  Blood transfusions for anemia or thrombocytopenia
In utero fetal surgery
  Relief of obstructive uropathy
  Repair of diaphragmatic hernia
  Thoracoamniotic shunt for large pleural effusions
Fetal gene therapy
  Hematopoietic stem-cell transplantation for hemoglobinopathy
    or immunodeficiency

TABLE 4-2
INDICATIONS FOR PRENATAL TESTING AND/OR REFERRAL TO A GENETIC COUNSELOR

Age ≥35 at delivery for a singleton pregnancy
Age ≥31 at delivery for a twin pregnancy
Abnormal serum screening
>2 miscarriages, stillbirths, or neonatal deaths
Previous child with congenital malformations or mental retardation
Previous child with a chromosomal abnormality
Maternal history, family history, or previous child with a known genetic disease
Maternal chromosomal abnormality such as a balanced translocation
Maternal illness that can cause fetal malformations (e.g., diabetes, phenylketonuria)
Maternal congenital malformation (e.g., congenital heart disease)
Exposure to teratogen (e.g., medication)
Known carrier of a genetic disease (e.g., cystic fibrosis)
Infection during pregnancy (rubella, toxoplasmosis, cytolomegavirus)

High-Risk Ethnic Groups

Ashkenazi Jew (Tay–Sachs, Gaucher, Canavan)	French Canadian (Tay–Sachs)
Black African (sickle cell disease)	Arab (sickle cell disease)
Indo-Pakistani (sickle cell disease)	Asian (thalassemias)
Caucasian (cystic fibrosis)	Cajun (Tay–Sachs)
Mediterranean (sickle cell disease, thalassemias)	

INDICATIONS FOR GENETIC COUNSELING OR PRENATAL TESTING

The American College of Obstetricians and Gynecologists (ACOG) recommends the use of a questionnaire to screen for genetic risk factors in routine practice.[1] The fundamental goal of genetic counseling is to provide information to the patient and her family to allow for decision making based on facts. In addition, increasing numbers of "wrongful birth" cases have made genetic counseling a part of standard medical care.[2] It is appropriate to refer a patient for genetic counseling when she has a risk factor for a fetal abnormality, a family history of a genetic problem, or when an invasive prenatal diagnostic procedure is planned (Table 4-2). In addition, many genetic conditions are amenable to DNA analysis and can be tested for if a family history is present (Table 4-3).

COMMON SCREENING TESTS

Hemoglobinopathies

The hemoglobinopathies that are amenable to carrier detection and prenatal detection include sickle cell disease and α- and β-thalassemia. ACOG recommends

TABLE 4-3
CONDITIONS AMENABLE TO DNA ANALYSIS

α_1-Antitrypsin deficiency	α-Thalassemia
Adult polycystic kidney disease, type 1	β-Thalassemia
Canavan disease	Congenital adrenal hyperplasia
Cystic fibrosis	DiGeorge syndrome
Duchenne muscular dystrophy	Familial Alzheimer disease
Familial hypercholesterolemia	Familial polyposis coli
Fragile X syndrome	Gardner syndrome
Hemoglobin Sc	Hemophilia A (factor IX deficiency)
Huntington disease	Marfan syndrome
Multiple endocrine neoplasia, Types I and IIa	Myotonic dystrophy
Neurofibromatosis, Types I and II	Norrie disease
Ornithine transcarbamylase deficiency	Phenylketonuria
Retinoblastoma	Sickle cell disease
Spinal muscular atrophy	Tay–Sachs disease
von Hippel–Lindau syndrome	Wiskott–Aldrich syndrome

that all pregnant women at risk (Table 4-2) be screened with hemoglobin electrophoresis.[3] The Sickledex or other forms of solubility testing are no longer thought to be appropriate for screening because they may fail to identify important hemoglobin abnormalities. In addition, women at risk for either of the thalassemias should be screened with a red-cell mean corpuscular volume (MCV). In women with a low MCV, no evidence of iron deficiency, and normal hemoglobin electrophoresis, further DNA testing should be pursued to identify possible α-thalassemia.

When a woman is identified as carrying a mutant hemoglobin gene, her partner should also be tested. If both prospective parents are carriers of the same abnormality, they should be counseled regarding the 25% risk of having an affected child. In addition, combinations of hemoglobin abnormalities can also produce seriously affected children. DNA-based prenatal diagnosis of the fetus should be offered.

Tay–Sachs Disease

Tay–Sachs disease is a recessively inherited disorder of lysosomal storage due to a deficiency of the enzyme hexosaminidase, which results in accumulation of GM_2 ganglioside, neurologic deterioration and eventual death. There is a high incidence of Tay–Sachs disease in Ashkenazi Jews, who have a carrier frequency of 1 in 27 persons. French Canadians and Cajuns are also at increased risk. Routine screening of these high-risk populations is recommended.[4] Since the introduction of carrier-screening programs, the number of affected infants born with Tay–Sachs disease to Ashkenazi Jewish parents has been reduced by 90%.[5] During pregnancy, enzyme assays are unreliable; thus, ideally carrier screening should be offered preconceptually. If testing is needed during pregnancy, DNA-based tests are available that allow precise definition of the carrier state.[6] If both parents are found to be carriers, CVS (chorionic villus sampling) or amniocentesis is recommended to identify affected fetuses.

Canavan Disease

Canavan disease is an untreatable, progressive neurologic disease due to a deficiency of the enzyme aspartoacyclase that usually results in death in the first decade of life. Ashkenazi Jews have a 1 in 40 carrier frequency of this autosomal recessive condition. DNA-based screening in this high-risk group is rec-

ommended preconceptually; however, testing can also be offered in early pregnancy.[7] If both partners are carriers of Canavan disease, then CVS or amniocentesis should be offered to determine whether the fetus is affected.

Gaucher Disease

Gaucher disease is the most common inherited disorder in individuals of Jewish ancestry. The carrier frequency is higher than for Tay–Sachs disease, on the order of 1 in 10 to 1 in 15.[8] The disease results from the deficiency of the enzyme glucocerebrosidase, which is important in lipid metabolism. There are three clinical subtypes of Gaucher disease, which vary in severity from mild to fatal. Ninety-nine percent of all Gaucher disease is Type 1, the nonneuronopathic form, which has the mildest clinical presentation. Enzyme-replacement therapy with modified human placental glucocerebrosidase has successfully ameliorated many of the symptoms of the disease.[9]

PCR (polymerase chain reaction)-based testing is available by blood test at any time, regardless of pregnancy.[10] Carrier testing should be considered in all individuals of Jewish ancestry and any individuals with a family history of Gaucher disease.

Cystic Fibrosis

Cystic fibrosis (CF) is the most common recessively inherited disorder among Caucasians of European ancestry, affecting approximately 1 in 1800 individuals. The carrier frequency in persons with Northern European ancestry is 1 in 20. The protean clinical manifestations of CF include chronic bronchitis, pulmonary infections, malabsorption caused by pancreatic dysfunction, meconium ileus, diabetes mellitus, and male sterility.

CF is caused by a chloride-channel defect. Seventy-five percent of mutations result from the loss of a phenylalanine amino acid residue at position 508 in the CF gene product,[11] known as the Δ F508 allele. However, over 600 mutations in the CF gene have been described.[12] The routine screening of asymptomatic individuals who have a negative family history for CF is currently controversial.[13] Although DNA tests are 100% specific, that is, all patients with a positive test are truly carriers, sensitivities vary by ethnic group.[12] In Caucasians, Ashkenazi Jews, Celtic Bretons, French Canadians, and some Native-Americans, sensitivities of 90% can be achieved. Thus, at present a negative test may be a false negative test in 10% of CF carriers. Sensitivities are much lower in Hispanics, African-Americans, and Asian–Americans. It is likely that, with increased public awareness of CF, many patients will request DNA analysis. Although the NIH consensus statement recommends universal prenatal testing,[12] this approach has not become the standard of care. While evidence suggests that screening may be cost effective in a Caucasian population and other populations where testing is sensitive, it is less clear that this approach would be effective in other ethnic groups due to the higher proportion of atypical mutations.[13] The American College of Obstetricians and Gynecologists is currently considering recommendations for practice.

Isoimmunization

All women currently undergo screening for blood-group sensitization during the course of routine prenatal care. If sensitization to an antigen that can cause fetal hemolytic disease is discovered (e.g., D, Kell, Kidd, and Duffy) the genotype of the father of the baby should be determined.[14] In the case of fathers heterozygous for RhD, fetal blood type can be determined by PCR testing with amniocentesis.[15,16] Prenatal diagnosis of fetal blood type in the case of other antigens is possible; however, diagnosis may require percutaneous umbilical-cord blood sampling (PUBS).

BRCA1 and BRCA2

BRCA1 and BRCA2 mutations confer an increased risk of breast and ovarian cancer on female carriers. Carriers of the BRCA1 gene mutation have a risk as high as 94% of either of these cancers developing by the age of 70.[17] In addition, there may be an increased risk of prostate and colon cancer in male carriers. As public awareness of this genetic mutation increases, obstetricians may be faced with requests for prenatal diagnosis from known carriers or families with a family history of breast or ovarian cancer. Because cancer does not generally develop in affected individuals before their adult years, prenatal diagnosis of BRCA1 or BRCA2 is fraught with ethical and management dilemmas. In general, testing is not recommended for individuals under the age of 18; thus, prenatal testing of the fetus is not recommended.

Maternal Serum Panel

Maternal serum triple marker screening using α-fetoprotein (MSAFP), human chorionic gonadotropin (HCG), and unconjugated estriol (μE_3) is currently recommended by the American College of Obstetricians and Gynecologists between 15 and 22 weeks of gestation for screening of low-risk singleton pregnancies for neural-tube defects and chromosomal abnormalities.[18] It should be stressed that testing is voluntary, and patients should be counseled regarding the purpose, limitations, and potential false positive results. Even patients who would not consider pregnancy termination may consider testing as there is a suggestion that prenatal diagnosis of spina bifida may improve neurologic outcome if diagnosis results in elective cesarean delivery.[19]

Screening for Neural-Tube Defects

α-Fetoprotein (AFP) function in the human fetus remains largely unknown. It is produced by the fetal liver and yolk sac and is the major serum protein early in fetal life. In some cases of fetal malformation, exposed fetal membrane and blood-vessel surfaces lead to elevated amniotic fluid levels of AFP, and in turn, maternal serum levels are elevated.

The first MSAFP screening program for detection of neural-tube defects began in 1975, and distribution curves for affected and unaffected pregnancies were developed.[20] Some overlap exists between the MSAFP levels of these two subsets. No cutoff level of MSAFP will completely separate affected and normal pregnancies, so the chosen cutoff point becomes a compromise between obtaining the highest detection rate and the lowest false positive rate possible. Results are reported as multiples of the median (MOM). Most centers have chosen 2.0 or 2.5 MOM as the cutoff values for screening, with a false positive rate of approximately 3 to 4%.

With these measures, screening programs have detected up to 90% of anencephalic fetuses and 80% of open spina bifida (2.0 MOM cutoff).[20] An additional benefit to screening for neural-tube defects is that almost all fetuses with gastroschisis and up to 70 to 80% of those with omphaloceles will also be detected.[21]

Interpretation and Adjustments

The optimal time for screening is from 16 to 18 weeks of gestation, although reference values are available for screening at from 13 to 21 weeks. Maternal weight,[22] race,[23] and insulin-dependent diabetes mellitus (IDDM)[24] all affect interretion of MSAFP levels, and this information should be provided with each sample so results can be compared to the appropriate mean. Women with elevated MSAFP results can be rescreened, as one-third to one-half of women with initially positive screens will have a negative second test. If, on retesting, a patient has an elevated MSAFP, an ultrasound examination should be performed to confirm dates, rule out twins or intrauterine fetal death, and search for anomalies. If menstrual dating is found to be inaccurate, then results should be recalculated based on the adjusted gestational age.

Ultrasonography for MSAFP Elevations

As methods of MSAFP screening were being developed, fetal ultrasonography was also improving. As equipment and experience of the sonographers improved, the detection rate of neural-tube defects increased. Open spina bifida is almost always associated with changes in intracranial anatomy viewed on ultrasound, including ventriculomegaly, deformation of the skull (lemon sign), and alterations in the cerebellum (banana sign).[25]

The reported detection rates for open spina bifida vary depending on the center, but generally range from 71 to 100%.[26,27] The detection rate for anencephaly should be 100% in all centers performing obstetrical ultrasound. ACOG now recommends that patients be counseled regarding a reduced risk of spina bifida based on the individual sensitivity of ultrasound at a given clinical center.[18] Patients should be counseled thoroughly, the ultrasound examination should be performed with high-resolution equipment by experienced examiners, no altered risk should be given if suboptimal views are obtained, and amniocentesis should be offered with nondirective counseling. In centers adept at diagnosing open spina bifida sonographically, amniocentesis can be reserved for patients with suspicious ultrasound findings, large MSAFP elevations despite a normal scan, or inability to adequately visualize fetal anatomy. In light of risk reductions of 90 to 95% in specialized centers, many patients may choose to forgo amniocentesis in the presence of a normal ultrasound exam.

At amniocentesis, AFP and acetylcholinesterase (AChE) should be routinely measured. AChE is a neural enzyme present in high concentrations in fetal cerebrospinal fluid and low concentrations in fetal serum. Presence of any detectable AChE in the amniotic fluid suggests an open neural-tube defect, gastroschisis, or, less commonly, omphalocele. AChE is absent in cases of nephrosis. False positive AChE and AFP can be found in cases of large fetal hemorrhage, recent intrauterine fetal death, involuting fetus of a multiple gestation or hemangiomas of placenta or cord.

Associated Disorders with MSAFP Elevations

Increased AFP has been associated with open neural-tube defects, gastroschisis, omphalocele, Finnish nephrosis, and large fetal hemorrhages. Disorders that have been associated with an elevated MSAFP are listed in Table 4-4.

Congenital nephrosis has a birth prevalence of 1 in 2600 per year in Finland and 1 in 40,000 in a non-Finnish population.[28] The diagnosis should be suspected regardless of ethnicity if MSAFP is elevated, AFP is markedly elevated, and AChE is negative.[29] This disease is inherited as an autosomal recessive trait and is at present untreatable. Affected fetuses appear normal on second-trimester ultrasound examination but die in early childhood, if not in utero. AFP levels are markedly elevated, with all measuring over 17 standard deviations above the mean.

An association between elevated MSAFP levels and placenta accreta and percreta has been reported.[30] A retrospective review found that 45% of patients with placenta accreta had elevated MSAFP levels when screened in the second trimester, whereas none of the controls had elevated values. Placental villi invading the myometrium and leading to mixing of

TABLE 4-4
CONDITIONS ASSOCIATED WITH ELEVATED MSAFP

Fetal

Poor gestational dates	Fetal death
Multiple gestation	Anencephaly
Neural-tube defects	Gastroschisis
Omphalocele	Renal agenesis
Congenital nephrosis (Finnish type)	Cloacal or bladder extrophy
	Pentalogy of Cantrell
Amniotic band sequence	Aplasia cutis
Epidermolysis bullosa	
Sacrococcygeal teratoma	

Placental

Abruption	Placenta accreta

Maternal

Maternal hepatoma	Maternal ovarian teratoma

maternal and fetal blood is a possible explanation. If MSAFP elevation is unexplained and the placenta is low lying, detailed examination of the placental site should be attempted.

Multiple Gestation

MSAFP levels in twins are approximately twice the median in singleton pregnancies, higher in triplet pregnancies, and even higher in quadruplet pregnancies,[31] suggesting that the level is related to the number of fetuses in utero. In one series of twin pregnancies discordant for neural-tube defects, MSAFP values ranged from 5.6 to 12.8 MOM.[32] On the basis of these findings, most, if not all, twins discordant for open neural-tube defects will be identified if twins with MSAFP levels >5.0 MOM have detailed evaluations.

Karyotype Analysis for MSAFP Elevations

Karyotype analysis in patients who undergo amniocentesis for MSAFP elevation is controversial. The incidence of chromosomal abnormalities detected by amniocentesis for elevated MSAFP has been reported as 1 in 78 to 1 in 114, which is clearly higher than the risk of a 35-year-old woman.[33-37] However, the types of abnormalities detected differ from the types associated with advanced maternal age, with trisomy 21 being an unusual finding, and sex chromosome aneuploidies and triploidy more common. Each center should determine a protocol on the basis of its own detection rates and patient population. However, karyotype testing should be considered in the presence of omphalocele or neural-tube defect, given the increased risk of chromosomal abnormality.

Risks Associated with MSAFP Elevations

"Unexplained elevations" of MSAFP have been found to be associated with various poor outcomes, including intrauterine growth restriction, low birth weight, placental abruption, perinatal loss, oligohydramnios, and preeclampsia.[38] While increased surveillance in the third trimester has been suggested, no guidelines exist for specific follow-up to change the risk or outcome. One possible strategy is to perform a follow-up ultrasound in the third trimester. Patients with intrauterine growth restriction or oligohydramnios can then be followed with appropriate antenatal surveillance.

Screening for Down Syndrome

Shortly after the introduction of MSAFP testing for neural-tube defects in the early 1980s, it was recognized that fetuses with Down syndrome (DS) had a lower mean MSAFP in the second trimester.[39,40] To improve sensitivity and specificity, unconjugated estriol and human chorionic gonadotropin have been added to second-trimester biochemical screening for DS. Like AFP, μE_3 is 25 to 30% lower in DS pregnancies,[41] while HCG has a median value twice that of normal controls.[41,42] The free β-subunit of HCG has been shown to be equivalent to total HCG in sensitivity and specificity.[43] Because these three markers—AFP, μE_3, and HCG—are all independent of maternal age and only weakly correlated with each other, they can be used in combination to estimate fetal DS risk.[42,44,45] As with AFP screening, the biochemical values are used in combination with maternal age to give an overall, patient-specific risk. Because the overall risk is calculated by combining the three assay results with maternal age, there is no definite "normal" or "abnormal" range for each marker. Therefore, it is not usually possible to estimate risk simply on the basis of knowing the three separate assay values. Most centers use a 1 in 270 risk of DS at midtrimester, the equivalent risk for a 35-year-old woman. This cutoff value generally results in a detection rate of 65%, with a false positive rate of 7 to 8%.[46] Other centers have elected to use a false positive rate of 5% as acceptable, which results in a 1 in 190 risk cutoff and a 61% detection rate.[45]

The protocol for triple marker screening is similar to MSAFP screening for DS, with testing being performed at 15 to 20 weeks of gestation. Because repeat testing may generate a falsely reassuring negative test, it is not recommended that testing be repeated for abnormally low MSAFP results. The exception to this is when the pregnancy is redated and the initial sample is found to have been drawn too early, rendering it uninterpretable. Maternal serum triple screening cannot be interpreted for multiple gestations.

Trisomy 18 Detection with Serum Screening

Mothers carrying fetuses affected with trisomy 18 have a characteristic triple screen pattern, with AFP, μE_3, and HCG all substantially lower than normal. Programs in which a separate protocol is used are able to detect 80% of trisomy 18, while identifying only

0.5% of women as high risk.[47] Thus, a majority of cases of trisomy 18 can be detected by triple screen without a substantial increase in the false positive rate.

Other Chromosomal Abnormalities Associated with an Abnormal Triple Panel

Two large series have indicated that women undergoing amniocentesis for an abnormal triple screening panel have a 2 to 4% risk for chromosomal abnormalities other than Down syndrome.[48,49] In both series, the risk was equivalent to the risk of Down syndrome. Abnormalities included other autosomal trisomies, structural abnormalities, and sex-chromosome abnormalities. Patients with an abnormal triple screen should be counseled that chromosomal abnormalities other than Down syndrome may be identified by amniocentesis. The clinical significance of some of these abnormalities may vary widely.

Screening in Women Older Than 35 Years of Age

Biochemical screening in older women has both advantages and limitations. Because age-based risk (Table 4-5) is used in the calculation, 26 to 34% of

patients older than age 35 will screen positive.[51,52] The detection rate for Down syndrome is between 75 and 89%. Thus, while a significant percentage of women over the age of 35 will be able to avoid the risks of amniocentesis, between 11 and 25% of cases of Down syndrome will be missed. Overall, the triple screen fails to detect 35 to 39% of chromosomal abnormalities in this population; however, a significant proportion of these are less serious sex-chromosome abnormalities. Ultrasound examination may reveal abnormalities that are not detected on triple screen, but the sensitivity of ultrasound in ruling out Down syndrome is controversial.

Biochemical screening in older patients remains controversial because of the previously described limitations. At present, amniocentesis should still be offered to all women older than 35 years of age, and patients who request biochemical screening should have detailed counseling about the limitations of this approach. While a negative triple screen may be reassuring to a patient who is averse to amniocentesis, counseling must stress both the high rate of positive triple screen results and that a negative result does not rule out either Down syndrome or other chromosomal abnormalities.

First-Trimester Maternal Serum Screening

Although triple marker screening has added greatly to our ability to detect chromosomal abnormalities, diagnosis under these circumstances generally occurs at 18 or 19 weeks of gestation or later. Several investigators have evaluated the efficacy of biochemical screening in the first trimester.[53-55] Early results are promising, indicating that a screening program combining maternal age, pregnancy-associated plasma protein A (PAPP-A) and HCG has detection rates for Down syndrome of 63 to 66%, with a false positive rate of 5%. This test performance is comparable to second-trimester serum screening and offers the advantage of diagnosis before 14 weeks. First-trimester serum screening does not screen for neural-tube defects. In combination with first-trimester ultrasound for nuchal translucency, which will be discussed in detail in the next section, detection rates may be higher. While at this time these technologies cannot be recommended to replace second-trimester screening, future developments in this area may improve our current screening strategies.

TABLE 4-5
RELATION BETWEEN MATERNAL AGE AND THE ESTIMATED RATE OF CHROMOSOMAL ABNORMALITIES

Age*	Risk of Down Syndrome	Risk of Chromosomal Abnormality
20	1/1667	1/526
25	1/1250	1/475
30	1/952	1/385
35	1/385	1/202
36	1/295	1/162
37	1/227	1/129
38	1/175	1/102
39	1/137	1/82
40	1/106	1/65
41	1/82	1/51
42	1/64	1/40
43	1/50	1/32
44	1/38	1/25
45	1/30	1/20
46	1/23	1/16
47	1/18	1/13
48	1/14	1/10
49	1/11	1/7

*Ages are at the expected time of delivery.
Data have been modified from Hook et al.[155]

PRENATAL DIAGNOSIS BY ULTRASOUND EXAMINATION

Since ultrasound was first introduced in the late 1950s, its use has become commonplace in many obstetric practices. Advances in technology and expertise have enhanced image quality and interpretation and made ultrasound the method of choice in imaging the fetus. In the past decade, ultrasound has been used increasingly in prenatal diagnosis and treatment.

In 1984 the members of the National Institutes of Health Consensus Development Conference (NIHCDC) reviewed the available literature to provide guidelines for obstetrical ultrasonography.[56] Clinical issues included indications for obstetrical ultrasound (i.e., routine screening versus targeted ultrasound) and ultrasound safety. The panel suggested certain situations in which ultrasound might be beneficial; these are listed in Table 4-6.

Most congenital anomalies occur sporadically in fetuses without known risk factors. For this reason, routine ultrasound as a screening tool is an attractive concept. Fetal malformations that have been diagnosed

---

TABLE 4-6
INDICATIONS FOR ULTRASONOGRAPHY*

Estimate gestational age for women with uncertain clinical dates or verify dates for women who are to undergo scheduled elective repeated cesarean delivery, indicated induction of labor, or other elective termination of pregnancy.

Evaluate fetal growth, for example, when the woman has an identified cause for uteroplacental insufficiency—severe preeclampsia, chronic hypertension, chronic renal disease, severe diabetes mellitus—or for other medical complications of pregnancy where fetal malnutrition (intrauterine growth retardation or macrosomia) is suspected.

Evaluate vaginal bleeding of undetermined cause.

Determine fetal presentation when the presenting part cannot be adequately determined in labor or the fetal presentation is variable in late pregnancy.

Multiple gestation suspected based on the detection of more than one fetal heartbeat pattern, fundal height larger than expected for dates, or previous use of fertility drugs.

Adjunct to amniocentesis.

Substantial discrepancy in uterine size compared with clinical dates.

Pelvic mass detected clinically.

Hydatidiform mole suspected on the basis of clinical signs of hypertension, proteinuria, or the presence of ovarian cysts felt on pelvic examination or failure to detect fetal heart tones with a Doppler ultrasonogram after 12 weeks of gestation.

Adjunct to cervical cerclage placement.

Ectopic pregnancy suspected or pregnancy occurring after tuboplasty or previous ectopic gestation.

Follow-up evaluation of placental location for identified placenta previa.

Adjunct to special procedures, such as fetoscopy, intrauterine transfusion, shunt placement, in vitro fertilization, embryo transfer, or chorionic villus sampling.

Fetal death suspected.

Uterine abnormality suspected—clinically significant leiomyoma or congenital structural abnormalities, such as uterus bicornis or uterus didelphys.

Locate intrauterine (contraceptive) device.

Ovarian follicle development surveillance.

Biophysical evaluation for fetal well-being after 28 weeks of gestation.

Observation of intrapartum events—version or extraction of second twin, manual removal of placenta.

Polyhydramnios or oligohydramnios suspected.

Abruptio placentae suspected.

Adjunct to external version from breech to vertex presentation.

Estimate fetal weight or presentation in premature rupture of membranes or premature labor.

Abnormal serum α-fetoprotein value for clinical gestational age.

Follow-up observation of identified fetal anomaly.

History of previous congenital anomaly.

Serial evaluation of fetal growth in multiple gestation.

Evaluate fetal condition in late registrants for prenatal care.

*From the National Institutes of Health Consensus Development Conference.[56]

TABLE 4-7
FETAL MALFORMATIONS THAT HAVE BEEN DIAGNOSED PRENATALLY BY ULTRASONOGRAPHY

Cranial and Intracranial
Agenesis of the corpus callosum
Anencephaly
Aqueductal stenosis
Arachnoid cyst
Choroid plexus cysts
Hydrocephalus
Dandy–Walker malformation
Exencephaly
Encephalocele
Holoprosencephaly
Iniencephaly
Microcephaly
Porencephalic cyst
Schizencephaly
Vein of Galen aneurysm

Craniofacial
Anophthalmia
Cyclopia
Cystic hygroma
Facial cleft
Goiter
Hypertelorism
Hypotelorism
Micrognathia
Microphthalmia
Teratoma

Spine
Hemivertebrae
Sacral agenesis
Sacrococcygeal teratoma
Spina bifida

Thoracic
Absent lungs
Bronchial atresia

Bronchogenic cyst
Cystic adenomatoid malformation
Diaphragmatic hernia
Hydrothorax
Pulmonary hypoplasia
Pulmonary sequestration

Gastrointestinal Tract
Anorectal atresia
Choledochal cyst
Cholelithiasis
Duodenal atresia
Enteric duplication cyst
Hepatic cyst
Hepatic neoplasm
Hirschsprung disease
Jejunoileal atresia
Meconium ileus
Meconium peritonitis
Mesenteric cyst
Persistent cloaca
Situs inversus
Tracheoesophageal fistula
Volvulus

Genitourinary System
Ambiguous genitalia
Bladder-outlet obstruction
Duplicated kidneys with ectopic
ureterocele
Multicystic kidney
Infantile polycystic kidney
Ovarian cyst
Pelvic kidney
Renal agenesis
Tumors—neuroblastoma
Ureteropelvic junction obstruction
Ureterovesical obstruction

Cardiovascular System
Atrioventricular septal defect—endocardial cushion defect
Cardiomyopathy
Coarctation of the aorta
Double-outlet right ventricle
Ebstein anomaly
Heterotaxy syndrome
Hypoplastic left ventricle
Hypoplastic right ventricle
Rhabdomyoma
Tetralogy of Fallot
Total anomalous pulmonary venous
return
Transposition of the great vessels
Valvular stenosis
Ventricular septal defect

Abdominal Wall and Trunk
Bladder exstrophy
Cloacal exstrophy
Ectopia cordis
Gastroschisis
Body-stalk anomaly
Omphalocele
Tumors—teratoma, melanoma
Urachal cyst

Extremities
Arthrogryposis
Limb dysplasias and shortening
Clinodactyly
Club feet
Polydactyly
Radial aplasia

---

prenatally by ultrasound are listed in Table 4-7. Some of these anomalies are more difficult to diagnose than others, whether because of technical factors such as cardiac defects, or lesion size such as small facial clefts. Others, such as choroid plexus cysts, depend on the gestational age of the fetus.

The accuracy of ultrasound in detecting certain lesions prenatally is difficult to assess because of differences in the extent of the malformation(s), quality of the equipment, and the expertise of the sonographer. Technical limitations, such as fetal position, amniotic fluid volume, and maternal habitus, will make some scans more difficult than others. The effi-

cacy of routine ultrasound in low- and high-risk pregnancies is discussed below.

Routine Ultrasound in Low-Risk Pregnancy

Although routine screening in pregnancy is recommended in other countries, including the United Kingdom,[57] Norway,[58] and Canada,[59] the NIHCDC did not endorse routine ultrasound screening, mainly because of a lack of evidence that it benefited the low-risk fetus. Other arguments against routine screening included appreciable cost and potential fetal harm.

Many studies have examined the use of ultrasound in low-risk pregnancy. Significantly higher rates of detection are seen in tertiary ultrasound units. Reported sensitivities range from 14 to 85% depending on the ultrasound center, and specificities are generally close to 99%.[60-68] This observation suggests that, in low-risk populations, ultrasound may be helpful in ruling out anomalies but is not very reliable in detecting them.[69] This information may prove useful in counseling patients regarding ultrasound's accuracy for detection of congenital malformations in the general population.

Ultrasound in High-Risk Pregnancies

Targeted studies appear much more accurate. In fetuses at high risk for anomalies (family history of an abnormality, and/or abnormal MSAFP, and/or a suspicious outside ultrasound), overall sensitivities of 95 to 99% and specificities of 91 to 99% have been reported in referral centers.[70-72] Ultrasound examination is recommended in high-risk pregnancies, although a normal ultrasound cannot guarantee a fetus free from abnormalities. Because of variations between ultrasound centers, each center must discuss detection rates with patients referred for specific indications.

Accuracy of Ultrasound in the Diagnosis of Congenital Heart Defects

Congenital heart disease is the most common congenital malformation, responsible for most deaths caused by congenital anomalies.[73] Yet cardiac defects are especially difficult to identify prenatally, and the accuracy of screening examinations is even more difficult to assess. The four-chamber view of the heart has been recommended as a screening tool to be incorporated into routine scans after 16 weeks of gestation in the hope of excluding most congenital heart disease. However, at present it appears that only 10% of congenital heart disease is actually detected prenatally.[74]

The sensitivity and specificity of the four-chamber view depends on the population screened and the experience of the sonographer. Several studies have specifically evaluated the accuracy of the four-chamber view in low-risk populations. The four-chamber view has been reported to detect between 36 and 64% of congenital heart disease.[75-78] Specificities approaching 100% were noted by all authors. In mixed populations,

sensitivities have been reported between 48 and 81%, again with excellent specificity.[79-81]

Fetal echocardiography, a more complex, detailed ultrasound examination of the fetal heart, is recommended only for patients at high risk for carrying fetuses with heart disease. In high-risk patients, scanned by skilled operators experienced in cardiac ultrasound, detection of congenital cardiac disease is much more accurate than in the general population. In one large series, sensitivity and specificity was reported as 92% and 99.7%, respectively.[82] Those who should be referred for fetal echocardiography include women with a family history of congenital heart disease, women with diabetes mellitus, a fetus with a suspected abnormality such as a structural defect or an arrhythmia, and women with exposure to a teratogenic medication. Referrals for an abnormal four-chamber heart have yielded the greatest numbers of prenatally detected congenital heart disease in fetal echocardiography centers. Chromosomal analysis should be considered in any fetus with a prenatally diagnosed cardiac anomaly.

Ultrasound Detection of Chromosomal Abnormalities

Fetuses with structural anomalies detected in utero have a high incidence of aneuploidy.[83-85] Despite this, detection of major malformations is a relatively insensitive tool to screen for chromosomal abnormalities, especially Down syndrome. Although most fetuses with trisomy 13 and 18 have major abnormalities detectable by ultrasound,[86,87] only about 30% of fetuses with DS have major structural malformations present.[88] Thus, special attention has been paid to subtle dysmorphology and evaluation of biometric measurements in an attempt to improve ultrasound detection of the fetus with DS.

Chromosomal Abnormalities in the Fetus with Major Malformations

Fetuses with prenatally detected structural abnormalities have a higher incidence of chromosomal aneuploidy than cases of similar abnormalities identified after birth.[85,89] This discrepancy is due in part to the fact that fetuses with malformations and chromosomal abnormalities have a high rate of intrauterine death.

The likelihood of chromosomal aneuploidy in the setting of fetal malformations depends on the type,

---

TABLE 4-8
SONOGRAPHIC FINDINGS IN CASES OF
CHROMOSOMAL ABNORMALITIES

Trisomy 21
  Duodenal atresia
  Tracheoesophageal fistula
  Esophageal atresia
  Atrioventricular canal defects
  Ventricular septal defects
  Atrial septal defects
  Hypoplasia of the middle quadrant of the fifth digit/clinodactyly
  Hydrothorax
  Nuchal fold >6 mm
Trisomy 18
  Intrauterine growth retardation
  Hydramnios
  Clenched hands with overlapping digits
  Clubfeet
  Rocker-bottom feet
  Ventricular septal defect
  Omphalocele
  Diaphragmatic hernia
  Choroid plexus cysts
Trisomy 13
  Holoprosencephaly (midline facial defect)
  Cleft lip and palate
  Ventricular septal defect, hypoplastic left ventricle
  Polydactyly
  Omphalocele
  Polycystic kidneys

---

number, and severity of the structural defects. In one series of 327 cases, the incidence of chromosomal abnormalities was 10% in fetuses with one malformation but 35% with two or more.[89] The frequency of chromosomal abnormalities is also highly dependent on the type of malformation, with specific defects indicating a high risk of a specific chromosomal aneuploidy (Table 4-8). Atrioventricular canal and duodenal atresia are highly associated with trisomy 21,[89,90] alobar holoprosencephaly with trisomy 13,[87,89] and cystic hygroma with Turner syndrome (monosomy X).[87,89]

Ultrasound Screening for Down Syndrome and Trisomy 18 in Cases without Major Malformations

Because only a third of fetuses with DS have major malformations detectable with prenatal ultrasound,[88] ultrasound diagnosis of subtle dysmorphology associated with DS has been used in an attempt to improve ultrasound detection of this disorder. Specific findings that have been associated with an increased risk of DS are discussed individually below. At present, there is

no consensus on the role of ultrasound screening for DS. Clearly, a percentage of DS fetuses can be identified by ultrasound, perhaps even in the first trimester. While the presence of certain subtle markers such as increased nuchal fold or combinations of markers can increase the risk of Down syndrome, there is no consensus on risk reduction in the absence of these markers. The subtlety of many of the findings of DS in the second trimester requires significant technical expertise if ultrasonographic screening is to be used. Patients need to be counseled on the limitations of ultrasound in the detection of DS; even in highly skilled hands a normal ultrasound cannot rule out a chromosomal abnormality.

The usefulness of various DS detection schemes depends on whether the markers are reliably obtained and whether they efficiently discriminate between fetuses with DS and normal fetuses. Many markers that may be associated with DS in high-risk populations may not be appropriate for screening in low risk populations. Thus, when an isolated finding that has been associated with Down syndrome is observed in a low-risk patient, the ideal management strategy remains controversial in many cases.

Second-Trimester Nuchal Fold

Eighty percent of infants with DS are noted to have redundant skin in the posterior neck.[91] This realization led to evaluation of nuchal fold measurements of ≥6 mm in the second trimester as a screening marker for DS.[92,93] Nuchal-fold measurement utilizes a transverse view through the fetal head, across the thalami at an angle that includes the cerebellum and occipital bone. The soft tissue posterior to the bone is measured. Care must be taken in measuring the nuchal fold because angling the transducer caudally can result in an incorrectly wide value and a false positive result. The nuchal fold is no longer sensitive and specific after 21 weeks of gestation.

The nuchal-fold measurement has been shown to have a sensitivity from 34 to 75%, with a low false positive rate.[93,94] The adjusted positive predictive value in one prospective study was 1 in 13; however, approximately half of the fetuses with increased nuchal fold thickness in this study had other findings as well.[93] Isolated nuchal-fold thickness is also associated with DS in a population without advanced maternal age or abnormal triple screen.[94] Thus, if an increased nuchal fold is noted, amniocentesis for karyotype should be considered.

Echogenic Bowel

While 7 to 12% of fetuses with DS will have echogenic bowel,[88,95] most fetuses with DS and echogenic bowel will have other sonographic findings.[95,96] However, review of several series of high-risk patients suggest that the estimated rate of chromosomal abnormalities in fetuses with isolated echogenic bowel may be as high as 1.4%.[95] In a low-risk population, the positive and negative predictive value of isolated echogenic bowel for chromosomal abnormalities is not known.

In addition, several studies have reported an increased risk of cystic fibrosis with the finding of echogenic bowel.[97,98] The prospective risk of cystic fibrosis in fetuses with isolated echogenic bowel has not been well established. Because there may be a significant risk of aneuploidy associated with isolated echogenic bowel, we currently offer amniocentesis for karyotype and cystic fibrosis testing to all women with echogenic bowel seen on sonographic evaluation to be as bright as bone. As echogenic bowel has also been associated with an increased risk of intrauterine growth restriction,[95-98] monitoring for growth abnormalities should be considered.

Minimal Intracranial Ventriculomegaly

Isolated minimal ventriculomegaly is identified when the atria of the lateral ventricles measure 10 to 15 mm. A review of the literature suggests that isolated ventriculomegaly is associated with a 2.7% risk of aneuploidy.[99] However, because a large proportion of reported cases occurred in high-risk women with advanced maternal age, the risk of aneuploidy in a low-risk pregnancy with isolated ventriculomegaly is not known. Although isolated mild ventriculomegaly often represents a normal variant, it has also been associated with absence of the corpus callosum, neural-tube defects, infection, and intracranial hemorrhage. Neurologic outcomes are highly variable, depending on the underlying cause and rate of progression of ventriculomegaly.

Every effort should be made to identify the corpus callosum or cavum septum pellucidum on ultrasound. Amniocentesis for viral studies and karyotype should be considered and maternal serum may also be sent for toxoplasmosis titers. Follow-up ultrasound examinations should be performed to assess progression of the ventriculomegaly.

Shortened Femur and Humerus Length

Infants with DS have, on average, shorter long bones than normal infants, a fact that has been used in prenatal ultrasound screening.[100-102] Most interest has focused on measurement of the fetal femur, as this is the long bone measured in virtually all routine obstetric ultrasound examinations after the first trimester. Investigators have looked at either the ratio of the biparietal diameter (BPD) to the femur length, the ratio of actual to expected femur length, femur–foot length ratios, or a femur length <5th percentile.

Several studies have described the usefulness of these measurements in predicting DS, and the results are conflicting.[103-107] The positive predictive value of a short femur has ranged from 1 in 21 to 1 in 644, the sensitivity from 12 to 68%, and the false positive rate from 2 to 15%.[104,107,108] Because of this high false positive rate even in the high-risk populations where this has been studied, use of shortened femur as a screening tool in a low-risk population may result in an unacceptably high amniocentesis rate.[108,109] Further, the difference in femur lengths between normal and DS fetuses was not statistically significant until after 17 weeks.[105] It appears that, although the femurs of DS fetuses are slightly shorter than those of normal fetuses, the limitations of ultrasound equipment are such that this small difference may not be of sufficient magnitude to permit sonographic discrimination in the second trimester.

If a shortened femur is detected, the remainder of the long bones, including the humerus, should be measured. Humerus length has also been noted to be short in patients with DS and in most series was found to be a more sensitive and specific marker.[107,110] In addition, shortened long bones can be associated with skeletal abnormalities, and follow-up ultrasound to document normal growth is recommended.

Pyelectasis

Pyelectasis, or minimal fetal hydronephrosis, has been shown to be present in 18 to 25% of fetuses with DS in the second trimester.[111,112] However, pyelectasis is also present in approximately 2.2% of normal second-trimester sonographic examinations,[113] rendering its value in screening unclear. Although there is an association between pyelectasis and DS, most studies have been performed in high-risk patients, who may have other sonographic findings. With isolated pyelectasis, the incidence of DS has been estimated at 1 in 340.[112] Thus, amniocentesis is not recommended in low-risk women with the finding of isolated pyelectasis.

In cases of pyelectasis not associated with chromosomal abnormalities, the majority will resolve. However, 9% will progress, and 4% will have functionally significant urologic lesions.[113] Thus, follow-up sonographic evaluation is recommended to rule out progression.

Choroid Plexus Cysts

Choroid plexus cysts are a common finding, occurring in approximately 1 to 3% of midtrimester sonographic evaluations. Given that 71% of fetuses with trisomy 18 have choroid plexus cysts, there is clearly an association.[114] However, most fetuses with this finding will be normal, and most fetuses with trisomy 18 will have other anomalies.

Two prospective series have shown a risk of chromosomal abnormalities in a fetus without other risk factors to be lower than the risk of fetal loss from amniocentesis.[115,116] Meta-analysis that combines smaller series gives an overall risk of trisomy 18 of 1 in 390 in a mixed population.[117] In women with advanced maternal age, abnormal triple screen, or other sonographic findings, the risks are likely higher. In one series, 10% of 38 high-risk women with an isolated choroid plexus cyst had trisomy 18 or 21.[115]

Because the risks are minimal in a low-risk population, women with an isolated choroid plexus cyst may decide after counseling that the risks of amniocentesis outweigh the risk of chromosomal abnormalities. Women with advanced maternal age, abnormal triple screen, or other sonographic findings should be considered for amniocentesis.

More than 95% of choroid plexus cysts resolve by 25 weeks of gestation, and persistence has not been associated with abnormal neurologic outcome[118]; thus, follow-up ultrasound is not recommended to document resolution. Further, resolution of a choroid plexus cyst does not reduce the risk of chromosomal abnormalities.

Echogenic Cardiac Focus

While an echogenic cardiac focus is associated with Down syndrome in the presence of other markers, evidence does not indicate a clinically significant increased risk of DS or other aneuploidies with an isolated finding of an echogenic cardiac focus in a low-risk pa-

tient.[119] Parents should be counseled that an echogenic focus does not represent a structural abnormality of the heart, nor is it associated with abnormal heart function.

Clinodactyly

While hypoplasia and/or clinodactyly of the middle phalanx of the fifth digit is present in approximately 60% of individuals with DS, it is also commonly present in the general population. Even at referral centers, screening for DS based on the finding of isolated clinodactyly would result in an unacceptably high false positive rate of 18%.[120] Thus, isolated clinodactyly is not an indication for amniocentesis.

First-Trimester Ultrasound Screening

As interest in earlier prenatal diagnosis increases, investigation of first-trimester prenatal diagnosis of chromosomal abnormalities has intensified. Because of the clear association between second-trimester nuchal thickening and aneuploidy, the utility of first-trimester nuchal thickening has been investigated.

Nuchal translucency appears to be most effective when measured between 10 and 13 weeks 6 days. Initial studies generally used cutoffs of greater than 3 mm; however, because the nuchal fold increases normally with increasing gestational age, the false positive rate at 13 weeks of gestation may be as high as 13%.[121] To reduce this false positive rate, studies have moved to a cutoff based on the actual crown-to-rump length. Theoretically, a cutoff of >95th percentile for gestational age will hold the false positive rate to 5%.

Initial results of this technique have been promising. The sensitivity of a nuchal fold measuring >95% for crown-to-rump length has been reported to be 82%, with a positive predictive value of 1 in 30 amniocenteses in a large prospective study.[122] However, other large studies have reported much lower sensitivities of 43 to 54%.[123,124] Detection rates are likely to be somewhat inflated because a proportion of abnormal fetuses that are detected in the first trimester will spontaneously abort prior to the second trimester.

Discrepancies between centers likely result from the technical difficulty in obtaining the correct view for first-trimester nuchal translucency, shown in Figure 4–1. As sonographers become more adept at obtaining accurate nuchal translucency measurements in the first trimester, the reliability of this technique in

Figure 4-1 First-trimester nuchal translucency measurement demonstrating correct view and caliper placement.

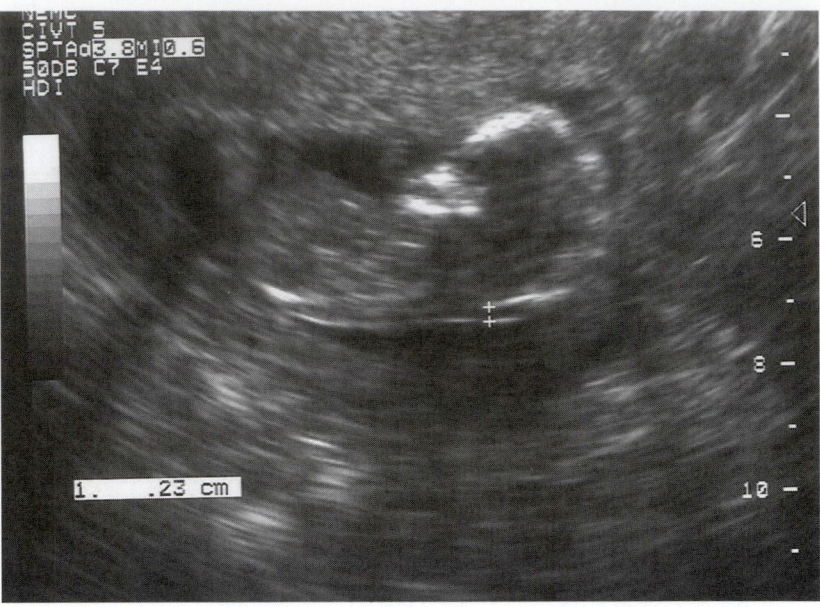

general use can be expected to improve. A large U.S. multicenter trial is currently under way to validate this technique and to evaluate the sensitivity and specificity of combining first-trimester nuchal translucency with first-trimester serum markers and to compare a first-trimester screening package with the current standard of midtrimester screening.

PRENATAL DIAGNOSIS PROCEDURES

Indications

The indications for invasive prenatal diagnostic procedures are summarized in Table 4-9. Amniocentesis or CVS is indicated when there is a need to obtain fetal material for cytogenetic, biochemical, or DNA studies.

**TABLE 4-9
INDICATIONS FOR PRENATAL
DIAGNOSTIC PROCEDURES**

Maternal age 35 or older at expected date of delivery
Abnormal maternal serum triple screen
Abnormal ultrasound examination
Either parent balanced translocation carrier
Family history of neural-tube defects
Family history of chromosomal abnormality
Family history of mendelian disorder amenable to DNA
  diagnosis
Family history of biochemical disorder

Amniocentesis

Midtrimester amniocentesis with ultrasound guidance is usually performed at 15 to 18 weeks of gestation in outpatient facilities. Chromosomal studies are carried out by culturing the few viable fetal cells present in amniotic fluid, and the results are generally available in 10 to 14 days. The safety and accuracy of midtrimester amniocentesis have been established in prospective collaborative studies.[22,125] Amniocentesis carries an estimated risk of fetal loss of 0.5 to 1.0%.[126,127] Culture failure occurs in less than 1% of cases. Repeat amniocentesis should be considered in cases of culture failure because of the increased risk of chromosomal abnormalities.[128]

In clinical circumstances where a more rapid analysis for common chromosomal abnormalities is desired, fluorescence in situ hybridization (FISH) probes are generally available for chromosomes 21, 13, 18, X, and Y with reliable results available in 2 to 3 days.[129] Samples obtained after 24 weeks are less likely to be informative; however, in cases where rapid chromosomal analysis is desired to aid intrapartum management, FISH may still be attempted.

Chromosomal mosaicism is the presence of two or more cell lines with different karyotypes in a single person. Mosaicism observed in amniocentesis samples does not necessarily mean that the fetus has mosaicism. The most common type of mosaicism detected by amniocentesis is pseudomosaicism.[130] Abnormal cell lines can arise during the culture process but are not present in the fetus.

True fetal mosaicism, diagnosed when the same abnormality is present on more than one coverslip, is rare (0.25%) but clinically important.[130] Whether true mosaicism is present is best resolved by karyotyping fetal lymphocytes obtained by percutaneous fetal blood sampling,[131] a method that provides results within 48 hours. Detailed ultrasound examination is also recommended to assess fetal growth and rule out structural anomalies. If both the ultrasound and the fetal blood sampling results are normal, the parents can be reassured that the major chromosomal abnormalities have been excluded.[131]

Early Amniocentesis

The Canadian Early and Mid-Trimester Amniocentesis trial results have indicated an increased risk of complications with amniocentesis performed between 11 and 13 weeks.[132] An estimated excess procedure-related risk of pregnancy loss of 1.8% was seen as well as an increased risk of amniotic fluid loss and talipes equinus compared to women undergoing amniocentesis between 15 and 17 weeks. The increased risk of talipes equinus and amniotic fluid loss were also seen in a prospective study comparing early amniocentesis to chorionic villus sampling.[133] However, the power of this study was not sufficient to demonstrate an increased risk of pregnancy loss compared to CVS. Amniotic fluid leakage was not associated with neonatal respiratory distress but did confer an increased risk of miscarriage and was associated with an increased risk of talipes equinus. The risks of amniocentesis between 13 and 15 weeks have not been extensively studied. Given these findings, amniocentesis prior to 15 weeks should not be offered routinely. However, in the rare case where the risks of chromosomal abnormality are high and CVS is either technically difficult or unavailable, early amniocentesis may be a reasonable option given informed consent regarding the risks.

Chorionic Villus Sampling

Chorionic villi may be obtained by aspiration through a transcervical catheter or transabdominal needle with ultrasound guidance. The choice is based on the location of the placenta and the operator's preference and experience. The main advantage of CVS over amniocentesis is the earlier availability of results, as the procedure is generally performed between 9 and 12 weeks of gestation. Initial results are available in 24 to 48 hours, and final results from cultured cells in 10 to 14 days. An additional advantage of CVS is that more tissue is obtained than by amniocentesis, which can be useful when DNA analysis or enzymatic diagnosis is necessary. However, for assays for which amniotic fluid is essential, such as measurement of the AFP concentration, amniocentesis must be used.

Current accumulated data on the safety of CVS indicate an overall loss rate of 2.5 to 3%.[134] Some of these losses are likely due to natural attrition of abnormal pregnancies. The National Institute of Child Health and Human Development compared transcervical CVS with amniocentesis and found that the procedure-related rate of fetal loss with CVS exceeded that for amniocentesis by 0.8%.[135] Reduction of the risks of CVS over time suggest that the experience of the operator may be crucial in achieving optimal safety. Evidence has suggested that there is no increased risk of limb-reduction defects after CVS over the base-line population risk in over 130,000 procedures.[134]

The greater frequency of contamination by maternal cells and false evidence of mosaicism in chorionic villus samples contribute to the reduced cytogenetic accuracy of this procedure as compared with amniocentesis. However, maternal cell contamination is uncommon in experienced cytogenetic laboratories with a reported incidence of approximately 2%.[136] Evidence of mosaicism occurs in less than 1% of cases[134] and is usually due to confined placental mosaicism.[137] When mosaicism is reported, further testing by amniocentesis is warranted to rule out fetal mosaicism. The clinical disadvantages of increased risk and potential diagnostic error with CVS must be weighed against the disadvantage of the later timing of amniocentesis.

Percutaneous Umbilical-Blood Sampling (PUBS)

Blood can be obtained from the umbilical cord under ultrasound guidance beginning at approximately 18 weeks of gestation. Access to the fetal circulation permits the prenatal evaluation of many fetal hematologic abnormalities, including isoimmunization, fetal hemoglobinopathies, thrombocytopenia, and coagulation factor abnormalities.[138] Fetal blood can be used for the prenatal diagnosis of some inborn errors of metabolism and permits the assessment of viral, bacterial, and parasitic infections by serologic testing and culture.[138] Fetal blood sampling may clarify whether chromosomal mosaicism detected by cytogenetic analysis of amniotic fluid cells or chorionic villi is truly present.[131] The need for rapid karyotyping when congenital abnormalities are suspected is the most common reason for fetal blood sampling in the United States.

Cytogenetic results from short-term fetal-lymphocyte cultures are usually available within 48 to 72 hours. The rate of fetal loss after PUBS is about 1 to 2% more than the background risk to the particular fetus.[138,139] Because many of the fetuses studied have severe congenital malformations, the background loss rate is high in comparison with that for the population undergoing amniocentesis or CVS. Because PUBS entails a substantially greater risk of pregnancy loss than amniocentesis, it should be reserved for situations in which rapid diagnosis is essential or in which diagnostic information cannot be obtained by safer means.

Fetal Biopsy

Fetal biopsy was initially performed by fetoscopy but is now performed with ultrasound guidance. Certain genetic skin disorders, such as epidermolysis bullosa, require fetal-skin sampling. Fetal muscle biopsy has been used to diagnose Duchenne muscular dystrophy in a family in which DNA studies were uninformative.[140] It is difficult to assess the safety and accuracy of fetal biopsy because experience with these procedures is limited. Patients should be made aware of their investigational nature. Rapid advances in DNA technology can be expected to elucidate the molecular basis of many diseases that now require fetal biopsy. As such knowledge is accumulated, the need for these procedures will decline.

Preimplantation Genetic Diagnosis

The development of techniques for the diagnosis of genetic diseases before implantation at 6 days after fertilization provides couples with two new options: (1) avoidance of implantation of affected fetuses and (2) identification of affected fetuses before organogenesis to permit gene therapy. This technique is generally available only in specialized centers and is not routinely offered. However, preimplantation diagnosis is ideal for high-risk couples who want to avoid having an affected child—for example, carriers of a balanced translocation. Preimplantation diagnosis may also be considered when the mother carries an X-linked disorder, when both parents carry an autosomal recessive condition amenable to DNA-based diagnosis, or when one of the parents carries an autosomal dominant condition amenable to DNA-based diagnosis. Preimplantation techniques have been used to diagnose thalassemias,[141] Marfan syndrome,[142] unbalanced translocations,[143] familial adenomatous polyposis coli,[144] cystic fibrosis,[145] and myotonic dystrophy,[146] as well as to select female fetuses in cases of X-linked disorders.

Analysis of Fetal Cells and DNA Circulating in Maternal Blood

Current screening strategies for DS rely on maternal age, serum markers, and ultrasound findings to identify high-risk populations for definitive diagnosis by amniocentesis. False positive rates must be kept low in screening programs to minimize fetal losses due to amniocentesis. Because these limitations reduce the detection rate for DS, there is great interest in the development of noninvasive methods for prenatal diagnosis. One approach under investigation has been to isolate the rare fetal nucleated cells circulating in maternal peripheral blood because these cells are a source of fetal chromosomes and DNA.[147,148] Successful isolation and identification of fetal cells in maternal blood would permit detection of chromosomal abnormalities as part of routine prenatal care without fetal risk.

While the presence of fetal cells in the maternal bloodstream has been demonstrated repeatedly, techniques to reliably distinguish fetal cells from maternal cells are still being refined. If the fetal karyotype is normal, the average number of fetal cells in 16 ml of maternal blood is 19.[148] Although many techniques have been used, the most widely studied method involves differentiation between maternal and fetal cells based on the presence of fetal hemoglobin. Even one fetal cell can yield enough DNA for diagnostic testing.[149] These techniques have already been used to diagnose fetal sex, HLA type,[150] Duchenne muscular dystrophy,[151] Rh status,[152] and orthinine transcarbamylase deficiency.[153] They have also been used to exclude β-thalassemia and sickle cell disease.[154] While not widely available yet, these techniques are currently being evaluated in clinical trials by the National Institute of Child Health and Human Development.

Diagnosis of fetal RhD status has also been reported by directly testing fetal DNA isolated from maternal serum.[155] In 45 women in the second and third trimester, testing was both 100% sensitive and specific but could not be used reliably in the first trimester because low levels of fetal DNA may yield a false negative result. This technique avoids the complicated process of cell sorting, and thus will likely be a less expensive option in certain cases. However, this technique cannot be used when the target gene is present in both the mother and the fetus because the origin of the DNA cannot be distinguished at this time. Thus, this technique may be limited in its application in noninvasive prenatal diagnosis.

REFERENCES

1. American College of Obstetricians and Gynecologists. Antenatal diagnosis of genetic disorders. ACOG Technical Bulletin No. 108, 1987:1.
2. Shaw MW. To be or not to be? That is the question. Am J Hum Genet 1984;36:1.
3. American College of Obstetricians and Gynecologists. Genetic screening for hemoglobinopathies. Committee Opinion No. 168, February 1996.
4. American College of Obstetricians and Gynecologists. Screening for Tay-Sachs disease. Committee Opinion No. 162, November 1995.
5. Sandhoff K, Conzelmann E, Neufeld EF, et al. The GM$_2$ gangliosidosis. In: Scriver CR, Beaudet AL, Sly WS, Valle D, eds. The metabolic basis of inherited disease. 6th ed. New York: McGraw-Hill, 1989:1807.
6. Triggs-Raine BL, Feigenbaum ASJ, Natowicz M, et al. Screening for carriers of Tay–Sachs disease among Ashkenazi Jews. N Engl J Med 1990;323:6.
7. American College of Obstetricians and Gynecologists. Screening for Canavan disease. Committee Opinion No. 212, November 1998.
8. Sidransky E, Ginns EI. Clinical heterogeneity among patients with Gaucher's disease. JAMA 1993;269:1154.
9. Barton NW, Brady RO, Dambrosia JM. Replacement therapy for inherited enzyme deficiency—macrophage-targeted glucocerebrosidase for Gaucher's disease. N Engl J Med 1991;324:1464.
10. Mistry PK, Smith SJ, Ali M, et al. Genetic diagnosis of Gaucher's disease. Lancet 1992;339:889.
11. Kerem B-S, Rommens JM, Buchanan JA, et al. Identification of the cystic fibrosis gene: genetic analysis. Science 1989;245:1073.
12. Genetic testing for cystic fibrosis. NIH Consensus Statement. 1997 April 14–16;15:1.
13. Vintzeileos AM, Ananth CV, Smulian JD, Fisher AJ, Day-Salvatore D, Beazoglou T. A cost-effectiveness analysis of prenatal carrier screening for cystic fibrosis. Obstet Gynecol 1998;91:529.
14. American College of Obstetrics and Gynecology. Management of isoimmunization in pregnancy. Educational Bulletin No. 227, August 1996.
15. Rossiter JP, Blakemore KJ, Kickler TS, et al. The use of polymerase chain reaction to determine fetal RhD status. Am J Obstet Gynecol 1995;171:1047.
16. Lighten AD, Overton TG, Sepulveda W, Warwick RM, Fisk NM, Bennett PR. Accuracy of prenatal determination of RhD type status by polymerase chain reaction with amniotic cells. Am J Obstet Gynecol 1995; 173:1182.
17. Easton DF, Ford D, Bishop DT, and the Breast Cancer Linkage Consortium. Breast and ovarian cancer incidence in BRCA-1 mutation carriers.
18. American College of Obstetrics and Gynecology. Maternal serum screening. Educational Bulletin No. 228, September 1996.
19. Luthy DA, Wardinsky T, Shurtloff DB, et al. Cesarean section before the onset of labor and subsequent motor function in infants with meningomyelocele diagnosed antenatally. N Engl J Med 1991;324:662.
20. Report of the U.K. Collaborative Study in relation to neural tube defects: maternal serum alpha fetoprotein measurements in antenatal screening for anencephaly and spina bifida in early pregnancy. Lancet 1977;1:1323.
21. Palomaki GE, Hill LE, Knight GJ, et al. Second-trimester maternal serum alpha-fetoprotein levels in pregnancies associated with gastroschisis and omphalocele. Obstet Gynecol 1988;71:906.
22. Wald N, Cuckle H, Boreham J, et al. The effect of maternal weight on maternal serum alpha-fetoprotein levels. Br J Obstet Gynaecol 1981;88:1094.
23. Baumgarten, A. Racial differences and biological significance of maternal serum alpha-fetoprotein. Lancet 1986; 2:573.
24. Wald NJ, Cuckle H, Boreham J, et al. Maternal serum alpha-fetoprotein and diabetes mellitus. Br J Obstet Gynaecol 1979;86:101.
25. Nicolaides KH, Campbell S, Gabbe S, et al. Ultrasound screening for spina bifida: cranial and cerebellar signs. Lancet 1986;2:72.
26. Whitehead N, MacMahon W, Fernhogff P, et al. Follow-up of elevated maternal serum alpha-fetoprotein levels: ultrasonography only or amniocentesis? Am J Obstet Gynecol 1991;164:1688.
27. Nadel AS, Green JK, Holmes LB, et al. Absence of need for amniocentesis in patients with elevated levels of maternal serum alpha-fetoprotein and normal ultrasonographic examinations. N Engl J Med 1990;323:557.
28. Ryyanen M, Seppala M, Kuusela P, et al. Antenatal screening for congenital nephrosis in Finland by maternal serum alpha-fetoprotein. Br J Obstet Gynaecol 1983; 90:437.
29. Hogge WA, Hogge JS, Schnatterly PT, et al. Congenital nephrosis: detection of index cases through maternal serum alpha-fetoprotein screening. Am J Obstet Gynecol 1992;167:1330.

30. Zelop C, Nadel A, Frigoletto FD, et al. Placenta accreta/percreta/increta: a cause of elevated maternal serum alpha-fetoprotein. Obstet Gynecol 1992;80:693.

31. Wald N, Cuckle H, Stirrat G. Maternal serum alpha-fetoprotein levels in triplet and quadruplet pregnancy. Br J Obstet Gynaecol 1978;85:124.

32. Ghosh A, Woo JSK, Rawlinson HA, et al. Prognostic significance of raised serum alpha-fetoprotein levels in twin pregnancies. Br J Obstet Gynaecol 1982;89:317.

33. Gosden C, Buckton K, Fotheringham Z, et al. Prenatal fetal karyotyping and maternal serum alpha-fetoprotein screening. BMJ 1981;282:255.

34. Bobrow M, Lindenbaum RH, Seabright M, et al. Karyotyping amniotic fluids from patients with high serum alpha-fetoprotein. Lancet 1981;1:606.

35. Warner AA, Pettenati MJ, Burton BK. Risk of fetal chromosomal anomalies in patients with elevated maternal serum alpha-fetoprotein. Obstet Gynecol 1990;75:64.

36. Barth WH, Frigoletto FD, Krauss MD, et al. Ultrasound detection of fetal aneuploidy in patients with elevated maternal serum alpha-fetoprotein. Obstet Gynecol 1991; 77:897.

37. Feuchtbaum LB, Cunningham G, Waller DK, Lustig LS, Tompkinson DG, Hook EB. Fetal karyotyping for chromosomal abnormalities after an unexplained elevated maternal serum alpha-fetoprotein screening. Obstet Gynecol 1995;86:248.

38. Simpson JL, Elias S, Morgan CD, et al. Does unexplained second-trimester (15 to 20 weeks gestation) maternal serum α-fetoprotein elevation presage adverse perinatal outcome? Am J Obstet Gynecol 1991;164:829.

39. Merkatz IR, Nitowsky HM, Macri JN, et al. An association between low maternal serum alpha-fetoprotein and fetal chromosomal abnormalities. Am J Obstet Gynecol 1984;148:886.

40. Cuckle HS, Wald NJ, Lindenbaum RH. Maternal serum alpha-fetoprotein measurement: a screening test for Down's syndrome. Lancet 1984;1:926.

41. Wald NJ, Cuckle HS, Densem JW, et al. Maternal serum screening for Down's syndrome in early pregnancy. BMJ 1986;297;883.

42. Wald NJ, Cuckle HS. Biochemical screening. In: Brock DJH, Rodeck CH, Ferguson-Smith MA, eds. Prenatal diagnosis and screening. London: Churchill Livingstone, 1992:566.

43. Knight GJ, Palomaki GE, Neveux LM, Fodor KK, Haddow JE. hCG and the free beta-subunit as screening tests for Down syndrome. Prenat Diagn 1998;18:235.

44. Wald NJ, Cuckle HS, Densem JW, et al. Maternal serum unconjugated oestriol as an antenatal screening test for Down's syndrome. Br J Obstet Gynaecol 1988;95:344.

45. Haddow JE, Palomaki GE, Knight GJ, et al. Prenatal screening for Down's syndrome with use of maternal serum markers. N Engl J Med 1992;327:588.

46. The New England Regional Genetics Group Collaborative Study of Down Syndrome Screening. Combining maternal serum alpha-fetoprotein measurements and age to screen for Down syndrome in pregnant women under age 35. Am J Obstet Gynecol 1989;160:575.

47. Canick JA, Palomaki GE, Osathanondh R. Prenatal screening for trisomy 18 in the second trimester. Prenat Diagn 1990;10:546.

48. Benn PA, Horne D, Briganti S, Greenstein RM. Prenatal diagnosis of diverse chromosome abnormalities in a population of patients identified by triple-marker testing as screen positive for Down syndrome. Am J Obstet Gynecol 1995;173:496.

49. Sheridan E, Williams J, Caine A, Morgan R, Mason G, Mueller RF. Counseling implications of chromosomal abnormalities other than trisomy 21 detected through a maternal serum screening programme. Br J Obstet Gynecol 1997;104:42.

50. Hook EB, Cross PK, Schreinemachers DM. Chromosomal abnormality rates at amniocentesis and in live-born infants. JAMA 1983;249:2034.

51. Haddow JE, Palomaki GE, Knight GJ, Cunningham GC, Lustig LS, Boyd PA. Reducing the need for amniocentesis in women 35 years of age or older with serum markers for screening. N Engl J Med 1994;330:1114.

52. Wenstrom, KD, Desai R, Owen J, DuBard MB, Boots L. Comparison of multiple-marker screening with amniocentesis for the detection of fetal aneuploidy in women >35 years old. Am J Obstet Gynecol 1995;173:1287.

53. Haddow JE, Palomaki GE, Knight GJ, Williams J, Miller WA, Johnson A. Screening of maternal serum for fetal Down syndrome in the first trimester. N Engl J Med 1998;338:955.

54. Wald NJ, George L, Smith D, Densem JW, Petterson K. Serum screening for Down syndrome between 8 and 14 weeks of pregnancy. International Prenatal Screening Research Group. Br J Obstet Gynaecol 1996;103:407.

55. Wheeler DM, Sinosich MJ. Prenatal screening in the first trimester of pregnancy. Prenat Diagn 1998;18:537.

56. Diagnostic ultrasound imaging in pregnancy. Bethesda, MD: Department of Health and Human Services, Publication No. 84-667, 1984.

57. Routine Ultrasound Examination in Pregnancy. London: Royal College of Obstetricians and Gynecologists, 1984.

58. Norwegian Institute for Hospital Research (Department of Social Affairs). Ultrasound in pregnancy: consensus statement, 1986. Int J Technol Assess Health Care 1987; 3:463.

59. Canadian Task Force Periodic Health Examination. 1992; Update(2) Routine prenatal.

60. Lys F, DeWals P, Borlee-Grimee I, et al. Evaluation of routine ultrasound examination for the prenatal diagnosis of malformation. Eur J Obstet Gynecol Reprod Biol 1989;30:101.

61. Li TM, Greenes RA, Weisburg M, et al. Data assessing the usefulness of screening obstetrical ultrasonography for detecting fetal and placental abnormalities in uncomplicated pregnancy: effects of screening a low-risk population. Med Decis Making 1988;8:48.

62. Levi S, Crouzet P, Schapps JP, et al. Ultrasound screening for fetal malformations. Lancet 1989;1:678.

63. Rosendahl H, Kivinen S. Antenatal detection of congenital malformations by routine ultrasonography. Obstet Gynecol 1989;73:947.

64. Sollie JE, Van Geijn HP, Arts NFT. Validity of a selective policy for ultrasound examination of fetal congenital anomalies. Eur J Obstet Gynecol Reprod Biol 1988; 27:125.

65. Shirley IM, Bottomley F, Robinson VP. Routine radiographer screening for fetal abnormalities by ultrasound in

an unselected low risk population. Br J Radiol 1992; 65:564.

66. Luck C. Value of routine ultrasound scanning at 19 weeks: a four year study of 8849 deliveries. BMJ 1992; 304:1474.

67. Chitty LS, Hunt GH, Moore J, et al. Effectiveness of routine ultrasonography in detecting fetal structural abnormalities in a low risk population. BMJ 1992; 303:1165.

68. Crane JP, LeFevre ML, Winborn RC, et al. A randomized trial of prenatal ultrasonographic screening: impact on the detection, management, and outcome of anomalous fetuses: the RADIUS Study Group. Am J Obstet Gynecol 1994;171:392.

69. Pitkin RM. Screening and detection of congenital malformation. Am J Obstet Gynecol 1991;164:1045.

70. Campbell S, Pearce JM. The prenatal diagnosis of fetal structural anomalies by ultrasound. Clin Obstet Gynecol 1983;10:475.

71. Manchester DK, Pretorius DH, Avery C, et al. Accuracy of ultrasound diagnoses in pregnancies complicated by suspected fetal anomalies. Prenat Diagn 1988;8:109.

72. Sabbagha RE, Sheikh Z, Tamura RK. Predictive value, sensitivity, and specificity of ultrasonic targeted imaging for fetal anomalies in gravid women at high risk for birth defects. Am J Obstet Gynecol 1985;152:822.

73. Allan LD, Crawford DC, Chita SK, et al. Prenatal screening for congenital heart disease. BMJ 1986;292:1717.

74. Allan LD. Cardiac ultrasound scanning. In: Drife JO, Donnai D, eds. Antenatal diagnosis of fetal anomalies. London: Springer-Verlag, 1991:97.

75. Rosendahl H, Kivinen S. Antenatal detection of congenital malformations by routine ultrasonography. Obstet Gynecol 1989;73:947.

76. Shirley IM, Bottomley F, Robinson VP. Routine radiographer screening for fetal abnormalities by ultrasound in an unselected low risk population. Br J Radiol 1992; 65:564.

77. Luck C. Value of routine ultrasound scanning at 19 weeks: a four year study of 8849 deliveries. BMJ 1992; 304:1474.

78. Chitty LS, Hunt GH, Moore J, et al. Effectiveness of routine ultrasonography in detecting fetal structural abnormalities in a low risk population. BMJ 1992; 303:1165.

79. Vergani P, Mariani S, Ghidini A, et al. Screening for congenital heart disease with the four-chamber view of the fetal heart. Am J Obstet Gynecol 1992;167:1000.

80. Achiron R, Glaser J, Gelernter I, et al. Extended fetal echocardiographic examination for detecting cardiac malformations in low risk pregnancies. BMJ 1992; 304:671.

81. Brocks V, Bang J. Routine examination by ultrasound for the detection of fetal malformations in a low risk population. Fetal Diagn Ther 1991;6:37.

82. Copel JA, Pilu G, Green J, et al. Fetal echocardiographic screening for congenital heart disease: the importance of the four-chamber view. Am J Obstet Gynecol 1987; 157:648.

83. Palmer CG, Miles JH, Howard Peebles PN, et al. Fetal karyotype following ascertainment of fetal anomalies by ultrasound. Prenat Diagn 1987;7:551.

84. Williamson RA, Weiner CP, Patil S. Abnormal pregnancy sonogram: selective indication for fetal karyotype. Obstet Gynecol 1987;69:15.

85. Wladimiroff JW, Sachs ES, Reuss A, et al. Prenatal diagnosis of chromosomal abnormalities in the presence of fetal structural defects. Am J Med Genet 1988;29:289.

86. Bundy AL, Saltzman DH, Pober B, et al. Antenatal sonographic findings in trisomy 18. J Ultrasound Med 1986; 5:361.

87. Benacerraf BR, Miller WA, Frigoletto FD. Sonographic detection of fetuses with trisomy 13 and 18: accuracy and limitations. Am J Obstet Gynecol 1988;158:404.

88. Nyberg DA, Resta RG, Luthy DA, et al. Prenatal sonographic findings of Down syndrome: review of 94 cases. Obstet Gynecol 1990;76:370.

89. Rizzo N, Pittalis MC, Pilu G, et al. Prenatal karyotype in malformed fetuses. Prenat Diagn 1990;10:17.

90. Copel JA, Cullen M, Green JJ, et al. The frequency of aneuploidy in prenatally diagnosed congenital heart disease: an indication for fetal karyotyping. Am J Obstet Gynecol 1988;158:409.

91. Hall B. Mongolism in newborn infants. Clin Pediatr 1966;5:4.

92. Toi A, Simpson GF, Filly RA. Ultrasonically evident fetal skin thickening: is it specific for Down syndrome? Am J Obstet Gynecol 1987;156:150.

93. Crane JP, Gray DL. Sonographically measured nuchal skinfold thickness as a screening tool for Down syndrome: results of a prospective clinical trial. Obstet Gynecol 1991;77:533.

94. Benacerraf BR, Laboda LA, Frigoletto FD. Thickened nuchal fold in fetuses not a risk for aneuploidy. Radiology 1992;184:239.

95. Bromley B, Doubliet P, Frigoletto FD, Krauss C, Estroff JA, Benacerraf BR. Is fetal hyperechoic bowel on second-trimester sonogram an indication for amniocentesis? Obstet Gynecol 1994;83:647.

96. Scioscia AL, Pretorius DH, Budorick NE, et al. Second-trimester echogenic bowel and chromosomal abnormalities. Am J Obstet Gynecol 1992;167:889.

97. Dicke JM, Crane JP. Sonographically detected hyperechoic fetal bowel: significance and implications for pregnancy management. Obstet Gynecol 1992;80:778.

98. MacGregor SN, Tamura R, Sabbagha R, Brenhofer JK, Kambich MP, Pergament E. Isolated hyperechoic fetal bowel: significance and implications for management. Am J Obtet Gynecol 1995;173;1254.

99. Vergani P, Locatelli A, Strobelt N, et al. Clinical outcome of mild ventriculomegaly. Am J Obstet Gynecol 1998; 178:218.

100. FitzSimmons J, Droste S, Shepard T, et al. Long-bone growth in fetuses with Down syndrome. Am J Obstet Gynecol 1989;161:1174.

101. Lockwood C, Benacerraf BR, Krinsky A, et al. A sonographic screening method for Down syndrome. Am J Obstet Gynecol 1987;157:803.

102. Benacerraf BR, Gelman R, Frigoletto FA. Sonographic identification of second trimester fetuses with Down's syndrome. N Engl J Med 1987;317:1371.

103. Cuckle H, Wald N, Quinn J, et al. Ultrasound femur length measurement in the screening for Down syndrome. Br J Obstet Gynaecol 1989;96:1373.

104. Lockwood CJ, Lynch L, Berkowitz RL. Ultrasonographic screening for the Down syndrome fetus. Am J Obstet Gynecol 1991;165:349.

105. Platt LD, Medearis AL, Carlson DE, et al. Screening for Down syndrome with the femur length/biparietal diameter ratio: a new twist of the data. Am J Obstet Gynecol 1992;167:124.

106. Lynch L, Berkowitz GS, Chitkara U, et al. Ultrasound detection of Down syndrome: is it really possible? Obstet Gynecol 1989;73:267.

107. Nyberg DA, Resta RG, Luthy DA, et al. Humerus and femur length shortening in the detection of Down's syndrome. Am J Obstet Gynecol 1993;168:534.

108. Grandjean H, Sarramon MF, et al. Femur/foot length ratio for the detection of Down syndrome: results of a multicenter prospective study. Am J Obstet Gynecol 1995;173:16.

109. Borrell A, Costa D, Ojuel J, Martinez JM, Seres A, Margarit E, Fortuny A. Limited effectiveness of femur and humerus shortening as markers of Down syndrome in early midtrimester fetuses. Fetal Diagn Ther 1997;12:156.

110. Rodis JF, Vintzileos AM, Fleming AD, et al. Comparison of humerus length with femur length in fetuses with Down syndrome. Am J Obstet Gynecol 1991;165:1051.

111. Benacerraf BR, Mandell J, Estroff JA, et al. Fetal pyelectasis: a possible association with Down syndrome. Obstet Gynecol 1990;76:58.

112. Corteville JE, Dicke JM, Crane JP. Fetal pyelectasis and Down syndrome: is genetic amniocentesis warranted? Obstet Gynecol 1992;79:770.

113. Morin L, Cendron M, Crombleholme TM, Garmel SH, Klauber GT, D'Alton ME. Minimal hydronephrosis in the fetus: clinical significance and implications for management. J Urol 1996;155:2047.

114. Fitzsimmons J, Wilson D, Pascoe-Mason J, Shaw CM, Cyr DR, Mack LA. Choroid plexus cysts in fetuses with trisomy 18. Obstet Gynecol 1989;73:257.

115. Reinsch RC. Choroid plexus cysts—association with trisomy: prospective review of 16,059 patients. Am J Obstet Gynecol 1997 176:1381.

116. Morcos CL, Platt LD, Carlson DE, Gregory KD, Greene NH, Korst LM. The isolated choroid plexus cyst. Obstet Gynecol 1998;92:232.

117. Gross SJ, Shulman LP, Tolley EA, et al. Isolated fetal choroid plexus cysts and trisomy 18: a review and meta-analysis. Am J Obstet Gynecol 1995;172:83.

118. DiGiovanni LM, Quinlan MP, Verp MS. Choroid plexus cysts: infant and early childhood developmental outcome. Obstet Gynecol 1997;90:191.

119. Bromley, B, Lieberman E, Shipp TA, Richardson M, Benacerraf BR. Significance of an echogenic intracardiac focus in fetuses at high and low risk for aneuploidy. J Ultrasound Med 1998;17:127.

120. Benacerraf BR, Harlow BL, Frigoletto FD. Hypoplasia of the middle phalanx of the fifth digit: a feature of the second trimester fetus with Down syndrome. J Ultrasound Med 1990;9:389.

121. Scott F, Boogert A, Sinosich M, et al. Establishment and application of a normal range for nuchal translucency across the first trimester. Prenat Diagn 1996;16:629.

122. Snijders RJM, Noble P, Sebire N, Souka A, Nicolaides KH, et al. UK Multicentre project on assessment of risk of trisomy 21 by maternal age and fetal nuchal-translucency thickness at 10–14 weeks of gestation. Lancet 1998;351:343.

123. Taipale P, Hiilesmaa V, Salonen R, Ylostalo P. Increased nuchal translucency as a marker for fetal chromosome defects. N Engl J Med 1997;337:1654.

124. Hafner E, Schuchter K, Liebhart E, Philipp K. Results of routine fetal nuchal translucency measurement at weeks 10-13 in 4233 unselected pregnant women. Prenat Diagn 1998;18:29.

125. Simpson NE, Dallaire L, Miller JR, et al. Prenatal diagnosis of genetic disease in Canada: report of a collaborative study. Can Med Assoc J 1976;115:739.

126. Working party on amniocentesis: an assessment of the hazards of amniocentesis. Br J Obstet Gynaecol 1978;85(Suppl):12.

127. Tabor A, Philip J, Madsen M, et al. Randomized controlled trial of genetic amniocentesis in 4606 low-risk women. Lancet 1986;1:1287.

128. Reid R, Sepulveda W, Kyle PM, Davies G. Amniotic fluid culture failure: clinical significance and association with aneuploidy. Obstet Gynecol 1996;87:588.

129. D'Alton ME, Malone FD, Chelmow D, Ward BE, Bianchi DW. Defining the role of fluorescence in situ hybridization on uncultured amniocytes for prenatal diagnosis of aneuploidies. Am J Obstet Gynecol. 1997;176:769.

130. Hsu LYF, Perlis TE. United States survey on chromosome mosaicism and pseudomosaicism in prenatal diagnosis. Prenat Diagn 1984;4:97.

131. Gosden C, Nicolaides KH, Rodeck CH. Fetal blood sampling in investigation of chromosome mosaicism in amniotic fluid cell culture. Lancet 1988;1:613.

132. Canadian Early and Mid-Trimester Amniocentesis Trial Group. Randomised trial to assess safety and fetal outcome of early and midtrimester amniocentesis. Lancet 1998;351:242.

133. Sundberg K, Bang J, Smidt-Jensen S, et al. Randomised study of risk of fetal loss related to early amniocentesis versus chorionic villus sampling. Lancet 1997; 350:697.

134. Kuliev A, Jackson L, Froster U, et al. Chorionic villus sampling safety: report of the World Health Organization. Am J Obstet Gynecol 1996;174:807.

135. Rhoads GG, Jackson LG, Schlesselman SE, et al. The safety and efficacy of chorionic villus sampling for early prenatal diagnosis of cytogenetic abnormalities. N Engl J Med 1989;320:609.

136. Ledbetter DH, Martin AO, Verlinsky Y, et al. Cytogenetic results of chorionic villus sampling: high success rate and diagnostic accuracy in the United States collaborative study. Am J Obstet Gynecol 1990;162:495.

137. Kalousek DK, Dill FJ, Pantzar T, et al. Confined chorionic mosaicism in prenatal diagnosis. Hum Genet 1987;77:163.

138. Shulman LP, Elias S. Percutaneous umbilical blood sampling, fetal skin sampling, and fetal liver biopsy. Semin Perinatol 1990;14:456.

139. Daffos F, Capella-Pavlovsky M, Forestier F. Fetal blood sampling during pregnancy with use of a needle guided by ultrasound: a study of 606 consecutive cases. Am J Obstet Gynecol 1985;153:655.

140. Evans MI, Greb A, Kunkel LM, et al. In utero fetal muscle biopsy for the diagnosis of Duchenne muscular dystrophy. Am J Obstet Gynecol 1991;165:728.

141. Kuliev A, Rechitsky S, Verlinsky O, et al. Preimplantation diagnosis of thalassemias. J Assist Reprod Genet 1998; 15:219.

142. Blaszczyk A, Tang YX, Dietz HC, et al. Preimplantation genetic diagnosis of human embryos for Marfan syndrome. J Assist Reprod Genet 1998;15:281.

143. Munne S, Scott R, Sable D, Cohen J. First pregnancies after preconception diagnosis of translocations of maternal origin. Fertil Steril 1998;69:675.

144. Ao A, Wells D, Handyside AH, Winston RM, Delhanty JD. Preimplantation diagnosis of inherited cancer: familial adenomatous polyposis coli. J Assist Reprod Genet 1998; 15:140.

145. Handyside AH, Lesko JG, Tarin JJ, et al. Birth of a normal girl after in vitro fertilization and preimplantation diagnostic testing for cystic fibrosis. N Engl J Med 1992; 327:905.

146. Sermon K, Lissens W, Joris H, et al. Clinical application of preimplantation diagnosis for myotonic dystrophy. Prenat Diagn 1997;17:925.

147. Bianchi DW, Flint AF, Pizzimenti MF, Knoll JH, Latt SA. Isolation of fetal DNA from nucleated erythrocytes in maternal blood. PNAS 1990; 87;3279.

148. Bianchi DW, Williams JM, Sullivan LM, Hanson FW, Klinger KW, Shuber AP. PCR quantitation of fetal cells in maternal blood in normal and aneuploid pregnancies. Am J Hum Genet 1997;61:822.

149. Takabayashi H, Kuwabara S, Ukita T, Ikawa K, Yamafuji K, Igarashi T. Development of non-invasive fetal DNA diagnosis from maternal blood. Prenat Diagn 1995;16:74.

150. Geifman-Holtzman O, Holtzman EJ, Vadnaid TJ, Phillops VE, Capeless EL, Bianchi DW. Detection of fetal HLA-DQa sequences in maternal blood: a gender independent technique of fetal cell identification. Prenat Diagn 1995; 15:261.

151. Sekizawa A, Kimura T, Sasaki M, Nazamura S, Kobayshi R, Sato T. Prenatal diagnosis of Duchenne muscular dystrophy using a single fetal nucleated erythrocyte in maternal blood. Neurology 1996;46:1350.

152. Sekizawa A, Watanabe A, Kimura T, Saito H, Yamihara T, Sato T. Prenatal diagnosis of the fetal RhD blood type using a single fetal nucleated erythrocyte from maternal blood. Obstet Gynecol 1996;87:501.

153. Watanabe A, Sekizawa A, Taguchi A, et al. Prenatal diagnosis of orthinine transcarbamylase deficiency by using a single nucleated erythrocyte from maternal blood. Hum Genet 1998;102:611.

154. Cheung MC, Goldberg JD, Golbus MS, Kan YW. Prenatal diagnosis of sickle cell anemia and thalassemia by analysis of fetal cells in maternal blood. Nat Genet 1996; 14:264.

155. Lo YMD, Hjelm NM, Fidler C, et al. Prenatal diagnosis of fetal RhD status by molecular analysis of maternal plasma. N Engl J Med 1998;339:1734.

Chapter 5
Infections in Pregnancy

Patrick Duff

Five Key Points

- The most common cause of urinary-tract infections in pregnant women is *Escherichia coli*.

- Intrapartum and postpartum infections are typically caused by multiple aerobic and anaerobic microorganisms.

- The maternal viral infections that pose the greatest risk to the developing fetus are rubella, cytomegalovirus, human immunodeficiency virus, and parvovirus.

- Perinatal transmission of hepatitis B can be almost entirely prevented by administration of hepatitis B immune globulin and hepatitis B vaccine to the neonate.

- The frequency of perinatal transmission of human immunodeficiency virus infection can be dramatically reduced by administration of optimal combination chemotherapy to the mother prior to and during delivery.

The purpose of this chapter is to review in detail the major maternal and perinatal infections that the obstetrician confronts in clinical practice. The first portion of the chapter focuses primarily on bacterial infections of the lower and upper genital tract. The second portion considers the viral, bacterial, and protozoal infections that pose special risks to the fetus.

VAGINAL INFECTIONS

Candidiasis

Candidiasis is responsible for approximately 25 to 30% of all cases of vaginitis.[1] The three principal organisms that cause symptomatic infection are, in descending order of frequency: *Candida albicans, C. tropicalis,* and *C. glabrata.* Candidiasis is not usually a sexually transmitted disease. Yeast are part of the nor-

mal vaginal flora in many women, and symptoms develop only when overgrowth of these organisms occurs. Several conditions predispose to symptomatic moniliasis, including recent antibiotic or corticosteroid therapy, diabetes, use of oral contraceptives, pregnancy, and immunodeficiency states. Serious systemic infections are uncommon unless the patient is receiving hyperalimentation or is immunocompromised.

Infected patients usually report vaginal and vulvar pruritus and a white, curd-like vaginal discharge. The vaginal pH is typically below 4.5. The vaginal mucosa and vulva may be erythematous and edematous; punctate, erythematous satellite lesions may be present on the lateral aspect of the vulva and medial aspect of the thighs. Figure 5-1 presents an algorithm for the diagnosis of vaginal infection.

The simplest test for confirmation of diagnosis is microscopic examination of a potassium hydroxide

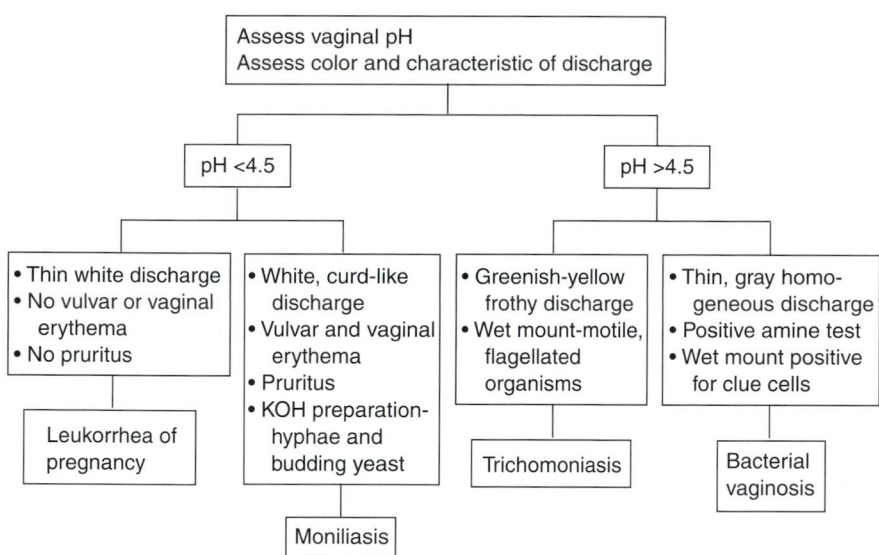

Figure 5-1 Algorithm for diagnosis of vaginal infection

preparation for hyphae, pseudohyphae, and budding yeast. Cultures are indicated only for patients who have persistent clinical findings and a negative microscopic examination and for those with recurrent infections who have had poor responses to treatment.

For uncomplicated Candida infections, topical therapy for 3 to 7 days with agents such as miconazole, terconazole, clotrimazole, and butoconazole is usually highly effective.[1] Treatment of women with persistent or recurrent infection is more problematic. These patients should be counseled about preventive measures such as avoidance of bubble baths, use of cotton undergarments, and close attention to perineal hygiene. In particularly refractory cases, administration of systemic antimicrobials such as ketoconazole or fluconazole should be considered because of their greater activity against reservoirs of yeast in the gastrointestinal tract. Neither drug has been studied extensively in pregnancy. However, fluconazole appears to have a more favorable toxicity profile. Fluconazole may be administered as a single 150-mg oral dose for treatment of the acute infection. In selected cases, weekly oral doses of 100 mg for 3 to 6 months may be necessary to suppress recurrent candidiasis. An alternative regimen for refractory cases is clotrimazole vaginal suppositories, 500 mg weekly. Boric acid should not be used in pregnancy because of possible teratogenic effects.[1,2] Similarly, the lack of substantive data supporting the safety of itraconazole in pregnancy and during lactation precludes its use until after delivery is complete and the infant no longer is breast-feeding.

Trichomoniasis

Trichomoniasis, a sexually transmitted disease caused by the protozoan *Trichomonas vaginalis*, is responsible for approximately 25% of cases of vaginitis. The organism is highly contagious; virtually 100% of women who have sexual contact with an infected partner contract the disease. Trichomoniasis has not been conclusively and consistently associated with serious maternal or neonatal complications.[1,3]

The usual symptoms of trichomoniasis are vaginal pruritus, superficial dyspareunia, frequency, dysuria, and a malodorous, yellow-green, frothy vaginal discharge. The vaginal mucosa is typically erythematous, and punctate hemorrhages may be present on the cervix ("strawberry cervix"). The pH of the vagina is usually in the range of 5 to 7 (see Figure 5-1).

The most useful test for rapid confirmation of infection is direct visualization of the flagellated organisms in a saline preparation (wet mount). The sensitivity of this test is 60 to 80%, depending on the size of the inoculum and the thoroughness with which the slide is inspected.[1,3] The Papanicolaou smear has similar sensitivity, but it is not as readily available to the office-based practitioner. *T. vaginalis* can be cultured on specialized media; however, culture is expensive and time-consuming, and is rarely indicated in clinical practice.

Metronidazole is the only antibiotic available in the United States that has consistent activity against *T. vaginalis*. Treatment efficacy is at least 95% if the patient is compliant and her sexual partner is treated concurrently. Absolute resistance of the organism to metronidazole is uncommon, and relative resistance can usually be overcome by administering the drug in higher doses for longer periods.

Metronidazole can be given in three oral dosage regimens: a single dose of 2 g; 250 mg three times daily for 7 days; or 500 mg twice daily for 7 days. The former dosage schedule improves compliance and reduces expense.[1,4]

In laboratory models, metronidazole has been associated with both mutagenicity and carcinogenecity. Although these effects have not been documented in humans, use of the drug in pregnancy, especially in the first trimester, still raises theoretical concerns. Accordingly, if the patient is relatively asymptomatic, treatment may be delayed until organogenesis is complete.[5]

Bacterial Vaginosis

Bacterial vaginosis (BV) is responsible for approximately 45% of cases of vaginitis.[1] It is a polymicrobial infection, and the predominant pathogens are anaerobes, *Gardnerella vaginalis,* Mobiluncus species, and genital mycoplasmas.[6] BV usually results from disturbances in the normal vaginal ecosystem caused by hormonal changes, pregnancy, or antibiotic administration. The

principal feature of this alteration in vaginal flora is a marked decrease in the Lactobacillus species that produce hydrogen peroxide and a corresponding increase in anaerobic organisms. In some instances, BV can result from sexual contact with an infected partner. In contrast to trichomoniasis and candidiasis, symptomatic BV in pregnancy has been associated with several serious maternal complications, including preterm labor, preterm premature rupture of membranes (PROM), chorioamnionitis, and puerperal endometritis.[7-10]

The most prominent clinical manifestation of BV is a thin, gray, homogeneous, malodorous vaginal discharge. Vulvar or vaginal pruritus is uncommon, and the vaginal pH is characteristically >4.5. When vaginal secretions are mixed with several drops of a 10% potassium hydroxide (KOH) solution, a pungent fishy odor is produced ("whiff test" or amine test). This same effect may be reproduced when vaginal secretions mix with seminal fluid. On microscopic examination of a saline preparation or Gram stain, the normal Lactobacillus flora is largely replaced by multiple small bacilli and cocci. Motile, comma-shaped Mobiluncus species and clue cells are present (Figure 5-2). The latter are vaginal epithelial cells whose outer surfaces are coated with multiple bacterial morphotypes. Culture

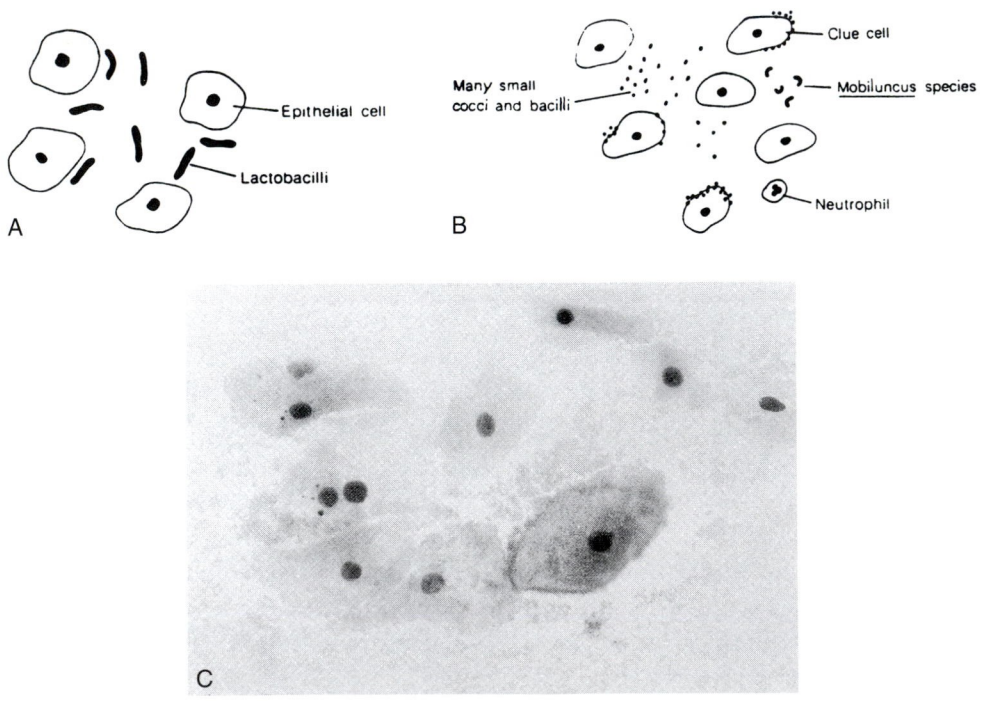

Figure 5-2 A. Schematic drawing of a normal vaginal smear. B. Schematic drawing of vaginal smear from a patient with bacterial vaginosis. C. Gram stain shows characteristic clue cell in a patient with bacterial vaginosis.

TABLE 5-1
TREATMENT OF BV IN PREGNANCY

Status of Patient	Drug	Dose	Approximate Cost of Treatment*
Low risk of preterm delivery	Oral metronidazole	250 mg PO tid for 7 days	$6.00
	Oral clindamycin	300 mg PO bid for 7 days	$22.00
	Metronidazole vaginal gel, 0.75%	1 applicatorful daily for 5 days	$33.00
High risk of preterm delivery	Oral metronidazole	250 mg PO tid for 7 days	$6.00
	Oral clindamycin	300 mg PO bid for 7 days	$22.00

TID = three times daily; BID = two times daily.

*1998 charges to patient at University of Florida outpatient pharmacy

of vaginal secretions is not indicated in routine clinical practice because isolation of a single organism such as *G. vaginalis* or Mobiluncus species is neither a necessary nor a sufficient condition for the diagnosis of BV (Figure 5-1).[11-13]

Because of the potential serious sequelae associated with BV, symptomatic low-risk and all high-risk pregnant patients (i.e., those with a history of preterm delivery, preterm PROM in the present pregnancy, or weight less than ideal body weight) should be screened for this condition and treated once the diagnosis is established. Concurrent treatment of the woman's sexual partner(s) has not been shown to improve outcome or prevent recurrences. The value of routine screening for BV in asymptomatic, low-risk patients has not been established.

As outlined in Table 5-1, low-risk women with BV may be treated with one of three regimens. High-risk women should be treated only with systemic antibiotics. Treatment of high-risk patients significantly reduces the risk of preterm delivery.[4,14-16]

ENDOCERVICAL INFECTIONS

Chlamydia

Chlamydia trachomatis can cause localized infection of the urethra, endocervix, and rectum. It also is responsible for most cases of perihepatitis (Fitz–Hugh–Curtis syndrome). Conjunctivitis or pneumonia may develop in infants delivered to infected women. The former complication occurs in up to 50% of infants delivered to infected mothers; the latter complication affects 3 to 18% of infants.[17]

C. trachomatis cannot be cultivated in artificial media, and isolation in tissue culture is relatively expen-

sive and time-consuming. Fortunately, less expensive, rapid nucleic acid probes such as polymerase chain reaction (PCR) and ligase chain reaction (LCR) are sufficiently sensitive to justify their clinical use for identification of chlamydial infection. In high-risk populations, the sensitivity and specificity of these tests exceed 90%. The latter method is particularly attractive because it seems to be equally accurate for both urine and endocervical specimens.[18,19]

Although tetracycline and doxycycline have the greatest activity against *C. trachomatis*, these drugs should not be used in pregnancy because of their potential harmful effects on fetal teeth. From the perspective of cost, ease of compliance, tolerability, and efficacy, the agent of choice in pregnancy is azithromycin powder, 1 g in a single dose.[20,21] Alternative regimens include erythromycin base, 500 mg four times daily for 7 days; erythromycin base, 250 mg four times daily for 14 days; erythromycin ethylsuccinate, 800 mg four times daily for 7 days; erythromycin ethylsuccinate, 400 mg four times daily for 14 days; or amoxicillin, 500 mg three times daily for 7 days.[4,22] The latter drugs are more likely than azithromycin to cause nausea, vomiting, or diarrhea. Moreover, the multidose, 7- to 14-day regimens do not facilitate patient compliance. Neonates delivered to infected mothers should receive prophylaxis with tetracycline or erythromycin ophthalmic preparations and be observed for evidence of an ensuing respiratory tract infection.

Gonorrhea

Gonorrhea is caused by the gram-negative, intracellular diplococcus *Neisseria gonorrhoeae*. The infection is transmitted primarily by sexual contact. It also may be transmitted perinatally from mother to infant and cause serious ophthalmic injury.

In pregnant women, gonorrhea may be manifested as an asymptomatic to mildly symptomatic localized infection of the urethra, endocervix, or rectum. Local infection may increase the risk of preterm labor and preterm PROM and predispose to intrapartum and postpartum infection. Gonorrhea also may present as a disseminated infection.[23] The most common manifestation of disseminated gonococcal infection is arthritis, typically affecting several small- to medium-sized joints. The next most common manifestation is a diffuse violaceous, papular skin rash. Less common, but potentially more serious, sequelae of disseminated infection include meningitis, pericarditis, endocarditis, and perihepatitis (Fitz–Hugh–Curtis syndrome).

The most reliable and inexpensive test for confirmation of gonococcal infection is culture of the organism on selective agar such as Thayer–Martin medium. Gram stain and nucleic acid probes are helpful when positive, but their sensitivity varies widely.[24,25] The newer LCR assay appears to offer greater sensitivity than the earlier generation of nucleic acid probes and permits simultaneous testing of samples for both *C. trachomatis* and *N. gonorrhoeae*.[26]

The drugs of choice for treating localized gonococcal infections in pregnancy are ceftriaxone, 125 mg intramuscularly in a single dose, and cefixime, 400 mg in a single oral dose.[4] Ceftriaxone is the preferred agent for treatment of disseminated infection and should be administered in a dose of 1 g intravenously or intramuscularly every 24 hours until a clinical response has been achieved. Tetracyclines and quinolones should not be used in pregnancy because of their injurious effects on fetal teeth and cartilage, respectively. Patients who are allergic to β-lactam antibiotics may be treated with a single 2-g intramuscular dose of spectinomycin. Treatment of the neonate with either silver nitrate or tetracycline ophthalmic preparations is effective in preventing most cases of ophthalmia neonatorum.[4]

URINARY-TRACT INFECTIONS

Acute Urethritis

Acute urethritis (acute urethral syndrome) is usually caused by one of three organisms: *Escherichia coli*, *N. gonorrhoeae*, or *C. trachomatis*.[27] Coliform organisms are part of the normal vaginal and perineal flora and may be introduced into the urethra during intercourse or when wiping after defecation. *N. gonorrhoeae* and *C. trachomatis* are sexually transmitted pathogens.

Affected patients typically experience frequency, urgency, and dysuria. Hesitancy, dribbling, and a mucopurulent urethral discharge may be present. On microscopic examination, the urine usually has white cells, but bacteria are not consistently present. Urine cultures may have low colony counts of coliform organisms, and examination of the urethral discharge may be positive for gonorrhea and chlamydia.

Most patients with acute urethritis warrant empiric treatment before the results of microbiologic tests are available. Infections caused by coliforms will usually respond to the antibiotics described below for treatment of asymptomatic bacteriuria and cystitis. If gonococcal infection is suspected, the patient should be treated with single doses of either oral cefixime, 400 mg, or intramuscular ceftriaxone, 125 mg. The former is approximately one-third the cost of the latter. If the patient is allergic to β-lactam antibiotics, an effective alternative is spectinomycin, administered intramuscularly in a single dose of 2 g. If chlamydial infection is suspected, the patient should be treated with azithromycin powder, 1 g orally. The sexual partners of patients with gonorrhea or chlamydia also should be treated with similar regimens.[4]

Asymptomatic Bacteriuria and Acute Cystitis

The prevalence of asymptomatic bacteriuria in pregnancy is 5 to 10%, and the majority of cases antedate the onset of pregnancy. The frequency of acute cystitis in pregnancy is 1 to 3%. Some cases of cystitis arise de novo; others develop as a result of failure to identify or treat asymptomatic bacteriuria.[27]

E. coli is responsible for 80 to 90% of cases of initial infections and 70 to 80% of recurrent cases. *Klebsiella pneumoniae* and Proteus species also are important pathogens, particularly in patients who have a history of recurrent infection, and each organism is responsible for 5 to 10% of infections. Approximately 3 to 7% of infections will be caused by gram-positive organisms such as group B streptococci, enterococci, and staphylococci.[27]

All pregnant women should be tested at their first prenatal appointment for preexisting asymptomatic bacteriuria. Although culture has been the gold standard for diagnosis of urinary-tract infection (UTI), the rapid dipstick tests for nitrites and leukocyte esterase have very good sensitivity and certainly could be used as a cost-saving measure in lieu of culture for the initial screening of asymptomatic, low-risk women.[28] If the initial screening test is negative, the likelihood of the patient subsequently developing an asymptomatic infection is 5% or less. If the test is positive, prompt treatment is necessary to prevent ascending infection.[27,29]

Patients with acute cystitis usually have symptoms of frequency, dysuria, urgency, suprapubic pain, hesitancy, and dribbling. Gross hematuria may be present, but fever and systemic symptoms are uncommon. In symptomatic patients, microscopic examination of the urine shows white cells and bacteria. The leukocyte esterase and nitrite tests will usually be positive if urine has been incubating in the bladder for several hours. When a urine culture is obtained, a catheterized sample is preferred because it minimizes the probability that urine will be contaminated by vaginal flora. In a symptomatic patient, particularly when urine is obtained by catheterization, a colony count of $\geq 10^2$/ml should be considered indicative of infection.[30]

Asymptomatic bacteriuria and acute cystitis characteristically respond well to short courses of oral antibiotics. Single-dose therapy is not as effective in pregnant women as in nonpregnant patients. However, a 3-day course of treatment appears to be comparable to a 7- to 10-day regimen, at least for an initial infection. The longer courses of therapy are more appropriate for patients with recurrent infections.[31]

When sensitivity tests are available (e.g., in patients with asymptomatic bacteriuria), they may be used to guide antibiotic selection. When empiric treatment is indicated, the choice of antibiotics must be based on established patterns of susceptibility. In recent years, 20 to 30% of strains of E. coli have developed resistance to ampicillin; thus, this drug should not be used when the results of sensitivity tests are unknown.[32] In addition, even if the organism is sensitive to ampicillin, other drugs are less likely to cause adverse effects such as monilial vaginitis and antibiotic-induced diarrhea. Two such agents are trimethoprim (160 mg) plus sulfamethoxazole (800 mg) (one tablet orally twice daily) and nitrofurantoin monohydrate-sustained release (100 mg orally twice daily).[27,31] Quinolone antibiotics are highly effective against most uropathogens, but they are contraindicated in pregnancy because of teratogenic effects on fetal cartilage. The combination agent, amoxicillin–clavulanate (875 mg orally twice daily), also has excellent activity against the broad range of uropathogens. However, the drug is very expensive and should be reserved for complicated UTIs caused by organisms resistant to less expensive antibiotics.

For patients who have an initial infection and experience a prompt response to treatment, a urine culture for test of cure is probably unnecessary. Cultures during, or immediately after, treatment are indicated for patients who respond to therapy poorly or who have a history of recurrent infection. During subsequent clinic appointments, the patient's urine should be screened for nitrites and leukocyte esterase.[28] If either of these tests is positive, repeat urine culture and retreatment are indicated.

Acute Pyelonephritis

The incidence of pyelonephritis in pregnancy is 1 to 2%. The vast majority of cases develop as a consequence of undiagnosed or inadequately treated lower-urinary-tract infection. Two major physiologic changes occur during pregnancy that predispose to ascending infection of the urinary tract. First, the high concentration of progesterone secreted by the placenta has an inhibitory effect on ureteral peristalsis. Second, the enlarging gravid uterus often compresses the ureters, particularly the right, at the pelvic brim, thus creating additional stasis. Stasis, in turn, facilitates migration of bacteria from the bladder into the ureters and renal parenchyma.[29]

Approximately 75 to 80% of cases of pyelonephritis occur on the right side; 10 to 15% are left-sided, and a slightly smaller percentage are bilateral. E. coli is again the principal pathogen. K. pneumoniae and Proteus species also are important causes of infection, particularly in women with recurrent episodes of pyelonephritis. Highly virulent gram-negative bacilli, such as Pseudomonas, Enterobacter, and Serratia, are unusual isolates except in immunocompromised patients. Gram-positive cocci do not usually cause upper-tract infection. Anaerobes also are unlikely pathogens unless the patient is chronically obstructed or has an indwelling bladder or ureteral catheter.[29]

The usual clinical manifestations of acute pyelonephritis in pregnancy are fever, chills, flank pain and tenderness, frequency, urgency, hematuria, and dysuria. Patients also may have signs of preterm labor, septic shock, and adult respiratory distress syndrome (ARDS). The urine dipstick test is usually positive for leukocyte esterase and nitrites. Urine colony counts greater than 10^2 colonies/ml from a specimen obtained by catheterization confirm the diagnosis of infection.

Pregnant patients with pyelonephritis may be considered for outpatient therapy if their disease manifestations are mild, they are hemodynamically stable, and they have no evidence of preterm labor.[33] If an outpatient approach is adopted, the patient should be treated with agents that have a high level of activity against the common uropathogens. Acceptable oral agents include amoxicillin–clavulanate, 875 mg twice daily, or trimethoprim (160 mg) plus sulfamethoxazole (80 mg) twice daily for 7 to 10 days. Alternatively, a visiting nurse could administer a parenteral agent such as ceftriaxone, 2 g intramuscularly or intravenously, once daily.

Pregnant patients who appear to be seriously ill or who show any signs of preterm labor should be hospitalized for intravenous antibiotic therapy.[29] They should receive appropriate supportive treatment and be monitored closely for complications such as sepsis and ARDS. One of the best choices for empiric intravenous antibiotic therapy is cefazolin, 1 g every 8 hours.[32] For hospitalized patients, this drug is less expensive to administer than the newer broader-spectrum cephalosporins or penicillins and has an equivalent spectrum of activity against the coliform organisms most likely to be responsible for infection. If the patient is critically ill or is at high risk for a resistant organism, a second antibiotic, such as gentamicin (1.5 mg/kg every 8 hours) or aztreonam (500 mg to 1 g every 8 to 12 hours) should be administered, along with cefazolin, until the results of susceptibility tests are available.[27]

By the end of 72 hours of treatment, almost 95% of patients will be afebrile and asymptomatic. The two most likely causes of treatment failure are a resistant microorganism or urinary-tract obstruction.[34] The latter condition is best diagnosed with renal ultrasonography and typically results from a stone or physical compression of the ureter by the gravid uterus.

Once the patient has begun to defervesce and her clinical examination has improved, she may be discharged from the hospital. Oral antibiotics should be prescribed to complete a total of 7 to 10 days of therapy. Selection of a specific oral agent should be based on considerations of efficacy, toxicity, and expense.[27]

Recurrent UTI will develop later in pregnancy in approximately 20 to 30% of pregnant patients with acute pyelonephritis.[29] The most cost-effective way to reduce the frequency of recurrence is to administer a daily prophylactic dose of an antibiotic, such as sulfisoxazole, 1 g, or nitrofurantoin monohydrate-sustained release, 100 mg.[27] Patients receiving prophylaxis should have their urine screened for bacteria at each subsequent clinic appointment. They also should be questioned about recurrence of symptoms. If symptoms recur, or the dipstick test for nitrites or leukocyte esterase is positive, a urine culture should be obtained to determine if retreatment is necessary.

Figure 5-3 presents a simplified algorithm for the management of pyelonephritis in pregnancy.

CHORIOAMNIONITIS

Chorioamnionitis (amnionitis, intraamniotic infection) occurs in approximately 1 to 5% of term pregnancies.[35] In patients with preterm delivery, the frequency of infection may approach 25%.[36] Chorioamnionitis is usually an ascending infection caused by organisms that are part of the normal vaginal flora. The principal pathogens are Bacteroides and Prevotella species, *E. coli*, anaerobic gram-positive organisms (Peptococci species and Peptostreptococci species), and group B streptococci. Several clinical risk factors for chorioamnionitis have been identified. The most important are young age, low socioeconomic status, nulliparity, extended duration of labor and ruptured membranes, multiple vaginal examinations, and preexisting infections of the lower genital tract such as bacterial vaginosis and group B streptococcal infection.

The diagnosis of chorioamnionitis can usually be established on the basis of the clinical findings of maternal fever and maternal and fetal tachycardia, in the absence of other localizing signs of infection.[35] Laboratory confirmation of the diagnosis of chorioamnionitis is not routinely necessary in laboring, term patients. However, in preterm patients who are being evaluated for tocolysis or corticosteroids, laboratory assessment may be necessary to confirm the diagnosis of intrauterine infection. In this clinical context, amniotic fluid should be obtained by transabdominal amniocentesis and tested for leukocyte esterase, glucose concentration (abnormal <15 mg/dl), and Gram stain.[37-40] Amniotic fluid cultures require a minimum of 48 to 72 hours before results are available and, thus, they are not of immediate value in making clinical

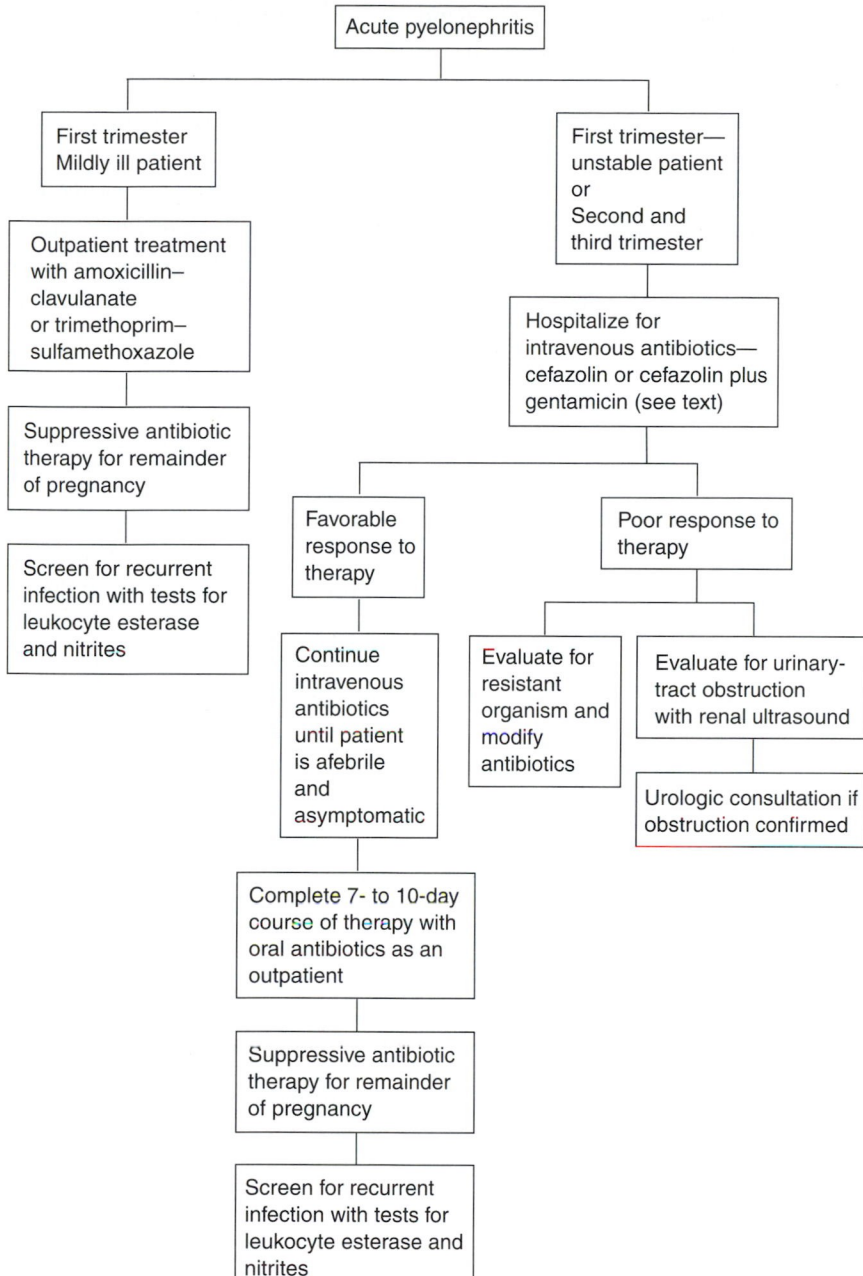

Figure 5-3 Management algorithm for acute pyelonephritis in pregnancy

decisions. The most sensitive test for diagnosis of chorioamnionitis is detection of elevated concentrations of interleukin-6 in the amniotic fluid. However, this test is not yet adapted for the rapid turnaround necessary for clinical decision making.[41]

Both the mother and infant may experience serious complications when chorioamnionitis is present. Bacteremia occurs in 3 to 12% of infected women. When cesarean delivery is required, wound infections develop in 3 to 8% of women, and approximately 1% develop a pelvic abscess. Fortunately, maternal death due to infection is exceedingly rare.[35]

Five to 10% of neonates delivered to mothers with chorioamnionitis have pneumonia and/or bacteremia. The predominant organisms responsible for these infections are group B streptococci and *E. coli*. Meningitis occurs in 1% or less of term infants and in a slightly higher percentage of preterm infants. Mortality due to infection ranges from 1 to 4% in term neonates but may approach 15% in preterm infants because of the confounding effects of other complications such as hyaline membrane disease and intraventricular hemorrhage.[24]

To prevent maternal and neonatal complications, parenteral antibiotic therapy should be initiated as soon as the diagnosis of chorioamnionitis is made, unless delivery is imminent. Three separate investigations have demonstrated that mother–infant pairs who receive prompt intrapartum treatment have better outcomes than patients treated after delivery.[42-44] The principal benefits of early treatment include decreased frequency of neonatal bacteremia and pneumonia and decreased duration of maternal fever and hospitalization.

The most extensively tested intravenous antibiotic regimen for treatment of chorioamnionitis is the combination of ampicillin (2 g every 6 hours) or penicillin (5 million units every 6 hours) plus gentamicin (1.5 mg/kg every 8 hours). These antibiotics specifically target the two organisms most likely to cause neonatal infection: group B streptococci and *E. coli*.[35] With rare exceptions, gentamicin is preferred to tobramycin or amikacin because it is available in an inexpensive generic formulation. Amikacin should be reserved for immunocompromised patients who are particularly likely to be infected by highly virulent, drug-resistant aerobic gram-negative bacilli. In patients who are allergic to β-lactam antibiotics, vancomycin (500 mg every 6 hours or 1 g every 12 hours), erythromycin (500 mg to 1 g every 6 hours), or clindamycin (900 mg every 8 hours) can be substituted for ampicillin or penicillin.

If a patient with chorioamnionitis requires cesarean delivery, a drug with activity against anaerobic organisms should be added to the antibiotic regimen postoperatively. Either clindamycin (900 mg every 8 hours) or metronidazole (500 mg every 12 hours) is an excellent choice for this purpose.[24,35] The latter agent is less expensive.

Extended-spectrum cephalosporins, penicillins, and carbapenems also provide excellent coverage against the bacteria that cause chorioamnionitis. Less information is available concerning the effectiveness of these drugs as compared with the ampicillin or penicillin-plus-gentamicin regimen. In addition, the toxicity profile for the fetus and neonate has not been as well delineated, and the drugs usually are more expensive than the combination regimens because they are not yet available in generic formulations.

As a general rule, parenteral antibiotics should be continued until the patient has been afebrile and asymptomatic for approximately 24 hours. Once an adequate clinical response has been achieved, antibiotics may be discontinued and the patient discharged. A course of oral antibiotics administered as an outpatient is rarely indicated.[24,35]

Chapman and Owen[45] have described an interesting approach to treatment of chorioamnionitis. They evaluated 109 women who had vaginal deliveries complicated by intrapartum infection. They assigned 55 women to receive a single intravenous dose of cefotetan (2 g) in the recovery room and 54 women to receive intravenous cefotetan (2 g) every 12 hours for a minimum of 48 hours. The principal outcome variable was length of postpartum hospitalization. The median interval from delivery to discharge was 24 hours lower in the single-dose group (33 hours vs. 57 hours, $p = 0.0001$). The incidence of failed therapy was 11% (6/55) in the single-dose group, as compared with 3.7% (2/54) in the multidose group. Although this observed difference was not statistically significant, a much larger sample size would be necessary to confidently conclude that no clinically meaningful difference in treatment effect exists.

Patients with chorioamnionitis are at increased risk for dysfunctional labor. Approximately 75% require oxytocin for augmentation of labor, and up to 30 to 40% require cesarean delivery, usually for failure to progress in labor.[24,46] While chorioamnionitis by itself should not be regarded as an indication for cesarean delivery, affected patients need close monitoring during labor to ensure that uterine contractility is optimized. In addition, the fetus also needs close surveillance. Fetal heart rate abnormalities such as tachycardia and decreased variability occur in over three-fourths of cases, and additional tests such as vibroacoustic stimulation, scalp stimulation, or scalp pH assessment may be necessary to evaluate fetal well-being.

PUERPERAL ENDOMETRITIS

The frequency of puerperal endometritis in women having vaginal delivery is approximately 1 to 3%. In women having a scheduled cesarean delivery prior to the onset of labor and rupture of membranes, the frequency of endometritis ranges from 5 to 15%. When cesarean delivery is performed after an extended period of labor and ruptured membranes, the incidence of infection is 30 to 35% without antibiotic prophylaxis and 15 to 20% with prophylaxis. In highly indigent patient populations, the frequency of infection may be almost double the figures cited above.[47]

Endometritis is a polymicrobial infection caused by microorganisms that are part of the normal vaginal flora. These bacteria gain access to the upper genital tract, peritoneal cavity, and, occasionally, the bloodstream as a result of vaginal examinations during labor and manipulations during surgery. The most common pathogenic bacteria are group B streptococci, anaerobic gram-positive cocci (Peptococci species and Peptostreptococci species), aerobic gram-negative bacilli (predominantly *E. coli, K. pneumoniae,* and Proteus species), and anaerobic gram-negative bacilli (principally Bacteroides and Prevotella species). *C. trachomatis* is not a common cause of early onset puerperal endometritis but has been implicated in late-onset infection. Similarly, the genital mycoplasmas are uncommon pathogens in patients with puerperal endometritis.[47]

The principal risk factors for endometritis are cesarean delivery, young age, low socioeconomic status, extended duration of labor and ruptured membranes, and multiple vaginal examinations. In addition, preexisting infection or colonization of the lower genital tract (gonorrhea, group B streptococci, bacterial vaginosis) and invasive internal monitoring also predispose to ascending infection.[24,47]

Affected patients typically have a fever of 38°C or higher within 36 hours of delivery. Other clinical findings include malaise, tachycardia, lower abdominal pain and tenderness, uterine tenderness, and discolored, malodorous lochia. A small number of patients also may have an inflammatory mass in the broad ligament, posterior cul-de-sac, or retrovesicular space.

The initial differential diagnosis of puerperal fever should include endometritis, atelectasis, pneumonia, viral syndrome, pyelonephritis, and appendicitis. Distinction among these disorders usually can be made on the basis of physical examination and a limited number of laboratory tests such as white-cell count, urinalysis and culture, and, in select patients, chest x-ray films. Endometrial cultures rarely are of value in making clinical decisions and should not routinely be obtained. Blood cultures are indicated only in patients who are immunocompromised or at increased risk for bacterial endocarditis or who fail to respond to initial therapy.[24,47]

Patients who have mild to moderately severe infections, particularly after vaginal delivery, can be treated with short intravenous courses of single agents such as the extended-spectrum cephalosporins and penicillins. Single-agent therapy with the carbapenem antibiotics (imipenem–cilastatin or meropenem) or combination antibiotic regimens should be considered for more severely ill patients, particularly those who are indigent and in poor general health and those who have had cesarean deliveries.[24,47,48] Table 5-2 lists several antibiotic regimens that are of proven efficacy and reasonable cost.

Once antibiotics are begun, approximately 90% of patients will defervesce within 48 to 72 hours. When the patient has been afebrile and asymptomatic for approximately 24 hours, parenteral antibiotics should be discontinued and the patient should be discharged. As a general rule, an extended course of oral antibiotics is not necessary following discharge.[49] There are at least two notable exceptions to this rule. First, patients who have had a vaginal delivery and who defervesce within 24 hours are candidates for early discharge. In these individuals, a short course of an oral antibiotic such as amoxicillin–clavulanate (875 mg twice daily) may be substituted for continued parenteral therapy. Second, patients who have had a

TABLE 5-2 COST-EFFECTIVE ANTIBIOTIC SELECTION FOR TREATMENT OF PUERPERAL ENDOMETRITIS		
Severity of Infection	**Antibiotic**	**Intravenous Dose**
Mild to moderate	Ampicillin–sulbactam	3 g q6h
	Ticarcillin–clavulanate	3.1 g q6h
	Cefotaxime	1–2 g q8h
	Cefotetan	2 g q12h
	Ceftizoxime	2 g q8–12h
Severe (especially after cesarean delivery)	Imipenem-cilastatin	500 mg q6h
	Meropenem	1 g q8h
	Clindamycin	900 mg q8h
	plus gentamicin	7 mg/kg/IBW q24h
	Penicillin	5 million units q6h
	plus metronidazole	500 mg q12h
	plus gentamicin	7 mg/kg/IBW q24h

IBW = ideal body weight.

staphylococcal bacteremia require a more extended period of administration of parenteral and oral antibiotics with specific antistaphylococcal activity (i.e., 10–21 days depending on the severity of the patient's illness and the response to therapy).[50]

Patients who fail to respond to the antibiotic therapy outlined above usually have one of two problems. The first is a resistant organism. The second major cause of treatment failure is a wound infection. Infected wounds should be opened completely to provide drainage. If extensive cellulitis at the margin of the incision is present,

an antibiotic with specific coverage against staphylococci, such as nafcillin sodium (500 to 1000 mg q4h), should be added to the treatment regimen.

When changes in antibiotic therapy do not result in clinical improvement and no evidence of wound infection is present, the following disorders should be considered: pelvic abscess, septic pelvic vein thrombophlebitis, drug fever, mastitis, and recrudescence of connective-tissue disease.[47] Figure 5-4 presents an algorithm for the evaluation and treatment of a patient with persistent postpartum fever.

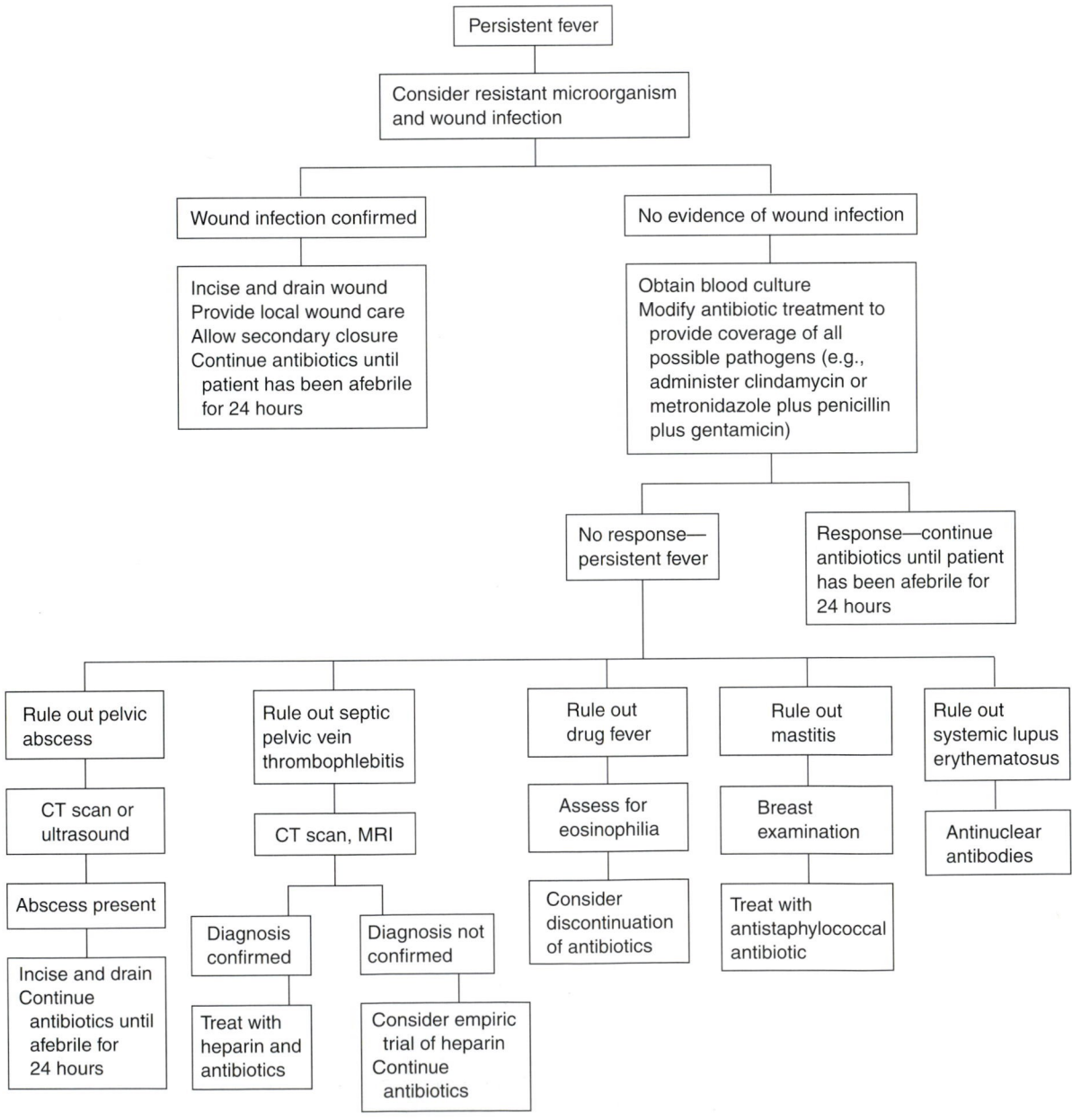

Figure 5-4 Algorithm for evaluation and management of a patient with persistent post-partum fever

Prevention of Puerperal Endometritis

Prophylactic antibiotics are clearly of value in reducing the frequency of postcesarean endometritis, particularly in women having surgery after an extended period of labor and ruptured membranes. The most appropriate agent for prophylaxis is a limited-spectrum (first-generation) cephalosporin, such as cefazolin. Cefazolin should be administered in an intravenous dose of 1 g immediately after the neonate's umbilical cord is clamped. A second dose should be given 8 hours after the first dose in exceptionally high-risk patients, especially when operating time is prolonged beyond 1 hour. In other patients, a single dose is usually adequate. Although extended-spectrum penicillins and cephalosporins are effective for prophylaxis, they offer no advantage over cefazolin and are severalfold more expensive. Moreover, widespread use of these drugs for prophylaxis may ultimately limit their usefulness for treatment of established infections.[51]

For patients who have an immediate hypersensitivity to β-lactam antibiotics, the most reasonable alternative is to administer a single dose of clindamycin (900 mg) plus gentamicin (1.5 mg/kg). Although these antibiotics are commonly used for treatment of overt infections, their administration is still warranted in penicillin-allergic patients who are at high risk for postoperative infection.

CYTOMEGALOVIRUS INFECTION

Epidemiology

Cytomegalovirus (CMV) is a double-stranded DNA virus that replicates within the nucleus of an infected cell. Humans are its only known host. Like herpes simplex virus, CMV may remain latent in host cells after the initial infection. Recurrent infection is usually due to reactivation of endogenous latent virus rather than reinfection with a new strain of virus.

CMV is not highly contagious, and, therefore, close personal contact is required for infection to occur. Horizontal transmission may result from transplantation of an infected organ or blood, from sexual contact, or from contact with contaminated saliva or urine. Vertical transmission may occur as a result of transplacental infection, exposure to contaminated genital tract secretions during delivery, or breastfeeding. The incubation period of the virus ranges from 28 to 60 days, with a mean of 40 days.[52]

Among young children, the most important risk factor for infection is close contact with playmates, particularly in the setting of day care. Infected children clearly pose a risk of transmitting virus to adult day-care workers. Small children also pose a risk to members of their own family.[53] In addition to acquiring infection from young children, adolescents and adults may develop infection as a result of sexual contact. CMV infection is endemic among homosexual men and heterosexuals with multiple partners. Additional risk factors for infection include lower socioeconomic status, history of abnormal cervical cytology, birth outside of North America, first pregnancy at less than 15 years, and coinfection with other sexually transmitted diseases such as trichomoniasis.[52,54]

Most children who acquire CMV infection are asymptomatic. When clinical manifestations are present, they include malaise, fever, lymphadenopathy, and hepatosplenomegaly. Similarly, most immunocompetent adults with primary or recurrent CMV are asymptomatic or have mild symptoms suggestive of mononucleosis. Severe respiratory infection due to CMV may occur in patients with immunodeficiency disorders such as HIV infection.

Diagnosis

The diagnosis of CMV infection can be confirmed by isolation of virus in tissue culture. The highest concentration of CMV is usually present in urine, seminal fluid, saliva, and breast milk. Techniques such as immunofluorescence staining and polymerase chain reaction permit identification of viral antigen within 24 hours.[52]

Serologic methods also are helpful in establishing the diagnosis of CMV infection provided that the reference laboratory is skilled in performing such tests. In the acute phase of infection, virus-specific IgM antibody is present in serum. IgM titers usually decline rapidly over a period of 30 to 60 days but can remain elevated for many months. There is no absolute IgG titer that clearly differentiates acute from recurrent infection. However, a fourfold or greater change in the IgG titer is consistent with recent acute infection.

Obstetric Considerations

As a result of exposure to either young children or an infected sexual partner, approximately 50 to 80% of adult women in the United States have serologic evidence of past CMV infection. Unfortunately, the presence of antibody is not perfectly protective against vertical transmission, and, thus, pregnant women with both recurrent and primary infection pose a special risk to their fetus. Fetal and neonatal CMV infection may occur at three distinct times: antepartum, intrapartum, and postpartum.[55]

Antepartum or congenital infection poses the greatest risk to the fetus and results from hematogenous dissemination of virus across the placenta. Dissemination may occur with both primary and recurrent (reactivated) infection but is much more likely in the former setting. Approximately 1 to 4% of uninfected women seroconvert during pregnancy. In women who acquire primary infection, 40 to 50% of the fetuses will be infected. The overall risk of congenital infection is greatest when maternal infection occurs in the third trimester, but the probability of severe fetal injury is highest when maternal infection occurs in the first trimester.[52,56]

Of infected fetuses delivered to mothers with primary infection, 5 to 18% are overtly symptomatic at birth. The most common clinical manifestations are hepatosplenomegaly, intracranial calcifications, jaundice, growth restriction, microcephaly, chorioretinitis, and hearing loss. The most frequent laboratory abnormalities are thrombocytopenia, hyperbilirubinemia, and elevated serum transaminase concentrations. Approximately 30% of severely infected infants die. Eighty percent of the survivors have major morbidity such as mental retardation, ocular abnormalities, or sensorineural hearing loss.[52,57] Approximately 85 to 90% of infected infants are asymptomatic at birth. Ten to 15% subsequently develop hearing loss, chorioretinitis, or dental defects within the first 2 years of life.[52,57]

Pregnant women who experience recurrent or reactivated CMV infection are much less likely to transmit infection to their fetus. Fowler et al.[58] studied 125 women with serologic evidence of primary infection and 64 with recurrent infection. In the former group, 18% of infants were symptomatic at birth. An additional 7% developed at least one major sequela within 5 years of follow-up. Two percent died, 15% had sensorineural hearing loss, and 13% had IQs less than 70. In contrast, none of the infants delivered to mothers with recurrent infection were symptomatic at birth. During the period of surveillance, 8% had at least one sequela, but none

had multiple defects. The most common sequela was hearing loss.

Overall, approximately 1% of infants (40,000) born in the United States each year have congenital CMV infection. Approximately 3000 to 4000 infants are symptomatic at birth, and an additional 4000 to 6000 subsequently have neurologic or developmental problems in the first years of life. CMV infection is now the principal cause of hearing deficits in children. Public health officials estimate that the annual cost of caring for children with congenital CMV is $1.86 billion.[59]

Perinatal CMV infection may occur during delivery as a result of exposure to infected genital-tract secretions. At the time of delivery, up to 10% of pregnant women may be shedding CMV in cervical secretions or urine. Twenty to 60% of exposed fetuses may subsequently shed virus in their pharynx or urine. The incubation period for this form of infection ranges from 7 to 12 weeks, with an average of 8 weeks. Fortunately, infected infants rarely have serious sequelae of infection acquired during delivery. In addition, infants who acquire CMV infection as a result of breast feeding also are very unlikely to sustain serious injury.[52,56-59]

Identification of virus in amniotic fluid is the most sensitive and specific test for diagnosing congenital infection.[24,52,60] However, identification does not necessarily delineate the severity of fetal injury, an issue that obviously is of great importance in counseling parents about the prognosis for their infants. Fortunately, detailed sonography is invaluable in providing information about severity of fetal impairment. The principal sonographic findings suggestive of serious fetal injury include microcephaly, ventriculomegaly, intracerebral calcifications, hydrops, growth restriction, and oligohydramnios. In addition, unusual findings that may also indicate a severely infected infant include fetal heart block, intraabdominal echodensities, meconium peritonitis, renal dysplasia, and isolated serous effusions. Ultrasound examination may be normal early in the course of fetal infection. Therefore, fetuses at risk should have repeat examinations to determine if anomalies are apparent.[52]

A vaccine for CMV is not available. Antiviral agents such as ganciclovir and foscarnet have moderate activity against CMV, but their use is limited primarily to treatment of severe infections in immunocompromised patients. Accordingly, obstetrician−gynecologists should focus most of their attention on educating patients about preventive measures.

One of the most important interventions is helping patients understand that CMV infection can be a sexually transmitted disease and that sexual promiscuity significantly increases an individual's risk of acquiring the infection. Individuals who have multiple sexual partners should be counseled that latex condoms provide an effective barrier to transmission of CMV. Another important intervention is educating health care workers, day-care workers, elementary schoolteachers, and mothers of young children about the importance of simple infection control measures such as handwashing and proper cleansing of environmental surfaces. Obstetricians and pediatricians must be consistently aware of the importance of transfusing only CMV-free blood products to fetuses, neonates, pregnant women, and immunocompromised patients and of screening potential donors of organs and semen for CMV infection. Finally, health-care workers must adhere to the principles of universal precautions when treating patients and handling potentially infected body fluids.

For several reasons, routine prenatal screening for CMV infection is not recommended. First, laboratory resources may be overwhelmed if all pregnant women were screened. Second, if laboratories do not ensure a high level of quality control, the interpretation of serologic tests may be confusing and may lead to incorrect, and irreversible, interventions such as pregnancy termination. Third, neither antiviral chemotherapy nor immunoprophylaxis is available to protect the fetus or neonate. Accordingly, screening should be limited to women who have symptoms suggestive of acute CMV infection, who have had definite occupational exposure to CMV, or who are immunocompromised.

GROUP B STREPTOCOCCAL INFECTION

Epidemiology

Fifteen to 30% of pregnant women harbor group B streptococci (*Streptococcus agalactiae*) in their lower genital tract or rectum. This organism is one of the two leading causes of early-onset neonatal infection. The prevalence of neonatal group B streptococcal infection is 1 to 2 per 1000 live births, and approximately 10,000 to 12,000 cases of neonatal streptococcal septicemia occur each year in the United States. The

annual economic cost of neonatal group B streptococcal infection is approximately $1 billion.[61]

Neonatal group B streptococcal infection can be divided into early-onset and late-onset infection. Approximately 80 to 85% of cases are early in onset and result almost exclusively from vertical transmission from a colonized mother. Early-onset infection presents primarily as a severe pneumonia or overwhelming septicemia. In preterm infants, the mortality from early-onset group B streptococcal infection approaches 25%.[24,61] In term infants, the mortality is lower, averaging approximately 5% in some investigations.[24,61] Late-onset infection occurs as a result of both vertical and horizontal transmission. It is manifested by bacteremia, meningitis, and pneumonia. The mortality from late-onset infection is approximately 5 to 10% for both preterm and term infants.[24,61]

Obstetric Considerations

Unfortunately, obstetric interventions have proven ineffective in preventing late-onset neonatal infection. Therefore, the remainder of this discussion focuses on early-onset infection. Major risk factors for early-onset infection include preterm labor, especially when complicated by preterm premature rupture of membranes (PROM); intrapartum maternal fever (chorioamnionitis); prolonged rupture of membranes, defined as more than 12 to 18 hours; and previous delivery of an infected infant. Approximately 25% of pregnant women have at least one risk factor for group B streptococcal infection. The neonatal attack rate in colonized patients is 40 to 50% in the presence of a risk factor and 5% or less in the absence of a risk factor. In infected infants, neonatal mortality approaches 30 to 35% when a maternal risk factor is present but is 5% or less when there are no risk factors.[24,61]

Several obstetric complications occur with increased frequency in pregnant women who are colonized with group B streptococci. The organism is an important cause of chorioamnionitis and postpartum endometritis.[62] It also may cause postcesarean wound infection, usually in conjunction with other aerobic and anaerobic bacilli and staphylococci. Group B streptococci also are responsible for approximately 2 to 3% of lower UTIs in pregnant women but usually do not cause pyelonephritis. Group B streptococcal UTI, in turn, is a risk factor for preterm PROM and preterm labor. Thomsen et al.[63] reported a study of 69 women at 27 to 31 weeks of gestation who had streptococcal UTIs. Patients were assigned to treatment with either penicillin or placebo. Treated patients had a significant reduction in the frequency of both preterm PROM and preterm labor. Other investigations have confirmed the association between group B streptococcal colonization, preterm labor, and preterm PROM.[24,64] Women with the latter complication who are colonized with group B streptococci tend to have a shorter latent period and higher frequency of chorioamnionitis and puerperal endometritis than noncolonized women.[65]

The definitive standard for the diagnosis of group B streptococcal infection is bacteriologic culture. A special nutrient broth (Todd–Hewitt broth) or selective blood agar is the preferred medium. Specimens for culture should be obtained from the lower vagina, perineum, and perianal area, using a cotton swab.

In recent years, considerable research has been devoted to assessment of rapid diagnostic tests for the identification of colonized women. Although the rapid diagnostic tests have reasonable sensitivity in identifying heavily colonized patients, they have poor sensitivity in identifying lightly and moderately colonized patients. This latter finding severely limits the usefulness of the rapid diagnostic tests in clinical practice.[65]

Several different strategies have been proposed for the prevention of neonatal group B streptococcal infection. No strategy is perfectly applicable in all clinical situations, and none can prevent all cases of neonatal infection. However, the guidelines recommended by the Centers for Disease Control and Prevention (CDC)[66] represent a reasonable approach to this difficult clinical problem. The essential components of the CDC recommendations are summarized in Table 5-3.

The two antibiotics that have been studied most extensively for intrapartum prophylaxis are intravenous penicillin (5 million units initially, then 2.5 million units q4h) and ampicillin (2 g initially, then 1 g q4h). In patients who are allergic to penicillin, alternative regimens include erythromycin (500 q6h), clindamycin (900 mg q8h), and vancomycin (500 mg q6h).[66] Neonatal outcome is maximized when antibiotics are administered at least 4 hours prior to delivery.[67]

Rosenstein and Schuchat[68] have assessed the theoretical impact of the CDC recommendations. They studied four areas in North America with an aggregate of 186,000 births per year. They assumed that cultures at 35 to 37 weeks would identify 87%

TABLE 5-3
CDC GUIDELINES FOR PREVENTION OF NEONATAL GROUP B STREPTOCOCCAL INFECTION

Patients with preterm labor or preterm premature rupture of membranes should be screened for group B streptococcal infection. Colonized patients should be treated with prophylactic antibiotics intrapartum.

All other patients should be screened for infection at 35 to 37 weeks of gestation.

Patients who have a positive culture at 35 to 37 weeks should be treated with prophylactic antibiotics intrapartum, regardless of whether or not a risk factor is present.

If the colonization status of a patient is unknown, intrapartum prophylaxis should be administered if any of the following risk factors are present:
   Prematurity
   Rupture of membranes >18 hours
   Intrapartum infection (maternal fever)
   History of previous infant with group B streptococcal infection

---

of women who were actually colonized at delivery and that antibiotic prophylaxis would prevent 95% of cases of neonatal infection. They identified 246 infected neonates, 80% of whom were born at term. Death occurred in 3% of term infants and 15% of preterm infants. The universal screening approach would have prevented 78% of cases of neonatal infection compared to 41% for the risk-factor–based approach.

HEPATITIS

Hepatitis is one of the most common and most highly contagious viral infections. At present, six distinct types of hepatitis virus have been identified: A, B, C, D, E, and G. Each type of hepatitis has a slightly different clinical implication for the pregnant woman and her fetus.

Hepatitis A

Epidemiology

Hepatitis A is responsible for 30 to 35% of cases of hepatitis in the United States.[69] This RNA virus is transmitted by person-to-person contact through fecal–oral contamination. Poor hygiene, poor sanitation, and intimate personal contact facilitate transmission. Epidemics frequently result from common exposure to contaminated food and water. In the United States, individuals at particular risk for hepatitis A are those who have recently immigrated from, or traveled to, developing nations of the world where the disease is endemic. Drug abusers, homosexual men, and children in day-care centers also are at increased risk for acquiring hepatitis A.

The incubation period of hepatitis A ranges from 15 to 50 days, with a mean of 28 to 30 days. The highest concentration of viral particles is in fecal material. The virus is not normally excreted in urine or other body fluids.

Some patients with hepatitis A are relatively asymptomatic. When symptoms do occur, they typically include malaise, fatigue, anorexia, nausea and vomiting, and right-upper-quadrant pain. The characteristic physical findings of acute hepatitis A are jaundice, hepatic tenderness, darkened urine, and acholic stools.

Diagnosis

The most useful diagnostic test for hepatitis A is identification of IgM-specific antibody.[69] IgM antibody usually is detectable 25 to 30 days following the initial exposure and persists in the serum for up to 6 months. IgG antibody is detectable within 35 to 40 days of exposure and persists indefinitely, thus conferring lifelong immunity. In addition, the serum concentration of alanine aminotransferase (ALT), aspartate aminotransferase (AST), and bilirubin are usually moderately to markedly elevated. Liver biopsy is rarely indicated to confirm the diagnosis of viral hepatitis. When performed, it characteristically shows extensive hepatocellular injury and a prominent inflammatory infiltrate.

Obstetric Considerations

Fortunately, acute hepatitis A is usually a self-limited illness, and only supportive care is required for the vast majority of patients. Recovery is typically complete within 4 to 6 weeks. Fulminant hepatitis, coagulopathy, or encephalopathy develop in fewer than 0.5% of affected patients.[69]

Infected patients should be advised of the need for sound nutrition, and physical activity should be limited to prevent upper abdominal trauma. Drugs with potential hepatotoxicity (e.g., erythromycin, isoniazid, acetaminophen, and α-methyldopa) should be avoided. Sexual and household contacts should receive immunoprophylaxis with a single intramuscular dose of immunoglobulin, 0.02 ml/kg within 2 weeks of exposure. In addition, they also should receive the formalin-inactivated hepatitis A vaccine. The vaccine is highly immunogenic and is safe for use in pregnancy.[70,71]

Two vaccine preparations are now available: Havrix (SmithKline Beecham) and Vaqta (Merck & Co.). The appropriate dose of Havrix is 1 ml intramuscularly; the corresponding dose of Vaqta is 0.5 ml. A second dose of the vaccine should be administered in 6 to 12 months if the patient has continuing exposure to infection. The only contraindication to the vaccine is allergy to alum (contained in both vaccines) or the preservative 2-phenoxyethanol (present in Havrix). The vaccine can be administered at the same time as other inactivated vaccines but should not be administered concurrently with live vaccines.[71]

As a general rule, unless the pregnant women becomes severely ill, hepatitis A does not pose a serious risk to the fetus. Perinatal transmission of infection is exceedingly rare, and a chronic carrier state does not exist. An infant delivered to an acutely infected mother should receive immunoglobulin to prevent horizontal transmission of infection after delivery.[70,72]

Hepatitis B

Epidemiology

Approximately 40 to 45% of all cases of hepatitis in the United States are caused by hepatitis B virus. Over 300,000 new cases of hepatitis B occur annually, and about 1.25 million Americans are chronic viral carriers. The frequencies of acute and chronic hepatitis B in pregnancy are 1 to 2 in 1000 and 5 to 15 in 1000, respectively.[69]

Hepatitis B is caused by a DNA virus, and the intact virus is termed the Dane particle. The virus has three major structural antigens: surface antigen (HB_sAg), core antigen (HB_cAg), and e antigen (HB_eAg). Transmission of hepatitis B occurs primarily as a result of parenteral injection, sexual contact, and perinatal exposure. Certain population groups have an increased prevalence of hepatitis B: Asians, Eskimos, drug addicts, transfusion recipients, dialysis patients, residents and employees of long-term–care facilities, prisoners, and recipients of tattoos.[69]

Following an acute infection caused by hepatitis B virus, less than 1% of patients contract fulminant hepatitis and die. Eighty-five to 90% experience complete resolution of their physical findings and develop protective levels of antibody. Ten to 15% become chronically infected; of these, 15 to 30% subsequently have chronic active or persistent hepatitis or cirrhosis, and a small percentage have hepatocellular carcinoma.

Chronic liver disease is particularly likely to occur in patients who remain seropositive for HB_eAg and who simultaneously become infected with the hepatitis D or C virus.[69,73,74]

Diagnosis

The diagnosis of acute hepatitis B is confirmed by detection of the surface antigen and IgM antibody to the core antigen.[69] Identification of HB_eAg is indicative of an exceptionally high viral inoculum and active viral replication. Patients who have chronic hepatitis B infection have persistence of the surface antigen in the serum and liver tissue. Some individuals, particularly Asians, also remain seropositive for HB_eAg.

Obstetric Considerations

Patients with acute and chronic hepatitis B infection pose a major threat of transmission to other household members, especially their sexual partners. In addition, infected women also may transmit infection to their fetus. Perinatal transmission occurs primarily as a result of the infant's exposure to infected blood and genital secretions during delivery. In the absence of immunoprophylaxis for the neonate, perinatal transmission occurs in 10 to 20% of women who are seropositive for HB_sAg and almost 90% in women who are seropositive for both Hb_sAg and HB_eAg.[69,74]

Fortunately, a combination of passive and active immunization is highly effective in preventing both horizontal and vertical transmission of hepatitis B infection. All individuals who have had household or sexual exposure to another person with hepatitis B infection should be tested to determine if they have antibody to the virus. If they are seronegative, they should immediately receive immunoprophylaxis with hepatitis B immunoglobulin (HBIG), 0.06 ml/kg intramuscularly. They then should receive the hepatitis B vaccination series. Similarly, infants delivered to seropositive mothers should receive HBIG, 0.5 ml intramuscularly, immediately after birth. They then should begin the hepatitis B vaccination series within 12 hours of birth.[69,74]

At present, two recombinant hepatitis B vaccines are available, Recombivax-HB and Engerix-B. Both products are composed of inactivated portions of the surface antigen and are prepared by recombinant DNA technology. Neither poses a risk of transmission of a blood-borne pathogen, and both are safe for administration during pregnancy to patients at risk.[69,75]

Neonatal immunoprophylaxis is approximately 85 to 95% effective in preventing neonatal hepatitis B infection. In view of the extremely favorable results of immunoprophylaxis, the Centers for Disease Control and Prevention (CDC) recommend universal hepatitis B vaccination for all infants.[74] Dosage recommendations vary depending on the mother's serostatus. Infants born to seronegative mothers require only the vaccine. Infants born to seropositive mothers should receive both the vaccine and HBIG. Therefore, obstetricians must continue to screen all of their patients for hepatitis B at some point during pregnancy. Selective screening on the basis of acknowledged risk factors will fail to identify 30 to 50% of seropositive women.

Patients infected with hepatitis B virus also may transmit infection to medical and nursing personnel who care for them. Each year approximately 12,000 American health-care workers contract hepatitis B as a result of an occupational injury such as a needle stick or splash to a mucous membrane. Health-care workers can protect themselves from hepatitis in three principal ways. First, they should be vaccinated for hepatitis B. Second, they should encourage all young adults and other individuals who have a specific risk factor to receive the hepatitis B vaccine. Third, they should consistently follow universal precautions to prevent sharp injuries and splashes to exposed mucous membrane or skin surfaces.[74,76]

Conversely, health-care workers who are infected with hepatitis B also pose a risk to others. They, too, must observe safeguards to prevent horizontal transmission of infection to their patients. Long-term treatment with high doses of interferon alpha may induce remission in approximately 50% of patients. Unfortunately, relapses frequently occur after the medication is discontinued, and responses are sustained in only 15 to 25% of patients.[69,73]

Hepatitis D

Epidemiology

Hepatitis D (delta hepatitis) is caused by an RNA virus that is dependent on coinfection with the hepatitis B virus for replication. Hepatitis D has an external coat of hepatitis B surface antigen and an internal delta antigen that is encoded by its own genome. The epidemiology of hepatitis D is similar to that of hepatitis B.[77]

Acute hepatitis D occurs in two forms: coinfection and superinfection. Coinfection represents the simultaneous occurrence of acute hepatitis B and D. It is usually a self-limited disorder and rarely leads to chronic liver disease. Superinfection occurs when acute hepatitis D develops in a patient who is a chronic hepatitis B carrier. Approximately 20 to 25% of hepatitis B carriers ultimately become superinfected with the delta virus, and chronic liver disease subsequently develops in about 80% of these individuals. Unfortunately, almost 25% ultimately die of hepatic failure.[77,78]

Diagnosis

The clinical manifestations of acute hepatitis D are similar to those of any acute viral hepatitis. The diagnosis of acute coinfection is confirmed by detection of delta antigen in hepatic tissue or serum and IgM-specific antibody in serum. In addition, the tests for Hb_sAg and HB_cAb-IgM are positive. In patients with superinfection, serologic tests reflect acute hepatitis D (positive antigen, positive IgM antibody) and chronic hepatitis B infection (positive surface antigen and HB_cAb-IgG). Patients with chronic hepatitis D usually have detectable serum levels of IgG-specific antibody for the delta virus and are seropositive for Hb_sAg. Unfortunately, IgG antibody does not eradicate the delta viremia, and the antigen still can be identified in serum and hepatic tissue.[69]

Obstetric Considerations

Patients with acute hepatitis D should receive the general supportive care outlined for hepatitis A. Patients with chronic infection should be monitored periodically for worsening hepatic function or coagulopathy. Long-term treatment with high doses of interferon alpha may induce remission in approximately 50% of patients. Unfortunately, relapses frequently occur after the medication is discontinued, and responses are sustained in only 15 to 25% of patients.[69]

Perinatal transmission of hepatitis D virus has been reported. Fortunately, however, transmission is uncommon because the neonatal immunoprophylaxis for hepatitis B is almost uniformly effective against hepatitis D.[69]

Hepatitis C

Epidemiology

Hepatitis C is a single-stranded RNA virus whose incubation period is 5 to 10 weeks. The principal risk factors for hepatitis C are intravenous drug abuse, transfusion, and sexual intercourse.[69,79] In a survey by Osmond and co-workers,[80] two-thirds of a selected population of drug abusers were seropositive for hepatitis C. In a similar survey of patients attending a sexually transmitted disease (STD) clinic in San Francisco, Weinstock et al.[81] found the prevalence of hepatitis C to be 7.7%. Approximately 90% of all cases of posttransfusion hepatitis are due to hepatitis C, and 2.5 to 15% of patients who receive multiple transfusions become infected with this virus. Hepatitis C is particularly likely to result in chronic liver disease. Biochemical evidence of hepatic dysfunction develops in approximately 50% of infected patients. Of these, about 20% subsequently have chronic active hepatitis or cirrhosis.[69]

Diagnosis

Approximately 75% of patients with hepatitis C are asymptomatic. The diagnosis is confirmed by identification of anti-C antibody. Initial screening for this antibody should be performed with an enzyme immunoassay (EIA). A positive EIA should be followed with a recombinant immunoblot assay (RIBA).[69] The present RIBA is able to detect four specific viral antigens. If at least two antigens are identified, the test is considered positive; if only one antigen is identified, the test is indeterminant. The present generation of laboratory assays does not precisely discriminate between IgM and IgG antibody. Moreover, antibody may not be detectable until up to 22 weeks after the onset of clinical illness. Direct detection of antigen also is possible with PCR. High titers of hepatitis C RNA correlate with increased infectivity.[82]

Obstetric Considerations

In a general obstetric population, the prevalence of hepatitis C is 1 to 3%. The principal factors that identify an obstetric patient at high risk for hepatitis C are concurrent sexually transmitted diseases, such as hepatitis B and HIV infection; multiple sexual partners; and history of multiple transfusions or intravenous drug abuse.[83] In selected series, the frequency of perinatal transmission of hepatitis C infection has ranged from 5 to 44%. Transmission is particularly likely to occur if the mother has high titers of hepatitis C RNA or is coinfected with the human immunodeficiency virus (HIV). Transmission is ≤ 5% in the absence of these risk factors.

A vaccine for hepatitis C is not available. Passive immunization with immunoglobulin (0.06 ml/kg intramuscularly) should be administered following percutaneous exposure to a person with hepatitis C. The benefit of immunoprophylaxis for the neonate has not been proven in controlled clinical trials. Although interferon alpha has shown some activity against the virus, relapses occur in 44 to 80% of patients within 6 to 12 months of discontinuation of therapy.[69]

Hepatitis G

Hepatitis G (HGV or GBV-C) is a recently discovered single-stranded RNA virus that is related to hepatitis C. It can cause acute and persistent infections in humans, but the disease is usually mild and the clinical significance of infection is uncertain. Persistent infection is usually not associated with biochemical evidence of ongoing hepatic injury. Hepatitis G appears to be more prevalent, but less virulent, than hepatitis C. Coinfection with hepatitis A, B, and C and HIV is common.[84,85] A chronic carrier state with hepatitis G may develop, and perinatal transmission has been documented. Feucht et al.[86] studied nine women who had HGV viremia by PCR. Vertical transmission occurred in three cases. Two of the mothers were coinfected with HIV and one with HCV.

Hepatitis G nucleic acid can be identified in serum by PCR. An enzyme-linked immunosorbent assay (ELISA) for the envelope protein of the virus also has been developed. At present, no immunoprophylactic agent or antiviral chemotherapy for hepatitis G is available.[84,85]

Hepatitis E

Epidemiology

Hepatitis E is an RNA virus that may cause both an icteric and anicteric form of infection. The virus is transmitted by the fecal–oral route, and the epidemiology of hepatitis E is similar to that of hepatitis A. The incubation period ranges from 2 to 9 weeks, with a mean of 45 days. Hepatitis E is rare in the United States but is endemic in developing countries.[87,88] In these countries, maternal mortality has been alarmingly high, ranging from 10 to 20%. Extreme poverty, coexisting medical illnesses, malnutrition, and poor prenatal care are at least partially responsible for the poor maternal prognosis. The only cases of hepatitis E in the United States have occurred in patients who traveled to countries where the disease was endemic.[89]

Diagnosis

Three new diagnostic tests are available for confirmation of hepatitis E infection. Virus-like particles can be identified in the stool of infected patients by electron microscopy. These particles will agglutinate when combined with serum from the patient. In addition, a fluorescent antibody blocking assay and Western blot assay are now available.[90]

Obstetric Considerations

Patients with acute hepatitis E should be treated as described previously for patients with hepatitis A. Once a patient has recovered from the acute illness, a chronic carrier state does not develop, and perinatal transmission usually does not occur. However, Khuroo et al.[91] described eight mothers in whom hepatitis E developed in the third trimester. Six of their infants had clinical and/or serologic evidence of hepatitis E. Two infants had hypothermia and hypoglycemia and died within 24 hours of birth.

HERPES SIMPLEX VIRUS INFECTION

Epidemiology

Herpes simplex (HSV), a double-stranded DNA virus, is transmitted by direct, intimate contact. Following the initial infection, the virus remains dormant in neuronal ganglia and may reactivate at later times. Two strains of the virus have been identified: HSV-1 and HSV-2. The former causes primarily oropharyngeal infection and the latter, genital-tract infection. Approximately 0.5 to 1.0% of women have an overt herpetic infection during pregnancy. About 400 cases of neonatal herpes occur annually in the United States, and the estimated incidence of neonatal infection ranges from 1 in 7500 to 1 in 30,000 live births.[92,93]

HSV infections are classified as primary, nonprimary first episode, and recurrent on the basis of historical and clinical findings and serologic testing.[94] Approximately 20 to 40% of Americans are seropositive for HSV; up to 80% of these individuals do not have a history of an overt primary infection.

The onset of HSV infection is usually heralded by a prodrome of neuralgias, paresthesias, and hypesthesias, followed by an eruption of painful vesicles in either the orolabial area or genitalia. The vesicles typically rupture, forming a shallow-based ulcer and then form a dry crust. Some vesicles become secondarily infected and evolve into frank pustules. Ultimately, the vesicles heal without scarring.

In patients experiencing a primary HSV infection, vesicles may be present for up to 3 weeks. Systemic symptoms may be moderately severe, and local complications such as urinary retention may occur. In recurrent infections, overt vesicles are fewer in number and less painful and typically persist for 14 days or less. In some patients, particularly those who are immunocompromised, HSV infection may be widely disseminated, affecting extensive areas of skin, mucosal membranes, and visceral organs. HSV also may cause a severe ocular infection, meningitis, encephalitis, and ascending myelitis.

Diagnosis

Several laboratory tests may be used to confirm the diagnosis of HSV infection. Cytologic preparations show characteristic multinucleated giant cells and intranuclear inclusions. PCR assays are extremely sensitive in detecting low concentrations of viral DNA. Serology is especially useful in classifying the initial herpetic episode as primary versus non-primary first episode.[94] In the former, no antibody is detected. In the latter, antibody to either HSV-1 or HSV-2 is present. Serologic testing is rarely indicated in patients who experience recurrent HSV infection.

Until the advent of PCR assays, viral isolation in tissue culture was considered the standard for confirmation of diagnosis. Viral isolation is usually possible within 72 to 96 hours of inoculation of the tissue culture. The highest rate of isolation (85 to 90%) is achieved when clinical specimens are obtained from fresh vesicles or pustules. Vesicular fluid should be aspirated with a fine needle into a tuberculin syringe, and ulcers should be scraped vigorously with a cotton-tipped applicator.[95]

Obstetric Considerations

Severe primary HSV infection has been associated with spontaneous abortion, preterm delivery, and intrauterine growth restriction. Isolated case reports also have been published documenting in utero infection even in the presence of intact membranes. However, the greatest risk to the fetus occurs when overt HSV infection is present at the time of labor. In this situation, the principal mechanism of infection is direct contact with infected vesicles during the process of vaginal birth.[93,94,96]

The frequency of neonatal infection depends on whether the mother has primary or recurrent infection. In the setting of a primary infection, the viral inoculum in the genital tract is high, and maternal antibody is not present. Approximately 40% of neonates delivered vaginally to mothers with primary infection will become infected. In the absence of antiviral chemotherapy, almost half of these infants die, and 35 to 40% experience severe neurologic morbidity such as chorioretinitis, microcephaly, mental retardation, seizures, and apnea. In women who have recurrent symptomatic HSV infection, the risk of neonatal infection following vaginal delivery is 5% or less. In women who are asymptomatically shedding HSV in the genital tract at the time of delivery, the risk of neonatal infection is $\leq$ 1%. At any given time, approximately 10% of women with a prior history of HSV may asymptomatically shed virus.[96-98]

Neonatal HSV infection may take many forms. In its simplest manifestation, it may appear as a localized abscess at the site of attachment of a scalp electrode or as isolated mucocutaneous lesions. In its more severe forms, it may present as widely disseminated mucocutaneous lesions, visceral infection, meningitis, and encephalitis. In such instances, mortality may approach 50 to 60%, and up to half of the survivors may have persistent morbidity.[92,94]

Clinical management of HSV infection has changed dramatically in recent years. Most notably, surveillance cultures of the genital tract in patients with a history of HSV infection have proven ineffective in preventing neonatal HSV infection and have resulted in many unnecessary cesarean deliveries.[99-101] Accordingly, the following simplified guidelines have now been recommended by the Infectious Diseases Society for Obstetrics and Gynecology and endorsed by ACOG.[102,103] At the time of the patient's initial prenatal appointment, she should be questioned about a history of HSV infection. If the history is positive, the patient should be asked about prodromal symptoms at the time she is admitted for delivery and examined thoroughly for cervical, vaginal, and vulvar lesions. If no prodromal symptoms or overt lesions are present, vaginal delivery should be anticipated. If symptoms or lesions are present, cesarean delivery should be performed. Cesarean delivery is indicated even in the presence of ruptured membranes of extended duration because operative delivery significantly decreases the size of the viral inoculum to which the infant is exposed.

Mothers with symptomatic infection do not need to be isolated from their infants or other patients. They should wash their hands carefully before handling the infant and shield the baby from any contact with vesicular lesions. Breast-feeding is permissible as long as no skin lesions are present directly on the breast.

In addition to the guidelines presented above, clinicians should be aware of possible indications for use of acyclovir during pregnancy. Immunocompromised patients with disseminated infections require hospitalization for treatment with intravenous acyclovir. Oral acyclovir, 400 mg three times daily for 5 to 7 days, should be considered for immunocompetent patients who have severe herpetic infection, especially near term. In addition, prophylactic treatment with oral acyclovir, 400 mg twice daily, may be appropriate in women with frequent recurrent infections in pregnancy near term. Acyclovir is classified by the FDA as a category C drug.[104,105] To date, the Acyclovir Registry has reported no increase in the frequency of adverse effects in infants exposed in utero to this antiviral agent.[106] There are limited data regarding the use of alternative agents such as valacyclovir and famciclovir during pregnancy, although both are classified as pregnancy category B drugs by the FDA.

HUMAN IMMUNODEFICIENCY VIRUS INFECTION

Epidemiology

HIV infection is caused by an RNA retrovirus that has a unique ability to attack the host's CD4 lymphocytes. The principal viral strain responsible for disease in the United States is HIV-1. HIV-2 is a related strain that is endemic in Africa, Portugal, and France. HIV-2 infection is uncommon in the United States except in individuals who have traveled to endemic areas or had sexual contact or shared needles with persons from endemic areas.[107]

HIV infection occurs in a continuum that can be divided into four major stages. Stage one is the acute retroviral infection that develops several weeks after exposure to the virus.[108] In this stage, the patient has clinical manifestations similar to mononucleosis. Over a period of several weeks, the acute episode resolves, and the patient enters the latent phase of illness. During the latent phase, the patient is asymptomatic, but viral replication persists in protected sanctuaries such as lymphatic tissue. The duration of the latent phase is approximately 5 to 10 years. Inexorably, the viral inoculum progressively increases, and the patient enters the symptomatic stage, characterized by mild to moderately severe symptoms such as fever, malaise, fatigue, anorexia, nausea, vomiting, diarrhea, weight loss, and generalized lymphadenopathy. Neurologic manifestations may be quite prominent and debilitating, particularly peripheral neuropathy and dementia. Opportunistic infections, of course, are the hallmark of HIV infection. Among the most common are *Pneumocystis carinii* pneumonia, disseminated *Mycobacterium avium* complex (MAC) infection, pulmonary tuberculosis, toxoplasmosis, candidiasis, and CMV infection. Genital herpes, hepatitis B, C, and D, and syphilis are common concurrent STDs. Ultimately, the patient develops the acquired immunodeficiency syndrome (AIDS). Once symptomatic HIV infection develops, the patient's life expectancy is usually ≤5 years. Unusual malignancies may occur during this stage of illness, particularly Kaposi sarcoma and non-Hodgkin lymphoma.[109,110]

At present, approximately 550,000 to 600,000 Americans have AIDS or have died from AIDS. An additional 1 to 1.5 million are infected with the virus but are not yet in the terminal stage of their illness. In the United States, approximately 15 to 20% of cases of HIV infection occur in women. Almost 75% of infected women are African-American or Hispanic. In women, the two most important mechanisms of HIV infection are intravenous drug abuse and heterosexual contact with a high-risk male. In the general obstetric population in the United States, the frequency of HIV infection is approximately one per 1000. However, in some inner-city populations, the prevalence of infection is as high as 1.0 to 1.5%.[109-111]

Heterosexual transmission is increasing in importance as a mechanism of spread of HIV infection. Several sexual practices have been shown to increase substantially the risk of transmission of infection. Of these, the most important is unprotected intercourse with multiple partners. Receptive anal intercourse also is an important risk factor. In addition, sexually transmitted diseases, particularly those that cause genital ulcers, also are important risk factors for HIV infection. Finally, use of illicit intravenous drugs and crack cocaine, contact with a noncircumcised male, and intercourse during menses are important independent risk factors for HIV infection.[109,110]

Diagnosis

The diagnosis of HIV infection can be confirmed by direct culture of virus from peripheral blood lymphocytes and monocytes and by detection of viral antigen by PCR. Infected patients usually have a decreased number of CD4 cells and an inverted CD4:CD8 ratio. Serum immunoglobulin levels also are elevated.

The principal diagnostic test is identification of virus-specific antibody. The initial serologic screening test should be an enzyme-linked immunosorbent assay (ELISA) or an enzyme immunoassay (EIA). These tests are highly sensitive, inexpensive, and readily suited for screening large numbers of patients. If the initial ELISA or EIA is positive, the test should be repeated. If the second test is positive, a confirmatory test such as the Western blot or immunofluorescent assay (IFA) should be performed. These tests detect specific viral antigens such as p24 (viral core), gp41 (envelope), and gp120/160 (envelope). If a patient has two positive ELISAs or EIAs, followed by a confirmatory Western blot or IFA, the likelihood of a false positive result is extremely low.[112]

As a general rule, patients in the United States should be routinely tested only for HIV-1 infection. Testing for HIV-2 is indicated if the patient has had sexual contact or has shared needles with a partner from an area of the world where HIV-2 infection is endemic. Testing also should be done if the patient has recently traveled to an endemic area or received a blood transfusion or nonsterile injection in such a locale. In addition, testing also should be performed in individuals who have clinical evidence of HIV infection, but in whom serologic tests for HIV-1 are nonconfirmatory. Screening for HIV-2 infection may be done with a specific EIA and Western blot. In addition, a commercial EIA is now available that simultaneously screens for HIV-1 and HIV-2.[113]

Obstetric Considerations

More than 90% of all cases of HIV infection in children are due to perinatal transmission. Perinatal transmission occurs primarily as a result of intrapartum exposure to infected maternal blood and genital-tract secretions although hematogenous dissemination in the antepartum period also may occur.[114] The frequency of vertical transmission of HIV infection varies from a low range of 5 to 10% to a high range of 50 to 60%. The average frequency in most investigations has been 20 to 30% in the absence of any obstetric intervention.[115,116] Factors that increase the likelihood of vertical transmission are summarized in Table 5-4.

Studies of obstetric outcomes in patients with HIV infection are difficult to interpret because affected

TABLE 5-4
FACTORS THAT INCREASE THE RISK OF VERTICAL TRANSMISSION OF HIV INFECTION

Risk Factor	Presumed Mechanism
HIV-1 vs. HIV-2	Risk is much greater with HIV-1, presumably as a result of greater virulence of HIV-1
History of previous child with HIV infection	Higher viral inoculum in mother
Mother with AIDS	Higher viral inoculum, decreased immunocompetence of the mother
Preterm delivery	Decreased neonatal immunocompetence
Decreased maternal CD4 count	Impaired maternal immunity
High viral load	Denotes higher rate of viral replication and greater infectivity
Firstborn twin	With vaginal delivery, firstborn twin has more prolonged exposure to infected blood and genital tract secretions
Chorioamnionitis	Placental vasculitis facilitates hematogenous dissemination of virus
Intrapartum blood exposure, e.g., episiotomy, vaginal laceration, forceps delivery	Greater contact with infected blood and genital secretions
Rupture of membranes	Increases probability of exposure to genital-tract secretions

oocyst, which is disrupted in the animal's intestine, releasing the invasive trophozoite. The trophozoite then is disseminated throughout the animal's body, ultimately forming cysts in brain and muscle.

Human infection occurs when infected meat is ingested or when food is contaminated by cat feces via flies, cockroaches, or fingers. Infection rates are highest in areas of poor sanitation and crowded living conditions. Stray cats and domestic cats that eat raw meat are most likely to carry the parasite.[160]

Approximately 40 to 50% of adults in the United States have antibodies to this organism, and the prevalence of antibody is highest in lower socioeconomic populations. The frequency of seroconversion during pregnancy is 5% or less, and approximately 3 in 1000 infants show evidence of congenital infection. Clinically significant congenital toxoplasmosis occurs in approximately 1 in 8000 pregnancies. Toxoplasmosis is more common in Western Europe, particularly France.[161]

Most infections in humans are asymptomatic. Even in the absence of symptoms, however, patients may have evidence of multiorgan involvement, and clinical disease can follow a long period of asymptomatic infection. Symptomatic toxoplasmosis usually presents as an illness similar to mononucleosis.

In contrast to infection in the immunocompetent host, toxoplasmosis can be a devastating infection in the immunosuppressed patient. Because immunity to *T. gondii* is cell-mediated, patients with HIV infection and those treated with long-term immunosuppressive therapy after organ transplantation are particularly susceptible to new or reactivated infection. In these patients, central nervous system dysfunction is the most common manifestation of infection. Findings typically include encephalitis, meningoencephalitis, and intracerebral mass lesions. Pneumonitis, myocarditis, and generalized lymphadenopathy also commonly occur.[120]

Diagnosis

The diagnosis of toxoplasmosis can be confirmed by serologic and histologic methods.[160] Serologic tests indicative of an acute infection include detection of IgM-specific antibody, demonstration of an extremely high IgG antibody titer, and documentation of IgG seroconversion from negative to positive. Clinicians should be aware that serologic assays for toxoplasmosis are not well standardized. When initial laboratory tests appear to indicate that an acute infection has occurred, serologic tests should be repeated in an experienced reference laboratory.

The best tissue for identification of *T. gondii* is a lymph node or brain biopsy specimen. Histologic preparations can be examined by light and electron microscopy. For light microscopy, specimens should be stained with either Giemsa or Wright stain.

Obstetric Considerations

Congenital infection can occur if acute toxoplasmosis develops during pregnancy. Chronic or latent infection is unlikely to cause fetal injury except perhaps in an immunosuppressed patient. Approximately 40% of neonates born to mothers with acute primary toxoplasmosis show evidence of infection. Congenital infection is most likely to occur when maternal infection develops in the third trimester. Less than half of affected infants are symptomatic at birth. The major clinical manifestations of congenital toxoplasmosis include rash, hepatosplenomegaly, ascites, fever, chorioretinitis, periventricular calcifications, ventriculomegaly, seizures, mental retardation, and uveitis.[161]

The most valuable tests for antenatal diagnosis of congenital toxoplasmosis are ultrasound, cordocentesis, and amniocentesis.[161] Ultrasound findings suggestive of infection include ventriculomegaly, intracranial calcifications, microcephaly, ascites, hepatosplenomegaly, and growth restriction. Fetal blood samples can be tested for IgM-specific antibody after 20 weeks of gestation. Fetal blood and amniotic fluid can be inoculated into mice, and the organism can subsequently be recovered from the blood of infected animals. In addition, Hohlfeld et al.[162] have identified a specific gene of *T. gondii* in amniotic fluid using PCR. In their investigation, 34 of 339 infants had congenital toxoplasmosis confirmed by serologic testing or autopsy. All amniotic fluid samples from affected pregnancies were positive by PCR, and test results were available within 1 day of specimen collection.

When acute toxoplasmosis occurs during pregnancy, treatment of the mother is imperative because it has been shown to reduce the risk of congenital infection and decrease the late sequelae of infection. Pyrimethamine, one of the drugs of choice in nonpregnant patients, is not recommended for use during the first trimester of pregnancy because of possible teratogenicity. Sulfonamides such as sulfadiazine can be used alone, but single-agent therapy appears to be less effective than combination therapy. In Europe, spiramycin, a macrolide antibiotic, has been used extensively in pregnancy with excellent success. It is available for use in the United States on special request to the CDC.[161,162]

The largest series of pregnancies at risk for congenital toxoplasmosis was reported by Daffos et al.[161] These authors followed 746 pregnant women who had serologically confirmed primary toxoplasmosis. Infection was diagnosed antenatally in 39 fetuses by umbilical-cord blood sampling. All mothers were treated during pregnancy with spiramycin. Mothers who had infected infants were also treated with pyrimethamine plus either sulfadoxine or sulfadiazine. Twenty-four of the 39 pregnancies were terminated. Of the remaining 15 pregnancies carried to term, 13 neonates were clinically well during a 3-month observation period, and 2 infants had chorioretinitis.

Early aggressive treatment of the infected neonate is an alternative to in utero therapy. Guerina and co-workers[163] have reported the results of a large screening project for neonatal toxoplasmosis in Massachusetts and New Hampshire. Over 600,000 infants were tested, and congenital infection was confirmed in 52. Detailed physical examination in 48 children showed abnormalities of the central nervous system in 19 (40%). After the infants were treated with combinations of pyrimethamine, sulfadiazine, and leucovorin for 1 year, only one child had a persistent neurologic defect (hemiplegia). Subsequently, four other children were found to have ophthalmologic abnormalities at ages 1 to 6. One child had a macular lesion, and three had minor retinal scars. Thus, early treatment reduces, but does not completely eliminate, the late sequelae of congenital toxoplasmosis.

In the treatment of the pregnant patient, prevention of acute toxoplasmosis is of paramount importance. Pregnant women should be advised to avoid contact with stray cats or cat litter. They should always wash their hands after preparing meat for cooking and should never eat raw or rare meat. Fruits and vegetables also should be washed carefully to remove possible contamination by oocysts.

VARICELLA

Epidemiology

The varicella–zoster virus (V–Z virus), a DNA organism, is a member of the herpes virus family. Humans are the only known source of infection. Natural varicella infection occurs primarily during early childhood. Less than 10% of cases occur in individuals over 10 years of age; however, older patients account for more than 50% of all fatalities due to varicella. Varicella is transmitted by direct contact and respiratory droplets. The virus is highly infectious, and approximately 95% of susceptible household contacts become infected following exposure. The incubation period is 10 to 14 days. Patients are infectious from 1 day before the outbreak of the rash until all of the cutaneous lesions have dried and crusted over. Immunity to varicella is usually lifelong.[164]

Herpes zoster infection occurs as a result of reactivation of latent virus infection in a patient who has already had varicella. Because of the presence in the host of virus-specific antibody, herpes zoster is usually a much less serious disorder than varicella and rarely poses a major risk to either the mother or her baby unless the former is immunocompromised. However, acute varicella may develop in susceptible patients when they are exposed to individuals with herpes zoster, and, therefore, they must be counseled appropriately about this risk.[164]

The usual clinical manifestations of varicella are fever, malaise, and rash. The characteristic skin lesions usually begin as pruritic macules, which appear in crops. The macules progress to papules, then to vesicles, and finally to crusts. The lesions initially appear on the trunk and then spread centripetally to the extremities.

In immunocompetent children serious complications of varicella are exceedingly rare. However, in adults, two life-threatening sequelae may develop: encephalitis and pneumonia. The former occurs in 1% or less of patients; the latter may develop in up to 20% of patients. Prior to the development of acyclovir, the mortality associated with varicella pneumonia in pregnancy approached 40%.[164,165]

Diagnosis

The diagnosis of varicella is usually made by clinical examination. In problematic cases, the virus can be isolated in tissue culture, and cytologic preparations may show multinucleated giant cells and eosinophilic intranuclear inclusions. Serologic assays are of primary value in assessing a patient's susceptibility to varicella immediately following exposure.[166] The two most useful antibody assays are the fluorescent anti-membrane antibody test (FAMA) and the ELISA. Both assays show sustained elevations, usually lifelong, following natural infection.

Obstetric Considerations

The optimal approach to maternal varicella infection is prevention. All women of reproductive age should be assessed for immunity to varicella, ideally before they attempt to become pregnant. Susceptible patients, particularly those who are likely to be exposed to varicella either at home or in the workplace, should be offered the new varicella vaccine. Varivax (Merck) is a live attenuated vaccine that is highly immunogenic. Individuals older than 12 years should receive two subcutaneous doses of the vaccine, 4 to 8 weeks apart. Vaccine recipients should use effective contraception for 3 months after immunization. The vaccine can be administered simultaneously with the MMR immunization, but it should not be given in conjunction with blood or blood products. In addition,

the vaccine is contraindicated in patients who are pregnant, who have immunodeficiency disorders, or who have received high-dose systemic steroids within 30 days of vaccination.[167]

If the patient presents for medical care when she is pregnant, she should be questioned about varicella immunity at the time of her first prenatal appointment. If she is uncertain about prior infection, an IgG varicella serology test should be performed. If the serology is positive, the patient can be reassured that she is immune and that she and her fetus are not at risk should subsequent exposure occur. If the serology is negative, the patient should be counseled to avoid exposure to individuals who may have varicella or herpes zoster.

Unfortunately, however, the more common situation that the obstetrician encounters is a pregnant patient who has been exposed acutely to an individual who has chickenpox. The management algorithm for this scenario is summarized in Figure 5-9. The patient should first be questioned about immunity to

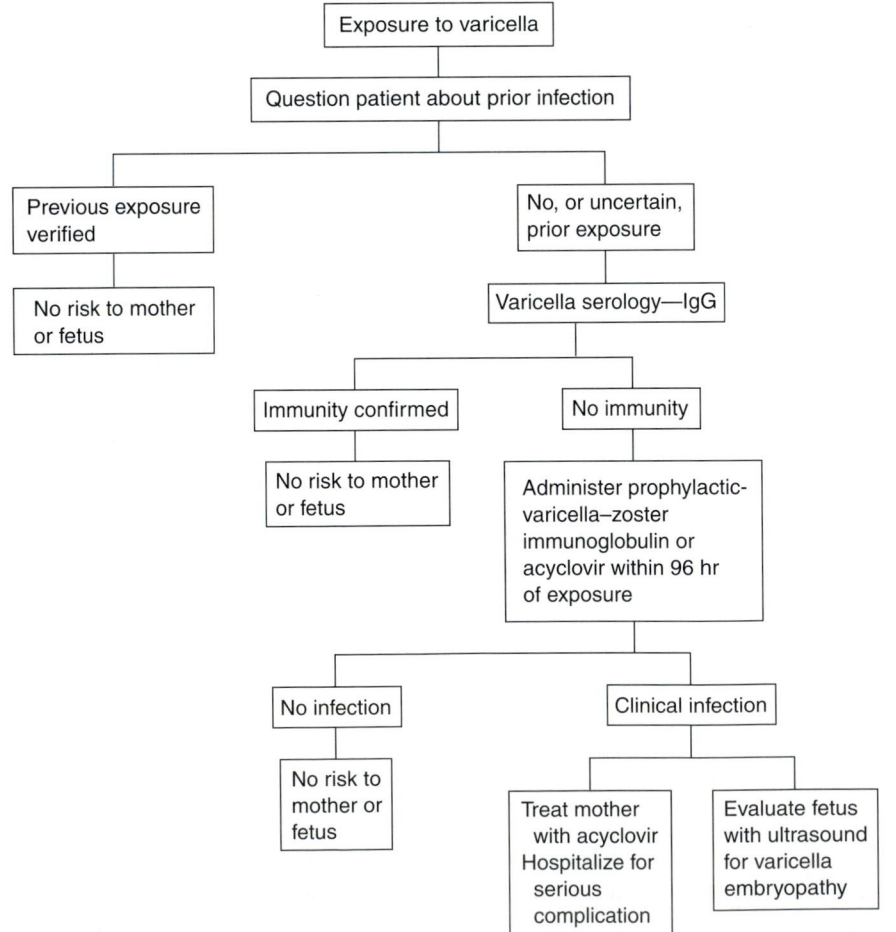

Figure 5-9 Algorithm for management of varicella exposure during pregnancy

varicella. If immunity cannot be documented by history, an IgG serology should be obtained and the result should be reviewed within 24 to 48 hours of exposure. If the serology is positive, the patient can be reassured that her fetus is not at risk. If the serology is negative, the patient should receive varicella–zoster immunoglobulin (VZIG).[164,168,169] This preparation is 60 to 80% effective in preventing infection if given within 96 hours of exposure. The dose of VZIG is one vial (125 units) per 10 kg of actual body weight, up to a maximum of five vials. In problematic cases, if waiting for the varicella serology will delay administration of VZIG for more than 96 hours after exposure, the immunization should be given without confirmatory serology. An alternative method of prophylaxis is administration of oral acyclovir, 800 mg, five times daily, for 5 to 7 days.[170]

Susceptible exposed patients should be counseled to report immediately if clinical manifestations of infection appear. Investigations in both children and adults have shown a definite benefit in treating affected patients early in the course of the disease with therapeutic doses of oral acyclovir, 800 mg, five times daily, for 7 to 10 days, or until all lesions have begun to crust over.[171,172] If signs of encephalitis or pneumonia develop, or if the patient is immunocompromised, she should be hospitalized immediately for treatment with intravenous acyclovir, 500 mg/m^2 every 8 hours.

Congenital varicella results primarily from hematogenous dissemination of virus across the placenta. Ascending infection following rupture of membranes is possible but extremely unlikely. Congenital infection may lead to spontaneous abortion, intrauterine fetal death, and varicella embryopathy. The latter disorder is manifested by multiple abnormalities such as cutaneous scars, limb hypoplasia, muscle atrophy, malformed digits, psychomotor retardation, microcephaly, cortical atrophy, cataracts, chorioretinitis, and micropthalmia.[164]

Fortunately, two investigations have demonstrated a relatively low frequency of anomalies even following exposure in the first half of pregnancy. Pastuszak et al.[173] reported a study of 106 women with varicella in the first 20 weeks of gestation. The frequency of varicella embryopathy was 1.2%, and the prevalence of preterm birth was 14%. Subsequently, Enders and co-workers[174] published the largest prospective study of varicella in pregnancy. They observed a 2% incidence of congenital infection when maternal varicella occurred at 13 to 20 weeks of gestation. The frequency of congenital infection was only 0.4% when maternal infection occurred before 13 weeks of gestation.

The presence of varicella virus in the fetal compartment can be identified by detection of virus-specific IgM antibody and elevated total IgM antibody in cord blood. Virus also can be cultured in amniotic fluid and identified by PCR in placental tissue. Unfortunately, identification of viral DNA, virus-specific antibody, or even the virus itself does not accurately predict the degree of fetal injury. For this purpose ultrasonography is the preferred diagnostic method. Sonographic findings suggestive of fetal varicella include polyhydramnios; hydrops; hyperechogenic foci in the abdominal organs, particularly the liver; cardiac malformations; limb deformities; microcephaly; and intrauterine growth restriction.[164]

The final major complication of varicella infection in pregnancy is neonatal varicella. Infection of the neonate occurs in 10 to 20% of infants whose mothers have acute varicella within the period from 5 days before to 2 days after delivery. Infection usually results from hematogenous dissemination of virus across the placenta at a time when no maternal antibody is present to provide passive immunity to the fetus. Less commonly, neonatal varicella results from postnatal exposure to the mother or another infected person.[164]

The clinical course of neonatal varicella can be variable in progression and severity. The infant usually becomes symptomatic within 5 to 10 days of delivery. Some neonates have only scattered skin lesions and no systemic signs of illness. Others have a biphasic course, initially presenting with a cluster of skin lesions, followed by more widespread dissemination. Still others have a more severe acute illness associated with extensive cutaneous lesions and visceral infection. The most common life-threatening complication is pneumonia. In reports published before the widespread availability of acyclovir, the mortality associated with neonatal varicella was 20 to 30%.[164]

To prevent neonatal varicella, an effort should be made to delay delivery until 5 to 7 days after the onset of maternal illness. If delay is not possible, the neonate should receive VZIG (one vial, 125 units) immediately after birth. An important additional preventive measure is isolation of the infant from the mother until all vesicular lesions likely to come in contact with the infant have crusted over.[164,169]

REFERENCES

1. Sobel JD. Vaginitis. N Engl J Med 1997;337:1896.

2. Sobel JD. Recurrent vulvovaginal candidiasis. N Engl J Med 1986;315:1455.

3. Thomason JL, Gelbart SM. Trichomonas vaginalis. Obstet Gynecol 1989;74:536.

4. 1998 guidelines for treatment of sexually transmitted diseases. MMWR 1998;47:(Suppl) 1.

5. Robbie M, Sweet RL. Metronidazole use in obstetrics and gynecology: a review. Am J Obstet Gynecol 1983;145:865.

6. Eschenbach DA, Hillier S, Critchlow C, Stevens C, DeRouen T, Holmes KK. Diagnosis and clinical manifestations of bacterial vaginosis. Am J Obstet Gynecol 1988; 158:819.

7. Martius J, Krohn MA, Hillier SL, Stamm WE, Holmes KK, Eschenbach DA. Relationships of vaginal Lactobacillus species, cervical Chlamydia trachomatis, and bacterial vaginosis to preterm birth. Obstet Gynecol 1988;71:89.

8. Gravett MG, Hummel D, Eschenbach DA, Holmes KK. Preterm labor associated with subclinical amniotic fluid infection and with bacterial vaginosis. Obstet Gynecol 1986;67:229.

9. Hillier SL, Nugent RP, Eschenbach DA, et al. Association between bacterial vaginosis and preterm delivery of a low-birth-weight infant. N Engl J Med 1995;333:1737.

10. Clark P, Kurtzer TA, Duff P. The role of bacterial vaginosis in peripartum infections. Infect Dis Obstet Gynecol 1994;2:179.

11. Thomasen JL, Gelbart SM, Anderson RJ, Walt AK, Osypowski PJ, Broekhuizen FF. Statistical evaluation of diagnostic criteria for bacterial vaginosis. Am J Obstet Gynecol 1990;162:155.

12. Nugent RP, Krohn MA, Hillier SL. Reliability of diagnosing bacterial vaginosis is improved by a standardized method of Gram stain interpretation. J Clin Microbiol 1991;29:297.

13. Spiegel CA, Amsel R, Holmes KK. Diagnosis of bacterial vaginosis by direct Gram stain of vaginal fluid. J Clin Microbiol 1983;18:170.

14. McGregor JA, French JI, Parker R, et al. Prevention of premature birth by screening and treatment for common genital tract infections: results of a prospective controlled evaluation. Am J Obstet Gynecol 1995;173:157.

15. Morales WJ, Schorr S, Albritton J. Effect of metronidazole in patients with preterm birth in preceding pregnancy and bacterial vaginosis: a placebo-controlled, double-blind study. Am J Obstet Gynecol 1994;171:345.

16. Hauth JC, Goldenberg RL, Andrews WW, et al. Reduced incidence of preterm delivery with metronidazole and erythromycin in women with bacterial vaginosis. N Engl J Med 1995;333:1732.

17. Alexander ER, Harrison HR. Role of Chlamydia trachomatis in perinatal infection. Rev Infect Dis 1983; 5:713.

18. Mercer LJ, Robinson DC, Sahm DF, Lawrie MJ, Hajj SN. Comparison of chemiluminescent DNA probe to cell culture for the screening of Chlamydia trachomatis in a gynecology clinic population. Obstet Gynecol 1990; 76:114.

19. Lee HH, Chernesky MA, Schachter J, et al. Diagnosis of Chlamydia trachomatis genitourinary infection in women by ligase chain reaction assay of urine. Lancet 1995;345:213.

20. Martin DH, Mroczkowski TF, Dalu ZA, et al. A controlled trial of a single dose of azithromycin for the treatment of chlamydia urethritis and cervicitis. N Engl J Med 1992;327:921.

21. Bush MR, Rosa C. Azithromycin and erythromycin in the treatment of cervical chlamydial infection during pregnancy. Obstet Gynecol 1994;84:61.

22. Crombleholme WR, Schachter J, Grossman M, Landers DV, Sweet RL. Amoxicillin therapy for Chlamydia trachomatis in pregnancy. Obstet Gynecol 1990;75:752.

23. Al-Suleiman SA, Grimes EM, Jonas HS. Disseminated gonococcal infections. Obstet Gynecol 1983;61:48.

24. Duff P. Maternal and perinatal infections. In: Gabbe SG, Niebyl JR, Simpson JL, eds. Obstetrics: Normal and problem pregnancies. 3rd ed. New York: Churchill Livingstone, 1996;1193.

25. Grimes DA. Gonorrhea and chlamydial infections. ACOG Technical Bulletin, No. 89, November 1985.

26. Smith KR, Ching S, Lee H, et al. Evaluation of ligase chain reaction for use with urine for identification of Neisseria gonorrhoeae in females attending a sexually transmitted disease clinic. J Clin Microbiol 1995;33:455.

27. Duff P. Urinary tract infections. Primary Care Update Ob Gynecol 1994;1:12.

28. Robertson AW, Duff P. The nitrite and leukocyte esterase tests for the evaluation of asymptomatic bacteriuria in pregnant patients. Obstet Gynecol 1988;71:878.

29. Duff P. Pyelonephritis in pregnancy. Clin Obstet Gynecol 1984;27:17.

30. Stamm WE, Counts GW, Running KR, et al. Diagnosis of coliform infection in acutely dysuric women. N Engl J Med 1982;307:463.

31. Stamm WE, Hooton TM. Management of urinary tract infections in adults. N Engl J Med 1993;329:1328.

32. Dunlow S, Duff P. Prevalence of antibiotic-resistant uropathogens in obstetric patients with acute pyelonephritis. Obstet Gynecol 1990;76:241.

33. Millar LK, Wing DA, Paul RH, Grimes DA. Outpatient treatment of pyelonephritis in pregnancy: a randomized controlled trial. Obstet Gynecol 1995;86:560.

34. Cunningham FG, Morris GB, Mickal A. Acute pyelonephritis of pregnancy: a clinical review. Obstet Gynecol 1973;43:112.

35. Gibbs RS, Duff P. Progress in pathogenesis and management of clinical intraamniotic infection. Am J Obstet Gynecol 1991;164:1317.

36. Armer TL, Duff P. Intraamniotic infection in patients with intact membranes and preterm labor. Obstet Gynecol Surv 1991;46:589.

37. Kirshon B, Rosenfeld B, Mari G, Belfort M. Amniotic fluid glucose and intraamniotic infection. Am J Obstet Gynecol 1991;164:818.

38. Romero R, Jimenez C, Lohda AK, et al. Amniotic fluid glucose concentration: a rapid and simple method for the detection of intraamniotic infection in preterm labor. Am J Obstet Gynecol 1990;163:968.

39. Gauthier DW, Meyer WJ, Bieniarz A. Correlation of amniotic fluid glucose concentration and intraamniotic

infection in patients with preterm labor or premature rupture of membranes. Am J Obstet Gynecol 1991; 165:1105.

40. Hoskins IA, Johnson TRB, Winkel CA. Leukocyte esterase activity in human amniotic fluid for the rapid detection of chorioamnionitis. Am J Obstet Gynecol 1987;157:730.

41. Romero R, Yoon BH, Mazor M, et al. The diagnostic and prognostic value of amniotic fluid white blood cell count, glucose, interleukin-6, and Gram stain in patients with preterm labor and intact membranes. Am J Obstet Gynecol 1993;169:805.

42. Sperling RS, Ramamurthy RS, Gibbs RS. A comparison of intrapartum versus immediate postpartum treatment of intra-amniotic infection. Obstet Gynecol 1987;70:861.

43. Gilstrap LC, Leveno KJ, Cox SM, et al. Intrapartum treatment of acute chorioamnionitis: impact on neonatal sepsis. Am J Obstet Gynecol 1988;159:579.

44. Gibbs RS, Dinsmoor MJ, Newton ER, et al. A randomized trial of intrapartum versus immediate postpartum treatment of women with intra-amniotic infection. Obstet Gynecol 1988;72:823.

45. Chapman SJ, Owen J. Randomized trial of single-dose versus multiple-dose cefotetan for the postpartum treatment of intrapartum chorioamnionitis. Am J Obstet Gynecol 1997;177:831.

46. Duff P, Sanders R, Gibbs RS. The course of labor in term patients with chorioamnionitis. Am J Obstet Gynecol 1983;147:391.

47. Duff P. Pathophysiology and management of postcesarean endomyometritis. Obstet Gynecol 1986;67:269.

48. Duff P. Antibiotic selection in obstetric patients. Infect Dis Clin North Am 1997;11:1.

49. Milligan DA, Brady K, Duff P. Short-term parenteral antibiotic therapy for puerperal endometritis. J Matern Fetal Med 1992;1:60.

50. Duff P. Staphylococcal infections. In: Gleicher N, ed. Principles and practice of medical therapy in pregnancy. 2nd ed. New York: Appleton & Lange, 1992:518.

51. Duff P. Prophylactic antibiotics for cesarean delivery: a simple cost-effective strategy for prevention of postoperative morbidity. Am J Obstet Gynecol 1987;157:794.

52. Duff P. Cytomegalovirus infection in pregnancy. Infect Dis Obstet Gynecol 1994;2:146.

53. Adler SP. Cytomegalovirus and child day care. N Engl J Med 1989;321:1290.

54. Betts RF. Cytomegalovirus infection epidemiology and biology in adults. Semin Perinatol 1983;7:22.

55. Chandler SH, Alexander ER, Holmes KK. Epidemiology of cytomegaloviral infection in a heterogeneous population of pregnant women. J Infect Dis 1985;152:249.

56. Adler SP. Cytomegalovirus and pregnancy. Curr Opin Obstet Gynecol 1992;4:670.

57. Stagno S, Pass RF, Dworsky ME, et al. Congenital cytomegalovirus infection. N Engl J Med 1982;306:995.

58. Fowler KB, Stagno S, Pass RF, et al. The outcome of congenital cytomegalovirus infection in relation to maternal antibody status. N Engl J Med 1992;326:663.

59. Dobbins JG, Stewart JA, Demmler GJ. Surveillance of congenital cytomegalovirus disease, 1990–1991. MMWR 1992;41:35.

60. Donner C, Liesnard C, Content J, et al. Prenatal diagnosis of 52 pregnancies at risk for congenital cytomegalovirus infection. Obstet Gynecol 1993;82:481.

61. American College of Obstetrics and Gynecologists: Group B streptococcal infections in pregnancy. ACOG Technical Bulletin, No. 170. July 1992.

62. Yancey MK, Duff P, Kublis P, Clark P, Frentzen BH. Risk factors for neonatal sepsis. Obstet Gynecol 1996; 87:188.

63. Thomsen AC, Morup L, Hansen KB. Antibiotic elimination of group-B streptococci in urine in prevention of preterm labor. Lancet 1987;1:591.

64. Newton ER, Clark M. Group B streptococcus and preterm rupture of membranes. Obstet Gynecol 1988; 71:198.

65. Yancey MK, Armer T, Clark P, Duff P. Assessment of rapid identification tests for genital carriage of group B streptococci. Obstet Gynecol 1992;80:1038.

66. Prevention of perinatal group B streptococcal disease: a public health perspective. MMWR 1996;45 (Suppl):1.

67. DeCueto M, Sanchez M-J, Sanpedro A, Miranda J-A, Herruzo A-J, Rosa-Fraile M. Timing of intrapartum ampicillin and prevention of vertical transmission of group B streptococcus. Obstet Gynecol 1998;91:112.

68. Rosenstein NE, Schuchat A. Opportunities for prevention of perinatal group B streptococcal disease: a multistate surveillance analysis. Obstet Gynecol 1997; 90:901.

69. Duff P. Hepatitis in pregnancy. ACOG Technical Bulletin, November 1992.

70. Centers for Disease Control. Protection against viral hepatitis: recommendations of the Immunization Practices Advisory Committee. MMWR 1990;39:1.

71. Duff B, Duff P. Hepatitis A vaccine: ready for prime time. Obstet Gynecol 1998;91:468.

72. Syndman DR. Hepatitis in pregnancy. N Engl J Med 1985;313:1398.

73. Hoofnagle JH, DiBisceglie AM. The treatment of chronic viral hepatitis. N Engl J Med 1997;336:347.

74. Centers for Disease Control. Hepatitis B virus: a comprehensive strategy for eliminating transmission in the United States through universal vaccination: recommendations of the Immunization Practices Advisory Committee (ACIP). MMWR 1991;40:1.

75. Lemon SM, Thomas DL. Vaccines to prevent viral hepatitis. N Engl J Med 1997;336:196.

76. Jagger J, Hunt EH, Brand-Elnaggar J, Pearson RD. Rates of needle-stick injury caused by various devices in a university hospital. N Engl J Med 1988;319:284.

77. Rizzetto M. The delta agent. Hepatology 1983;3:729.

78. Jacobson IM, Dienstag JL, Werner BG, et al. Epidemiology and clinical impact of hepatitis D virus (delta) infection. Hepatology 1985;5:188.

79. Lynch-Salamon DI, Combs CA. Hepatitis C in obstetrics and gynecology. Obstet Gynecol 1992;79:621.

80. Osmond DH, Padian NS, Sheppard HW, Glass S, Shiboski SC, Reingold A. Risk factors for hepatitis C virus positivity in heterosexual couples. JAMA 1993; 269:361.

81. Weinstock HS, Bolan G, Reingold AL, Polish LB. Hepatitis C virus infection among patients attending a

clinic for sexually transmitted diseases. JAMA 1993; 269:392.

82. Lau JY, Davis GL, Kniffen J, et al. Significance of serum hepatitis C virus RNA levels in chronic hepatitis C. Lancet 1993;341:1501.

83. Bohman VR, Stettler RW, Little BB, Wendel GD, Sutor LJ, Cunningham FG. Seroprevalence and risk factors for hepatitis C virus antibody in pregnant women. Obstet Gynecol 1992;80:609.

84. Alter MJ, Gallagher M, Morris TT, et al. Acute non-A-E hepatitis in the United States and the role of hepatitis G virus infection. N Engl J Med 1997;336:741.

85. Alter HJ, Nakatsuji Y, Melpolder J, et al. The incidence of transfusion-associated hepatitis G virus infection and its relation to liver disease. N Engl J Med 1997;336:747.

86. Feucht HH, Zollner B, Polywka S, Laufs R. Vertical transmission of hepatitis G. Lancet 1996;347:615.

87. Velazquez O, Stetler HC, Avila C, et al. Epidemic transmission of enterically transmitted non-A, non-B hepatitis in Mexico, 1986–1987. JAMA 1990;263:3281.

88. Wong DC, Purcell RH, Sreenivasan MA, Prasad SR, Pavri KM. Epidemic and endemic hepatitis in India: evidence for a non-A, non-B hepatitis virus aetiology. Lancet 1980;2:876.

89. Centers for Disease Control. Hepatitis E among U.S. travelers, 1989–1992. MMWR 1993;42:1.

90. Favorov MO, Fields HA, Puray MA, et al. Serologic identification of hepatitis E virus infections in epidemic and endemic settings. J Med Virol 1992;36:246.

91. Khuroo MS, Kamili S, Jameel S. Vertical transmission of hepatitis E virus. Lancet 1995;345:1025.

92. Cook CR, Gall SA. Herpes in pregnancy. Infect Dis Obstet Gynecol 1994;1:298.

93. Stone KM, Brooks CA, Guinan ME, Alexander ER. National surveillance for neonatal herpes simplex virus infections. Sex Transm Dis 1989;16:152.

94. Brown ZA, Vontver LA, Benedetti J, et al. Effects on infants of a first episode of genital herpes during pregnancy. N Engl J Med 1987;317:1246.

95. Cone RW, Hobson AC, Brown Z, et al. Frequent detection of genital herpes simplex virus DNA by polymerase chain reaction among pregnant women. JAMA 1994; 272:792.

96. Whitley R, Arvin A, Prober C, et al. Predictors of morbidity and mortality in neonates with herpes simplex virus infections. N Engl J Med 1991;324:450.

97. Brown ZA, Benedetti J, Ashley R, et al. Neonatal herpes simplex virus infection in relation to asymptomatic maternal infection at the time of labor. N Engl J Med 1991;324:1247.

98. Prober CG, Sullender WM, Yasukawa LL, Au DS, Yeager AS, Arvin AM. Low risk of herpes simplex virus infections in neonates exposed to the virus at the time of vaginal delivery to mothers with recurrent genital herpes simplex virus infections. N Engl J Med 1987;316:240.

99. Prober CG, Hensleigh PA, Boucher FD, Yasukawa LL, Au DS, Arvin AM. Use of routine viral cultures at delivery to identify neonates exposed to herpes simplex virus. N Engl J Med 1988;318:887.

100. Arvin AM, Hensleigh PA, Prober CG, et al. Failure of antepartum maternal cultures to predict the infant's risk of exposure to herpes simplex virus at delivery. N Engl J Med 1986;315:796.

101. Randolph AG, Washington AE, Prober CG. Cesarean delivery for women presenting with genital herpes lesions: efficacy, risks, and costs. JAMA 1993;270:77.

102. Gibbs RS, Amstey MS, Sweet RL, et al. Management of genital herpes infection in pregnancy. Obstet Gynecol 1988;71:779.

103. Gibbs RS, Mead PB. Preventing neonatal herpes— current strategies. N Engl J Med 1992;326:946.

104. Whitley RJ, Gramm JW. Acyclovir: a decade later. N Engl J Med 1992;327:782.

105. Randolph AG, Hartshorn RM, Washington AE. Acyclovir prophylaxis in late pregnancy to prevent neonatal herpes: a cost-effectiveness analysis. Obstet Gynecol 1996; 88:603.

106. Centers for Disease Control. Pregnancy outcomes following systemic prenatal acyclovir exposure—June 1, 1984–June 30, 1993. MMWR 1993;42:806.

107. O'Brien TR, George JR, Holmberg SD. Human immunodeficiency virus type 2 infection in the United States. JAMA 1992;267:2775.

108. Schacker T, Collier AC, Hughes J, Shea T, Corey L. Clinical and epidemiologic features of primary HIV infection. Ann Intern Med 1996;125:257.

109. Duff P. HIV infection in women. Primary Care Update OB/GYNs 1996;3:45.

110. Minkoff HL. Human immunodeficiency virus infections in pregnancy. ACOG Educational Bulletin No. 232, January 1997.

111. Guinan ME, Hardy A. Epidemiology of AIDS in women in the United States. JAMA 1987;257:2039.

112. Robertson ES. AIDS testing in the 1990s. Primary Care Update for OB/GYNs 1996;3:50.

113. O'Brien TR, Holmberg SD. Human immunodeficiency virus type 2 infections in the United States. JAMA 1992; 267:2775.

114. Landesman SH, Kalish LA, Burns DN, et al. Obstetrical factors and the transmission of human immunodeficiency virus type 1 from mother to child. N Engl J Med 1996; 334:1617.

115. Italian Multicenter Study. Epidemiology, clinical features, and prognostic factors of paediatric HIV infection. Lancet 1988;2:1043.

116. European Collaborative Study. Mother-to-child transmission of HIV infection. Lancet 1988;2:1039.

117. Connor EM, Sperling RS, Gelber R, et al. Reduction of maternal-infant transmission of human immunodeficiency virus type[1] with zidovudine treatment. N Engl J Med 1994;331:1173.

118. Carpenter CCJ, Cooper DA, Fischl MA, et al. Antiretroviral therapy in adults. Updated recommendations of the International AIDS Society—USA panel. JAMA 2000; 283:381.

119. Minkoff H, Augenbraun M. Antiretroviral therapy for pregnant women. Amer J Obstet Gynecol 1997;176:478.

120. 1997 USPHS/IDSA guidelines for the prevention of opportunistic infections in persons infected with human immunodeficiency virus. MMWR 1997;46 (Suppl):1.

120a. Mandelbrot L, LeChanadec J, Berrebi A, et al. Perinatal HIV-1 transmission. Interaction between zidovudine prophylaxis and mode of delivery in the French perinatal cohort. JAMA 1998;280:55.

120b. The international perinatal HIV group. The mode of delivery and the risk of vertical transmission of human immunodeficiency virus type 1. N Engl J Med 1999; 340:977.

121. Dunn DT, Newell ML, Ades AE, Peckham CS. Risk of human immunodeficiency virus type 1 transmission through breastfeeding. Lancet 1992;340:585.

122. Kumar ML. Human parvovirus B_{19} and its associated diseases. Clin Perinatol 1991;18:209.

123. Thurn J. Human parvovirus B_{19}: historical and clinical review. Rev Infect Dis 1988;10:1005.

124. Centers for Disease Control. Risks associated with human parvovirus B_{19} infection. MMWR 1989;38:81.

125. Cartter ML, Farley TA, Rosengren S, et al. Occupational risk factors for infection with parvovirus B_{19} among pregnant women. J Infect Dis 1991;163:282.

126. Gillespie SM, Cartter ML, Asch S, et al. Occupation risk of human parvovirus B_{19} infection for school and day-care personnel during an outbreak of erythema infectiosum. JAMA 1990;263:2061.

127. Rodis JF, Hovick TJ, Quinn DL, et al. Human parvovirus infection in pregnancy. Obstet Gynecol 1988;72:733.

128. Rodis JF, Quinn DL, Gary W, et al. Management and outcomes of pregnancies complicated by human B_{19} parvovirus infection: a prospective study. Am J Obstet Gynecol 1990;163:1168.

129. Public Health Laboratory Service Working Party on Fifth Disease. Prospective study of human parvovirus (B_{19}) infection in pregnancy. BMJ 1990;300:1166.

130. Peters MT, Nicolaides KH. Cordocentesis for the diagnosis and treatment of human fetal parvovirus infection. Obstet Gynecol 1990;75:501.

131. Pryde PG, Nugent CE, Pridjian G, et al. Spontaneous resolution of nonimmune hydrops fetalis secondary to human parvovirus B_{19} infection. Obstet Gynecol 1992; 79:859.

132. Humphrey W, Magoon M, O'Shaughnessy R. Severe nonimmune hydrops secondary to parvovirus B_{19} infection: spontaneous reversal in utero and survival of a term infant. Obstet Gynecol 1991;78:900.

133. Fairley CK, Smoleniec JS, Caul OE, Miller E. Observational study of effect of intrauterine transfusions on outcome of fetal hydrops after parvovirus B_{19} infection. Lancet 1995;346:1335.

134. Conry JA, Torok T, Andrews I. Perinatal encephalopathy secondary to in utero human parvovirus B-19 (HPV) infection, abstracted. Neurology 1993;43:A346.

135. Brown KE, Green SW, deMayolo JA, et al. Congenital anaemia after transplacental B_{19} parvovirus infection. Lancet 1994;343:895.

136. Rodis JF, Rodner C, Hansen AA, Borgida AF, Deoliveira I, Rosengren SS. Long-term outcome of children following maternal human parvovirus B19 infection. Obstet Gynecol 1998;91:125.

137. Sautter RL, Crist AE, Johnson LM, LeBar WD. Comparison of five methods for the determination of rubella immunity. Infect Dis Obstet Gynecol 1994; 1:188.

138. American College of Obstetricians and Gynecologists.

rubella and pregnancy. ACOG Technical Bulletin No. 171. August 1992.

139. Centers for Disease Control. Rubella and congenital rubella syndrome—United States, January 1, 1991–May 7, 1994. MMWR 1994;43:391.

140. Miller E, Cradock-Watson JE, Pollock TM. Consequences of confirmed maternal rubella at successive stages of pregnancy. Lancet 1982;2:781.

141. Centers for Disease Control: Rubella prevention: recommendations of the Immunization Practices Advisory Committee (ACIP). MMWR 1990;39:1.

142. Munro ND, Smithells RW, Sheppard S, Holzel H, Jones G. Temporal relations between maternal rubella and congenital defects. Lancet 1987;2:201.

143. McIntosh EDG, Menser MA: A fifty-year follow-up of congenital rubella. Lancet 1992;340:414.

144. Bart SW, Stetler HC, Preblud SR, et al. Fetal risk associated with rubella vaccine: an update. Rev Infect Dis 1985;7:S95.

145. National Vaccine Advisory Committee. The measles epidemic: the problems, barriers, and recommendations. JAMA 1991;266:1547.

146. Atkinson WL, Hadler SC, Redd SB, Orenstein WA. Measles surveillance—United States, 1991. MMWR 41(55–6):1992;41:1.

147. Hersh BS, Markowitz LE, Maes EF, et al. The geographic distribution of measles in the United States, 1980 through 1989. JAMA 1992;267:1936.

148. Atmar RL, Englund JA, Hammill H. Complications of measles during pregnancy. Clin Infect Dis 1992; 14:217.

149. Centers for Disease Control. Measles prevention: supplementary statement. MMWR 1992;38:11.

150. Christensen PE, Schmidt H, Bang HO, et al. An epidemic of measles in Southern Greenland, 1951. Acta Med Scand 1953;148:430.

151. Eberhart-Phillips JE, Frederick PD, Baron RC, Mascola L. Measles in pregnancy: a descriptive study of 58 cases. Obstet Gynecol 1993;82:797.

152. Stein SJ, Greenspoon JS. Rubeola during pregnancy. Obstet Gynecol 1991;78:925.

153. Centers for Disease Control. Measles prevention: recommendations of the Immunization Practices Advisory Committee (ACIP). MMWR 1989;3811.

154. Hook EW, Marra CM. Acquired syphilis in adults. N Engl J Med 1992;326:1060.

155. Rolfs RT, Nakashima AK. Epidemiology of primary and secondary syphilis in the United States, 1981 through 1989. JAMA 1990;264:1432.

156. Ricci JM, Fojaco RM, O'Sullivan MJ. Congenital syphilis: the University of Miami/Jackson Memorial Medical Center experience, 1986-1988. Obstet Gynecol 1989;74:687.

157. Wendel GD, Sanchez PJ, Peters MT, et al. Identification of *Treponema pallidum* in amniotic fluid and fetal blood from pregnancies complicated by congenital syphilis. Obstet Gynecol 1991;78:890.

158. Ziaya PR, Hankins GDV, Gilstrap LC, Halsey AB. Intravenous penicillin desensitization and treatment during pregnancy. JAMA 1986;256:2561.

159. Klein VR, Cox SM, Mitchell MD, Wendel GD. The

Jarisch-Herxheimer reaction complicating syphilotherapy in pregnancy. Obstet Gynecol 1990;75:375.

160. Krick JA, Remington JS. Toxoplasmosis in the adult—an overview. N Engl J Med 1978;298:550.

161. Daffos F. Prenatal management of 746 pregnancies at risk for congenital toxoplasmosis. N Engl J Med 1998; 318:271.

162. Hohlfeld P, Daffos F, Costa JM, et al. Prenatal diagnosis of congenital toxoplasmosis with a polymerase-chain reaction test on amniotic fluid. N Engl J Med 1994; 331:695.

163. Guerina NG, Hsu HW, Meissner HC, et al. Neonatal serologic screening and early treatment for congenital *Toxoplasma gondii* infection. N Engl J Med 1994;330:1858.

164. Chapman S, Duff P. Varicella in pregnancy. Semin Perinatol 1993;17:403.

165. Smego R, Asperilla MO. Use of acyclovir for varicella pneumonia during pregnancy. Obstet Gynecol 1991; 78:1112.

166. McGregor JA, Mark S, Crawford GP, Levin MJ. Varicella zoster antibody testing in the care of pregnant women exposed to varicella. Am J Obstet Gynecol 1987; 157:281.

167. Duff P. Varicella vaccine. Infect Dis Obstet Gynecol 1996;4:63.

168. Duff P. Varicella in pregnancy: five priorities for clinicians. Infect Dis Obstet Gynecol 1994;1:163.

169. Prevention of varicella. Recommendations of the Advisory Committee on Immunization Practices (ACIP). MMWR 1996;45(Suppl):1.

170. Asano Y, Yoshikawa T, Suga S, et al. Postexposure prophylaxis of varicella in family contact by oral acyclovir. Pediatrics 1993;92:219.

171. Wallace MR, Bowler WA, Murray NB, Brodine SK, Oldfield EC. Treatment of adult varicella with oral acyclovir: a randomized, placebo-controlled trial. Ann Intern Med 1992;117:358.

172. Dunkle LM, Arvin AM, Whitley RJ, et al. A controlled trial of acyclovir for chickenpox in normal children. N Engl J Med 1991;325:1539.

173. Pastuszak AL, Levy M, Schick B, et al. Outcome after maternal varicella infection in the first 20 weeks of pregnancy. N Engl J Med 1994;330:901.

174. Enders G, Miller E, Cradock-Watson J, et al. Consequences of varicella and herpes zoster in pregnancy: prospective study of 1739 cases. Lancet 1994;343:1547.

Chapter 6
Medical Complications of Pregnancy

CARDIAC DISEASE

Mark Landon

Five Key Points

- Cardiac function changes dramatically in pregnancy. Heart rate increases by 10 to 20%; cardiac output increases by 30 to 50%.

- Mitral stenosis is the most common manifestation of rheumatic heart disease in pregnancy. Atrial fibrillation is the most likely arrhythmia to be associated with this cardiac lesion.

- Patients with small atrial and ventricular septal defects generally have uncomplicated pregnancies.

- Patients with pulmonary hypertension have a significant increase in the risk of maternal mortality.

- Pregnant patients with Marfan syndrome are at increased risk for mortality from aortic dissection. Hypertension accentuates this risk.

Cardiac disease complicating pregnancy is a challenging clinical problem. Cardiovascular changes of normal pregnancy may impose a tremendous risk for women with certain categories of heart disease. Patients known to have only minimal limitation of their activity while not pregnant can suddenly experience worsening of their symptoms during gestation. Maternal mortality is increased with several cardiac conditions. The fetus is also at risk when maternal cardiac status deteriorates. Cardiac failure resulting in the delivery of poorly oxygenated blood to the pregnant uterus can critically affect fetal growth and viability. Therefore, an understanding of hemodynamic changes that occur during gestation becomes extremely im-

portant when planning therapy for the pregnant patient with heart disease

CARDIOVASCULAR CHANGES OF PREGNANCY

An expanded maternal plasma volume is responsible for most of the increase in blood volume found in pregnancy. This increase begins in the first trimester and accelerates to levels 50% above the nonpregnant mean by 32 weeks of gestation.[1] Women with a multiple gestation usually show even greater increments in their plasma volume. It was once believed that plasma volume declined in later pregnancy. These data

TABLE 6-1
CIRCULATORY ADJUSTMENTS DURING
NORMAL PREGNANCY

	Initial Increase	Peak
Blood volume	By 6 weeks	↑ 40% (avg) by 32 wk
Plasma volume	By 6 weeks	↑ 50% (avg) by 32 wk
Red-cell volume	Progressively after first trimester	↑ 20% by term

were derived from studies performed in the supine position, resulting in diminished preload. Studies performed in the left lateral position have documented that plasma volume remains stable from 32 weeks of gestation until delivery (Table 6-1).

The plasma volume expansion of normal pregnancy is mediated by hormonal factors. Plasma renin activity rises sharply secondary to estrogen-augmented hepatic production of renin substrate. Progesterone competitively blocks the action of aldosterone at the renal tubule. In spite of this, sodium and water are gradually retained, resulting in a 6- to 8-liter expansion of total body water. Two-thirds of this increase (4 to 6 liters) is distributed extracellularly, which clinically is manifested as edema of normal pregnancy.

Red-cell mass increases from 16 weeks of gestation until term and may reach values 20% above the average nonpregnant mean. Hematocrit declines as a dilutional anemia results during the second trimester because of the proportionately greater rise in plasma volume. Later in pregnancy, hemoglobin levels increase as erythropoiesis continues, while plasma volume stabilizes. Overall, blood volume rises an average of 40% over nonpregnant levels.[2]

Cardiac output rises early in pregnancy and reaches levels approximately 30 to 50% over base-line levels by 20 to 24 weeks of gestation.[3] Output measurements are greatly affected by changes in maternal position. Cardiac output measured in the left lateral position falls slightly during the last trimester of pregnancy.[4] In supine subjects studied during the second half of gestation, cardiac output is significantly decreased because of diminished venous return. Collateral vessels serve to ensure adequate return of blood to the right side of the heart. Insufficient collateral circulation will result in hypotension if the supine position is maintained for a prolonged period. This vasovagal-like syndrome has been termed the "supine hypotensive syndrome of pregnancy." Symptoms of hypotension and bradycardia are usually promptly relieved by placing the patient in the left lateral position.

The increased cardiac output observed early in pregnancy can be attributed to a larger stroke volume. Robson and colleagues have documented a rise in stroke volume by the 8th week of pregnancy, with maximal levels reached by midgestation.[4] As pregnancy advances, heart rate rises 10 to 20%, while cardiac output remains unchanged or falls. It follows, therefore, that stroke volume exhibits a progressive modest decline.

Volume changes alone are not responsible for the increased cardiac output found in pregnancy. Studies of the pulmonary vasculature reveal no change in pulmonary artery diastolic pressure during gestation.[5] This important index of cardiac function reflects left ventricular filling pressure. For end-diastolic volume to increase without a change in end-diastolic pressure, left ventricular enlargement must be present. Using echocardiographic techniques, it has been demonstrated that the diameter of the left ventricle increases in early pregnancy.[6] End-diastolic volume thus increases without an increased filling pressure, resulting in an increased stroke volume. Estrogens also enhance ventricular contractility and further increase stroke volume and output. Echocardiographic studies performed during pregnancy have revealed a decrease in the preejection period and an increase in left ventricular ejection time, reflecting an increase in left ventricular contractility.[7]

Normal pregnancy is accompanied by a slight decline in systolic blood pressure and a modest decrease in diastolic values. Mean systemic blood pressure declines at midpregnancy and features a somewhat widened pulse pressure. The decline in systemic blood pressure follows that of total vascular resistance, which, in turn, is accompanied by a progressive rise in cardiac output. The low-resistance circulation (diminished afterload) created by midpregnancy is believed to be hormonally modulated and is characterized by a refractoriness to vasopressors such as angiotension. Women in whom a decline in systemic blood pressure in early gestation fails to occur are more likely to have pregnancy-induced hypertension.

Labor produces significant changes in the cardiovascular system. With each uterine contraction as much as 500 ml of blood is squeezed from the uterus to the maternal circulation. As a result of this autotransfusion, systemic venous pressure rises. Right ventricular pressure then rises, and cardiac output increases about 20% in the supine position. Mean arterial pressure is thus increased and is followed by a reflex bradycardia.

Maternal pain and anxiety result in increased adrenergic stimulation, which is accompanied by a rise in blood pressure and tachycardia, particularly during the second stage of labor. It follows that anesthesia can greatly influence these hemodynamic changes. Epidural anesthesia may attenuate the normal increase in cardiac output and heart rate because it acts as an analgesic as well as a peripheral vasodilator, reducing venous return to the heart. These changes result in a diminished preload or ventricular end-diastolic volume. Similar effects may be observed with spinal anesthesia, particularly if a patient is not adequately hydrated prior to its administration. However, regional anesthesia can be used safely in most patients with cardiac disease. For women undergoing cesarean delivery, consideration of potentiating right-to-left shunting with diminished preload must be weighed against the risk of myocardial depression by general anesthetic agents, as well as acute hypertension associated with intubation and extubation.

Both epidural and spinal anesthesia may produce a fall in cardiac output and blood pressure prior to elective cesarean delivery. Hypotension usually can be corrected by employing left lateral uterine displacement and infusing appropriate intravenous fluids. Correction of hypotension with ephedrine is inadvisable in patients who cannot tolerate tachycardia.

After vaginal delivery, because of the reduction in caval compression and an increase in blood volume following uterine contraction, circulating cardiac output may rise 10 to 20%. A bradycardia often ensues, which lasts for a few days. After cesarean delivery, which is accompanied by greater blood loss, cardiac output and blood pressure may temporarily decrease.

DIAGNOSIS OF CARDIAC DISEASE

Pregnancy is often accompanied by physiologic changes that may be confused with underlying cardiac disease. Symptoms and clinical signs associated with heart disease are often present in a normal pregnancy. Pregnant women commonly experience fatigue, shortness of breath, orthopnea, and peripheral edema. These findings are similar to those present in congestive heart failure. The following symptoms, however, should suggest the presence of underlying cardiac disease: (1) any progressive limitation of physical activity

---

TABLE 6-2
MANIFESTATIONS OF CARDIAC DISEASE

History
  Progressive or severe dyspnea
  Dyspnea at rest
  Paroxysmal nocturnal dyspnea
  Angina or syncope with exertion
  Hemoptysis
Physical examination
  Loud systolic murmur or click
  Diastolic murmur
  Cardiomegaly, including parasternal heave
  Cyanosis or clubbing
  Persistent jugular venous distension
  Features of Marfan syndrome
Electrocardiogram
  Dysrhythmia

---

due to worsening dyspnea; (2) chest pain that accompanies exercise or increased activity; or (3) syncope preceded by palpitations or physical exertion (Table 6-2).

Physical examination of the heart and cardiovascular system are altered by normal physiologic changes, which can be confused with underlying heart disease. Systolic outflow murmurs, believed to represent pulmonic flow, are observed in 90% of pregnant women. In addition to this type of murmur, other systolic flow murmurs are often auscultated in the neck (brachiocephalic arteries), and a continuous mammary souffle may be heard over the breast in late pregnancy. Diastolic murmurs are uncommon; when present, they require further evaluation. Venous distention and accompanying peripheral edema are found in the majority of pregnancies. While neck veins may become pronounced, normal venous pulsations should occur. If absent, further evaluation is required.

Several techniques used to investigate cardiac function may be modified by pregnancy. Chest films will often demonstrate cardiomegaly and increased pulmonary vascular markings. EKG findings may aid in the preliminary diagnosis of valvular disease or anatomic defects if chamber hypertrophy is identified. Myocardial ischemia should not be confused with the ST-segment depression and flattening of T waves in the precordial leads, which may be present in normal pregnant women. Premature atrial and ventricular beats are also common in pregnancy.

Echocardiography is the preferred technique for detection and management of cardiac abnormalities during pregnancy. M-mode echocardiography has documented that the internal dimensions of the left ventricle, ejection fraction, and stroke volume are all increased in pregnant women after the first trimester.[8,9] Less commonly, modified stress testing and cardiac catherization are used in evaluating pregnant women.

GENERAL MANAGEMENT PRINCIPLES

Pregnant women with cardiac disease should be followed by both a cardiologist and an obstetrician. It is preferable to identify cardiac disease *prior* to pregnancy, so that appropriate counseling regarding risks and outcome may be undertaken. Certain conditions are associated with such high maternal mortality rates that pregnancy may not be advised (Table 6-3). Patients with mitral lesions may elect to undergo cardiac catheterization and valve replacement earlier in their illness if contemplating pregnancy.

It is important to define precisely the nature of a patient's cardiac disease. This information will enable the physician to appropriately assess the risks of pregnancy not only for the mother but for her fetus as well. For most congenital defects, a multifactorial pattern of inheritance exists, with risk to the fetus of developing structural disease varying according to the site of the specific lesion.

There is debate regarding the need for antibiotic prophylaxis during labor and delivery with valvular lesions. Although the efficacy of antibiotic prophylaxis against infective endocarditis has not been proven, the low risk of drug toxicity when weighed against the dangers of endocarditis makes such prophylaxis a consideration. Manual removal of the placenta is an absolute indication for antibiotic prophylaxis in patients with structural heart disease. For some patients, including those with prosthetic valves, mortality rates are particularly high should they become infected. These women should certainly receive prophylaxis for cesarean delivery. Prophylaxis usually includes the intravenous administration of aqueous penicillin G and an aminoglycoside at the start of true labor, with continuation every 8 hours until one dose has been given after delivery. Vancomycin may be substituted in patients who are allergic to penicillin.

Antibiotic prophylaxis for rheumatic fever should be used in patients with a positive history, especially if they demonstrate valvular disease. The American Heart Association recommends a monthly injection of 1.2 million units of penicillin G benzathine. Alternative regimens include daily oral administration of penicillin or erythromycin.

Anticoagulation may be required in individuals with prosthetic valves as well as in those with arrhythmias who may be at risk for thrombus formation. Patients with mitral stenosis and associated atrial fibrillation should also be anticoagulated. Pregnancy will influence the type of anticoagulation therapy to be used. Oral anticoagulants are contraindicated, as fetal exposure to coumadin during the first 2 months of gestation may result in malformations.[5] Heparin does not cross the placenta and, thus, is the preferred anticoagulant.

Cardiac function in patients with valvular disease should be assessed regularly. When function deteriorates and the patient fails to respond to medical treatment, cardiac surgery may become necessary. Ideally, cardiac surgery should be undertaken early in gestation, but preferably following fetal organogenesis. Open heart surgery has been associated with a low maternal mortality rate and improved fetal survival. In 68 cases using cardiopulmonary bypass, Becker and colleagues reported one maternal death and an 80% fetal salvage rate.[10,11]

TABLE 6-3
MATERNAL MORTALITY RISK ASSOCIATED WITH SPECIFIC CARDIAC DISEASES

Group I—Mortality <1%
  Atrial septal defect (uncomplicated)
  Ventricular septal defect (uncomplicated)
  Patent ductus arteriosus (uncomplicated)
  Pulmonic/tricuspid disease
  Corrected tetralogy of Fallot
  Porcine valve
  Mitral stenosis (mild)
Group II—Mortality 5–15%
  Mitral stenosis with atrial fibrillation
  Artificial valve
  Mitral stenosis (moderate to severe)
  Aortic stenosis
  Coarctation of aorta, uncomplicated
  Uncorrected tetralogy of Fallot
  Previous myocardial infarction
Group III—Mortality 25–50%
  Pulmonary hypertension
  Coarctation of aorta (complicated)
  Marfan syndrome with aortic involvement
  Eisenmenger syndrome

Adapted from Clark SL. Structural cardiac disease in pregnancy. In: Clark SL, Cotton DB, Hankins GDV, Phelan JP, eds. Critical care obstetrics. Blackwell Scientific Publications 1991:115.

TABLE 6-4
RECOMMENDED REGIMEN FOR ANTIBIOTIC PROPHYLAXIS

For labor and delivery	Ampicillin 2.0 g IM or IV plus gentamicin 1.5 mg/kg IM or IV given in active labor; one follow-up dose given 8 hours later and postpartum
Oral regimen for minor or repetitive procedures in low-risk patients	Amoxicillin 3.0 g orally 1 hour before procedure and 1.5 g 6 hours later
Penicillin-allergic patients	Vancomycin 1.0 g IV slowly over 1 hour, plus gentamicin 1.5 mg/kg IM or IV given 1 hour before procedure; repeat once 8 hours later.

IM = intramuscularly; IV = intravenously.

Derived from Shulman ST, Amren DP, Bisno AL, et al. Prevention of bacterial endocarditis. Circulation 1984;70(6):1125A; and Dajani AS, Bisno A, Chung KK. Prevention of bacterial endocarditis: recommendations by the American Heart Association. JAMA 1990;264:2919.

SPECIFIC VALVULAR DISEASES

Mitral Stenosis

Mitral stenosis is the most common form of rheumatic heart disease found in pregnancy. It can be an isolated lesion or it can accompany aortic or right-sided valvular lesions. In patients in whom rheumatic disease develops, mitral insufficiency often precedes the development of stenosis. Symptoms develop over time, when a reduction in cardiac output causes patients to become easily fatigued. Obstruction to left atrial outflow produces a rise in atrial pressure and, eventually, pulmonary capillary wedge pressure. Pulmonary congestion and right ventricular failure are seen 5 to 10 years after the onset of symptoms.[12] Patients generally remain asymptomatic until the valve area decreases to less than 2.5 cm^2. In patients with a valve area of less than 1 cm^2, mild exercise will produce symptoms. In symptomatic patients, the maternal mortality rate during pregnancy is sufficiently high to recommend surgical correction prior to pregnancy.

The augmented cardiac output of pregnancy, including tachycardia and increased circulatory volume, impose a tremendous stress on patients with significant mitral disease. Increases in cardiac output and shortened diastolic filling time may raise the diastolic gradient across the mitral valve, thereby elevating left atrial and pulmonary capillary pressure. In women with significant lesions, dyspnea is often present by 20 weeks of gestation, when resting cardiac output has reached its maximum.

Symptoms of reduced cardiac output should be treated with limitation of activity and cautious diuresis.

Atrial fibrillation must be aggressively treated. In hemodynamically stable patients, digitalis is initially used to slow the ventricular rate prior to cardioversion. As the size of the left atrium increases, there is a possibility that mural thrombus formation may occur. The patient should be anticoagulated with heparin if left atrial enlargement is present or if atrial fibrillation develops.

When medical measures do not alleviate symptoms, valve commissurotomy or replacement must be considered. Commissurotomy is reserved for women with isolated mitral disease who do not have significant regurgitation and who have limited calcification of the mitral valve. Percutaneous, mitral balloon valvuloplasty has been performed successfully during pregnancy.[13,14] In pregnant women with pure mitral stenosis characterized by simple commissural or commissural-band stenosis, balloon valvuloplasty is a desirable procedure in light of the risks associated with more extensive surgery. Valve replacement has become more popular with improved understanding of maternal and fetal physiology during cardiopulmonary bypass. It does, however, carry a higher risk of maternal and fetal mortality as compared with valvotomy.

Labor and delivery can challenge a patient with mitral stenosis. Patients with significant disease require invasive hemodynamic monitoring. Pulmonary capillary wedge pressure and cardiac output can be determined by the use of the Swan–Ganz catheter. The volume of fluids administered should be monitored carefully during both labor and the immediate postpartum period. Clark et al. have emphasized that, because pulmonary capillary wedge pressure does not accurately reflect left ventricular filling pressures in women with mitral stenosis, such patients often require high-normal wedge pressure in order to maintain cardiac output.[15] Patients should be given oxygen and should labor in the semi-Fowler position. Although epidural anesthesia is the preferred anesthetic technique, a decline in cardiac output has been associated with its use.[16] Ventricular rate must be monitored closely to avoid tachycardia, which may result in decreased cardiac output. Stenosis of the mitral valve is accompanied by a relatively fixed stroke volume, which may not rise with an increase in heart rate. Rapid heart rates further decrease diastolic filling time and elevate left atrial pressure. If sinus tachycardia becomes excessive (>140 bpm), the use of anesthetics to alleviate pain or cautious use of propranolol may be employed. Patients who receive epidural anesthesia should be carefully observed for hypotension, which may precipitate tachycardia. In patients delivering vaginally, the second stage of labor should be shortened by outlet forceps or vacuum extraction. A large bolus of intravenous oxytocin should be avoided, as it may precipitate hypotension.

The postpartum period represents the most hazardous time for women with mitral stenosis. A rise in wedge pressure is common, and careful attention must be given to changes in cardiac output that accompany fluid shifts following delivery. In general, a requirement for frequent administration of diuretics is to be anticipated.

Aortic Stenosis

Aortic stenosis is uncommonly encountered during pregnancy. Valvular thickening resulting from acute rheumatic disease does not typically occur for several decades following the acute disease, and symptoms generally are delayed until the 5th or 6th decade of life. Similarly, many patients a with congenital bicuspid aortic valve do not become symptomatic until after their childbearing years. Symptoms of angina, dyspnea, or syncope in patients with aortic stenosis signal significant decompensation, with mortality rates approaching 50% within 5 years. Women with such symptoms should be promptly evaluated. If significant left ventricular dysfunction is present and the valve area is less than 1 cm^2, pregnancy is contraindicated. Commissurotomy or heterograft prosthetic valve replacement are options for management.

Obstruction to left ventricular outflow and reduction in cardiac output are responsible for the symptoms associated with aortic stenosis. Physical exertion may result in relative ischemia of the cerebral and coronary vessels, producing syncope and angina. With longstanding aortic stenosis, left ventricular hypertrophy occurs as a compensatory mechanism and further increases the oxygen requirements of the heart and the propensity for anginal episodes. A rise in left atrial pressure is needed to fill the hypertrophied left ventricle. This requirement may be reflected in elevated pulmonary vascular pressures, leading to progressive dyspnea. Critical aortic stenosis creates a narrow window of appropriate fluid loading. Small decreases in preload due to hemorrhage or regional anesthesia may result in decreased cardiac output and accompanying hypotension.[17] Small increases in intravascular volume may produce significant increases in filling pressures, resulting in pulmonary edema.

The goal of treatment is thus to maintain filling pressures within the narrow therapeutic window and to avoid tachycardia.[19] The high mortality rate previously reported in association with pregnancy termination in women with aortic stenosis may reflect the occurrence of hypovolemia, which decreases venous return and left ventricular filling. This effect is poorly tolerated, as an adequate end-diastolic volume is necessary in the face of increased filling pressures and a fixed afterload or impedance to outflow. Some reports have emphasized the use of noninvasive techniques to secure a diagnosis and provide physiologic assessment in women with aortic stenosis, and maternal mortality now is much less common.[19,20] Severe lesions that fix cardiac output may, however, become symptomatic during the second half of gestation. Valve replacement or valvotomy has been successfully undertaken, as has percutaneous balloon aortic valvuloplasty in cases refractory to medical management.

Regional anesthesia, with its attendant risk for reducing preload or end-diastolic volume, must be used with great caution during labor and delivery. Hypotension can be avoided by the use of left lateral uterine displacement and appropriate fluid administration. A fall in blood pressure produces tachycardia, which may aggravate the condition of compromised patients. Tachycardia reduces the ventricular filling time and further reduces cardiac output. Central monitoring employing a Swan–Ganz catheter is encouraged in all symptomatic patients, as well as in those who have physical or diagnostic signs suggesting significant valve obstruction. Hypovolemia poses a greater risk than fluid overload; accordingly, wedge pressures should be maintained in an elevated range of 16 to 18 mm Hg to protect against unexpected blood loss.

Mitral Regurgitation

Mitral regurgitation may follow rheumatic fever or occur in association with idiopathic hypertrophic subaortic stenosis or mitral-valve prolapse. Mitral-valve prolapse is probably the most common cause of regurgitation in women of childbearing age.

Symptoms of left-sided failure generally develop later in life in women with mitral regurgitation than in patients with pure mitral stenosis. Reduced ventricular output leads to fatigue and dyspnea results from pulmonary congestion. In the final stage of this disease, patients with elevated pulmonary arteriolar pressure will have right-sided failure.

Pregnancy is generally well tolerated in patients with minimal mitral insufficiency. The typical decrescendo systolic murmur is diminished during pregnancy, as the fall in peripheral vascular resistance reduces, allowing more forward flow and less regurgitation across the mitral valve. Atrial enlargement and fibrillation may develop in patients with longstanding disease. The risk for arrhythmias may be increased during pregnancy. Therefore, reduction of left ventricular afterload may become an important therapeutic maneuver in patients with impaired cardiac output.

During labor and delivery, patients with significant mitral insufficiency may benefit from central monitoring to direct fluid and drug therapy. Pain may be associated with an increase in blood pressure due to enhanced sympathetic activity. If systemic vascular resistance also rises, pulmonary congestion may follow. Epidural analgesia is recommended to prevent this occurrence.

Aortic Regurgitation

Aortic regurgitation often coexists with mitral disease following rheumatic fever. Occasionally, aortic regurgitation is seen with a congenital bicuspid valve or in association with a collagen vascular disease such as rheumatoid arthritis or systemic lupus erythematosus. Dilatation of the aortic root is responsible for regurgitation found in patients with Marfan syndrome.

Most patients with aortic insufficiency experience symptoms of failure during the fourth or fifth decade of life. Progressive left ventricular dilatation results

from a state of chronic volume overload. In compensated cases, left ventricular end-diastolic pressure remains normal for several years. Pregnancy is complicated by episodes of failure in less than 10% of cases.[21] Restriction of activity along with treatment with digitalis, diuretics, and agents that reduce afterload should be instituted should symptoms of cardiac failure develop. Patients with aortic regurgitation due to endocarditis may require valve replacement.[22] Heterograft valves are preferred in pregnancy because they do not require that the patient be anticoagulated.[22]

The decrease in systemic vascular resistance observed during pregnancy may reduce the amount of regurgitant flow and the intensity of the regurgitant murmur. The stress of labor and delivery, however, may precipitate left-sided ventricular dysfunction. Afterload reduction has been successfully employed when vascular resistance remains high. Epidural anesthesia is recommended for vaginal delivery and may serve to prevent peripheral vasoconstriction. Bradycardia is poorly tolerated in patients with significant aortic regurgitation. Slowing of the heart rate increases the duration of ventricular diastole and regurgitation across the valve.

Congenital Lesions

Left-to-right shunting may occur through septal defects of the atrium or ventricle or with patent ductus arteriosus. Surgical correction of these lesions is often performed during infancy and childhood. Patients treated successfully in childhood may be followed for varying periods of time as long as their disease is stable. However, the hemodynamic changes of pregnancy may result in cardiovascular decompensation even after years of apparently good health.[23] During pregnancy, right-sided and left-sided resistance decrease in a similar manner; therefore, the degree of shunting is not significantly altered. Small defects can be expected to result in a good pregnancy outcome. In patients in whom pulmonary hypertension leading to shunt reversal has developed (Eisenmenger syndrome), maternal mortality rates of up to 50% have been reported.

Ventricular Septal Defect

Small ventricular septal defects (VSDs) are common and often close spontaneously in early life, whereas large defects discovered in childhood are most often surgically repaired. The small group of patients with uncorrected large VSDs are themselves growth-restricted and may experience frequent respiratory infections.

Patients with small VSDs generally tolerate pregnancy well. The degree of left-to-right shunting is not significantly affected if base-line pulmonary vascular resistance is not altered. However, hemodynamic changes of pregnancy, including an increased circulating blood volume and tachycardia, may increase left-to-right shunting to a critical level. Once pulmonary vascular resistance rises, right ventricular failure develops and reverse shunting with cyanosis may occur.

Increases in systemic vascular resistance, which accompany the stress of labor, may increase the degree of left-to-right shunting. Continuous epidural anesthesia should be used with caution because lowering of systemic pressure may not be tolerated by all patients. Women with significant pulmonary hypertension exhibit a right-to-left shunt, and a further fall in arterial PO_2 will occur if systemic vascular resistance is markedly reduced. The development of cyanosis generally signals right-to-left shunting. If cyanosis develops during labor, oxygen should be administered and steps taken to increase vascular resistance. Invasive hemodynamic monitoring is required to guide therapy.

Atrial Septal Defect

Atrial septal defect (ASD) is a common congenital heart lesion found in the adult population. The most common defect in the adult population is the ostium secundum defect. This defect may be associated with mitral-valve prolapse. Primum defects are generally corrected during childhood, but may have residual mitral regurgitation associated with them. Interatrial shunting through a typical ASD produces greater pulmonary blood flow relative to the systemic circulation. This change is generally well tolerated unless pulmonary hypertension is present. In general, right-sided failure and arrhythmias are not observed until the fourth or fifth decade of life.

No specific therapy is required in most pregnant women with ASD. Prophylactic antibiotics are often administered, although the risk of bacterial endocarditis is low, and routine anticoagulation is not recommended. Patients with no complications may be treated during labor and delivery without invasive monitoring. Epidural anesthesia is a well-accepted analgesic technique. It avoids marked increases in systemic vascular resistance which would augment left-to-right shunting.[21]

Patent Ductus Arteriosus

Persistent ductus arteriosus results in blood flow throughout the cardiac cycle from the higher pressure aorta to the lower pressure pulmonary artery. This effect increases pulmonary blood flow, with resulting enlargement of the pulmonary vasculature and left-sided chambers of the heart. Most women with patent ductus arteriosus (PDA) have their lesion corrected during childhood. As with an ASD, patients with a small ductus tolerate pregnancy well and usually have a benign clinical course until middle age.

Large PDAs are associated with growth restriction, chronic respiratory infections, and congestive heart failure during childhood and early adulthood. Pulmonary hypertension develops in affected patients, which is associated with significant mortality during gestation. The increase in left ventricular volume and workload that accompanies pregnancy results in left-sided failure, which further exacerbates preexisting pulmonary congestion. For this reason, therapeutic termination of pregnancy is generally indicated if significant right-to-left shunting is detected early in gestation. The risk for congenital heart disease in the offspring of women with PDA ranges from 4 to 11%.

Tetralogy of Fallot

This congenital anomaly consists of right-ventricular-outflow obstruction, VSD, right ventricular hypertrophy, and an overriding aorta. Right-to-left shunting is usually present, resulting in cyanosis. Patients with uncorrected tetralogy of Fallot have reduced life expectancy; thus, pregnancy with this condition has been uncommon. With uncorrected lesions, spontaneous abortions and intrauterine growth restriction are frequently observed.

The outcome for women with corrected lesions has improved remarkably. In a report of 31 pregnancies in 27 patients, all ended in live births at term, and few maternal complications were reported.[24] However, an increased incidence of growth restriction occurred.

Women with an uncorrected tetralogy usually will experience cardiac failure during pregnancy. Polycythemia and diminished peripheral oxygen saturation are poor prognostic signs. Echocardiographic assessment should be used to document ventricular function as well as the degree of shunting present. During pregnancy, the potential for increased right-to-left shunting exists due to a decline in systemic vascular resistance. The hypoxia associated with an uncorrected lesion can present a therapeutic challenge.

During labor and delivery, invasive monitoring may be necessary for the prompt recognition of cardiac failure. Increases in cardiac output observed during labor may raise pulmonary vascular tone and increase shunting to the left side of the heart. Venous return should be carefully maintained because a fall in blood volume may limit the ability of the right ventricle to perfuse the lungs. Right ventricular function will also depend on the degree of ventricular obstruction. Continuous delivery of oxygen is imperative.

In women with shunting, relief of pain during labor and delivery is best managed with systemic medications, inhalation analgesia, or pudendal block. Epidural or spinal anesthesia should be employed with caution because of the potential for hypotension resulting from decreases in vascular resistance and venous return. Ephedrine should be carefully administered in patients with right-sided failure, as it may produce a rise in pulmonary vascular resistance. In most cases, general anesthesia is preferred for cesarean delivery.

Complications may arise in the postpartum period, and hypovolemia should be promptly identified and corrected because the decline in systemic resistance will increase right-to-left shunting and cyanosis. A low threshold for blood replacement is prudent.

Eisenmenger Syndrome

Eisenmenger syndrome is defined as right-to-left or bidirectional shunting at either the atrial or ventricular level, combined with elevated pulmonary vascular resistance. Maternal mortality rates range from 12 to 70%, and fetal mortality rates approach 50%. Because of these risks, termination of pregnancy is recommended in patients with Eisenmenger syndrome complicated by significant pulmonary hypertension. Women who continue pregnancy require strict limitation of activity and consideration for anticoagulation.

The amount of right-to-left shunting observed in patients with this disorder will be dependent on the degree of pulmonary hypertension present and the relationship between pulmonary and systemic vascular resistances. Right ventricular failure is deleterious because it limits pulmonary blood flow and may increase right-to-left shunting. Cyanosis, chest pain, syncope, and hemoptysis are all symptoms associated with poor prognosis.

Monitoring with a right heart catheter is essential for management during labor and delivery. Hypovolemia and inadequate preload should be avoided by using uterine displacement. Controversy exists regarding the use of epidural anesthesia in patients with Eisenmenger syndrome because a fall in systemic vascular resistance could result in greater right to left shunting and cyanosis. Oxygen has proved to be an effective pulmonary vasodilator and can result in increased peripheral oxygen saturation. Epidural morphine has been used in a patient with pulmonary hypertension. This technique provides good analgesia with little effect on systemic blood pressure.[25] Serial determinations of arterial oxygen concentrations should be made when epidural anesthesia is administered. A fall in PO_2 despite oxygen support should prompt discontinuance of this anesthetic technique. Cesarean delivery offers no advantage over vaginal delivery in women with Eisenmenger syndrome.[26]

Obstructive Lesions

Coarctation of the Aorta

Severe coarctation is usually surgically corrected during infancy. Whereas early studies reported a significant risk for maternal mortality, management in the last two decades rarely results in maternal death.[27]

Patients at greatest risk are those with associated cardiac lesions or aneurysms of the aorta or circle of Willis. Coarctation should be suspected when a large difference in blood pressure is found between measurements in the upper extremities and legs. Because the constriction is often located at the level of the left subclavian artery, there may be isolated hypertension when blood pressure is determined in the right arm.

Following repair of coarctation, antihypertensive therapy should be prescribed to prevent any risk of aortic dissection. Women with repair performed during childhood should be carefully evaluated for aortic narrowing. If significant obstruction of the aorta is present, left ventricular compromise may be exacerbated during pregnancy. As with aortic stenosis, stroke volume is relatively fixed in these patients, so that normal compensatory mechanisms such as tachycardia may not be sufficient to maintain an adequate cardiac output. Hypotension during labor and postpartum should therefore be avoided. Appropriate precautions should be taken against infective endocarditis.

Surgical repair during pregnancy should be limited to cases of aortic dissection. Neurologic symptoms should be carefully evaluated as well. As stated earlier, it is not uncommon to find cerebral berry aneurysms in association with coarctation of the aorta.

Developmental Cardiac Lesions

Marfan Syndrome

Marfan syndrome is an autosomal dominant disorder of connective tissue with cardiac manifestations, including weakness of the aortic root and wall. Mitral valve prolapse is a component of this disease in 90% of cases. Certain families with Marfan syndrome have isolated skeletal deformities in the absence of disease of the aorta or aortic valve.[28]

Patients with Marfan syndrome should receive genetic counseling and be made aware of the risks of pregnancy with their particular condition. As cardiac manifestations may be minimal or absent, study of the cardiovascular system of these patients is key for counseling women about the dangers of pregnancy. Transesophageal echocardiographic measurement of the width of the aorta has been helpful in selecting patients at greatest risk for aortic dissection, although serial measurements of aortic root diameter may occasionally fail to detect a patient at risk for dissection.[29] Dilatation of the aorta >40 mm poses a significant risk for aortic dissection.[30] A review of the literature in this report substantiates that mortality rates of up to 50% exist with Marfan disease in pregnancy and generally reflect cases in which significant maternal cardiovascular disease existed prior to conception.

The risk for aortic dissection is influenced by superimposed hypertension. The most prominent symptom of dissection is excruciating chest pain. Painless dissection has been described and may be accompanied by hypertension and tachycardia. β-blockade and sodium nitroprusside infusion are the preferred medical therapy in such cases. Hypotension follows if the dissection is large or if it ruptures. A loud murmur of aortic insufficiency may be auscultated. Emergency surgical correction is required in patients with progressive dissection.

The management of patients with Marfan disease includes efforts to minimize hypertension as well as the contractile force transmitted to the aortic wall. β-blockade using propranolol may be efficacious. Regional anesthesia for labor and delivery is generally well tolerated.[31]

Mitral Valve Prolapse

Mitral valve prolapse (MVP) is the most common congenital heart lesion found in young women of childbearing age. The incidence in this population is approximately 12%.[32] Histologic examination of the mitral valve leaflets reveals myxomatous degeneration. MVP is associated with skeletal deformities including pectus excavatum and a high arched palate and is observed in patients with Marfan syndrome and Ehler–Danlos syndrome. The dysfunctional characteristic of MVP is abnormal prolapse of one or both mitral leaflets into the left atrium during ventricular systole. Most women with MVP are asymptomatic, whereas others experience palpitations, atypical chest pain, and syncope.

Most women with MVP have uneventful pregnancies. The increased intravascular volume of pregnancy which increases left ventricular end diastolic volume may result in less prolapse of the mitral valve leaflets.

Debate still exists as to whether routine antibiotic prophylaxis is warranted during pregnancy in patients with MVP. The American Heart Association has advised that antibiotics are not necessary in most patients undergoing routine vaginal or cesarean delivery.[33] Other authors suggest treating only those patients who have mitral regurgitation.

Idiopathic Hypertrophic Subaortic Stenosis (IHSS)

IHSS or asymmetric septal hypertrophy (ASH) is an autosomal dominant cardiac lesion which exhibits variable penetrance. Genetic counseling should be undertaken in affected individuals. In addition, prenatal ultrasonographic diagnosis has been reported.[34] IHSS manifests as obstruction to left ventricular flow secondary to a hypertrophied interventricular septum and outflow tract. The symptoms at presentation are similar to those of aortic stenosis and include dyspnea, angina, and syncope.

During ventricular systole, contraction of the myocardium results in narrowing of the outflow tract. Conditions which increase left ventricular end diastolic volume will improve this condition. Pregnancy, which is marked by an increased circulating blood volume, may initially result in improvement in outflow tract obstruction. As gestation advances, the fall in systemic vascular resistance, and diminished preload due to reduced venous return resulting from compression of the vena cava may exacerbate the symptoms found in patients with IHSS. Patients may thus develop ventricular failure and supraventricular tachycardias during pregnancy.[35] These may be found in association with left atrial distention resulting from coexisting mitral regurgitation. Maternal death has been rarely reported in patients with IHSS.[36,37]

Management of patients with IHSS should include (1) avoidance of inotropic agents such as digitalis which increase obstruction and precipitate failure; (2) maintenance of the left lateral decubitus position during labor; (3) restriction of the use of diuretics or drugs that decrease systemic vascular resistance; and (4) prompt recognition and treatment of arrhythmias.[38] As in the nonpregnant state, β-blockade can be helpful when symptoms arise during pregnancy or labor. The use of forceps to minimize Valsalva efforts which might increase outflow obstruction has been suggested.[38]

OTHER CARDIAC DISEASES

Peripartum Cardiomyopathy

Peripartum cardiomyopathy has classically been defined as congestive failure with cardiomyopathy found in the last month of pregnancy or in the first five months postpartum.[39,40] A hypocontractile myocardium with left-sided failure develops in women who have no previous history of cardiac disease. The overwhelming majority of women present with cardiac failure in the first three months postpartum.[39] The lesion is more common among older black multiparas particularly in association with twins or preeclampsia.

The etiology of this disease is unknown despite multiple theories, suggesting an autoimmune process, viral infection, and genetic predisposition. Histologic examination of the myocardium reveals muscular hypertrophy surrounded by interstitial edema and chronic inflammatory infiltrate.[41] It has been postulated that viral myocardial infections could trigger an autoimmune myocarditis. Therapy with steroids and azathioprine has thus been attempted, although this management should probably be restricted to cases in which the diagnosis has been established by endomyocardial biopsy. Primary therapy of peripartum cardiomyopathy includes bed rest, sodium restriction, digitalis, and diuretics.[42] Thromboembolic complications stemming from mural thrombi are a feared complication. Anticoagulation may be necessary,

particularly in patients with massively enlarged cardiac chambers.

It is clear that the prognosis for women with this disease can be predicted by the size of the heart several months after the diagnosis has been made. Approximately 50% of affected women will continue to have symptoms of failure and cardiomegaly beyond six months. These women should be advised against pregnancy as the incidence of recurrent disease is high with mortality rates approaching 100 percent.[43] If a viral etiology has been established with return to normal size and function, the recurrence risk is believed to be minimal.[44]

Ischemic Cardiac Disease

Coronary artery disease is uncommon in women during the reproductive years. Delayed childbearing and increased rates of smoking for some women may lead to an increase in the frequency of ischemic cardiac disease during pregnancy. The incidence of myocardial infarction during pregnancy is approximately 1 in 10,000.[45] Chronic hypertension has been documented in one third of women who suffer a myocardial infarction during pregnancy; however, mortality rates for these women do not appear to be greater than those without an elevation in blood pressure.[46] Whereas cigarette smoking and diabetes mellitus are other recognized risk factors for atherosclerosis, maternal age exceeding 35 years is the most consistent characteristic in pregnant women suffering a myocardial infarction.[47]

Coronary atherosclerosis is usually etiologic in pregnant women with a myocardial infarction; however, coronary artery spasm and embolism may also limit oxygen availability to the myocardium and can produce angina as well as infarction. Acute myocardial infarction has been described following ergonovine administration for uterine bleeding.[48]

Chest pain suggesting myocardial ischemia requires medical attention, even in seemingly low risk pregnant women. Anginal episodes should be evaluated with electrocardiography and exercise stress testing if clinical suspicion is high. Thallium nucleotide imaging of coronary blood flow is associated with limited radiation exposure (estimated 780 mrad), yet it has rarely been performed during pregnancy. Two-dimensional echocardiography may be of some value in detecting wall motion abnormalities during chest pain. If myocardial ischemia is strongly suggested, then interruption of pregnancy should be considered. If pregnancy is continued and symptoms do not abate with cessation of smoking and prescribed rest, then medical therapy including nitrates, β-blockers, or calcium channel blockers should be initiated. Repeated severe anginal episodes may necessitate coronary angiography with consideration for angioplasty or even bypass surgery during pregnancy.[49]

Two-thirds of myocardial infarctions occur during the third trimester. For affected women, the mortality rate has been reported to be 45% compared to 23% in patients suffering an infarction during the first two trimesters.[46] Hankins and colleagues reported that approximately 20% of pregnant women died at the time of infarction, and mortality occurred in 50% of patients who delivered within 2 weeks of the event. In contrast, these authors found no deaths among 34 women without recurrent infarction who delivered more than two weeks postinfarction. Unexplained fetal death was reported in five of these cases. The preponderance of infarctions during the third trimester and the increased risk of maternal mortality when delivery occurs within two weeks of infarction suggest that the hemodynamic burdens of late pregnancy and delivery are particularly hazardous to women with coronary artery disease.[47]

The management of myocardial infarction during pregnancy is essentially the same as in the nonpregnant individual. Patients should be admitted to the coronary or medical intensive care unit. Development of cardiac failure, arrhythmias, or recurrent angina warrants consideration of termination of pregnancy in women less than 24 weeks of gestation. An effort should be made to allow a period of healing and recovery before initiating labor. In women with no further symptoms, pregnancy can be allowed to progress to fetal maturity. During labor and delivery, pain should be minimized in order to decrease myocardial oxygen consumption. Conduction anesthesia is recommended and may reduce the normal anticipated increase in cardiac output. Invasive hemodynamic monitoring is often employed. Cesarean delivery should be reserved for obstetric indications as it does not improve maternal survival rates. There is continued debate as to whether women with a previous myocardial infarction should attempt pregnancy.[50]

REFERENCES

1. Scott DE. Anemia in pregnancy. Obstet Gynecol Annu 1972;1:219.

2. Metcalfe J, Ueland K. Maternal cardiovascular adjustment to pregnancy. Prog Cardiovasc Dis 1974;16:363.

3. Metcalfe J, McAnulty JH, Ueland K. Cardiovascular physiology. Clin Obstet Gynecol 1981;24:693.

4. Robson S, Hunter S, Boys RJ, et al. Serial study of factors influencing changes in cardiac output during human pregnancy. Am J Physiol 1989;256:H-1060.

5. Barry WH, Crossman W. Cardiac catheterization. In: Braunwald E. ed. Heart disease: a textbook of cardiovascular medicine, Vol. I, Philadelphia, WB Saunders Co., 1980.

6. Katz R, Karliner JS, Resnik R. Effects of a natural volume overload state (pregnancy) on left ventricular performance in normal human subjects. Circulation 1978;58:434.

7. Sadaniantz A, Kocheril AG, Emans S, et al. Cardiovascular changes in pregnancy evaluated by two-dimensional and Doppler echocardiography. Am J Soc Endocardiol 1992; 2:253.

8. Rubler S, Damini PM, Pinto ER. Cardiac size and performing during pregnancy estimated with echocardiography. Am J Cardiol 1977;40:534.

9. Vered Z, Poler SM, Gibson P, et al. Non-invasive detection of the morphologic and hemodynamic changes during normal pregnancy. Clin Cardiol 1991;14:327.

10. Becker RM. Intracardiac surgery in pregnant women. Ann Thoracic Surg 1983;36:463.

11. Strickland RA, Oliver WC, Chatigian RC, et al. Anesthesia cardiopulmonary bypass and the pregnant patient. Mayo Clin Proc 1991;66:411.

12. Rapaport E. Natural history of aortic and mitral valve disorders. Am J Cardiol 1982;35:221.

13. Ribeiro PA, Fawzy ME, Awad M. Balloon valvotomy for pregnant patients with severe pliable mitral stenosis using the Inoue technique with total abdominal and pelvic shielding. Am Heart J 1992;125:1558.

14. Kultursay H, Turkoglu C, Akin, et al. Mitral balloon valvuloplasty with transesophageal echocardiography without using fluoroscopy. Cathet Cardiovasc Diagn 1992;27:317.

15. Clark SL, Phelan J, Greenspoon J. Labor and delivery in the presence of mitral stenosis: central hemodynamic observations. Am J Obstet Gynecol 1985;152:982.

16. Ducey JP, Ellsworth SM. The hemodynamic effects of severe mitral stenosis and pulmonary hypertension during labor and delivery. Intensive Care Med 1989;15:192.

17. Szekely P, Turner R, Snaith L. Pregnancy and the changing pattern of rheumatic heart disease. Br Heart 1973; 35:1293.

18. Easterling TR, Chadwick HS, Otto CM, Benedetti TJ. Aortic stenosis in pregnancy. Obstet Gynecol 1988; 72:113.

19. Arias F, Pineda J. Aortic stenosis and pregnancy. J Repro Med 1978;20:229.

20. Lao TT, Sermer M, MaGee L, et al. Congenital aortic stenosis and pregnancy—a reappraisal. Am J Obstet Gynecol 1993;169:540.

21. Sullivan JM, Ramanathan KB. Management of medical problems in pregnancy—Severe cardiac disease. N Engl J Med 1985;313:304.

22. Westaby S, Parry AJ, Forfar JC. Reoperation for prosthetic valve endocarditis in the third trimester of pregnancy. Ann Thoracic Surg 1992;53:263.

23. Jackson GM, Dildy GA, Varner MW, et al. Severe pulmonary hypertension in pregnancy following successful

repair of ventricular septal defect in childhood. Obstet Gynecol 1993;82:6805.

24. Singh H, Bolton PJ, Oakley CM. Pregnancy after surgical correction of Tetralogy of Fallot. BMJ 1982;285:168.
25. Abboud JK, Raya J, Noueihed R. Intrathecal morphine for relief of labor pain in a parturient with severe pulmonary hypertension. Anesthesiology 1983;59:477.
26. Gleicher N, Midwall J, Hockberger D. Eisenmenger's syndrome and pregnancy. Obstet Gynecol Surv 1979;34:721.
27. Deal K, Wooley CF. Coarctation of the aorta and pregnancy. Ann Intern Med 1973;78:706.
28. Pyeritz RE, McKusick VA. The Marfan syndrome: diagnosis and management. N Engl J Med 1979;300:722.
29. Rosenblum N, Grossman A, Gabbe SG. Failure of serial echocardiographic studies to predict dissection in a pregnant women with Marfan's syndrome. Am J Obstet Gynecol 1983;146:470.
30. Pyeritz RE. Maternal and fetal complications of pregnancy in the Marfan syndrome. Am J Med 1982;71:784.
31. Gordon CF, Johnson MD. Anesthetic management of the pregnant patient with Marfan syndrome. J Clin Anesth 1993;5:248.
32. Devereux RB, Kramer-Fox R, Kligfield P. Mitral valve prolapse: causes, clinical manifestations, and management. Ann Intern Med 1989;111:305.
33. Dajani AS, Bisno A, Chung KJ. Prevention of bacterial endocarditis. JAMA 1990;264:2919.
34. Stewart PA, Buis-Lein T, Verivey RA, Wladimiroff JW. Prenatal ultrasonic diagnosis of familial asymmetric septal hypertrophy. Prenat Diagn 1986;6:249.
35. Turner GD, McGarry K, Oakley CM. Management of pregnancy with hypertrophic cardiomyopathy. BMJ 1979; 1:1749.
36. Shah DM, Sunderji SG. Hypertrophic cardiomyopathy and pregnancy: report of a maternal mortality and review of literature. Obstet Gynecol Surv 1985;40:444.
37. Pellicca F, Cianfrocca C, Gaudio C, et al. Sudden death during pregnancy in hypertrophic cardiomyopathy. Eur Heart J 1992;13:241.
38. Kolibash AJ, Ruiz DE, Lewis RP. Idiopathic hypertrophic subaortic stenosis in pregnancy. Ann Intern Med 1975; 82:791.
39. Walsh JJ, Burch GE. Postpartal heart disease. Arch Intern Med 1961;108:817.
40. DeMakis JG, Rahimtoola SH. Peripartum cardiomyopathy. Circulation 1971;44:964.
41. DeMakis JG, Rahimtoola SH, Sutton GC. Natural course of peripartum cardiomyopathy. Circulation 1971;44:1053.
42. Julian DG, Szekely P. Peripartum cardiomyopathy. Prog Cardiovasc Dis 1985;27:223.
43. St. John Sutton M, Cole P, Plappert M. Effects of subsequent pregnancy on left ventricular function in peripartum cardiomyopathy. Am Heart J 1991;121:1776.
44. Carvalho A, Brandao A, Martinez EE, et al. Prognosis in peripartum cardiomyopathy. Am J Cardiol 1989;64:540.
45. Ginz B. Myocardial infarction in pregnancy. J Obstet Gynaecol Br Commonw 1970;77:610.
46. Hussaini MH. Myocardial infarction during pregnancy: report of two cases with a review of the literature. Postgrad Med J 1971;47:660.
47. Hankins GDV, Wendel GD, Leveno KJ, et al. Myocardial infarction during pregnancy: a review. Obstet Gynecol 1985;65:139.
48. Liao JK, Cockrill BA, Yurchak PM. Acute myocardial infarction after ergonovine administration for uterine bleeding. Am J Caurdiol 1991;68:823.
49. Majdan JF, Walinsley P, Cowchock SF, et al. Coronary artery bypass surgery during pregnancy. Am J Cardiol 1983;52:1145.
50. Frenkel Y, Barkai G, Brisin L, et al. Pregnancy after myocardial infarction: are we playing safe? Obstet Gynecol 1991;77:822.

PULMONARY DISEASE

Philip Samuels

Five Key Points

- Respiratory tract infection is the most common cause for an exacerbation of asthma in pregnancy. The most appropriate initial treatment for a pregnant patient with mild asthma is an inhaled beta β_2-agonist.

- The most common clinical manifestation of pulmonary embolism in pregnancy is dyspnea. The diagnosis is best established by a ventilation/perfusion scan of the lung. Pulmonary angiography should be reserved for problematic cases.

- The most common cause of bacterial pneumonia in pregnancy is *Streptococcus pneumoniae*.

- Isoniazid is the most effective agent for prevention of reactivated tuberculosis. Active disease in pregnancy should be treated with at least two antibiotics, usually isoniazid and rifampin.

- Cystic fibrosis is the most common autosomal recessive disorder in the Caucasian population.

ASTHMA

Epidemiology

Asthma is the most common obstructive pulmonary disease that coexists with pregnancy. It is observed in 0.4 to 1.3% of pregnant women.[1,2] A study at Johns Hopkins Hospital reported a 1% incidence of asthma complicating pregnancy and a 0.15% incidence of severe asthma requiring hospitalization during gestation.[3] Pregnancy can have a variable effect on the course of asthma. Data compiled from nine studies published between 1953 and 1976 demonstrated that 49% of pregnant patients had no change in the course of their asthma, 29% showed improvement, and 22% showed exacerbation of their disease.[4-7] A 1989 study from the United Kingdom demonstrated that asthma improved in 69% of pregnant women,

worsened in 9%, and showed no change in 22%.[8] With advances in therapy and the use of more selective β-agonist inhalers, these results are probably now much better.

Nonetheless, asthma continues to be a major problem for adolescents who become pregnant. Apter and coinvestigators[9] studied 28 pregnancies in 21 adolescents. There were 56 exacerbations of asthma, including 22 hospitalizations and 20 emergency room visits. In 64% of the pregnancies, systemic corticosteroids were required.[2] These investigators found that the two most frequent factors associated with exacerbations of asthma included respiratory tract infections (59%) and noncompliance with medical regimens (27%). Williams[10] noted that approximately one-third of patients with asthma reacted differently in subsequent pregnancies irrespective of the sex of the fetus.

Perinatal Outcome

Data indicate that the risk of perinatal morbidity and mortality is minimally increased in the patient with asthma, especially if adequate medical care is received. Sims and coworkers[11] observed a small increase in the number of growth-restricted newborns in mothers receiving oral steroid therapy. In the study of Apter et al.[9] there was only one premature infant and no cases complicated by intrauterine growth restriction (IUGR).

Mabie and coworkers[12] compared outcomes in 200 pregnancies in 142 patients with asthma with a control group of 22,651 without asthma. They found no difference in prematurity, IUGR, or perinatal mortality. Most of the patients had mild asthma, and 12% experienced exacerbations during labor. They also found that the rate of postpartum exacerbations was higher in those who had undergone cesarean delivery.

Perlow and colleagues[13] retrospectively studied 183 patients with asthma. Patients with steroid-dependent asthma showed a higher incidence of gestational diabetes, preterm labor, premature rupture of the membranes, and preterm delivery. These factors were also increased somewhat in patients with non–steroid-dependent asthma on long-term medications. Cesarean delivery, growth restriction, and delivery of very-low-birth-weight infants were not increased. The authors concluded that perinatal outcome is compromised in patients with asthma who take long-term medications.

Schatz et al.[14] published a prospective case-control study of 486 patients with asthma. They found that, in well-controlled, actively treated patients, there was no increase in perinatal complications. They attributed this to aggressive management of the asthma.

Treatment

The goals in treating asthma during pregnancy are (1) reduction in the number of asthmatic attacks, (2) prevention of status asthmaticus, and (3) assurance of adequate maternal and fetal oxygenation. Patients receiving allergen desensitization may continue this treatment throughout pregnancy.[15] The Centers for Disease Control and Prevention (CDC) recommends that patients with chronic bronchial asthma receive the influenza immunization and the pneumococcal vaccine.[16] These are killed vaccines and can be administered safely during pregnancy.

Inhaled β-agonists have become the mainstay of short- and long-term therapy for asthma in pregnancy. The most widely used of these agents are albuterol and metaproterenol. Salmeterol, a long-acting beta-agonist, can be used twice daily on a regular basis. Albuterol can be used to supplement this. Anticholinergic inhalers are also used. This therapy can be used on an as-needed basis for patients with severe disease. In a fairly large study, no adverse pregnancy outcome was seen in women who used β-agonist inhalers in the first trimester.[17] The most common side effects seen with these agents include cardiac arrhythmias and tachycardia, but this is uncommon.

In addition to inhaled β-agonists, many patients require inhaled glucocorticoids. This therapy has helped control asthma on an outpatient basis.[18,19] Several agents of varying potencies and duration of action are available. The main side effect is oropharyngeal candidiasis, but this is minimized if a spacer device is used with the inhaler. Cromolyn is another antiinflammatory agent that may be used during pregnancy. It prevents mast-cell degranulation. It is not as powerful as glucocorticoids and works more slowly. It is usually used as adjunctive therapy and may be administered with β-agonists, anticholinergics, and glucocorticoids.

The use of aminophylline has dramatically declined during pregnancy, but some obstetricians still use it because of their familiarity with this agent. Cyclic adenosine monophosphate (cAMP), which produces relaxation of the bronchi, is released when β_2-receptors are stimulated by agonists. cAMP is metabolized by phosphodiesterase. Aminophylline derivatives inhibit phosphodiesterase and, therefore, increase circulating levels of cAMP. Aminophylline crosses the placenta but has shown no harmful effects to the fetus.[20-22]

Oral or parenteral corticosteroids should be employed when the aerosolized forms are inadequate. Although administration of glucocorticoids to pregnant rabbits has been associated with cleft palate,[23] these medications have not proven to be teratogenic in humans.

Schatz and colleagues[24] found no evidence of neonatal adrenal suppression in 71 infants born to mothers receiving a daily average of 8.2 mg of prednisone during gestation. In another report, neonatal adrenal insufficiency was not observed in infants whose mothers received up to 60 mg of prednisone daily throughout pregnancy.[25]

The lack of fetal and neonatal effects associated with maternal glucocorticoid ingestion is probably due to the small amount of administered glucocorticoid that actually reaches the fetal compartment. A fetus is exposed to only 10 to 30% of the prednisone ingested by the mother because most of the drug is inactivated by placental 11-β-ol-dehydrogenase.[26,27] Of the small amount of prednisone that actually reaches the fetus, even a smaller fraction will be metabolized by the fetus to the active form of the drug, prednisolone. When selecting a corticosteroid for use during pregnancy, it is important to look at the ratio of glucocorticoid to mineralocorticoid activity as well as the amount of drug that crosses the placenta. Prednisone and methylprednisolone are excellent choices because they have minimal mineralocorticoid effects and cross the placenta poorly.

Status asthmaticus requires immediate therapeutic intervention. During this period of acute treatment, the patient should receive a 30 to 40% concentration of humidified oxygen and should be well hydrated. Subcutaneous catecholamines should be administered. Because it has both α- and β-agonist activities, epinephrine can theoretically decrease uterine blood flow and thus decrease fetal oxygenation during this critical period. There is no evidence, however, that epinephrine has deleterious effects on the fetus. Terbutaline, a β_2-agonist that is more selective than epinephrine, is a better first-line drug in pregnancy. If the patient does not improve rapidly after the subcutaneous administration of catecholamines, intravenous corticosteroids should be administered. Methylprednisolone in a dose of 100 mg every 6 to 8 hours, or hydrocortisone in a dose of 100 mg every 4 hours, should be given until the asthma attack clears. Nebulized β-agonists should also be used. Rarely, intravenous aminophylline in a loading dose of 5 mg/kg, followed by 0.6 mg/kg/hr, can be used in the poorly responsive patient.

In the unusual patient who is resistant to these measures and has a falling PO_2, endotracheal intubation should be considered. This procedure should be undertaken only under the guidance of a pulmonary specialist, anesthesiologist, or intensivist.

Acute asthma attacks are unusual during labor. If they occur, however, they should be treated in the usual fashion. Epidural anesthesia is preferred for labor, vaginal delivery, and/or cesarean delivery. General anesthesia carries the risks of atelectasis and subsequent pulmonary infection.[28] If the patient has been receiving oral corticosteroids during pregnancy, intravenous dosages should be used for labor and delivery. Generally, 100 mg of hydrocortisone every 4 to 6 hours, or 100 mg of methylprednisolone administered intravenously at 6- to 8-hour intervals during labor and for 24 hours after delivery, should suffice. Thereafter, the patient should resume her maintenance dose of oral glucocorticoids.

PULMONARY EMBOLUS

Epidemiology

Pulmonary embolus complicates between 0.09 and 0.7 in 1000 pregnancies.[29,30] Prompt diagnosis and treatment are imperative, as untreated pulmonary emboli during pregnancy carry a 12.8% mortality rate, while treatment lowers this to 0.7%.[31] If untreated, more than one-third of these patients will have recurrent emboli.[32] The vast majority of pulmonary emboli arise from thrombophlebitis of the deep femoral and pelvic veins. The reported incidence of deep venous thrombosis during pregnancy is 0.4 in 1000.[29] This figure is six times the frequency in nonpregnant women.[33] In a review by Weiner,[34] the incidence of deep venous-thrombosis in pregnancy was 0.36%.

It is now common for patients in preterm labor to be aggressively treated with prolonged bed rest. This approach places these patients at an increased risk for thrombophlebitis and pulmonary embolism. Girz and Heiselman[35] report a case of a fatal pulmonary embolus that occurred during tocolysis. It is prudent, therefore, to administer prophylactic, low-dose heparin to patients who are at prolonged bed rest. Pneumatic compression boots may be used instead with equal results.

The patient with an acute pulmonary embolus usually presents with chest pain and dyspnea. Occasionally, a pleural friction rub may be auscultated. Chest x-ray films are often normal, but arterial blood-gas values usually show a decreased PO_2 and a slightly more decreased PCO_2. Hypercapnia bodes a poor outcome.[35] Massive pulmonary emboli are easily diagnosed. Hypotension and cardiovascular collapse often complicate such cases. In contrast, patients with small emboli only may have subtle signs and symptoms. It is imperative to establish the proper diagnosis in affected patients, as these small clots may be the harbinger of a massive embolus.

Certain acquired disorders of coagulation place the patient at increased risk for thrombophlebitis and pulmonary embolism. Congenital deficiency of antithrombin III is an autosomal dominant trait. The prevalence is approximately 1 in 3500 individuals. Pregnancy in these patients is often complicated by thrombophlebitis.[36] Protein C deficiency is another autosomal dominant trait. During pregnancy, there may be up to a 25% risk of deep venous thrombosis in those with a protein C deficiency.[36] In congenital deficiencies of protein S, a vitamin K–dependent inhibitor of hemostasis, there is a high incidence of thrombophlebitis.[36] Researchers have found that up to 5% of the population carry a mutation of factor V, known as the factor V Leiden mutation.[37,38] This causes activated protein C resistance. Heterozygotes for this disorder have a 5- to 10-fold increased risk for thrombosis, and homozygotes have a 40 times increased risk. In patients with a prior history of deep venous thrombosis, levels of protein C, protein S, and antithrombin III should be assessed prior to pregnancy, as gestation causes changes that may make the results confusing or unreliable. Since factor V Leiden mutation is detected by DNA analysis, pregnancy does not alter test results.

Diagnosis

Although impedance plethysmography is still occasionally used to detect lower-extremity thrombosis, Doppler study with compression sonography has made testing much more accurate. Its positive predictive value is 94%, as compared with 83% for impedance plethysmography.[39] A more recent study by Spritzer et al.[40] shows the usefulness and excellent sensitivity of magnetic resonance imaging in detecting thrombosis above the knee. The usefulness of this in pregnancy is questionable.

The diagnosis of pulmonary embolus must be established radiographically. Adequate technique is essential so that fetal exposure to ionizing radiation is minimized. Pulmonary ventilation/perfusion (V/Q) scans are useful in diagnosing pulmonary embolism only if chest x-ray films are normal. Calculations have shown that the maximum fetal radiation exposure from this study is 50 mrem.[41] These isotopes are excreted through the maternal urinary tract, and the fetus receives 85% of its radiation exposure from the maternal bladder. Frequent micturition should, therefore, theoretically lower fetal exposure.[41] If necessary, a Foley catheter can be used to empty the bladder. A large study showed that "high probability" V/Q scans with clinical symptoms carried a high likelihood that the patient actually had a pulmonary embolus.[42]

If the V/Q scan is equivocal or if the patient's chest x-ray films are abnormal, selective pulmonary angiography should be undertaken immediately. In experienced hands, the procedure carries a morbidity of less than 1%. Abdominal shielding should be used during the procedure. The increased plasma volume and vasodilatation that occur during pregnancy should make the procedure faster and technically easier than in the nonpregnant patient. Spiral CT scanning is becoming widely used in diagnosing of pulmonary embolus because this technique obviates the small risk of invasive angiography.

Ginsberg and colleagues[43] have carefully looked at radiation exposure from various procedures during pregnancy. Their review suggests that there is a small but undefined increase in the risk of childhood cancer following radiation exposures of less than 5 rad. They believe that, with careful use of available procedures, the diagnosis of venous thrombosis is possible with fetal exposure below 0.5 rad. Furthermore, in diagnosing pulmonary embolism, it is possible to keep fetal radiation exposure below 0.05 rad.[43] Because the risk to the fetus from such exposure is small in both relative and absolute terms, the diagnostic procedure should be undertaken without hesitation when indicated.

Treatment

Once the diagnosis is established, therapy should be initiated without delay. Anticoagulation with heparin is the treatment of choice. Heparin, a large, negatively charged protein with a molecular weight of 20 kd, does not cross the placenta.[44] The main complication of heparin therapy is maternal bleeding. This complication can be minimized, however, with meticulous attention to dosage and frequent monitoring of the activated partial thromboplastin time (APTT). Hemorrhage, nevertheless, appears to complicate the course of between 8 and 33% of patients anticoagulated with heparin.[45-47] Other potential complications of heparin therapy include osteopenia, alopecia, urticaria, bronchoconstriction secondary to histamine release, and idiosyncratic thrombocytopenia.[48] Platelet counts should be checked weekly during the first 2 weeks of therapy. Bone demineralization can occur if more than 22,000 units of heparin are administered daily for more than 20 weeks.

An initial loading dose of 80 units/kg should be administered intravenously, followed by a continuous infusion of 18 units/kg/h. When calculating these doses, an adjusted body weight should be used. This is calculated as follows:

Adjusted body weight = [ideal body weight + (0.3)(actual body weight − ideal body weight)].

The required maintenance dose of heparin infusion can show large interpatient variation, but the APTT should be kept approximately twice the upper limit of normal. This intravenous regimen should be continued for 7 to 10 days in a stable patient.

For the remainder of the pregnancy, patients should receive enough subcutaneous heparin to keep the APTT at 1.5 to 2 times the upper limit of normal. The usual patient requires 7500 to 12,000 units of heparin two to three times daily. Although less convenient, the thrice-daily dosing keeps the level more constant. Doses must be individualized to keep the APTT at the desired prolongation. As clotting factors change during pregnancy, the APTT should be determined regularly and dosages of subcutaneous heparin adjusted accordingly.[49] In the stable patient, therapy can be stopped for labor and delivery. If necessary, heparin can be reversed with protamine sulfate. Heparin therapy can be restarted safely several hours after delivery.

Coumadin can be used in the postpartum period. Although only small amounts cross into breast milk, its use in the breast-feeding mother remains controversial. Regardless of the therapy, the patient needs to remain anticoagulated for 8 to 12 weeks after delivery, at which time clotting factors should have returned to normal. After that, therapy must be individualized.

Low-molecular-weight heparin is gaining in popularity because of its longer half-life and because there is no need to monitor therapy with tests such as the APTT. Unfortunately, its longer half-life has been associated with bleeding into the epidural space after conduction anesthesia in nonpregnant patients. The only way to determine if an individual is anticoagulated with low-molecular-weight heparin is to check factor X activity. This time-consuming and expensive coagulation assay is not readily or rapidly available in most institutions. Some insurers and physicians are advocating the initial outpatient treatment of uncomplicated pulmonary embolus with low-molecular-weight heparin. At present, it is safest to continue using conventional unfractionated heparin begun in an inpatient setting. In pregnancy at least, low-molecular-weight heparin should probably be reserved for the patient who has hypersensitivity to the beef and/or pork components of fractionated heparin.

Oral anticoagulants should not be used during gestation. These drugs are vitamin K antagonists that readily cross the placenta and are teratogenic when used in early pregnancy. In the first trimester, these drugs are associated with facial dysmorphism, hypoplastic digits, stippled epiphyses, and mental retardation.[50,51] In midtrimester, optic atrophy, faulty brain development, and developmental retardation may occur.[50] In addition, the fetus is anticoagulated by these drugs, which can result in severe fetal hemorrhage in the event of trauma or preterm labor.

There is no universal consensus on treatment of the patient with thrombophlebitis in a prior pregnancy. If the patient had never experienced a pulmonary embolus, many individuals would give the patient prophylactic heparin, beginning with a dose of 5000 units twice daily and increasing the dose each trimester until the patient is receiving 10,000 units twice daily. Many authors believe that some form of anticoagulant therapy is necessary because the incidence of recurrent thromboembolic disease is 4 to 12%.[53,54] There is no consensus about whether women with a pulmonary embolus in the past need heparin prophylaxis or actual anticoagulation. In general, we advise anticoagulation under careful supervision.

PNEUMONIA

Bacterial Pneumonia

The most common cause of bacterial pneumonia in pregnant women is *Streptococcus pneumoniae*, and most affected patients are smokers.[35] The clinical hallmarks of pneumococcal pneumonia are sudden onset, productive cough, purulent sputum, tachypnea, and fever with shaking chills. The diagnosis should be made on the basis of chest x-ray films, Gram stain of the sputum, and cultures of blood and sputum. Chest x-ray films usually reveal lobar consolidation and air bronchograms. Gram stain shows numerous leukocytes and gram-positive diplococci.

Patients with pneumococcal pneumonia complicating pregnancy should initially be hospitalized and treated with 600,000 units of aqueous penicillin G intravenously four times daily. Parenteral treatment should continue for several days after defervescence.

The therapy can then be changed to oral penicillin or ampicillin (500 mg four times daily). Treatment should be continued for a total of 10 to 14 days. For patients who are allergic to penicillin, either a cephalosporin or erythromycin can be used. It should be noted, however, that 10 to 15% of patients who are allergic to penicillin will also react to cephalosporins.

A vaccine consisting of the capsular antigens from *S. pneumoniae* has been used to prevent pneumococcal infections. It should be used during pregnancy in special circumstances, such as the patient about to undergo splenectomy[56] and in the immunosuppressed patient.

Mycoplasma Pneumonia

Mycoplasma pneumonia is caused by *Mycoplasma pneumoniae*, a small organism lacking a cell wall. It, therefore, does not respond to therapy with penicillin or cephalosporins. This form of pneumonia is common in young adults. In contrast to the sudden onset of pneumococcal pneumonia, patients with mycoplasma pneumonia usually have a slow, gradual onset of symptoms with a nonproductive cough. The diagnosis is usually made clinically. On chest x-ray films, infiltrates are diffuse and patchy and can be either unilateral or bilateral. Antibodies to mycoplasma can be used to confirm the diagnosis. One must consider mycoplasma pneumonia in any patient whose clinical symptoms are not responding to penicillin or cephalosporins. During pregnancy, the treatment of mycoplasma pneumonia consists of the administration of erythromycin for 10 to 14 days. Azithromycin can also be used. The latter medication may cause less gastrointestinal distress than erythromycin but is more expensive. Tetracycline and its derivatives should be avoided.

Gram-Negative Infections

In immunocompromised patients, patients with alcoholism, and heavy smokers, pneumonia secondary to *Haemophilus influenzae* and *Klebsiella pneumoniae* may occur. Pneumonia caused by these organisms requires immediate hospitalization and therapy with intravenous antibiotics.

Viral Pneumonia

In recent years, there has been resurgence of pneumonia due to influenza A. It is uncertain whether this is due to a true increase in the disease or to an increased ability to diagnosis it. Patients need supportive therapy if this complication develops, and maternal deaths have been reported.[57,58] Of interest, the routine administration of influenza vaccine to pregnant women is now recommended by the CDC. Unvaccinated pregnant women who are exposed to influenza A should receive amantadine. The prophylactic dose is 200 mg in a single or divided dose daily for 10 days. If administered immediately after exposure, it can prevent 70 to 90% of infections. Some authors believe that it can decrease the duration of illness and severity of symptoms if used within 48 hours of the onset of symptoms. In this instance, the patient should take 200 mg daily until symptoms have been dissipated for 24 hours.[59] If influenza A pneumonia develops, the physician must be vigilant for the development of a superinfection with *Staphylococcus aureus*.

Varicella affects very few adults, but in up to 25% of those who contract the disease varicella pneumonia may develop.[60,61] The mortality rate of varicella pneumonia in pregnancy approached 30% in the era prior to the availability of effective antiviral agents such as acyclovir. The likelihood of developing pneumonia during primary varicella infection appears to be increased in the third trimester and in smokers. It should be treated aggressively with supportive therapy and intravenous acyclovir in a dose of 7.5 mg/kg every 8 hours. The use of this medication has been shown to decrease mortality rates by one-half.[62]

Concluding Perspective

Even with improved technology and antibiotics, Madinger and coworkers[63] believe that the maternal and fetal outcomes have not improved dramatically in patients with pneumonia. They retrospectively reviewed 250 cases of pneumonia during pregnancy that occurred among 32,170 patients. Medical complications included bacteremia in 16%, empyema in 8%, atrial fibrillation in 4%, and respiratory failure necessitating intubation and ventilation in 20%. Preterm labor occurred in 44% of the patients and preterm delivery in 36%. One patient with cystic fibrosis died. Perinatal mortality included one stillbirth and two neonatal deaths. There is a significant correlation between underlying maternal disease, maternal medical complications, and preterm delivery in the pregnant woman with pneumonia.[6]

TUBERCULOSIS

Epidemiology

Tuberculosis is a pulmonary infection caused by the acid-fast bacillus *Mycobacterium tuberculosis*. There has been a decline in the frequency of tuberculosis in the United States over the past 50 years. Most obstetricians do not consider this diagnosis when a pregnant patient presents with lethargy and respiratory symptoms. However, as more women enter the United States from developing nations, there has been a resurgence of tuberculosis in the pregnant population, primarily in urban areas. Furthermore, the increasing number of individuals with human immunodeficiency virus infection has also led to an increase in tuberculosis complicating pregnancy. Unfortunately, much of the tuberculosis is becoming multidrug resistant.

Diagnosis

Pregnancy should not be a deterrent to the accurate diagnosis and treatment of tuberculosis. Tuberculin skin testing with subcutaneous administration of intermediate-strength purified protein derivative (PPD) is the mainstay of testing for tuberculosis in the United States. In high-risk areas, it should be administered at the first prenatal visit. Carter and Mates[64] found that most women with tuberculosis were asymptomatic and would have missed diagnosis and thus treatment if they had not undergone PPD testing. A positive PPD only means that the patient has been previously exposed to tuberculosis and that there are dormant organisms present. Less than 10% of patients with a positive PPD and an intact immune system will have active disease. This method, however, has several drawbacks. Only 80% of patients with reactivation of tuberculosis will have positive tests. In addition, any patient who has previously received the bacille Calmette–Guérin (BCG) vaccine may have a positive tuberculin skin test for a number of years after vaccination. Although this vaccine is rarely used in the United States, it is administered routinely in countries where tuberculosis is endemic.

If the differential diagnosis of tuberculosis is entertained in a patient presenting with respiratory and constitutional symptoms, chest radiography with abdominal shielding should be immediately performed. Chest x-ray films should also be obtained without delay if the patient's previously negative tuberculin skin test becomes positive, if it cannot be determined when a patient's skin test became positive, or if a patient has persistent respiratory or constitutional symptoms.[65] Without abdominal shielding, the radiation exposure to the fetus from a single chest x-ray examination is minimal, approximately 2.5 mrad. With abdominal shielding, the exposure is even less.[66,67]

The definitive diagnosis of tuberculosis is based on identifying *M. tuberculosis* by culture or by acid-fast or fluorescent stain of the sputum. First morning sputum specimens obtained on three consecutive days are usually the best source for cultures and stain. If the patient is not able to produce a sputum sample voluntarily, production can be elicited by having the patient inhale aerosolized hypertonic saline. Any patient having a positive smear for acid-fast bacilli should be started on antituberculous chemotherapy while awaiting the results of the cultures and drug-sensitivity tests. Sensitivity testing is crucial because of the emergence of multidrug-resistant tuberculosis.

Treatment

When adequate treatment is implemented, tuberculosis appears to have no adverse effect on pregnancy, and, conversely, pregnancy does not alter the natural history of the disease.[68-70] Highly effective chemotherapeutic agents have been developed for the treatment of tuberculosis (Table 6-5).[71] Although the prognosis for tuberculosis during pregnancy is excellent, severe complications such as miliary, renal, and meningeal tuberculosis have been described.[72] Treatment should be started empirically when the diagnosis is strongly suspected, but should be individualized when sensitivities are available. Standard therapy for pregnancy is isoniazid in a single dose of 300 mg and rifampin, 600 mg/day.[11] If a resistant strain is suspected, ethambutol should be added.[73] This therapy should be continued for 9 months.

Isoniazid prophylaxis is usually recommended for patients under the age of 35 years whose tuberculin skin test has recently converted (within 2 years) but do not have active disease. Such prophylaxis is discouraged during pregnancy but may be begun during the postpartum period. The major adverse effects of isoniazid include hepatitis, peripheral neuropathy, and hypersensitivity reactions. Transient elevations of the serum transaminases are seen in approximately 20% of patients. Transaminase levels should, therefore, be monitored monthly. If they reach five times the upper limit of normal, the drug should be discontinued. If

	TABLE 6-5	
MEDICATIONS COMMONLY USED TO TREAT PULMONARY TUBERCULOSIS		
Medication	**Daily Dosage**	**Potential Maternal Toxicities**
Isoniazid	300 mg in a single oral dose	Peripheral neuropathy (prevented with oral pyridoxine), hepatic dysfunction with elevated transaminaes
Ethambutol	15 mg/kg/day in a single oral dose	Optic neuritis
Para-aminosalicylic acid	10–12 g/day in two to three divided oral doses	Diverse gastrointestinal symptoms
Rifampin	600 mg/day in a single oral dose	Gastrointestinal disturbance, hepato-toxicity, orange discoloration of body fluids
Streptomycin	15 mg/kg/day in a single intramuscular injection	Ototoxicity, nephrotoxicity
Kanamycin	20 mg/kg/day in a single intramuscular injection	Ototoxicity, nephrotoxicity

these guidelines are followed, serious isoniazid hepatitis can be avoided.[74] Peripheral neuropathy appears to be related to a deficiency of pyridoxine (vitamin B_6). Patients taking isoniazid should receive a 25- to 50-mg supplement of pyridoxine daily to prevent this complication.

Isoniazid has been studied extensively during pregnancy, and there appears to be no increase in congenital malformations.[75] Only one study noted a small excess of nonspecific congenital anomalies in patients taking this drug, but certainly no associated syndrome was observed.[76]

Ethambutol also appears safe for use during pregnancy and has not been associated with an increase in congenital anomalies.[77] In doses higher than those usually recommended (>15 mg/kg/day), ethambutol can produce retrobulbar neuritis. This finding has not been observed in abortuses or in neonates of mothers receiving this medication.[77,78]

If possible, streptomycin should be avoided during pregnancy. In one report, more than 10% of the offspring of patients treated with streptomycin during pregnancy showed damage to cranial nerve VIII.[75] This precaution also holds true for kanamycin, capreomycin, and viomycin.[79]

Rifampin inhibits DNA-dependent RNA polymerase. It readily crosses the placenta and could theoretically injure the fetus. One study reported a 3 to 4% incidence of severe congenital malformations associated with use of rifampin during pregnancy.[75] However, this figure is not significantly higher than the expected background rate of malformations. Para-aminosalicylic acid was once commonly used during pregnancy. Because it is associated with severe gastrointestinal side effects, it is no longer recommended for the pregnant woman who is already prone to nausea and vomiting. Its use has not been associated with congenital malformations.

Transplacental passage of tuberculosis is extremely rare. Most perinatal infections occur when a mother with active tuberculosis handles her neonate.[80] The risk to the child of contracting tuberculosis from a mother with active disease during the first year of life may be as high as 50%.[81] Daily administration of isoniazid chemoprophylaxis should be given to the newborn for the length of the mother's treatment.[79] This therapy obviously requires a great deal of motivation on the part of the parent to make certain that the child receives the medication.

CYSTIC FIBROSIS

Cystic fibrosis (CF) is an autosomal recessive disorder, the gene for which was first cloned in 1989. It is a disease of mucous glands of the digestive, respiratory, and reproductive tracts. With advances in antibiotic therapy and respiratory care, the life span of patients with CF has increased greatly over the past 20 years; therefore, many of these patients are reaching the reproductive age. The genes responsible for CF have been identified and many differing mutations have been identified. Prenatal and carrier testing is readily available.

Some women with CF have impaired fertility. Because of poor absorption from the gastrointestinal tract, some patients may have poor nutrition and delayed menarche or anovulatory cycles. Others have decreased or thickened cervical mucus. Once patients become pregnant, it is imperative to maintain a good nutritional status to help them throughout the pregnancy. Patients need approximately an additional 300 kcal/day to meet the energy needs of pregnancy.[82] It is important to stress a healthy diet to these patients.

Patients who have progressive deterioration of their pulmonary status, with hypoxemia and/or hypercapnia, are not good candidates for pregnancy. Corkey et al. described two patients whose pulmonary function declined greatly during pregnancy.[83] Cohen et al.[84] reported congestive heart failure in 13% of 129 pregnancies in 100 women with CF. In that series, 18% of the women died within 24 months of delivery. However, this study was published almost 20 years ago; with the changes in antibiotic therapy and respiratory care, the current risk is not nearly as high.

It is important that the patient understand her needs during pregnancy. Her pulmonary status, as well as her cardiovascular status, must be monitored constantly. Frequent pulmonary function tests are crucial because these patients have many respiratory infections, especially with *Pseudomonas aeruginosa*, and must undergo repeated antibiotic therapy throughout pregnancy. Whereas such therapy previously required prolonged hospital stays, most individuals can now be treated on an outpatient basis.

In summary, with careful attention to cardiac and pulmonary status, as well as proper nutritional counseling, patients with CF can carry to term with minimal difficulty if their disease is not too severe. A multidisciplinary team (pulmonologist, respiratory therapist, maternal–fetal medicine specialist, obstetrician) is essential. The patient must realize that she may be hospitalized several times throughout the pregnancy. Because of recurrent maternal infections and poor nutritional status, the fetus is at risk for growth restriction.

REFERENCES

1. Greenberger PA, Patterson R. Management of asthma during pregnancy. N Engl J Med 1985;312:897.
2. de Swiet M. Diseases of the respiratory system. Clin Obstet Gynecol 1977;4:287.
3. Hernandez E, Angle CS, Johnson JWC: Asthma in pregnancy: current concepts. Obstet Gynecol 1980;55:739.
4. Turner ES, Greenberger PA, Patterson R. Management of the pregnant asthmatic patient. Ann Intern Med 1980; 94:905.
5. Hiddleson HJH. Bronchial asthma and pregnancy. NZ Med J 1964;63:521.
6. Gordon M, Niswander KR, Berendes H, Kantor AG. Fetal morbidity following potentially anoxigenic obstetric conditions. VII. Bronchial asthma. Am J Obstet Gynecol 1970; 106:421.
7. Schaefer G, Silverman F. Pregnancy complicated by asthma. Am J Obstet Gynecol 1961;82:182.
8. White RJ, Coutts II, Gibbs CJ, MacIntyre C. A prospective study of asthma during pregnancy and the puerperium. Respir Med 1989;83:103.
9. Apter AJ, Greenbeger PA, Patterson R. Outcomes of pregnancy in adolescents with severe asthma. Arch Intern Med 1989;149:2571.
10. Williams DA. Asthma in pregnancy. Acta Allergy 1967; 22:311.
11. Sims CD, Chamberlin CVP, de Swiet M. Lung function tests in bronchial asthma during and after pregnancy. Br J Obstet Gynaecol 1976;88:434.
12. Mabie WC, Barton JR, Wasserstrum N, Sibai BM. Clinical observations in asthma in pregnancy. J Matern Fetal Med 1992;1:45.
13. Perlow JH, Montgomery D, Morgan MA, et al. Severity of asthma and perinatal outcome. Am J Obstet Gynecol 1992;167:963.
14. Schatz M, Zeiger RS, Hoffman CP, et al. Perinatal outcomes in the pregnancies of asthmatic women: a prospective controlled analysis. Am J Respir Crit Care Med 1995; 151:1170.
15. Metzger WJ, Turner E, Patterson R. The safety of immunotherapy during pregnancy. J Allergy Clin Immunol 1978;61:268.
16. Centers for Disease Control and Prevention: Prevention and control of influenza. MMWR 1984;33:253.
17. Schatz M, Zeiger RS, Harden KM, et al. The safety of inhaled beta-agonist bronchodilators during pregnancy. J Allergy Clin Immunol 1988;82:686.
18. Barnes PJ. A new approach to the treatment of asthma. N Engl J Med 1989;221:1517.
19. Kerstjens JAM, Brand PLP, Hughes MD, et al. A comparison of bronchodilator therapy with or without inhaled corticosteroid therapy for obstructive airways disease. N Engl J Med 1992;327:1413.
20. Greenberger P, Patterson R. Safety of therapy for allergic systems during pregnancy. Ann Intern Med 1978; 89:234.
21. Weinstein AM, Dubin BD, Podleski WK, et al. Asthma in pregnancy. JAMA 1979;241:1161.
22. Nelson MM, Forfar JO. Associations between drugs administered during pregnancy and congenital abnormalities of the fetus. BMJ 1971;1:523.
23. Fainstat TP. Cortisone-induced congenital cleft palate in rabbits. Endocrinology 1954;55:502.
24. Schatz M, Patterson R, Zeitz S, et al. Corticosteroid therapy for the pregnant asthmatic patient. JAMA 1975; 233:804.
25. Weinberger SE, Weiss ST, Coatan WR, et al. Pregnancy and the lung. Am Rev Respir Dis 1980;121:559.
26. Beitins R, Baynard F, Ances IG et al. The transplacental passage of prednisone and prednisolone in pregnancy near term. J Pediatr 1972;81:936.

27. Levitz M, Jansen V, Dancis J. The transfer and metabolism of corticosteroids in the perfused human placenta. Am J Obstet Gynecol 1978;132:363.

28. Marx GF. Obstetric anesthesia in the presence of medical complications. Clin Obstet Gynecol 1974;17:165.

29. Aaro LA, Jiergens JL. Thrombophlebitis associated with pregnancy. Am J Obstet Gynecol 1971;109:1128.

30. Treffers BL, Fluiderkoper GH, Weehink GH, Kloosterman GJ. Epidemiological observations of thromboembolic disease during pregnancy and in the puerperium in 56,022 women. Int J Gynaecol Obstet 1983;21:327.

31. VillaSanta U. Thromboembolic disease in pregnancy. Am J Obstet Gynecol 1965;93:142.

32. Barritt DW, Jorden SC. Anticoagulant drugs in the treatment of pulmonary embolism: a controlled trial. Lancet 1960;1:1309.

33. Skibsted L, Wadt J, Nissen F. Thrombectomy of acute iliofemoral venous thrombosis during pregnancy. Surg Gynecol Obstet 1989;169:50.

34. Weiner CP. Diagnosis and management of thromboembolic disease during pregnancy. Clin Obstet Gynecol 1985;28:107.

35. Girz BA, Heiselman DE. Fatal intrapartum pulmonary embolus during tocolysis. Am J Obstet Gynecol 1988;158:145.

36. Conrad J, Horellou MJ, VanDreden P, et al. Thrombosis and pregnancy in congenital deficiencies in AT-III protein C or protein S: study of 78 women. Thromb Haemost 1990;63:319.

37. Hooper WC, Evatt BL. The role of activated protein C resistance in the pathogenesis of venous thrombosis. Am J Med Sci 1998;316(2):120.

38. Dizon-Tounson DS, Nelson LM, Jang H, Varner MW, Ward K. The incidence of factor V Leiden mutation in an obstetric population and its relationship to deep vein thrombosis. Am J Obstet Gynecol 1997;176:883.

39. Heijboer H, Buller HR, Lensing AW, et al. A comparison of real-time compression ultrasonography with impedance plethysmography for the diagnosis of deep vein thrombosis in symptomatic patients. N Engl J Med 1993;329:1365.

40. Spritzer CE, Evans AC, Kay JJ. Magnetic resonance imaging of deep venous thrombosis in pregnant women with lower extremity edema. Obstet Gynecol 1995;85:603.

41. Macus CS, Mason GR, Kuperus JH, Mena I. Pulmonary imaging in pregnancy: maternal risk and fetal dosimetry. Clin Nucl Med 1985;10:1.

42. The PIOPED Investigators. Value of the ventilation/perfusion scan in acute pulmonary embolism: results of the prospective investigation of pulmonary embolism diagnosis (PIOPED). JAMA 1990;273:2753.

43. Ginsberg JS, Hirsh J, Rainbow AJ, Coates G. Risks to the fetus of radiologic procedures used in the diagnosis of maternal venous thromboembolic disease. Thromb Haemost 1989;61:189.

44. Qaso LA, Juergens JL. Thrombophlebitis associated with pregnancy. Am J Obstet Gynecol 1971;109:1128.

45. Gervin AS. Complications of heparin therapy. Surg Gynecol Obstet 1975;140:789.

46. Hall JG. Pauli RM, Wilson KM. Maternal and fetal sequelae of anticoagulation during pregnancy. Am J Med 1978;68:122.

47. Walker AM, Jick H. Predictors of bleeding during heparin therapy. JAMA 1980;244:1209.

48. Merrill LK, VerBurg DJ. The choice of long term anticoagulants for the pregnant patient. Obstet Gynecol 1976;47:711.

49. Spearing GS, Fraser I, Turner G, Dixon G. Long term self administered subcutaneous heparin in pregnancy. BMJ 1978;1:1457.

50. Stevenson R, Burton DM, Ferlavto GJ, Taylor HA. Hazards of oral anticoagulants during pregnancy. JAMA 1980;243:1549.

51. Sgavi WL, Hall JG. Multiple congenital anomalies associated with oral anticoagulants. Am J Obstet Gynecol 1977;127:191.

52. Harrod MJE, Sherrod PS. Warfarin embryopathy in siblings. Obstet Gynecol 1981;57:673.

53. Howell R, Fidler J, Letsky E, et al. The risks of antenatal subcutaneous heparin prophylaxis: a controlled trial. Br J Obstet Gynaecol 1983;90:1124.

54. Lao TT, de Swiet M, Letsky E, et al. Prophylaxis of thromboembolism in pregnancy: an alternative. Br J Obstet Gynaecol 1985;92:202.

55. Hopwood HG. Pneumonia in pregnancy. Obstet Gynecol 1965;25:875.

56. Austrian R. Pneumococcal vaccine: development and prospects. Am J Med 1979;67:546.

57. McKinney P, Volkert P, Kaufman R. Fatal swine influenza pneumonia during late pregnancy. Arch Intern Med 1990;150:213.

58. Kort BA, Cefalo RC, Baker VV. Fatal influenza A pneumonia in pregnancy. Am J Perinatol 1986;3:179.

59. Mostow SR. Prevention, management and control of influenza: role of amantadine. Am J Med 1987;82(Suppl 6a):35.

60. Cox SM, Cunningham FG, Luby J. Management of varicella pneumonia complicating pregnancy. Am J Perinatol 1990;7:100.

61. Esmonde TF, Herdman G, Anderson G. Chickenpox pneumonia: an association with pregnancy. Thorax 1989;44:812.

62. Haake DA, Zakowski PC, Haake DL, Bryson YJ. Early treatment with acyclovir for varicella pneumonia in otherwise healthy adults: retrospective controlled study and review. Rev Infect Dis 1990;12:788.

63. Madinger NE, Greenspoon JS, Ellrodt AG. Pneumonia during pregnancy: has modern technology improved maternal and fetal outcome? Am J Obstet Gynecol 1989;161:657.

64. Carter EJ, Mates S. Tuberculosis during pregnancy: the Rhode Island experience, 1987–1991. Chest 1994;106:1466.

65. Weinstein L, Murphy T. The management of tuberculosis during pregnancy. Clin Perinatol 1974;1:395.

66. Bonebarak CR, Noller KL, Loehnen CP, et al. Routine chest roentgenography in pregnancy. JAMA 1978;240:2747.

67. Swartz HM, Reichling BA. Hazards of radiation exposure for pregnant women. JAMA 1978;239:1907.

68. Schaefer G, Zervoudakis IA, Fuchs FF, David S. Pregnancy in pulmonary tuberculosis. Obstet Gynecol 1975;46:706.

69. DeMarch AP. Tuberculosis in pregnancy: five to ten year review of 215 patients in their fertile age. Chest 1975; 68:800.

70. Maccato ML. Pneumonia and pulmonary tuberculosis in pregnancy. Obstet Gynecol Clin North Am 1989;16:417.

71. Hamadeh MA, Glassroth J. Tuberculosis in pregnancy. Chest 1992;101:1114.

72. Golditch IM. Tuberculous meningitis in pregnancy. Am J Obstet Gynecol 1971;110:1144.

73. Centers for Disease Control and Prevention. Initial therapy for tuberculosis in the era of multi-drug resistance: recommendations of the Advisory Council for the Elimination of Tuberculosis. MMWR 1993;42:1.

74. Byrd RB, Horn BR, Solomon DA, Griggs GA. Toxic effects of isoniazid in tuberculosis chemoprophylaxis. JAMA 1979;241:1239.

75. Sider DF, Layde PM, Johnson MW, Lyne HA. Treatment of tuberculosis during pregnancy. Am Rev Respir Dis 1980;122:65.

76. Heinonen OP, Slone D, Shapiro S. Birth defects and drugs in pregnancy. Littleton, MA: Publishing Sciences Group, 1977.

77. Sewitt T, Nebel L, Terracina S, Ankarman S. Ethambutol in pregnancy: observations on embryogenesis. Chest 1974; 66:25.

78. Brobowitz ID. Ethambutol in pregnancy. Chest 1974;66:20.

79. Robinson GC, Cambon KG. Hearing loss in infants of tuberculous mothers treated with streptomycin in pregnancy. N Engl J Med 1964;271:949.

80. Perinatal prophylaxis of tuberculosis. Lancet 1990; 336:1479.

81. Kendig EL Jr. The place of BCC vaccine in the management of infants born of tuberculous mothers. N Engl J Med 1969;281:520.

82. Rush D, Johnstone FD, King JC. Nutrition and pregnancy. In: Burrows GN, Ferris TF, eds. Medical complications during pregnancy. 3rd ed. Philadelphia: Saunders, 1988.

83. Corkey CW, Newth CJ, Corey M, et al. Pregnancy in cystic fibrosis: a better prognosis in patients with pancreatic function? Am J Obstet Gynecol 1981;140:737.

84. Cohen LF, deSant'Agnese PA, Friedlander L. Cystic fibrosis and pregnancy: a national survey. Lancet 1980; 2:842.

GASTROINTESTINAL DISEASE

Mark Landon

Five Key Points

- The symptoms of peptic ulcer disease usually improve during pregnancy.
- Antacids remain a first line of choice for therapy of peptic ulcer disease during pregnancy. H_2 antagonists and proton pump inhibitors are employed in unresponsive cases.
- Most cases of pancreatitis in pregnancy are due to gallstones.
- If inflammatory bowel disease is in remission at the onset of pregnancy, the prognosis for mother and fetus is usually excellent.
- Pregnant patients with symptomatic inflammatory bowel disease should be treated with medical therapy as in the nonpregnant state.

PEPTIC ULCER DISEASE

Symptoms of peptic ulcer appear to improve during pregnancy. In a survey of pregnant women with a previous history of peptic ulcer disease, 44% became asymptomatic and 44% demonstrated a marked improvement in symptoms.[1] The remaining 12% remained the same or experienced worsening symptoms during gestation. Of those interviewed, nearly half experienced recurrent symptoms by 3 months postpartum, and 75% had relapsed by 6 months after delivery. A low rate of hospitalization for peptic ulcer disease can be expected for pregnant women, as none of the 175 women hospitalized for advanced symptoms of ulcer disease were found to be pregnant.[2] Factors that might improve the clinical course of patients with peptic ulcer disease during pregnancy include progesterone-induced lower ouput of gastric acid as well as increased gastric mucus production. The placenta is rich in histaminase, which may inactivate histamine or block its action at the level of the parietal cell. This effect may be responsible for a decline in gastric acid output in patients who exhibit hyperacidity in the nonpregnant state.[3]

The interplay of acid secretion and mucosal resistance is believed to be important in the pathogenesis of peptic ulceration. Infection of the stomach and duodenum with *Helicobacter pylori* has been implicated as a significant factor as well. This organism is found in nearly all patients with duodenal ulceration, although it is unknown whether pregnancy alters its frequency.

Pregnant women will commonly report dyspepsia; this is often attributed to gastric reflux ("heartburn") in the lower esophagus. Heartburn usually responds to antacid therapy and adopting a semirecumbent position when supine. This regimen will often bring relief to patients with underlying peptic ulcer disease as well, and further diagnostic procedures are rarely needed. In patients with significant pain that is unresponsive to antacid regimens, endoscopic examination of the upper gastrointestinal tract should be performed. Barium studies should, in most cases, be avoided in gravid women, as endoscopy obviates the need for this procedure, which does pose some potential risk to the developing fetus.

The primary medical treatment for the symptomatic patient with peptic ulcer disease during pregnancy is as in the nonpregnant state—antacid therapy and diet. Administration of antacid 1 hour after meals and at bedtime usually provides relief of symptoms and promotes ulcer healing. In refractory cases, a dose may be added at 3 hours after meals. Patients with peptic ulcer disease should be maintained on a diet that avoids caffeine, salicylates, ethanol, or any gastric stimulant that aggravates their condition.

H$_2$ antagonists (cimetidine and ranitidine) as well as proton pump inhibitors remain a second-line choice for therapy in pregnancy.[4] Because antiandrogenic effects found in animal experiments with cimetidine have not been associated with ranitidine, this agent is preferred during gestation. Elective treatment of *Helicobacter pylori* with antibiotics and bismuth subsalicylate is generally recommended following delivery and during breast-feeding.[5]

ACUTE PANCREATITIS

The true incidence of pancreatitis complicating pregnancy is difficult to ascertain. Approximately 1% of cases of acute pancreatitis occur in pregnant women.[6] An incidence of 1 in 1066 pregnancies to 1 in 2888 deliveries has been reported.[7,8] Whereas maternal mortality approached 50% in the past, this is now an uncommon event, especially if the diagnosis is established promptly.[7] Most cases of pancreatitis during pregnancy are associated with gallstones. McKay et al. noted that 18 of 20 patients in whom pancreatitis developed while they were pregnant or within 5 months postpartum had cholelithiasis.[6] In nonpregnant individuals, alcoholism is by far the most common causative factor. Other causes for pancreatitis include infection, previous surgery, preeclampsia, hyperparathyroidism, thiazide ingestion, and penetrating duodenal ulcer. Many cases are idiopathic.

The clinical presentation of pancreatitis is not significantly altered in pregnancy. The disease may occur at any stage of gestation but is more common in the third trimester and puerperium. Epigastric pain, which may radiate to the flanks or shoulders, along with abdominal tenderness and nausea or vomiting, should prompt appropriate laboratory investigation. Mild fever and leukocytosis may be present. Plain films of the abdomen may simply reveal an adynamic ileus. Ultrasound imaging is of limited value, so that if significant pancreatic necrosis is suspected, computed tomographic (CT) imaging becomes preferable.

In most cases, this radiologic study is unnecessary because the diagnosis is made by laboratory evaluation.

In evaluating the pregnant patient in whom pancreatitis is suspected, the differential diagnosis includes most causes of abdominal pain in young women, including peptic ulcer disease with or without perforation, acute cholecystitis, biliary colic, and intestinal obstruction. Specific tests employed to corroborate the diagnosis of pancreatitis rely on the measurement of pancreatic enzymes, primarily amylase. Elevated values should suggest pancreatitis, although they may be present with other conditions such as cholecystitis, intestinal obstruction, peptic ulcer disease, hepatic trauma, and ruptured ectopic pregnancy.

In most cases, acute pancreatitis resolves spontaneously within a few days. In less than 10% of cases, the illness is complicated, and such patients are best treated in a teritary-care setting, which can provide an intensive-care environment. Pancreatic secretory activity should be reduced by keeping the patient on parenteral nutrition. Nasogastric suction is reserved for those with persistent nausea and vomiting. Meperidine is the drug of choice for analgesia because, unlike morphine, it does not constrict the sphincter of Oddi. Fluid and electrolyte replacement and serial assays of hemoglobin, white-cell count, amylase, liver enzymes, glucose, and calcium are essential. In advanced cases, hypocalcemia may be present, and calcium replacement is necessary. Patients who have been unable to eat for longer than 1 week may benefit from intravenous alimentation.

Percutaneous aspiration of pancreatic exudate is important in refractory cases. This CT-guided procedure may be necessary to distinguish between sterile and infected pancreatic necrosis. For infected cases, surgical drainage of the pancreatic exudate is necessary.

INFLAMMATORY BOWEL DISEASE

Ulcerative colitis (UC) and Crohn disease (CD) or regional enteritis are idiopathic disorders that have their peak incidence in the reproductive age group. UC is a disease of the colon or rectum, marked by acute attacks of bloody stools, diarrhea, cramping abdominal pain, weight loss, and dehydration. The prevalence of UC in the female population under 40 years of age is 40 to 100 per 100,000.[9] CD is considerably less common than UC, with an incidence of

2 to 4 per 100,000. The average age of onset is between 20 and 30 years. CD, in contrast to UC, tends to run a more subacute and chronic course, with symptoms including fever, diarrhea, and cramping abdominal pain.[10] Because CD may involve only the colon, histologic differentiation from UC can be important.

Ulcerative Colitis

A good outcome can generally be expected in pregnancies complicated by UC. In a group of 102 patients treated with therapies including steroids, sulfasalazine, or both, a spontaneous abortion rate of only 11% was recorded in 216 women followed over a 20-year period.[11] Women with quiescent disease at conception have a slightly greater chance of successfully reaching term as compared with patients whose disease is active during pregnancy. The proportion of low-birth-weight babies and the incidence of anomalies appear to be similar to those in the general population. Pregnancy also has little effect on disease activity. Of 129 pregnancies in which colitis was quiescent at the time of conception, 90 (70%) of the patients remained free of symptoms throughout pregnancy and the puerperium.[11] In women of reproductive age, DeDombal et al. found a 45% chance of recurrent disease developing in any given year.[12]

Crohn Disease

Unlike women with UC, some patients with CD and large-bowel disease appear to be subfertile. It has been suggested that temporary infertility may be related to the activity of the disease.[13] Khosla et al. described infertility in 112 patients with CD and reported a 12% rate, similar to that seen in the general population.[14] A case-control study indicated that the number of offspring of women with CD was 57% of that of paired controls.[15]

Studies describing the effect of CD on pregnancy suggest minimal if any increased risk to mother or fetus. In Crohn's original report, 53 patients with regional ileitis had 84 pregnancies, and 75 (89%) infants survived.[16] More recent studies confirm these excellent results, with full-term delivery rates of 73 to 83%.[17,18]

Active CD poses a greater risk of spontaneous abortion.[14,17,18] A higher spontaneous rate of loss can be expected in patients with active disease at the time of conception and in patients with severe disease.[14] Women in whom disease first develops during pregnancy also are at increased risk for unfavorable outcomes.

The effect of pregnancy on CD is similar to that reported for patients with UC. Most patients have no change in disease activity, whereas 15% have been reported to improve and 10% worsen during pregnancy.[12] If a woman conceives while CD is in remission, she is just as likely to remain in remission as a nonpregnant patient. Maintenance on medication does not affect the relapse rate. Conflicting data exist as to whether postpartum flare-ups are increased. Overall, the risk of exacerbation during pregnancy is not higher than that in the nonpregnant population.[15]

Treatment of Inflammatory Bowel Disease during Pregnancy

The general treatment of inflammatory bowel disease is not altered greatly by pregnancy. All women should be followed closely so that the activity of their disease may be assessed and psychological support can be provided. Dietary counseling for patients with UC should emphasize proper nutritional intake. Patients with mild disease may respond to a low-roughage diet or the exclusion of milk products if they are lactose-intolerant. In contrast, patients with CD often benefit from low-residue diets, presumably because the caliber of their small bowel may be limited by inflammation.

The initial therapy for episodes of diarrhea generally includes narcotics such as codeine and diphenoxylate. Long-term use of narcotics should be avoided, as it may incite toxic megacolon in patients with UC. When simple measures are unsuccessful in quieting an attack, sulfasalazine and systemic steroids should be administered. The safety of both of these drugs has been well established in pregnancy. The active metabolite of sulfasalazine, 5-aminosalicylic acid, and its N-acetyl derivative are also favored treatments. Both sulfasalazine and 5-ASA can be given safely to nursing mothers.[19]

Steroids are indicated in patients who do not respond to simple supportive measures. Steroid retention enemas may be effective for mild to moderate distal colitis or proctitis. Patients with severe disease should initially be treated with high doses of intravenous hydrocortisone or its equivalent. Oral prednisone can then be substituted and tapered as the attack subsides. The safety of corticosteroids and sulfasalazine in pregnancy associated with inflammatory bowel disease was addressed in a national survey.[19] In examining 287 pregnancies, Mogadam et al. found no adverse effects that could be attributed to these drugs.

Patients with severe disease who become profoundly dehydrated require hospitalization and intravenous fluids. The development of significant hypoalbuminemia, coupled with inadequate caloric intake, may require the institution of parenteral hyperalimentation. The benefits of such nutritional therapy include diminished gastrointestinal secretion and motility, potential relief of partial obstruction, closure of fistulas, and renewal of immunocompetence.

Although most acute episodes of inflammatory bowel disease respond to medical treatment, operative intervention will occasionally be necessary to treat perforation, obstruction, or patients unresponsive to standard therapies. While elective surgery for medically intractable disease or recurrent dysplastic lesions of the colon is best accomplished following pregnancy, patients who have undergone definitive surgical procedures for UC during pregnancy seem to fare well. Surgery during pregnancy does pose a significant risk of preterm delivery, probably because of the amount of uterine manipulation required during efforts to reach the distal colon. Surgery should not be delayed, however, in cases of perforation or complete obstruction.[20]

Ileostomy function during pregnancy is normal in most cases. Of 84 term pregnancies reported by Hudson, intestinal obstruction occurred in just 7 cases.[21] Of 17 cesarean deliveries performed in his series, all were done for obstetrical indications. Similarly, Gopal and colleagues described 82 pregnancies in 66 women following colostomy or ileostomy. Stomal dysfunction responded to conservative measures in all but three women, who required surgery for intestinal obstruction.[22] Complications from an episiotomy have been uncommon in patients previously operated on for UC. Data are not available for CD. However, the higher rate of perineal involvement in these patients should warrant a thorough evaluation before contemplating vaginal delivery.

REFERENCES

1. Clark DH. Peptic ulcer in women. BMJ 1953;1:1259.
2. Vessley MP, Villard-Mackintoch L, Painter R. Oral contraceptives and pregnancy in relation to peptic ulcer. Contraception 1992;46:349.
3. Clark DH, Tankel HI. Gastric acid and plasma histaminase during pregnancy. Lancet 1954;2:886.
4. Lewis JH, Weingold AB. The use of gastrointestinal drugs during pregnancy and lactation. Am J Gastroenterol 1985;80:912.
5. Baron TH, Ramirez B, Richter JE. Gastrointestinal motility disorders during pregnancy. Ann Intern Med 1993;118:306.
6. McKay AJ, O'Neill J, Imrie CW. Pancreatitis, pregnancy, and gallstones. Br J Obstet Gynaecol 1980;87:47.
7. Corlett RC, Mishell DR. Pancreatitis in pregnancy. Am J Obstet Gynecol 1972;113:281.
8. Wilkinson EJ. Acute pancreatitis in pregnancy: a review of 98 cases and a report of 8 new cases. Obstet Gynecol Surv 1973;28:5281.
9. Kirsner JB, Shorter RG. Recent developments in nonspecific inflammatory bowel disease. N Engl J Med 1982; 306:775.
10. Sorokin JJ, Levine SM. Pregnancy and inflammatory bowel disease: a review of the literature. Obstet Gynecol 1983;62:247.
11. Willoughby CP, Truelove SC. Ulcerative colitis and pregnancy. Gut 1980;21:469.
12. DeDombal FT, Watts JM, Watkinson G. Ulcerative colitis and pregnancy. Lancet 1965;2:599.
13. DeDombal FT, Burton IL, Goligher JC. Crohn's disease and pregnancy. BMJ 1972;3:550.
14. Khosla R, Willoughby CP, Jewell DP. Crohn's disease and pregnancy. Gut 1984;25:52.
15. Mayberry JF, Weterman IT. European survey of fertility and pregnancy in women with Crohn's disease: a case control study by European collaborative group. Gut 1986;27:821.
16. Crohn BB, Yarnis, Korelitz BI. Regional ileitis complicating pregnancy. Gastroenterology 1956;31:615.
17. Haagen Nielsen O, Andreasson B, Bondesen B, Jacobsen O, Jarnum S. Pregnancy in Crohn's disease. Scand J Gastroenterol 1984;19:724.
18. Woolfson K, Cohen Z, McLeod RS. Crohn's disease and pregnancy. Dis Colon Rectum 1990;33:869.
19. Mogadam M, Dibbins MO, Korelitz BI, Ahmed SW. Pregnancy and inflammatory bowel disease: effect of sulfasalazine and corticosteroids on fetal outcome. Gastroenterology 1981;80:72.
20. Anderson JB, Turner GM, Williamson RCN. Fulminant ulcerative colitis in late pregnancy and the puerperium. Proc R Soc Med 1987;80:492.
21. Hudson CN. Ileostomy in pregnancy. Proc R Soc Med 1972;65:281.
22. Gopal KA, Amshel AL, Shonberg IL, et al. Ostomy and pregnancy. Dis Colon Rectum 1985;28:912.

Noninfectious Hepatobiliary Diseases

Philip Samuels

Five Key Points

- Acute fatty liver of pregnancy must be differentiated from fulminant hepatitis and HELLP syndrome. Patients with acute fatty liver require prompt delivery.

- Cholestasis of pregnancy is distinguished by intense, persistent pruritus, mild hyperbilirubinemia, and pronounced elevation of the serum concentration of alkaline phosphatase.

- Pregnancy does not adversely affect hepatic graft function or survival.

- Pregnancy predisposes to cholelithiasis and subsequent cholecystitis.

- If performed in the second trimester, cholecystectomy is associated with minimal maternal and fetal morbidity.

ACUTE FATTY LIVER

Epidemiology

Acute fatty liver is a rare condition of unknown cause that has an incidence of between 1 in 6692 and 1 in 15,900 pregnancies.[1-3] Before 1970, the published mortality rate for both mother and infant was approximately 85%.[4] Since 1975, maternal survival has increased to >90%, with neonatal survival related mostly to gestational age at time of delivery. These improved outcomes have been attributed to early recognition of the disorder, followed by prompt delivery and improved neonatal care.[1,5-7] With its usual onset in the third trimester, acute fatty liver often first presents as nausea and vomiting,[1,7,8] followed by severe abdominal pain and headache. Within a few days jaundice appears, the patient becomes somnolent and, if untreated, eventually comatose. Hematemesis and spontaneous bleeding result when hypoprothrombinemia and disseminated intravascular coagulation (DIC) develop. Oliguria, metabolic acidosis, and eventually anuria occur in approximately 50% of patients with acute fatty liver of pregnancy if not treated promptly.[9] Rather than liver failure, DIC, renal failure, profound hypoglycemia, and occasionally pancreatitis are the most often cited immediate causes of death.[2,8,9] Two cases of liver rupture associated with acute fatty liver have also been reported.[10,11] Although the cause of the occasional accompanying stillbirth has not been definitively delineated, Mose and Shah[2] suggest that uteroplacental insufficiency may be the cause of fetal distress and fetal death in acute fatty liver. The primary differential diagnoses in cases of acute fatty liver include fulminant hepatitis and the liver dysfunction associated with the HELLP syndrome (hemolysis, elevated liver enzymes, and low platelet count) or preeclampsia.[12-14]

Etiology

The cause of acute fatty liver remains elusive. Brown et al.[15] theorize that there is a spectrum of disease that includes the whole range from mild preeclampsia to acute fatty liver of pregnancy. Grimbert and colleagues[16] investigated the effects of excessive estradiol and progesterone on liver mitochondria in mice. The resulting mitochondrial changes are similar to those seen in acute fatty liver of pregnancy, leading the authors to conclude that imbalance of these hormones may contribute to the development of this pregnancy complication. Treem and co-workers[17] note the similarities in clinical presentation and histologic appearance of the liver in pregnant women with acute fatty liver and in children with metabolic defects in the intramitochondrial β-oxidation pathway. They report a case that suggests that acute fatty liver may be a result of a defect in fatty acid oxidation. Two case reports suggest that similar metabolic defects may be responsible for acute fatty liver.[18,19]

Clinical Diagnosis

Malaise, nausea with vomiting, and epigastric and/or right upper quadrant pain are usually present. The problem is that many of these symptoms are nonspecific and do not become suspicious until the disease process is advanced. The duration of these prodromal symptoms and signs is variable. In a study of 14 cases over 8 years, Usta et al.[7] reported a mean gestational age of 34.5 weeks, with a range of 28 to 39 weeks. Four patients had hepatic encephalopathy, three had pulmonary edema, and three had ascites.[7] Reyes et al.[3] reported lethargy and jaundice as main presenting symptoms and signs in 11 patients with acute fatty liver of pregnancy in Chile. Unusual findings included 7 patients with pruritus, 2 of whom experienced it

weeks before the clinical onset of disease. Patients may also be febrile or present with hepatorenal syndrome.[20] By the time the diagnosis is made, patients often manifest a clinical coagulopathy manifested by hypoprothrombinemia and hypofibrinogenemia.

Laboratory Diagnosis

Because clinical signs are so nonspecific, whenever there is a suspicion of acute fatty liver, the obstetrician should embark on a laboratory evaluation (Table 6-6). In acute fatty liver of pregnancy, serum transaminase levels are elevated but usually remain below 500 IU/liter.[5,21] In acute hepatitis, however, these levels are frequently above 1000 IU/liter. In liver dysfunction associated with preeclampsia or the HELLP syndrome, the transaminases are often in the same range as in acute fatty liver of pregnancy but are occasionally higher. As a result of DIC, the prothrombin time and activated partial thromboplastin time (APTT) are often prolonged. The prothrombin time is usually increased before the APTT because it reflects early depletion of the vitamin K–dependent clotting factors synthesized in the liver. This change is not usually seen in preeclampsia/HELLP. A decreased fibrinogen level is accompanied by an elevation in fibrin degradation products and the D-dimer. Although the serum bilirubin level is elevated, it usually remains below 5 mg/dl but may rarely rise as high as 10 mg/dl.

A liver biopsy specimen will reveal pericentral microvesicular fatty change. There is little inflammatory-cell infiltration or hepatic necrosis. Periportal areas are usually preserved.[21] This picture is very different from fulminant hepatitis, in which hepatocellular necrosis is significant. Special staining and electron microscopy show no evidence of viral particles in acute fatty liver of pregnancy. The diagnosis can be made on frozen

TABLE 6-6
DIFFERENTIAL DIAGNOSIS OF LIVER DISEASE IN PREGNANCY

	Serum Transaminase Levels (IU/liter)	Bilirubin Level (mg/dl)	Coagulopathy	Serum Bile Acids
Acute hepatitis	>1000	>5	−	Normal
Acute fatty liver	<500	<5	+	Normal
Intrahepatic cholestasis	<300	<5, mostly direct	−	Greatly increased
HELLP	>500	<5	+	Normal
Drug-induced hepatitis	<500	<5	−	Normal

section of the liver biopsy material using oil red O stain.[6] This staining is very sensitive but not specific for acute fatty liver of pregnancy. Similar staining is also seen in patients with severe preeclampsia and the HELLP syndrome. Barton and colleagues[22] believe that electron microscopy is more beneficial in establishing a definitive diagnosis, but this test is really only of research interest. However, liver biopsy should virtually never be needed to make the diagnosis of acute fatty liver. This procedure is extremely dangerous due to the severe coagulopathy that usually accompanies this disorder. If biopsy is essential to make the diagnosis and establish a plan of treatment, fresh-frozen plasma can be administered to correct the coagulopathy before performing the procedure.

Goodacre and colleagues[23] as well as Mabie and colleagues[24] believe that diagnosis of acute fatty liver of pregnancy can occasionally be made using computed tomographic (CT) scanning. The finding of decreased attenuation over the liver is compatible with fatty infiltration. Usta et al.[7] found that CT scanning resulted in a large number of false negative diagnoses. Thus, a negative scan does not rule out fatty liver of pregnancy. This finding was corroborated by Van Le and Podrasky.[25] In their study of five patients with acute fatty liver, none had an abnormal CT scan, and only one had an abnormal right-upper-quadrant ultrasound examination. CT scanning is not part of the usual work-up of acute fatty liver. The use of magnetic resonance imaging in establishing this diagnosis has not been studied.

Management

Once the diagnosis has been established, delivery should be accomplished as quickly and as safely as possible.[26] Important supportive measures must first be initiated to ensure maternal well-being. The patient's coagulopathy, if severe, must be corrected with fresh-frozen plasma. If more-concentrated fibrinogen is needed, cryoprecipitate can be administered. Intravenous fluids containing adequate glucose should be given to prevent profound hypoglycemia, which can be fatal in this disorder. If there is not a severe coagulopathy or the coagulopathy has been corrected, invasive hemodynamic monitoring may be instituted, if necessary, before delivery.

Delivery soon after diagnosis is paramount, and vaginal delivery is preferable. If the patient's cervix is unfavorable, cervical ripening agents may be employed

to maximize the likelihood of a vaginal delivery. However, cesarean delivery is warranted if it appears that delivery cannot be effected in a timely fashion and the patient's condition is deteriorating. If the patient's coagulopathy has been corrected, epidural anesthesia is the best choice. Spinal anesthesia can also be used. Regional anesthesia is preferable because it allows adequate assessment of the patient's level of consciousness. General anesthesia should be avoided if possible because of the hepatotoxicity of some anesthetic agents. Narcotic doses must be adjusted, as these drugs are metabolized by the liver.

Early diagnosis and delivery afford both mother and neonate an excellent chance for survival.[5,6] If delivery is effected before hepatic encephalopathy and renal failure develop, patients usually improve rather rapidly.[5-7,9,12] However, Ockner and colleagues[27] have reported a case in which a patient with biopsy-proven acute fatty liver and negative studies for hepatitis did not improve postpartum. After orthotopic liver transplantation, the multisystem failure rapidly reversed.[27] Amon et al.[20] also reported a successful postpartum liver transplant in a patient with acute fatty liver and severe preeclampsia. There is little risk of recurrence of acute fatty liver in subsequent pregnancies[9] although Barton et al.[22] and Schoeman et al.[19] have reported such cases.

INTRAHEPATIC CHOLESTASIS OF PREGNANCY

Epidemiology

Intrahepatic cholestasis is characterized by intense persistent pruritus and mild jaundice during the last trimester of pregnancy. However, it can occur earlier in gestation.[28,29] The disease is reported to affect up to 10% of pregnancies in Chile.[30] Gonzalez et al.[31] determined the prevalence of intrahepatic cholestasis of pregnancy in Chile to be 4.7% in singleton pregnancies. In twin pregnancies, the incidence was 20.9%. The disease is also common in the Swedish population.[32,33] Berg et al.[33] reported the incidence in Sweden to be between 1 and 1.5%. In their study, the incidence of intrahepatic cholestasis of pregnancy had a distinct seasonal variation, peaking in November. This disorder is much less common in the United States. In 1987, Wilson[34] reported the first case of intrahepatic cholestasis of pregnancy in an African-American. Intrahepatic cholestasis tends to recur in subsequent pregnancies, but the severity may vary from one pregnancy to the next. In their Chilean study, Gonzalez et al.[31] found a recurrence rate of 70.5% in singleton pregnancies.

Clinical Manifestations

In patients with intrahepatic cholestasis, pruritus that gradually worsens at night usually develops insidiously. As the disease progresses, the patient experiences bothersome pruritus virtually continuously. Approximately 2 weeks later after the initial onset of the disease, clinical jaundice develops in 50% of cases. The jaundice is usually mild, soon plateaus, and remains constant until delivery. The pruritus worsens with onset of jaundice, and the patient's skin can become excoriated. The symptoms usually abate within 2 days after delivery. The differential diagnosis must include viral hepatitis and gallbladder disease. To differentiate, there is usually no abdominal discomfort (as seen in hepatitis) or nausea and vomiting (as seen in gallbladder disease).

Laboratory Diagnosis

Serum alkaline phosphatase levels are increased 5- to 10-fold over the upper limit of normal in intrahepatic cholestasis of pregnancy. Bilirubin is elevated, but usually not above 5 mg/dl; most is the direct conjugated form. If intrahepatic cholestasis lasts for several weeks, liver dysfunction may result in decreased vitamin K resorption or decreased prothrombin production, leading to a prolongation of the prothrombin time. Serum transaminase levels are usually normal or moderately elevated, remaining well below the levels associated with viral hepatitis. Serum cholesterol and triglyceride levels are also usually markedly elevated.

The serum bile acids (chenodeoxycholic acid, deoxycholic acid, and cholic acid) are increased. The levels are often more than 10 times the normal concentration. These acids are deposited in the skin and probably cause the extreme pruritus.[35] The degree of pruritus, however, is not always related to the serum level of bile acids.[36] To make the diagnosis of intrahepatic cholestasis of pregnancy, the fasting levels of serum bile acids should be at least three times the upper limit of normal. Elevation of serum bile acids alone cannot be used to make the diagnosis; the patient must also have clinical symptoms. Wojcicka-Jagodzinska and colleagues[37] reported that carbohydrate

metabolism is disturbed in patients with intrahepatic cholestasis of pregnancy. Therefore, these patients should be screened for gestational diabetes when the diagnosis of cholestasis is made.

Perinatal Outcome

The risk of preterm birth and fetal death appears to be increased in patients suffering from intrahepatic cholestasis of pregnancy,[28,38] but this issue remains somewhat controversial. While the preterm birth rate has been reported to be between 30 and 60% by some investigators, another study noted no increase in preterm delivery or fetal loss.[39] Fisk and Storey[40] studied 83 pregnancies complicated by intrahepatic cholestasis over a 10-year period. Meconium staining occurred in 45% of the pregnancies, spontaneous preterm labor occurred in 44%, and intrapartum fetal distress complicated 22%. In the 86 pregnancies studied, 2 stillbirths occurred, and 1 neonate died soon after birth. The overall perinatal mortality in this group of patients was 35 per 1000. Nonstress tests and serial ultrasonography to assess amniotic fluid volume failed to predict fetal compromise.[40] Early intervention was indicated in 49 pregnancies, 12 because of suspected fetal distress. In light of this study, antepartum fetal surveillance should be undertaken in pregnant women with intrahepatic cholestasis of pregnancy. It may also be prudent to induce labor at term and, of course, at the first sign of any fetal compromise.[40]

Management

Treatment is aimed at reducing the intense pruritus. Diphenhydramine, hydroxyzine, and other antihistamines may help, but are often of little use, especially in advanced cases. Cholestyramine resin has proven effective in some cases. Cholestyramine is an anion-binding resin that interrupts the enterohepatic circulation and reduces the resorption of bile acids. A total of 8 to 16 g/day in three to four divided doses is often helpful in relieving pruritus. It is most effective if started as soon as the pruritus is noted, before it becomes severe. It often takes up to 2 weeks to work. Because cholestyramine also interferes with vitamin K absorption, the prothrombin time should be checked at least weekly in the beginning of therapy. If cholestyramine therapy is prolonged, parenteral vitamin K should be administered. When the prothrombin time returns to normal, the frequency of injections can be decreased.

Cholestyramine interferes with absorption of other medications, so timing of the dosage is important. Cholestyramine causes a sensation of bloating and often results in constipation. If the patient cannot tolerate cholestyramine, antacids containing aluminum may be used to bind bile acids. Phenobarbital, in a dose of up to 90 mg daily given at bedtime, can occasionally be helpful. Phenobarbital induces hepatic microsomal enzymes, increasing bile salt secretion and bile flow.[41-43] This medication usually takes more than 2 weeks to become effective. Phenobarbital should not be given within 2 hours of cholestyramine, or the phenobarbital will be bound and excreted without being absorbed. The key to treating pregnancy-induced cholestasis is to begin therapy as soon as the diagnosis is made.

Low doses of dexamethasone have also been used with some success in treating pregnancy-induced cholestasis. When pruritus is intolerable, delivery may be undertaken as soon as fetal lung maturity has been documented. Jaundice usually disappears within several days after delivery. The patient should be counseled that the condition may recur during subsequent pregnancies.[31] It is also important to note that some patients may manifest symptoms of intrahepatic cholestasis when taking oral contraceptives.[33]

PREGNANCY AND LIVER TRANSPLANTATION

Pregnancy in the patient whose liver has undergone transplantation is becoming more common in perinatal centers. Laifer and colleagues[44] reported the results of eight pregnancies in women with liver transplants. Seven of the eight patients conceived between 3 weeks and 24 months after transplantation. Six had live births, and one electively terminated her pregnancy. Pregnancy-induced hypertension developed in five patients, including three with severe preeclampsia. The six infants born to these women were delivered between 26 and 37 weeks.[44] Five of the six infants survived, and none had structural anomalies. One patient underwent orthotopic liver transplantation at 26 weeks of gestation after presenting in hepatic coma from fulminant hepatitis B. She was delivered on postoperative day 7 because of fetal distress. Laifer et al.[44] concluded that pregnancy does not appear to have a deleterious effect on hepatic graft function or

survival. All eight of the patients in their series survived without permanent sequelae. As in the case of patients with a renal allograft, liver transplant recipients should continue their immunosuppressive medications throughout pregnancy. Furthermore, they should wait several years before conception to make certain that liver function is acceptable and that there are no signs of rejection.

GALLBLADDER DISEASE

Cholelithiasis is responsible for approximately 7% of cases of jaundice occurring during gestation.[45] Pregnancy appears to increase the likelihood of gallstone formation but not the risk of developing acute cholecystitis.[46-48] Pregnancy markedly alters gallbladder function. Ultrasound studies performed after 14 weeks of gestation have shown that gallbladder emptying in the fasting state is decreased, and the percentage of emptying is decreased, thus leaving more residual contents that becomes sludge.[47]

Once the diagnosis of cholelithiasis is confirmed, attacks of biliary colic should be treated symptomatically during gestation. Ultrasound examination of the gallbladder and biliary tract will aid in the diagnosis of these patients. Hiatt and colleagues[49] report that ultrasound successfully confirmed the presence of gallstones in 18 of 26 patients. In the same series, ultrasound also demonstrated dilated intrahepatic ducts in one of two patients with surgically proven choledocholithiasis. Before resorting to surgery, attempts should be made to treat these patients medically. Attacks usually respond to intravenous hydration, parenteral analgesics, and antibiotics. Nasogastric suction is occasionally needed. Lockwood and associates[50] have also used total parenteral nutrition. Their patient did well, with no fetal or maternal morbidity.

If possible, cholecystectomy should be postponed until after delivery. In their study of 26 patients, Hiatt and coworkers[49] found it necessary to perform cholecystectomy and cholangiography on 19 women, with four requiring bile-duct explorations. They noted that only two of seven patients who presented in the first trimester with cholecystitis carried their pregnancies to term. If ascending cholangitis develops, cholecystectomy should not be postponed. Cholecystectomy should also be performed if common bile duct obstruction occurs or severe pancreatitis develops. Certainly, surgery should not be delayed if an acute abdomen develops. In these instances, temporizing will only increase perinatal and maternal risks.[46] If cholecystectomy is performed in the second or third trimester, fetal mortality is less than 5%.[48] If pancreatitis secondary to biliary tract stones remains untreated, however, the fetal mortality approaches 60%.[48]

Dixon and colleagues[51] reviewed their experience with 44 patients and found that conservative management of cholecystitis was followed by recurrent episodes of biliary-tract symptoms requiring multiple hospitalizations. Cholecystectomy performed in the second trimester was associated with little maternal morbidity, no fetal loss, and a substantial reduction of total hospital days. Baillie and colleagues[52] demonstrated that they were able to avoid cholecystectomy in five pregnant women by performing endoscopic sphincterotomy. Four of these patients had acute cholangitis, and one had pancreatitis. All five women delivered healthy infants at term. Their experience indicates that endoscopic retrograde cholangiopancreatography and sphincterotomy can be safely performed in pregnancy.[52] Before such treatment can be routinely recommended, more studies need to be conducted with this technique.

Laparoscopic cholecystectomy has been performed successfully in early pregnancy.[53] If the uterus is below the umbilicus, the procedure should be safe. However, the abdomen should be insufflated to the lowest possible pressure and fetal heart tones should be auscultated intermittently during the case, especially if surgery is prolonged.

Gallbladder rupture has been reported as a rare complication of pregnancy.[54,55] This event may occur because gastrointestinal symptoms are often confusing in pregnancy, thus delaying appropriate diagnosis. Surgeons may be reluctant to operate on a pregnant patient even though her gallbladder disease warrants intervention. Such delays can have devastating consequences.[54] As obstetricians, it is our duty to help establish the proper diagnosis and, if therapy is out of our field of expertise, to encourage our colleagues to undertake appropriate therapy in a manner that is most beneficial to mother and fetus.

REFERENCES

1. Castro MA, Goodwin TM, Shaw KJ, et al. Disseminated intravascular coagulation and antithrombin III depression in acute fatty liver of pregnancy. Am J Obstet Gynecol 1996;174:211.

2. Mose KJ Jr, Shah DM. Acute fatty liver of pregnancy: etiology of fetal distress and fetal wastage. Obstet Gynecol 1987;69:482.

3. Reyes H, Sandoval L, Wainstein A, et al. Acute fatty liver of pregnancy: a clinical study of 12 episodes in 11 patients. Gut 1994;35:101.

4. Nash DT, Dale JT. Acute yellow atrophy of liver in pregnancy. NY State J Med 1971;71:458.

5. Hou SH, Levin S, Ahola S, et al. Acute fatty liver of pregnancy: survival with early cesarean section. Dig Dis Sci 1984;29:449.

6. Ebert EC, Sun EA, Wright SH, et al. Does early diagnosis and delivery in acute fatty liver of pregnancy lead to improvement in maternal and infant survival? Dig Dis Sci 1984;29:453.

7. Usta IM, Barton JR, Amon EA, et al. Acute fatty liver of pregnancy: an experience in the diagnosis and management of fourteen cases. Am J Obstet Gynecol 1994; 171:1342.

8. Purdie JM, Walters BN. Acute fatty liver of pregnancy: clinical features and diagnosis. Aust NZ J Gynaecol 1988; 28:62.

9. Shaffer EA. Liver disease in pregnancy. Curr Probl Obstet Gynecol 1984;7:15.

10. Minuk GY, Lui RC, Kelly JK. Rupture of the liver associated with acute fatty liver of pregnancy. Am J Gastroenterol 1987;82:457.

11. Roh LS. Subcapsular hematoma in fatty liver of pregnancy. J Forensic Sci 1986;31:1509.

12. Riley CA, Romero R, Duff TP. Hepatic dysfunction with disseminated intravascular coagulation in toxemia of pregnancy: a distinct clinical syndrome. Gastroenterology 1981; 80:1346.

13. Brown MS, Reddy KR, Hensley GT, et al. The initial presentation of fatty liver of pregnancy mimicking acute viral hepatitis. Am J Gastroenterol 1987;82:554.

14. Riley CA, Latham PS, Romero R, Duffy TP. Acute fatty liver of pregnancy: a reassessment based on observations in nine patients. Ann Intern Med 1987;106:703.

15. Brown MA, Pasaris G, Carlton MA. Pregnancy-induced hypertension and acute fatty liver of pregnancy: atypical presentations. Am J Obstet Gynecol 1990;164:154.

16. Grimbert S, Fisch C, Deschamps D, et al. Effects of female sex hormones on mitochondria: possible role of acute fatty liver of pregnancy. Am J Physiol 1995;268:6107.

17. Treem WR, Rinaldo P, Hale DE, et al. Acute fatty liver of pregnancy and long-chain 3-hydroxyacyl-coenzyme A dehydrogenase deficiency. Hepatology 1994;19:339.

18. Sims HF, Brackett JC, Powell CK, et al. The molecular basis of pediatric long chain 3-hydroxyacyl-CoA dehydrogenase deficiency associated with maternal acute fatty liver of pregnancy. Proc Natl Acad Sci USA 1995;92:841.

19. Schoeman MN, Batey RG, Wilcken B. Recurrent acute fatty liver of pregnancy associated with a fatty-acid oxidation defect in the offspring. Gastroenterology 1991; 100:544.

20. Amon E, Allen SR, Petrie RH, Belew JE. Acute fatty liver of pregnancy associated with preeclampsia: management of hepatic failure with postpartum liver transplantation. Am J Perinatol 1991;8:278.

21. Snyder RR, Hankins GD. Etiology and management of acute fatty liver of pregnancy. Clin Perinatol 1986;13:813.

22. Barton JR, Sibai BM, Mabie WC, Shanklin DR. Recurrent acute fatty liver of pregnancy. Am J Obstet Gynecol 1990;163:534.

23. Goodacre RL, Hunter DJ, Millward S, et al. The diagnosis of acute fatty liver of pregnancy by computed tomography. J Clin Gastroenterol 1988;10:680.

24. Mabie WC, Dacus JV, Sibai BM, et al. Computed tomography in acute fatty liver of pregnancy. Am J Obstet Gynecol 1988;158:142.

25. Van Le L, Podrasky A. Computed tomographic and ultrasonographic findings in women with acute fatty liver of pregnancy. J Reprod Med 1990;35:815.

26. Bacq Y, Riely CA. Acute fatty liver of pregnancy: the hepatologist's view. Gastroenterologist 1993;1:257.

27. Ockner SA, Brunt EM, Cohn SM, et al. Fulminant hepatic failure caused by acute fatty liver of pregnancy treated by orthotopic liver transplantation. Hepatology 1990;11:59.

28. Furhoff AK, Hellstrom K. Jaundice in pregnancy: follow-up study of the series of women originally reported by L. Thorling. I. The pregnancies. Acta Med Scand 1973; 193:259.

29. Rencoret R, Aste H. Jaundice during pregnancy. Med J Aust 1973;1:167.

30. Reyes H, Gonzalez MC, Rabalta J, et al. Prevalence of intrahepatic cholestasis of pregnancy in Chile. Ann Intern Med 1978;88:487.

31. Gonzalez MC, Reyes H, Arrese M, et al. Intrahepatic cholestasis of pregnancy in twin pregnancies. J Hepatol 1989;9:84.

32. Rannevik G, Jeppson S, Kullinder S. Effect of oral contraceptives on the liver in women with recurrent cholestasis during previous pregnancies. J Obstet Gynaecol Br Commonw 1972;79:1128.

33. Berg B, Helm G, Petersohn L, Tryding N. Cholestasis of pregnancy: clinical and laboratory studies. Acta Obstet Gynecol Scand 1986;65:107.

34. Wilson JA. Intrahepatic cholestasis of pregnancy with marked elevation of transaminases in a black American. Dig Dis Sci 1987;32:665.

35. Engstrom J, Hellstrom J, Posse N, Sjoball J. Recurrent cholestasis of pregnancy: treatment with cholestyramine of one case with an unusually early onset. Acta Obstet Gynecol Scand 1970;49:29.

36. Ghent CN, Bloomer JR, Koatska G. Elevations in skin tissue levels of bile acids in humans with cholestasis: relation to serum levels and to pruritus. Gastroenterology 1977;73;125.

37. Wojcicka-Jagodzinska J, Kuczynska-Sicinska J, Czajkowski K, Smolarcyzk R. Carbohydrate metabolism in the course of intrahepatic cholestasis in pregnancy. Am J Obstet Gynecol 1989;161:959.

38. Johnson WG, Baskett TF. Obstetric cholestasis: a 14 year review. Am J Obstet Gynecol 1979;143:299.

39. Johnson P, Samsioe G, Gustafsson A. Studies in cholestasis of pregnancy with special reference to clinical aspects and liver function tests. Acta Obstet Gynecol Scand, Suppl 1975;54:77.

40. Fisk NM, Storey GN. Fetal outcome in obstetric cholestasis. Br J Obstet Gynaecol 1988;95:1137.

41. Espinoza J, Barnaf L, Schnaidt E. The effect of phenobarbital on intrahepatic cholestasis of pregnancy. Am J Obstet Gynecol 1974;119:234.

42. Bloomer JR, Bower JL. Phenobarbital effects in cholestasis liver disease. Ann Intern Med 1975;82:310.

43. Laatikinen T. Effect of cholestyramine and phenobarbital on pruritus and serum bile acid levels in cholestasis of pregnancy. Am J Obstet Gynecol 1978;132:501.

44. Laifer SA, Darby MJ, Scantlebuty VP, et al. Pregnancy and liver transplantation. Obstet Gynecol 1990;76:1083.

45. Riley CA, Romero R, Duffy TP. Hepatic dysfunction with disseminated intravascular coagulation in toxemia of pregnancy: a distinct clinical syndrome. Gastroenterology 1981;80:1346.

46. Kammerer WS. Nonobstetric surgery during pregnancy. Med Clin North Am 1979;63:1157.

47. Bennion LJ, Grundy SM. Risk factors for the development of cholelithiasis in man. N Engl J Med 1978; 299:1221.

48. Printen KJ, Ott RA. Cholecystectomy during pregnancy. Am Surg 1978;44:432.

49. Hiatt JR, Hiatt JC, Williams RA, Klein SR. Biliary disease in pregnancy: strategy for surgical management. Am J Surg 1986;151:263.

50. Lockwood C, Stiller RJ, Bolognese RJ. Maternal total parenteral nutrition in chronic cholecystitis: a case report. J Reprod Med 1987;32:785.

51. Dixon NP, Faddis DM, Silberman H. Aggressive management of cholecystitis during pregnancy. Am J Surg 1987; 154:292.

52. Baillie J, Cairns SR, Putman WS, Cotton PB. Endoscopic management of choledocholithiasis during pregnancy. Surg Gynecol Obstet 1990;171:1.

53. Penton ON, Nagy AG, Scudamore CH, Panton RJ. Laparoscopic cholecystectomy: a continuing plea for routine cholangiography. Surg Laparosc Endosc 1995;5:43.

54. Petrozza JC, Mastrobattista JM, Monga M. Gallbladder perforation in pregnancy. Am J Perinatol 1995;12:339.

55. Behera A, Gupta NM. Haemoperitoneum and haemobilia due to cystic artery tear associated with gallbladder perforation in acute cholecystitis complicating pregnancy: case report. Eur J Surg 1991;157:619.

RENAL DISEASE

Philip Samuels

Five Key Points

- **Asymptomatic bacteriuria is present in 5 to 10% of pregnant women, acute cystitis in 1 to 3%, and acute pyelonephritis in 1 to 2%. Pyelonephritis is an important cause of sepsis and preterm labor.**

- **Most renal and ureteral stones that develop during pregnancy will pass spontaneously.**

- **In patients with chronic renal disease, the presence of hypertension is the best predictor of adverse pregnancy outcome.**

- **Angiotensin converting enzyme inhibitors and angiotensin antagonists are teratogenic and should not be used to treat hypertension in pregnancy.**

- **Preeclampsia is the most common complication of pregnancy in a patient who has had a renal transplant.**

ASYMPTOMATIC BACTERIURIA AND ACUTE PYELONEPHRITIS

The diagnosis of asymptomatic bacteriuria (ASB) is based on a clean-catch voided urine culture revealing greater than 100,000 colonies per ml of a single organism.[1] Between 1.2 and 5% of young girls will demonstrate ASB at some time before puberty.[2] After puberty, with the onset of sexual activity, the prevalence of ASB may increase to 10%.[2] Of women with ASB, approximately 35% have bacteria arising from the kidneys rather than from the lower urinary tract. These patients are at special risk for developing pyelonephritis.

All pregnant women should be screened for bacteriuria at the first prenatal visit. It is important to diagnose and treat ASB in pregnancy. If left untreated, a symptomatic urinary tract infection (UTI) will develop in up to 40% of these patients.[3,4] Recognition and appropriate therapy for ASB can eliminate 70% of acute UTIs in pregnancy. Nonetheless, symptomatic cystitis or pyelonephritis develops in 2% of pregnant women with negative urine cultures. This group accounts for 30% of the cases of acute UTI that develop during gestation.

Escherichia coli is the organism responsible for most cases of ASB. Patients can therefore be safely treated with nitrofurantoin, ampicillin, cephalosporins, and short-acting sulfa drugs. Sulfa compounds should be avoided near term, as they can displace bilirubin from albumin-binding sites and can lead to hyperbilirubinemia in the newborn. Nitrofurantoin should not be used in mothers with glucose-6-phosphate dehydrogenase deficiency, as it can result in a hemolytic crisis. If the fetus has this enzyme deficiency, it may also experience hemolysis. Therapy for ASB should range from 3 days for the initial infection to 7 to 10 days for recurrent infection. The patient should have another culture performed 1 to 2 weeks after discontinuing therapy. Approximately 15% of patients will experience a reinfection and/or will not respond to initial therapy. Therapy should be reinstituted after careful microbial sensitivity testing. Patients with recurrent UTI during pregnancy and those with a history of pyelonephritis should undergo radiologic evaluation of the upper urinary tract. This procedure should be delayed until the patient is at least 3 months postpartum so that the anatomic and physiologic changes of pregnancy can regress. Of the women in the above categories, 20% will have a structural abnormality, but most of these abnormalities will have no clinical significance.

Occasionally, it is difficult to distinguish severe cystitis from pyelonephritis. Although the drugs used for treatment are similar, pyelonephritis requires initial parenteral antibiotics. Sandberg and co-investigators[5] studied symptomatic UTI in 174 women. They found that C-reactive protein was elevated in 91% of pregnant women with acute pyelonephritis and in only 5% of women with cystitis. Occurring in approximately 1 to 2% of all pregnancies, pyelonephritis is an important source of maternal morbidity. Pyelonephritis is the most common nonobstetric cause of hospitalization during pregnancy.[6] Recurrent pyelonephritis has been implicated as a factor in fetal death and intrauterine growth restriction (IUGR). There also appears to be an association between acute pyelonephritis and preterm labor.[7,8] If pyelonephritis is aggressively treated, it does not increase the likelihood of premature delivery or delivery of a low-birth-weight infant.[9]

Acute pyelonephritis should be initially treated on an inpatient basis, with intravenous antibiotics. Empiric therapy should be begun as soon as the presumptive diagnosis is made. Therapy can be tailored to the specific organism after results of sensitivity testing have been obtained approximately 48 hours later. Because septicemia may occasionally result from pyelonephritis, blood cultures should be obtained if patients do not respond rapidly to initial antibiotic therapy. *E. coli* is the most common organism isolated in pyelonephritis. During gestation, the right side is most affected, as engorged vessels may inhibit ureteral drainage of the kidney. Generally, a broad-spectrum first-generation cephalosporin is the initial therapy of choice, as in many locations, *E. coli has* developed resistance to ampicillin. Fan and co-investigators[9] reviewed 107 cases of pyelonephritis in 103 pregnant women. They reported that 33% were resistant to ampicillin and 13% to first-generation cephalosporins. If resistance to more common therapies is encountered, a later-generation cephalosporin or an aminoglycoside can safely be administered. However, peak and trough aminoglycoside levels should be monitored.

The serum creatinine and blood urea nitrogen (BUN) levels should be followed as well. During the febrile period, acetaminophen should be employed to keep the patient's temperature below 38°C. Small doses of acetaminophen will not mask the fever and symptoms in a patient who is unresponsive to treatment.

Intravenous antibiotic therapy should be continued for 24 to 48 hours after the patient becomes afebrile and costovertebral angle tenderness disappears. After the cessation of intravenous therapy, oral antibiotics should be continued to complete a 10- to 14-day course of treatment. On termination of therapy, the patient should be monitored for recurrent infection on a regular basis with culture or rapid tests for nitrites and leukocyte esterases. After an episode of acute pyelonephritis, antibiotic suppression should be implemented and continued for the remainder of pregnancy. Nitrofurantoin, 100 mg once daily, is an acceptable regimen for suppression.

In a study by van Dorsten and colleagues,[10] the overall frequency of positive urine cultures following hospitalization for pyelonephritis was 38%. Nitrofurantoin suppression reduced the rate to 8%. Nitrofurantoin did not lower the rate of positive cultures if the inpatient antibiotic selection was inappropriate or if the culture was positive at time of discharge.[10] Today, there is increased pressure to treat pyelonephritis as an outpatient condition. Although this is discouraged, it is possible if daily nursing contact is maintained during the acute phase of the disease and appropriate laboratory parameters are followed. The major responsibility for the patient's care still rests with the physician, not with the home health care agency.

Cunningham and co-workers[11] noted that pulmonary injury resembling adult respiratory distress syndrome (ARDS) can occur in patients with acute pyelonephritis. Clinical manifestations of this complication usually occur 24 to 48 hours after the patient is admitted for pyelonephritis.[11,12] Some of these patients will require endotracheal intubation, mechanical ventilation,[13] and positive-end-expiratory pressure (PEEP). This ARDS-type picture probably results from endotoxin-induced alveolar capillary membrane injury. Towers et al. found pulmonary injury in 11 of 130 patients with pyelonephritis.[14] A fever of greater than 40°C, a maternal heart rate above 110, and a gestation longer than 20 weeks placed the patient at increased risk for pulmonary injury.

Austenfeld and Snow[15] studied 64 pregnancies in 30 women who had previously undergone ureteral reimplantation for vesicoureteral reflux. During pregnancy, 57% of these women had at least one UTI and 17% had more than one UTI or an episode of pyelonephritis.[15] Therefore, these patients need close surveillance throughout pregnancy.

UROLITHIASIS

The prevalence of urolithiasis during pregnancy is 0.03%, with an incidence no higher than that in the general population.[16] Colicky abdominal pain, recurrent UTI, and hematuria suggest urolithiasis. If the diagnosis is suspected, intravenous pyelography should be undertaken, limiting this study to the minimum number of exposures necessary to make the diagnosis. It is important, however, to take the proper number of x-ray films using the appropriate technique to gain the necessary information. Ultrasound can often be used to establish the diagnosis. Newer ultrasound flow studies can actually follow flow from the ureter to the bladder and detect obstruction without the use of ionizing radiation. Urine microscopy can often detect crystals and help distinguish the type of stone before it is passed. For any patient suspected or proved to have renal stones, serum calcium, phosphorus, and magnesium levels should be measured. It is important to rule out hyperparathyroidism. Serum urate should also be determined.

Because of the physiologic hydroureter characteristic of pregnancy, most patients with symptomatic urolithiasis will spontaneously pass their stones. Treatment should be conservative, consisting of hydration and narcotic analgesia for pain relief.[17] Occasionally, urologic intervention, including procedures such as ureteroscopy or percutaneous nephrostomy, will be necessary.

Recurrent UTI with urease-containing organisms causes precipitation of calcium phosphate in the kidney that may lead to the development of staghorn calculi. Surgery is rarely indicated in these patients, especially during gestation. Patients with staghorn calculi should have frequent urine cultures, and bacteriuria should be treated aggressively. Recurrent infections can lead to chronic pyelonephritis, with resultant loss of kidney function.

GLOMERULONEPHRITIS

Acute glomerulonephritis is uncommon during pregnancy, with an estimated incidence of 1 per 40,000 pregnancies.[18] The low incidence results from the fact that poststreptococcal glomerulonephritis rarely occurs in adults. It is mentioned here because acute glomerulonephritis can be difficult to distinguish from preeclampsia. Periorbital edema, a striking clinical feature of acute glomerulonephritis, is often seen in preeclampsia. Hematuria, red-cell casts in the urine sediment, and depressed serum complement levels indicate glomerular disease. Treatment of acute glomerulonephritis in pregnancy is similar to that for the nonpregnant patient. Blood pressure control is essential, and careful attention to fluid and electrolyte balance is imperative. Sodium intake should be restricted during the acute disease. Serum potassium levels must also be carefully monitored.

Packham and co-workers[19] reviewed 395 pregnancies in 238 women with primary glomerulonephritis. Only 51% of their infants were born at term. In addition, there was a 20% fetal loss rate, 15% after 20 weeks of gestation. IUGR was noted in 15% of the live-born fetuses. Maternal renal function deteriorated in 15% of pregnancies. Hypertension was recorded in 52% of the pregnancies, developing before 32 weeks of gestation in 26%. This blood pressure elevation was not an exacerbation of previously diagnosed hypertension. Eighteen percent of the women who developed de novo hypertension in pregnancy remained hypertensive postpartum. Increased proteinuria was recorded in 59% of these pregnancies and was irreversible in 15%.[19] The highest incidence of fetal and maternal complications occurred in patients with primary focal and segmental hyalinosis and sclerosis. The lowest incidence of complications was observed in non-IgA diffuse mesangial proliferative glomerulonephritis.[19]

Packham and co-workers[20] also studied 33 pregnancies in 24 patients with biopsy-proven membranous glomerulonephritis. Fetal loss occurred in 24% of pregnancies, preterm delivery in 43%, and a full-term liveborn infant in only 33%. Hypertension was noted in 46% of these pregnant women. Thirty percent of patients had proteinuria in the nephrotic range in the first trimester.[20] The presence of heavy proteinuria during the first trimester correlated with a poor fetal and maternal outcome.[20]

Jungers et al.[21] described 69 pregnancies in 34 patients with IgA glomerulonephritis. The fetal loss rate in this group was 15%. Preexisting hypertension was statistically associated with poor fetal outcome. Hypertension at the time of conception also correlated with a deterioration of maternal renal function during pregnancy. Hypertension in the first pregnancy was highly predictive of recurrence of hypertension in a subsequent pregnancy.[21] Kincaide-Smith and Fairley[22] analyzed 102 pregnancies in 65 women with IgA glomerulonephritis. They noted that hypertension occurred in 63% of pregnancies, with 18% being severe. They also observed a decrease in renal function in 22% of these women.

Abe[23] retrospectively studied 240 pregnancies in 166 women with preexisting glomerular disease between 1976 and 1988. Eight percent of the pregnancies resulted in spontaneous abortion, 6% resulted in stillbirth, and 86% were liveborn. Most losses occurred in women with glomerular filtration rates (GFRs) less than 70 ml/min and preexisting hypertension. Even though the majority of women with renal insufficiency had good pregnancy outcomes, the long-term prognosis of the kidney disease was worse if the GFR was less than 50 ml/min and the serum creatinine was more than 1.5 mg/dl.[23] Renal complications were worse in patients with membranoproliferative glomerulonephritis, with hypertension developing in 29% and a long-term decrease in renal function developing in 33%.

Imbasciati and Ponticelli[24] summarized six studies that included a total of 906 pregnancies in 558 women with preexisting glomerular disease. This review has the limitations of including patients from a wide span of years and varying geographic locations. Nonetheless, broad generalizations can be made. The overall perinatal mortality was 13%. Hypertension, renal insufficiency, and proteinuria in the nephrotic range were the strongest prognostic factors for a poor pregnancy outcome. Hypertension persisted in 3 to 12% of patients in whom hypertension developed for the first time during pregnancy. In 3% of these 166 women, the course of their glomerular disease accelerated after pregnancy.

CHRONIC RENAL DISEASE

Chronic renal disease can be silent until its advanced stages. Because obstetricians routinely examine the patient's urine for the presence of protein, glucose, and ketones, they may be the first to suspect chronic renal disease. Any pregnant woman with more than trace proteinuria should collect a 24-hour urine specimen for creatinine clearance and total protein excretion. Creatinine clearance is elevated in pregnancy. During the first trimester, it may exceed 140 ml/min. Before pregnancy, 24-hour urinary protein excretion should not exceed 0.2 g. During gestation, quantities up to 0.3 g/day may be normal. Moderate proteinuria

(less than 2 g/day) is usually seen in glomerular disease. New onset of proteinuria in the third trimester, of course, should be considered preeclampsia until proven otherwise.

Microscopic examination of the urine can reveal much about the patient's renal status. If renal disease is suspected, a catheterized specimen should be obtained. More than one to two red cells per high-power field or any red-cell casts are indicative of renal disease. Red cells usually indicate glomerular disease or collagen vascular disease. Less frequently they suggest trauma, malignant hypertension, or tumor. Increased numbers of white cells (more than one or two per high-power field) or the appearance of white-cell casts is usually indicative of acute or chronic infection. Cellular casts are found in the presence of renal tubular dysfunction, and hyaline casts suggest significant proteinuria. A single bacterium seen in an unspun catheterized urine specimen is suggestive of significant bacteriuria, and a follow-up culture should be performed.

The obstetrician can easily be misled when relying solely on the BUN and serum creatinine to assess renal function. A 70% decline in creatinine clearance, an indirect measure of GFR, can be seen before a significant rise in the BUN or serum creatinine occurs. In fact, little change in the serum creatinine or the BUN is seen until the creatinine clearance falls to ≤50 ml/min. Below that level, small decrements in creatinine clearance can lead to large increases in the BUN and creatinine levels. A single creatinine clearance value less than 100 ml/min is not diagnostic of renal disease. An incomplete 24-hour urine collection is the most frequent cause of this finding. An abnormal clearance rate should, therefore, be restudied.

Serum urate is an often overlooked but helpful parameter in detecting renal dysfunction. Excretion of uric acid is dependent not only on glomerular filtration but also on tubular secretion. An elevated serum urate level in the presence of normal BUN and serum creatinine levels may, therefore, implicate tubular disease. A solitary increase in uric acid may also signify impending or early preeclampsia.

EFFECT OF PREGNANCY ON RENAL FUNCTION IN CHRONIC RENAL DISEASE

Although base-line creatinine clearance is decreased in patients with chronic renal insufficiency, it should still increase during gestation. A moderate fall in creatinine clearance is often observed during late gestation in patients with renal disease. This decrease is typically more severe in patients with diffuse glomerular disease. It usually reverses after delivery.

The long-term effect of pregnancy on renal disease remains controversial. If the patient's serum creatinine is less than 1.5 mg/dl, pregnancy should have little effect on the long-term prognosis of the patient's kidney disease. However, pregnancy is associated with an increased incidence of pyelonephritis in patients with chronic renal disease. There are few data concerning the long-term effect of pregnancy on renal disease in women with true renal insufficiency. Occasionally, some patients with a base-line serum creatinine level greater than 1.5 mg/dl will experience a significant decrease in renal function during gestation that does not improve during the postpartum period.[24-26] This deterioration occurs more frequently in women with diffuse glomerulonephritis. However, it is not possible to predict which patients with renal insufficiency will experience a permanent reduction in renal function.

If renal function significantly deteriorates during gestation, termination of pregnancy may not reverse the process. Therefore, abortion cannot be routinely recommended for patients who become pregnant and whose base-line serum creatinine level exceeds 1.5 mg/dl. Ideally, patients with chronic renal disease should be thoroughly counseled before conception about the possible consequences of pregnancy.

Severe hypertension is the greatest threat to the pregnant patient with chronic renal disease. Left uncontrolled, profound hypertension can lead to intracerebral hemorrhage as well as deteriorating renal function. In most pregnancies complicated by chronic renal dysfunction, some degree of hypertension is present.[25-27] Approximately 50% of these patients will have worsening hypertension as pregnancy progresses, and diastolic blood pressures of 110 mm Hg or greater will develop in about 20% of cases.[28] Patients with diffuse proliferative glomerulonephritis and nephrosclerosis are at greatest risk for the development of severe hypertension. Blood pressure control is the cornerstone of successful treatment of chronic renal disease in pregnancy.

Worsening proteinuria is common during pregnancy complicated by chronic renal disease and often reaches the nephrotic range.[28] In general, massive proteinuria does not indicate an increased risk for mother or fetus.[24] Low serum albumin, however, has been correlated with low birth weight.[29]

EFFECT OF CHRONIC RENAL DISEASE ON PREGNANCY

Despite pessimistic reports from many years ago, more than 85% of women with chronic renal disease will have a surviving infant if renal function is well preserved. However, if hypertension is not controlled and if renal function is not well preserved, there is still a high likelihood of pregnancy loss.[19] Antepartum fetal surveillance and advances in neonatal care have made great strides in improving perinatal outcome in these patients. One study reported a total fetal loss rate of 13.8%, including miscarriage, stillbirths, and neonatal deaths.[27] This is not different from the general population. Imbasciati and Ponticelli[27] summarized three studies that included 81 pregnancies in 78 women with serum creatinine concentrations less than 1.4 mg/dl. The perinatal loss rate was only 9%. Nevertheless, 33% of the infants were growth-restricted, and 50% were born preterm secondary to either maternal or fetal indications. Disturbingly, 33% of the women showed acceleration of their renal disease after delivery.

The outlook for women with severe renal insufficiency whose base-line serum creatinine level is more than 1.5 mg/dl is less clear. This is due to in part to the limited number of reported pregnancies in such patients as well as to the large number who undergo elective abortion. One study reported no surviving infants when the maternal BUN was greater than 60 mg/dl.[30] However, other investigations have found that about 80% of such pregnancies resulted in surviving infants.[27,31] The reported incidence of preterm birth ranges from 20 to 50%.[28,32]

SURVEILLANCE AND TREATMENT

A 24-hour urine collection for creatinine clearance and total protein excretion should be obtained as soon as the pregnancy is confirmed. These parameters should be monitored monthly. The patient should be seen about once every 2 weeks until 32 weeks of gestation and weekly thereafter. These are general guidelines, and more frequent visits may be necessary in individual cases. Control of hypertension is critical in treating patients with chronic renal disease. β-Blockers, calcium-channel blockers, α-blockers, clonidine, and hydralazine can be used to treat blood pressure effectively as long as the dosages are monitored carefully. Angiotensin-converting–enzyme (ACE) inhibitors should be avoided during pregnancy. These drugs have been associated with irreversible renal dysplasia with resulting fetal and neonatal oliguria/anuria.[33,34] Furthermore, congenital anomalies, including microcephaly and encephalocele,[33] have been encountered in fetuses born to mothers using ACE inhibitors. The use of diuretics in pregnancy is controversial.[35] For massive debilitating edema, a short course of diuretics can be helpful. Electrolytes must be monitored carefully. Salt restriction does not appear to be beneficial once edema has developed. However, salt restriction should be instituted without hesitation in pregnant women with true renal insufficiency.

Fetal growth should be assessed with serial ultrasonography because growth restriction is common in women with chronic renal disease. Antepartum fetal heart rate testing should be started around 28 weeks of gestation.[36] Obstetricians should have a low threshold for hospitalizing patients with chronic renal disease. Increasing hypertension and decreasing renal function warrant immediate hospitalization. A sudden deterioration of renal function may be due to infection, dehydration, electrolyte imbalance, or obstruction. The timing of delivery must be individualized. Maternal indications for delivery include uncontrollable hypertension, the development of superimposed preeclampsia, and decreasing renal function after fetal viability has been reached. Fetal indications are dictated by the assessment of fetal growth and fetal well-being.

Renal biopsy is rarely indicated during pregnancy. It is never indicated after 34 weeks of gestation, when delivery of the fetus and subsequent biopsy would be a safer alternative. Excessive bleeding secondary to the greatly increased renal blood flow has been reported by some,[37] but not all,[38] observers. If coagulation indices are normal and blood pressure is well controlled, morbidity should be no greater than that observed in the nonpregnant patient.[39] Packham and Fairley[40] reported a series of 111 renal biopsies performed in 104 pregnant women over a 20-year period. The complication rate was 4.5%. The most likely clinical dilemma necessitating renal biopsy in a pregnant woman would be the development of nephrotic syndrome and increasing hypertension between 22 and 30 weeks of gestation. In this case, renal biopsy may distinguish chronic renal disease from preeclampsia and have a significant impact on the treatment plan.

PREGNANCY IN THE RENAL TRANSPLANT RECIPIENT

Pregnancy following renal transplantation is common. Many previously anovulatory patients begin ovulating postoperatively and regain fertility as renal function normalizes.[41] Many transplant recipients have failed to realize they are pregnant until well into the second trimester.

On learning of pregnancy, a patient's natural impulse is to stop taking all medications. The importance of continuing immunosuppresive therapy cannot be overemphasized to recipients of renal allografts. Glucocorticoids, especially prednisone, are metabolized in the placenta by 11β-ol-dehydrogenase, with only limited amounts reaching the fetus. No studies have documented an increased rate of malformations. Adrenocortical insufficiency has been only rarely reported in infants born to mothers taking glucocorticoids.[42] Nevertheless, a pediatrician should be present at the delivery and should be aware of this possibility.

Azathioprine cannot be activated in the fetus because of its lack of inosinate pyrophosphorylase.[43] Azathioprine has been shown to cause decreased levels of IgG and IgM as well as a smaller thymic shadow on chest x-ray films in exposed neonates.[44] The long-term implications of this treatment are not yet known. IUGR has been reported in infants born to mothers receiving azathioprine.[45] These risks are outweighed, however, by the potentially disastrous consequences of allograft rejection that may occur if the patient stops her medication.

Cyclosporins and Neoral (cyclosporin) appear to be relatively safe for use during gestation, but do present some risks. Patients on cyclosporins may develop arterial hypertension secondary to its interference with the normal hemodynamic adaptation to pregnancy.[46] Cyclosporins cross the placenta, but there is no evidence of teratogenesis.[47,48] Intrauterine growth restriction, in the absence of maternal hypertension, has been reported in a patient taking cyclosporine during pregnancy.[49] Most women taking cyclosporins have had no complications attributable to the drug, and the risk of allograft rejection certainly outweighs the fetal risk of the medication. Therefore, the medication should be continued throughout gestation.

Davison[50] reviewed 1569 renal transplants in 1009 women. He found that 22% of the women elected to abort their pregnancies, 16% had a spontaneous abortion, and 8% experienced perinatal deaths.

Furthermore, he observed that 45% of the surviving pregnancies were delivered preterm and 22% were complicated by intrauterine growth restriction.[50] Three percent of the infants were born with major malformations, a rate no different from expected in the background population. Preeclampsia complicated 30% of the pregnancies, but, as previously noted, the diagnosis is difficult to make in a patient who may already have hypertension and proteinuria. Importantly, allograft rejection was suspected in 9% of these women, and this figure is no different from that expected in a nonpregnant population. Also, the long-term rejection rate was the same as for women who had not experienced a pregnancy.

During pregnancy, renal allograft recipients must be carefully monitored for signs of rejection even though the rate is no greater than that expected in the nonpregnant population. Unfortunately, the clinical hallmarks of rejection—fever, oliguria, tenderness, and decreasing renal function—are not always exhibited by the pregnant patient. Occasionally, rejection may mimic pyelonephritis or preeclampsia, which occurs in approximately one-third of renal transplant patients. In these cases renal biopsy is indicated to distinguish rejection from preeclampsia. Rejection has been known to occur during the puerperium, when maternal immunocompetence returns to its prepregnancy level.[51]

Infection can be disastrous for the renal allograft. Therefore, urine cultures should be obtained regularly during pregnancy, and bacteriuria should be aggressively treated. It is crucial to remember that the allograft is denervated, and the patient may experience no pain with pyelonephritis. The only symptoms may be fever and nausea.

Renal function, as determined by 24-hour creatinine clearance and protein excretion, should also be assessed regularly. Approximately 15% of transplant recipients will exhibit a significant decrease in renal function in late pregnancy.[52] This condition usually, but not always, reverses after pregnancy. Proteinuria develops in about 40% of patients near term, but most often disappears soon after delivery unless significant hypertension is present.

As in patients with chronic renal disease, serial ultrasonography should be used to assess fetal growth, and antepartum fetal heart rate testing should be started at approximately 28 weeks of gestation. About 50% of renal allograft recipients will deliver preterm. Preterm labor, preterm rupture of membranes, and

IUGR are common. Vaginal delivery should be accomplished when possible, with cesarean delivery reserved for obstetric indications. Allograft recipients may have an increased frequency of cephalopelvic disproportion from pelvic osteodystrophy,[53] resulting from prolonged renal disease with hypercalcemia or extended steroid use. However, the transplanted kidney rarely obstructs vaginal delivery despite its pelvic location.

Although there have been many successful pregnancies in renal allograft recipients, no group has devised precise criteria for when it is safe to conceive after transplantation. Lindheimer and Katz, the leading authorities on renal disease in pregnancy, suggest waiting 2 years after a cadaver transplant and 1 year after graft from a living donor.[54] They also suggest that serum creatinine level be less than 1 to 5 mg/μl.

ACUTE RENAL FAILURE IN PREGNANCY

Acute renal failure (ARF) is defined as a urine output of less than 400 ml in 24 hours. To make the diagnosis ureteral and urethral obstruction must be excluded. The incidence of ARF during pregnancy is approximately 1 per 10,000. It is seen most frequently in septic first-trimester abortions and in cases of sudden severe volume depletion resulting from hemorrhage caused by placenta previa, placental abruption, or postpartum uterine atony.[55] It is also observed in the marked volume contraction associated with severe preeclampsia and with acute fatty liver of pregnancy.[56,57]

The incidence of ARF in pregnancy has decreased over the years. Stratta and colleagues[58] reported 81 cases of pregnancy-related ARF between 1958 and 1987, accounting for 9% of the total number of ARF cases needing dialysis during that interval. In these 81 ARF cases, 11.6% experienced irreversible renal damage, the majority of which were due to severe preeclampsia/eclampsia.[58]

Renal ischemia is the common denominator in all cases of ARF. With mild ischemia, quickly reversible prerenal failure results. With more prolonged ischemia, acute tubular necrosis occurs. This process is also reversible, as glomeruli are not affected. Severe ischemia, however, may produce acute cortical necrosis. This pathology is irreversible. Stratta and colleagues[59] have reported 17 cases of ARF occurring over 15 years, and all were due to preeclampsia/eclampsia. Cortical necrosis occurred in 29.5% of the cases.[59] Whether or not ARF was associated with cortical necrosis did not appear to be related to chronological age, parity, gestational age at which preeclampsia developed, duration of preeclampsia prior to delivery, or eclamptic seizures. The only statistically significant factor associated with the appearance of cortical necrosis was placental abruption.[59] In another study, Turney and co-workers[60] demonstrated that acute cortical necrosis, which occurred in 12.7% of their patients with ARF, had a 100% mortality rate within 6 years.

Sibai and colleagues[61] studied the remote prognosis in 31 consecutive cases of ARF in patients with hypertensive disorders of pregnancy. Eighteen of the 31 patients had "pure" preeclampsia, while 13 pregnancies had other hypertensive disorders and renal disease. Five percent of the 18 patients with pure preeclampsia required dialysis. Of the other 13 women, 42% required dialysis. The majority of pregnancies in both groups were complicated by placental abruption and hemorrhage.[61] All 16 surviving patients in the pure preeclampsia group had normal renal function on long-term follow-up. Conversely, 9 of the 11 patients without preeclampsia required long-term dialysis, and four ultimately died of end-stage renal disease.[61]

Clinically, patients with reversible ARF first experience a period of oliguria of variable duration. Polyuria then occurs. It is important to recognize that BUN and serum creatinine levels continue to rise early in the polyuric phase. During the recovery phase, urine output approaches normal. In these patients, it is important to monitor electrolytes frequently and to treat any imbalance carefully.

The main goal of treatment is the elimination of the underlying cause. Volume and electrolyte balance must receive careful attention. To assess volume requirements, invasive hemodynamic monitoring is useful. This is especially true during the polyuric phase. Central hyperalimentation may also be required if renal failure is prolonged.

Acidosis occurs frequently in cases of ARF. Therefore, arterial blood-gas levels should be monitored. Acidosis must be treated promptly to prevent hyperkalemia, which may develop rapidly and can be fatal. Absolute restriction of potassium intake should be instituted immediately. Sodium bicarbonate, used to treat acidosis, may overload the patient with sodium and water. In this case, peritoneal dialysis or hemodialysis may be instituted. The main indications for dialysis in ARF of pregnancy are hypernatremia, hyperkalemia, severe acidosis, volume overload, and worsening uremia.

REFERENCES

1. Kass E. Asymptomatic infections of the urinary tract. Trans Assoc Am Physicians 1956;60:56.
2. Kunin C. The natural history of recurrent bacteriuria in schoolgirls. N Engl J Med 1970;282:1443.
3. Savage W, Hajj S, Kass E. Demographic and prognostic characteristics of bacteriuria in pregnancy. Medicine (Baltimore) 1967;46:385.
4. Whalley P. Bacteriuria of pregnancy. Am J Obstet Gynecol 1967;97:723.
5. Sandberg T, Likin-Janson G, Eden CS. Host response in women with symptomatic urinary tract infection. Scand J Infect Dis 1989;21:67.
6. Plattner MS. Pyelonephritis in pregnancy. J Perinatol Neonat Nursing 1994;8:20.
7. Brumfitt W. The significance of symptomatic and asymptomatic infection in pregnancy. Contrib Nephrol 1981; 25:23.
8. Gilstrap L, Leveno K, Cunningham F, et al. Renal infection and pregnancy outcome. Am J Obstet Gynecol 1981; 141:709.
9. Fan YD, Pastorek JG II, Miller JM Jr, Mulvey J. Acute pyelonephritis in pregnancy. Am J Perinatol 1987;4:324.
10. van Dorsten JP, Lenke RR, Schifrin BS. Pyelonephritis in pregnancy: the role of in-hospital management and nitrofurantoin suppression. J Reprod Med 1987;32:895.
11. Cunningham FG, Lucas MJ, Hankins GD. Pulmonary injury complicating antepartum pyelonephritis. Am J Obstet Gynecol 1987;156:797.
12. Pruett K, Faro S. Pyelonephritis associated with respiratory distress. Obstet Gynecol 1987;69:444.
13. Goorman G, Schlaeffer E, Kopernic G. Adult respiratory distress syndrome as a complication of acute pyelonephritis during pregnancy. Eur J Obstet Gynecol Rep Biol 1990;36:75.
14. Towers CV, Kaminskas CM, Garite TJ, et al. Pulmonary injury associated with antepartum pyelonephritis: can at risk patients be identified? Am J Obstet Gynecol 1991; 164:974.
15. Austenfeld MS, Snow BW. Complications of pregnancy in women after reimplantation for vesicoureteral reflux. J Urol 1988;140:1103.
16. Harris R, Dunnihoo D. The incidence and significance of urinary calculi in pregnancy. Am J Obstet Gynecol 1967; 99:237.
17. Strong D, Murchison R, Lynch D. The management of ureteral calculi during pregnancy. Surv Gynecol Obstet 1978;146:604.
18. Nadler N, Salinas-Madrigal L, Charles A, Pollack V. Acute glomerulonephritis during late pregnancy. Obstet Gynecol 1969;34:277.
19. Packham DK, North RA, Fairley KF, et al. Primary glomerulonephritis and pregnancy. Q J Med 1989;71:537.
20. Packham DK, North RA, Fairly KF, et al. Membranous glomerulonephritis and pregnancy. Clin Nephrol 1988; 30:487.

21. Jungers P, Forget D, Houillier P, et al. Pregnancy in IgA nephropathy, reflux nephropathy, and focal glomerular sclerosis. Am J Kidney Dis 1987;9:334.

22. Kincaid-Smith P, Fairley KF. Renal disease in pregnancy: three controversial areas: mesangial IgA nephropathy, focal glomerular sclerosis (focal and segmental hyalinosis and sclerosis), and reflux nephropathy. Am J Kidney Dis 1987; 9:328.

23. Abe S. An overview of pregnancy in women with underlying renal disease. Am J Kidney Dis 1991;17:112.

24. Imbasciati E, Ponticelli C: Pregnancy and renal disease: predictors for fetal and maternal outcome. Am J Nephrol 1991;11:353.

25. Bear R. Pregnancy in patients with renal disease: a study of 44 cases. Obstet Gynecol 1976;48:13.

26. Hou S. Pregnancy in women with chronic renal disease. N Engl J Med 1985;321:839.

27. Hou S, Grossman S, Madias N. Pregnancy in women with renal disease and moderate renal insufficiency. Am J Med 1985;78:185.

28. Katz A, Davison J, et al. Pregnancy in women with kidney disease. Kidney Int 1980;18:192.

29. Studd J, Blainey J. Pregnancy and the nephrotic syndrome. BMJ 1969;1:276.

30. Mackay E. Pregnancy and renal disease: a ten year study. Aust NZ J Obstet Gynaecol 1963;3:21.

31. Kincaid-Smith P, Fairley K, Bullen M. Kidney disease and pregnancy. Med J Aust 1967;11:1155.

32. Surian M, Imbasciati E, Banfi G, et al. Glomerular disease and pregnancy. Nephron 1984;36:101.

33. Piper JM, Ray WA, Rosa FW. Pregnancy outcome following exposure to angiotensin-converting enzyme inhibitors. Obstet Gynecol 1992;80:429.

34. Hulton SA, Thomspon PD, Cooper PA, Rothberg AD. Angiotensin-converting enzyme inhibitors in pregnancy may result in neonatal renal failure. S Afr Med J 1990; 78:673.

35. Sibai B, Grossman R, Grossman H. Effects of diuretics on plasma volume in pregnancies with long term hypertension. Am J Obstet Gynecol 1984;150:831.

36. Sanchez-Casajuz A, Famos I, Santos M. Monitorization fetal en el transcurso de hemodialissi durante el embarazo. Rev Clin Esp 1978;149:187.

37. Schewitz L, Friedman E, Pollak V. Bleeding after renal biopsy in pregnancy. Obstet Gynecol 1965;26:295.

38. Lindheimer M, Spargo B, Katz A. Renal biopsy in pregnancy-induced hypertension. J Reprod Med 1975;15:189.

39. Lindheimer M, Fisher K, Spargo B, Katz A. Hypertension in pregnancy: a biopsy study with long term followup. Contrib Nephrol 1981;25:71.

40. Packham D, Fairley KF. Renal biopsy: indications and complications in pregnancy. Br J Obstet Gynaecol 1987; 94:935.

41. Merkatz I, Schwartz G, David D, et al. Resumption of female reproductive function following renal transplantation. JAMA 1971;216:1749.

42. Penn I, Makowski E, Harris P. Parenthood following renal transplantation. Kidney Int 1980;18:221.

43. Saarikoski S., Sappala M. Immunosuppression during pregnancy: transmission of azathioprine and its metabolites from mother to fetus. Am J Obstet Gynecol 1973; 115:1100.

44. Cote C, Meuwissen H, Pickering R. Effects on the neonate of prednisone and azathioprine administered to the mother during pregnancy. J Pediatr 1974;85:324.

45. Scott J. Fetal growth retardation associated with maternal administration of immunosuppressive drugs. Am J Obstet Gynecol 1977;128:668.

46. Ponticelli C, Montagnino G. Causes of arterial hypertension in kidney transplantation. Contrib Nephrol 1987; 54:226.

47. Derfler K, Suhuller A, Herold C, et al. Successful outcome of a complicated pregnancy in a renal transplant recipient taking cyclosporin A. Clin Nephrol 1988;29:96.

48. Salamalekis EE, Mortakis AE, Phocas I, et al. Successful pregnancy in a renal transplant recipient taking cyclosporin A: hormonal and immunological studies. Int J Gynaecol Obstet 1989;30:267.

49. Pickerell MD, Sawers R, Michael J. Pregnancy after renal transplantation: severe intrauterine growth retardation during treatment with cyclosporin A. BMJ 1988;1:825.

50. Davison J. Renal transplantation and pregnancy. Am J Kidney Dis 1987;9:374.

51. Parson V, Bewick M, Elias J, et al. Pregnancy following renal transplantation. J R Soc Med 1979;72:815.

52. Davison J, Lindheimer M. Pregnancy in women with renal allografts. Semin Nephrol 1984;4:240.

53. Huffer W, Kuzela D, Popovtzer M. Metabolic bone disease in chronic renal failure. II. Renal transplant patients. Am J Pathol 1975;78:385.

54. Lindheinmer MD, Katz AI. Pregnancy in the renal transplant patient. Am J Kidney Dis 1992;19:173.

55. Davison J: Renal disease. In: de Swiet M, ed. Medical disorders in obstetric practice. Oxford: Blackwell, 1984: 236.

56. Pertuiset N, Grunfeld JP. Acute renal failure in pregnancy. Baillieres Clin Obstet Gynaecol 1987;1:873.

57. Grunfeld JP, Pertuiset N. Acute renal failure in pregnancy: 1987. Am J Kidney Dis 1987;9:359.

58. Stratta P, Canavese C, Dogliani M, et al. Pregnancy-related acute renal failure. Clin Nephrol 1989;32:14.

59. Stratta P, Canavese C, Colla L, et al. Acute renal failure in preeclampsia-eclampsia. Gynecol Obstet Invest 1987; 24:225.

60. Turney JH, Ellis CM, Parson FM. Obstetric acute renal failure 1956–1987. Br J Obstet Gynaecol 1989;96:679.

61. Sibai BM, Villar MA, Mabie BC. Acute renal failure in hypertensive disorders of pregnancy: pregnancy outcome and remote prognosis in thirty-one consecutive cases. Am J Obstet Gynecol 1990;162:777.

Hematologic Disorders

Philip Samuels

Five Key Points

- Iron deficiency is the most common cause of anemia in pregnancy. Folate deficiency is most likely to occur in women who have a multiple gestation or hemoglobinopathy or who abuse alcohol or take antiseizure medications.

- Sickle-cell anemia is the most common hemoglobinopathy in African-Americans. The thalassemias are more common in women of Mediterranean or Asian ethnicity.

- The most common cause of mild to moderate thrombocytopenia (platelet count 50,000 to 150,000 per mm^3) in pregnancy is gestational thrombocytopenia. Severe preeclampsia and idiopathic thrombocytopenic purpura are the more likely causes of severe thrombocytopenia (platelet count <50,000 per mm^3). Thrombotic thrombocytopenic purpura and hemolytic–uremic syndrome also must be considered in the differential diagnosis of severe thrombocytopenia.

- The most appropriate initial therapy for idiopathic thrombocytopenic purpura is administration of glucocorticoids. Intravenous immune globin, plasmapharesis, and splenectomy should be reserved for patients in whom medical therapy fails. Patients with thrombotic thrombocytopenic purpura should be treated with plasma exchange.

- Neonatal alloimmune thrombocytopenia is associated with an approximately 25% risk of intracranial hemorrhage and a 5 to 10% risk of mortality.

HEMATOLOGIC COMPLICATIONS OF PREGNANCY

Iron-Deficiency Anemia

A low hemoglobin is the most common hematologic complication seen in pregnancy, but seldom requires consultation. During a singleton pregnancy, maternal plasma volume gradually expands by approximately 50% (1000 ml). The total red-cell mass also increases, but only by approximately 25% (300 ml).[1] It is not surprising, therefore, that hemoglobin and hematocrit levels usually fall during gestation. These changes are not necessarily pathologic, but rather represent a physiologic alteration of pregnancy. By 6 weeks postpartum, in the absence of excessive blood loss during the puerperium, hemoglobin and hematocrit levels have returned to normal.

Approximately 50% of pregnant women are anemic, by definition, with a hematocrit less than 32%. The incidence of anemia changes with epidemiologic differences in the population studied. Approximately 75% of anemias that occur during pregnancy are secondary to iron deficiency.[1] A physiologic anemia becomes pathologic when the patient's iron stores are insufficient to mount a reticulocytosis. Patients at particular risk include those with poor nutrition and those with frequent pregnancies without an adequate interval to replenish iron stores. Ho and co–investigators[2] performed elaborate hematologic evaluations of 221 normal full-term gravidas in Taiwan. None of the studied patients received an added hematinic during gestation. In the previously nonanemic patients, 23 (10.4%) developed clinical anemia after a full-term pregnancy. In 22 of 23 women with a diminished hematocrit, the anemia was secondary to iron deficiency.[2] Among the 198 nonanemic women at term, 92 (46.5%) showed evidence of iron depletion even though they had a normal hematocrit.[2]

To distinguish the normal physiologic changes of pregnancy from those of pathologic iron deficiency anemia, one must understand the iron requirements of pregnancy (Table 6-7) and the proper use of hematologic laboratory parameters. Approximately 65% of stored iron is in the circulating red cells.[1,3-5] In the adult woman, additional iron stores are located in the bone marrow, liver, and spleen in the form of ferritin. Ferritin comprises approximately 25% (500 mg) of the 2-g iron stores found in the normal woman. Circulating ferritin in the serum mirrors total body stores. If the dietary iron intake is poor, the interval between pregnancies is short, or delivery is complicated by hemorrhage, pathologic iron-deficiency anemia readily develops. The first pathologic change to occur in iron-deficiency anemia is the depletion of iron stores in the bone marrow, liver, and spleen, resulting in a depressed serum ferritin level. The serum iron level falls, as does the percentage saturation of transferrin. The total iron-binding capacity rises, as this is a reflection of the amount of unbound transferrin. A fall in the hematocrit follows. Microcytic, hypochromic red cells are released into the circulation.

Care must be taken when using laboratory parameters to establish the diagnosis of iron deficiency anemia during gestation. A serum iron concentration less than 60 mg/dl with less than 16% saturation of transferrin is suggestive of iron deficiency. An increase in total iron-binding capacity, however, is not reliable, as 15% of pregnant women without iron deficiency will have an increase in this parameter.[6] Serum ferritin levels normally decrease mildly during pregnancy. They can, however, change 25% from one day to the next. Nevertheless, a significantly reduced ferritin concentration is indicative of iron-deficiency anemia and is the best parameter with which to judge the degree of iron deficiency. If a patient has been iron-deficient for an extended period and begins taking iron, her serum iron level can rise before she has repleted her iron stores. Again, serum ferritin is the best parameter to measure total body iron stores.

Whether all women should receive prophylactic iron during pregnancy remains controversial. Long[8] believes that physiology is responsible for much of the decrease in hematocrit, and that, unless the patient is symptomatic or the hematocrit level is very low, iron supplementation is unnecessary. In pregnancy, iron absorption from the duodenum increases, providing 1.3 to 2.6 mg of elemental iron daily in patients with ideal dietary habits.[9,10] In patients who do not show clear signs of iron-deficiency anemia, it is uncertain whether prophylactic iron leads to increased hemoglobin levels at term. Iron prophylaxis is safe, and with the exception of dyspepsia and constipation, side effects are few. One 325-mg tablet of ferrous sulfate daily provides adequate prophylaxis. It contains 60 mg of elemental iron, 10% of which is absorbed. If the iron is not needed, it will not be absorbed and will be excreted in the stool. Most iron tablets provide roughly equivalent amounts of elemental iron. No particular preparation offers a significant advantage over another.

One iron tablet three times daily is recommended for the pregnant patient with iron-deficiency anemia. To ensure maximum absorption, iron should be ingested about 30 minutes before meals. When taken in this manner, however, dyspepsia and nausea are more common. Therefore, therapy must be individualized to maximize patient compliance. It is uncertain whether or not this thrice-daily recommendation has

TABLE 6-7
IRON REQUIREMENTS IN PREGNANCY

Source	Approximate Iron Requirement
Increased maternal red-cell mass	450 mg
Fetus and placenta	360 mg
Blood loss from vaginal delivery	190 mg
Lactation	1 mg/day

any scientific foundation. In reality, twice-daily iron should provide adequate therapy. If isolated iron-deficiency anemia is present, one should see a dramatic reticulocytosis approximately 2 weeks after the initiation of therapy. Because iron absorption is pH-dependent, taking iron with ascorbic acid (vitamin C) may increase duodenal absorption. Conversely, taking iron with antacids, a common occurrence, will decrease absorption.

Folate Deficiency

Folic acid, a water-soluble vitamin, is found in green vegetables, peanuts, and liver. These foods, in general, are not the most sought after by pregnant women. Folate stores are located primarily in the liver and are usually sufficient for 6 weeks. After 3 weeks of a diet deficient in folate, the serum folate level falls. During pregnancy, folate deficiency is the most common cause of megaloblastic anemia; vitamin B_{12} deficiency is extremely rare. The daily folate requirement in the nonpregnant state is approximately 50 μg, but this rises three- to fourfold during gestation.[11] Fetal demands increase the requirement, as does the decrease in the gastrointestinal absorption of folate during pregnancy.[12]

Folate deficiency is not a cause of significant perinatal morbidity. Maternal morbidity, however, may result from the anemia, especially if the patient also suffers from significant blood loss during the puerperium. Prenatal vitamins that require a prescription contain 1 mg of folic acid. Most nonprescription prenatal vitamins contain 0.8 mg of folic acid. These amounts are more than adequate to prevent and treat folate deficiency. Women with significant hemoglobinopathies, patients ingesting anticonvulsants, women carrying a multiple gestation, and women with frequent conception may require more than 1 mg of supplemental folate daily. Importantly, those at risk of giving birth to a child with a neural-tube defect should take 4 mg of folic acid daily from 1 month before conception through the first trimester. If the patient is folic acid–deficient, her reticulocyte count will be depressed. Within 3 days after the administration of sufficient folic acid, reticulocytosis usually occurs. Folic acid deficiency should also be considered when an anemic patient has unexplained thrombocytopenia and leukopenia. These findings rapidly reverse and the hematocrit should rise as much as 1% per day after 1 week of folate replacement.

Iron deficiency is frequently coexistent with folic-acid deficiency. If a patient with folate deficiency does not develop a significant reticulocytosis within 1 week after administration of sufficient replacement therapy, appropriate tests for iron deficiency should also be performed.

Hemoglobinopathies

Hemoglobin is a tetrameric protein composed of two pairs of polypeptide chains with a heme group attached to each.[13] The normal adult hemoglobin A_1 comprises 95% of hemoglobin. It consists of two α-chains and two β-chains. The remaining 5% of hemoglobin usually consists of hemoglobin A_2 (containing two α-chains and two δ-chains) and/or hemoglobin F (with two α-chains and two γ-chains). In the fetus, hemoglobin F declines during the third trimester of pregnancy, usually disappearing several months after birth. Hemoglobinopathies occur when there is a change in the structure of a peptide chain or a defect in the ability to synthesize a specific polypeptide chain. The patterns of inheritance are usually straightforward. The prevalence of the most common hemoglobinopathies is listed in Table 6-8.

Hemoglobin S

Hemoglobin S, a variant of hemoglobin A, is present in patients with sickle-cell disease (hemoglobin SS) and sickle-cell trait (hemoglobin AS). A single substitution of valine for glutamic acid at the sixth position in the β-polypeptide chain causes clinically significant changes in the physical characteristics of this hemoglobin. At low oxygen tensions, red cells containing hemoglobin S assume a sickle shape. Sludging in small vessels occurs, resulting in microinfarction of the affected organs. Sickle cells have a life span of 5 to 10 days, as compared with 120 days for a normal

TABLE 6-8
PREVALENCE OF HEMOGLOBINOPATHIES IN PREGNANCY

Hemoglobinopathy	Frequency in Adult African-Americans
Sickle-cell trait	8.3%
Sickle-cell disease	0.14%
Hemoglobin SC disease	0.13%
Hemoglobin S/β-thalassemia	0.06%

red cell. Sickling is most often triggered by hypoxia, acidosis, or dehydration.

Approximately 1 of 12 adult African-Americans is heterozygous for hemoglobin S and, therefore, has sickle-cell trait. These individuals generally have 35 to 45% hemoglobin S and are asymptomatic. The child of two individuals with sickle-cell trait has a 50% probability of inheriting the trait and a 25% probability of actually having sickle-cell disease. One of every 625 African-American children born in the United States is homozygous for hemoglobin S, and the frequency of sickle-cell disease among adult African-Americans is 1 in 708.[14] All at-risk patients should be screened for hemoglobin S at their first prenatal visit. Patients with a positive screen should undergo hemoglobin electrophoresis. Women identified as having sickle-cell trait are not at increased risk for poor perinatal outcome. Prenatal diagnosis of sickle-cell disease can be performed by DNA analysis with the polymerase chain reaction (PCR) and Southern blotting.[15,16] PCR amplification of DNA fragments allows a more rapid laboratory diagnosis. Hemoglobin S can also be identified by hemoglobin electrophoresis and DNA analysis of fetal blood.[17] Wang et al.[18] reported on 500 prenatal diagnoses of sickle-cell disease, 196 using only Southern blotting and 304 using PCR. PCR greatly shortened the time interval from sampling to diagnosis and resulted in an overall fourfold increase in identification of affected fetuses.

Painful vasoocclusive episodes involving multiple organs are the clinical hallmark of sickle-cell anemia. The most common sites for these episodes are the extremities, joints, and abdomen. Vasoocculsive episodes can also occur in the lung, resulting in pulmonary infarction. Analgesia, oxygen, and hydration are the therapeutic foundations for these painful crises. Sickle-cell disease can affect virtually all organ systems. Osteomyelitis is common, and osteomyelitis caused by Salmonella is found almost exclusively in these patients. The risk of pyelonephritis is significantly increased. Sickling may also occur in the renal medulla, where oxygen tension is reduced, resulting in papillary necrosis. These patients also exhibit renal tubular dysfunction and hyposthenuria. Because of chronic hemolysis and decreased red-cell survival, patients with sickle-cell anemia often have some degree of hyperbilirubinemia and jaundice. Cholelithiasis is seen in about 30% of cases.[19,20] Because of chronic anemia, high-output cardiac failure can occur.

Many pregnancies complicated by sickle-cell anemia are associated with poor perinatal outcomes. The rate of spontaneous abortion may be as high as 25%.[21,22] Perinatal mortality is approximately 15%.[23-25] In a report by Seoud and co-workers,[26] the perinatal mortality rate was 10.5%. Much of this poor perinatal outcome is related to preterm birth. Approximately 30% of infants born to mothers with sickle-cell disease have birth weights below 2500 g.[22] In the report by Seoud et al.,[26] the mean birth weight was 2443 g. In a multicenter study, Smith et al.[27] reported that 21% of infants born to mothers with sickle-cell disease were small for gestational age. It has been hypothesized that sickling in the uterine vessels may lead to decreased fetal oxygenation and intrauterine growth restriction.[28] Increased levels of hemoglobin F in the mother may spare her from painful crises during pregnancy and may theoretically have a protective effect on the neonate. Morris et al.[29] studied 270 singleton pregnancies in 175 women with sickle-cell disease. The overall fetal wastage rate was 32.3%. Mothers with high hemoglobin F levels had a significantly lower perinatal mortality rate.

Stillbirth rates of 8 to 10% have been described in patients with sickle-cell anemia.[22] These fetal deaths occur not only during crises but also unexpectedly. Careful antepartum fetal testing must, therefore, be conducted. Anyaegbunam and co-workers[30] studied Doppler flow velocimetry in patients with hemoglobinopathies. They showed abnormal systolic/diastolic ratios for the uterine or umbilical arteries in 88% of patients with hemoglobin SS, as compared with 7% with hemoglobin AS and 4% with hemoglobin AA. This study implies that Doppler studies may play a useful role in the care of the mother with hemoglobin SS. Serial ultrasound evaluations also are of value in assessing fetal growth.

Although maternal mortality is rare in patients with sickle-cell anemia, maternal morbidity is great. Infections are common, occurring in 50 to 67% of women with hemoglobin SS. The most common source of infection is a UTI. Patients with hemoglobin AS are also at greater risk for a UTI and should be screened regularly. Pulmonary infection and infarction are also common, and patients with sickle-cell anemia should receive pneumococcal vaccine before pregnancy. Any infection demands prompt attention because fever, dehydration, and acidosis will result in further sickling and painful crises. The incidence of pregnancy-induced hypertension is increased in patients with sickle-cell anemia and may complicate up to one-third of pregnancies.[23,27]

The care of the pregnant patient with sickle-cell anemia must be individualized and meticulous. These patients will benefit from care in a medical center experienced in treating the multitude of problems that can complicate such pregnancies. From early gestation, good dietary habits should be promoted. A folic acid supplement of at least 1 mg/day should be administered as soon as pregnancy is confirmed. Although hemoglobin and hematocrit levels are decreased, iron supplements must not be routinely given. Serum iron and ferritin levels should be checked monthly and iron supplementation started only when these levels are diminished. Abudu and co-workers[31] found that serum ferritin values were significantly higher in pregnant women with hemoglobin SS disease than in those with hemoglobin AA. They concluded that the physiologic changes of pregnancy in patients with hemoglobin SS did not result in an iron-deficient state and that the use of prophylactic iron supplementation in these patients appears unjustified.

The role of transfusion in pregnancies complicated by sickle-cell disease is controversial. Prophylactic exchange transfusions were often used in the past, but they have fallen out of favor today. Although prophylactic exchange transfusions improved the maternal sense of well-being, they did not change perinatal morbidity and mortality.[32,33] Transfusions are recommended when sickle-cell crises cannot be controlled by conservative therapy. They are also recommended when patients have extensive constitutional symptoms such as shortness of breath or the inability to function at home.

Vaginal delivery is preferable for patients with sickle-cell disease; cesarean delivery should be reserved for obstetric indications. Patients should labor in the left lateral recumbent position and receive supplemental oxygen. While adequate hydration should be maintained, fluid overload must be avoided. Conduction anesthesia is recommended because it provides excellent pain relief and can be used for cesarean delivery if necessary.

Hemoglobin SC Disease

Hemoglobin C is another β-chain variant in which lysine is substituted for glutamic acid in the sixth position. Clinically significant hemoglobin SC disease occurs in 1 in 833 African-Americans.[14] Women with both S and C hemoglobin suffer less morbidity in pregnancy than do patients with only hemoglobin S.[18,21,34] As in sickle-cell disease, however, there is an increased incidence of early spontaneous abortion and pregnancy-induced hypertension.[21,22,34]

Because patients with SC disease may exhibit only mild symptoms, the hemoglobinopathy may remain undiagnosed until the patient suffers a crisis during pregnancy. These crises may be marked by sequestration of a large volume of red cells in the spleen accompanied by a sudden, dramatic fall in hematocrit.[34,35] Because these patients have increased splenic activity, they may be mildly thrombocytopenic throughout pregnancy. During gestation, patients with hemoglobin SC should receive the same program of prenatal care outlined for women with hemoglobin SS.

Thalassemia

Thalassemia results from a defect in the rate of globin-chain synthesis. Any of the polypeptide chains can be affected. The disease may range from minimal suppression of synthesis of the affected chain to its complete absence. Either α- or β-thalassemia can occur. Heterozygous patients are often asymptomatic. Thalassemia can be detected by prenatal diagnosis. Wainscoat and co-workers[36] were able to offer prenatal diagnosis to 19 of 25 families with a potential for β-thalassemia using linkage analysis of restriction-fragment–length polymorphisms (RFLP). Focharoen and co-workers[37] have been able to diagnose β-thalassemia in the second trimester by in vitro protein synthesis. They also detected α-thalassemia by gene amplification in the first trimester.

Homozygous α-thalassemia results in the formation of tetramers of β-chains known as hemoglobin Bart. This hemoglobinopathy can result in hydrops fetalis. Ghosh and co-investigators[38] reported their experience with 26 Asian women who were at risk for giving birth to a fetus with homozygous α-thalassemia. Six of the 26 fetuses were affected. In two of the six cases, progressive fetal ascites appeared before 24 weeks of gestation. In the remaining four cases, there was evidence of intrauterine growth restriction by 28 weeks of gestation.

β-Thalassemia is the most common form of thalassemia. In the homozygous state, synthesis of hemoglobin A_1 may be completely suppressed. In this condition, electrophoresis shows only hemoglobin F and hemoglobin A_2. The homozygous state of β-thalassemia is known as thalassemia major. Patients with this disorder are transfusion-dependent and have marked hepatosplenomegaly and bone changes secondary to increased hematopoiesis. These individuals usually die from infection or cardiovascular complications before they reach childbearing age. Successful full-term pregnancies have been reported.[39] The few patients who do become pregnant generally exhibit severe anemia and congestive heart failure. Prenatal care is dependent on transfusion therapy similar to that used in the care of the patient with sickle-cell disease.

Patients with the heterozygous state are often asymptomatic. They are detected by an increase in their level of hemoglobin. Patients with thalassemia minima have microcytosis, but are asymptomatic. Those with thalassemia intermedia exhibit splenomegaly and significant anemia and may become transfusion-dependent during pregnancy. Their anemia can be significant enough to produce high-output cardiac failure.[40] If these patients have not undergone splenectomy, they are at risk for a hypersplenic crisis.[41] Also, extramedullary hematopoiesis may impinge on the spine, resulting in neurologic symptoms.[42]

These patients should follow a treatment program similar to that for patients with sickle-cell disease. As in the case of sickle-cell disease, iron supplementation should be given only if necessary, as indiscriminate use of iron can lead to hemochromatosis. White and co-workers[43] have shown that patients with β-thalassemia usually have a much higher ferritin concentration than normal patients.[43] Although routine iron therapy is not necessary, folic acid supplementation appears important in β-thalassemia carriers. Leung and co-investigators[44] showed that the daily administration of folate significantly increased the predelivery hemoglobin concentration in both nulliparous and multiparous patients.

Asymptomatic thalassemia carriers need no special testing. As in the case of sickle-cell disease, antepartum fetal evaluation is essential in patients with thalassemia who are anemic. They should undergo frequent ultrasonography to assess fetal growth, as well as nonstress testing to evaluate fetal well-being.

Occasionally, individuals will inherit two hemoglobinopathies, such as sickle-cell thalassemia (hemoglobin S thal). The prevalence of this disorder among adult African-Americans is 1 in 1172.[45] The clinical course is variable. If minimal suppression of β-chain synthesis occurs, patients may be free of symptoms. However, with total suppression of β-chain synthesis, a clinical picture similar to that of sickle-cell disease will develop. The course of these patients during pregnancy is quite variable, and their therapy must be individualized.

PREGNANCY-ASSOCIATED THROMBOCYTOPENIA

The widespread use of automated blood counts has resulted in the discovery of thrombocytopenia coexisting with pregnancy in many patients. Affecting approximately 3 to 7% of pregnancies, thrombocytopenia is the most frequent hematologic complication of pregnancy resulting in consultation with a hematologist. Platelet counts generally fall slightly, due to hemodilution and increased turnover, as gestation progresses. However, platelet counts do not usually fall below the normal range. In pregnancy, the vast majority of cases of mild to moderate thrombocytopenia are caused by gestational thrombocytopenia.[46] This form of thrombocytopenia has little chance of causing maternal or neonatal problems.[47] The common and rare causes of thrombocytopenia in the pregnant woman at term are shown in Table 6-9. Until

---

TABLE 6-9
CAUSES OF PREGNANCY-ASSOCIATED THROMBOCYTOPENIA

Major causes
  Gestational thrombocytopenia
  Severe preeclampsia
    HELLP syndrome
  Immune thrombocytopenic purpura (ITP)
  Disseminated intravascular coagulation
    Abruptio placenta
    Sepsis
    Following severe hemorrhage
    Retained dead fetus
Rare causes
  Human immunodeficiency virus (HIV) infection
  Lupus anticoagulant/antiphospholipid antibody syndrome
  Systemic lupus erythematosus (SLE)
  Thrombotic thrombocytopenic purpura (TTP)
  Hemolytic–uremic syndrome (HUS)
  Type IIB von Willebrand disease
  Other autoimmunity diseases
  Folic acid deficiency

the late 1980s, it was assumed that all patients with an unexplained low platelet count had immune thrombocytopenic purpura (ITP), a recognized cause of neonatal thrombocytopenia. Unfortunately, traditional platelet antibody testing cannot distinguish among gestational thrombocytopenia, ITP, and thrombocytopenia accompanying preeclampsia.[48,49] However, the distinction between these disorders is important because each of these diagnoses has specific maternal and neonatal implications and management differs.

Gestational Thrombocytopenia

Patients with gestational thrombocytopenia usually present with mild (platelet count, 100,000 to 149,000/mm^3) to moderate (platelet count, 50,000 to 99,000/mm^3) thrombocytopenia.[50] These patients require no therapy, and the fetus appears to be at negligible risk of being born with profound thrombocytopenia (platelet count, <50,000/mm^3) or a bleeding diathesis. This distinct entity was first suggested, but not specifically defined, in a study published in 1986 by Hart et al.[51] In this investigation, 28 of 116 pregnant women (24%) who were evaluated prospectively during an 8-month period in 1983 had platelet counts <150,000/mm^3 at least once during pregnancy. In 17 patients who were followed after delivery, platelet counts returned to normal. Platelet-associated IgG (a positive direct test) was present in 79% of these 28 women, and 61% had serum antiplatelet IgG (a positive indirect test). None of these women had positive antibodies after delivery. Hart et al.[51] were actually describing gestational thrombocytopenia before the condition had been recognized as a distinct entity. Furthermore, they were the first to demonstrate that conventional platelet antibody testing cannot distinguish gestational thrombocytopenia from ITP.[51]

Samuels et al.[48] also investigated 74 mothers with gestational thrombocytopenia. Forty-six (62%) of these patients had circulating antiplatelet IgG in their plasma (a positive indirect test). These women gave birth to two neonates with thrombocytopenia, but both had platelet counts >50,000/mm^3 and there were no bleeding complications. Burrows and Kelton[50,52,53] have further shown, in a large series, that there is little risk to the mother or neonate in cases of gestational thrombocytopenia. Studies[48,50,52] have

convincingly demonstrated that gestational thrombocytopenia is an entity distinct from ITP.

The decrease in platelet count that occurs in gestational thrombocytopenia is not merely due to dilution of platelets with increasing blood volume. It appears to be due to an acceleration of the normal increase in platelet destruction that occurs during pregnancy.[46] The increase in platelet-associated IgG seen in these patients may merely reflect immune complexes adhering to the platelet surface rather than specific antiplatelet antibodies. Pregnant women who have gestational thrombocytopenia do not require any special therapy during the puerperium unless their platelet counts fall below 20,000/mm^3 or if there is clinical bleeding with a platelet count below 50,000/mm^3.

Immune Thrombocytopenia Purpura

ITP only affects 1 to 3 per 1000 pregnancies. In 1954, Peterson and Larson[54] were the first to recognize that profound thrombocytopenia (platelet count <50,000/mm^3) may develop in infants born to women with ITP. In 1973, Territo et al.[55] made the first effort to predict which infants were at increased risk for being born with profound thrombocytopenia. They demonstrated, in a small number of patients, that fetuses born to mothers with platelet counts <100,000/mm^3 were at highest risk. Many larger studies have since shown that this arbitrary cutoff, while generally true, is not useful in individual cases. Subsequently, a number of efforts have been made to use noninvasive parameters to assess the risk of severe neonatal thrombocytopenia, including the administration of maternal glucocorticoids, history of splenectomy, and the presence of maternal antiplatelet antibodies. However, none of these has shown the desired positive or negative predictive values.[56-60]

In general, pregnancy does not precipitate new-onset ITP or change its severity. However, individual patients may experience exacerbations of ITP during pregnancy; the disease usually improves postpartum.[48,61,62] Harrington et al.[63] were the first to demonstrate that this disorder was humorally mediated. Cines and Schreiber[64] developed the first platelet antiglobulin test, a radioimmunoassay, in 1979. This type of testing is now mostly performed by enzyme-linked immunoassay (ELISA) or flow cytometry. New assays have shown that these autoantibodies may be directed against specific platelet surface glycoproteins, including the IIb/IIIa and Ib/IX complexes.[65] After the platelets are coated with antibody, they are removed from circulation by binding to the Fc receptors of macrophages in the reticuloendothelial system, especially the spleen. Approximately 90% of women with ITP will have platelet-associated IgG.[64] Unfortunately, this finding is not specific for ITP; studies have shown that these tests are also positive in women with gestational thrombocytopenia and preeclampsia.[48,49]

To make the issue more confusing, the pathogenesis of ITP in children and adults usually differs. Childhood ITP often follows a viral infection and clinically presents with petechiae and bleeding.[66] This form of ITP is generally self-limited and disappears over time. Conversely, adults have milder bleeding and easy bruisability and are often diagnosed after a prolonged period of subtle symptoms. Adult ITP usually runs a chronic course, and long-term therapy is often necessary. Many pregnancies occur when women are in their late teens and early 20s. In these women with a history of ITP, it may be difficult to ascertain whether the patient has childhood ITP or early adult ITP. Also, no study has shown whether the risk of neonatal thrombocytopenia is similar in both forms of ITP.

ITP is different from other causes of thrombocytopenia in pregnancy because of the aforementioned risk of profound neonatal thrombocytopenia. Before 1990 it was assumed that all patients with unexplained thrombocytopenia during gestation had ITP. It was only after 1990 that gestational thrombocytopenia became recognized as a distinct entity.[47,48] Thus, the earlier studies of ITP may have included at least some cases of gestational thrombocytopenia, making it difficult to determine the true incidence of neonatal thrombocytopenia in women with ITP.

In 1980, Scott et al.[67] were the first to institute direct fetal platelet determination in a series of women with ITP by using fetal scalp sampling. However, this procedure requires operator skill, an engaged fetal vertex, and a dilated cervix. Ghidini et al.[68] subsequently described the use of cordocentesis to assess fetuses at risk for thrombocytopenia. They found a 1.4% risk of perinatal death in fetuses undergoing the procedure at ≥28 weeks of gestation. Bleeding from the needle insertion site in the cord occurred in up to 41% of cases but usually stopped in less than 60 seconds. Complication rates certainly will be higher when this procedure is performed by less-experienced operators. Furthermore, cordocentesis is expensive when including the price of the procedure, the physician consultation fee, the ultrasound guidance, and the fetal monitoring that must accompany the procedure. Indeed, the risks, associated costs, and low rate at which profoundly thrombocytopenic infants are identified do not justify the routine use of cordocentesis in all mothers with ITP.

In a meta-analysis, Burrows and Kelton[69] found a 14.6% incidence of profound thrombocytopenia in infants born to mothers with ITP. However, this meta-analysis did not take into account that many of the studies did not exclude patients with gestational thrombocytopenia. Therefore, the risks of profound thrombocytopenia may very well be greater than their reported incidence. These authors also reported a neonatal morbidity rate of 24 per 1000 with few serious complications. This may be an underestimation due to the reasons cited above.

THROMBOTIC THROMBOCYTOPENIC PURPURA AND HEMOLYTIC–UREMIC SYNDROME

These two conditions are characterized by microangiopathic hemolytic anemia and severe thrombocytopenia. Pregnancy does not predispose a patient to these conditions, but they should be considered when evaluating the pregnant woman with profound thrombocytopenia. Thrombotic thrombocytopenic purpura (TTP) is characterized by a pentad of findings, which is shown in Table 6-10.[70,71] The complete pentad occurs in 40% of patients, but approximately 75% present with the triad of microangiopathic hemolytic anemia, thrombocytopenia, and neurologic changes.[72] Pathologically, these patients have thrombotic occlusion of arterioles and capillaries[70] in multiple organs. In many ways, the pathophysiology

---

TABLE 6-10
PENTAD OF FINDINGS IN THROMBOTIC THROMBOCYTOPENIC PURPURA*

Microangiopathic hemolytic anemia[†]
Thrombocytopenia[†]
Neurologic abnormalities[†]—confusion, headache, paresis, visual hallucinations, seizures
Fever
Renal dysfunction

---

*The classic pentad is only found in 40% of patients.
[†]These three findings are present in 74% of patients.[72]

mirrors that of severe preeclampsia. Weiner[73] has published an extensive literature review concerning TTP. In this series of 45 patients, the disease developed antepartum in 40; in 58% it occurred before 24 weeks of gestation. The mean gestational age at onset of symptoms was 23.5 weeks, and the fetal and maternal mortality rates were 80 and 44%, respectively.[73] This series included many patients who contracted the disease before plasma infusion/exchange therapy was used for treating TTP.

TTP may be confused with early-onset severe preeclampsia. In preeclampsia, antithrombin III levels are frequently low, and this is not the case with TTP.[74] Therefore, this test may be a useful discriminator between these two disorders.

Although the hemolytic–uremic syndrome (HUS) has many features in common with TTP, it usually has its onset in the postpartum period. Patients with HUS display the triad of microangiopathic hemolytic anemia, acute nephropathy, and thrombocytopenia. HUS is rare in adults, and the thrombocytopenia is usually milder than that seen in TTP, with only 50% of patients having platelet counts $<100,000/mm^3$ at the time of diagnosis. Thrombocytopenia worsens as the disease progresses.[75] Many patients with HUS have chronic renal disease.[71] The majority of cases of HUS occurring in pregnancy develop at least 2 days after delivery.[71,76] Maternal mortality may exceed 50% in postpartum HUS.

EVALUATION OF THROMBOCYTOPENIA DURING PREGNANCY AND THE PUERPERIUM

Before deciding on a therapeutic regimen for the patient with thrombocytopenia, the obstetrician must evaluate the patient and attempt to ascertain the cause of her low platelet count. Important management decisions are dependent on arriving at an accurate diagnosis. A complete medical history is crucial. It is essential to learn whether the patient has previously had a depressed platelet count or a clinical bleeding diathesis. It is also important to know whether these clinical conditions occur coincidentally with pregnancy. A complete medication history should be elicited because certain medications, such as heparin, can result in maternal thrombocytopenia. The obstetric history should focus on whether there have been any maternal or neonatal bleeding problems in the past. Excessive bleeding from an episiotomy site or

cesarean delivery incision, a need for blood component therapy, easy bruising, or bleeding from intravenous sites during labor should alert the physician to the possibility of thrombocytopenia in the previous pregnancy. The obstetrician should also question whether the infant had any bleeding diathesis or if there was any problem following a circumcision. The obstetrician should also ask pertinent questions to determine whether severe preeclampsia or HELLP syndrome is the cause of her thrombocytopenia. All thrombocytopenic pregnant women should be carefully evaluated for the presence of risk factors for human immunodeficiency virus (HIV) infection because this infection can cause an ITP-like syndrome.

An accurate assessment of gestational age should also be carried out, because some of the causes of thrombocytopenia in pregnancy are dependent on gestational age. A thorough physical examination of the patient should also be performed. The physician should look for ecchymoses or petechiae. Blood pressure should be determined to ascertain whether the patient has impending preeclampsia. The physician should also look for petechiae at the site of placement of the sphygomomanometer. If HELLP syndrome is developing, scleral icterus may be present. The eye grounds should be examined for evidence of arteriolar spasm or hemorrhage.

It is imperative that a peripheral blood smear be examined by an experienced hematologist or pathologist whenever a case of thrombocytopenia is diagnosed for the first time during pregnancy. This individual must determine if microangiopathic hemolysis is present. This specialist can also rule out platelet clumping, which will result in a factitious thrombocytopenia. Other laboratory evaluations should be performed as necessary to rule out preeclampsia and/or HELLP syndrome, as well as disseminated intravascular coagulopathy. If a diagnosis of ITP is entertained, appropriate platelet antibody testing should be performed. After determining the cause of thrombocytopenia, the physician can better determine whether or not therapy or obstetric intervention is warranted.

THERAPY FOR THROMBOCYTOPENIA DURING PREGNANCY

Gestational Thrombocytopenia

Gestational thrombocytopenia usually requires no special therapy. In patients with mild to moderate thrombocytopenia and no antenatal or antecedent history of thrombocytopenia, no intervention is necessary. If the maternal platelet count drops below 75,000/mm³, the patient may still have gestational thrombocytopenia, but there are not enough published data on mothers with counts this low to determine if there are any maternal or fetal risks. These patients, therefore, should be treated as if they have de novo ITP. Although approximately 4% of patients have gestational thrombocytopenia, less than 1% of patients with gestational thrombocytopenia have platelet counts <100,000/mm³.[53]

Immune Thrombocytopenic Purpura

Treatment of ITP during pregnancy and the puerperium requires attention to both mother and fetus. As in other cases of thrombocytopenia, maternal therapy needs to be instituted only if there is evidence of a bleeding diathesis or to prevent a bleeding complication if surgery is anticipated. There is usually no spontaneous bleeding unless the platelet count falls below 20,000/mm³; surgical bleeding does not usually occur until the platelet count is below 50,000/mm³. The conventional forms of increasing the platelet count in the patient with ITP include glucocorticoid therapy, intravenous immune globulin, and/or splenectomy.

If the patient is having a bleeding diathesis or if the platelet count is below 20,000/mm³, there is usually a need to increase the platelet count in a relatively short time. Although oral glucocorticoids can be used, intravenous glucocorticoids usually work more rapidly. Any steroid that has a glucocorticoid effect can be used. However, hematologists have the most experience with methylprednisolone. It can be given intravenously, and it has very little mineralocorticoid effect. It is important to avoid steroids with strong mineralocorticoid effects because these agents can disturb electrolyte balance and cause fluid retention, resulting in hypertension. The usual dose of methylprednisolone is 1.0 to 1.5 mg/kg of total body weight intravenously daily in two to three divided doses. It usually takes about 2 days to see a response, but the maximum effect may not be evident until 10 days. Even though methylprednisolone has little mineralocorticoid effect, serum electrolytes should be assessed when patients are receiving large intravenous doses of this steroid. There is little chance that methylprednisolone will cause neonatal adrenal suppression

because very little crosses the placenta. The drug is metabolized by placental 11β-ol-dehydrogenase to an inactive 11-keto metabolite.

After the platelet count has risen satisfactorily in response to intravenous methylprednisolone, the regimen can be changed to oral prednisolone. The usual dose is 60 to 100 mg/day. It can be given in a single dose, but there is less gastrointestinal upset with divided doses. The dose can then be tapered rapidly to 30 to 40 mg/day, and then decreased more slowly to maintain the platelet count at about 100,000/mm³. If oral prednisolone is used for initial therapy, the usual starting dose is 1 mg/kg of total body weight.

The response rate to glucocorticoids is about 70%. If the patient has been taking glucocorticoids for a period of at least 2 to 3 weeks, she may have adrenal suppression and should receive increased doses of steroids during labor and delivery in order to avoid an adrenal crisis. Also, if the patient has been on glucocorticoids for some time, she may experience significant side effects, including fluid retention, hirsutism, acne, striae, poor wound healing, gestational diabetes, and monilia vaginitis. In rare circumstances, patients on long-term steroids during gestation can develop osteoporosis or cataract formation. However, the chance of any fetal or neonatal side effects from these glucocorticoids is remote.

Although glucocorticoids are the mainstays of treatment, up to 30% of patients will not respond to these medications. In this instance, the next treatment is intravenous immunoglobulin. The usual dose is 04. g/kg/day for 3 to 5 days. However, it may be necessary to use as much as 1 g/kg/day. The response usually begins in 2 to 3 days and peaks in 5 days. The length of this response is variable, so the timing of therapy is extremely important. If the obstetrician wants a peak platelet count for delivery, therapy should be instituted about 5 to 8 days before the planned delivery. Although intravenous immunoglobulin is very expensive, it should be used before contemplating splenectomy, as some patients with ITP will experience remission after delivery.[47]

Splenectomy should be reserved for those who do not respond to medical treatment. In extremely urgent cases of life-threatening bleeding or nonresponse, splenectomy can be safely performed at the time of cesarean delivery after extending a midline incision cephalad.

Platelet transfusions are indicated when there is clinically significant bleeding and while awaiting other therapies to become effective. Each "pack" of platelets will increase the platelet count by approximately 10,000/mm^3. The half-life of these platelets is extremely short because the same antibodies and reticuloendothelial-cell clearance rates that affect the mother's endogenous platelets will similarly affect the transfused platelets.

While treating maternal thrombocytopenia is fairly straightforward, the need for evaluation of the fetal platelet count remains controversial. Although Cooke et al.[76] and Kelton[61] have attempted to show that there is no risk in delivering a profoundly thrombocytopenic fetus vaginally, these meta-analyses are only generalizations. There is no one series large enough from which to draw firm conclusions concerning mode of delivery of the profoundly thrombocytopenic fetus.

Five to 38% of fetuses born to mothers with ITP will have platelet counts <50,000/mm^3. Several studies have tried to determine if administering glucocorticoids to the mother may raise the fetal platelet count in utero.[56,57,59] Although the study by Karapatkin et al.[59] was promising, other studies have not corroborated these findings. Furthermore, studies have shown that splenectomy has no bearing on neonatal platelet counts. The study by Samuels et al.[48] demonstrated that 19.2% of patients with ITP who received no therapy gave birth to profoundly thrombocytopenic infants, as compared with 22.7% of those receiving prednisone alone, 23% of those who had undergone a splenectomy and received prednisone, and 17.8% of those who had undergone only splenectomy. The rate of profound neonatal thrombocytopenia was not significantly different among any of these groups. Even if there is not a difference in perinatal morbidity between vaginal and cesarean delivery, there are advantages of knowing whether a fetus is at risk of being born with a platelet count <50,000/mm^3. The use of scalp electrodes and vacuum extractors are examples of interventions that should be avoided in the profoundly thrombocytopenic fetus. Furthermore, because of the potential neonatal morbidity, it might be safest if the profoundly thrombocytopenic infant were delivered in a tertiary-care setting. Cordocentesis is the only method currently available to determine the fetal platelet count accurately before the onset of labor, and it is both expensive and invasive. Furthermore, it carries an inherent risk of fetal complications. Fear of an adverse outcome in the setting of a neonate with an unknown platelet count has led obstetricians to overuse invasive testing as well as surgical deliveries.

In summary, the treatment of thrombocytopenia during gestation depends on its cause. The obstetrician need not act on the mother's platelet count unless it is <20,000/mm^3, or unless it is <50,000/mm^3 with evidence of clinical bleeding, or if surgery is anticipated. In these cases, the treatment will depend on the diagnosis. Furthermore, whether delivery needs to be expedited or can be delayed also depends on the cause of thrombocytopenia. The fetal/neonatal platelet count need only be considered if the mother clearly has ITP or, in the case of presumed gestational thrombocytopenia, when the platelet count is <75,000/mm^3. The key to treating these patients is to accurately determine the cause for the thrombocytopenia and to approach the patient and her fetus rationally.

Management of Thrombotic Thrombocytopenic Purpura and Hemolytic–Uremic Syndrome

Before the use of plasma exchange, maternal–fetal outcomes in cases complicated by TTP were uniformly poor.[73] The first cases treated with plasma exchange for TTP during pregnancy were reported in 1984.[77] One report described a patient who had previous fetal deaths from chronic TTP and experienced a successful pregnancy when treated with aspirin, dipyridamole, and plasma infusion.[78] There are no large series of patients with TTP in pregnancy. However, it does appear through case reports that the prognosis has improved greatly with plasma infusion and plasma exchange.

HUS has been much more difficult to treat. Only a few case reports have appeared. Supportive therapy remains the mainstay of treatment. Dialysis is often necessary, with close attention to fluid management. Platelet-function inhibitors have also been used in two cases during pregnancy.[79,80] Plasma infusion and plasma exchange can be attempted, but the results have not been as good as in cases of TTP.[81] Vincristine has been used with some success.

Neonatal Alloimmune Thrombocytopenia

In neonatal alloimmune thrombocytopenia, a rare disorder, the mother lacks a specific platelet antigen and antibodies to this antigen develop. The disease is somewhat analogous to Rh isoimmunization but involves platelets. If the fetus inherits this antigen from its father, maternal antibody can cross the placenta, resulting in severe neonatal thrombocytopenia. The mother, however, will have a normal platelet count. Deaver and co-investigators[82] reviewed 58 cases of neonatal alloimmune thrombocytopenia. The overall mortality rate was 9%, and the total incidence of suspected intracranial hemorrhage was 28%. The mortality rate was 24% for the firstborn infant and only 5% for subsequent offspring. The improved outcome in the latter group appeared to be related to more frequent use of cesarean delivery and to earlier use of corticosteroids in these children because obstetricians and pediatricians were expecting the disease.[82] The most common antibodies noted in these patients are anti-PLA 1 and BAK antibodies.[83] Transfusion of maternal platelets into the neonate also improved outcome in these cases. After birth or in utero the child can be transfused with the mother's platelets since she lacks the antigen that would lead to platelet destruction by circulating antibodies. Bussel and colleagues[84] have demonstrated that the antenatal use of intravenous immunoglobulin may help to prevent thrombocytopenia in infants at risk for neonatal alloimmune thrombocytopenia. These investigators administered 1 g/kg/week to at-risk mothers and observed no toxicity. The concomitant use of glucocorticoids has not been shown to boost the effect of the intravenous immunoglobulin.[85] Because of the frequency with which very low platelet counts are encountered in these fetuses, there is a small risk of fetal exsanguination with cordocentesis.[86]

REFERENCES

1. Pitkin RM. Nutritional influences during pregnancy. Med Clin North Am 1977;61:3.
2. Ho CH, Yuan CC, Yeh SH. Serum ferritin, folate, and cobalamin levels and their correlation with anemia in normal full-term pregnant women. Eur J Obstet Gynecol Reprod Biol 1987;26:7.
3. DeLeeuw NKM, Lowenstein L, Hsieh YS. Iron deficiency and hydremia or normal pregnancy. Medicine (Baltimore) 1966;45:291.
4. Chopa J, Noe E, Matthew J, et al. Anemia in pregnancy. Am J Public Health 1967;57:857.
5. Holly RG. Dynamics of iron metabolism in pregnancy. Am J Obstet Gynecol 1965;93:370.
6. Carr MC. Serum iron/TIBC in the diagnosis of iron deficiency anemia during pregnancy. Obstet Gynecol 1971;38:602.
7. Boued JL. Iron deficiency: assessment during pregnancy and its importance in pregnant adolescents. Am J Clin Nutr 1994;59:5025.
8. Long PJ. Rethinking iron supplementation during pregnancy. J Nurse Midwifery 1995;40:36.
9. Zuspan FP, Long WN, Russell JK, et al. Anemia in pregnancy. J Reprod Med 1971;6:13.
10. Pritchard JA. Changes in the blood volume during pregnancy and delivery. Anesthesiology 1965;26:393.
11. Rothman D. Folic acid in pregnancy. Am J Obstet Gynecol 1970;108:49.
12. Giles C, Ball EW. Iron and folic acid deficiency in pregnancy. BMJ 1965;1:656.
13. Lambert EK, Bloom RN, Kosby M. Pregnancy in patients with hemoglobinopathies and thalassemias. J Reprod Med 1977;19:193.
14. Motulsky AG. Frequency of sickling disorders in US blacks. N Engl J Med 1973;288:31.
15. Lynch JR, Brown JM. The polymerase chain reaction: current and future clinical applications. J Med Genet 1990;27:2.
16. Husain SM, Kalavathi P, Anandraj MP. Analysis of sickle cell gene using polymerase chain reaction and restriction enzyme Bsu 361. Ind J Med Res 1995;101:273.
17. Posey YF, Shah D, Ulm JE, et al. Prenatal diagnosis of sickle cell anemia: hemoglobin electrophoresis versus DNA analysis. Am J Clin Pathol 1989;92:347.
18. Wang X, Seeman C, Chen T, et al. Experience with 500 prenatal diagnoses of sickle cell disease. Prenat Diagn 1994;14:851.
19. Barret-Connor E. Cholelithiasis in sickle cell anemia. Am J Med 1968;45:889.
20. Cameron JL, Moddrey WC, Ziridema GD, et al. Biliary tract disease in sickle cell anemia: surgical considerations. Ann Surg 1971;174:702.
21. Charache S, Scott J, Niebyl J, Bonds D. Management of sickle cell disease in pregnant patients. Obstet Gynecol 1980;55:407.
22. Fort AA, Morrison JC, Berreras L, et al. Counseling the patient with sickle cell disease about reproduction: pregnancy outcome does not justify the maternal risk. Am J Obstet Gynecol 1971;111:391.
23. Horger EO III. Sickle cell and sickle cell-hemoglobin disease during pregnancy. Obstet Gynecol 1972;39:873.
24. Milner PF, Jones BR, Dobler J. Outcome of pregnancy in sickle cell anemia and sickle cell-hemoglobin C disease. Am J Obstet Gynecol 1980;138:239.
25. Fessas P, Loukopoulos D. Beta thalassaemias. Clin Hematol 1974;3:411.
26. Seoud MA, Cantwell C, Nobles G. Levy OL. Outcome of pregnancies complicated by sickle cell disease and sickle c hemoglobinopathies. Am J Perinatol 1994; 11:187.
27. Smith JA, England M, Bellevue R, et al. Pregnancy in sickle cell disease: experience of the cooperative study of sickle cell disease. Obstet Gynecol 1996;87:199.
28. Fiakpui EF, Moron EM. Pregnancy in sickle hemoglobins. J Reprod Med 1973;11:28.
29. Morris JS, Dunn DT, Poddorr D, Serjeant GR. Hematological risk factors for pregnancy outcome in Jamaican

women with homozygous sickle cell disease. Br J Obstet Gynaecol 1994;101:770.

30. Anyaegbunam A, Langer O, Brustman L, et al. The application of uterine and umbilical artery velocimetry to the antenatal supervision of pregnancies complicated by maternal sickle hemoglobinopathies. Am J Obstet Gynecol 1988;159:544.

31. Abudu OO, Macaulay K, Oluboyede OA. Serial evaluation of iron stores in pregnant Nigerians with hemoglobin SS or SC. J Natl Med Assoc 1990;82:41.

32. Koshy M, Burd L. Wallace D, et al. Prophylactic red-cell transfusions in pregnant patients with sickle cell disease: a randomized cooperative study. N Engl J Med 1988; 319:1447.

33. Tuck SM, James CE, Brewster EM, et al. Prophylactic blood transfusion in maternal sickle cell syndromes. Br J Obstet Gynecol 1987;94:121.

34. Fullerton WT, Hendrickse J, Williams W, et al. Hemoglobin SC: clinical course. In: Jonxis JHP, ed. Abnormal hemoglobins in Africa: a symposium. Oxford: Blackwell Scientific, 1965:215.

35. Solanki DL, Keltter GG, Castro O. Acute splenic sequestration crises in adults with sickle cell disease. Am J Med 1986;80:985.

36. Wainscoat JS, Work S, Sampietro M, et al. Feasibility of prenatal diagnosis of beta thalassaemia by DNA polymorphisms in an Italian population. Br J Haematol 1986; 62:495.

37. Focharoen S, Winichagoon P, Thonglairoam V. Prenatal diagnosis of thalassemia and hemoglobinopathies in Thailand: experience from 100 pregnancies. Southeast Asian J Trop Med Public Health 1991;22:16.

38. Ghosh A, Tan MH, Liang ST, et al. Ultrasound evaluation of pregnancies at risk for homozygous alpha-thalassaemia-1. Prenat Diagn 1987;7:307.

39. Mordel N, Birkenfeld A, Goldfarb AN, Rachmilewitz EA. Successful full-term pregnancy in homozygous beta-thalassemia major: case report and review of the literature. Obstet Gynecol 1989;73:837.

40. Necheles T. Obstetric complications associated with haemoglobinopathies. Clin Hematol 1973;2:497.

41. Savona-Ventura C, Bonello F. Betathalassemia syndromes in pregnancy. Obstet Gynecol Surv 1994;49:129.

42. Singounas EG, Sakas DE, Hadley OM. Paraplegia in a pregnant thalassemic woman due to extramedullary hematopoesis: successful management with transfusions. Surg Neurol 1991;36:210.

43. White JM, Richard R, Jelenski G, et al. Iron state in alpha and beta thalassaemia trait. J Clin Pathol 1986; 39:256.

44. Leung CF, Lao TT, Chang AM. Effect of folate supplement on pregnant women with beta-thalassaemia minor. Eur J Obstet Gynecol Reprod Biol 1989;33:209.

45. Schmidt RM. Laboratory diagnosis of hemoglobinopathies. JAMA 1973;224:1276.

46. McRae KR, Samuels P, Schreiber AAAD. Pregnancy-associated thrombocytopenia: pathogenesis and management. Blood 1992;80:2697.

47. Aster RH. Gestational thrombocytopenia: a plea for conservative management. N Engl J Med 1990;323:264.

48. Samuels P, Bussel JB, Braitman LE, et al. Estimation of the risk of thrombocytopenia in the offspring of pregnant women with presumed thrombocytopenic purpura. N Engl J Med 1990;323:229.

49. Samuels P, Main EK, Tomaski A, et al. Abnormalities in platelet antiglobulin tests in preeclamptic mothers and their neonates. Am J Obstet Gyencol 1987;107:109.

50. Burrows RF, Kelton JG. Incidentally detected thrombocytopenia in healthy mothers and their infants. N Engl J Med 1988;319:142.

51. Hart D, Dunetz C, Nardi M, et al. An epidemic of maternal thrombocytopenia associated with elevated antiplatelet antibody in 116 consecutive pregnancies: relationship to neonatal platelet count. Am J Obstet Gynecol 1986; 154:878.

52. Burrows RF, Kelton JG. Fetal thrombocytopenia and its relation to maternal thrombocytopenia. N Engl J Med 1993;329:1463.

53. Burrows RF, Kelton JG. Low fetal risks in pregnancies associated with idiopathic thrombocytopenia purpura. Am J Obstet Gynecol 1990;163:1147.

54. Peterson OH Jr, Larson P. Thrombocytopenic purpura in pregnancy. Obstet Gyencol 1954;4:454.

55. Territo J, Finkelstein J, Oh W, et al. Management of autoimmune thrombocytopenia in pregnancy and in the neonate. Obstet Gynecol 1973;51:590.

56. Carloss HW, MacMillan R, Crosby WH. Management of pregnancy in women with immune thrombocytopenic purpura. JAMA 1980;244:2756.

57. Noriega-Guerra L, Aviles-Miranda A, de la Cadena OA, et al. Pregnancy in patients with autoimmune thrombocytopenic purpura. Am J Obstet Gynecol 1979;133:439.

58. Heys RFI. Childbearing and idiopathic thrombocytopenic purpura. J Obstet Gynaecol Br Commonw 1966; 73:205.

59. Karapatkin M, Porges RF, Karapatkin S. Platelet counts in infants of women with autoimmune thrombocytopenia: effects of steroid administration to the mother. N Engl J Med 1981;305:936.

60. Cines DB, Dusak B, Tomaski A, et al. Immune thrombocytopenic purpura and pregnancy. N Engl J Med 1982; 306:826.

61. Cines DB. Idiopathic thrombocytopenic purpura complicating pregnancy. Medical Grand Rounds 1984;3:344.

62. Kelton JG, Inwood MJ, Narr RM, et al. The prenatal prediction of thrombocytopenia in infants of mothers with clinically diagnosed immune thrombocytopenia. Am J Obstet Gynecol 1982;144:449.

63. Harrington WJ, Minnich V, Arimura G. The autoimmune thrombocytopenias. In: Tascantinss LM, ed. Progress in hematology. New York: Grune and Stratton, 1956:166.

64. Cines DB, Schreiber AD. Immune thrombocytopenia: use of a Coombs antiglobulin test to detect IgG and C3 on platelets. N Engl J Med 1979;300:106.

65. He R, Reid DM, Jones CE, Shulman NR. Spectrum of Ig classes, specificities, and titers of serum antiglycoproteins in chronic idiopathic thrombocytopenic purpura. Blood 1994;83:1024.

66. Yeager AM, Zinkham WH. Varicella-associated thrombocytopenia: clues to the etiology of childhood idiopathic

thrombocytopenic purpura. John Hopkins Med J 1980;146:270.

67. Scott JR, Cruikshank DR, Kochenour NK, et al. Fetal platelet counts in the obstetric management of immunologic thrombocytopenic purpura. Am J Obstet Gynecol 1980;136:495.

68. Ghidini A, Sepulveda W, Lockwood CJ, Romero R. Complications of blood sampling. Am J Obstet Gynecol 1993; 168:1339.

69. Burrows RF, Kelton JG. Pregnancy in patients with idiopathic thrombocytopenic purpura: assessing the risks for the infant at delivery. Obstet Gynecol Survey 1993;458:781.

70. Moschowitz E. Hyaline thrombosis of the terminal arterioles and capillaries: a hitherto undescribed disease. Proc NY Pathol Soc 1924;24:21.

71. Miller JM, Pastorek JG. Thrombotic thrombocytopenic purpura and the hemolytic uremic syndrome in pregnancy. Clin Obstet Gynecol 1991;34:64.

72. Ridolfi RL, Bell WR. Thrombotic thrombocytopenic purpura: report of 25 cases and a review of the literature. Medicine (Baltimore) 1981;60:413.

73. Weiner CP. Thrombotic microangiopathy in pregnancy and the postpartum period. Semin Hematol 1987;24:71.

74. Weiner CP, Kwaan HC, Xu C, et al. Antithrombin III activity in women with hypertension during pregnancy. Obstet Gynecol 1985;65:301.

75. Nield GH. Haemolytic uraemic syndrome. Nephron 1991;59:194.

76. Cooke RL, Miller RC, Katz VL, et al. Immune thrombocytopenic purpura in pregnancy: a reappraisal of management. Obstet Gynecol 1991;78:578.

77. Lian ECY, Byrnes JJ, Harkness DR. Two successful pregnancies in a woman with chronic thrombotic thrombocytopenic purpura. Int J Obstet Gynecol 1989;29:359.

78. Ezra Y, Mordel N, Sadovsky E, et al. Successful pregnancies of two patients with relapsing thrombotic thrombocytopenic purpura. Int J Obstet Gynecol 1989;29:359.

79. Ponticelli C, Rivolta E, Imbasciatti E, et al. Hemolytic uremic syndrome in adults. Arch Intern Med 1980; 140:353.

80. Beattie TJ, Murphy AV, Willoughby MLN, Belcj JJF. Prostacyclin infusion in haemolytic-uraemic syndrome of children. BMJ 1981;283:470.

81. Olah KS, Gee H. Postpartum haemolytic uraemic syndrome precipitated by antibiotics. Br J Obstet Gynaecol 1990;97:83.

82. Deaver JE, Leppert PC, Zaroulis CG. Neonatal alloimmune thrombocytopenic purpura. Am J Perinatol 1986; 3:127.

83. Okada N, Oda M, Sano T, et al. Intracranial hemorrhage in utero due to fetomaternal Bak(a) incompatibility. Nippon Ketsueki Gakkai Zasshi 1988;51:1086.

84. Bussell JB, McFarland JG, Berkowtiz R. Antenatal treatment of fetal alloimmune cytopenias. Blut 1989;59:136.

85. Menell JS, Bussel JB. Antenatal management of thrombocytopenias. Clin Perinatol 1994;21:591.

86. Paidas AH, Berkowitz RL, Lynch L, et al. Alloimmune thrombocytopenia: fetal and neonatal losses related to cordocentesis. Am J Obstet Gynecol 1995;172:475.

Neurologic Disorders

Philip Samuels

Five Key Points

- Pregnant women with a seizure disorder are at increased risk for having an infant with a congenital anomaly.

- Subarachnoid hemorrhages in pregnancy are most likely to result from rupture of a berry aneurysm or bleeding from an arteriovenous malformation.

- The most common symptoms of multiple sclerosis are visual disturbance, motor weakness, and loss of coordination. The disease is best diagnosed by magnetic resonance imaging.

- Pregnancy outcome is not adversely affected by pseudotumor cerebri.

- Carpal-tunnel syndrome in pregnancy should be treated conservatively by placement of splints on the volar surface of the affected hand.

SEIZURE DISORDERS

Affecting approximately 1% of the general population, seizure disorders are the most frequent major neurologic complication encountered in pregnancy. Seizure disorders may be divided into acquired and idiopathic. Acquired seizures, which account for less than 15% of all seizures, may result from trauma, infection, space-occupying masses, or metabolic disorders. Over 85% of seizure disorders are classified as idiopathic, meaning that no causative agent or inciting incident can be identified. Idiopathic seizures can be divided into types such as tonic–clonic, partial complex with or without generalization, myoclonic, focal, or absence.

Although initial therapy is usually based on the type of seizure experienced, patients may respond differently to each medication. Therefore, it is not unusual to encounter a patient who may be taking any of the major antiepileptic medications. Some patients take more than one medication. Furthermore, patients may be placed on a certain medication because they did not tolerate the side effects of another anticonvulsant (Table 6-11). Because of the stigma surrounding epilepsy and the misunderstandings of many patients and physicians, the treatment of the pregnant patient with a seizure disorder can create quite a challenge for the obstetrician. In addition, because many patients with epilepsy have been seizure-free on their medications, they may not have been evaluated by a neurologist in several years. The obstetrician and neurologist must work closely together to safely guide the patient through her pregnancy. Through this cooperation, the vast majority of pregnant women with seizure disorders can have a successful pregnancy with minimal risk to mother and fetus.

Effects of Epilepsy on Oral Contraceptives

Women with seizure disorders should seek care from an obstetrician/gynecologist as soon as they become

TABLE 6-11
POSSIBLE ADVERSE EFFECTS OF ANTICONVULSANTS

Drug	Maternal Effects	Fetal Effects
Phenytoin	Nystagmus, ataxia, hirsutism, gingival hyperplasia, megaloblastic anemia	Possible teratogenesis and carcinogenesis, coagulopathy, hypocalcemia
Phenobarbital	Drowsiness, ataxia	Possible teratogenesis, coagulopathy, neonatal depression, withdrawal
Primidone	Drowsiness, ataxia, nausea	Possible teratogenesis, coagulopathy, neonatal depression
Carbamazepine	Drowsiness, leukopenia, ataxia, mild hepatotoxicity	Possible craniofacial and neural-tube defects
Valproic acid	Ataxia, drowsiness, alopecia, hepatotoxicity, thrombocytopenia	Neural-tube defects and possible craniofacial and skeletal defects
Trimethadione	Drowsiness, nausea	Strong teratogenic potential
Ethosuximide	Nausea, hepatotoxicity, leukopenia, thrombocytopenia	Possible teratogenesis

sexually active. Contraception may present a challenge to women with epilepsy, and the use of oral contraceptives may require special adjustments. Antiepileptic medications that induce hepatic microsomal enzymes—such as phenytoin, phenobarbital, and carbamazepine[1]—have been associated with contraceptive failure. The increased hepatic enzymatic activity induced by these medications may lead to rapid clearance of these contraceptive hormones. Patients on anticonvulsants who are taking low-dose oral contraceptives may have more breakthrough bleeding[2] and may be at increased risk for unplanned pregnancy.[3,4] This rapid clearance does not appear to be induced by valproate or benzodiazepines.[1]

Effect of Pregnancy on Epilepsy

The classic teaching is that between 30 and 50% of patients will show an increase in seizure frequency during pregnancy. This finding was confirmed in the landmark study of Knight and Rhind[5] of 153 pregnancies in 59 patients between 1953 and 1973. In that study, 45% of the patients showed an increase in seizure frequency during pregnancy, while 50% had no change and 4.8% experienced a decrease. However, anticonvulsant levels could not be readily measured until the mid-1970s. When the study of Knight and Rhind was performed, anticonvulsant doses were increased by physicians only when patients had breakthrough seizures. An important finding from that study was that patients who had frequent seizures prior to gestation tended to have exacerbations during pregnancy.[5] Virtually all patients who experienced more than one seizure each month

had worsening of their epilepsy during pregnancy, whereas few patients with no seizure activity for over 9 months experienced exacerbation of epilepsy during pregnancy.

With the introduction of new medications and the ability to monitor anticonvulsant levels, the number of patients with uncontrolled seizures has diminished. Patients with more frequent seizures, however, still tend to have exacerbations of seizure activity during pregnancy. In a large classic study by Schmidt et al.,[6] 63% of patients had no change or a decrease in seizure frequency during pregnancy, while 37% of patients had an increase in seizure frequency. Importantly, in 34 of the 50 patients who showed an increase in seizure frequency during pregnancy, the increase was associated with noncompliance with drug regimens or sleep deprivation. This observation is critical because many women stop taking all medications as soon as they suspect they are pregnant. Furthermore, the usual physical and emotional stresses of pregnancy may result in sleep deprivation. In a study by Tanganelli and Regesta,[7] seizure frequency either did not change or improved in 82.6% of pregnancies. This better outcome than that in older studies is due to the ability to effectively monitor anticonvulsant levels.

In summary, we now have the means to monitor anticonvulsant levels in patients frequently, and we have a larger array of medications to control seizures. We also understand that sleep deprivation can be a catalyst for seizures. With patient cooperation and close surveillance, seizure frequency should remain the same or even improve in most epileptic patients during a closely monitored pregnancy.

Effects of Pregnancy on the Anticonvulsant Medications

Levels of anticonvulsant medications can change dramatically during pregnancy. They usually decrease in total concentration as pregnancy progresses. Many factors, including altered protein binding, delayed gastric emptying, nausea and vomiting, changes in plasma volume, and changes in the volume of distribution, can affect the levels of anticonvulsant medications. Without some understanding of this subject, it is difficult to treat the patient with epilepsy correctly. A few crucial points are summarized below.

Because many patients experience nausea and vomiting in the first trimester, drug levels may fall. If this decline in serum drug concentration leads to increased seizure activity, nausea must be aggressively treated or anticonvulsant drugs must be given parenterally. Clinicians must also realize that, due to variable protein binding, total drug levels may not represent free active drug. This observation is especially true of phenytoin. If breakthrough seizures occur in a patient taking phenytoin, free phenytoin levels should be determined. For other medications, protein binding is not as high, but in case of breakthrough seizures, drug levels should be pushed to the upper limits of normal unless the patient experiences clinical signs of toxicity.

All anticonvulsants interfere with folic acid metabolism, and patients on anticonvulsants may actually become deficient in folic acid. Folic acid deficiency has been associated with neural-tube defects and other congenital malformations.[8,9] Because organogenesis occurs during the first weeks after conception, folic acid supplementation should be begun before pregnancy. Increasing folic acid ingestion, however, increases the activity of hepatic microsomal enzymes and thus the clearance of anticonvulsant medications. Therefore, levels should be checked frequently after folic acid therapy is implemented.

Neonatal hemorrhage due to a decrease in the production of vitamin K–dependent clotting factors (II, VII, IX, X) in the fetal liver, has been reported in infants born to mothers taking phenobarbital, phenytoin, and primidone.[10] In one series,[10] 8 of 16 infants exposed to these medications had a cord-blood coagulation pattern indicative of vitamin K deficiency. These infants responded to vitamin K infusion. Bleyer and Skinner[11] reviewed a case of their own and another 21 cases of hemorrhagic disease

following anticonvulsant therapy that have appeared in the literature. They reached the conclusion that these cases were due to deficiencies of vitamin K–dependent clotting factors and recommended that, at birth, infants should be given 1 mg of vitamin K intramuscularly. This recommendation is now followed by virtually all U.S. hospitals.

Effect of Epilepsy on Pregnancy

The majority of women with seizure disorders who become pregnant will have an uneventful pregnancy with an excellent outcome. There appear, however, to be several pregnancy complications that are more prevalent in the mother with epilepsy than in the general population. In a review of all birth certificates for infants born in the state of Washington, Yerby and co-workers[12] identified 200 births to mothers with seizure disorders. They found that mothers with seizure disorders were 2.66 times more likely to have had a previous fetal death after 20 weeks of gestation than the control population. The increased incidence of stillbirth also has been confirmed in other studies.[5,13,14]

Because of the long duration of most of these studies, many patients were pregnant during the 1970s and early 1980s. With the increased use of ultrasound to identify growth restriction, malformations, and oligohydramnios, many of the stillborn fetuses may have been identified as being at risk and might have undergone antepartum fetal testing and intervention before the fetal death occurred. These studies also were not stratified by medications taken, dosages, drug levels, or seizure activity during pregnancy. Hiilesmaa et al.,[15] in a study of 150 pregnant women with seizure disorders, found no difference in perinatal mortality between patients and controls. This was a more recent study in which antepartum fetal surveillance was applied.

Yerby and colleagues[12] also found an increased incidence of preeclampsia in women with seizure disorders, and this finding has been confirmed in other large retrospective studies.[5,13] Hiilesmaa et al.,[15] however, found no difference in the rate of preeclampsia between pregnant women with epilepsy and pregnant controls. Yerby et al.[12] also showed a 2.79-fold increase in low-birth-weight infants. In a carefully performed study in Italy, Matroiacovo and co-workers[16] found that the mean birth weight in neonates born to women with epilepsy was 107 g lower than controls but still fell within the normal range for gestational age.

Yerby and colleagues[12] found a significant decrease in 1- and 5-minute Apgar scores. This may be attributed to the fetal effect of maternal depressant medications such as phenobarbital. They also demonstrated an increased rate of cesarean delivery in patients with a seizure disorder. Conversely, Hiilesmaa et al.[15,17] found no increase in preterm labor, bleeding, pregnancy-induced hypertension, operative vaginal delivery, or cesarean delivery rates.

In summary, there may be an increased risk of stillbirths in women with seizure disorders. The cause of this complication is not readily apparent but may be due to factors that are easily detectable today (such as intrauterine growth restriction) that were not detected when older studies were conducted. The incidence of preeclampsia may be higher in mothers with seizure disorders. The vast majority of pregnancies, however, will be uncomplicated, with no increase in complications over the expected rate. Nonetheless, because of these few potential problems, the obstetrician should be more vigilant for pregnancy-related complications in pregnant women with seizure disorders and use antepartum fetal surveillance when appropriate.

Effects of Anticonvulsant Medications on the Fetus

There is little doubt that anticonvulsant medications are associated with an increase in congenital malformations, but the magnitude of this risk and the association of certain anomalies with specific drugs remains debatable. Hanson and Smith[18] identified a specific fetal hydantoin syndrome in five neonates in 1975. They noted growth and performance delays, craniofacial abnormalities (including clefting), and limb anomalies, including hypoplasia of nails and distal phalanges. Hanson et al.[19] later reported that 7 to 11% of infants exposed to phenytoin had this recognizable pattern of malformations and that 31% of exposed fetuses had at least some aspects of the syndrome. Conversely, Gaily et al.[20] reported no evidence of the hydantoin syndrome in 82 women exposed in utero to phenytoin. Some of the patients had hypertelorism and hypoplasia of the distal phalanges, but none had the complete hydantoin syndrome as described by Hanson et al.[19]

Since the original reports by Hanson and colleagues, many studies have reported congenital malformations in infants born to mothers taking anticonvulsant medications. These reports typify the discrepancies that fill the medical literature concerning this subject and make the subject so confusing to physician and patient. There are studies that report that each of the commonly used anticonvulsant medications (phenytoin, phenobarbital, carbamazepine, valproate, and primidone) is the worst teratogen, yet there are other studies that report that each of these medications has a weak teratogenic potential. It is most important, therefore, to treat the patient with the medication that best controls her seizures.

Another example of discrepancies and the need for more research is the incidence of facial clefting among infants born to mothers with epilepsy. This is one of the more common anomalies found in these neonates. In a study by Friis et al.,[21] patients with untreated epilepsy had an incidence of facial clefting 2.7 times the expected rate, whereas infants of mothers treated with anticonvulsants had 4.7 times the expected rate of clefting. They concluded that epilepsy itself may increase the risk for cleft lip, with anticonvulsant medications increasing the risk even more. A study by Kelly et al.[22] demonstrated that the association between epilepsy and facial clefting is, in large part, due to shared causal determinants that are probably both genetic and environmental in origin. They believe that the role of anticonvulsant medications in this association seems to be overestimated and probably represents only a modest additive influence.

In a landmark multiinstitutional study, Nakane et al.[23] examined 902 pregnancies in mothers with idiopathic epilepsy. The overall rate of congenital malformations was 7.2%. The rate was 8.7% in the mothers who received anticonvulsant medications during pregnancy and 1.9% in nonmedicated mothers. Looking only at liveborn infants, 9.9% had malformations (11.5% in the medicated group and 2.3% in the nonmedicated group). The incidence of malformations in mothers receiving anticonvulsant therapy was, therefore, about five times that of the nonmedicated group.[23] The predominant malformations were cleft lip and/or palate (3.14%) and cardiovascular malformations (2.95%). These authors also noted that, as the number of anticonvulsant medications used in combination during pregnancy increased, the incidence of fetal malformations rose dramatically.[23] The malformation rate was less than 5% when one medication was used and was greater than 20% when four medications were used. In this study, only 15% of patients were treated with a single antiepileptic medication.[23]

Kaneko et al. examined various drug combinations and the incidence of malformations.[24] The overall malformation rate was 14%, but, in patients who were receiving a single medication, the malformation rate was only 6.5%.[25] The malformation rate for those treated with multiple medications was 15.6%. There was no dose-dependent increase in the incidence of malformations associated with any individual medication. In this study there was also no relationship between the type of defect and the individual anticonvulsant. Kaneko et al.[26] subsequently published a follow-up study that showed a malformation rate of only 6.3%. The lower rate of malformations may be attributable to the increase in patients receiving monotherapy. In the earlier study,[24] 16.1% of patients received a single medication, whereas 63.4% received a single medication in the later study.[26] This observation confirms the impression that more neurologists are treating patients with a single agent. Now that anticonvulsant levels can be easily measured, single medications can be given at higher doses to make certain that therapeutic levels are achieved, thus lessening the need for multiple medications.

Dravet et al.[27] studied 227 women participating in a prospective study between 1984 and 1988. There was a 7% rate of malformation among infants born to mothers taking antiepileptic medications as compared with 1.36% in the control group. Therefore, fetuses exposed in utero to anticonvulsants had a relative risk of 6.9 of being born with a congenital malformation. In this study, the frequency of spina bifida was 17 times more than would be expected in the general population, and heart defects were 9.6 times greater than expected. Cleft lip, with or without cleft palate, was 8.4 times more frequent than expected in the general population.

A study by Koch et al.[28] had a different emphasis. It showed no difference between the rate of malformations in mothers receiving polytherapy and mothers receiving a single medication. Infants born to mothers with epilepsy, regardless of therapy, had twice as many major malformations as infants born to the control population. The number of minor anomalies was approximately three times greater in infants born to mothers receiving anticonvulsant medication than in the control group. In the mothers receiving monotherapy, those taking valproate had the highest rate of minor malformations.[28] Gaily and Granstrom[29] also investigated minor anomalies in children of mothers with epilepsy. They proposed that there was no specific syndrome for a specific medication (i.e., the fetal hydantoin syndrome). Instead, they argued that many of these minor malformations may be linked to epilepsy and to anticonvulsant medications in general.[29]

Teenagers are often treated with valproate because of its low-side-effect profile. However, it has been reported to be associated with specific anomalies. In 1984, DiLiberti et al. reported a specific fetal valproate syndrome.[30] They found a consistent facial phenotype in all seven children studied and other anomalies in four. This finding was confirmed by Ardinger and colleagues[31] in 1988. Lindhout and Schmidt[32] confirmed the association between neural-tube defects and valproate exposure in utero, with a 1.5% risk of an infant being born with a neural-tube defect if the mothers took valproate in the first trimester. Lindhout et al.[25] also studied 34 cases of neural-tube defects in mothers taking anticonvulsant medications. In 33 of 34 cases, mothers were exposed to either valproate or carbamazepine. Whereas anencephaly and lumbosacral neural-tube defects occur with equal frequency in the general population, these studies strongly suggest that carbamazepine and valproate are specifically associated with lumbosacral neural-tube defects.

Many obstetricians believe that carbamazepine is safer to use during pregnancy than other antiepileptic medications, but this is not necessarily the case. In 1989, Jones et al.[33] reported a pattern of minor craniofacial defects, fingernail hypoplasia, and developmental delay in infants exposed in utero to carbamazepine. Rosa[34] has also shown that there is a 1% risk of spina bifida in infants of mothers taking carbamazepine. Because this spectrum of defects (except spina bifida) is similar to that in the fetal hydantoin syndrome, Jones et al.[33] hypothesized that, as both drugs are metabolized through an arene oxide pathway, perhaps an epoxide intermediary is the teratogenic agent. Fetuses with low levels of epoxide hydrolase are exposed to higher levels of epoxide intermediaries, and this effect may lead to an increase in malformations. Conversely, fetuses with high enzyme levels clear epoxides rapidly, minimizing exposure to the potential teratogens. Phenytoin, phenobarbital, and, to a lesser extent, carbamazepine are metabolized through this pathway.[35]

There has been much debate over whether epilepsy itself and/or the use of antiepileptic medications is associated with psychomotor delays or mental retardation. In the landmark study by Nelson and Ellenberg,[13] an IQ below 70 was seen in 65.2 per 1000 7-year-old children in the seizure group as compared with 34 per 1000 in the age-matched control group, a statistically significant difference. Before generalizations can be made, many confounding factors must be evaluated, including other anomalies and social environment. In a review by Granstrom and Gaily,[36] none of the major antiepileptic medications appeared to carry special risk for mental retardation. They suggest, however, that polytherapy and inherited defects in antiepileptic medication metabolism in the fetus increase the risk for mental retardation. This study is important because these researchers stress that other factors associated with maternal epilepsy, such as seizures during pregnancy, inherited brain disorders, and a nonoptimal psychosocial environment, can also affect a child's psychomotor development.[36] In summary, there appears to be a small, undefined risk of a slightly lower IQ in infants born to mothers with epilepsy. It does not appear that any particular medication results in a higher risk of this outcome.

Preconceptual Counseling for Women with Seizure Disorders

It is imperative, but not usually possible, to counsel the patient with epilepsy prior to pregnancy. A personal and family history should be taken. The clinician must stress that the patient has a greater than 90% chance of having a successful pregnancy resulting in a normal newborn. A detailed history of medication use and seizure control should be obtained. The patient must be informed that, if she has frequent seizures before conception, this pattern will probably continue or even worsen. If she has frequent seizures, she should delay conception until control is better, even if this entails a change of medication. The obstetrician must stress that controlling seizures is of primary importance and that the patient will need to take whatever medication(s) is necessary to achieve this goal throughout her pregnancy. If the patient has had no seizures during the past 2 to 5 years, an attempt may be made to withdraw antiepileptic medications. Withdrawal should be accomplished over a 1- to 3-month period. Up to 50% of patients will relapse and need to restart their medications. This withdrawal should be attempted only if the patient is completely seizure-free and only in cooperation with a neurologist. During the period of withdrawal, patients should refrain from driving.

Ideally, it is best to have the patient take a single medication during pregnancy. If the patient is on multiple medications, she should be slowly changed to monotherapy if possible. As the other medications are gradually withdrawn, the serum concentration of the remaining medication should be monitored frequently to be certain the level remains therapeutic. The patient should refrain from conceiving until seizures have been well controlled for several months on the single medication. The patient must also be counseled that she should get adequate rest and sleep during pregnancy, as sleep deprivation is associated with increased seizure frequency. Again, driving should be curtailed during any major medication change.

The choice of antiepileptic medication depends on the seizure type. As the foregoing literature review has shown, there are studies claiming teratogenesis for each of the major anticonvulsant medications, yet there are also studies showing that each medication individually may not be particularly teratogenic. The most important point is to control maternal seizures. The anticonvulsant that does the best job of controlling seizures is the one that should be used.

Folic acid supplementation may help to prevent neural-tube defects.[9] Supplementation should begin at least 1 month prior to planned conception and continued throughout pregnancy.[37] Anticonvulsant levels should be checked frequently after implementing or increasing folic acid administration, as this cofactor in metabolism leads to lower anticonvulsant levels.[37] The vitamin D supplement in prenatal vitamins also is important for these patients because anticonvulsants, particularly phenytoin, may interfere with the conversion of 25-hydroxycholecalciferol to 1,25-dihydroxycholecalciferol, the active form of vitamin D.

Whether or not they ask, all mothers with idiopathic epilepsy wonder if their child will have epilepsy. There is a surprising paucity of data in this area. Children of parents without seizures have a 0.5 to 1% risk for epilepsy. The infant born to a mother with a seizure disorder of unknown cause has a four times greater chance of idiopathic epilepsy than the general population.[38] Interestingly, it appears that epilepsy in the father does not increase a child's risk of a seizure disorder developing.[39]

Care during Pregnancy

Once the patient becomes pregnant, it is of the utmost importance to establish accurate gestational dating to prevent any confusion about adequacy of fetal growth in later gestation. The patient's anticonvulsant level should be followed periodically and dosages adjusted to keep the patient seizure-free. It takes several half-lives for a medication to reach a steady state (Table 6-12). Drugs like phenobarbital have extremely long half-lives, and the levels should not be checked too frequently. If levels are measured before the drug reaches a steady state and the dosage is increased, the

TABLE 6-12
ANTICONVULSANTS COMMONLY USED DURING PREGNANCY

Drug	Therapeutic Level (mg/liter)	Usual Dosage for Nonpregnant Women	Half-Life (hours)
Carbamazepine	4–10 mg/liter	600–1200 mg/day in three or divided doses	Initially 36 mg/liter chronic therapy 16 mg/liter
Phenobarbital	15–40 mg/liter	90–180 mg/day in two or three divided doses	100 mg/liter
Phenytoin	10–20 mg/liter total; 1–2, free	300–500 mg/day in single or divided doses	Avg 24 mg/liter
Primidone	5–15 mg/liter	750–1500 mg/day in three divided doses	8 mg/liter
Valproic acid	50–100 mg/liter	550–2000 mg/day in three or divided doses	Avg. 13 mg/liter

medication level will eventually become toxic to the patient. Drug levels should be determined immediately before the next dose (trough levels) in order to assess if dosing is adequate. If the patient is showing signs of toxicity, determination of peak level may be helpful, especially in drugs with shorter half-lives.

At approximately 16 to 18 weeks of gestation, the patient should undergo blood testing for maternal serum α-fetoprotein (MSAFP) to detect a neural-tube defect. At 18 to 22 weeks, the patient should also have a comprehensive ultrasound examination performed by an experienced sonographer to search for congenital malformations. A fetal echocardiogram should then be obtained at 20 to 23 weeks to evaluate for cardiac malformations, which are among the more common malformations of women taking any antiepileptic medications.[31,32,34,40,41]

As previously noted, there may be an increased risk for intrauterine growth restriction for fetuses exposed in utero to anticonvulsant medications. If the patient's weight gain and fundal growth appear appropriate, regular ultrasound examinations for fetal weight assessment are probably unnecessary. If, however, there is any question of fundal growth or if the patient's habitus precludes adequate assessment of this clinical parameter, serial ultrasonography for fetal weight assessment and amniotc fluid volume should be performed.

In older retrospective studies, there appears to be an increased risk of stillbirth in mothers taking anti-convulsant medications.[5,12,14] In one prospective study, however, this complication was not seen.[15] As previously noted, in the studies that showed an increase in stillbirths, factors such as intrauterine growth restriction or oligohydramnios were not identified prenatally. With modern surveillance and the frequent use of ultrasonography, many of these risk factors can be detected before the fetus faces imminent risk. Nonstress testing, therefore, is not necessary in all mothers with seizure disorders. It should be limited to those who have medical or obstetric complications that place the patient at increased risk for delivering a stillborn baby.

If at all possible, the patient should be maintained on a single medication, and drug levels should be drawn at appropriate intervals to make certain that the patient is receiving enough medication. This is particularly important if the patient is experiencing breakthrough seizures. If possible, free levels of the anticonvulsant medication should be measured, especially in the case of phenytoin. A brief seizure during pregnancy does not appear to be deleterious to the fetus.[16] It is best to use the lowest dose of a single medication that will keep the patient seizure-free. This, however, must be individualized. For instance, if the patient usually experiences seizures during the day and drives, it is important to make certain that the patient remains seizure-free. For this type of patient, drug dosages should be increased if levels fall. If, on the other hand, the patient only has brief partial complex seizures that do not generalize and occur only during her sleep, it is optimal to keep the medications at the lowest serum concentration that will keep her seizure-free. The key to managing anticonvulsants in pregnancy is individualization of therapy.

Early hemorrhagic disease of the newborn can occur in infants exposed to anticonvulsants in utero, and this complication appears to be due to a deficiency of the vitamin K–dependent clotting factors II, VII, IX, and X. The use of vitamin K in the third trimester, in an attempt to prevent the rare complication of immediate neonatal hemorrhagic disease, is somewhat controversial but becoming more common. Although some advocate administering 10 to 20 mg of vitamin K orally each day to mothers during the final 1 or 2 months of pregnancy, this is certainly not the standard of care. There appears to be no adverse effect of administering this vitamin, but, on the other hand, its utility has not been clearly demonstrated. Very little hemorrhagic disease of the newborn is seen today; this is probably because virtually all infants receive 1 mg of vitamin K intramuscularly at birth.

Labor and Delivery

Vaginal delivery is the route of choice for the mother with a seizure disorder. If the mother has frequent seizures that are brought on by the stress of labor, she may undergo cesarean delivery after stabilization. Fortunately, this phenomenon is rare. Seizures during labor may cause transient fetal bradycardia.[15] The fetal heart rate should be given time to recover. If it does not, then one must assume fetal distress and/or placental abruption and deliver by cesarean. Because stress often exacerbates seizure disorders, an epidural anesthetic can benefit many laboring patients with epilepsy.

Management of anticonvulsant medications during a prolonged labor presents a challenge. During labor, oral absorption of medications is erratic; if the patient vomits it is almost negligible. Phenytoin or phenobarbital medications may be administered parenterally. An anticonvulsant level should be obtained first to help ascertain the appropriate dosage. Phenobarbital may be given intramuscularly, and phenytoin may be given intravenously. If the patient's phenytoin level is normal, the usual daily dose may be administered intravenously. The introduction of phosphenytoin has made this type of administration much easier. Because of the long half-life of phenobarbital, if the patient's serum level is therapeutic, a 60- to 90-mg intramuscular dose will probably be sufficient to maintain the patient through labor and delivery.

The main problem arises if the patient is taking carbamazepine. This medication is not manufactured in a parenteral form. Oral administration may be attempted, but, if the patient has seizures or a preseizure aura, she may be loaded with a therapeutic dose of phenytoin to carry her through labor. Benzodiazepines may also be used for acute seizures, but one must remember that they can cause early neonatal depression as well as maternal apnea.[42]

Prenatal diagnostic techniques are not perfect. Even if the infant appears to have no anomalies on ultrasound, an experienced pediatrician should be present at the delivery of the infant born to a mother taking anticonvulsant medications.

Postpartum Period

The levels of anticonvulsant medications must be monitored frequently during the first few weeks postpartum because they can rapidly rise. If the patient's medication dosages were increased during pregnancy, they will need to be decreased rather rapidly after delivery, eventually reaching prepregnancy doses. All of the major anticonvulsant medications cross into breast milk. The levels vary from 18 to 79% of the plasma levels.[42,43] The use of these medications, however, is not a contraindication to breast-feeding. Primidone, phenobarbital, and benzodiazepines may have a sedative effect on the fetus, and withdrawal symptoms have been described during the intervals between feedings. Should the infant exhibit these types of symptoms, breast-feeding should be discontinued. The main reason to avoid breast-feeding is if the mother's seizures are exacerbated by sleep deprivation. She then must decide whether she wants to stop breast-feeding, supplement with formula, or supplement with breast milk obtained by pumping.

All methods of contraception are available to women with idiopathic seizure disorders. The majority of women are able to take oral contraceptives without any adverse effects.[44] Oral contraceptive failures are more common in women taking anticonvulsants. Such failures are due to the fact that all of the major anticonvulsant medications induce hepatic enzymes, which then metabolize steroid hormones faster.[44,45] These patients may, therefore, require oral contraceptives with higher dosages of estrogens. However, the amount of enzyme induction varies, and oral contraceptive doses must be individualized.

In conclusion, the majority of women with idiopathic epilepsy will have an uneventful pregnancy with an excellent outcome. To optimize neonatal outcome, the patient should take only one medication and, when possible, use the lowest dose effective in keeping her free of seizures. Simple interventions such as taking folic acid from the time of conception, taking prenatal vitamins containing vitamin D, and giving the infant vitamin K at birth will help to optimize the neonatal outcome. There is an increase in congenital malformations in infants exposed to anticonvulsant medications in utero. The majority of infants exposed to these medications, however, will have no malformations. With modern techniques for prenatal diagnosis, including ultrasound and maternal serum marker screening, many of these malformations can be detected early. The majority of women with epilepsy will labor normally and have spontaneous vaginal deliveries.

MIGRAINE HEADACHE

Headaches are extremely common in women, and the majority of migraine headaches occur in women of child-bearing age. Between 15 and 20% of pregnant women are affected by migraine headaches.[46] Migraines can be classified as those with aura (other neurologic signs and symptoms) and those without aura. The headaches, which are associated with vasodilation of the cerebral vasculature, vary in duration. They are frequently accompanied by photosensitivity and nausea. Migraines with aura may be accompanied by sensations in the extremities and other lateralizing signs, sometimes making them difficult to distinguish from transient ischemic attacks.

Migraine symptoms tend to improve during pregnancy.[47,48,49] Friedman and Merritt 48 found that more than 80% of their patients reported improvement of migraine symptoms, with some experiencing no headache at all during pregnancy. Granella and co-workers[50] found that migraines disappeared during pregnancy in 67% of cases. Two studies found that patients who experienced severe migraines near the time of their menses actually improved the most during pregnancy.[49,50] Chen and co-workers[51] identified 508 women with a history of migraine from the Collaborative Perinatal Project of the National Institute of Neurological and Communicative Disorders and Stroke. They found that patients with migraines smoked more heavily and had a longer smoking history than did their headache-free peers. They also found that in nonsmokers migraine was often associated with allergies.[51]

Chancellor and colleagues[52] followed nine patients whose migraines first occurred during pregnancy at various gestational ages. They were followed for more than 4 years after pregnancy, and the prognosis for headache was excellent. In four of the nine patients complications of pregnancy developed, including preeclampsia in two.[52]

Supportive therapy is recommended for patients who experience migraine attacks during gestation. Both narcotic and nonnarcotic analgesics can be used as necessary. The use of nonsteroidal antiinflammatory agents should be limited in late pregnancy because, when used over a long period, they can cause premature closure of the ductus arteriosus with resultant tricuspid regurgitation and/or oligohydramnios. Nonetheless, they can be used for brief periods under physician supervision. When pain is severe, parenteral narcotics may be used.

Antiemetic therapy, either orally or parenterally, is an important adjunct in treating migraines. For those with frequent migraines, prophylaxis can be employed but may take several weeks to become effective. β-Blockers and calcium-channel blockers may be safely administered during pregnancy for prophylaxis against migraine headaches. The tricyclic antidepressants and selective serotonin reuptake inhibitors can also be used safely for prophylaxis during pregnancy but take weeks to become effective. Four percent lidocaine, administered intranasally, also has been shown to relieve migraine symptoms acutely.[53,54] However, up to 40% of treated patients experience relapses.[54]

Ergotamine should be avoided during pregnancy. Previous reports have suggested that it may cause birth defects that have a vascular disruptive cause. Hughes and Goldstein[55] report a case in which an infant showed evidence of early arrested cerebral maturation and paraplegia. They hypothesize that ergotamine, acting either alone or in synergy with propranolol and caffeine, produced fetal vasoconstriction that resulted in tissue ischemia and subsequent malformation.[55] It is important to note that this cause is strictly theoretical. In addition, ergots are uterotonic and have an abortifacient potential. Sumatriptan, a serotonin receptor agonist, is very successful in treating migraines. It has a potential for vasoconstriction and has not been studied in pregnancy. It should only be used if the physician believes that the potential benefit clearly outweighs the risk. Table 6-13 shows medications commonly used to treat migraines.

Dietary factors may precipitate migraine attacks. Careful history may identify foods that should be avoided, including those containing monosodium glutamate, red wine, cured meats, and strong cheeses containing tyramine. Relative hypoglycemia and alcohol can also trigger migraine attacks.

CORTICAL VENOUS THROMBOSIS

The chief symptoms in patients with cortical venous thrombosis are headache, lethargy, and vomiting. Hemiplegia may occur, and seizure activity is common.[56,57] This disorder occurs most frequently during the immediate postpartum period and may be attributed to a hypercoagulable state.[58] An incidence of 1 in 10,000 pregnancies was reported in one study.[59] With the availability of CT and MRI, accurate diagnosis is possible. The actual incidence may be higher, as patients may be asymptomatic. Many patients with cortical venous thrombosis show signs of seizure activity, and affected patients should be treated with phenytoin.[56] The patient should receive a loading dose of 10 mg/kg followed by 300 to 500 mg orally each day. Phenytoin levels should be checked frequently to make certain that they are therapeutic and that phenytoin toxicity does not develop. Some

TABLE 6-13
MEDICATIONS COMMONLY USED TO TREAT MIGRAINES

Medication	Class	Use	Dosage	Route of Administration	Safe for Pregnancy
Acetaminophen	Pain reliever	Acute pain	4 gm/day maximum	po or pr	Yes
Codeine	Narcotic	Acute pain	30–90 mg q 3–4 h	po	Yes
Meperidine	Narcotic	Acute pain	25–100 mg q 3–6 h	po, IM, or IV	Yes
Ibuprofen	Nonsteroidal	Acute pain	2400 mg/day in divided doses	po	Do not use in late pregnancy
Prochloroperazine	Phenothiazine	Nausea	5–25 mg q 2–8 h depending on route	po, pr, IM, or IV	Yes
Promethazine	Phenothiazine	Nausea	12.5–50 mg q 2–8 h depending on route	po, pr, IM, or IV	Yes
Butalbital (50 mg), acetaminophen (325 mg) caffeine (40 mg)	Sedative, pain reliever, vasoconstrictor	Acute migraine	2 tablets every 4 h, not to exceed 6 tablets daily	po	Yes
Isometheptene mucate (65 mg), Dichloraphenazone (100 mg), Acetaminophen (325 mg)	Vasoconstrictor, sedative, pain reliever	Acute migraine	2 capsules immediately followed by one hourly for no more than 5 capsules in 12 hours	po	Yes
Caffeine	Vasoconstrictor	Acute pain	500 mg in 50 ml IV solution—may repeat	po or IV	Yes
Sumatriptin	Vasoconstrictor	Acute pain	300 mg/day po max 6 mg sq X 2/day max	po or subcutaneous	Probably not
Ergotamine with caffeine	Vasoconstrictor	Acute pain	2 mg/200 mg (po), then 1 mg/100 mg q 1/2 h for 6 tab/day max; or 2 mg/100 mg pr and repeat once in 1 h	po or pr	No
Nortriptyline	Tricyclic	Prophylaxis	25–100 mg qhs	po	Yes
Amitriptyline	Tricyclic	Prophylaxis	50–150 mg qhs	po	Yes
Fluoxetine	SSRI	Prophylaxis	24–40 mg qhs	po	Probably
Propranolol	β-blocker	Prophylaxis	80–120 mg bid	po	Caution for IUGR
Nadolol	β-blocker	Prophylaxis	20–80 mg qd	po	Caution for IUGR
Atenolol	β-blocker	Prophylaxis	25–100 mg qd	po	Caution for IUGR
Carbamazepine	Membrane stabilizer	Prophylaxis	Up to 1200 mg/day in three divided doses	po	Risk of NTD, ? other problems

neurosurgeons are advocating expectant management and do not routinely give anticonvulsants. Whether these patients need prophylactic anticoagulation in a subsequent pregnancy remains debatable. Clearly, if the patient has an underlying hypercoagulable state, anticoagulation should be undertaken in a future pregnancy.

SUBARACHNOID HEMORRHAGE

Epidemiology

The rate of subarachnoid hemorrhage complicating pregnancy is approximately 1 per 10,400.[60] With the increase in cocaine abuse occurring across the country, this incidence is probably higher, as the associated increase in vasospasm associated with this drug may lead to bleeding from preexisting berry aneurysms and arteriovenous (AV) malformations.[61]

Most subarachnoid hemorrhages that occur in pregnant patients are caused by either rupture of a berry aneurysm or bleeding from a congenital AV malformation. Most berry aneurysms are located in the vessels of the circle of Willis or those arising from it.

Robinson and co-workers[62] evaluated 26 patients with spontaneous subarachnoid hemorrhage during pregnancy and found that approximately one-half were caused by berry aneurysms and one-half by AV malformations. They observed that AV malformations were more common in patients below the age of 25 years and usually bled before 20 weeks of gestation. Conversely, berry aneurysms were more likely to occur in patients over the age of 30 years and usually bled in the third trimester.[62] Pregnancy appears to increase the risk of bleeding from an AV malformation. The maternal mortality rate associated with an untreated AV malformation is reported to be 33%. This figure, however, is based on old data, and the rate is most certainly significantly lower today.

Diagnosis and Treatment

Any patient with localized signs of cerebral or meningeal irritation must be thoroughly evaluated. If the clinical examination is suggestive of intracranial hemorrhage, MRI or a CT scan should be performed. If necessary, contrast dyes may be used. MRI angiography may also be a valuable study. The dyes employed in CT scanning contain nonradioactive iodine, but the chance of inducing a fetal goiter is small. If there is no sign of increased intracranial pressure on scanning, a spinal fluid examination should be performed to look for blood and rule out infection. If there is evidence of bleeding, angiography may be indicated. Cerebral angiography can be safely used to pinpoint the origin of cerebral bleeding. Subarachnoid hemorrhages, whether caused by AV malformations or berry aneurysms, should be treated surgically when possible. Surgery under hypothermia or hypotension appears to cause no adverse fetal effects. The fetal heart rate should be monitored. If fetal bradycardia occurs, blood pressure should be raised sufficiently to normalize the fetal heart rate.[63]

The patient who has undergone corrective surgery for an aneurysm or AV malformation should be allowed to deliver vaginally. Because the Valsalva maneuver can increase intracranial pressure,[62] epidural anesthesia is recommended. Interestingly, Szabo and colleagues[64] have reported that moderate increases in blood pressure do not cause spontaneous hemorrhage in nonpregnant patients with intracranial AV malformations. If the aneurysm or AV malformation has not been surgically corrected, some authors have advocated elective cesarean delivery after documentation of fetal lung maturity.[62] Laidler and colleagues[65] have reviewed the advantages of regional anesthesia in these patients.

As pregnancy has a deleterious effect on AV malformations, patients with inoperable lesions should be counseled about the dangers of future childbearing. Previously, permanent sterilization was encouraged.[62] With improved imaging techniques, the patient should be thoroughly evaluated before any recommendations are made for permanent sterilization.

Venous-venous (VV) malformations are low-pressure phenomena. Affected pregnancies usually progress to term, and patients deliver vaginally without any hemorrhagic event or complications.

MULTIPLE SCLEROSIS

Multiple sclerosis (MS) is a demyelinating disease that attacks men and women with equal frequency. The onset of symptoms usually occurs between the ages of 20 and 40 years. In the United States, the disease is more common in those residing above 40 degrees north latitude. The prevalence for those living in the southern United States is 10 per 100,000, while it is approximately 50 per 100,000 in those living in the northern states.[66]

In the past, the diagnosis of MS was often made years after the initial onset of sensory symptoms. With the advent of MRI scanning, the diagnosis is now being made earlier. The onset is usually subtle. Common presenting symptoms include weakness of one or both lower extremities, visual complaints, and loss of coordination. Because the disease primarily affects the white matter of the central nervous system, symptoms attributable to disruption of gray matter are uncommon. The disease is characterized by exacerbations and remissions. Less than one-third of patients show steady progression of their disease after its onset.

It is impossible to predict the long-range prognosis of a patient with MS. About one-half of patients are still able to work at their usual profession 10 years after the onset of the illness. After 20 years, however, only about one-third remain employed. In a study of 185 women with MS, Weinshenker and colleagues[58] showed that there was no association between long-term disability and (1) total number of term pregnancies, (2) the timing of pregnancy relative to the onset of MS, or (3) the worsening of MS in relation to a pregnancy. The average life expectancy in patients with MS is also impossible to predict. Patients may live with the disease for more than 25 years. When death occurs, it is usually attributable to infection.

MS and pregnancy can coexist without unusual complications. Liebowitz and colleagues[68] found no decrease in fertility and no increase in perinatal mortality in patients with MS. Their study suggested that pregnancy does not predispose a patient to MS but that patients with "premorbid" disease are more likely to have the onset of early symptoms during pregnancy.

In fact, Runmanker and Andersen[69] demonstrated that the risk of onset of MS is reduced during gestation while the risk of onset during the postpartum period was no different than during the nonpregnant state. Furthermore, these investigators demonstrated a lower risk of onset of MS in parous than in nulliparous patients. Of 170 pregnant patients with MS studied by Millar and coworkers,[70] relapses occurred in only 45, the majority during the puerperium and postpartum periods. Birk and co-investigators[71] carefully followed pregnancies in eight women with MS. None of the women worsened during pregnancy.

However, six of the eight women experienced relapses within the first 7 weeks after delivery.

Frith and McLeod[72] studied 85 pregnancies and found no increased risk of relapse during pregnancy. They noted that most of the relapses that did occur during pregnancy took place in the third trimester. In another series, Frith and McLeod[73] reported that relapses occurred most frequently in the last trimester and also in the first 3 months postpartum. In a large study, Nelson and colleagues[74] analyzed 191 pregnancies in women with nonprogressive MS. The exacerbation rate during the 9-month postpartum period was 34%, three times the rate during the 9 months of pregnancy. The rate was highest in the 3 months immediately following delivery and stabilized after the sixth postpartum month.[74] The exacerbation rates were the same in breast-feeding and non–breast-feeding women.

Berbardi and colleagues showed a decreased risk of relapse during the 9 months of pregnancy and the first 6 months postpartum.[75] Worthington et al.[76] found more frequent relapses only in the first 6 months postpartum. Long-term prognosis was unaffected by pregnancy.[76] Verdru et al.[77] demonstrated that pregnancy delayed the onset of long-term disability. In patients with at least one pregnancy after the onset of disease, the mean time to dependence on a wheelchair was 18.6 years, as compared with 12.5 years for other women.[77] This study did not take into account the severity of the disease. Perhaps more-symptomatic women never became pregnant.

Late in the course of multiple sclerosis, women may be wheelchair-dependent and thus become more susceptible to asymptomatic urinary-tract infections during pregnancy. Therefore, they should be screened routinely. If the patient has a significant sensory deficit as a result of MS, there may be little pain associated with labor. It might be difficult, therefore, for the patient to discern when labor begins. Uterine contractions occur normally, but voluntary expulsive efforts may be hindered in the second stage of labor. Delivery by forceps or vacuum extraction may be indicated. Bader and colleagues[78] report that women with MS who receive epidural anesthesia for vaginal delivery do not have a significantly higher incidence of exacerbation of their MS postpartum than those receiving only local anesthesia.

PSEUDOTUMOR CEREBRI

Pseudotumor cerebri may complicate as many as 1 in 870 births.[79] The association of this disorder with pregnancy, oral contraceptive use, and obesity remains controversial.[80-81] More than 95% of patients with pseudotumor cerebri present with headaches, and 15% have diplopia. Papilledema is found in virtually all patients.[82] To establish the diagnosis, one must demonstrate elevated cerebrospinal fluid (CSF) pressure, normal CSF composition, and the absence of an intracranial mass on MRI or CT scan.[83]

Pregnancy outcome appears to be unaffected by the illness.[80,82] There is no increase in fetal wastage or congenital anomalies.[80] Koppel and colleagues[84] reported a case of pseudotumor cerebri that presented in a 15-year-old primigravida following eclampsia. It lasted for 3 weeks. Wheatley and colleagues[85] noted a case of pseudotumor cerebri occurring in the pregnancy of a diabetic woman. They caution that it is important to make the distinction between symptoms of pseudotumor cerebri and visual impairment caused by diabetic retinopathy, as the treatments are different.[85] Thomas[86] described a case of pseudotumor cerebri occurring in two consecutive pregnancies in a woman with hemoglobin SC. In both instances, symptoms resolved following delivery and both infants were born at term.

Most patients respond well to conservative treatment.[79] The main objectives of treatment are relief of pain and preservation of vision. The patient should be followed closely with visual acuity and visual field determinations at intervals indicated by the clinical condition. In patients with mild disease, analgesics may be adequate. If pain persists, diuretics may be used. Acetazolamide, a carbonic anhydrase inhibitor, will reduce CSF production in many patients.[87] The usual dose is 500 mg twice daily. In more difficult cases, prednisone in doses of 40 to 60 mg daily may provide improved results.[79] Patients may be treated for 2 weeks, with the dose being tapered over the next month.[80] Serial lumbar punctures to reduce CSF pressure are rarely necessary today. Surgical approaches are reserved for patients with refractory disease, in whom rapid visual deterioration occurs. Surgical procedures usually shunt CSF from the spinal canal into the abdominal cavity.

Pseudotumor cerebri is not an indication for cesarean delivery. A review of the literature reveals that 73% of the reported patients delivered vaginally.[82] Cesarean delivery should be undertaken only for obstetric indications. Both epidural and spinal anesthesia, when expertly administered, can be safely used in patients with pseudotumor cerebri.[88] The Valsalva maneuver, which can increase CSF pressure, should be avoided when possible, and the second stage of labor should be shortened by outlet forceps or vacuum extraction. The recurrence rate for pseudo-tumor cerebri is between 10 and 12% in nonpregnant patients. Pregnancy does not appear to predispose to a recurrence.[80]

CARPAL-TUNNEL SYNDROME

The medial border of the carpal tunnel consists of the pisiform and hamate bones, and its lateral border consists of the scaphoid and trapezium bones. They are covered on the palmar surface by the flexor retinaculum. The median nerve and flexor tendons pass through this carpal tunnel, which has little room for expansion. If the wrist is extremely flexed or extended, the volume of the carpal tunnel is further reduced. In pregnancy, weight gain and edema can produce the carpal-tunnel syndrome that results from compression of the median nerve. Wallace and Cook[89] first reported the association between carpal-tunnel syndrome and pregnancy in 1957. Although 20% of pregnant women report pain on the palmar surface of the hand, the incidence of true carpal-tunnel syndrome in pregnancy remains unknown. Commonly, the syndrome consists of pain, numbness, and/or tingling in the distribution of the median nerve in the hand and wrist. This distribution includes the thumb, index finger, long finger, and radial side of the ring finger on the palmar aspect. These sensations often waken the patient. Compressing the median nerve and percussing the wrist and forearm with a reflex hammer (Tinel maneuver) often exacerbates the pain. In severe cases, weakness and decreased motor function can occur.

McClennan and co-workers[90] studied 1216 consecutive pregnancies. Of these patients, 427 (35%) reported hand symptoms. Fewer than 20% of these 427 women described the classic carpal-tunnel syndrome. No patient required operative intervention. Most symptoms were bilateral and commenced in the third trimester of pregnancy. Ekman-Ordeberg et al.[81] found a 2.3% incidence of carpal-tunnel syndrome in a prospective study of 2538 pregnancies. The syndrome appeared to be more common in primigravidas with generalized edema. Conservative therapy with splinting of the wrist at night completely relieved symptoms in 46 of 56 patients. Of the remaining 10, three required surgery before delivery. Wand[92] retrospectively studied 40 women with carpal-tunnel syndrome that developed in pregnancy and 18 women with carpal-tunnel syndrome that developed in the puerperium. He confirmed that the syndrome occurs most frequently in primigravidas

over the age of 30 years. All cases that developed before delivery occurred during the third trimester and resolved within 2 weeks after delivery. In the cases that developed during the puerperium in women who breast-fed their infants, the symptoms lasted longer, a mean of 5.8 months.[92] In another series, Wand[93] studied 27 women in whom carpal-tunnel syndrome developed during the puerperium. The condition was associated with breast-feeding in 24 of these women. Symptoms lasted an average of 6.5 months in the breast-feeding women. Only two of these patients required surgical decompression.[93]

Supportive and conservative therapies are usually adequate for the treatment of carpal-tunnel syndrome. Symptoms usually subside in the postpartum period as total body water returns to normal. Splints placed on the volar surface of the hand, which keep the wrist in a neutral position and maximize the capacity of the carpal tunnel, often provide dramatic relief. Local injections of glucocorticoids may also be used in severe cases. In an uncontrolled series, Ellis[94] reported that pyridoxine in a dose of 100 to 200 mg daily for 12 weeks can provide relief in a large percentage of patients with carpal-tunnel syndrome. However, before this therapy can be recommended, controlled trials need to be undertaken.

Surgical correction of this syndrome should not be delayed in patients with deteriorating muscle tone and motor function. Electromyography can be used to confirm this deterioration. Decompression surgery for carpal-tunnel syndrome is a simple procedure that can be safely carried out during pregnancy using local anesthesia, an axillary block, or a Bier block. With new endoscopic procedures, the procedure is even less invasive. It is important to warn patients that carpal-tunnel syndrome can recur in future pregnancies.[95]

REFERENCES

1. Cramer JA, Jones EE. Reproductive function in epilepsy. Epilepsia 1991;32(Suppl 6):S19.
2. Back DJ, Bates M, Bowden A, et al. The interaction of phenobarbital and other anticonvulsants with oral contraceptive steroid therapy. Contraception 1980;22:495.
3. Coulam CB, Annegers JF. Do anticonvulsants reduce the efficacy of oral contraceptives? Epilepsia 1979;20:519.
4. Janz D, Schmidt D. Anti-epileptic drugs and failure of oral contraceptives. Lancet 1974;1:1113.
5. Knight AH, Rhind EG. Epilepsy and pregnancy: a study of 153 pregnancies in 59 patients. Epilepsia 1975;16:99.
6. Schmidt D, Canger R, Avanzini G, et al. Change of seizure frequency in pregnant epileptic women. J Neurol Neurosurg Psychiatry 1983;46:751.
7. Tanganelli P, Regesta G. Epilepsy, pregnancy, and major

birth anomalies: an Italian prospective, controlled study. Neurology 1992;42(Suppl 5):89.

8. Ogawa Y, Kaneko S, Otani K, Fukushima Y. Serum folic acid in epileptic mothers and their relationship to congenital malformations. Epilepsy Res 1991;8:75.

9. Milunsky A, Jick H, Jick SS, et al. Multivitamin/folic acid supplementation in early pregnancy reduces the prevalence of neural tube defects. JAMA 1989;262:2847.

10. Mountain KR, Hirsh J, Gallus AS. Neonatal coagulation defect due to anticonvulsant drug treatment in pregnancy. Lancet 1970;1:265.

11. Bleyer WA, Skinner AL. Fatal neonatal hemorrhage after maternal anticonvulsant therapy. JAMA 1976;235:626.

12. Yerby M, Koepsell T, Daling J. Pregnancy complications and outcomes in a cohort of women with epilepsy. Epilepsia 1985;26:631.

13. Nelson KB, Ellenberg JH. Maternal seizure disorder, outcome of pregnancy, and neurologic abnormalities in the children of women with epilepsy. Neurology 1982; 32:1247.

14. Kallen B. A register study of maternal epilepsy and delivery outcome with special reference to drug use. Acta Neurol Scand 1986;73:253.

15. Hiilesmaa VK, Bardy A, Teramo K. Obstetric outcome in women with epilepsy. Am J Obstet Gynecol 1985; 152:499.

16. Matroiacovo P, Bertollini R, Licata D. Fetal growth in the offspring of epileptic women: results of an Italian multicentric cohort study. Acta Neurol Scand 1988;78:110.

17. Hiilesmaa VK, Teramo K, Granstrom ML. Fetal head growth retardation associated with maternal antiepileptic drugs. Lancet 1981;1:165.

18. Hanson JW, Smith DW. The fetal hydantoin syndrome. J Pediatr 1975;87:285.

19. Hanson JW, Myrianthopoulos NC, Sedgwick Harvey MA, Smith DW. Risks to the offspring of women treated with hydantoin anticonvulsants, with emphasis on the fetal hydantoin syndrome. J Pediatr 1976;89:662.

20. Gaily E, Granstrom ML, Hiilesmaa V, Bardy A. Minor anomalies in offspring of epileptic mothers. J Pediatr 1988;112:520.

21. Friis ML, Holm NV, Sindrup EH, et al. Facial clefts in sibs and children of epileptic patients. Neurology 1986;36:346.

22. Kelly TE, Rein M, Edwards P. Teratogenicity of anticonvulsant drugs. Am J Med Genet 1984;19:451.

23. Nakane Y, Okuma T, Takahashi R, et al. Multi-institutional study on the teratogenicity and fetal toxicity of antiepileptic drugs: a report of a collaborative study group in Japan. Epilepsia 1980;21:663.

24. Kaneko S, Otani K, Fukushima Y, et al. Teratogenicity of antiepileptic drugs: analysis of possible risk factors. Epilepsia 1988;29:459.

25. Lindhout D, Omtziget JGC, Cornel MC. Spectrum of neural-tube defects in 34 infants prenatally exposed to antiepileptic drugs. Neurology 1992;42(Suppl 5):111.

26. Kaneko S, Otani K, Kondo T, et al. Malformation in infants of mothers with epilepsy receiving antiepileptic drugs. Neurology 1992;42(Suppl 5):68.

27. Dravet C, Julian C, Legras C, et al. Epilepsy, antiepileptic drugs, and malformations in children of women with epilepsy: a French prospective cohort study. Neurology 1992;42 (Suppl 5):75.

28. Koch S, Losche G, Jager-Roman E, et al. Major and minor birth malformations and antiepileptic drugs. Neurology 1992;42(Suppl 5):83.

29. Gaily E, Granstrom ML. Minor anomalies in children of mothers with epilepsy. Neurology 1992;42(Suppl 5):128.

30. DiLiberti JH, Farndon PA, Dennis NR, Curry CJR. The fetal valproate syndrome. Am J Med Genet 1984;19:473.

31. Ardinger HH, Atkin JF, Blackston RD, et al. Verification of the fetal valproate syndrome phenotype. Am J Med Genet 1988;29:171.

32. Lindhout D, Schmidt D. In-utero exposure to valproate and neural tube defects. Lancet 1986;2:1392.

33. Jones KL, Lacro RV, Johnson KA, Adams J. Pattern of malformations in the children of women treated with carbamazepine during pregnancy. N Engl J Med 1989; 320:1661.

34. Rosa FW. Spina bifida in infants of women treated with carbamazepine during pregnancy. N Engl J Med 1991; 324:674.

35. Finnell RH, Buehler BA, Kerr BM, et al. Clinical and experimental studies linking oxidative metabolism to phenytoin-induced teratogenesis. Neurology 1992; 42(Suppl 5):25.

36. Gaily E, Kantola-Sorbu E, Granstrom ML. Intelligence of children of epileptic mothers. J Pediatr 1988;113:677.

37. Dansky LV, Andermann E, Rosenblatt D, et al. Anticonvulsants, folate levels, and pregnancy outcome: a prospective study. Ann Neurol 1987;21:176.

38. Granstrom ML, Gaily E. Psychomotor development in children of mothers with epilepsy. Neurology 1991; 42(Suppl 5):144.

39. Blandfort M, Tsuboi T, Vogel F. Genetic counseling in the epileptics. Hum Genet 1987;76:303.

40. Bronshtein M, Zimmer EZ, Gerlis LM, et al. Early ultrasound diagnosis of fetal congenital heart defects in high-risk and low-risk pregnancies. Obstet Gynecol 1993; 82:225.

41. Wigton TR, Sabbagha RE, Tamura RK, et al. Sonographic diagnosis of congenital heart disease: comparison between the four chamber view and multiple cardiac views. Obstet Gynecol 1993;82:219.

42. Yerby MS. Problems and management of the pregnant woman with epilepsy. Epilepsia 1987;28(Suppl 3):S29.

43. Kaneko S, Sato T, Suzuki K. The levels of anticonvulsants in breast milk. Br J Clin Pharmacol 1974;7:624.

44. Mattson RH, Cramer JA, Darney PD, Naftolin F. Use of oral contraceptives by women with epilepsy. JAMA 1986; 256:238.

45. Orme MLE. The clinical pharmacology of oral contraceptive steroids. Br J Clin Pharmacol 1982;14:31.

46. Callaghan P. The migraine syndrome in pregnancy. Neurology 1968;18:197.

47. Somerville B. A study of migraine in pregnancy. Neurology 1972;22:824.

48. Friedman AP, Merritt HH. Headache, prognosis and treatment. Philadelphia: FA Davis, 1959.

49. Lance JW, Anthony MD. Some clinical aspects of migraine. Arch Neurol 1966;15:356.

50. Granella F, Sances G, Zanferrar C, et al. Migraine without aura and reproductive life events: a clinical epidemiological study of 1300 women. Headache 1993;33:385.

51. Chen TC, Leviton A, Edelstein S, Ellenberg JH. Migraine

and other diseases in women of reproductive age: the influence of smoking on observed associations. Arch Neurol 1987;44:1024.

52. Chancellor AM, Wroe SJ, Cull RE. Migraine occurring for the first time in pregnancy. Headache 1990;30:224.

53. Maizels M, Scott B, Cohen W, Chen W. Intranasal lidocaine for treatment of migraine: a randomized, double-blind, controlled trial. JAMA 1996;276:319.

54. Kudrow L, Kudrow DB, Sandweiss JH. Rapid and sustained relief of migraine attacks with intranasal lidocaine: preliminary findings. Headache 1995;35:79.

55. Hughes HE, Goldstein DA. Birth defects following maternal exposure to ergotamine, beta blocker, and caffeine. J Med Genet 1988;25:396.

56. Estanol B, Rodriguez A, Counte G, et al. Intracranial venous thrombosis in young women. Stroke 1979; 10:680.

57. Krayenbuhl HA. Cerebral venous and sinus thrombosis. Clin Neurosurg 1967;14:1.

58. Weinshenker BG, Hader W, Carriere W, et al. The influence of pregnancy on disability from multiple sclerosis: a population-based study in Middlesex County, Ontario. Neurology 1989;39:1438.

59. Abraham J, Rios PS, Inbaraj SG, et al. An epidemiological study of hemiplegia due to stroke in south India. Stroke 1970;1:477.

60. Miller HJ, Hinkley CM. Berry aneurysms in pregnancy: a ten year report. South Med J 1970;63:279.

61. Henderson CE, Torbey M. Rupture of intracranial aneurysm associated with cocaine use during pregnancy. Am J Perinatol 1988;5:142.

62. Robinson JL, Hall CJ, Sevzimer CB. Arterial venous malformations, aneurysms, and pregnancy. J Neurosurg 1974; 41:63.

63. Minielly R, Yuzpe AA, Drake CC. Subarachnoid hemorrhage secondary to ruptured cerebral aneurysm in pregnancy. Obstet Gynecol 1979;53:64.

64. Szabo MD, Crosby C, Sundaram P, et al. Hypertension does not cause spontaneous hemorrhage of intracranial arteriovenous malformations. Anesthesiology 1989;70:761.

65. Laidler JA, Jackson IJ, Redfern N. The management of cesarean section in a patient with an intracranial arteriovenous malformation. Anaesthesia 1989;44:490.

66. McAlpine D, Lunisden CE, Acheson ED. Multiple sclerosis, a reappraisal. 2nd ed. Williams & Wilkins, Baltimore, 1972.

67. Bansal BC, Prakash C, Gupta RR, Brahmanandam KRV. Study of serum lipid and blood fibrinolytic activity in cases of cerebral venous/venous sinus thrombosis during the puerperium. Am J Obstet Gynecol 1974;119:1079.

68. Liebowitz U, Antonovosky A, Katz R, et al. Does pregnancy increase the risk of multiple sclerosis? J Neurol Neurosurg Psychiatry 1967;30:354.

69. Runmanker B, Andersen O. Pregnancy is associated with a lower risk of onset and a better prognosis in multiple sclerosis. Brain 1995;118:253.

70. Millar JHD, Allison RS, Cheeseman EA. Pregnancy as a factor in influencing relapse in disseminated multiple sclerosis. Brain 1959;82:417.

71. Birk K, Ford C, Smeltzer S, et al. The clinical course of multiple sclerosis during pregnancy and the puerperium. Arch Neurol 1990;47:738.

72. Frith JA, McLeod JC. Pregnancy and multiple sclerosis. J Neurol Neurosurg Psychiatry 1988;51:595.

73. Frith JA, McLeod JG. Pregnancy and multiple sclerosis: an Australian perspective. Clin Exp Neurol 1987;24:1.

74. Nelson LM, Franklin GM, Jones MC. Risk of multiple sclerosis exacerbation during pregnancy and breastfeeding. JAMA 1988;259:3441.

75. Berbardi S, Grasso MG, Bertollini R, et al. The influences of pregnancy on relapses of multiple sclerosis: a cohort study. Acta Neurol Scand 1991;84:403.

76. Worthington J, Jones R, Crawford M, Fort A. Pregnancy and multiple sclerosis—a 3 year prospective study. J Neurol 1994;241:228.

77. Verdru P, Theys P, Beartrijs M, et al. Pregnancy and multiple sclerosis: the influence on longterm disability. Clin Neurol Neurosurg 1994;96:38.

78. Bader Am, Hunt CO, Datta S, et al. Anesthesia for the obstetric patient with multiple sclerosis. J Clin Anesth 1988;1:21.

79. Katz VL, Peterson R, Cefalo RC. Pseudotumor cerebri and pregnancy. Am J Perinatol 6:442, 1989.

80. Peteson CM, Kelly JV. Pseudotumor cerebri in pregnancy: case reports and literature reviewed. Obstet Gynecol Surv 1985;50:323.

81. Ireland B, Corbett JJ, Wallace RB. The search for causes of idiopathic intracranial hypertension: a preliminary case-control study. Arch Neurol 1990;47:315.

82. Koontz WL, Herbert WNP, Cefalo R. Pseudotumor cerebri in pregnancy. Obstet Gynecol 62:325, 1983

83. Donaldson JO. Neurology in pregnancy. Philadelphia: Saunders, 1978.

84. Koppel BS, Kaunitz AM, Tuchman AJ. Pseudotumor cerebri following eclampsia. Eur Neurol 1990;30:6.

85. Wheatley T, Clark JD, Edwards OM, Jordan K. Retinal haemorrhages and papilloedema due to benign intracranial hypertension in a pregnant diabetic. Diabetic Med 1986; 3:482.

86. Thomas E. Recurrent benign intracranial hypertension associated with hemoglobin SC disease in pregnancy. Obstet Gynecol 1986;67:7S.

87. Rubin RC, Henderson ES, Ommaya AK, et al. The production of cerebrospinal fluid in man and its modification by acetazolamide. J Neurosurg 1966;25:430.

88. Palop R, Choed-Amphai E, Miller R. Epidural anesthesia for delivery complicated by benign intracranial hypertension. Anesthesiology 1979;50:159.

89. Wallace JT, Cook AW. Carpal tunnel syndrome in pregnancy. Am J Gynecol 1957;73:1333.

90. McClennan HG, Oats JN, Walstab JE. Survey of hand symptoms in pregnancy. Med J Aust 1987;147:542.

91. Ekman-Ordeberg G, Salgeback S, Ordeberg G. Carpal tunnel syndrome in pregnancy: a prospective study. Acta Obstet Gynecol Scand 1987;66:233.

92. Wand JS. Carpal tunnel syndrome in pregnancy and lactation. J Hand Surg 1990;15:93.

93. Wand JS. The natural history of carpal tunnel syndrome in lactation. J R Soc Med 1989;82:349.

94. Ellis JM. Treatment of carpal tunnel syndrome with vitamin B6. South Med J 1987;80:882.

95. Tobin SM. Carpal tunnel syndrome in pregnancy. Am J Obstet Gynecol 1967;97:493.

COLLAGEN VASCULAR DISEASES

Philip Samuels

Five Key Points

- Systemic lupus erythematosus (SLE) is characterized by many clinical findings, including skin lesions, arthralgias and arthritis, nephritis, neurologic and psychiatric abnormalities, renal disease, and pericarditis.
- Exacerbations of SLE in pregnancy should be treated with glucocorticoids.
- Obstetric patients with a history of adverse pregnancy outcome (severe intrauterine growth restriction, recurrent losses, stillbirth) who test positive for the lupus anticoagulant and anticardiolipin antibodies should be treated with low-dose aspirin and heparin.
- Aspirin is the mainstay of therapy for pregnant patients with rheumatoid arthritis.
- Maternal myasthenia gravis poses a risk of neonatal myasthenia because of transplacental passage of antibodies that block transmission through the myoneural junction.

Collagen vascular diseases occur more commonly in women and often have their onset during the childbearing years. Although these diseases are infrequent, they will be seen in the pregnant population. Immune diseases encompass a large group of diseases, but this section will cover the more common collagen vascular diseases: systemic lupus erythematosus, rheumatoid arthritis, and myasthenia gravis. Patients with symptoms consistent with collagen vascular diseases can be screened with certain laboratory tests. These tests are outlined in Tables 6-14 and 6-15.

SYSTEMIC LUPUS ERYTHEMATOSUS

Systemic lupus erythematosus (SLE) is a chronic disease characterized by exacerbations and remissions. It can involve a large number of body systems. Therefore, diagnosis is difficult, and definitive diagnosis is often delayed. The prevalence of SLE is approximately 1 in 1000 in the general population. In women of childbearing years, the prevalence is greater than 1 in 500. In African-American women in childbearing years, the prevalence is as high as 1 in 245.[1,2] The diagnosis of SLE is based on fulfillment of specific criteria set forth by the American Rheumatism Association, which can be found in any rheumatology textbook.

Clinical Manifestations

The disease is often insidious in onset. Skin lesions are the hallmark of 80% of patients with SLE. The lesions may include the classic butterfly (malar) rash, hair loss, or raised (discoid) lesions. Patients with skin lesions often experience photosensitivity. In 90% of patients with SLE, arthralgias with some arthritis are common. Roughly half of patients experience nephritis, neurologic, or psychiatric symptoms.

TABLE 6-14
AUTOANTIBODIES OF CLINICAL SIGNIFICANCE
TO THE OBSTETRICIAN

Antibody	Disease
Antinuclear antibodies (ANA)	All collagen diseases
Anti-double-stranded DNA antibodies	Very sensitive and specific for SLE
Antiextractable nuclear antibodies (includes anti-Sm, anti-RNP, anti-SSA, anti-SSB)	SLE, Sjögren syndrome, other collagen vascular diseases
Antimicrobial antibodies	Hashimoto thyroiditis
Antineutrophil cytoplasmic antibodies (ANCA)	Wegener granulomatosis, polyarteritis nodosa
Antimitochondrial antibodies	Primary biliary cirrhosis
Antiscleroderma (SCL)-70 antibodies	Scleroderma and progressive systemic sclerosis
Anti-PM-1	Polymyositis
Anti-RANA	Rheumatoid arthritis
Antiplatelet antibodies (direct and indirect)	Immune thrombocytopenic purpura

The most serious abnormalities that occur in SLE include renal and cardiac lesions. The renal lesions include glomerulonephritis (proliferative or membranous) and mesangial nephritis. Proteinuria, varying in severity, is found in patients with glomerulonephritis. Proteinuria can often be a marker of disease activity. The neurologic symptoms of SLE may include seizures or peripheral neuropathy. The psychiatric features often include a psychotic episode. The most common cardiac manifestation is pericarditis.

Laboratory Diagnosis

More than 90% of patients with SLE exhibit significant titers of antinuclear antibodies (ANAs). In 80 to 90% of patients, an autoantibody will be directed against double-stranded DNA. Ten percent of patients with SLE will have anti-DNA antibodies but not ANAs. Therefore, when the index of suspicion is high,

tests for identification of double-stranded DNA antibodies should be obtained even when the ANA count is negative.

Anti-DNA antibodies can be divided into subclasses. The high-affinity antibodies are seen more commonly in patients with renal involvement, while the low-affinity antibodies are seen in milder forms of the disease. Extractable nuclear antibodies can be subdivided into antibodies against ribonuclear proteins (anti-RNP, anti-SM), anti-SSA, and anti-SSB. Anti-RNP antibodies are seen in 26% of patients with SLE; anti-SM antibodies are found in 28% of these patients. Anti-SSA and anti-SSB antibodies, more commonly found in patients with Sjögren's syndrome, are present in 25% and 12% of patients with SLE, respectively. These antibodies have been associated with fetal and neonatal heart block in a small number of patients. Antihistone antibodies are seen in approximately 50% of patients with SLE. They are present in over 90% of patients with drug-induced lupus and are, therefore, useful in making this diagnosis.

The Effect of Pregnancy on SLE

It is debatable whether pregnancy acutely affects SLE activity.[3,4] Mintz and colleagues[5] found an increased risk of lupus exacerbation during pregnancy and the postpartum period. All patients responded to glucocorticoid therapy. Other studies, however, have not shown an increased risk of flare-ups.[6-8] The most convincing study in this respect was a prospective study performed by Lockshin,[6] who concluded that there is no need for prophylactic glucocorticoids in pregnant patients with SLE who have not previously required steroids.

Maternal morbidity and mortality are increased in the patient with SLE. Most maternal deaths occur

TABLE 6-15
SIGNIFICANCE OF DIFFERENT PATTERNS OF ANTINUCLEAR ANTIBODIES

ANA Pattern	Differential Diagnosis
Homogeneous	Often seen in false positive tests. May be associated with almost any collagen vascular disease, as well as chronic active hepatitis and drug-induced lupus. This pattern does very little to help the clinician refine a diagnosis.
Speckled	SLE, rheumatoid arthritis, Sjögren syndrome, mixed connective-tissue disease
Nucleolar	Scleroderma, progressive systemic sclerosis, SLE, Sjögren syndrome
Centromere	Scleroderma, CREST syndrome

during the puerperium as a result of pulmonary hemorrhage or lupus pneumonitis.[9,10] Pneumonitis is due to vasculitis in the lungs and may result in pulmonary hypertension and eventual death. Cardiac tamponade has also been reported in postpartum patients with SLE.[11] Clinicians must also realize that patients who are immunosuppressed from long-term glucocorticoid therapy are at increased risk for secondary opportunistic infection during pregnancy.

Women with lupus nephritis must be aware of the small but significant risk of permanent deterioration of renal function during pregnancy, an effect that occurs in up to 10% of patients.[12] Others have suggested a higher rate of deterioration of renal function during pregnancy, perhaps as high as 50%.[13] However, the sample size in these studies was small. The largest summary of studies reported a 7.1% incidence of permanent renal dysfunction and a 30.2% incidence of transient renal dysfunction during gestation.[14] In this review, the transient renal deterioration usually occurred in the third trimester. Clinicians must also remember that poor pregnancy outcome is associated with active lupus nephropathy.[15] A serum creatinine of at least 1.5 mg/dl, a blood urea nitrogen (BUN) level greater than 50 mg/dl, and a creatinine clearance of less than 50 ml/min are indicative of poor pregnancy outcome.[15,16]

Most maternal–fetal medicine specialists advise patients with SLE not to conceive during the time of increased lupus activity. Increased lupus activity is associated with increased flare-ups during pregnancy. The best study supporting this observation was performed by Mintz and colleagues.[5] In general, a patient's disease should be quiescent for about 6 months prior to conception. Hayslett and Lynn[17] observed that pregnancy outcome was good in 92% of women whose lupus had been in remission for at least 6 months prior to conception.

It may be difficult to differentiate a lupus flare-up from preeclampsia because they have similar signs and symptoms. Both disorders often present with proteinuria, edema, and hypertension. To make the issue more confusing, patients with lupus nephropathy are at an increased risk for superimposed preeclampsia developing during gestation. It is difficult, but essential, to make the distinction between these two phenomena. The therapy for the two are at different ends of the therapeutic spectrum. The treatment for preeclampsia is delivery, while the treatment for lupus nephritis is administration of glucocorticoids and possibly azathioprine. Complement levels may be helpful in making the distinction. However, complement levels normally rise during pregnancy so a patient's complement level may have fallen from a previous determination but still be within normal limits. Base-line complement levels, therefore, are important in these patients. Obviously, if the diagnosis of preeclampsia is made, obstetric intervention is required. If preeclampsia develops very early in pregnancy, it can result in major neonatal morbidity and/or mortality. Accordingly, it is essential to distinguish between the two conditions, even to the point of performing a renal biopsy to distinguish between SLE and preeclampsia.

SLE can have adverse effects on pregnancy in each trimester. In the first trimester the spontaneous abortion rate is increased, with an incidence somewhere between 16 and 40%.[18-21] The risk of abortion is not necessarily related to disease activity.[5] In one study, patients with Sjögren's syndrome were compared with patients with SLE, and both were compared with controls. The relative risk of fetal loss was elevated in patients with Sjögren's syndrome and those with SLE.[22] In the third trimester, intrauterine growth restriction (IUGR) is more frequent in patients with SLE.[23] There is a high risk of prematurity in infants born to mothers with SLE, usually because of associated conditions such as IUGR, chronic hypertension, and preeclampsia. It also appears that preterm premature rupture of the membranes may be responsible for a significant percentage of the preterm births that occur in women with SLE.[24] Johnson et al. found that 39% of those delivering prematurely had experienced preterm premature rupture of the membranes.[25] This complication was not related to the effect of glucocorticoid treatment, level of disease activity, or level of abnormal antibodies. In this investigation, preterm premature rupture of the membranes was the most frequent cause of preterm delivery.

Since the late 1980s, the lupus inhibitor (lupus anticoagulant) and anticardiolipin (antiphospholipid) antibodies have been the subject of intense research and speculation. The identification of lupus inhibitors is often confusing. No single assay can be used to identify these substances, and different reference laboratories use different coagulation assays to make the diagnosis. The initial screening test should be identification of a prolonged activated partial thromboplastin time (APTT) using platelet-poor plasma. However, a sensitive reagent must be used to avoid false negative results. Other commonly used coagulation assays include the tissue thromboplastin inhibition test, the Kaolin clotting time, and the dilute Russell viper venom time. The hexagonal antibody test has also shown promising results. This variety of tests makes it difficult for the critical reader to compare different studies concerning the role of lupus inhibitor in pregnancy outcome. As patients' insurance carriers change and require the physician to use different laboratories, patients may have tests repeated in various laboratories, thus confusing the diagnosis even more.

There is also confusion surrounding the difference between anticardiolipin antibodies and antiphospholipid antibodies. Antiphospholipid antibodies encompass many phospholipids—cardiolipin is merely one of these. Although many clinicians may use the terms interchangeably, the lupus inhibitor and anticardiolipin antibodies are distinct entities. The correlation between the two is imperfect.[25] Different researchers have shown that these antibodies are causes of poor pregnancy outcomes.[26-31]

Although several therapy options have been investigated, none have really been tested in a controlled fashion. Shortly after the discovery of the relationship between lupus inhibitor, anticardiolipin antibodies, and pregnancy loss, university centers began to treat patients with prednisone and low-dose aspirin. Several studies have shown that heparin gives better results with fewer side effects. The standard of care now appears to be treatment of patients with heparin and low-dose aspirin throughout gestation. Some authors have used intravenous immunoglobulin with moderate success, but this form of therapy is very expensive. At present, low-molecular-weight heparin is gaining in popularity, but its price is prohibitively expensive. Its principal advantages as compared with conventional heparin are once-daily dosing and less frequent need for monitoring of anticoagulant effect.

The Effects of SLE on Pregnancy

In contrast to the study of Le Thi Huong et al.,[23] Leu and Lan[32] found that anti-SSA antibodies were associated with growth restriction in pregnancies complicated by SLE. The presence of these antibodies, however, did not affect perinatal mortality.

Treatment of patients with the lupus inhibitor and anticardiolipin antibodies remains controversial but is becoming more uniform. The mainstay of therapy is now low-dose aspirin and subcutaneous heparin. Gattenby et al.[33] showed a dramatic improvement in patients receiving only aspirin therapy for elevated anticardiolipin antibodies. In patients with elevated antibodies and SLE, the fetal wastage rate dropped from 88 to 55%. In those with elevated antibodies alone, the rate of loss fell from 79 to 25%.[33] Balasch and co-workers[34] studied 65 consecutive women with two or more spontaneous abortions. Seven (10.7%) were found to have anticardiolipin antibodies. Four of the seven women (57.1%) carried to term after being treated with low-dose aspirin alone. While the number of patients treated with aspirin alone is small, it appears that this therapy offers at least some benefit in patients who have anticardiolipin antibodies.

Heparin therapy was initially instituted in treating this disorder because infarctions were found in the placentas of patients with anticardiolipin antibodies. Rosove et al.[35] initiated heparin therapy at a mean gestational age of 10.3 weeks in 14 women with prior adverse pregnancy outcomes. The daily dosage ranged from 10,000 to 36,000 units. Live births occurred in 14 of 15 pregnancies (93.3%) with a mean gestational age of 36.1 weeks and a mean birth-weight percentile of 57%.[35] Heparin is now frequently used to treat patients with antiphospholipid antibodies. Low dose heparin has fewer side effects than prednisone, which was previously used to treat this array of disorders. Prednisone is associated with increased striae, induction of gestational diabetes mellitus, poor wound healing, increased frequency of candida infections, candidiasis, fluid retention, aseptic necrosis, cataracts, and other complications, especially when used in high doses. Branch et al.[36] found equivalent fetal survival when using heparin and aspirin; prednisone and aspirin; or heparin, prednisone, and aspirin. Maternal side effects were much less frequent with heparin and low-dose aspirin. This study included 82 pregnancies in 54 women. It showed that the diagnosis of SLE, a history of preeclampsia, a history of thrombosis, a false positive test for syphilis, and the titer of IgG anticardiolipin antibody did not correlate with the outcome of the current pregnancy.[36] The number of prior fetal deaths did correlate significantly with outcome in the current pregnancy. Some individuals are using low-molecular-weight heparin to treat lupus inhibitor/antiphospholipid antibodies. The benefits and drawbacks of this therapy are discussed in this chapter in the section on treatment of pulmonary embolism.

Intravenous immunoglobulin is currently being used by some in treating difficult patients with lupus inhibitor and/or antiphospholipid antibodies. Its mechanism of action is not entirely understood, but it may bind to receptors, preventing the binding of these deleterious antibodies. The correct dosage and dosage interval have not been delineated. Branch et al.[36] have used intravenous immunoglobulin with some success. Kaaja et al.[37] used high-dose immunoglobulin in conjunction with low-dose aspirin in four patients with good results. This therapy, however, remains experimental.

Anticardiolipin antibodies and the lupus inhibitor are associated with in vitro anticoagulation, but in vivo they are associated with thrombosis. Seropositive patients, therefore, are probably at some risk for thrombosis during gestation.[38-41] Mizoguchi et al.[40] described a 34-year-old woman with lupus inhibitor who had had six recurrent pregnancy losses without an intervening live birth. During her subsequent pregnancy, she developed multiple brain infarctions and hemiparesis. Rallings and co-workers[41] reported a 28-year-old primigravida in whom an acute anteroseptal myocardial infarction developed; she died during gestation. She had had a history of thromboembolism. The only serologic abnormality noted was an elevated level of IgG anticardiolipin antibody.

Our approach is to individualize therapy of patients with lupus inhibitor and antiphospholipid antibodies. We take the patient's history and laboratory results into account when making decisions regarding therapy. Unfortunately, patients are occasionally tested for this syndrome after having only one spontaneous abortion. If a patient has equivocal or weakly positive testing, we discourage therapy. For the patient whom we feel truly has this syndrome, we usually prescribe low-dose aspirin and heparin. We start the heparin dosing at 5000 units twice daily and increase to 10,000 units twice daily by term. Low-molecular-weight heparin is reserved for patients with sensitivity to the pork and beef components of fractionated heparin. The key in treating these patients is to make certain they understand the potential side effects of the prescribed medication regimen and that they undergo the proper fetal and maternal surveillance throughout pregnancy.

Neonatal Manifestations of SLE

Complete congenital heartblock, an infrequent complication of SLE, can be diagnosed prenatally. In the mid-trimester. a fetal heart rate of about 60 bpm with no baseline variability is indicative of congenital heart block. The patient should immediately undergo fetal echocardiography to rule out an associated congenital cardiac malformation. Doppler studies can also confirm an atrioventricular dissociation. Fetal echocardiography can usually be carried out at 20 to 24 weeks of gestation and even earlier in the asthenic patient. Affected fetuses usually show no evidence of congestive heart failure or hydrops. Nonetheless, they should be followed with serial ultrasonography every 1 to 2 weeks to determine if heart failure has developed. Complete congenital heart block in the fetus of a mother with SLE appears to be the result of immune complex deposition in fetal cardiac tissue as demonstrated by Litsey and co-workers.[42] Scott and colleagues[43] identified the anti-SSA(Ro) antibody in 83% of mothers delivering infants with complete congenital heart block. Anti-SSB(La) antibodies were found in a smaller but significant number of these mothers. Scheib and Waxman[44] have shown that these antibodies bind to fetal cardiac tissue. Derksen and Meilof[45] found that the presence, but not the titer, of anti-SSA antibody correlated with development of complete congenital heartblock.

Le Thi Huong[23] found manifestations of neonatal lupus in 3 of 22 infants whose mothers had anti-SSA antibody. Two had cutaneous manifestations and one had complete heart block. The titer of antibody did not appear to be related to the disease course. Conversely, Leu and Lan[32] found that patients with high-titer anti-SSA antibody had a greater chance of having a neonate with manifestations of lupus. Three of 257 women with this antibody gave birth to an infant with complete congenital heart block.[32] All three had high antibody titers.

In the absence of structural cardiac anomalies, the neonatal mortality rate for infants born with complete congenital heartblock is approximately 5%. In the studies of Vetter and Rashkad[46] and Esscher and Scott[47] the mortality rate was 20 to 30% if a structural abnormality was also found. With advances in pediatric cardiac surgery, the mortality rate is probably considerably lower now. Infants born to mothers with SLE may exhibit erythematous skin lesions of the face, scalp, and upper thorax.[23,48,49] These lesions usually disappear by 12 months of age.

Maternal and Fetal Surveillance

Because of the increased risk of adverse pregnancy outcome, the obstetrician caring for the patient with

SLE should insist on close maternal and fetal surveillance. Any patient with a history of SLE should undergo preconceptional counseling. Patients should have an examination of their urine sediment and a 24-hour urine collection for creatinine clearance and total protein excretion in early pregnancy to determine the extent of any renal compromise. They should have tests performed to detect the presence of the lupus inhibitor, anticardiolipin antibodies, anti-SSA(Ro) antibodies, and anti-SSB(La) antibodies. As previously described, these findings are associated with poorer pregnancy outcome. If indicated, therapy should be initiated after fully informing the patient of the risks and benefits to both her and the fetus. If anti-SSA or anti-SSB antibodies are present, fetal echocardiography should be performed in the second trimester to rule out complete congenital heart block.

Because of the risks of IUGR and preterm birth, accurate gestational dating is imperative in the patient with SLE. Menstrual dating should be confirmed by ultrasonography at the first prenatal visit. At 18 to 20 weeks of gestation an additional ultrasound examination should be performed to confirm gestational age, ascertain appropriate fetal growth, and make certain that fetal anatomy is normal. IUGR in patients with SLE is usually asymmetric. However,[23] Fine et al.[12] showed that symmetric IUGR can also occur. Because of the risk of IUGR and stillbirth, serial ultrasound examinations should be performed monthly after 20 weeks of gestation, with special attention to growth of the fetal abdomen, head, and femur.[50] The obstetrician should also be attentive to the volume of amniotic fluid, as decreased amniotic fluid can be the harbinger of fetal compromise and stillbirth.

At 28 weeks of gestation, weekly antepartum fetal heart rate testing should be initiated using the nonstress test. Antepartum fetal heart rate testing has been shown to improve fetal outcome in patients with systemic lupus erythematosus.[51] Carroll[52] has shown that Doppler blood flow velocimetry may be useful in following the gravida with lupus inhibitor. In that study, abnormal umbilical artery systolic/diastolic ratios were found in five of six women with the lupus inhibitor who delivered growth-restricted fetuses. Ariyuki et al.[53] have similarly demonstrated that Doppler may be a useful adjuvant in caring for the patient with SLE.

Despite the sophisticated array of laboratory studies that are available to follow patients with SLE, the patient's clinical status remains of prime importance.

There is no substitute for careful monitoring of maternal blood pressure and weight gain. An increase in blood pressure and rapid weight gain may be the earliest signs of superimposed preeclampsia, which is common in patients with SLE. They can also be the harbinger of a lupus flare.[54] Twenty-four hour urine collections for creatinine clearance and total protein excretion should be carried out regularly. Serum creatinine, BUN, and uric acid levels should be determined whenever these urine collections are performed. A rise in serum uric acid may also be a sign of impending preeclampsia. During a normal pregnancy, complement levels rise. A fall in the third or fourth components (C3 or C4) or a fall in total hemolytic complement (CH50) has been associated with an impending exacerbation of SLE.[55-57] Because complement levels tend to rise during pregnancy, a single complement determination is of no value. A downward trend in complement levels, however, may be significant, even though the level may still be within normal limits.

The timing of delivery is important and should be individualized. All too often, preterm delivery is performed merely to allay physician and patient anxiety. The obstetrician should strive for a vaginal delivery. If the patient is taking glucocorticoids or if there is any evidence of lupus exacerbation, peripartum steroids should be administered parenterally in stress doses. In the patient who undergoes cesarean delivery, intravenous steroids should be continued for 48 hours postoperatively because adequate gastrointestinal absorption cannot be guaranteed until normal bowel function returns. Steroids should be tapered slowly and with great care in the postpartum period to prevent an exacerbation of SLE.[13,58]

Drug Therapy for SLE during Pregnancy

Patients with SLE are often hesitant to take their prescribed medications during pregnancy for fear of fetal effects. Many obstetricians are also reluctant to prescribe these medications for similar reasons. It is important for the obstetrician to be aware of the benefits and risks of medications used to treat SLE. Any steroid that has mineralocorticoid activity exacerbates interstitial fluid retention. The obstetrician should therefore choose a steroid with minimal mineralocorticoid activity and maximum glucocorticoid activity. Steroid use, in combination with pregnancy, may worsen acne and striae. Corticosteroid administration can also lead to gastrointestinal discomfort and ulceration.

Long-term corticosteroid administration has been associated with bone demineralization. For the pregnant woman who is taking increased corticosteroids only during pregnancy, the actual risk is unknown. There is also a risk of cataract formation with long-term corticosteroid administration. The induction of gestational diabetes from glucocorticoid administration is a distinct possibility. Approximately 3% of all pregnancies are complicated by gestational diabetes.[59] We perform 1-hour, 50-g oral-glucose screening tests at 20, 28, and 32 weeks of gestation in patients on long-term glucocorticoids. We also test for diabetes later in gestation if there is any evidence of fetal macrosomia.

Pregnant women are often more concerned about the effects of the medication on their fetus than they are about the effects on themselves. The long-term ingestion of corticosteroids has not been associated with teratogenesis in humans. An increase in the background incidence of cleft palate has been seen in rats and rabbits exposed to long-term corticosteroids but never in humans. Neonatal adrenal suppression is a theoretical consideration in patients taking corticosteroids, but it has only rarely been reported. Nonetheless, the pediatrician should be informed when a mother has been taking corticosteroids antenatally.

Only a fraction of the steroids ingested by a pregnant woman reach the fetus. Prednisone, the most widely used glucocorticoid during gestation, is metabolized by the mother to its active form, prednisolone. An 11β-hydroxy radical is responsible for prednisolone's physiologic activity. The placenta has an abundance of the enzyme 11β-ol dehydrogenase, which converts the active glucocorticoid to an inactive 11-keto metabolite. Depending on the study, only 10 to 50% of a dose of prednisone and only one-sixth of a dose of hydrocortisone reach the fetus.[62-65]

To minimize potential fetal effects, prednisone should be the oral glucocorticoid of choice.[66] Both methylprednisolone and hydrocortisone are satisfactory for intravenous use when needed. Methylprednisolone has less mineralocorticoid effect and should create fewer maternal side effects.

Occasionally, azathioprine, a derivative of 6-mercaptopurine, will be required to ameliorate a patient's disease activity. Between 64 to 93% of an administered dose appears in fetal blood 2.5 to 6 hours after intravenous administration Azathioprine has not been

shown to be teratogenic in humans, although congenital malformations have been observed in animal models. Long-term azathioprine use during pregnancy has been associated with neonatal lymphopenia, lower serum IgG and IgM levels, and a decreased thymic shadow on x-ray films.[67] All of these changes have reversed with time. Scott[68,69] reported an increased incidence of IUGR in infants born to mothers who took azathioprine during pregnancy.

RHEUMATOID ARTHRITIS

Rheumatoid arthritis is an autoimmune disease with a population prevalence of approximately 20 per 1000. Its crippling chronic form occurs in about 0.35% of the population. The onset of the disease is usually between the ages of 20 and 60 years, and women are two to three times more commonly affected than men. The diagnosis of rheumatoid arthritis is based on guidelines set forth by the American Rheumatism Association.

Clinical Manifestations

Articular involvement is the hallmark of rheumatoid arthritis. The most common finding is an erythematous, warm, swollen metacarpophalangeal joint. The proximal interphalangeal and wrist joints may also be involved. Less frequently, metatarsophalangeal and shoulder joints are affected. Over time, cartilage destruction occurs. Carpal-tunnel syndrome is a frequent concomitant of rheumatoid arthritis.

Extraarticular features of rheumatoid arthritis are found in patients with the most joint involvement and the highest titers of rheumatoid factor. Rheumatoid nodules, which occur in 20% of affected patients, can appear in the heart and lungs and along any extremity. Pericarditis, myocarditis, and endocarditis are occasionally seen in patients with rheumatoid arthritis. Unlike SLE, rheumatoid arthritis rarely involves the kidneys. It is important to note that, after 10 years of disease, more than 50% of patients are still able to work, and 15% will have a complete remission.

Laboratory Findings

Rheumatoid factors, IgM and IgG antibodies directed against the Fc fragment of IgG, are the hallmark laboratory finding of rheumatoid arthritis, but are not pathognomonic for this disorder. More-severe disease is seen with higher titers of rheumatoid factor. Antinuclear antibodies are also found in approximately 20% of patients with rheumatoid arthritis.

Effects of Pregnancy on Rheumatoid Arthritis

Hench[77] observed that many patients with rheumatoid arthritis experienced remissions during pregnancy. Persellin[78] noted that in pregnant women with rheumatoid arthritis, 74% underwent remission during the first trimester, 20% in the second trimester, and 5% in the third trimester. In this series, however, 90% of patients experienced a postpartum exacerbation of their disease. Approximately 25% of these flare-ups occurred in the first 4 weeks postpartum.[78] In a review, Klipple and Cecere[79] reported that approximately 70% of patients with rheumatoid arthritis experienced substantial improvements in disease activity during pregnancy. Most of these patients no longer required medications. This remission, however, was short lived, with more than 90% of women relapsing within 6 to 8 months postpartum.[80]

Quinn and colleagues[80] studied 24 pregnant women with rheumatoid arthritis, 21 of whom had minimal disease activity during pregnancy. Nineteen of these 21 women had significant flare-ups during the puerperium. These researchers noted that IgM rheumatoid factor levels increased during flares. Nelson and colleagues[81] investigated HLA antigens in patients with rheumatoid arthritis and their offspring, as this autoimmune disorder has a known HLA class II antigen association. They found that amelioration of rheumatoid arthritis during gestation was associated with a disparity in HLA class II antigens between mother and fetus. They suggested that the maternal immune response to paternal HLA antigens may play a role in the remission in this disease that is often seen during pregnancy.[81] Lasink and coworkers[82] examined the onset of rheumatoid arthritis in relation to pregnancy in 135 patients. They concluded that pregnancy may delay the clinical onset of disease in patients in whom rheumatoid arthritis will ultimately develop.

Effect of Rheumatoid Arthritis on Pregnancy

Rheumatoid arthritis appears to have no adverse effects on pregnancy.[79,83,84] Spector and Silman[85] examined pregnancy outcomes in 195 women with rheumatoid arthritis and 462 controls. They found no increase in spontaneous abortions or stillbirths in patients with rheumatoid arthritis.

To avoid pain and joint damage, care should be taken when positioning the patient with severe articular involvement on the delivery table. This precaution is especially true if the patient has epidural or spinal anesthesia because a joint can be damaged without the patient feeling pain. Obstetric anesthesiologists must also be cautious during rapid sequence induction of general anesthesia and intubation of patients with spinal involvement of rheumatoid arthritis. Subluxation of the atlanto-occipital joint is possible, with devastating consequences.

Effects of Medications Used to Treat Rheumatoid Arthritis

Salicylates

Acetylsalicylic acid (aspirin) and its derivatives remain the mainstay for the treatment of rheumatoid arthritis in pregnancy. Salicylate used throughout pregnancy may be associated with a prolonged gestation, long labor, increased blood loss at delivery and postpartum hemorrhage.[86,87] When a mother has been taking large doses of aspirin or another antiinflammatory agent, a bleeding time should be performed on the neonate before circumcision is performed. Salicylates have been shown to be teratogenic in animals but not in humans. Despite these potential problems, antiinflammatory agents remain the drug of choice in treating the pain and stiffness associated with rheumatoid arthritis during gestation.

NSAIDs

The newer nonsteroidal antiinflammatory drugs (NSAIDs) also are used in the treatment of rheumatoid arthritis. They have both analgesic and antiinflammatory properties. Indomethacin, an older agent, when used in late pregnancy, can cause premature closure of the fetal ductus arteriosus leading to tricuspid regurgitation and pulmonary hypertension. Closure of the ductus arteriosus appears to be gestational-age-dependent. These drugs, therefore, should be discontinued before 32 weeks of gestation if possible. NSAIDs can also cause changes in the fetal renal blood flow, resulting in oligohydramnios. It is unclear how long it takes these changes to occur, and the effects of drugs other than indomethacin have not been fully delineated. Physicians caring for patients taking these medications, therefore, should check the amniotic fluid index frequently. Chrysotherapy, penicillamine, and immunosuppressive agents have also been used to treat rheumatoid arthritis during pregnancy. These should be used only if the proposed benefits are significant. There is a paucity of data concerning the use of these agents during pregnancy.

MYASTHENIA GRAVIS

Although its prevalence is only 1 in 25,000 in the general population, myasthenia gravis occasionally coexists with pregnancy.[88] Women are twice as frequently affected as men and have an earlier onset of the disease, with a peak incidence occurring between the ages of 20 and 30 years. Even though 60% of patients with myasthenia gravis have enlargement of the thymus, only 8% have a malignant thymoma.[89] Thymectomy improves symptoms in up to two-thirds of patients, but most still need additional medical therapy.[90] If the patient presents for prepregnancy counseling and is symptomatic despite large doses of medication, thymectomy should be undertaken before attempting pregnancy.

Myasthenia gravis in pregnancy has been extensively studied by Plauche.[91] In a review of 314 pregnancies in 217 patients with myasthenia, he found no change in the myasthenic status throughout pregnancy, the puerperium, or the postpartum period in 31.5% of patients. Exacerbations occurred in 40.8% of patients during pregnancy, including 30.6% during the puerperium. Another 28% showed a remission of their myasthenia during gestation.[91]

A team approach is necessary for proper treatment of the patient with myasthenia gravis. The neurologist and/or rheumatologist are not always familiar with the medications used by the obstetrician in treating complications of pregnancy. Conversely, because of the infrequency with which obstetricians see myasthenia gravis, they are commonly unfamiliar with the interactions between these medications and the disease. Magnesium sulfate, for example, is absolutely contraindicated in the patient with myasthenia because it accentuates the neuromuscular blockade that is characteristic of the disease.[92,93] Cohen and coworkers[94] reported a near maternal death from administration of magnesium to a patient with myasthenia. Catanzarite and coinvestigators[92] described a respiratory arrest in a patient with myasthenia in preterm labor who was treated with ritodrine and dexamethasone. Although glucocorticoids generally

ameliorate myasthenic symptoms, they may initially result in increased weakness in 25 to 80% of patients. Catanzarite and colleagues[92] proposed that this paradoxic effect, coupled with the hypokalemia caused by the ritodrine, led to the crisis they reported.

Patient Management

Most patients with myasthenia gravis will be taking acetylcholinesterase inhibitors when they become pregnant. These medications are generally safe to use during gestation and do not readily cross the placenta. Dosage adjustments, however, are frequently necessary because of the physiologic changes in vascular volume, renal blood flow, and hepatic function during pregnancy. Because myasthenia gravis is a disease of striated muscle, the smooth muscle of the uterus is generally not affected. The first stage of labor progresses normally. The second stage of labor involves voluntary pushing and the use of skeletal and pelvic girdle musculature.[95] These maternal expulsive efforts may be impaired because of myasthenia, and the obstetrician must be prepared to perform an operative vaginal delivery. Cesarean delivery should be reserved for obstetric indications. Patients are apt to undergo myasthenic crisis during labor, and the oral medications normally used have variable gastrointestinal absorption during this time. Therefore, parenteral acetylcholinesterase inhibitors should be used during labor.

Anesthesia and analgesia during labor in the patient with myasthenia gravis present special challenges for the obstetric anesthesiologist. Although they are extremely sensitive to narcotics, patients with myasthenia gravis may be given these medications if carefully monitored.[96] Epidural anesthesia decreases the requirement of parenteral narcotics, prevents fatigue, and provides excellent anesthesia.[16] However, if general anesthesia is elected for cesarean delivery, nondepolarizing muscle relaxants should be used with great care, if at all. Patients with myasthenia are sensitive to these agents, and a prolonged response is usually seen.[95] It is also imperative to remember that certain inhalation agents may exacerbate myasthenia.

If a puerperal infection develops, aminoglycosides should be used with extreme caution. These agents can block the motor end-plate and cause a myasthenic crisis.[16]

Occasionally, myasthenia will be exacerbated during pregnancy. In such cases, therapy with extremely large doses of acetylcholinesterase inhibitors yields little response. These patients can be treated with plasmapheresis. After plasmapheresis, symptoms usually improve and the dose of acetylcholinesterase inhibitors can often be temporarily reduced. The procedure should be carried out with the patient in the left lateral position with the uterus tilted off the inferior vena cava. It should be performed relatively slowly, with careful attention to maternal blood pressure. If plasmapheresis is being performed after 24 weeks of gestation, continuous fetal monitoring should be employed.

Neonatal Myasthenia Gravis

Neonatal myasthenia occurs in 10 to 25% of infants born to mothers with myasthenia gravis.[97-100] In his review series, Plauche[91] reported a 20.2% incidence of neonatal myasthenia, with a 2.1% stillbirth rate and a 3.8% neonatal mortality rate. This study reviewed cases over a 40-year period, and with modern neonatal care, the neonatal mortality rate today is assuredly considerably lower. Neonatal myasthenia does not begin at birth but is usually evident within the first 2 days of life. It lasts an average of 3 weeks but can persist up to 15 weeks.[100] Symptoms usually include a weak cry, poor sucking effort, and, rarely, respiratory distress. Neonatal myasthenia is thought to be secondary to transplacental passage of IgG antibodies directed against acetylcholine receptors on skeletal muscles.

REFERENCES

1. Fessel WJ. Systemic lupus erythematosus in the community. Incidence, prevalence, outcome and first symptoms: the high prevalence in black women. Arch Intern Med 1974;134:1027.
2. Estes D, Christian CL. The natural history of systemic lupus erythematosus by prospective analysis. Medicine 1971;50:85.
3. Garsenstein M, Pollak VE, Karik RM. Systemic lupus erythematosus and pregnancy. N Engl J Med 1962; 276:165.
4. Zurier RB. Systemic lupus erythematosus and pregnancy. Clin Rheum Dis 1975;1:613.
5. Mintz G, Nitz J, Gutierrez G, et al. Prospective study of pregnancy in systemic lupus erythematosus: results of a multidisciplinary approach. J Rheumatol 1986;13:732.
6. Lockshin MD. Lupus erythematosus and allied disorders in pregnancy. Bull NY Acad Med 1987;63:797.
7. Lockshin MD, Reinitz E, Druzin ML, et al. Lupus pregnancy; case-control prospective study demonstrating

8. Lockshin MD. Pregnancy does not cause systemic lupus erythematosus to worsen. Arthritis Rheum 1989;32:665.
9. Ainslie WH, Britt K, Moshipur JA. Maternal death due to lupus pneumonitis in pregnancy. Mt. Sinai J Med 1979;46:494.
10. Leikin JB, Arof HM, Pearlman LM. Acute lupus pneumonitis in the postpartum period: a case history and review of the literature. Obstet Gynecol 1986;68:295.
11. Averbuch M, Bojko A, Levo Y. Cardiac tamponade in the early postpartum period as the presenting and predominant manifestation of systemic lupus erythematosus. J. Rheumatol 1986;13:444.
12. Fine LG, Barnett EV, Danovitch GM, et al. Systemic lupus erythematosus in pregnancy. Ann Intern Med 1981;94:667.
13. Mackey E. Pregnancy and renal disease: a ten-year study. Aust NZ J Obstet Gynaecol 1963;3:21.
14. Ramsey-Goldman R. Pregnancy in systemic lupus erythematosus. Rheum Dis Clin North Am 1988:14.
15. Houser MT, Fish AJ, Tagatz GE, et al. Pregnancy and systemic lupus erythematosus. Am J Obstet Gynecol 1980;138:409.
16. Foldes FF, McNall PG. Myasthenia gravis: a guide for anesthesiologists. Anesthesiology 1962;23:837.
17. Hayslett JP, Lynn RI. Effect of pregnancy in patients with lupus nephropathy. Kidney Int 1980;18:207.
18. Fraga A, Mintz G, Orozco J, et al. Sterility and fertility rates, fetal wastage and maternal morbidity in systemic lupus erythematosus. J Rheumatol 1974;1:1293.
19. Castillo JD, Engback L. The nature of the neuromuscular block produced by magnesium. J Physiol 1954;124:370.
20. Kitzmiller JL. Autoimmune disorders; maternal, fetal and neonatal risks. Clin Obstet Gynecol 1978;21:385.
21. Zurier RG, Argyros T, Urman J, et al. Systemic lupus erythematosus: management during pregnancy. Obstet Gynecol 1978;51:178.
22. Julkunen H, Kaaja R, Kurki P, et al. Fetal outcome in women with primary Sjogren's syndrome: a retrospective case-control study. Clin Exp Rheumatol 1995;13:65.
23. Le Thi Huong D, Wechsler B, Piette JC, et al. Pregnancy and its outcome in systemic lupus erythematosus. Q J Med 1994;87:721.
24. Johnson MJ, Petri M, Witter FR, Repke JT. Evaluation of preterm delivery in a systemic lupus erythematosus pregnancy clinic. Obstet Gynecol 1995;86:396.
25. Rosove MH, Brewer PM, Runge A, Hirji K. Simultaneous lupus anticoagulant and anticardiolipin assays and clinical detection of antiphospholipids. Am J Hematol 1989;32:148.
26. Lockwood CJ, Romero R, Feinber RF. The prevalence and biologic significance of lupus anticoagulant and anticardiolipin antibodies in a general obstetric population. Am J Obstet Gynecol 1989;161:369.
27. Hanly JG, Gladman DD, Rose TH, et al. Lupus pregnancy, a prospective study of placental changes. Arthritis Rheum 1988;31:358.
28. Hedfors E, Lindahl G, Lindblad S. Anticardiolipin antibodies during pregnancy. J Rheumatol 1987;14:160.
29. Hokkanen E. Myasthenia gravis. Ann Clin Res 1969;1:94.

30. Lubbe WF, Butler WS, Palmer SJ, et al. Lupus anticoagulant in pregnancy. Br J Obstet Gynaecol 1984;97:357.

31. Branch DW, Scott JR, Kochenour NK, et al. Obstetric complications associated with the lupus anticoagulant. N Engl J Med 1985;313:1322.

32. Leu LY, Lan JL. The influence on pregnancy of anti-SSA/Ro antibodies in systemic lupus erythematosus. Chi Mien I Hsueh Tsa Chih 1992;25:12.

33. Gatengy PA, Cameron K, Shearman RP. Pregnancy loss with phospholipid antibodies: improved outcome with aspirin containing treatment. Aust NZ J Obstet Gynaecol 1989;29:294.

34. Balasch J, Font J, Lopez-Soto A, et al. Antiphospholipid antibodies in unselected patients with repeated abortion. Hum Reprod 1990;5:43.

35. Rosove MH, Tabsh K, Wasserstrum N, et al. Heparin therapy for pregnant women with lupus anticoagulant or anticardiolipin antibodies. Obstet Gynecol 1990;75:630.

36. Branch DW, Silver RM, Blackwell JL, et al. Outcome of treated pregnancies in women with antiphospholipid syndrome: an update of the Utah experience. Obstet Gynecol 1992;80:614.

37. Kaaja R, Julkunen H, Ammala P, et al. Intravenous immunoglobulin treatment of pregnant patients with recurrent pregnancy losses associated with antiphospholipid antibodies. Acta Obstet Gynaecol Scand 1993;72:63.

38. Unander AM, Norberg R, Hahn L, et al. Anticardiolipin antibodies and complement in ninety-nine women with habitual abortion. Am J Obstet Gynecol 1987;156:114.

39. Chamley LW, Pattison NS, McKay EJ. IgM lupus anticoagulants can be associated with recurrent fetal loss of thrombic episodes. Thromb Res 1990;58:343.

40. Mizoguchi K, Kakisako S, Tanaka M, et al. Lupus anticoagulant as a risk factor for cerebral infarction and habitual abortions. Kurume Med J 1989;36:113.

41. Rallings P, Exner T, Abraham R. Coronary artery vasculitis and myocardial infarction associated with antiphospholipid antibodies in a pregnant woman. Aust NZ J Med 1989;19:347.

42. Litsey S, Noonan J, O'Connor W, et al. Maternal connective tissue disease and congenital heart block. N Engl J Med 1985;312:98.

43. Scott JS, Maddison PJ, Tayler PV, et al. Connective-tissue disease, antibodies to ribonucleoprotein and congenital heart block. N Engl J Med 1983;309:209.

44. Scheib JS, Waxman J. Congenital heart block in successive pregnancies: a case report and evaluation of risk with therapeutic consideration. Gynecol 1989;73:481.

45. Derksen RH, Meilof JF. Anti-Ro/SS-A and anti La/SS-B autoantibody levels in relation to systemic lupus erythematosus disease activity and congenital heart block; a longitudinal study comprising two consecutive pregnancies in a patient with systemic lupus erythematosus. Arthritis Rheum 1992;45:953.

46. Vetter VL, Rashkad WJ. Congenital complete heart block and connective tissue disease. N Engl J Med 1983; 309:236.

47. Esscher E, Scott JS. Congenital heart block and maternal systemic lupus erythematosus. BMJ 1979;1:1235.

48. Lockshin MD, Gibofsky A, Peebles CL, et al. Neonatal lupus erythematosus with heart block: family study of a patient with anti-SS-A and SS-B antibodies. Arthritis Rheum 1983;26:210.

49. McCuiston CH, Schoch EP. Possible discoid lupus erythematosus in a newborn infant: report of case with subsequent development of acute systemic lupus erythematosus in mother. Arch Dermatol Syphilol 1954;70:782.

50. McGee CD, Makowski EL. Systemic lupus erythematosus in pregnancy. Am J Obstet Gynecol 1970;107:1008.

51. Adams D, Druzin MI, Edersheim T, et al. Condition specific antepartum testing: systemic lupus erythematosus and associated serologic abnormalities. Am J Reprod Immunol 1992;28:159.

52. Carroll BA. Obstetric duplex sonography in patients with lupus anticoagulant syndrome. J Ultrasound Med 1990;9:17.

53. Ariyuki Y, Hata T, Kitao M. Reverse end-diastolic umbilical artery velocity in a case of intrauterine fetal death at 14 weeks' gestation. Am J Obstet Gynecol 1993; 169:1621.

54. Buyon JP, Cronstein BN, Morris M, et al. Serum complement values (C_3 and C_4) to differentiate between systemic lupus activity and preeclampsia. Am J Med 1986; 81:194.

55. Tozman ECS, Urowitz MB, Gladman DD. Systemic lupus erythematosus and pregnancy. J Rheumatol 1980; 7:624.

56. Zulman MI, Talal N, Hoffman GS, et al. Problems associated with the management of pregnancies in patients with systemic lupus erythematosus. J Rheumatol 1980; 7:37.

57. Zurier RG, Argyros T, Urman J, et al. Systemic lupus erythematosus: management during pregnancy. Obstet Gynecol 1978;51:178.

58. Bongiovanni AM, McPadden AJ. Steroids during pregnancy and possible fetal consequences. Fertil Steril 1960; 11:181.

59. Freinkel N. Gestational diabetes, 1979: philosophical and practical aspects of a major health problem. Diabetes Care 1980;3:399.

60. Fainstat T. Cortisone-induced congenital cleft palate in rabbits. Endocrinology 1954;455:502.

61. Giannopoulos G, Tulchinsky D. The influence of hormones on fetal lung development. In: Ryan KJ, Tulchinsky D, eds. Maternal-fetal endocrinology. Philadelphia: Saunders, 1988:310.

62. Ballard PL, Granberg P, Ballard RA. Glucocorticoid levels in maternal and cord serum after prenatal betamethasone therapy to prevent respiratory distress syndrome. J Clin Invest 1975;56:15.

63. Blanford AT, Pearson-Murphy BE. In vitro metabolism of prednisolone, dexamethasone, betamethasone, and cortisol by the human placenta. Am J Obstet Gynecol 1977; 137:264.

64. Osathanondh R, Tulchinsky D, Kamali H, et al. Dexamethasone levels in treated pregnant women and newborn infants. J Pediatr 1977;90:617.

65. Beirins IZ, Bayard F, Ances IG, et al. The transplacental passage of prednisone and prednisolone in pregnancy near term. J Pediatr 1972;81:936.

66. Gabbe SG. Drug therapy in autoimmune disease. Clin Obstet Gynecol 1983;26:635.

67. Cote CJ, Meuwissen HJ, Pickering RJ. Effects on the neonate of prednisone and azathioprine administered to the mother during pregnancy. J Pediatr 1974;85:324.

68. Scott JR. Fetal growth retardation associated with maternal administration of immunosuppressive drugs. Am J Obstet Gynecol 1977;128:668.

69. Scott JR. Immunologic diseases in pregnancy. Prog Allergy 1977;23:321.

70. Davison JM, Lindheimer MD. Pregnancy in renal transplant recipients. J Reprod Med 1982;27:613.

71. Turnam GR. Rheumatoid arthritis. Clin Obstet Gynecol 1983;26:560.

72. Masi AT, Maldonade-Cocco JA, Kaplan SB, et al. Prospective study of the early course of rheumatoid arthritis in young adults: comparison of patients with and without rheumatoid factor positivity at entry and identification of variables correlating with outcome. Semin Arthritis Rheum 1976;5:299.

73. Gordon DA, Stein JL, Broder I. The extrarticular features of rheumatoid arthritis: a systemic analysis of 127 cases. Am J Med 1973;54:445.

74. Hurd ER. Extraarticular manifestations of rheumatoid arthritis. Semin Arthritis Rheum 1979;8:151.

75. Hollingsworth JW, Saykaly RJ. Systemic complications of rheumatoid arthritis. Med Clin North Am 1977;61:217.

76. Rodman GP, ed. Primer on the rheumatic diseases. JAMA 1973;suppl 224:661.

77. Hench PS. The ameliorating effect of pregnancy on chronic atrophic (infectious) rheumatoid arthritis, fibrositis and intermittent hydrarthrosis. Proc Mayo Clin 1938;13:161.

78. Persellin RH. The effect of pregnancy on rheumatoid arthritis. Bull Rheum Dis 1977;27:922.

79. Klipple GL, Cecere FA. Rheumatoid arthritis and pregnancy. Rheum Dis Clin North Am 1989;15:213.

80. Quinn C, Mulpeter K, Casey EB, Feighery CF. Changes in levels of IgM RF and alpha 2 PAG correlate with increased disease activity in rheumatoid arthritis during the puerperium. Scand J Rheumatol 1993;22:273.

81. Nelson JL, Hughes KA, Smith AG, et al. Maternal-fetal disparity in HLA class II alloantigens and the pregnancy-induced amelioration of rheumatoid arthritis. N Engl J Med 1993;329:466.

82. Lasink M, de Boer A, Kijkmans BA, et al. The onset of rheumatoid arthritis in relation to pregnancy and childbirth. Clin Exp Rheumatol 1993;11:171.

83. Kaplan D, Diamond H. Rheumatoid arthritis and pregnancy. Clin Obstet Gynecol 1965;8:286.

84. Betson JR, Dorn RV. Forty cases of arthritis and pregnancy. J Int Coll Surg 1964;42:521.

85. Spector TD, Silman AJ. Is poor pregnancy outcome a risk factor in rheumatoid arthritis? Ann Rheum Dis 1990;49:12.

86. Bulmash JM. Rheumatoid arthritis and pregnancy. Obstet Gynecol Annu 1979;8:223.

87. Bulmash JM. Systemic lupus erythematosus and pregnancy. Obstet Gynecol Annu 1978;7:153.

88. Kurtzke JF. Epidemiology of myasthenia gravis. Adv Neurol 1978;19:545.

89. Hokkanen E. Myasthenia gravis. Ann Clin Res 1969;1:94.

90. Havard CW, Fonseca V. New treatment approaches to myasthenia gravis. Drugs 1990;39:66.

91. Plauche WC. Myasthenia gravis. Clin Obstet Gynecol 1983;26:594.

92. Catanzarite VA, McHargue AM, Sandberg EC, et al. Respiratory arrest during therapy for premature labor in a patient with myasthenia gravis. Obstet Gynecol 1984;64:819.

93. Castillo JD, Engbaek L. The nature of the neuromuscular block produced by magnesium. J Physiol 1954;124:370.

94. Cohen BA, London RS, Goldstein PJ. Myasthenia gravis and preeclampsia. Obstet Gynecol 1976;48:35.

95. McNall PG, Jafarnia MR. Management of myasthenia gravis in obstetrical patients. Am J Obstet Gynecol 1965;92:518.

96. Rolbin SH, Levinson G, Shnider SM, et al. Anesthetic considerations for myasthenia gravis and pregnancy. Anesth Analg 1978;57:441.

97. Barlow CF. Neonatal myasthenia gravis. Am J Dis Child 1981;135:209.

98. Donaldson JO, Penn AS, Lisak RP, et al. Antiacetylcholine receptor antibody in neonatal myasthenia gravis. Am J Dis Child 1981;135:222.

99. Namba T, Brown SB, Grob D. Neonatal myasthenia gravis: report of two cases and review of the literature. Pediatrics 1970;45:488.

100. Scott JR. Immunologic diseases in pregnancy. Prog Allergy 1977;23:321.

Diabetes Mellitus and Other Endocrine Diseases

Mark Landon

Key Points

- Perinatal mortality for pregnancy complicated by diabetes mellitus has decreased from approximately 65% before the discovery of insulin to 2 to 5% at present.
- The actions of human placental lactogen are primarily responsible for the diabetogenic effect of pregnancy.
- Congenital malformations are the most common cause of perinatal mortality in infants of insulin-dependent diabetic mothers. The two most common malformations are cardiac defects and neural-tube defects.
- The most common cause of hypothyroidism in pregnant women is previous treatment for hyperthyroidism. The most common cause of hyperthyroidism in pregnancy is Graves disease.
- Pregnant patients with symptomatic pituitary microadenomas can be safely treated with bromocriptine.

DIABETES MELLITUS

Perinatal mortality for pregnancy complicated by diabetes mellitus has been reduced from approximately 65% before the discovery of insulin to 2 to 5% at present. This dramatic improvement in perinatal outcome has been largely attributed to clinical efforts resulting in improved maternal glycemic control. When optimal care is provided for the diabetic woman, the perinatal mortality rate excluding major congenital malformations is equivalent to that observed in normal pregnancies.

The failure to establish optimal glycemic control, as well as other less well understood metabolic factors, continue to result in significant perinatal morbidity. For this reason, both clinical and basic laboratory investigations concerning the cause and prevention of congenital malformations, macrosomia, and intrauterine

death have become a focus in recent years. In spite of these concerns, the outlook for most diabetic women contemplating pregnancy remains excellent. Such optimism is now incorporated into a more realistic appreciation of the impact that diabetic vascular complications can have on pregnancy, as well as the effect that pregnancy may have on these disease processes. The modern management of pregnancy in a diabetic woman requires an organized team approach. Using this model, successful pregnancies have become the norm for women with complicated diabetes.

Pathophysiology

During normal pregnancy, maternal metabolism must adjust to provide adequate nutrition for both the mother and the growing fetoplacental unit. Early in pregnancy, glucose homeostasis is affected by an increase in estrogen and progesterone, which leads to β-cell hyperplasia and increased insulin secretion.[1] The heightened peripheral utilization of glucose results in a 10% reduction in maternal glucose levels by the end of the first trimester. A decrease in hepatic glucose production accompanies this phenomenon, such that insulin-dependent diabetic women commonly experience periods of hypoglycemia in the first trimester. Availability of gluconeogenic amino acids is reduced, whereas levels of fatty acids, triglycerides, and ketones are increased. This state of accelerated starvation during fasting marked by increased fat catabolism and a decline in maternal glucose production allows utilization of fat stores for energy.[2] As pregnancy progresses, fasting levels of insulin rise from approximately 5 mU/liter to 8 mU/liter at term.[3] Fasting hypoglycemia may also appear in late pregnancy as the conceptus increases its glucose utilization.

Lipids continue to serve as an important maternal fuel as pregnancy advances. Despite the accelerated starvation of the fasting state, early in pregnancy, fat storage actually increases. A rise in the production of human placental lactogen (HPL), a polypeptide hormone produced by the syncytiotrophoblast, promotes lipolysis in adipose tissue. The release of glycerol and fatty acids reduces both maternal glucose and amino acid utilization and, in doing so, spares these fuels for the fetus.

Rising levels of HPL and other "contra-insulin" hormones modify maternal glucose and amino acid utilization. The actions of HPL are largely responsible for the diabetogenic state of pregnancy. Blood glucose levels are thus greater in response to an oral or intravenous carbohydrate load than in the nonpregnant state. In normal pregnancy, glucose homeostasis is maintained by an augmented amount of insulin response to counterbalance its decreased sensitivity.[4]

With placental growth, larger amounts of contra-insulin factors such as HPL are synthesized. A woman with overt diabetes requires additional insulin therapy as pregnancy progresses. Her increased insulin requirement, approximately 30% over the prepregnancy dose, is roughly equivalent to the endogenous increase seen in a normal gestation. If the pregnant woman has borderline pancreatic reserve, it is possible that her endogenous insulin production will be inadequate, resulting in gestational diabetes mellitus. Unlike known insulin-requiring patients, obese patients with gestational diabetes mellitus (GDM), with limited β-cell reserve but presumed peripheral insulin resistance, may experience large increases in both their insulin secretion and requirement during pregnancy. Normal pregnancy results in approximately a 44% decline in insulin sensitivity, as compared with a 56% decline in pregnancies complicated by GDM.[5] Insulin may inadequately suppress hepatic glucose production in late pregnancy in women with GDM, indicating that in GDM hyperglycemia results from insulin resistance arising from several metabolic changes.[5]

The placenta also controls the transport of nutrients to the fetal compartment. Substrate supply to the fetus depends on the specific modes of transfer. Glucose transport across the placenta occurs by carrier-mediated facilitated diffusion. Glucose levels in the fetus are directly proportional to maternal plasma glucose concentrations. Glucose is the primary fuel used by the fetus for protein and fat synthesis. The degree of placental transfer of glucose and other fuels is also affected by placental metabolism. Further modification of the transfer of carbohydrate may be influenced by placental insulin and insulin-like growth factor receptors. The placenta is essentially impermeable to protein hormones such as insulin, glucagon, growth hormone, and HPL. In addition to glucose transfer, many amino acids are actively transported across the placenta to the fetal compartment. This process contributes to a diminution in maternal amino acid levels in the fasting state. Ketoacids appear to diffuse freely across the placenta and may serve as an important fetal substrate during periods of maternal starvation.

Fetal glucose levels are normally maintained within a narrow range reflecting the regulation of maternal carbohydrate homeostasis. During pregnancy in the insulin-dependent diabetic woman, periods of hyperglycemia lead to fetal hyperglycemia. Persistent elevations of glucose and likely amino acids can stimulate the fetal pancreas, resulting in β-cell hyperplasia and fetal hyperinsulinemia.[6]

Perinatal Morbidity and Mortality

Fetal Death

Although relatively uncommon today, fetal death still may complicate the pregnancies of women who do not receive optimal care. Such losses have been observed most often after the 36th week of pregnancy in patients with vascular disease, poor glycemic control, hydramnios, fetal macrosomia, or preeclampsia. In women with vascular complications fetal growth restriction and intrauterine death may occur as early as the second trimester.

The precise cause of stillbirths in pregnancies complicated by diabetes remains unknown. Because extramedullary hematopoiesis is a feature commonly observed in stillborn infants of women with insulin-dependent diabetes mellitus (IDDM), chronic intrauterine hypoxia has been cited as a likely cause of these intrauterine fetal deaths.[7] Reduced uterine blood flow is thought to contribute to the increased incidence of intrauterine growth restriction (IUGR) observed in pregnancies complicated by diabetic vasculopathy. Investigations using radioactive tracers have also suggested a relationship between poor maternal metabolic control and reduced uteroplacental blood flow.[8] Ketoacidosis and preeclampsia, two factors known to be associated with an increased incidence of intrauterine deaths, may further decrease uterine blood flow. In diabetic ketoacidosis, hypovolemia and hypotension caused by dehydration may reduce flow through the intervillous space, while in preeclampsia, narrowing and vasospasm of spiral arterioles may result.

There is considerable evidence linking fetal hyperinsulinism and hypoxia in utero.[9] Hyperinsulinemia in the fetus produces an increase in oxygen consumption and a decrease in arterial oxygen content.[10] Persistent maternal–fetal hyperglycemia occurs independently of maternal uterine blood flow, which may not be increased enough to allow for enhanced oxygen delivery in the face of increased metabolic demands. Thus, hyperinsulinemia in the fetus of the diabetic mother appears to increase the metabolic rate and oxygen requirement in the face of several factors such as hyperglycemia, ketoacidosis, preeclampsia, and maternal vasculopathy, which can reduce placental blood flow and fetal oxygenation.

Congenital Malformations

With the reduction in intrauterine deaths and a marked decrease in neonatal mortality related to hyaline membrane disease (HMD) and traumatic delivery, congenital malformations have emerged as the most important cause of perinatal loss in pregnancies complicated by IDDM. In the past, these anomalies were responsible for approximately 10% of all perinatal deaths. At present, however, malformations account for 30 to 50% of perinatal mortality.[11] Neonatal deaths

TABLE 6-16 FREQUENCY OF CONGENITAL MALFORMATIONS IN INFANTS OF DIABETIC MOTHERS		
Reference	No. of Malformations/ Total No.	Percent
Albert et al.[12]	29/289	10.0
Ylinen et al.[13]	11/142	7.7
Mills et al.[11]	25/279	9.0
Greene[14]	35/451	7.7
Steel et al.[15]	12/239	7.8
Fuhrmann et al.[16]	22/292	7.5
Simpson et al.[17]	9/106	8.5
Kitzmiller et al.[18]	13/194	6.7

now exceed stillbirths in pregnancies complicated by IDDM, and fatal congenital malformations account for this changing pattern.

Most studies have documented a two- to sixfold increase in major malformations in infants of insulin-dependent diabetic mothers. At the Ohio State University Diabetes in Pregnancy Program, we have observed 29 congenital anomalies in 289 (10%) women with IDDM enrolled from 1987 through 1993.[12] Similar figures were obtained in the Diabetes in Early Pregnancy Study in the United States.[11] The incidence of major anomalies was 2.1% in 389 control patients and 9.0% in 279 women with IDDM. In general, the incidence of major malformations in worldwide studies of offspring of mothers with IDDM has ranged from 5 to 10% (Table 6-16).

Malformations in IDDM have an impact on most organ systems, and, thus, the teratogenic insult occurs before the seventh week of gestation. Central nervous system malformations, particularly anencephaly, open spina bifida, and holoprosencephaly, are increased 10-fold.[19] Cardiac anomalies, especially ventricular septal defects and complex lesions such as transposition of the great vessels, are increased 5-fold. The congenital defect thought to be most characteristic of diabetic embryopathy is sacral agenesis or caudal dysplasia.

Impaired glycemic control and associated derangement in maternal metabolism appear to contribute to abnormal embryogenesis. The notion of excess glucose as the single teratogenic agent in diabetic pregnancy has thus been replaced with the view of a multifactorial cause[20] (Table 6-17). Maternal hyperglycemia has been proposed by most investigators as the primary teratogenic factor, but hyperketonemia, hypoglycemia, somatomedin inhibitor excess, and excess free oxygen radicals have also been

TABLE 6-17
POTENTIAL FACTORS ASSOCIATED WITH TERATOGENESIS IN PREGNANCY COMPLICATED BY DIABETES MELLITUS

Hyperglycemia
Excess of ketone bodies
Somatomedin inhibition
Arachidonic acid deficiency
Free oxygen radical excess

suggested. The profile of a woman most likely to have an infant with congenital anomalies would include a patient with poor periconceptional control, longstanding diabetes, and vascular disease.

Macrosomia

Excessive fetal growth may predispose the fetus of a woman with IDDM to shoulder dystocia, traumatic birth injury, and asphyxia injury. Newborn adiposity appears to be a significant risk factor for childhood obesity and Type II diabetes.

While macrosomia has been defined as a birth weight in excess of 4000 to 4500 g, it is preferable to categorize infants as large for gestational age (a birth weight above the 90th percentile) using population-specific growth curves. According to these definitions, macrosomia may complicate 25 to 50% of pregnancies complicated by GDM and 40% of IDDM pregnancies. A birth weight greater than 4500 g occurs 10 times more often in diabetic women than in a non-diabetic control population.[21]

Fetal macrosomia in IDDM is reflected by increased adiposity, muscle mass, and organomegaly. The disproportionate increase in the size of the trunk and shoulder compared with the head may contribute to the increased risk of shoulder dystocia.

The concept that maternal hyperglycemia leading to fetal hyperglycemia and hyperinsulinemia results in excessive fetal growth and adipose deposition was first advanced by Pedersen.[23] The Pederson hypothesis has been supported by measurement of excess insulin in amniotic fluid and cord blood. Both are increased in the amniotic fluid of insulin-treated diabetic women at term.[24] The results of several clinical series have validated the Pederson hypothesis inasmuch as improved maternal glycemic control has been associated with a decline in the incidence of macrosomia.[25,26] Landon and colleagues, using daily capillary glucose values obtained during the second and third trimesters

in insulin-dependent women, reported a rate of 9% for macrosomia when mean values were less than 110 mg/dl, as compared with 34% when less than optimal control was achieved.[27] Jovanovic-Peterson et al. have suggested that 1-hour postprandial glucose measurements correlate best with the frequency of macrosomia.[28] After controlling for other factors, these authors noted that the strongest prediction for birth weight was third-trimester nonfasting glucose measurements. The persistent high frequency of macrosomia in diabetic pregnancy may be explained by the inability of diabetic women to achieve true physiologic glucose levels, particularly in the postprandial state. Alternatively, individual fetal response, including the possibility of varying glucose transport activity and thus β-cell stimulus, may explain why macrosomia continues to occur in patients with seemingly well-controlled diabetes.[29]

Hypoglycemia

Neonatal hypoglycemia, a blood glucose level below 35 to 40 mg/dl during the first 12 hours of life, results from a rapid drop in plasma glucose concentrations following clamping of the umbilical cord. Hypoglycemia is particularly common in macrosomic newborns, in which rates exceed 50%. With near physiologic control of maternal glucose levels during pregnancy, overall rates of 5 to 15% have been reported.[30,31] The degree of hypoglycemia is influenced by maternal glucose control during the latter half of pregnancy and by maternal glycemia control during labor and delivery. Poor maternal glucose control can result in fetal β-cell hyperplasia, leading to exaggerated insulin release following delivery.

Respiratory Distress Syndrome

Maternal diabetes appears to affect fetal pulmonary development. Experimental animal studies have primarily detailed the effects of hyperglycemia and hyperinsulinemia on pulmonary surfactant biosynthesis. Both of these factors are involved in delayed pulmonary maturation in the fetuses of women with IDDM.[32] Insulin can interfere with substrate availability for surfactant biosynthesis and may also modulate the normal timing of glucocorticoid-induced pulmonary maturation.[33,34]

Clinical studies investigating the effect of maternal diabetes on fetal lung maturation have produced conflicting data. Modern management protocols that have resulted in good glucose control and delayed delivery until lung maturity has been established have made respiratory distress syndrome (RDS) a less common occurrence than in the woman with IDDM. In women with well-controlled diabetes who deliver at term, the risk of RDS is no higher than that observed in the general population.[35,36] Kjos et al. studied the outcome of 526 diabetic gestations delivered within 5 days of amniotic fluid fetal lung maturation testing and reported hyaline membrane disease in 5 neonates (0.95%), all of whom were delivered prior to 34 weeks of gestation.[35] Mimouni et al. compared outcomes of 127 women with IDDM with matched controls and concluded that diabetes in pregnancy as currently managed is not a direct risk factor for the development of RDS.[36] Yet, cesarean delivery not preceded by labor or associated with prematurity, both of which are increased in diabetic pregnancies, clearly increase the likelihood of neonatal respiratory disease.[36]

Classification of Maternal Diabetes

The age at onset of diabetes, the duration of the disease and the presence of vasculopathy can significantly influence perinatal outcome.[37] Priscilla White's pioneering work at the Joslin Clinic led to a classification system that has been widely applied to pregnant women with diabetes.[37] A modification of this system is used today. The White classification facilitates evaluation of pregnant women with diabetes and formulation of a plan of management (Table 6-18).

Class A_1 diabetes mellitus, a subset of GDM, includes patients who have demonstrated carbohydrate intolerance during a 100 g 3-hour oral glucose-tolerance test; however, their fasting and 2-hour postprandial glucose levels are maintained by dietary regulation alone. If the fasting or postprandial glucose levels are elevated, patients are designated Class A_2. Insulin is most often required for these women.

The International Workshop Conferences on Gestational Diabetes sponsored by the American Diabetes Association in cooperation with the American College of Obstetricians and Gynecologists have recommended that the term gestational diabetes rather than Class A diabetes be used to describe women with carbohydrate intolerance of variable severity with onset or recognition during the present pregnancy.[38,39] The term gestational diabetes fails to specify whether the patient requires dietary adjustment alone or treatment with diet and insulin. This distinction is important because patients who are normoglycemic while fasting have a significantly lower perinatal mortality rate as well as a risk for subsequent diabetes. Women with gestational diabetes that requires insulin are at greater risk for a poor perinatal outcome than those controlled by diet alone.

Patients requiring insulin are designated by the letters B, C, D, R, F, and T. Class B patients are those whose onset of disease occurs after age 20. They have had diabetes for less than 10 years and have no vascular complications. Included in this subgroup of patients are those who have been previously treated with oral hypoglycemic agents. Class C diabetes includes patients who have the onset of their disease between the ages of 10 and 19 or have had the disease for 10 to 19 years. Vascular disease is not present. Class D represents women whose disease is of 20 years' duration or more, whose onset occurred before age 10, or who have benign retinopathy. The

TABLE 16-18
MODIFIED WHITE CLASSIFICATION OF DIABETES IN PREGNANCY

Class	Diabetes Onset Age (yr)		Duration (yr)	Vascular Disease	Insulin Need
Gestational diabetes					
A_1	Any		Any	0	0
A_2	Any		Any	0	+
Pregestational diabetes					
B	>20		<10	0	+
C	10–19	or	10–19	0	+
D	<10	or	>20	+	+
F	Any		Any	+	+
R	Any		Any	+	+
T	Any		Any	+	+
H	Any		Any	+	+

latter includes microaneurysms, exudates, and venous dilation.

Nephropathy

Renal disease develops in 25 to 30% of women with IDDM, with a peak incidence after approximately 16 years of diabetes.[40] Class F describes the 5 to 10% of pregnant patients with underlying renal disease. This includes those with reduced creatinine clearance and/or proteinuria of at least 400 mg in 24 hours measured during the first 20 weeks of gestation. In our experience, two factors present prior to 20 weeks of gestation appear to be predictive of adverse perinatal outcome in these women (e.g., preterm delivery, low birth weight, or preeclampsia)—Proteinuria >3.0 g/24 hr and serum creatinine >1.5 mg/dl.

In a series of 45 Class F women, 12 women had such risk factors.[41] Preeclampsia developed in 92% with a mean gestational age at delivery of 34 weeks, as compared with an incidence of preeclampsia of 36% in 33 women without these risk factors who reached an average gestational age of 36 weeks.[41] Remarkably, perinatal survival was 100% in this series, and no deliveries occurred prior to 30 weeks of gestation.

The treatment of the diabetic woman with nephropathy requires considerable expertise. Although controversial, some nephrologists recommend a modified reduction in protein intake for pregnant women with nephropathy. Control of hypertension in pregnant women with diabetic nephropathy is crucial to prevent further deterioration of kidney function and to optimize pregnancy outcome. We cautiously use diuretics when patients are extremely nephrotic, as this group may be prone to volume-dependent forms of hypertension. Angiotensin-converting–enzyme inhibitors, which reduce intraglomerular pressure and dramatically improve proteinuria in nonpregnant diabetic patients, are contraindicated during pregnancy because they may damage the fetal kidney.

Pregnancy does not appear to produce a permanent worsening of diabetic renal disease.[42,43] Proteinuria generally increases, and pregnancy-induced hypertension may often develop. Following delivery, proteinuria declines in the majority of cases. In a series of 45 Class F women, 26 (58%) had more than a 1-g increase in proteinuria, and by the third trimester, 25 (56%) excreted more than 3.0 g/24 hours.[41] In the vast majority of cases, protein excretion returned

to base-line levels following gestation. Changes in creatinine clearance during pregnancy are variable in Class F patients. Kitzmiller, in reviewing 44 patients from the literature, noted that about one-third of women had an expected rise in creatinine clearance during gestation, as compared with one-third who had a decline of more than 15% by the third trimester.[42] Of interest, most patients with a severe reduction in creatinine clearance (<50 ml/min) at the onset of pregnancy do not demonstrate a further reduction in first-trimester clearance during pregnancy.[42] However, a decline in renal function can be anticipated in 20 to 30% of cases. Several authors have suggested that any deterioration of renal function after pregnancy is probably consistent with the natural course of diabetic nephropathy and is not related to pregnancy per se.[42]

With improved survival of diabetic patients following renal transplantation, increasing numbers of kidney recipients have now achieved pregnancy (Class T). Fortunately, episodes of renal allograft rejection have been uncommon. Prednisone and azathioprine were administered throughout gestation. An increase in fetal loss and superimposed preeclampsia and preterm delivery has been observed.

Retinopathy

Class R diabetes is used to describe women with proliferative retinopathy. Pregnancy does not affect the prevalence of retinopathy.[44] In Klein et al.'s prospective series of 1717 pregnant diabetic women, pregnancy was associated with a greater than twofold independent risk for progression of retinopathy.[45] Laser photocoagulation therapy during pregnancy has helped maintain many pregnancies to a gestational age at which neonatal survival is likely.

In a series of 172 patients, including 40 cases with background retinopathy and 11 with proliferative changes, new-onset proliferative retinopathy developed in only one patient during pregnancy.[46] Progression to proliferative retinopathy during pregnancy rarely occurs in women with background retinopathy or those without any eye ground changes.[47] Of 561 women in these two categories, neovascularization developed in only 17 (3.0%) during gestation.[47] In contrast, 23 of 26 (88.5%) with untreated proliferative disease experienced worsening retinopathy during pregnancy. Thus, identification and treatment of proliferative retinopathy prior to pregnancy is critical for women of reproductive age who have longstanding diabetes.

Pregnancy may increase the prevalence of some background changes,[48] and retinopathy may progress despite strict metabolic control. Two studies have confirmed the development of both nonproliferative and proliferative changes with rapid normalization of glucose control in early pregnancy.[49,50] In a subset of 140 women without proliferative retinopathy at base line followed in the Diabetes in Early Pregnancy Study, progression of retinopathy was seen in 10.3, 21.1, 18.8, and 54.8% of patients with no retinopathy, microaneurysms only, mild nonproliferative retinopathy, and moderate-to-severe nonproliferative retinopathy at base line, respectively. Elevated glycosylated hemoglobin at base line and the magnitude of improvement of glucose control through week 14 was associated with a higher risk of progression of retinopathy.[49] Whether improving control or simply suboptimal control itself contributes to a deterioration of background retinopathy remains uncertain. Fortunately, most patients who require laser photocoagulation will respond to this therapy and should therefore be treated promptly. However, women who demonstrate severe florid disk neovascularization that is unresponsive to laser therapy during early pregnancy may be at great risk for deterioration of their vision. Termination of pregnancy should be considered in this group of patients.

Coronary Artery Disease

Class H diabetes refers to the presence of diabetes of any duration associated with ischemic myocardial disease. There is evidence that the small number of women who have coronary artery disease are at an increased risk of dying during gestation, particularly women who suffer an infarction during pregnancy.[51] For these cases, the maternal mortality rate is approximately 50%.[51] A high index of suspicion for ischemic heart disease should be maintained in women with longstanding diabetes, since anginal symptoms may be minimal and infarction may thus present as congestive heart failure.[52] While there are a few reports of successful pregnancies following myocardial infarction in diabetic women, cardiac status should be carefully assessed early in gestation or preferably prior to pregnancy. The decision to undertake a pregnancy in a woman with IDDM and coronary artery disease needs to be made only after serious consideration.

The potential for morbidity and mortality must be thoroughly reviewed with the patient and her family.

Detection of Diabetes in Pregnancy

Ninety percent of the cases of diabetes in pregnancy represent women with GDM. Patients with GDM are at significant risk for glucose intolerance developing later in life. O'Sullivan has reported that more than 50% of these patients become diabetic after years of follow-up.[53] The likelihood for subsequent diabetes apparently increases when GDM is diagnosed in early pregnancy and when insulin is required for treatment.

GDM is a state restricted to pregnant women whose impaired glucose tolerance is discovered during pregnancy. Because, in most cases, patients with GDM have normal fasting glucose levels, some challenge of glucose tolerance must be performed. Traditionally, obstetricians relied on historical and clinical risk factors to select patients in whom GDM was most likely to develop. This group included patients with a family history of diabetes or those whose past pregnancies were marked by an unexplained stillbirth or the delivery of a malformed or macrosomic infant. Interestingly, over half of all patients who exhibit abnormal glucose tolerance lack the risk factors mentioned above. In a series of 6214 women, Coustan and colleagues reported that using historical risk factors and an arbitrary cutoff age of 30 years for screening would miss 35% of cases of GDM.[54]

The American College of Obstetricians and Gynecologists has suggested that, whereas selective screening for GDM may be appropriate in some clinical settings, such as teen clinics (low-risk populations), universal screening may be more appropriate in other settings (high-risk populations).[55] Similarly, the American Diabetes Association has endorsed selective screening in that the risk for GDM is sufficiently low in lean women less than age 25 as to obviate the need for testing this group.[56] It should be noted that in some countries, experts have questioned the benefit of GDM screening programs altogether.[57] As O'Sullivan's original work, which established the criteria for the diagnosis of GDM, failed to evaluate its association with perinatal outcome, many have questioned the overall significance of this diagnosis. In fact, two studies have addressed the relationship between mild degrees of carbohydrate tolerance and rates of neonatal macrosomia. In a study of 3637 women without GDM, Sermer and colleagues demonstrated a graded increase in adverse outcomes (including large infants) with increasing maternal carbohydrate intolerance.[58] Sacks et al. also identified fasting and 2-hour glucose values as independent risk factors for macrosomia in a multivariate analysis of over 3500 pregnant women. However, no clinically meaningful glucose threshold for macrosomia could be identified, and they concluded that the criteria for GDM will continue to be established by consensus.[59]

The 50-g glucose challenge may be performed in the fasting or fed state, yet sensitivity is improved if the test is performed in the fasting state.[60,61] A plasma value between 135 and 140 mg/dl is commonly used as a threshold for performing a 3-hour oral glucose-tolerance test (OGTT). Coustan et al. have demonstrated that 10% of women with GDM will have screening test values between 130 and 139 mg/dl.[60] This study indicated that the sensitivity of screening is increased from 90% to nearly 100% if universal screening is employed using a threshold of 130 mg/dl.[54] With lowering the threshold of screening tests, further diagnostic testing increases from 14% (140 mg/dl) to 23% (130 mg/dl), which is accompanied by an approximate 12% increase in the overall cost to diagnose each case of GDM.

Using the plasma cutoff of 135 to 140 mg/dl, one can expect approximately 15 to 20% of patients with an abnormal screening value to have an abnormal 3-hour OGTT. The OGTT, rather than the intravenous test, is favored because it is probably more physiologic and assesses the gastrointestinal factors involved in insulin secretion. The oral test also appears to be more sensitive and has been well standardized. The criteria for establishing the diagnosis of gestational diabetes are listed in Table 6-19. The U.S.

National Diabetes Data Group criteria represent a theoretic conversion of O'Sullivan's thresholds in whole blood. Carpenter and Coustan prefer to use another modification of these data, which is supported by a comparison of the old Somogyi–Nelson method and current plasma glucose oxidase assays.[63] Recently, the Fourth International Workshop Conference of GDM suggested a further modification of the Carpenter–Coustan criteria.[56] It has been demonstrated that less-stringent criteria are associated with as much perinatal morbidity and fetal macrosomia as subjects diagnosed by the National Diabetes Data Group Criteria.[64] Regardless of the criteria employed, the patient must have a normal fasting value and two abnormal postprandial glucose determinations to be designated as Class A_1.

Women who demonstrate one abnormal value on the diagnostic 3-hour OGTT are also at apparent increased risk for fetal macrosomia.[65] Langer and colleagues[65] prefer to identify and treat such patients as having GDM. Other authors have suggested repeating the OGTT later in pregnancy in women who initially demonstrate one abnormal value, reserving the diagnosis for women with two subsequent abnormal values. In a study of 106 women with one abnormal OGTT value at approximately 30 weeks of gestation, in whom the OGTT was repeated one month later, gestational diabetes developed in 34%.[66]

Treatment of the Insulin-Dependent Patient

Clinical efforts aimed at optimizing maternal glycemic control are primarily responsible for the decline in perinatal death seen in IDDM pregnancies over the past few decades. Blood-glucose self-monitoring combined with aggressive insulin therapy aided in improving maternal glycemic status. Patients should be taught to monitor their glucose levels using glucose-oxidase impregnated test strips and a portable glucose reflectance meter.[67] Conventional insulin therapy should be abandoned in favor of intensive therapy consisting of multiple injections or subcutaneous pump therapy. Patients are instructed on dietary composition, insulin action, recognition and treatment of hypoglycemia, adjusting insulin dosage for exercise and sick days, as well as monitoring for hyperglycemia and potential ketosis. Intensive insulin therapy is essentially an attempt to simulate physiologic insulin requirements. Insulin administration is provided for both basal needs and meals, and rapid adjustments are

TABLE 6-19
SCREENING TESTS FOR GESTATIONAL DIABETES

Screening Test 50-g, 1-hour		Plasma Glucose (mg/dl) 130–140	
Oral 100-g GTT*	NDDG	Carpenter[62]	Fourth International Workshop[56]
Fasting	105	95	95
1-hour	190	180	180
2-hour	165	155	160
3-hour	145	140	140

Diagnosis of gestational diabetes is made when any two values are met or exceeded.

*NDDG = National Diabetes Data Group

made in response to glucose measurements. Frequent blood-glucose self-monitoring is fundamental to achieve the therapeutic objective of physiologic glucose control. Glucose determinations are made in the fasting state and before lunch, dinner, and bedtime. Postprandial and nocturnal values are also helpful. Patients are instructed on an insulin dose for each meal and at bedtime if necessary. Mealtime insulin needs are determined by the composition of the meal, the premeal glucose measurement, and the level of activity anticipated following the meal. Basal or intermediate-acting insulin requirements are determined by periodic 2 a.m. to 4 a.m. glucose measurements as well as late afternoon values, which reflect morning NPH or Lente action. During pregnancy, many diabetic women develop the self-management skills that are essential to an intensive insulin therapy regimen. In addition, patients are encouraged to contact their physician at any time if questions should arise concerning the management of their diabetes. During early pregnancy, patients are instructed to report their glucose values by telephone on a weekly (minimum) basis.

Insulin therapy must be individualized, with dosage determinations tailored to diet and exercise. Beef and pork insulin have largely been replaced by semisynthetic human insulin preparations. Since human insulin is far less immunogenic than animal insulin, it is preferred for pregnant women, especially those receiving insulin for the first time. Human insulin may have a more rapid onset and shorter duration of action, factors that must be considered when changing patients to these preparations.

Insulin is generally administered in two to three injections. We prefer a three-injection regimen, although most patients initially present taking a combination of intermediate-acting and short-acting insulin before dinner and breakfast. As a general rule, the amount of intermediate-acting insulin will exceed the short-acting component by a 2:1 ratio. Patients usually receive two-thirds of their total dose with breakfast and the remaining third in the evening as a combined dose with dinner or split into components with short-acting insulin at dinnertime and intermediate-acting insulin at bedtime in an effort to minimize periods of nocturnal hypoglycemia. Some women may also require a small dose of short-acting insulin before lunch, thus constituting a four-injection daily regimen.

There has now been considerable experience with open-loop continuous subcutaneous insulin infusion (CSII) pump therapy during pregnancy. The pump is a battery-powered unit that may be worn like a beeper during most daily activities. These systems provide continuous short-acting insulin therapy via a subcutaneous infusion. The basal infusion rate and bolus doses to cover meals are determined by frequent self-monitoring of blood glucose levels. The basal infusion rate is generally close to 1 unit per hour.

Diet therapy is critical to successful regulation of maternal diabetes. A program consisting of three meals and several snacks is employed for most patients. Dietary composition should be 50 to 60% carbohydrate, 20% protein, and 25 to 30% fat with less than 10% saturated fats, up to 10% polyunsaturated fatty acids, and the remainder derived from monosaturated sources.[68] Caloric intake is established based on prepregnancy weight and weight gain during gestation. Weight reduction is not advised. Patients should consume approximately 35 kcal/kg of ideal body weight. Obese women may be treated with an intake as low as 1600 calories per day; if ketonuria develops, this allowance may be increased.

The presence of maternal vasculopathy should be thoroughly assessed early in pregnancy. The patient should be evaluated by an ophthalmologist familiar with diabetic retinopathy. Ophthalmologic examinations should be performed during each trimester and repeated more often if retinopathy is detected. Baseline renal function is established by assaying a 24-hour urine collection for creatinine clearance and protein. An electrocardiogram and urine culture should also be obtained.

Antepartum Fetal Evaluation

Improved understanding of the importance of maternal glycemic control has played a major role in reducing stillbirths in diabetic pregnancies. Currently, antepartum fetal monitoring tests are used primarily to reassure the obstetrician and avoid unnecessary premature delivery. These biophysical techniques have few false negative results, and, in a patient with well-controlled diabetes who exhibits no vasculopathy or significant hypertension, reassuring antepartum testing allows the fetus to benefit from further maturation in utero.

Daily maternal assessment of fetal activity serves as a screening technique in a program of fetal surveillance. To date, few studies have applied this method to a large number of women with diabetes mellitus. While the false negative rate with maternal monitoring of

her usual morning insulin dose should be withheld. If her surgery is not performed early in the day, one-third to one-half of the patient's intermediate-acting dose of insulin may be administered. Epidural anesthesia is preferred because an awake patient is more alert to the early signs of hypoglycemia. Following surgery, glucose levels should be monitored every 2 hours, and an intravenous solution containing 5% dextrose should be administered.

Following delivery, insulin requirements are usually significantly lower than during pregnancy. The objective of "tight control" used in the antepartum period can be relaxed; glucose values of 150 to 200 mg/dl are acceptable. Patients delivered vaginally, who are able to eat a regular diet, are given one-third to one-half of their end-of-pregnancy dose of NPH insulin the morning of the first postpartum day. Frequent glucose determinations should be used to guide insulin dosage. If the patient has been given supplemental regular insulin in addition to the morning NPH dose, the amount of NPH insulin on the following morning is increased in an amount equal to two-thirds of the additional regular insulin. Most patients are stabilized on this regimen within a few days after delivery.

Treatment of the Patient with Gestational Diabetes

Primary treatment of GDM consists of nutritional counseling and dietary intervention. The optimal diet should provide caloric and nutrient needs to sustain pregnancy while minimizing postprandial hyperglycemia. Women with GDM rarely require hospitalization for dietary instruction and management. Once the diagnosis is established, patients should begin a dietary program of 2000 to 2500 kcal daily.[77] This represents approximately 35 kcal/kg of present pregnancy weight. Jovanovic-Peterson and Peterson have noted that a diet composed of 50% to 60% carbohydrate will cause excessive weight gain and postprandial hyperglycemia and require insulin therapy in 50% of patients.[78] For this reason, several groups have studied the use of calorie-restricted diets. Significant ketonuria may develop in patients on a restricted diet, which may have a detrimental effect on fetal neurologic development. A diet of at least 1800 kcal is preferred since it improves glycemic control and does not increase serum ketone levels.[79] Similar results have been reported by Jovanovic-Peterson and Peterson,

who recommend 30 kcal/kg of present pregnant weight for normal weight women, 24 kcal/kg for overweight women, and 12 kcal/kg for morbidly obese women.[80] These authors indicate that moderate calorie restriction with modification of the carbohydrate component may be advised in obese women with GDM.

Once the patient with GDM is placed on an appropriate diet, surveillance of blood-glucose levels is necessary to be certain that good glycemic control has been established. Weekly assessment of fasting or postprandial glucose levels should be performed at clinic or office visits. Some clinicians prefer to have patients perform daily blood-glucose self-monitoring, which in two retrospective studies has been associated with a decline in macrosomia at the expense of nearly half of all women requiring insulin therapy.[81] Our approach is to provide women with GDM with a reflectance meter; however, if after a few weeks, both fasting and postprandial measurements are within the normal range, the frequency of testing can be reduced accordingly.

Both ADA and ACOG have recommended that fasting plasma glucose levels be maintained below 105 mg/dl and 2-hour postprandial values below 120 mg/dl in women with GDM. If a patient repeatedly exceeds these thresholds, insulin therapy is indicated. The use of the above cutoffs for initiating insulin treatment is based on data regarding increased perinatal morbidity when such values are exceeded in women with preexisting diabetes. It is unclear whether these thresholds are appropriate for instituting insulin in women with GDM.

In addition to aggressive insulin therapy and hypocaloric diet regimens, exercise has been studied as an alternative primary treatment for GDM. Such an approach is beneficial for non-insulin-dependent nonpregnant diabetic patients in whom physical training increases insulin sensitivity. Fasting and postprandial insulin concentrations and glucose excursions are lowered in both obese and physically fit individuals who exercise. This effect apparently is sustained up to 5 to 7 days after the last training session.

Bung and colleagues[82] also conducted a prospective study of the utility of exercise in the treatment of GDM. These authors studied 41 women with GDM who manifested elevated fasting glucose levels, which would normally require insulin therapy. In the final analysis, 17 women completed a supervised bicycle ergometry training program, as compared with

TABLE 6-20
ANTEPARTUM FETAL SURVEILLANCE FOR INSULIN-DEPENDENT DIABETES MELLITUS

Ultrasonography at 4- to 6-week intervals
Maternal assessment of fetal activity, daily at 28 weeks
Nonstress test weekly at 28 weeks (high risk)
Nonstress test twice weekly at 32 weeks (low risk)
Contraction stress test or biophysical profile if NST nonreactive
Lung profile if elective delivery prior to 38 to 39 weeks

fetal activity is low (~1%), the false positive rate may be as high as 60%.

The nonstress test (NST) has become the preferred method to assess antepartum fetal well-being in the patient with diabetes mellitus.[69] If the NST is nonreactive, a contraction stress test or biophysical profile should be performed. Fetal heart rate monitoring should be initiated early in the third trimester, usually by 32 weeks of gestation (Table 6-20). An apparent increased fetal death rate exists within 1 week of a reactive NST in pregnancies complicated by IDDM as compared with other high-risk gestations.[70] If the NST is to be used as the primary method of antepartum heart rate testing, it should be performed at least twice weekly once the patient reaches 32 weeks of gestation. In women with vascular disease or poor control, in whom the incidence of abnormal tests and intrauterine deaths is greater, testing may be indicated earlier and more frequently.

It is important to include not only the results of antepartum fetal testing but to weigh all the clinical features involving mother and fetus before a decision is made to intervene for suspected fetal distress, especially if this decision may result in a preterm delivery. In reviewing nine series involving 993 diabetic patients, an abnormal test of fetal condition led to delivery 5% of the time.[71] It appears that outpatient testing protocols work well in insulin dependent patients. Whether such testing is required for all patients with insulin dependent diabetes mellitus remains debatable.[72] However, women whose diabetes is poorly controlled, as well as those with hypertension or vasculopathy that may be associated with fetal growth restriction require a program of antepartum fetal surveillance.

Ultrasound is a valuable tool in evaluating fetal growth, estimating fetal weight, and detecting malformations. A determination of maternal serum α-fetoprotein (MSAFP) at 16 weeks of gestation

should be employed in association with a detailed ultrasound study at 15 to 20 weeks in an attempt to detect neural-tube defects and other anomalies. MSAFP levels are lower in diabetic women than in the nondiabetic population.[73] A lower threshold for the upper limit of normal may thus be preferable in pregnancies complicated by diabetes mellitus in order to help detect spina bifida and other major malformations that are increased in this population. Fetal echocardiography should be performed at 20 to 22 weeks of gestation to identify possible cardiac anomalies. A review of the prenatal diagnosis experience in 289 women with IDDM in the Ohio State University Diabetes in Pregnancy Program revealed 29 anomalies, 12 of which were cardiac, 14 noncardiac, and 3 combined.[12] Twelve of 15 (80%) cardiac and 10 of 17 (59%) noncardiac lesions were identified prenatally. When considering cardiac defects alone, a glycosylated hemoglobin cutoff for these anomalies could not be identified. Thus, detailed cardiac imaging should be offered to all women with IDDM to assist in the detection of cardiac lesions.

Ultrasound examinations should be repeated during the third trimester at 4- to 6-week intervals to assess fetal growth. The detection of fetal macrosomia, the leading risk factor for shoulder dystocia, is important in the selection of patients who are best delivered by cesarean. An increased rate of cephalopelvic disproportion and shoulder dystocia, accompanied by significant risk of traumatic birth injury and asphyxia, have been consistently associated with the vaginal delivery of large infants. The risk of such complications rises exponentially when birth weight exceeds 4 kg and is greater for the fetus of a diabetic mother as compared with a fetus of similar weight whose mother does not have diabetes.[74] Recommended fetal weight cut-offs for cesarean section in the setting of maternal diabetes have ranged between 4000 and 4500 g. Despite its limitations, sonographic measurement of the fetal abdominal circumference has proved most helpful in predicting fetal macrosomia.[75]

Timing and Mode of Delivery

As a goal, delivery should be delayed until term, when fetal maturation has taken place, provided that the patient's diabetes is well controlled and antepartum surveillance remains normal. In practice, elective induction of labor is often planned at 38 to 40 weeks of gestation in patients with well-controlled diabetes and no vascular disease. Patients with vascular disease are delivered prior to term only if hypertension worsens, fetal growth restriction occurs, or there is concern regarding glycemic control. Before elective delivery prior to 38 to 39 weeks of gestation, an amniocentesis should be performed to document fetal pulmonary maturity. Although the value of the lecithin:sphingomyelin (L:S) ratio has been questioned in pregnancies complicated by diabetes mellitus, as mentioned earlier, many series report a reassuringly low incidence of respiratory distress syndrome (RDS) with a mature ratio.[36] The acidic phospholipid, phosphatidylglycerol (PG), is the final marker of fetal pulmonary maturation. Fetal hyperinsulinemia may be associated with the delayed appearance of PG and an increased incidence of RDS. Landon et al.[27] have correlated the appearance of PG in amniotic fluid with maternal glycemic control during gestation.

RDS may occur in the IDDM with a mature L:S ratio but absent PG. Therefore, caution should be used in planning the delivery of patients with an L:S ratio of 2.0 and absent PG. Most important, the clinician must be familiar with the laboratory analysis of amniotic fluid in his or her institution and the neonatal outcome for the IDDM at various L:S ratios in the presence or absence of PG. This information must be factored against the risks to the fetus or mother of prolonging gestation.

The route of delivery for the diabetic patient remains controversial. Cousins,[76] in reviewing the literature on IDDM pregnancy, noted a cesarean delivery rate of approximately 45%. This figure represents the practice trends of most U.S. obstetricians and perinatologists.[69] Cesarean delivery is usually favored when fetal distress has been suggested by antepartum heart rate monitoring. If a patient reaches 38 weeks of gestation with a mature fetal lung profile and is at significant risk for intrauterine death because of poor control or a history of a prior stillbirth, an elective delivery should be planned. Elective cesarean delivery should be performed if the cervix is not favorable for induction or if the infant is believed to be excessively large.

During labor, continuous fetal heart rate monitoring is required. Labor should be allowed to progress as long as a normal rate of cervical dilatation, followed by descent in the second stage, is documented. The risk for shoulder dystocia in a fetus with macrosomia and IDDM is greater than for the large, normal infant. Despite attempts to select patients with excessive fetal size for elective cesarean delivery, ar-

rest of dilation despite adequate labor or an arrest of descent should alert the physician to the possibility of cephalopelvic disproportion. About 25% of macrosomic infants (≥4000 g) delivered after a prolonged second stage will have shoulder dystocia. It follows that cesarean delivery is favored over midpelvic operative delivery in most cases of maternal diabetes.

Glucose Regulation during Labor and Delivery

As neonatal hypoglycemia is, in part, related to maternal glucose levels during labor, it is important to maintain maternal plasma glucose levels at physiologic levels. The patient should be allowed nothing by mouth after midnight of the evening before induction or elective cesarean delivery, and the usual bedtime dose of insulin should be administered. On arrival to labor and delivery, the patient's capillary glucose level should be assessed with a bedside reflectance meter. Continuous infusion of both insulin and glucose are then administered based on maternal glucose levels (Table 6-21). Ten units of regular insulin may be added to 1000 ml of solution containing 5% dextrose. An infusion rate of 100 to 125 ml/hr (1 unit/hr) will, in most cases, result in good glucose control. Glucose levels should be recorded hourly and the infusion rate adjusted accordingly. It may be necessary to increase the insulin infusion during the second stage of labor because increased catecholamine secretion may worsen glucose control.

When cesarean delivery is to be performed, it should be scheduled for early morning. This simplifies intrapartum glucose control and allows the neonatal team to prepare for the care of the newborn. The patient should be given nothing by mouth, and

---

TABLE 6-21
INSULIN MANAGEMENT DURING LABOR AND DELIVERY

Usual dose of intermediate-acting insulin given at bedtime
Morning dose of insulin withheld
Intravenous infusion of normal saline begun
Once active labor begins or glucose levels fall below
  70 mg/dl, infusion changes from saline to 5% dextrose
  at 100–125 cc/hr
Glucose levels checked hourly using a portable reflectance
  meter allowing for adjustment in the infusion rate
Regular (short-acting) insulin administered beginning at
  1.0 units/hr by intravenous infusion if glucose levels exceed
  140 mg/dl

Chapter 7
Hypertensive Disorders during Pregnancy

Robert S. Egerman

Five Key Points

- **Hypertensive disorders in pregnancy may be classified as pregnancy-induced hypertension, preeclampsia/eclampsia, chronic hypertension, and chronic hypertension with superimposed pregnancy-induced hypertension or preeclampsia.**
- **Chronic hypertension complicates 1 to 3% of all pregnancies. Most cases are due to essential hypertension.**
- **The most common adverse effects of chronic hypertension in pregnancy are intrauterine growth restriction and superimposed preeclampsia.**
- **Antihypertensive agents commonly used during pregnancy include alpha methyldopa, nifedipine, and labetalol.**
- **The most common causes of maternal death in patients with severe preeclampsia/eclampsia are cerebrovascular accident, hemorrhage, and pulmonary edema.**

Hypertension affects 7 to 10% of all pregnancies. Acute complications may be suffered by the pregnant woman and subsequent fetal morbidity and mortality may be incurred. Complications of hypertension account for 15% of all maternal deaths in the U.S.[1]

Hypertensive disease during pregnancy can be divided into preexisting or chronic hypertension and pregnancy-induced hypertension. Within the category of pregnancy-induced hypertension are preeclampsia, chronic hypertension with superimposed preeclampsia, and gestational hypertension.

NORMAL BLOOD PRESSURE FOR PREGNANCY

A physiologic change in blood pressure is expected during pregnancy. In 259 normal pregnant women undergoing ambulatory blood pressure monitoring, Brown et al. reported a slight increase in blood pressure throughout gestation.[2] In measurements between 9 and 17 weeks of gestation, systolic and diastolic pressures (±SD) were 111±5 and 65±4 mm Hg, respectively. By the third trimester (at 31 to 40 weeks), both values increased, 115 ± 8 mm Hg systolic and 70 ± 6 mm Hg diastolic. During sleep, blood pressure decreased by 14 to 16 mm Hg systolic and 13 to 14 mm Hg diastolic. Ambulatory pressures record 12 mm higher for systolic and 6 mm higher for diastolic measurements as compared with conventional sphygmomanometric measurements.

CHRONIC HYPERTENSION

Diagnosis and Evaluation

With the release of the Sixth Report from the National Committee on the Prevention, Detection, Evaluation, and Treatment of High Blood Pressure, hypertension has been categorized into subsets as listed in Table 7-1.[3]

Chronic hypertension complicates 1 to 3% of pregnancies. As in the nonpregnant state, most hypertension during pregnancy is primary or essential hypertension. Since women of childbearing age are relatively young, an effort should be made to ensure that a secondary cause is not present. Chronic hypertension is typically diagnosed before 20 weeks of gestation.

The evaluation begins with historical information regarding prior hypertension and assessment of the extent of the previous work-up and therapy. Use of medications and recreational drugs, as well as a review of systems for target-organ involvement, is included. The severity of organ damage depends on the degree and duration of hypertension. A history of either scleroderma or polyarteritis nodosa portends a particularly poor prognosis for both the mother and the fetus.

The physical examination should be focused on causes of secondary hypertension and identification of target-organ damage. Renovascular disease, renal parenchymal disease, aortic coarctation, hyperthyroidism, Cushing syndrome, pheochromocytoma, and primary aldosteronism are conditions to consider. Identification of a pheochromocytoma is particularly important since maternal mortality is extremely high if the condition is not diagnosed before the onset of labor.

Blood pressure measurements should be taken in the seated position at the level of the patient's heart, with an appropriately sized sphygmomanometer cuff. The fifth Korotkoff sound, phase V (absence of sound), should be used for the determination of the diastolic value instead of the phase IV Korotkoff sound

TABLE 7-1
CLASSIFICATION OF BLOOD PRESSURE

Category	SBP (mm Hg)	DBP (mm Hg)
Optimal	<120	<80
Normal	120–129	80–84
High normal	130–139	85–89
Chronic hypertension		
Stage I	140–159	90–99
Stage II	160–179	100–109
Stage III	≥180	≥110

SBP = systolic blood pressure; DBP = diastolic blood pressure.

(muffling). If the patient is hypertensive, blood pressure measurements should be recorded in both arms at the initial visit. The diagnosis of hypertension should be established on the basis of at least two elevated blood pressures on at least two separate occasions.

Funduscopic examination should be performed to confirm the absence of papilledema or hemorrhage. The thyroid gland should be carefully palpated. The heart should be auscultated for murmurs and the lungs for rales. The flanks and abdomen should be examined for bruits and the peripheral pulses for their intensity and concordance.

Renal function should be assessed by determination of the serum creatinine level and a 24-hour urine collection for protein and creatinine clearance. A decreased serum potassium is suggestive of hyperaldosteronism. Levels of an antinuclear antibody or thyroid-stimulating hormone can be obtained if systemic lupus erythematosus or hyperthyroidism is suspected. A urinalysis should be performed and the sediment examined. A urine culture and sensitivity also should be ordered since a lower-urinary-tract infection can ascend into the kidneys and worsen existing renal disease. A complete blood count should also be obtained. Patients with longstanding hypertension or a concomitant comorbid condition should undergo electrocardiography. If a pathologic murmur is auscultated, echocardiography should be performed.

Perinatal Outcome with Chronic Hypertension

A higher frequency of small-for-gestational age (SGA) infants can be expected from pregnancies complicated by chronic hypertension. In a study by McCowan et al. (in which SGA was defined as <5%), of 155 women whose pregnancies were complicated by pure chronic hypertension without superimposed preeclampsia, more than twice as many hypertensive women delivered SGA infants (10.9%) as compared with controls (4.1%).[4] When diastolic blood pressure was severely elevated ($\geq$110 mm Hg), patients were at increased risk for superimposed preeclampsia and delivery before 32 weeks of gestation. Sibai and Anderson reported that, in women whose diastolic pressures were >110 mm Hg in the first trimester, the uncorrected perinatal mortality was as high as 25%.[5]

An increase in placental abruption is seen in pregnancies complicated by hypertensive disease. The frequency of this complication is from 0.5 to 10%, and abruption leads to significant perinatal morbidity and mortality. Interestingly, medical treatment of chronic hypertension does not affect the frequency of abruption, superimposed preeclampsia, or preterm delivery.[6]

Superimposed Preeclampsia

Perinatal outcome depends on the severity of the maternal hypertension and the presence of superimposed preeclampsia. In Sibai and Anderson's series of 44 women with severe chronic hypertension, pregnancy outcome was considerably worse (perinatal mortality, abruption, maternal renal compromise) in women in whom superimposed preeclampsia developed.[5] Distinguishing superimposed preeclampsia from exacerbation of chronic hypertension is difficult, and any clinical symptom suggesting preeclampsia should be carefully addressed. Superimposed preeclampsia should be suspected whenever hypertension worsens in association with peripheral and periorbital edema and proteinuria. Twenty-four-hour urine protein excretion greater than 1 g or an elevated uric acid of $\geq$6 mg/dl is suggestive of superimposed preeclampsia, as are abnormal liver-function tests, thrombocytopenia, or altered coagulation tests. If the underlying source of hypertension is related to systemic lupus erythematosus, falling component levels or increased anti-dS DNA titers may be useful in diagnosing a lupus flare. Severe superimposed preeclampsia usually is an indication for delivery in pregnancies greater than 28 weeks of gestation.[7] Further management is addressed below.

Choice of Antihypertensive Medication

Treatment of chronic hypertension is necessary to prevent maternal cardiovascular, cerebrovascular, renal, and retinal injury, even though treatment will not change the frequency of superimposed preeclampsia or abruption. In Sibai et al.'s series of 211 patients with mild chronic hypertension, half experienced a decrease in mean arterial pressure, one-third remained unchanged, and the remainder experienced an increase.[8] A severe exacerbation was seen in 4% whose blood pressure dropped, in 16% whose blood pressure remained unchanged, and in 32% whose blood pressure increased. Most women with mild hypertension do not require medication during pregnancy. Patients should receive medication if the diastolic pressure exceeds 105 mm Hg or the systolic pressure equals or exceeds 160 mm Hg. Once therapy is initiated, the goal is to keep the diastolic pressure less than 100 mm Hg and the systolic pressure less than 150 mm Hg. Women with diabetes or renal disease will benefit from a diastolic pressure <90 mm Hg.[7]

Pregnancy restricts the choice of antihypertensive agents because of potential teratogenicity and concern for alteration in uterine blood flow. Commonly used drugs include α-methyldopa (a centrally acting α_2-receptor stimulant that decreases norepinephrine release), labetalol (a β- and α_1-receptor blocker), nifedipine (a dihydropyridine calcium-channel blocker), and hydralazine (an arteriolar dilator).

α-Methyldopa has been used extensively during pregnancy, with no adverse fetal or neonatal effects reported from its use. It has limited efficacy and should be used when the degree of hypertension is not severe. Abnormal liver-function tests and a Coombs-positive hemolytic anemia are possible adverse effects. The initial dose is 250 mg three to four times per day. Total maximum daily dose is 2 g. Drowsiness, fatigue, orthostasis, and dry mouth may be experienced while taking this medication.

β-Blocking agents cause a slowing of the heart, vasodilation, and a decrease in cardiac output. Adverse effects include bronchoconstriction (precluding their use in patients with asthma) and hypoglycemia (must be used with caution in patients with insulin-dependent diabetes). Fetal growth restriction and oligohydramnios have been reported with their use, in addition to neonatal bradycardia and hypoglycemia.

Calcium-channel blockers inhibit cellular calcium influx by blocking voltage-dependent calcium channels. Of the many groups of these agents, the dihydropyridines have been used most widely during pregnancy.[9] Nifedipine has been used for the treatment of chronic hypertension and pregnancy-induced hypertension. Headache, fatigue, swelling, and reflex tachycardia are potential side effects. Rarely, pancytopenia or hepatitis may result from its use. A typical dose is 10 to 30 mg four times per day, up to a maximal total daily dose of 120 mg. A once-daily, long-acting preparation is available, and therapy can be initiated at 30 to 60 mg.[10] Calcium-channel blockers should be used with extreme caution, if at all, in combination with magnesium sulfate because of the potential for severe hypotension and respiratory depression. The use of nifedipine for management of hypertensive crises is under scrutiny.

Hydralazine is a smooth-muscle relaxant that causes vasodilation. It is frequently used as an intravenous bolus for intrapartum hypertensive emergencies. Side effects include reflex tachycardia, orthostatic hypotension, a lupus syndrome, and neonatal thrombocytopenia. It is best used as an adjuvant agent.[7] An oral preparation is available, and the initial dose is 10 mg four times per day. Dosage can be increased to a maximum of 300 mg per day.

Some pharmacologic agents have the potential for adverse perinatal outcome. Ganglionic blockers may cause meconium ileus. Angiotensin-converting–enzyme (ACE) inhibitors have been associated with fetal renal tubular dysgenesis, oligohydramnios, fetal growth restriction, anuria, and fetal hypotension. Similar concerns are postulated for the angiotensin II receptor blockers. Thiazide diuretics, although commonly used in the nonpregnant individual, can deplete intravascular volume and can cause electrolyte abnormalities, hyperglycemia, and hemorrhagic pancreatitis. Neonatal effects include growth restriction, electrolyte abnormalities, and thrombocytopenia.

Patient and Fetal Surveillance

Sonography should be performed in the latter part of the second trimester and repeated as indicated in the third trimester to assess fetal growth. Weekly antenatal fetal heart rate testing should begin at 34 weeks of gestation if the patient is not on antihypertensive medication. If the patient is taking medication, twice-weekly testing should be initiated at 32 weeks of gestation. Assessment of amniotic fluid volume should be performed weekly as well. Fetal assessment should be initiated sooner if the fetus is growth-restricted or

if the mother has a comorbid condition such as diabetes or systemic lupus erythematosus.

If the cervix is favorable at 38 to 39 weeks of gestation, labor should be induced. If the cervix is unfavorable, fetal surveillance should be continued, awaiting the onset of spontaneous labor or a more favorable cervix. In no instance should the pregnancy be prolonged beyond 42 weeks. If growth restriction and oligohydramnios are present, delivery may be indicated even prior to term.

The development of superimposed preeclampsia alters the aforementioned management. If the patient is at 37 weeks of gestation or greater, she should be delivered. Otherwise, the patient should be hospitalized and carefully evaluated. Subsequent management and timing of delivery will be determined by the severity of the preeclampsia. Consultation with a perinatologist is frequently helpful.

GESTATIONAL HYPERTENSION

Gestational hypertension is an ambiguous entity. Generally, if hypertension develops after 20 weeks, the diagnosis is preeclampsia. Occasionally, given no other evidence of preeclampsia, the patient may be exhibiting gestational hypertension. Many of these patients have underlying chronic hypertension or the early development of preeclampsia. If the diagnosis remains gestational hypertension, the outcome of the pregnancy is good without pharmacotherapy.[11]

PREECLAMPSIA

Diagnosis and Evaluation

Preeclampsia is a condition unique to pregnancy that affects many organ systems. The pathophysiology is poorly understood despite a prolific volume of literature published on this subject. The underlying perturbation involves endothelial-cell disruption and vasospasm. Brain, liver, kidneys, and placenta are particularly vulnerable. Low oncotic pressure, decreased intravascular volume, third spacing of fluid, and activation of the coagulation system can be seen. Preeclampsia is classically described as a triad of hypertension, edema, and proteinuria; however, any one or more of these findings may be absent. Interestingly, one-fifth of women with eclampsia have diastolic pressures <90 mm Hg or absent proteinuria and one-third have no edema.[12]

Preeclampsia jeopardizes both the mother and the fetus. Predominant maternal risks include seizures (eclampsia), coagulopathy, hemorrhage, pulmonary edema, cerebrovascular accident, abruption, renal failure, and death. The fetus is at risk for growth restriction, asphyxia, and death.

Predisposing Factors

Extremes of age, African-American ancestry, or a familial history of preeclampsia are predisposing factors. Medical complications (obesity, diabetes, renal disease, chronic hypertension, thyroid disease, sickle-cell anemia, and collagen vascular disease), as well as obstetric complications (multiple or molar gestations), also place the pregnant woman at risk for preeclampsia.

Mild Preeclampsia

Mild preeclampsia is defined as systolic blood pressure ≥140 mm Hg but <160 mm Hg, or diastolic ≥90 mm Hg but <110 mm Hg. Older criteria using increases in diastolic pressure of 15 mm Hg and systolic pressure of 30 mm Hg over base line are insensitive and should not be used to diagnose preeclampsia given the large number of healthy pregnant women who may experience such an increase. Proteinuria is ≥300 mg/24 hours but <5 g. Uric acid and hematocrit may be increased because of decreased renal perfusion and hemoconcentration from low intravascular volume, respectively. The presence of hemolytic anemia constitutes severe disease.

The patient should be questioned regarding neurologic or abdominal symptoms. Laboratory assessment should include a complete blood count, liver-function battery, and creatinine and uric acid levels. Sonography should be performed to determine the adequacy of fetal growth and amniotic fluid volume.

Outpatient Management

Bed rest is commonly prescribed. The patient should be evaluated twice weekly and questioned regarding symptoms. Blood pressure, maternal weight, urine protein, and antenatal testing should be obtained at these visits. Amniotic fluid assessment is a part of our fetal surveillance. Platelet count should be assessed periodically, and fetal growth should be determined sonographically at 3- to 4-week intervals. The patient should be instructed to record and report fetal movements as well as symptoms of severe preeclampsia. Abnormal laboratory analysis, urinary protein ≥1 g on 24-hour urine collection, diastolic blood pressure >100 mm Hg, abnormal fetal growth, or poor compliance with outpatient management warrant hospitalization.

Delivery of a patient with mild preeclampsia should be performed if the patient has a favorable cervix at or beyond 37 weeks of gestation. The decision as to when to induce labor in the presence of an unfavorable cervix is based on the degree of maternal hypertension, proteinuria and other laboratory abnormalities, and assessment of fetal well-being. Delivery should be considered in any patient with mild preeclampsia, regardless of the status of the cervix, by 40 weeks of gestation because of maternal concerns as well as the potential for uteroplacental insufficiency.

Severe Preeclampsia

Severe preeclampsia is defined as systolic blood pressure ≥160 mm Hg or diastolic ≥110 mm Hg. In addition, an array of organ involvement constitutes additional criteria for severe preeclampsia. These abnormalities are listed in Table 7-2.

Conservative Management

All patients with severe preeclampsia should be admitted to the hospital; those beyond 34 weeks of gestation should be delivered. The urgency of delivery depends on the stability of the mother and the fetus. A current protocol at our institution is to perform amniocentesis for fetal lung maturity if the patient is between 32 and 34 weeks of gestation. If the fetus is mature, then the patient is delivered.

TABLE 7-2
CRITERIA FOR THE DIAGNOSIS OF SEVERE PREECLAMPSIA

Hypertension (systolic ≥160 mm Hg, diastolic ≥110 mm Hg)
Proteinuria (>5 g in 24-hour collection)
Pulmonary edema
Neurologic symptoms or seizures
Epigastric or right upper quadrant pain
HELLP syndrome
Oliguria (<500 ml in 24 hours)
Increased creatinine
Fetal growth restriction or oligohydramnios

Alternatively, if pulmonary maturity is not demonstrated, glucocorticoids are administered and the fetus is delivered 48 hours later. Patients who are between 24 and 32 weeks of gestation may be candidates for conservative treatment. Pregnancies <24 weeks carry a poor prognosis (6.7% neonatal survival);[13] conservative treatment would not be likely to extend the pregnancy significantly, while placing the mother at significant risk. Therefore, delivery is indicated. Conversely, conservative management is more likely to be of significant benefit to the fetus at 24 to 27 weeks of gestation. Sibai et al. observed a 75% rate of neonatal survival for patients treated conservatively as compared with 35% survival when patients were delivered immediately.[13]

Blood pressure should be controlled with either parenteral labetalol or hydralazine (see below), and magnesium sulfate should be administered for seizure prophylaxis. Ideally, blood pressure should be maintained between 140 and 150 mm Hg systolic and between 90 and 100 mm Hg diastolic. Glucocorticoids should be administered to promote fetal lung maturity, and the patient and the fetus should be intensively monitored. Continuous electronic fetal monitoring should be implemented during the first 24 hours. Strict attention should be paid to clinical manifestations of neurologic or hepatic disease. Laboratory assessment should be performed to assess renal, hepatic, and hematologic function. Maternal or fetal deterioration mandates delivery regardless of the patient's gestational age or fetal pulmonary status.

After the initial 24- to 48-hour period of stabilization, blood pressure should be controlled to keep systolic and diastolic values in the aforementioned range, typically with divided doses of nifedipine (40 to 120 mg/day). Daily antenatal testing should be performed. Tests of renal, hepatic, and hematologic function should be obtained every 2 to 3 days, depending on the maternal status.

HELLP Syndrome

HELLP syndrome (hemolysis, elevated liver function, and low platelet count) affects up to 10% of pregnancies complicated by severe preeclampsia and eclampsia. HELLP syndrome is a hallmark of a critical illness.[16]

At the University of Tennessee, Memphis, patients who are diagnosed with HELLP syndrome typically have the following laboratory abnormalities[17]: hemolysis—abnormal peripheral smear, total bilirubin >1.2 mg/dl; serum lactate dehydrogenase >600 U/liter; elevated liver enzymes—serum aspartate aminotransferase >70 U/liter; serum lactate dehydrogenase >600 U/liter; low platelet count—platelets <100,000/μl.

Variations exist in that patients may display one or more aspects of the syndrome. Disseminated intravascular coagulation (DIC) tends to complicate HELLP syndrome when patients experience placental abruption, vaginal bleeding, or subcapsular hepatic hematoma.[18] DIC and abruption have been strongly associated with antepartum fetal death.

Patients generally deliver preterm, although delivery of patients with preeclampsia is not necessarily curative, as up to 30% of patients have manifestations of HELLP syndrome within 48 hours after delivery.[18] Malaise, fatigue, and nonspecific complaints (90%) are experienced a few days before presentation. Fifty percent of patients have nausea, vomiting, and/or headache. An equal percentage experience abdominal pain.[18]

Weight gain and edema were present in over 50% of patients in Sibai's series.[18] Blood pressure was elevated to the severe range (systolic ≥160 mm Hg or diastolic ≥110 mm Hg) in two-thirds of patients, yet diastolic blood pressure was <90 mm Hg in 15%. Proteinuria of ≥2+ on dipstick testing was observed in 85% of patients, minimal proteinuria (1+) in 9%, and no proteinuria in 6%.[18]

Liver function abnormalities may be normal initially despite abdominal complaints, only to become elevated postpartum. Platelet nadirs and transaminase elevations commonly occur after delivery.

Among pregnancies complicated by HELLP syndrome, DIC (21%), acute renal failure (7.7%), pulmonary edema (6%), liver hematoma (0.9%), and retinal detachment (0.9%) can occur. The maternal mortality rate is approximately 1%.[19,20] Interestingly, neonatal outcome is apparently no worse with HELLP syndrome as compared with outcomes from pregnancies complicated by severe preeclampsia or partial HELLP syndrome.[21]

The general intrapartum management of preeclampsia is discussed below. Nuances specific for patients with HELLP syndrome include delivery for fluid overload, worsening hypertension, or coagulopathy. Right-upper-quadrant or epigastric pain presages rupture of a liver hematoma, potentially with subsequent vascular collapse. These symptoms are indications for prompt delivery. The type of anesthesia employed depends on the coagulation status of the patient; regional anesthesia is contraindicated if a coagulopathy is present.

If the patient is beyond 30 to 32 weeks of gestation, labor may be induced. Cervical ripening agents may be useful if the cervix is unfavorable. Before 30 weeks of gestation, a prolonged labor can be anticipated; therefore, cesarean delivery should be considered. If the platelet count is <50,000/μl, platelets should be given at the time of the skin incision, and additional platelets should be administered during uterine closure if the tissue oozes.

At delivery, manipulation of the liver should be avoided. If blood is in the peritoneal cavity, the liver must be considered a potential source. Immediate management of a suspected ruptured liver hematoma includes adequate exposure, pressure with laparotomy packs, resuscitation with large volumes of blood products and fluids, and prompt surgical consultation. Embolization of the branch of the hepatic artery supplying the involved segment may be beneficial. If an unruptured hematoma is discovered on ultrasound or computed tomography, and the patient is hemodynamically stable, attempts at evacuation of the hematoma should be avoided. Postpartum, the patient requires continued observation in an intensive-care unit, and the general or vascular surgical service should be notified.

When closing the abdomen, a subfascial, intraperitoneal, closed suction drain should be placed. The intraperitoneal drain will reveal intraperitoneal hemorrhage from either the operative field or the liver after abdominal closure.

Finally, atypical presentations are not uncommon; however, the clinician must be vigilant in distinguishing between HELLP syndrome and thrombotic thrombocytopenic purpura/hemolytic uremic syndrome, as well as systemic lupus erythematosus.[22]

Intrapartum

Patients should be evaluated and monitored carefully in the labor and delivery unit. Preterm infants or patients with complicated courses should be referred to tertiary care center. Magnesium sulfate should be used for seizure prophylaxis, administered typically as a 6-g intravenous loading dose over 20 minutes, then continued at 2 g per hour. Adjustment in dose may be needed for patients with renal compromise or decreased urine output. Therapeutic levels are 4 to 8 mg/dl, respiratory depression at 15 mg/dl, and

dysrhythmias and cardiac arrest at 20 to 30 mg/dl. Caution must be used in the administration of this drug to avoid an inadvertent overdose.

Hypertension should be treated during labor to prevent the loss of cerebral autoregulation, followed by maternal cerebrovascular or encephalopathic complications. Uncontrolled hypertension can lead to congestive heart failure and renal failure. The goal is to maintain the mean arterial pressure between 105 and 125 mm Hg. Typically this goal can be achieved by treating systolic pressures ≥165 mm Hg or diastolic values ≥105 mm Hg. Caution should be used so as to not lower the mean arterial blood pressure to the point that uteroplacental perfusion is compromised.

Several agents may be used to acutely control blood pressure intrapartum. Labetalol in bolus doses should be given as a slow intravenous push. A response should be seen within 10 minutes. The protocol at the University of Tennessee, Memphis, is to begin with 20 mg, and, if necessary, increase to 40 mg, then to 80 mg at 10-minute intervals if a response is not seen. A total of 300 mg may be given.[23] Hydralazine is an alternative agent that is administered in 5-mg bolus doses at 20-minute intervals up to a total of 30 mg. The response to hydralazine may be unpredictable. Hypotension can occur if the patient is intravascularly depleted. For unresponsive hypertension, nitroprusside can be administered as a continuous infusion beginning with 0.5 μg/kg/min, increasing by 0.25 μg/kg/min every 5 minutes up to a total of 5 μg/kg/min. The patient needs to be carefully observed for cyanide toxicity while on this medication.

Eclampsia

Eclampsia is the new onset of convulsions or coma during pregnancy. It is rare during the first 20 weeks of gestation.[12] Cerebral vasospasm, hemorrhage, edema, or encephalopathy can be responsible for the seizure. Seizures are typically accompanied by hypertension, although the blood pressure need be only mildly elevated. Many times the patient will report a frontal or occipital headache; however, in 20% of cases the seizure occurs without premonitory symptoms.[12] Half of all seizures occur before labor, 25% intrapartum, and the remainder postpartum. Late postpartum eclampsia may occur as late as 2 weeks after delivery.

Seizure activity typically lasts for only 60 to 90 seconds. Maintaining an open airway is of paramount importance during the seizure. The patient's blood pressure should be stabilized, and she should be evaluated for the presence of a coagulopathy. Magnesium sulfate should be the initial anticonvulsant. Intravenous amobarbital (250 mg) can be administered over 3 minutes for persistent convulsions; alternatively, sodium pentothal may be used (50 mg initially, then titrated in 25-mg boluses to 100 mg if needed). Caution must be exercised in the administration of sedatives or tranquilizers so as to not depress maternal gag reflexes and contribute to aspiration. If the patient is undelivered, she should be stabilized first and then delivered. The fetal heart rate typically responds to the convulsion with bradycardia, decelerations, and loss of variability. These alterations are usually transient. With an unstable patient, a frantic cesarean delivery for fetal distress is imprudent.

Postictal depression is common after an eclamptic event, but focal neurologic deficits occur in a small percentage of patients. Computed tomography is useful in the evaluation of intracranial hemorrhage or cerebral edema.

Postpartum

Patients remain at risk postpartum for the complications of preeclampsia/eclampsia. Patients with mild preeclampsia should be treated with intravenous magnesium sulfate for 12 hours after delivery; those with severe preeclampsia should be treated for 24 hours. Fluid intake should be restricted to 100 ml/hr, and blood pressure should be controlled as outlined previously. In women with chronic hypertension who are older or obese, careful attention must be paid to the development of congestive heart failure and pulmonary edema. Affected patients should be treated with intravenous furosemide and supplemental oxygen. An echocardiogram should be obtained.

The majority of antihypertensive agents discussed previously are acceptable for lactating women. Thiazide diuretics may inhibit lactation.[24]

Prediction of Preeclampsia

A means of predicting preeclampsia would be beneficial in selecting patients for more intensive observation, treatment, and study. The rollover test has poor reproducibility, and angiotensin II infusions are too complex to be used as a clinical screen. Ambulatory blood pressure monitoring, although cumbersome,

may have future utility when a hyperbaric index is used to increase the sensitivity and specificity of routine blood pressure measurements.[25]

Prevention

Prevention of preeclampsia has received considerable attention. Historically, a low-sodium diet has been prescribed. However, in a randomized clinical trial of nulliparous women, sodium restriction to ≤50 mmol had no effect on maternal blood pressure or obstetric outcomes (birth weight, gestational age, or mortality).[26]

The issue of calcium supplementation has been more controversial. The postulated mechanism of calcium supplementation is suppression of parathyroid hormone, which results in decreased free intracellular cytoplasmic calcium and reduced muscular activity. Belizán et al. reported that women receiving 2 g of elemental calcium after the 20th week of gestation had significantly less hypertensive disease than the control group (9.8 vs. 14.8%, respectively).[27] In a large multicenter trial, Levine et al. assigned 4589 nulliparous women to either 2 g of elemental calcium or placebo beginning at 13 to 21 weeks of gestation.[28] No differences were seen between the study and control groups in the frequencies of preeclampsia (6.9% and 7.3%) or pregnancy-associated hypertension (15.3% and 17.3%).

Similarly, low-dose aspirin has been studied as a means to reduce the incidence of preeclampsia. Despite the initial enthusiasm for this agent, a large multicenter trial of women at high risk for preeclampsia produced disappointing results.[29] Patients included had either insulin-dependent diabetes, chronic hypertension, multiple gestations, or a history of preeclampsia. Women were enrolled between 13 and 26 weeks of gestation and randomized to either 60 mg of aspirin or placebo. The frequency of preeclampsia in the study group ($n = 1254$) was 18%, not significantly different from the frequency in the control group ($n = 1249$) of 20%. In comparing the four subgroups, similar frequencies of preeclampsia were seen in the study and control subjects. Furthermore, there was no reduction in the frequency of perinatal loss, preterm birth, or SGA.

Finally, neither supplementation with magnesium aspartate nor fish oil has demonstrated a decrease in the incidence of preeclampsia.[30,31] Until the etiology of preeclampsia is better understood, it is unlikely that an effective prophylactic agent will emerge.[32]

REFERENCES

1. American College of Obstetricians and Gynecologists. Hypertension in pregnancy. ACOG Technical Bulletin no. 219, January 1996.
2. Brown MA, Robinson AR, Bowyer L, et al. Ambulatory blood pressure monitoring in pregnancy: what is normal? Am J Obstet Gynecol 1998: 836.
3. National Heart, Lung, and Blood Institute National High Blood Pressure Education Program. Sixth report of the Joint National Committee on Prevention, Detection, Evaluation, and Treatment of High Blood Pressure. Bethesda, MD: NIH Publication No. 98–4080, 1997.
4. McCowan LME, Buist RG, North RA, Gamble G. Perinatal morbidity in chronic hypertension. Br J Obstet Gynaecol 1996;103:123.
5. Sibai BM, Anderson GD. Pregnancy outcome of intensive therapy in severe hypertension in first trimester. Obstet Gynecol 1986:67:517.
6. Sibai BM, Mabie WC, Shamsa F, Villar MA, Anderson GD. A comparison of no medication versus methyldopa or labetalol in chronic hypertension during pregnancy. Am J Obstet Gynecol 1990;162:960.
7. Sibai BM, Usta IM. Chronic hypertension in pregnancy. In: Sciarra JJ, ed., Gynecology and obstetrics. Philadelphia: Lippincott/Harper & Row, 1995:1.
8. Sibai BM, Abdella TN, Anderson GD. Pregnancy outcome in 211 patients with mild chronic hypertension. Obstet Gynecol 1983;8:19.
9. Lewis R, Belfort M, Sibai B. The role of calcium channel blockers in the treatment of women with preeclampsia. Fetal Matern Med Rev 1996;8:19.
10. Physicians' Desk Reference. 52nd ed. Montvale, NJ: Medical Economics Company, 1998, p. 2200.
11. Sibai BM. Treatment of hypertension in pregnant women. N Engl J Med 1996;335:257.
12. Sibai BM. Eclampsia VI. Maternal-perinatal outcome in 254 consecutive cases. Am J Obstet Gynecol 1990; 163:1049.
13. Sibai BM, Akl S, Fairlie F, Moretti M. A protocol for managing severe preeclampsia in the second trimester. Am J Obstet Gynecol 1990;163:733.
14. Moodley J, Rajagopal M. Maternal and perinatal outcome associated with hypertensive crises of pregnancy. Hypertens Preg 1998;17:43.
15. Sibai M, Mercer BM, Schiff E, Friedman SA. Aggressive versus expectant management of severe preeclampsia at 28 to 32 weeks' gestation: a randomized controlled trial. Am J Obstet Gynecol 1994;171:818.
16. Weinstein L. Syndrome of hemolysis, elevated liver enzymes, and low platelet count: a severe consequence of hypertension in pregnancy. Am J Obstet Gynecol 1982; 142:159.
17. Sibai BM, Taslimi MM, El-Nazer A, et al. Maternal-perinatal outcome associated with the syndrome of hemolysis, elevated liver enzymes, and low platelets in severe preeclampsia-eclampsia. Am J Obstet Gynecol 1986;155:501.
18. Sibai BM. The HELLP syndrome (hemolysis, elevated liver enzymes, and low platelets): much ado about nothing? Am J Obstet Gynecol 1990;162:311.
19. Sibai BM, Ramadan MK. Acute renal failure in pregnancies complicated by hemolysis, elevated liver enzymes, and low platelets. Am J Obstet Gynecol 1993;168:1682.
20. Sibai BM, Ramadan MK, Usta I, Salama M, Mercer BM, Friedman SA. Maternal morbidity and mortality in 442 pregnancies with hemolysis, elevated liver enzymes, and low platelets (HELLP syndrome). Am J Obstet Gynecol 1993;169:1000.
21. Abramovici D, Friedman SA, Mercer BM, Audibert F, Kao L, Sibai BM. Neonatal outcome in severe preeclampsia at 24–36 weeks' gestation: does the HELLP (hemolysis, elevated liver enzymes, and low platelets) syndrome matter? Am J Obstet Gynecol 1999;180:221.
22. Egerman RS, Witlin AG, Friedman SA, Sibai BM. Thrombotic thrombocytopenic purpura and hemolytic uremic syndrome in pregnancy: review of 11 cases. Am J Obstet Gynecol 1996;175(4pt1):950.
23. Mabie WC, Gonzalez AR, Sibai BM, Amon E. A comparative trial of labetalol and hydralazine in the acute management of severe hypertension complicating pregnancy. Obstet Gynecol 1987;70:328.
24. Briggs GG, Freeman RK, Yaffe SJ. Chlorothiazide. In: Briggs GG, Freeman RK, Yaffe SJ, eds. Drugs in pregnancy and lactation. 4th ed. Baltimore: Williams & Wilkins, 1994:161.
25. Hermida RC, Ayala DE, Mojón AR, et al. Blood pressure excess for the early identification of gestational hypertension and preeclampsia. Hypertension 1998;31(ptI):83.
26. Knuist M, Bonsel GJ, Zondervan HA, Treffers PE. Low sodium diet and pregnancy-induced hypertension: a multicentre randomised controlled trial. Br J Obstet Gynaecol 1998;105:430.
27. Belizán JM, Villar J, Gonzalez L, Campodonico L, Bergel E. Calcium supplementation to prevent hypertensive disorders of pregnancy. N Engl J Med 1991;325:1399.
28. Levine RJ, Hauth HC, Curet LB, et al. Trial of calcium to prevent preeclampsia. N Engl J Med 1997;337:69.
29. Caritis S, Sibai B, Hauth J, et al. Low-dose aspirin to prevent preeclampsia in women at high risk. N Engl J Med 1998;338:701.
30. Sibai BM, Villar MA, Bray E. Magnesium supplementation during pregnancy: a double-blind randomized controlled clinical trial. Am J Obstet Gynecol 1989;161:115.
31. Salvig JD, Olsen SF, SEcher NJ. Effects of fish oil supplementation in late pregnancy on blood pressure: a randomised controlled trial. Br J Obstet Gynaecol 1996; 103:529.
32. Sibai BM. Prevention of preeclampsia: a big disappointment! Am J Obstet Gynecol 1998:179;1275.

Chapter 8

Emergencies during Pregnancy: Trauma and Nonobstetric Surgical Conditions

Jennifer Gunter
Mark D. Pearlman

Five Key Points

- **Pregnant women are at increased risk for anesthesia-related deaths, primarily due to aspiration of gastric contents.**

- **The incidence of congenital anomalies is not increased in women exposed to general and regional anesthetics, even in the first trimester of pregnancy.**

- **Appendectomy is the most common nonobstetric surgery performed during pregnancy, followed by cholecystectomy for gallstones.**

- **The most common causes of trauma during pregnancy are motor vehicle accidents and domestic violence.**

- **Abruptio placentae is the leading cause of fetal loss resulting from trauma during pregnancy.**

Surgical conditions complicate 0.5 to 2% of pregnancies, and trauma complicates 6 to 7%.[1,2] The accurate diagnosis and management of trauma or a surgical illness during pregnancy requires the coordinated care of obstetricians, surgeons, anesthesiologists, radiologists, and often other specialists to optimize outcome for both the woman and her fetus. When a pregnant patient is injured or a nonobstetric surgical condition develops, definitive care should not be delayed or avoided on the basis of the pregnancy, as both maternal and fetal outcomes may be compromised. The most common cause of maternal morbidity and mortality from nonobstetric surgical conditions is related to delays in instituting appropriate medical and surgical care. The importance of avoiding delays in the management of surgical conditions during pregnancy has long been recognized, for it was in 1908 that Babler issued his statement that "the mortality of appendicitis complicating pregnancy is the mortality of delay."[3] The most important question that should be asked when treating the pregnant woman who has a surgical condition is, "How would I treat this patient if she were not pregnant?"

While any surgical illness may develop during pregnancy, some conditions are more common among women of reproductive age and are therefore more likely to occur during pregnancy. An understanding of maternal and fetal physiology is essential to provide the specialized care required by a pregnant patient with trauma or a surgical illness. This chapter will focus on the challenges specific to the diagnosis and management of the most common nonobstetric surgical conditions in the pregnant patient with regard to both maternal and fetal well being. Management of trauma or surgical conditions must begin with consideration and understanding of the altered anatomy and physiology of pregnancy. Accurate interpretation of normal changes in maternal cardiovascular, pulmonary, genitourinary, and gastrointestinal physiology is critically important in making a correct diagnosis and initiating the most appropriate therapy.

GENERAL CONSIDERATIONS

The most common nonobstetric surgery performed in pregnancy involves the abdomen or pelvis, accounting for approximately 60% of procedures. In 1989 Mazze and Kallen published data from the Swedish health registries regarding outcome after nonobstetric surgery during pregnancy.[1] Surgery for a nonobstetric condition was performed in 5405 of 720,000 pregnancies, with abdominal surgery accounting for 25% of procedures, gynecologic and urologic surgery for 19% of cases, and laparoscopy another 16% of procedures. Urologic disease requiring surgery during pregnancy is uncommon and is not considered further in this chapter.

The most common nonobstetric cause for surgery during pregnancy is suspected appendicitis.[1,4] Other common surgical conditions that may be encountered during pregnancy include biliary-tract disorders, pancreatitis, and adnexal mass or torsion.[5,6] While gastrointestinal and gynecologic disorders are the most common surgical conditions during pregnancy, other nonobstetrical surgical illnesses may occur. The principles that apply to the diagnosis and management of abdominal and gynecologic conditions may be applied to almost all surgery during pregnancy.

When considering surgery in a pregnant patient for nonobstetric indications it is important to consider the physiologic and anatomic changes of pregnancy. These changes may interfere with diagnosis and treatment and may affect the choice or timing of a surgical procedure and the type of anesthetic. It is also important to consider the effect of surgical and medical treatment on the fetus. Important fetal considerations include spontaneous abortion,

teratogenicity, premature labor and delivery, fetal distress, and intrauterine death.

Physiologic and Anatomic Changes of Pregnancy

Delays in the diagnosis and management of surgical conditions are more common during pregnancy for a variety of reasons. Physiologic changes of pregnancy may mimic or mask surgical disorders, especially those involving abdominal or pelvic structures. Abdominal pain, anorexia, nausea, and vomiting may normally occur during pregnancy; however, these are also symptoms associated with gastrointestinal surgical conditions. Physiologic dyspnea is common during pregnancy and may be misinterpreted by both physician and patient as being of a cardiac or pulmonary origin.[7] Conversely, care should be taken not to dismiss shortness of breath as resulting from normal pregnancy without an appropriate evaluation.

The physical findings, particularly of abdominal or pelvic disorders, may be altered during pregnancy. A thorough abdominal examination may be difficult, especially at later gestational ages, and the enlarging uterus may also interfere with the identification of abdominal or pelvic masses. The cephalic migration of the appendix during pregnancy has been well described and may increase the difficulty in diagnosing appendicitis. In 1932, Baer et al. first described the gradual displacement of the placenta from McBurney's point during early pregnancy upward to the level of the iliac crest or higher (Figure 8-1).[7]

The cardiac, vascular, and hematologic changes of normal pregnancy may mimic or mask evidence of cardiovascular compromise. The resting pulse rate increases approximately 10 to 15 beats per minute during pregnancy, and brachial artery blood pressure decreases, reaching the nadir in the second trimester.[8] Maternal blood volume increases by about 40 to 45% during pregnancy, which may delay the signs and symptoms of hypovolemia; therefore, caution must be exercised in estimating blood loss in a pregnant patient.[8]

During the evaluation of a pregnant patient, care should be taken with maternal positioning, especially beyond 20 weeks of gestation, as the pregnant uterus may compress the vena cava and decrease venous return, resulting in a decrease in cardiac output and in hypotension. Limiting the time spent in the supine position and placing the patient in the left lateral

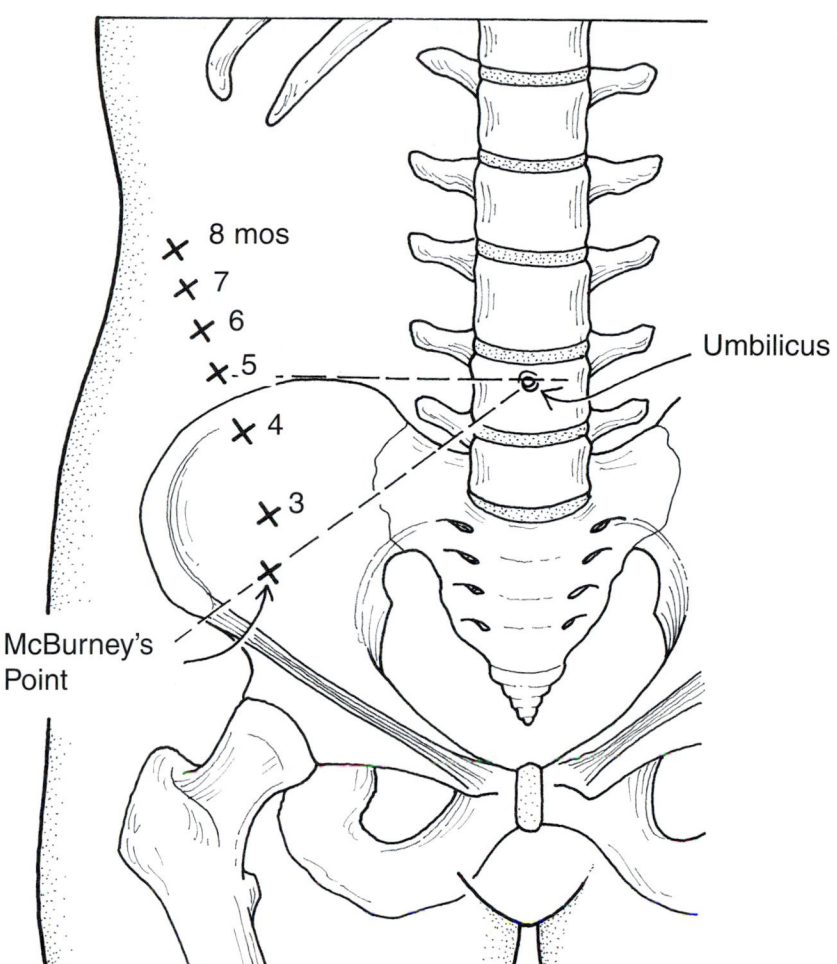

Figure 8-1 Position of appendix at various gestational ages. *Adapted from Baer, et al.* [7]

position or displacing the uterus will help to minimize this occurrence.

Laboratory investigations used in the diagnosis and management of surgical disorders may be altered in pregnancy. Changes in the white-cell count, which are useful in the diagnosis of intraabdominal inflammatory conditions, may be more difficult to interpret in the gravid patient. The white-cell count may vary during pregnancy, and a leukocytosis of up to 12,000/mm^3 may be normal.[8] Laboratory tests used to evaluate the liver and gallbladder may also be abnormal. The plasma albumin concentration decreases by the third trimester to an average of 3.0 g/dl, and total alkaline phosphatase will almost double by the end of a pregnancy due to the production of this enzyme by the placenta.[8]

Diagnostic Procedures

Imaging techniques are a vital tool in the diagnosis of a variety of surgical disorders. Multiple imaging methods are now available, including ultrasound, ionizing radiation, and magnetic resonance imaging. When ordering a diagnostic procedure, the clinician must consider the potential pregnancy-induced alterations in sensitivity and specificity of the test, as well as the maternal and fetal risks of the procedure.

Ultrasound

Ultrasound is frequently used in the diagnosis of many gastrointestinal and gynecologic disorders. Diagnostic ultrasound employs high-frequency sound waves for real-time imaging, and there are no known adverse maternal or fetal effects from this imaging technique during pregnancy.[9,10] Ultrasound is useful for imaging the liver, biliary tree, and adnexal structures and in identifying peritoneal fluid. Compression ultrasound of the appendix has also been described for diagnosing appendicitis in pregnancy; however, the sensitivity of this procedure for diagnosing appendicitis in pregnancy may be somewhat reduced.[11,12]

Ionizing Radiation

Ionizing radiation, used in conventional radiography and computed tomographic (CT) scanning, produces significant energy that can potentially damage DNA, resulting in tissue damage, mutation, and cancer.[8,13] The dose of ionizing radiation from x-ray imaging is measured in rad, and exposure to less than 5 rad during pregnancy is not associated with an increase in fetal anomalies or pregnancy loss.[14] With appropriate lead shielding, x-ray examination of body parts such as the head, limbs, or chest of the pregnant woman results in minute doses of radiation to the fetus, well below the 5-rad guideline. Plain x-ray films of the abdomen deliver a higher dose of ionizing radiation to the fetus, and a single abdominal film will result in a fetal dose of approximately 100 mrad.

Fluoroscopy and CT scanning are extremely useful diagnostic procedures that may result in higher fetal doses than conventional x-ray examination, depending on the body part imaged. When calculating fetal radiation exposure from fluoroscopy, it is important to consider the fluoroscopy time, the number of x-ray films, and the distance of the body part from the uterus.[8] One common indication for fluoroscopy in pregnancy is endoscopic retrograde cholangiopancreatography (ERCP) for the management of choledocholithiasis. Endoscopic management of choledocholithiasis can be accomplished in pregnancy with lead shielding and little or even no fluoroscopy time, thus minimizing fetal radiation exposure.[15,16]

Cranial CT scanning is commonly performed during pregnancy and delivers a fetal dose of less than 0.05 rad.[8] CT scanning of the abdomen delivers a higher dose of radiation to the fetus, but this is dependent on the number and thickness of the slices, and, as with any procedure involving ionizing radiation, imaging closer to the uterus increases the fetal dose.[8] It is frequently helpful to consult a radiation physicist to estimate fetal dosimetry.

Magnetic Resonance Imaging

Magnetic resonance imaging (MRI) is not associated with any known adverse fetal effects and avoids the risks associated with ionizing radiation. Long-term data on the use of MRI during pregnancy are limited; therefore, it is not currently recommended for use in the first trimester.[14]

Discussing imaging techniques for a pregnant patient with the radiologist is of utmost importance as acceptable alternatives not associated with ionizing radiation may be available. If ionizing radiation is the only alternative, radiation doses can be calculated, especially when multiple x-ray films, fluoroscopy, or CT scanning are required. With good communication between the obstetrician and radiologist, it is usually possible to stay well within the 5-rad limit of fetal exposure to ionizing radiation. It is of equal importance that concerns about fetal effects from radiation exposure not interfere with maternal evaluation.[14]

Anesthesia

Maternal outcome after a surgical procedure is generally not affected by the pregnancy; however, pregnant women are at increased risk for anesthesia-related deaths.[17] Pregnancy delays gastric emptying and decreases the resting tone of the lower esophageal sphincter, resulting in an increased risk of pulmonary aspiration of gastric contents.[8,17] Aspiration of gastric contents with subsequent pneumonitis is the most common cause of death from anesthesia in pregnancy, and is associated with at least 25% of all anesthesia-related deaths.[18,19] Administering antacids prior to induction of general anesthesia reduces mortality from pulmonary aspiration of gastric contents.[19] Pregnant women are also at increased risk for failed intubation, which is the another leading cause of anesthesia-related deaths in pregnancy.[17,20]

Epidural and spinal anesthetics may also be used for a variety of nonobstetric surgical procedures during pregnancy. The concern with both epidural and spinal anesthetics is the sympathetic blockade with resulting peripheral vasodilation and venous pooling.[17,19] The pregnant woman needs to be well hydrated prior to initiating regional anesthesia in order to avoid maternal hypotension, uterine hypoperfusion, and possibly fetal hypoxia. Prehydration, careful monitoring of maternal blood pressure, heart rate, oxygen saturation, and fetal monitoring will help prevent this complication.

Apart from the risks of anesthesia, maternal morbidity and mortality from surgery are related to complications such as perforation of a viscus, peritonitis, and other infections.[21-23] The risk of these complications increases with delays in diagnosis and surgical intervention.

Fetal Considerations

Fetal risks from nonobstetric surgery during pregnancy have raised many concerns, including possible teratogenicity, intrauterine death, fetal hypoxia and acidosis, and premature labor and delivery. However, several large studies have failed to show an increase in congenital malformations or stillbirths among pregnant women exposed to general anesthesia, including nitrous oxide, even with exposure in the first trimester.[1,2,24] Similarly, no increase in the incidence of spontaneous abortion has been identified with the use of general anesthesia in early pregnancy, although one study has shown a slight increase in the spontaneous abortion rate in the first and second trimester after operative gynecologic procedures.[21] Because early pregnancy loss is so common, with 15 to 20% of clinically recognized pregnancies aborting in the first or early second trimester, it is difficult to attribute a first-trimester loss to either a surgical procedure or the associated anesthetic. For this reason, it is advisable to document fetal viability before and after any surgical procedure.[25] Surgery performed in early pregnancy will not significantly increase the risk of spontaneous abortion; however, surgical complications, such as peritonitis or perforated viscus, will significantly increase the risk of fetal loss.[26]

The majority of nonobstetric surgery is performed in early pregnancy, with 41% of procedures occurring in the first trimester. Thirty-five percent of procedures are performed in the second trimester and 24% in the third trimester.[1] The major fetal risk from surgery at a more advanced gestational age is the morbidity and mortality associated with premature labor and delivery. An increase in the risk of premature delivery with appendectomy after 23 weeks of gestation was documented by Mazze and Kallen in 1991.[4] In this study the incidence of preterm delivery was 22% within 1 week of appendectomy; however, pregnancies that continued past the first postoperative week had no further increase in the rate of premature delivery. Uterine manipulation should be avoided or reduced as much as possible to decrease uterine irritability and subsequent premature labor.[27] The risk of premature labor is lowest with prompt diagnosis and management of surgical conditions but increases when complications arise, either from the surgery or the underlying disorder. Perioperative infections are associated with the greatest risk of premature labor and delivery.[22,23,26]

In addition to routine monitoring of maternal vital signs and oxygenation, close monitoring of uterine activity and fetal well-being should be performed. Tocolysis may also be considered after 22 weeks of gestational age to reduce the risk of preterm labor and delivery with intraabdominal and pelvic surgery. Intraoperative fetal heart rate monitoring should be considered if the fetus is viable. A Doppler device or ultrasound transducer wrapped in a sterile plastic bag may be used for this purpose.[27] The risk of intraoperative fetal compromise can be minimized by placing a wedge under the patient's right flank—which displaces the uterus to the left, thereby avoiding supine hypotension—and by carefully monitoring and replacing any maternal fluid losses.

Surgical Approaches

When considering abdominal or pelvic surgery in pregnancy for a nonobstetric indication, the obstetrician or surgeon must decide if laparotomy or laparoscopy is the preferred procedure. Many studies have documented the relative safety of laparotomy during pregnancy.[1,2,4,26]

Laparoscopy is being performed more frequently as an alternative to laparotomy for gynecologic and general surgery during pregnancy.[1,24] The most common laparoscopic procedures performed during pregnancy are cholecystectomy, adnexal surgery, and appendectomy.[28] Data published in 1989 by Mazze and Kallen from several Swedish health-care registries revealed that 16% of all nonobstetric surgery during pregnancy were laparoscopic procedures.[1] More recent publications suggest that number may be increasing.[24]

Studies on pregnant baboons have shown no significant change in maternal or fetal parameters at insufflation pressures of 10 mm Hg with carbon dioxide; however, significant cardiovascular and respiratory changes were seen in both the gravid baboon and fetus at pressures of 20 mm Hg.[28,29] Decreases in placental perfusion, fetal acidosis, and cardiovascular changes have also been identified in pregnant ewes with carbon dioxide insufflation pressures over 15 mm Hg.[30,31]

No increased risk of fetal malformations has been identified with laparoscopy during pregnancy, and fetal outcome appears to be the same with either laparoscopy or laparotomy.[24,28] The use of diagnostic laparoscopy and operative laparoscopy for appendicitis, cholecystectomy, and adnexal surgery in pregnancy is well supported in the literature; however, data to support the use of laparoscopy after 20 weeks of gestation are somewhat limited.[24,32-35] Laparoscopy has some advantages over laparotomy, including less postoperative pain and shorter hospital stays, but longer operative times may be encountered with laparoscopic approaches, dependent, in part, on the skill of the operator. The available data suggest that laparoscopy is a safe alternative to laparotomy during pregnancy before 20 weeks, provided that insufflation pressures are kept below 15 mm Hg. Other considerations include avoidance of cervical and uterine instrumentation and excessive uterine manipulation, and the use of an open laparoscopic technique with advancing gestational age to avoid uterine puncture with the Veress needle or trocar.

COMMON SURGICAL DISORDERS DURING PREGNANCY

The differential diagnosis of abdominal pain during pregnancy includes both obstetric and nonobstetric conditions. The common nonobstetric illnesses requiring surgery during pregnancy are disorders that are more frequent among women of reproductive age (Table 8-1). The differential diagnosis of abdominal pain must also include obstetric conditions; the common pregnancy-related causes of abdominal pain are listed in Table 8-2.

Appendicitis

Appendicitis complicates about 0.1% of pregnancies, and appendectomy is the most common nonobstetric surgery during pregnancy.[4] The preoperative diagnosis of appendicitis is correct in approximately 64% of

TABLE 8-1 COMMON NONOBSTETRIC CAUSES OF ABDOMINAL PAIN IN PREGNANCY

Appendicitis
Biliary-tract disease
   Cholelithiasis
   Cholecystitis
   Choledocholithiasis
Pancreatitis
Intestinal obstruction
Adnexal events
   Mass
   Torsion
Pyelonephritis

TABLE 8-2 COMMON OBSTETRICAL CAUSES OF ABDOMINAL PAIN	
First Trimester	**Second and Third Trimesters**
Ectopic pregnancy	Preterm labor
Spontaneous abortion	Severe preeclampsia
	Acute fatty liver
	Placental abruption
	Uterine rupture
	Chorioamnionitis
	Round ligament pain

cases, with appendicitis confirmed in 1 in 1500 deliveries.[4,23] Appendicitis occurs with equal frequency in all three trimesters; however, both maternal and fetal complications increase as the pregnancy advances secondary to delays in diagnosis and surgical intervention.[5,23]

Diagnosis

The diagnosis of appendicitis may be more difficult during pregnancy for a variety of reasons. Common symptoms of appendicitis such as abdominal pain, anorexia, nausea, and vomiting are also symptoms associated with pregnancy.[5,22,23] A distinction should be made regarding the duration of these symptoms, as the new onset of nausea and vomiting is much more suspect than that which has been present since early pregnancy.

The most common sign of appendicitis in both the pregnant and nonpregnant patient is abdominal pain; however, the differential diagnosis of abdominal pain in the pregnant patient includes many obstetric and nonobstetric conditions (see Tables 8-1 and 8-2). The location of abdominal pain with appendicitis typically varies during pregnancy. Early in the first trimester, pain from appendicitis commonly localizes in the right lower quadrant at McBurney's point. However, as the gestation advances and the appendix is displaced to a more lateral and superior location by the enlarging uterus, the point of maximal tenderness moves in this direction, often reaching the right upper quadrant, or the flank by the third trimester (see Figure 8-1).[5,7] While right-sided abdominal pain is more common, back or flank pain may be present with a retrocecal appendix, and diffuse abdominal pain may indicate peritonitis or appendiceal rupture.[5,23] Rebound tenderness and guarding, which are common physical findings of appendicitis in a nonpregnant patient, are elicited less frequently during pregnancy, especially in the third trimester, possibly due to increased attenuation and laxity of the muscles of the anterior abdominal wall.[5,23,36]

Laboratory tests and diagnostic imaging may be less useful in the diagnosis of appendicitis in a pregnant patient. Leukocytosis is common with appendicitis, but as previously discussed, the normal white-cell count increases up to $12,000/mm^3$ during pregnancy.[8] Changes in the white blood cell differential count, such as granulocytosis or an increase in the number of immature forms, may be more helpful in the diagnosis during pregnancy.

Diagnostic imaging, particularly ultrasound, may be helpful in diagnosing appendicitis during pregnancy. The presence of a noncompressible appendix with a diameter of >6 mm and no evidence of peristalsis is highly suggestive of appendicitis.[11,12,37] Ultrasound may also identify an appendiceal abscess or assist in excluding other conditions, such as ectopic pregnancy or adnexal pathology. Ultrasound is most valuable in early pregnancy because advancing uterine size makes visualization of the abdominal and pelvic organs increasingly difficult.

Management

Once appendicitis has been diagnosed in a pregnant woman, every effort should be made to avoid delays in surgical treatment. In early pregnancy, especially if the diagnosis is still in question, a laparoscopic approach may be preferred. Laparoscopic appendectomy can be performed safely before 20 weeks if a surgeon skilled in the procedure is available.[28,38]

Laparotomy is the preferred approach for appendicitis in the following clinical situations: after 20 weeks of gestation, when appendiceal rupture or abscess is suspected, when a laparoscopic approach is not technically feasible, or when a surgeon skilled in laparoscopic appendectomy is not available.[28] For patients with localized tenderness, a muscle-splitting incision over the point of maximum tenderness is appropriate.[5,23] A midline incision for suspected appendicitis is preferred by some, especially in view of the 36% incidence of incorrect diagnosis at the time of laparotomy.[4] A midline incision is indicated for patients with poorly localized or atypical pain, suspected rupture or abscess formation, or in late pregnancy for exposure in case rapid delivery of the fetus is required.[5,23,36]

The use of prophylactic broad-spectrum antibiotics is indicated for appendectomy regardless of

approach. Postoperative antibiotics are indicated in cases with peritonitis, perforation, or abscess formation; however, there is no benefit from postoperative antibiotics with uncomplicated appendicitis.[36,39]

When diagnosed and managed correctly, appendicitis has few maternal complications and a low risk of fetal loss. Delay in the surgical treatment of appendicitis dramatically increases both maternal and fetal risks, and perinatal mortality may reach as high as 20% with perforative appendicitis.[40] It is generally preferable to err on the side of performing more appendectomies during pregnancy, removing a percentage of normal appendices, because a missed or delayed diagnosis of appendicitis has such serious ramifications for both mother and fetus.[24,40]

Biliary-Tract Disease

Biliary-tract disease is the second most common nonobstetric surgical condition during pregnancy.[5,41] The incidence of biliary tract disease during pregnancy ranges from 0.03 to 0.16 percent.[42] The majority of biliary-tract disease in pregnancy is due to gallstones: cholecystitis, choledocholithiasis, and gallstone pancreatitis.[5] Gallstone pancreatitis is the most common cause of pancreatitis during pregnancy.[43]

Biliary-tract disorders are common among women of reproductive age and are four times more common in women than in men.[16] The incidence of gallstone disease is even higher during pregnancy because biliary physiology is altered in pregnancy.[42,43] The formation of cholesterol gallstones is due to incomplete emptying of the gallbladder in pregnancy, which results in large residual volumes in the gallbladder by the third trimester, increasing the development of cholesterol crystals.[41] Postpartum ultrasound of the biliary system indicates a 26.2% incidence of biliary sludge as compared with 4% 1-year postpartum.[44] Pregnancy-related factors that may also contribute to a lithogenic environment are an increase in the size of the bile acid pool and increased biliary cholesterol concentration.[45,46]

Diagnosis

Symptoms of biliary-tract disease typically include anorexia, nausea, vomiting, and dyspepsia, which may also occur normally during pregnancy. Symptoms not typically associated with a normal pregnancy but which may be seen with biliary-tract disease include precipitation of gastrointestinal complaints by fatty foods and epigastric or right-upper-quadrant pain.

Patients with acute cholecystitis or choledocholithiasis generally have a leukocytosis that is greater than expected during pregnancy. Fever is also common.[5,47] An elevated alkaline phosphatase level should be considered normal during pregnancy; however, elevations of serum amylase are usually seen only with gallstone pancreatitis.[47]

Ultrasound is extremely useful in the diagnosis of biliary-tract disease during pregnancy and should be performed early in the evaluation if there are symptoms suggestive of gallstone disease or pancreatitis. Ultrasound findings suggestive of biliary-tract disease include gallstones and sludge within the gallbladder, thickening of the wall of the gallbladder, edema or fluid around the gallbladder, and dilatation of the common bile duct.[5] Inflammatory changes may sometimes be identified with gallstone pancreatitis.[16]

Management

The initial management of cholelithiasis and cholecystitis in pregnancy is medical. Most patients will have resolution of symptoms with gastrointestinal-tract rest, intravenous fluids, analgesics and, if necessary, nasogastric suction. With a persistent fever, leukocytosis, or suspected acute cholecystitis, intravenous antibiotics may be appropriate.[5,47] Fetal monitoring should be used, depending on gestational age. Up to 84% of patients with acute cholelithiasis and cholecystitis in pregnancy will be managed successfully with this form of conservative therapy.[47] Patients who respond to medical treatment may have a cholecystectomy performed postpartum.

Surgical management of biliary-tract disease in pregnancy may be necessary. Conservative therapy of cholelithiasis or cholecystitis in pregnancy fails in approximately 15% of cases, and for these patients operative intervention is required.[47] Repeated attacks of biliary colic and acute cholecystitis, despite aggressive conservative therapy, are also an indication for cholecystectomy in pregnancy. Pregnant patients with symptomatic cholelithiasis or cholecystitis are at high risk of recurrence during pregnancy, and up to 58% of patients may have recurrent episodes during pregnancy; 27% require two or more hospitalizations.[48] If there is no resolution or worsening of symptoms by the fourth hospital day, or if three or more episodes occur within the same trimester, operative intervention should be considered.[47] Complications of gallstone

disease, specifically choledocholithiasis, pancreatitis, and ascending cholangitis, are also indications for surgery during pregnancy.[46]

Open cholecystectomy has been well described during pregnancy and is associated with low maternal and fetal risks. Maternal and fetal outcomes are best when the procedure is performed in the second trimester.[5] There are increasing reports of the safety of laparoscopic cholecystectomy during pregnancy, especially in the first and second trimesters. However, with advancing uterine size an open laparoscopic technique is preferable to avoid uterine puncture.[15,16]

Choledocholithiasis and gallstone pancreatitis are indications for exploration of the common bile duct. The incidence of common-bile-duct stones is not increased significantly during pregnancy; however, in one series 50% of patients required exploration of the common bile duct on the basis of intraoperative cholangiograms.[46,48] Exploration of the common bile duct during pregnancy is associated with a greater maternal morbidity and a higher fetal loss rate.[5] Endoscopic management of choledocholithiasis and gallstone pancreatitis ERCP and retrograde sphincterotomy in pregnancy has been described.[15,16,46] With careful lead shielding, no radiography, and limited use of fluoroscopy, these techniques can be used with minimal fetal exposure to ionizing radiation.[15] Endoscopic sphincterotomy without use of fluoroscopy has recently been described during pregnancy for gallstone pancreatitis.[16]

Adnexal Disorders

Surgical evaluation of an adnexal mass is the most common major gynecologic procedure during pregnancy; approximately 1 in 1000 pregnancies are complicated by adnexal surgery.[49] Prompt diagnosis and appropriate management of ovarian neoplasms is vital, as complications are more frequent during pregnancy and increase both maternal and fetal risks. Adnexal torsion is the fifth most common cause of emergency gynecologic surgery, and the risk of adnexal torsion is increased during pregnancy, particularly in the presence of preexisting adnexal pathology.[50,51] Other complications of ovarian neoplasms to be considered during pregnancy are pelvic impaction, hemorrhage, rupture, and obstructed labor.[52] Ovarian malignancy, while uncommon during pregnancy, must also be considered in the differential diagnosis of an adnexal mass. Of all ovarian lesions that require surgery during pregnancy, 2 to 4% will be malignant.[52,53]

Ovarian cysts are frequently identified in early pregnancy; most are small and are not associated with an increased complication rate. However, 1 of 328 pregnancies is complicated by an ovarian mass large enough to cause concern.[52,54] The majority of adnexal masses during pregnancy are functional cysts, either corpus luteum or follicular cysts, and are less than 6 cm in diameter.[49,52] These functional cysts are generally identified early in the first trimester and usually resolve by 14 to 18 weeks of gestation.[52,53] In one study, only 7% of ovarian lesions requiring surgery were functional, and no functional cysts were identified when surgery was delayed until 18 weeks of gestation.[53]

The common adnexal lesions of reproductive age are also the most common neoplasms requiring surgery during pregnancy. Benign cystic teratoma is the most frequent histologic diagnosis of an adnexal mass during pregnancy, with serous cystadenoma and mucinous cystadenoma diagnosed in 25% and 12% of cases, respectively.[53] Other less common causes of adnexal lesions in pregnancy are para-ovarian cyst, endometriosis, and ovarian malignancy.[53]

Diagnosis

The diagnosis of an adnexal mass during pregnancy is often difficult because most lesions are asymptomatic. However, complications of adnexal lesions are frequently symptomatic. Torsion, hemorrhage, and rupture may cause symptoms and signs of peritoneal irritation, presenting with abdominal or pelvic pain, nausea, and vomiting. In one series of adnexal torsion, 97% of patients presented with abdominal pain.[51] Identification of a pelvic mass may be more difficult during pregnancy due to the enlarged uterus, especially as the pregnancy advances. In the first trimester and early second trimester it may be possible to identify an adnexal mass on pelvic examination. However, as the uterine size increases, the ovaries become abdominal structures, making palpation very difficult.[52]

A higher index of suspicion for adnexal pathology should be maintained for patients who have conceived with ovarian stimulation, especially in the case of ovarian hyperstimulation syndrome (OHSS). Gonadotropin therapy may produce multiple follicular and lutein cysts, which may persist under the influence of endogenous human chorionic gonadotropin.[55] The risk of torsion of a hyperstimulated

ovary in pregnancy is significant. In a report by Mashiach et al., adnexal torsion developed in 16% of pregnant women with OHSS.[55]

Laboratory investigations are of little benefit in the asymptomatic adnexal mass in pregnancy. Nonspecific findings such as leukocytosis may be seen with torsion, hemorrhage, and rupture. Hemorrhage or rupture of an ovarian lesion may cause a decrease in hemoglobin and hematocrit. Usually, this is not a significant finding, unless there is ongoing active bleeding.

Ultrasound is extremely useful in the identification and evaluation of an adnexal mass during pregnancy. Ultrasound can also distinguish between simple cystic lesions, septate lesions, and masses with internal echoes or solid components. Simple cystic lesions smaller than 6 cm are usually functional; however, functional cysts up to 11 cm have been identified during pregnancy.[52] Lesions with internal septations, solid components, surface irregularities, and papillae are less likely to be functional.

Color Doppler sonography may be used in the diagnosis of adnexal torsion. Findings that are suggestive of ovarian torsion are an absence or severe alteration of arterial or venous flow and diminished or no flow within the twisted adnexa.[56-58] Other ultrasound findings that are suggestive of adnexal torsion in the appropriate clinical setting are ovarian enlargement (greater than 10 to 14 cm), and the presence of a mass (Figure 8-2).[56,57] The diagnosis of adnexal torsion is confirmed at surgery. Typically the adnexa is engorged, edematous, dark in color, and may have focal areas of hemorrhage (see Figure 8-2).

The majority of adnexal lesions in pregnancy are functional and will resolve sonographically by 14 to 18 weeks of gestation.[52] If an asymptomatic adnexal mass is diagnosed in the first trimester the patient should be carefully observed and an ultrasound study should be repeated at 16 to 18 weeks of gestation. If the mass has resolved, then no further intervention is required. However, if it remains unchanged or increases in size, surgical intervention is appropriate.[52] The optimal time for exploration of an adnexal mass in pregnancy appears to be approximately 18 weeks of gestation, as almost all functional cysts will have resolved, the risk of spontaneous abortion is low, and the uterus is still small enough to permit adequate surgical exposure.[52] Surgical intervention for persistent adnexal lesions is recommended in pregnancy, even though the risk of malignancy is low, as

Figure 8-2 Adnexal torsion at 12 weeks of gestational age. A. Ultrasound of multiseptate mass. *(Courtesy of J. Gunter, J. Rosenthal)* B. Appearance of tuboovarian torsion at laparoscopy. *(Courtesy of J. Gunter, W. Hobart)*

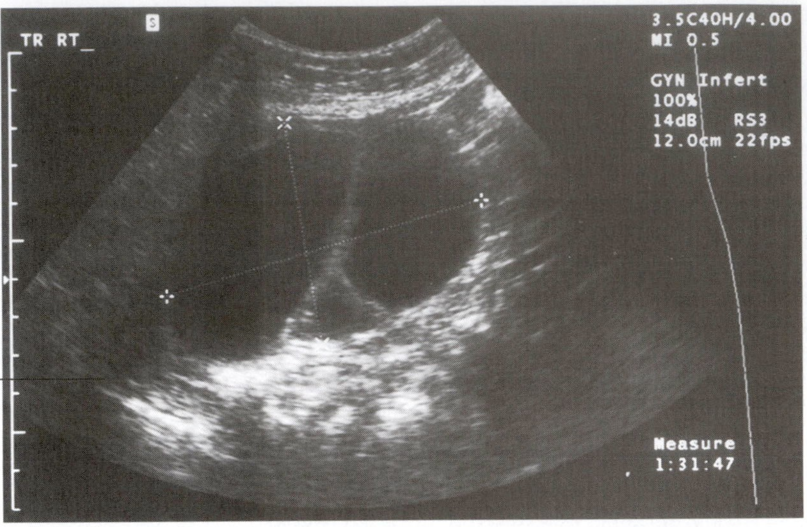
TR RT
3.5C40H/4.00
MI 0.5
GYN Infert
100%
14dB RS3
12.0cm 22fps
Measure
1:31:47
Transverse scan, lower right quadrant
A
Right
Left

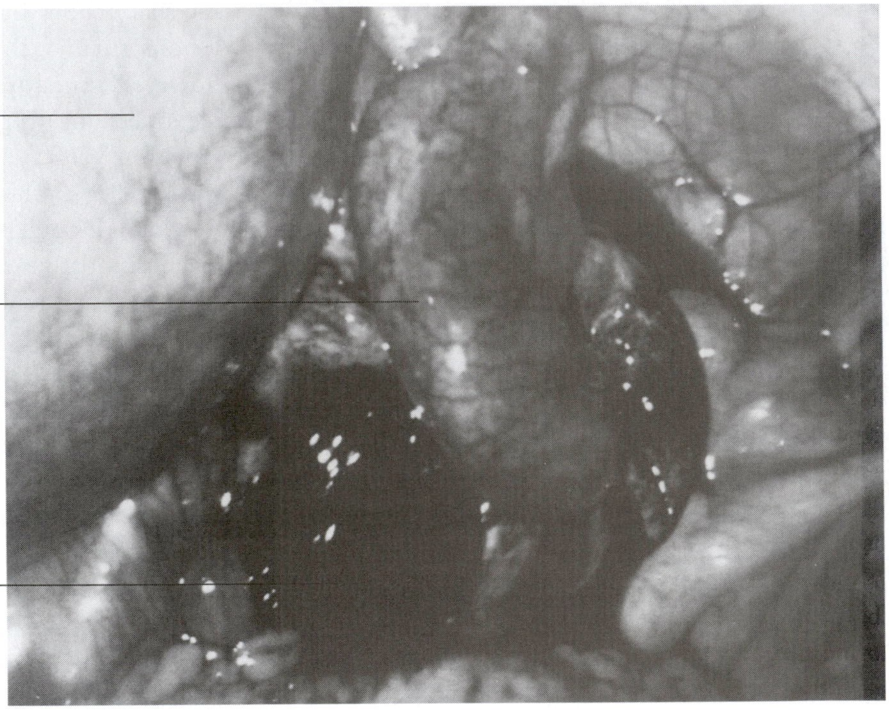
Uterus
Fallopian tube
Adnexal mass
B

potential complications such as hemorrhage, torsion, rupture, and necrosis will increase maternal and fetal morbidity.

Management

Surgical intervention for adnexal lesions is appropriate in the first trimester if a complication such as peritonitis, rupture, hemorrhage, torsion, infarction, or infection is suspected. A mass larger than 10 cm, or one with internal septations or varying echogenicity, is unlikely to resolve and may require removal before 16 to 18 weeks of gestation. If ovarian cystectomy or oophorectomy is performed in the first trimester, some investigators recommend progesterone supplementation, as the corpus luteum may be removed or damaged, thus affecting progesterone production. The use of supplemental progesterone is controversial and there are no clear guidelines for indication or dosage. Although it is believed that the corpus luteum may be not be required after 7 weeks, most authors still recommend the use of supplemental progesterone after adnexal surgery for up to 10 to 12 weeks.[59]

If an acute adnexal event such as torsion, rupture, or hemorrhage with hemodynamic instability is suspected, delays in surgical management will adversely affect both maternal and fetal outcome. Prompt management of adnexal torsion is vital to avoid ischemic necrosis and loss of the affected ovary, and expedient surgical exploration of suspected rupture or hemorrhage will reduce maternal blood loss and subsequent complications such as peritonitis.

Adnexal torsion may be managed with untwisting of the ovary via laparoscopy or laparotomy.[60-62] Simple untwisting or, if indicated, detorsion with cyst aspiration or cystectomy may be performed. Long-term follow-up of these patients indicates that the majority of ovaries can be salvaged in this manner. Detorsion of the ovary has been performed even if the adnexa appears necrotic, as ovarian function has been demonstrated to return in approximately 94% of patients.[62,63]

The type of surgical procedure performed in the pregnant woman with an adnexal mass depends on the gestational age at the time of surgery, size of the mass, potential for malignancy, and operator experience. A laparoscopic approach for the evaluation of adnexal lesions under 20 weeks is appropriate, especially when the diagnosis is in question. The differential diagnosis of an adnexal mass with abdominal or pelvic pain in pregnancy includes adnexal torsion, rupture, hemorrhage, appendicitis, ectopic pregnancy, and tubo-ovarian abscess; preoperative diagnosis of these conditions may be difficult. In one study, only 27% of cases involving adnexal torsion were correctly identified preoperatively.[51] After a diagnostic laparoscopy, the definitive surgery may be completed laparoscopically if possible or converted to a laparotomy.

Indications for laparotomy include hemodynamic instability, suspected malignancy, large size of the mass, gestational age, and operator experience. A laparotomy may be the appropriate initial operative route depending on the clinical situation. After 18 to 20 weeks of gestational age laparoscopy becomes more difficult, operator experience may be limited, and excessive uterine manipulation is more difficult to avoid.[28] Therefore, surgical exploration of an adnexal mass at later gestations is probably best accomplished with a laparotomy through a midline incision. The use of prophylactic antibiotics for adnexal surgery in pregnancy is not indicated unless the patient is febrile or an intraabdominal or pelvic infection is suspected.

TRAUMA DURING PREGNANCY

Trauma during pregnancy is remarkably common, complicating between 6 and 7% of all pregnancies.[64] This accounts for 240,000 to 280,000 episodes of trauma during pregnancy each year in the United States alone. Two separate patients need to be considered in treating the pregnant trauma victim; however, they are inextricably linked and the axiom that "what's good for the mother is good for the fetus" holds true. Treatment of the pregnant trauma victim requires the collaborative efforts of a number of specialists. Incorporating an obstetrician into the team caring for the injured pregnant woman is important in all cases, and the obstetrician must be prepared to assist other specialists in trauma care in prioritizing maternal and fetal care.

The physiologic and anatomic changes during pregnancy that modify trauma care are numerous and were reviewed in the first section of this chapter. Physiologic changes in blood pressure, pulse, hemoglobin, and hematocrit and the supine hypotension syndrome are all important to recognize in treating the pregnant trauma victim so that accurate assessment of intravascular volume is optimized. The supine hypotension syndrome is particularly important in pregnant trauma victims because they are frequently put in the supine position, especially if there is concern for neck injury. Appropriate displacement of the uterus off the aorta and inferior vena cava should be performed as an initial priority, along with establishment of an airway and repletion of intravascular volume.

Patterns of Injury during Blunt Abdominal Trauma

Blunt abdominal trauma is the most common type of injury during pregnancy, accounting for more than 95% of trauma during pregnancy.[64] Approximately two-thirds of all cases of trauma during pregnancy result from motor vehicle crashes, with the remaining third being equally split between falls and direct assaults to the abdomen.[64-66] Direct assaults to the abdomen frequently result from domestic violence. According to the American College of Obstetricians and Gynecologists, approximately 2 million to 4 million women are assaulted each year by their male partners.[67] A review of physical abuse of pregnant women by Gazmararian et al. found that over the past two decades the prevalence of physical abuse during pregnancy ranged from 1 to 20% of the pregnant population of the United States.[68] Risk factors for physical abuse include single marital status, lower level of education, unemployment, unplanned pregnancy, substance abuse, and emotional problems. Unfortunately, many of these factors contribute to the fact that approximately 60% of abused pregnant women stay with their abusers throughout the pregnancy and, thus, remain at continued risk for injury.

Specific Injuries during Pregnancy

Placental Abruption

Placental abruption accounts for 50 to 70% of all fetal losses due to trauma.[69] Life-threatening maternal injuries are much more likely to result in placental abruption than non-life-threatening injuries (Table 8-3). However, because 90% or more of injuries are relatively minor, most placental abruptions are due to minor trauma.

The mechanism of placental abruption due to trauma was first hypothesized by Crosby et al.[70] In

their model using pregnant baboons in car crashes (Figure 8-3), they demonstrated a significant increase in intrauterine pressure during the crash sequence. Because of the presumed difference in elasticity of the uterus and placenta, they theorized that, when shear forces at the uteroplacental interface exceeded a certain threshold, uteroplacental separation occurred. However, other studies have examined the elastic differences in the uterus and placenta, and it is uncertain whether the differences between these two tissues are sufficient to explain most traumatic abruptions (Ashton-Miller, JA, Pearlman, MD: unpublished data). An alternative theory is that the wave which is generated within the amniotic fluid at the time of the sudden deceleration can create pressure differences within the amniotic fluid and uteroplacental interface that can cause placental separation. Regardless of the mechanism, placental abruptions can and do occur even after seemingly minor trauma, leading to the important observation that all truncal trauma during the second half of pregnancy should be evaluated.

Hurd and co-workers published an important observational study on the frequency of signs and

TABLE 8-3
IMMEDIATE ADVERSE FETAL OUTCOME FOLLOWING BLUNT ABDOMINAL TRAUMA

Study	no. (%)	AP, no. (%)	DFI, no. (%)	Fetal Loss, no. (%)
Rothenberger[76]				
LT	18 (22)	4 (22.2)	1 (5.6)	6 (33)
NLT	64 (78)	3 (4.7)	2 (3.1)	4 (6.3)
Pearlman[72]				
LT	2	2 (100)	0 (0)	1 (50)
NLT	83	3 (2.4)	0 (0)	9 (0)
Willams[66]				
LT	2 (2.4)	1 (50)	0 (0)	1 (50)
NLT	82 (9.8)	1 (1.2)	0 (0)	0 (0)
Elliot[78]				
LT	10 (32.2)	5 (50)	0 (0)	5 (50)
NLT	21 (67.8)	1 (4.8)	2 (6.5)	1 (6.7)
Goodwin[65]				
LT	—	—	—	—
NLT	205 (100)	0 (0)	0 (0)	2 (1)
Rose[82]				
LT	—	—	—	—
NLT	32 (100)	0 (0)	0 (0)	1 (3.3)
Total				
LT	32 (6.2)	12 (37.5)*	1 (3.1)	12 (40.6)*
NLT	487 (93.8)	8 (1.6)	4 (0.8)	8 (1.6)

*P < 0.0001 by Fischer's exact test.

AP = abruptio placentae: DFI = direct fetal injury; LT = life-threatening injuries, maternal mortality excluded; NLT = non-life-threatening injuries.

Modification from Pearlman et al.[69]

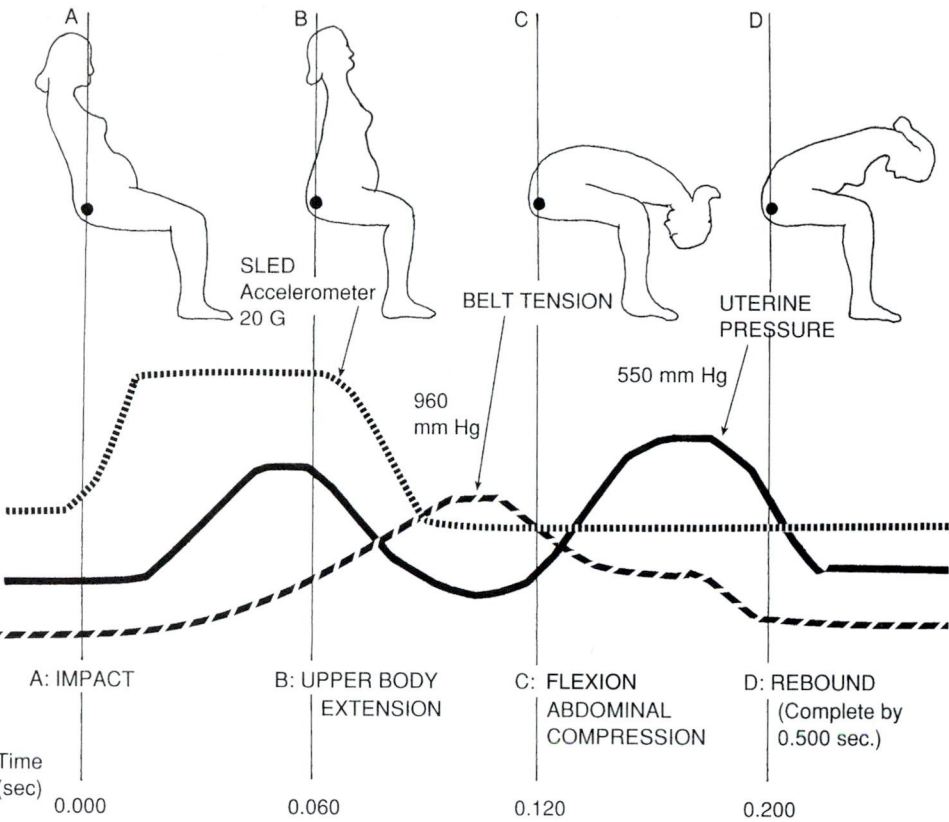

Figure 8-3 Impact sequence. Relationship between body motion, uterine pressure, and belt tension. *Modified from Crosby WM et al. Impact injuries in pregnancy. Am J Obstet Gynecol. 1968;101:102. In: Hankins CVD. Operative obstetrics. Stamford, CT: Appleton & Lange, 1995, Fig. 35-3, p. 655,*

symptoms in abruptio placentae due to all causes.[71] However, none of these signs and symptoms had sufficient sensitivity to reliably evaluate the pregnant trauma victim. Several controlled studies evaluated the sensitivity of uterine activity monitoring in diagnosing abruptio placentae.[65,66,72] All of these studies concluded that monitoring for a short time following trauma during pregnancy yielded high sensitivity and was a good screening tool for evaluating the pregnant trauma victim for abruptio placentae. The ACOG Educational Bulletin recommends a 4-hour monitoring period following trauma in the second half of pregnancy.[75] The finding of more than three uterine contractions in any 1 hour, uterine tenderness, abnormal fetal heart tracing, ruptured amniotic membranes, vaginal bleeding, or other severe maternal injuries require continued in-hospital observation and monitoring. In women who have frequent uterine contractions following trauma in the second half of pregnancy, continued observation for a 24-hour period is suggested. Using this policy, women who do not have immediate adverse outcomes have preg-

nancy outcomes similar to those of uninjured women.[72] Because placental abruption associated with trauma is often concealed, clinically significant hypofibrinogenemia has been found in two-thirds of women with traumatic placental abruption, as compared with one-third of women with nontraumatic placental abruption.[73]

While uterine contractions are common following trauma, a majority of women will have spontaneous abatement of contractions.[65,72] Uterine contractions are a sensitive but nonspecific finding of placental abruption. Virtually all patients who suffer traumatic placental separation will have uterine contractions, but only 12.5% of women with contractions have placental abruption.[72] Premature delivery following trauma is uncommon in the absence of placental abruption. Tocolytics are usually not indicated in this setting.[72] Magnesium sulfate is the preferred agent if tocolytics are necessary. β-Mimetics may increase the pulse rate and dilate the peripheral vasculature, making assessment for hemorrhage more difficult. Similarly, calcium-channel blockers may cause maternal hypotension and decrease uterine blood flow, effects that obviously are undesirable in the face of possible maternal hemorrhage.

Uterine Rupture

Compared to placental abruption, uterine rupture occurs much less commonly and almost always results from direct intense abdominal trauma. Approximately 0.6% of cases of trauma in pregnancy will be complicated by uterine rupture.[64] Because severe and unusual cases of trauma during pregnancy are more commonly reported, the actual incidence is likely lower than this. Factors that predispose to uterine rupture in labor also increase the possibility of traumatic uterine rupture, such as prior uterine scar, hydramnios, and multiple gestation. However, traumatic uterine rupture can occur in the absence of any predisposing cause and should be suspected when the mechanism of injury (direct abdominal impact) is associated with abdominal pain. The presentation may be very similar to abruptio placentae, with abdominal pain and tenderness, nonreassuring fetal heart tones, or fetal death.

Uterine rupture is extremely rare in the first trimester because the pelvis protects the uterus from direct injury. Beyond 12 weeks of gestation, the uterus becomes an abdominal organ and is more susceptible to direct injury. Uterine injury can range from lacerations of the serosa; complete disruption of the myometrial wall, with or without extrusion of the fetus, placenta, or umbilical cord into the abdominal cavity; avulsion of the uterine vasculature with intraperitoneal or retroperitoneal hemorrhage; or complete uterine avulsion. This latter injury has been described in association with poor placement of a lap belt.[74] Approximately 75% of full-thickness uterine ruptures involve the fundus. Clinical signs in this circumstance can provide assistance in making the diagnosis. Signs of peritoneal irritation, such as guarding, rigidity, distention, and rebound tenderness may be present. Because of the attenuation and gradual stretching of the parietal peritoneum, these findings are sometimes less common during pregnancy. An abnormal lie determined by the Leopold maneuver or abdominal x-ray films, particularly if the fetal extremities are extended, is another clue that the fetus has been extruded outside the uterine cavity. Finally, the fundus may be difficult to palpate if there is significant fundal disruption.

Adjunctive tests in establishing the diagnosis are useful if uterine rupture is suspected. As previously mentioned, abdominal radiography may demonstrate an abnormal fetal lie or extended fetal extremities. In addition, the finding of free air in the abdomen is highly suggestive, although this is not a specific finding, as ruptured viscus can also cause this abnormality. Peritoneal lavage is both safe and accurate in diagnosing intraabdominal hemorrhage at any gestational age, but it is not specific in localizing the cause of intraperitoneal hemorrhage.[76]

Both CT scanning and MRI have been used to detect intraabdominal or retroperitoneal hemorrhage. Ultrasound has also been used to diagnose intraperitoneal hemorrhage, although the accuracy of ultrasound during pregnancy for this indication has not been determined.

At the time of laparotomy, the finding of uterine rupture does not necessarily require hysterectomy. Smith and others demonstrated not only successful repair of uterine rupture due to trauma during pregnancy, but also good outcome in a subsequent pregnancy.[77] In the absence of life-threatening hemorrhage or significant uterine vascular injury, salvage of the uterus is possible, even with extensive lacerations. Subsequent pregnancy should be managed by repeat cesarean delivery.

Direct Fetal Injury

While fetal death due to direct fetal injury is described in the literature, it is a distinctly less common cause of fetal death than abruptio placentae, maternal hypovolemic shock, or pelvic fracture.[78,79] Of these uncommon fetal injuries, fetal skull and brain injury appear to be the most common. The mechanism most frequently described is fracture of the maternal pelvis in later gestation, when the fetal head is engaged. Unusual cases of fetal injury have also been described. For example, in one case a newborn had paraplegia and contractures resulting from a motor vehicle accident prior to birth.[80] Other cases of fetal brain injury with survival have been described.

Pelvic Fractures

Pelvic fractures may result from trauma and often present unique potential complications for the pregnant woman. Because of the extensive vascular hypertrophy of pregnancy, significant retroperitoneal and intraperitoneal hemorrhage resulting in hypovolemic shock may occur as a result of pelvic fracture during pregnancy. Also, because of the magnitude of force required to cause pelvic fracture, abruptio placentae, direct fetal injury or uterine rupture are also possible. Urinary-tract injuries are also common in patients with pelvic fracture. In general, vaginal delivery still is possible even with a recent pelvic fracture. Exceptions to this management plan include unstable pelvic fractures or pelvic fractures that have healed in a way that results in obstruction of the birth canal. Published reports demonstrate that more than 80% of women who have had a pelvic fracture can deliver vaginally.[81]

Fetal–Maternal Hemorrhage (FMH)

In 1985, Rose and colleagues described the incidence of fetal–maternal hemorrhage following trauma during pregnancy as assessed by the Kleihauer–Betke assay.[82] In this study, fetal–maternal hemorrhage was demonstrated four times more frequently in the trauma group as compared with a control group of uninjured pregnant women. Among the nine pregnancies with documented fetal–maternal hemorrhage, three demonstrated an adverse fetal effect presumed to be due to the hemorrhage. After this small published experience, several larger series were performed.[65,72] While the frequency of fetal–maternal hemorrhage is about fourfold higher in trauma victims as compared with uninjured controls, adverse fetal outcomes fortunately are rare events. Furthermore, the Kleihauer–Betke assay does not appear to be a useful predictive test for fetal complications because of the slow turnaround time, poor correlation between positive assays and fetal outcome, and the availability of more sensitive indicators of fetal compromise (e.g., fetal heart rate monitoring). However, because of the fourfold increased risk of fetal–maternal hemorrhage resulting from trauma, Rh-negative women are at increased risk for alloimmunization. Therefore, Kleihauer–Betke testing may have a role in Rh-negative women to evaluate those at risk for Rh alloimmunization and to identify those who need additional doses of Rh immune globulin.

Management of Blunt Abdominal Trauma

For the most part, treatment priorities for the pregnant trauma victim are similar to those for the non-pregnant woman. Two notable exceptions are that supine positioning should be avoided in the second half of pregnancy, and attention to fetal assessment must await primary stabilization of the injured woman. Treatment priorities include establishing a patent airway, providing oxygenation, and maintaining circulatory volume. The lateral decubitus position is preferred. However, in cases in which neck stabilization is a priority and the supine position must be maintained, the uterus should be displaced either manually or by insertion of a wedge beneath the patient's right hip. Investigators have demonstrated that there is a close correlation of low maternal serum bicarbonate level with fetal death, underlying the importance of establishing and maintaining adequate maternal oxygenation and circulatory volume.[83] Once emergency resuscitative measures have been instituted, a systematic search for maternal injuries, fractures, and external bleeding should be performed.

Evaluation of the fetus should await the institution of emergency resuscitation and the evaluation for significant maternal injuries. Findings of abdominal distention, tenderness, and peritoneal irritation require immediate evaluation. Evidence of hypovolemia should prompt aggressive resuscitation and exploratory laparotomy. Because of the possibility of multiple different sources of bleeding, it is preferable that both a trauma surgeon and an obstetrician are present at the laparotomy. Documentation of fetal viability and gestational age is important, and, if time permits, some assessment of fetal well-being can be invaluable for decision making during intraoperative management.

In the more stable patient with signs and symptoms suggestive of intraperitoneal hemorrhage, peritoneal lavage is both safe and accurate even in late gestation.[76] A peritoneal dialysis catheter should be inserted by an open technique, taking care to direct the catheter laterally away from the uterus. Aspiration of blood is an indication to perform exploratory laparotomy.

If exploratory laparotomy is necessary, the need for concurrent cesarean delivery depends on several factors. Laparotomy itself is not an indication for cesarean, and factors to consider include gestational age, fetal condition assessed by intrapartum evaluation, extent of uterine injuries, and whether the large uterus hinders adequate treatment or evaluation of other intraabdominal organs.

Tetanus immunization is another important aspect of care for the trauma patient. If a wound is contaminated,

250 units of human tetanus immunoglobulin should be given intravenously. In addition, combined tetanus/diphtheria toxoid (0.5 ml) should be administered if tetanus immunization status is unknown, the patient's immunization series is incomplete, or more than 10 years have elapsed since the last tetanus immunization was given. For severe contaminated wounds, tetanus/diphtheria toxoid should be given if the time since the last immunization was more than 5 years.

For women who are injured in the second half of pregnancy and who do not have life-threatening injuries, routine electronic fetal monitoring is strongly recommended.[65,66,72,75] Several studies have demonstrated that the use of electronic monitoring is the best predictor of placental abruption and may also assist in diagnosing uterine rupture. In one study, abruptio placentae was not present if uterine contractions were not detected or if the frequency was less than every 10 minutes during the first 4 hours of monitoring.[72] Importantly, about 12% of those who had frequent uterine contractions were subsequently found to have placental abruption. In these cases, abnormal fetal tracings were common, including fetal tachycardia and late decelerations. Thus, the isolated finding of uterine contractions should heighten one's awareness of the possibility of uteroplacental separation. If four or more uterine contractions are noted during any 1 hour of monitoring during the initial 4-hour monitoring period, continued monitoring for a minimum of 24 hours is recommended. In the presence of uterine contractions without abruptio placentae, the typical course would be for diminution in the frequency of contractions during the 4-hour monitoring period. Shorter and longer durations of monitoring from 2 to 24 hours have been recommended and used successfully in other studies. In the absence of uterine contractions or other ominous signs such as uterine tenderness, bleeding, or signs of fetal compromise, the patient can be discharged after the monitoring period. It is rare to have abruptio placentae occur remote from the time of injury, and case reports of "delayed abruption" may represent delayed diagnosis.[84]

Penetrating Trauma

The most common penetrating injuries are knife and gunshot wounds and may be associated with aggravated assaults, suicide attempts, or attempts to cause abortion. When the uterus is injured by penetrating wounds, the fetus is more likely to be injured than the woman. The fetus sustains injury in two-thirds of penetrating injuries, while visceral injuries to the mother are seen in only 20 percent.[85] Awwad and colleagues have reported a unique experience with high-velocity penetrating wounds of the pregnant uterus, collecting data in Lebanon over 16 years.[85] Among 14 women with penetrating injury, two died. From their experience, the authors presented three key observations: (1) visceral injuries were present when the entrance wound was in either the upper abdomen or back, (2) when the entry wound site was anterior and below the uterine fundus, visceral injuries were absent in all six affected women, and (3) perinatal death ensued in half the cases, due to either maternal shock, uteroplacental insufficiency, or direct fetal injury.

The disparate risk for the woman and her fetus following penetrating trauma results from at least two factors. First, the likelihood of injury to an intraabdominal organ is directly proportional to the size of that organ. In late pregnancy, the uterus occupies a large proportion of the intraabdominal volume, which places the uterus and its contents at significant risk for injury. Second, the mass of the myometrium, amniotic fluid, fetus, and placenta act as a "shield" against injury to maternal intraabdominal organs. A projectile penetrating the abdominal cavity and uterus transfers energy to the tissues through which it is passing. The loss of kinetic energy to the surrounding tissue slows the velocity of the bullet, with the bullet often coming to rest within the uterus. This effect has been confirmed in clinical series with injuries isolated to the uterus in more than two-thirds of cases.[84-88] Thus, when the uterus is injured by penetrating wounds, the fetus is more likely to be injured.

As the uterus enlarges, the abdominal viscera are forced upward, occupying a smaller volume in the upper abdomen. While the uterus does "protect" abdominal viscera by diminishing missile velocity and displacing the viscera, penetrating wounds that enter or exit above the uterus can create very complex wounds, with the possibility of multiple entry and exit wounds in the bowel. High-velocity projectiles can penetrate through the entire uterus, causing serious injury to organs posterior to the uterus (e.g., the aorta and sigmoid colon).

Essentially three decisions must be made in the management of penetrating wounds during pregnancy: (1) whether to perform exploratory laparotomy, (2) whether to deliver the fetus, and (3) if delivery is planned, which method should be used.

The first decision, whether to explore, is readily apparent if there is obvious hypovolemia and hemoperitoneum, but it is usually more difficult because many of these women are hemodynamically stable. Most authors agree that pregnant women who suffer gunshot wounds to the abdomen should have their abdomens explored.[72,88] As a bullet enters the abdominal cavity, it can be deflected by abdominal structures. This can dramatically alter its path, making it impossible to accurately predict the course of the bullet once it has entered the body. As the bullet is deflected, it tends to tumble, which creates more extensive damage to internal organs than the small entry wound might suggest. In addition, high-velocity projectiles create shock waves, and temporary cavitation can damage tissue well outside the actual path of the projectile.

Knife wounds to the uterus are much less likely to result in extrauterine injuries, and overall their prognosis is much better as compared with gunshot wounds. The decision to perform laparotomy in the pregnant woman with an abdominal stab wound must be individualized. Stab wounds to the upper abdomen are more likely to cause visceral injury than lower abdominal stab wounds, and exploration is necessary in most cases of upper abdominal wounds. Although stab wounds to the lower abdomen have been successfully managed without laparotomy, several considerations must be addressed.[89] In nonpregnant patients, stab wounds do not penetrate the peritoneum in about one-third of the cases. Unless a large extraperitoneal vessel is lacerated—for example, the inferior epigastric artery—these extraperitoneal wounds generally do not need exploration. However, distention and attenuation of the abdominal wall during pregnancy may make it more susceptible to peritoneal penetration. A fistulogram of the wound can be performed to determine whether there has been peritoneal penetration. Demonstration of spillage into the gastrointestinal or urinary tract requires surgical intervention. Intravenous pyelography or retrograde cystourethrography are useful if injury to the urethra or bladder is suspected. Amniocentesis has been suggested to determine whether there is blood or bacteria within the amniotic fluid. The presence of bloody amniotic fluid alone, however, is not an indication for delivery, particularly for the very immature fetus. Likewise, growth of a few colonies of bacteria from the amniotic fluid in the clinically uninfected uterus does not mandate delivery.

The uterine vessels are lateral and somewhat posteriorly placed during pregnancy, which makes them unlikely to be injured by stab wounds. However, longer blades or entry through the lateral abdominal wall may lacerate uterine vessels. Because of the increased blood flow to the uterus (600 ml/min at term) evidence of hypovolemia is usually quickly apparent if there is uterine vascular injury. If there is any question about intraperitoneal bleeding, peritoneal lavage is a simple and accurate method of establishing whether there is a hemoperitoneum.[74] If the uterus has been penetrated, there is significant risk for fetal or placental injury. It is very difficult to assess the extent of fetal injury unless the fetus has died. The decision to intervene in a pregnancy where uterine perforation is known or suspected can be difficult. There is little reason to intervene if the fetus is not viable, unless the uterus must be emptied to adequately explore or repair maternal injuries. While some authors have proceeded with cesarean delivery when uterine stab wounds were found at exploration, most of the fetal wounds were either superficial or of such severity that immediate delivery would not have affected the outcome. Finally, tetanus prophylaxis as previously outlined should be administered to pregnant women who suffer penetrating injuries.

Thermal Injury

On the basis of experience with 50 pregnant women who had been burned, Matthews recommended that women in the second or third trimester with burns over 50% of their body should be delivered immediately because otherwise maternal death is almost certain, and the fetal survival rate is not improved by waiting.[90,91] He emphasized that if the fetus is not delivered, the maternal prognosis is markedly worse than for a nonpregnant woman suffering otherwise comparable burns. Conversely, two subsequent reports suggested that pregnancy did not alter maternal outcome as compared with the outcome for nonpregnant women of similar age.[92,93] Jain and Garg[93] found abortion to be common in the first trimester and most often caused by septicemia. Rayburn and colleagues[94] and Akhtar and co-workers[95] observed that fetal survival usually parallels the percentage of burned surface area and survival of the mother. For instance, there was a 50% maternal and fetal loss in the group who had burns over 40 to 60% of their body-surface area, as compared with 11% fetal and a

0% maternal loss rate with burns over 20 to 40% of body-surface area. Again, pregnancy did not alter maternal survival, whereas adequate shock management and early excision with grafting reduced mortality. Rode and associates[96] conducted a multicenter retrospective review of five South African burn centers and reported similar results from 33 women with an average burn area of 30%. Maternal mortality was 70% for burns exceeding 50% of body-surface area. Cesarean delivery was reserved for the unusual case when the gravely ill woman's condition jeopardized the viable fetus.

Thus, for severely burned women, fetal prognosis is poor. Usually the woman enters labor spontaneously within a few days to a week and often gives birth to a stillborn infant. Contributory factors are hypovolemia, pulmonary injury, septicemia, and the intensely catabolic state.

REFERENCES

1. Mazze RI, Kallen B. Reproductive outcome after anesthesia and operation during pregnancy: a registry study of 5405 cases. Am J Obstet Gynecol 1989;161:1178.
2. Duncan PG, Pope WDB, Cohen MM, et al. Fetal risk of anesthesia and surgery during pregnancy. Anesthesiology 1986;64:790.
3. Babler EA. Perforative appendicitis complicating pregnancy. JAMA 1908;51:1310.
4. Mazze RI, Kallen BK. Appendectomy during pregnancy: a Swedish registry study of cases. Obstet Gynecol 1991; 77:835–840.
5. Fallon WF, Newman JS, Fallon GL, et al. The surgical management of intra-abdominal inflammatory conditions during pregnancy. Surg Clin North Am 1995;75:15.
6. Coleman MT, Trianfo VA, Rund DA. Nonobstetric emergencies in pregnancy: trauma and surgical conditions. Am J Obstet Gynecol 1997;177:497.
7. Baer JL, Reis RA, Arens RA. Appendicitis in pregnancy with changes in position and axis of the normal appendix in pregnancy. JAMA 1932;98:1359.
8. Maternal adaptations to pregnancy. In: Cunningham FG, MacDonald PC, Gant NF et al., eds. Williams obstetrics. Norwalk, CT: Appleton & Lange, 1997:191.
9. American Institute of Ultrasound in Medicine (AIUM). AIUM bioeffects considerations for the safety of diagnostic ultrasound. J Ultrasound Med 1988;7:S1.
10. American College of Obstetricians and Gynecologists. Ultrasonography in pregnancy. ACOG Technical Bulletin no. 187. December 1993.
11. Lim HK, Bae SH, Seo GS. Diagnosis of acute appendicitis in pregnant women: value of sonography. AJR 1992; 159:539.
12. Hansen GC, Toot PJ, Lynch CO. Subtle ultrasound signs of appendicitis in a pregnant patient. J Reprod Med 1993; 38:223.
13. Hall EJ. Scientific view of low level radiation risks. Radiographics 1991;11:509.
14. American College of Obstetricians and Gynecologists. Guidelines for diagnostic imaging during pregnancy. Committee Opinion 158. September 1995.
15. Baillie J, Carins SR, Putnam WS, et al. Endoscopic management of choledocholithiasis during pregnancy. Surg Gynecol Obstet 1990;171:1.
16. Rai R, Kalloo AN. Biliary tract disease in pregnancy. J Soc Obstet Gynaecol Can 1997;19:1075.
17. American College of Obstetrics and Gynecologists. Obstetric analgesia and anesthesia. ACOG Technical Bulletin 225. July 1996.
18. Atrash HK, Koonin LM, Lawson HW, et al. Maternal mortality in the United States, 1979–1986. Obstet Gynecol 1990;76:1055.
19. Analgesia and anesthesia. In: Cunningham FG, MacDonald PC, Gant NF, et al., eds. Williams obstetrics. Norwalk, CT: Appleton & Lange, 1997:379.
20. Samsoon GLT, Young JRB. Difficult tracheal intubation: a retrospective study. Anesthesia 1987;42:487.
21. Tamir IL, Bongard FS, Klein SR. Acute appendicitis in the pregnant patient. Am J Surg 1990;160:571.
22. Horowitz MD, Gomez GA, Santiesteban R, et al. Acute appendicitis during pregnancy. Arch Surg 1985; 120:1362.
23. Babaknia A, Parsa H, Woodruff JD. Appendicitis during pregnancy. Obstet Gynecol 1977;50:40.
24. Reedy MB, Kallen B, Keuhl TJ. Laparoscopy during pregnancy: a study of five fetal outcome parameters with use of the Swedish Health Registry. Am J Obstet Gynecol 1997;177:673.
25. American College of Obstetricians and Gynecologists. Early pregnancy loss. ACOG Technical Bulletin no. 212. September 1995.
26. Saunders P, Milton PJD. Laparotomy during pregnancy: an assessment of diagnostic accuracy and fetal wastage. BMJ 1973;21:165.
27. Sharp HT. Gastrointestinal surgical conditions during pregnancy. Clin Obstet Gynecol 1994;37:306.
28. Reedy M., Uy K, Thompson E, Rayburn W. Laparoscopy during pregnancy: a safe alternative to laparotomy? Contemp Obstet Gynecol 1998;April:75.
29. Reedy MB, Galan HL, et al. Laparoscopic insufflation in the gravid baboon: maternal and fetal effects. J Am Assoc Gynecol Laparosc 1995;2:83.
30. Barnard JM, Chaffin D, Droste S, et al. Fetal response to carbon dioxide pneumoperitoneum in the pregnant ewe. Obstet Gynecol 1995;85:669.
31. Hunter JG, Swanstrom L, Thornburg K. Carbon dioxide pneumoperitoneum induces fetal acidosis in a pregnant ewe model. Surg Endosc 1995;9:272.
32. Eldering SC. Laparoscopic cholecystectomy in pregnancy. Am J Surg 1993;165:625.
33. Morrell DG, Mullins JR, Harrison PB. Laparoscopic cholecystectomy during pregnancy in symptomatic patients. Surgery 1992;112:856.
34. Morice P, Louis-Sylvestre C, Chapron C, Dubuisson JB. Laparoscopy for adnexal torsion in pregnant women. J Reprod Med 1997;42:435.
35. Shaley E, Rahav D, Romano S. Laparoscopic relief of

adnexal torsion in early pregnancy: case reports. Br J Obstet Gynaecol 1990;97:853.

36. Cunningham FG, McCubbin JH. Appendicitis complicating pregnancy. Obstet Gynecol 1975;45:415.

37. Jeffery RB Jr, Laing FC, Lewis FR. Acute appendicitis: high resolution real-time ultrasound findings. Radiology 1987;163:11.

38. Schreiber JH. Laparoscopic appendectomy in pregnancy. Surg Endosc 1990;4:100.

39. McCorriston CC. Nonobstetrical abdominal surgery during pregnancy. Am J Obstet Gynecol 1963;86:593.

40. Mahmoodian S. Appendicitis complicating pregnancy. South Med J 1992;85:19.

41. Braverman DZ, Johnson ML, Kern F Jr. Effects of pregnancy and contraceptive steroids on gallbladder function. N Eng J Med 1980;302:362.

42. Swisher SG, Schmit PJ, Hunt KK, et al. Biliary disease during pregnancy. Am J Surg 1994;168:576.

43. Wilkinson EJ. Acute pancreatitis in pregnancy: a review of 98 cases and a report of 8 new cases. Obstet Gynecol Surv 1973;28:281.

44. Valdivieso V, Covassubias C, Siegel F, et al. Pregnancy and cholelithiasis: pathogenesis and natural course of gallstones diagnoses in early puerperium. Hepatology 1993;17:1.

45. Kern F, Everson GT, DeMark B, et al. Biliary lipids, bile acids, and gallbladder function in the human female: effects of pregnancy and the ovulatory cycle. J Clin Invest 1981;68:1229.

46. Scott LD. Gallstone disease and pancreatitis in pregnancy. Gastroenterol Clin North Am 1992;4:803.

47. Landers D, Carmona, Crombleholme W, Lim R. Acute cholecystis in pregnancy. Obstet Gynecol 1987;69:131.

48. Dixon NP, Faddis DM, Silberman H. Aggressive management of cholecystitis during pregnancy. Am J Surg 1987;154:292.

49. American College of Obstetricians and Gynecologists. Cancer of the ovary. ACOG Technical Bulletin no. 141. May 1990.

50. Hibbard LT. Adnexal torsion. Am J Obstet Gynecol 1985;152:456.

51. Baker TE, Copas PR. Adnexal torsion: a clinical dilemma. J Reprod Med 1995;40:447.

52. Cancer in pregnancy. In: Disia PJ, Creasman NT, eds. Clinical gynecologic oncology. St. Louis: Mosby Year Book 1993:544.

53. Struyk APHB, Tretters PE. Ovarian tumors in pregnancy. Acta Obstet Gynecol Scand 1984;63:421.

54. Grimes WH Jr, Bartholemew RA, Colvin ED, et al. Ovarian cyst complicating pregnancy. Am J Obstet Gynecol 1954;68:594.

55. Mashiach S, Bider D, Moran O, et al. Adnexal torsion of hyperstimulated ovaries in pregnancies after gonadotropin therapy. Fertil Steril 1990;53:76.

56. American College of Obstetricians and Gynecologists. Gynecologic ultrasonography. ACOG Technical Bulletin no. 215. November 1995.

57. Fleischer AC, Stein SM, Cullinan JA et al. Color Doppler sonography of adnexal torsion. J Ultrasound Med 1995;14:523.

58. Tepper R, Lerner-Geva L, Zalel Y, et al. Adnexal torsion: the contribution of color Doppler sonography to

diagnosis and post-operative follow-up. Eur J Obstet Gynecol Reprod Biol 1995;62:121.

59. Grant, WM. Adnexal masses. In: Hankins GDV, Clark SL, Cunningham FG, Gilshrap LC, eds. Operative obstetrics. Norwalk, CT: Appleton & Lange 1995:405.

60. Iwabe T, Harada T, Miura H, et al. Laparoscopic unwinding of adnexal torsion caused by ovarian hyperstimulation. Hum Reprod 1994;9:2350.

61. Gordon JD, Hopkins KL, Jeffery RB, et al. Adnexal torsion: color Doppler diagnosis and laparoscopic treatment. Fertil Steril 1994;61:383.

62. Oelsner G, Bider D, Goldenberg M, et al. Long-term follow-up of the twisted adnexa managed by detorsion. Fertil Steril 1993;60:976.

63. Shalev E, Bustan M, Yarom I, et al. Recovery of ovarian function after laparoscopic detorsion. Hum Reprod 1995;10:2965.

64. Pearlman MD, Tintinalli JE. Blunt trauma during pregnancy. N Eng J Med 1990;323:1609.

65. Goodwin TM, Breen MT. Pregnancy outcome and fetomaternal hemorrhage after non-catastrophic trauma. Am J Obstet Gynecol 1990;162:665.

66. Williams JK, McClain L, Rosemurgy AS, Colorado NM. Evaluation of abdominal trauma in the third trimester of pregnancy: maternal and fetal considerations. Obstet Gynecol 1990;75:33.

67. American College of Obstetricians and Gynecologists. Automobile passenger restraints for children and pregnant women. ACOG Technical Bulletin No. 151. January 1991.

68. Gazmararian JA, Lozorick S, Spitz AM, Ballard TJ, Saltzman LE, Marks JS. Prevalence of violence against pregnant women. JAMA 1996;275:1915.

69. Pearlman MD, Tintinalli JE. Evaluation and treatment of the gravida and fetus following trauma during pregnancy. Obstet Gynecol Clin North Am 1991;18:371.

70. Crosby WM, Snyder RG, Snow CC, Hanson PG. Impact injuries in pregnancy. 1. Experimental studies. Am J Obstet Gynecol 1968;101:100.

71. Hurd WW, Miodovnik M, Hertzberg V, Lavin JP. Selective management of abruptio placentae: a prospective study. Obstet Gynecol 1983;61:467.

72. Pearlman MD, Tintinalli JE, Lorenz RP. A prospective controlled study of outcome after trauma during pregnancy. Am J Obstet Gynecol 1990; 162:1502.

73. Stettler RW, Lutich A, Pritchard JA, Cunningham FG. Traumatic placental abruption: a separation from traditional thought. Presented at the Annual Clinical Meeting of the American College of Obstetricians and Gynecologists, Las Vegas, May 1992.

74. McCormick RD. Seat belt injury: case of complete transection of the pregnant uterus. J Am Osteopath Assoc 1968;67:1139.

75. American College of Obstetricians and Gynecologists. Trauma during pregnancy. ACOG Technical Bulletin no. 161. November 1991.

76. Rothenberger DA, Quattlebaum FW, Zabel J, Fischer RP. Diagnostic peritoneal lavage for blunt trauma in pregnant women. Am J Obstet Gynecol 1977;129:479.

77. Smith A, LeMire WA, Hurd WW, Pearlman MD. Repair of the traumatically ruptured gravid uterus: a report of

two cases resulting in subsequent viable pregnancies. J Reprod Med 1994; 39:825.

78. Elliot M. Vehicular accidents and pregnancy. Aust NZ J Obster Gynecol 1966;6:279.

79. Stafford PA, Biddinger PW, Zumwalt RE. Lethal intrauterine fetal trauma. Am J Obstet Gynecol 1998; 159:485.

80. Weyerts LK, Jones MC, James HE. Paraplegia and congenital contractures as a consequence of intrauterine trauma. Am J Med Genet 1992;43:751.

81. Madsen LV, Jensen J, Christensen ST. Parturition and pelvic fracture. Follow-up of 34 obstetric patients with a history of pelvic fracture. Acta Obstet Gynecol Scand 1983;62:617.

82. Rose PG, Strohm PL, Zuspan FP. Fetomaternal hemorrhage following trauma. Am J Obstet Gynecol, 1985; 152:844.

83. Scorpio RJ, Esposito TJ, Smith LG, Gens DR. Blunt trauma during pregnancy. Factors affecting fetal outcome. J Trauma 1992;32:213.

84. Lavin JP Jr, Miodovnik M. Delayed abruption after maternal trauma as a result of an automobile accident. J Reprod Med 1981;26:621.

85. Buchsbaum HJ. Penetrating injury of the abdomen. In: Buchsbaum HJ, ed. Trauma in pregnancy. Philadelphia: Saunders, 1979: 82.

86. Awwad JT, Axar GB, Aouad AT, Raad J, Karqam KS. Postmortem cesarean section follow maternal blast injury: case report. J Trauma 1994;36:260.

87. Franger AL, Buchsbaum JH, Peacemen AM. Abdominal gunshot wounds in pregnancy. Am J Obstet Gynecol 1989;160:1124.

88. Kirshon B, Young R, Gordon AN. Conservative management of abdominal gunshot wound in a pregnant woman. Am J Perinatol 1988;5(3):232.

89. Grubb DK. Non-surgical management of penetrating uterine trauma in pregnancy: a case report. Am J Obstet Gynecol 1992;166:583.

90. Matthews RN. Obstetric implications of burns in pregnancy. Br J Obstet Gynecol 1982;89:603.

91. Matthews RN. Old burns and pregnancy. Br J Obstet Gynaecol 1982;89:610.

92. Amy BW, McManus WF, Goodwin CW, Mason A, Pruitt BA. Thermal injury in the pregnant patient. Surg Gynecol Obstet 1985;161:209.

93. Jain ML, Garg AK. Burns with pregnancy: a cased review of 25 cases. Burns 1993;19:166.

94. Rayburn W, Smith B, Feller I, Varner M, Cruikshank D. Major burns during pregnancy: effects on fetal well-being. Obstet Gynecol 1984;63:392.

95. Akhtar MA, Mulawkar PM, Kulkarni HR. Burns in pregnancy: effect on maternal and fetal outcomes. Burns 1994; 20:351.

96. Rode H, Millar AJW, Cywes S, et al. Thermal injury in pregnancy—the neglected tragedy. South Afr Med J 1990; 77:346.

Chapter 9
Multiple Gestation

John A. Read

Five Key Points

- The frequency of multiple gestation has increased significantly over the past two decades, primarily because of assisted reproductive technologies.

- Early diagnosis is essential. Attention to details and use of established protocols from specialized twin clinics can improve outcome.

- Preterm birth and growth disorders are the major contributors to morbidity and mortality in multiple gestations.

- There are a number of problems specific to multiple gestation that warrant consultation with a maternal–fetal medicine specialist.

- Vaginal delivery is possible in the majority of cases if twin A is in a cephalic presentation and no unusual complications are present. Patients with higher-order multiple gestations are best delivered by cesarean in a tertiary-care facility.

Multiple gestation has always generated a great fascination. The birth and survival of multiples, especially of more than two, was thought of as uncommon. The use of a variety of methods of assisted reproductive technology, including ovulation-induction agents, multiple embryo transfers during in vitro fertilization, and a rising pregnancy rate among older women has resulted in a changing pattern of multiple births.[1] Between 1973 and 1990, the rates of twin and triplet births have increased 2 and 7 times, respectively, versus singletons.

After prospective parents get over the initial shock, surprise and excitement, they must come to grips with the reality that they face a potentially very complicated and difficult pregnancy. Multiple gestation remains one of the highest-risk situations for the fetus and neonate despite recent advances in perinatal and neonatal care.

Unfortunately, it is often the obstetric practitioner who underestimates the complex and potentially serious consequences of a multifetal pregnancy. There is a long list of significantly increased complications for both mother and fetus/neonate in these pregnancies (Table 9-1). As a result of these complicating factors, it was formerly noted that, although twins accounted for only about 1% of pregnancies, they were responsible for approximately 10% or more of preterm deliveries and 25% of deaths among premature infants. The perinatal mortality has, in general, remained one order of magnitude higher (10×) for twins versus singletons and is approximately doubled for triplets over twins. While the perinatal mortality has declined

---

TABLE 9-1
INCREASED RISKS ASSOCIATED WITH MULTIPLE PREGNANCY

Maternal	Fetal/Neonatal
Abruptio placenta	Abortion/vanishing twin
Anemia	Birth trauma
Cesarean delivery	Congenital anomalies
Hemorrhage: antepartum/ intrapartum	Cord entanglement/prolapse
	Discordant growth
Hydramnios/oligohydramnios	Twin-to-twin transfusion syndrome
Hyperemesis gravidarum	Intrauterine growth restriction
Operative delivery	Intrauterine fetal death of one or more fetuses
Pregnancy-induced hypertension	Low birth weight
Premature labor/delivery	Malpresentation
Preterm premature rupture of membranes	Increased neonatal morbidity and mortality

---

from the 13 to 15% range for twins in the 1960s[2], it still remains in the 8 to 10% range[3,4] unless care is given in specialized twin clinics. Our own experience suggests that a 1 to 2% rate is attainable in this setting.

The focus of this chapter will be on the management of twin gestations with reference to higher-order multiples where appropriate. The challenge to those who render obstetric care to these patients is to provide a rational and careful plan of management that addresses the multitude of sources for increased morbidity and mortality in these high-risk cases.

INCIDENCE AND ETIOLOGY

Traditionally, the incidence of twin gestations in the United States has been cited at 1 in 80 to 1 in 100 pregnancies (Table 9-2). Over the past two decades in particular, several factors have resulted in an increase in the rate of multiple births, and new information has altered our appreciation of the true background rate. Jewell and Yip[5] reported that the rates of twin and triplet births rose 19 and 100%, respectively, during the 1980s. In 25% of cases this increase was ascribed to increases in maternal age and the rest to the widespread use of fertility-enhancing technologies

in older and more educated white women. Luke[1] also has detailed the rising rate between the 1970s and '90s.

In the past, all references citing the incidence of multiple birth had referred to births and recognized abortions. Newer evidence indicates that the incidence of multiple conceptions is much higher. In a series of 1000 consecutive first-trimester ultrasounds, Landy et al.[6] showed a 5.4% incidence of multiple gestation if early pregnancy gestational sacs were counted and a 3.3% incidence if only fetal poles with cardiac activity were included.

Dizygotic twins are the result of fertilization of two ova, where the production of two or more ova may result from either endogenous or exogenous influences. There are a number of recognized clinical associations with "fraternal" twinning. Previous baseline racial incidence in the United States may vary from a low of approximately 1 in 140 in Asians to a high of 1 in 70 in African-Americans, with the incidence in Caucasians approximately 1 in 100. In some families there seems to be an increased incidence, especially through maternal members of the family tree. As previously noted, increasing age and parity may increase the risk of multiple gestation. An increase in circulating gonadotropins, which may occur spontaneously or as a result of increased body weight, may increase the frequency of multiple ovulation.

Assisted reproductive technology and the use of "fertility drugs" must always prompt an investigation for multiple gestation. Callahan et al.[7] have reported that by 1991, 35% of twin and 77% of higher-order multiple-gestation pregnancies were the result of assisted-reproduction techniques. The use of clomiphene citrate is associated with approximately a 5%

TABLE 9-2
FREQUENCY OF MULTIFETAL GESTATIONS

	"Natural"	1970s	1990s
All twins	1:80 births	1:55	1:43
Monozygotic twins	1:250		
Triplets	1:6400	1:3323	1:1341
Quadruplets	1:512,000		>10–20×*

*Increased, but possibly much offset by fetal reduction procedures.

incidence of twins, with occasional higher-order multiples. The use of human menopausal gonadotropins can result in a rate of over 20% multiple gestations, frequently of higher order. However, in well-managed cases a 10% incidence can be expected, with three-fourths being twins.[8] In addition to ovulation induction, in vitro fertilization (IVF) and gamete intrafallopian transfer (GIFT) procedures have significantly raised the incidence of multiple gestations, especially of higher order. Ho et al[9] reported that 88% of the triplet pregnancies in their unit resulted from ovulation induction and artificial fertilization. Specifically for triplets, Lipitz et al.[10] have reported that 6.6% were spontaneous, 15.1% were clomiphene-induced, 52.8% were the direct result of gonadotropins, and 25.5% resulted from IVF procedures. In a review of 71 quadruplet pregnancies from the 1980s, Collins and Bleyl[11] found that 94% followed ovulation-induction therapy.

The reason for monozygotic twinning is unclear. The splitting of an early embryo has been likened to a teratogenic event, which besides producing two genetically identical individuals, may result in many other unfavorable consequences. At one time monozygotic twins represented approximately one-third of all twins. Because these gestations have remained at a constant rate, uninfluenced by the factors responsible for the presence of dizygotic (and higher) multiples, the proportion of these "identical" twins may be significantly less. The suggestion has been made, however, that ovulation induction may also increase the incidence of monozygotic twins.[12]

The presence of diamnionic–monochorionic or monoamnionic–monochorionic placentation virtually is 100% predictive of monozygosity. In addition the incidence of monozygosity has been reported as 15% in separate dichorionic placentas and 23% where fused dichorionic placentas are found.[13] In addition, confirmation requires, at a minimum, concordance of sex and blood type, and DNA testing may be necessary to prove conclusively that the neonates are identical.

DIAGNOSIS AND EARLY GESTATION

The optimal management of all high-risk pregnancies, and especially multiple gestations, begins with the first prenatal visit. If various perinatal strategies likely to improve outcome are to be successful, the diagnosis should be made as early as possible. The basic prenatal database, comprised of a complete and accurate menstrual history, including information regarding the certainty, regularity, and normalcy of the last menses, other bleeding, and the use of contraceptive measures, is important. Notation of any historical factors that suggest the increased possibility of multiples such as family history, racial extraction, increased age or parity, and use of infertility agents must be noted.

Clinical Methods of Diagnosis

While there are a number of clinical clues to the diagnosis of multiple gestation, they unfortunately suffer from a great lack of sensitivity. Before the widespread availability of ultrasound in the 1970s, it was generally reported that as many as two-thirds or more of twin gestations were not diagnosed until labor, and half of these were not identified until after delivery of the first infant. A large-for-dates fundal height (>2 cm above expected) or a rapid increase in uterine size should always make one consider the diagnosis of a multiple gestation. It is our experience, however, that the average gestation at which the fundus is ≥3 cm is not until 25 to 26 weeks of gestation, and this measurement can be confused by factors such as maternal obesity, inaccurate menstrual dates, late prenatal care, intrauterine growth restriction (IUGR) in both twins, and the failure of the obstetric care provider to consider the diagnosis. Multiple gestation should be the first consideration in the differential diagnosis of a large-for-dates uterus. The auscultation of two or more fetal heart rates (separate places and rates) can be diagnostic, but often is not possible until well into the third trimester. While associated with twin gestations, excessive anemia, maternal weight gain, and fetal activity are individually not very sensitive indicators.

α-Fetoprotein

The routine use of maternal serum α-fetoprotein (MSAFP) screening would seem to be valuable in the diagnosis of multiple gestation since, in addition to other abnormalities, the presence of more than one fetus could often result in elevated levels. Using what would be considered a normal median for twin pregnancies of 2 to 2.5 MOM as a screening cutoff, Johnson et al. identified twins as a cause of elevated MSAFP in 10 to 20% of patients.[14] While these authors predicted a 56% sensitivity using 2.5 MOM, only 40% of the twins in their study were detected. In another study, the institutional median for twin gestation was 1.75 MOM and an elevated level was arbitrarily set at 3.5 MOM.[15] A discordant value of amniotic fluid AFP has been found significantly more often in twins of opposite sexes, suggesting that discordant amniotic fluid AFP is more common in dizygous twins.[16] The authors of this study found that, no matter what the zygosity, acetylcholinesterase was identical in all amniotic fluid samples of twins and thus not helpful for diagnosis.

Ultrasound Diagnosis

If one believes that the early diagnosis of multiple gestation is the most important element in the reduction of perinatal morbidity and mortality with specialized care, then routine screening with ultrasound should not be controversial. With today's ultrasound equipment the competent ultrasonographer should make the correct diagnosis virtually 100% of the time. Diagnosis is only the first of multiple uses for ultrasound (Table 9-3) in current high-level management of multiple-fetus pregnancies.

Using the equipment available in the 1970s, Persson et al.[17] correctly detected 98% of twin gestations with screening at 20 weeks. These patients were placed on home bed rest until 28 weeks and then hospitalized. The perinatal mortality rate for 28 weeks or greater was only 6 per 1000. In my first experience with a special twin clinic and the introduction of screening ultrasound between 1980 and 1982 at Tripler Army Medical Center, the diagnosis of twins was made before 24 weeks in 87.5% of cases after the institution of screening as opposed to 45.5% prior to routine screening (ultrasound by indication only). In the screening group the diagnosis was made prior to

---

TABLE 9-3
USES OF ULTRASOUND IN MULTIPLE GESTATION

Diagnosis
Assessment of gestational age
Determination of amnion/chorion status
Survey for anomalies
Invasive procedures (amniocentesis/chorionic villus sampling)
Fetal lie and presentation
Determination and analysis of fetal growth
Biophysical profile
Doppler flow studies
Intrapartum treatment

---

clinical suspicion 85% of the time versus 36% before routine screening was instituted. In a nonrandomized study reported in 1985 by Hughey and Olive,[18] 94% of twins were diagnosed by the 24th week, compared with 68% for unscreened controls. More importantly, the frequency of unfavorable outcomes was reduced from 60% to 25% in the routinely screened patients. Compared with universal identification in the screened group of the RADIUS study,[19] 37.7% of the control group were not identified until after 26 weeks and 13.1% were not scanned until admission for delivery. An additional argument for screening all pregnancies with ultrasound relative to multiple gestations is the increased incidence of associated congenital anomalies, placental and membrane abnormalities, and need for early accurate dating of the pregnancy for the identification and management of growth disturbances.

Vanishing Twin

With the high-resolution ultrasound now available, especially when used vaginally, one is able to confirm the diagnosis of intrauterine pregnancy at a very early gestational age. Often one will see more than one, or what appears to be more than one, gestational sac. In a review stimulated by reports of apparently disappearing sacs and embryos, Landy et al.[6] reported on 1000 first-trimester ultrasounds. As previously noted, the incidence of multiple gestation was much higher than expected. The more usual rate of multiples was accounted for by the phenomenon of the "vanishing twin." The loss, or vanishing, rate approximates 50% if all suspected diagnoses are included (i.e., number of early "sacs"), but was at least 21.2% if only documented embryos are included. It was further noted that there was a higher incidence of first-trimester bleeding in these multiple pregnancies (18.5%) than in singleton pregnancies (7.2%). These observations led to the conclusion that the incidence of multiple pregnancies is much higher than previously expected and that many episodes of first-trimester bleeding, perhaps 5%, may be associated with the loss of one conceptus. Dickey et al.[20] reported that, when two viable embryos were present, the probability of delivering two infants was 90% if the mother was under age 30 and 84% if over age 30. For triplets the rates were 90% and 44%, respectively.

Since the prognosis for the remaining fetus is excellent and there may be at least some emotional trauma associated with the loss of a twin, the diagnosis of vanishing twin should not be made until after two embryos are identified with certainty. Fluid collections, subchorionic bleeding and certain anatomic and artifactual situations may mimic a second or third gestation. Jauniaux et al.[21] reported finding postpartum evidence in half of the cases reviewed.

The prognosis for a multiple gestation diagnosed in the first trimester may be further aided by the recognition of early discordant growth. Kol et al.[22] reported that 5% of initially viable embryos after assisted reproduction underwent spontaneous fetal death and that the incidence increased if there was significant intrafetal size variation. When reviewing cases with continued viability, Weissman et al.[23] found major congenital anomalies in all of 5 cases when the crown-to-rump length differed by 5 or more days. Benson et al.[24] found that the vanishing twin phenomenon was not observed when two heartbeats were still observed after 8 weeks of gestation, an observation that agrees with the prognosis for first-trimester abortion in singleton pregnancies.

Status of the Amnion(s), Chorion(s), and Placenta

It has long been recognized that zygosity and status of the placenta and membranes have important implications in the management and outcome of multiple gestations. First, there is a wide range of perinatal mortality based on membrane status alone, with a high in the range of 50% with monoamniotic/monochorionic status and a rate approximating that in singletons with a diamniotic/dichorionic configuration. In addition, there are differences in anomaly rates and special developmental problems in monozygotic gestations. Genetic counseling and management of discordant growth and anomalies, fetal death in utero, and possible multifetal reduction in higher-order multiples depend greatly on information about zygosity and placentation.

The vast improvement in sonographic equipment has greatly facilitated the correct prediction of amnionicity and chorionicity (Table 9-4). The first sonographic criteria were offered in 1985 by Barss et al.[25] and included observations of placental number, presence and thickness of the septum, and separation of gestational sacs in early gestation. Winn et al.[26] reported that, when using a cutoff of 2-mm thickness of the dividing membrane, the accuracy in predicting monochorionic and dichorionic twinning was 82% and 95%, respectively. Subsequent review[27] shows that measuring membrane thickness has a high interobserver and intraobserver variability that depends on multiple factors, including the subject, the site of sampling, and the chorionicity and that this variability explains the suboptimal accuracy with this method, especially in the second and third trimesters. Using a classification of chorionicity based on the number of layers seen in the dividing membrane, D'Alton and Dudley[28] found a predictive accuracy of 100% for dichorionic twins when three or four layers were seen, and 94.4% for monochorionic when only two layers were visualized (Figure 9-1). Using a high-frequency (10 MHz) abdominal transducer, Vayssiere et al.[29] were able to correctly diagnose all of 12 diamniotic/monochorionic pregnancies where the membrane was visualized, and they recommended this technique as the first-line method of diagnosis.

The presence of a triangular projection of placental tissue extending between the layers where the intertwin membranes approach the placenta (Figure 9-2)

TABLE 9-4
ULTRASONOGRAPHIC CRITERIA FOR DETERMINATION OF AMNIONICITY, CHORIONICITY, AND ZYGOSITY

Ultrasound Observation	Status
Two or more separate placentas	Diamniotic/dichorionic
"Thick" intervening membrane	Diamniotic/dichorionic
"Thin" intervening membrane	Likely diamniotic/monochorionic
No intervening membrane visualized	Possibly monoamniotic/monochorionic
Multiple layers (4 vs. 2) in membrane	Most likely diamniotic/dichorionic
Presence of "twin peak" or "lambda" sign	Most likely diamniotic/dichorionic
"T" insertion of thin membrane	Likely diamniotic/monochorionic
Two yolk sacs in early gestation	Diamniotic
Different fetal sexes	Diamniotic/dichorionic and dizygotic

Figure 9-1 Ultrasound demonstrates a thin, two-layered membrane suggestive of a monochorionic/diamniotic placenta.

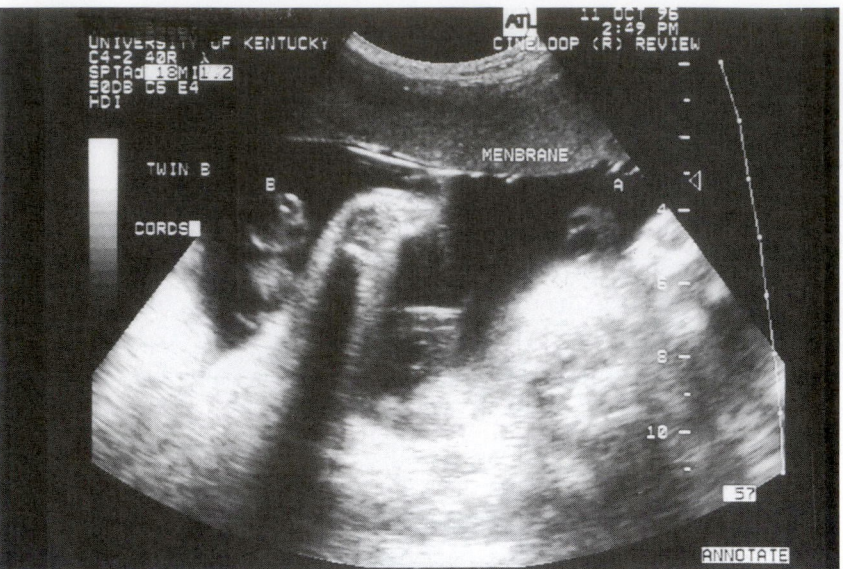

has been called the "twin peak" sign by Finberg[30] and the "lambda sign" by Bessis and Papernik.[31] In the former study, a retrospective analysis found the sign in all of 15 cases, while in the latter case the finding was present in 20 of 24 diamniotic cases and none of 6 monochorionic placentas. Wood et al.[32] have provided a prospective study of this phenomenon showing a sensitivity for dichorionicity of 94%, a specificity of 88%, a positive predictive value of 97%, and a negative predictive value of 78%. They also concluded that real-time assessment was superior. In a recent evaluation, Sepulveda et al.[33] have added the factor of gestational age to the evaluation of these signs. They concluded that at 10 to 14 weeks, the presence or absence of the lambda or twin peak sign

is 100% predictable of dichorionicity and monochorionicity, respectively. At 16 to 20 weeks this sign is indicative of dichorionicity but its absence does not rule out dizygosity.

As to the diagnosis of a monoamniotic/monochorionic situation, there are a great number of referrals that turn out to be false positive. This is due in part to the office ultrasound equipment in use and also to extreme difficulty of diagnosis in some situations. There are a number of basic prerequisites for this diagnosis: (1) a single placenta, (2) no membrane seen, (3) same-sex fetuses, (4) adequate amniotic fluid, and (5) free movement of the fetuses, which excludes a stuck twin.[34] The pitfalls that result in a low diagnostic accuracy have been reviewed.[35] Suggestions for

Figure 9-2 Lamba or twin peak sign (arrowhead) denotes dichorionic/diamniotic placenta.

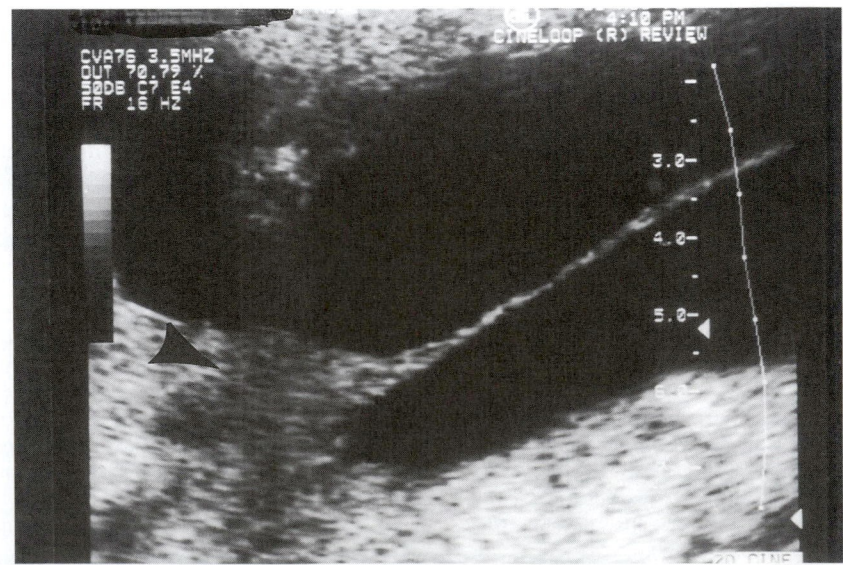

improving poor ultrasound accuracy have included computed tomographic amniography. Data have suggested improved accuracy when using first-trimester ultrasonography. The presence of two yolk sacs was found to confirm diamnionicity in the first trimester prior to visualization of the amniotic membrane.[36] Serial ultrasound examination should be employed whenever a monoamniotic pregnancy is suspected.

Determination of Gestational Age

The accurate determination of gestational age is critical, considering the high incidence of prematurity and growth disturbances in multiple pregnancies. Because clinical parameters and sometimes menstrual history are often confusing, ultrasound should be the standard for dating the pregnancy. In the first trimester, the crown-to-rump length performed between 8 and 10 weeks can be as accurate as ±3 days when done with a vaginal probe. In general, before the third trimester the growth rate for twins is similar to that of singletons.[37] The use of multiple parameters and standard tables should ordinarily suffice prior to 22 to 24 weeks, especially if correlated with the clinical history. If a small amount of size discordance is noted, it has been our practice to use the larger of the multiples to estimate or confirm gestational age, considering the overall high incidence of IUGR. In a report using IVF pregnancies to assess the accuracy of midtrimester biometry, Chervenak et al.[38] were able to derive a gestational dating formula that is applicable to both singleton and multiple pregnancies prior to 22 weeks. Gestational age calculations based on the larger multiple slightly overestimated (0.8 day), while those estimates using the mean or the smaller fetus underestimated by 0.32 or 1.29 days, respectively. While noting that the head circumference was the best single measurement, Chervenak and co-workers[38] recommended using the simple average of gestational age in twins and adding 1 day to this in triplets. In addition, a careful search for a fetal growth disorder, anomalies, or a measurement error is recommended if there is more than 1 week difference.

Finally, if the patient is not evaluated until the third trimester, the use of ultrasound parameters is always circumspect. Even if both or all fetuses agree, there is still the potential for considerable error. If late dating or confirmation of menstrual dates is required, specific curves for twins should be employed[39] and correlated with the clinical and ultrasonographic picture.

PRENATAL DIAGNOSIS

The task of genetic counseling and prenatal diagnosis in multiple gestations is more complicated for a number of reasons (Table 9-5). Both the counseling and the performance of any invasive procedure carry degrees of difficulty and risk. For this reason, patients with a need for genetic counseling and/or invasive prenatal diagnostic procedures should be referred to specialists who are experienced in these areas.

Prospective parents of multiples must understand that there is an increased risk of fetal anomalies in multiple gestations, especially with monozygotic twinning. In addition, some abnormalities, such as neural-tube defects and congenital heart disease, carry an increased risk for any siblings, including the other twin, and must be meticulously sought in the apparently normal twin. These anomalies are sometimes concordant but are most often discordant, and careful consideration as to what will be done with the results is important. Many parents are reluctant to sacrifice or possibly sacrifice a normal twin for the purposes of terminating an abnormal fetus, while others will terminate the pregnancy or attempt selective termination. These difficult choices are why some parents will refuse all prenatal diagnostic studies.

Since both the rate of dizygotic twinning and the risk of aneuploidy increases with maternal age, the need for genetic counseling and prenatal diagnosis will be more frequent in these cases. In the case of a monozygotic gestation, the identical genetic constitution means that, except in rare instances, both fetuses will be normal or abnormal. In these cases the risk of aneuploidy equals the same age-related risk as a singleton pregnancy.

On the other hand, the majority of multiple pregnancies are dizygotic, and each fetus has a separate

---

TABLE 9-5
PROBLEMS WITH PRENATAL DIAGNOSIS IN MULTIPLE GESTATIONS

Increased associated rate of congenital anomalies
Increased rate of multiple gestation and aneuploidy with increasing maternal age
Complicated risk calculations for counseling
Correct determination of zygosity
Ability to sample all fetuses
Ability to determine that all fetuses were sampled
Increased base-line loss rate of pregnancies before 28 weeks
Possible increased loss rate with CVS and amniocentesis
Difficulties with interpretation of MSAFP and/or triple screen

Figure 9-3 Risk of live-born child with Down syndrome versus maternal age in singleton and twin gestations. *Adapted with permission from Rodis et al.[40]*

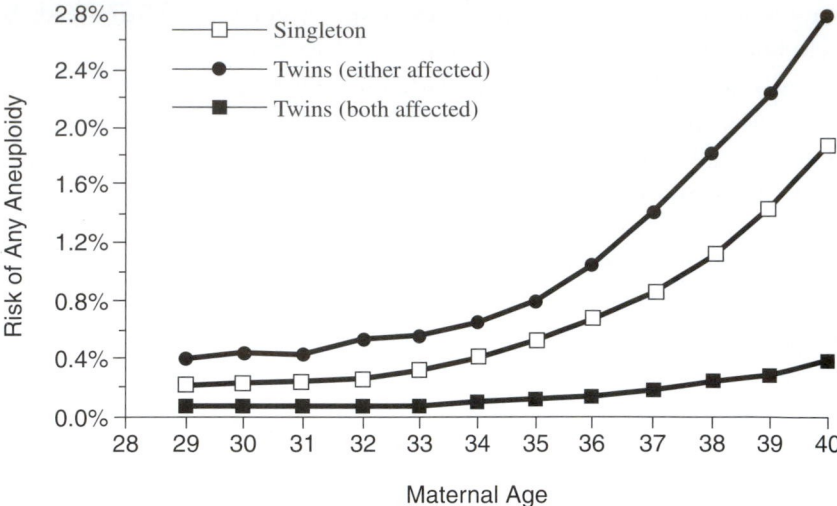

age-related risk of aneuploidy. When counseling is given, both the risk of either or both twins being abnormal must be considered. The formulas applicable to these calculations have been nicely presented by Rodis et al.[40] For unknown zygosity, the best overall estimate of the risk of one affected fetus would be $5/3x$ (x = the age-related risk of fetal aneuploidy). Using various assumptions, it was calculated that a 33-year-old has a risk at either amniocentesis or delivery of Down syndrome in one twin equal to or greater than a 35-year-old and that for all chromosomal anomalies the age drops to 31 to 32 years (Figures 9-3 and 9-4). Meyers et al.[41] refined these calculations using birth data (percentage of dizygosity at various ages) and concluded that invasive prenatal

diagnosis should be offered to all women with twin gestations at age 31.

Invasive Diagnostic Procedures

When considering invasive diagnostic procedures, there are a number of considerations that complicate matters in multiple gestation:

1. The zygosity(ies) of the pregnancy. The methods for this determination have been previously discussed and are far from totally accurate, considering that up to 30% of monozygotic twins are diamniotic/dichorionic. When performing invasive procedures for genetic diagnosis, all diamniotic/

Figure 9-4 Risk of live-born child with any chromosomal abnormality versus maternal age in singleton and twin gestations. *Adapted with permission from Rodis et al.[40] Reprinted with permission from the American College of Obstetricians and Gynecologists.*

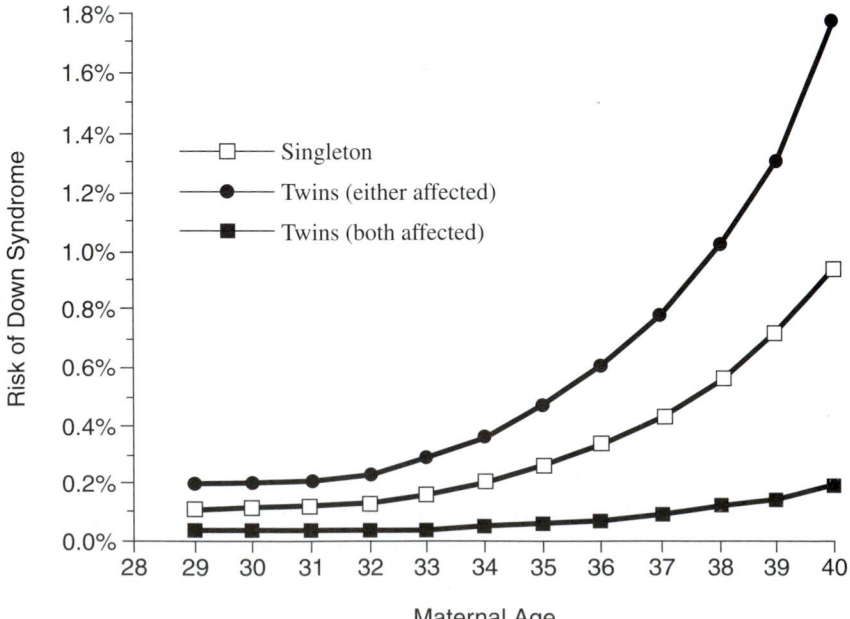

dichorionic fetuses must be sampled. In addition, it can be argued that regardless of zygosity all fetuses should be sampled due to the possibility of posttwinning mitotic nondisjunction.

2. The ability to sample all fetuses. Sometimes, because of the positions of the fetuses and their placentas, it is difficult to obtain a sample. This is especially true for higher-order multiples. When the technique of chorionic villus sampling (CVS) is employed, both vaginal and abdominal approaches may be necessary. Amniocentesis may present the same problems, with risks increasing for transplacental and cross-membrane approaches.

3. The ability to be sure, in fact, that all fetuses were sampled. Expert ultrasound guidance is needed with both CVS and amniocentesis. Careful identification of the chorion frondosum sites and approach from different locations (abdominal and vaginal when necessary) to different areas on opposite sides of the dividing membrane are needed. Care must be taken that only one frondosum is sampled.

With amniocentesis, the number and location of sacs must be determined. After the sac has been successfully entered and sufficient fluid has been removed for testing, approximately 3 ml of sterile diluted indigo carmine dye (blue) should be injected into the sac. The second sac should then be entered under ultrasound guidance and fluid removed. If the fluid is blue, either the first sac was reentered, or the gestation is monoamniotic. The technique of injecting sterile air bubbles into the first sac has also been employed. While greatly improved ultrasound equipment may possibly obviate the need for the above techniques, even in very experienced hands there is always a small percentage of blue second aspirations.

Because of the possibility of discordant outcomes for both chromosomal and biochemical abnormalities and the possibility of selective termination for abnormalities, the location of fetuses and placentas must be mapped carefully and noted in the record. In this way a second procedure can be avoided. However, sometimes when an abnormal result is obtained with CVS, a confirmatory amniocentesis should be performed because of the possibility of discordant fetal/trophoblastic findings.

4. The increased base-line loss rate associated with multiple gestations must be weighed against the possibly higher loss rates after both CVS and amniocentesis. In a large series collected over many years, Anderson et al.[42] found a pregnancy loss rate with amniocentesis of 3.6% for twins, as compared with 0.6% for singletons. In general, all postamniocentesis loss rates reported are higher for twins than singletons, but the question remains whether this is due to the inherent risks in multiple gestations. In a case-control study, Ghidini et al.[43] found that, despite the maternal age being older in the 101 cases versus 108 controls, the fetal loss rate was similar (3.5% and 3.2%, respectively: relative risk, 1.07 [95% confidence interval, 0.3 to 3.5]). They also had no losses within 3 weeks of the procedure and concluded that second-trimester amniocentesis in twin pregnancy was apparently not associated with excess loss. Wapner et al.[44] reported a comparison of amniocentesis and CVS with a loss rate in the entire pregnancy from sampling to 28 weeks of 2.9% for amniocentesis and 3.2% for CVS (p not significant). They concluded that, in the hands of experienced operators, CVS in twin gestations was at least as safe as amniocentesis. In light of a significant body of evidence, it is important for counseling purposes that the patient understands that, overall, there may be a slightly increased postprocedure loss rate in twins as compared with singletons.

Difficulties with Screening

The difficulties encountered with maternal serum α-fetoprotein screening have been detailed previously. As to serum screening for Down syndrome in twins, one would expect less sensitivity than in singletons because, no matter how the "normal" values for twins are manipulated, there will always be the contribution of the normal twin averaged with the abnormal. At this time there are no prospectively derived data describing sensitivity and specificity of serum screening for Down syndrome in twins.

ANTEPARTUM MANAGEMENT

That multiple gestation has multiple fetal, neonatal, and maternal hazards is unquestioned by anyone providing obstetrical care. While perinatal morbidity and mortality have improved, rates for multiple gestation have continued at nearly an order of magnitude higher than singletons. Moreover, while the rates of perinatal mortality have improved from the 12.4% reported by

Kohl and Casey[45] from a study of 6503 sets of twins delivered at 32 hospitals between 1961 and 1972, the perinatal mortality rates for the 1980s were still in the range of 7% or greater.[46,47]

Multifetal pregnancies will benefit from improved perinatal technology and intensive neonatal care only if such care begins early in the pregnancy. The perinatal mortality rate of 0.6% reported by Persson et al. in the 1970s[17] for twin pregnancies at 28 weeks or greater remains a milestone. The use of universal ultrasound screening at 20 weeks, followed by home bed rest to 28 weeks, was the mainstay of this approach. The simple provision of early prenatal care can make a tremendous difference in these cases. Kovacs et al.[48] reported a fetal loss rate of 2.3% in patients with twins receiving prenatal care before 27 weeks, as opposed to 13.4% when no prenatal care was received. Gardner et al.[49] found that, where "appropriate" antepartum care was given, the perinatal mortality rate fell from 16% to 6.8%, and the mean birth weight increased from 2007 g to 2546 g.

Intensive Antepartum Care

It is now the belief of many, supported by personal experience and data, that when the diagnosis of a multiple gestation is established, the high-risk nature of the pregnancy calls for specialized and intensive antepartum care. For optimal results, mothers carrying multiples should be cared for by practitioners who are thoroughly familiar with the problems and subtleties of management in these cases. This may require the general obstetrician to seek periodic consultation with a specialist in maternal–fetal medicine, and, if complications arise, transfer the care of the patient to a level III facility. My experience since 1980 and that of several authors suggests that optimal care can be delivered in a special "twin clinic."

The concept of specialized intensive care has grown over the years from the work and observations of many clinicians and investigators. It may have started with the work of Persson and Grennert in Malmo, Sweden,[50] where 90% of pregnancies were screened with ultrasound and 90% of twins were diagnosed early. These pregnancies were followed with a program featuring special antenatal supervision and hospital bed rest after 28 weeks. The resultant perinatal mortality was reported as 0.5% as opposed to 8% for the patients in the control group. Using a specific program of prenatal care with ultrasound scanning,

early leave from work, and home visits by midwives, Papiernik et al.[51] found a reduced rate of very-low-birth-weight infants and early preterm births. The perinatal mortality rate was 2.6%. O'Connor et al.,[52] on the other hand, showed that hospital rest during the third trimester could be replaced by intensified antenatal care in a special twin clinic without negative effects. Beginning in the late 1970s, patients in this twin clinic were encouraged to rest at home, avoid smoking, and use extra iron and folate supplements. Cervical examinations were performed at least every 2 weeks, and uterine contraction monitoring with tocodynamometry was performed at each visit. Gestational age, as well as fetal growth, was assessed with ultrasound, and hospital admissions were reserved for IUGR, medical complications, preeclampsia, and premature labor. Beginning in 1980 and continuing to the present, we have taken this basic approach, with the addition over time of antepartum fetal heart rate testing and improved ultrasound monitoring, modified home bed rest and weekly visits after 20 to 24 weeks, use of tocolytics as indicated, screening for vaginal infections, and ultrasound cervical evaluation. Our perinatal mortality rate has ranged from slightly over 3% to, more recently, 1%. In a multidisciplinary specialized twin clinic that emphasized constant evaluation by a single main caregiver under the supervision of a maternal–fetal medicine specialist and with special attention to preterm birth prevention education, individualized modified maternal activity, quality nutrition, and tracking of women who did not attend the clinic, Ellings and Newman[4] have attained a perinatal mortality rate of 1%.

An outline of special twin clinic recommendations is found in Table 9-6. Several aspects of this care will be discussed in the following sections.

Preterm Birth Prevention

History

Multifetal pregnancy carries an independently high risk for prematurity; more than 50% of these pregnancies will conclude prior to 37 weeks. In fact, women with multiple gestation have the highest population-attributable risk for preterm labor.[53] It is important to recognize, however, that many other factors also can increase the risk. A history of preterm delivery or preterm labor has a significant risk of recurrence in subsequent pregnancies. The presence of uterine structural anomalies, cervical surgery or

TABLE 9-6
PROTOCOL FOR SPECIALIZED MANAGEMENT OF MULTIPLE PREGNANCY

Area of Concern	Gestational Age	Clinical Intervention	Result/Comment
Early diagnosis	5–24 weeks	Consider risk factors	Optimizes management with early diagnosis
		Ultrasound examination for those at risk and size > dates	If not screening must be attentive to risk factors and size/date discrepancy
		Consider universal screening	
		Determine zygosity/placentation	Valuable for risk assessment and subsequent management
Counseling	10–23 weeks		
Genetics		MSAFP screening	Anomalies increased
		Age adjusted for aneuploidy	Advanced maternal age lowered
		Targeted ultrasound	Detection of early discordance or anomalies important
Nutrition		Extra iron and folate given	Anemia very common: follow hemoglobin/hematocrit findings
		Early weight gain emphasized	Important for overall growth
		Weight gain of 40–45 lb	Nutrition has large influence on fetal growth in multiples
Lifestyle		Reduced activity after 20 wk	Consider modified bed rest after 24 weeks/stop working
Other		Smoking cessation	Negative effect on fetal growth plus other complications
Cervical incompetence	16–24 weeks	Check cervix (digital and ultrasound) by 20 weeks for twins; earlier for triplets and above	Important to detect early silent effacement/dilatation
			Cerclage only with indications
Growth disturbances	20–36 weeks	Ultrasound for growth every 4 wk after 20 wk, every 2 after 30 wk	Plot all growth parameters serially
IUGR one or more fetuses		Bed rest, possibly hospitalize noncompliant patient	Consider Doppler studies
Twin-to-twin transfusion: (polyhydramnios/ oligohydramnios)		Bed rest on diagnosis Amniocentesis	Maximize intrauterine support
Premature labor	24 weeks–term	Patient education for self-monitoring	Limit of 4–6 contractions/hr.
		Frequent uterine activity monitoring (1–2/wk)	Multiples often don't notice contractions well. Consider home uterine activity monitoring in triplets or more.
		Frequent cervical exams and ultrasound for cervical length	Changes in cervical length, funneling, or "cervical score" give increased risk
		Screen for infection	Decrease premature labor/rupture of membranes
		Bed rest	Less uterine activity
		Tocolytics	Careful but liberal use
Preeclampsia	24 wk–term	Frequent blood pressure and urine protein monitoring	Multiples are at several times risk; also nulliparity and chronic hypertension additive
		Low-dose aspirin (80 mg)	Possibly reduced risk?
		Bed rest	

US = ultrasound

lacerations, or a history of multiple pregnancy terminations should also alert the clinician. If there is a history of recurrent urinary-tract infections or pyelonephritis, increased surveillance is suggested. A patient with a history of vaginal discharge or recurrent vaginitis should be examined frequently because of the association of certain vaginal infections such as bacterial vaginosis with premature labor and preterm premature rupture of the membranes. A history of bleeding during the pregnancy also increases the risk of preterm delivery. Finally, because of the associations of smoking with preterm birth, low birth weight, and placental abruption, patients who use tobacco need to be strongly counseled and assisted to quit.

Patient Education

While preterm labor and delivery is extremely common in multifetal gestations, with twins and triplets having preterm delivery rates on the order of 51% and 91%, respectively,[54] most parents do not initially appreciate this risk. Patients must be informed that not only will they not go to full term (40 weeks), but that preterm birth and low birth weight represent the greatest challenges in the management of their pregnancy. Unless they are well informed, these women are often unaware of or discount early signs and symptoms of premature labor such as prodromal uterine contractions. It is often said, and indeed confirmed by personal experience, that mothers carrying multiples do not notice uterine activity as well as those with a singleton pregnancy. Thus, it is all the more important that the patient pay careful attention to possible premonitory symptoms such as increased lower pelvic pressure, low back pain or ache, increased vaginal discharge, or simply a change in frequency of Braxton–Hicks contractions. The patient must not be discouraged from promptly contacting her caregiver if she has suspicions of preterm labor. Early diagnosis can permit obstetrical interventions before advanced cervical dilation has occurred. Office personnel answering patient telephone inquiries must be aware of the special circumstances of multiple gestation, and patients should be empowered to request evaluation.

Other educational aspects that should be addressed include prenatal nutrition, modifications in lifestyle, multiple methods used in monitoring of the pregnancy, treatment of premature labor, and the treatment and prognosis for the premature newborn. Prepared childbirth classes and support groups for parents with multiple gestation should be encouraged.

Nutritional Aspects of Multiple Gestation

Second only to prematurity, intrauterine growth restriction is a major contributor to morbidity and mortality in multiple gestations. Not only are infants smaller in multiple gestations, but the greater the number of infants, the smaller they will be on average.[55] Because of the increased competition for limited maternal resources, maternal nutrition has a larger influence on fetal growth in multiple as compared with singleton gestations. Brown and Schloesser[56] found that infant birth weights increased linearly with prenatal weight gain for women who entered pregnancy underweight or at normal weight, but not in obese women. Furthermore, they calculated a mean weight gain that resulted in birth weights in the range which gave the least perinatal mortality (3000 to 3500 g). For underweight women, this weight gain was nearly 45 lb, while approximately 41 lb was optimal for normal-weight women.

The pattern of weight gain has also been determined to be of importance. Using multiple regression models, Luke et al.[57] reported that the pattern of early low weight gain (<0.85 lb per week before 24 weeks) and late low weight gain (<1 lb per week after 24 weeks) was negatively associated with intrauterine growth. In a later report[58] critical periods of weight gain also were associated with the gravida's prepregnant weight status. Twin birth weight is significantly associated with weight gain before 20 weeks in underweight women, before 20 and after 28 weeks in overweight women, and during the entire gestation of normal-weight women. The largest effect was in underweight women at less than 20 weeks of gestation.

The above findings again underscore the need for early diagnosis of twin gestation and proper patient education. Improvement in birth weights from proper nutrition has a great potential to improve outcomes at a minimum of cost. While optimal weight gain and recommended dietary allowances (RDAs) have not been established for higher-order multiples, it is reasonable to assume that optimal weight gains will be higher. In addition, it is reasonable to suggest RDAs of 50 to 100% higher for all multiple gestations.

Bed Rest and Other Lifestyle Modifications

It is the belief of many clinicians who manage multiple-fetus pregnancies that a reduction in activity and an increase in time spent in the lateral recumbent position are important ingredients for improving outcomes. Furthermore, since most perinatal mortality occurs before the third trimester, it would seem important to begin a program of limited activity at midgestation. The duration, amount, and location of this inactivity is somewhat controversial, and a number of parameters may be the most important consideration in any individual case. Patients with multiple fetuses are advised to cease strenuous activity and/or employment at some time after 20 weeks of gestation in many high-risk clinics. This is thought to be especially critical in cases of higher-order multiples. Bed rest will improve uterine blood flow and increase birth weight up to 10%. In addition, it has been shown to decrease uterine activity.[59]

A number of retrospective studies have demonstrated benefits of bed rest. Komaromy and Lampe,[60] in a 1977 study of third-trimester (after 26 to 27 weeks) hospital-rested versus non-rested twin pregnancies found a significant increase in gestational age at delivery from 35 to 37.5 weeks, and in mean birth weight from 1972 to 2581 g. The perinatal mortality in these cases was reduced from 21.7% to 5.9%, and the incidence of birth weight <2500 g from 77 to 40%. Jeffrey et al. had earlier reported[61] that bed rest decreased perinatal mortality in twin gestations of less than 30 weeks as compared with regular activity. They noted an overall increase in birth weight and a decrease in the frequency of small-for-gestational-age infants. However, since 58% of the mortality occurred prior to 30 weeks, it was concluded that earlier diagnosis was needed, and rest from the time of diagnosis should be considered. In a study from an Air Force hospital, Gilstrap et al.[46] compared women pregnant with twins who were hospitalized prior to 28 weeks with a group not hospitalized until after 28 weeks or until a pregnancy complication or labor occurred. They found an improvement in perinatal mortality from 8.5% to 2% in the patients treated with early hospitalization.

The value of hospitalization for bed rest has been questioned, however. O'Connor et al.[52] demonstrated that third-trimester bed rest at home and in the hospital were equivalent. Persson et al.,[17] employing home rest from 20 to 28 weeks, achieved a very low perinatal mortality rate. Two randomized prospective studies from Scotland and Australia published in 1990,[62,63] using subjects with twin pregnancies entered at 26 to 30 and 28 to 30 weeks, respectively, did not show a decrease in perinatal mortality with hospitalization. The second study did show an improvement in fetal growth. In addition, a meta-analysis of prospective trials[64] found that both preterm delivery and neonatal death were increased with routine hospitalization, but that there was a decrease in maternal hypertension. Newman et al.[65] have also shown that routine hospitalization for triplets is also unnecessary.

Because of the potential for significant perinatal mortality in multiple gestations, especially in the middle to late second trimester, many still believe that a program of modified activity begun before the 24th week is beneficial. This intervention can be accomplished at home, where any program of bed rest is obviously modified. The suggested advantages are increases in gestational age at birth and birth weight,

decreases in perinatal mortality, and possible prevention or delay in onset of preeclampsia. Home rest may prevent hospitalizations and is certainly less expensive than hospitalization. While conditioning may deteriorate, it should not be as pronounced as with enforced hospital rest, and it is probably easier and less stressful for the patient to be at home. While it has been our practice to keep patients out of the hospital if possible, there are certainly indications for hospitalization. These include progressive cervical effacement and dilation, preterm labor, increasing IUGR or discordant growth, and hypertension or other medical/obstetric complications.

As for sexual intercourse, it has been our practice to suggest refraining after 20 weeks. We also suggest a leave of absence from work after the 24th week. The presence of complications and financial hardship may modify this recommendation. Newman and Ellings[66] have suggested that it is important to evaluate the work issue carefully, and they have listed certain indications to cease employment (Table 9-7).

Monitoring of the Cervix and Uterine Activity

Preterm labor and delivery is a major challenge in multiple gestations. The finding that cervical changes, including those consistent with cervical incompetence, can occur by the middle of the second trimester, coupled with the observation that mothers expecting multiples may not perceive uterine activity well, suggest that a cervical examination be performed frequently beginning at 20 weeks. This practice is even more important in higher-order multiples and should begin earlier. Whenever the cervix is examined, the characteristics of length, consistency, station, position, dilation, and the status of the lower segment should be recorded. Holbrook et al.[67] reported that, by using

---

TABLE 9-7
INDICATIONS FOR PATIENTS WITH MULTIPLE GESTATION TO DISCONTINUE WORK

Work that involves prolonged standing or heavy lifting
Work on heavy or other industrial machinery
Work involving continuous or repetitive low-level exertion or intermittent high-level exertion
Military duty
Work in uncomfortable environment: high stress, cold, hot, dampness, toxic exposure
Presence of more than two fetuses
Prior history of singleton preterm birth

regular cervical monitoring, they were frequently able to observe abnormal cervical changes prior to the onset of uterine contractions. While there might be concern that these examinations could precipitate premature rupture of the membranes and premature labor, there is evidence that this is not the case.[68]

Using the concept of a cervical score as described by Houlton et al.,[69] where the value is obtained by taking the cervical length (0 to 3 cm) minus the dilation, Neilson et al.[70] attempted to better predict preterm labor in twin gestations. They made three specific observations: (1) The lower the score, the shorter the mean time before delivery, although there were many cases in which "ripe" cervixes existed several weeks before delivery. (2) The cervical score itself was a better predictor than changes in score. (3) A group at high risk for preterm delivery could be identified (score −2 or less before 34 weeks). Newman et al.[71] applied this scoring system to patients at a special twin clinic at the Medical University of South Carolina in an attempt to confirm its value. They found that a score of zero or less before 34 weeks was 75% predictive of preterm delivery and, alternatively, that only 2 of 78 patients with positive scores delivered in less than 1 week.

There have been a number of investigators who have looked at the role of cervical length assessment with ultrasound as a predictor of preterm birth in twin gestations. Examples of cervical-length measurements are shown in Figure 9-5. The use of endovaginal cervical-length measurements has been shown to have a much better interobserver reliability than digital examination.[72] In the multicenter NICHHD Maternal–Fetal Medicine Units study of preterm birth prediction,[73] a cervical-length measurement of ≤25 mm at 24 weeks was consistently associated with preterm birth at less than 32, 35, and 37 weeks. While this association at 28 weeks was not strong, the presence of a positive test for fetal fibronectin at both 28 and 30 weeks was strongly associated with preterm birth at less than 32 weeks. Imseis et al.[74] found that a transvaginal ultrasonographic measurement of the cervix of >35 mm at 24 to 26 weeks in twin gestations identified those at low risk of delivery before 34 weeks. Our own preliminary data show that, when patients delivering before or after 35 weeks are compared: (1) The mean cervical lengths before 23 weeks are similar. (2) After 23 weeks the cervical lengths are shorter in the early delivery group. (3) There is a significant difference in the interval change between 20 and 28 weeks in early versus late delivery groups. (4) Funneling of the cervix (Figure 9-6) was present in nearly half of the early delivery group at 24 weeks versus 8% in the late group. (5) In predicting delivery before 35 weeks, sensitivity and specificity for cervical length of <34 mm at 24 weeks were 35% and 85%, respectively (Positive Predictive Value = 63%; Negative Predictive Value = 64%).[75] We believe that, by using ultrasound assessment of cervical length, the clinician may be alerted to those multiple gestations at even higher risk of preterm delivery.

Over many years in our twin clinic, we have observed that patients may have considerable cervical

Figure 9-5 Assessment of length of cervical canal (arrow) by endovaginal ultrasound.

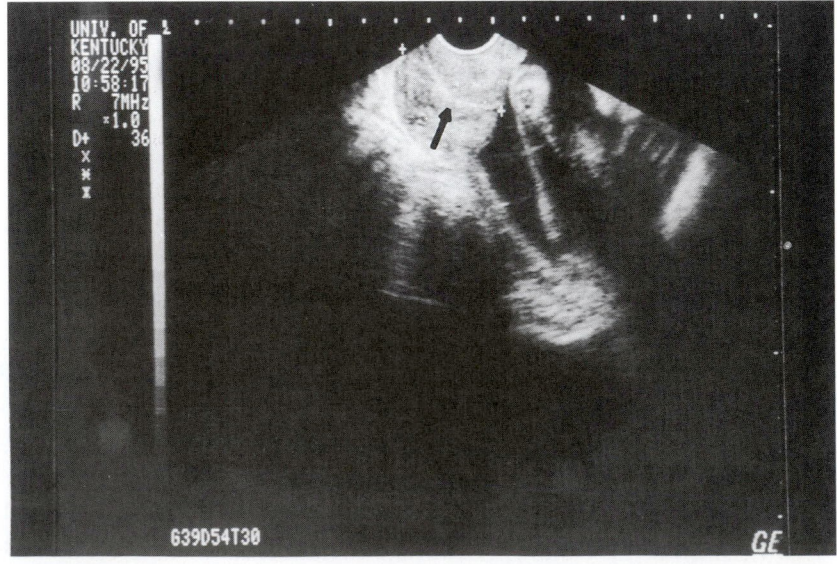

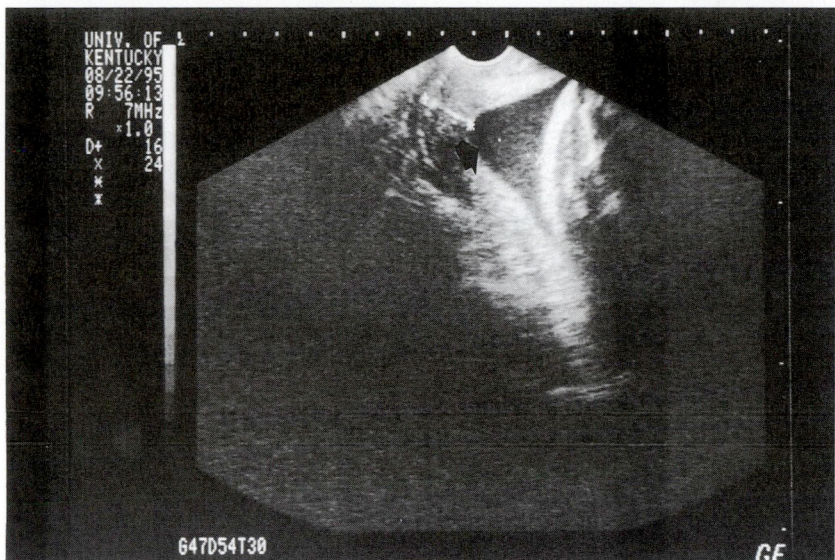

Figure 9-6 Endovaginal ultrasound demonstrates funneling (arrowhead) and shortening of the cervical canal.

change yet be unaware of significant uterine activity. This inability of many patients to differentiate significant from nonsignificant contractions suggests that some form of regular monitoring of uterine activity might be beneficial. Tocodynamometric correlation with cervical change in asymptomatic patients has shown that weekly or more frequent tocodynamometry after 24 weeks can permit early detection of premature labor. Newman et al.[76] demonstrated a progressive increase in the frequency of uterine activity after 23 weeks in twin gestations, while this rise did not occur until after 36 weeks in singletons. There is controversy about the location and frequency of these observations. Using home uterine activity monitoring, Knuppel et al.[77] diagnosed preterm labor earlier in a monitored than in an unmonitored group and used tocolysis resulting in fewer preterm births. In a prospective study, Dyson et al.[78] found that home uterine monitoring improved pregnancy outcomes as compared with a group treated with intensive education and routine palpation of uterine activity by a clinician and another group that received standard obstetric care. Home uterine activity monitoring can be expensive and, while it may be of benefit in certain situations, it has not been proven essential. It is our own experience that weekly tocodynamometry after 24 weeks combined with patient education, weekly cervical examinations, and ultrasonographic cervical assessment, provides excellent results. One must pay close attention to subtle cervical changes and the presence of uterine activity. Clinical judgment can then be used regarding institution of tocolytic

therapy, more frequent office visits, or home uterine activity monitoring.

Prophylactic Tocolysis

Since more than half of multiple gestations are complicated by preterm labor and delivery, and since spontaneous uterine activity begins earlier and is significantly greater throughout pregnancy,[76] it has been an attractive idea to use tocolytic drugs prophylactically. Indeed, some small studies have suggested a clinical benefit. Skjaerris and Aberg[79] used terbutaline versus placebo in 50 patients and showed a significant reduction in the incidence of preterm labor and the total number of days hospitalized for preterm labor. However, they did not find a significant difference in birth weight or pregnancy duration. In another study of 60 patients, O'Leary[80] found an increase in birth weight and time gained from entry until delivery with bed rest plus oral terbutaline versus bed rest plus placebo. Others have not found a benefit.[81,82] In addition, the picture is clouded by the use of other agents such as NSAIDs and calcium-channel blockers, which have not been systematically studied. Since there are no large prospective, randomized trials in multiple gestations, the consensus would be not to use tocolytic drugs prophylactically. Rather, they should be used only in patients with clear evidence of regular uterine activity or cervical change.

The presence of uterine irritability (high-frequency–low-amplitude uterine contractions >6/hr)[83] (Figure 9-7) is associated with a significant increase in preterm delivery in general, and an even greater increase with

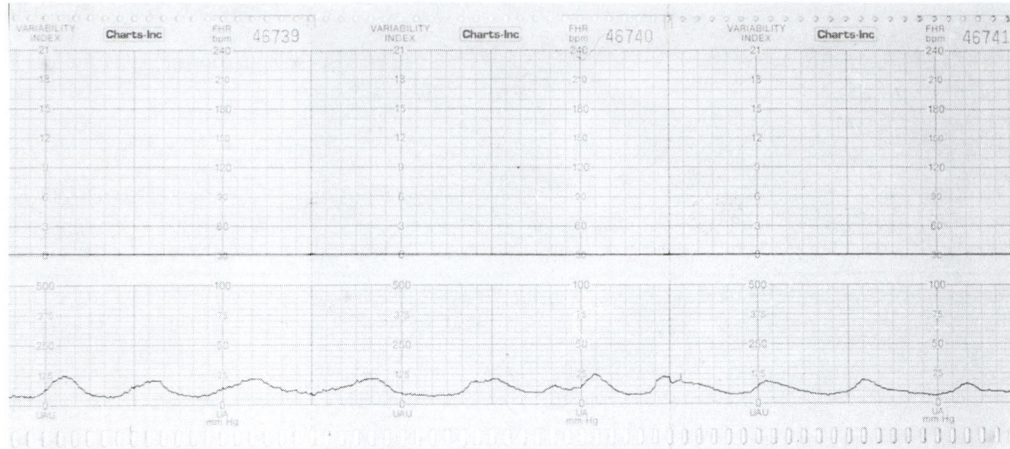

Figure 9-7 Tocodynamometry shows high-frequency–low-amplitude uterine activity.

multiple gestations. The use of frequent tocody-namometry along with digital and sonographic examinations of the cervix should identify the patients most likely to benefit from oral outpatient tocolytic therapy. This "indicated prophylaxis" may be employed when frequent uterine activity is unresponsive to rest and hydration and in the presence of gradual changes in the cervix occurring in association with uterine irritability. Inpatient intravenous tocolytics are indicated for true preterm labor prior to 34 to 35 weeks. Whenever tocolytics might be indicated, obviously other surveillance must be intensified.

Use of Cervical Cerclage

There has been a long held common belief that many early deliveries in multiple gestations resulted from an incompetent cervix. The logic behind this belief had to do with larger intrauterine volumes, hormones, early cervical softening, and other unspecified factors. As previously noted, painless cervical change does occur more often in multiple gestations. However, is this finding due to cervical incompetence? There are to date no trials that have demonstrated a benefit for prophylactic cerclage in multiples. In fact, Sinha et al.[84] found a higher incidence of premature labor and cervical damage in the treatment group. Even in triplet pregnancies,[85] no benefit has been demonstrated for elective cerclage.

Michaels et al.,[86] using a combination of cervical length, dilatation, and funneling, found an incidence of incompetent cervix of 13.7% in twins. None of the cerclage patients delivered before 29 weeks, and the perinatal mortality rate and incidence of low birth weight was significantly less in this group versus

controls. However, the criteria were somewhat subjective. Our own experience indicates that the presence of funneling before 24 weeks leads to an increase in preterm deliveries. Furthermore, it is a common observation that higher-order multiples are even more likely to experience cervical incompetence. Accordingly, we believe that early evaluation of the cervix using both digital and ultrasound methods is indicated, at 20 weeks in twins and earlier in higher-order multiples. If the clinical diagnosis of incompetent cervix is made, cerclage is indicated.

Monitoring Fetal Growth

After preterm birth, abnormal fetal growth (IUGR or discordance) is the most important contributor to perinatal mortality in multiple gestations. Since abnormalities of growth may occur in nearly half of twin gestations, and IUGR, when present, can increase the perinatal mortality rate (relative risk, 4.8),[87] it is important to monitor fetal growth. The clinical monitoring of fetal growth can often be difficult even in singleton pregnancies for which there are existing clinical standards. Although certain risk factors may alert the clinician to growth problems in multiple pregnancies (poor weight gain, smoking, failure of fundal height growth or sudden rapid growth, and patient noncompliance), problems with fetal lie, discordance, and general lack of good clinical standards confuse the picture. Use of serial ultrasonographic assessment and plotting of fetal biometric parameters are the most reliable means of detecting abnormalities or of reassuring normalcy of fetal growth.

The challenge over time has been both to accurately determine fetal growth and to find the best way to do so. As the pregnancy advances in gestational age, the number of fetuses increases, or the fetal lie is other than cephalic, the technical difficulty in growth assessment increases. In noncephalic presentations, molding of the head (dolichocephaly) may invalidate the use of the biparietal diameter (BPD) in calculations. In one report, the femur length and abdominal circumference were obtainable in 96 to 99% of fetuses, but accurate BPD measurements were possible in only 79%.[39] With improving equipment and skill of the ultrasonographer, we believe that the BPD can be obtained in nearly all cases, although the use of the BPD alone is not a sensitive enough predictor of IUGR or discordance unless extreme differences exist. Chitkara et al.[88] obtained a diagnostic accuracy of greater than 90% for IUGR in twins by using estimated fetal weight, where abdominal circumference was the single measurement most predictive of IUGR. The interpair difference in estimated fetal weight has also been found to be the best predictor of discordant fetal growth,[89] with an interpair abdominal circumference difference of 20 mm or more being significant.

Before abnormal patterns of fetal growth can be determined, one must ask what is the normal pattern of fetal growth in twins. Earlier work[37] suggested a slowing of both BPD and abdominal circumference growth in twins during the last trimester. This observation has led to a recommendation that growth charts specifically derived for twin pregnancies be used for assessing growth in twin pregnancies. In addition, one report suggests that chorionicity[90] needs to be considered and specific nomograms be used for monochorionic versus dichorionic twins to accurately identify growth-restricted fetuses. On the other hand, one can argue that there is no intrinsic reason for a twin fetus not to grow in the same way as a singleton sibling. If twin growth curves are smaller it must be a consequence of the intrauterine environment and represent growth restriction. In a survey of 19,600 normal infants, Luke et al.[91] reported no significant difference in twin and singleton growth until after 36 weeks. Accordingly, use of singleton growth curves will avoid missing possible abnormal growth patterns that might be clinically significant.

Two abnormal patterns of growth that occur in twin gestation are IUGR in one or both twins and discordant growth, which may or may not involve IUGR. In order to detect abnormal patterns, a detailed assessment of each fetus is required. Serial ultrasound measurements of the biparietal diameter, head circumference,

abdominal circumference, and femur length must be taken. Any number of formulas to determine an estimated fetal weight are available, valid and fairly equivalent with an accuracy of up to ±15%. The data obtained should then be plotted on longitudinal growth charts to facilitate assessment of growth patterns and concordance between the fetuses. It has been our practice to perform ultrasonography for growth parameters every 4 weeks until 28 weeks and every 2 to 3 weeks thereafter.

Discordance in growth between fetuses is defined as greater than 20% in weight based on the weight of the larger fetus. Significant discordance is reported to occur in 23% of twin pregnancies.[39] Discordant growth may arise whenever any factor that affects fetal growth is applied unequally to the fetuses. Possible causes for discordant growth included suboptical placental implantation site, presence of an abnormal cord insertion, differences in sex, placental crowding, anomalies in one fetus, or twin-to-twin transfusion. Significant differences may exist when both twins are in the normal range of growth or when only one fetus is outside the normal range. Management will be discussed in a subsequent section.

Antepartum Fetal Surveillance

FETAL KICK COUNTS. As a first screening effort, all pregnant women should be instructed in fetal movement or kick counting. This method of antepartum fetal surveillance is easily taught, and the only cost involved is the second level of testing it might engender. Long experience tells us that by the middle to end of the second trimester, most mothers of twins cannot only appreciate fetal movement but can also tell which fetus is moving. These observations may be enhanced by the frequent use of ultrasound with which the mother can relate to the location and lie of the fetuses. While there are no good trials of the efficacy of fetal kick counts in multiple gestations, when the patient states that one fetus is not moving as well as the other or general fetal movement is significantly decreased, the clinician should pay careful attention. Personal experience suggests that problems such as IUGR, oligohydramnios, anomalies, and abnormal fetal heart rate patterns often seem to be associated with a decrease in perceived fetal movement. On the other hand, obesity or hydramnios may decrease the perception of fetal movements, and higher-order multiples make the discernment of each fetus's movements almost impossible to identify. There are several protocols for fetal kick count or movement assessment. The "count to ten" method[92] seems to be easily understood and performed.

FETAL HEART RATE TESTING. The first-line mode of fetal heart rate testing should be the nonstress test (NST). This mode of testing is easily and reliably performed in the office or by visiting home nurses in a short time and for little cost. It is less costly than the contraction stress test (CST), especially when oxytocin must be used, and it has, at least, the theoretical advantage of not producing contractions. The indications for fetal heart rate testing in multiple-gestation pregnancies are the same as for singletons, with the additions of fetal death or anomalies in one fetus and growth discordance of greater than 20%.

A number of authors have noted that NST results are equally predictive in multiple and singleton pregnancies.[93-96] In Blake et al.'s study[96] the perinatal mortality rate in nonreactive fetuses was six times that in reactive ones, and the overall perinatal mortality rate was close to that of singletons. In a study of 665 twin gestations, Sherman et al.[97] found 10 pregnancies with death of one or both twins in cases managed without NSTs, and only one fetal death in patients receiving NSTs. The reduction, however, was not statistically significant because of a small sample size.

When the standard NST is nonreactive, fetal vibratory acoustic stimulation can be used to obtain a reactive test. Sherer et al.[98] performed acoustic stimulation on twins undergoing an NST. In these cases they found that the fetal heart rate accelerations were synchronous in all cases, as opposed to their earlier work[99] with spontaneous accelerations, in which fetal heart rate accelerations were noted to coincide within 15 seconds of each other only 57% of the time.

When the NST is nonreactive in one or more fetuses, it is prudent to proceed to the biophysical profile.[100] A score of 8 to 10 is reassuring; a score of 4 to 6 should prompt evaluation for delivery and retesting in 4 to 6 hours; and scores of 0 to 2 indicate immediate delivery if both fetuses are considered salvageable. Lodeiro et al.,[101] using a maximum score of 12, reported on the use of the biophysical profile (BPP) in 49 twin gestations. They found that a reactive NST was associated with a score of 8 or more and good pregnancy outcome in all cases. They felt, as we do, that there is no benefit to performing a BPP

if the NST is reactive, but that when one or both fetuses are nonreactive, "fetal biophysical profile scoring appears to differentiate well the sleeping from the asphyxiated fetus."[101] While the BPP is not needed as a first-line test with twins, it may be the only reasonable first approach to antepartum testing in higher-order multiples. Because of multiple and earlier growth and other problems in these cases, testing should be started much earlier.

There is some debate about the proper amniotic fluid volume to use when scoring the test. In singletons, most investigators today would use an amniotic fluid index (AFI) of 5 cm or more to score as normal. Several authors[102-104] have attempted to establish normal sonographic ranges of amniotic fluid in twin pregnancies. The best technique to measure amniotic fluid volume has yet to be established or validated. Moreover, Magann et al.[105] have reported that the summated (four-quadrant) AFI is a poor predictor of intertwin differences in amniotic fluid and cannot identify those at risk for oligohydramnios or hydramnios. Of note is that subjectively decreased or borderline amniotic fluid volumes in either or both twins are often the indication to begin antepartum heart rate testing in our clinic. Feeling that each twin needs a separate evaluation, we also use in our ultrasound reports a modified AFI for each fetus in which the two largest pockets (head and tail) are added together. While this assessment seems to correlate well with other measures, one would expect that the lower limit of normal would be somewhat less than in singletons.

One of the major challenges faced by the clinician managing a multiple-gestation pregnancy is what to do when faced with non-reassuring tests. This task is even more difficult when one fetus is normal and the pregnancy is at only 26 to 32 weeks. Prior to 32 weeks, relative immaturity of the fetus may lead to an increase in nonreactive NSTs (possibly a false positive result). On the other hand, these earlier gestations are most at risk for serious complications of prematurity such as intraventricular hemorrhage, cerebral palsy, and chronic lung disease. By using an integrated approach that combines multiple testing methods, including the biophysical profile, ultrasound growth estimates, and possibly umbilical artery Doppler studies (S:D ratio), the clinician may avoid iatrogenic prematurity and its consequences. Devoe and Ware[106] suggest from their data that, when combinations of abnormal results occur, such as abnormal growth on ultrasound and abnormal Doppler studies or nonreactive NST and abnormal Doppler studies, fetal compromise is highly likely and delivery is indicated.

FETAL LUNG MATURITY STUDIES. Often the indications for intervention in multiple pregnancy are not clear-cut and the gestational age is in a gray zone for fetal maturation (32 to 36 weeks). Several available methods can reliably predict pulmonary maturity. While there are many false negative results, the knowledge of lung maturity or the presence of a very immature fetus may significantly affect the management scheme. Leveno et al.[107] reported that lecithin:sphingomylein ratios, unless borderline, were similar in numerical and predictive value to those of singletons and that fetal lung maturation occurred several weeks earlier in twins. This observation has led to the willingness to seek confirmation of fetal lung maturity at earlier gestational ages in multiple gestations. Other studies have suggested that there is no difference in fetal lung maturation between twins and singletons[108] and that overall twins do not mature earlier than singletons.[109] Since clinical studies have shown that pulmonary maturity studies are similar in concordant twins, either sac could be sampled. Where discordance is significant, the sac of the larger, presumably unstressed, twin should be sampled, or both sacs.

MANAGEMENT OF PREGNANCY COMPLICATIONS

There are a number of pregnancy complications that are unique to the management of multiple gestations, and others that occur much more frequently with multiples. These potential complications need to be anticipated and managed promptly. In many of these cases, consultation with a subspecialist in maternal-fetal medicine should be obtained.

Premature Labor

Preterm delivery has been reported to occur at a rate 12 times that of singleton gestations.[110] Furthermore, as discussed earlier, in higher-order multiples nearly all cases are delivered prior to 37 weeks, with the average gestation at delivery decreasing with an increasing number of fetuses (Figure 9-8). Data from the United States[111] shows that 51% of twins and 91% of triplets were born before 37 weeks. Preterm labor can often be difficult to diagnose even in singleton pregnancies. With not only the degree of difficulty in diagnosis increased, but also the bias to treat early in multiple gestations due to the high frequency of early deliveries, the situation is compounded. Also, because of the risks involved, especially at early gestational ages, various levels of uterine activity have been used to define a threshold for treatment even without cervical change. The often used threshold of 4 contractions per hour suggested by Newman et al.[76] was derived from singleton gestations. In multiple gestations there is no uniformly accepted definition of uterine activity that clearly predicts premature labor, although it is generally thought to be less than in singletons. Thus, the diagnosis of preterm labor and the decision to administer tocolytics must be influenced by several factors, including gestational

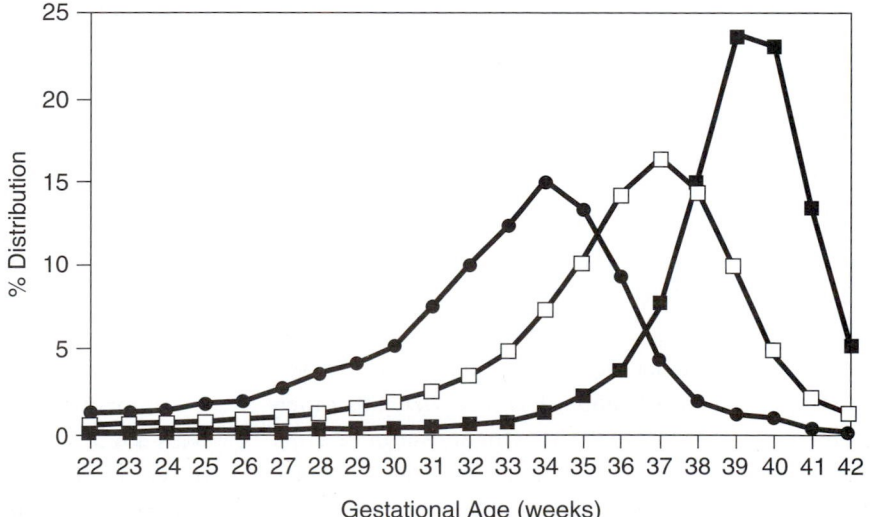

Figure 9-8 Distribution of gestational age at birth for singletons (■, 1995), twins (□, 1991–1999), and triplets (●, 1991–1995) in the United States. *Reprinted with permission from Keith et al.* [54]

age, fetal well-being, subtle cervical changes, prior episodes of preterm labor, and a history of preterm delivery. Although the use of prophylactic tocolytics is not recommended, in gestations prior to 34 weeks a liberal policy of early tocolytic intervention may be justified.

The same contraindications to the use of tocolytic therapy apply for multiple births as for singletons, including fetal distress, significant unexplained vaginal bleeding, chorioamnionitis, and advanced dilatation. In addition, specific contraindications for multiples would be severe size discordancy after 32 weeks, anomalies incompatible with survival in both twins, fetal death of both twins, and fetal lung maturity documented after 32 to 34 weeks. Additional maternal contraindications include significant pregnancy-induced hypertension or medical conditions that might make tocolytic therapy hazardous. The decision to employ tocolytics, the particular agent, the route of administration, and the duration of therapy is open to discussion. Gestational age and a number of other factors may affect these choices. Since many of these situations are unclear, perinatal consultation is recommended.

Although the techniques and management of tocolytic use in multiple gestations are basically the same as in singleton gestations, there are some special considerations worth noting. Multiple gestations will normally have a much larger increase in intravascular volume and a greater cardiac output. As a result, careful monitoring of fluid status is important. Because of the relatively larger uterus the frequency of supine hypotension is increased; thus patient positioning is important. The higher incidence of pregnancy-induced hypertension may complicate or contraindicate tocolytic use. Differing fetal status, both in growth parameters and amniotic fluid volume, may preclude the use of tocolytics, especially indomethacin. Finally, the prospect of earlier lung maturity may suggest assessment with amniocentesis, especially if the gestation is more than 33 weeks, rather than aggressive tocolysis.

The use of β-mimetic agents for tocolysis has been compared between multiple gestations and singleton pregnancies. Rayburn et al.[112] found that neither the physiologic consequences nor the incidence of undesirable cardiovascular side effects differed in the two groups. While it has been widely recognized that there is an association between β-mimetic use in multiple gestations and pulmonary edema, we believe that the incidence and severity of this problem can be reduced

or eliminated with careful attention to vital signs, fluid balance, and avoidance of overhydration.

The concern regarding side effects with β-mimetics has led most clinicians to use magnesium sulfate as the first-line tocolytic agent. Magnesium sulfate use also has been compared between singletons and twin gestations,[113] and no differences were noted in rates of complications. The conclusion was that guidelines for prescribing intravenous magnesium sulfate to inhibit preterm labor in singletons are equally safe and effective for twin pregnancies. We have observed that the infusion rate may need to be higher due to the increased blood volume and renal clearance in multiple gestations. Attention to vital signs and fluid balance is important with magnesium sulfate because both cardiorespiratory depression and pulmonary edema may occur, especially with higher rates and extended duration of infusion.

The use of indomethacin for tocolysis in twins is an attractive option in patients with polyhydramnios. Lange et al.[114] reported its use where initially fluid was at least adequate in both sacs and the pregnancy was less than 32 completed weeks. The amniotic fluid volumes were found to decrease in all cases, and the pregnancies were successfully prolonged. Because of concern for the effects of prostaglandin inhibition on the fetal ductus arteriosus, care must be taken at later gestational ages. Pregnancies in which indomethacin is used must be carefully monitored for the onset of oligohydramnios. Furthermore, its use is contraindicated if one twin already has oligohydramnios because of the potential to further compromise that fetus.

The use of oral agents such as terbutaline and nifedipine following intravenous tocolysis is controversial. While the use of these agents is of questionable efficacy in singletons, we have personally found them quite helpful as previously discussed.

Discordant Growth and IUGR

The use of ultrasound for the monitoring of growth was previously discussed. It has long been recognized that when there were significant differences between the weights of twin pairs or higher-order multiples, there was a higher incidence of IUGR and a higher perinatal mortality rate. Erkkola et al.[115] reported that a weight difference of 25% or more was associated with a 6.5 times relative risk of stillbirth as compared to lesser differences. Thus, the early diagnosis of discordancy and/or IUGR is important because not only can fetal surveillance be started for the fetuses at risk, but hopefully a program of measures to improve fetal growth (bed rest, diet modification, smoking cessation) can be implemented.

At what level of intertwin difference should discordance be diagnosed? O'Brien et al.[116] made several excellent observations when analyzing discordancy and growth restriction in twin births. First, it was noted that, when the intertwin difference was expressed as a percentage of the weight of the larger twin, the 90th percentile of the difference was fairly stable between 20 and 25%. Second, differences of greater than 20 to 25% were associated with a single fetus with IUGR more than 50% of the time. When the difference in weight exceeded 20 to 25%, at least two-thirds of the fetuses were growth-restricted. A more recent study[117] of premature twin births revealed that it was at 30% difference that significantly higher incidences of fetal death (25%), congenital anomalies (37.5%), small-for-gestational-age infants (32%), Apgar scores <7 at 5 minutes (33.3%), and periventricular leukomalacia (16.7%) occurred despite a 79% cesarean rate in this group. It was also noted that all deaths in the 30% group were of the small infants. With these data in mind, and considering problems in diagnostic accuracy with ultrasound, we and many others have chosen a 20% difference to initiate antepartum testing.

One practical difficulty in management of this problem is the variability in ultrasound estimates of fetal weight of ±10 to 15% no matter which formulas are used. While the BPD difference alone has been generally recognized not to be a good predictor of discordance (unless significantly different—a late finding in IUGR), an abdominal circumference difference of 20 mm or more has been found[118] to have a positive predictive value of 83% for the prediction of twin discordancy of greater than 20%. The estimated fetal weight was found to have a better sensitivity (92.9%), but not as good a positive predictive value (72%). A study by Caravello et al.[119] concluded that these popular methods of predicting growth discordance have limited accuracy when held to the 25% difference standard. In addition, it has been reported that crown-to-rump differences in early pregnancy do not correlate with birth-weight differences in either monochorionic or dichorionic pregnancies.[120] Of note is the fact that the risk of true discordance seems to be greater in second twins and possibly in female fetuses of unlike-sex pairs.[121]

Once the diagnosis of discordancy is made, there are several essential considerations regarding the course of the discordance. The chorionicity, gestational age, and estimated weight percentiles of each twin need to be determined as precisely as possible. The presence of separate placentas and/or unlike sexes indicates dichorionicity and virtually rules out twin-to-twin transfusion. If the discordance occurs early in a dichorionic pair, a careful survey for anomalies must be conducted and consideration given to genetic testing even if anomalies or advanced maternal age are not present. The pattern of growth is important, as previously concordant, average-growth fetuses experiencing third-trimester discordance suggests IUGR from causes extrinsic to the fetus. The presence of unequal umbilical artery Doppler studies with an abnormal flow in the smaller twin suggests a problem with placental perfusion.

After the determination of discordance has been made, the fetal response to various therapeutic measures intended to improve the intrauterine environment must be followed by serially plotting growth curves. Knowing the gestational age allows one to follow with minimal concern a set of discordant twins that, for example, are at the 30th and 80th percentiles for weight. As the estimated weight of either or both twins approaches the 10th percentile and amniotic fluid volume appears compromised, the intensity of antepartum testing must be increased. At term, when the lighter twin has reached 2500 g or more, discordancy becomes less of a risk factor.[122] There is evidence to support the conclusion that discordance as an isolated finding does not warrant intervention, especially in preterm twins less than 32 completed weeks.[123] Delivery should not be considered until adequate weights (>2000 g) are attained unless there are signs of fetal distress on antepartum testing.

Twin-Twin Transfusion

A special case of discordancy occurs in monochorionic twinning. Since nearly all cases of monozygotic twins have vascular connections, this twin-to-twin transfusion syndrome (TTTS) is thought to result from unbalanced shunting of blood flow through one or more arteriovenous anastomoses in the placenta. The classical observation was of poor growth and oligohydramnios in the donor twin and polycythemia, hydrops, and hydramnios in the recipient.

The traditional criteria were based on the neonatal findings of a >20% difference in birth weight in same-sex twins, demonstration of interfetal vascular connections with a monochorionic placenta, and a >5 g/dl hemoglobin difference.

Both the criteria for diagnosis and the cause of this syndrome have been recently questioned. Danskin and Nielson observed that neither birth–weight differences of >20% nor hemoglobin differences >5 g/dl occurred more frequently in monozygotic gestations.[124] In addition, when cordocentesis has been performed[125] significant hemoglobin differences were confirmed in less than half the cases. The presence of a velamentous insertion of the cord in the smaller twin has been reported in 64% of monozygotic cases, where significant intertwin weight differences exist, suggesting a more complex explanation for the syndrome.[126] Saunders et al.[127] have suggested that the syndrome may develop as a consequence of uteroplacental insufficiency affecting the donor twin. The presence of a velamentous cord insertion makes the umbilical circulation vulnerable to compression (Figure 9-9), and this increased resistance in the placental circulation leads to increased shunting to the

Figure 9-9 Twin-to-twin transfusion syndrome. A. Velamentous insertion of cord was observed with color-flow Doppler. B. Velamentous insertion was confirmed at delivery by gross examination of the placenta. C. Placenta showed unequal sharing of blood flow; smaller twin was on the right (dark area). The umbilical-cord hematocrits were 18% in the smaller twin and 74% in the larger twin.

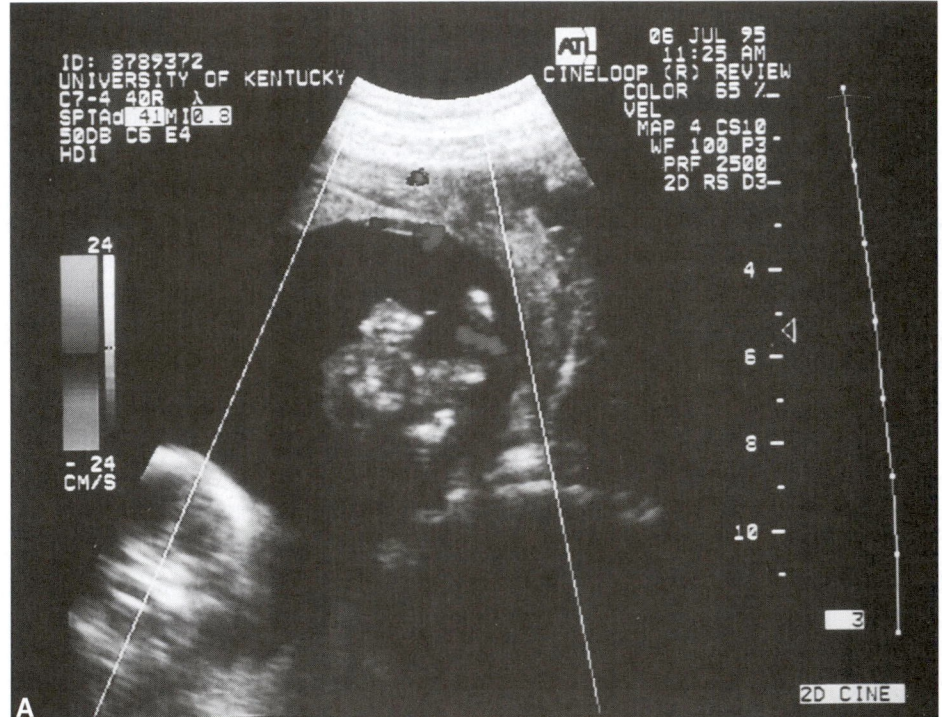

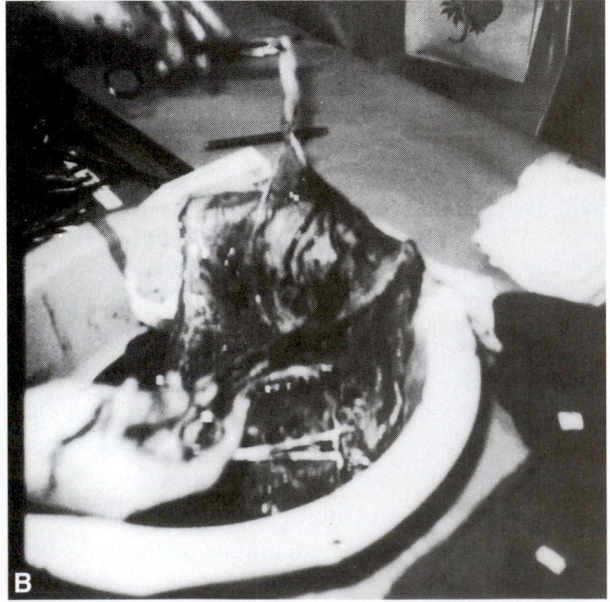

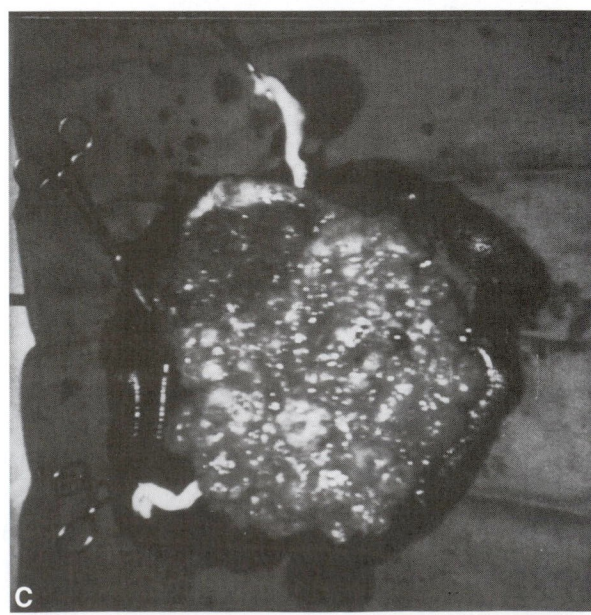

TABLE 9-8
ULTRASONOGRAPHIC CRITERIA FOR DIAGNOSIS OF TWIN-TO-TWIN TRANSFUSION SYNDROME

Marked growth discordance (>20% or 1.5 weeks)
Same-sex twins
Monochorionic placenta (by ultrasound criteria)
Presence of polyhydramnios in one sac
Presence of significant oligohydramnios (stuck twin) in other sac

---

recipient twin through common vascular channels. These twins also often have unequal sharing of placental mass. As the amniotic fluid volume in the recipient sac becomes larger due to increased renal blood flow and urine output, the increased intrauterine pressure further compromises flow in the velamentous cord. This observation may explain much of the success with therapeutic amniocentesis. In only one report, for reasons yet unexplained, a preponderance of female fetuses[128] with this syndrome (89%) has been noted. Umbilical-artery Doppler velocimetry results have also given differing pictures. It has been reported that abnormal S:D ratios correlate with adverse outcome and IUGR,[129] with the S:D ratios usually elevated in the donor twins, but also possibly abnormal in the recipient. In a group of older fetuses diagnosed only by hemoglobin differences at birth, the S:D ratios have been reported as concordant.[130]

With more recent information in mind and allowing for therapeutic possibilities, it is clear that the diagnosis of TTTS must be made using antepartum ultrasound criteria (Table 9-8). The differentiation of severe, moderate, and mild TTTS[131] can be made on grounds of timing of onset (<20, >24 weeks, at birth), degree of oligohydramnios/polyhydramnios found, and percentage of fetal weight discordance. This classification is important because there is a great difference in prognosis and therapy in these cases. The differences in severity may, in fact, be reflected in conflicting outcomes reported for various therapeutic measures.

Treatment methods attempted with the diagnosis of twin-to-twin transfusion syndrome can be measured against a perinatal mortality rate of up to 100% in the early and severe cases without intervention. Severe polyhydramnios at midpregnancy has previously been fatal to both fetuses despite a number of attempted therapies. Cheschier and Seeds[132] reported that, when this complication occurred before 26 weeks, all fetuses died. When this diagnosis is made,

bed rest is prescribed. Using repeated aggressive amniocentesis, Elliot et al.[133] reported a perinatal survival rate of 79%. Important factors in this investigation included early diagnosis and removal of large volumes (mean 1683 ml, with range of 225 to 5000 ml) of amniotic fluid so that no pocket greater than 8 cm remained. Reisner et al.[134] reported a survival increase from 40% in a nonintervention cohort as compared with a 74% survival using serial amniocentesis, while Dennis and Winkler[135] found an 82% survival in the treated group versus 50% in the untreated group. With amniocentesis or any therapeutic intervention, it seems that a rate-limiting step for success is the ability to carry the pregnancy past approximately 28 weeks, as many perinatal deaths are from complications of prematurity.

At present, laser coagulation of communicating vessels on the placenta is an experimental technique with major technical difficulties and limitations. De Lia et al.[136] reported a series of 35 patients referred for this surgery. Nine of the patients were eliminated, and the 26 who underwent the procedure had a posterior placenta. The survival rate was 53% in the treated group, with 96% of fetuses developing normally. Ville et al.[137] reported a survival rate of 55%, which is comparable to that reported for serial amniocentesis, but suggest that intact survival may be better. Larger-scale comparisons need to be performed, but, in any case, it is important that patients are counseled in a realistic manner and any therapy chosen is begun early.

Monoamniotic Twins

Monozygotic twin gestations wherein embryo splitting occurs between 8 and 13 days postconception result in monoamniotic/monochorionic placentation. This occurs in approximately 1% of monozygotic twinning. Because there is a common amniotic sac in these pregnancies, the twins incur the additional risk of cord entanglement, which has been reported to result in a 40 to 60% perinatal mortality. Prior to high-resolution ultrasound, this problem was not diagnosed in utero and thus was not a clinical management problem. The ability to diagnose this condition, outlined previously, has resulted in a great many suggestions for management.

Rodis et al.[34] recommended intense fetal surveillance from 25 to 32 weeks of gestation, after which time cesarean delivery should be undertaken. This approach must be tempered by the understanding that this can be a difficult diagnosis with many false positive results, especially in the latter part of pregnancy,[138] and that increased morbidity and mortality can result from unnecessary early intervention.

With improved ultrasound equipment, this diagnosis can be made more reliably, and even the presence of cord entanglement detected[139] using color-flow Doppler. Antepartum surveillance can thus be tailored to meet the perceived risk and much expensive hospitalization avoided. Two reports[140,141] have shown a plateau effect for fetal death in these cases at 30 and 32 weeks. Twins that were alive at 30 to 32 weeks had outcomes no different from monochorionic/diamniotic controls, thus showing no advantage to early delivery. Thus, with accurate antepartum diagnosis, appropriately intensive fetal surveillance, and properly timed delivery, the survival in monoamniotic twins has improved greatly. This was the conclusion in a 10-year review[142] citing a 92% survival rate. Lastly, cesarean delivery can possibly be avoided in selected cases in which cord entanglement does not seem to exist and both twins are adequately monitored and without distress.

Presence of Fetal Anomalies Specific to Twinning

The rate of congenital anomalies in twins is 1.5 to 2 times that of singletons[42] and is most frequent in monozygotic gestations. The process of monozygotic twinning itself produces multiple possibilities for abnormal development due to partial, unequal, or abnormal separation of the embryo. The two major anomalies unique to twins—acardiac twinning and conjoint twinning—occur in monozygotic gestations.

Acardiac twinning occurs at a rate of approximately 1 in 30,000 to 1 in 40,000 pregnancies, or approximately 1% of monozygotic twins. These malformed fetuses have either no heart at all or very rudimentary cardiac tissue and can be classified according to severity. In the most severe form, acardiac amorphous, there is no significant resemblance to a human fetus. The acardiac acephalus has varying degrees of fetal development without development of cephalic structures and is the most common. A paracephalic acardiac possesses degrees of headlike structures (Figure 9-10). The diagnosis is made in a monochorionic gestation when a nonviable anomalous fetus continues to grow. The acardiac twin obviously

requires a normal "pump" twin to supply its circulation, which occurs through a mechanism known as twin reverse arterial perfusion (TRAP) sequence. This reversed flow has been documented using Doppler ultrasound.[143]

A large series of these cases has been reviewed by Moore et al.,[144] detailing the problems that occur in these pregnancies. Hydramnios was a common finding (40%) and had a strong association with preterm labor and delivery and congestive heart failure in the pump twin. They also found that the incidence of congestive failure was related to the weight ratio of the pump twin to recipient twin; the larger the acardiac relative to the normal twin, the worse the prognosis. If the acardiac mass was less than 50% of the normal twin, the negative predictive values for hydramnios and preterm delivery were both 83%.[144] The overall survival was approximately 45%, with perinatal mortality mainly due to preterm delivery.

A number of possible therapies has been suggested,

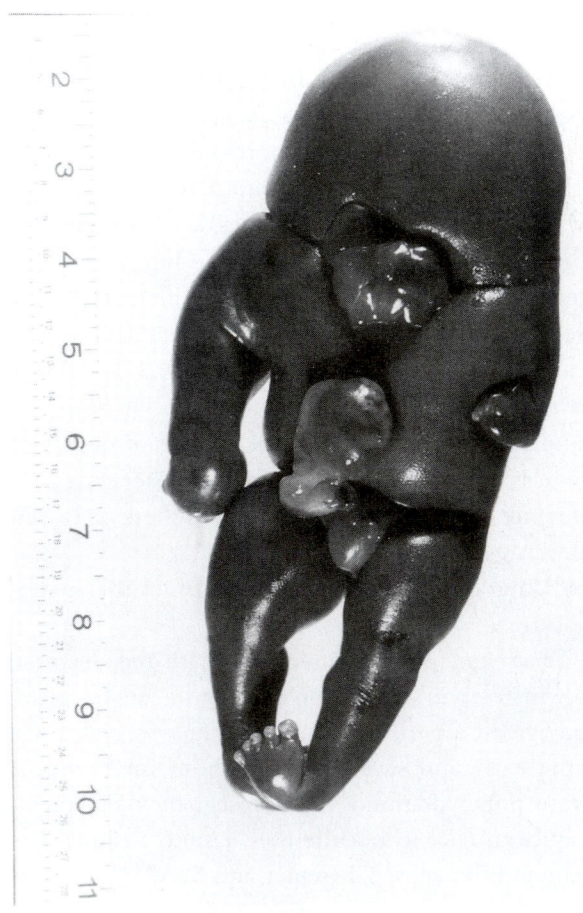

Figure 9-10 Paracephalic acardiac twin.

including the use of digoxin[145] and indomethacin.[146] In a review of reported invasive procedures, Arias et al.[147] have concluded that fetal surgery is the best available treatment for acardiac twinning. They recommend endoscopic laser surgery prior to 24 weeks and umbilical-cord ligation thereafter, as pump twin mortality was only 13.6% in these cases, as compared with an expected 50%. As to case selection, it should be pointed out that where flow to the acardiac twin is decreasing or absent, or the acardiac fetal mass is very small as compared with the pump twin,[144] invasive techniques may be avoided.

Conjoint twinning results from the late and incomplete division of the embryonic disk at day 13 to 15 after conception. This occurs in approximately 1 in 100,000 pregnancies. These gestations are classified by the areas joined together: chest (thoracopagus), head (craniopagus), abdomen (omphalopagus), or body with two heads (dicephalus) (Figure 9-11). With modern ultrasonographic equipment, these pregnancies can be diagnosed quite early. At the time of diagnosis, it is important to first identify the point and degree of attachment, as the sharing of vital organs and large amounts of anatomy has a poor to hopeless prognosis. Second, the presence of associated anomalies may confer lethality even when small attachments exist.

Because of hydramnios, preterm labor is often present. It has been the consensus that, unless the gestation is very small and previable or unsalvageable due to abnormalities, a cesarean delivery should be performed to prevent maternal and fetal damage.

Presence of a Single Anomalous Fetus

As already noted, the rate of congenital anomalies in multiple gestations is increased. When the specific twinning abnormalities are eliminated, most are structural abnormalities as would be seen in any pregnancy. While occasionally both or all fetuses may be affected, in most cases only one fetus is abnormal. Depending on the severity of the anomaly, a dilemma is presented to both the parents and to those treating the pregnancy. The options available include termination of the entire pregnancy, selective termination of the anomalous fetus,[148] and continuation of the entire pregnancy. Besides concerns for the psychological and emotional health of the family faced with this dilemma, the risks involved and which option has the best outcome for the normal fetus must be determined.

The use of selective feticide is limited when the gestational age at diagnosis is late or the pregnancy is monochorionic. In addition, some authors have reported loss rates as high as 10 to 12% after the procedure.[148] On the other hand, it is known that an anomalous fetus raises the rate of premature delivery in singletons, and this risk has been confirmed also in multiple gestations.[149,150] The report by Alexander et al.[150] indicates that, while twins complicated by a major anomaly delivered, on average, 2 weeks earlier, the outcomes for the normal twins were similar to those seen in otherwise uncomplicated twin gestations. In addition, Lipitz et al.[151] reported 14 cases with one normal twin and one anencephalic fetus and noted a generally favorable outcome for the normal fetus. When faced with this situation, the clinician must be ready to provide counseling regarding all possible options.

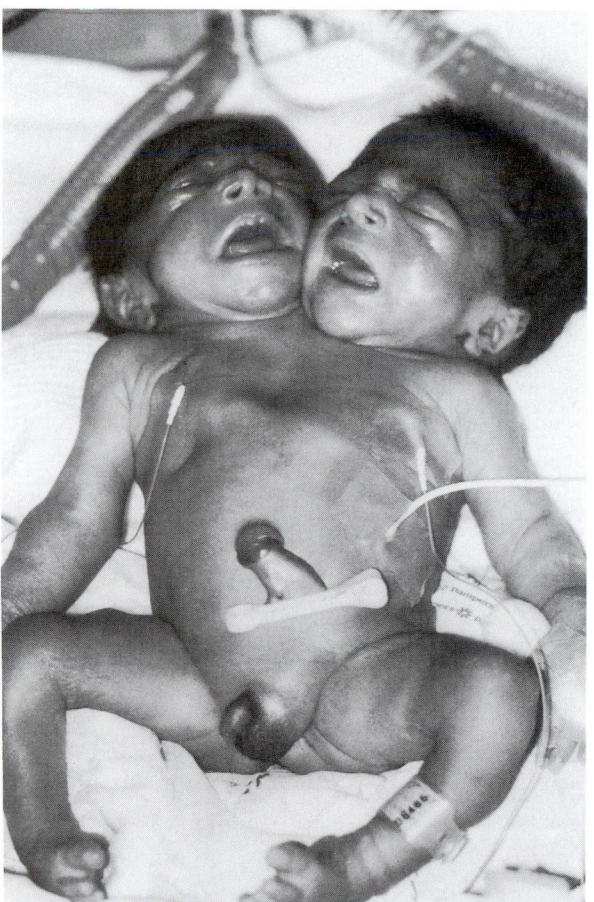

Figure 9-11 Dicephalic conjoined twins. The presence of multiple circulatory anomalies resulted in the death of the infants on the first day of life.

Single Intrauterine Demise after 20 Weeks

As previously discussed, the spontaneous loss of a single member of a multiple gestation early in gestation is quite common and probably has little consequence. Rates of loss during the second half of pregnancy have ranged from 0.5 to 6.8%, with a mean of 2 to 3%.[152] Death of a single fetus occurs approximately three times as often in monochorionic as in dichorionic gestations.[153] Furthermore, the death of one fetus has generally been associated with an increase in preterm delivery of the surviving fetus. In a 1985 review by Enbom[154] of 39 reported cases, significant morbidity and mortality was cited in 46% and was due to prematurity, preeclampsia, fetal distress, and, in monochorionic gestations, disseminated intravascular coagulation and organ damage in the surviving twin.

When the death of one member of a multiple gestation is discovered, it is important to ascertain the chorionicity involved and the cause of the death. There is a significant incidence of structural anomalies in the dead twin (25%),[155] and a careful survey of the surviving fetus for anomalies is indicated. In the case of monochorionic gestations, surveillance for damage to the surviving fetus such as central nervous system, pulmonary, or other infarcts, is important (Figure 9-12). Intensive fetal monitoring should be undertaken, and, in the absence of fetal distress, pregnancies less than 32 weeks should be managed conservatively, as premature delivery may carry higher risks.

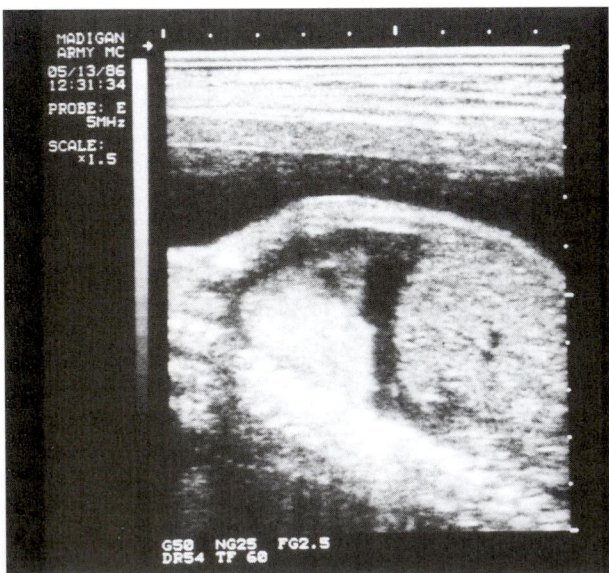

Figure 9-12 Hydropic changes in the surviving fetus following the intrauterine death of one twin. At birth, the infant had multiple organ infarcts and subsequently died.

This conservative course of action is justified, in part, because the timing and nature of the injury to the surviving twin is uncertain. Hypotension in the acute state and chronic serial embolization may be responsible for these injuries. Acute anemia, postulated to be from acute hemorrhage into the dead recipient twin, has been documented using fetal blood sampling.[156] Moreover, a conservative course of action is justified by the generally recognized inability to prevent complications in the survivor (stillbirth, multicystic encephalomalacia, renal cortical necrosis, pulmonary infarct) after the other twin's death even if nearly immediate intervention is employed. Because of the potential for chronic events to produce damage, a reasonable course of action in monochorionic gestations would be to deliver at or beyond 32 weeks when fetal lung maturity is documented. In the case of dizygotic twins with a single death, treatment should be individualized. Antepartum fetal surveillance should be intensified, and fetal lung maturity should be assessed prior to delivery. No adverse maternal effects due to conservative management have been noted,[155] and decisions about delivery should be based on the usual obstetric considerations.

Pregnancy-Induced Hypertension

The incidence of pregnancy-induced hypertension is increased three to five times in twin gestations. In addition, onset of disease may occur early in multiple as compared with singleton gestations. The rate of severe preeclampsia is significantly increased in triplet as compared with twin pregnancies,[157] although the overall rate of preeclampsia is not. A review of birth certificate records from Washington[158] found a nearly fourfold increased risk of preeclampsia in twins. The use of bed rest has been associated with a decrease in preeclampsia,[64] and early recognition of this condition and employment of rest may decrease the severity. While low-dose aspirin may not be beneficial in low-risk pregnancies to prevent preeclampsia, it may reduce the incidence in twin gestations.[159] Large clinical trials are still needed to confirm efficacy. The detailed management of preeclampsia is reviewed elsewhere in this textbook.

Postdates in Multiples

Several observations have led to the belief that twins become "postdates" much earlier than singletons.

First is the fact that the average length of gestation is only 36 to 37 weeks instead of 40 weeks. Second, fetal growth plateaus at 34 to 35 weeks and the placenta "matures" much earlier. Third is the clinical observation that amniotic fluid often decreases much earlier in multiple as compared with singleton gestation. Finally, a general observation made in the past, before antepartum fetal heart rate monitoring, is that the incidence of intrauterine death increased after 37 to 38 weeks. Luke[160] demonstrated that the lowest fetal death rate for twins occurs at 36 to 38 weeks. These observations have led many to consider twins as "postdates" after 38 weeks. However, with close antepartum surveillance, is this still true? Stone et al.[161] have compared morbidity and mortality in twin gestations delivered between 36 to 38 weeks (n = 210) versus those delivered after 38 weeks (n = 147). There was no difference in neonatal outcome between the two groups except for an increased frequency of hyperbilirubinemia and hypoglycemia in the younger twins. In this group of patients monitored antepartum,

they concluded that, in the face of "adequate intrauterine growth and amniotic fluid, elective delivery at 38 weeks does not appear to be indicated."[161]

INTRAPARTUM MANAGEMENT

Just as the management of multiple gestations can be complex and open to many opinions, so are the optimal pathways for intrapartum management (Figure 9-13). Much discussion can be generated given the possibility of various presentations, degrees of prematurity, and other complications. Despite early diagnosis and excellent antepartum care, the obstetrician may be faced with a number of new complicating factors. In addition to higher incidences of prematurity, premature rupture of the membranes, and malpresentation, the clinician may also be faced with IUGR, discordant growth, fetal abnormalities, polyhydramnios, oligohydramnios, placenta previa, or abruptio placentae. Maternal diabetes or preeclampsia may complicate the overall management, and cord

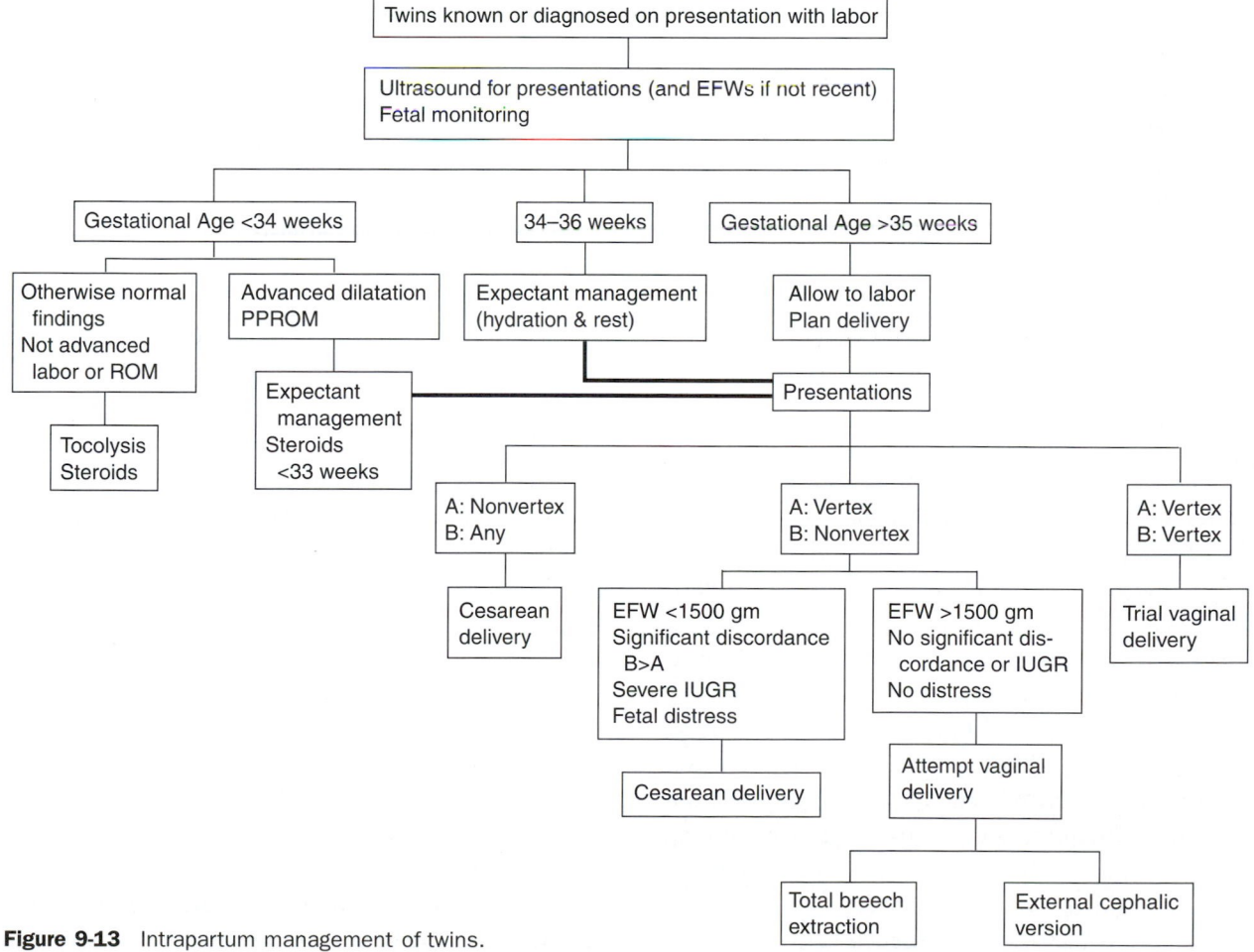

Figure 9-13 Intrapartum management of twins.

prolapse or hemorrhage may occur at the time of delivery. It is important to have a clear understanding of the delivery process in multiple gestations and the potential complications if these complications are to be prevented or managed effectively.

Initial Labor Evaluation

Early diagnosis of multiple gestation and confirmation of gestational age greatly facilitate planning and improve outcome. Although much less common today due to the widespread use of ultrasound, there still is the occasional multiple gestation that is not diagnosed until the onset of labor or intrapartum. At the time of admission, the presentations should be confirmed and the estimated weights reassessed. Data show that fetal presentation can often change between the last ultrasound and the time of labor.[162] A complete blood count and blood type/Rh and antibody screen should be obtained. Because of the increased risk of postpartum hemorrhage, blood can be typed and screened and held in the blood bank. Urine should be checked for protein, and additional evaluation for preeclampsia should be carried out. Besides noting the dilation, effacement, position, and consistency of the cervix and the station of the presenting part, the clinician should determine the adequacy of the pelvis. Fetal monitoring should be initiated. In addition to contraction frequency, it is important to monitor both fetuses adequately during the labor, as the well-being of one does not ensure that of the other. Furthermore, the possibility of fetal compromise is more common than in singletons.

Conduct of Labor

The course of labor in twin gestations is similar to that for singletons, with the average length of labor being longer for nulliparas than for multiparas. Because the cervix is frequently somewhat advanced in Bishop score at the onset of labor,[76] it comes as no surprise that the latent phase in multiple gestations is often shorter than for singletons.[163]

The active phase of labor, however, can often be longer than in a singleton gestation. The prolongation in these cases has been attributed to dysfunction from uterine overdistention and to crowding of presenting parts in the pelvis. The more frequent use of regional anesthetics and the higher incidence of prematurity may also contribute to a lengthened active phase.[164] The judicious use of oxytocin for augmentation can safely correct dysfunctional labor. In addition, oxytocin can be safely used to induce labor. Direct monitoring of intrauterine pressure will help to prevent uterine hyperstimulation.

As mentioned previously, it is important that both twins be adequately monitored. This is usually accomplished with a scalp electrode on twin A and an external monitor on twin B. When a nonreassuring fetal heart rate pattern is encountered, the management may be somewhat hampered. Only twin A is assessable for scalp stimulation or fetal scalp blood sampling. The finding of fetal heart rate acceleration in response to vibroacoustic stimulation is acceptable for ensuring the well-being of either fetus.[164]

After the delivery of the first twin, the second twin may be at risk for distress from decreased placental perfusion or premature separation of the placenta. Prior to widespread use of electronic fetal monitoring, the consensus in the literature was that a delay of more than 8 to 10 minutes in the delivery of twin B was associated with a poor outcome. With the use of fetal heart rate and contraction monitoring it has been shown that a time restriction for the delivery interval is not necessary.[165] With the addition of real-time ultrasound in the delivery room, both fetal position and status can be determined. There is no set time limit beyond which cesarean delivery must be performed. Moreover, the use of cesarean delivery for the second twin should be performed only in unusual circumstances, such as fetal distress with rapid vaginal delivery not possible.

When the patient has had a prior cesarean delivery the consensus previously held that a repeat cesarean delivery was indicated. Experience from a number of locations indicates that, under the proper circumstances, patients with a prior low transverse incision are candidates for a trial of labor. Miller et al.[166] have reported a large experience in twins with prior cesarean deliveries who were delivered vaginally without uterine rupture and without an increase in maternal or perinatal morbidity or mortality.

Management of Delivery

The delivery of twins can be one of the more stressful experiences for an obstetrician due to the rapid decision making and high level of skill often required. The successful delivery of healthy twins also produces great satisfaction. In these cases careful preparation and flexibility in action with changing conditions distinguish the thoughtful clinician. To be optimally

TABLE 9-9		
DELIVERY ROOM REQUIREMENTS FOR VAGINAL DELIVERY OF TWINS		
Place	Delivery room with cesarean delivery capability— not labor/delivery room	
People	Obstetrician skilled in twin deliveries	
	Assistant for obstetrician	
	Anesthesiologist/nurse-anesthetist	
	Obstetric nursing team	
	Pediatric/neonatal team	
Equipment	Fetal monitor with twin capability	
	Ultrasound machine	
	Anesthesia equipment and monitors	
	Appropriate forceps and vacuum extractor	
	Warmer for each infant	
	Suction bulbs (2) and DeLee Suction Traps (2)	
	Two different sets of clamps for umbilical cords	
	Heparinized labeled syringes for cord gasses	
	Syringes/tubes (labeled) to collect cord blood	
Drugs	Oxytocin	
	Methylergonovine	
	15-methylprostaglandin $F_{2\alpha}$	
Available	Blood: minimum type and screen 2 units	

prepared, a number of items must be assembled (Table 9-9) prior to delivery. The delivery should be planned in a location where a rapid cesarean delivery can be performed and with all the essentials to support the needs of both mother and infants.

Because of increasing concern for the possibility of fetal injury due to malpresentation or prematurity, a considerable controversy arose over past decades regarding the choice of delivery route in twins. Much of this debate centers on the presentation of the second twin and a decreasing experience with both breech and operative vaginal deliveries. The percentages of various presentations reported by different authors[157,161] are remarkably similar. Slightly more than 80% of twins will have the first present as a vertex. In slightly more than half of these, the second twin is also vertex. In slightly less than 20%, the first twin is not a cephalic presentation. Overall, approximately 60% of cases will thus have one or both twins as a nonvertex presentation. Chervenak et al.[167] have grouped these presentations into three general categories and proposed systematic management plans for each category: (1) vertex A/vertex B, (2) vertex A/nonvertex B, and (3) nonvertex A. In the following discussions it must be realized that management protocols are only guidelines for action and counseling. Patients should be given full and detailed information regarding the risks and benefits of each approach as well as alternatives when expected and unexpected events occur.

Vertex Twin A/Vertex Twin B

The presence of cephalic presentations in both fetuses should permit a vaginal delivery in most cases. The general consensus is that this is safe regardless of gestational age or fetal weight unless other obstetric or medical indications warrant an operative abdominal delivery,[164] although there are some suggestions that fetuses under 1000 g might benefit from cesarean delivery.[168] The use of intrapartum ultrasound and continuous fetal heart rate monitoring should be considered standard for monitoring the status of twin B during and after the delivery of twin A. Once the first twin is delivered, the second should be guided into the pelvis by an experienced assistant and maintained in a cephalic presentation with gentle abdominal pressure. This is done to prevent twin B from assuming an abnormal lie and, at the same time, to reduce the possibility of the cord preceding the head into the pelvis. Uterine activity should be monitored, and, if contractions fail to resume promptly, oxytocin should be initiated.

An amniotomy should not be performed on the second twin until the head is engaged in the pelvis. An amniotomy performed too early may result in cord prolapse. After safe amniotomy, a scalp electrode can be applied, and the remainder of the second stage managed as a singleton delivery. In the event of fetal distress, an immediate delivery is indicated and the obstetrician must quickly decide between use of forceps, use of vacuum extraction, or cesarean delivery. Internal podalic version and difficult forceps deliveries should be avoided.

Umbilical-cord blood for acid–base status and other tests should be obtained. The draining of cord blood from twin A should be avoided prior to the delivery of twin B on the chance that intertwin vascular connections might exist and the intravascular volume of twin B might be diminished.

Vertex A/Nonvertex B

This combination of presentations represents the most controversial area of intrapartum management with multiple gestation. Because of the fear of excess morbidity and possible mortality in the second twin delivered from other than a vertex presentation, some have advocated routine cesarean delivery in these cases.[169] Worry about head entrapment, cord prolapse, and other problems common to singleton breeches, combined with a growing inexperience with management of breech delivery, may have contributed to this belief. That routine cesarean is not always necessary and perhaps not desirable considering maternal morbidity is supported by a growing body of evidence. Acker et al.[170] demonstrated no significant difference in low 5-minute Apgar scores between second twins weighing 1500 g or more delivered by breech extraction versus cesarean. In addition, since approximately 30% of second twins with an unstable lie convert to vertex after the first twin delivers, many also suggest individualizing the approach for each patient. Since external cephalic version in term singleton breeches has returned to wide use, the suggestion that it could be employed to convert the second twin to vertex for delivery was made.[171] There are thus two alternatives for delivery of twin B: external cephalic version and vaginal breech delivery.

Chervenak et al.[171] reported that a planned external cephalic version of the second twin was successful in 71% of transverse and 73% of breech presentations. As always this should be attempted only in a room with cesarean capability and preferably under epidural anesthesia. It should be done in a gentle manner under direct guidance and monitoring with real-time ultrasound. A forward or backward roll is acceptable, usually employing the shortest distance. Once the fetus is in the vertex position, gentle pressure should be used to hold this position until the head is engaged in the pelvis and membranes can safely be ruptured. If distress occurs during the attempt at version, the obstetrician must decide if cesarean delivery or total breech extraction is to be performed. If distress occurs after successful version, the choice must be made between vacuum, forceps, or cesarean delivery. If the second twin is much larger than the first, external version may be the best choice, as entrapment of the larger head is a theoretical problem. However, the large size of the second twin may reduce the probability of successful version.[171]

The second option is a vaginal breech delivery of twin B. This option may be considered when the usual criteria for vaginal breech delivery are met,[172] except that CT pelvimetry is probably not necessary unless there is an unproven or clinically small pelvis and the breech twin is larger than 3000 g. In addition, head extension is usually not a problem. A skilled obstetrician and a willing patient are also needed. Several studies[173-175] have supported vaginal breech delivery of the second twin, concluding that cesarean offers no advantage. While it has been recommended[164] that any second twin less than 1500 g or less than 34

weeks of gestation in the nonvertex position be delivered by cesarean, no firm evidence supports this recommendation. Breech-extracted second twins between 750 and 2000 g as compared with twins delivered by cesarean showed no significant differences in any measure of neonatal outcome.[176,177]

As the experience with total breech extraction has been compared to external cephalic version, important observations have been made.[170-172] External version has been associated with a higher failure rate of vaginal delivery. Moreover, version was associated with complications of fetal distress, cord prolapse, and compound presentation not otherwise seen. In our experience, version attempt has resulted in most of the cases of cesarean delivery for the second twin that have occurred recently. As a result, total breech extraction is our first choice in these cases.

As with any twin delivery, total breech extraction is performed in the cesarean delivery room with ultrasound guidance and fetal monitoring. If the buttocks is the presenting part, the mother can push. If, in the majority of cases, it is a footling presentation both feet must be grasped tightly before rupturing the membranes. The membranes can then be ruptured and the breech delivered, taking special care to keep the head flexed. Piper forceps should be kept near, although they are needed infrequently. Uterine manipulation of the second twin does not appear to increase the incidence of postpartum infection, nor does the time interval between deliveries.[178]

Nonvertex Twin A

When the first twin is other than vertex, cesarean delivery appears to be the preferred approach. It must be recognized that this recommendation is based on a paucity of data in the modern era. Much of the support for this position is based on the belief that the second twin may interfere with the flexion of twin A's head during the breech delivery or that interlocking of fetal heads, a rare but potentially dangerous complication, might occur. A group of 24 breech–vertex twins has been reported.[179] There were no differences in Apgar scores or neonatal morbidity and mortality as compared with 35 cases delivered abdominally. Further research is needed before a change in recommendations is considered.

Anesthesia Considerations

Regional lumbar epidural anesthesia is, in our opinion, the best choice for the delivery of twins. There are several reasons for this recommendation: (1) Preterm fetuses may be more susceptible to the respiratory and neurologic depressant effects of narcotics, sedatives, and general anesthesia. (2) The mother's pulmonary functional residual capacity is already decreased over that of a singleton gestation. This effect may lead[180] to an increased susceptibility to rapid desaturation during anesthesia induction. (3) Not only does an epidural provide better labor anesthesia, but it also aids in preventing uncontrolled bearing down by the mother. This effect may permit a smoother delivery over a relaxed perineum. (4) As previously mentioned, epidural anesthesia facilitates external cephalic version or intrauterine manipulation necessary to effect the delivery of the second twin. (5) The presence of an epidural anesthesia avoids the need for a rapid induction of general anesthesia should an emergent cesarean delivery be needed. Because of the propensity for mothers of twins to experience supine hypotension, excellent hydration and careful positioning is needed during both labor and delivery.

Delivery of Higher-Order Multiples

It is the general consensus that, due to the difficulties encountered in monitoring three or more fetuses and the great variety of presentations encountered, these gestations are best delivered by cesarean. While there are small retrospective reports of safe vaginal deliveries in higher-order multiple gestations, no prospective randomized trials exist. Because the infants obtained from these deliveries are often very premature or have many problems that require skilled neonatal care, the delivery of these cases should take place in tertiary-care centers.

REFERENCES

1. Luke B. The changing pattern of multiple births in the United States: maternal and infant characteristics, 1973 and 1990. Obstet Gynecol 1994;84:101.
2. Naeye RL, et al. Twins: causes of perinatal death in 12 United States and one African city. Am J Obstet Gynecol 1978;131:267.
3. Chervenak FA, et al. Twin gestation, antenatal diagnosis and perinatal outcome in 385 consecutive pregnancies. J Reprod Med 1984;29:727.
4. Ellings J, et al. Reduction in very low birth weight deliveries and perinatal mortality in a specialized, multi-disciplinary twin clinic. Obstet Gynecol 1993;81:387.
5. Jewell SE, Yip R. Increasing trends in plural births in the United States. Obstet Gynecol 1995;85:229.
6. Landy HJ, Weiner S, Corson SL. The "vanishing twin": ultrasonic assessment of fetal disappearance in the first trimester. Am J Obstet Gynecol 1986;155:14.
7. Callahan TL, et al. The economic impact of multiple-gestation pregnancies and the contribution of assisted-reproduction techniques to their incidence. N Engl J Med 1994;331:244.
8. Mishell DR, Davajan V, eds. Infertility, contraception and reproductive endocrinology. 2nd ed. Montvale, NJ: Medical Economics, 1986.
9. Ho ML, Chen JY, Ling UP, et al. Changing epidemiology of triplet pregnancy: etiology and outcome over twelve years. Am J Perinatol 1996;13:269.
10. Lipitz S, Seidman DS, Alcaley M, et al. The effect of fertility drugs and in-vitro methods on the outcome of 106 triplet pregnancies. Fertil Steril 1993;60(6):1031.
11. Collins MS, Bleyl JA. Seventy-one quadruplet pregnancies: management and outcome. Am J Obstet Gynecol 1990;162:1384.
12. Derom C, Vlietinck R, Derom R, et al. Increased monozygotic twinning rate after ovulation induction. Lancet 1987;8544:1236.
13. Strong SJ, Corney G. The placenta in twin pregnancy. Oxford: Pergamon Press, 1967.
14. Johnson JM, Harman CR, Evans JA, et al. Maternal serum alphafetoprotein in twin pregnancy. Am J Obstet Gynecol 1990;162:1020.
15. Hong S, Berkowitz G, Wang W, et al. Unexplained elevated maternal serum alpha-fetoprotein levels and pregnancy outcome in twins. Obstet Gynecol 1996;88:337.
16. Drugan A, Sokol RJ, Syner FN, et al. Clinical implications of amniotic fluid alpha-fetoprotein in twin pregnancy. J Reprod Med 1989;34:977.
17. Persson PH, Grennert L, Gunnser G, Kullander S. On improved outcome in twin pregnancies. Acta Obstet Gynecol Scand 1979;58:3.
18. Hughey MJ, Olive DL. Routine ultrasound screening for the detection and management of twin pregnancies. J Reprod Med 1985;30:427.
19. LeFevre ML, Bain RP, Ewigman BG, et al. A randomized trial of prenatal ultrasonographic screening: impact on maternal management and outcome. Am J Obstet Gynecol 1993; 169:483.
20. Dickey RP, Olar TT, Curole DN, et al. The probability of multiple births when multiple gestational sacs or viable embryos are diagnosed at first trimester ultrasound. Hum Reprod 1990;5(7):880.
21. Jauniaux E, Elkazen N, Leroy F, et al. Clinical and morphologic aspects of the vanishing twin phenomenon. Obstet Gynecol 1988;72:577.
22. Kol S, Levron J, Lewit N, et al. The natural history of multiple pregnancies after assisted reproduction: is spontaneous fetal demise a clinically significant phenomenon? Fertil Steril 1993;60:127.
23. Weissman A, Achiron R, Lipitz S, et al. The first trimester growth-discordant twin: an ominous prenatal finding. Obstet Gynecol 1994;84:110.
24. Benson CB, Doubilet PM, Laks MP. Outcome of twin gestations following sonographic demonstration of two heartbeats in the first trimester. Ultrasound Obstet Gynecol 1993;3:343.
25. Barss VA, Benacerraf BR, Frigoletto FD. Ultrasonographic determination of chorion type in twin gestation. Obstet Gynecol 1985;66:779.

26. Winn HN, Gabrielli S, Reece A, et al. Ultrasonic criteria for the prenatal diagnosis of placental chorionicity in twin gestations. Am J Obstet Gynecol 1989;161:1540.

27. Stagiannis KD, Sepulveda W, Southwell D, et al. Ultrasonic measurement of the dividing membrane in twin pregnancy during the second and third trimesters: a reproducibility study. Am J Obstet Gynecol 1995; 173:1546.

28. D'Alton ME, Dudley DK. The ultrasonographic prediction of chorionicity in twin gestation. Am J Obstet Gynecol 1989;160:557.

29. Vayssiere CF, Heim N, Camus E, et al. Determination of chorionicity in twin gestations by high-frequency abdominal ultrasonography: counting the layers of the dividing membrane. Am J Obstet Gynecol 1996; 175:1529.

30. Finberg H. The twin peak sign: reliable evidence of dichorionic twinning. J Ultrasound Med 1992;11:571.

31. Bessis R, Papernik E. Echographic imagery of amniotic membranes in twin pregnancies. In: Twin research 3: twin biology and multiple pregnancy. New York: Liss, 1981:183.

32. Wood SL, St. Onge R, Connors G, Elliot PD. Evaluation of the twin peak or lambda sign in determining chorionicity in multiple pregnancy. Obstet Gynecol 1996; 88:6.

33. Sepulveda W, Sebire NJ, Hughes K, et al. Evolution of the lambda or twin-chorionic peak sign in dichorionic twin pregnancies. Obstet Gynecol 1997;89:439.

34. Rodis JF, Vintzileos AM, Campbell WA, et al. Antenatal diagnosis and management of monoamniotic twins. Am J Obstet Gynecol 1987;157:1255.

35. Strohbehn K, Dattel BJ. Pitfalls in the diagnosis of non-conjoined monoamniotic twins. J Perinatol 1995;15:484.

36. Bromley B, Benacerraf B. Using the number of yolk sacs to determine amnionicity in early first trimester chorionic twins. J Ultrasound Med 1995;14:415.

37. Socol ML, Tamura RK, Sabbagha RE, et al. Diminished biparietal diameter and abdominal circumference growth in twins. Obstet Gynecol 1984;64:235.

38. Chervenak FA, Skupski DW, Romero R, et al. How accurate is fetal biometry in the assessment of fetal age? Am J Obstet Gynecol 1998;178:678.

39. Rodis JF, Vintzileos AM, Campbell WA, et al. Intrauterine fetal growth in concordant twin gestations. Am J Obstet Gynecol 1990;162:1025.

40. Rodis JF, Egan JFX, Craffey A, et al. Calculated risk of chromosomal abnormalities in twin gestations. Obstet Gynecol 1990;76:1037.

41. Meyers C, Adam R, Dungan J, Prenger V. Aneuploidy in twin gestations: when is maternal age advanced? Obstet Gynecol 1997:89:248.

42. Anderson RL, Goldberg JD, Golbus MS. Prenatal diagnosis in multiple gestation: 20 years experience with amniocentesis. Prenat Diagn 1991;11:263.

43. Ghidini A, Lynch L, Hicks C, et al. The risk of second-trimester amniocentesis in twin gestations: a case control study. Am J Obstet Gynecol 1993;169:1013.

44. Wapner RJ, Johnson A, Davis G, et al. Prenatal diagnosis in twin gestations: a comparison between second-trimester amniocentesis and first-trimester chorionic villus sampling. Obstet Gynecol 1993;82:49.

45. Kohl SG, Casey G. Twin gestation. Mt Sinai J Med 1975;42:523.

46. Gilstrap LC, Hauth JC, Hankins GVD, Beck A. Twins: prophylactic hospitalization and ward rest at early gestational age. Obstet Gynecol 1987;69:578.

47. Andrews WW, Leveno KJ, Sherman ML, et al. Elective hospitalization in the management of twin pregnancies. Obstet Gynecol 1991;77:826.

48. Kovacs BW, Kirschbaum TH, Paul RH. Twin gestations. I. Antenatal care and complications. Obstet Gynecol 1989;74:313.

49. Gardner MO, Amaya MA, Sakakini J Jr. Effects of prenatal care on twin gestation. J Reprod Med 1990; 35:519.

50. Persson PH, Grennert L. Towards a normalization of the outcome of twin pregnancy. Acta Genet Med Gemellol 1979;28:341.

51. Papiernik E, Mussy MA, Vial M, Richard A. A low rate of perinatal deaths for twin births. Acta Genet Med Gemellol 1985;34:201.

52. O'Connor MC, Arias E, Royston JP, Dalrymple IJ. The merits of special antenatal care for twin pregnancies. Br J Obstet Gynaecol 1981;88:222.

53. Heffner LJ, Sherman CB, Speizer FE, Weiss ST. Clinical and environmental predictors of preterm labor. Obstet Gynecol 1993;81:750.

54. Keith LG, Cervantes A, Oleszczuk JJ, Papiernik E. Multiple births and preterm delivery. Prenat Neonat Med 1998;3:125.

55. Caspi E, Ronen J, Schreyer P, Goldberg MD. The outcome of pregnancy after gonadotrophin therapy. Br J Obstet Gynaecol 1976;83:967.

56. Brown JE, Schloesser PT. Prepregnancy weight status, prenatal weight gain, and the outcome of term twin gestations. Am J Obstet Gynecol 1990;162:182.

57. Luke B, Minogue J, Witter FR, et al. The ideal twin pregnancy: patterns of weight gain, discordancy, and length of gestation. Am J Obstet Gynecol 1993;169:588.

58. Luke B, Gillespie B, Min SJ, et al. Critical periods of maternal weight gain: effect on twin birth weight. Am J Obstet Gynecol 1997;177:1055.

59. Moore TR, Iams JD, Creasy RK, et al. Diurnal and gestational patterns of uterine activity in normal human pregnancy. Obstet Gynecol 1994;83:517.

60. Komaromy B, Lampe L. The value of bed rest in twin pregnancies. Int J Gynecol Obstet 1977;15:262.

61. Jeffrey RL, Bowes WA, Delaney JJ. Role of bed rest in twin gestation. Obstet Gynecol 1974;43:822.

62. MacLennan AH, Green RC, O'Shea R, et al. Routine hospital admission in twin pregnancy between 26 and 30 weeks' gestation. Lancet 1990;335:267.

63. Crowther CA, Verkuyl DAA, Neilson JP, et al. The effects of hospitalization for rest on fetal growth, neonatal morbidity and length of gestation in twin pregnancy. Br J Obstet Gynaecol 1990;97:872.

64. Crowther CA. Hospitalization for bedrest in multiple pregnancy (Cochrane Review). In: The Cochrane Library, Issue 1, 1999. Oxford: Update Software.

65. Newman RB, Hamer C, Miller MC. Outpatient triplet management: a contemporary review. Am J Obstet Gynecol 1989;161:547.

66. Newman RB, Ellings J. Antepartum management of the

multiple gestation: the case for specialized care. Semin Perinatol 1995;19:387.

67. Holbrook RH, Falcon J, Herron M, et al. Evaluation of the weekly cervical examination in a preterm birth prevention program. Am J Perinatol 1987;4:240.

68. Bivins HA, Newman RB, Ellings JM, et al. Risk of antepartum cervical examination in multifetal pregnancies. Am J Obstet Gynecol 1993;169:22.

69. Houlton MCC, Marivate M, Philpott RH. Factors associated with preterm labor and changes in the cervix before labour in twin pregnancy. Br J Obstet Gynecol 1982;89:190.

70. Neilson JP, Verkuyl DAA, Crowther CA, Bannerman C. Preterm labor in twin pregnancies: prediction by cervical assessment. Obstet Gynecol 1988;72:719.

71. Newman RB, Godsey RK, Ellings JM, et al. Quantification of cervical change: relationship to preterm delivery in multifetal gestation. Am J Obstet Gynecol 1991;165:264.

72. Goldberg J, Newman RB, Rust PE. Interobserver reliability of digital and endovaginal ultrasonographic cervical length measurements. Am J Obstet Gynecol 1997;177:853.

73. Goldenberg RL, Iams JD, Miodovnik M, et al. The preterm birth prediction study: risk factors in twin gestations. Am J Obstet Gynecol 1996;175:1047.

74. Imseis HM, Albert TA, Iams JD. Identifying twin gestations at low risk for preterm birth with a transvaginal ultrasonographic cervical measurement at 24–26 weeks gestation. Am J Obstet Gynecol 1997;177:1149.

75. Fontenot MT, Read JA, Ulmer S, et al. Significance of cervical length by transvaginal sonography in twin gestation. Abstract. In: Am J Obstet Gynecol 1997;176:S10.

76. Newman RB, Gill PJ, Katz M. Uterine activity during pregnancy in ambulatory patients: comparison of singleton and twin gestations. Am J Obstet Gynecol 1986;154:530.

77. Knuppel RA, Lake MF, Watson DL, et al. Preventing preterm birth in twin gestation: home uterine activity monitoring and perinatal nursing support. Obstet Gynecol 1990;76:24S.

78. Dyson DC, Crites YM, Ray DA, et al. Prevention of preterm birth in high-risk patients: the role of education and provider contact versus home uterine monitoring. Am J Obstet Gynecol 1991;164:756.

79. Skjaerris J, Aberg A. Prevention of prematurity in twin pregnancy by orally administered terbutaline. Acta Obstet Gynecol Scand Suppl 1982;108:39.

80. O'Leary JA. Prophylactic tocolysis of twins. Am J Obstet Gynecol 1986;154:904.

81. O'Connor MC, Murphy H, Dalrymple IJ. Double blind trial of ritodrine and placebo in twin pregnancy. Br J Obstet Gynaecol 1979;86:706.

82. Ashworth MF, Spooner SF, Verkuyl DAA, et al. Failure to prevent preterm labour and delivery in twin pregnancy using prophylactic oral salbutamol. Br J Obstet Gynaecol 1990;97:878.

83. Roberts WE, Perry KG, Naef RW, et al. The irritable uterus: a risk factor for preterm birth? Am J Obstet Gynecol 1995;172:138.

84. Sinha DP, Nandalsumar VL, Brough AK, Beebujann MS. Relative cervical incompetence in twin pregnancy: as-

sessment and efficacy of cervical suture. Acta Genet Med Gemellol 1979;28:327.

85. Mordel N, Zajicek G, Benshushan A, et al. Elective suture of uterine cervix in triplets. Am J Perinatol 1993;10:14.

86. Michaels WH, Schreiber FR, Padgett RJ, et al. Ultrasound surveillance of the cervix in twin gestations: management of cervical incompetency. Obstet Gynecol 1991;78:739.

87. Guaschino S, Spinillo A, Stola E, Pesando PC. Growth retardation, size at birth and perinatal mortality in twin pregnancy. Int J Gynecol Obstet 1987;25:399.

88. Chitkara U, Berkowitz GS, Levine R, et al. Twin pregnancy: routine use of ultrasound examinations in the prenatal diagnosis of intrauterine growth retardation and discordant growth. Am J Perinatol 1985;2:49.

89. Storlazzi E, Vintzileos AM, Campbell WA, et al. Ultrasonic diagnosis of discordant fetal growth in twin gestations. Obstet Gynecol 1987;69:363.

90. Ananth CV, Vintzileos AM, Shen-Schwarz S, et al. Standards of birth weight in twin gestations stratified by placental chorionicity. Obstet Gynecol 1998;91:917.

91. Luke B, Minogue J, Witter FR. The role of fetal growth restriction and gestational age on length of hospital stay in twin infants. Obstet Gynecol 1993;81:949.

92. Moore TR, Piacquadio K. A prospective evaluation of fetal movement screening to reduce the incidence of antepartum fetal death. Am J Obstet Gynecol 1989;160:1075.

93. Patkos P, Boucher M, Broussard PM, et al. Factors influencing nonstress test results in multiple gestations. Am J Obstet Gynecol 1986;154:1107.

94. Bailey D, Flynn AM, Kelly J, O'Connor M. Antepartum fetal heart rate monitoring in multiple pregnancy. Br J Obstet Gynaecol 1980;87:561.

95. Devoe LD, Azor H. Simultaneous nonstress fetal heart rate testing in twin pregnancy. Obstet Gynecol 1981;58:450.

96. Blake GD, Knuppel RA, Ingardia CJ, et al. Evaluation of nonstress fetal heart rate testing in multiple gestations. Obstet Gynecol 1984;63:528.

97. Sherman SJ, Kovacs BW, Medearis AL, et al. Nonstress test assessment of twins. J Reprod Med 1992;37:804.

98. Sherer DM, Abramowicz JS, D'Amico ML, et al. Fetal vibratory acoustic stimulation in twin gestations with simultaneous fetal heart rate monitoring. Am J Obstet Gynecol 1991;164:1104.

99. Sherer DM, Nawrocki MN, Peco NE, et al. The occurrence of simultaneous fetal heart rate accelerations during nonstress testing. Obstet Gynecol 1990;76:817.

100. Manning FA, Baskett TF, Morrison I, Lange I. Fetal biophysical profile scoring: a prospective study in 1,184 high-risk patients. Am J Obstet Gynecol 1981;140:289.

101. Lodeiro JG, Vintzileos AM, Feinstein SJ, et al. Fetal biophysical profile in twin gestations. Obstet Gynecol 1986;67:824.

102. Watson WJ, Harlass FE, Menard MK, et al. Sonographic assessment of amniotic fluid in normal twin pregnancy. Am J Perinatol 1995;12:122.

103. Chau AC, Kjos SL, Kovacs BW. Ultrasonic measurement of amniotic fluid volume in normal diamniotic twin pregnancies. Am J Obstet Gynecol 1996;174:1003.

104. Porter TF, Dildy GA, Blanchard JR, et al. Normal values for amniotic fluid index during uncomplicated twin pregnancy. Obstet Gynecol 1996;87:699.

105. Magann EF, Chauhan SP, Whitworth NS, et al. The accuracy of summated amniotic fluid index in evaluating amniotic fluid volume in twin pregnancies. Am J Obstet Gynecol 1997;177:1041.

106. Devoe LD, Ware DJ. Antenatal assessment of twin gestation. Semin Perinatol 1995;19:413.

107. Leveno KJ, Quirk JG, Whalley PJ, et al. Fetal lung maturation in twin gestation. Am J Obstet Gynecol 1984; 148:405.

108. Winn HN, Romero R, Roberts A, et al. Comparison of fetal lung maturation in preterm singleton and twin pregnancies. Am J Perinatol 1992;9:326.

109. Friedman SA, Schiff E, Lu K, et al. Do twins mature earlier than singletons? Results from a matched cohort study. Am J Obstet Gynecol 1997;176:1193.

110. Rush R, Kierse M, Howat P, et al. Contribution of preterm delivery to perinatal mortality. BMJ 1976;2:965.

112. Keith LG, Cervantes A, Mazela J, et al. Multiple births and preterm delivery. Prenat Neonat Med 1998;3:125.

112. Rayburn W, Piehl E, Schork MA, Kirscht J. Intravenous ritodrine therapy: a comparison between twin and singleton gestations. Obstet Gynecol 1986;67:243.

113. Hales KA, Matthews JP, Rayburn WF, Atkinson BD. Intravenous magnesium sulfate for premature labor: comparison between twin and singleton gestations. Am J Perinatol 1995;12:7.

114. Lange IR, Harman CR, Ash KM, et al. Twin with hydramnios: treating premature labor at source. Am J Obstet Gynecol 1989;160:552.

115. Erkkola R, Ala-Mello S, Piiroinen O, et al. Growth discordancy in twin pregnancies: a risk factor not detected by measurements of the biparietal diameter. Obstet Gynecol 1985;66:203.

116. O'Brien WF, Knuppel RA, Scerbo JC, Rattan PK. Birth weight in twins: an analysis of discordancy and growth retardation. Obstet Gynecol 1986;67:483.

117. Cheung VYT, Bocking AD, Dasilva OP. Preterm discordant twins: what birthweight difference is significant. Am J Obstet Gynecol 1995;172:955.

118. Hill LM, Guzick D, Chenevey P, et al. The sonographic assessment of twin growth discordancy. Obstet Gynecol 1994;84:501.

119. Caravello JW, Chauhan SP, Morrison JC, et al. Sonographic examination does not predict twin growth discordance accurately. Obstet Gynecol 1997;89:529.

120. Sebire NJ, D'Ercole C, Soares W, et al. Intertwin disparity in fetal size in monochorionic and dichorionic pregnancies. Obstet Gynecol 1998;91:82.

121. Blickstein I, Weissman A. Birth weight discordancy in male-first and female-first pairs of unlike-sexed twins. Am J Obstet Gynecol 1990;162:661.

122. Blickstein I, Shoham-Schwartz Z, Lancet M. Growth discordancy in appropriate for gestational age, term twins. Obstet Gynecol 1988;72:582.

123. Talbot GT, Goldstein RF, Nesbitt T, et al. Is size discordancy an indication for delivery of preterm twins? Am J Obstet Gynecol 1997;177:1050.

124. Danskin F, Nielson JP. Twin to twin transfusion syndrome: what are appropriate diagnostic criteria? Am J Obstet Gynecol 1989;161:365.

125. Bruner JP, Rosemond RL. Twin-to-twin transfusion syndrome: a subset of the twin oligohydramnios-polyhydramnios sequence. Am J Obstet Gynecol 1993; 169:925.

126. Fries MH, Goldstein RB, Kilpatrick SJ, et al. The role of velamentous cord insertion in the etiology of twin-twin transfusion syndrome. Obstet Gynecol 1993:81:569.

127. Saunders NJ, Snijders RJM, Nicolaides KH. Therapeutic amniocentesis in twin-twin transfusion syndrome appearing in the second trimester of pregnancy. Am J Obstet Gynecol 1992;166:820.

128. Nores J, Athanassiou A, Elkadry E, et al. Gender differences in twin-twin transfusion syndrome. Obstet Gynecol 1997;90:580.

129. Gaziano EP, Knox GE, Bendel RP, et al. Is pulsed Doppler velocimetry useful in the management of multiple-gestation pregnancies? Am J Obstet Gynecol 1991; 164:1426.

130. Giles WB, Trudinger BJ, Cook CM, Connelly AJ. Doppler umbilical studies in the twin-twin transfusion syndrome. Obstet Gynecol 1990;76:1097.

131. Elliot JP. Amniocentesis for twin-twin transfusion. Contemp OB-GYN 1992;Aug:30.

132. Cheschier NC, Seeds JW. Polyhydramnios and oligohydramnios in twin gestations. Obstet Gynecol 1988; 71:882.

133. Elliott JP, Urig MA, Clewell WH. Aggressive therapeutic amniocentesis for treatment of twin-twin transfusion syndrome. Obstet Gynecol 1991;77:537.

134. Reisner DP, Mahony BS, Petty CN, et al. Stuck twin syndrome: outcome in thirty-seven consecutive cases. Am J Obstet Gynecol 1993;169:991.

135. Dennis LG, Winkler CL. Twin-to-twin transfusion syndrome: aggressive therapeutic amniocentesis. Am J Obstet Gynecol 1997;177:342.

136. De Lia JE, Kuhlmann RS, Harstad TW, Cruikshank DP. Fetoscopic laser ablation of placental vessels in severe previable twin-twin transfusion syndrome. Am J Obstet Gynecol 1995;172:1202.

137. Ville Y, Hecher K, Gagnon A, et al. Endoscopic laser coagulation in the management of severe twin-to-twin transfusion syndrome. Br J Obstet Gynecol 1998; 105:446.

138. Watson WA, Valea FA, Seeds JW. Sonographic evaluation of growth discordance and chorionicity in twin gestation. Am J Perinatol 1991;8:342.

139. Aisenbrey GA, Catanzarite VA, Hurley TJ, et al. Monoamniotic and pseudomonoamniotic twins: sonographic diagnosis, detection of cord entanglement, and obstetric management. Obstet Gynecol 1995;86:218.

140. Carr SR, Aronson MP, Coustan DR. Survival rates in monoamniotic twins do not decrease after 30 weeks gestation. Am J Obstet Gynecol 1990;163:719.

141. Tessen JA, Zlatnik FJ. Monoamniotic twins: a retrospective controlled study. Obstet Gynecol 1991;77:832.

142. Rodis JF, McIlveen PF, Egan JFX, et al. Monoamniotic twins: improved perinatal survival with accurate prenatal diagnosis and antepartum fetal surveillance. Am J Obstet Gynecol 1997;177:1046.

143. Pretorius DH, Leopold GR, Moore TR, et al. Acardiac twin: report of Doppler sonography. J Ultrasound Med 1988;7:413.

144. Moore TR, Gale S, Benirschke K. Perinatal outcome of forty-nine pregnancies complicated by acardiac twinning. Am J Obstet Gynecol 1990;163:907.

145. Platt LD, DeVore GR, Bieniarz A, et al. Antenatal diagnosis of acephalus acardia: a proposed management scheme. Am J Obstet Gynecol 1983;146:857.

146. Ash K, Harman CR, Gritter H. TRAP sequence—successful outcome with indomethacin treatment. Obstet Gynecol 1990;76:960.

147. Arias F, Sunderji S, Gimpelson R, Colton E. Treatment of acardiac twinning. Obstet Gynecol 1998;91:818.

148. Evans MI, Dommergues M, Wapner RJ, et al. Efficacy of transabdominal multifetal pregnancy reduction: collaborative experience among the world's largest centers. Obstet Gynecol 1993;82:61.

149. Malone FD, Craigo SD, Chelmow D, D'Alton ME. Outcome of twin gestations complicated by a single anomalous fetus. Obstet Gynecol 1996;88:1.

150. Alexander JM, Ramus R, Cox SM, Gilstrap LC. Outcome of twin gestations with a single anomalous fetus. Am J Obstet Gynecol 1997;177:849.

151. Lipitz S, Meizner I, Yagel S, et al. Expectant management of twin pregnancies discordant for anencephaly. Obstet Gynecol 1995;86:969.

152. Carlson NJ, Towers CV. Multiple gestation complicated by the death of one fetus. Obstet Gynecol 1989;73:685.

153. Cherouny PH, Hoskins IA, Johnson TRB, Niebyl JR. Multiple pregnancy with late death of one fetus. Obstet Gynecol 1989;74:318.

154. Enbom JA. Twin pregnancy with intrauterine death of one twin. Am J Obstet Gynecol 1985;152:424.

155. Kilby MD, Govind A, O'Brien PMS. Outcome of twin pregnancies complicated by a single intrauterine death: a comparison with viable twin pregnancies. Obstet Gynecol 1994;84:107.

156. Okamura K, Murotsuki J, Tanigawara S, et al. Funipuncture for evaluation of hematologic and coagulation indices in the surviving twin following co-twin's death. Obstet Gynecol 1994;83:975.

157. Mastrobattista JM, Skupski DW, Monga M, et al. The rate of severe preeclampsia is increased in triplet as compared to twin gestations. Am J Perinatol 1997;14:263.

158. Coonrod DV, Hickok DE, Zhu K, et al. Risk factors for preeclampsia in twin pregnancies: a population-based cohort study. Obstet Gynecol 1995;85:645.

159. Caspi E, Raziel A, Sherman D, et al. Prevention of pregnancy-induced hypertension in twins by early administration of low-dose aspirin: a preliminary report. Am J Reprod Immunol 1994;31:19.

160. Luke B. Reducing fetal deaths in multiple births: optimal birth weights and gestational ages of infants of twin and triplet births. Acta Genet Med Gemellol 1996;45:333.

161. Stone J, Bianco A, Lockwood CJ, et al. Does the morbidity of twin gestations after 36 weeks increase with advancing gestational age? Prenat Neonat Med 1998;3:235.

162. Divon MY, Marin MJ, Pollack RN, et al. Twin gestation: fetal presentation as a function of gestational age. Am J Obstet Gynecol 1993;168:1500.

163. Friedman EA, Sachtleben MR. The effect of uterine overdistention on labor. I. Multiple pregnancy. Obstet Gynecol 1964;23:164.

164. Adams DM, Chervenak FA. Intrapartum management of twin gestation. Clin Obstet Gynecol 1990;33:52.

165. Rayburn WF, Lavin JP, Miodovnik M, Varner MW. Multiple gestation: time interval between delivery of the first and second twins. Obstet Gynecol 1984;63:502.

166. Miller DA, Mullin P, Hou D, Paul RH. Vaginal birth after cesarean section in twin gestation. Am J Obstet Gynecol 1996;175:194.

167. Chervenak FA, Johnson RE, Youcha S, et al. Intrapartum management of twin gestation. Obstet Gynecol 1985;65:119.

168. Zhang J, Bowes WA, Grey TW, McMahon MJ. Twin delivery and neonatal and infant mortality: a population based study. Obstet Gynecol 1996;88:593.

169. Cetrulo CL. The controversy of mode of delivery in twins: the intrapartum management of twin gestation (part I). Semin Perinatol 1986;10:39.

170. Acker D, Lieberman M, Holbrook H, et al. Delivery of the second twin. Obstet Gynecol 1982;59:710.

171. Chervenak FA, Johnson RE, Berkowitz RL, Hobbins JC. Intrapartum external version of the second twin. Obstet Gynecol 1983;62:160.

172. Christian SS, Brady K, Read JA, Kopelman JR. Vaginal breech delivery: a five year prospective evaluation of a protocol using computed tomographic pelvimetry. Am J Obstet Gynecol 1990;163:848.

173. Gocke SE, Nageotte M, Garite T, et al. Management of the nonvertex second twin: primary cesarean section, external version, or primary breech extraction. Am J Obstet Gynecol 1989;161:111.

174. Wells SR, Thorp JM, Bowes WA Jr. Management of the nonvertex second twin. Surg Gynecol Obstet 1991;172:383.

175. Chauhan SP, Roberts WE, McLaren RA, et al. Delivery of the nonvertex second twin: breech extraction versus external cephalic version. Am J Obstet Gynecol 1995;173:1015.

176. Davison L, Easterling TR, Jackson JC, Benedetti TJ. Breech extraction of low-birth-weight second twins: can cesarean be justified? Am J Obstet Gynecol 1992;166:497.

177. Chauhan SP, Washburne JF, Martin JN, et al. Intrapartum assessment by house staff of birth weight among twins. Obstet Gynecol 1993;82:523.

178. Alexander JM, Gilstrap LC, Cox SM, Ramin SM. The relationship of infection to method of delivery in twin pregnancy. Am J Obstet Gynecol 1997;177:1063.

179. Blickstein I, Weissman A, Ben-Hur H, et al. Vaginal delivery of breech-vertex twins. J Reprod Med 1993;38:879.

180. Redick LF. Anesthesia for twin delivery. Clin Perinatol 1988;15:107.

Chapter 10

Isoimmunization

Richard O'Shaughnessy
Melanie Kennedy

Five Key Points

- The most common cause of fetal red-cell isoimmunization is anti-D. Immunization typically occurs as a result of a previous pregnancy.

- Isoimmunized patients should be monitored with serial antibody titers, ultrasound examination, and amniocentesis for determination of amniotic fluid bilirubin concentration (ΔOD450). Cordocentesis is indicated when ΔOD450 concentrations are in high zone II or zone III on the Liley graph.

- Hydropic fetuses should be delivered or treated with intravascular transfusion.

- Rh-immune globulin is highly effective in preventing anti-D isoimmunization.

- Alloimmune thrombocytopenia is diagnosed by direct assessment of the fetal platelet count. The disorder is best treated by fetal platelet transfusion and administration of intravenous immune globulin to the mother.

Maternal isoantibodies directed against fetal red cells and platelets can cause significant fetal disease. These antibodies, derived from prior exposure to foreign red cells and platelets, can induce fetal anemia and thrombocytopenia, respectively. Effective therapeutic strategies are available, and the skilled obstetrician should be knowledgeable in the diagnosis and management of isoimmune fetal anemia and alloimmune fetal thrombocytopenia. The term isoimmunization is equivalent to the term alloimmunization; by convention, we refer to isoimmune fetal anemia and alloimmune thrombocytopenia. Both processes are mediated by isoantibodies (alloantibodies). This chapter will focus on clinical approaches to detection and treatment of these important problems.

ISOIMMUNE FETAL ANEMIA (ERYTHROBLASTOSIS FETALIS–HEMOLYTIC DISEASE OF THE NEWBORN) (EBF–HDN)

Definition

The term erythroblastosis fetalis was introduced by Diamond et al. in 1932 and refers to the fetal pathologic finding of an increase in circulating immature red cell forms as the fetus strives to maintain a normal hemoglobin concentration in the face of unrelenting hemolytic anemia.[1] At that time, investigators were not aware of the isoimmune nature of the problem, but in the intervening years, the immunologic nature of this disease became evident, and we are aware now that the fetal anemia is due to the destruction of fetal red cells by maternal isoantibodies that transverse the placenta. [2] Erythroblastosis fetalis (EBF) refers to the fetal disease; hemolytic disease of the newborn (HDN) refers to the same disease during the newborn period.

Types of EBF-HDN

The most common type of erythroblastosis fetalis is due to ABO incompatibility between mother and fetus. This is almost always a very mild form of erythroblastosis fetalis. It usually occurs in type O mothers with hemolysis in the type A or B fetus due to the placental transport of naturally occurring anti-A or anti-B antibodies. There are isolated case reports of severe fetal anemia and hydrops fetalis due to ABO incompatibility, but this is not a condition that generally causes severe fetal disease and does not require antenatal detection or monitoring.[3] This self-limited disease is primarily a problem for the neonatal practitioner when the newborn demonstrates jaundice.

The severest form of erythroblastosis fetalis is due to Rh isoimmunization, which refers to an aggressive form of fetal hemolytic anemia due to antibodies directed against the D antigen on the red cell. The presence or absence of the D antigen confers Rh positivity or negativity, respectively. The D antigen is the most immunogenic of the red-cell antigens and induces the most severe form of fetal hemolytic anemia. This severe disease led to the development of passive immunization with Rh immune globulin in the late 1960s.

The other antigens expressed by the Rh locus (C, c, E, e), in addition to many other red-cell antigens, are sufficiently immunogenic to induce clinically significant fetal hemolysis. In most cases the fetal hemolytic anemia is not as severe as in Rh disease. Nonetheless, very severe forms of erythroblastosis fetalis due to isoantibodies other than anti-D can occur and require careful monitoring. More than 40 other red-cell antigens can induce maternal isoantibodies and the hemolytic response of erythroblastosis fetalis. Several of these incompatibilities have been associated with disease that is severe enough to cause intrauterine death[4] (Table 10-1). Anti-D, anti-Kell, anti-c anti-Fy^a, and anti-Jk^a are the most problematic in causing severe disease.[5,6]

Cause

The cause of maternal isoimmunization and subsequent erythroblastosis fetalis is maternal exposure to foreign red cells, except in the case of naturally occurring alloantibodies of the ABO system. The antibody response that occurs following exposure to foreign red cells leads to a lifelong isoimmunization.

The leading cause of maternal isoimmunization is fetal–maternal hemorrhage through the placenta. The clinically obvious opportunities for fetal–maternal hemorrhage include delivery, spontaneous and therapeutic abortion, and amniocentesis. Other traumatic events can lead to disruption of the fetal–maternal interface at the placenta with resultant fetal-to-maternal hemorrhage. Bowman and colleagues[7] found the presence of fetal–maternal hemorrhage in 75% of pregnant women when assessed by the Kleihauer–Betke technique. Using more sensitive flow cytometric techniques, fetal–maternal hemorrhage

---

TABLE 10-1
BLOOD GROUP SYSTEMS ASSOCIATED WITH EBF-HDN

Blood Group System	Antigens
Rhesus	D, C, c, E, e
Kell	K, k, Ko, Kp^a, Kp^b, Js^a, Js^b
Duffy	Fy^a, Fy^b, Fy^3
Kidd	Jk^a, Jk^b, Jk^3
MNS	M, N, S, s, U, Mi^a, Mt^a, Vx, Mur, Hil, Hut
Lutheran	Lu^a, Lu^b
Diego	Di^a, Di^b
Xg	Xga
P	PP$_1$p^k(Tj^a)
Public antigens	Yt^a, Yt^b, Lan, En^a, Ge, Jr^a, Co^a, Co^{a-b-}
Private antigens	Batty, Becker, Berrens, Biles, Evans, Gonzales, Good, Heibel, Hunt, Jobbins, Radin, Rm, Ven, Wright^a, Wright^b, Zd

Modified from American College of Obstetricians and Gynecologists.[6]

is detected in nearly all pregnancies.[8] In their study, Bowman et al. discovered that the frequency and volume of fetal–maternal hemorrhage increases as the pregnancy progresses.[7] In 60% of cases the fetal–maternal hemorrhage was less than 0.1 ml. In only 0.25% of cases was the hemorrhage greater than 30 ml. Of importance was the fact the fetal–maternal hemorrhage was not invariably associated with clinically evident events in the mother. Thus, silent fetal–maternal hemorrhages occur throughout pregnancy. This important observation has led to the use of Rh immunoglobulin prophylaxis in all Rh-negative women during pregnancy instead of only those with obvious opportunities for fetal–maternal bleeding.

The leading cause of isoimmunization for antibodies other than anti-D is donor blood transfusion. When a woman in her reproductive years receives a donor unit of red cells, she accepts approximately a 1% risk that she will be exposed to a foreign red-cell antigen that will induce an isoimmune response. Standard blood banking techniques do not include matching for most red-cell antigens that can induce significant isoimmunization. The risk of subsequent EBF-HDN is much higher if her sexual partner or one of his blood relatives is the donor.[9,10] Another potential cause for EBF is exposure to foreign red cells through shared needles by drug abusers.

Incidence

When Rh-negative women were prospectively studied (prior to the availability of Rh immune globulin [RhIg] immunoprophylaxis), approximately 16% of those who carried and delivered an Rh-positive fetus had active immunization.[11] The majority of that risk was found to occur at the time of delivery, the time at which most fetal–maternal hemorrhage occurs. Approximately half of the cases (8%) of isoimmunization is detected by 6 months postpartum, but 8% may not be detected until the onset of the next pregnancy. Approximately 2% of the cases of isoimmunization occur during the incident pregnancy, usually after 28 weeks of gestation. Clinically significant maternal red-cell isoimmunization is therefore rare during the first pregnancy. It usually requires exposure over one or more pregnancies to provide a significant opportunity for the isoimmunization to occur. However, there is a great degree of individual variation in responsiveness to antigenic exposure in the development of active immunization. Some women may form high antibody titers in response to immeasurably small amounts of fetal–maternal hemorrhage in the first pregnancy. Others may not form active antibody even when exposed to a large volume of foreign red cells, such as might occur with inadvertent transfusion of mismatched blood.[12]

ABO incompatibility between mother and fetus confers a degree of protection to the mother in reducing the risk of alloimmunization.[11] The fetal cells in the mother's blood are destroyed by the maternal ABO antibodies prior to their detection as Rh-incompatible.

The frequency of Rh isoimmunization in the general obstetric population continues to be a point of significance for the clinician. The introduction of Rh immune globulin has significantly reduced the number of cases of Rh disease from approximately 45 cases per 10,000 live births in 1968 to a current level of approximately 10 cases per 10,000 live births.[13] While the use of Rh immune globulin has had a significant impact in reducing the frequency of this problem, a gap in the use of this protective passive immunization, especially in women experiencing miscarriage, has allowed persistence of this significant problem.

Isoantibodies Other Than Anti-D

Isoantibodies other than anti-D are associated with significant erythroblastosis fetalis. They are detected by the same mechanism of screening for alloantibodies in the serum of all pregnant women. Isoantibodies of the immunoglobulin class G can cross the placenta, and, in some instances, cause fetal hemolytic anemia. It is important for the clinician to use a laboratory that will give a reliable interpretation of the routine antibody screen. A positive antibody screen may indicate the possibility of significant disease, and it is important for the laboratory to notify the clinician of the presence of significant isoantibodies. Table 10-1 lists the isoantibodies other than anti-D that are associated with fetal hemolytic anemia. Nearly 50% of the new isoimmunizations seen at our program are due to antibodies other than anti-D.

In many cases a positive maternal antibody screen is not associated with fetal hemolytic disease. This situation occurs when the maternal antibody response is preponderantly IgM, and the antibodies cannot cross the placenta. A common cause of a positive maternal antibody screen that does not result in fetal hemolytic anemia is the anti-Lewis antibodies (anti-Le-^{a} and anti-Le^b), which are generally IgM. Again, the reference laboratory should be consulted for definition of the antibody and its potential association with EBF.

Fetal Effects of Erythroblastosis Fetalis

The fetus responds to the presence of red-cell isoantibodies with a hemolytic anemia. These antibodies attach to the fetal red cell, leading to destruction via the reticuloendothelial system. The hemolytic anemia can vary from mild to severe. In most cases the fetus can compensate by generating new red cells. Our experience and that of others[14] indicates that in approximately 80% of cases, the fetus can respond to the hemolysis by increasing and maintaining red-cell production and maintain a normal hemoglobin.

Approximately 20% of fetuses cannot compensate for the hemolytic anemia, and significant anemia develops. Failure to compensate depends somewhat on the antibody involved and the fetal reserve. The most aggressive of the isoimmunizations is due to Rh-D antigen. Other forms of fetal hemolytic anemia often associated with fetal decompensation include isoimmunization to anti-c and anti-Kell. However, many isoantibodies can induce significant erythroblastosis fetalis and require careful monitoring.

The fetal ability to respond is highly variable. It is not clear what leads to fetal failure in utero. The fetus recruits medullary and extramedullary sites for red-cell regeneration, but in some cases the fetal response is insufficient. Data suggest that some component of the fetal anemia with Kell immunization is due to suppression of the active bone marrow response to the hemolytic anemia. Vaughan and colleagues found that serum from 22 women with anti-Kell antibodies inhibited the growth of Kell-positive erythroid progenitor cells from cord blood and concluded that erythroid suppression rather than hemolysis is the predominant mechanism producing fetal anemia in Kell-isoimmunized pregnancies.[15] Data from our institution suggest that the fetal anemia in Kell isoimmunization is, nonetheless, largely a hemolytic process.[16]

Fetuses who decompensate tend to demonstrate a common pathophysiology in utero, usually ending with hydrops fetalis. This dramatic finding is evident on ultrasound and to the examining eye of the clinician following birth. It is manifested by a diffuse tissue edema secondary to severe fetal anemia. The hydropic change includes widespread tissue edema, ascites, and pericardial and pleural effusions, in addition to placentomegaly and polyhydramnios. Data from Nicolaides et al.[17] and Forestier et al.[18] indicate that fetuses affected with erythroblastosis fetalis demonstrate hydropic change in utero when the fetal hemoglobin deficit reaches approximately 7 g/dl. The time course for the fetus affected with erythroblastosis fetalis to decompensate and hydrops to develop in utero is not known.

The Neonatal Effects of EBF-HDN

After the newborn is delivered, the separation from the maternal circulation leads to potential additional danger due to accumulation of the hemolytic pigment bilirubin. In utero, the placenta serves to clear unconjugated bilirubin, but ex utero this hemolytic product can accumulate and cause irreversible brain damage (kernicterus). Exchange transfusion and phototherapy are available to the neonatologist to correct hyperbilirubinemia; exchange transfusion also can normalize neonatal hemoglobin and reduce antibody concentration.

Diagnosis

The diagnosis of erythroblastosis fetalis requires determination of major blood group, Rh type, and antibody screen on all pregnant patients as part of routine prenatal laboratory testing. If the mother has a positive antibody screen, the antibody must be identified to determine potential for causing erythroblastosis fetalis. If a maternal antibody is associated with erythroblastosis fetalis, and if paternity is certain, the father's blood type should be obtained. The father determines the fetal antigenic incompatibility; ascertaining the paternal type can be helpful to the clinician to assess the risk of significant fetal disease. If the father is heterozygous for the antigen in question, there is a 50% chance that the fetus is unaffected. If paternity is not certain, it is best to assume that the fetus is affected.

Fetal Blood Typing

Fetal cells from amniocentesis or chorionic villus sampling can be tested by the polymerase chain reaction (PCR) to detect the genes that encode the antigenic components of the Rh locus, the Kell antigens (K1, K2), the Duffy antigens (Fy^a, Fy^b), and the Kidd antigens (Jk^a, Jk^h) and thereby determine the fetal blood type.[20-25] If the fetus proves to be antigen-negative, then it will be unaffected by the maternal isoantibody. Users of this technique must be aware that the presence of a gene does not necessarily correspond to the expression of the encoded antigen on the cell surface. Also, new variant alleles may not be identified with these assays. Nonetheless, fetal blood genotyping represents a safe and reliable way to determine fetal blood type in most cases. Cordocentesis, safe after 18 weeks of gestation, must be done at this time for typing red-cell antigens.

Fetal antigen typing by sampling fetal cells in the mother's blood has been done in a research setting but is technically demanding and not yet available clinically.[26] In a subsequent study, Lo and colleagues[27] extracted fetal DNA from maternal plasma of 57 RhD-negative pregnant women. Thirty-nine fetuses were RhD-positive; 18 were RhD-negative. The results of RhD PCR analysis of maternal plasma obtained in the second and third trimester were completely concordant with the fetal blood type determined by serologic methods on cord blood. Analysis of maternal blood in the first trimester was not so accurate. The authors concluded that fetal RhD genotyping can be done rapidly and reliably with analysis of maternal plasma beginning in the second trimester.

Monitoring for Erythroblastosis Fetalis

When a diagnosis of erythroblastosis fetalis is made, it is important to monitor the fetus in utero, recognizing that in most cases the fetus will compensate for the hemolytic anemia. Monitoring can ensure that the fetus is responding and compensating for the hemolytic disease. The fetus should be monitored in conjunction with laboratories and clinicians who have experience with these rare conditions. In most cases, the primary care doctor can consult with a perinatologist and co-treat the patient.

The primary monitoring techniques available to the clinician include the maternal serologic response, measuring the concentration of isoantibodies in the mother's blood; amniocentesis, measuring the fetal hemolytic pigment in amniotic fluid; and cordocentesis, measuring the fetal hemolytic indexes directly. Some have advocated exclusive monitoring with cordocentesis since the fetal hematocrit, reticulocyte count, direct antiglobulin test, and bilirubin level can be measured directly, giving a thorough, if momentary, assessment of the fetal condition in utero.[28] This information, while valuable, is obtained at a risk of approximately 1% of fetal death associated with the cordocentesis procedure. Because of the comparatively high risk of cordocentesis, we favor primary monitoring with less risky, indirect testing.

Other noninvasive techniques are available to the clinician to monitor the fetus in utero. The most important is ultrasound. Ultrasound defines the presence of hydropic changes, which indicate life-threatening fetal decompensation. Ultrasound markers may indicate impending fetal hydrops in utero, but not reliably so. Cardiomegaly, polyhydramnios, increased placental thickness, increased liver size, increased diameter of the umbilical vein, and pericardial effusion are markers that anticipate fetal failure.[29] Unfortunately, however, monitoring with ultrasound imaging of the fetus alone is not consistently sensitive in predicting fetal hydropic decompensation in utero.[17]

Other biophysical measurements can be valuable to the clinician. Doppler velocimetry, especially measuring the velocity of blood flow in the middle cerebral artery or splenic artery of the fetus, has shown significant promise in the noninvasive diagnosis of fetal anemia.[30,31] Biophysical scoring, maternal perception of daily fetal movement, and, finally, nonstress testing are also valuable. The technique of nonstress testing may demonstrate a sinusoidal pattern in fetuses affected by severe hemolytic anemia[32,33] (Figure 10-1). All noninvasive monitoring techniques described above can be used by the clinician to assess fetal compensation in utero.[34] These techniques are in addition to the primary monitoring tools of serology, amniocentesis, and cordocentesis, which have been proven effective over time. In addition, serology and amniocentesis offer the advantage that they can often be performed by the primary care physician with the samples sent for analysis and interpretation to the laboratory of the consultant. The monitoring techniques have been developed primarily for the management of RhD isoimmunization, but are useful, also, for monitoring of EBF caused by other isoantibodies.[16,19, 35-37]

Data from our institution indicate that anti-Kell anemia is largely a hemolytic process and that traditional monitoring methods of antibody titer and amniotic fluid spectrophotometry developed for Rh isoimmunization are effective in monitoring Kell

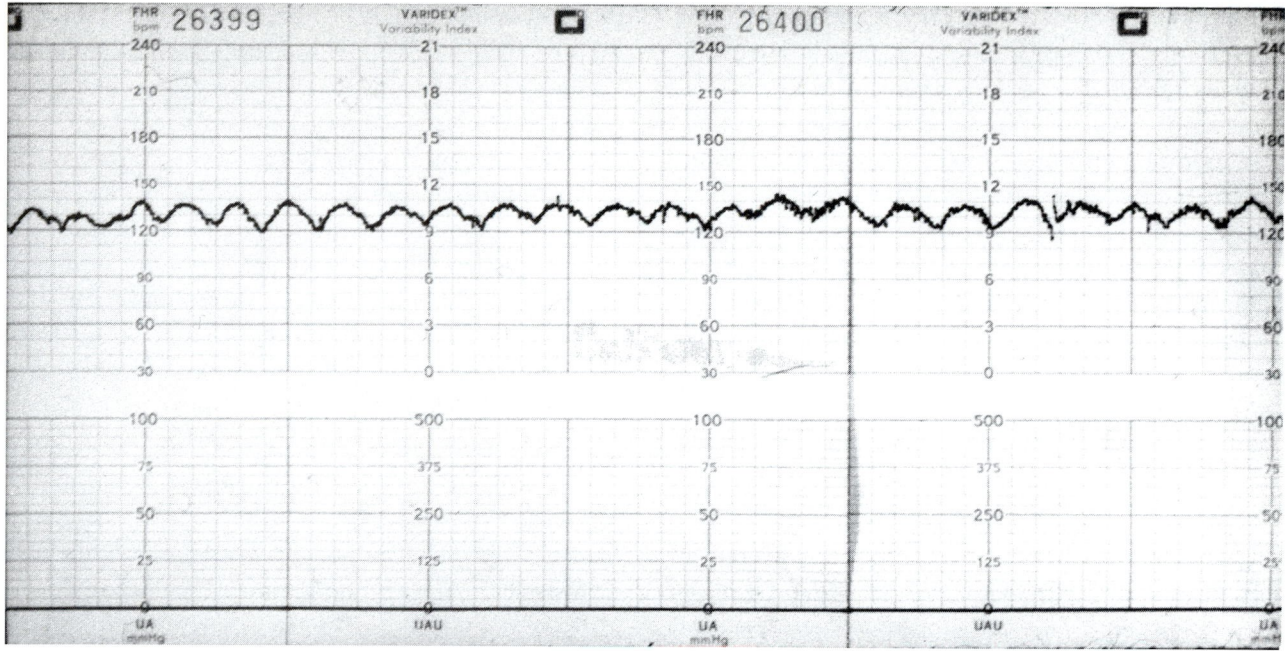

Figure 10-1 Sinusoidal fetal heart rate pattern noted on nonstress monitoring of fetal heart rate at 34 weeks of gestation in a pregnancy complicated by RhD isoimmunization. Delivery by cesarean section followed shortly thereafter. Cord hemoglobin at birth was 4.0 g/dl.

isoimmunization. In 21 Kell-isoimmunized pregnancies with Kell-positive fetuses, all of the severely affected fetuses had maternal titers ≥1/32. The affected fetuses had higher cord bilirubin and demonstrated higher amniotic fluid change in optical density at 450 nm (ΔOD450) than unaffected fetuses.[16] Nevertheless, it appears that some component of the fetal anemia in Kell isoimmunization is due to suppression of hematopoiesis rather than hemolysis, and special care should be taken in monitoring these cases.[15,19,39]

History of Erythroblastosis Fetalis

In the absence of a prior pregnancy with a fetus or newborn affected with EBF, monitoring should begin with maternal serologic evaluation and proceed to amniocentesis or cordocentesis only if the antibody titer becomes higher than threshold values. If there is a history of an affected pregnancy, then the history must be taken into account in anticipating the severity of disease and determining appropriate methods for monitoring. Prior affected pregnancies may be indicated by history of hydrops fetalis or need for intrauterine transfusion (IUT), or more mild disease with jaundice or anemia in the newborn.

If the prior pregnancies include severely affected fetuses or newborns (i.e., hydrops fetalis, need for IUT), then that degree of severity should be anticipated in the current pregnancy. If hydrops has occurred in the past, there is a 90% chance that it will recur in subsequent pregnancies, assuming that the fetus is antigen-positive.[14] If prior pregnancies include mild or moderate disease, then EBF may recur at the same degree or become progressively worse in subsequent pregnancies.

When there is a history of prior EBF, fetal monitoring must usually begin with amniocentesis. The antibody titer is often not reflective of the severity of fetal disease in subsequent immunized pregnancies. Only if the history is of mild disease, with one of the more benign antibodies (e.g., anti-M) in low titer (≤1/4) can titer be relied on to reflect the severity of fetal disease in subsequent affected pregnancies. In most cases it is safer to proceed to the next level of indirect fetal assessment, amniocentesis.

Serology

The immune response of the pregnant woman affected by erythroblastosis fetalis can be monitored by the measurement of the antibody concentration in her serum.[40] Using the indirect antiglobulin (Coombs) technique, the laboratory technologist can detect the presence of IgG isoantibodies. The antibody concentration can be measured using the titration technique, in which serial dilutions of maternal serum are mixed with appropriate red cells to determine the highest dilution of maternal serum associated with visible agglutination of the red cells. Other methods are available to more precisely quantitate maternal antibody concentration but are not routinely employed in the United States.

The titer of antibody in the mother's blood is generally proportional to the severity of fetal disease. Allen et al.[41] found a linear correlation between maternal anti-D antibody titer and the likelihood of fetal death due to EBF. Moreover, they found that history of a severely affected fetus in a prior pregnancy, when combined with antibody titer in the current pregnancy, gave a more powerful prediction of fetal death than antibody titer alone. In a study of 260 Rh-immunized pregnancies reported by Bowell et al.,[42] the maternal anti-D titer, similarly, correlated inversely with cord hemoglobin and directly with cord bilirubin at birth. Finally, Nicolaides and Rodeck found a negative correlation between maternal antibody concentration and fetal hemoglobin obtained by cordocentesis in 237 pregnancies with Rhesus isoimmunization.[43] They also found that, when maternal anti-D antibody concentration was less than 15 IU/ml, there were no cases of severe fetal anemia.

The antibody titer, then, is a marker of fetal disease severity, albeit a very indirect one. The usefulness of antibody titration has been questioned.[44] The antibody titer measures only disease activity at that time. Serial antibody titers must usually be done at monthly intervals to provide an adequate ongoing picture of disease activity. The antibody level is most indicative of fetal status in the first immunized pregnancy. In subsequent pregnancies, the maternal antibody response may not be as informative. As stated previously, if there is a history of prior affected newborns with anemia or jaundice, or history of a severely affected fetus (e.g., hydrops fetalis, stillborn, required fetal transfusions), then antibody titer should not be relied on to monitor fetal well-being. In the first immunized pregnancy, as long as the antibody titer remains less than 1/32, the so-called "critical titer," nothing else needs to be done to monitor the fetus.

If the antibody titer is ≥1/32, or if there is a history of an affected newborn, then the titer of antibody cannot be relied on to predict the severity of fetal disease. In these cases, amniocentesis is needed.

The concept of a critical titer represents a screening cutoff point and has been useful primarily for serologic monitoring of anti-D isoimmunization.[45] The literature does not clearly support serologic monitoring for other red-cell isoimmunization, but our experience and that of others has been that antibody titer correlates with the severity of fetal disease even in non-Rh isoimmunization.[16,19,35-37,47]

Other laboratory assays of maternal serum have been used, still primarily in a research setting, to monitor fetal disease severity through maternal blood testing.[48,50,51] The antibody-dependent cell-mediated cytotoxicity (ADCC) and monocyte monolayer assays incorporate marker red cells with maternal serum in a cellular response assay. These tests currently are not clinically useful in monitoring fetal condition.[52]

Amniocentesis

Amniocentesis measures the concentration of bilirubin-like hemolytic pigments using scanning spectrophotometry with measurement of $\Delta OD450$. The magnitude of deviation from the base line measures the concentration of hemolytic pigment and is another indirect marker of disease severity. Contaminants in the amniotic fluid such as blood or meconium can interfere with an interpretation of amniotic fluid spectrophotometry. Polyhydramnios may dilute the hemolytic pigment and interfere with determining the relationship of $\Delta OD450$ to fetal anemia.

Liley correlated $\Delta OD450$ with cord hemoglobin at birth in 101 pregnancies and found that amniotic fluid analysis reliably separated severely affected fetuses from those less severely affected.[53,54] His data were valid as early as 28 weeks of gestation (Figure 10-2). Like Liley, we used the graphic display of $\Delta OD450$ versus gestational age and found that the amniotic fluid concentration of hemolytic pigment reliably separated the anemic from the nonanemic fetus, with an area of overlap in between, as early as 20 weeks of gestation.[55] We used a modified Liley graph developed by MacPherson and colleagues[56] based on data from Ohio State University in the 1960s (Figure 10-3). In 91 women with nonhydropic fetuses in utero affected with EBF measured from

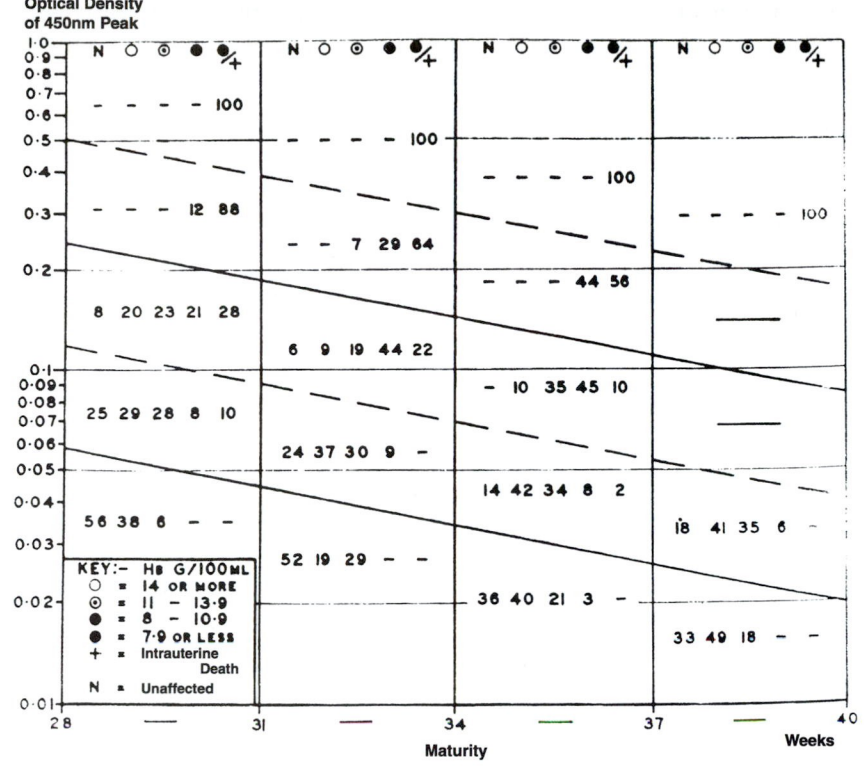

Figure 10-2 Percentage probability of the various grades of affliction for the peak size in a single specimen. Amniotic fluid spectrophotometry correlated with severity of disease in 101 pregnancies. *Reprinted from Liley,[54] with permission.*

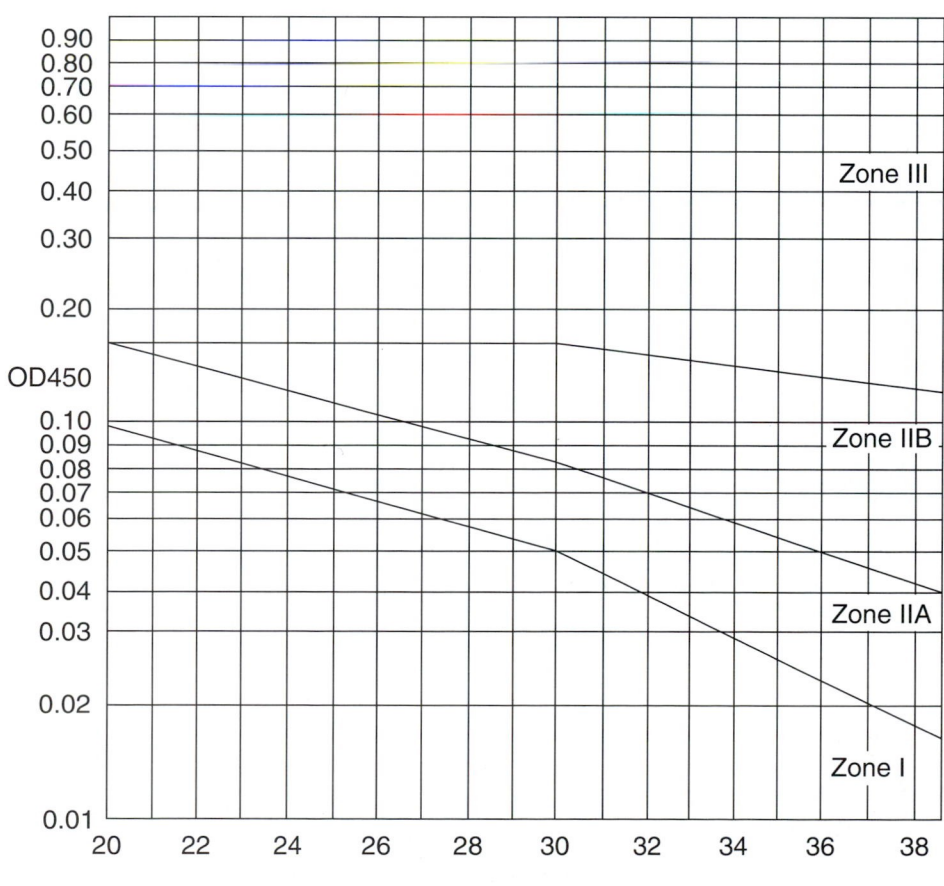

Figure 10-3 ΔOD450 by weeks of gestation (Liley curve), as modified for use at the Ohio State University Hospital. Zone I = Consistent with an unaffected or mildly affected infant; Zone IIA = Consistent with a mildly to moderately affected infant; Zone IIB = Consistent with a moderately to severely affected infant; and Zone III = Consistent with a severely affected infant.

1977 to 1987, the ΔOD450 in amniotic fluid from patients who had begun amniocentesis prior to 28 weeks of gestation was correlated with severity of disease.[55] In 79 cases RhD isoimmunization was present. A variety of antibodies were responsible for the other 12 cases of EBF (4 anti-E; 2 anti-C; 2 anti-K; 1 anti-M; 1 anti-Fy[a]). These 91 women underwent 445 amniocenteses. Amniotic fluid ΔOD450 was correlated with severity of disease as measured by cord hemoglobin at birth, intrauterine fetal death (6 fetuses), or the need for IUT (17 patients). The figure indicates that those fetuses with more severe disease (cord hemoglobin $\leq$10.9 g/dl, intrauterine fetal death, or need for IUT) could be reliably separated from those with milder disease (cord hemoglobin $\geq$11 g/dl or unaffected) on a graphic display of amniotic fluid ΔOD450 using three zones (Figure 10-4). The degree of separation of these two populations was not complete. An area of overlap occurred such that in the midzone it was impossible with any single value to discriminate the more severely from the less severely affected patients.

Our data, along with Liley's, have shown that amniotic fluid spectrophotometric measurement of hemolytic pigment in amniotic fluid is a reliable method to measure the severity of EBF as early as 20 weeks of gestation. Queenan and colleagues[57] have shown also that the concentration of hemolytic pigment in the amniotic fluid is reflective of the severity of fetal disease as early as 14 weeks of gestation. When amniocentesis is employed as a monitoring technique, it is important to sample sequentially.[58] In Zone I, sampling can be repeated every 4 weeks. In Zone II, sampling should be repeated at 1- to 2-week intervals to establish the trend of values. A trend of falling ΔOD450 values in the midzone is favorable.

The continuing clinical usefulness of amniotic fluid spectrophotometry has been called into question.[59] It must be recognized that this test is only an indirect assessment of fetal anemia and that amniotic fluid contaminants or polyhydramnios may interfere with interpretation. In most instances, however, amniocentesis is an effective and reliable means of evaluating the severity of fetal anemia.

Cordocentesis

If amniotic fluid spectrophotometry falls in Zone III, simple confirmation should be done within 1 week and then further planning made for delivery or more detailed fetal diagnosis with cordocentesis and intervention with delivery or fetal transfusion. If the ΔOD450 trend plateaus or climbs into high Zone II or Zone III, and if the fetus is too early for delivery, then

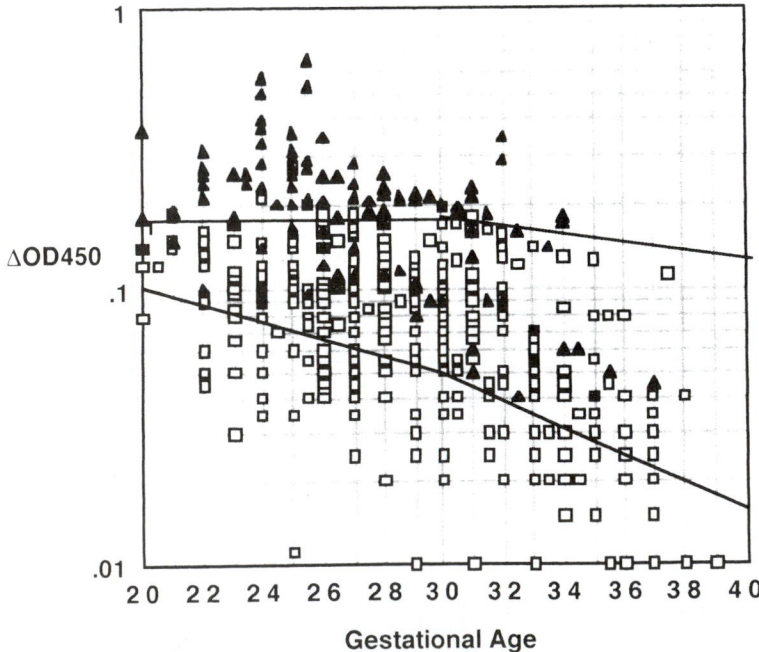

Figure 10-4 Amniotic fluid ΔOD450 from 20 weeks of gestation until delivery in 445 amniocenteses from 91 women with nonhydropic fetuses affected by EBF.

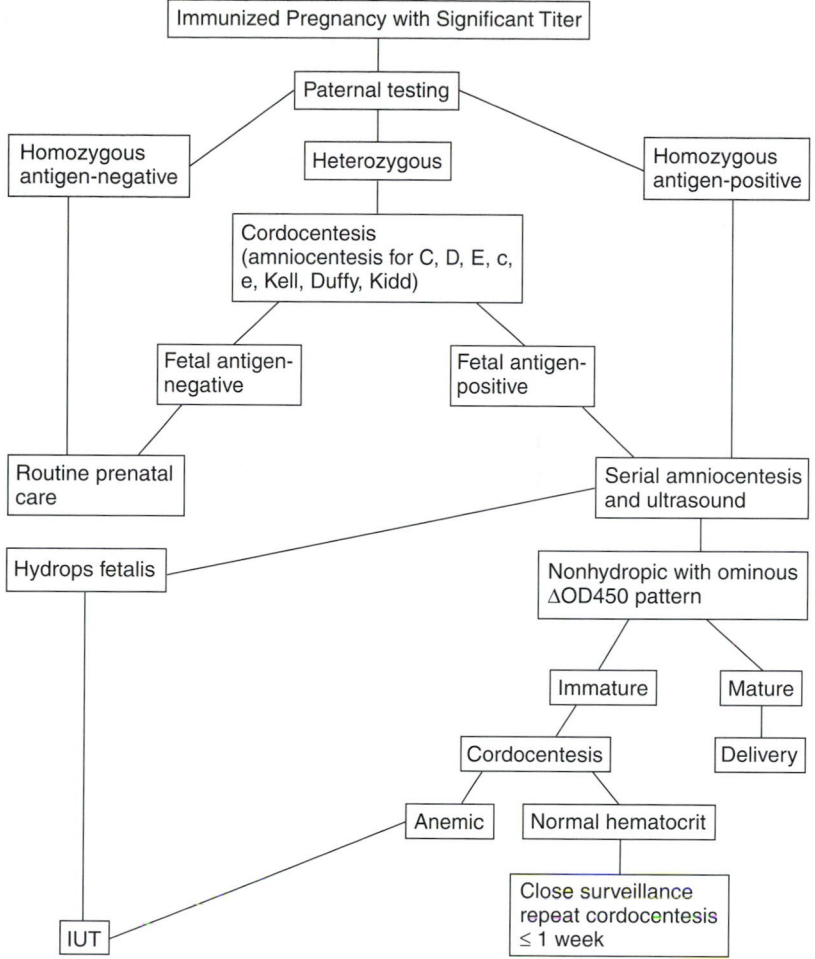

Figure 10-5 Management algorithm for erythroblastosis fetalis.

cordocentesis should be used. In the fetus at risk, the presence of hydropic change, polyhydramnios, or blood or meconium staining of amniotic fluid will render amniotic fluid interpretation meaningless, and cordocentesis will be necessary. This technique will directly measure the fetal hemolytic indexes and indicate the next step in management.

As stated before, because cordocentesis offers a direct assessment of fetal condition, it has been proposed as a primary monitoring tool.[28] Cordocentesis, however, is not readily available in many instances and is riskier for the fetus than the indirect testing of maternal serology and amniocentesis. Therefore, we favor primary monitoring with indirect testing. The management algorithm shown in Figure 10-5 will indicate cases in which cordocentesis should be used. Transplacental amniocentesis or cordocentesis should

be avoided if possible, since the resultant fetal–maternal hemorrhage can increase the intensity of the antibody response.

Fetal Transfusion

The first fetal transfusions were done by the intraperitoneal technique using fluoroscopic guidance. In 1963, Liley showed that fetal intraperitoneal transfusion with absorption of red cells into the circulation via peritoneal lymphatics was effective in preventing fetal death in the severely affected fetus with erythroblastosis fetalis.[54] Improvements in technology now allow intravascular transfusion of the severely affected fetus.[46,60-62] Both intravascular and intraperitoneal techniques are effective in the nonhydropic fetus. When fetal ascites is present, intraperitoneal transfusion is ineffective. Intravascular techniques allow more careful monitoring of transfusion volume and fetal hemoglobin, ensuring that the fetal hemoglobin level is maintained within the normal range. Intravascular transfusion can start as early as 18 weeks of gestation and continue until fetal maturity and cervical ripening are present to allow vaginal delivery. After 34 weeks of gestation, however, testing for fetal maturity should be performed, and strong consideration should be given to the option of delivery rather than further fetal transfusions.

Fetal exchange transfusion is not usually used.[63] The fetal placenta easily accommodates the volume of simple transfusion, so exchange transfusion is not needed in most cases. Combined techniques using both intraperitoneal and intravascular transfusions are advocated by some.[64] Antigen-negative packed red cells are used for transfusion. It is preferable to use the mother's blood for fetal transfusion, if possible.[65] The mother can successfully donate multiple units of blood for use in fetal transfusions. However, maternal red cells must be washed before use to remove the antibody that causes EBF.

Fetal transfusion therapy should be performed only in centers with extensive experience in using these techniques.[66,67] Fetal transfusion is necessary in approximately 10% of cases of erythroblastosis fetalis. When monitoring confirms that significant fetal anemia is present (fetal hemoglobin less than 10 g/dl), then fetal transfusions should be instituted. The fetal hematocrit will drop approximately 1% per day following transfusion, and repeat transfusions are necessary at 2- to 3-week intervals to maintain the fetal hematocrit in the normal range of 30 to 50%. If necessary, it is possible to prolong the interval between transfusions[64,68] even further by administering larger volumes of blood to the fetus intravascularly or in combination with intraperitoneal transfusion. It is important to avoid excessive transfusion, because volume overload and sludging may be injurious to the fetus.[69,70]

Neonatal Outcome

Using current monitoring and therapeutic techniques, one should anticipate a survival rate >90% for fetuses requiring transfusion. There is no evidence of adverse outcome for survivors. Doyle and colleagues[71] performed sensorineural testing at 2 years of age on 38 children who had undergone a program of fetal

transfusion for severe erythoblastosis fetalis and found no evidence of impairment, in comparison with a control group of 60 normal children. Hudon et al.[72] followed 40 survivors of fetal transfusion therapy up until 5 years of age and found normal developmental testing. They and others concluded that normal developmental outcome can be expected for children treated with IUT.[72-74]

Following multiple transfusions in utero, the newborn may demonstrate a suppressed bone marrow and will need continued monitoring for delayed neonatal anemia at about 4 to 6 weeks after delivery.[75,76] Treatment of the newborn with erythropoietin may enhance bone marrow responsiveness and decrease the need for late neonatal transfusion.

Other Therapies

Other therapies are available to the clinician in treating this severe disease, but none have proven to be particularly effective.[77] Treatment of the mother by plasmapheresis, the administration of antigen orally, and the use of promethazine, phenobarbital, corticosteroids, intravenous immunoglobulin (IVIG) and stem-cell transplantation have been tried as forms of therapy. IVIG therapy administered to the mother or the fetus has shown some benefit, but has not been dramatically effective in ameliorating the fetal hemolytic response.[49,78-82] Further testing of IVIG therapy is warranted, especially as adjunctive treatment of early-onset severe disease. Trials of stem-cell transplantation have not been proven to be effective.[83] Anderson and Cordero showed that corticosteroids reduced the ΔOD450 in amniotic fluid, but there was no clear indication that the fetal condition improved in utero concomitantly.[84] It is important for the clinician who administers corticosteroids to the mother of a fetus affected with erythroblastosis fetalis not to rely on the ΔOD450 measurements as indicators of fetal status in utero. In these situations cordocentesis will be warranted to monitor disease severity. Plasmapheresis can reduce the concentration of maternal antibody and may be adjunctive therapy in severe early disease before fetal transfusion can be performed, but this is rarely necessary.[85]

Strategies to alter the maternal immune response by the oral administration of antigen[86] or to suppress the hemolytic effect in utero with maternally administered promethazine[87] have not been effective. Phenobarbital administered antenatally to the mother may enhance the bilirubin-conjugating ability of the neonatal hepatic enzymes, but this, too, has not been demonstrated to be of significant additional benefit.

The remarkable effectiveness of fetal transfusion therapy has reduced the stimulus to devise other means of treatment for these affected fetuses. In very severely affected cases with recurrent early fetal death, preimplantation blastomere biopsy may be employed if the father is heterozygous.[88] In vitro fertilization with blastomere biopsy and transfer of antigen-negative embryos is available for these difficult cases. Also, artificial insemination from an antigen-negative donor will ensure an unaffected fetus.

Prevention of Rh Isoimmunization, Rh Immune Globulin (RhIg)

In 1968 Rh immune globulin (RhIg) was licensed for postpartum use. The exact mechanism of action of RhIg remains unclear, but administration of appropriate doses at appropriate times can prevent the primary immune response of Rh-negative women bearing Rh-positive infants to produce anti-D.[89,90] The use of postpartum RhIg reduces the incidence of alloimmunization by 90%, from 12 to 16% for each pregnancy, to 1.5 to 2%. Introduction of prophylactic antepartum use of RhIg at 28 weeks, as well as at delivery, further reduces the incidence of immunization from 1.5 to 2% to 0.2%. RhIg is prepared from human volunteers; modern processing virtually precludes transmission of blood-borne disease.

Male volunteer studies provided the scientific assurance that the primary immune response could be prevented by passively administered antibody. Studies established that 20 μg of purified anti-D was more than adequate to prevent immunization by 1 ml of Rh-positive red cells (not whole blood).[12] Thus, a 300-μg dose of RhIg will prevent immunization by 15 ml of red cells, or about 30 ml of whole blood. The volume of fetal–maternal hemorrhage during labor and delivery is usually much less than 15 ml, so nearly all deliveries are adequately protected. For first-trimester abortions, a dose of 50 μg is adequate since the fetal blood volume is less than 5 ml whole blood. During pregnancy, causes of transplacental hemorrhage include amniocentesis, external cephalic version, antepartum obstetric hemorrhage, and maternal abdominal trauma. Massive hemorrhage ($>$30 ml) must be recognized for adequate doses of RhIg to be administered. The most commonly used test to quantitate these bleeds is the Kleihauer–Betke acid elution stain. RhIg should be administered as soon as possible after exposure, but within 72 hours to provide maximum benefit. In situations in which RhIg administration is delayed for longer than 72 hours, some protective benefit is achieved with dosing as late as 2 weeks or more following exposure.[91]

In Canada, Bowman noted that a small number (2%) of women were being sensitized, apparently during the pregnancy, even though the women were adequately treated postpartum.[77] Bowman did an extended trial using a 300-μg dose of RhIg at 28 to 34 weeks (and later at 28 weeks only) to Rh-negative women without anti-D in their serum. This injection was followed by a postpartum dose of 300 μg to the women who delivered an Rh-positive infant. His results showed a further decrease in incidence of immunization to 0.2%. He also showed that antepartum RhIg did not harm the infant. The half-life of passively administered anti-D (RhIg) is approximately 25 days, so the administration of a 300-μg dose should provide adequate protection in a normal pregnancy for about 12 weeks. If delivery does not occur by then, a second dose of RhIg should be given to prevent possible enhancement, or augmentation, of the immune response. When the level of anti-D is low, a small amount of red cells may apparently increase the chance of isoimmunization. Therefore, if RhIg is given prior to 28 weeks and/or gestation is postterm, another dose is recommended antepartum. An example is RhIg given following a midtrimester genetic amniocentesis. These women require a second dose 12 weeks later and a third dose postpartum if an Rh-positive infant is delivered (Table 10-2 and Figure 10-6).

All pregnant women must have accurate blood typing done at an early prenatal visit. Having these initial tests done at the delivery hospital reduces the chances of errors after delivery. Each woman given RhIg prior to delivery should receive a card indicating that fact and should receive a postpartum injection unless the infant is Rh-negative. The hospital blood bank must be notified that antepartum RhIg has been administered. The presence of circulating anti-D may lead to the inaccurate conclusion of active immunization rather than passively acquired antibody. Withholding RhIg when indicated postpartum increases the risk of a primary immune response. Considerable confusion can surround the postpartum period when antepartum RhIg has been given. The danger is that RhIg will be inappropriately withheld.

TABLE 10-2
INDICATIONS FOR ADMINISTRATION OF RHIG*

Abortions, spontaneous or induced	
First trimester	50 μg
After first trimester	300 μg
Full term delivery of Rh-positive infant	300 μg
Stillbirths (unless fetus proven to be RhD-negative	300 μg
Amniocentesis	
Genetic followed by	300 μg
Second dose 12 weeks later	300 μg
Third dose for Rh-positive infant	300 μg
Second or third trimester	300 μg
Possibly second dose 12 weeks later and/or at delivery	300 μg
Transplacental fetal–maternal hemorrhages	300 μg
Threatened abortion	
External cephalic version	
Antepartum hemorrhage	
Maternal abdominal trauma	
Antepartum prophylactic about 28 weeks	300 μg
Must be followed by second dose at delivery if infant is Rh-positive	300 μg

Maternal blood sample must be evaluated for possible excessive fetal–maternal hemorrhage (>30 ml fetal whole blood in maternal circulation): 300-μg dose for 30 ml fetal whole blood. Calculate appropriate dose based on volume of fetal hemorrhage.

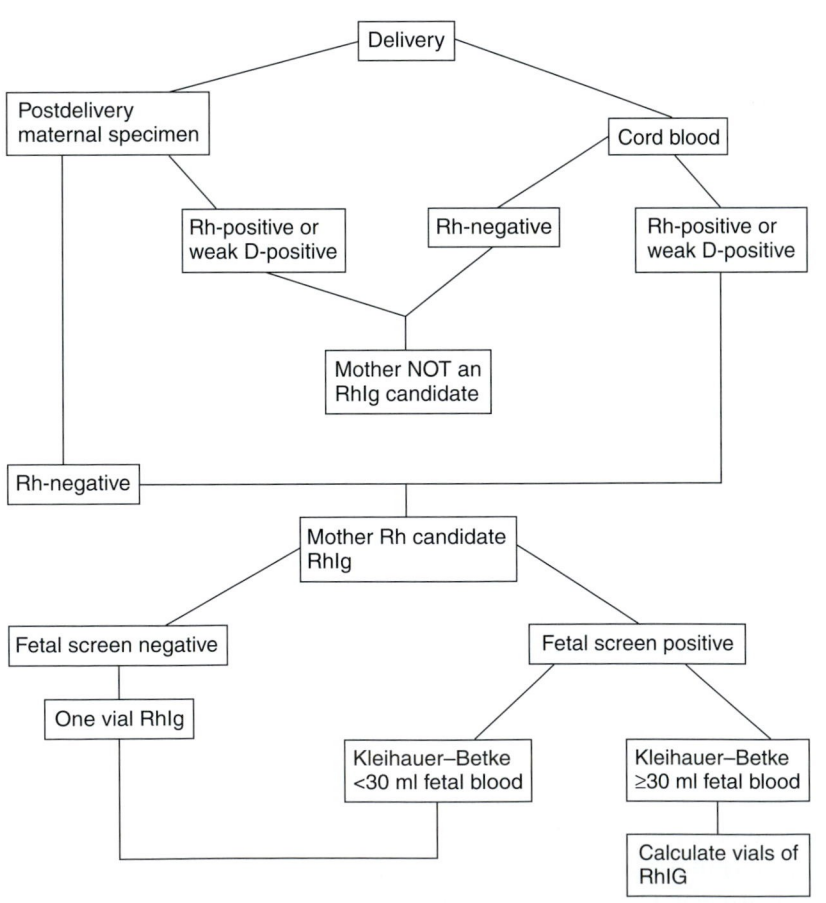

Figure 10-6 RhIg work-up.

ALLOIMMUNE THROMBOCYTOPENIA (FETAL OR NEONATAL ALLOIMMUNE THROMBOCYTOPENIA) [FAIT OR NAIT]

Definition

Analagous to EBF-HDN, alloimmune thrombocytopenia affecting the fetus and newborn is caused by specific antibodies against platelet antigens inherited from the father but absent in the mother.

Antigen Systems

The most common antigen involved in FAIT/NAIT is PlA1 (HPA-1a), which is also associated with the most severe disease.[92] Infrequently, KO (HPA-2), Bak (HPA-3), Pen/Yuk (HPA-4), or Br (HPA-5) are involved. These antigens are platelet-specific and represent specific polymorphisms in the platelet membrane glycoproteins.[93]

Cause

In the case of FAIT/NAIT, the alloimmune antibody may arise in the first pregnancy (25% primiparous PlA1 negative women in one report[94]) and cause severe thrombocytopenia in the fetus and newborn. In fact, the diagnosis is usually discovered at birth, when the newborn presents with petechiae, ecchymoses, or even intracranial hemorrhage. The mother generally will be found to be negative for PlA1 and have anti-PlA1 antibody; the father may be heterozygous or homozygous for PlA. The next pregnancy will be at risk, depending on the zygosity of the father.

The antibodies may be first detected early in pregnancy. In the large natural history study by Williamson et al.,[94] antibodies were detected as early as 17 weeks, paralleling the development of fetal platelet antigens[95] and B3 integrin on the syncytiotrophoblast.[96] For white populations, 2 to 3% of men and women are PlA1-negative, or about 1 in 40 women. Nearly all of their partners will be incompatible. The ability of the mother to produce anti-PlA1 is strongly associated with the HLA class II antigen, DRB3*0101,[94,97] and this association has been explored for screening women at risk. In an observational study by Williamson et al.,[94] only 12% of PlA1-negative women had anti- PlA1, and about one-fourth of these had transient antibodies. About 2.5% of the pregnancies in PlA1-negative women resulted in severely thrombocytopenic newborns (platelet count $<10 \times 10^9$), with another 2.5% mildly thrombocytopenic. Thus, about 1 in 1000 pregnancies will be affected by FAIT/NAIT.[98] About half of the affected neonates are born to primiparas, and the recurrence rate is high (50% if the father is heterozygous and a virtual certainty if he is homozygous). Seventy percent of affected infants are born with platelet counts lower than 50,000/μl and approximately 20% have intracranial hemorrhages, half of which occur before the onset of labor.[99]

Fetal Effects of Alloimmune Thrombocytopenia

Thrombocytopenia develops in the fetus as a result of the transfer across the placenta of the alloimmune platelet-specific antibody and subsequent destruction of platelets. The thrombocytopenia may be mild or quite severe. The most severe complications are intrauterine fetal death and intracranial hemorrhage as early as 20 weeks of gestation.[100]

As with EBF-HDN, the fetal ability to respond to the platelet destruction is highly variable. Platelets are produced in the bone marrow and in extramedullary sites, leading to stress on the hematopoietic system.

Neonatal Effects of FAIT/NAIT

Intracranial hemorrhage is the most feared complication in the neonatal period. The risk is inversely proportional to the platelet count and increases significantly at levels $<20,000/\mu$l with greater risk at levels $<10,000/\mu$l.

Diagnosis

Most cases are diagnosed at birth, after the effects of thrombocytopenia (petechiae, ecchymoses, and intracranial hemorrhage) are noted. In addition, the history of a previous child with thrombocytopenia can alert the obstetrician to a probable subsequent affected pregnancy. Another clinical setting in which serologic screening for platelet alloantibodies is indicated is when fetal hydrocephaly or intracranial hemorrhage is detected by ultrasound imaging. Routine prenatal typing for platelet antigens or screening for alloimmune platelet antibodies is not yet readily available, although this has been proposed.[101]

In neonatal cases, if future pregnancies are anticipated, the mother, father, and infant should be typed for platelet antigens at a referral laboratory. Genomic testing can determine the zygosity of the father and the potential for future affected pregnancies. The mother should be tested for alloimmune platelet antibodies. Currently, antibody titers are not standardized or routinely performed, although the report from Williamson et al.[94] found that titers of 1:32 or greater were associated with more severe thrombocytopenia.

When a history of a previous affected pregnancy is present, the mother should be tested for platelet alloantibodies. If this test is not readily available, the mother and father should be typed for platelet antigens. The genotype of the fetus can be determined by amniocentesis as early as 18 weeks of gestation.[102] Care must be taken to determine that detected antibodies are truly platelet-specific. Other antibodies, such as HLA, can give positive reactions in some assays but do not have clinical significance for thrombocytopenia.[103] If there is a history of antenatal intracranial hemorrhage (ICH) in a previously affected sibling, then the risk of recurrent ICH is high, especially if that ICH occurred early in pregnancy.[104]

Monitoring for FAIT/NAIT

Monitoring should begin at about 20 weeks of gestation, as fetal thrombocytopenia and ICH may occur by this point, and because cordocentesis and transfusion become technically possible. The monitoring techniques include cordocentesis to determine fetal platelet count and provide transfusion and ultrasound to detect hemorrhage. Ultrasound alone is not sufficient.

Therapy for FAIT

Vaginal delivery can be traumatic, but routine elective cesarean section will not solve the problem, since half of the intracranial hemorrhages occur before the onset of labor. In affected pregnancies it is necessary to monitor the fetus for thrombocytopenia and to treat the thrombocytopenia with fetal platelet transfusions, maternal IVIG, or both.[103] The optimal treatment for pregnancies complicated by FAIT remains to be determined.

Cordocentesis is used to monitor the platelet count. Because of the risk of hemorrhage and possible exsanguination, cordocentesis should only be attempted if platelet concentrates compatible with the mother's antibody are available.[105] The surest source is the mother herself; she can donate by plateletpheresis. The platelets are then washed to remove antibody and suspended in saline. If the fetus is thrombocytopenic, the platelets can be infused at the time of cordocentesis.

If platelet transfusions are used as the sole therapy, they must be repeated weekly, because the platelet life span is 8 to 10 days.[106,107] This form of treatment necessitates weekly cordocenteses, with the attendant complications, and logistical problems for the mother, if she is the platelet donor.

Another approach is to administer intravenous immune globulin (IVIG) weekly to the mother[92,99,104] once cordocentesis has shown the fetus to be affected. The mechanism by which maternally administered IVIG increases the fetal platelet count is not understood. Some investigators have failed to demonstrate any benefit from maternal IVIG therapy.[108,109] The IVIG dose used most successfully is 1 g/kg/week, with the platelet count monitored by cordocentesis, about 4 to 6 weeks later to ascertain response. If the thrombocytopenia does not respond after 4 to 6 weeks of IVIG therapy, the addition of prednisone, 60 mg orally each day, has been shown to be beneficial. Although IVIG is not effective in all cases, the incidence of fetal ICH in treated patients is much lower than expected. In a randomized trial of 54 affected pregnancies, Bussel et al.[99] found that 70% responded to maternal IVIG alone and 80% to IVIG + prednisone ("salvage regimen"). There were no cases of ICH. Some failures occurred even when IVIG was combined with weekly platelet transfusions. Administering IVIG directly to the fetus has not been uniformly successful.[38,110]

The fetal platelet count should be determined before delivery, and platelets transfused if the count is $<50,000/\mu l$. Delivery may be vaginal if the fetal platelet count is $50,000/\mu l$ or greater. Figure 10-7 outlines a management strategy for FAIT. This algorithm assumes that the threshold value of $50,000/\mu l$ is necessary for fetal hemostasis sufficient to allow vaginal delivery. Individual fetuses may be fully hemostatic, however, at lower platelet counts.

Therapy for NAIT

The newborn's platelet count must be monitored and platelet transfusions given to keep the count

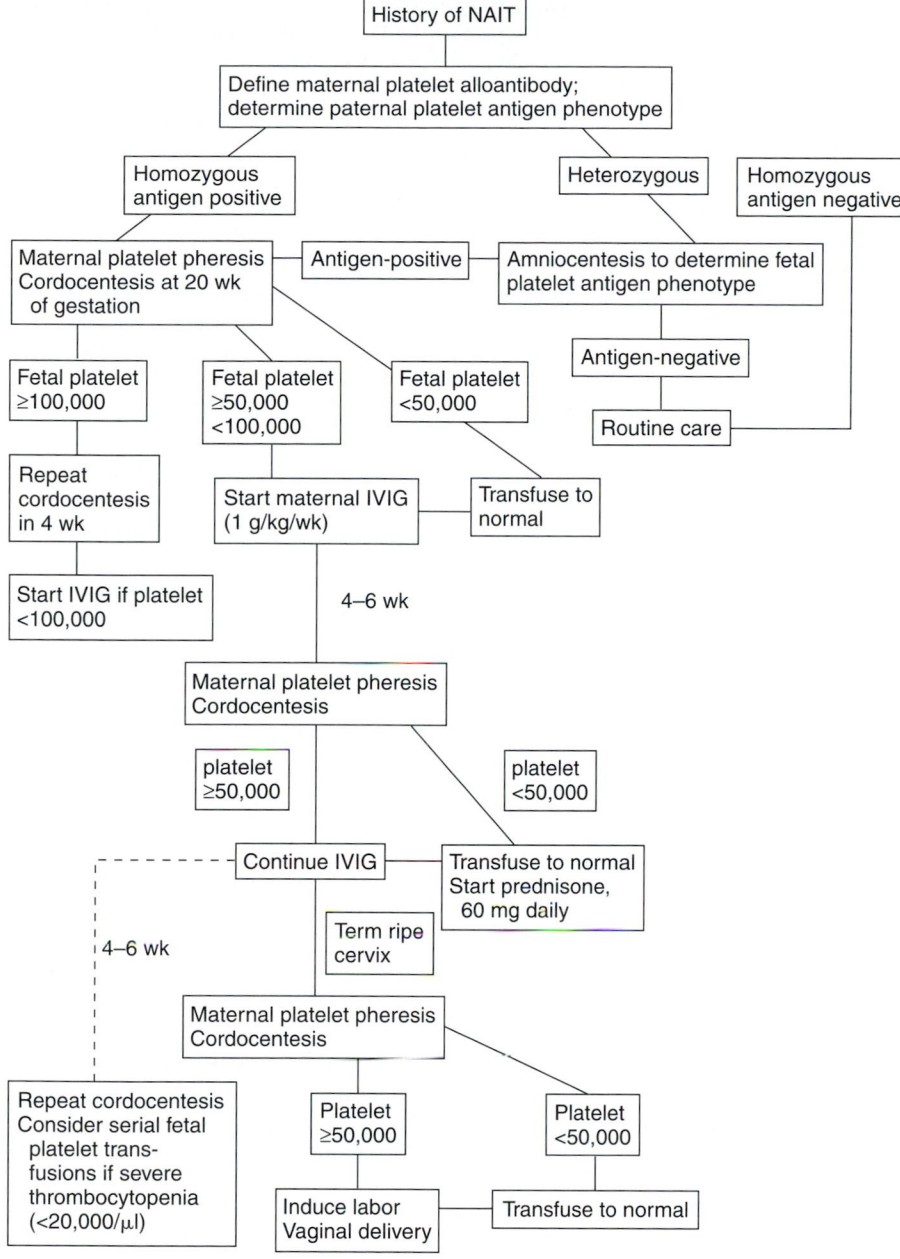

Figure 10-7 Suggested management of pregnancy with FAIT/NAIT.

>20,000/μl. Generally, thrombocytopenia disappears during the first week of life but occasionally persists for several weeks. Ultrasound is used to detect intracranial hemorrhages. When intracranial hemorrhages are detected, there is risk of permanent brain damage.

REFERENCES

1. Diamond LK, Blackfan KD, Baty JM. Erythoblastosis fetalis and its association with universal edema of the fetus, icterus gravis neonatorum and anemia of the newborn. J Pediatr 1932;1:269.

2. Levine P, Katzin EM, Burnham L. Isoimmunization in pregnancy: its possible bearing on the etiology of erythroblastosis fetalis. JAMA 1941;116:825.

3. Stiller JR, Herzlinger R, Siegel S, Whetham JCG. Fetal ascites associated with ABO incompatibility: case report and review of the literature. Am J Obstet Gynecol 1996; 175:1371.

4. Weinstein L. Irregular antibodies causing hemolytic disease of the newborn: a continuing problem. Clin Obstet Gynecol 1982;25:321.

5. Filbey D, Hanson U, Wesstrom G. The prevalence of red cell antibodies in pregnancy correlated to the outcome of the newborn: a 12 year study in central Sweden. Acta Obstet Gynecol Scand 1995;74:687.

6. American College of Obstetricians and Gynecologists. ACOG Educational Bulletin no. 227, August 1996.

7. Bowman JM, Pollock JM, Penston LE. Fetomaternal transplacental hemorrhage during pregnancy and after delivery. Vox Sang 1986;51:117.

8. Medearis AL, Hensleigh PA, Parks DR, Herzenberg LA. Detection of fetal erythrocytes in maternal blood postpartum with the fluorescence activated cellsorter. Am J Obstet Gynecol 1984;148:290.

9. Kanter MH, Hodge SE. Risk of hemolytic disease of the newborn as a result of directed donations from relatives. Transfusion 1989;29:620.

10. Kennedy M, O'Shaughnessy R, Waheed A, Hewitt M, Krugh P. Hemolytic disease of the newborn caused by a husband's directed donation for joint surgery. J Bone Joint Surg Am 1999;81(8):1170.

11. Woodrow JC. Rh immunization and its prevention. Series Haematol 1970;3.

12. Pollack W, Ascari WQ, Kochesky RJ, et al. Studies on Rh prophylaxis. I. relationship between doses of anti-Rh and size of antigenic stimulus. Transfusion 1971;11:333.

13. Chavez G, Mulinare J, Edmonds L. Epidemiology of Rh hemolytic disease of the newborn in the United States. JAMA 1991;265:3270.

14. Bowman JM. The management of Rh-isoimmunization. Obstet Gynecol 1978;52:1.

15. Vaughan J, Manning M, Warwick R, Letsky E, Murray N, Roberts I. Inhibition of erythroid progenitor cells by anti-Kell antibodies in fetal alloimmune anemia. N Engl J Med 1998;338:798.

16. McKenna D, Nagaraja H, O'Shaughnessy R. Management of pregnancies complicated by anti-kell isoimmunization at the Ohio State University. Obstet Gynecol 1999;5:667.

17. Nicolaides K, Soothill PW, Clewell W, et al. Fetal hemoglobin measurement in the assessment of red cell immunization. Lancet 1988;1:1073.

18. Forestier R, Daffos R, Galacteros F, Bardakjian J, Rainaut M, Beuzard Y. Hematological values of 163 normal fetuses between 18 and 30 weeks of gestation. Pediatr Res 1986;20:342.

19. Bowman JM, Pollock JM, Manning FA, et al. Maternal Kell blood group alloimmunization. Obstet Gynecol 1992;79:239.

20. Bennett P, Le Van Kim C, Colin Y, et al. Prenatal determination of fetal RhD type by DNA amplification. N Engl J Med 1993;329:607.

21. Le Van Kim C, Mouro K, Brossard Y, Chavinie J, Cartron J, Colin Y. PCR-based determination of Rhc and RhE status of fetuses at risk of Rhc and RhE haemolytic disease. Fr J Haematol 1994;88:193.

22. Hessner M, McFarland J, Endean D. Genotyping of KEL1 and KEL2 of the human Kell blood group system by the polymerase chain reaction with sequence-specific primers. Transfusion 1996;36:495.

23. Hessner MJ, Atkinson BA, Johnson ST, et al. Development of an ASPCR for prenatal genotyping of the RhC/c and RhE/e antigen systems. Am J. Obstet Gynecol 1997;176:Abstract 27.

24. Hessner MJ, Pircon, RA Johnson ST, Luhm RA. Prenatal genotyping of Jk^a and Jk^b of the human Kidd blood group system by allele-specific polymerase chain reaction. Prenat Diagn 1998;18:1225.

25. Hessner MJ, Pircon RA, Johnson ST, Luhm RA. Prenatal genotyping of the Duffy blood group system by allele-specific polymerase chain reaction. Prenat Diagn 1999;19(1):41.

26. Lo Y, Bowell PJ, Selinger M, et al. Prenatal determination of fetal RhD status by analysis of peripheral blood of Rhesus negative mothers. Lancet 1993;341:1147.

27. Lo Y, Hjelm NM, Fidler C, et al. Prenatal diagnosis of fetal RhD status by molecular analysis of maternal plasma. N Engl J Med 1998;339:1734.

28. Weiner CP, Williamson RA, Wenstrom KD, Sipes SL, Grant SS, Widness JA. Management of fetal hemolytic disease by cordocentesis. Am J Obstet Gynecol 1991; 165(3):546.

29. Frigoletto F, Greene M, Benacerraf B, Barss V, Saltzman D. Ultrasonographic fetal surveillance in the management of the isoimmunized pregnancy. N Engl J Med 1986; 315:430.

30. Mari G, Andrignolo A, Abuhamad AZ, et al. Diagnosis of fetal anemia with Doppler ultrasound in the pregnancy complicated by maternal blood group immunization. Ultrasound Obstet Gynecol 1995;5:400.

31. Bahado-Singh R, Oz U, Deren O, et al. A new splenic artery doppler velocimetric index for prediction of severe fetal anemia associated with Rh alloimmunization. Am J Obstet Gynecol 1999;180:49.

32. Visser GHA. Antepartum sinusoidal and decelerative heart rate patterns in Rh disease. Am J Obstet Gynecol 1982;143:538.

33. Ouzounian J, Alsulyman O, Monteiro H, Songster G. The nonreactive nonstress test: predictive value for neonatal anemia in the isoimmunized pregnancy. Obstet Gynecol 1996;88:364.

34. Moise K. Changing trends in the management of red blood cell alloimmunization in pregnancy. Arch Pathol Lab Med 1994;118:421.

35. De Young-Owens A, Boyle J, Kennedy M, O'Shaughnessy R, Rose R. Anti-M isoimmunization: management and outcome at the Ohio State University from 1969–1995. Obstet Gynecol 1997; 90:962.

36. Strohm PL, Iams JD, Kennedy MS. Hemolytic disease of the newborn from Anti-E. J Reprod Med 1988; 33:404.

37. Bowman J. Hemolytic disease (erythroblastosis fetalis). In: Creasy R, Resnick R, eds. Maternal fetal medicine. Philadelphia: Saunders, 1999;736.

38. Bowman J, Harman, C, Mentigolou S, Pollock J. Intravenous fetal trransfusion of immunoglobulin for alloimmune thrombocytopenia. Lancet 1992;340:1034.

39. Vaughan J, Warwick R, Letsky E, Nicolini U, Rodeck C, Fisk N. Erythropoietic suppression in fetal anemia because of Kell alloimmunization. Am J Obstet Gynecol 1994;171:247.

40. Judd WJ, Luban N, Ness P, Silberstein L, Stroup M, Widman F. Prenatal and perinatal immunohematology: recommendations for serologic management of the fetus, newborn infant and obstetric patient. Transfusion 1990; 30:175.

41. Allen FH, Diamond LK, Jones AR. Erythroblastosis fetalis. IX. The problems of stillbirth. N Engl J Med 1954;251:453.

42. Bowell P, Wainscoat J, Peto T, Gunson H. Maternal anti-D concentrations and outcome in rhesus haemolytic disease of the newborn. BMJ 1982;285:327.

43. Nicolaides K, Rodeck C. Maternal serum anti-D antibody concentration in the assessment of rhesus isoimmunization. BMJ 1992;304:1155.

44. van Dijk G, Dooren M, Overbeeke M. Red cell antibodies in pregnancy: there is no "critical titer." Transfusion Med 1995;5:199.

45. Gottval T, Hilden J. Concentration of anti-D antibodies in Rh(D) alloimmunized pregnant women, as a predictor of anemia and/or hyperbilirubinemia in their newborn infants. Acta Obstet Gynecol Scand 1997;76:733.

46. Bang J, Bock J, Trolle D. Ultrasound guided fetal intravenous transfusion for severe rhesus hemolytic disease. BMJ 1982;284:373.

47. Gordon M, Kennedy M, O'Shaughnessy R, Waheed A. Severe hemolytic disease of the newborn due to anti-Js^B. Vox Sang 1995;69:140.

48. Contreras M, Garner S, Silva M. Prenatal testing to predict the severity of hemolytic disease of the fetus and newborn. Curr Op Hematol 1996;3:480.

49. Alonso J, Decaro J, Marrero A, Lavalle E, Martell M, Cuadro J. Repeated direct fetal intravascular high-dose immunoglobulin therapy for the treatment of Rh hemolytic disease. J Perinat Med 1994;22:415.

50. Garner S, Gorick B, Lai W, et al. Prediction of the severity of haemolytic disease of the newborn. Vox Sang 1995;68:169.

51. Larson P, Thorp J, Miller R, Hoffman M. The monocyte monolayer assay: a noninvasive technique for predicting the severity of in utero hemolysis. Am J Perinatol 1995;12:157.

52. Moise K, Perkins J, Sosler S, et al. The predictive value of maternal serum testing for detection of fetal anemia in red blood cell alloimmunization. Am J Obstet Gynecol 1995;172:1003.

53. Liley A. Liquor amnii analyses in the management of the pregnancy complicated by rhesus sensitization. Am J Obstet Gynecol 1961;82:1359.

54. Liley AW. Intrauterine transfusion of foetus in haemolytic disease. BMJ 1963;2:1107.

55. O'Shaughnessy R. Amniotic fluid spectrophotometry is useful after twenty weeks gestation in the care of pregnancies complicated by red blood cell isoimmunization. Am J Obstet Gynecol 1991;164:256.

56. MacPherson C. unpublished data, 1965.

57. Queenan JT, Tomai TP, Ural SH, King JC. Use of amniotic fluid optical density in evaluation of erythroblastosis fetalis. Am J Obstet Gynecol 1993;168:1370.

58. Liley A. Errors in the assessment of hemolytic disease from amniotic fluid. Am J Obstet Gynecol 1963;86:485.

59. Nicolaides K, Rodeck C, Mibashan R. Have Liley charts outlived their usefulness? Am J Obstet Gynecol 1986; 155:90.

60. Berkowitz R, Chitkara U, Goldberg J, Wilkins I, Chervenak F, Lynch L. Intrauterine intravascular transfusions for severe red blood cell isoimmunization: ultrasound-guided percutaneous approach. Am J Obstet Gynecol 1986; 155:574.

61. de Crespigny LCh, Robinson HP, Quinn M, Dole L, Ross A, Cauchi M. Ultrasound guided fetal blood transfusion for severe rhesus isoimmunization. Obstet Gynecol 1985;66:529.

62. Rodeck C, Nicolaides K, Warsof S, Fysh W, Gamsu H, Kemp J. The management of severe rhesus isoimmunization by fetoscopic intravascular transfusions. Am J Obstet Gynecol 1984;150:769.

63. Grannum P, Copel J, Plaxe S, Scioscia A, Hobbins J. In utero exchange transfusion by direct intravascular injection in severe erythroblastosis fetalis. N Engl J Med 1986;315:1431.

64. Moise K, Carpenter R, Kirshon B, Deter R, Sala J, Cano L. Comparison of four types of intrauterine transfusion: effect on fetal hematocrit. Fetal Ther 1989;4:126.

65. El-Azeem S, Samuels P, Rose R, Kennedy M, O'Shaughnessy R. The effect of the source of transfused blood on the rate of consumption of transfused red blood cells in pregnancies affected by red blood cell alloimmunization. Am J Obstet Gynecol 1997;177:753.

66. Schumacher B, Moise K. Fetal transfusion for red blood cell alloimmunization in pregnancy. Obstet Gynecol 1996;88:137.

67. Skupski D, Wolf C, Bussel J. Fetal transfusion therapy. Obstet Gynecol Surv 1996;51:181.

68. Inglis S, Lysikiewicz A, Sonnenblick A, Streltzoff J, Bussel J, Chervenak F. Advantages of larger volume, less frequent intrauterine red blood cell transfusions for maternal red cell alloimmunization. Am J Perinatol 1996;13:27.

69. Dildy G, Smith L, Moise K, Cano L, Hesketh D. Porencephalic cyst: a complication of fetal intravascular transfusion. Am J Obstet Gynecol 1991;165:7.

70. Selbing A, Stangerberg M, Westgren M, Rahman F. Intrauterine intravascular transfusions in fetal erythroblastosis: the influence of net transfusion volume on fetal survival. Acta Obstet Gynecol Scand 1993;72:20.

71. Doyle L, Kelly E, Rickards A, Ford G, Callanan C. Sensorineural outcome at 2 years for survivors of erythroblastosis treated with fetal intravascular transfusions. Obstet Gynecol 1993;81:931.

72. Hudon L, Moise KJ, Hegemier SE, et al. Long-term neurodevelopmental outcome after intrauterine transfusion for treatment of fetal hemolytic disease. Am J Obstet Gynecol 1998;179:858.

73. Grab D, Paulus W, Bommer A, Buck G, Teriade R. Treatment of fetal erythroblastosis by intravascular transfusions: outcome at 6 years. Obstet Gynecol 1999;93:165.

74. Janssens H, de Hann M, van Kamp I, Brand R, Hanbai H, Veen S. Outcome for children treated with fetal intravascular transfusions because of severe blood group antagonism. J Pediatr 1997;131:373.

75. Dallacasa P, Ancora G, Miniero R, et al. Erythropoietin course in newborns with Rh hemolytic disease transfused and not transfused in utero. Pediatr Res 1996; 40:357.

76. Saade G, Moise K, Belfort M, Hesketh D, Carpenter R. Fetal and neonatal hematologic parameters in red cell alloimmunization: predicting the need for late neonatal transfusions. Fetal Diagn Ther 1993;8:161.

77. Bowman J. Antenatal suppression of Rh alloimmunization. Clin Obstet Gynecol 1991;34:296.

78. Deka D, Buckshee K, Kinra G. Intravenous immunoglobulin as primary therapy or adjuvant therapy to

intrauterine fetal blood transfusion: a new approach in the management of severe Rh-immunization. J Obstet Gynaecol Res 1996;22:561.

79. Dooren M, Kamp I, Scherpenisse J, et al. No beneficial effect of low-dose fetal intravenous gammaglobulin administration in combination with intravascular transfusion in severe Rh D haemolytic disease. Vox Sang 1994; 66:253.

80. Margulies M. High-dose gamma globulin (IVIG) followed by intrauterine transfusion (IVT): a new alternative treatment of severe fetal hemolytic disease. J Perinat Med 1997;25:85.

81. Margulies M, Voto L, Mathet E, Margulies M. High-dose intravenous IgG for the treatment of severe Rhesus alloimmunization. Vox Sang 1991;61:181.

82. Porter T, Silver R, Jackson G, Branch D, Scott J. Intravenous immune globulin in the management of severe Rh D hemolytic disease. Obstet Gynecol Surv 1997;52:193.

83. Thilogantham B, Nicolaides K. Intrauterine bone marrow transplantation at 12 weeks gestation. Lancet 1993; 342:243.

84. Anderson CW, Cordero L. Changes in amniotic fluid optical density at 450 Mμ in Rh-sensitized patients after maternal hydrocortisone treatment. Am J Obstet Gynecol 1980;137:820.

85. Robinson E, Tovey L. Intensive plasma exchange in the management of severe Rh Disease. Br J Haematol 1980; 45:621.

86. Bierme SJ, Blanc M, Abbol M, et al. Oral Rh treatment for severely immunized mothers. Lancet 1979;1:604.

87. Gusdon JP, Caudle MR, Herbst GA et al. Phagocytosis and erythroblastosis: I. modification of the neonatal response by promethazine hydrochloride. Am J Obstet Gynecol 1976;125:224.

88. Van den Veyver IB, Chong SS, Cota J, et al. Single-cell analysis of the RhD blood type for use in preimplantation diagnosis in the prevention of severe hemolytic disease of the newborn. Am J Obstet Gynecol 1995;172:533.

89. Hartwell EA. Use of Rh immune globulin. ASCP practice parameter. Am J Clin Pathol 1998;110:281.

90. Urbaniak SJ, ed. Consensus conference on AntiD prophylaxis. Br J Obstet Gynaecol 1998;105(Suppl 18).

91. Samson D, Mollison PL. Effect on primary Rh immunization of delayed administration of anti-Rh. Immunology 1975;28:349.

92. Bussel J, Berkowitz R, McFarland J. Maternal IVIG in neonatal alloimmune thrombocytopenia. Br J Haematol 1997;96:186.

93. Garraty G. Platelet immunology—similarities and differences with red cell immunology. Immunohematology 1995;11:112.

94. Williamson LM, Hackett G, Rennie J, et al. The natural history of fetomaternal alloimmunization to the platelet-specific antigen HPA-la(P1^{A1}, Zw^a) as determined by antenatal screening. Blood 1998;92:2280.

95. Gruel Y, Boizard B, Daffos F, Forestier F, Caen J, Wautier JL. Determination of platelet antigens and glycoproteins in the human fetus. Blood 1986;68:488.

96. Zhou Y, Fisher SJ, Janatpour M, et al. Human cytotrophoblasts adopt a vascular phenotype as they differentiate: a strategy for successful endovascular invasion. J Clin Invest 1997;99:2139.

97. de Waal LP, van Dalen CM, Engelfriet CP, von dem Borne AEGK. Alloimmunization against the platelet-specific Zw^a antigen, resulting in neonatal alloimmune thrombocytopenia or posttransfusion purpura, is associated with the supertypic DRw52 antigen including DR3 and DRw6. Hum Immunol 1986;17:45.

98. Dreyfus M, Kaplan C, Verdy E, et al. Frequency of immune thrombocytopenia in newborns: a prospective study. Blood 1997;89:4402.

99. Bussel J, Berkowitz R, Lynch L, et al. Antenatal management of alloimmune thrombocytopenia with intravenous γ-globulin: a randomized trial of the addition of low-dose steroid to intravenous γ-globulin. Am J Obstet Gynecol 1996;174:1414.

100. Giovangrandi Y, Daffos F, Kaplan C. Very early intracranial hemorrhage in alloimmune thrombocytopenia. Lancet 1990;2:310.

101. Flug F, Karpatkin M, Karpatkin S. Should all pregnant women be tested for their platelet PLA (Zw, HPA-1) phenotype? Br J Haematol 1994;86:1.

102. McFarland, Aster R, Bussel J, Gianopoulos J, Derbes R, Newman P. Prenatal diagnosis of neonatal alloimmune thrombocytopenia using allele-specific oligonucleotide probes. Blood 1991;78:2276.

103. Johnson J, Ryan G, al-Musa A, Farkas S, Blanchette V. Prenatal diagnosis and management of neonatal alloimmune thrombocytopenia. Semin Perinatol 1997;21:45.

104. Bussel J, Zabusky B, Berkowitz R, McFarland J. Fetal alloimmune thrombocytopenia. N Engl J Med 1997; 37:22.

105. Paidas MJ, Berkowitz RL, Lynch L, et al. Alloimmune thrombocytopenia: fetal and neonatal losses related to cordocentesis. Am J Obstet Gynecol 1995;172:475.

106. Murphy M, Pullon H, Metcalfe P, Chapman J, Jenkins E, Waters A, et al. Management of fetal alloimmune thrombocytopenia by weekly in utero platelet transfusions. Vox Sang 1990;58:45.

107. Nicolini U, Rodeck C, Kochenour N, Greco P, Fist N, Letsky E. In-utero platelet transfusion for alloimmune thrombocytopenia. Lancet 1988;2:506.

108. Giers G, Hoch J, Bauer H, et al. Therapy with intravenous immunoglobulin G during pregnancy for fetal alloimmune thrombocytopenic purpura. Prenat Diagn 1996;16:495.

109. Mir N, Samson D, House M, Kovar I. Failure of antenatal high-dose immunoglobulin to improve fetal platelet count in neonatal allo-immune thrombocytopenia. Vox Sang 1988;55:188.

110. Zimmerman R, Huch A. In-utero fetal therapy with immunoglobulin for alloimmune thrombocytopenia. Lancet 1992;340:606.

Chapter 11

Evaluation and Treatment of the Patient with a Stillborn Fetus

Isabelle Wilkins
Lynda Hudon

Five Key Points

- Between 20 and 40% of all stillbirths can be explained by an underlying fetal cause.
- Abruptio placentae has become the leading cause of fetal death, accounting for 15% of all deaths.
- Most of the unexplained fetal deaths are not associated with maternal risk factors.
- Gross autopsy of the fetus and placenta is the most useful examination in determining the cause of death and should be performed in all cases of stillbirths.
- Antenatal testing in women with a previous stillbirth should begin at 32 to 34 weeks of gestation.

Although overall perinatal mortality has decreased significantly over the past three decades in industrialized countries, fetal death remains an obstetrical catastrophe that cannot easily be predicted or prevented.[1] Because approximately 35% of all stillbirths remain unexplained, the treatment and counseling of these patients can be frustrating.

DEFINITION AND INCIDENCE

Perinatal mortality statistics can be rather confusing because of differences between countries in categorizing fetal death and stillbirth. According to the World Health Organization, the perinatal period extends from 22 weeks of gestation (or 500 g) through 28 completed days of life while the neonatal period is from birth through 7 completed days of life.[2,3] In contrast, the American College of Obstetricians and Gynecologists (ACOG) uses birth and 28 days of life to define the boundaries of the neonatal period. In 1995, ACOG recommended that death in fetuses weighing more than 500 g be reported and included in perinatal mortality statistics. A variety of requirements for gestational age (above 20 or 28 weeks) and birth weights (from 350 to 1000 g) are still currently used in different health systems.[4]

The fetal death rate is usually expressed as the number of fetal deaths per 1000 births, but this statistic may be hidden in the overall perinatal death rate and not readily available. The proportion of perinatal deaths reported as fetal deaths varies from 33% to 68% throughout the world.[2]

Over the past three decades, the total fetal death rate has decreased by 64%: it fell from 11.5 per 1000 births in 1960 to 5.1 in the 1980s.[1]

RISK FACTORS

In a retrospective study, Copper et al.[5] identified several risk factors associated with an increased risk of stillbirth. Several maternal demographics were found to be significantly associated with a higher risk of fetal death. A prepregnancy maternal weight greater than 85 kg was associated with a 2-fold increase in fetal death, whereas black women had a 1.6-fold increased risk. Smoking and single marital status were also associated with a significant rise in the rate of stillbirth. Fretts and Usher[6] found that women older than 35 had a 2.2-fold increase in the risk of unexplained fetal death. The unexplained fetal death rate was 1 in 440 births in women 35 years of age or older, as compared with 1 in 1000 births in women younger than 35. Alessandri et al.[7] reported that mothers with unexplained stillbirths had a significantly higher average weekly weight gain as compared with controls. They also reported that pregnancies ending in unexplained stillbirth were less likely to have had medical and obstetrical complications, had less hypertension and antihypertensive medication, and had a greater weight gain as compared with pregnancies with live births. Stillbirths account for a small proportion of all births, so it is understandable that most of the obstetrical and medical complications occur in pregnancies with a live birth. Copper et al.[5] reported that the only maternal conditions significantly associated with an increased risk of fetal death were hemoglobinopathy (sixfold increase), Rh sensitization (eightfold increase), and chorioamnionitis (sixfold increase). Because the first two conditions are rarely found in the population, they are associated with less than 2% of all stillbirths. Isolated polyhydramnios, excluding major fetal abnormalities, is associated with a ninefold increased risk of stillbirth. Maternal infection, usually chorioamnionitis, is associated with a high proportion of all stillbirths (9.4%). Some factors associated with an increased risk of preterm delivery such as previous preterm delivery, first-trimester bleeding, short cervical length, and a history

of a cervical conization are also associated with an increased risk of stillbirth.

CAUSES OF FETAL DEATH (Table 11-1)

Fetal Causes

Between 20 and 40% of all stillbirths can be explained by an apparent underlying fetal cause. Congenital structural anomalies, intrauterine growth restriction, chromosomal anomalies, nonimmune hydrops fetalis, and alloimmunization are among the most common fetal causes of stillbirth.

Congenital Anomalies

Depending on the series, 25 to 50% of all stillborn fetuses with congenital anomalies have a genetic cause.[8,9] Pauli and Reiser[9] have categorized fetal death on the basis of presumptive cause: it was found to be sporadic in 29% of the cases, chromosomal in 25%, multifactorial in 12%, mendelian (single gene disorder) in 4.7%, environmental in 3.6%, and unclassified in 26%. A large proportion of the multiple anomaly syndromes could not be precisely identified. Trisomy 21, monosomy X (Turner syndrome), and trisomy 18 were found to be the most common chromosomal abnormalities among stillborn fetuses. Although the overall incidence of chromosomal defects among stillbirths was 5.6% in their series, it can be as high as 8% according to other series.[8] The most common structural anomalies are central

---

TABLE 11-1
CAUSES OF FETAL DEATH

Fetal causes (20 to 40%)
   Congenital anomalies
   Intrauterine growth restriction
   Chromosomal anomalies
   Alloimmunization
   Nonimmune hydrops fetalis
Placental causes (20 to 25%)
   Abruption
   Cord accident
   Placenta previa
   Twin-to-twin transfusion syndrome
Maternal causes (10%)
   Chorioamnionitis
   Hypertension
   Diabetes
   Postterm pregnancy
   Antiphospholipid syndrome
Unexplained (25 to 35%)

nervous system anomalies (48%), followed by cardiac and gastrointestinal anomalies (approximately 9% each).

Deaths due to lethal anomalies have declined with the increased use of antenatal ultrasound, largely because the neonatal deaths of anencephalic infants have been replaced by terminations of pregnancy before viability. Although genetic prenatal diagnosis in women older than 35 will decrease the perinatal mortality rate due to structural and chromosomal anomalies in this specific population, it will not significantly decrease the overall perinatal mortality rate, since most of these anomalies occur in younger women. For this reason, prenatal screening of all pregnancies in the second trimester using multiple serum markers (α-fetoprotein, human chorionic gonadotropin, and unconjugated estriol) and ultrasound will help reduce the perinatal mortality rate by increased terminations of anomalous fetuses.[10]

Intrauterine Growth Restriction

Despite the fact that fetal deaths secondary to intrauterine growth restriction have declined by 60% over the past three decades, it is still the second most common cause of fetal death after abruptio placentae.[1] Nonanomalous growth-restricted fetuses have a 10-fold increased risk of death, the majority of which occur before 36 weeks of gestation. Alessandri et al.[7] found that 54.6% of unexplained antepartum stillbirths had low birth weight. The authors did not specifically categorize all fetuses as being growth-restricted and may have included in their series preterm fetuses that were adequate for gestational age.

Severe intrauterine growth restriction secondary to placental insufficiency can result in stillbirth. The most common causes of placental insufficiency are uncontrolled chronic hypertension, pregnancy-induced hypertension, antiphospholipid syndrome, maternal vascular disease, chronic renal failure, and smoking.

Red-Cell Alloimmunization

Perinatal mortality secondary to red-cell alloimmunization has decreased significantly over the past two decades. The perinatal mortality fell from 18 per 10,000 births to 0.7 to 1.5 per 10,000 between 1975 and 1992.[1,11] Although Rh immune globulin can prevent alloimmunization in Rh-negative women, red-cell alloimmunization to non-Rh antigens such as Kell, Kidd, and Duffy continues to be a problem.

Multiple Gestation

The advancements in assisted reproductive techniques are thought to be partially responsible for the rising incidence in multiple gestations, which have a significantly increased risk for fetal death. Although this risk is greater in monozygotic multiple gestations, due in part to vascular placental communications causing twin-to-twin transfusion syndrome, dizygotic multiple gestations still remain at higher risk as compared with singleton pregnancies. The incidence of intrauterine death of a twin is between 3 and 7%.[12-14]

Placental and Umbilical Cord Causes

Abruptio placentae has become the leading cause of fetal death, accounting for 15% of all cases.[1] Copper et al.[5] reported that placental abruption is the obstetrical condition associated with the highest risk of stillbirth (12.4-fold increase). In contrast, severe antepartum hemorrhage in the presence of placenta previa is a rare cause of fetal death.

In the series by Fretts and Usher,[1] nuchal cord loops and knots were associated with 21% of the unexplained fetal deaths, but these were also present in 28% of all live births during the same period. Alessandri et al.[7] found a 6.5-fold increased risk of fetal death with cord abnormalities such as twisting and spiraling. Fetal death can also be associated with cord prolapse, cord occlusion/constriction, and vasa previa.[15] Tumors of the umbilical cord are rare; the most common type is the hemangioma. There is a high incidence of fetal abnormality and fetal death in cases of cord hemangiomas although no consistent abnormality has been reported in these cases.[16]

Maternal Causes

Infections

The fetal death rate secondary to maternal intrauterine infection has remained unchanged for the past three decades. Copper et al.[5] found that chorioamnionitis was associated with a sixfold increased risk for stillbirth and was responsible for 9.4% of all stillbirths. Among the possible causes of stillbirth due to infections, *Chlamydia trachomatis*, *Ureaplasma urealyticum*, *Mycoplasma hominis*, group B streptococci, *Listeria monocytogenes*, rubella virus, Coxsackie B virus, cytomegalovirus, varicella and Herpes simplex viruses 1 and 2, *Candida albicans*, and *Toxoplasma gondii* have all been reported to be associated with stillbirth. Bacterial and viral infections, as opposed to mycotic and parasitic infections, are the most commonly identified causes of stillbirth secondary to fetal sepsis. Ascending infection from the vagina or endocervix to the amniotic cavity constitutes the predominant route for prenatal infection. Prenatal infection with group B streptococci has been identified as a major cause of neonatal death, and the prevention strategies based on risk factors or third-trimester universal screening are effective in the prevention of neonatal sepsis but not fetal sepsis leading to stillbirth. Although rare, fulminant intraamniotic infection with *Listeria monocytogenes* in patients with intact membranes has been reported to cause fetal death through transplacental infection.[17,18]

Maternal Diseases

Most of the unexplained fetal deaths are not associated with maternal risk factors. Maternal diabetes and hypertension are together associated with 5 to 8% of all stillbirths.[6,7] Women with gestational diabetes controlled with diet alone do not have an increased risk for fetal death.[19] The fetal death rate is significantly elevated in patients with insulin-dependant diabetes as compared with nondiabetic patients, although Fretts and Usher[1] found that the incidence has been reduced to 16 per 1000 births over the past three decades. This decrease can probably be explained by better prenatal care for diabetic patients. In the report by Fretts and Usher,[1] approximately half of the otherwise unexplained fetal deaths were attributed to maternal diabetes. It is unclear why insulin-dependent diabetics have an excessive stillbirth rate, but it is known that sudden fetal death rarely occurs when maternal glycemic control is optimized. Fetal polycythemia, hyperglycemia associated with hypoxemia, or hyperinsulinemia causing increased metabolic rate and oxygen requirements may be involved in the causal relationship. These metabolic changes occur because of suboptimal maternal glycemic control.

Uncontrolled chronic hypertension has been associated with placental insufficiency, intrauterine growth restriction, and an increased incidence of preeclampsia. Severe preeclampsia can also be associated with placental abruption, intrauterine growth restriction, and fetal death.

The relationship between pregnancy loss and the antiphospholipid syndrome has been explored by many authors.[20-22] The association of antiphospholipid syndrome with increased perinatal mortality remains controversial, in part due to the various definitions that have been used to describe the syndrome. In addition, antiphospholipid antibodies are found with some frequency in asymptomatic women with uncomplicated pregnancies. Placental infarcts and thromboses, intrauterine growth restriction, recurrent spontaneous abortions, and multiple pregnancy loss have all been strongly associated with antiphospholipid syndrome.[20] In the report by Oshiro and co-workers,[20] more than 80% of the women with antiphospholipid antibodies experienced at least one fetal death, and over 50% had at least two fetal deaths. The incidence of anticardiolipin antibodies and lupus anticoagulant in women with normal pregnancies was 1.5 and 3.8%, respectively. Infante-Rivard and associates[21] reported that women with one spontaneous abortion or one fetal death were not more likely than women with normal pregnancy outcome to have either a positive test for lupus anticoagulant or anticardiolipin antibodies. The odds ratio for the association between lupus anticoagulant and fetal loss in patients with no previous fetal loss was 1.36 (95% confidence interval, 0.75 to 2.43). This finding contrasts with other studies consisting of case series of women with recurrent pregnancy loss who showed a stronger association between anticardiolipin antibodies, lupus anticoagulant, and pregnancy loss.

Uterine Rupture

Because offering a trial of labor after a previous low-transverse cesarean delivery is now considered to be the standard of care, the cause and incidence of uterine rupture has changed over the past decade. Peripartum uterine rupture, as well as uterine rupture secondary to maternal trauma, are now responsible for almost 3% of all stillbirths.[7]

Other Maternal Causes

Cocaine use has been associated with severe abruptio placentae, while other illicit drugs may be associated with intrauterine growth restriction, placental insufficiency, and inconsistent prenatal care.

Postterm pregnancies are responsible for approximately 1 to 1.8% of all stillbirths.[5,23] The risk of having a stillbirth decreases as gestation progresses to 40 completed weeks. The highest stillbirth rate in term patients is in nulliparous women at 38 weeks of gestation (2.7%). In multiparous women, the risk does not increase after 40 weeks (1.5%), whereas there is a slightly increased risk of stillbirth for primigravidas in the postterm period (2.26%).[23] A major concern and criticism of most studies on prolonged pregnancies is the validity of the dating criteria. Early ultrasound assessment has been accepted as an accurate method of verifying gestational age. Approximately 7.5% of all pregnancies reach 42 weeks by menstrual dating alone, as compared with 2.6% when dating is based on early ultrasound examination.[24]

UNEXPLAINED FETAL DEATH

Although an appropriate work-up for fetal death should minimize the proportion of stillbirths falling in this category, between 25 and 35% of all fetal deaths will remain unexplained despite adequate evaluation and investigation. Fretts and Usher[6] reported that the risk of fetal death in women older than 35 years of age was double the rate in younger women.

There may be an association between unexplained stillbirth and gestational age greater than 40 weeks as reported by Yudkin et al.,[25] although the majority of all stillbirths occur before 28 weeks of gestation.[5] The risk of unexplained stillbirth at 33 to 34 weeks was reported to be 23 per 1000 births as compared with 0.4 per 1000 at 39 to 40 weeks and 1.2 per 1000 at 41 weeks and later.

MANAGEMENT OF FETAL DEATH

Diagnosis

Suspicion of an intrauterine fetal death raised by decreased or absent fetal movements as reported by the patient or by absent heart tones on auscultation should prompt an immediate ultrasound evaluation. Unless severe oligohydramnios or morbid maternal obesity are present, transabdominal ultrasound should easily confirm the diagnosis of fetal death. The transvaginal ultrasound approach or the use of color Doppler can be useful in those situations. The absence of heart activity and fetal movements should be documented. Some ultrasound findings can help to grossly identify the time elapsed since fetal death. Oligohydramnios, skin edema, ascites, intraluminal bowel gas, or overlapping sutures of the calvarium are signs of maceration. The fetal presentation, the presence of macrosomia or any fetal congenital anomaly that can potentially cause significant dystocia (e.g., severe hydrocephalus, prune-belly syndrome, sacrococcygeal

teratoma) are useful information for the physician in order to plan the delivery.

Delivery

The diagnosis of fetal death is a devastating event for the pregnant patient and her family. Although spontaneous labor and delivery will occur within 2 weeks in approximately 80 to 90% of cases, the latency period can be longer in preterm stillbirths. Most patients will find a long latency period unacceptable and will ask for a rapid induction of labor; others will need some time to cope with the emotional aspects of a stillbirth. Because medical complications secondary to a retained dead fetus will generally not occur for several weeks, a latency period aimed at awaiting spontaneous labor remains a safe option if acceptable for the patient. One situation in which expectant management can be indicated is in the case of fetal death of one twin. In that case, expectant management until fetal lung maturity of the surviving twin is attained can avoid additional morbidity attributable to prematurity (see "Management of Fetal Death in Multiple Gestations," below).

Vaginal delivery is the preferred mode of delivery. Cesarean delivery is rarely indicated and should be reserved for selected cases. Placenta previa, placenta accreta or percreta, placental abruption causing maternal hemodynamic instability, and uterine rupture are situations in which a dead fetus needs to be delivered by cesarean. Patients with multiple previous cesarean deliveries or a previous classical cesarean should be carefully counseled about the risk of uterine rupture before they consent to a vaginal delivery. Some types of congenital anomalies can cause severe dystocia and preclude a vaginal delivery. In some cases, such as severe fetal hydrocephalus or bladder obstruction with a megabladder, decompression under ultrasound guidance prior to delivery can allow a vaginal birth.

Because the majority of fetal deaths occur before 28 weeks, cervical ripening is necessary and is an important part of the induction of labor.[5] There are several safe and efficient methods to achieve cervical ripening. The same methods as in viable pregnancies can be used, although, because fetal distress is not an issue, fetal heart rate monitoring is unnecessary. Uterine contraction monitoring may still be indicated to document uterine hyperstimulation.

Induction of labor may be accomplished with intravenous oxytocin or vaginal prostaglandin E_1 analog or E$_2$. Because of the relative myometrial resistance to oxytocin, high doses (up to 300 mU per minute) are usually necessary to achieve uterine contractions in a second-trimester stillbirth. High-dose oxytocin administered in small volumes of intravenous fluid, in addition to the use of laminaria tents, usually leads to successful vaginal delivery.

Because the antidiuretic effect of oxytocin is clinically demonstrable at a dose of 40 mIU per minute, close monitoring of serum electrolytes as well as fluid balance is important. Fluid overload and hyponatremia can be avoided with careful monitoring. Baseline serum electrolytes are indicated and should be checked at least every 24 hours.

Delivery of an early-second-trimester intrauterine fetal death can also be successfully performed with intraamniotic injection of prostaglandin F$_{2\alpha}$, hypertonic saline, or hyperosmolar urea or with surgical dilatation and extraction. Surgical dilatation and extraction does not carry additional maternal morbidity when performed by an experienced physician.

Evaluation

The purpose of a careful evaluation of a stillbirth is to determine the cause of death and to identify the risk of recurrence for a future pregnancy. A detailed family and obstetrical history will help to identify dominant or recessive genetic disorders that may explain fetal death. A history of maternal illnesses, medications or drug exposure can also be helpful in determining the cause of death. Figure 11-1 presents a simplified algorithm for evaluation of a stillborn fetus.

Examination of the Fetus and Placenta

Examination of the fetus and placenta immediately after delivery is too often forgotten by the delivering physician. Gross examination of the fetus can help determine the time elapsed since death. Corneal clouding, reddening of the skin with desquamation in the face, back, and abdominal areas limited to less than 5% of the body surface are seen 12 hours or more after death. Brown skin discoloration with moderate to severe desquamation is seen 24 hours or more after death, while increased joint mobility is usually seen more than 48 hours after the time of death. Observations concerning the presence of cord loops, knots, cord prolapse, appearance of the amniotic fluid, and gross placental findings (signs of abruption, accessory lobes, velamentous cord insertion, meconium staining) should be recorded in the patient's medical

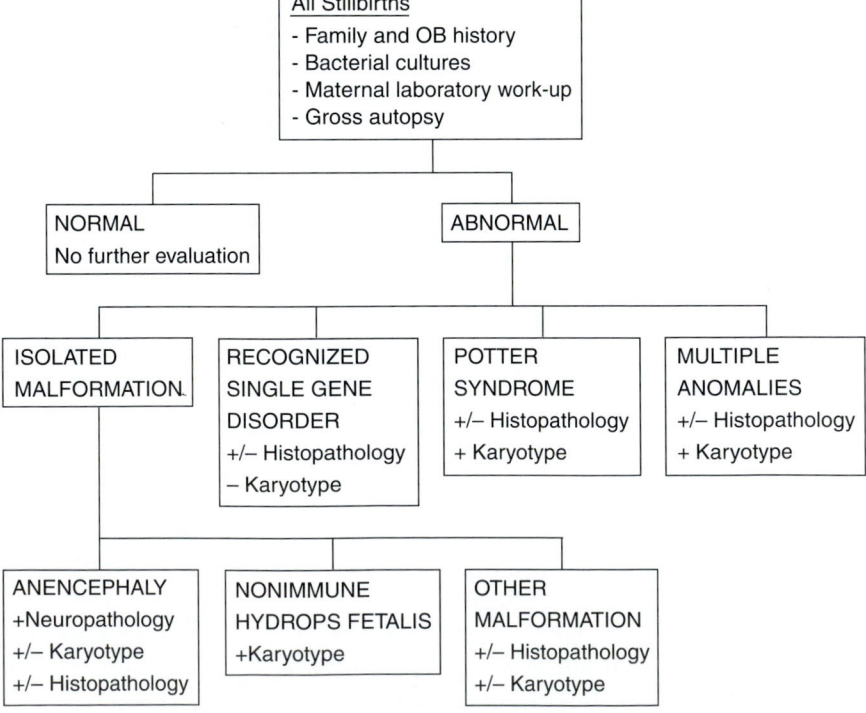

Figure 11-1 Evaluation of a stillborn: diagnostic and management algorithm. *From Mueller R, Sybert VP, Johnson J, Brown ZA, Chen WJ. Evaluation of a protocol for post-mortem examination of stillbirths. N Engl J Med 1983;309:586.*

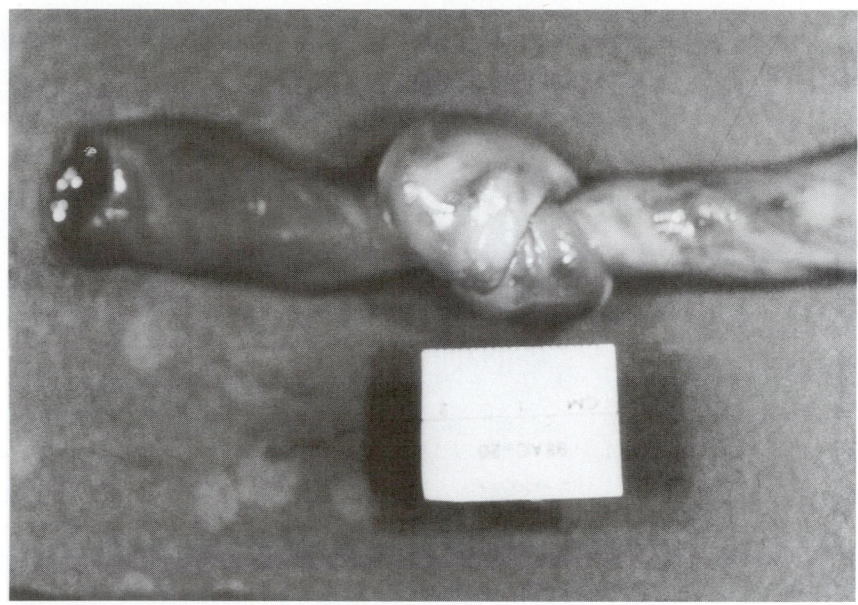

Figure 11-2 The true knot in this umbilical cord was thought to be responsible for a term fetal death. *Courtesy of Edwina Popek, M.D., Department of Pathology, Baylor College of Medicine, Houston, TX.*

chart (Figures 11-2 to 11-4). Obvious congenital malformations should be recorded. Any dysmorphic features should lead to cytogenetic studies to rule out chromosomal abnormalities. The foot length, as measured from the big toe to the heel, can be used to determine gestational age in case other indexes are altered by hydrops fetalis, growth restriction, or massive maceration (Table 11-2).

Gross Autopsy

In a retrospective study on the postmortem evaluation of 124 stillbirths or early neonatal deaths, Mueller et al.[8] found that the most useful examination was the gross autopsy and recommended that gross postmortem examination, including evaluation of the placenta, be performed in all cases of stillbirth. No specific cause for loss of apparently normal

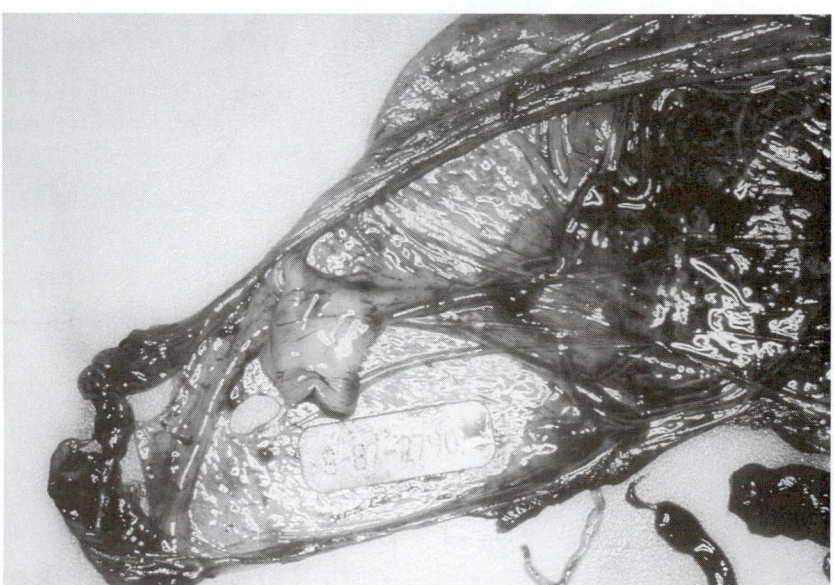

Figure 11-3 The velamentous insertion of this umbilical cord was associated with vasa previa, causing fetal exsanguination and death. *Courtesy of Edwina Popek, M.D., Department of Pathology, Baylor College of Medicine, Houston, TX.*

Figure 11-4 Top. Massive placental abruption causing fetal death. Bottom. Close-up view of extensive area of placental abruption. *Courtesy of Edwina Popek, M.D., Department of Pathology, Baylor College of Medicine, Houston, TX.*

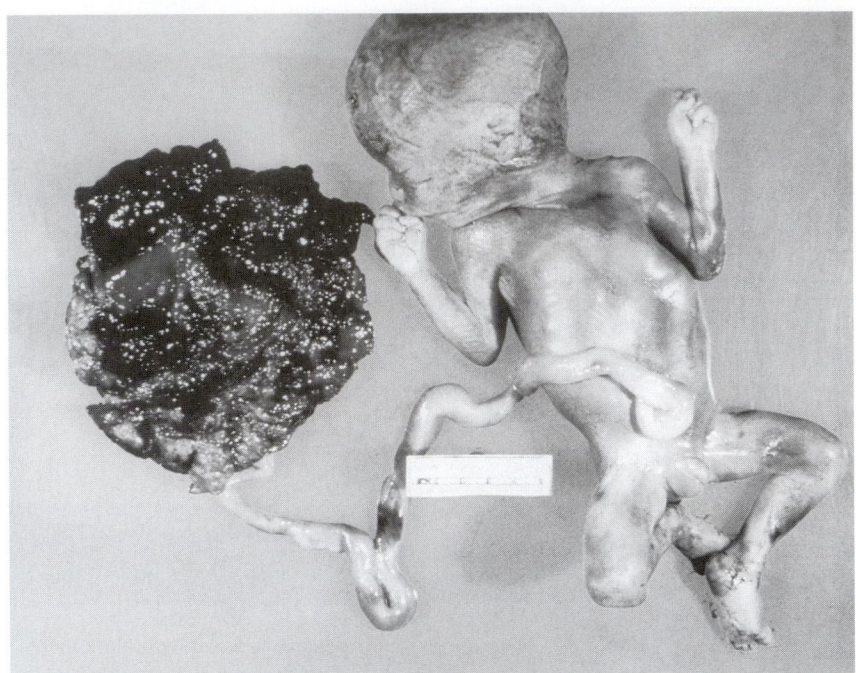

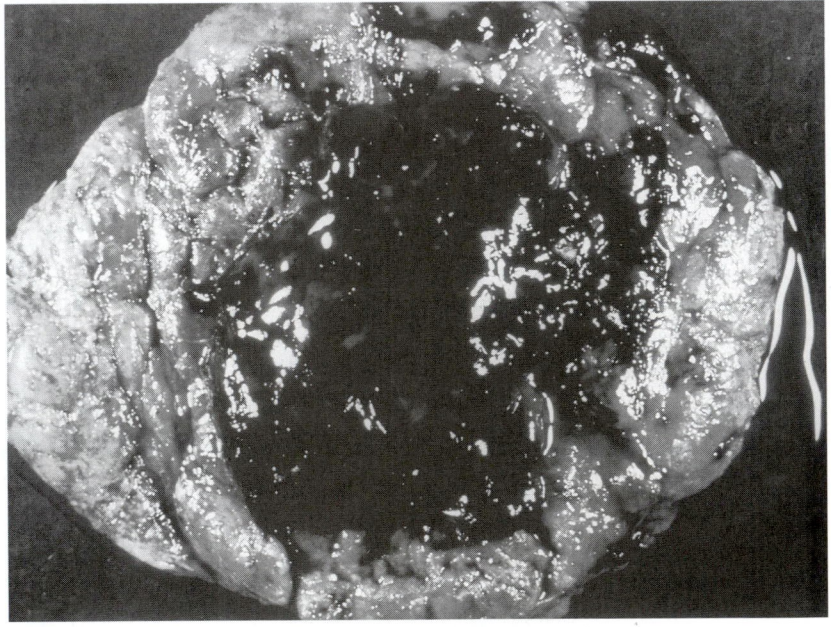

pregnancies was found based on histopathological study alone in this series. The usefulness of the autopsy can be evaluated when comparing the cause of death based on clinical impressions with the gross autopsy findings. In a study by Saller et al., the clinical diagnosis was confirmed by an autopsy in 26 to 29% of the cases.[26] The cause of death was changed according to the autopsy findings in 30% of the cases while the autopsy findings were inconclusive in 38% of the cases. In 18 to 24% of the cases, the gross autopsy alone disclosed the main cause of death and

had direct implications for future pregnancies in 4% of the cases.[8,26,27] Even in cases in which the cause of fetal death seems obvious (e.g., anencephaly), accurate diagnosis as well as prediction of the risk of recurrence will be possible only with more extensive evaluation. For example, a case of anencephaly with polydactyly may be due to the Meckel–Gruber syndrome, an autosomal recessive disorder with a 25% risk of recurrence; can have a multifactorial cause with a risk of recurrence of 3 to 5%; or may be due to trisomy 13 with a 1% chance of recurrence. Pictures

TABLE 11-2
MEASUREMENTS OF STILLBORN: GESTATIONAL AGE VERSUS MEAN FOOT LENGTH

Gestational Age (weeks)	Toe-to-Heel Length (cm; mean ±SD)
20	3.6±0.7
21	3.8±0.1
22	4.0±0.4
23	4.2±0.5
24	4.4±0.3
25	4.6±0.4
26	4.8±0.7
27	5.0±0.5
28	5.2±0.6
29	5.4±0.8
30	5.7±0.7
31	5.9±0.7
32	6.1±1.1
33	6.3±0.7
34	6.5±0.6
35	6.7±0.4
36	6.9±1.1
37	7.1±1.2
38	7.3±0.8
39	7.5±0.5
40	7.7±0.8
41	7.9±0.8
42	8.1±1.1

Adapted from Sung CJ, Singer DB. Fetal growth and maturation. In: Wigglesworth JS, Singer DB, eds. Textbook of fetal and perinatal pathology. Boston: Blackwell Scientific, 1991:35.

and x-ray films are commonly part of the gross evaluation of the stillborn in order to document and describe dysmorphic features and skeletal disorders.

KARYOTYPE

Most authors agree that fetal karyotype is not indicated in all cases of fetal death (see Figure 11-1). Indications for cytogenetic studies include multiple congenital anomalies, growth restriction, dysmorphic features, a family history of congenital anomalies or genetic disorders, nonimmune hydrops fetalis, a history of recurrent pregnancy losses, or a parent with a known balanced translocation.[3,8]

In more than 25% of cases, postmortem cytogenetic studies are unsuccessful in obtaining chromosome analysis. Bacterial contamination of the tissue samples is common and is one of the main reason for culture failure. For this reason, in cases in which fetal karyotyping is indicated, genetic amniocentesis before delivery can be offered in order to obtain successful cytogenetic studies in more than 99% of cases.[28]

If no predelivery studies have been performed, cytogenetic studies are best done on tissues sampled immediately after delivery. If the fetus is not macerated, a skin biopsy is the best choice. After local disinfection with alcohol, approximately 1 cm of skin should be excised and submitted for culture of fibroblasts. Cord blood or fetal blood obtained by cardiac puncture immediately after birth is an excellent option in cases of recent fetal death, although this will be unsuccessful if the blood is coagulated. In cases of macerated fetuses, more than one type of tissue should be sent, such as skin, pericardium, lung, and umbilical cord. Amnion stripped from the placenta will usually grow without any contamination by maternal cells.

If the results of chromosome studies are abnormal, further testing of the family may be necessary. For certain diagnoses, family studies are necessary to provide accurate estimates of recurrence risks. Both chromosomal translocation and autosomal dominant disorders can be inherited or can occur de novo, and evaluation of the family is essential to determine which is the case.

Cultures

Maternal cervical and vaginal cultures should be done as soon as possible after the diagnosis of fetal death. Ascending infection, especially in cases of ruptured membranes, is associated with up to 9.4% of all stillbirths.[5] Cervical cultures for gonorrhea, chlamydia, and aerobic bacteria as well as vaginal and anal culture for group B streptococci should be part of the routine evaluation. Bacterial aerobic and anaerobic cultures of the maternal and fetal placental surfaces should also be included as part of the routine investigation.

If an amniocentesis is performed for cytogenetic studies, amniotic fluid should also be processed for bacterial aerobic and anaerobic cultures, as well as viral cultures. Identification of viral DNA in amniotic fluid by polymerase chain reaction (PCR) is a very sensitive diagnostic technique but not widely available at present.

Maternal Evaluation

In a 1993 Technical Bulletin, ACOG suggested a basic maternal work-up for all pregnancies with stillbirths (Table 11-3).[4] A random serum glucose, activated partial thromboplastin time, complete blood count with platelet count, antibody screen, VDRL, Kleihauer–Betke test, and urine toxicology were suggested to rule out the most common maternal causes

TABLE 11-3
DIAGNOSTIC EVALUATION OF A STILLBORN FETUS

Prior to delivery
  Kleihauer–Betke test
  Blood type and antibody screen
  Activated partial thromboplastin time, complete blood count
    with platelet count
  Serum glucose
  VDRL
  Urine toxicology
  Cervical and vaginal cultures
    Chlamydia
    Gonorrhea
    Group B streptococci
  Selected cases
    Serology for toxoplasmosis, cytomegalovirus
    Thyroid function tests
    Anticardiolipin antibody and lupus anticoagulant
After delivery
  Placenta
    Gross examination
    Bacterial cultures (maternal and fetal surfaces)
    Histopathological examination
  Fetus
    Physical examination
    Gross autopsy
    Karyotype if indicated (fetal blood, skin fibroblast, amnion)
    Metabolic studies if indicated (skin fibroblast)

of stillbirth. Other authors, in addition to this work-up, have proposed maternal serologic analysis for toxoplasmosis and cytomegalovirus.[28] Thyroid-function tests should be performed in selected cases in which there is a clinical suspicion of a thyroid disorder. Infante-Rivard et al.[21] have suggested that testing for anticardiolipin antibodies and lupus anticoagulant is not cost effective in patients with no history of multiple pregnancy loss.

Other Studies

The finding of nonimmune hydrops fetalis in a stillborn fetus warrants additional studies. The most common causes of nonimmune hydrops are chromosomal anomalies, congenital heart defects, other major structural congenital anomalies, congenital infections with cytomegalovirus and syphilis, and fetal anemia from conditions such as α-thalassemia and parvovirus infection. Some of the more common causes of fetal anemia, like red-cell alloimmunization or massive fetal–maternal hemorrhage, will be identified with routine laboratory studies, while other conditions like glucose-6-phosphatase dehydrogenase deficiency require additional analyses. A small but significant proportion of the storage diseases can present with

nonimmune hydrops fetalis. Some of these specific disorders include sialidosis, galactosialidosis, sialic acid storage disorder, Niemann–Pick disease types A and C, I-cell disease, and GM_1 gangliosidosis. Appropriate enzymatic and DNA studies can be obtained from amniotic fluid, chorionic villi, or skin fibroblasts.[29]

MANAGEMENT OF FETAL DEATH IN MULTIPLE GESTATION

Multiple gestations are at significantly increased risk for fetal death. The incidence of intrauterine fetal death of one twin is between 3 and 7%, depending on the series.[12-14] The most common causes for fetal death of one twin are cord accidents, twin-to-twin transfusion syndrome, placental abruption, and congenital anomalies. Weight discrepancy between twins is a risk factor for stillbirth. Approximately 50% of the twin pregnancies complicated by fetal death are monochorionic.

Early death of one twin, usually in the first trimester or early second trimester, is not typically associated with increased maternal or co-twin morbidity. After the first half of pregnancy, fetal death in monochorionic twins has been associated with increased perinatal morbidity, especially neurologic sequelae, as compared with dichorionic twin pregnancies. This effect is probably due to the presence of vascular anastomoses in the placental circulation. Vascular communications are almost universal in monochorionic placentation and are associated with transfusion between twins.[30] It is hypothesized that at the time of death of one twin, hypoperfusion and severe hypotension in the surviving twin is responsible for the resulting neurologic morbidity or death.[31]

Because the main cause of perinatal mortality in twins is prematurity, expectant management of twin gestations with the death of one twin is the most reasonable option, despite concern about morbidity and even mortality in the surviving twin. Early delivery of the surviving twin will not improve neurologic prognosis because the injury usually occurs at the time of death of the co-twin.

After fetal death in one twin has been confirmed, a targeted ultrasound should be performed to rule out congenital anomalies, twin-to-twin transfusion syndrome, placental abruption, and growth restriction in the surviving twin. The maternal evaluation consists of the same basic work-up described earlier for fetal death in singletons. Maternal conditions such as diabetes or hypertension should be under optimal control.

The maternal hazard of disseminated intravascular coagulation (DIC) is stressed by many authors, although no recent series has reported DIC in cases of fetal death managed expectantly. The 25% risk of DIC estimated by Landy et al.'s series[32] has probably been overemphasized. Although controversial, initial maternal coagulation studies at the diagnosis of fetal death, followed by studies every 1 to 4 weeks depending on the symptoms and the time elapsed since death, are reasonable. As for singleton pregnancies with intrauterine fetal death, it seems likely that maternal coagulation changes occur after 3 to 4 weeks.[3]

Pregnancies complicated by fetal death in one twin should be managed expectantly unless the pregnancy is at term. Weekly steroids to promote lung maturation are indicated until 34 weeks. Twice-weekly fetal testing using nonstress tests and/or biophysical profile are indicated.[13] Hospitalization of patients with preterm labor, placental abruption, premature rupture of the membranes, and uncontrolled diabetes or hypertension is indicated. Patients without additional risk factors can be followed on an outpatient basis. Delivery past 34 weeks, preferably at term, or at documentation of lung maturity will avoid unnecessary neonatal morbidity due to prematurity.

The mode of delivery remains controversial, but elective cesarean delivery does not seem to improve the prognosis of the surviving twin. An individualized approach should be based on the obstetrical conditions, the presence of obstetrical complications such as preeclampsia or placental abruption, and the presentations of the twins. Cesarean delivery should be reserved for obstetrical indications. Vaginal delivery should be favored if the surviving twin is the presenting one and is in a cephalic presentation. When the stillborn fetus is thought to be macerated and of low birth weight by ultrasound evaluation, the mode of delivery should be decided as if the surviving twin was a singleton pregnancy.

COUNSELING FOR FUTURE PREGNANCY

The determination of the cause of death will be extremely helpful for counseling. A follow-up visit 2 to 3 months after delivery should be planned to discuss the results of the tests performed. More precise identification of the cause of death will usually help the parents to cope with the emotional issues related to fetal death. In addition, the follow-up visit will help to evaluate and diagnose severe anxiety and depression in the parents in order to be able to offer adequate referral.

The risk of recurrence depends on the cause of death. Many of the causes of stillbirth are sporadic and thus do not have an increased risk of recurrence. Cases of dominant conditions or chromosomal anomalies warrant a genetic evaluation of the parents. The risk of recurrence is not the same in the case of a de novo mutation versus a balanced translocation in one parent. It was once believed that the risk for recurrent stillbirth in a couple with one previous stillbirth was twice the risk of the general population. However, this figure was derived from studies with a heterogeneous group of pregnancy losses and does not apply to a specific diagnosis. In the majority of the cases in which an anomaly is detected, there is an increased risk of recurrence for that disorder only.

MANAGEMENT OF A PREGNANCY AFTER A PREVIOUS FETAL DEATH

A prenatal evaluation of the woman who has experienced a previous fetal death should be done. The cause, as well as the timing, of the previous stillbirth will dictate specific evaluation and management strategies.

In the case of a previous child with a structural anomaly, prenatal diagnosis should be offered with a second-trimester targeted ultrasound. Fetal echocardiography, if available, should be offered in the case of a previous heart defect. Amniocentesis is indicated for the antenatal diagnosis of chromosomal anomalies. In some cases of recessive metabolic disorders, like Gaucher or Tay–Sachs disease or GM_1 gangliosidosis, DNA analysis of amniotic fluid can be used for prenatal diagnosis. In the case of a sensitized Rh-negative mother with a heterozygous Rh-positive father of the child, fetal RhD status can be determined on amniotic fluid using PCR technology.[34]

Some maternal conditions warrant preconceptional and early prenatal care in order to decrease the risk of fetal death. Preconceptional optimal glycemic control in the diabetic patient is important, although it is common for a diabetic patient to seek prenatal care once she is already pregnant. Optimal glycemic control should be emphasized throughout the pregnancy in every diabetic patient, but most of all in cases of previous stillbirth. Adequate blood pressure control should also be achieved in the chronically hypertensive patient, although Sibai et al.[35] reported no decrease in fetal death in a randomized control trial comparing placebo to labetalol and α-methyldopa.

Treatment of low-risk pregnant women with positive antiphospholipid antibodies cannot be justified on the basis of the available evidence. Low-risk patients include those with positive antiphospholipid antibodies who had zero to two spontaneous abortions, with only one of these being a fetal death (past 12 weeks), and no history of complications such as thrombocytopenia, thrombosis, or early-onset preeclampsia.[36] Low-dose aspirin in addition to heparin therapy seems beneficial in patients with antiphospholipid antibodies in the following situations: previous late fetal death or severe intrauterine growth restriction accompanied by pathologic evidence of placental infarctions, two or more previous intrauterine fetal deaths with or without placental infarctions, and significantly elevated anticardiolipin antibody titers.[37] Low-dose aspirin seems to be the cornerstone of the treatment. There is no consensus establishing the doses of heparin that should be used.[38] Patients with previous thrombosis should be fully anticoagulated, while patients without previous thrombotic events but who have an indication for heparin therapy have been treated with prophylactic or therapeutic doses of heparin by different investigators.[37-39]

The patient already sensitized to red-cell antigens should ideally be followed by a perinatologist. Previous obstetrical history, antibody quantification, paternal genotype for the specific antigen involved, targeted ultrasound to detect early hydrops fetalis, fetal cerebral artery velocities to detect early anemia, amniocentesis for fetal blood typing as well as measurements of optical density at 450 nm are methods to evaluate and follow sensitized patients. To date, intrauterine transfusion is the only treatment available for hemolytic disease of the fetus secondary to red-cell alloimmunization.

Antenatal testing should begin at 32 to 34 weeks with nonstress tests and biophysical profile as indicated in high-risk patients.[4] Because the majority of fetal deaths occur before 34 weeks, the impact of antenatal testing on the incidence of stillbirths will probably not be significant.[5] The timing and mode of delivery should be based on obstetrical conditions and the presence of complications. As a general rule, the patient with a previous unexplained stillbirth should be delivered at term. She should not be allowed to go postterm because of the increased risk of stillbirth.

REFERENCES

1. Fretts RC, Boyd ME, Usher RG, Usher HA. The changing pattern of fetal death, 1961–1988. Obstet Gynecol 1992;79:35.
2. Howell EM, Blondel B. International infant mortality rates: bias from reporting differences. Am J Public Health 1994;84:850.
3. American College of Obstetricians and Gynecologists. Perinatal and infant mortality statistics. ACOG Committee Opinion. 1995;167.
4. American College of Obstetricians and Gynecologists. Diagnosis and management of fetal death. ACOG Technical Bulletin 1993;176.
5. Copper RL, Goldenberg RL, Dubard MB, Davis RO. Risk factors for fetal death in white, black, and Hispanic women. Obstet Gynecol 1994;84:490.
6. Fretts RC, Usher RH. Causes of fetal death in women of advanced maternal age. Obstet Gynecol 1997;89:40.
7. Alessandri LM, Stanley FJ, Garner JB, Newnham J, Walters BNJ. A case-control study of unexplained antepartum stillbirths. Br J Obstet Gynaecol 1992;99:711.
8. Mueller R, Sybert VP, Johnson J, Brown ZA, Chen WJ. Evaluation of a protocol for postmortem examination of stillbirths. N Engl J Med 1983;309:586.
9. Pauli RM, Reiser CA. Wisconsin stillbirth service program. II. Analysis of diagnoses and diagnostic categories in the first 1,000 referrals. Am J Med Genet 1994;50:135.
10. Burton BK, Prins GS, Verp MS. A prospective trial of prenatal screening for Down syndrome by means of maternal serum α-fetoprotein, human chorionic gonadotropin, and unconjugated estriol. Am J Obstet Gynecol 1993;169:526.
11. Hussey R, Clarke C. Deaths from Rh haemolytic disease in England and Wales in 1988 and 1989. BMJ 1991;303:445.
12. Fusi L, Gordon H. Twin pregnancy complicated by single intrauterine death: problems and outcome with conservative management. Br J Obstet Gynaecol 1990;97:511.
13. Burke MS. Single fetal demise in twin gestation. Clin Obstet Gynecol 1990;33:69.
14. Kilby MD, Govind A, O'Brien SP. Outcome of twin pregnancies complicated by a single intrauterine death: a comparison with viable twin pregnancies. Obstet Gynecol 1994;84:107.
15. Hallak M, Pryde PG, Qureshi F, Johnson MP, Jacques SM, Evans MI. Constriction of the umbilical cord leading to fetal death: a report of three cases. J Reprod Med 1994;39:561.
16. Sondergaard G. Hemangioma of the umbilical cord. Acta Obstet Gynecol Scand 1994;73:434.
17. Benirschke K, Robb JA. Infectious causes of fetal death. Clin Obstet Gynecol 1987;30:284.
18. Naeye RL. Causes of perinatal mortality in the US Collaborative Perinatal Project. JAMA 1977;238:228.
19. Landon MB, Gabbe SG. Fetal surveillance in the pregnancy complicated by diabetes mellitus. Clin Perinatol 1993;20:549.
20. Oshiro BT, Silver RM, Scott JR, Yu G, Branch W. Antiphospholipid antibodies and fetal death. Obstet Gynecol 1996;87:489.

21. Infante-Rivard C, David M, Gauthier R, Rivard GE. Lupus anticoagulants, anticardiolipin antibodies, and fetal loss: a case-control study. N Engl J Med 1991;325:1063.

22. Scott JR, Rote NS, Branch DW. Immunologic aspects of recurrent abortion and fetal death. Obstet Gynecol 1987; 70:645.

23. Ingemarsson I, Kallen K. Stillbirths and rate neonatal deaths in 76,761 postterm pregnancies in Sweden, 1982–1991: a register study. Acta Obstet Gynecol Scand 1997;76:658.

24. Boyd ME, Usher RH, McLean GH, Kramer MS. Obstetric consequences of postmaturity. Am J Obstet Gynecol 1988;158:334.

25. Yudkin PL, Wood L, Redman CWG. Risk of unexplained stillbirth at different gestational ages. Lancet 1987;1:1192.

26. Saller DN, Lesser KB, Harrel U, Rogers BB, Oyer CE. The clinical utility of the perinatal autopsy. JAMA 1995; 273:663.

27. Cartlidge PHT, Danwson AT, Stewart JH, Vujanic GM. Value and quality of perinatal and infant postmortem examinations: cohort analysis of 400 consecutive deaths. BMJ 1995;310:155.

28. Ahlenius I, Floberg J, Thomassen P. Sixty-six cases of intrauterine fetal death: a prospective study with an extensive test protocol. Acta Obstet Gynecol Scand 1995; 74:109.

29. Curry CJR, Honore LH. A protocol for the investigation of pregnancy loss. Clin Perinatol 1990;17:723.

30. Robertson EG, Neer KJ. Placental injection studies in twin gestation. Am J Obstet Gynecol 1983;147:170.

31. Rydhstroem H. Pregnancy with stillbirth of both twins. Br J Obstet Gynecol 1996;103:25.

32. Landy HJ, Weiner S, Corson SL, Batzer FR, Bolognese RJ. The vanishing twin: ultrasonographic assessment of fetal disappearance in the first trimester. Am J Obstet Gynecol 1989;155:14.

33. Pritchart JA. Fetal death in utero. Obstet Gynecol 1959; 14:573.

34. Lighten A, Overton T, Sepulveda W, Warwick RM, Fisk NM, Bennett PR. Accuracy of prenatal determination of RhD type status by polymerase chain reaction using amniotic cells in RhD-negative women. Am J Obstet Gynecol 1995;173:1182.

35. Sibai BM, Mabie WC, Shasma F, Villar MA, Anderson GD. A comparison of no medication versus methyldopa or labetalol in chronic hypertension complicating pregnancy. Am J Obstet Gynecol 1990;162:960.

36. Cowchock S, Reece E. Do low-risk pregnant women with antiphospholipid antibodies need to be treated? Am J Obstet Gynecol 1997;176:1099.

37. Black K, Echer M, Librizzi R. Prevention of recurrent fetal loss caused by antiphospholipid syndrome. J Perinatol 1996;16:181.

38. Piette J, Karmochkine M, Papo T, Du L, Frances C, Wechsler B. Treatment of the antiphospholipid syndrome. Clin Rev Allerg Immunol 1995;13:73.

39. Cowchock S. Prevention of fetal death in the antiphospholipid antibody syndrome. Lupus 1996;5:467.

Chapter 12

Pregnancy Termination

Gregory J. Locksmith

Five Key Points

- Abortion, one of the most frequently performed operations in the United States, has very low morbidity and mortality rates.

- Accurate dating of the pregnancy is essential before performing any abortion.

- Ripening the cervix preoperatively facilitates timely completion of the abortion and probably lowers the risk of cervical laceration and uterine perforation.

- Studies have demonstrated that medical abortion, using mifepristone plus a prostaglandin or methotrexate plus a prostaglandin, is effective and highly acceptable up to 8 weeks of gestation.

- The main advantages of surgical abortion are that it is faster and, up to 16 weeks, safer. The advantages of medical abortion are that it is not an invasive procedure and that it can be administered more easily and more discreetly.

Termination of pregnancy is one of the most frequently performed operations in the United States. Although the number of legal abortions reported to the Centers for Disease Control and Prevention (CDC) has declined over the past several years, 321 abortions per 1000 live births were reported in 1994.[1]

The change in the legal status of abortion in 1973 resulted in greater access to abortion services, refinements in abortion techniques, and lower fatality rates. The most recent case fatality rates reported to CDC are 0.8 per 100,000 induced legal abortions.[1] The risk of death increases with gestational age, the type of procedure being performed, and the type of anesthesia. Morbidity and mortality rates associated with first-trimester abortion are approximately one-tenth those of second-trimester abortion. At equal gestational ages, surgical abortion is associated with lower morbidity and mortality than medical methods.

General anesthesia increases risk as compared with local anesthesia.[2,3]

INDICATIONS FOR ABORTION

The only condition necessary for termination of a pregnancy is the informed consent of the patient. In some circumstances, physicians should recommend termination of a desired pregnancy. Certain medical conditions pose a serious threat to a woman's health if her pregnancy were to be continued past the first trimester. Examples of such disorders include primary or secondary pulmonary hypertension, Marfan syndrome complicated by a dilated aortic root, cardiomyopathy, invasive carcinoma of the cervix, severe renal insufficiency, and thrombotic thrombocytopenic purpura. Fetal indications for pregnancy termination include major congenital malformations, chromosomal abnormalities, inherited metabolic defects, exposure to known teratogens, and rupture of membranes before the fetus is viable.[4]

The physician's responsibility is to educate the patient about the relative risks and benefits of abortion versus continuation of pregnancy as they apply specifically to her. Although physicians also have a duty to make recommendations, ultimately the choice of whether or not to terminate a pregnancy is the woman's. Some women are willing to face a large amount of risk in order to have a child; others would not be willing to accept even a relatively small risk.

SURGICAL ABORTION

First Trimester

According to CDC statistics,[1] in 1993 and 1994, 88% of legal abortions in the United States were performed before 15 weeks of gestation, and 52 to 54% were performed before 9 weeks. In 1994, all first-trimester abortions reported to CDC were curettage procedures. Most of them were performed in free-standing abortion clinics or in medical offices. These settings offer the advantages of lower cost and simplified logistics, with medical standards comparable to those of a hospital. Typically, the procedures are performed under local anesthesia with or without conscious sedation.

Approach to the Patient

Although the vast majority of women seeking abortion services can have the procedure performed safely at an outpatient center, some historical factors warrant that the patient have the abortion performed in a hospital. Examples of such disorders are symptomatic cardiac or respiratory disease, hemoglobinopathies, coagulopathies, uterine anomalies, myomata, previous complications resulting from first-trimester abortion, and mental disorders that would preclude patient cooperation during the procedure.[5] Accurate dating of the pregnancy is extremely important. Pelvic ultrasound is an excellent complement to physical examination in determining the size, shape, and position of the uterus. Laboratory evaluation should include the measurement of serum hemoglobin and hematocrit, and determination of the patient's Rh status type.

The informed consent process should include a description of the procedure, its associated risks, and the alternatives. The physician should provide the woman with referral opportunities for prenatal care and adoption services and should document in the medical record that all the elements of informed consent were satisfied.

Suction Curettage

Although surgical abortion in the first trimester can be completed either by sharp or suction curettage, the suction method is favored because is it more effective and safer.[6] Suction curettage is limited to pregnancies between 7 and 12 weeks gestation. Before 7 weeks it has been discouraged, mainly because of concern about rigid cannulae producing inadequate uterine evacuation.[7] After 14 weeks the fetus is too large to allow evacuation by suction. Excellent textbooks[5,8] provide detailed descriptions of the proper technique for suction curettage abortion. This section will highlight some key technical points for optimizing efficacy and limiting the morbidity and discomfort of the operation.

The choice of instruments depends somewhat on operator preference, but some instruments clearly are superior to others. Unless the cervix is going to be ripened preoperatively, dilators should be closely graduated and finely tapered to ensure use of the least amount of force possible. Pratt and Denniston dilators meet these criteria. Hank dilators are not finely tapered, and Hegar dilators meet neither of the criteria. The operating table should have padded knee crutches to support the patient's legs comfortably while she is in the lithotomy position. Foot slings and stirrups without knee support do not provide adequate comfort.[5]

Preoperative Preparation

The woman should empty her bladder voluntarily before starting the procedure. Some women will benefit from parenterally administered conscious sedation. Standard premedications (Table 12-1) for suction abortion are narcotic analgesics plus benzodiazepines. Optional agents include promethazine (12.5–25 mg) for nausea and atropine (0.4 mg) to prevent vasovagal responses to cervical manipulation. Because of the risk of respiratory depression with narcotics and benzodiazepines, pulse, blood pressure, and peripheral oxygen saturation should be monitored throughout the procedure and until the recovery period is over.

TABLE 12-1
STANDARD INTRAVENOUS MEDICATIONS FOR CONSCIOUS SEDATION DURING SUCTION CURETTAGE ABORTION

Agent	Dose
Benzodiazepines	
Midazolam (Versed)	1–3 mg
Diazepam (Valium)	2–10 mg
Narcotic analgesics	
Meperidine (Demerol)	25–100 mg
Fentanyl	30–100 mcg
Morphine	2–10 mg
Butorphanol (Stadol)	1–4 mg
Antiemetics	
Promethazine (Phenergan)	12.5–25 mg

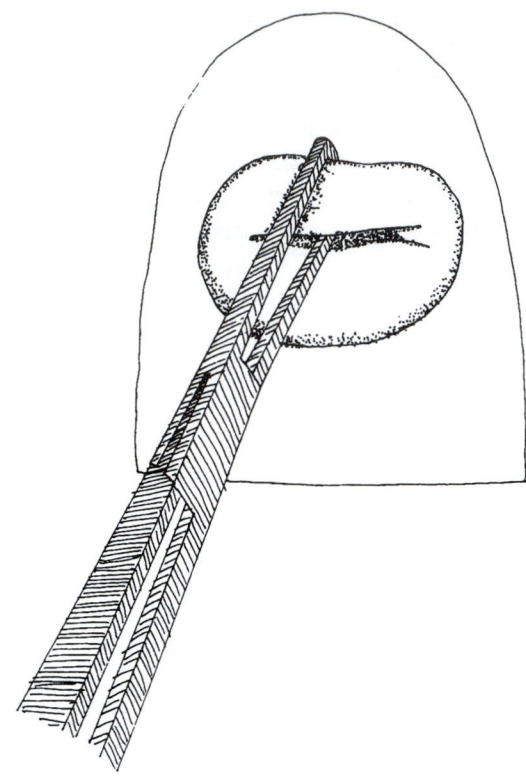

Figure 12-1 Technique for proper vertical placement of the tenaculum on the cervix.

Several steps can prevent introducing infection into the sterile intrauterine environment. The vagina and cervix should be washed with antiseptic solution. Scrubbing the vulva, however, is not necessary and causes discomfort for the patient. Although sterile instruments are required and sterile gloves are recommended, caps, gowns, masks, and drapes are unnecessary. Despite the use of sterile gloves, the surgeon should refrain from touching any portion of an instrument that will enter the uterus.

The majority of suction curettage abortions are performed with a paracervical block, but general anesthesia is acceptable and used frequently. General anesthesia provides better pain control but is more expensive and is associated with a higher risk of hemorrhage, uterine trauma, and death.[2,3] Local anesthesia, although safer overall, is complicated more frequently by convulsions and postoperative fevers.[2]

A paramount principle of the paracervical block technique is to administer the smallest volume of the most dilute concentration of anesthetic agent that is effective. The addition of epinephrine to the anesthetic (1:200,000) may lower the risk of toxicity by slowing the rate of systemic absorption but can cause tachycardia. Some experts[4] recommend against its use as a supplement to local anesthesia.

The initial injection of local anesthesia should be made at the 12-o'clock position, just before applying the tenaculum. The tenaculum can be manipulated to expose other areas of the cervix to facilitate injecting the remainder of the anesthetic. Most practitioners inject at various sites around the cervix submucosally at the cervicovaginal junction. Wiebe[9] demonstrated superior anesthetic effect with injections deep into the cervical stroma; however, this technique may increase

the risk of intravascular injection. Some experts[5,6] recommend waiting at least 2 to 3 minutes after administering a paracervical block before proceeding with the abortion. Wiebe and Rawling[10] did not find a significant improvement in pain control associated with waiting, but insufficient numbers and improper randomization of subjects weakened their conclusions.

The tenaculum should be placed high on the cervix at 12 o'clock with one end in the endocervical canal and the other end on the anterior ectocervix (Figure 12-1). Vertical placement, as opposed to horizontal placement, reduces the risk of tearing through the cervix during dilation.[6] To further reduce the risk of cervical laceration, Darney[5] recommends using the Bierer atraumatic tenaculum. Sounding the uterus provides no more useful information than a careful bimanual examination and increases the risk of uterine perforation. Therefore, it is not recommended.

Cervical Dilation

Starting with the smallest dilator that will enter the canal easily, the cervix should be dilated to 1 mm less than the diameter of the selected suction cannula.

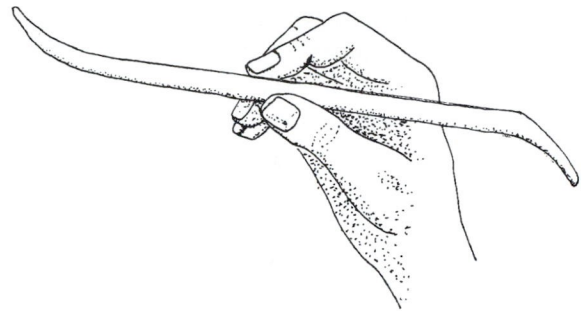

Figure 12-2 Proper technique for holding the dilator during advancement through the cervix.

Pratt dilators are labeled by their circumference in millimeters, but suction cannulae are labeled by their diameter. To obtain the approximate diameter of the Pratt dilator, divide the circumference by 3. Skipping over dilators to save time is not advised because it increases the likelihood of using excessive force, raising the risk of cervical trauma and uterine perforation. Maintaining hold of the dilator between the index finger and thumb during advancement is another measure to limit the force applied to the cervix (Figure 12-2).

To eliminate the need for forceful dilation, osmotic dilators, mifepristone (RU 486), or prostaglandins can be used preoperatively to ripen the cervix (Table 12-2). Osmotic dilators (laminaria tents, Lamicel, Dilapan) are inexpensive and might reduce the risk of cervical trauma[11] and uterine perforation[12]; however, they require trained personnel to insert and occasionally fragment or produce a false track during manipulation.[13] Mifepristone has proven effectiveness[14] and relatively few side effects,[15] but it is expensive and not yet available in many countries. The prostaglandin analog gemeprost is effective but expensive, unstable at room temperature, and causes abdominal pain, nausea, vomiting, and diarrhea.[16,17] Misoprostol, another prostaglandin analog, probably is the best agent overall for priming the cervix. It has superior efficacy versus placebo[18] and similar efficacy but fewer side effects than gemeprost.[17] In a study comparing misoprostol and mifepristone,[19] no significant differences in efficacy or incidence of side effects were found in 100 subjects. Misoprostol is inexpensive, stable at room temperature, and can be administered orally or vaginally. The advantage of the oral route is that women can take the drug at home, without supervision, the night before the operation.

Uterine Evacuation

The rigid cannulae for standard suction curettage range from 6 to 14 mm in diameter. A rule of thumb is to select the size that is 1 mm less than the gestational age of the pregnancy in weeks. Although smaller cannulae require less dilation, they are associated with prolonged operating time and increased risk of incomplete abortion. Straight cannulae tend to cause less pain when rotated but the angulated forms provide easier access to cornual areas, particularly when the uterus is retroflexed or anteroflexed.[5]

A negative pump pressure of 50 to 70 mm Hg provides the optimal balance between efficacy and trauma. Completeness of the evacuation is confirmed

TABLE 12-2
ADVANTAGES AND DISADVANTAGES OF DIFFERENT CERVICAL RIPENING DEVICES AND AGENTS

Ripener	Advantages	Disadvantages

Osmotic dilators
  Laminaria
  Lamicel
  Dilapan
	Effective, inexpensive, no systemic side effects	Requires experienced personnel to insert, can fragment or break
		Sometimes difficult to remove

Mifepristone	Effective, favorable side effect profile	Expensive, not widely available
Prostaglandins Gemeprost	Effective	Expensive, high incidence of gastrointestinal side effects, strict storage requirements
Misoprostol	Effective, inexpensive, can be taken orally or vaginally	Some side effects but less than with gemeprost

with a sharp curette to explore the walls of the uterine cavity in systematic fashion. The endometrium should feel gritty. A slick area suggests retained products of conception. Retained tissue is removed more effectively and safely by suction than by sharp curettage. At the end of the procedure, the uterus should be contracted firmly, and no more than a trickle of blood should be emanating from the external os.

After the procedure is completed, the aspirated tissue should be sent for pathological examination or inspected carefully by the surgeon. Once blood is washed away, the tissue should be floated in water or white vinegar to facilitate identification of villi. Recognition is optimized by viewing the tissue under a dissecting microscope or in a glass dish over a horizontal x-ray viewing box. If villi are not identified and previous ultrasound has not confirmed an intrauterine pregnancy, a diagnostic work-up for ectopic pregnancy should be initiated.

Postoperative Care

The recovery period should last for at least 30 minutes. Before discharge, all Rh-negative patients should be given 50 μg of Rh immune globulin for abortions performed at or before 12 weeks of gestation. Patients should be instructed to watch for an increase in bleeding, pain, or fever. Specifically instructing the woman to take her temperature daily for 3 to 5 days is a prudent measure. Scheduling the postoperative visit for 1 week rather than 4 weeks after the procedure enables the physician to detect delayed complications earlier in their course and thereby reduce morbidity.

Early Suction Curettage

Minisuction and menstrual regulation are terms used to describe an adaptation of suction curettage for termination of pregnancy through 6 to 7 weeks. This procedure requires a 6- to 7-mm flexible cannula connected to a 50- to 60-cc, self-locking syringe with a pinch valve. The procedure commonly was termed menstrual regulation because it was performed in the past without confirmation of pregnancy. The current standard of care, however, is to obtain a sensitive β-human chorionic gonadotropin (β-HCG) assay before performing any procedure that has the potential to terminate a pregnancy. Care also should be taken to confirm that the gestational age is 7 weeks or less from the last menstrual period.

The cervix can be anesthetized locally and dilated with 4 or 5 mm cannulae or dilators. The smaller cannulae, although useful for dilating the cervix, are not large enough to evacuate the uterus reliably.[4] After inserting the cannula and creating suction by releasing the pinch valve, the uterus is evacuated using the same principles as for suction curettage.

The primary risks of suction abortion at less than 8 weeks are the misdiagnosis of ectopic pregnancy and inadequate uterine evacuation. After the procedure is completed, the aspirated tissue should be inspected carefully to confirm removal of the conceptus.[7] If no villi or gestational sac can be identified, either of these outcomes are possible, and the physician should obtain serum β-HCG titers and perform vaginal ultrasounds as appropriate until the correct diagnosis is made.

Second Trimester

Although the vast majority of legal pregnancy terminations are performed in the first trimester, midtrimester terminations comprise a noteworthy proportion of the total number of abortions. Abortions frequently are performed in the second trimester for fetal chromosomal or structural anomalies. An even stronger determinant of the need for late abortion, however, is young age. In 1994, 26% of abortions performed for women less than 15 years of age, 17% for those aged 16 to 19 years, 12% for those 20 to 24, and 9% for those 25 or older were performed after 12 weeks.[1] Lack of ready access to abortion services probably is the primary reason for the delay among younger women.[4] The proportion of second-trimester abortions performed surgically is inversely related to gestational age. In 1994, curettage accounted for 99% of all abortions performed at 13 to 15 weeks gestation, 90% at 16 to 20 weeks, and 83% after 20 weeks.[1]

Dilation and Evacuation (D&E)

Fetuses beyond 14 weeks cannot be evacuated by suction cannulae and must be removed from the uterus manually with grasping forceps (D&E). Surprisingly, the morbidity and mortality rates of D&E throughout most of the second trimester are lower than those for medically induced abortion. Other advantages of D&E include greater convenience and lower expense. The safety of D&E, however, requires that the surgeon possess a high level of experience and skill in performing the procedure. The second-trimester uterus has a thinner lower segment and a greater blood supply. The fetus is more difficult to extract through the cervix. As compared with first-trimester pregnancy terminations, mid- and late-term abortions account for a disproportionately large percentage of serious complications and fatalities. Whereas the mortality rate for abortions performed before 9 weeks is approximately 0.5 per 100,000 procedures, this figure rises to 7.8 per 100,000 for abortions performed between 16 and 20 weeks.[20]

Approach to the Patient

Contraindications to D&E are the same as for first-trimester suction curettage with some notable additions. Individual physicians have various upper limits of gestational age beyond which they will not perform D&E. Accurate determination of gestational age is of paramount importance. Errors in judging the duration of pregnancy have been responsible for many abortion complications.

Up to 16 to 18 weeks, D&E is associated with fewer complications than medically induced abortion. After this time, the morbidity and mortality of the methods are relatively equal.[6] The advantages of D&E notwithstanding, a significant number of women will opt for medical termination. A notable group in this category are women with a desired pregnancy but a dead or anomalous fetus.[21]

Preoperative Preparation

The standard equipment for D&E is similar to that for suction curettage with some notable exceptions. Sopher and Bierer forceps are preferable to standard sponge forceps for evacuating the uterus. In addition, intraoperative ultrasound improves operator efficiency by permitting visual negotiation of the uterine cavity and identification of the fetus and placenta.

Adequate preoperative cervical dilation is essential. Either hydrophilic dilators or prostaglandins are effective. The cervical canal must be dilated to 12 mm in the early second trimester and to 20 mm for pregnancies beyond 18 weeks.[22] Achieving the required dilation for more advanced pregnancies with hydrophilic dilators sometimes requires a two- or three-stage process over 24 to 48 hours, during which dilators are removed and replaced with a progressively larger quantity.

D&E, unlike suction curettage, requires preoperative uterotonic agents to facilitate evacuation. Darney[22] recommends adding 5 units of vasopressin per 15 ml of anesthetic to the paracervical block. This measure not only increases uterine tone, but the vasoconstrictive action reduces intraoperative blood loss and systemic absorption of the anesthetic. Vasopressin should never be given intravenously and is contraindicated in women with hypertension or other risk factors for stroke. Alternatively, oxytocin (40 to 100 units/liter in crystalloid solution) can be infused intraoperatively.

Uterine Evacuation

After ascertaining that the grasping forceps are able to pass through the cervical canal, the membranes are ruptured and the amniotic fluid aspirated completely using a large suction cannula. Draining the fluid allows the uterus to contract before starting the evacuation process. This maneuver reduces blood loss and advances the fetus toward the cervix so that it is more easily grasped. It also may reduce the risk of amniotic fluid embolus.

In general, fetal extraction should be attempted before removing the placenta. Fetal lie is an important factor influencing the ease with which D&E can be completed, particularly at later gestational ages. Breech and cephalic presentations allow for the most rapid evacuation. Transverse presentations are problematic, and conversion to a breech using the grasping forceps is recommended.[22] Nearly all extractions can be accomplished from the lower portion of the uterus if the amniotic fluid has been drained and the cervix is dilated adequately. Occasionally, a low-lying placenta will compromise evacuation of the fetus. In this instance, removing the placenta first will likely lead to less blood loss than attempting to extract the fetus first.[23]

The entire fetus and most of the placenta usually can be removed with the forceps. Small remaining placental fragments can be removed with suction. Ultrasound visualization of a midline uterine "stripe" confirms complete evacuation. If significant amounts of tissue cannot be removed easily, the surgeon should discontinue the operation and administer intravenous oxytocin for 2 to 3 hours while closely monitoring the woman for bleeding. After this time the retained tissue usually is visible at the internal os and removed easily.[6]

Complications of Surgical Abortion

Hemorrhage

Hemorrhage is often defined imprecisely; thus, reported rates associated with surgical abortion vary widely. The rate of blood transfusion associated with first-trimester suction curettage in a large, multicenter study was 0 per 170,000 cases.[24] In another survey of 11,747 D&E procedures,[25] excessive bleeding was found to occur in 9 per 1000 cases. Risk factors for hemorrhage include the use of general anesthesia, excessive operating time, and, with D&E, placenta previa[23] and placenta accreta.[26]

Excessive intraoperative or postoperative bleeding can be attributed to uterine atony, retained products of conception, uterine trauma resulting in laceration of a pelvic blood vessel, or coagulopathy. When hemorrhage occurs, the surgeon initially should determine the cause of bleeding by performing a bimanual examination and gently exploring the uterine cavity. A soft and floppy but intact uterus generally is due to uterine atony. Bimanual uterine massage and administration of parenteral uterotonic agents (Table 12-3) usually will correct the problem.

The incidence of retained tissue is 0.3 per 1000 to 6 per 1000[24,27,28] in the first trimester. This complication should be suspected in the presence of immediate or delayed bleeding or postabortal infection. The bleeding often does not decrease after administering uterotonic agents. During exploration with a sharp curette, the uterine cavity usually feels asymmetric or lacks a gritty surface. The treatment for retained tissue is reaspiration with the largest cannula that passes through the cervix. Prophylactic antibiotics should be administered to women who present more than 12 hours after the procedure. If no tissue is obtained, ultrasound of the endometrial cavity can assist in localizing the retained products.

Uterine Perforation

During first-trimester suction curettage, the risk of uterine perforation is 0.1 per 1000 to 2 per 1000.[24,27,28] The usual site of perforation is at the midfundus and results from failure to identify a retroverted or retroflexed uterus before dilating the cervix. Less common but more hazardous are perforations of the lower uterine segment or cervix. These usually occur during forcible cervical dilation. Lateral perforations are particularly worrisome because they can be associated with injury to a branch of the uterine artery. Preoperative cervical ripening, eliminating uterine sounding, and carefully ascertaining the uterine position before dilating the cervix should reduce the risk of perforation.

If perforation occurs during first-trimester suction curettage, the operator should stop the procedure and determine the location and extent of injury. If the perforation is fundal and occurs before the uterine evacuation has begun, the procedure usually can be completed under ultrasound guidance. If complicated by hemorrhage or suspected injury to abdominal organs, prompt laparotomy is required.

Perforation occurs in 4 per 1000 D&E procedures.[25] Risk factors include underestimation of the gestational age and inadequate cervical dilation. Perforation often results during D&E when the operator fails to negotiate properly an anteriorly positioned uterus and advances the forceps horizontally through the posterior lower uterine segment. Perforations in this area are troublesome because they often are associated with injury to the rectosigmoid colon. Staying mindful of uterine position, using intraoperative ultrasound, and resisting the temptation to grasp material that is deep inside the uterine cavity can reduce this risk. If the extraction can be completed within the low portion of the uterine cavity, just inside the internal os, the risk of perforation at any location is reduced.[22]

Awake patients sometimes note a sudden increase in abdominal pain if perforation occurs. If perforation is suspected, the uterine cavity should be explored using a uterine sound. Once perforation is confirmed, the abortion should be discontinued. Unlike perforations complicating first-trimester abortions, those associated with D&E almost always require surgical exploration of the abdominal cavity. Completing the abortion transabdominally via the uterine perforation is preferable to proceeding transvaginally and risking further trauma to abdominal organs or blood vessels.

TABLE 12-3
STANDARD UTEROTONIC AGENTS

Agent	Dose	Route
Oxytocin	40 units in 1000 cc crystalloid solution	Rapid intravenous infusion
Methylergonovine	0.2 mg	Intramuscular
(15S)-15-methyl prostaglandin $F_{2\alpha}$ tromethamine (Hemabate)	250 μg	intramuscular $F_{2\alpha}$

The choice of skin incision should be based on the level of suspicion for bowel injury. A vertical midline incision is indicated if bowel repair is required.

Cervical Laceration

Cervical injury is one of the more commonly reported complications of surgical abortion. Depending on how it is defined, the rates vary from 0.01 to 1%.[11,24,28] Cervical trauma can occur internally or externally, rarely is serious, and usually is associated with forceful dilation and general anesthesia. External lacerations typically are a consequence of the tenaculum tearing through the cervix. At worst, external lacerations result in persistent bleeding that can be repaired with a single hemostatic suture. Internal lacerations can extend into the uterine corpus and through the entire thickness of the wall. A lateral laceration can extend to a branch of the uterine artery and result in serious hemorrhage.

Eliminating predisposing factors minimizes the risk of cervical trauma. Preoperative cervical ripening most effectively obviates the need for forceful dilation. Using finely tapered and closely graduated dilators and local anesthesia are helpful if ripening cannot be performed. Vertical placement of the tenaculum reduces the risk of external cervical lacerations.

Acute Hematometra

Acute hematometra has an incidence ranging from 1 per 1000 to 5 per 1000.[28,29] It typically occurs after abortions performed at 11 to 14 weeks and results from a combination of uterine atony and a rapidly closing cervix. Women with this condition often complain of severe cramping and weakness within 2 hours of the abortion. Typical physical signs are mild vaginal bleeding, tachycardia, diaphoresis, and a tender and distended uterus. Treatment consists of prompt dilation and suction evacuation of the clot and blood, followed by administration of a uterotonic agent.

Syncopal Episodes

Syncope can occur during abortion as a vasovagal reaction to cervical stimulation, as a result of hyperventilation, or as a reaction to local anesthesia. Vasovagal syncope, produced by manipulation or dilation of the cervix, can result in severe bradycardia and hypotension. Placing the patient in Trendelenburg position and giving intravenous atropine (0.6 mg) usually provides relief.[5] Prophylactic administration of atropine intravenously or with the paracervical block

should be considered in patients thought to be at high risk for this complication.

Toxic reactions to local anesthetic agents generally occur from excessive intravascular absorption or direct intravascular injection of the agent. Patients with toxic reactions to local anesthetics will note an immediate sensation of tinnitus and perioral numbness, sometimes accompanied by paresthesias, lightheadedness, and syncope. Severe reactions can result in seizures, sinus bradycardia, atrioventricular block, and asystole. Treatment is supportive and is aimed at maintaining respiration and circulation. Seizures should be controlled by administration of intravenous diazepam.

The duration of the toxic reaction usually is self-limited and depends on the rapidity with which the anesthetic agent is cleared from the bloodstream. The ester chloroprocaine is metabolized rapidly by cholinesterase in the plasma and has a half-life in the bloodstream of 21 seconds. The amide lidocaine, although less expensive and less allergenic, is metabolized in the liver at a much slower rate, with a half-life of 1.6 hours.[30]

Infection

Postabortal infection often is the result of retained products of conception. Its incidence is reported to be 1 per 1000 to 5 per 1000 with first-trimester procedures[24,27,28] and 1 to 2% with D&E.[25] Peterson et al.[25] reported that as gestational age increased from 13 to 21 weeks, the rate of postoperative fever increased from 0.5% to 1.6%. Women with postabortal endometritis generally present 2 to 3 days after the operation with a fever greater than 100°F. Typical symptoms are uterine tenderness, fever, and malodorous vaginal discharge. Increased vaginal bleeding can occur with or without retained tissue.

Similar to pelvic inflammatory disease, the spectrum of postabortal infection typically is polymicrobial. Mild cases of endometritis can be treated with oral, broad-spectrum antibiotics. More serious cases should be managed in the hospital with broad-spectrum parenteral agents and repeat curettage. Table 12-4 lists recommended antimicrobial regimens for postabortal infection based on the severity of illness.

Clostridial sepsis, although once a common complication of illegal abortion, rarely complicates legally performed abortions. A distinguishing presentation of clostridia sepsis is tachycardia that is out of proportion to fever. An upright x-ray examination of the

TABLE 12-4
RECOMMENDED ANTIMICROBIAL REGIMENS FOR POSTABORTAL SEPSIS

Agent	Dose	Route	Frequency	Duration
Mild infection				
Amoxicillin/clavulanic acid (Augmentin)	875 mg	Oral	Twice daily	7–10 days
Ciprofloxacin plus metronidazole	500 mg 500 mg	Oral	Twice daily	7– 10 days
Moderate infection				
Cefotetan	1 g	Intravenous	Every 12 hours	Until afebrile for 24 hours
Ampicillin/sulbactam (Unasyn)	1.5–3.0 g	Intravenous	Every 6 hours	Until afebrile for 24 hours
Severe infection				
Gentamicin plus	7 mg/kg/of ideal body weight	Intravenous	Once daily	Until afebrile for 48 hours
Clindamycin plus	900 mg	Intravenous	Every 8 hours	
Penicillin G	5 million units	Intravenous	Every 4 to 6 hours	
Imipenem-cilastatin	500 mg	Intravenous	Every 6 hours	Until afebrile for 48 hours

IBW = ideal body weight

abdomen may show gas bubbles in the uterus, and a Gram stain of cervical secretions or curetted tissue demonstrates large, gram-positive rods. Patients with clostridia sepsis should improve with high-dose penicillin but require close monitoring. If hemolysis or persistent hemodynamic instability develops, prompt hysterectomy is required.[6]

The benefit of prophylactic antibiotics is well established. In a large cohort study, Park et al.[31] found that prophylactic antibiotics were the single most protective factor for reducing the rate of febrile complications after suction curettage abortion (relative risk, 0.36; 95% confidence interval, 0.18 to 0.70). Oral doxycycline has a broad spectrum of activity and excellent bioavailability and is the most commonly recommended agent. Various dosage and timing schedules are used in practice. A short postoperative course of doxycycline probably results in less nausea and vomiting; however, the two largest prospective clinical trials demonstrating the effectiveness of antibiotic prophylaxis used 400 mg of doxycycline given as a single preoperative dose[32] or 100 mg given 1 hour preoperatively and 200 mg given 30 minutes postoperatively.[33]

Cervical Stenosis and Asherman Syndrome

Cervical stenosis is a late complication of suction curettage and has a reported incidence of 1 in 1000 to 2 in 1000.[24] Its cause is not well defined. Women with this condition note amenorrhea or hypomenorrhea with cyclic pelvic pain. Dilation under paracervical anesthesia corrects the problem.

Asherman syndrome (intrauterine synechiae) occurs less commonly after abortion than does cervical stenosis. Although usually preceded by an endometrial infection, it can occur in the absence of any other complication, presumably as a result of overly aggressive curettage. Asherman syndrome should be suspected in women with amenorrhea or hypomenorrhea without cyclic pelvic pain. Treatment involves hysteroscopic lysis of the intrauterine adhesions.

MEDICAL ABORTION

First Trimester

Until recently, virtually all legal first-trimester abortions were performed surgically. Surgical abortion, although very safe and effective, has some disadvantages. The procedure is expensive and requires a certain amount of training and expertise. Moreover, various legal, economic, geographic, and social conditions worldwide impede access to abortion services. The development of medications to induce abortion, therefore, has created considerable interest. Mifepristone (RU 486) and methotrexate are now available. Evidence demonstrates that these agents, when combined with a prostaglandin, induce abortion effectively and safely in early pregnancy.

Not only does the availability of medical methods of pregnancy termination increase access to legal abortion, but it also expands a woman's choices. Between 20 to 60% of women, if given a choice, would prefer medical abortion over suction curettage.[34,35] Several papers have compared the methods directly. In a large, partly randomized Scottish study,[34] 2% of women randomized to the vacuum aspiration group stated after the procedure that they would opt for a different method in the future. Of those randomized to the medical abortion group, 21% said they would opt for a different method. Almost all of those dissatisfied with medical abortion, however, were between 50 and 63 days of gestation; very few of those at less than 50 days were dissatisfied. Another paper[36] from the same study found that the efficacy rate and degree of pain were equal in subjects at less than 50 days of gestation. From 50 to 63 days, medical abortion was less effective (93% vs. 98%) and more painful.

An important conclusion from many of the studies comparing medical and surgical abortion is that choice is an extremely important factor in determining a woman's satisfaction with a particular method. Among the women in the Scottish study who chose their abortion method, satisfaction between the two groups (medical vs. surgical) was equal. The Scottish group later reported that 85 to 90% of their subjects would be willing to pay extra to have the complete range of abortion options.[37]

Mifepristone (RU 486)

Mifepristone antagonizes the action of progesterone. This action has various effects on the pregnant uterus, such as endothelial vascular damage in the endometrium,[38] increased prostaglandin synthesis,[39] and decreased prostaglandin metabolism.[39] These effects result in decidual necrosis, detachment at the decidual–chorionic interface, and increased myometrial contractility.[40]

Mifepristone became licensed in France for use as a medical abortifacient in 1988. Since then, the United Kingdom, Sweden, and China have approved its use. The U.S. Food and Drug Administration recently has judged it safe and effective as an abortifacient, and full approval is expected.[41]

Originally used as a single agent to induce delayed menses, mifepristone is 75 to 85% effective in terminating documented pregnancies aged within 10 days of missed menses.[42,43] Mifepristone plus gemeprost is 97% efficacious within 11 days of missed menses.[44] Another potential use for mifepristone as a single agent is to induce expulsion in early nondeveloping pregnancies. In a double-blind, placebo-controlled trial,[45] a single 600-mg dose of mifepristone induced spontaneous expulsion within 5 days of administration in 82% of subjects versus an expulsion rate of 8% for those receiving placebo. In a separate trial[46] that included a similar group of patients, 56 of 59 (95%) had a timely and complete abortion after being given mifepristone plus misoprostol 48 hours later.

For normally developing pregnancies beyond 42 days, the failure rate of mifepristone alone is unacceptably high. When combined with a low dose of prostaglandin, however, success rates exceed 90%.[41] A large cohort study[47] performed in the United States demonstrated success rates of 92% in pregnancies at 49 days or less, 83% in those at 50 to 56 days, and 77% in gestations at 57 to 63 days from previous menses.

The usual recommended mifepristone dose has been 600 mg, once orally. A large WHO-sponsored trial[48] compared 200-, 400-, and 600-mg doses of mifepristone, all followed by 1 mg of gemeprost, and found no difference in the rates of success. A smaller study[49] also showed equal efficacy for 200- versus 600-mg doses when combined with 600 μg of misoprostol. Moreover, no difference in efficacy has been noted between sequential 25-mg doses and a single 600-mg dose of mifepristone.[50]

Common side effects associated with mifepristone are nausea and vomiting, fatigue, abdominal pain, lightheadedness, anorexia, headache, and breast tenderness.[51] Gastrointestinal symptoms are more frequent with the addition of a prostaglandin. Teratogenicity is a concern in cases of failed medical abortion in which a woman decides to continue the pregnancy, but the teratogenic risk of mifepristone is unknown.

Methotrexate

Although effective and well tolerated by women who have taken it as an abortifacient, mifepristone is not available yet in the United States or in many other countries, and it is relatively expensive. However, physicians can offer methotrexate as an alternative. Methotrexate is cytotoxic to trophoblastic cells. Experimental protocols have used a dose of 50 mg per square meter of body surface area. At this relatively low dose, methotrexate has very few side effects.

Methotrexate is less expensive than mifepristone, is more readily available in most parts of the world, and has been found to have similar efficacy.[52]

At gestations less than 42 days, methotrexate appears to be effective as a single agent.[53] Used before 57 days, the combination of methotrexate plus misoprostol is highly effective. In a randomized, controlled trial, Creinin and Vittinghoff[54] demonstrated that intramuscular methotrexate plus vaginal misoprostol induced abortion in 90% of subjects versus 47% in those given misoprostol alone. Creinin et al.[55] subsequently reported that methotrexate (50 mg) administered once orally, followed by vaginal misoprostol, was 91% effective in inducing abortion in women up to 49 days of gestation.

As with mifepristone, the effectiveness of methotrexate diminishes with advancing gestational age.[56] The timing of the dose of misoprostol also influences efficacy. A small, prospective randomized trial[57] demonstrated that methotrexate followed by misoprostol 7 days later was more effective than a regimen with misoprostol given 3 days later (98 vs. 83%; $p = 0.033$).

The overall efficacy of methotrexate plus misoprostol is similar to that of mifepristone plus prostaglandin, but the methotrexate combination works more slowly. With methotrexate regimens, uterine emptying can take as long as 2 weeks. Potential advantages of this slower onset of action, however, are less severe uterine cramping, a lower risk of hemorrhage, plus the opportunity for the woman to self-administer misoprostol and abort at home.

Side effects attributed to methotrexate include nausea, vomiting, diarrhea, headache, lightheadedness, subjective fever or chills, and stomatitis.[54,55] Teratogenicity also is a concern with methotrexate; however, as with mifepristone, its true potential is unknown.

Prostaglandins

Prostaglandins originally were used for first-trimester abortion as single agents.[58] However, these regimens never gained popularity because the dose of prostaglandin required to achieve satisfactory results was associated with an unacceptably high incidence of severe nausea and vomiting, diarrhea, and abdominal pain. Adding mifepristone or methotrexate improves efficacy and allows a smaller dose of prostaglandin to be used, resulting in fewer side effects and less pain. In a partly randomized trial[59] of 301 women requesting termination of pregnancy ≤56 days of amenorrhea, those given mifepristone plus gemeprost aborted more frequently (98 vs. 87%; $p = 0.0004$) and required less analgesic medication (55 vs. 76%; $p = 0.0001$) than those given gemeprost alone.

For women with an anembryonic gestation or early embryonic death, pretreatment with mifepristone or methotrexate might be unnecessary.[60] In theory, the purpose of methotrexate or mifepristone is to weaken the attachment of the pregnancy to the uterus. In women with an abnormally developing pregnancy, support of the decidual lining, presumably, already is unstable. Whether misoprostol alone is any less effective than misoprostol plus pretreatment in these women is unknown.

Three different prostaglandins have been used in trials. Sulprostone, a prostaglandin (PG) E_2 analog that was administered intramuscularly, is not used currently because of concerns about cardiovascular collapse in women with preexisting heart disease. Gemeprost is a PGE_1 analog that is administered as a vaginal suppository. Misoprostol is a PGE_1 analog marketed as an oral agent for peptic ulcer disease. When combined with mifepristone, the success rates of misoprostol and gemeprost are similar,[61] but gemeprost has been found to cause expulsion more quickly.[62] Misoprostol, however, is much less expensive and does not require the strict storage conditions necessary for gemeprost.

The optimal dose for misoprostol for inducing abortion in the first trimester probably is 800 μg given once vaginally. Although dividing the dose into 400-μg increments given 2 hours apart has been associated with lower rates of vomiting and diarrhea, it is also associated with lower efficacy.[63] In a prospective, randomized trial[64] of 270 pregnant women up to 63 days of gestation, vaginal and oral misoprostol (800 μg) were compared after pretreatment with mifepristone. The vaginal misoprostol group had a higher overall abortion rate (95% vs 87%; $p = 0.03$), a higher abortion rate within 4 hours (93% vs. 78%; $p < 0.001$), and a lower rate of vomiting (31% vs. 44%; $p = 0.002$).

The superior efficacy of the vaginal route might be due to enhanced bioavailability. In a pharmacokinetic study that included 10 pregnant and 10 nonpregnant women, Zieman et al.[65] demonstrated that the systemic bioavailability of vaginally administered misoprostol is three times higher than that of orally administered misoprostol. Although peak serum levels were lower and were reached more slowly with vaginal administration, they were sustained for a much longer time (Fig. 12-3). Recommended regimens for

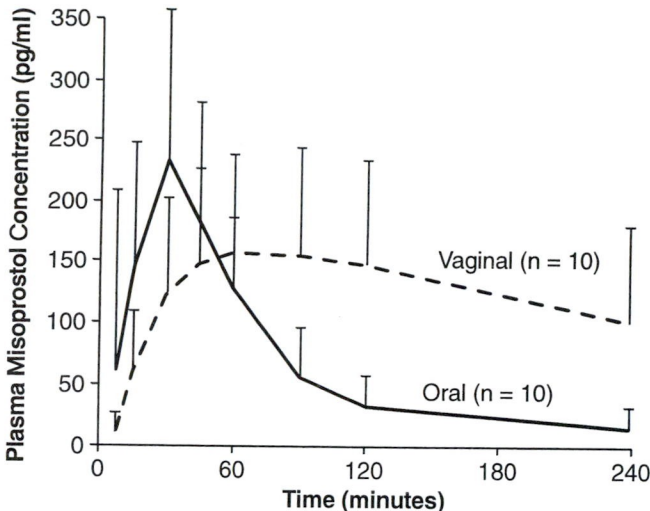

Figure 12-3 Mean plasma concentrations of misoprostol acid over time with oral (solid line) and vaginal (dotted line) administration. *Reprinted with permission from the American College of Obstetricians and Gynecologists.*

medical induction of abortion in the first trimester are listed in Table 12-5.

Medical Abortion in the Second Trimester

Abortion is induced medically in the second trimester by two principal means: hypertonic instillation (saline and urea), and uterotonic agents (prostaglandins and oxytocin). The hypertonic agents are administered percutaneously into the amniotic cavity. Oxytocin is administered as an intravenous infusion, and the prostaglandins are administered systemically or into the amniotic cavity.

Hypertonic Instillation

Amnioinfusion of hypertonic saline or urea is used less frequently now than in the past. The method requires amniocentesis and is associated with a relatively slow time to abortion. In one study,[66] the addition of

TABLE 12-5
RECOMMENDED MEDICAL REGIMENS FOR INDUCING ABORTION IN THE FIRST TRIMESTER

Regimen A	Mifepristone (RU 486), 200 mg orally, followed in 36–48 hours by misoprostol, 800 μg vaginally
Regimen B	Methotrexate, 50 mg/m² of patient's body surface area intramuscularly, followed in 7 days by misoprostol, 800 μg vaginally

oxytocin reduced the time to abortion from approximately 35 hours to 25 hours but also increased the risk of uterine perforation. In another study,[67] intraamniotic urea plus prostaglandin produced shorter times to abortion and fewer complications than hypertonic saline alone.

Hypertonic saline instillation has been associated with several very serious complications. Cardiovascular collapse, pulmonary and cerebral edema, and renal failure occur with inadvertent intravascular injection. These complications are avoided by performing the instillation under real-time ultrasound guidance and allowing the solution to infuse by gravity drainage rather than by pump.[5] Disseminated intravascular coagulation (DIC) can occur despite perfect technique.

Intraamniotic Prostaglandins

In the past, prostaglandins were administered intravenously to induce abortion, but this route was associated with a high incidence of vomiting and diarrhea. Administering the agent into the amniotic cavity reduces these side effects. The commercially available preparation for intraamniotic administration is (15S)-15-methylprostaglandin F$_{2\alpha}$ (carboprost tromethamine, Hemabate). The recommended dose is 1 mg given very slowly. If the cervix is treated with osmotic dilators before prostaglandin instillation, the time to abortion is reduced, successful abortion is more likely after a single dose, and the risk of cervical trauma is lowered.[68]

Systemic Prostaglandins

Therapeutic prostaglandin levels are achieved via many routes of administration, including intramuscular, oral, and intravaginal. Of these routes, the transvaginal route combines the greatest efficacy with the lowest incidence of complications and side effects. Of the various prostaglandin preparations, dinoprostone (PGE$_2$) suppositories, gemeprost suppositories, and misoprostol tablets are the most thoroughly evaluated.

A small study[69] that compared misoprostol (200 μg intravaginally every 12 hours) with dinoprostone (20 mg intravaginally every 3 hours) found no difference in efficacy but significantly lower rates of fever, vomiting, and diarrhea in the group receiving misoprostol. The most dramatic finding in this study was the average cost of treatment per patient ($315 for dinoprostone and $1 for misoprostol). Another study[70] compared two regimens of intravaginal misoprostol (100 μg every 6 hours and 200 mg every 12 hours) and intravaginal gemeprost (1 mg every 3 hours). No significant difference was found between the groups in the total rate of abortion (complete plus incomplete). The rate of complete abortion was highest in the twice-daily misoprostol group and, of the successful abortions, the time to completion was lowest in the gemeprost group. Gastrointestinal side effects were lowest in the misoprostol groups.

Pretreatment with laminaria[71] or mifepristone[72] reduces the time to abortion in the second trimester. In a study that compared intravaginal gemeprost alone and gemeprost plus pretreatment with an osmotic dilator or mifepristone,[73] the group that received pretreatment with mifepristone had the shortest induction-to-abortion intervals and the lowest rate of gastrointestinal side effects. No difference in efficacy or time to abortion exists between 600- and 200-mg doses of mifepristone when given 36 to 48 hours before intravaginal misoprostol in the second trimester.[74]

A study that compared vaginal and oral misoprostol, each dosed at 200 μg every 3 hours, demonstrated a shorter time to delivery in the vaginal administration group (9 hours versus 13 hours) and no difference in side effects.[75] In another study, in which all subjects received an initial loading dose of vaginal misoprostol (600 mg) after pretreatment with mifepristone, no significant differences in mean induction-to-abortion time or in side effects were found between vaginal and oral misoprostol, both given at a dose of 400 μg every 3 hours.[76]

High-Dose Oxytocin

Oxytocin administered at doses less than 40 mU per minute is unlikely to induce labor in the second trimester. In 1991, a group from the University of Alabama at Birmingham[77] published a retrospective report of their experience with a concentrated oxytocin infusion protocol (Table 12-6), demonstrating similar efficacy and fewer side effects than dinoprostone suppositories. In a subsequent prospective randomized trial from the same center,[78] the group receiving high-dose oxytocin had an 80% success rate versus an 86% rate for those who received dinoprostone ($p = 0.48$). The mean time to delivery was 13 hours in each group. Side effects such as fever, nausea, vomiting, diarrhea, and hypotension were significantly lower in the oxytocin group.

Complications of Medical Abortion

All methods of medical abortion share the same complications. The largest drawback of medically induced abortion is the relatively high rate of incomplete expulsion of the entire pregnancy: failed abortion, incomplete abortion, or retained placenta. Several studies[36,79-81] have found greater amounts of blood loss

---

TABLE 12-6
BIRMINGHAM PROTOCOL FOR HIGH-DOSE OXYTOCIN FOR SECOND-TRIMESTER TERMINATION

1. Add 50 units oxytocin to 500 ml 5% dextrose in lactated Ringer's solution or 5% dextrose in normal saline and infuse over 3 hours.
2. Infuse maintenance intravenous fluids at 125 cc/hr for 1 hour.
3. Add 100 units oxytocin to 500 ml 5% dextrose in lactated Ringer's solution or 5% dextrose in normal saline and infuse over 3 hours.
4. Infuse maintenance intravenous fluids at 125 cc/hr for 1 hour.
5. Add 150 units oxytocin to 500 ml 5% dextrose in lactated Ringer's solution or 5% dextrose in normal saline and infuse over 3 hours.
6. Infuse maintenance intravenous fluids at 125 cc/hr for 1 hour.
7. Add 200 units oxytocin to 500 ml 5% dextrose in lactated Ringer's solution or 5% dextrose in normal saline and infuse over 3 hours.
8. Infuse maintenance intravenous fluids at 125 cc/hr for 1 hour.
9. Add 250 units oxytocin to 500 ml 5% dextrose in lactated Ringer's solution or 5% dextrose in normal saline and infuse over 3 hours.
10. Infuse maintenance intravenous fluids at 125 cc/hr for 1 hour.
11. Add 300 units oxytocin to 500 ml 5% dextrose in lactated Ringer's solution or 5% dextrose in normal saline and infuse over 3 hours.

If delivery is not imminent, change to another method to induce delivery.

From Winkler et al.[77] with permission.

with medical abortion as compared with surgical abortion. Less common but more serious complications include uterine rupture and DIC.

Failed and Incomplete Abortion

Incomplete expulsion of the fetus or placenta can result in excessive blood loss and infection. When prostaglandins have not produced abortion within a reasonable time, high-dose oxytocin can be used as second-line therapy. If the physician has sufficient experience, D&E is probably the most convenient method for the patient. In fact, D&E is performed more easily after failed medical abortion than as a primary procedure because the cervix is already dilated, the uterus is contracted, and the fetus usually is in the lower uterus.

Uterine Rupture

During labor, fetal expulsion takes place along the path of least resistance. Rarely, this path is not through the cervix. Expulsion into the abdominal cavity can occur through the anterior or posterior lower uterine segment. Expulsion into the vagina can occur through a rent in the cervix above the external os or as a result of annular detachment of the cervix.

An analysis of over 2000 second-trimester abortions[82] using extraamniotic or intraamniotic prostaglandins found the incidence of uterine trauma to be 0.17%. Pretreatment of the cervix with laminaria or prostaglandins should reduce the risk of uterine rupture during medical abortion but is not completely protective. Risk factors for uterine rupture include previous uterine surgery, multiparity, and polyhydramnios. Physicians should select their patients carefully. Those for whom labor at term is contraindicated should not undergo labor for termination of pregnancy in an earlier trimester. Amnioreduction should be considered before inducing midtrimester abortion in patients with severe polyhydramnios. If an experienced operator is available to perform the procedure, D&E is preferable in women with previous low transverse cesarean scars or in multiparous women. The safety of the commonly used doses of abortifacients for second-trimester termination is proven only up to 24 weeks.

REFERENCES

1. Koonin LM, Smith JC, Ramick M, Strauss LT, Hopkins FW. Abortion surveillance—United States, 1993 and 1994. MMWR 1997;46(SS-4):37.

2. Grimes DA, Schulz KF, Cates W, Tyler CW. Local versus general anesthesia: which is safer for suction curettage abortion? Am J Obstet Gynecol 1979;135:1030.

3. Peterson HB, Grimes DA, Cates W, Rubin GL. Comparative risk of death from induced abortion at <12 weeks' gestation performed with local versus general anesthesia. Am J Obstet Gynecol 1981;141:763.

4. Stubblefield PG. Pregnancy termination. In: Gabbe SG, Niebyl JR, Simpson JL, eds. Obstetrics: normal and problem pregnancies. 3rd ed. New York: Churchill Livingstone, 1996:1249.

5. Darney PD. First-trimester elective abortion. In: Darney PD, ed. Office and ambulatory surgery. Oradell, NJ: Medical Economics, 1987:158.

6. Grimes DA. Surgical management of abortion. In: Thompson JD, Rock JA, eds. TeLindes operative gynecology. 7th ed. Philadelphia: Lippincott, 1992:317.

7. Kaunitz AM, Rovira EZ, Grimes DA, Schulz KF. Abortions that fail. Obstet Gynecol 1985;66:533.

8. Hern WM. Abortion practice. 2nd ed. Philadelphia: Lippincott, 1990.

9. Wiebe ER. Comparison of the efficacy of different local anesthetics and techniques of local anesthesia in therapeutic abortions. Am J Obstet Gynecol 1992; 167:131.

10. Wiebe ER, Rawling M. Pain control in abortion. Int J Gynecol Obstet 1995;50:41.

11. Schulz KF, Grimes DA, Cates W. Measures to prevent cervical injury during suction curettage abortion. Lancet 1983;1:1182.

12. Grimes DA, Schulz KF Cates WJ. Prevention of uterine perforation during curettage abortion. JAMA 1984; 251:2108.

13. Johnson N. Intracervical tents: usage and mode of action. Obstet Gynecol Survey 1989;44:410.

14. World Health Organization. The use of mifepristone (RU-486) for cervical preparation in first trimester pregnancy termination by vacuum aspiration. Br J Obstet Gynecol 1990;97:260.

15. Gupta JK, Johnson J. Should we use prostaglandins, tents, or progesterone antagonists for cervical ripening before first trimester abortion? Contraception 1992;46:489.

16. Kuah KB. Predilation of the cervix in first trimester termination of pregnancy: a comparative study of the prostaglandin analogue, 16,16 dimethyl-trans-delta^{2}PGE$_1$, methyl ethyl ester (Cervagem®) and mechanical dilation. Aust NZ J Obstet Gynecol 1993;33:162.

17. Ngai SW, Yeung KCA, Lao T, Ho PC. Oral misoprostol versus vaginal gemeprost for cervical dilation prior to vacuum aspiration in women in the sixth to twelfth week of gestation. Contraception 1995;51:347.

18. Ngai SW, Tang Os, Lao T, Ho PC, Ma HK. Oral misoprostol versus placebo for cervical dilatation before vacuum aspiration in first trimester pregnancy. Hum Reprod 1995;10:1220.

19. Ngai SW, Yeung KCA, Lao T, Ho PC. Oral misoprostol versus mifepristone for cervical dilatation before vacuum aspiration in first trimester nulliparous pregnancy: a double blind prospective randomised study. Br J Obstet Gynecol 1996;103:1120.

20. Grimes DA. Second-trimester abortions in the United States. Fam Plann Perspec 1984;16:260.

21. Shulman LP, Ling FW, Meyers CM, Shanklin DR, Simpson JL, Elias S. Dilation and evacuation for second-trimester genetic pregnancy termination. Obstet Gynecol 1990;75:1037.

22. Darney PD. Second-trimester elective abortion. In: Darney PD, ed. Office and ambulatory surgery. Oradell, NJ: Medical Economics, 1987:194.

23. Thomas AG, Alvarez M, Friedman F, Brodman ML, Kim J, Lockwood C. The effect of placenta previa on blood loss in second-trimester pregnancy termination. Obstet Gynecol 1994;84:58.

24. Hakim-Elahi E, Tovell HMM, Burnhill MS. Complications of first-trimester abortion: a report of 170,000 cases. Obstet Gynecol 1990;76:129.

25. Peterson WF, Berry N, Grace MR, Gulbrandson CL. Second-trimester abortion by dilatation and evacuation: an analysis of 11,747 cases. Obstet Gynecol 1983;62:185.

26. Rashbaum WK, Gates EJ, Jones J, Goldman B, Morris A, Lyman WD. Placenta accreta encountered during dilation and evacuation in the second trimester. Obstet Gynecol 1995;85:701.

27. Hodgson JE, Portmann KC. Complications of 10,453 consecutive first-trimester abortions: a prospective study. Am J Obstet Gynecol 1974;120:802.

28. Wulff GJL, Freiman SL. Elective abortion: complications seen in a free-standing clinic. Obstet Gynecol 1977; 49:351.

29. Sands RX, Burnhill MS, Hakim-Elahi E. Postabortal uterine atony. Obstet Gynecol 1974;43:595.

30. Hardman JG, Limbird LE, eds. Goodman and Gilman's: The pharmacological basis of therapeutics. 9th ed. New York: McGraw-Hill, 1990:339, 754.

31. Park TK, Flock M, Schulz KF, Grimes DA. Preventing febrile complications of suction curettage abortion. Am J Obstet Gynecol 1985;152:252.

32. Darj E, Stralin EB, Nilsson S. The prophylactic effect of doxycycline on postoperative infection rate after first-trimester abortion. Obstet Gynecol 1987;70:755.

33. Levallois P, Rioux JE. Prophylactic antibiotics for suction curettage abortion: results of a clinical controlled trial. Am J Obstet Gynecol 1988;158:100.

34. Henshaw RC, Naji SA, Russell IT, Templeton AA. Comparison of medical abortion with surgical vacuum aspiration: women's preferences and acceptability of treatment. BMJ 1993;307:714.

35. Winikoff B. Acceptability of medical abortion in early pregnancy. Fam Plann Perspec 1995;27:142, 185.

36. Henshaw AC, Naji SA, Russell IT, Templeton AA. A comparison of medical abortion (using mifepristone and gemeprost) with surgical vacuum aspiration: efficacy and early medical sequelae. Hum Reprod 1994;2167.

37. Howie FL, Henshaw RC, Naji SA, Russell IT, Templeton AA. Medical abortion or vacuum aspiration? Two year follow up of a patient preference trial. Br J Obstet Gynaecol 1997;104:829.

38. Johannisson E, Oberholzer M, Swahn ML, Bydgeman M. Vascular changes in the human endometrium following the administration of the progesterone antagonist RU 486. Contraception 1989;39:103.

39. Brooks J, Holland P, Kelly R. Comparison of antiprogestin stimulation of uterine prostaglandin synthesis in vitro. Prostaglandins Leukot Essent Fatty Acids 1990; 40:191.

40. Swahn ML, Bydgeman M. The effect of the antiprogestin RU 486 on uterine contractility and sensitivity to prostaglandin and oxytocin. Br J Obstet Gynaecol 1988; 95:126.

41. Grimes DA. Medical abortion in early pregnancy: a review of the evidence. Obstet Gynecol 1997;89:790.

42. Grimes DA, Mishell DR, David HP. A randomized clinical trial of mifepristone (RU486) for induction of delayed menses: efficacy and acceptability. Contraception 1992;46:1.

43. Couzinet B, LeStrat N, Silvestre L, Schiason G. Late luteal administration of the antiprogesterone RU486 in normal women: effects of menstrual cycle events and fertility control in a long-term study. Fertil Steril 1990; 54:1039.

44. World Health Organization Task Force on Post-ovulatory Methods of Fertility Regulation. Menstrual regulation by mifepristone plus prostaglandin: results from a multicentre trial. Hum Reprod 1995;10:308.

45. Lelaidier C, Baton-Saint-Mleux C, Fernandez H, Bourget P, Frydman R. Mifepristone (RU 486) induces embryo expulsion in first trimester non-developing pregnancies: a prospective randomized trial. Hum Reprod 1993;8:492.

46. El-Rafaey H, Hinshaw K, Henshaw R, Smith N, Templeton A. Medical management of missed abortion and anembryonic pregnancy. BMJ 1992;305:1399.

47. Spitz IM, Bardin CW, Benton L, Robbins A. Early pregnancy termination with mifepristone and misoprostol in the United States. N Engl J Med 1998;338:1241.

48. World Health Organization Task Force on Post-ovulatory Methods of Fertility Regulation. Termination of pregnancy with reduced doses of mifepristone. BMJ 1993;307:532.

49. McKinley C, Thong KJ, Baird DT. The effect of dose of mifepristone and gestation on the efficacy of medical abortion with mifepristone and misoprostol. Hum Reprod 1993;8:1502.

50. World Health Organization. Pregnancy termination with mifepristone and gemeprost: a multicenter comparison between repeated doses and a single dose of mifepristone. Fertil Steril 1991;56:32.

51. Tang GWK, Lau OWK, Yip P. Further acceptability evaluation of RU486 and ONO 802 as abortifacient agents in a Chinese population. Contraception 1993;48:267.

52. Hausknecht RU. Methotrexate and misoprostol to terminate early pregnancy. N Engl J Med 1995;333:537.

53. Creinin MD. Methotrexate for abortion at <42 days gestation. Contraception 1993;48:519.

54. Creinin MD, Vittinghoff E. Methotrexate and misoprostol vs misoprostol alone for early abortion. JAMA 1994; 272:1190.

55. Creinin MD, Vittinghoff E, Schaff E, Klaisle C, Darney PD, Dean C. Medical abortion with oral methotrexate and vaginal misoprostol. Obstet Gynecol 1997;90:611.

56. Creinin MD. Methotrexate and misoprostol for abortion at 57–63 days gestation. Contraception 1994;50:511.

57. Creinin MD, Vittinghoff E, Galbraith S, Klaisle C. A randomized trial comparing misoprostol three and seven days after methotrexate for early abortion. Am J Obstet Gynecol 1995;173:1578.

58. Karim SMM, Filshie GM. Therapeutic abortion using prostaglandin F_{2alpha}. Lancet 1970;1:157.

59. Norman JE, Thong KJ, Rodger MW, Baird DT. Medical abortion in women of ≤56 days amenorrhoea: a comparison between gemeprost (a PGE_1 analogue) alone and mifepristone and gemeprost. Br J Obstet Gynaecol 1992; 99:601.

60. Creinin MD, Moyer R, Guido R. Misoprostol for medical evacuation of early pregnancy failure. Obstet Gynecol 1997;89:768.

61. Baird DT, Sukcharoen N, Thong KJ. Randomized trial of misoprostol and cervagem in combination with a reduced dose of mifepristone for induction of abortion. Hum Reprod 1995;10:1521.

62. Peplow PV. RU486 combined with PGE_1 analog in voluntary termination of early pregnancy—a comparison of recent findings with gemeprost and misoprostol. Contraception 1994;50:69.

63. El-Rafaey H, Templeton A. Early abortion induction by a combination of mifepristone and oral misoprostol: a comparison between two dose regimens of misoprostol and their effect on blood pressure. Br J Obstet Gynaecol 1994;101:792.

64. El-Rafaey H, Rajasekar D, Abdalla M, Calder L, Templeton A. Induction of abortion with mifepristone (RU 486) and oral or vaginal misoprostol. N Engl J Med 1995;332:983.

65. Zieman M, Fong SK, Benowitz NL, Bankster D, Darney PD. Absorption kinetics of misoprostol with oral or vaginal administration. Obstet Gynecol 1997;90:88.

66. Berger GS, Edelman DA, Kerenyi TD. Oxytocin administration, instillation-to-abortion time, and morbidity associated with saline instillation. Am J Obstet Gynecol 1975;121:941.

67. Binkin NJ, Schulz KF, Grimes DA, Cates W. Urea-prostaglandin versus hypertonic saline for instillation abortion. Am J Obstet Gynecol 1983;146:947.

68. Osathonondh R. Conception control. In: Ryan KJ, Barbieri R, Berkowitz RS, eds. Kistner's Gynecology. 5th ed. St. Louis: Year Book, 1989:480.

69. Jain JK, Mishell DR. A comparison of intravaginal misoprostol with prostaglandin E_2 for termination of second-trimester pregnancy. N Engl J Med 1994;331:290.

70. Nuutila M, Toivonen J, Ylikorkala O, Halmesmäki E. A comparison between two doses of intravaginal misopros-tol and gemeprost for induction of second trimester abortion. Obstet Gynecol 1997;90:896.

71. Bydgeman M, Christensen NJ. Termination of second-trimester pregnancy by laminaria and intramuscular injections of 15-methyl PGF_{2alpha} or 16-phenoxy-17,18,19,20-tetranor PGE_2 methyl sulfonamide: a randomized study. Acta Obstet Gynecol Scand 1983;62:535.

72. Rodger MW, Baird DT. Pretreatment with mifepristone (RU 486) reduces interval between prostaglandin administration and expulsion in second trimester abortion. Br J Obstet Gynaecol 1990;97:41.

73. Thong KJ, Baird DT. A study of gemeprost alone, dilapan or mifepristone in combination with gemeprost for the termination of second trimester pregnancy. Contraception 1992;46:11.

74. Webster D, Penney GC, Templeton A. A comparison of 600 and 200 mg mifepristone prior to second trimester abortion with the prostaglandin misoprostol. Br J Obstet Gynaecol 1996;103:706.

75. Ho PC, Ngai SW, Liu KL, Wong GCY, Lee SWH. Vaginal misoprostol compared with oral misoprostol in termination of second-trimester pregnancy. Obstet Gynecol 1997;90:735.

76. El-Rafaey H, Templeton A. Induction of abortion in the second trimester by a combination of misoprostol and mifepristone: a randomized comparison between two misoprostol regimens. Hum Reprod 1995;10;475.

77. Winkler CL, Gray SE, Hauth JC, Owen J, Tucker JM. Mid-second-trimester labor induction: concentrated oxytocin compared with prostaglandin E_2 vaginal suppositories. Obstet Gynecol 1991;77:297.

78. Owen J, Hauth JC, Winkler CL, Gray SE. Midtrimester pregnancy termination: a randomized trial of prostaglandin E_2 versus concentrated oxytocin. Obstet Gynecol 1992;167:1112.

79. Holmgren K. Women's evaluation of three early abortion methods. Acta Obstet Gynecol Scand 1992;71:616.

80. Thonneau P, Poirel H, Fougeyrollas B, et al. A comparative analysis of fall in haemoglobin following abortions conducted by mifepristone (600 mg) and vacuum aspiration. Hum Reprod 1995;1512.

81. Chan YF, Ho PC, Ma HK. Blood loss in termination of early pregnancy by vacuum aspiration and by combination of mifepristone and gemeprost. Contraception 1993; 47:85.

82. Hill NCW, Mackenzie IZ. 2308 second trimester terminations using extra-amniotic saline or intra-amniotic prostaglandin E_2: an analysis of efficacy and complications. Br J Obstet Gynaecol 1989;96:1424.

Chapter 13

Preterm Delivery

Alice R. Goepfert

Five Key Points

- Preterm birth is the leading cause of perinatal morbidity and mortality in the United States.

- Approximately a third of all preterm births are associated with preterm premature rupture of membranes.

- The principal complications experienced by preterm infants are intraventricular hemorrhage, hyaline-membrane disease, necrotizing enterocolitis, sepsis, and thermal instability.

- Bacterial vaginosis is associated with a twofold increase in the risk of preterm delivery. However, the single most important risk factor for preterm delivery is a history of a previous spontaneous preterm delivery.

- For most patients with preterm premature rupture of membranes at <32 weeks of gestation, expectant management is preferred. At gestational ages >32 weeks, delivery is usually indicated if fetal lung maturity can be confirmed.

Preterm birth is the leading cause of perinatal morbidity and mortality in the United States today. Prematurity also contributes significantly to major long-term neonatal morbidity, including chronic lung disease, hearing and visual impairment, developmental delay, and cerebral palsy. Furthermore, of those infants born prior to term in whom major handicaps do not develop, there are a proportionately larger number with more subtle intellectual and behavioral problems noted during long-term follow-up.[1,2] Births prior to 37 weeks of gestation are considered premature; however, the greatest morbidity and mortality occur in infants born prior to 32 weeks of gestation.[3] Regionalization of perinatal care and advances in neonatal care during the past several decades have reduced the perinatal morbidity and mortality associated with prematurity. Unfortunately, the preterm birth rate has actually increased.[4]

Approximately 45% of preterm deliveries occur following spontaneous labor, and 30% follow preterm premature rupture of membranes. The remainder of preterm deliveries are iatrogenic, secondary to fetal or maternal indications.[5] Much progress has been made in the past decade in determining the cause of spontaneous preterm labor and preterm premature rupture of membranes. However, a better understanding of the pathogenesis of these complications of pregnancy is necessary before we can accurately identify the majority of women at risk and develop effective therapy to prevent preterm birth.

DEFINITIONS

In the older literature, the concept of prematurity versus low birth weight was not well defined. An infant born weighing less than 2500 g is not necessarily premature. As many as one-third of these low-birth-weight infants are actually growth-restricted rather than preterm, and the morbidities associated with these two conditions are not necessarily the same.[6] Although the distinction continues to be a problem in some developing nations, in the United States today most pregnancies can be accurately dated by correlating menstrual history with biochemical tests for pregnancy and early ultrasound measurement of fetal size.

A preterm birth is one that occurs prior to 37 weeks of gestation, regardless of fetal size. Births that occur before 20 weeks of gestation are termed "abortions" rather than preterm deliveries. Low-birth-weight (LBW) infants weigh less than 2500 g at birth, very-low-birth-weight (VLBW) infants weigh less than 1500 g, and extremely-low-birth-weight (ELBW) infants weigh less than 1000 g. These terms have been useful when describing morbidity and mortality associated with certain groups of infants. However, with infants surviving at lower gestational ages and birth weights, the term ELBW is being largely replaced in the current literature by the actual birth weights.

PERINATAL MORBIDITY AND MORTALITY

All infants born at less than 37 weeks of gestation are at risk for a variety of complications due to prematurity, including intraventricular hemorrhage (IVH),

respiratory distress syndrome (RDS), bronchopulmonary dysplasia (BPD), necrotizing enterocolitis (NEC), sepsis, patent ductus arteriosus (PDA), thermal instability, apnea and bradycardia, and retinopathy of prematurity (ROP). However, as the gestational age and birth weight decrease, particularly at <28 weeks or <1000 g, the mortality rate, as well as the incidence and severity of these morbidities, greatly increases. Long-term neurologic sequelae such as mental retardation, cerebral palsy, seizure disorders, blindness, and deafness continue to be a major concern with extreme prematurity. The prevalence of serious long-term morbidity in these infants remains high.[3,7-9] A summary of the range of survival rates for infants born between 23 and 29 weeks of gestation taken from the literature and from our experience at the University of Alabama is presented in Table 13-1.[8-14]

When faced with the potential delivery of an extremely premature infant, the concept of intact survival becomes very important to the obstetrician responsible for making management plans and counseling parents about options. Intact survival is generally defined as survival without major morbidity (such as grade 3 or 4 IVH, grade 3 or 4 ROP, NEC requiring surgery, oxygen dependence at discharge from the hospital, and seizures) and obviously decreases with gestational age or birth weight. As noted in Table 13-1, only 10% of infants surviving a preterm birth at 23 weeks of gestation survive intact, as compared with at least 50% of infants surviving delivery at 27 completed weeks of gestation. Tables 13-2 and 13-3 present morbidity and mortality statistics according to gestational age and birth weight from our own center during a recent 1-year period.[10]

TABLE 13-1
SURVIVAL BY GESTATIONAL AGE* (1989–1996)[8-14]

Weeks of Gestation	% Survival (range)	% Intact† survival (range)
23	(15–46)	(10)
24	(43–55)	(15–28)
25	(59–84)	(34–47)
26	(71–88)	(40–63)
27	(79–96)	(50)
28	(88–91)	(54)
29	(95)	(71)

*By best obstetric estimate.
†Without major morbidity.

Following PROM, labor often begins within a relatively short time. However, the duration of the latency period varies inversely with gestational age. Over 90% of women with PROM at term have spontaneous labor within 24 hours.[92] Yet PROM occurring between 28 and 34 weeks of gestation is associated with spontaneous labor within 24 hours in only 50% of women and labor within 1 week in 90% of women.[93,94] Prior to 26 weeks of gestation, approximately 50% of women will have spontaneous labor within 1 week of PROM.[91,95]

Pulmonary hypoplasia is a rare complication when PROM occurs after 26 weeks of gestation. In this group, the primary concerns relate to infection and other morbidity and mortality associated with prematurity. The most serious infection-related neonatal complications in preterm infants include sepsis and pneumonia.

Although uncommon, risk of stillbirth resulting from cord compression in pregnancies managed expectantly must also be considered. Maternal morbidity is largely infection-related but also includes retained placenta and abruptio placentae.

Expectant Management

The approach to management of pPROM depends on a number of factors, including the gestational age and presence of clinically evident intrauterine infection, associated preterm labor, or nonreassuring fetal status. The crucial factors to be determined in the initial evaluation of a woman with suspected pPROM are outlined in Table 13-11. Essential to the counseling and management of women with pPROM is knowledge of maternal, fetal, and neonatal risks. In general, decisions regarding management should be guided by weighing the relative risks of prematurity versus infection-associated morbidity. Specific approaches to management remain controversial. However, there is a consensus that, in the absence of overt infection or evidence of fetal compromise, expectant

---

TABLE 13-11
INITIAL EVALUATION OF PATIENT WITH POSSIBLE PRETERM PROM

Confirm the diagnosis of PROM by sterile speculum exam
Determine the gestational age
Rule out maternal and/or fetal infection
Rule out labor
Rule out fetal distress

---

management is appropriate when the pregnancy is remote from term. In this scenario, the risks of prematurity generally outweigh the maternal or fetal/neonatal risks associated with infection. There is also agreement that because the prematurity risks are low, delivery is usually indicated when PROM occurs at or near term. What remains uncertain, however, is at what gestational age the pendulum of risk swings dictating a shift from expectant management to labor induction. No clear gestational age cutoff has been established, and opinions vary regarding management of pPROM in the intermediate gestational age range (32 to 34 weeks).

One approach to clinical decision making in this group of pregnancies involves assessment of vaginal pool amniotic fluid for evidence of fetal lung maturity. The test for fetal lung maturity generally recommended for amniotic fluid obtained from the vagina is the presence of phosphatidylglycerol (PG). Vaginal fluid is often contaminated by blood, mucus, and other substances; however, the PG test is unaffected. If the lungs are mature, a decision to deliver can be made; if immature, expectant management may be prudent. A clinical decision protocol based on this approach, which may be used to guide management, is summarized in Figure 13-2. One study compared expectant management to labor induction in women with pPROM and a mature amniotic fluid test between 32 and 36 weeks.[96] In this study, expectant management did not improve neonatal outcome and was associated with increased maternal infection-related morbidity compared to women whose pregnancies were managed with labor induction.

Multiple prospective randomized clinical trials of prophylactic antibiotics in the expectant management of women with pPROM have been published, and most show an increase of 5 to 7 days in the latency period in treated patients with no increase in maternal or neonatal morbidity and mortality.[97-103] In addition, two meta-analyses also demonstrated reduced rates of maternal and neonatal infection with antibiotic treatment versus placebo or expectant management alone.[104,105] A large multicenter trial of antibiotics in pPROM from the NICHD Maternal–Fetal Medicine Units Network also demonstrated a prolonged latency period and decreased composite perinatal morbidity with the use of antibiotics versus placebo.[106] These same benefits were evident when antibiotics were used in women with pPROM who also received corticosteroid therapy.[107] The antibiotic

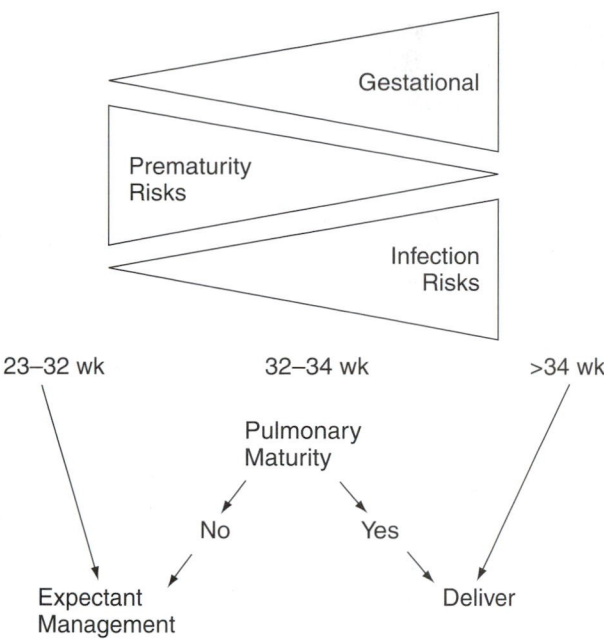

Figure 13-2 Management of preterm premature rupture of membranes.

TABLE 13-12
EXPECTANT MANAGEMENT OF PPROM AT UAB

Document PROM by sterile speculum examination
Rule out preterm labor by tocodynamometry
Hospitalization with limited activity
Observe closely for signs of infection
Avoid digital examinations
Daily fetal monitoring (nonstress tests)
Broad-spectrum antibiotics
Corticosteroids if <32 weeks and no evidence of infection
No tocolytic therapy

regimen and the duration of treatment are variable among studies; however, broad-spectrum antibiotics that include coverage for group B streptococci appear to be the best choice. At our center, we currently use a combination of ampicillin or amoxicillin and erythromycin or azithromycin for 10 days, with retreatment in labor with our standard group B streptococcal prophylaxis protocol.

Antenatal corticosteroid use in women with pPROM continues to be a source of some controversy. However, more recent data, which include antibiotic therapy in conjunction with corticosteroid therapy in pPROM, demonstrate reductions in respiratory distress syndrome more comparable to studies in women with intact membranes.[108] The NIH Consensus Development Panel convened a conference on antenatal corticosteroids in 1994 and recommended their use in women with pPROM prior to 32 weeks of gestation in the absence of intrauterine infection.[109] The available data indicate that the benefits of corticosteroids in reducing the incidence of respiratory distress syndrome and intraventricular hemorrhage outweigh the risk in these very preterm infants. Due to the potential risks to the fetus and mother and unknown benefits with repeated courses of corticosteroids, it appears reasonable to limit use to one course in women with pPROM.

Tocolytic therapy in women with pPROM has been shown to prolong the latency period only on a short-term basis[110,111] and may be reasonable in women without evidence of infection or advanced preterm labor with the goal of administering antenatal corticosteroids and antibiotics or for transport to a tertiary-care center. An outline of the expectant management protocol for women with pPROM used at our center is presented in Table 13-12.

REFERENCES

1. Hack M, Taylor HG, Klein N, Eiben R, Schatschneider C, Mercuri-Minich N. School-age outcomes in children with birth weights under 750 g. N Engl J Med 1994; 331:753.
2. Halsey CL, Collin MF, Anderson CL. Extremely low birth weight children and their peers: a comparison of preschool performance. Pediatrics 1993;91:807.
3. Robertson PA, Sniderman SH, Laros RK Jr, et al. Neonatal morbidity according to gestational age and birth weight from five tertiary care centers in the United States, 1983 through 1986. Am J Obstet Gynecol 1992; 166:1629.
4. Ventura SJ, Martin JA, Mathews TJ, Clarke SC. Advance report of final natality statistics, 1994. Monthly Vital Stat Rep 1996;44(11):Suppl:75.
5. Tucker JM, Goldenberg RL, Davis RO, Copper RL, Winkler CL, Hauth JC. Etiologies of preterm birth in an indigent population: is prevention a logical expectation? Obstet Gynecol 1991;77:343.
6. Lugo G, Cassidy G. Intrauterine growth retardation: clinicopathologic findings in 233 consecutive infants. Am J Obstet Gynecol 1971;109:615.
7. Copper RL, Goldenberg RL, Creasy RK, et al. A multicenter study of preterm birth weight and gestational age specific mortality. Am J Obstet Gynecol 1993;168:1993.
8. Fanaroff AA, Wright LL, Stevenson DK, et al. Very-low-birth-weight outcomes of the National Institute of Child Health and Human Development Neonatal Research Network, May 1991 through December 1992. Am J Obstet Gynecol 1995;173:1423.
9. Piecuch RE, Leonard CH, Cooper BA, Kilpatrick SJ, Schlueter MA, Sola A. Outcome of infants born at 24–26 weeks' gestation. II. Neurodevelopmental outcome. Obstet Gynecol 1997;90:808.

10. Dr. Carlo, unpublished data, University of Alabama at Birmingham, 1995–1996.

11. Hack, M, Wright L, Shankaran S, et al. Very-low-birth-weight outcomes of the National Institute of Child Health and Human Development Neonatal Network, November 1989 to October 1990. Washington, DC: Government Printing Office, 1991.

12. Bottoms SF, Paul RH, Iams JD, et al. Obstetric determinants of neonatal survival: influence of willingness to perform cesarean delivery on survival of extremely low-birth-weight infants. Am J Obstet Gynecol 1997; 176:960.

13. Kilpatrick SJ, Schlueter MA, Piecuch R, Leonard CH, Rogido M, Sola A. Outcome of infants born at 24 to 26 weeks' gestation. I. Survival and cost. Obstet Gynecol 1997;90:803.

14. Stevenson DK, Wright LL, Lemons JA, et al. Very low birth weight outcomes of the National Institute of Child Health and Human Development Neonatal Research Network, January 1993 through December 1994. Am J Obstet Gynecol 1998;179:1632.

15. Meis PJ, Ernest JM, Moore ML, Michielutte R, Sharp PC, Buescher PA. Regional program for prevention of premature birth in northwestern North Carolina. Am J Obstet Gynecol 1987;157:550.

16. Meis PJ, Michielutte R, Peters TJ, et al. Factors associated with preterm birth in Cardiff, Wales. II. Indicated and spontaneous preterm birth. Am J Obstet Gynecol 1995; 173:597.

17. Andrews WW, Goldenberg RL, Hauth JC. Preterm labor: emerging role of genital tract infections. Infect Agents Dis 1995;4:196.

18. Romero R, Mazor M. Infection and preterm labor. Clin Obstet Gynecol 1988;31:553.

19. Mead PB. Epidemiology of bacterial vaginosis. Am J Obstet Gynecol 1993;169:446.

20. Goldenberg RL, Klebanoff MA, Nugent R, Krohn MA, Hillier S, Andrews WW. Bacterial colonization of the vagina during pregnancy in four ethnic groups. Am J Obstet Gynecol 1996;174:1618.

21. Watts DA, Krohn MA, Hillier SL, Eschenbach DA. The association of occult amniotic fluid infection with gestational age and neonatal outcome among women in preterm labor. Obstet Gynecol 1992;79:351.

22. Cassell G, Hauth JC, Andrews W, Cutter G, Goldenberg R. Chorioamnion colonization: correlation with gestational age in women delivered following spontaneous labor versus indicated delivery. Am J Obstet Gynecol 1993;168:425.

23. Hillier SL, Martins J, Krohn M, Kiviat N, Holmes KK, Eschenbach DA. A case-control study of chorioamnion infection and histologic chorioamnionitis in prematurity. N Engl J Med 1988;319:972.

24. Hillier SL, Krohn MA, Cassen E, Easterling TR, Rabe LK, Eschenbach DA. The role of bacterial vaginosis and vaginal bacteria in amniotic fluid infection in women in preterm labor with intact fetal membranes. Clin Infect Dis 1995;20(Suppl 2):276.

25. Eschenbach DA, Gravett MG, Chen KC, Hoyme UB, Holmes KK. Bacterial vaginosis during pregnancy: an association with prematurity and postpartum complications. Scand J Urol Nephrol Suppl 1984;86:213.

26. Kurki T, Sivonen A, Renkonen OV, Savia E, Ylikorkala O. Bacterial vaginosis in early pregnancy and pregnancy outcome. Obstet Gynecol 1992;80:173.

27. Riduan JM, Hillier SL, Utomo B, Wiknjosastro G, Linnan M, Kandun N. Bacterial vaginosis and prematurity in Indonesia: association in early and late pregnancy. Am J Obstet Gynecol 1993;169:175.

28. Hillier SL, Nugent RP, Eschenbach DA, et al. Association between bacterial vaginosis and preterm delivery of a low-birth-weight infant. N Engl J Med 1995; 333:1737.

29. Morales WJ, Schorr S, Albritton J. Effect of metronidazole in patients with preterm birth in preceding pregnancy and bacterial vaginosis: a placebo-controlled, double-blind study. Am J Obstet Gynecol 1994;171:345.

30. Hauth JC, Goldenberg RL, Andrews WW, DuBard MB, Copper RL. Reduced incidence of preterm delivery with metronidazole and erythromycin in women with bacterial vaginosis. N Engl J Med 1995;333:1732.

31. Klebanoff M, Carey JC, and the NICHD Maternal-Fetal Medicine Units Network. Metronidazole did not prevent preterm birth in asymptomatic women with bacterial vaginosis. Am J Obstet Gynecol 1999;180:S2.

32. Shiono PH, Klebanoff MA, Graubard BI, Berendes HW, Rhoads GG. Birth weight among women of different ethnic groups. JAMA 1986;255:48.

33. Wen SW, Goldenberg RL, Cutter G, Hoffman H, Cliver SP. Intrauterine growth retardation and preterm delivery: prenatal risk factors in an indigent population. Am J Obstet Gynecol 1990;162:213.

34. Kramer MS. Determinants of low birth weight: methodological assessment and meta-anlysis. Bull World Health Organ 1987;65:663.

35. Kleinman JC, Kessel SS. Racial difference in low birth weight: trends and risk factors. N Engl J Med 1987; 317:749.

36. Adams MM, Read JA, Rawlings JS, Harlass FB, Sarno AP, Rhodes PH. Preterm delivery among black and white enlisted women in the United States Army. Obstet Gynecol 1993;81:65.

37. Meis PJ, Goldenberg Rl, Mercer B, et al. The preterm prediction study: significance of vaginal infections. Am J Obstet Gynecol 1995;173:1231.

38. Hay PE, Lamont RF, Taylor-Robinson D, Morgan DJ, Ison C, Pearson J. Abnormal bacterial colonization of the genital tract and subsequent preterm delivery and late miscarriage. BMJ 1994;308:295.

39. McGregor JA, French JI, Parker R, et al. Prevention of premature birth by screening and treatment for common genital tract infections: results of a prospective controlled evaluation. Am J Obstet Gynecol 1995;173:157.

40. Papiernik E, Kaminski M. Multifactorial study of the risk of prematurity at 32 weeks of gestation: a study for the frequency of 30 predictive charicteristics. J Perinat Med 1974;2:30.

41. Creasy RK, Gummer BA, Liggins GC. System for predicting spontaneous preterm birth. Obstet Gynecol 1980;55:692.

42. Owen J, Goldenberg RL, Davis RO, Kirk KA, Copper RL. Evaluation of a risk scoring system as a predictor of preterm birth in an indigent population. Am J Obstet Gynecol 1990;163:873.

43. Collaborative Group on Preterm Birth Prevention. Multicenter randomized, controlled trial of preterm birth prevention program. Am J Obstet Gynecol 1993;169:352.

44. Hueston WJ, Knox MA, Eilers G, Pamwels J, Lonsdorf D. The effectiveness of preterm-birth prevention educational program for high-risk women: a meta-analysis. Obstet Gynecol 1995;86:705.

45. Carr-Hill RA, Hall MH. The repetition of spontaneous preterm labour. Br J Obstet Gynaecol 1991;164:921.

46. Kristensen J, Langhoff-Ross J, Kristensen FB. Implications of idiopathic preterm delivery for previous and subsequent pregnancies. Obstet Gynecol 1995;86:800.

47. Goldenberg RL, Mayberry SK, Copper RL, DuBard MB, Hauth JC. Pregnancy outcome following a second-trimester loss. Obstet Gynecol 1993;81:444.

48. Anderson BM, Turnbull AC. Relationship between length of gestation and cervical dilation, uterine contractility, and other factors during pregnancy. Am J Obstet Gynecol 1969;105:1207.

49. Bouyer J, Papiernik E, Dreyfus J, Collin D, Winisdoerffer B, Gueguen S. Maturation signs of the cervix and prediction of preterm birth. Obstet Gynecol 1986;68:209.

50. Papiernik E, Bouyer J, Collin D, Winisdoerffer G, Dreyfus J. Precocious cervical ripening and preterm labor. Obstet Gynecol 1986;67:238.

51. Holcomb WL Jr, Smeltzer JS. Cervical effacement: variation in belief among clinicians. Obstet Gynecol 1991;78:43.

52. Sonek JD, Iams JD, Blumenfeld M, Johnson F, Landon M, Gabbe S. Measurement of cervical length in pregnancy: comparison between vaginal ultrasonography and digital examination. Obstet Gynecol 1990;76:172.

53. Anderson HF. Transvaginal and transabdominal ultrasonography of the uterine cervix during pregnancy. J Clin Ultrasound 1991;19:77.

54. Anderson HF, Nugent CE, Wanty SD, Hayaski RH. Prediction of risk for preterm delivery by ultrasonographic measurement of cervical length. Am J Obstet Gynecol 1990;163:859.

55. Iams JC, Paraskos J, Landon MB, Teteris JN, Johnson FF. Cervical sonography in preterm labor. Obstet Gynecol 1994;84:40.

56. Tongsong T, Kamprapauth P, Srisomboon J, Nanapirak C, Piyamongkol N, Sirichotiyakul S. Single transvaginal sonographic measurement of cervical length early in the third trimester as a predictor of preterm delivery. Obstet Gynecol 1995;86:184.

57. Timor-Tritsch IE, Boozarjomehri F, Masakowski Y, Monteagudo A, Chao CR. Can a "snapshot" sagittal view of the cervix by transvaginal ultrasonography predict active preterm labor? Am J Obstet Gynecol 1996;174:990.

58. Iams JD, Goldenberg RL, Meis PJ, et al. The length of the cervix and the risk of spontaneous preterm delivery. N Engl J Med 1996;334:567.

59. Beckmann CA, Beckmann CRB, Stanziano GJ, Bergauer NK, Marth CB. Accuracy of maternal perception of preterm uterine activity. Am J Obstet Gynecol 1996;174:672.

60. Grimes DA, Schulz FK. Randomized controlled trials of home uterine activity monitoring: a review and critique. Obstet Gynecol 1992;79:137.

61. Sachs BP, Hellerstein S, Freeman R, Frigolleto F, Hauth JC. Home monitoring of uterine activity: does it prevent prematurity? N Engl J Med 1991;325:1374.

62. US Preventive Services Task Force. Home uterine activity monitoring for preterm labor: policy statement. JAMA 1993;270:369.

63. American College of Obstetrics and Gynecology. Home uterine activity monitoring. ACOG Committee Opinion no 172, May 1996:6.

64. Wapner RJ, Cotton DB, Artal R, Librizzi RJ, Ross MG. A randomized multicenter trial assessing a home uterine activity monitoring device used in the absence of daily nursing contact. Am J Obstet Gynecol 1995; 172:1026.

65. The Collaborative Home Uterine Monitoring Study Group. A multicenter randomized controlled trial of home uterine monitoring: active versus sham device. Am J Obstet Gynecol 1995;173:1120.

66. Colton T, Kayne JL, Zhang Y, Heeren T. A meta-analysis of home uterine activity monitoring. Am J Obstet Gynecol 1995;173:499.

67. Dyson DC, Crites YM, Ray DA, Armstrong MA. Prevention of preterm birth in high-risk patients: the role of education and provider contact versus home uterine monitoring. Am J Obstet Gynecol 1991;164:756.

68. Dyson DC, Danbe KH, Bamber JA, et al. Monitoring women at risk for preterm labor. N Engl J Med 1998;338:15.

69. Nugent RP, Krohn MA, Hillier SL. Reliability of diagnosing bacterial vaginosis is improved by a standardized method of Gram stain interpretation. J Clin Microbiol 1991;29:297.

70. Amsel RP, Totten PA, Spiegel CA, et al. Non-specific vaginitis: diagnostic and microbial and epidemiological associations. Am J Med 1983;74:14.

71. Matsurra H, Hakomori S. The oncofetal domain of fibronectin defined by monoclonal antibody FDC-6: its presence in fibronectins from fetal and tumor tissues and its absence in those from normal adult tissues and plasma. Proc Natl Acad Sci USA 1985;82:6517.

72. Feinberg RJ, Kliman HJ, Lockwood CJ. Is oncofetal fibronectin a trophoblast glue for human implantation? Am J Pathol 1991;138:537.

73. Lockwood CJ, Senyei AE, Dische MR, et al. Fetal fibronectin in cervical and vaginal secretions as a predictor of preterm delivery. N Engl J Med 1991;325:669.

74. Lockwood CJ, Feinberg RK, Kilman H, Garite TJ, Senyei AE. Cervicovaginal oncofetal fibronectin in preterm labor patients: a result of chorion extracellular matrix degradation. Am J Obstet Gynecol 1991;164:374. Abstract.

75. Goldenberg RL, Mercer BM, Meis RJ, Copper RL, Das A, McNellis D. The preterm prediction study: fetal fibronectin testing and spontaneous preterm birth. Obstet Gynecol 1996;87:643.

76. Goldenberg RL, Thom E, Moawad AH, Johnson F, Roberts J, Caritis SN. The preterm prediction study: fetal fibronectin, bacterial vaginosis, and peripartum infection. Obstet Gynecol 1996;87:656.

77. Goldenberg RL, Iams JD, Mercer BM, et al. The preterm prediction study: the value of new vs. standard risk factors in predicting early and all spontaneous preterm births. Am J Public Health 1998;88:233.

78. King JF, Grant A, Keirse MJNC. Beta-mimetics in preterm labour: an overview of the randomized controlled trials. Br J Obstet Gynaecol 1988;95:211.

79. Copper RL, Goldenberg RL, Davis RO, et al. Warning symptoms, uterine contractions, and cervical examination findings in women at risk of preterm delivery. Am J Obstet Gynecol 1990;162:748.

80. Iams JD, Johnson FF, Parker M. A prospective evaluation of the signs and symptoms of preterm labor. Obstet Gynecol 1994;84:227.

81. Iams JD, Casal D, McGregor JA, et al. Fetal fibronectin improves the accuracy of diagnosis of preterm labor. Am J Obstet Gynecol 1995;173:141.

82. Peaceman AM, Andrews WW, Thorp JM, et al. Fetal fibronectin as a predictor of preterm birth in patients with symptoms: a multicenter trial. Am J Obstet Gynecol 1997;177:13.

83. Murakawa H, Utimi T, Hasegawa I, Tanaka K, Fuzimori R. Evaluation of threatened preterm delivery by transvaginal ultrasonographic measurement of cervical length. Obstet Gynecol 1993;82:829.

84. Gomez R, Galasso M, Romero R, et al. Ultrasonographic examination of the cervix is better than cervical digital examination as a predictor of preterm delivery in patients with preterm labor and intact membranes. Am J Obstet Gynecol 1994;171:956.

85. Iams JD, Parakos J, Landon MB, Teteris JN, Johnson FF. Cervical sonography in preterm labor. Obstet Gynecol 1994;84:40.

86. Crane JMG, Van den Hof M, Armson BA, Liston R. Transvaginal ultrasound in the prediction of preterm delivery: Singleton and twin gestations. Obstet Gynecol 1997;90:357.

87. French JI, McGregor JA. The pathophysiology of premature rupture of the membranes. Semin Perinatol 1996; 20:344.

88. Richards DS. Complications of prolonged PROM and oligohydramnios. Clin Obstet Gynecol 1998;41:817.

89. Kilbride HW, Yeast J, Thibeault DW. Defining limits of survival: lethal pulmonary hypoplasia after midtrimester premature rupture of membranes. Am J Obstet Gynecol 1996;175:675.

90. Pena SDJ, Shokier MHK. Syndrome of camptodactyly, multiple ankylosis, facial anomalies, and pulmonary hypoplasia: a lethal condition. J Pediatr 1974;85:373.

91. Schucker JL, Mercer BM. Midtrimester premature rupture of the membranes. Semin Perinatol 1996;20:389.

92. Gunn GC, Mishell DR, Morton DG. Premature rupture of the fetal membranes: a review. Am J Obstet Gynecol 1970;106:469.

93. Mead PB. Management of the patient with premature rupture of the membranes. Clin Perinatol 1980;7:243.

94. Garite TJ, Freeman RK, Linzey EM, et al. Prospective randomized study of corticosteroids in the management of premature rupture of the membranes and the premature gestation. Am J Obstet Gynecol 1981;141:508.

95. Taylor J, Garite TJ. Premature rupture of membranes before fetal viability. Obstet Gynecol 1984;4:615.

96. Mercer BM, Crocker LG, Boe NM, Sibai BM. Induction versus expectant management in preterm rupture of the membranes with mature amniotic fluid at 32 to 36 weeks: a randomized trial. Am J Obstet Gynecol 1993; 169:775.

97. Amon E, Lewis, Sibai B, et al. Antibiotic prophylaxis in preterm PROM: a prospective randomized study. Am J Obstet Gynecol 1988;159:539.

98. Morales W, Angel J, O'Brien W, et al. Use of ampicillin and corticosteroids in PROM: a randomized study. Obstet Gynecol 1989;73:721.

99. McGregor JA, French JI, Seo K. Antimicrobial therapy in preterm premature rupture of the membranes: results of a prospective, double-blind, placebo-controlled trial of erythromycin. Am J Obstet Gynecol 1991; 165:632.

100. Christmas JT, Cox SM, Gilstrap LC, et al. Expectant management of preterm ruptured membranes: effects of antimicrobial therapy. Obstet Gynecol 1992;80:759.

101. Blanco J, Iams J, Artal R, et al. Multicenter double-blind prospective random trial of ceftizoximes: placebo in women with preterm premature ruptured membranes. Am J Obstet Gynecol 1993;168:378.

102. Lockwood CJ, Costigan K, Ghidine A, et al. Double blind placebo-controlled trial of piperacillin prophylaxis in preterm membrane rupture. Am J Obstet Gynecol 1993;169:970.

103. Owen J, Groome LJ, Hauth JC. Randomized trial of prophylactic antibiotic therapy after preterm amnion rupture. Am J Obstet Gynecol 1993;169:976.

104. Mercer BM, Arheart KL. Antimicrobial therapy in expectant management of preterm premature rupture of the membranes. Lancet 1995;346:1271.

105. Egarter C, Leitich H, Karas H, et al. Antibiotic treatment in preterm premature rupture of membranes and neonatal morbidity: a metaanalysis. Am J Obstet Gynecol 1996;174:589.

106. Mercer BM, Miodovnik M, Thurnau GR, et al. Antibiotic therapy for reduction of infant morbidity after preterm premature rupture of the membranes: a randomized controlled trial. JAMA 1997;278:989.

107. Lovett SM, Weiss JD, Diogo MJ, Williams PT, Garite TJ. A prospective double-blind, randomized, controlled clinical trial of ampicillin-sulbactam for preterm premature rupture of membranes in women receiving antenatal corticosteroid therapy. Am J Obstet Gynecol 1997; 176:1030.

108. Lewis DF, Brody K, Edwards MS, et al. Preterm premature ruptured membranes: a randomized trial of steroids after treatment with antibiotics. Obstet Gynecol 1996; 88:801.

109. National Institutes of Health. National Institutes of Health Consensus Development Conference Statement: Effect of corticosteroids for fetal maturation on perinatal outcomes, February 28-March 2, 1994. Am J Obstet Gynecol 1995;173:246.

110. Christensen KK, Ingemarsson I, Leideman T, Solum H, Svenningsen N. Effect of ritodrine on labor after premature rupture of the membranes. Obstet Gynecol 1980; 55:187.

111. Weiner CP, Renk K, Klugman M. The therapeutic efficacy and cost-effectiveness of aggressive tocolysis for premature labor associated with premature rupture of the membranes. Am J Obstet Gynecol 1988;159:216.

Chapter 14

Antepartum Hemorrhage

B. Denise Raynor

Five Key Points

- Third-trimester bleeding occurs in up to 4% of all pregnancies. The two most common causes are abruptio placentae and placenta previa.

- The principal risk factors for placenta previa are increased maternal age, increased parity, smoking, previous induced or spontaneous abortion, uterine anomaly, and prior cesarean delivery.

- The definitive diagnostic test for placenta previa is ultrasonography.

- The principal risk factors for abruptio placentae are hypertension, trauma, preterm premature rupture of membranes, smoking, cocaine abuse, and prior history of abruption.

- The fetal and neonatal mortality associated with vasa previa exceeds 50%.

Antepartum hemorrhage, or third-trimester bleeding, is an important obstetric complication, occurring in up to 4% of pregnancies. Approximately 30% of cases are caused by placental abruption, and another 20% can be attributed to placenta previa[1] (Table 14-1).

TABLE 14-1
CAUSES OF ANTEPARTUM HEMORRHAGE

Life-threatening
  Placental abruption
  Placenta previa
  Trauma
  Uterine rupture
Other
  Labor
  Infection
    Cervicitis
    Vaginitis
  Malignancy
  Vasa previa

The remaining 50% are either unexplained or result from cervical dilatation accompanying labor or lesions in the cervix or vagina. Thus, about half of the women who present with antepartum bleeding may have a potentially life-threatening cause, and, while the maternal mortality rate from obstetrical hemorrhage has fallen in recent years, hemorrhage remains a leading cause of maternal death. It is, therefore, incumbent on the physician evaluating any pregnant woman with antepartum bleeding to diagnose a life-threatening cause and anticipate emergency measures needed for the care of both mother and fetus.

PLACENTA PREVIA

Definition

Placenta previa is defined as placental implantation over the cervical os. Previas can be classified by the extent to which the cervical os is covered (Figure 14-1). In

Figure 14-1 Types of placenta previa.
T: = total; P: = partial; M: = marginal;
L: = low-lying.

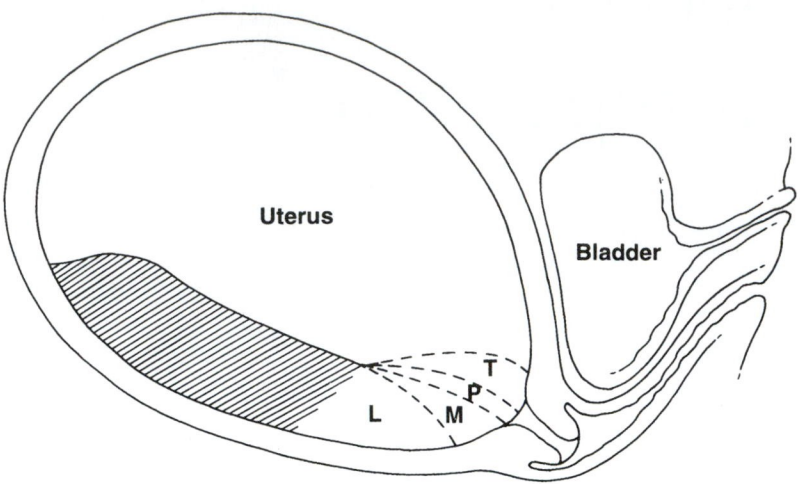

total or complete previa, the cervical os is covered completely by the placenta. If the placenta is centered over the cervix, it is known as a central previa. When the cervical os is only partially covered by the edge of the placenta, a partial previa occurs. A marginal placenta previa is present when the placental edge extends to the internal os but does not cover it. While not technically categorized as a placenta previa, a low-lying placenta is one that extends near the cervix but does not encroach on the internal os. A low-lying placenta may be difficult to distinguish from a marginal placenta previa and can also be a cause of antepartum bleeding, although usually not major hemorrhage with significant complications.

Incidence

The incidence of placenta previa is about 1 in 200 to 1 in 250 births.[2] Approximately one-third of diagnosed cases are partial previas, while the reported frequency of total placenta previa varies from 20 to 43%.[2,3] The diagnosis of previa at delivery is much less common than earlier in gestation. During the second trimester, placenta previa is present on ultrasound examination in 5 to 15% of pregnancies.[3] Ninety percent of these will resolve by term.[4] Resolution is somewhat dependent on the type of previa diagnosed; a total previa will remain into the third trimester in 26% of patients, while a partial previa persists in only one-tenth as many patients.[5] However, if placenta previa is diagnosed or persists after 30 weeks of gestation, a previa is more likely to be present at delivery.[6] While the probability that a previa will disappear by the third trimester is high in asymptomatic

patients, previas associated with bleeding are less likely to resolve.

Historically, the process of resolution of low-lying placentas and placenta previas has been attributed to "placental migration." A more plausible explanation is the combination of differential growth of the lower uterine segment and villous atrophy of placental tissue near the cervical edge. However, pregnancies complicated by a diagnosis of placenta previa in the second trimester that later resolve remain at increased risk for preterm delivery, intrauterine growth restriction, and placental abruption.[7]

Risk Factors

Both advanced maternal age and multiparity are associated with an increased risk of placenta previa; whether these factors are independent remains unclear.[2,3,8] Additional factors include smoking, which doubles the risk,[9] and previous induced or spontaneous abortion, which increases the risk by 30%[10] (Table 14-2).

The single most important risk factor for placenta previa is previous cesarean delivery. The incidence of placenta previa increases linearly with the number of

TABLE 14-2 RISK FACTORS FOR PLACENTA PREVIA
Prior cesarean delivery
Smoking
Previous spontaneous or induced abortion
Advanced maternal age
Multiparity

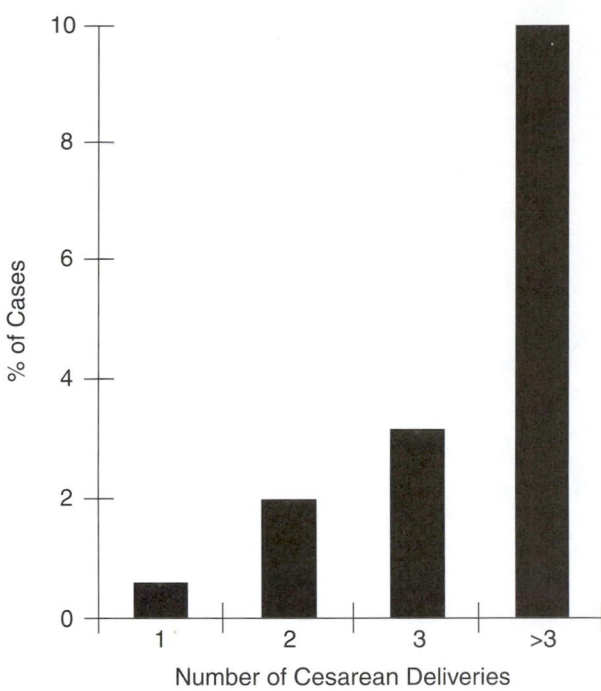

Figure 14-2 The incidence of placenta previa in women with previous cesarean delivery.

previous cesarean deliveries, rising from less than 1% with one, to 10% with four or more[8] (Figure 14-2). One hypothesis for this relationship is the failure of scar tissue in the lower uterine segment to support differential growth, not allowing the "migration" of a placenta that has implanted near the cervix in early gestation. In this setting, many of the placenta previas noted in the second trimester would not resolve.

Diagnosis

Placenta previa presents classically with painless vaginal bleeding. Bleeding results from detachment of placental tissue as the lower uterine segment lengthens and the subsequent inability of the lower segment to contract and constrict vessels to stop the bleeding. While 70% of women with placenta previa will present with painless bleeding, 20% will have uterine contractions as well. The other 10% will be diagnosed by incidental ultrasound or at the time of cesarean delivery.[11]

The first episode of bleeding occurs before 30 weeks of gestation in about one-third of the patients, and another third will not bleed until after 36 weeks, with the peak incidence for the first episode around 34 weeks.[12] A marginal, partial, or low-lying placenta may not cause bleeding until the onset of labor at term. The initial bleeding episode usually resolves spontaneously and is rarely fatal. A characteristic pattern of intermittent bleeding usually develops.

Ultrasound examination provides the most accurate diagnosis of placenta previa (Figure 14-3). Traditionally, obstetricians have relied on transabdominal ultrasound, which has a reported accuracy of greater than 90%.[13,14] However, the false positive rate is about 5%.[3,14] The most common cause for a false positive diagnosis is an overdistended bladder, which lengthens the appearance of the cervix and compresses the anterior uterine wall against the posterior wall (Figure 14-4). Other causes of false positive diagnoses

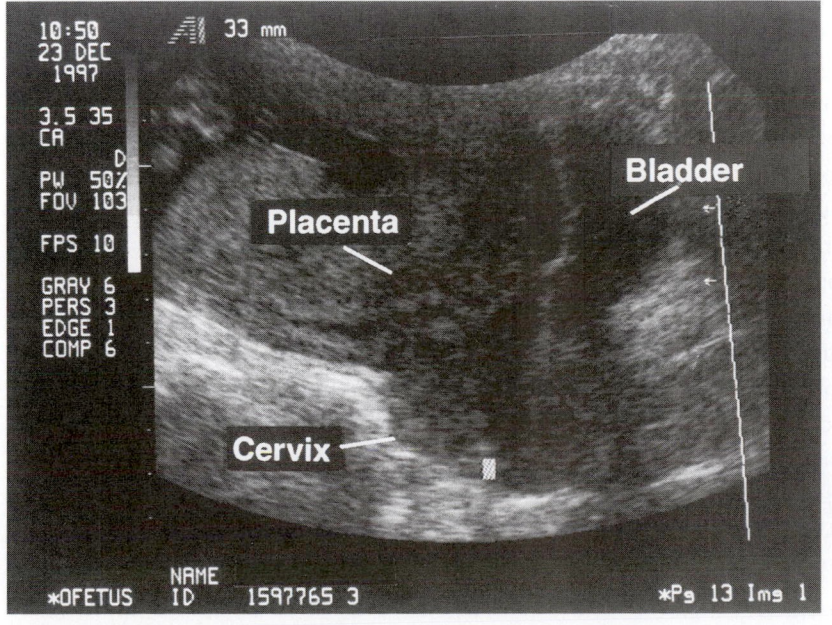

Figure 14-3 Transabdominal ultrasound of placenta previa. *Courtesy of Brenda Griffin, R.D.M.S., Grady Perinatal Center, Atlanta.*

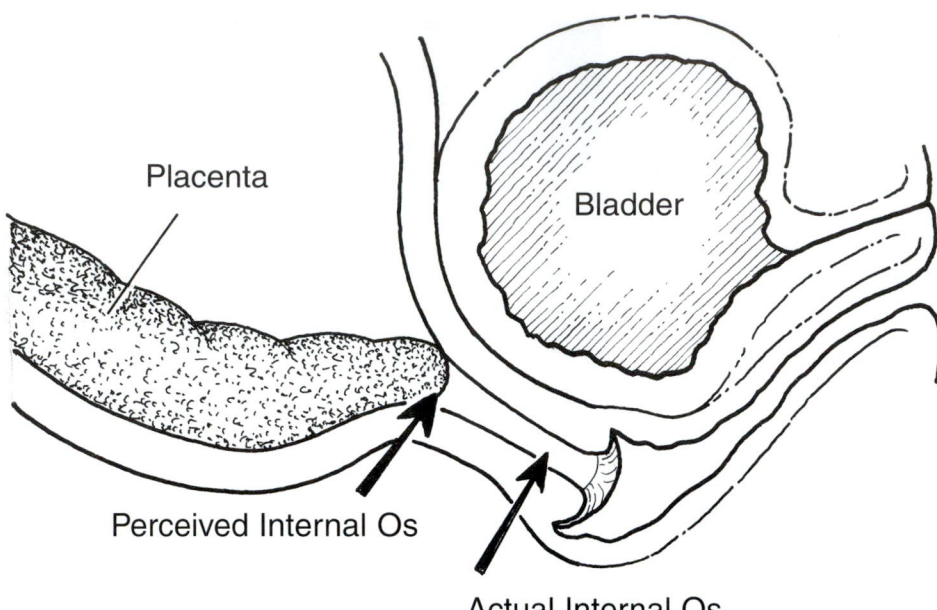

Figure 14-4 False positive diagnosis of placenta previa with an overdistended bladder. The cervix appears longer and the actual internal os is inferior to the perceived cervical os.

include a uterine contraction or fibroid that pushes an anterior placenta against the posterior wall, a posterior placenta that obscures visualization of the cervical os, and a blood clot in the lower uterine segment.

The false negative rate for transabdominal ultrasound diagnosis of previa is about 7% but may be as high as 20%.[3,14,15] False negative diagnoses are more likely due to shadowing of the cervix by the fetal head, particularly in the late third trimester, or a posterior placenta that obscures the os.

Despite several studies demonstrating the safety of the transvaginal approach,[15-18] many physicians consider transvaginal ultrasound contraindicated in the evaluation of antepartum bleeding. Transvaginal ultrasound has much higher sensitivity and specificity than the transabdominal approach. In a comparison of transabdominal and transvaginal ultrasound diagnosis of placenta previa, Farine et al. found that the positive predictive value for transabdominal ultrasound was 38%, as compared with 71% for transvaginal; the negative predictive values were 80% and 100%, respectively.[15] The transabdominal approach failed to diagnose previa in 5 cases, while 22 cases without previa, considered positive by the transabdominal scan, were correctly diagnosed transvaginally. Transvaginal examination failed to identify 10 cases, which were also missed transabdominally; all were marginal previas.

Many physicians fear that the vaginal probe may be inadvertently inserted through the cervix and into the placenta previa, causing hemorrhage. Timor-Tritsch and Yunis have shown that the minimum and mean angles between the vaginal transducer and the axis of the cervix are 44 and 63.8 degrees, respectively.[18] Since the vaginal probe is straight and inflexible, it is physically impossible to insert the probe into the cervical canal unless the two are aligned. Because the transducer is both straight and rigid, it cannot be compared to a finger, which can be manipulated into almost any angle and clearly has a much smaller diameter than a vaginal probe. In addition, the probe should be inserted under direct visualization, which allows evaluation of the anatomy. The focal length for a 6.5- to 7.5-MHz transducer is 2 to 3 cm; any closer to the cervix would yield an unfocused, blurry image.

For those who remain wary of the safety of transvaginal ultrasound, the translabial or transperineal approach is a useful alternative[19] (Figure 14-5). In a study of patients in the third trimester with either an inconclusive examination or the diagnosis of placenta previa by transabdominal ultrasound, transperineal ultrasound was able to successfully visualize the cervix relative to the placenta in all patients as well as to correctly exclude placenta previa in all inconclusive diagnoses and correctly identify 9 of 10 previas. The

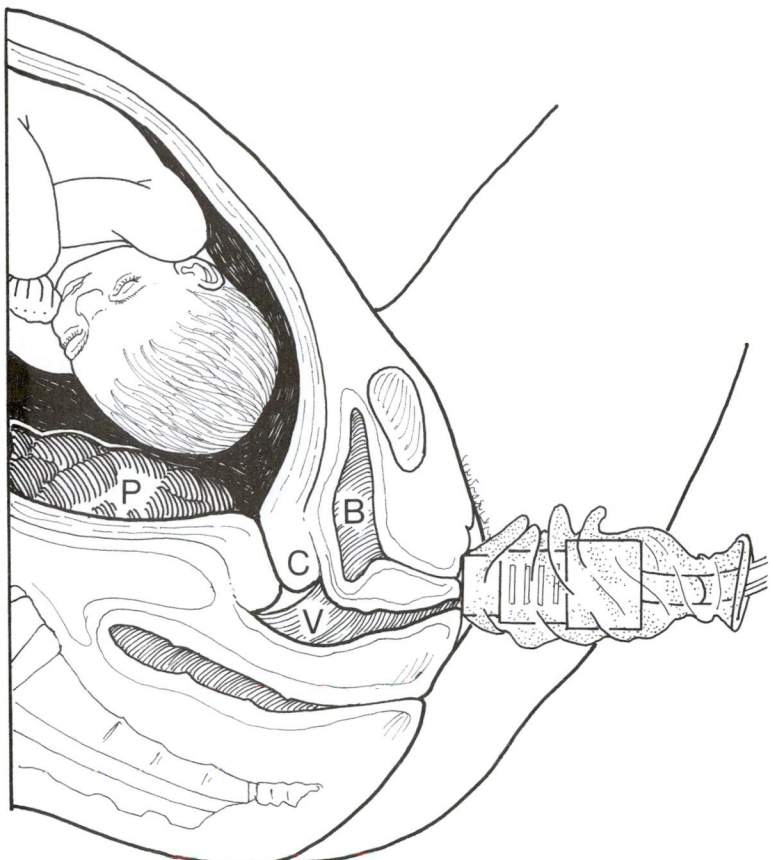

Figure 14-5 The technique for translabial or transperineal ultrasound. The probe is placed on the anterior labia. H = fetal head; P= placenta; C = cervix; B = bladder; V = vagina.

10th case was a marginal placenta previa; the infant delivered vaginally and the original diagnosis was not confirmed. To perform transperineal ultrasound, a curvilinear abdominal transducer is placed on the anterior labia (Figures 14-5 and 14-6).

Complications

Any one of the variations of placenta accreta has an important association with placenta previa. Placenta accreta is defined as an abnormally adherent placenta

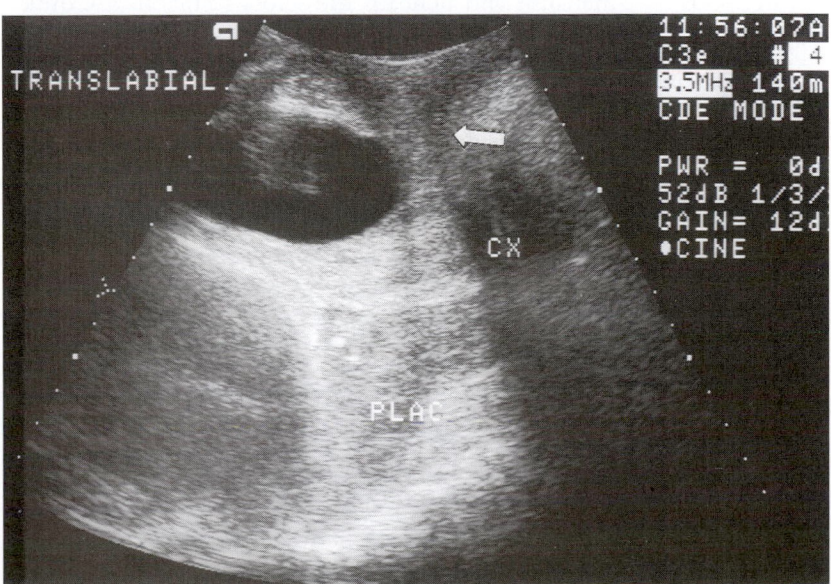

Fig 14-6 Transperineal image of placenta previa. The vagina is oriented vertically (arrow), while the cervix is oriented horizontally. CX = cervix; PLAC = placenta. *Courtesy of Laura Gray-Sorton, R.D.M.S., Grady Perinatal Center, Atlanta.*

that is directly attached to the myometrium because of inadequate development of the fibrinoid layer (Nitabuch layer) and the absence of the decidua basalis. In placenta increta, the placenta actually invades the myometrium. In placenta percreta, placental tissue penetrates the myometrium and may even pierce the serosa. Accreta/increta/percreta may be classified as total, involving all of the placenta; partial, involving several cotyledons; or focal, involving only one cotyledon. The incidence of placenta accreta in women with placenta previa is 5%.[8] Conversely, the reported incidence of placenta previa in all patients with placenta accreta varies from 34 to 64%,[20,21] and 43 to 60% of patients with accreta have a uterus previously scarred by cesarean delivery.[8,20]

The presence of a uterine scar from a prior cesarean delivery significantly increases the risk of accreta, and the proportion increases linearly with the number of cesarean deliveries.[8] The incidence of accreta in women with placenta previa and one prior cesarean is 24%; for women with a previa and four or more cesareans, it is 67% (Figure 14-7).[8] In view of the high cesarean delivery rate over the past three decades, this statistic is alarming. The incidence of placenta accreta combined with previa has risen from 2 per 1000 in 1952 to 101 per 1000 in 1985.[8]

Several studies in the '90s found the overall incidence of placenta previa accreta to range from 10 to 25%.[22-24] However, in women with prior cesareans, the incidence is almost 40%.[22,23]

While placenta accreta has been diagnosed on antenatal ultrasound, prenatal diagnosis is uncommon.[25,26] Ultrasound findings are often subtle and not easily identified without careful investigation. Thinning or absence of the sonolucent myometrial area between the placenta and the hyperechoic interface of the uterine serosa and the posterior bladder wall is characteristic. An additional finding is a thinned, distorted, or broken uterovesical interface found in placenta percreta. One ultrasound series was able to correctly identify all placenta percretas, but falsely diagnosed accreta in 4 of 16 cases. Two of these false positive diagnoses were uterine scar dehiscences with placental tissue visible through the opening at cesarean delivery.[26]

ABRUPTIO PLACENTAE

Definition

Abruptio placentae, or placental abruption, is the premature separation of a normally implanted placenta from the uterus. Typically, the process of abruption begins with bleeding from arterial vessels in the basal layer of the decidua. The decidua is split by this hemorrhage, leaving only a thin layer attached to the placenta. As the hematoma expands, it compresses and ultimately destroys placental tissue. The identification of a clot with a depression in the maternal surface of the placenta following delivery confirms the diagnosis of abruption. The process may be self-limited or may continue, with the blood going in any of several directions. Extravasation of blood into the myometrium and beneath the serosa results in a Couvelaire uterus, which has a bluish, dark red, or purplish cast. Once the blood reaches the edge of the placenta, it can pass through the membranes into the amniotic cavity, creating "port wine" fluid that is pathognomonic of abruption. Blood can also remain trapped between the placenta and the uterine wall; this is known as a concealed abruption. Finally, blood may become trapped between the decidua and membranes and eventually pass through the cervix into the vagina. Since blood may be lost in any one of several areas, maternal blood loss may be far in excess of that appreciated by the amount of vaginal bleeding observed.

Placental abruption can be localized to three sites: retroplacental, between the placenta and the myometrium; preplacental, between the placenta and amniotic fluid; and subchorionic, between the placenta

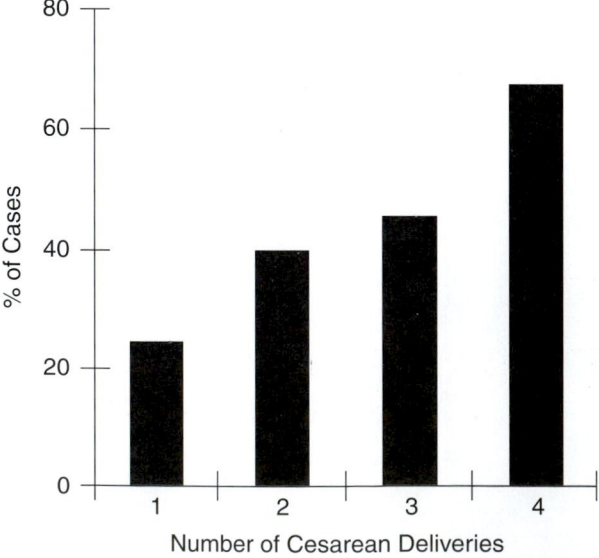

Figure 14-7 The incidence of placenta accreta in women with placenta previa and previous cesarean delivery.

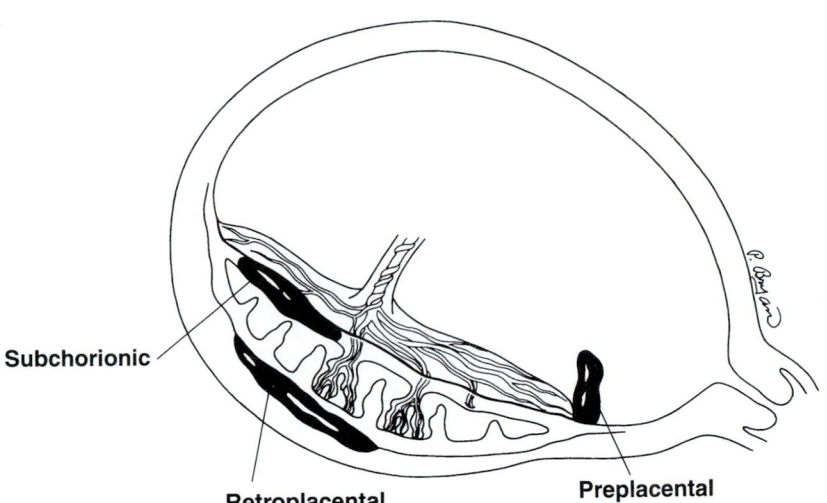

Fig 14-8 Sites of placental abruption hematoma formation.

and the membranes (Fig 14-8). Retroplacental hematomas have the worst prognosis for fetal survival; a clot larger than 50% is associated with a 50% fetal mortality. By comparison, the fetal mortality is 10% with a subchorionic bleed of similar volume.[27]

The severity of an abruption can be classified into three grades (Table 14-3). Grade 1 is characterized by minimal vaginal bleeding and uterine irritability. Maternal blood pressure, serum fibrinogen level, and fetal heart rate patterns are all normal. In Grade 2, bleeding is mild to moderate. Uterine contractions are present and some may be tetanic; the uterus may be tender. While supine maternal blood pressure is normal, maternal tachycardia occurs and postural blood pressure changes may be detected. Serum fibrinogen levels are usually between 150 and 250 mg/dl. Nonreassuring fetal heart rate tracings suggesting fetal distress are seen. With Grade 3, bleeding is moderate to severe, tetanic contractions are present and the uterus is very tender. Maternal hypotension is present and fetal death has occurred. Maternal fibrinogen is lower than 150 mg/dl and may be accompanied by thrombocytopenia and coagulation abnormalities.

Pathologic examination of placentas from pregnancies complicated by abruption demonstrates vascular abnormalities. Sixty percent have inadequate physiologic transformation of the spiral arteries; 33% have vascular occlusion of myometrial arteries with surrounding hemorrhage.[28] These findings are similar to those seen in preeclampsia and some cases of preterm delivery, both of which are associated with placental separation.

Incidence

Because of variation in diagnostic criteria, the incidence of abruption varies from 1 in 75 to 1 in 225 deliveries.[29-31] Some of this variation may also be accounted for by differences in studied populations. A Swedish study reported a 1 in 225 incidence, while a study from the University of Tennessee found an incidence of 1 in 90.[30,31] Grade 3 abruption accounts for 15% of cases; the remaining cases are about equally divided between Grade 1 and Grade 2. About 15% of abruptions result in fetal death, with another 15% causing neonatal death.[29]

TABLE 14-3
CLASSIFICATION OF PLACENTAL ABRUPTION

Grade	Bleeding	Contractions	Blood Pressure	Heart Rate	Fibrinogen, mg/dl	Fetal Heart Rate
1	Minimal	Minimal	Normal	Normal	Normal	Normal
2	Mild to moderate	Sometimes tetanic	Normal	Increased	150–250	Decelerations
3	Moderate to severe; may be concealed	Tetanic	Decreased	Increased	<150	Intrauterine fetal death

Risk Factors

The most common risk factor for the development of placental abruption is hypertension, both chronic and pregnancy-induced (Table 14-4). Women with preeclampsia are 1.9 times more likely to have an abruption than normotensive women; women with chronic hypertension are 3.1 times more likely.[34] The risk is particularly high with Grade 3 abruption. Almost 50% of abruptions associated with fetal death are in mothers with hypertensive disorders, equally divided between chronic hypertension and preeclampsia/eclampsia.[33] Preeclampsia is associated with 14% of mild and 25% of moderate abruptions.[34] This relationship is probably the result of the vascular placental disease present in both categories of hypertensive disease.

Blunt maternal trauma represents an increasingly important cause of placental abruption. Motor vehicle accidents now account for 36% of maternal deaths in this country, helping to make trauma the leading nonobstetric cause of maternal death.[35] One in 12 pregnancies is complicated by physical trauma.[36] Abruption may develop in as many as half of the patients with major trauma injuries.[37] In automobile accidents, lap seatbelts can cause a shearing effect from alterations in uterine shape. These changes in shape occur with rapid forward propulsion and recoil from vehicle deceleration and impact. The placenta is unable to conform to changes in uterine shape and position, resulting in placental separation.[38]

With the increasing public awareness of domestic violence, physical assault is another major contributor to trauma. One study of pregnant women in the inner city found 1 in 12 women was a victim of battery.[39] Physical abuse is not confined to any socioeconomic setting and the reported incidence varies from 4 to

---

TABLE 14-4
RISK FACTORS FOR PLACENTAL ABRUPTION

Hypertension, chronic and pregnancy-induced
Trauma
Substance abuse
  Tobacco
  Cocaine
Previous abruption
Overdistended uterus
  Multiple gestation
  Polyhydramnios
Preterm rupture of membranes

17% in a study involving both urban and rural sites.[40] Even with apparently minor injuries, placental separation will occur in up to 6% of victims.[41,42] The prevalence of abuse emphasizes the importance of questioning patients with antepartum bleeding about possible physical abuse, even in the absence of physical signs.

Preterm rupture of membranes has been reported to increase the incidence of abruption within 24 hours of rupture. The incidence is about 6%.[43,44] A meta-analysis found a pooled odds ratio of 3.05 for abruption after premature rupture of membranes.[32] Rapid decompression of polyhydramnios, either by membrane rupture or amniocentesis, has also been associated with abruption. In the case of twins, abruption may follow the delivery of the first twin with rapid delivery of the second twin. In this setting, a retroplacental hematoma may not have time to form, complicating the ability to make the diagnosis. The actual incidence of abruption in twin gestations is difficult to determine.

Smoking has also been linked to an increased incidence of abruptio placentae.[45,46] One study attributed as many as 40% of cases to cigarette abuse.[45] Abruption may be related to placental vascular changes that result from the vasoconstrictive effects of nicotine.

Cocaine abuse is another risk factor for abruptio placentae; reported odds ratios vary from 1.5 to 9.8.[47,48] This heightened risk seems to be independent of adequacy of prenatal care and other substance abuse.[48] Although placental pathology has not demonstrated consistent abnormalities associated with use of this drug, the hypothetical mechanism for the elevated risk is cocaine-induced vasoconstriction and vascular damage.

Once a woman has had an abruptio placentae, she has a significantly increased risk of recurrence. The reported incidence of recurrence varies from 5 to 17%, 30 times the risk for the general population.[1,31-33] After two abruptions, the recurrence risk is 25%. Not uncommonly, women who have suffered a fetal death with abruption will have another catastrophic abruption; 30% of subsequent pregnancies will result in a stillbirth.[1] As yet, there appears to be no obstetrical intervention that can consistently prevent this unfortunate outcome. Many of these women will have an uneventful antepartum course with normal antepartum fetal testing within 24 hours of an abruption.[49]

Earlier studies have suggested an association between placental abruption, advanced maternal age, and parity. Two large studies have challenged these findings and found no relationship between these factors and abruptio placentae.[50,51]

Diagnosis

The classic presenting symptoms of abruption are vaginal bleeding, uterine tenderness, and painful, tetanic uterine contractions. While 80% of patients will present with vaginal bleeding, the remainder have concealed abruption and show no evidence of vaginal bleeding. About two-thirds of patients will have uterine tenderness or back pain. The tenderness may be localized to the area of placental detachment or generalized over the uterus. Back pain may be associated with a posterior placenta. Frequent uterine contractions or uterine hypertonus are seen in about one-third of cases[29] (Figure 14-9). Importantly, with minimal or absent vaginal bleeding, women may be misdiagnosed with preterm labor. This error may result in fetal death, serious maternal blood loss, and coagulopathy.

When abruption is suspected to result from trauma, bleeding may be absent and the abruption is more likely to be concealed. In this setting, however, placental separation is usually associated with frequent contractions and often accompanied by a nonreassuring fetal heart rate tracing. Twenty percent of trauma patients with contractions separated by 10 minutes or less were found to have abruption.[42] Symptoms of abruption usually develop within 4 hours of the traumatic event.

Traditional teaching has held that ultrasonography is not useful in the diagnosis of abruption. Only 24% of cases of confirmed placental abruption were identified sonographically in one study.[52] However, technologic advances in ultrasound imaging have improved the diagnostic accuracy for abruption to about 50%.[53] Still, while ultrasound may be helpful in identifying abruption, a negative sonographic examination cannot rule it out. For the patient with antepartum hemorrhage without evidence of placenta previa, placental abruption must remain high in the index of suspicion.

Difficulty in sonographic diagnosis of abruption is related to the evolution of the bleeding process itself. Acute hemorrhage will appear either hyperechoic or isoechoic with the placenta; frequently, this appears on ultrasound as a thickened placenta. Sometimes, an ill-defined retroplacental collection may be seen.[54] A preplacental hematoma, however, may be visualized floating in the amniotic fluid while attached to the placenta. During the resolution of the hematoma, it will appear more hypoechoic within 1 week and then sonolucent by the following week.[55] This changing image may be confused with a myoma, chorioangioma, or an accessory lobe of placenta. A clot that extends down to the cervical os may be misinterpreted as a placenta previa.

Gestational age at diagnosis has important implications for prognosis. Subchorionic or retroplacental

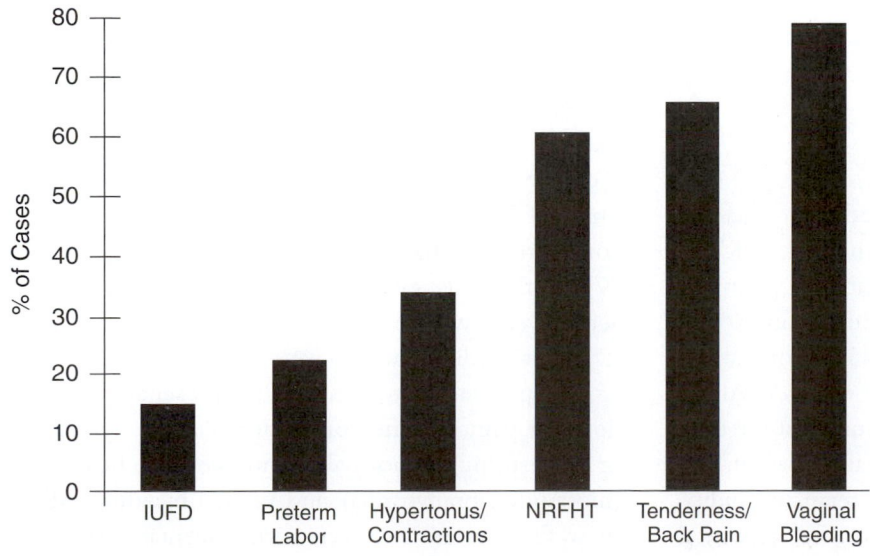

Figure 14-9 The occurrence of signs and symptoms associated with placental abruption.[29] IUFD = intrauterine fetal death; NRFHT = nonreassuring fetal heart tracing.

hematomas are common findings on ultrasound examinations performed in the second trimester. If the bleeding is seen prior to 20 weeks, 82% of patients will deliver at term. However, if bleeding occurs after 20 weeks, the percentage of patients who deliver at term is reduced to 27%.[53] Occasionally, chronic abruption may develop and patients may experience recurrent episodes of bleeding, often accompanied by uterine contractions.

Complications

Placental abruption associated with intrauterine fetal death is complicated by disseminated intravascular coagulopathy (DIC) in about 30% of women. DIC is less common with less severe degrees of abruption.[56,57] DIC is also a more common complication in abruption associated with trauma; coagulopathy occurs twice as often as in nontraumatic abruption.[58] Since maternal fibrinogen concentrations are normal in Grade 1 abruptions, DIC does not develop in these patients. The development of DIC is the result of thromboplastin released from the site of placental injury initiating intravascular activation of the extrinsic clotting cascade, eventually depleting platelets, factor V, and factor VIII. Fibrinogen is converted to fibrin, causing fibrinogen levels to decline and fibrin degradation products to rise. While hypofibrinogemia is the most sensitive indicator of abruption-associated DIC, other laboratory abnormalities include elevated fibrin degradation products, D-dimers and thrombocytopenia.

Acute renal failure is an infrequent complication of abruptio placentae, usually the result of maternal hypovolemia. Acute tubular necrosis develops in the majority of affected patients, although acute cortical necrosis has been reported.[59]

Neonatal Outcome

The perinatal mortality rate associated with placental abruption has been reported to be as high as 30%.[60,61] The principal causes of perinatal death are prematurity, fetal hemorrhage, and anoxia. More than 20% of abruptions present before 28 weeks and a comparable number present between 28 and 30 weeks.[62] About half of the stillbirths have already occurred at the time of admission to the hospital. Neonates that survive appear to have a high rate of long-term morbidity. Fourteen percent of neonates born after placental

abruption had significant neurologic deficits in their first year in one study.[30] Another study found an association between abruption and cerebral palsy in low-birth-weight infants.[63] A trend toward worsening neonatal outcome with increasing severity of abruption, although not statistically significant due to small sample size, was also observed.

A higher incidence of small-for-gestational-age neonates has been noted in pregnancies complicated by placental abruption. Hibbard and Jeffcoate reported that 81% of neonates born before 36 weeks following abruption were less than the mean birth weight for gestational age.[1] Whether this observation is independent of other risk factors for abruption, such as smoking, substance abuse, and hypertension, all of which are associated with fetal growth restriction, remains unclear.

UTERINE RUPTURE

While uterine rupture is generally considered an intrapartum event, it should be considered in the differential diagnosis of antepartum bleeding, particularly when associated with preterm labor or uterine contractions. The high rate of cesarean delivery has significantly increased the number of women who are at risk for uterine rupture, even though this complication is rare. When rupture is defined as a uterine scar separation associated with hemorrhage and/or fetal distress, the reported incidence is 0.5 to 0.8%.[64-66] Uterine rupture occurs somewhat more often with two or more prior cesareans, for which the incidence is 1.1 to 1.8%.[64,67] Although the vast majority of cesarean deliveries in recent obstetrical practice are performed through low transverse incisions, vertical or classical incisions are still used in some situations, such as preterm malpresentations, multiple gestations, and emergency deliveries. Classical incisions are more likely to rupture, with an incidence as high as 12%.[68] Rupture of classical incisions can occur prior to the onset of labor in one-third of patients, and not uncommonly will happen several weeks prior to term.[69] When clinically evident, these ruptures are usually acute events with significant associated fetal and maternal morbidity.

Symptomatic uterine rupture presents with abdominal pain, uterine contractions (either hypotonic or hypertonic), abnormalities in the fetal heart rate (most often bradycardia), and vaginal bleeding. All of these findings are also seen with placental abruption.

However, with rupture, vaginal bleeding is not the most common sign. In two series of catastrophic rupture, vaginal bleeding was present in 2 of 8 and 4 of 12 women.[70,71] The most common findings with uterine rupture were abnormal fetal heart patterns and abdominal pain.

VASA PREVIA

Vasa previa is an extremely rare cause of antepartum hemorrhage and is the only instance of fetal rather than maternal hemorrhage discussed in this chapter. With a vasa previa, there is a velamentous insertion of the cord, and the fetal vessels cross the membranes without the protection of Wharton's jelly. The vessels lie below the presenting fetal part and frequently traverse the cervical os. The incidence of vasa previa is 1 in 3000 pregnancies.

In the presence of vasa previa, rupture of membranes causes rupture of the fetal vessels, resulting in acute vaginal bleeding and an associated abrupt change in the fetal heart rate pattern. Usually, the initial fetal heart response will be tachycardia, followed by bradycardia. A high index of suspicion is crucial for the diagnosis; rapid diagnosis and immediate delivery are imperative to avoid fetal death. Since the fetal blood volume is small, even a small amount of vaginal bleeding can cause significant fetal anemia and even exsanguination. Fetal mortality exceeds 50%.[72] Additional neonatal morbidity may result from vessel compression from the presenting part, compromising fetal oxygenation.

Prenatal diagnosis of vasa previa has been reported.[73-75] Color Doppler has been a useful adjunct in the visualization of blood vessels crossing the cervical os and the actual site of cord insertion. Patients at risk are those with low-lying placenta, placenta previa, velamentous-cord insertion, and succenturiate lobes. Prenatal diagnosis of vasa previa should prompt the decision to deliver by scheduled cesarean.

In some instances, the vessels may be palpated on cervical examination or visualized on speculum examination. The Apt test is helpful in diagnosing the fetal origin of vaginal bleeding. The test is based on the susceptibility of adult oxyhemoglobin to alkali, which produces globin hematin with a brownish-yellow color. To perform the Apt test, one part of vaginal fluid is mixed with 5 to 10 parts of water. The tube is centrifuged for 2 minutes. If the supernatant is pink, 5 parts of supernatant are mixed with 1 part of 0.25 N (1%) sodium hydroxide. This mixture is then centrifuged for 2 minutes. Fetal blood will produce a pink color, while maternal blood will be a brownish-yellow. Although the Apt test is simple and rapid, the reagents frequently are not available in modern labor and delivery suites. Other tests that may be helpful are examination of a Wright stain of the bloody fluid for nucleated red cells, which are normally present in fetal blood but rare in maternal blood.

MANAGEMENT OF ANTEPARTUM HEMORRHAGE

Blood Loss and Volume Changes

Any pregnant women who presents with antepartum bleeding at 24 weeks or more of gestation should be quickly evaluated for the amount and source of blood loss. Blood loss may be considerably higher than is initially apparent, for a number of reasons. First, obstetricians usually underestimate blood loss. Second, bleeding, in the case of abruption, may be concealed in several intrauterine sites. Third, hypertensive disease may accompany bleeding, and an apparently normotensive patient may become hypertensive with fluid resuscitation. Most importantly, the normal physiologic cardiovascular adaptations of pregnancy alter maternal response to blood loss and hypovolemia, obscuring signs that are apparent in the nonpregnant patient. Understanding these changes is important in the assessment of maternal volume status.

Maternal blood volume increases significantly during the first and second trimesters and, by the end of the second trimester, it is 1000 to 2000 ml higher than the prepregnant blood volume. In the average 135-lb patient, blood volume is about 6 liters at 30 weeks. Maternal cardiac output increases by 40 to 45% and total peripheral resistance falls to its nadir in the second trimester. These physiologic changes help prepare the gravida for an anticipated blood loss at uncomplicated vaginal delivery of 500 ml. Clearly, most women delivered by cesarean, in which true blood loss is about 1000 ml, can tolerate a larger deficit without signs of volume depletion.

A brief review of the normal physiologic response to hemorrhage is helpful in this context as well. When 1 liter of blood is rapidly lost, vasoconstriction of both the arterial and venous circulation acts to redistribute blood flow to essential organs. After about 4 hours, interstitial fluid is shunted into the intravascular space in an attempt to replace lost blood volume. This fluid shift can replace as much as 30% of that lost with hemorrhage.

Since a pregnant woman can physiologically adapt to considerable blood loss, it is not until she has lost 1200 to 1500 ml, or 20 to 25% of the total blood volume, that physical signs of hypovolemia will appear. Tachycardia is usually the first response, often accompanied by postural blood pressure changes. These signs correlate with those seen in a Grade 2 abruption. Once blood loss reaches 2000 ml, or about 30% of blood volume, patients will show frank hypotension, as in Grade 3 abruption.

While hemoglobin and hematocrit are the usual laboratory parameters used to estimate blood loss, they may not reflect the current status. With acute bleeding, the hematocrit may not change for at least 4 hours. Conversely, administration of large amounts of intravenous fluids may significantly lower the hematocrit.

General Measures

Evaluation of the patient with antepartum bleeding should begin with the placement of a large-bore (16-gauge) intravenous catheter and rapid infusion of crystalloid solution (Table 14-5). Blood should be drawn for hemoglobin, hematocrit, platelet count, fibrinogen, fibrin-degradation products, prothrombin time, partial thromboplastin time, and type and cross match for at least 4 units of blood. Also, a Kleihauer–

TABLE 14-5
MANAGEMENT OF ANTEPARTUM HEMORRHAGE: GENERAL MEASURES

16-gauge intravenous line
Rapid infusion of crystalloid solution
Type and cross for 4 units of packed red cells
Laboratory
  Hemoglobin and hematocrit
  Fibrinogen
  Platelet count
  Prothrombin time/partial thromboplastin time
  "Clotting tube"
  Kleihauer–Betke for Rh-negative unsensitized patients
Continuous electronic fetal monitoring
Ultrasound
  Previa
  Abruption
  Placental location
  Fetal presentation
Notify anesthesia department

Betke test should be ordered for Rh-negative women. An additional red-top tube should be drawn for the "clot test," which may be useful to estimate fibrinogen levels before laboratory information is available. If no clot forms in 6 minutes, or if a clot forms and dissolves in 30 minutes, then fibrinogen levels are below 150 mg/dl and a coagulation defect is present.

Continuous fetal monitoring to evaluate fetal heart rate patterns and uterine activity should be started as soon as possible. Ultrasound examination should be performed to identify placenta previa or abruption. Fetal presentation and the position of the placenta should also be noted at the time of ultrasound examination. For patients of unknown gestational age, a femur length measurement may be a quick and helpful guide. If previa can be excluded, speculum examination should be performed to confirm that blood is coming from above the cervical os and to inspect the cervix for dilation.

Placenta Previa

If previa is suspected but not confirmed by transabdominal ultrasound, the transvaginal or transperineal approach should be used. If the diagnosis is still in doubt, the presentation is vertex, hemorrhage is not life-threatening, and delivery is anticipated, the double-setup examination may be useful. The double setup should be performed in an operating room that is prepared for an immediate cesarean delivery. A gentle speculum examination may demonstrate placental tissue in the cervical os. Otherwise, the obstetrician should proceed to digital palpation of the vaginal fornices, using ultrasound information to guide palpation to the most likely areas. If the head is palpable throughout the lower segment, then vaginal delivery may be feasible. If, however, the fornices feel full or boggy, previa is likely. Finally, if the other elements of the examination are not conclusive, the fingers may be carefully introduced into the cervical os. If hemorrhage occurs, the obstetrician should proceed immediately to cesarean delivery.

If placenta previa is confirmed by sonography and the patient is at term, she should be delivered by cesarean if the previa is complete. Patients at 34 to 36 weeks of gestation also should be considered for delivery if fetal lung maturity is confirmed. Patients at less than 34 weeks of gestation should, in general, be managed expectantly, awaiting the development of fetal lung maturity.[76-79]

For patients between 24 and 34 weeks of gestation with stable fetal heart rate patterns, expectant management is the preferred strategy. Maternal blood loss should be replaced as needed to maintain a hematocrit of 30 to 35%, providing a safe margin against a large hemorrhage and optimizing fetal oxygen supply. Blood should be available at all times in anticipation of the need for transfusion. Even in the face of a large hemorrhage, maternal and neonatal outcomes have been good with expectant management. However, 20% of women managed expectantly still deliver by 32 weeks.[3]

Corticosteroids should be administered, not only to enhance fetal lung maturity, but also to decrease the incidence of intraventricular hemorrhage and necrotizing enterocolitis, important complications seen in very preterm neonates.[79] Controversy remains about the use of multiple weekly doses of steroids during a prolonged course; currently, there are few data on the safety and efficacy of use.

Since about 20% of patients with placenta previa present with uterine contractions; some patients may be considered for tocolysis. Magnesium sulfate is the usual agent of choice. Betamimetics such as ritodrine or terbutaline may cause maternal hypotension in the face of maternal hypovolemia. Betamimetics also cause maternal and fetal tachycardia, which may complicate assessment of maternal and fetal status. Some patients may require long-term intravenous tocolysis and experience either recurrent contractions or bleeding with attempts to wean the magnesium sulfate. Even intravenous tocolysis over several weeks has been well tolerated.

Another controversial issue involves hospitalization for bed rest as opposed to outpatient management. Initially, one study suggested that hospitalization was cost effective if the total costs of maternal and neonatal hospitalization were considered.[80] Later studies challenged this finding.[81,82] The recent emphasis on decreasing health care costs has tended to favor outpatient management. However, a number of factors have a bearing on management decisions. Initial hospitalization of at least 72 hours is advisable since almost one-third of candidates for delayed delivery will need to be delivered in that time interval. In addition, 50% of the patients in whom expectant management fails require delivery because of excessive bleeding with or without contractions.[3] At our institution, we consider factors such as the availability of support to ensure compliance with bed rest at home, the availability of transportation, and distance from the hospital. Since we care for a primarily indigent patient population, the vast majority of our patients are hospitalized until delivery.

Amniocentesis to confirm fetal lung maturity after 35 weeks should be performed and delivery by cesarean planned. One-quarter to one-third of expectantly managed gestations will achieve 36 weeks of gestation. Since newborns born by emergency cesarean tend to be more anemic than those born after elective section, optimal management is scheduled cesarean before the onset of labor or during an incidence of recurrent bleeding.[3]

The fact that fetal blood loss may be occurring with maternal bleeding should also be kept in mind. At least one-third of neonates born to mothers who required antepartum transfusion will themselves require transfusion following delivery.[3] All Rh-negative unsensitized mothers should be given Rh immune globulin with bleeding. A Kleihauer–Betke test should also be performed to detect the infrequent patient with fetal–maternal hemorrhage in excess of 30 ml. The Kleihauer–Betke test will quantitate the amount of blood loss and allow calculation of the appropriate dose of immune globulin. A positive indirect Coombs test 48 hours after treatment will document dosing adequacy. Testing should be repeated after each bleeding episode.

Prior to cesarean delivery, knowledge of the position of the placenta as determined by ultrasound is important for decision making about the uterine incision. If the placenta is posterior or does not extend anteriorly into the lower segment, a low transverse incision can be made. However, if the placenta is anterior, a vertical incision should be made at or above the placental edge, rather than through the placenta. Sometimes, the appearance of a vascular and boggy lower segment will provide a guide to placental position. An incision through the placenta can extend more easily into the uterine arteries. Of equal importance is the risk of fetal and maternal hemorrhage following placental laceration, which may be severe, increasing the possibility of neonatal anemia. In addition, delivery may be more complicated and delayed because of difficulty in locating and grasping the presenting part, further increasing the risk of fetal bleeding.

All patients with placenta previa are at risk for intraoperative hemorrhage because increased bleeding after placental separation may result from the poorer contractility of the lower uterine segment. Therefore, the issue of hysterectomy for uterine atony should be addressed prior to surgery.

Placenta Accreta

A prudent approach to patients with placenta previa and one or more previous cesareans is to discuss the risks of accreta, to discuss the desire for further fertility, and to counsel patients preoperatively for possible hysterectomy. At least two-thirds of women with a placenta previa and placenta accreta will require hysterectomy at delivery.[3] Hysterectomy offers the least morbidity and the best chance of survival.[21] However, if uterine preservation is important and maternal bleeding is not excessive, a number of different techniques can be attempted to control bleeding. When the diagnosis of complete accreta is confirmed or suspected, and placental separation has not taken place, bleeding may be minimal and the placenta can be left in place. The umbilical cord should be ligated close to the cord insertion and antibiotics administered. The use of methotrexate has been suggested, but whether this treatment will improve outcome has not been established. Similar therapy in abdominal pregnancy may increase the risk of infection through rapid necrosis of placental tissue.[83] If the placenta has been removed, a simple approach is tight packing of the lower uterine segment with removal of the packing transvaginally in 12 hours.[84] Uterine curettage may be successful in controlling bleeding due to accreta. Another technique is an interrupted circular suture on the serosal surface of the uterus around the lower segment above and below the transverse incision.[85] Alternatively, the bleeding sites may be oversewn and oxytocics and antibiotics given. This technique is more successful with a focal accreta. Another possibility is localized uterine resection. Bilateral uterine artery and hypogastric artery ligation may be attempted; angiographic arterial embolization is an additional option.

Abruptio Placentae

If placenta previa and other causes of antepartum hemorrhage have been eliminated, placental abruption becomes the most likely diagnosis. Assessment of maternal volume status is critical, since bleeding may be concealed. Continuous fetal monitoring is also imperative, since distress will develop in as many as 60% of fetuses.

Maternal serum fibrinogen concentration is a critical indicator in placental abruption because hypofibrinogenemia can provide a guide to estimate blood loss and maternal volume status as well as the presence of coagulation abnormalities. When fibrinogen has fallen from the normal 450 mg/dl to less than 300 mg/dl, a Grade 2 abruption has occurred and coagulation abnormalities are present; most of these women will require transfusion. With serum fibrinogen below 150 mg/dl, maternal blood loss has been greater than 2000 ml and DIC is present. Both groups of patients will require 1 to 2 liters of rapid isotonic crystalloid replacement while awaiting blood for transfusion. A Foley catheter should be inserted for monitoring of urine output, an additional indicator of volume status. If urine output falls below 30 ml per hour, an additional fluid bolus of 250 to 500 ml should be attempted. If urine output does not respond, consideration should be given to invasive monitoring to provide better information on intravascular volume. In the absence of maternal cardiac disease, severe preeclampsia or acute renal failure, a central venous catheter is adequate. Because of the potential for coagulopathy, the catheter should probably be placed in the antecubital rather than the subclavian or internal jugular veins. Normal cardiovascular pressure (CVP) should be 4 to 7 cm H_2O, but more importantly, the level should fall in response to fluid administration. If the CVP is less than 7, but urine output is still inadequate, the CVP should be replaced by a pulmonary artery catheter to evaluate additional cardiac or renal complications.

In most cases, delivery is the treatment of choice for placental abruption. The method of delivery remains controversial. With mild abruption, vaginal delivery should be possible. Even before the use of continuous fetal monitoring, there was no increase in perinatal mortality with vaginal delivery in these cases, regardless of the length of labor.[34] In more severe cases, labor may be attempted if bleeding is not excessive and the fetal heart rate patterns appear stable. In some instances, labor may be fairly rapid. During labor, careful attention should be paid to fetal heart rate patterns for evidence of nonreassuring changes. Amniotomy and fetal scalp electrode application should be performed as soon as possible. An intrauterine pressure catheter may be useful for reliable monitoring of uterine activity. Oxytocin may be used to stimulate or augment contractions. Maternal urine output should be monitored with an indwelling

Foley catheter, and serial hematocrits should be obtained every 2 to 3 hours. Unfortunately, since fetal distress will develop in up to 60% of these cases, cesarean delivery may be required for fetal indications. However, as long as the fetus is not compromised, no arbitrary limit need be placed on the length of labor, even in the face of falling platelet or fibrinogen values. With continuous fetal monitoring and replacement of coagulation factors, neonatal and maternal outcome with vaginal delivery are good.

When intrauterine fetal death has occurred, vaginal delivery is desirable. Fetal death is often accompanied by DIC; in this setting, maternal survival is the paramount issue. The most important concerns are to reestablish maternal blood volume and correct coagulation abnormalities. Once these problems have been addressed, attention can be turned to the issues of delivery. The widely held belief that coagulopathy cannot be corrected until the uterus has been evacuated has led some physicians to argue that cesarean delivery is always necessary. In fact, surgery on these patients is fraught with difficulty. Generalized bleeding will occur from all surgical incisions when the fibrinogen level is lower than 150 mg/dl or the platelet count is lower than 40,000/mm^3, and control of hemorrhage may be difficult. In contrast, vaginal delivery is usually not associated with excessive bleeding because uterine bleeding is controlled by the mechanical contraction of myometrial fibers rather than being dependent on coagulation factors. Moreover, if postpartum hemorrhage does occur, the bleeding is easily detected vaginally. On the other hand, postoperative intraabdominal, retroperitoneal, or incisional bleeding is less evident. With vaginal delivery, episiotomy should be avoided, if possible, since the incision may bleed extensively. If episiotomy must be done, careful attention should be paid to hemostasis and closure. Even with induction times extending beyond 18 hours, maternal outcomes are good if maternal volume and coagulation status are well maintained.[51]

Postpartum hemorrhage from uterine atony does not occur more frequently with abruption. Even a Couvelaire uterus usually responds normally to oxytocics, and hysterectomy is not required.

When placental abruption occurs in the preterm pregnancy, bleeding is not brisk, and the fetus is not compromised, tocolysis and delayed delivery may be considered. Magnesium sulfate is the best choice, avoiding the maternal cardiovascular changes associated with betamimetic agents. The gestation can be significantly extended without adverse maternal or fetal complications in more than half of the patients.[86,87] The decision to delay delivery should consider the benefit to fetal survival and the severity of the abruption. However, delayed delivery may even be possible with severe abruption. There are case reports of second-trimester abruption complicated by DIC treated with blood-product replacement in which live fetuses were later delivered.[88,89]

Fetal–maternal hemorrhage can also occur with placental abruption. Therefore, the Kleibauer–Betke test should be performed on Rh-negative unsensitized mothers. The average volume lost is about 12 ml. A larger bleed is uncommon but is more likely when abruption is associated with trauma.[58] Rh immune globulin should be given if expectant management is successful or as usual postpartum. A positive indirect Coombs test performed 48 hours after administration will indicate if the dose was adequate.

REFERENCES

1. Hibbard BM, Jeffcoate TN. Abruptio placentae. Obstet Gynecol 1966;27:155.
2. Brenner W, Edelman D, Hendricks C. Characteristics of patients with placenta previa and results of "expectant management." Am J Obstet Gynecol 1978;132:180.
3. Cotton D, Ead J, Paul R, Quilligan E. The conservative aggressive management of placenta previa. Am J Obstet Gynecol 1980;17:687.
4. Wexler P, Gottesfeld KR. Early diagnosis of placenta previa. Obstet Gynecol 1979;54:231.
5. Zelop C, Bromley B, Frigoletto FJ, Benacerraf B. Second trimester sonographically diagnosed placenta previa: prediction of persistent previa at birth. Int J Gynaecol Obstet 1979;33:287.
6. Corneau J, Shaw L, Marcell CC, Lavery JP. Early placenta previa and delivery outcome. Obstet Gynecol 1983;61:577.
7. Newton ER, Barss V, Cetrulo CL. The epidemiology and clinical history of asymptomatic midtrimester placenta previa. Am J Obstet Gynecol 1984;48:743.
8. Clark SL, Koonings PP, Phelan JP. Placenta previa/accreta and prior cesarean section. Am J Obstet Gynecol 1985;66:89.
9. Williams MA, Mittendorf R, Lieberman E, Monson RR, Scholenbaum SC, Genest DR. Cigarette smoking during pregnancy in relation to placenta previa. Am J Obstet Gynecol 1991;165:29.
10. Taylor VM, Kramer MD, Vaugh TL, Peacock S. Placenta previa in relation to induced and spontaneous abortion: a population-based study. Obstet Gynecol 1993;82:82.
11. Benedetti TJ. Obstetric hemorrhage. In: Gabbe SG, Niebyl JR, Simpson JL, eds. Obstetrics: normal and problem pregnancies. New York: Churchill Livingstone, 1996: 511.
12. Crenshaw C, Jones DE, Parker RT. Placenta previa: a survey of twenty years experience with improved perinatal

survival by expectant therapy and cesarean delivery. Obstet Gynecol Surv 1973;28:461

13. Bowie JD, Rochester D, Cadkin AV, Cooke WT, Kunzman A. Accuracy of placental localization by ultrasound. Radiology 1978;128:177.

14. Sunden B. Placentography by ultrasound. Acta Obstet Gynecol Scand 1970;49:179.

15. Farine D, Fox HE, Jacobson S, Timor-Tritsch IE. Vaginal ultrasound for diagnosis of placenta previa. Am J Obstet Gynecol 1988;59:566.

16. Leerentveld RA, Gilberts E, Arnold M, Wladimiroff WJ. Accuracy and safety of transvaginal sonographic placental localization. Obstet Gynecol 1990;76:759.

17. Laing FC. Placenta previa: avoiding false negative diagnosis. J Clin Ultrasound 1981;9:109.

18. Timor-Tritsch IE, Yunis RA. Confirming the safety of transvaginal sonography in patients suspected of placenta previa. Obstet Gynecol 1993;81:742.

19. Hertzberg BS, Bowie JD, Carroll BA, Kliewer MA, Weber TM. Diagnosis of placenta previa during the third trimester: role of transperineal sonography. Am J Roentgenol 1992;159:83.

20. Read J, Cotton D, Miller F. Placenta accreta: changing clinical aspects and outcome. Obstet Gynecol 1980;56:31.

21. Fox H. Placenta accreta 1945–1969. Obstet Gynecol 1979;54:231.

22. Chattopadhyay SK, Kharif H, Sherbeeni MM. Placenta praevia and accreta after previous caesarean section. Eur J Obstet Gynecol Reprod Biol 1993;52:151.

23. Miller DA, Chollet JA, Goodwin TM. Clinical risk factors for placenta previa–placenta accreta. Am J Obstet Gynecol 1997;177:210.

24. Hong TH, Shau WY, Hsieh CC, Chiu TH, Hsu JJ, Hsieh TT. Risk factors for placenta accreta. Obstet Gynecol 1999;93:545.

25. Hoffman-Tretin J, Koeningsberg M, Rabin A, Anyaebunam A. Placenta accreta. Additional sonographic observations. J Ultrasound Med 1992;11:326.

26. Finberg HJ, Williams JW. Placenta accreta: prospective sonographic diagnosis in patients with placenta previa and prior cesarean. J Ultrasound Med 1992;11:333.

27. Nyberg DA, Mack LA, Benedetti TJ, et al. Placental abruption and placental hemorrhage: correlation of sonographic findings with fetal outcome. Radiology 1987;35:357.

28. Domissee J, Tiltman A. Placental bed biopsies in placental abruption. Br J Obstet Gynaecol 1992;99:651.

29. Hurd WW, Miodovnik M, Hertzberg V, Lavin JP. Selective management of abruptio placentae: a prospective study. Obstet Gynecol 1983;61:467.

30. Abdella TN, Sibai BM, Hays JM, Anderson GD. Perinatal outcome in abruptio placentae. Obstet Gynecol 1984;63:365.

31. Karegard M, Gennser G. Incidence and recurrence rate of abruptio placentae in Sweden. Obstet Gynecol 1986;67:523.

32. Anath CV, Savitz DA, Williams MA. Placental abruption and its association with hypertension and prolonged rupture of membranes: a methodologic review and meta-analysis. Obstet Gynecol 1996;88:309.

33. Pritchard J, Mason R, Corley M, Pritchard S. Genesis of severe placental abruption. Am J Obstet Gynecol 1970;108:22.

34. Golditch IM, Boyce NE. Management of abruptio placentae. JAMA 1970;212:288.

35. Varner MW. Maternal mortality in Iowa from 1952 to 1986. Surg Obstet Gynecol 1989;168:555.

36. American College of Obstetricians and Gynecologists. Trauma in pregnancy. ACOG Technical Bulletin no. 161, November 1991.

37. Pearlman MD, Tintinalli JE, Lorenz RP. Blunt trauma during pregnancy. N Engl J Med 1990;323:1609.

38. Depp R. Cesarean delivery. In: Gabbe SG, Niebyl JR, Simpson JL, eds. Obstetrics: normal and problem pregnancies. New York: Churchill Livingstone, 1996: 633.

39. Helton AS, McFarlane J, Anderson ET. Battered women and pregnancy: a prevalence study. Am J Public Health 1987;77:1337.

40. Centers for Disease Control and Prevention. Physical violence during the 12 months preceding childbirth—Alaska, Maine, Oklahoma, and West Virginia, 1990–1991. MMWR 1994;43:132.

41. Goodwin TM, Breen MT. Pregnancy outcome and fetomaternal hemorrhage after noncatastrophic trauma. Am J Obstet Gynecol 1990;162:665.

42. Pearlman MD, Tintinalli JE, Lorenz RP. A prospective controlled study of outcome after trauma during pregnancy. Am J Obstet Gynecol 1990;162:173.

43. Vintzileos AM, Campbell WA, Nochimson DJ, Weinbaum PJ. Preterm premature rupture of the membranes: a risk factor for the development of abruptio placentae. Am J Obstet Gynecol 1987;156:1234.

44. Gonen R, Hannah ME, Milligan JE. Does prolonged preterm premature rupture of the membranes predispose to abruptio placenta? Obstet Gynecol 1989;74:347.

45. Naeye RL. Abruptio placentae and placenta previa: frequency, perinatal mortality, and cigarette smoking. Obstet Gynecol 1980;55:701.

46. Voigt LF, Hollenbach KA, Krohn MA, Daling JR, Hickok DE. The relationship of abruptio placentae with maternal smoking and small for gestational age infants. Obstet Gynecol 1990;75:771.

47. Hoskins IA, Friedman DM, Freiden FJ, Ordorica SA, Young BK. Relationship between antepartum cocaine abuse, abnormal umbilical artery Doppler velocimetry, and placental abruption. Obstet Gynecol 1991;78:279.

48. Slutsker L. Risks associated with cocaine use during pregnancy. Obstet Gynecol 1992;79:778.

49. Green JR. Placenta previa and abruptio placentae. In: Creasy RK, Resnick R, eds. Maternal-fetal medicine: principles and practice. Philadelphia: Saunders, 1994:611.

50. Krohn M, Voight L, McKnight B, Daling JR, Starzyk P, Benedetti TJ. Correlates of placental abruption in birth certificate data. Br J Obstet Gynaecol 1987;94:333.

51. Naeye RL, Harkness WL, Utts J. Abruptio placentae and perinatal death: a prospective study. Am J Obstet Gynecol 1977;128:740.

52. Scholl JS. Abruptio placentae: Clinical management in nonacute cases. Am J Obstet Gynecol 156:40, 1987.

53. Benedetti TJ. Obstetric hemorrhage. In: Gabbe SG, Niebyl JR, Simpson JL, eds. Obstetrics: normal and problem pregnancies. New York: Churchill Livingstone, 1996: 508.

54. Spirt BA, Gordon LP. Sonography of the placenta. In: Fleischer AC, Manning FA, Jeanty P, Romero R, eds. Sonography in obstetrics and gynecology: principles

and practice. Stamford, CT: Appleton and Lange, 1996: 198.

55. Nyberg, DA, Cyr DR, Mack LA et al. Sonographic spectrum of placental abruption. Am J Roentgenol 1987; 148:161.

56. Obstetrical hemorrhage. In: Cunningham FG, MacDonald P, Gant NF, Leveno KJ, Gilstrap LC, eds. Williams obstetrics. Stamford CT: Appleton and Lange, 1993:830.

57. Green JR. Placenta previa and abruptio placentae. In: Creasy RK, Resnick R, eds. Maternal-fetal medicine: principles and practice. Philadelphia: Saunders, 1994:615.

58. Critical care and trauma. In: Cunningham FG, MacDonald P, Gant NF, Leveno KJ, Gilstrap LC, eds. Williams obstetrics. Stamford, CT: Appleton and Lange, 1993:1075.

59. Grunfeld JP, Pertuiset N. Acute renal failure in pregnancy: 1987. Am J Kidney Dis 1987;9:359.

60. Lowe TW, Cunningham FG. Placental abruption. Clin Obstet Gynecol 1990;33:406.

61. Saftlas A, Olson D, Atrash HK, Rochat R, Rowley D. National trends in the incidence of abruptio placentae. 1979–1987. Obstet Gynecol 1991;78:1081.

62. Blair RG. Abruption of placenta: a review of 189 cases occurring between 1965 and 1969. J Obstet Gynaecol Br Commonw 1973;89:244.

63. Spinilli A, Fazzi E, Stronati E, et al. Severity of abruptio placenta and neurodevelopmental outcome in low birth weight infants. Early Hum Dev 1993;35:44.

64. Miller DA, Diaz FG, Paul RH. Vaginal birth after cesarean: a 10-year experience. Obstet Gynecol 1994;84:255.

65. Flamm BL, Newman LA, Thomas SJ et al. Vaginal birth after cesarean delivery: results of a 5-year multicenter collaborative study. Obstet Gynecol 1990;76:750.

66. Flamm BL, Goings J, Yunbao L, Wolde-Tsadik G. Elective repeat cesarean delivery versus trial of labor: a prospective multicenter study. Obstet Gynecol 1994;83:927.

67. Leung AS, Farmer RM, Leung EK, et al. Risk factors associated with uterine rupture during trial of labor after cesarean delivery: a case controlled study. Am J Obstet Gynecol 1993;168:1358.

68. Rosen MG, Dickinson JC, Westhoff CL. Vaginal birth after cesarean: a meta-analysis of morbidity and mortality. Obstet Gynecol 1991;77:465.

69. Pritchard JA. Injuries to the birth canal. In: Pritchard JA, MacDonald PS, Gant NF, eds. Williams obstetrics. Norwalk, CT: Appleton-Century-Crofts, 1985: 545.

70. Jones RO, Nagashima AW, Hartnett-Goodman MM, Goodlin RC. Rupture of low transverse cesarean scars during trial of labor. Obstet Gynecol 1991;77:815.

71. Scott JR. Mandatory trial of labor after cesarean delivery: an alternative viewpoint. Obstet Gynecol 1991;77:811.

72. Torrey E. Vasa previa. Am J Obstet Gynecol 1952;63:146.

73. Nelson LH, Malone PJ, King M. Diagnosis of vasa previa with transvaginal and color flow Doppler ultrasound. Obstet Gynecol 1990;76:506.

74. Harding JA, Lewis DF, Major CA, et al. Color flow Doppler: a useful instrument in the diagnosis of vasa previa. Am J Obstet Gynecol 1990;163:1566.

75. Obstetrical hemorrhage. In Cunningham FG, MacDonald P, Gant NF, Leveno KJ, Gilstrap LC, eds. Williams obstetrics. Stamford, CT: Appleton and Lange, 1993: 840.

76. Keirse MJNC. New perspectives for the effective treatment of preterm labor. Am J Obstet Gynecol 1995; 173:618.

77. Copper RL, Goldenberg RL, Creasy RK, et al. A multicenter study of preterm birth weight and gestational age-specific neonatal mortality. Am J Obstet Gynecol 1993; 168:78.

78. Gross, I. Hormonal therapy for prevention of respiratory distress syndrome. In: Polin RA, Fox WM, eds. Fetal and neonatal physiology. Philadelphia: Saunders, 1992: 1003.

79. National Institute of Health Consensus Development Conference on the Effect of Corticosteroids for Fetal Maturation on Perinatal Outcomes. Consensus Development Conference statement. Bethesda, MD: National Institutes of Health, 1994.

80. d'Angelo L, Irwin L. Conservative management of placenta previa: a cost benefit analysis. Am J Obstet Gynecol 1984;149:320.

82. Mouer J. Placenta previa: antepartum conservative management inpatient vs outpatient. Am J Obstet Gynecol 1994;170:1685.

83. Droste S, Keil K. Expectant management of placenta previa: cost benefit analysis of outpatient treatment. Am J Obstet Gynecol 1994;170:1254.

84. Rahman MS, Al-Suleiman SA, Rahman J, et al. Advanced abdominal pregnancy. Obstet Gynecol 1982;59:366.

85. Druzin ML. Packing of lower uterine segment for control of postcesarean bleeding in instances of placenta previa. Surg Gynecol Obstet 1989;169:543.

86. Cho JY, Kim SJ, Cha KY, Kay CW, Kim MI, Cha KS. Interrupted circular suture: bleeding control during cesarean delivery in placenta previa accreta. Obstet Gynecol 1991; 78:876.

87. Saller DJ. Tocolysis in the management of third trimester bleeding. J Perinatol 1990;10:125.

88. Combs C, Nyberg D, Mack L, et al. Expectant management after sonographic diagnosis of placental abruption. Am J Perinatol 1992;9:170.

89. Montaeiro AA, Onocencio AC, Jorge CS. Placental abruption with disseminated intravascular coagulopathy in the second trimester of pregnancy with fetal survival. Br J Obstet Gynaecol 1987;94:811.

Chapter 15
Postdate Pregnancy

Cesar Rosa

Five Key Points

- The frequency of postdate pregnancy is 5 to 10%. Accurate dating decreases the incidence to approximately 2%.

- Fetal macrosomia is increased in postdate pregnancies, increasing the risk for operative deliveries, birth canal injury, cesarean birth, and shoulder dystocia.

- Postdate fetuses have a higher incidence of meconium in the amniotic fluid. Oligohydramnios is also more common.

- A higher incidence of nonreassuring fetal heart tracings and perinatal morbidity and mortality mandate antepartum testing for patients who are beyond 41 completed weeks of gestation.

- When the estimated gestational age is reliable and the cervix is favorable, labor should be induced at 41 to 42 weeks of gestation. When the cervix is unfavorable and delivery is indicated, a cervical ripening agent should be administered.

Human gestation lasts an average of 280 days. A term pregnancy is one that lasts between 37 to 42 completed weeks of gestation. A postdate or postterm pregnancy lasts over 42 weeks, or 294 days from the first day of the last menstruation. Approximately 90% of all pregnancies will be delivered by the 42nd completed week of gestation, with 50% delivering by the due date, and the other 40% by the end of the 42nd week.[1] The likelihood that a woman will deliver on her due date is about 5%, and approximately 4% of all pregnancies will deliver after 43 weeks of gestation[2] (Figure 15-1).

For the expectant mother, not having her child by the estimated date of delivery may lead to significant anxiety due to unmet expectations. Importantly, as the gestation progresses beyond 41 weeks, the likelihood of perinatal complications increases.[3,4]

In some clinics, postdate pregnancy is the most common antepartum complication. It is often the most common indication for antepartum fetal testing and is a frequent indication for induction of labor.[5] Hence, because of the increased fetal risk, and because of the increased resource utilization, it is important to develop a management plan that will optimize the maternal and fetal outcome, with the wisest expenditure of resources.

INCIDENCE

Depending on the population under consideration and on the dating criteria used, the incidence of pregnancies that remain undelivered after 42 weeks will vary from approximately 3 to 10%. In a review of 15,226 births delivered in Montreal, Canada, Usher

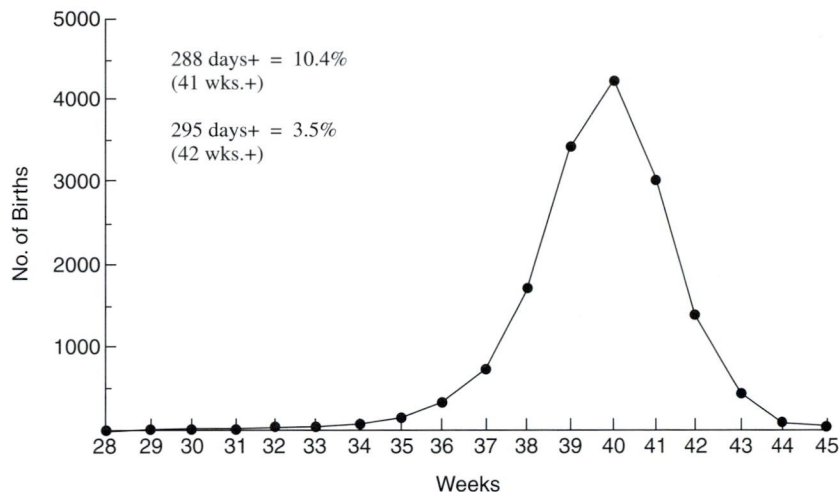

288 days+ = 10.4%
(41 wks.+)

295 days+ = 3.5%
(42 wks.+)

Figure 15-1 Distribution of births in relation to length of gestation. *From McClure Brown JC. Postmaturity. Am J Obstet Gynecol 1963;85:573. Reprinted by permission.*

and colleagues reported that, when gestational age was precisely confirmed, only 4.4% of pregnancies that reached 39 weeks exceeded 293 days of gestation.[4] In assessing a subset of the above cohort, the authors observed that, although 7.5% of all pregnancies reached 42 weeks by menstrual dating, only 2.6% did so when dating was based on early ultrasound. When the diagnosis of postdates was restricted to patients in whom both menstrual and early ultrasound dates exceeded 293 days, the incidence was only 1.1%.[4] These data suggest that the majority of presumed prolonged pregnancies are actually a consequence of a prolonged follicular phase or delayed ovulation.[6]

ETIOLOGY

The reason for postdate pregnancy is not known, although it is reasonable to surmise that the explanation lies in the mechanism for the initiation of human parturition. A number of naturally occurring anomalies have been associated with prolonged pregnancies and may offer some insight into the cause of this phenomenon. One example is the fact that anencephalic fetuses without pituitary glands have prolonged gestation, in contrast to anencephalics with developed pituitary glands.[2] In addition, 10 of 19 postterm fetuses deemed to have died from congenital malformations had adrenal gland hypoplasia.[7]

Another naturally occurring condition leading to prolonged pregnancies is placental sulfatase deficiency, an X-linked disorder occurring in approximately 1 in 2000 to 1 in 6000 newborns. The newborns are affected with ichthyosis, a skin disorder characterized

by hyperkeratosis and associated with corneal opacities, pyloric stenosis, and cryptorchidism. The placenta is unable to hydrolyze the estrogen precursors dihydroepiandrosterone sulfate (DHEA-S) or 16 α-hydroxy-DHEA-S; hence the maternal serum estrogens concentration is abnormally low. Most pregnancies with placental sulfatase deficiency used to be detected by finding abnormally low maternal urinary or serum estriol when evaluating patients for placental function due to postdate pregnancy. These patients usually fail to go in labor, and many require cesarean delivery.[8] More recently, given the wide utilization of maternal serum unconjugated estriol as part of the multiple-marker screening for fetuses with Down syndrome, placental sulfatase deficiency has been identified earlier in pregnancy.[9-11]

The common denominator in the above conditions is an abnormally low level of maternal estrogens. Although the steroid hormones have no direct effect on the contractility of the uterus, they exert a regulatory influence through their action on protein synthesis and the synthesis of cell-surface receptors.[12] Hence, one may hypothesize that the reason for some postdate pregnancies may be related to an alteration of the physiologic mechanisms that control the onset of labor.

MORBIDITY

Possibly due to the lack of reliable ways to date pregnancies, the clinical relevance of a prolonged pregnancy remained unrecognized until 1902 when Ballantyne described the problem of postdate pregnancy for the first time in modern obstetric terms.[2]

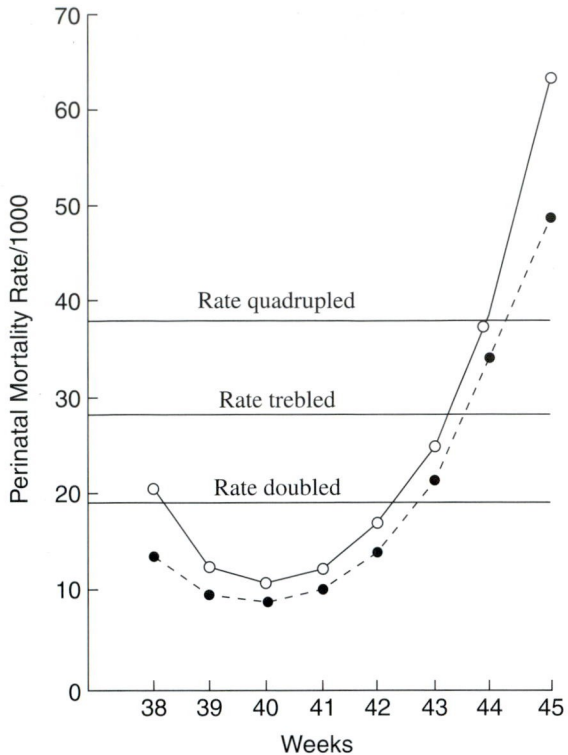

Figure 15-2 Relationship of perinatal mortality to length of gestation. Solid line = preeclampsia excluded; dotted line = preeclampsia, congenital malformations, and antepartum hemorrhage excluded. *From McClure Brown JC. Postmaturity. Am J Obstet Gynecol 1963;85:573. Reprinted by permission.*

In one of the earlier and most-often-quoted articles, McClure Browne reported a twofold increase in perinatal mortality after 42 weeks of gestation.[13] The increased mortality was evident after excluding preeclampsia, congenital malformations, and antepartum hemorrhage (Figure 15-2). Other more recent series have corroborated an increased incidence of perinatal morbidity and mortality in the postdate neonate.[3,4]

Fetal Morbidity

Clifford described the postmature or dysmature infant as withered, meconium-stained, fragile, with long nails and peeling skin. The placentas were described as small, and the infants were noted to be at risk for hypoglycemia, thermal instability, and meconium aspiration.[14] The small placentas lead to placental insufficiency, driving the fetus to use its own energy stores in the liver and adipose tissues. The result is a neonate with little subcutaneous fat and some degree of fetal weight restriction. Due to poor placental function, the amniotic fluid may be decreased, resulting in increased risk of cord compression and passage of meconium. In utero aspiration of thick meconium may lead to meconium aspiration syndrome. Uteroplacental insufficiency may result in nonreassuring fetal heart rate patterns and even fetal death.

Fortunately, the postmaturity syndrome is present in only 10 to 20% of postdate pregnancies.[5] The later intellectual development of postterm infants appears normal except for those with perinatal asphyxia or severe neonatal problems.[15] Interestingly, the postmaturity syndrome also has been described in pregnancies 38 to 41 weeks in duration.[16]

Postdate pregnancies are frequently associated with decreased amniotic fluid. Although highly variable, in normal pregnancies the amniotic fluid reaches a mean volume of 750 ml at approximately 22 weeks of gestation. This volume is maintained relatively constant until approximately 39 weeks of gestation, when it decreases sharply.[17] Other investigators have documented a maximum of 1000 to 1200 ml at 38 weeks of gestation, with a rapid decrease to an average of 300 ml at 42 weeks.[6]

The reduced amniotic fluid volume increases the risk of cord compression, leading to reflex passage of meconium.[18] The incidence of fetal distress in postdate pregnancies with normal amniotic fluid is low, indicating that a determination of the amount of amniotic fluid should be useful in the evaluation of the postdate fetus.[19,20] In fact, Leveno and colleagues described a prospective study of 727 postdate pregnancies in which 59 patients were delivered via cesarean due to fetal distress.[21] The majority of those patients had fetal heart tracings consistent with cord compression, and the incidence of oligohydramnios in that subgroup was high. The authors concluded that the pathophysiology of fetal distress in prolonged pregnancies is oligohydramnios leading to cord compression, rather than uteroplacental insufficiency.[21]

Meconium staining occurs in approximately 25 to 30% of postdate pregnancies, a rate that is two times higher than for term pregnancies.[22] The presence of meconium is associated with the meconium aspiration syndrome, pulmonary hypertension, and an increased risk for assisted ventilation.[23-25] Because many postdate pregnancies have reduced amniotic fluid, the meconium often is thicker, which increases the probability and severity of meconium aspiration syndrome. Given the demonstrated benefit of nasal and oropharyngeal suctioning of the infant while on the mother's perineum,[26] the presence of meconium should be suspected in the patient who has scant fluid on rupture of membranes during labor. At the time of birth, suction devices must be available for prompt suctioning of the neonate with meconium-stained fluid.

The worst perinatal outcome can be anticipated in fetuses who are postdate and growth-restricted.[19,27] A review of all deliveries occurring in Sweden over 6 years documented that there was a significant rise in the odds ratio for fetal death from 41 weeks on (odds ratio 2.9 at 43 weeks). The odds ratio for fetal mortality at 43 weeks was 10.0 when growth restriction was present.[28]

Considering the likelihood of diminished placental function in postdate pregnancies, the intuitive thought may be that there would be a high risk of fetal growth restriction in these pregnancies. The fact is, however, that the most common growth disturbance encountered in postdate pregnancies is macrosomia.[4] The fetus continues to gain weight into the postdate period, and the percentage of postterm infants weighing >4000 g at birth is twice that at term (16% vs. 8%).[14,29] In some studies the incidence of fetal macrosomia in postdate pregnancy has been as high as 25%.[22]

Macrosomic fetuses experience a higher incidence of difficult deliveries, including shoulder dystocia, clavicular and humeral fracture, and brachial plexus injury.[29–31] The relative probability of shoulder dystocia in fetuses over 4000 g has been reported to be 11 times greater than average.[32] In their review of the outcome of macrosomic infants born in California, Lipscomb and colleagues reported an 18.5% incidence of shoulder dystocia among infants weighing over 4500 g.[33] Up to 20% of these infants experience nerve injuries, and in the minority of cases, these may lead to permanent handicap.[32] Importantly, the perinatal mortality in infants experiencing shoulder dystocia ranges from 21 per 1000 to 290 per 1000.[31]

A neonatal risk that needs to be acknowledged is that of iatrogenic damage. Although mostly a hypothetical possibility, induction for postdate pregnancy in a patient with uncertain dates may result in neonatal morbidity due to prematurity. In addition, induction of labor when the cervix is not favorable results in long labor with depletion of fetal reserve, increasing the likelihood of fetal intolerance of labor and subsequent cesarean delivery.[34]

Maternal Morbidity

The main risk for the mother with a postdate pregnancy is that of operative delivery, whether associated with spontaneous or induced labor. Because of the higher incidence of macrosomic fetuses, these parturients have a higher incidence of cesarean delivery and operative vaginal delivery.[22] The likelihood of vaginal sidewall, cervical, and perineal lacerations increases with operative deliveries.[34,35] Women with postdate pregnancies also have a high frequency of unfavorable Bishop scores, making induction of labor more difficult.[36] In addition, there is a higher incidence of nonreassuring fetal heart tracings, leading to cesarean delivery for fetal distress.[22]

Even after controlling for induction of labor and the size of the infant, the incidence of cesarean delivery is increased in postdate pregnancies due to increased uterine dysfunction.[35] The risk of cesarean delivery is higher among nulliparas.[37] With cesarean delivery, as opposed to vaginal delivery, the risk of postpartum infection, hemorrhage, wound complications, pulmonary embolism, prolonged hospital stay, and maternal mortality is increased.[38,39]

MANAGEMENT

Dating the Pregnancy

Given the lower incidence of postdate pregnancy when the dating of the pregnancy is precise,[4] the most important component of a global management strategy is the accurate and meticulous documentation of gestational age. With the advent of assisted reproductive techniques, we can now ascertain to the hour when fertilization occurs. One may anticipate that in a few years, when a large number of these precisely timed pregnancies are available for review, the information obtained will yield a more precise range for the duration of normal pregnancies.

The most readily available and possibly the single best predictor of the actual gestational age is the date of the last menstrual period (LMP). There are two obvious shortcomings: the biologic variation and unpredictability of the ovulation date in relation to the LMP[6] and the fact that up to 40% of patients are uncertain about the date of their LMP.[40]

The following may be used to corroborate the LMP-based gestational age: a positive serum human chorionic gonadotropin at 5 weeks of gestation; fetal heart tones documented with an electronic device (Doppler device) at 10 weeks of gestation; and fetal heart tones auscultated with a nonelectronic stethoscope at 18 to 20 weeks.[41] Of the traditional obstetric landmarks, a bimanual examination consistent with gestational age in the first 12 weeks of gestation is probably the most dependable. Other landmarks of limited help in documenting the gestational age are the fundal height at the level of the umbilicus at approximately 20 weeks of gestation and maternal perception of fetal activity (quickening) at approximately 18 weeks of gestation.

Probably the most widely used resource for the accurate dating of pregnancies is obstetric sonography. Modern equipment is widely available in most obstetric practices in this country, providing an easy and safe method for pregnancy dating. In the first trimester of pregnancy a crown-to-rump length (CRL) determination is accurate to within 5 days of the actual gestational age in 95% of cases.[42] Beyond 12 weeks, and because of the normal ventral curvature of the fetus, the CRL is no longer reliable. From approximately 14 to 20 weeks of gestation, a biparietal diameter determination will be within 7 to 10 days of the actual gestational age. Beyond 24 weeks of gestation, the confidence intervals may be as wide as ±2 weeks, so sonography loses its value as a dating method.[43]

Sweeping the Amniotic Membranes

Sweeping, or stripping, the amniotic membranes off the inner surface of the lower uterine segment may help to induce labor by causing a release of prostaglandins from the amniotic–decidual interphase. The first reference to this method in the modern medical literature is by Swann in 1958.[44] He described how this maneuver probably evolved as an alternative to the more commonly used method of rupturing the amniotic membranes for induction of labor.

To date, there are ten articles in the literature reporting on the effectiveness of sweeping the membranes as a method to accelerate the onset of labor and decrease the proportion of postdate pregnancies.[44-53] Of the seven reports that included randomization of the study population,[47-53] six showed that sweeping the membranes was effective in accelerating the onset of labor as compared with the control groups. Of the seven studies that evaluated the incidence of postdate pregnancy,[47-53] all documented a lower incidence in the study groups. In the seven

randomized studies,[47-53] four included weekly vaginal examinations and sweeping of the membranes commencing at 38 weeks,[47,50,51,53] two included a single examination with sweep at ≥40 weeks,[49,52] and one included a single examination at 41 weeks.[48] None of these studies documented any increase in infection, premature rupture of membranes (PROM), or other complications in the groups undergoing sweeping of the membranes. Although a β error is possible, the seven studies quoted above include 466 patients in the experimental groups and 452 in the control groups. The similar complication rates in the two groups fail to support any concern that sweeping the membranes increases the incidence of PROM or maternal infection.

Outlined below is a suggested protocol for practitioners who wish to perform sweeping of the membranes to induce labor and/or to reduce the incidence of posterm pregnancy. First, the practitioner should ensure that the patient is ≥39 weeks of gestation as determined by reliable dating criteria. Sonography performed earlier during the pregnancy, or prior to the intervention, should document normal placentation. The fetal presentation should be cephalic, or if breech, the patient should have been evaluated and counseled for a vaginal delivery of the breech-presenting infant. There should be no contraindication for a vaginal birth. After counseling the patient, the procedure should be performed using a sterile examination glove. If the cervical canal admits an examining finger, the finger should be introduced beyond the internal os and the amniotic membranes swept from the decidua for at least 2 cm beyond the internal os using a circular motion. If the cervical canal does not admit the examining finger, then vigorous massage of the cervix may be performed. The procedure is almost universally painful. The patient should be informed about the procedure, and she should be empowered to stop the attempt at sweeping the membranes if it proves to be too painful for her. In addition to the discomfort associated with the procedure, the patient should be advised of the possibility that she may experience vaginal bleeding or spotting. The procedure may be repeated at the time of the following prenatal visit if spontaneous labor does not occur.

Antenatal Testing

Although by definition a pregnancy is not postdate until 42 weeks, due to the gradual but measurable increment in perinatal mortality after 41 weeks, it is prudent to commence antenatal testing at 41 completed weeks of gestation.[54-56] In addition to the available clinical data, other evidence that supports commencing antenatal testing at 41 weeks is the demonstration that umbilical-cord plasma erythropoietin is elevated in neonates born at 41 weeks and beyond as compared with neonates born at 37 to 40 weeks. The cord erythropoietin is thought to be an indicator of decreased fetal oxygenation, and it increases as the pregnancy advances beyond 41 weeks.[57]

A number of methods have been described for the antenatal evaluation of the fetus at risk for fetal death or poor outcome. The contraction stress test (CST) is associated with a false negative rate of <1 in 1000 live births.[58] Although highly effective in reducing the perinatal mortality rate, it is a time-consuming test, and it is contraindicated in patients with preterm labor and placenta previa. In addition, the frequency of equivocal tests in postdate patients may reach 35 to 40%.[22] When the test is negative, the patient does not require testing for 1 week. However, equivocal tests should be repeated in 24 hours.[22]

The nonstress test (NST) offers the advantage of being a quicker test with no known contraindications. The relative disadvantage is that the NST needs to be performed twice weekly to achieve a false negative rate of 1.9 in 1000.[59] A negative NST performed weekly has a false negative rate of 6 in 1000.[59,60]

The biophysical profile (BPP), described by Manning et al. in 1980, uses real-time sonography to assess the fetus.[61] The test consists of five parameters that are assigned a score of 0 or 2. The five components of the BPP are amniotic fluid volume, fetal tone, fetal motion, fetal breathing activity, and the NST. When applied weekly to postdate patients, the false negative rate of the BPP is similar to that of a weekly NST (approximately 7 per 1000).[61] Hence, when performing surveillance on postdate pregnancies, the BPP should also be performed twice weekly.

The modified biophysical profile (mBPP), introduced in 1982, consists of an NST and a determination of amniotic fluid volume.[60] When performed twice weekly on a group of 8038 postdate patients, this test was associated with a false negative rate of 1.12 per 1000.[62] Because in patients with postdate pregnancies oligohydramnios may develop relatively soon after documentation of a normal amniotic fluid index (AFI) (i.e., 3 to 4 days), it is important to perform the amniotic fluid determination twice weekly in patients with postdate pregnancies.[63] Given the

relative simplicity of the test and its low false negative rate, the mBPP has been adopted by many as the antepartum test of choice.

An area of controversy is the level of amniotic fluid that constitutes oligohydramnios and at what point the relative amount of amniotic fluid predicts a poor neonatal outcome. Initially, the adequacy of the amniotic fluid volume was based on the dimension of the deepest vertical pocket of fluid, and thresholds of 1 to 3 cm were used.[64] At present, most clinicians use the AFI to assess the adequacy of the amniotic fluid level. An AFI >8 cm is normal, 5 to 8 cm is borderline, and <5 cm is oligohydramnios.[65]

Induction of Labor

One management strategy is to induce labor on all patients when they reach 41 weeks of estimated gestational age. A relative disadvantage of this strategy is the fact that a significant number of patients with postdate pregnancies have a cervix that is unfavorable for induction.[36] This fact presents a dilemma: should postdate patients have their labors induced despite an unfavorable cervix, thus risking a higher cesarean delivery rate? Or should these patients be followed with antepartum monitoring until they labor spontaneously or their cervix becomes favorable for induction?

Two randomized clinical trials have addressed this issue. The first, a Canadian multicenter collaborative study, reviewed the outcomes of 3407 women with uncomplicated pregnancies of ≥41 weeks of gestation.[66] The patients were randomized to induction at 41 weeks (using intracervical prostaglandin gel whenever the cervix was not favorable for induction), as compared with antenatal testing via daily fetal kick counts and NST with fluid assessment three times per week. The cesarean delivery rate for the induction rate was significantly lower (21.2% vs. 24.5%, $p = 0.03$). The lower cesarean rate was due to a lower frequency of fetal distress in the induction group. Two stillbirths occurred in the expectantly managed group, as compared with none in the induction group, a nonsignificant difference. The authors concluded that induction of labor resulted in a lower cesarean delivery rate and that the neonatal mortality and morbidity were similar in the two groups.[65]

The second trial, sponsored by the National Institute of Child Health and Human Development Network of Maternal–Fetal Units, evaluated 440 patients with uncomplicated pregnancies at 41 weeks of gestation.[67] The patients were randomized to immediate induction of labor (n = 265) versus expectant management (n = 175). The group that underwent induction of labor was further randomized to include one group that received one dose of intracervical prostaglandin E_2 gel and a second group that received a placebo gel. The group that underwent expectant management had an NST and amniotic fluid determination two times per week. The incidence of adverse perinatal outcome was similar in both groups (1.5% vs. 1%, $p = >0.05$), and there were no differences in mean birth weights or frequency of macrosomia between the two groups ($p = >0.05$). There were no fetal deaths in either group. The prostaglandin gel was not more effective than placebo in ripening the cervix, and the cesarean delivery rates were similar in all groups (18% in the expectant management group, 23% in the prostaglandin-gel induction group, and 18% in the placebo-gel induction group). The authors concluded that, in light of similar outcomes, either management strategy was acceptable.[67]

In a review of 11 clinical trials investigating a policy of induction of labor at 41 weeks (including the Canadian multicenter study), Grant concluded that induction at 41 weeks resulted in a modest (14%) reduction in the cesarean delivery rate and a lower perinatal mortality rate (0.3 versus 2.5 per 1000) as compared with a plan of expectant management.[68] The author concluded that the available evidence suggests that induction of labor should be recommended to women with certain dates >41 weeks of gestation.

The American College of Obstetrician and Gynecologists Practice Patterns publication, an evidence-based review of the literature, states that it is not known whether induction or expectant management is preferable for an otherwise uncomplicated postdate pregnancy with a favorable cervix. It also states that there is good evidence that either induction or expectant management will result in a good outcome among postdate patients with an unfavorable cervix and without additional complications.[69]

One may conclude that the difference in outcome between routine induction at 41 weeks and expectant management with antepartum testing is sufficiently small that there is no overwhelming evidence in favor of either of the two treatment options. It is important to note that the above studies have not considered the patients' preference for any particular strategy. One needs to also consider that the preferred management strategy will be influenced by the population of patients served and by the facilities available.

Cervical Ripening

In an effort to improve the likelihood of a successful induction of labor, several appliances and chemicals have been used to promote cervical ripening. Hygroscopic cervical dilators and Foley catheters inserted in the cervical canal have achieved varying levels of success.[70] In addition, several prostaglandin preparations have been studied. Currently, there are two prostaglandins with a labeled indication for induction of labor: Prepidil (dinoprostone cervical gel, Upjohn, Kalamazoo, MI), a prostaglandin E_2 gel applied intracervically in a dose of 0.5 mg every 6 hours, and Cervidil (dinoprostone 10 mg, Forest Pharmaceuticals, St. Louis, MO), a vaginal insert designed to release the dinoprostone at approximately 0.3 mg/h over 12 hours. In addition, many hospital pharmacies prepare their own prostaglandin E_2 gels from 20-mg prostaglandin suppositories (Prostin E_2, Upjohn).[71]

Although the Maternal–Fetal Units trial found that prostaglandin E_2 gel application was not more effective than placebo in inducing labor,[67] other studies on women with postdate pregnancy have shown the prostaglandin gel to be effective.[72-74] The lack of a standard preparation, dose, and route of delivery are factors that limit the interpretation of the available data. A meta-analysis of the results of studies comparing prostaglandin therapy to placebo or no treatment, and comparing different prostaglandin preparations and routes of administration, showed that prostaglandin administered vaginally or intracervically appears to offer the best balance of effectiveness and safety. Prostaglandin E_2 was found to be preferable to prostaglandin $F_{2\alpha}$, based on effectiveness at lower doses.[75]

More recently, misoprostol, a synthetic prostaglandin E_1 analog marketed in the United States since 1988 for protection of the gastric mucosa in patients ingesting nonsteroidal antiinflammatory agents, has been promoted as a cervical-ripening and labor-inducing agent. Various trials comparing intravaginal misoprostol in varying doses with intracervical prostaglandin E_2 gel show that misoprostol is an effective agent for facilitating induction of labor.[76-78] A meta-analysis of eight studies that included 488 patients receiving misoprostol and 478 controls documented that the women receiving misoprostol had a lower cesarean delivery rate (odds ratio, 0.67, 95% confidence interval, 0.48–0.93) and a higher incidence of vaginal delivery within 24 hours of misoprostol administration (odds ratio, 2.64, 95% confidence interval, 1.87–3.71). The use of misoprostol was associated with a higher incidence of tachysystole but not hyperstimulation, and the mean interval from start of induction to delivery was 4.6 hours shorter.[79]

Because of the higher incidence of polysystole, misoprostol should be administered cautiously. The optimal dose appears to be between 25 and 50 μg every 3 hours.[80,81] A 100-μg tablet can be divided into two or four parts to obtain the 50- or 25-μg portions, respectively. The tablet fragment should be placed in the posterior vaginal fornix by the examining fingers. If fetal intolerance of labor occurs due to polysystole, the remaining fragment of the tablet should be removed from the vagina, the vagina irrigated with saline, and 0.25 mg of terbutaline administered subcutaneously. These maneuvers will resolve the uterine polysystole in the majority of patients. Prior to applying misoprostol, fetal well-being should be documented via a reassuring fetal heart tracing. In addition to being highly effective, misoprostol is also inexpensive, especially as compared with any of the commercially available prostaglandin E$_2$ preparations, and does not require refrigeration.

A number of serious complications have been reported in patients receiving misoprostol. Wing and colleagues reported on a clinical trial comparing misoprostol to oxytocin for induction of labor in women with a prior cesarean delivery.[82] Two of the patients receiving misoprostol experienced disruption of the prior uterine incision. Because of safety concerns, the trial was stopped after 38 patients had been enrolled. Of note, there was no documentation of the type of uterine scar in 13 of the patients. The two disruptions occurred in this subgroup.[82] Additionally, Bennett described a patient who received 25 μg of misoprostol every 3 hours for induction of labor and in whom a posterior uterine rupture developed that required hysterectomy as a life-saving procedure.[83] In a recent literature review, Plaut and colleagues concluded that misoprostol may increase the risk of uterine rupture in the patient with a scarred uterus. They identified uterine rupture in 5 of 89 patients with previous cesarean delivery who had labor induction with misoprostol. In their review, the uterine rupture rate in patients attempting vaginal birth after cesarean was significantly higher in those who received misoprostol, 5.6%, compared to 0.2% in those who did not receive misoprostol.[84] Insofar as misoprostol does not have induction of labor as one of its labeled indications,

it is important that the medication be administered under a well-defined clinical protocol.

CONCLUSIONS

Prevention of postdate pregnancy begins with accurate dating of gestational age. At 39 weeks of gestation, after normal placental location has been verified, weekly sweeping of the amniotic membranes has been shown to decrease the incidence of postterm pregnancy. Once the patient reaches 41 weeks of gestation, induction of labor should be undertaken in patients with a favorable cervix. Patients with an unfavorable cervix should be offered either induction of labor with the aid of a ripening agent such as intracervical prostaglandin E$_2$ or misoprostol, or initiation of antepartum testing. At this time, the most commonly recommended plan of testing is the modified fetal biophysical profile (NST and AFI) twice weekly. If the antenatal testing remains reassuring, the patient may be followed expectantly. At 42 weeks of gestation, induction of labor should be strongly considered unless the cervix remains markedly unfavorable.

REFERENCES

1. Treolar AE, Behn BG, Cowan DW. Analysis of gestational interval. Am J Obstet Gynecol 1967;99:34.
2. Resnik R. Post-term pregnancy. In: Creasy RK and Resnik R, eds. Maternal-fetal medicine. Philadelphia: Saunders, 1994:521.
3. Arias F. Predictability of complications associated with prolongation of pregnancy. Obstet Gynecol 1987;70:101.
4. Usher RH, Boyd ME, McLean FH, Kramer MS. Assessment of fetal risk in postdate pregnancies. Am J Obstet Gynecol 1988;158:259.
5. Rayburn WF, Motley ME, Stempel LE, Gendreau M. Antepartum prediction of the postmature infant. Obstet Gynecol 1982;60:148.
6. Resnik R. Postterm gestation. J Reprod Med 1988; 33:249.
7. Naeye RL. Causes of perinatal mortality: excess in prolonged gestations. Am J Epidemiol 1978;108:429.
8. The endocrinology of pregnancy. In: Speroff L, Glass RH, Kase NG, eds. Clinical gynecologic endocrinology and infertility. Baltimore: Williams & Wilkins, 1999:275.
9. Schleifer RA, Bradley LA, Richards DS, Ponting NR. Pregnancy outcome for women with very low levels of maternal serum unconjugated estriol on second-trimester screening. Am J Obstet Gynecol 1995;173:1152.
10. Bradley LA, Canick JA, Palomaki GE, Haddow JE. Undetectable maternal serum unconjugated estriol levels in the second trimester: risk of perinatal complications associated with placental sulfatase deficiency. Am J Obstet Gynecol 1997;176:531.

11. Reynolds JW, Burry K, Carlson CV. Fetoplacental steroid metabolism in prolonged pregnancies. Am J Obstet Gynecol 1986;154:74.

12. Fuchs AR, Fuchs F. Physiology and endocrinology of parturition. In: Gabbe SG, Niebyl JR, Simpson JL, eds. Obstetrics, normal and abnormal pregnancies. New York: Churchill Livingstone, 1996:111.

13. McClure Browne JC. Postmaturity. Am J Obstet Gynecol 1963;85:573.

14. Clifford SH. Postmaturity—with placental dysfunction. J Pediatr 1954;44:1.

15. Mannino F. Neonatal complications of postterm gestation. J Reprod Med 1988;33:271.

16. Sjostedt S, Engleson G, Rooth G. Dysmaturity. Arch Dis Child 1958;33:123.

17. Gilbert WM, Brace RA. Amniotic fluid volume and normal flows to and from the amniotic cavity. Semin Perinatol 1993;17:150.

18. Hon EH, Bradfield AH, Hess OW. The electronic evaluation of the fetal heart rate. V. The vagal factor in fetal bradycardia. Am J Obstet Gynecol 1961;82:291.

19. Crowley P, O'Herlihy C, Boylan P. The value of ultrasound measurement of amniotic fluid volume in the management of prolonged pregnancies. Br J Obstet Gynecol 1984;91:444.

20. Phelan JP, Platt LD, Yeh S-Y, et al. The role of ultrasound assessment of amniotic fluid volume in the management of the postdate pregnancy. Am J Obstet Gynecol 1985; 151:304.

21. Leveno KJ, Quirk JG, Cunningham FG, et al. Prolonged pregnancy. Am J Obstet Gynecol 1984;150:465.

22. Freeman RK, Garite TJ, Mondanlou H, Dorchester W, Rommal C, Devaney M. Postdate pregnancy: utilization of contraction stress testing for primary fetal surveillance. Am J Obstet Gynecol 1981;140:128.

23. Murphy JD, Vawler GF, Reid LM. Pulmonary vascular disease in fatal meconium aspiration. J Pediatr 1984; 104:762.

24. Carson BS. Suctioning the meconium stained infant. Am J Dis Child 1988;142:698.

25. Katz VL, Bowes WA Jr. Meconium aspiration syndromes: reflections on a murky subject. Am J Obstet Gynecol 1992;166:171.

26. Linder N, Aranda JV Tsur M, et al. Need for endotracheal intubation and suction in meconium-stained neonates. J Pediatr 1988;112:613.

27. Sachs BP, Friedman EA. Results of an epidemiologic study of postdate pregnancy. J Reprod Med 1986;31:162.

28. Divon MY, Haglund B, Nisell H, Otterblad PO, Westgreen M. Fetal and neonatal mortality in the postterm pregnancy: the impact of gestational age and fetal growth restriction. Am J Obstet Gynecol 1998;178:726.

29. Eden R, Seifert L, Winegar A, Spellacy WN. Perinatal characteristics of uncomplicated post-date pregnancies. Obstet Gynecol 1987;69:296.

30. Callenbach JC, Hall RT. Morbidity and mortality of advanced gestational age: post-term or postmature. Obstet Gynecol 1978;53:721.

31. Benedetti TJ, Gabbe SJ. Shoulder dystocia. A complication of fetal macrosomia and prolonged second stage of labor with midpelvic delivery. Obstet Gynecol 1978;52:526.

32. Acker DB, Sachs BP, Friedman EA. Risk factors for shoulder dystocia. Obstet Gynecol 1985;66:762.

33. Lipscomb KR, Gregory K, Shaw K. The outcome of macrosomic infants weighing at least 4500 grams: Los Angeles County and University of Southern California experience. Obstet Gynecol 1995;85:558.

34. Bishop EH. Pelvic scoring for elective induction. Obstet Gynecol 1964;24:266.

35. Boyd ME, Usher RH, McLean FH, Kramer MS. Obstetric consequences of postmaturity. Am J Obstet Gynecol 1988;158:334.

36. Harris BA, Huddleston JF, Sutliff G, Perlis HW. The unfavorable cervix in prolonged pregnancy. Obstet Gynecol 1983;62:171.

37. Arulkumaran S, Gibb DMF, Tamby Raja RL, Heng SH, Ratnam SS. Failed induction of labour. Aust NZ J Obstet Gynecol 1985;25:190.

38. Duff P. Pathophysiology and management of postcesarean endomyometritis. Obstet Gynecol 1986;67:269.

39. The Cesarean Birth Task Force. NIH consensus development statement on cesarean childbirth. Obstet Gynecol 1980;57:537.

40. Hall MH, Carr-Hill RA, Fraser C Campbell D, Samphier ML. The extent and antecedents of uncertain gestation. Br J Obstet Gynaecol 1985;92:445.

41. American College of Obstetricians and Gynecologists. Assessment of Fetal Lung Maturity. ACOG Educational Bulletin no. 230. November 1996.

42. Robinson HP, Fleming JEE. A critical evaluation of sonar "crown-rump length" measurements. Br J Obstet Gynaecol 1975;82:702.

43. American College of Obstetricians and Gynecologists. Ultrasonography in Pregnancy. ACOG Technical Bulletin no. 187. 1993.

44. Swann RO. Induction of labor by stripping membranes. Obstet Gynecol 1958;11:74.

45. Weissberg SM, Spellacy WN. Membrane stripping to induce labor. J Reprod Med 1977;19:125.

46. McColgin SW, Patrissi GA, Morrison JC. Stripping the fetal membranes at term—is the procedure safe and efficacious? J Reprod Med 1990;35:811.

47. McColgin SW, Hampton HL, McCaul JF, Howard PR, Andrew ME, Morrison JC. Stripping membranes at term: can it safely reduce the incidence of post-term pregnancies? Obstet Gynecol 1990;76:678.

48. El-Torey M, Grant JM. Sweeping of the membranes is an effective method of induction of labour in prolonged pregnancy: a report of a randomized trial. Br J Obstet Gynecol 1992;99:455.

49. Allott HA, Palmer CR. Sweeping the membranes: a valid procedure in stimulating the onset of labour? Br J Obstet Gynecol 1993;100:898.

50. Wiriyasirivaj B, Vutyavanich T, Ruandsri R-A. A randomized controlled trial of membrane stripping at term to promote labor. Obstet Gynecol 1996;87:767.

51. Berghella V, Rogers RA, Lescale K. Stripping of membranes as a safe method to reduce prolonged pregnancies. Obstet Gynecol 1996;87:927.

52. Crane J, Bennett K, Young D, Windrim R, Kravitz H. The effectiveness of sweeping membranes at term: a randomized trial. Obstet Gynecol 1997;89:586.

53. Magann EF, McNamara MF, Whitworth NS, Chauhan SP, Thorpe RA, Morrison JC. Can we decrease postdatism in women with an unfavorable cervix and a negative fetal fibronectin test by serial membrane sweeping? Am J Obstet Gynecol 1998;179:890.

54. Bochner CJ, Williams III J, Castro L, Medearis A, Hobel CJ, Wade M. The efficacy of starting postterm antenatal testing at 41 weeks as compared with 42 weeks of gestational age. Am J Obstet Gynecol 1988;159:550.

55. Guidetti DA, Divon MY, Langer O. Postdate fetal surveillance: is 41 weeks too early? Am J Obstet Gynecol 1989; 161:91.

56. Grubb DK, Rabelo YA, Paul RH. Post-term pregnancy: fetal death rate with antepartum surveillance. Obstet Gynecol 1992;79:1024.

57. Jazayeri A, Tsibris JCM, Spellacy WN. Elevated umbilical cord plasma erythropoietin levels in prolonged pregnancies. Obstet Gynecol 1998;92:61.

58. Lagrew DC, Freeman RK. Management of postdate pregnancy. Am J Obstet Gynecol 1986;154:8.

59. Boehm FH, Salyer S, Shah DM, Vaughn WK. Improved outcome of twice weekly nonstress testing. Obstet Gynecol 1986;67:566.

60. Eden RD, Gergely RZ, Schifrin BS, Wade ME. Comparison of antepartum testing schemes for the management of the postdate pregnancy. Am J Obstet Gynecol 1982;144:683.

61. Manning FA, Platt LK, Sipos L. Antepartum fetal evaluation: development of a fetal biophysical profile. Am J Obstet Gynecol 1980;136:787.

62. Grubb DK, Rabello YA, Paul RH. Post-term pregnancy: fetal death rate with antepartum surveillance. Obstet Gynecol 1992;79:1024.

63. Lagrew DC, Pircon RA, Nageotte M, Freeman RK, Dorchester W. How frequently should the amniotic fluid index be repeated? Am J Obstet Gynecol 1992;167:1129.

64. Eden RD. Postdate pregnancy: antenatal assessment of fetal well-being. Clin Obstet Gynecol 1989;32:235.

65. Rutherford SE, Phelan JP, Smith CV, Jacobs N. The four quadrant assessment of amniotic fluid volume: an adjunct to antepartum fetal heart rate testing. Obstet Gynecol 1987;70:353.

66. Hannah ME, Hannah WJ, Hellman J, Hewson S, Milner R, Willan A. Induction of labor as compared with serial antenatal monitoring in post-term pregnancy. N Engl J Med 1992;326:1587.

67. The National Institute of Child Health and Human Development Network of Maternal–Fetal Units. A clinical trial of induction of labor versus expectant management in postterm pregnancy. Am J Obstet Gynecol 1994;170:716.

68. Grant JM. Induction of labor confers benefits in prolonged pregnancy. Br J Obstet Gynaecol 1994;101:99.

69. American College of Obstetrician and Gynecologists. Management of postterm pregnancy. ACOG Practice Patterns no. 6. October, 1997.

70. O'Brien WF. Cervical ripening and labor induction: progress and challenges. Clin Obstet Gynecol 1995;38:221.

71. Sanchez-Ramos L, Farah LA, Kaunitz AW, Adair CD, Del Valle GO, Fuqua P. Preinduction cervical ripening with commercially available prostaglandin E_2 gel: a randomized, double-blind comparison with a hospital-compounded preparation. Am J Obstet Gynecol 1995;173:1079.

72. Rayburn W, Gosen R, Ramadei C, Woods R, Scott J Jr. Outpatient cervical ripening with prostaglandin E_2 gel in uncomplicated postdate pregnancies. Am J Obstet Gynecol 1988;158:1417.

73. Sawai SK, O'Brien WF, Mastrogiannis DS, Krammer J, Mastry MG, Porter GW. Patient administered outpatient intravaginal prostaglandin E_2 suppositories in post-date pregnancies: a double-blind, randomized, placebo-controlled study. Obstet Gynecol 1994;84:807.

74. Papageorgiou I, Tsionou C, Minaretzis D, Michalas S, Aravantinos D. Labor characteristics of uncomplicated prolonged pregnancies after induction with intracervical prostaglandin E_2 gel versus intravenous oxytocin. Gynecol Obstet Invest 1992;34:92.

75. Keirse MJNC. Prostaglandins in preinduction cervical ripening—meta-analysis of worldwide clinical experience. J Reprod Med 1993;38:89.

76. Wing DA, Jones MM, Rahall A, Goodwin M, Paul RH. A comparison of misoprostol and prostaglandin E_2 gel for preinduction cervical ripening and labor induction. Am J Obstet Gynecol 1995;172:1804.

77. Wing DA, Rahall A, Jones MM, Goodwin M, Paul RH. Misoprostol: an effective agent for cervical ripening and labor induction. Am J Obstet Gynecol 1995;172:1811.

78. Varaklis K, Gumina R, Stubblefield PG. Randomized controlled trial of vaginal misoprostol and intracervical prostaglandin E_2 gel for induction of labor at term. Obstet Gynecol 1995;86:541.

79. Sanchez-Ramos L, Kaunitz AW, Wears RL, Delke I, Gaudier FL. Misoprostol for cervical ripening and labor induction: a meta-analysis. Obstet Gynecol 1997;89:633.

80. Wing D, Paul RH. A comparison of differing dosing regimens of vaginally administered misoprostol for preinduction cervical ripening and labor induction. Am J Obstet Gynecol 1996;175:158.

81. Farah LA, Sanchez-Ramos L, Rosa C, Del Valle GO, Gaudier FL, Kaunitz AM. Randomized trial of two doses of the prostaglandin E_1 analog misoprostol for labor induction. Am J Obstet Gynecol 1997;177:364.

82. Wing D, Lovett K, Paul RH. Disruption of prior uterine incision following misoprostol for labor induction in women with previous cesarean delivery. Obstet Gynecol 1998;91:828.

83. Bennett BB. Uterine rupture during induction of labor at term with intravaginal misoprostol. Obstet Gynecol 1997; 89:832.

84. Plaut MM, Schwartz ML, Lubarsky SL. Uterine rupture associated with the use of misoprostol in the gravid patient with a previous cesarean section. Am J Obstet Gynecol 1999;180:1535.

Chapter 16

Abnormal Presentations

Michael K. Yancey

Five Key Points

- Malpresentation complicates approximately 5% of term deliveries and up to 10% of preterm deliveries.

- Malpresentation may be a manifestation of an underlying fetal or maternal abnormality or may merely represent a biologic variation in the otherwise normal fetus and mother.

- External cephalic version is a safe and cost-effective means of converting a breech or transverse presentation to a cephalic presentation.

- A selective trial of labor and attempted vaginal breech delivery is a reasonable alternative to cesarean delivery for the term or near-term fetus in a frank or complete breech presentation who cannot be converted to a cephalic presentation by external cephalic version.

- Attempts at vaginal delivery should be performed only by individuals who are experienced in vaginal breech delivery and practice in a facility with adequate ancillary resources.

The position of the fetus in relation to the birth canal during the course of labor is an important consideration for intrapartum management. The fetal lie refers to the position of the fetal longitudinal axis relative to the maternal axis. A longitudinal lie is when the fetus is in a cephalic or breech presentation; a transverse lie is when the fetal long axis is approximately 90 degrees from the maternal long axis (Figure 16-1). A difference of approximately 45 degrees is referred to as an oblique lie, which is generally considered unstable, as the fetus will always convert to a transverse or longitudinal lie during the course of labor. Malpresentation may also occur in the fetus in a cephalic presentation, or head-down longitudinal lie. The degree of flexion or extension of the fetal head is termed attitude, with the normal attitude characteristic of the

vertex presentation being complete flexion with the fetal chin lying against the fetal chest. If the fetal head is in a neutral or slightly extended position, the presentation is termed sinciput. Distinction of this is generally not clinically relevant, as the majority of fetuses will spontaneously convert to a vertex presentation as labor progresses. Moderate extension of the fetal head results in a brow presentation, while extreme extension can result in a face presentation. The approximate frequencies of these various malpresentations are listed in Table 16-1.

In consideration of fetal malpresentation, it is often helpful to consider the factors that may potentially influence fetal presentation. Given that the majority of fetuses are in a vertex presentation at delivery, determination of presentation is unlikely to be

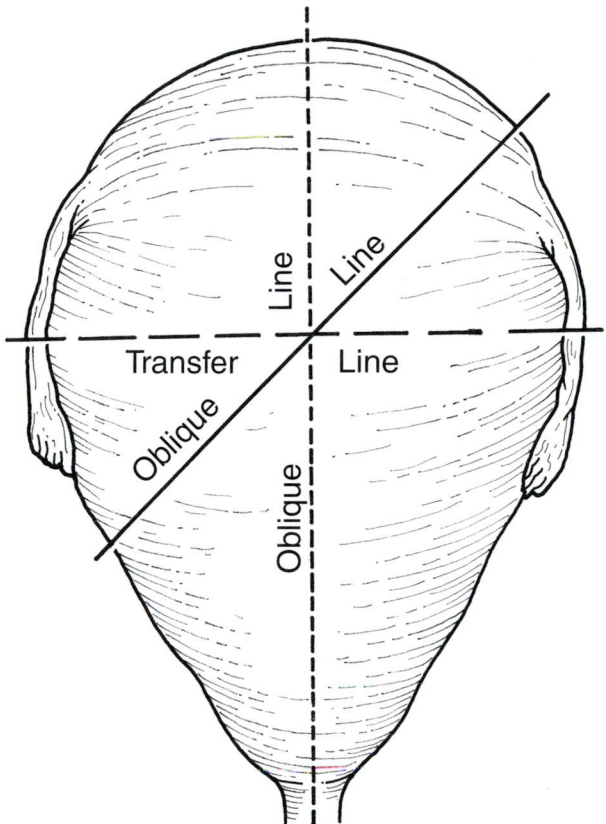

Figure 16-1 Fetal lie in relation to the maternal longitudinal axis. Longitudinal lies include breech and cephalic presentations.

a random event. Determination of fetal presentation is most likely primarily influenced by the general funnel shape of the uterine cavity, with the widest region in the uterine fundus. Since in general the near-term fetus has flexed hips, the breech and lower extremities occupy a greater amount of space than the fetal head; therefore, the fetus tends to be in a position that provides the best fit within the uterine confines—a vertex presentation. Accordingly, when caring for the parturient with a malpresenting fetus, the provider must carefully consider the following issues:

- Is the abnormal presentation merely a chance occurrence due to normal fetal activity within a relatively spacious uterine cavity and maternal pelvis, such as in the preterm fetus of a multiparous patient?
- Could the abnormal presentation be due to an intrinsic problem affecting fetal movement, such as a central nervous system defect or myotonic dystrophy? Alternatively, could there be a fetal anomaly causing alterations in the fetal contours or resting position, such as hydrocephaly and macrocephaly with the enlarged fetal head occupying the uterine

fundus, or an anterior fetal neck mass that could cause extreme extension resulting in a face presentation?
- Is the malpresentation a consequence of alterations in the contours of the intrauterine cavity from intrinsic or extrinsic factors? Intrinsic uterine factors include abnormal placental position or large uterine leiomyoma. Extrinsic factors affecting the contours of the uterine cavity potentially resulting in abnormal presentations include abnormalities of the pelvic architecture, such as a woman with a previous pelvic fracture, or the presence of a pelvic mass such as an ovarian neoplasm.

After consideration of these factors, the clinician may better assess management options in an effort to provide the safest delivery for both mother and fetus. Management options to consider for any parturient with a malpresenting fetus include three basic categories:

- Allow a trial of labor and attempt vaginal delivery of the malpresenting fetus.
- Attempt to convert the malpresentation to a vertex presentation.
- Abandon efforts at vaginal delivery in lieu of abdominal delivery.

Failure to carefully consider the various antecedent factors leading to fetal malpresentation may lead to the incorrect conclusion that perinatal outcome is principally affected by mode of delivery and can be improved by the liberal use of cesarean delivery, a tenet that has not been supported by evidence-based data for many of the various malpresentations.

This chapter will examine the various causes and management issues concerning fetal malpresentation, with emphasis on the management of labor and mode of delivery as it relates to perinatal outcome.

TABLE 16-1
APPROXIMATE DISTRIBUTION OF FETAL PRESENTATIONS AT DELIVERY

Presentation	Proportion	Incidence
Cephalic		
Vertex	95.5%	955 in 1000 births
Brow	0.1%	1 in 1000 births
Face	0.2%	1 in 500 births
Compound	0.15%	1 in 700 births
Breech	3.5%	1 in 30 births
Transverse	0.3%	1 in 300 births
Oblique	0.2%	1 in 500 births

MALPRESENTATION DUE TO DEFLEXION ATTITUDES

Deflexion of the fetal head early in the course of labor is a relatively infrequent occurrence. The soft tissue and bony elements of the pelvis tend to promote passage of the fetal head in a flexed attitude, with the smallest dimension of the fetal head presenting to the birth canal (Figure 16-2). The true incidence of fetuses with some degree of deflexion at the onset of labor is not currently known, as many such fetuses probably spontaneously convert to a normally flexed attitude (vertex presentation) as labor progresses. However, recognition of the persistent deflexion abnormality can alert the care provider to the increased likelihood of abnormal labor progression and the need for careful postnatal assessment of the neonate.

Face Presentation

Face presentation is caused by full extension of the fetal head with the fetal occiput lying against its upper back. This presentation is found in approximately 1 in 500 births.[1] Of all the various malpresentations discussed in this chapter, face presentation is associated with the highest incidence of serious underlying fetal abnormalities. Anencephaly, iniencephaly, and anterior fetal neck masses, such as a goiter or teratoma, may be present in up to 60% of fetuses with face presentation.[1-3] Other predisposing factors include contracted maternal pelvis, multiparity, prematurity, and macrosomia.[1,4] Prenatal diagnosis can be accomplished by the use of the Leopold maneuver, with the finding of a cephalic prominence on the same side of the maternal abdomen as the fetal back. Visual inspection of the maternal abdomen will demonstrate an elongated fetal contour due to the extended neck and unengaged head. In addition, a groove may be palpated between the fetal occiput and back. However, only approximately 5% of infants with face presentations are diagnosed prior to the onset of labor, with the majority diagnosed in the late active phase or second stage of labor.[1,5] This may be due in part to the fact that the majority of fetuses with face presentation initially present to the pelvic inlet in a brow presentation with subsequent extension of the head as descent occurs.

Diagnosis is principally accomplished by digital examination with palpation of fetal mouth, nose, and orbits. It may occasionally be difficult to differentiate a face presentation from a breech presentation, particularly in the patient diagnosed during the second stage of labor, when substantial facial edema may be

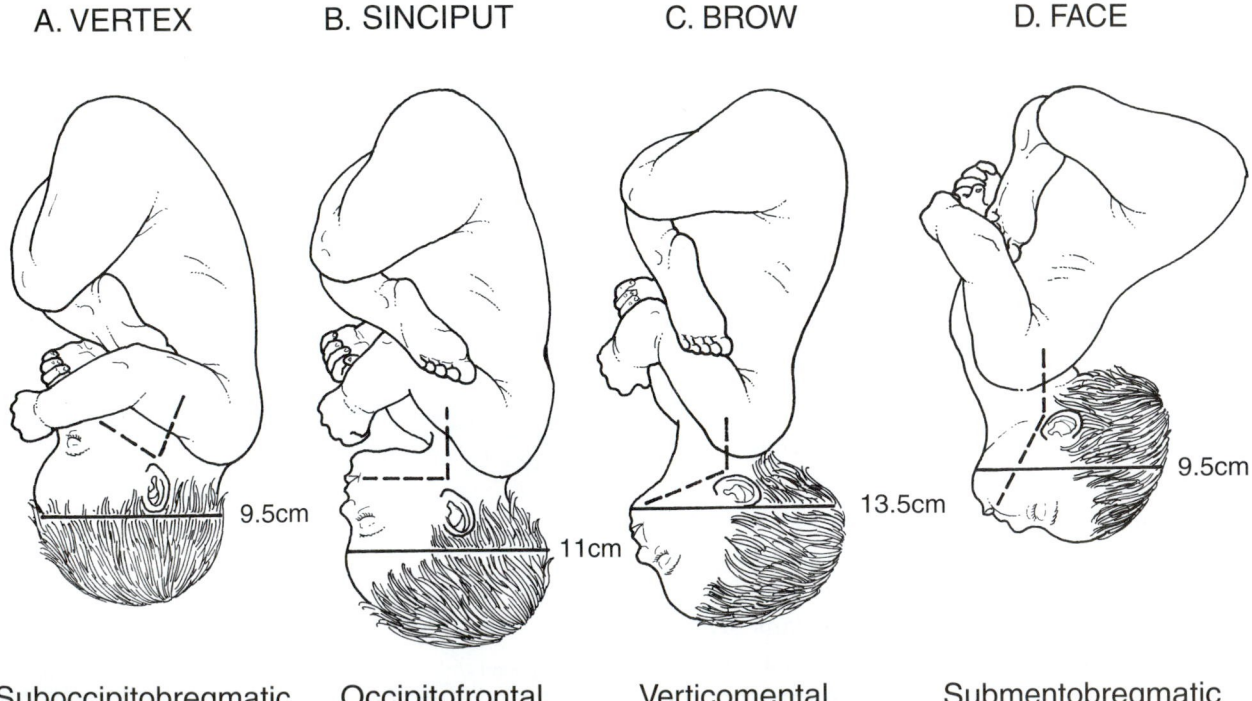

A. VERTEX	B. SINCIPUT	C. BROW	D. FACE
9.5cm	11cm	13.5cm	9.5cm
Suboccipitobregmatic	Occipitofrontal	Verticomental	Submentobregmatic

Figure 16-2 Types of cephalic presentations, with corresponding largest anteroposterior diameters that must traverse the birth canal.

present. One useful means is to examine the relationship between the orifice and bony prominences of the presenting part. A face presentation will have a triangular relationship between the mouth and adjacent malar eminences, while a breech presentation will be characterized by the presence of the anus at the midpoint of a straight line between the ischial tuberosities. Equivocal findings should prompt immediate intrapartum sonography. Given the relatively high frequency of lethal anomalies such as anencephaly, an intrapartum fetal anatomic survey of the cranial structures should be performed if not previously done during the antenatal period.

The course of labor for the fetus with a face presentation is often prolonged due to the relatively larger dimension of the fetal head presenting to the maternal pelvis in comparison to a vertex presentation.[6] There is an increased likelihood of cephalopelvic disproportion, and the cardinal movements of labor are impaired, most importantly flexion of the fetal head at the time of delivery. The point of reference for determining position of the fetal head relative to the maternal pelvis is the chin, or mentum. The prognosis for vaginal delivery depends on the orientation of the fetal head within the maternal pelvis. The most favorable prognosis for vaginal delivery is associated with a mentum anterior position. Fortunately, this is the most common orientation noted at the time of diagnosis, occurring in approximately 70% of cases, while 10% are mentum transverse orientation and 20% mentum posterior.[6] In the absence of fetal macrosomia or relative maternal pelvic contracture, the majority of infants with a mentum anterior face presentation will deliver either spontaneously or by assisted vaginal delivery. In addition, many infants with a mentum transverse orientation will undergo internal rotation and deliver from mentum anterior orientation. While approximately 25% of infants with a mentum posterior orientation will undergo spontaneous rotation to a mentum anterior position, those who remain in a persistent mentum posterior orientation are unlikely to deliver vaginally.[6,7] Overall, vaginal delivery occurs in approximately 70 to 80% of fetuses with a face presentation. Cesarean delivery can be difficult, particularly when done in the second stage. It is often helpful to have an assistant provide transvaginal elevation of the fetal head with both the surgeon and an assistant attempting to flex the head as it is raised from the pelvis. Flexion of the head prior to delivery through the uterine incision will

decrease the potential for extension of the incision and fetal cervical spine injury from hyperextension.

Attempts at manual conversion of the face presentation to a vertex presentation or delivery by internal podalic version are contraindicated, as such procedures are associated with extraordinarily high rates of fetal and maternal trauma.[7,8] Therefore, expectant management is recommended for the fetus with a face presentation in labor. While prolongation of labor is common, a continued trial of labor is a reasonable option as long as progress is made. Oxytocin augmentation should be considered only in situations in which labor is progressing abnormally, there is a hypocontractile uterine pattern, and there is no evidence of cephalopelvic disproportion.

Nonreassuring fetal heart patterns are more likely to be encountered in the fetus with a face presentation relative to a vertex presentation; therefore, continuous electronic monitoring is recommended. Fetal heart monitoring is ideally achieved through the use of an external device, as the placement of a fetal electrode can result in serious ocular injury or scarring of the fetal face. In situations in which external monitoring is inadequate, a fetal electrode may be carefully placed on the fetal chin or brow at or above the hairline. Prolongation of the second stage is common; however, continued efforts at vaginal delivery are recommended as long as progress is made. In the event of nonreassuring fetal heart monitoring, low or outlet forceps delivery may be attempted if the fetus is in a mentum anterior position and the operator has sufficient experience with this procedure. The use of a vacuum device is contraindicated.

Operative vaginal delivery is generally not recommended if the fetus is in a mentum transverse or posterior orientation. Vaginal delivery may result in marked facial edema and bruising and rarely laryngeal or tracheal edema due to pressure on these structures as the fetus traverses the birth canal.[9] Therefore, it is recommended that pediatricians skilled in neonatal intubation attend the delivery.

Brow Presentation

Deflexion of the fetal head to a neutral or partially extended position results in a brow presentation, which occurs in approximately in 1 in 1000 deliveries.[6,10] Similar to face presentations, this abnormality is likely an underrecognized occurrence in the early stages of labor, with many fetuses undergoing spontaneous flexion to assume a vertex presentation as the head descends through the birth canal. Diagnosis of a brow presentation prior to the onset of labor is unusual, with the majority being diagnosed in the late active phase or second stage of labor.[10,11] The diagnosis is typically determined by digital examination through a dilated cervix with palpation of the anterior fontanel, orbits, and upper nose. Associated factors include prematurity, extreme cephalopelvic disproportion, grand multiparity, and polyhydramnios.[6,11]

The point of reference on the fetal head is the frontal bone immediately anterior to the anterior fontanel, referred to as the frontum. The prognosis for vaginal delivery is most favorable in fetuses with a frontum anterior orientation.[11] Dystocia is common with brow presentation as the largest diameter of the fetal head; the verticomental diameter presents to the maternal pelvis (see Figure 16-2). Continued progress in labor and subsequent vaginal delivery typically occur only when there is a spontaneous conversion to either vertex or face presentation, or when the fetal head is relatively small in relation to the maternal pelvic capacity. Spontaneous conversion to a vertex or face presentation has been reported to occur in approximately two thirds of fetuses diagnosed with brow presentation in labor, and the majority of these will deliver vaginally.[6] However, if spontaneous conversion does not occur, the prognosis for successful vaginal delivery worsens, as less than half of fetuses with a persistent brow presentation will undergo spontaneous vaginal delivery, and protracted labor and secondary arrest disorders are common.

Attempts to convert a brow presentation to a vertex presentation with manual displacement of the vertex or manipulation with obstetric forceps are contraindicated due to the potential for serious traumatic injury to the fetus and mother. Therefore, expectant management and a carefully monitored trial of labor with minimal intervention is the recommended management for the majority of fetuses diagnosed with this condition. Persistent nonreassuring fetal heart rate patterns, secondary arrest disorders, or obvious cephalopelvic disproportion are best treated with expeditious cesarean delivery. Oxytocin should be used only when there is evidence of abnormal progression of labor and a hypocontractile uterine pattern.

Compound Presentation

A compound presentation occurs when there is an extremity lying adjacent to the presenting part, most

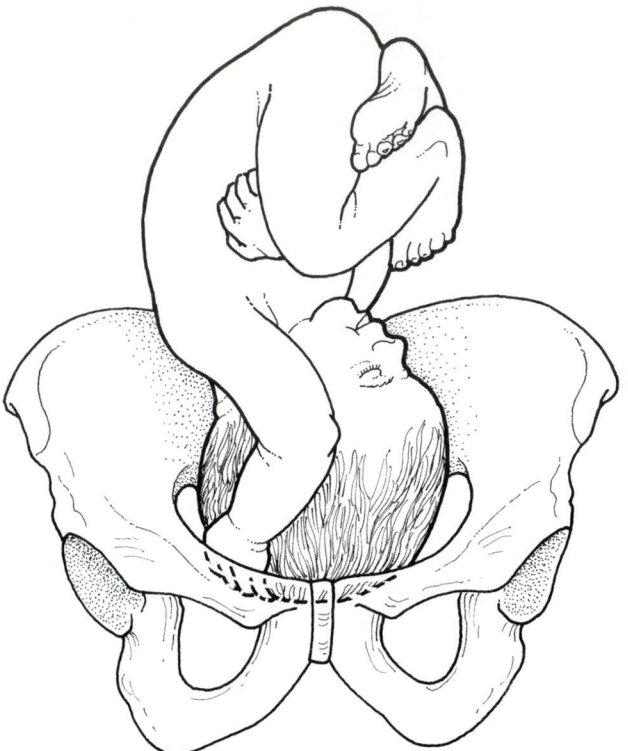

Figure 16-3 Compound presentation with the fetal hand and arm lying adjacent to the vertex. This is the most common type of compound presentation.

typically a fetus in a cephalic presentation with an upper extremity, or rarely, lower extremity immediately adjacent to the vertex (Figure 16-3). The incidence of compound presentation is approximately 1 in 700 deliveries; prematurity is the most common contributing factor.[6,12] An additional antecedent factor is an unstable lie or breech presentation prior to the onset of labor with preceding conversion to a vertex presentation either spontaneously or by external cephalic version.[13] Following rupture of the membranes, umbilical-cord prolapse occurs in 10 to 20% of cases.[6,12] Another potential cause of adverse perinatal outcome is trauma to the prolapsed extremity during the course of labor. Injuries to the extremity include soft-tissue damage, fractures of the long bones, neurologic injury, or ischemia due to compression of the vascular supply.

The diagnosis of this condition is not typically made until the active phase of labor. The probability that the fetus will spontaneously retract the extremity is related to the stage of labor at which the diagnosis is made, with eventual conversion to a vertex presentation occurring frequently when compound presentation is diagnosed in the latent or early active phase of labor. A persistent compound presentation is associated with vaginal delivery when the extremity is relatively small, such as when the fetal hand lies alongside the vertex, or in cases of a preterm fetus delivered to a mother with a normal or generous pelvic capacity. Vaginal delivery of a term or near-term fetus is unlikely when the fetal arm lies adjacent to the vertex. Efforts to manipulate the prolapsed extremity should not be attempted because of the risk for cord prolapse or trauma to the extremity. Oxytocin augmentation should be offered only judiciously to women who have evidence of protracted labor and a hypocontractile uterine pattern.

Transverse Presentation

When the fetal longitudinal axis crosses the maternal longitudinal axis, the fetus is deemed to be in a transverse or oblique lie (Figure 16-4). A transverse lie is present when the fetal longitudinal axis is perpendicular to the maternal axis, while an oblique lie occurs when the fetal axis lies approximately 45 degrees off the maternal axis. Prior to labor or rupture of membranes, the fetus in an oblique lie may rotate to a longitudinal lie and then back to an oblique or transverse lie, a situation often referred to as an unstable lie. A nonlongitudinal lie at the onset of labor or rupture of membranes can result in either the umbilical cord or an extremity prolapsing through the cervix or the fetus lying across the maternal pelvis with the midportion of the back adjacent to the pelvic inlet; these situations are not conducive to safe vaginal delivery. Transverse or oblique presentations are associated with umbilical-cord prolapse in approximately 20% of cases, the highest risk of any of the malpresentations.[6,14] Predisposing factors for a transverse or oblique lie include grand multiparity, prematurity, placenta previa, or extreme pelvic contracture. The overall incidence is approximately 1 in 300 deliveries, with a much higher incidence in preterm deliveries.[6,14] While suspicion of a transverse or oblique lie may be entertained following clinical examination with the Leopold maneuvers, definitive diagnosis is generally made with sonographic or radiographic studies. Following the onset of labor, the absence of a palpable presenting part should generate suspicion for a transverse or oblique lie. Only 25 to 50% of fetuses in a oblique or transverse lie are diagnosed prior to the onset of labor.[6,14,15] If the diagnosis is made prior to the onset of labor, a targeted sonographic examination should be performed to evaluate for major fetal malformations and to exclude placenta previa.

Following exclusion of patients with placenta previa or fetal malformations not conducive to vaginal delivery, consideration should be given to attempts at conversion of the term or near-term fetus to a longitudinal presentation by external cephalic version.[15] Alternatives to external cephalic version are expectant management and immediate delivery by cesarean.

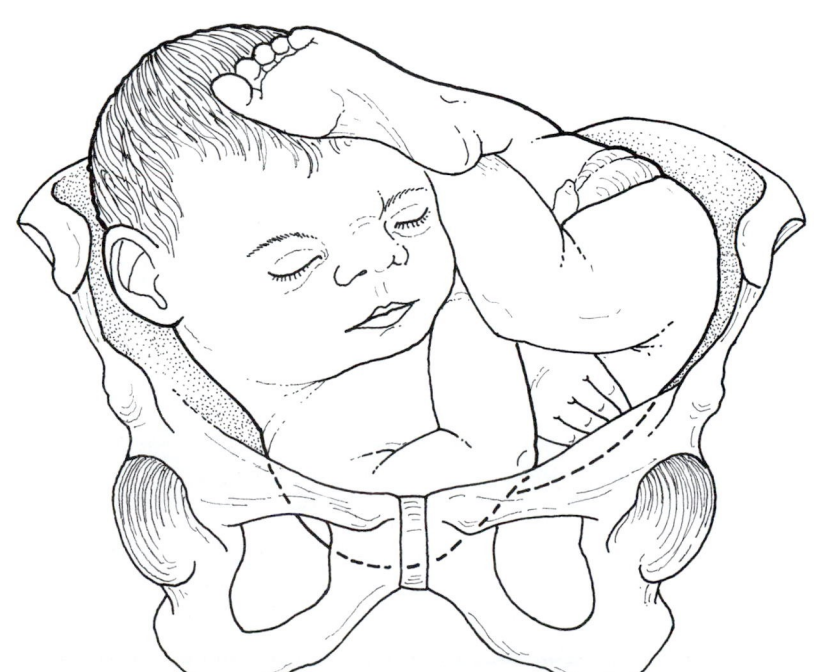

Figure 16-4 Transverse presentation with the fetal longitudinal axis perpendicular to the maternal longitudinal axis. Neglected labor in this situation can result in prolapse of the arm through the cervix.

Phelan and colleagues reported their observational experience with 29 patients diagnosed with a transverse lie at term managed expectantly.[16] Spontaneous conversion to either a vertex or breech presentation prior to the onset of labor occurred in 83% of cases. However, only 55% of the patients ultimately delivered vaginally, and the majority of cesarean deliveries were performed for persistent malpresentation. One patient suffered uterine rupture, and there were two cases of umbilical-cord prolapse and one neonatal death. Prospective trials of external cephalic version have described more favorable results; thus, it is recommended that the patient at term diagnosed with a transverse or oblique presentation be offered an attempt at external cephalic version.[17] If the fetus can be converted to a cephalic or breech presentation and the patient's cervix is favorable, labor may be induced. If the cervix is unfavorable for induction, close monitoring is provided to ensure that the fetus remains in a longitudinal lie. If the version attempt is unsuccessful, consideration should be given to immediate cesarean delivery.[15]

Due to the unacceptably high rates of fetal trauma, perinatal death and maternal morbidity, internal podalic version and breech extraction are not recommended in the singleton gestation with a transverse or oblique lie. If cesarean delivery is selected for the fetus in a transverse or oblique lie, careful preoperative and intraoperative consideration of the specific type of abdominal and uterine incisions should occur, as the lower uterine segment may be poorly developed in these circumstances. Intraoperative version to a longitudinal lie is occasionally useful, particularly if the fetus is in a back-down transverse lie.[18] If the version is successful, an upper-segment uterine incision may be avoided. If version is unsuccessful and the back-down transverse lie persists, a classic cesarean incision is usually indicated.

Breech Presentation

Breech presentation is a relatively common finding, with the incidence inversely related to the gestational age at the time of assessment (Table 16-2). Sonographic assessment in the late second trimester will demonstrate approximately 25% of fetuses in a breech presentation, a proportion that falls to less than 5% at term.[20] Similarly, breech presentation is encountered in approximately 20% of fetuses delivered at 25 to 28 weeks as compared with less than 3% at term.[19] There

are three basic types of breech presentation (Figure 16-5). The frank breech fetus has flexed hips and extended knees with the feet typically in the proximity of the vertex, occupying the uterine fundus. The fetus in a complete breech presentation has flexed hips and one or both knees flexed. The footling, or incomplete, breech presentation is defined as a fetus with one or both hips extended and the fetal foot or knee presenting to the cervical opening. At term, the frank breech presentation is the most common subtype, while footling breech presentation predominates in the preterm population (Table 16-3).[20,21]

Causative or predisposing factors for breech presentation are similar to those for other types of malpresentation and generally relate to abnormalities of fetal activity, fetal shape, or the contours or size of the intrauterine compartment. The incidence of breech presentation is increased in multiparous patients relative to nulliparous patients, likely due to increased laxity in the maternal abdominal and uterine musculature in the former. In addition, the incidence is increased if there is either oligohydramnios or polyhydramnios. Oligohydramnios results in restricted space for the fetus to move and reduces the likelihood that the preterm gestation will be able to spontaneously convert to a cephalic presentation by term. Conversely, excessive amounts of amniotic fluid may allow for increased fetal mobility with frequent alterations in presentation.

TABLE 16-2
PROPORTION OF SINGLETON GESTATIONS IN A BREECH PRESENTATION AT VARIOUS GESTATIONAL AGES

Gestational Age (wk)	Breech by Sonography (%)	Breech at Delivery (%)
25–28	27.8	21.3
29–32	14	8.2
33–36	8.8	5.4
37–40	6.7	2.6

Derived from Scheer and Nubar[19] and Hickok et al.[20]

TABLE 16-3
DISTRIBUTION OF TYPES OF BREECH PRESENTATION

	% Overall	% of Term	% of Preterm
Frank	60	70	40
Complete	10	10	10
Footling	30	20	50

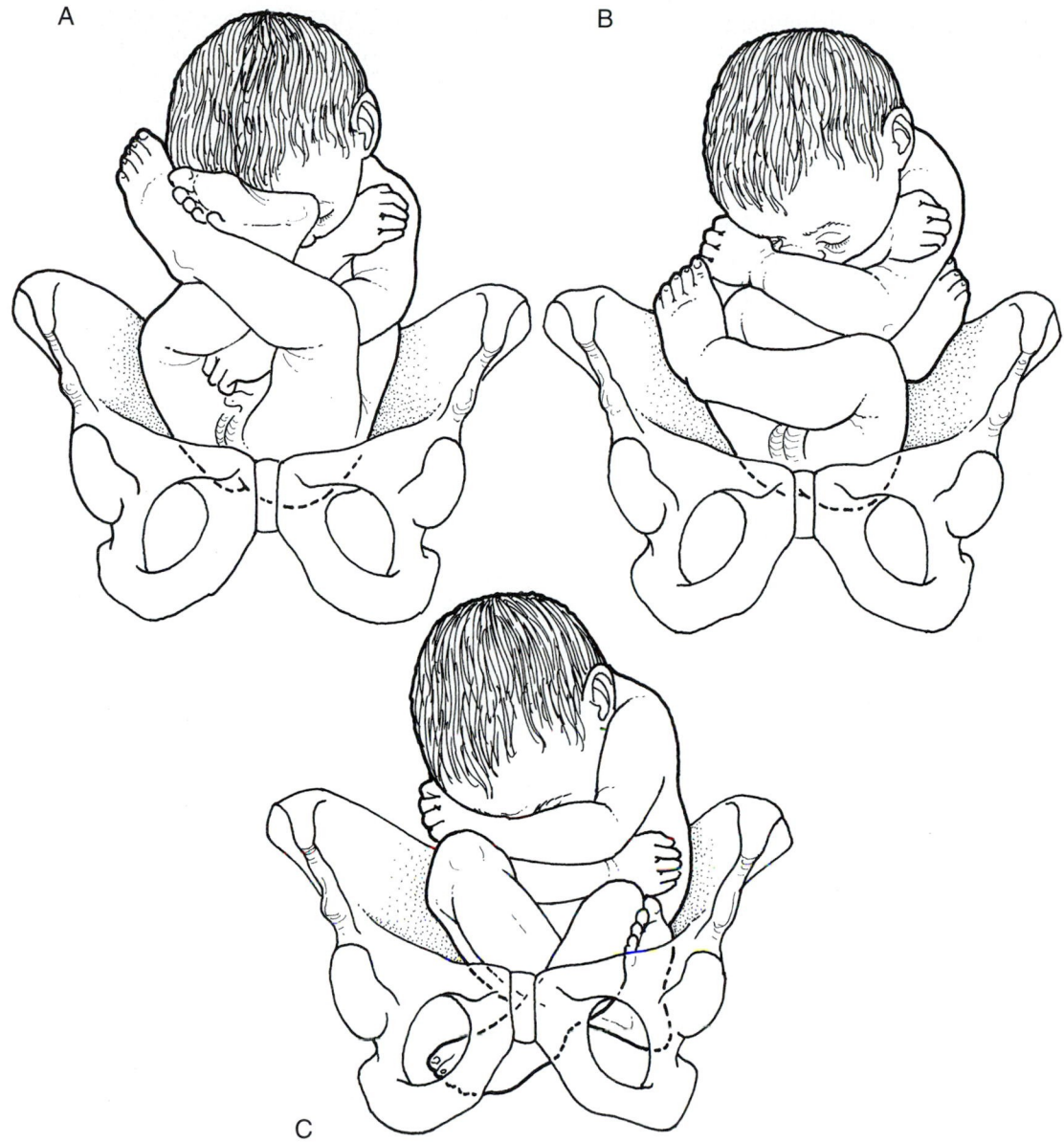

Figure 16-5 Types of breech presentation. A. Frank. B. Complete. C. Incomplete.

Breech presentation is a common finding in multiple gestations with one or both fetuses in a noncephalic presentation in approximately 60% of twin gestations. Uterine and placental factors may predispose to breech presentation with an increased incidence noted in women who have müllerian anomalies such as a septate uterus or uterine didelphys.[22] It has also been reported that placental implantation in the cornual–fundal position is a more common finding in breech as compared with cephalic presentations.[23] Maternal pelvic masses may impinge on the lower uterine segment, allowing less room for the fetal vertex to occupy, predisposing to breech presentation. Abnormal fetal tone or movement due to

neuromuscular disorders, such as myotonic dystrophy, or severe central nervous system abnormalities, such as anencephaly or hydrocephalus, are associated with increased risk for breech presentation.[24,25] Fetal aneuploidy is also associated with an increased incidence of breech presentation, possibly related to prematurity, decreased fetal size, and abnormal fetal activity.[24] However, in spite of the multitude of predisposing factors that have been previously described, the majority of term breech fetuses have no identified risk factor.

Diagnosis

The diagnosis of breech presentation can be confirmed through physical examination or imaging studies. The examination maneuvers described by Leopold have historically been used to identify the fetus with a malpresentation. Unfortunately, the positive predictive value of this technique is only approximately 30%, and at least 25% of breech-presenting fetuses at term are misdiagnosed as a cephalic presentation using this technique.[26] Another means of detecting the fetus in the breech presentation is by pelvic examination with palpation and identification of the presenting fetal part by digital examination through a dilated cervix. Unfortunately, these findings may also be misleading, particularly in the patient with minimal cervical dilation. In general, relying on physical examination techniques results in identification of approximately 60% of term breech presentations prior to labor.[27] Ultrasound is a highly sensitive and specific test for confirmation of fetal presentation, and it should be used liberally in women at term who are deemed to be at risk or have physical findings suggestive of malpresentation. Thorp and colleagues found that the routine use of Leopold maneuvers and the liberal use of sonography reduced the percentage of term breech fetuses with initial diagnosis in labor.[26] The detection of breech presentation prior to labor is a worthwhile clinical goal, as the patient may then undergo evaluation for underlying problems that might have resulted in the malpresentation and be appropriately counseled regarding management options.

Perinatal Outcome

In comparing the perinatal outcome of breech fetuses relative to infants delivered from a cephalic presentation, it becomes apparent that, regardless of the route of delivery, breech fetuses tend to have lower birth weights, decreased placental mass, a higher perinatal mortality rate, and an increased incidence of major congenital anomalies, aneuploidy, and subsequent cerebral palsy.[21,28-34] In addition, there is a higher incidence of adverse intrapartum events such as placental abruption, prolapse of the umbilical cord, low Apgar scores, and decreased umbilical-cord pH values.[9,29,35-37]

Specific complications of vaginal delivery include approximately a twofold increase in birth trauma relative to cephalic infants.[29,31,38,39] Injuries include peripheral-nerve damage, such as brachial plexus palsy, intracerebral hemorrhage due to rupture of superior cerebral bridging veins or posterior fossa bleeding from extension of lacerations to the tentorium into the lateral-strait sinuses. In fact, intracerebral hemor-

rhages are the most common cause of perinatal death in nonanomalous breech fetuses. Breech fetuses delivered vaginally also have been reported to have traumatic rupture of the liver or spleen, hemorrhage into the adrenal gland, spinal-cord injury, bruise or trauma to the kidney, bladder, or genitalia or musculoskeletal injuries, including long-bone fractures.[22,29,31,39] In addition, labor-arrest disorders are more common in breech as compared with cephalic infants, particularly in those weighing more than 3500 g, with cesarean delivery rates as high as 75% due to labor arrest.[39,40]

Effect of Mode of Delivery on Outcome for the Breech Fetus at Term

Schutte and colleagues analyzed 57,819 infants in the Netherlands and found an increased perinatal mortality rate for breech infants as compared with cephalic infants after correction for gestational age, congenital anomalies, and birth weight.[34] These authors concluded that "it may be that breech presentation may not be coincidental but rather a product of the quality of the infant so that the 'fittest' infants present by the vertex and the 'weakest' by the breech. If there is some truth in this supposition, it is unlikely that medical intervention based upon present knowledge can improve the outcomes of infants in breech presentation to the same level as that for infants in vertex presentation."[34] Nonetheless, there has been a dramatic shift in the percentage of breech fetuses delivered by cesarean over the past several decades, climbing from <10% to over 90% in many centers.[28,41]

However, the impact of mode of delivery on the perinatal outcome of the term fetus in a breech presentation remains one of the more contentious issues in contemporary obstetrics. Population-based studies have shown an increase in relative risk for perinatal mortality following vaginal delivery of the breech infant, even after controlling for birth weight and demographic factors.[22,42-44] But none of these studies controlled for the means of selection of infants for vaginal delivery over cesarean delivery or the specific intrapartum management methods used. Retrospective cohort studies have found conflicting results, with some investigations demonstrating an increased relative risk for poor perinatal outcome for breech fetuses delivered vaginally as compared with breech fetuses delivered abdominally,[22,45] while other similar studies have failed to detect any statistically significant differences.[27,46-49]

There are a multitude of factors that could have significant effects on perinatal outcome. Therefore, the ideal study method for attempting to determine the role of delivery route on neonatal health for the breech-presenting fetus would be a prospective randomized trial. While two prospective randomized trials have been reported, these trials have had inadequate sample sizes to provide sufficient power to exclude a clinically significant increase in perinatal mortality with selective vaginal delivery.[50,51] Collea et al. prospectively studied 208 women with fetuses in a frank breech presentation with estimated fetal weights of 2500 to 3800 g and no hyperextension of the fetal head.[50] One hundred fifteen of these patients were randomized to intended trial of labor, and these women subsequently underwent x-ray pelvimetry. Women who had adequate pelvimetry had a 82.6% vaginal delivery rate with no perinatal deaths; two infants suffered transient brachial plexus injuries. Gimovsky et al. studied 105 women with fetuses in a nonfrank presentation, randomizing 35 to cesarean delivery and 70 to attempted trial of labor.[51] Thirty-nine of the 70 women who were randomized to trial of labor had inadequate pelvimetry or had a failed trial of labor and underwent cesarean delivery, while the remaining 31 (44%) delivered vaginally without an increase in perinatal morbidity.

Unfortunately, it is highly unlikely that a large prospective randomized trial will be accomplished, as such a trial would require over 7000 patients in order to have sufficient power to exclude an excess perinatal mortality of 2 per 1000 neonates. Also, the counseling of patients for enrollment in a multicenter trial has proven to be extremely problematic and likely prohibitive for a large randomized trial.[52]

In the absence of a randomized trial with sufficient sample size, several authors have attempted to compare large cohorts of infants delivered by various routes through multiple regression analysis, with many concluding that the mode of delivery may not have a significant effect on perinatal outcome when other significant confounding variables are controlled through regression analysis. Oian et al. studied 580 breech infants and analyzed the effect of 56 variables on perinatal mortality.[53] Factors that were significantly associated with an increase in perinatal mortality rate were low birth weight, maternal diabetes, congenital anomalies, and a 5-minute Apgar scores of less than 7. Rosen and colleagues used multiple regression analysis in infants with a birth weight of less than 4 kg and concluded that the route of delivery for a breech-presenting fetus may not significantly affect outcome.[54] Croughan-Minihane studied the

long-term morbidity associated with breech presentation through multiple regression analysis in 1240 infants and determined that the route of delivery had no impact on neonatal asphyxia, intracranial hemorrhage, seizures, cerebral palsy, or developmental delays.[41] Danielian and colleagues similarly found no increase in long-term neurodevelopmental handicaps associated with vaginal breech delivery as compared with breech fetuses delivered by cesarean.[46] Finally, many authors have found no improvement in perinatal mortality rates associated with breech presentation over the past several decades in spite of a trend toward more liberal use of cesarean delivery.[28,47,53,55]

It is apparent that vaginal delivery of the breech fetus poses some increase in risk for adverse perinatal outcome due to fetal head entrapment, birth trauma, or asphyxia as compared with cesarean delivery.[29,36,56,57] Likewise, there is little question that cesarean delivery increases the likelihood of maternal morbidity and mortality as compared with vaginal delivery.[58] The preferred mode of delivery for the breech fetus should ideally have the lowest overall cumulative maternal and fetal risk.

The critical question at the heart of the controversy is the accurate delineation of risk associated with an intent to vaginally deliver the term fetus in a frank breech presentation without macrosomia, major anomaly, or hyperextended head. Cheng and Hannah pooled data from 24 studies published between 1966 and 1992 for analysis of perinatal mortality and morbidity with regard to the intended mode of delivery.[59] These authors concluded that, relative to cesarean delivery, the intent to deliver the breech-presenting fetus vaginally resulted in an almost fourfold increase in the corrected perinatal mortality rate (odds ratio, 3.89; 95% confidence interval, 2.22–6.69) and a nearly threefold increase in long-term morbidity (odds ratio, 2.88; 95% confidence interval, 1.04–7.97).

While this analysis provides some useful information, it is apparent that contemporary intrapartum management methods and expected perinatal outcome for all infants is not comparable to techniques and outcomes three decades ago. Indeed, including only the studies that used radiographic pelvimetry for selection of candidates and intrapartum fetal monitoring with exclusion of fetuses with hyperextended heads, the differences in corrected perinatal mortality and long-term morbidity were not statistically significantly different. Also, many of the included studies were retrospective, nonrandomized trials, thus increasing the potential for selection bias affecting the results. A meta-analysis of contemporary selective trials selected nine investigations for inclusion, two prospective randomized trials and seven cohort studies.[57] The authors found that the pooled increase in risk associated with a selective trial of labor was a 0.9% increase in injury and a 1.1% increase in either injury or perinatal death associated with a selected trial of labor. Excluding trials that contained fetuses delivered vaginally from a nonfrank breech presentation lowered the pooled increase in risk for serious injury to 0.6% and risk for injury or death to 1.0%. These results were heavily influenced by a single study that contributed the majority of adverse outcomes to the pooled results.[45]

In contrast to these meta-analysis investigations, which pooled results from studies spanning several decades with disparate management methods, there have been numerous studies reporting encouraging results with protocols for selective vaginal breech delivery.[40,47,60-65] After collectively considering the favorable published experience with such protocols and the results of the two prospective, randomized trials, a selective trial of labor and attempted vaginal breech delivery appears to be a reasonable option for the parturient with a fetus in the frank or complete breech presentation, an estimated fetal weight between 2000 and 4000 g, and adequate pelvimetry.[65]

Mode of Delivery for the Preterm Breech Fetus

While it appears that a selective trial of labor for the term breech fetus may be a reasonable option, there are fewer data that are supportive of the safety and efficacy of vaginal delivery of the preterm breech fetus. There are no prospective randomized trials that have demonstrated safety of this approach, and retrospective investigations suggest that there is a higher perinatal morbidity and mortality rate associated with vaginal breech delivery in infants with birth weights of less than 1500 g.[66-73] Potential reasons for this increase in morbidity and mortality include the higher frequency of nonfrank presentations in preterm fetuses with a greater risk of cord prolapse and subsequent asphyxial injury. Furthermore, preterm fetuses have an increase in the head-circumference-to-abdominal-circumference ratio, and the predominant nonfrank presentations provide less effective cervical dilation than the buttocks and legs of the frank breech; both factors, in turn, increase the risk of head entrapment.[66] Finally, the preterm fetus has a cerebral

vasculature with a greater propensity for traumatic rupture.

Interestingly, in spite of these differences, other retrospective studies have suggested that the mode of delivery may have minimal impact on neonatal outcome in the very-low-birth-weight breech fetus.[74-77] A likely explanation for the discrepant findings in these retrospective studies is the potential for selection bias in the management of these fetuses, as the parturient with a breech fetus expected to have a poor neonatal outcome is less likely to undergo cesarean delivery than is the woman whose fetus is expected to do well.[69] However, until further investigations provide more definitive results, cesarean delivery will probably remain the most appropriate mode of delivery in the nonanomalous very-low-birth-weight breech fetus (700 to 1500 g). Extremely-low-birth-weight fetuses (500 to 700 g) or the preterm breech fetus with a major anomaly are less likely to have their overall outcome improved by cesarean delivery. In addition, the majority of cesarean deliveries for extremely-low-birth-weight breech fetuses require vertical uterine incisions, a procedure that will have profound effects on future pregnancies. Therefore, the mode of delivery in such situations should be individualized according to the patient's desires and the clinical circumstances.

MANAGEMENT OF THE BREECH PRESENTATION

External Cephalic Version

As the proportion of breech fetuses who have been delivered vaginally has declined, so has the cumulative experience of practicing obstetricians in the methods of vaginal breech delivery. Residency training programs have likewise been faced with a decline in vaginal breech deliveries, and it is likely that many graduating residents now have only limited experience in vaginal breech delivery. Furthermore, even if training is adequate, the typical obstetrician may only perform two to three vaginal breech deliveries annually, a number that may not ensure proficiency. The only remaining delivery option for the breech-presenting fetus is a cesarean delivery, which increases maternal morbidity and is more costly than vaginal delivery. Thus, reducing the number of breech fetuses through the use of external cephalic version has emerged as perhaps the least controversial and most widely accepted management option.

The effectiveness of external cephalic version as a means of converting the breech fetus to a vertex presentation has been confirmed over the past several decades.[17,78] A review of prospective trials, including more than 1300 patients, found an overall success rate of approximately 65%.[17] Only 2% of the fetuses who underwent successful version returned to a breech presentation at delivery, as compared with control populations in which approximately 85% of breech fetuses at 37 to 38 weeks remained breech at delivery. Zhang and colleagues estimated that if external cephalic version is used extensively, cesarean delivery rates for malpresentation would be approximately 50% less, regardless of the management approach for breech fetuses in labor (selective trial of labor or universal cesarean delivery).[17] Using a hypothetical population of women with fetuses in a breech presentation, these authors estimated that a program using external cephalic version would result in a cesarean delivery rate of 36.7%, as compared with an 83.2% rate without external cephalic version. Gifford and colleagues performed decision analysis attempting to determine the most cost-effective approach to the management of the breech fetus at term.[79] These authors studied four alternative management strategies and found that external cephalic version followed by selective trial of labor for the remaining breech-presenting fetuses was the most cost-effective approach.

Complications of external cephalic version are unusual.[17,80] While fetal bradycardia occurs in approximately 20% of fetuses undergoing external version attempts, this usually spontaneously resolves and is not associated with further nonreassuring fetal testing.[17] Fetal distress requiring abdominal delivery occurs in less than 1% of breech-presenting fetuses and fetal–maternal hemorrhage occurs in approximately 6% of patients.[17]

Maternal conditions that are absolute contraindications to external cephalic version are placenta previa, ruptured membranes, and multiple gestation. Relative contraindications to attempts at external cephalic version include uterine anomalies such as a septate or bicornuate uterus, the presence of third-trimester bleeding, prenatal identification of a nuchal cord, or suspected fetal pelvic disproportion, which would make vaginal delivery unlikely even in the event that the fetus was in a vertex presentation. In addition, the fetus with suspected intrauterine growth restriction

or oligohydramnios may be a poor candidate for external cephalic version. The safety of external cephalic version in the woman with a prior cesarean delivery has not been extensively studied; however, a small series has been reported with no excess complications.[81]

The likelihood of successful external cephalic version is related to a multitude of factors. Lower success rates have been associated with primiparity, anterior placental implantation, maternal obesity, fetal macrosomia, frank breech presentation, back posterior fetal position, and engagement of the presenting part.[82-84]

In general, external cephalic version should be avoided in the preterm fetus for three principal reasons. (1) Expectant management of the preterm fetus in a breech presentation is associated with a spontaneous version rate of approximately 90% in breech infants between 28 and 36 weeks of gestation. (2) Preterm fetuses who undergo successful external cephalic version have a greater likelihood of returning to a breech presentation prior to the onset of labor than is the term fetus following successful version. (3) Performing external cephalic version procedures in preterm gestations will occasionally result in preterm delivery due to fetal distress or premature labor.[85] The procedure should be performed prior to 40 weeks of gestation as decreased success rates have been noted after 40 weeks.[17] Newman and colleagues reported a scoring system used for the prediction of success rate based on various maternal factors, providing a potential means of selecting appropriate candidates for version attempts (Table 16-4).[82]

While the ideal methods for external cephalic version have not been completely elucidated, the majority of reported series use rather similar protocols.[17,85-93] The patient should have a gestational age of at least 37 weeks and a previous sonographic examination to screen for major fetal anomalies and placenta previa. She should have an intravenous line placed, and fetal monitoring should be reassuring prior to the procedure.

At our facility, we generally perform these procedures in the morning after the patient has fasted for 8 hours to reduce the potential for aspiration in the unlikely event that fetal compromise requires an emergent abdominal delivery under general anesthesia. If a tocolytic agent is to be used, it should be administered approximately 15 to 30 minutes prior to the attempt to obtain maximum effect. The patient should be in a supine lateral tilt position with her hips and knees flexed slightly to relax abdominal musculature.

TABLE 16-4
NEWMAN SCORING INDEX FOR PREDICTION OF
SUCCESS OF EXTERNAL CEPHALIC VERSION

	Points		
	0	1	2
Parity	0	1	≥2
Dilation (cm)	≥3	1–2	0
Estimated fetal weight (g)	<2500	2500–3500	>3500
Placenta location	Anterior	Posterior	Lateral or fundal
Station	≥−1	−2	≤−3

Score	% Successful External Cephalic Version
0–2	0
3	14
4	35
5	60
6	64
7	68
8	80
9–10	100

Adapted from Newman.[82]

One or two operators may attempt the procedure. The first step is to attempt to elevate the breech from the maternal pelvis by gentle suprapubic pressure in a cephalad direction Figure 16-6A). The version is unlikely to be successful if this cannot be accomplished. Having an assistant attempt to elevate the breech from the pelvis through transvaginal pressure is usually not helpful. Once the breech has been elevated from the pelvis, either a forward or a backward roll technique can be used. Steady, gentle pressure is applied to the fetal poles in opposite directions to accomplish the rotation (Figure 16-6B) until the fetus is in a cephalic presentation (Figure 16-6C). If unsuccessful, rotation of the fetus in the opposite direction may be attempted. In the author's experience, persistence beyond 5 to 10 minutes is unlikely to achieve success.

Monitoring of the fetal condition during the attempt is an important safety consideration and can be easily accomplished with real-time sonography. The transducer can be held by the operator and used to apply pressure to one of the fetal poles, or held by an assistant. Efforts should temporarily cease if a fetal heart rate deceleration occurs; repetitive decelerations should prompt abandonment of the procedure. Fetal monitoring should continue for at least 30 minutes after the procedure, and the patient should be discharged only if fetal testing is reassuring. She should be instructed to return immediately if she notices vaginal bleeding, rupture of membranes, increase in abdominal pain or decreased fetal movement. Rh-negative women should receive Rh immune globulin for prophylaxis against isoimmunization.

Several investigators have studied methods aimed at improving the success rate of external cephalic version. The routine use of a tocolytic agent, such as ritodrine or terbutaline, in patients undergoing external cephalic version has been included in many previously reported protocols; however, randomized prospective trials have had conflicting results.[86,91] Given that β-mimetics are usually well tolerated for short-term use, it is reasonable to administer a single dose subcutaneously to nondiabetic parturients prior to the version attempt. Stimulation of fetal activity with fetal acoustic stimulation has also been reported to be efficacious, particularly in the fetus whose spine is in a direct anterior or posterior position.[94,95] In addition, there has been a small series reported using transabdominal amnioinfusion to improve the success rate of external cephalic version in breech-presenting fetuses with relative oligohydramnios.[96] Historically, the use of regional anesthesia or analgesia during external cephalic version attempts has been avoided because of concerns that such agents might allow excessive force to be used during the attempt and thereby increase the risk for placental abruption, fetal injury, and uterine rupture. However, two randomized trials of epidural analgesia during external cephalic version reported statistically significant increases in the success

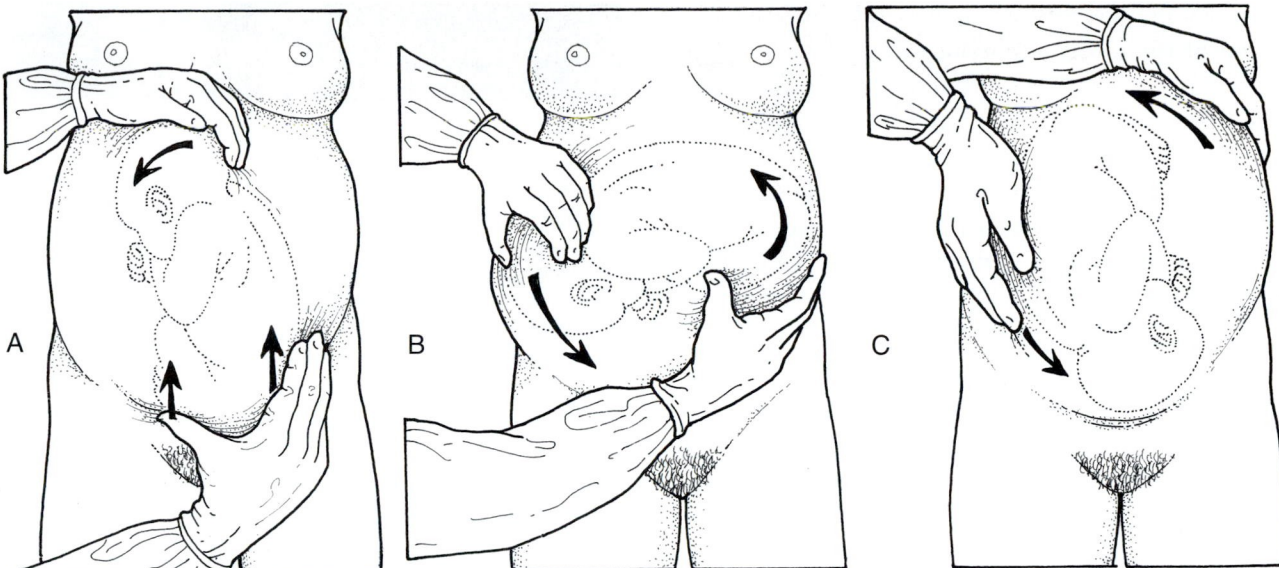

Figure 16-6 External cephalic version. The breech is elevated out of the maternal pelvis by suprapubic pressure (A), and then either clockwise or counterclockwise rotation of the fetal poles is attempted (B) until the fetus lies in a cephalic presentation (C).

rate without any adverse outcomes.[97,98] If epidural analgesia is used, it should be kept in mind that the purpose of the analgesia is to provide maternal abdominal wall relaxation, not to allow greater force to be used.

Suggested Methods for Selective Vaginal Delivery

Protocol elements that have been proposed for the selection of appropriate candidates for a trial of labor and vaginal breech delivery are primarily based on clinical intuition rather than on evidence-based data. The only clinical scoring method developed for the prediction of successful vaginal breech delivery is the Zatuchni–Andros index.[99] This index was based on clinical observations made at the time of admission in labor (Table 16-5). After exclusion of cases with cord prolapse, hyperextension of the fetal head, or congenital anomalies, all cases of perinatal morbidity were associated with a score of ≤3. While favorable results with the use of this scoring index have been reported,[65,100,101] a critical examination of the components of the score show that favorable consideration is given to multiparous women who present in labor with a gestational age of ≤37 weeks of gestation. However, nulliparity has not been demonstrated to be a risk factor for poor outcome. In addition, efforts by others to base selection criteria on obstetric history

and cervical status on admission have demonstrated an increased risk for poor perinatal outcome associated with vaginal breech delivery as compared with abdominal delivery.[102]

Retrospective case series have demonstrated that hyperextension of the fetal head is associated with an increased risk of perinatal morbidity and mortality in the breech fetus delivered vaginally.[103-106] This hyperextension of the fetal head occurs in approximately 5% of breech fetuses, and vaginal delivery may be associated with a high incidence of spinal cord injury.[103-106] These injuries occur predominantly in fetuses who have deflexion of greater than 90 degrees. Cervical spine injuries have also occurred in such fetuses delivered abdominally; thus, care must be taken even during cesarean delivery.

TABLE 16-5 ZATUCHNI–ANDROS INDEX

Points

	0	1	2
Parity	0		≥1
Gestational age (weeks)	≥39	38	≤37
Prior breech	0	1	2
Estimated fetal weight (lb)	>8	7–8	<7
Cervical dilation (cm)	≤2	3	≥4
Station	−3	−2	−1

Adapted from Zatuchni and Andros.[99]

In an attempt to select appropriate candidates for a trial of labor, it is important to assess the maternal pelvic dimensions in an effort to reduce the likelihood for entrapment of the fetal head. Radiographic pelvimetry has commonly been used for this, as clinical pelvimetry or the history of a previous delivery of a cephalic-presenting infant may be inadequate in identifying the woman with a contracted pelvis.[105,106] While some authors[65] have questioned the efficacy of routine radiographic pelvimetry, it is apparent that such methods are the only means available to the clinician for objective measurement of the upper planes of the maternal pelvis. However, while Van Loon and colleagues[107] found that the use of radiographic pelvimetry was associated with fewer emergency cesarean deliveries and an improvement in Apgar scores, there have been no randomized trials demonstrating a decrease in fetal head entrapment or improved perinatal outcome with radiographic pelvimetry. Nonetheless, many of the contemporary trials supporting the safety of selective vaginal breech delivery have employed radiographic pelvimetry as a means of selecting women with adequate pelvic dimensions.[47,61-64]

Historically, conventional radiographic pelvimetry has been used; however, this technique is technically difficult and results in approximately 1000 to 1100 mrad of radiation to the fetus.[61-63] Computed tomography (CT) has also been used to assess maternal pelvic dimensions, offers the benefits of reduced radiation exposure to the fetus, and is technically easier to interpret.[108] Magnetic resonance imaging (MRI) has been shown to provide excellent imagery of the pelvic dimensions with no radiation exposure to the fetus; however, the expense and limited availability of this method limits its usefulness.[107,109] At my institution, computed tomographic pelvimetry is used with critical thresholds established through a compilation of previous reports (Table 16-6).[35,61] Pelvimetry is deemed adequate if all measurements meet or exceed these limits. Use of these thresholds results in the exclusion of approximately 30% of women from a trial of labor on the basis of inadequate pelvimetry.

Given the usual error in estimations of fetal weight through the use of ultrasonographic fetal biometry, it would be reasonable to exclude fetuses with an estimated fetal weight of less than 2000 g from a trial of labor in order to avoid vaginal delivery of the fetus with an actual birth weight of 1500 g or less. At the time that fetal biometry is performed, sonographic

TABLE 16-6
THRESHOLD CRITERIA USED FOR COMPUTED TOMOGRAPHIC PELVIMETRY

Inlet	
Anteroposterior	≥10.0 cm
Transverse	≥11.5 cm
Mengert	≥90 (anteroposterior × transverse/145 × 100)
Midplane	
Interspinous	≥9.5 cm
Posterior Sagittal	≥4.0 cm

examination can be used to screen for the hyperextended fetal head or major congenital anomalies if an anatomic survey has not been previously performed. An upper weight limit of 3800 to 4000 g has been proposed based on reports of increased morbidity and lower probability of successful vaginal delivery in the macrosomic breech fetus.[39,44,110]

If the fetal weight is sufficient, no major anomalies are noted, the head is flexed, and the fetus is in a frank or complete breech presentation, consideration may be given to a selective trial of labor. The fetus in a footling or incomplete breech presentation is usually not considered a candidate for vaginal delivery because of a 10 to 15% risk of umbilical cord prolapse and an increased risk for fetal head entrapment due to inadequate dilation of the cervix by the presenting breech. If the above selection criteria are met, the patient should be thoroughly counseled regarding the risks, benefits, and alternatives of vaginal breech delivery with equal emphasis on both maternal and fetal concerns. Such counseling should be nondirective and not based principally on the care providers' personal experience or opinions. Following such counseling the patient may elect to have further consideration for a trial of labor and vaginal breech delivery. If her care providers lack adequate experience in this method of delivery, consideration should be given for referral to a colleague experienced in performing vaginal breech deliveries. At this point, it is recommended that the patient undergo radiographic assessment of pelvic dimensions in order to objectively determine if she is an appropriate candidate. If pelvimetry is deemed adequate and fetal head flexion is confirmed, she may be considered as a candidate for a trial of labor. Radiographic pelvimetry, particularly MRI or CT imaging, is often easier to obtain on a scheduled basis prior to the onset of labor. Evaluation for fetal head hyperextension may then be performed by sonography when the patient is evaluated at the on-set of labor.[111] Labor induction should be performed only for the usual obstetric indications. A history of prior cesarean delivery should not be considered a contraindication for attempted vaginal delivery.[112,113]

Principles of labor management are essentially the same as those used in the management of the cephalic presentation. Oxytocin may be used judiciously in patients with secondary arrest disorders and uterine hypocontractility. While epidural analgesia may pro-long the second stage and result in a slight increase in the risk for cesarean delivery due to second stage ar-rest,[40,114] beneficial effects include a decrease in un-controlled maternal pushing in the late active phase and second stage while allowing enhanced operator assistance.

There are three basic types of vaginal breech de-livery. Spontaneous breech delivery occurs when the fetus is expelled without any assistance or manipula-tion and typically occurs only in the precipitate de-livery of an extremely premature fetus. Assisted breech delivery includes partial breech extraction and total breech extraction. Partial breech extraction occurs when the infant delivers without interference or manipulation to the umbilicus, then the remainder of the fetus is delivered with operator assistance. A total breech extraction occurs when the entire body of the fetus is extracted by the operator and is typically per-formed only in multiple gestations following the de-livery of the first fetus. This latter situation is discussed in Chapter 9.

Two experienced obstetricians, an anesthetist, and a pediatrician should attend the delivery. One birth attendant should perform the breech delivery while the assistant supports the body of the fetus during ex-traction of the arms and head and attempts to main-tain flexion of the fetal head through suprapubic pres-sure. The breech fetus typically enters the pelvic inlet with the bitrochanteric plane oriented obliquely and then undergoes internal rotation to an anteroposte-rior position. A prolapsed leg will usually rotate ante-riorly. The anterior hip typically presents to the outlet before the posterior hip. While there is no evidence-based data to support the routine use of episiotomy, most experienced operators prefer to perform this procedure as the breech is crowning to allow greater room at the outlet for manipulation and extraction of the fetal legs, arms, and head. Maternal expulsive efforts should be allowed to proceed and achieve delivery of the breech and lower trunk

without interference. The delivery attendant's only role at this point is to encourage maternal expulsive efforts and monitor fetal well-being. Excessive trac-tion applied prematurely can result in deflexion of the fetal head with the occipital frontal diameter subse-quently presenting to the inlet, increasing the likeli-hood of fetal head entrapment. If sudden fetal com-promise is suspected during the second stage prior to the spontaneous delivery of the lower half of the fetus, the attendant is faced with the difficult decision of whether to attempt total breech extraction or to proceed with abdominal delivery. Total breech ex-traction should be attempted only by an experienced operator in the presence of an assistant who will be able to maintain fetal head flexion and an anesthetist who can administer appropriate anesthesia in a timely manner.

When the iliac crests become visible, the lower extremities may be delivered by inserting two fingers along the inner thigh until the popliteal fossa is reached. Pressure is applied to gently abduct the thighs away from the midline, flexing the knee and drawing the foot to the introitus where it can be easily deliv-ered (Figure 16-7). These steps are often referred to as the Pinard maneuver, which can also be performed in the rare situation when there is a need to extract the legs prior to delivery of the breech. Delivery of the leg and foot can be aided by rotating the fetal trunk 45 to 90 degrees counterclockwise for the right leg and clockwise for the left. Delivery of the lower extremities and hips is followed by external rotation with the fetal back directed toward the maternal symphysis. Rarely, rotation occurs in such a manner that the fetal back is oriented toward the maternal sacrum, a situation that requires the avoidance of traction on the fetal body to prevent extension of the fetal head.

Following delivery of the legs and lower trunk, the legs and pelvis should be wrapped in a towel and the attendant should hold the fetus as depicted in Figure 16-8A. Continued maternal expulsive efforts, occa-sionally aided by gentle traction, result in delivery of the chest and thorax. As the upper fetal trunk deliv-ers, the assistant should provide gentle suprapubic pressure to maintain head flexion, except in the rare situation when the fetal back has rotated to a poste-rior position. As the scapula and axilla become visi-ble, the attendant places two fingers over the shoul-der, sweeping down the humerus to flex the elbow while simultaneously rotating the fetal trunk 45 to

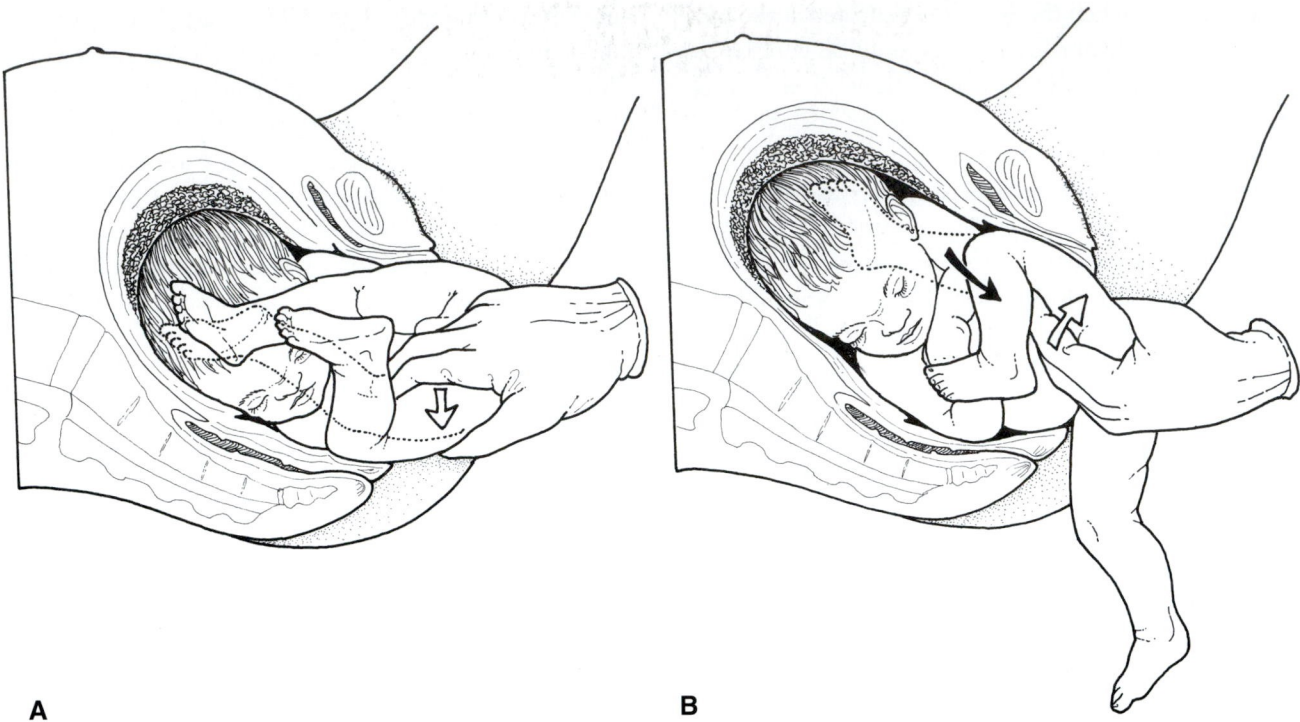

Figure 16-7 A. Extraction of the fetal legs is accomplished by externally rotating (adducting) the thighs to flex the knee, which causes the foot to descend to the introitus. B. Extraction can be facilitated by rotation of the fetal trunk toward the opposite hip (clockwise for the left leg and counterclockwise for the right leg).

90 degrees counterclockwise for the right arm and clockwise for the left (Figure 16-8B). The operator's fingers are used to splint the humerus as it is swept in a caudad direction across the chest and delivered (Figure 16-8C). The fetal trunk is then rotated in the opposite direction for delivery of the other arm (Figure 16-8D).

Occasionally, the fetal arms may be behind the neck; a position referred to as a nuchal arm (Figure 16-9). The rotational procedure described above is used, which usually results in the arm rotating anteriorly to lie against the fetal face. It may then be gently swept across the fetal chest with two of the operator's fingers serving as a splint as described above. If extraction of the arm is delayed until the upper shoulders are visible, a nuchal arm can be more difficult to reduce, as the head now occupies the lower birth canal, allowing less room for manipulation of the arm. When this situation is encountered, extraction can be facilitated by slightly elevating the head and shoulders in the birth canal. If both arms are behind the neck, the arm closest to the maternal symphysis is delivered first.

The delivery of the fetal head is perhaps the most technically challenging aspect of the vaginal breech delivery. In the typical circumstance in which the head is in an occiput anterior orientation, the birth attendant may perform a modified Mauriceau–Smellie–Veit maneuver by placing the infant's body over the ventral aspect of the operator's dominant arm with the two fingers on the maxilla in order to maintain head flexion. The nondominant hand grasps the shoulders and applies gentle downward traction while the fetal body is elevated toward the maternal abdomen (Figure 16-10). Traction is applied while the mother continues expulsive efforts and while suprapubic pressure is provided by the assistant. To avoid trauma to the fetal mouth and to facilitate maintenance of head flexion, the attendant's fingers should be placed on the maxilla immediately adjacent to the nares, rather than in the fetus's mouth, as originally described.

The alternative to the Mauriceau–Smellie–Veit maneuver is to use Piper forceps to allow controlled delivery of the fetal head. While the routine use of Piper forceps is unlikely to provide benefit to all

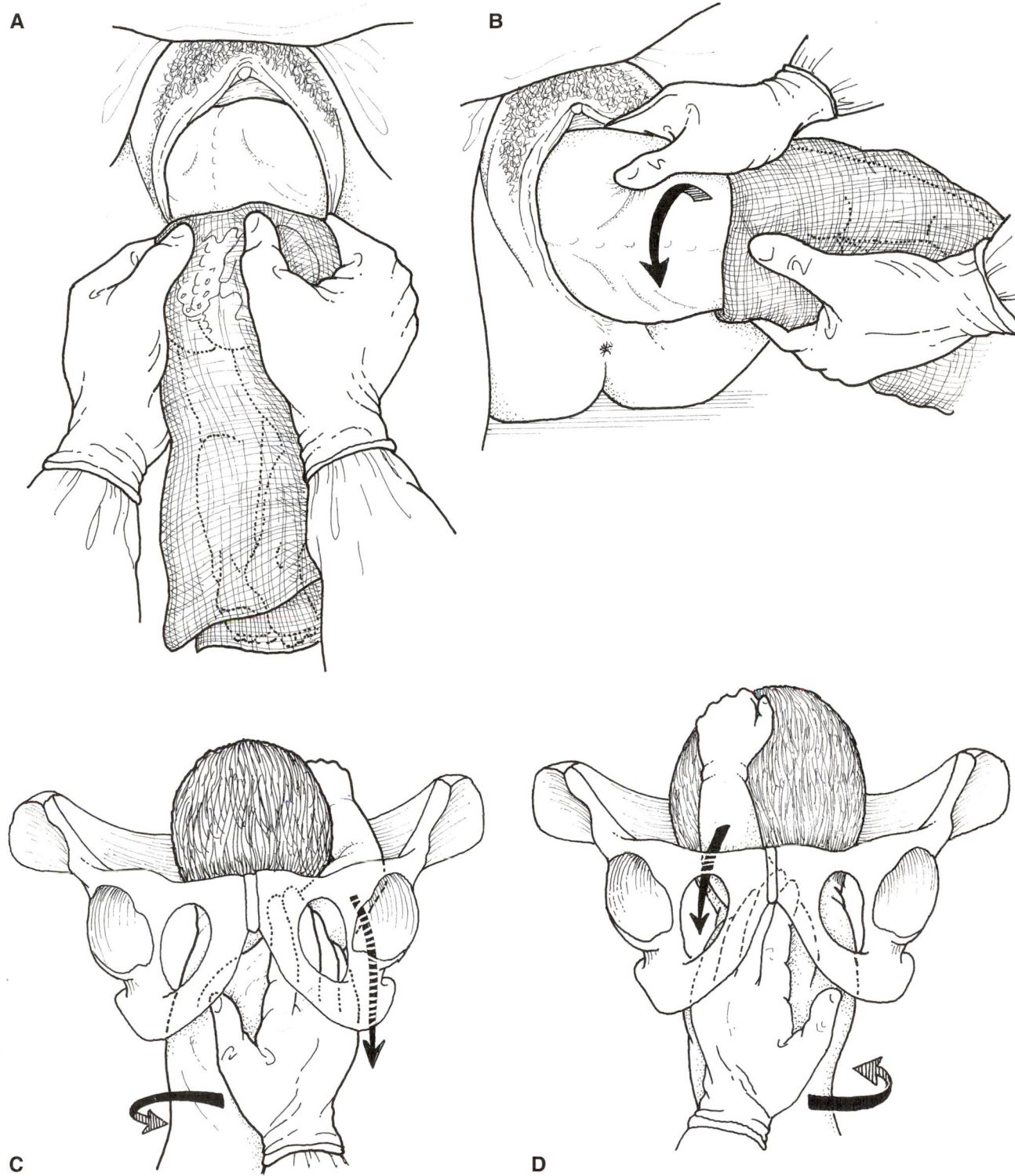

Figure 16-8 A. Following delivery of the fetal legs, the lower portion of the fetus is wrapped in a towel and the fetus is grasped with the operator's hands on the pelvic girdle, taking care not to grasp above the pelvis. B. As the scapula and axilla pass the introitus, the fetal trunk is rotated counterclockwise as two fingers of the attendant's right hand sweep over the right shoulder and down the ventral aspect of the arm. C. Gentle pressure on the lower arm in a posterior and caudad direction results in descent of the arm to the introitus. D. Following delivery of the right arm, the fetal trunk is rotated clockwise approximately 180 degrees with two fingers of the operator's left hand sweeping over the shoulder and down the humerus in a similar manner to deliver the left arm.

fetuses,
confide
the use
extracti
ceps is
requires
classic f
below t
tion for
kneelin
body, i
16–11).
gle of n
plane an
nal long

section or other perinatal care maneuvers? Am J Obstet Gynecol 1983;145:123.

78. Laros RK, Flanagan TA, Kilpatrick SJ. Management of term breech presentation: a protocol of external cephalic version and selective trial of labor. Am J Obstet Gynecol 1995;172:1916.

79. Gifford DS, Keeler E, Kahn KL. Reduction in cost and cesarean rate by routine use of external cephalic version: a decision analysis. Obstet Gynecol 1995;85:930.

80. Hofmeyr GJ. External cephalic version at term: how high are the stakes? Br J Obstet Gynaecol 1991;98:1.

81. Flamm BL, Fried MW, Lonky NM, Giles WS. External cephalic version after previous cesarean section. Am J Obstet Gynecol 1991;165:370.

82. Newman RB, Peacock B, Bandorsten P. Predicting success of external cephalic version at term. Am J Obstet Gynecol 1993;169:245.

83. Fortunato SJ, Mercer LJ, Guzick DS. External cephalic version with tocolysis: factors associated with success. Obstet Gynecol 1988;72:59.

84. Ferguson JE, Armstrong MA, Dyson DC. Maternal and fetal factors affecting success of antepartum external cephalic version. Obstet Gynecol 1987;70:722.

85. Kasule J, Chimbira TH, Brown IM. Controlled trial of external cephalic version. Br J Obstet Gynaecol 1985; 92:14.

86. Robertson AW, Kopelman JN, Read JA, Duff P, Magelssen DJ, Dashow EE. External cephalic version at term: is a tocolytic necessary? Obstet Gynecol 1987; 70:896.

87. Marchick R. Antepartum external cephalic version with tocolysis: a study of term singleton breech presentations. Am J Obstet Gynecol 1988;158:1339.

88. Scaling ST. External cephalic version without tocolysis. Am J Obstet Gynecol 1988;158:1424.

89. Van Veelen AJ, Van Cappellen AW, Flu PK, Straub MJ, Wallenburg HC. Effect of external cephalic version in late pregnancy on presentation at delivery: a randomized control trial. Br J Obstet Gynaecol 1989;96:916.

90. Hanss JW. The efficacy of external cephalic version and its impact on the breech experience. Am J Obstet Gynecol 1990;162:1459.

91. Fernandez CO, Bloom SL, Smulian JC, Ananth CV, Wendel GD Jr. A randomized placebo-controlled evaluation of terbutaline for external cephalic version. Obstet Gynecol 1997;90:775.

92. Van Dorsten JP, Schifrin BS, Wallace RL. Randomized control trial of external cephalic version with tocolysis in late pregnancy. Am J Obstet Gynecol 1981;141:417.

93. Hibbard LT, Schumann WR. Prophylactic external cephalic version in an obstetric practice. Am J Obstet Gynecol 1973;116:511.

94. Johnson RL, Strong TH, Radin TG, Elliott JP. Fetal acoustic stimulation as an adjunct to external cephalic version. J Reprod Med 1995;40:696.

95. Johnson RL, Elliott JP. Fetal acoustic stimulation, an adjunct to external cephalic version: a blinded, randomized crossover study. Am J Obstet Gynecol 1995;173:1369.

96. Benifla JL, Goffinet F, Darai E, Madelenat P. Antepartum transabdominal amnioinfusion to facilitate external cephalic version after initial failure. Obstet Gynecol 1994;84:1041.

97. Schoor SJ, Speights SE, Ross EL, et. al. A randomized trial of epidural anesthesia to improve external cephalic version success. Am J Obstet Gynecol 1997;177:1133.

98. Mancuso KM, Yancey MK, Murphy JA, Markenson GR. Epidural analgesia for cephalic version: a randomized trial. Obstet Gynecol 2000;95:648.

99. Zatuchni GI, Andros GJ. Prognostic index for vaginal delivery in breech presentation at term. Am J Obstet Gynecol 1965;93:237.

100. Zatuchni GI, Andros GJ. Prognostic index for vaginal delivery in breech presentation at term. Am J Obstet Gynecol 1967;98:854.

101. Mark C, Roberts PHR. Breech scoring index. Am J Obstet Gynecol 1968;101:572.

102. Barlov K, Larsson G. Results of a five year prospective study using a feto-pelvic scoring system for term singleton breech delivery after uncomplicated pregnancy. Acta Obstet Gynecol Scand 1986;65:315.

103. Caterini H, Langer A, Sama JC, Devanesan M, Pelosi MA. Fetal risk in hyperextension of the fetal head in breech presentation. Am J Obstet Gynecol 1975;126:632.

104. Daw E. Hyperextension of the head in breech presentation. Am J Obstet Gynecol 1974;119:564.

105. Ballas S, Toaff R, Jaffa AJ. Deflexion of the fetal head in breech presentation. Obstet Gynecol 1978;52:653.

106. Abroms IF, Bresnan MJ, Zuckerman JE, Fischer EG, Strand R. Cervical cord injuries secondary to hyperextension of the head in breech presentations. Obstet Gynecol 1973;41:369.

107. Van Loon AJ, Mantingh A, Serlier EK, Kroon G, Mooyaart EL, Huisjes HJ. Randomised controlled trial of magnetic-resonance pelvimetry in breech presentation at term. Lancet 1997;350:1799.

108. Kopelman JN, Duff P, Karl RT, Schipul AH, Read JA. Computed tomographic pelvimetry in the evaluation of breech presentation. Obstet Gynecol 1986;68:455.

109. Van Loon AJ, Mantingh A, Thijn CJ, Mooyaart EL. Pelvimetry by magnetic resonance imaging in breech presentation. Am J Obstet Gynecol 1990;163:1256.

110. Wolter DF. Patterns of management with breech presentation. Am J Obstet Gynecol 1976;125:733.

111. Fontenot T, Campbell B, Mitchell-Tutt E, et al. Radiographic evaluation of breech presentation: is it necessary? Ultrasound Obstet Gynecol 1997;10:338.

112. Sarno AP, Phelan JP, Ahn MO, Strong TH. Vaginal birth after cesarean delivery. Trial of labor in women with breech presentation. J Reprod Med 1989;34:831.

113. Ophir E, Oettinger M, Yagoda A, Markovits Y, Rojansky N, Shapiro H. Breech presentation after cesarean section: always a section? Am J Obstet Gynecol 1989;161:25.

114. Chadha YC, Mahmood TA, Dick MJ, Smith NC, Campbell DM, Templeton NA. Breech delivery and epidural analgesia. Br J Obstet Gynaecol 1992; 99:96.

115. Dufour P, Vinatier D, Puech F. The use of intravenous nitroglycerin for cervico-uterine relaxation: a review of the literature. Arch Gynecol Obstet 1997;261:1.

Chapter 17
Labor and Delivery: Normal and Abnormal

Gregory E. Chow
Michael K. Yancey

Five Key Points

- **Misoprostol has comparable efficacy to prostaglandin E$_2$ and has become an inexpensive alternative for labor induction in the patient with an unfavorable cervix.**

- **Early amniotomy and aggressive use of oxytocin has not been demonstrated to dramatically reduce the rate of cesarean delivery for dystocia in the United States.**

- **Episiotomy is useful in select cases but should not be performed on a routine basis.**

- **Shoulder dystocia is usually an unavoidable and unpreventable complication of vaginal delivery. Anticipation and preparation are the key elements in effective management of this potentially serious complication.**

- **Uterine inversion is an obstetric emergency that must be recognized and treated immediately to avoid hypovolemic shock.**

Labor and delivery (parturition) represent the culmination of a process that has long been regarded as the miracle of life. It is a normal physiologic function that, prior to the era of modern medicine, carried with it an element of mystery and confusion. While much of the veil of the processes of labor has been lifted, there are still areas in which our understanding of the physiology and course of labor remain obscure. Thus, the process of parturition continues to persist as one of the more enigmatic physiologic functions in humans.

In preparation for labor and, ultimately, delivery many changes must occur within the uterine and cervical tissues. While many of the physiologic changes are becoming clearer, translating this scientific knowledge into practice is sometimes a daunting challenge. Due to the extremely emotional nature of the process of childbirth, experimentation with new agents and techniques is fraught with many practical problems as well as ethical considerations. Because childbirth evokes such strong feelings, the science of obstetrics has always seemed to lag behind the art of obstetrics. Modern childbirth must simultaneously remain cost effective and appealing to patients who rightfully expect to have a wide array of choices in the methods and circumstances of this major life event. New techniques, which may have an excellent evidence-based foundation, often seem to do battle with the traditional methods of managing labor. Some of these traditions have survived decades or even centuries before being challenged by modern practitioners. Medicolegal aspects of labor management and patient autonomy often preclude the gathering of evidence-based data prior to widespread use. Electrical fetal monitoring is a perfect example of technology being put into use prior to being scrutinized by appropriate scientific trials. It is for this reason that there still remains much to be understood about the subtleties of the correct management of normal laboring patients.

There are many pathways that may result in the same desired outcome—the safe delivery of a healthy infant. Because this outcome is more often the rule than the exception, it is often difficult to ascertain a difference in outcomes of one intervention over another without the use of randomized control trials—an extremely difficult and expensive prospect in obstetrics. Modern labor management is often based on classic observational studies, as evidence-based data has only recently begun to accumulate for various intrapartum interventions.

In spite of the persistent questions about appropriate labor management, it is essential that the practitioner understand what is currently known about the usual progression of parturition. With this understanding, the labor attendant can recognize abnormalities as they develop and then make reasonable management decisions using an evidence-based approach. This chapter will discuss the factors and events that are important to define normal labor and delivery, as well as describe the deviation from these norms.

DEFINITION OF LABOR

The process of labor is defined as progressive change in the uterine cervix in response to repetitive uterine contractions. Labor may either be spontaneous, augmented, or artificially induced. It is immediately apparent in the definition that what connotes significant progressive change is largely subjective. While retrospective categorization of true and false labor is rather straightforward, prospectively differentiating true from false labor poses a much greater problem, and the clinician is often confronted with the question, "Is this patient truly in labor?" This question becomes especially pertinent when considering the normal progression of labor, because it emphasizes that some flexibility in clinical judgment is essential in the management of normal laboring patients. The need for flexibility in diagnosis takes on particular importance when managing the preterm gestation. At term, the issue becomes less critical as observation over time will usually make the diagnosis clear.

MECHANISM OF LABOR

Initiation of Labor

The precise mechanism for the initiation of spontaneous labor in humans is not yet fully understood, although the triggering process is likely to be an extremely complex system involving various hormones and tissues. This lack of a known trigger mechanism for labor results in our inability to accurately predict the onset of labor, term or preterm, or to effectively halt the process once it has started. Much of the current understanding of labor processes comes from work with animals.

Although primary differences in reproduction exist between humans and lower mammals, much of the primary understanding of the labor and parturition process comes from Liggins's classic early work performed in the sheep model.[1-3] This work not only drew attention to the fact that circulating hormones may be involved in the initiation of labor, but also provided insight into the cervical changes that occurred in preparation for labor. Some of the practice of modern obstetrics is directly drawn from early work with the sheep model, which has provided clues to important events occurring during parturition. This scientific work, of course, is not directly applicable to humans, but nevertheless has provided insight into some of the potential hormones and chemical mediators of labor, helping to circumvent some of the obvious ethical and technical difficulties with attempting to study labor in human subjects.

In the sheep model, there is a specific cascade of systemic hormonal events responsible for the initiation of labor. The key initial event that signals the onset of labor is the secretion of cortisol by the fetal adrenal cortex.[4] This initial increase in cortisol stimulates increased activity of placental 17α-hydroxylase which, in turn, catalyzes the conversion of progesterone to androgens and estrogens. The resulting fall in the levels of progesterone and subsequent rise in estrogen have multiple effects. First, the rise in serum estrogen levels causes an increase in the formation of gap junctions within the myometrial tissue of the ovine uterus.[5] Gap junctions are important cellular contact areas that allow electrical coupling of myometrial cells. This intercellular electrical communication is critical to the synchronization of muscular activity within the uterus. The coupling of more-efficient electrical and mechanical activity results in a net improvement in the coordination of contractility in the uterus and an increase in the intrauterine pressure generated during a contraction.

Secondly, there is an increase in the synthesis of prostaglandins. This increase is due to the fall in progesterone, which has both inhibitory and stimulatory effects on synthesis, and a rise in estrogen, which stimulates synthesis of prostanoids.[6] While it remains unclear whether an absolute fall in progesterone or an alteration of the relative ratio of estrogen : progesterone levels is the key element, the importance of progesterone in maintaining a quiescent uterus can be illustrated in species of mammals that are dependent on the corpus luteum. Corpus luteum–dependent mammals are those that rely on the production of progesterone throughout gestation for maintenance of the pregnancy. In many of these lower mammals, destruction of the corpus luteum plays an important role in the cause of abortion because of loss of progesterone's inhibitory effect on prostaglandin synthesis.

The family of prostaglandins (PGs) are synthesized from an obligate precursor, arachidonic acid (Figure 17-1). Through the actions of the enzyme cyclooxygenase, arachidonic acid is converted to two endoperoxides (PGG_2 and PGH_2). These are the parent compounds to all of the clinically important prostaglandin compounds biologically active during parturition. These endoperoxides give rise to $PGF_{2\alpha}$, PGE_2, and PGD_2. Two other biologically active prostaglandins are also produced through this enzymatic pathway; prostacyclin (PGI_2), through the actions of prostacyclin synthetase, and thromboxane A_2, through the actions of thromboxane synthetase.

Prostaglandin production in the ovine model occurs primarily within the uterus and cervix. The increase in formation of prostaglandins has myriad effects on uterine smooth muscle, endothelium, connective tissue, and vasculature. Prostaglandins affect the cervix by causing collagen catabolism and an end result of cervical ripening.[7]

In humans, while there is no evidence to support the fact that one specific hormonal event is responsible for the initiation of labor, significant data have shed light on the physiologic changes that occur in early labor, as well as the hormones involved in the initiation of these changes. Estrogen production by the combined mechanisms in the maternal and fetal compartments increases prior to the onset of spontaneous labor, regardless of gestational age.[8] This increase in estrogen production may be due to increased corticotropin-releasing hormone production within the uteroplacental unit and is associated with increases in uterine myometrial oxytocin receptor expression, increased gap junction formation, and increased prostaglandin synthesis in the uterine and cervical tissue.[9,10] Our understanding of the importance of the role of prostaglandin synthesis in the mechanism of labor has largely been expanded through Liggins's research on sheep, as it is apparent that prostaglandins are a key terminal effector of cervical remodeling and uterine activity. Therefore, spontaneous labor in humans is likely closely linked to alterations in steroid hormone production and metabolism, which eventually promotes myriad physiologic actions of prostaglandins on the reproductive organs, primarily the uterus and cervix.

INDUCTION OF LABOR

Preinduction Cervical Assessment and Preparation

Prostaglandins clearly play a pivotal role in the initiation of the normal labor process in humans. One of

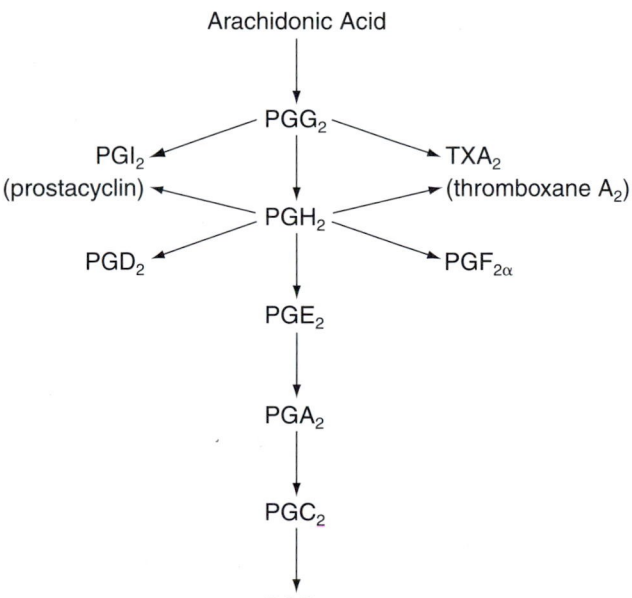

Figure 17-1 Basic pathway of prostaglandin (PG) synthesis. PGG_2 and PGH_2 are the parent compounds to the other clinically relevant prostaglandins.

TABLE 17-1
BISHOP'S CERVICAL SCORING CRITERIA

Score*	Dilation (cm)	Effacement (%)	Station†	Consistency	Position of Cervix
0	Closed	0–30	−3	Firm	Posterior
1	1–2	40–50	−2	Medium	Midposition
2	3–4	60–70	−1, 0	Soft	Anterior
3	≥5	≥80	+1, 2		

*A score of >9 is considered favorable.

†Station is represented on a −3 to +3 scale.

the key processes linked to prostaglandins is an alteration in the collagen matrix and water content of the cervix. These changes result in softening and effacement, a process referred to as ripening. Artificial ripening of the cervix is a method used commonly in preparation for labor induction in parturients whose cervix has not undergone natural ripening. Substantial improvement in the success of labor induction has been demonstrated when induction is initiated with a ripened cervix in contrast to an unripened cervix.[11] In 1964, Bishop[12] described a method that has allowed the clinician to grade the cervix in a quantitative fashion based on five criteria assessed by digital examination of the cervix (Table 17-1). The total Bishop score gives the practitioner an indication of the favorable quality of the cervix for induction.[12] In his series, Bishop found that a score of greater than 9 was associated with successful induction. While these data were obtained from the evaluation of multiparous women undergoing elective induction of labor, it has been extrapolated for use by many clinicians in nulliparous patients. A score of less than 6 is usually considered unfavorable.

Artificial cervical ripening can be accomplished through the use of exogenous prostaglandin preparations applied to the cervix or by promoting local endogenous prostaglandin production by mechanically disrupting the interface between the fetal membranes and the upper cervix. Methods commonly used to increase local prostaglandin production include placement of mechanical dilators into the cervical canal, digital sweeping of the membranes away from the cervix (stripping the membranes) or placement of a Foley catheter through the cervical canal and instilling sterile crystalloid solution through the catheter to elevate the fetal membranes away from the cervix and lower uterine segment. These methods cause release of arachidonic acid from the fetal membranes with subsequent endogenous prostaglandin production.

Exogenous PGE_2 preparations are commonly used for initiation of local cervical ripening and induction of labor. The effects of this agent on the cervix to induce cervical ripening have been well described.[13-17] Application of PGE_2 to the cervix results in histologic alterations similar to changes occurring with spontaneous cervical ripening. The main effect of using PGE_2 within the microhistologic structure of the cervix is to cause dissolution of collagen fibrils. There is considerable evidence that collagen, one of the major connective tissues of the cervix, supplies the cervix with the strength and integrity necessary to retain the products of conception until the time of parturition.[18] This dissociation of collagen brings about the changes in the physical characteristics within the cervix that allow it to dilate and soften.

PGE_2 has been FDA-approved to be administered in one of two fashions. It may be applied as an intracervical gel containing 0.25 mg of dinoprostone or an intravaginal insert with a controlled release of 10 mg of dinoprostone. The clinical indication for which PGE_2 is most commonly used is for the postdate pregnancy; however, it has clinical utility for all other indications for induction of labor as well. Several clinical trials have shown increased efficacy of cervical ripening with intracervical or intravaginal administration of PGE_2 as compared with placebo, or no treatment.[19-25]

Important prerequisites for the use of PGE_2 preparations are the ability to monitor uterine activity and fetal heart rate, a reassuring fetal heart tracing, and the capability for rapid delivery if nonreassuring fetal testing develops. Although infrequent, the primary side effect of PGE_2 when used for cervical ripening is uterine hyperstimulation. After administration, the patient typically remains recumbent for 1 hour and remains under observation with continuous monitoring of uterine activity and fetal heartbeat for at least 2 hours. Intracervical gel can be applied every 6 to

8 hours with up to three doses in a 24-hour period, while the vaginal insert is allowed to remain in place for 10 hours. Subsequent dosage depends on clinical factors such as cervical change and uterine activity.

Prostaglandins for Labor Induction

A new synthetic prostaglandin that is achieving wide acceptance for labor induction is misoprostol, a synthetic, methylated PGE_1 analog (Figure 17-2). Originally developed to treat gastrointestinal ulcers caused by nonsteroidal antiinflammatory drugs, numerous randomized control trials have been performed to evaluate its efficacy as a cervical ripening and labor-induction agent. Misoprostol has been shown to have comparable or improved efficacy to that of PGE_2 in the aspects of safety, successful induction, and side-effect profile.[26-31] The advantages of using this agent are the shorter interval from start of induction to delivery and a significant reduction in the cost of the medication. It is currently administered intravaginally or orally. The most frequently used dosages for oral or intravaginal administration range from 25 to 100 μg every 4 to 6 hours. Misoprostol is a potent agent, and

its major side effect noted is an increase in the incidence of tachysystole, which is usually defined as the occurrence of more than six contractions in a 10-minute time period. It differs from uterine hyperstimulation in that it is not associated with fetal heart rate abnormalities and typically requires no treatment. In addition, cases of uterine rupture have been reported in women receiving this agent. Thus, care must be used in selecting appropriate patients, and they should be monitored closely.[32] Comparative studies have failed to detect statistically significant differences between misoprostol and PGE_2 in the incidence of cesarean delivery, maternal side effects, or neonatal outcome. The optimal dosage and dosing interval have yet to be completely determined.

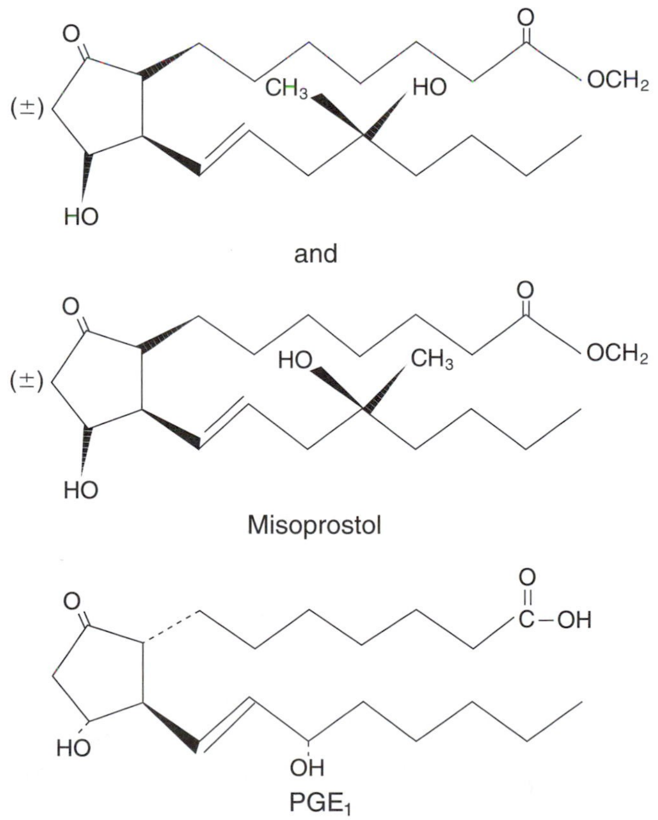

Oxytocin for Labor Induction

Oxytocin (Pitocin) has traditionally been one of the most commonly used agents for the induction of labor. Although it is probably not the primary hormonal signal in the initiation of spontaneous labor, it is very effective when used as an adjunct to other induction methods to augment labor.[33-35] Oxytocin is a hormone that contains eight amino acids, and it is produced by the posterior pituitary gland (Figure 17-3). In the circulation it has an effective half-life of 5 to 10 minutes. Pharmacologic preparations are available for administration by buccal, intranasal, intramuscular (IM), or intravenous (IV) routes; however, contemporary use for labor induction or augmentation is almost exclusively by the intravenous route. The primary effect of oxytocin on uterine myocytes is to increase free intracellular calcium and stimulate uterine contractions.

Oxytocin should be administered as an IV piggyback because of the potential side effects of excessive uterine activity and systemic hypotension associated with bolus infusion. Most commonly, 10 to 20 units are diluted in 1000 cc of an isotonic solution and administered at a rate of approximately 1 to 2 mU/min, with subsequent increases of 1 to 2 mU/min every 30 minutes until the desired contractile pattern is

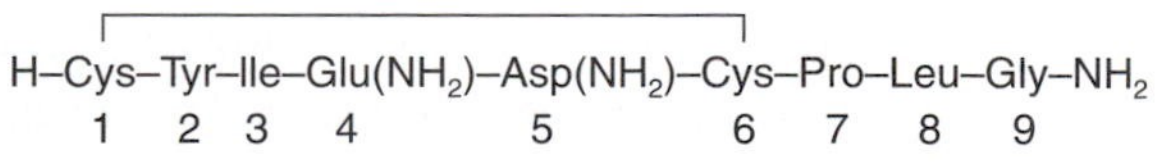

Figure 17-2 Structure of misoprostol (PGE_1 analog). Diastereomers of misoprostol are compared with PGE_1.

H–Cys–Tyr–Ile–Glu(NH_2)–Asp(NH_2)–Cys–Pro–Leu–Gly–NH_2
 1   2   3   4   5   6   7   8   9

Figure 17-3 Structure of oxytocin. The peptide consists of nine amino acids with a disulfide bond joining two cysteine amino acids.

reached. Although higher starting doses and more rapid increases in infusion rate have resulted in shorter duration of labor, there has been no consistent decrease in cesarean delivery.[36,37] These protocols have also been associated with a greater incidence of uterine hyperstimulation. There is still some debate about the optimal dosing regimen of oxytocin for maximal effectiveness and minimal untoward effects.

The side effects of oxytocin can be extremely serious. Excessive doses of oxytocin can cause uterine hyperstimulation, which can potentially result in impairment of fetal oxygenation and uterine rupture. Both oxytocin and antidiuretic hormone (ADH) are produced within the posterior pituitary and are structurally similar in five of eight amino acids. High doses of oxytocin may have an ADH effect that results in significant fluid retention and overload with prolonged administration. Therefore, fluid management should be closely monitored, especially in cases of prolonged induction and when doses exceed 40 mU/min.

Amniotomy

Amniotomy is a commonly used method for the induction of labor, particularly in the woman with a favorable cervix. This procedure was described as early as the 18th century as a method to facilitate labor. While amniotomy may be effective in initiating labor in some women, it is only occasionally used as the sole means of labor induction in contemporary obstetrics because the combined use of amniotomy and oxytocin administration have been demonstrated to be superior to either method alone.[38]

Amniotomy does initiate uterine activity in the term pregnancy. Disruption of the chorioamnion likely results in arachidonic acid conversion by the cyclooxygenase pathway to PGE_2, resulting in increased uterine activity.[39] In addition, reducing the intrauterine volume by allowing egress of amniotic fluid may allow an increase in contractile strength.

Amniotomy may also be used in conjunction with the other methods of labor induction. When used as an adjunct in this fashion, it is a highly successful means of induction.[40] It ideally should be performed in women with a favorable Bishop score, as performance of amniotomy in women with low cervical scores may increase the likelihood of intrapartum infection and prolonged induction. The indications for amniotomy are induction of labor, inability to monitor the fetal heart rate with external means, the need to evaluate the amniotic fluid, the need to administer

an amnioinfusion, and the need to directly assess uterine activity in women with protraction disorders. There are several contraindications to the performance of amniotomy. Amniotomy should not be performed if any of the following conditions have been previously diagnosed: placenta previa, vasa previa, funic presentation, abnormal fetal lie, prior classical cesarean incision, or active herpes simplex virus infection.

The actual mechanics of performing an amniotomy involve placement of a disposable plastic hook (amniohook) between the index and middle fingers of the examining hand. The hook of the instrument should be held between the fingers until the cervix is reached to prevent laceration of the vulva or vaginal side walls. Once the membranes are palpated, the hook is placed against them, and a small rent made through the chorioamniotic membrane to allow egress of the amniotic fluid (Figure 17-4). The hook is again held between the examiner's fingers and removed as the operator takes care to avoid puncturing the examining glove during the procedure.

In general, amniotomy should be avoided in a patient with an unengaged presenting part. In the situation in which the fetal head is not well applied to the cervix, stimulation of the fetal head by the examining finger may result in fetal movement coincident with rupture of the chorioamnion, increasing the risk for umbilical-cord prolapse. When an amniotomy must be performed in a patient with an unengaged presenting part, a second operator may hold the fetal head in place with a hand on the mother's abdomen, exerting pressure behind the fetus's neck as the amniotomy is performed. This maneuver will help to prevent movement of the head and subsequent prolapse of the umbilical cord.

The role of routine amniotomy in women already in spontaneous labor is debatable. Protocols for the active management of labor instituted by clinicians at the National Maternity Hospital in Dublin, Ireland, considered early amniotomy a critical element for augmentation of active-phase labor.[41] However, the potential for ascending infection may abolish any beneficial effects in hastening delivery.

LABOR PROGRESSION

First Stage

The progression of labor, measured by increasing cervical effacement and dilatation, along with descent of the presenting part in the birth canal, is markedly var-

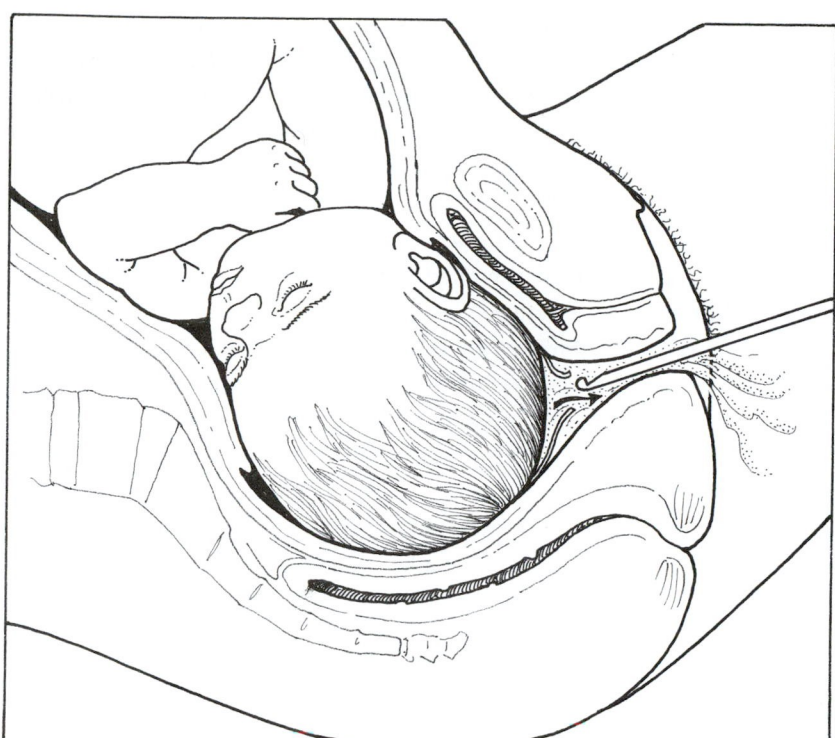

Fig. 17-4 Use of amniohook to artificially rupture the chorioamniotic membranes.

ied from individual to individual. Early spontaneous labor, particularly in the nulliparous patient, is often characterized by regular uterine contractions, with only minimal changes in the cervix over the span of several hours. In contrast, the multiparous patient may complete the entire labor process in several hours.

Based on the pioneering work by Friedman, with graphic depiction of changes in cervical dilatation, it became logical to divide labor into three stages (Table 17-2). The first stage begins with the onset of regular uterine activity resulting in progressive cervical change, and continues until the cervix is completely dilated. The first stage is subdivided into 2 phases: the latent phase and active phase. The latent phase of the first stage of labor is designated as the time from the onset of regular uterine activity resulting in cervical effacement and dilatation until the point of entry into the active phase of the first stage. The active phase is designated as the portion of labor in which the rate of cervical change is at its maximum slope. This ac-

tive phase begins as cervical dilatation accelerates and ends as the cervix becomes completely dilated. For the majority of patients, the active phase begins when the cervix is 3 or 4 cm dilated; however, from a practical standpoint, entry into active phase can only be determined retrospectively.

While the divisions of the first stage of labor can be fairly well defined when studied in a large population of parturients, it often is difficult to determine precisely when a particular patient's labor begins. Many women have episodic contractions in the weeks prior to actual labor. Cervical softening, effacement, and dilatation may be noted weeks or even months prior to delivery. The absence of a defining event can often lead to exasperation and frustration for both the patient and her care providers, occasionally resulting in well-intentioned, but unnecessary and potentially harmful, interventions.

The deceleration phase (the end of the active phase) is denoted as the period during which the

	TABLE 17-2 STAGES OF LABOR				
	First Stage		**Second Stage**	**Third Stage**
	Latent Phase	Active Phase		
Onset	Cervical dilatation	Maximal cervical dilatation/Time	Complete cervical dilatation	Delivery of baby
Completion	Active phase	Complete cervical dilatation	Delivery of baby	Delivery of placenta

slope (velocity of change) of cervical dilatation slows as the cervix becomes completely dilated. Some patients may appear to bypass this phase, prompting debate about the true existence of the deceleration phase. However, there are patients who clearly accelerate into the active phase of labor and then appear to have a slowing of the rate of cervical dilatation as the second stage approaches, most commonly at an approximate cervical dilatation of 8 to 9 cm. While the deceleration phase may give the impression of impending arrest, the majority of women continue to progress and eventually deliver vaginally.

Unfortunately, there are no absolute standards for assessing the adequacy of labor progression. Friedman studied the labor progress of a large cohort of women in order to determine guidelines for the progress of "normal" labor.[42] His investigations were critically important, and much of the management of labor in the modern era continues to be based on his observations. However, in evaluating these data, it is important to remember that they make inferences based on a statistical model, labeling women progressing at the 5th percentile to be abnormal. In clinical practice, progress below these thresholds should alert the practitioner to evaluate the patient for causes of inadequate progress and should not be used as an indication for immediately aborting labor and delivering the patient by cesarean delivery (or cesarean section).

The normal progression of labor, as described by Friedman, is depicted in Table 17-3. It is readily apparent that the standards of progression are quite different when comparing nulliparous and multiparous patients, with progress in labor typically more rapid in women who have previously had a vaginal delivery as compared with those who have not. However, there is no clear distinction between a woman who has had one child and women who have had more than one child. It is an incorrect assumption that with each succeeding child the labor course will progress with greater rapidity. The average time for a nulliparous woman to complete the first stage of labor is 11.8 hours, and 95% will complete the first stage of labor by 34.5 hours. In the multiparous woman, the average time to complete the first stage is 7.2 hours, and 95% will complete the first stage in less than 19.7 hours.

Subdividing the first stage of labor into latent and active phases can provide practical insight for monitoring a patient's course in labor. The parturient in the latent phase would not be anticipated to always have appreciable change in cervical effacement or dilatation over the span of several hours. However, the lack of appreciable change in women in the active phase of labor over the period of 2 to 3 hours should immediately prompt assessment of uterine contractility and should raise the possibility of relative cephalopelvic disproportion due to malpresentation, fetal macrosomia, or pelvic contracture. Conversely, in the patient who continues to make progress, albeit at a slower-than-average rate, intervention is not always needed, only vigilant surveillance. From the data by Friedman, 1.2 cm/hr and 1.5 cm/hr rates of change in the active phase for the nulliparous and multiparous woman represent the 95th percentile for progress. Failure to meet this standard may be indicative of abnormal labor.

In nulliparous women, it is quite typical for cervical dilatation to occur concurrently with descent of the vertex through the birth canal. The cervix is retracted laterally to a dilatation of approximately 6 to 7 cm, then descent of the fetus causes retraction of the cervix over the presenting part until complete dilatation is achieved. In multiparous women, the presenting part may remain at a high station until late in

---

TABLE 17-3
NORMAL PROGRESS OF FIRST STAGE OF LABOR

Group	Latent Phase, First Stage (hr)	Active Phase, First Stage (hr)	Deceleration Phase, First Stage (hr)
Nulliparous			
Mean	6.4	4.6	0.84
Standard deviation	5.1	3.6	1.0
Limit	20.1	11.7	2.7
Multiparous			
Mean	4.8	2.4	0.36
Standard deviation	4.9	2.2	0.3
Limit	13.6	5.2	0.86

Adapted from Friedman et al.[42]

the first stage; then a rapid change in station occurs, coincident with a strong maternal urge to push.

The ideal approach to the management of labor remains a contentious issue in modern obstetrics, with polarized factions advocating either expectant management with minimal intervention unless there is a clear protraction disorder, or active management of labor. This debate has been driven largely by the increase in the cesarean delivery rate in the United States over the past 25 years. The aggressive active management approach involves the early use of amniotomy and aggressive dosing of oxytocin in women with suboptimal uterine activity to hasten delivery and lower cesarean delivery rates. Data from the National Maternity Hospital in Dublin, Ireland, where this approach was pioneered, showed a marked decrease in the cesarean delivery rate for dystocia and shorter interval to delivery without a significant increase in maternal or perinatal complications with this management scheme.[43] While several investigators have found similar results when applying these methods in small populations, a large U.S. trial reported by Frigoletto and colleagues[44] demonstrated no statistically significant decrease in the cesarean delivery rate with such a protocol. Thus, without a clear benefit for active management protocols, amniotomy is recommended only for previously cited indications, and oxytocin augmentation is recommended only for women with protraction disorders and evidence of suboptimal uterine activity, such as less than 250 Montevideo units. (See "Protraction of the Active Phase," below, for an explanation of Montevideo units.)

Second Stage

The second stage of labor begins with complete dilation of the cervix and ends with delivery of the neonate. The interval for completion of this stage also depends on parity. The average time for nulliparous women to complete this stage is 1.1 hour; 95% of nulliparas deliver their babies within 2.0 hours in the absence of conduction anesthesia. The mean duration of the second stage for multiparous women is 0.39 hour, with 95% delivering within 1.1 hours. The use of conduction analgesia may prolong the second stage; the outer limits of normal for duration of the second stage are 2 hours for nulliparas and 3 hours for multiparas.

Progress during the second stage of labor is measured by descent of the fetal head through the birth canal. Station of the fetal head is measured by its relative position to the ischial spine, which is designated as 0 station. The pelvis is divided into five 1-cm increments cephalad to the ischial spine (−5 to 0 station) and caudad to the spine (0 to +5 station) (Figure 17-5). In the nulliparous patient, the usual station of the fetal head at the beginning of the second stage is 0 station or lower. From a practical standpoint, the maximum time interval for serial examinations during the second stage is approximately 1 hour, as the lack of appreciable descent during this span of time is usually indicative of inadequate maternal expulsive efforts, malpositioning of the fetal head, or cephalopelvic disproportion. Ideally, serial assessment is accomplished by the same examiner because molding of the fetal head and caput secundum formation may make progress, or lack thereof, difficult to detect with certainty. In general, as long as fetal assessment remains reassuring and progress is made, the patient is allowed to continue pushing in anticipation of vaginal delivery.

Cardinal Movements

The fetal head normally undergoes several changes in orientation as it traverses the pelvis during labor. These movements are referred to as the cardinal movements of labor and occur as the vertex negotiates the varying dimensions of the bony pelvis and soft tissues. These movements are engagement, internal rotation, flexion, descent, extension, external rotation (restitution), and expulsion (Figure 17-6). Even though these movements are listed separately, many are accomplished in a simultaneous fashion as the fetus passes through the birth canal. Abnormal labor progression may occur if these movements are impaired by malpositioning of the fetal head or constriction of the maternal pelvis.

Pelvimetry

Essential to the understanding of the progress of labor is the knowledge of the anatomy of the female pelvis. As the fetus must traverse the pelvis during the course of labor, the internal capacity of the bony pelvis is the absolute limiting dimension for safe passage of the fetus. The study of the dimensions of the female pelvis through which the fetus is transmitted during parturition is referred to as pelvimetry.

The female bony pelvis is composed of two innominate (hip) bones that are joined anteriorly by the

Fig. 17-5 The relationship of the fetal
head to station within the maternal pelvis.

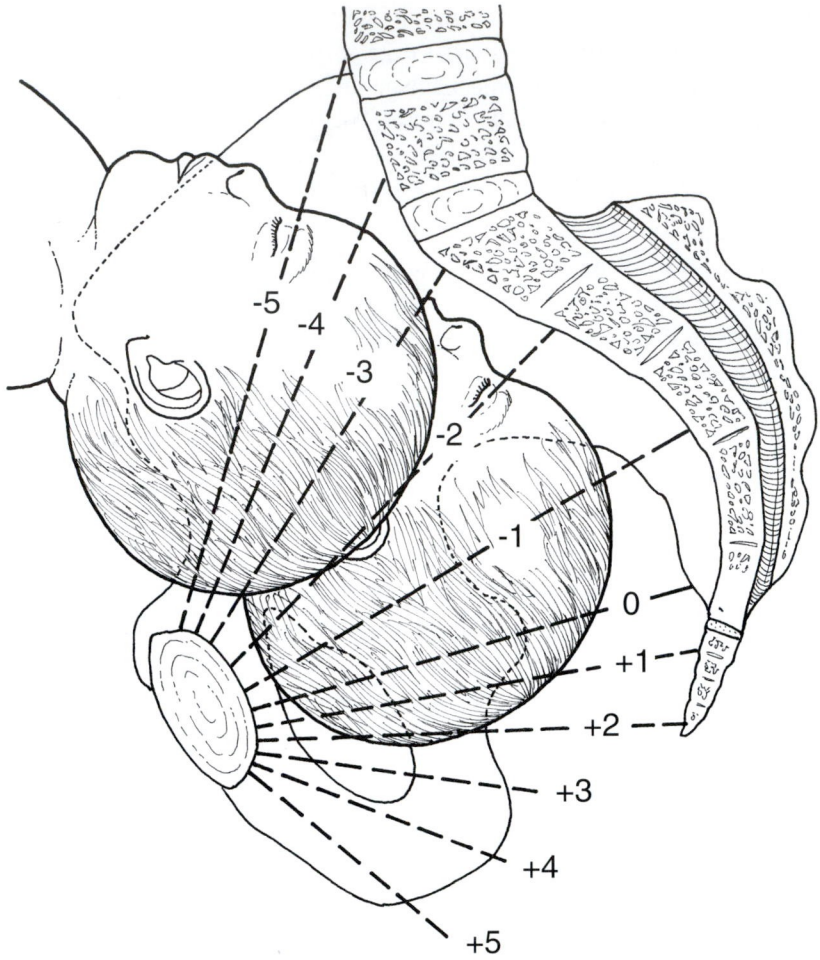

symphysis pubis and posteriorly by the sacrum and
coccyx. Each innominate bone is made up of three
portions; the ilium, ischium, and pubis (Figure 17-7).
The pelvic brim, which is formed by the symphysis
pubis, arcuate line of the ilium, and the ala of the
sacrum divides the pelvis into the true pelvis (caudad
to this line), and the false pelvis (cephalad to this line).
This pelvic brim is the inlet to the true pelvis, which
must have sufficient capacity for the fetal head to
engage into the birth canal.

For discussion of pelvic capacity, the birth canal
can be viewed as having three important transverse
planes: the inlet, midplane, and outlet (Figure 17-8).
The boundaries of these planes are defined by several
bony landmarks. The plane of the inlet is bounded by
the arcuate line, sacral promontory, and superior aspect of the pubic symphysis. The midplane extends
from the ischial spines to the inferior margin of the
pubic symphysis. The pelvic outlet extends from the
inferior portion of the symphysis pubis to the inferior aspect of the coccyx.

Based on the pioneering work by Caldwell and
Moloy, the general shape of the bony pelvis can be
divided into four general configurations: gynecoid,
anthropoid, platypelloid, and android.[45] The difference in the shapes of the pelvic inlet, midplane, and
outlet are such that the prognosis for spontaneous
vaginal delivery changes depending on the shape of the
pelvis. The prognosis is usually good for the gynecoid
and anthropoid pelvis and poor for the platypelloid
and android pelvis. While each of these different
types of female pelvis subtypes are described as separate entities, it is likely that the pelvic bony structure
for most women represents a composite or combination of the various dimensions of two or more of
these subtypes.

The gynecoid pelvis is the most common of the
pelvic subtypes and has a configuration most conducive to vaginal delivery (Figure 17-9). At the inlet,
the transverse diameter is slightly larger than the
anteroposterior diameter, allowing the fetal vertex to
enter the pelvis in a transverse orientation. As labor

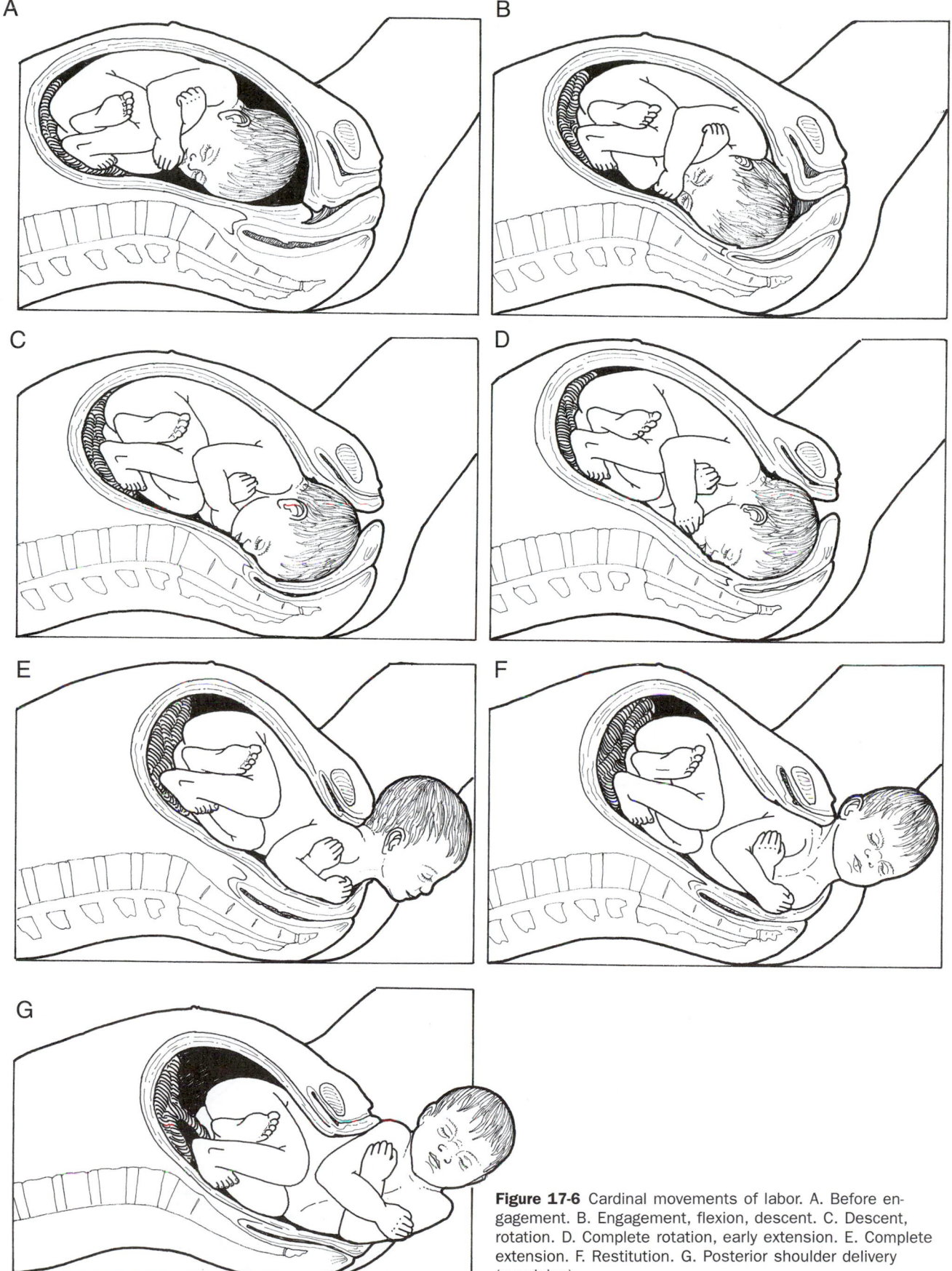

Figure 17-6 Cardinal movements of labor. A. Before engagement. B. Engagement, flexion, descent. C. Descent, rotation. D. Complete rotation, early extension. E. Complete extension. F. Restitution. G. Posterior shoulder delivery (expulsion).

Figure 17-7 The bony structure of the pelvis consists of two innominate bones (ilium, ischium, pubis) fused with the sacrum and coccyx posteriorly.

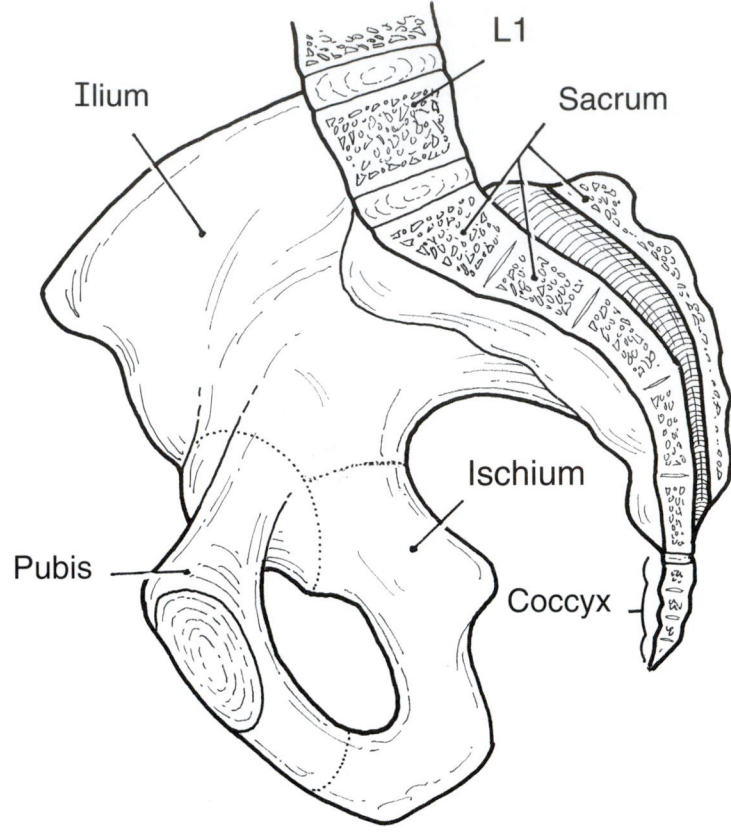

Figure 17-8 The important planes of the pelvis. Failure of the fetal head to negotiate these planes in the appropriate orientation may result in protraction and arrest disorders of labor.

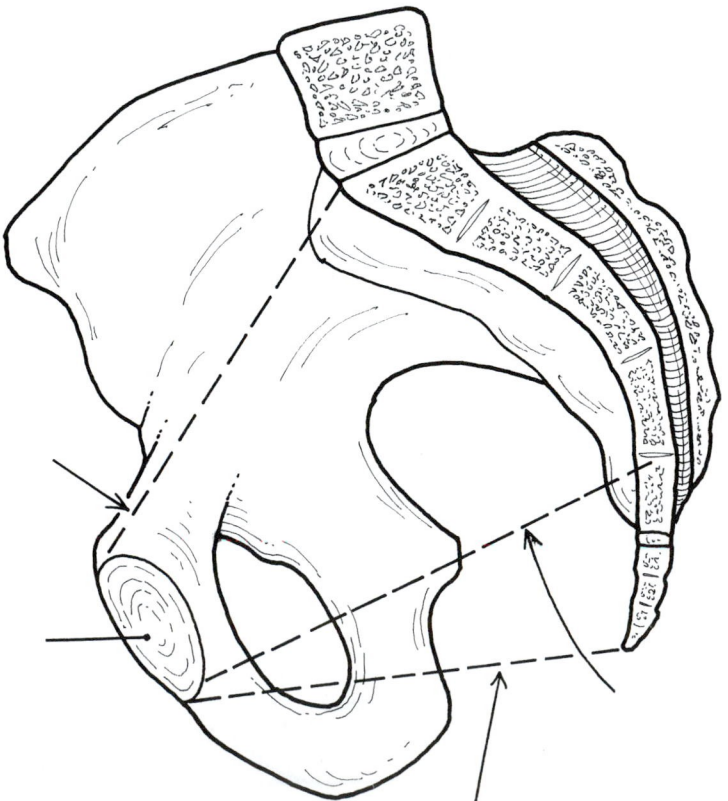

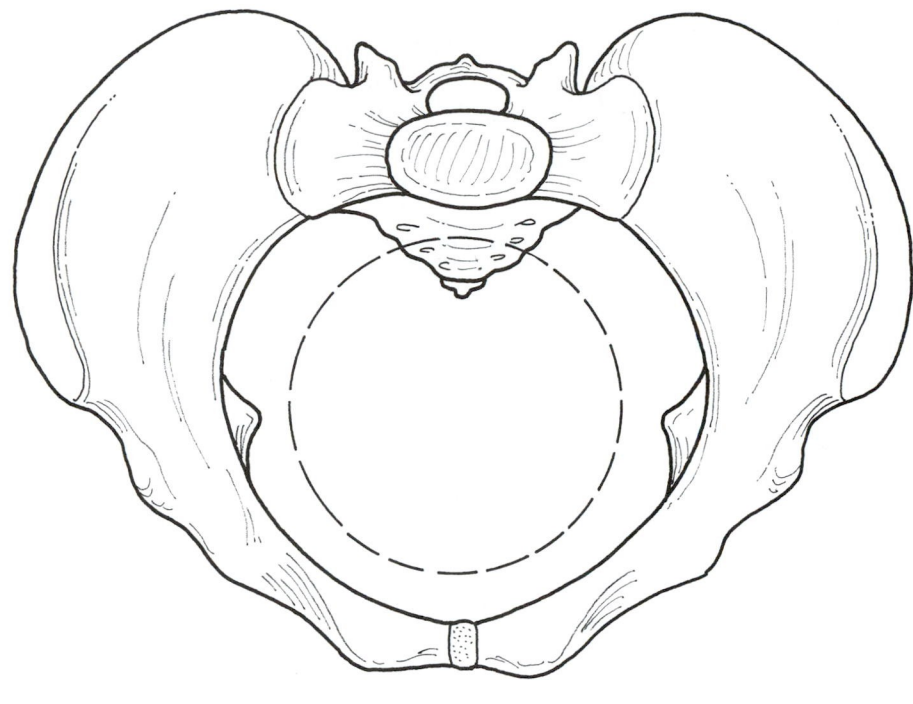

Figure 17-9 The gynecoid pelvis is the most common subtype of pelvis. Note the particularly rounded inlet with capacity in both the transverse and antero-posterior planes.

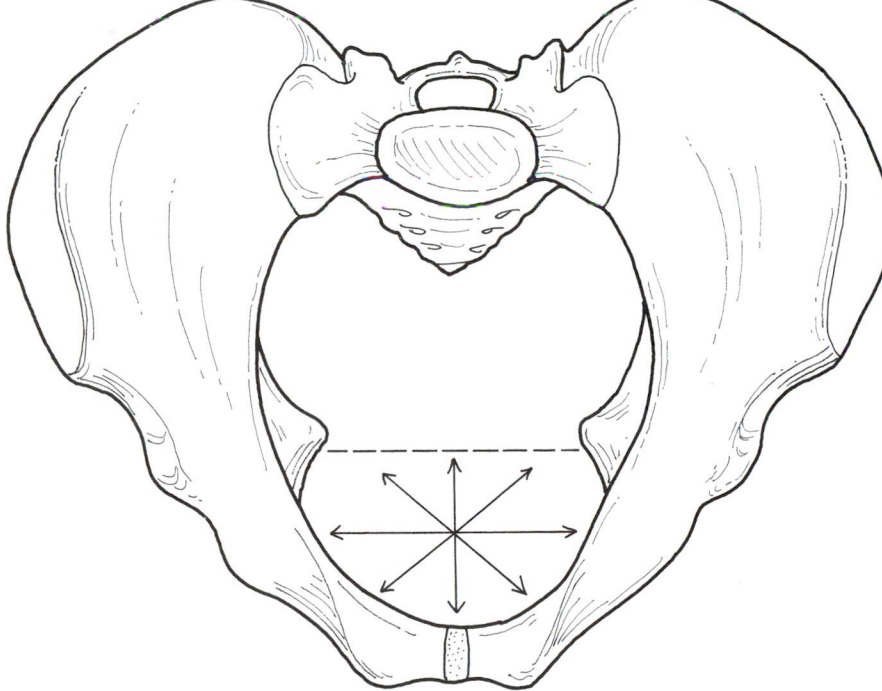

Figure 17-10 Anthropoid pelvis. Note the limited capacity of the anterior compartment. The anthropoid pelvis often predisposes to a persistent occiput posterior presentation.

progresses and the vertex descends, the interspinous diameter becomes the limiting dimension at the pelvic midplane. This limitation causes rotation to occur as the fetal vertex descends so that the sagittal suture lies in an anteroposterior position. Once internal rotation has occurred, it is unusual for the outlet to be constricted to a degree that prevents further progression in labor, precluding vaginal delivery.

In the anthropoid pelvis, the anterior portion of the pelvis has slightly less capacity than the gynecoid pelvis (Figure 17-10). As descent occurs, the occiput tends to rotate posteriorly to adopt an occiput posterior orientation within the pelvis. As long as the biparietal diameter has the ability to pass through the posterior compartment of the pelvis and through the level of the ischial spines, the prognosis for delivery is

Figure 17-11 The android pelvis is a contracted pelvis with convergent side walls and prominent ischial spines. Note the limited dimensions in the anteroposterior planes.

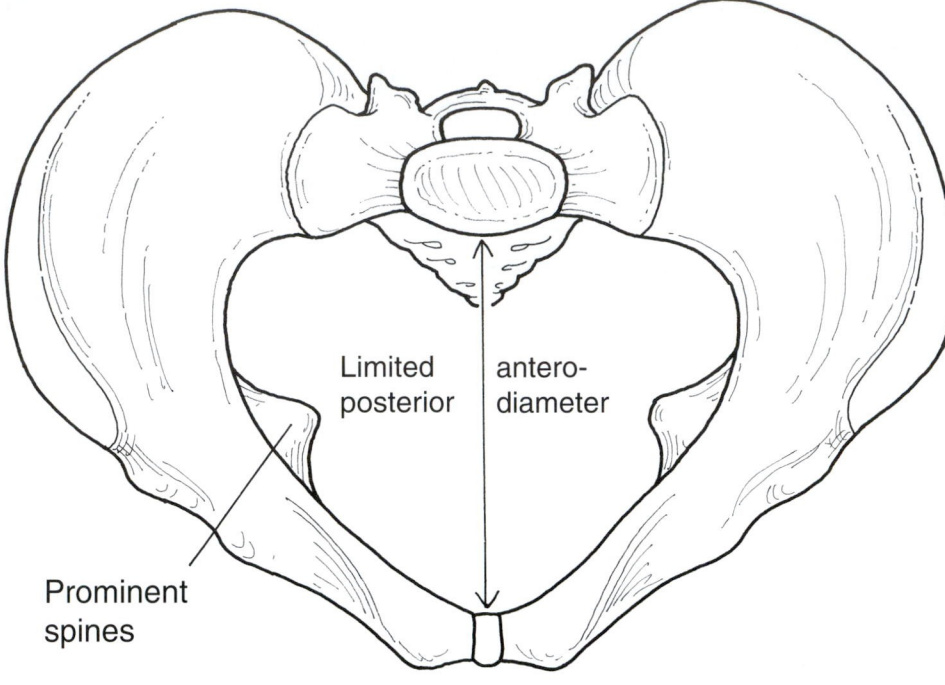

Limited posterior   antero-diameter

Prominent spines

Figure 17-12 The platypelloid pelvis is a contracted pelvis with limited dimensions in the anteroposterior planes. Predisposes to midpelvis transverse positions.

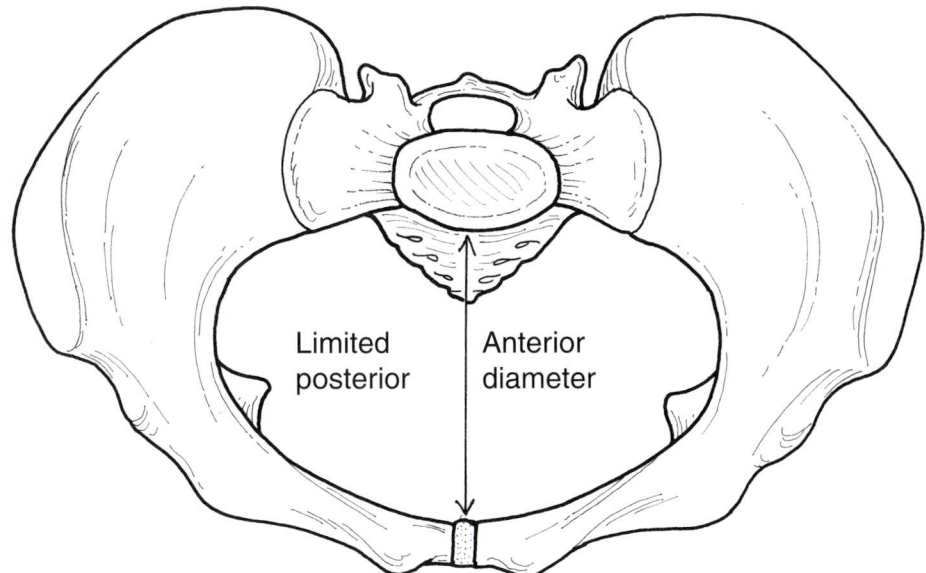

Limited posterior   Anterior diameter

good, even though the head will likely persist in an occiput posterior position at the time of delivery.

The android pelvis is commonly seen in males. This type of pelvis is severely constricted as the pelvic side walls converge toward the pelvic outlet (Figure 17-11). The dimensions of this pelvis may seriously inhibit the ability for the vertex to reach a point of engagement in the pelvis. The overall capacity of this pelvis is limited, and even if engagement does occur, the relatively shortened bispinous and posterior sagittal dimensions typically prevent descent through the midplane.

The platypelloid pelvis is significantly constricted, particularly in the anteroposterior dimensions, with the inlet having a flattened, oval appearance. While the transverse diameters may be adequate, the fetal vertex may not be able to engage into the pelvis because of the significant foreshortening of the anteroposterior diameter from the inlet through to the outlet (Figure 17-12). This type of pelvis predisposes to persistent occiput transverse positions.

Several pelvic dimensions can readily be measured during a physical examination and used to assess clinical adequacy of the pelvis. The three principal measurements are the obstetric conjugate, the interspinous diameter, and the subpubic angle (Figure 17-13). The obstetric conjugate is the distance from the sacral promontory to the nearest portion of the symphysis pubis and represents the portion of the inlet through which the greatest transverse diameter of the fetal head, the biparietal diameter, must pass. While it is impossible to measure the obstetric conjugate during clinical examination because the point of reference on the symphysis pubis is typically at the midpoint of the pubic bone, this dimension can be approximated by measuring the distance from the sacral promontory to the inferior aspect of the symphysis. This clinically measured diameter is known as the diagonal conjugate and is typically only 1.5 cm greater in length than the obstetric conjugate. An adequate distance for the diagonal conjugate is 11.5 cm, corresponding to an obstetric conjugate of 10.0 cm. The interspinous diameter can be measured by estimating the width between the ischial spines by digital palpation during the pelvic examination. The interspinous diamter is the smallest diameter of the midplane that the biparietal diameter of the fetus must traverse, and its minimal width for a term-sized fetus should be 10 cm. Finally, the subpubic angle reflects, to a degree, the dimensions of the outlet of the pelvis. An angle of less than 90 degrees may be indicative of a contracted pelvis; however, it is unusual for the outlet to be contracted without coexisting constriction of the inlet or midpelvis.

While assessment of the three pelvic dimensions described above are typically the most useful for determining adequacy of pelvic dimensions, assessment of other anatomic landmarks may also provide some clinically useful information. Prominence of the sacral promontory, a markedly prominent coccyx, or prominent ischial spines may portend difficulty for the passage of the fetal head through these dimensions. However, from a practical standpoint, the predictive value of clinical pelvimetry remains limited except in cases of extreme pelvic contracture or an excessively large fetus. Vaginal delivery in the parturient with an adequately sized gynecoid pelvis may be precluded by abnormal positioning of the fetal head or relatively large fetal size. Conversely, molding of the fetal head during the course of labor may allow a normal-sized fetus to negotiate a mildly constricted pelvis. Thus, it should be uncommon for a parturient to be excluded from a trial of labor based solely on the suspicion of inadequate pelvic capacity from clinical examination.

As clinical pelvimetry is inadequate in precisely assessing all of the important pelvic dimensions accurately and identifying patients likely to suffer cephalopelvic disproportion, investigations using radiographic methods have been done in an attempt to provide more accurate and clinically predictive information. Computed tomographic (CT) pelvimetry and conventional radiographic pelvimetry have both been explored. Unfortunately, while these methods are useful for obtaining reliable and reproducible information, their utility in labor management remains limited. The dynamic changes that occur in the pelvis during the course of labor and our inability to effectively estimate fetal size and adequately gauge the impact that soft tissues play during labor, combined with concerns about fetal radiation exposure, limit the clinical usefulness of radiographic methods. Thurnau and colleagues[46] have attempted to overcome some of these limitations through the development of a fetal–pelvic index, with fetal biometry compared to maternal pelvic dimensions as determined by conventional radiographic pelvimetry. These investigators found that the fetal–pelvic index was accurate in predicting which patients who would require a cesarean delivery for cephalopelvic disproportion. They then expanded the use of the fetal–pelvic index to study macrosomic infants, patients with abnormal labor patterns, and women attempting vaginal birth after previous cesarean delivery. The overall positive and negative predictive values of this index for all groups studied were 0.98 and 0.90, respectively. Unfortunately, the a priori decision to perform cesarean delivery based on a positive fetal–pelvic index eliminates the possibility of vaginal delivery for the small percentage of patients who will have a successful trial of labor. The widespread use of this method has been justifiably limited by concern regarding fetal radiation exposure and insufficient evidence-based data supporting the efficacy of this index in improving maternal and neonatal outcomes while reducing overall health-care costs. Accordingly, the use of radiologic pelvimetry in modern obstetrics is primarily limited to the use of CT pelvimetry when evaluating a patient for vaginal breech delivery as discussed in Chapter 16.[47]

Disorders of Labor Progression

Disorders of labor progression may occur during the first or second stage of labor. Protracted labor is de-

Figure 17-13 Anatomically important landmarks and pelvic dimensions. Clinically important pelvic dimensions include the diagonal conjugate, interspinous diameter
(A) and subpubic angle (B). Measurement
of these dimensions is important in the
assessment of pelvimetry.

A

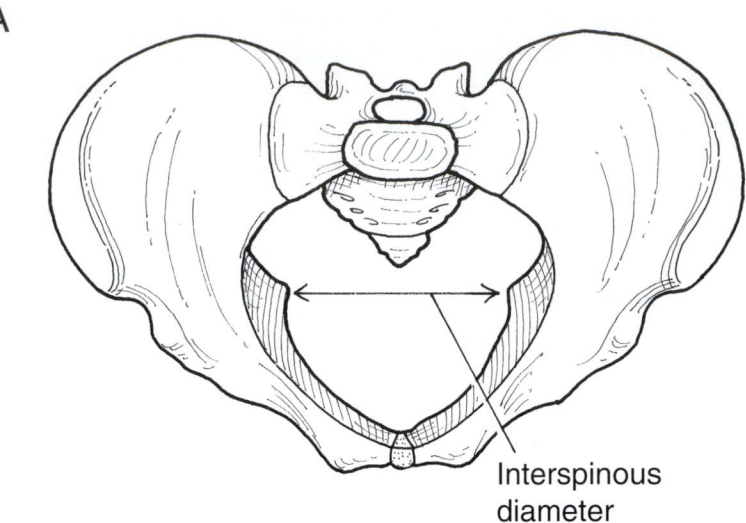

Interspinous
diameter

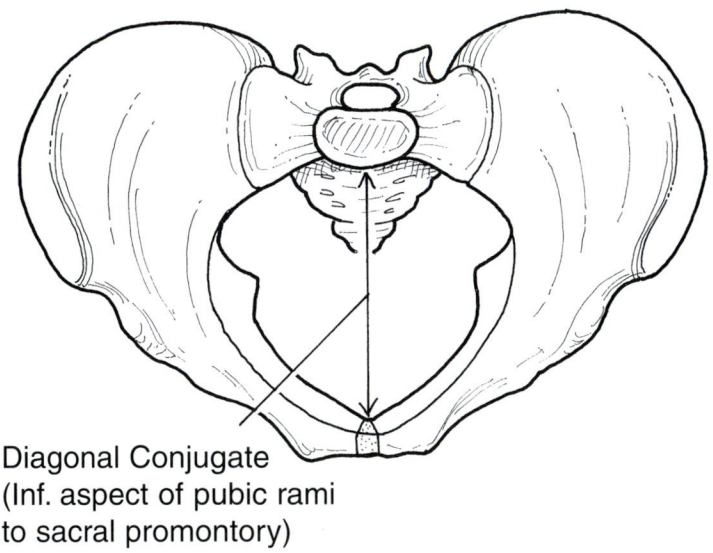

Diagonal Conjugate
(Inf. aspect of pubic rami
to sacral promontory)

B

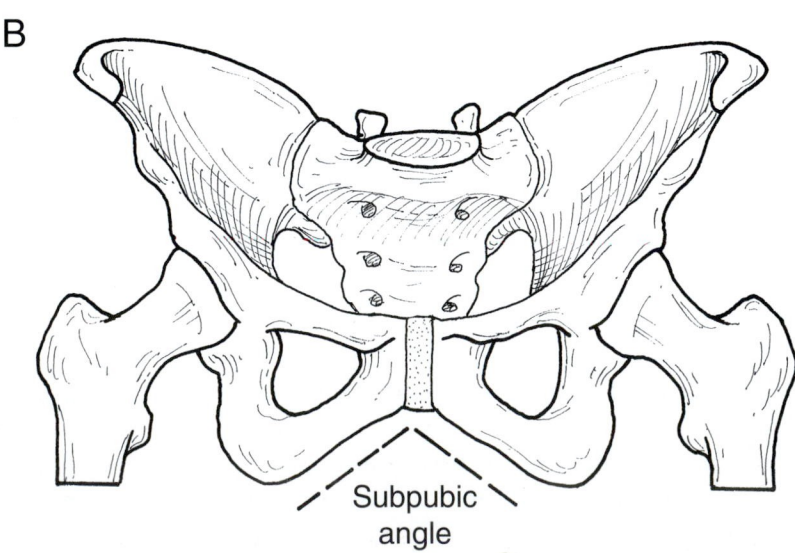

Subpubic
angle

fined as progress less than the anticipated minimal rate of change; arrested labor denotes the absence of appreciable progress in a given time interval. Temporal standards used to define protraction generally comply with the outer limits for progress described by Friedman.[42] Arrest of dilatation is defined as no apparent progression in cervical dilatation over a 2-hour period in the active phase of labor. Arrest of descent is defined as the lack of appreciable descent of the presenting part over a 1-hour period in the second stage of labor. Dystocia, a general term used to connotate arrest of dilatation or arrest of descent, is the leading indication for primary cesarean delivery in the United States today.[48] When evaluating a patient for any arrest disorder, the practitioner needs to be aware of the potentially myriad causes responsible for these problems, which can be broadly classified as uterine factors, cervical factors, cephalopelvic disproportion, and malposition.

Inadequate uterine contractility is the principal uterine factor and can often be corrected through the use of oxytocin. However, even with appropriate stimulation of the uterus, improved contractility may not occur due to intrinsic dysfunction of the uterus. Such dysfunction may be due to the lack of adequate uterine preparation prior to labor with inadequate gap junction formation and insufficient oxytocin receptors on the myocyte cell surface, a problem occasionally encountered in the patient with induced labor, particularly in a preterm gestation. Poor uterine contractility may also be due to extrinsic factors such as magnesium sulfate use, excessive analgesia during early labor, chorioamnionitis, or even the presence of large uterine fibroids.

Cervical factors also may contribute to protraction or arrest disorders. As discussed earlier, induction in an unprepared cervix may play a role in failure of induction. There is clearly a benefit to preparation of the cervix for labor, most likely because changes in the collagen composition of the cervix are clearly necessary for the cervix to properly dilate and permit passage of the fetus through the birth canal.[49] Cervical stenosis or scarring due to a prior conization may also be an important consideration when assessing cervical factors as a cause of labor abnormalities.

Cephalopelvic disproportion (CPD) refers to the inability of the fetal head to negotiate the pelvic dimensions and is a major contributor to disorders of labor progression. While extreme instances of CPD may be obvious, the majority of cases of CPD will become apparent only after the patient has had an unsuccessful trial of labor. Prior to the onset of labor, CPD may be suspected because of an apparently large fetus, yet labor may progress without difficulty to a normal spontaneous delivery. In contrast, the parturient with a normal-sized fetus and apparently normal pelvic dimensions may suffer arrested labor in the absence of uterine contractile dysfunction or fetal malposition.

Malpresentation can result in a relatively larger dimension of the fetal cranium than the suboccipitobregmatic diameter of a vertex presentation traversing the birth canal. Face and brow presentations are two such disorders and are discussed in the previous chapter. Malposition of the fetal head results in a relatively larger portion of the fetal head attempting to traverse through smaller segments of the birth canal, such as is seen in occiput posterior or transverse positions.

Protraction of the Latent Phase

Protraction of the latent phase of labor has not been associated with an increase in the risk for perinatal morbidity, mortality, or an increased risk for abdominal delivery. Therefore, the clinician should be sure that the remedy for the disorder does not in itself provide more harm than good. Overzealous and ill-timed attempts at hastening the progress of labor may initiate a cascade of events culminating in untoward events such as chorioamnionitis or cesarean delivery. Management options for latent-phase protraction disorders include expectant management, labor augmentation with oxytocin and/or amniotomy, or therapeutic rest with narcotic analgesia. Expectant management with continued observation can often result in the patient becoming progressively exhausted, with eventual requests for abandonment of labor and delivery by cesarean section. Augmentation with oxytocin and amniotomy may similarly increase the likelihood of cesarean delivery due to ascending infection or dysfunctional uterine contractility. Therefore, of these three options, therapeutic rest, accomplished through the administration of relatively large doses of narcotic analgesia (10 to 20 mg of morphine or an equivalent dose of an alternative agent) is often the most effective and humane course of action. In some cases, uterine activity will cease with sedation, evidence that the patient was not in true labor. However, approximately 85% of affected patients will awaken from sedation in active labor.[50]

If regular uterine contractions persist and there is no apparent progress, the patient may indeed have a

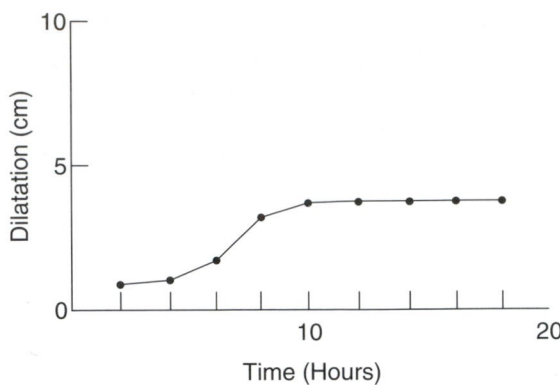

Figure 17-14 Latent-phase arrest.

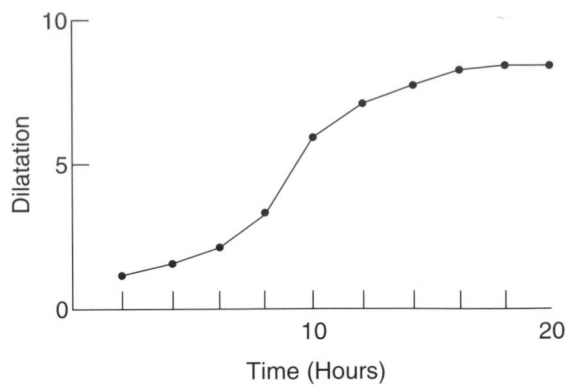

Figure 17-15 Protraction and arrest of the active phase.

latent-phase arrest. However, this is an extremely uncommon event, and cesarean delivery should be considered only after amniotomy has been performed, augmentation of labor as necessary has occurred, and further evaluation has shown no other reasons for failure to progress (Figure 17-14).

Protraction of the Active Phase

Protraction during the active phase is defined as an incremental change in cervical dilatation of less than 1.5 cm/hr in a multiparous patient, and 1.2 cm/hr in a nulliparous patient. When this diagnosis is made, a thorough evaluation for the possible causes should ensue. Again, augmentation with oxytocin is indicated if the uterine contractile pattern appears hypotonic. If membranes remain intact, an amniotomy should be performed. This action also allows the placement of an intrauterine pressure monitor to accurately assess uterine contractility. Caldeyro-Barcia et al.[51] described a method of quantifying uterine contractility by measuring the difference in pressure, in millimeters of mercury, generated by the uterus from base-line tone to the peak intensity of the contraction, then summating contraction intensity over a 10-minute period. This unit of measurement is commonly known today as the Montivideo unit, and the typical range generated in a 10-minute time frame during spontaneous labor varies from 150 to 250 Montivideo units. While this gives the practitioner some measure of intrauterine pressure, labor progress does not necessarily correlate linearly with the magnitude of Montivideo units. However, 250 Montivideo units is the desired goal for intrauterine pressure during augmented labor. Thus, measuring the intrauterine pressure in this fashion serves to reassure the clinician that contraction intensity and frequency are sufficient to effect cervical change. It also provides the practitioner

an objective measurement of uterine activity that can be used to adjust the dose of oxytocin for augmentation of dysfunctional labor. If the patient makes no progress in the active phase of labor for 2 hours or longer, despite active management, arrest of dilatation has occurred and cesarean delivery is usually indicated. Protraction and arrest disorders of the active phase are graphically depicted in Figure 17-15.

Second Stage Protraction and Arrest

Protraction of the second stage is defined as a rate of descent of the fetal head less than 2 cm/hr in a multiparous patient and less than 1 cm/hr in a nulliparous patient. Protraction may also be defined as a duration of the second stage for longer than 1 hour in the multipara or 2 hours in the nullipara. Regional anesthesia may prolong the duration of the second stage by approximately 1 hour, therefore, 2 hours and 3 hours are used for multiparous and nulliparous patients, respectively, in labor with regional anesthesia.[52] Cases for protraction or failure of the fetus to descend toward the outlet include cephalopelvic disproportion, inadequate uterine contractility, soft-tissue dystocia, distended bladder, obstruction of the birth canal by ovarian tumors or uterine leiomyomata, conduction anesthesia, malposition of the fetal head, maternal exhaustion, and ineffective expulsive efforts. Arrest of descent is diagnosed if there is no significant progress in descent of the vertex over 1 hour. Again, when this event occurs and all options for resolution have been exhausted, operative delivery should be strongly considered.

The choice between operative vaginal delivery and cesarean delivery should be based on considerations such as operator expertise, position and station of the fetal head, and perceived adequacy of the pelvis for safe passage of the fetus. The increased risk for

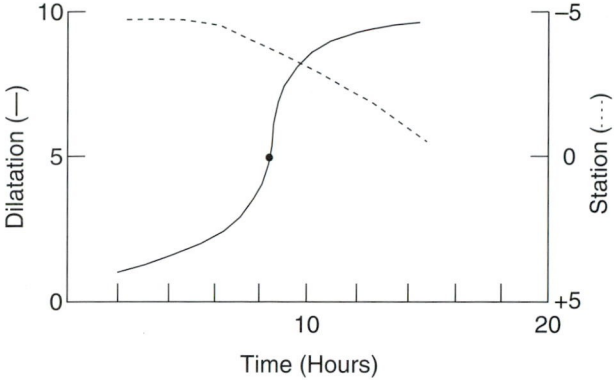

Figure 17-16 Protraction of the second stage.

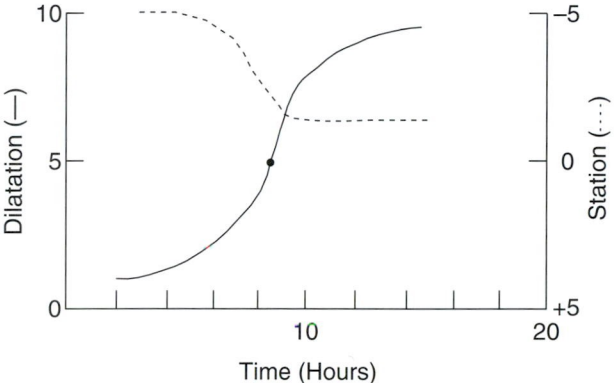

Figure 17-17 Arrest of the second stage.

fetal and maternal trauma observed following mid-forceps procedures indicates that abdominal delivery is the preferred route of delivery in a woman with midpelvic arrest.[53] Graphic illustrations of second stage protraction and arrest disorders are depicted in Figures 17-16 and 17-17.

DELIVERY

Spontaneous Vaginal Delivery

Vaginal delivery is the culminating event of a normal course of labor. It may occur naturally without assistance (common in many third-world countries) or with assistance from a birth attendant (typical in developed countries). Preparations for assisted vaginal delivery begin during the second stage of labor with careful examination to estimate the fetal size relative to the pelvic capacity and to determine the attitude and position of the fetal vertex. Review of the preceding course of labor and antenatal history may also provide useful clinical information and alert the obstetric or neonatal providers to special problems or

needs. Equipment needed for the care of the mother or neonate and all instruments essential for delivery should be readily available. Finally, the need for immediate resuscitation of the neonate cannot often be accurately predicted on the basis of intrapartum events; thus, delivery attendants should be prepared to provide immediate neonatal cardiorespiratory support at all deliveries.

As the fetal vertex descends under the pubic symphysis, the perineum and labia minora will naturally undergo distention and stretching. Many believe that this perineal distention decreases the likelihood of perineal and vaginal wall lacerations with the expulsion of the fetus. As the fetal head delivers by extension, support of the perineal body by the birth attendant can facilitate delivery and help prevent perineal lacerations. Once the fetal head is exposed to the bregma, a modified Ritgen maneuver can be performed to facilitate extension and expulsion of the fetal head. This maneuver is accomplished by placing several towel-covered fingers against the perineum and rectum, palpating the fetal chin and applying traction in an anteroinferior direction, reducing the perineal body over the fetal face and chin. The nasopharynx and oropharynx of the fetus are then cleared of mucus and amniotic fluid with gentle suction as the head naturally restitutes to a transverse orientation. Bulb suctioning is typically performed when there is no meconium staining of the amniotic fluid. When meconium staining is present, the use of a modified DeLee suction device attached to a mechanical vacuum source may provide more effective clearing of the fetal airway and reduce the risk of meconium aspiration syndrome.

The neck should be palpated to determine if a nuchal cord is present. If present, the umbilical cord should be looped over the fetal head or doubly clamped and transected. Excessive traction on the umbilical cord in an attempt to reduce a tight nuchal cord or failure to reduce the nuchal cord prior to delivery of the body can result in avulsion of the cord near the fetal umbilicus with subsequent fetal hemorrhage.

The delivery attendant should then place his or her hands against the fetal parietal bones and apply gentle downward pressure on the head while the mother bears down. The anterior shoulder should then be noted to pass underneath the symphysis. Following delivery of the anterior shoulder, the fetus should be gently lifted toward the pubis for delivery of the posterior shoulder. Some attendants prefer to not have the mother bear down during this portion of the delivery in an effort to avoid rapid expulsion and tearing of perineal tissue. Regardless of maternal bearing efforts, the perineal body should be carefully supported during delivery of the posterior shoulder in an effort to prevent injury to the perineum and vagina. Once the shoulders have cleared the introitus, the remainder of the baby will deliver spontaneously. The practitioner should attempt to control the expulsion of the baby throughout because rapid expulsion at any point in the delivery will predispose to vaginal injury. Care must also be taken to maintain a firm grasp of the infant as it exits the introitus.

Episiotomy and Repair

Occasionally, a "relaxing" incision, known as an episiotomy, is made to increase the caliber of the introitus to facilitate delivery. A mediolateral episiotomy divides the bulbocavernosus and superficial transverse perineal musculature (Figure 17-18). A midline episiotomy is made through the perineal body, separating the median raphe of the perineal body where the bulbocavernosus and superficial transverse perineal muscles insert. While a midline episiotomy usually extends half the distance between the posterior fourchette and the rectum, it may be extended to the level of the external anal sphincter. The major complications associated with episiotomy are infection, hematoma, extension into the anal musculature (third-degree laceration) or rectal mucosa (fourth-degree laceration), dehiscence, and fistula formation.

In the United States, the mediolateral episiotomy is not commonly used because of an increase in post-delivery pain, greater technical difficulty with repair, and increased blood loss as compared with midline episiotomy. Mediolateral episiotomy is generally reserved for women who have an underlying condition that could increase the potential for complications associated with deep perineal lacerations or lacerations

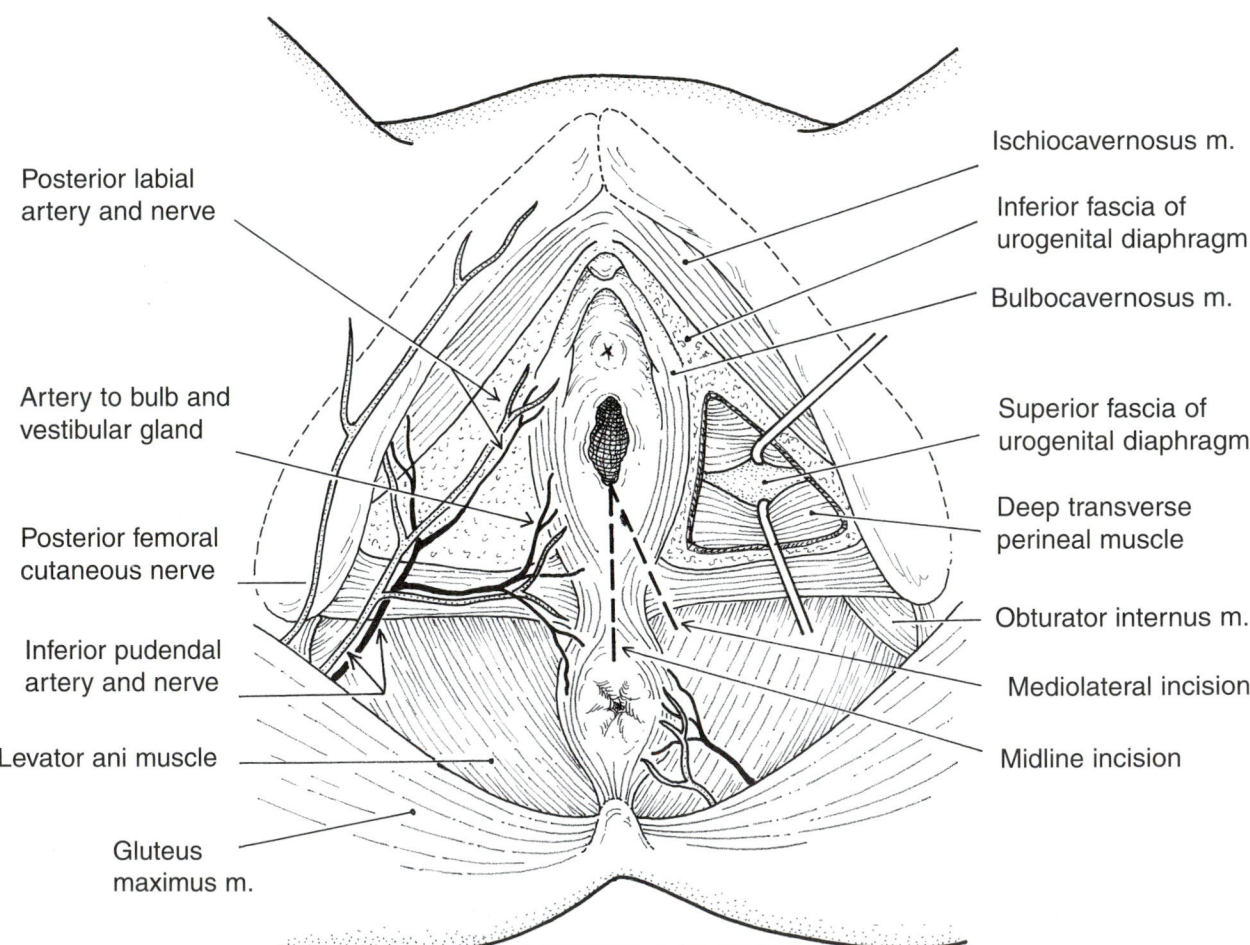

Fig. 17-18 Mediolateral and midline episiotomy with musculature of the urogenital diaphragm.

of the rectum, such as active inflammatory bowel disease, prior rectovaginal fistula, or prior major posterior perineal surgery.

While there is general agreement that some parturients require an episiotomy to hasten delivery in situations of sudden fetal compromise or the inability of maternal expulsive efforts to deliver the fetal head, there is considerable controversy regarding the beneficial effects of prophylactic episiotomy. The liberal or routine use of this procedure has been purported since the early part of this century to reduce the duration of the second stage, prevent birth canal lacerations, ease the reapproximation of separated tissues, and reduce pelvic musculature and nerve damage from overdistention of the birth canal, thereby decreasing the risk for future pelvic relaxation.[54] In examining contemporary evidence-based information, these alleged benefits are largely unsupported. Shortening of the second stage though the routine use of episiotomy has not been conclusively demonstrated and would not be anticipated to be a clinically significant benefit in the era of modern obstetrics when fetal monitoring is routinely performed throughout the second stage. Randomized trials have demonstrated that, while the liberal use of episiotomy is associated with a decrease in vaginal mucosal lacerations, there is an increase in the incidence of deep perineal lacerations.[55–57] Lastly, there are no adequately designed investigations demonstrating a decrease in pelvic muscle or nerve damage with the routine use of episiotomy. Thus, the only real benefit of routine episiotomy may be greater ease in reapproximation of birth canal lacerations or wounds, an effect that is likely of more benefit to the delivery attendant than the parturient. In the absence of data demonstrating a benefit in the reduction of pelvic relaxation, the detrimental acute effects of episiotomy have led some authors to suggest that use be restricted to situations with clear indications and that rates in excess of 30% are excessive.[58]

When midline episiotomy is performed, repair is typically accomplished by using a 2-0 or 3-0 absorbable suture. While there are many ways to repair this incision, the basic tenet of repair is to restore the normal anatomy of the perineum. The most common method for repair involves reapproximating vaginal mucosa and subcutaneous vaginal tissue from the vaginal apex of the incision to the hymenal ring. The perineal body is then reapproximated to the midline with either a simple interrupted suture or a continuous running suture. Finally, the subcutaneous

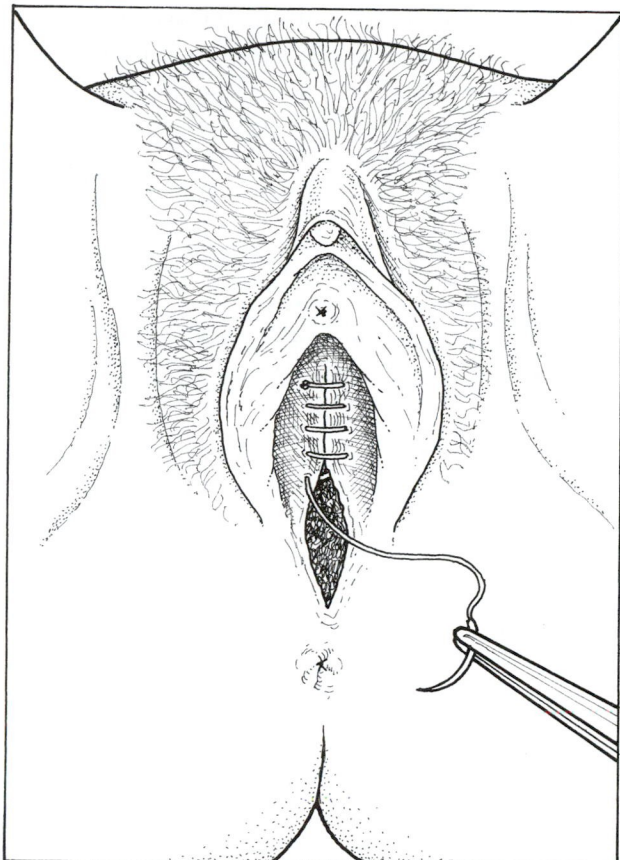

Figure 17-19 Repair of episiotomy. Restoration of the normal anatomy of the perineal body using absorbable suture material.

closure of the dermis completes the restoration of the perineal body (Figure 17-19). Rectal examination should always be performed before and after repair to exclude rectal injury or suture placement through the rectal mucosa, as unrecognized injuries may lead to rectovaginal fistula.

In the event of a third- or fourth-degree laceration, restoration of the normal anatomy requires meticulous attention to surgical technique. Some pelvic surgeons advocate repair, or at least supervision of repair, by the most experienced clinician available. Improper repair may predispose the patient to wound breakdown, infection, fistula formation, and possible late sequelae relating to pelvic floor weakness and rectal incontinence. While there is a paucity of data to support the postponement of repair until an expert in pelvic support is available to repair the perineal damage, there is no question that proper surgical restoration will avoid some immediate complications and potentially some late complications as well.

The repair of the fourth-degree perineal laceration should be approached by first visualizing the restoration of each layer of injured tissue from the rectal mucosa to the vaginal mucosa. Adequate exposure, hemostasis, and proper lighting are essential to properly repair these injuries. Typically, 4-0 absorbable suture is used to reapproximate the rectal mucosa. Whether the mucosa is united with one continuous suture or interrupted sutures is probably of little consequence. In either case, sutures should be placed close enough to each other to restore mucosal integrity along the entire length of the laceration and yet avoid devitalization of the mucosal and submucosal tissues. It is critical to have adequate mobilization of the wound edges so that the reapproximated tissue will not be under tension. Careful handling of the tissue will also help to prevent devascularization and tissue necrosis, both of which contribute to repair breakdown. A second layer imbricated over the first reinforces the rectal mucosa and relieves tension on the first suture line. This layer also serves to reapproximate the internal anal sphincter, a coalescence of smooth-muscle fibers that is extremely difficult to recognize.

For both third- and fourth-degree lacerations, 2-0 suture is used to reapproximate the external anal sphincter by opposing the torn muscle bellies and fascial capsules of the sphincter. Two or three separate interrupted sutures are sufficient to support the return of the external anal sphincter to its original position. Failure to adequately reapproximate the sphincter musculature can result in the patient suffering incontinence of flatus or feces. Finally, a continuous suture layer is placed in the subvaginal tissue to build a shelf over the rectovaginal space and the external anal sphincter. The remainder of the repair proceeds in the same fashion as the repair of the midline episiotomy.

Forceps-Assisted Delivery

Clinicians managing the second stage of labor will often be presented with cases in which either spontaneous or augmented labor and maternal expulsive efforts are inadequate to effect a spontaneous vaginal delivery. In addition, deterioration of the fetal or maternal condition may occasionally necessitate an expedited delivery. If the fetal head has descended into the lower portions of the birth canal, operative vaginal delivery is usually preferable to abdominal delivery. The use of forceps to assist vaginal delivery was described as early as the 17th century. The design of forceps has since evolved remarkably, and there are

a plethora of types available for use. Forceps fall into a few basic functional categories, and choice is often simply due to user preference.

A single blade of a pair of forceps has four basic parts; the handle, shank, pelvic curve, and cephalic curve (Figure 17-20). There are many variations in each of these parts that change the appearance of and tailor the forceps for use in specific circumstances. In general, forceps can be categorized as classic or specialized instruments. Classic forceps are primarily traction instruments to be used when the fetal head is in the lower portion of the pelvis and oriented in an anteroposterior position. There are two types of classic forceps, Simpson and Elliott, differentiated by the configuration of the shanks. Simpson forceps have parallel shanks and Elliott forceps have overlapping shanks. The parallel shanks of the Simpson forceps cause greater distention of the introitus as traction is applied, but also allow the operator to more easily perform an episiotomy. Specialized forceps are designed for a specific situation, such as Piper forceps for use in breech deliveries, or Kielland forceps, which are primarily a rotational instrument.

The cephalic curve refers to the portion of each blade that is curved to conform to the fetal head. Early obstetric forceps were designed as destructive instruments to crush the fetal head in situations of obstructed labor in order to preserve the mother's life; thus, they did not have a cephalic curve. Alterations of the cephalic curve primarily allow the forceps to conform to fetal heads with varying degrees of molding. For example, Simpson forceps have a gradual, elongated cephalic curve designed for traction on a molded fetal head. Tucker–McLane forceps have a shortened, more rounded cephalic curve, which is ideal for traction on an unmolded fetal head, typical of fetuses delivered to multiparous patients.

A fenestration (window) within the blade provides a better grip on the fetal head so that the blades will not slip during traction. This is particularly important with forceps that have a gradual cephalic curve, such as Simpson or Elliot forceps. If there were no fenestration in the blades of these instruments, much greater compressive forces would have to be applied to ensure against the blades slipping during traction. Forceps with a greater cephalic curve, such as Tucker–McLane, are less prone to slipping, and therefore, commonly are not fenestrated. Pseudofenestration is a modification that can be applied to any variety of forceps. The blade is solid, but has a depressed center region on the fetal side of the blade. This modification

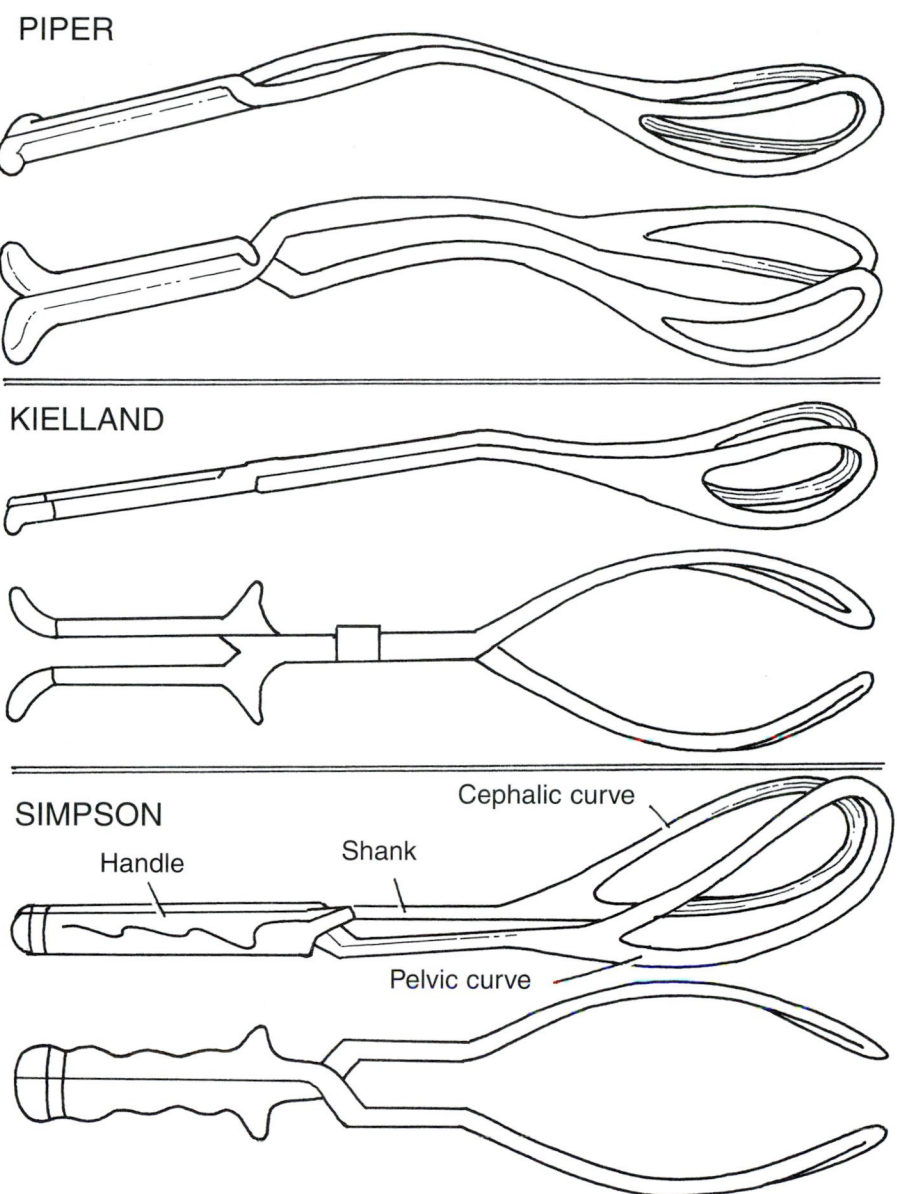

PIPER

KIELLAND

SIMPSON

Cephalic curve

Handle

Shank

Pelvic curve

Figure 17-20 Three examples of obstetric forceps: Kielland (rotational), Piper (assisted breech delivery), and Simpson (traction).

is particularly useful for rotational procedures with the depression in the fetal side of the blade providing excellent traction on the fetal head without excessive compressive forces, while the solid face of the maternal side of the blade reduces the potential for maternal vaginal laceration during placement or rotation.

The pelvic curve is the portion of the blade that conforms to the natural curve of the maternal pelvis. This is the normal arc through which the fetal vertex must pass to allow for delivery. This pelvic curve is a necessity in all traction-type forceps because it allows the operator to deliver the fetal vertex while following the natural curve of the pelvic outlet. Simpson and Elliot forceps have a pelvic curve, making them ideal traction forceps. In contrast, Kielland forceps are rotational forceps, without a significant pelvic curve.

The absence of the pelvic curve allows for easier placement when the fetal head is in a transverse position. Although traction can be performed with Kielland forceps, it becomes necessary to continually reorient the blades to adjust for the changing position of the vertex within the maternal pelvis as it negotiates the final cardinal movements of labor. Therefore, when a rotational procedure is performed with Kielland forceps, the forceps are often removed following completion of the rotation, and traction forceps are then applied to effect delivery.

Classic forceps can be easily applied with the vertex in an anteroposterior orientation. When the sagittal suture is more than 45 degrees off of the anteroposterior plane, application typically requires "wandering" the blade into proper position. Attempts to place classic forceps in this circumstance can result in severe vaginal lacerations and the inability to achieve a biparietal, bimalar application, particularly if the fetal head is in an asynclitic position. Thus, when the vertex is in a transverse or asynclitic orientation, the use of specialized forceps or a vacuum extractor may be required to assist delivery of the fetus. Kielland and Barton forceps are specialized forceps that can be used to effect delivery of the fetus with the vertex in a transverse position. Barton forceps consist of a hinged anterior blade, which is applied first, and a fixed posterior blade. This type of forceps is capable of generating an extreme amount of rotational force and is no longer in common use. Kielland forceps have a relatively small blade without a pelvic curve, which facilitates application to the fetal head in a transverse position. The anterior blade can be applied using one of three methods: (1) the blade can be directly applied, (2) the blade can be applied across the fetal face with the blade then "wandered" anteriorly, and (3) the anterior blade can be inserted in an inverted position underneath the symphysis with the blade then rotated 180 degrees. In addition, the sliding lock on Kielland forceps allows for a biparietal, bimalar application when the fetal head is in an asynclitic orientation.

Prior to the performance of an operative delivery, the operator must satisfy certain basic prerequisites in order to execute a safe operative vaginal delivery (Table 17-4). The Committee on Obstetrics and Maternal and Fetal Medicine of the American College of Obstetricians and Gynecologists has recommended that operative vaginal delivery be classified according to the station of the vertex and degree of rotation.[59] Current guidelines classify forceps operations as outlet, low, and mid. There is no current use for the classification of high forceps in modern obstetrics. For an operation to be classified as outlet forceps, the oper-

ator must visualize the fetal head at the introitus without manually separating the labia; the fetal skull must reach the pelvic floor; the sagittal suture must be in an anteroposterior diameter or right or left occiput anterior or posterior position no more than 45 degrees off of the anteroposterior plane. If the leading point is at or below +2 (cm) station, or the delivery requires more than a 45-degree rotation and does not meet criteria for outlet forceps, this delivery is classified as low forceps. Midforceps are defined as any in which where the leading point of the vertex is between 0 and +2 (cm) station.

The placement of classic forceps should begin with the proper positioning of the patient in the low lithotomy position. For low forceps and midforceps procedures, the bladder should be emptied if this has not been done recently. The application of each blade involves placement of the cephalic blade against the vertex, with the handle pointing in a direction perpendicular to the floor. The left blade (designated by the orientation of the patient's left side) is normally inserted first. The handle is held in the left hand as the right hand displaces the vaginal side wall from the fetal head. With the forceps being held with the handle pointing vertically and the flat portion of the blade resting against the crown of the fetal head, the handle is gently lowered while rotating the forceps 90 degrees counterclockwise. The blade remains flush against the vertex throughout the entire motion (Figure 17-21). Forceful application is not required as the weight of the forceps blade is sufficient to allow the instrument to fall into place.

The right blade should be applied in a similar fashion. Application efforts should cease immediately if bright red blood is noted or if the mother has a sudden onset of sharp pain in the vaginal area, as these likely signify a vaginal-wall laceration. If bleeding or pain occurs, the offending blade should be removed, cephalic position should be reassessed, and another attempt can then be made as appropriate.

Once both blades have been placed, the position of each blade should be rechecked in reference to the fetal vertex in order to ensure a bimalar, biparietal application (Figure 17-22). The sagittal suture of the calvarium should be approximately perpendicular to the plane of the shanks of each blade. The relation of the posterior fontanelle to each blade should be equidistant. In addition, there should be no more than one fingerbreadth distance between the end of the blade and the calvarium. Finally, the blades should be applied

---

TABLE 17-4
PREREQUISITES FOR OPERATIVE VAGINAL DELIVERY

Complete cervical dilatation
Ruptured membranes
Known rotation of vertex in relation to anteroposterior axis
Engaged fetal head
Estimated fetal weight
Assessment of clinical pelvimetry
Adequate maternal analgesia
Experience in application and use
Capability for emergency abdominal delivery

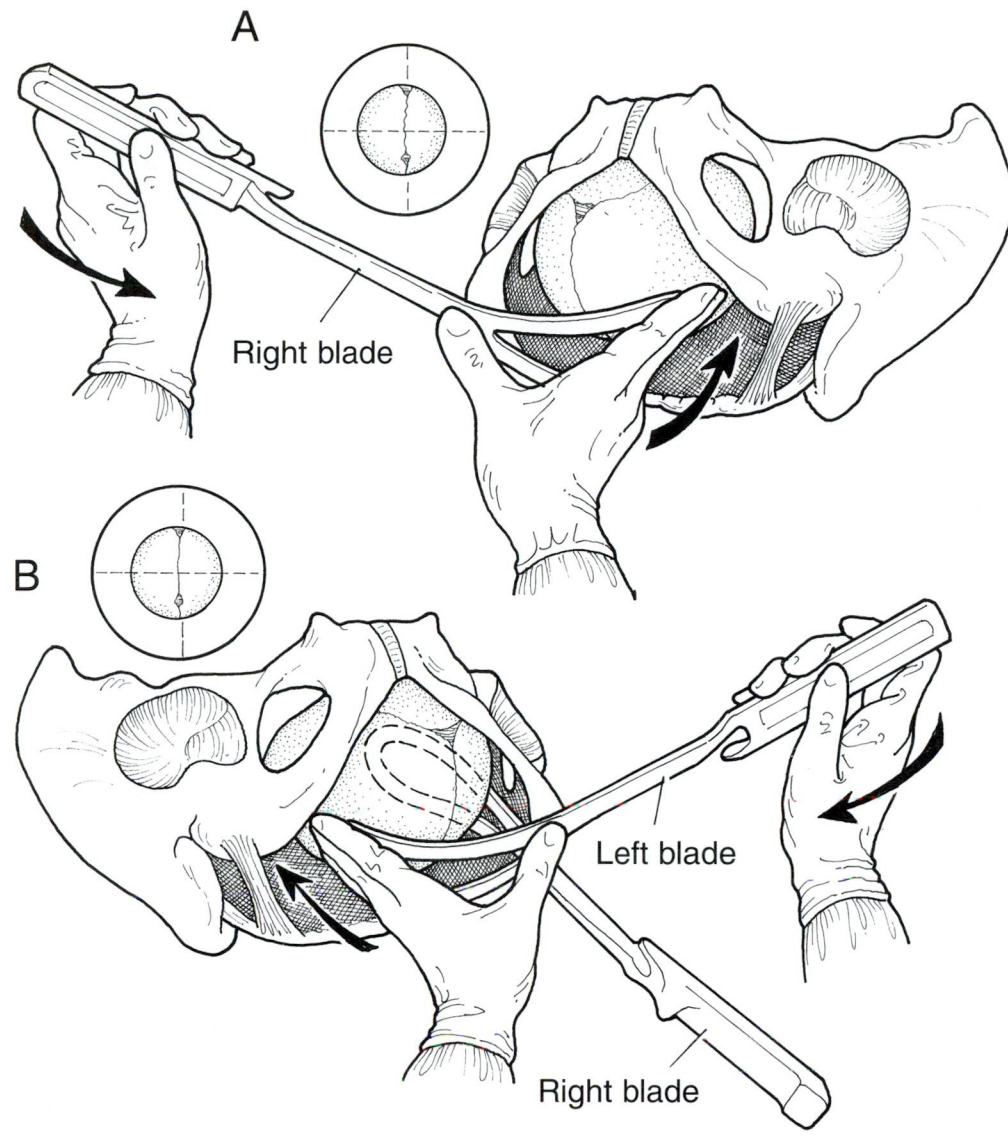

A

Right blade

B

Left blade

Right blade

Figure 17-21 Proper placement of forceps blades. Note the orientation of the blade to the fetal head prior to (A) and after (B) placement.

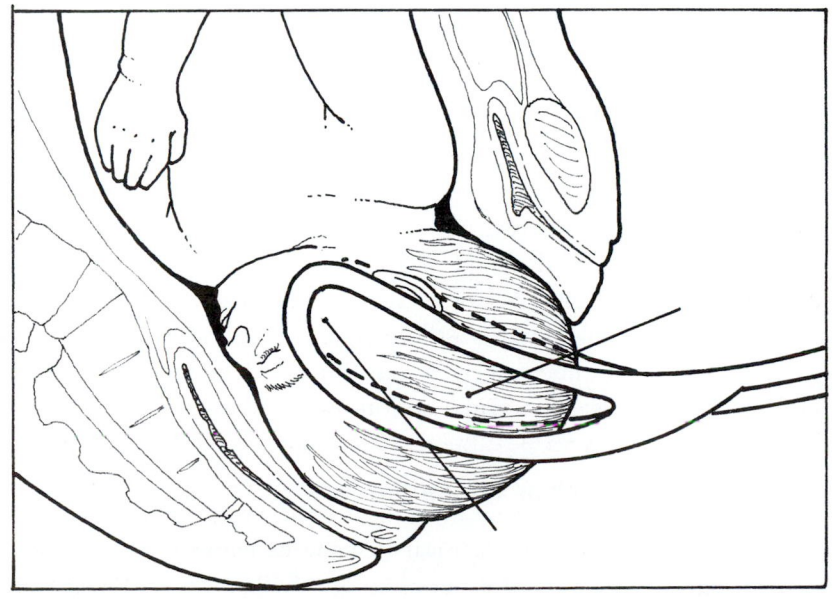

Figure 17-22 Bimalar/biparietal application. Correct forceps application with both blades in contact with the malar prominences and parietal bones.

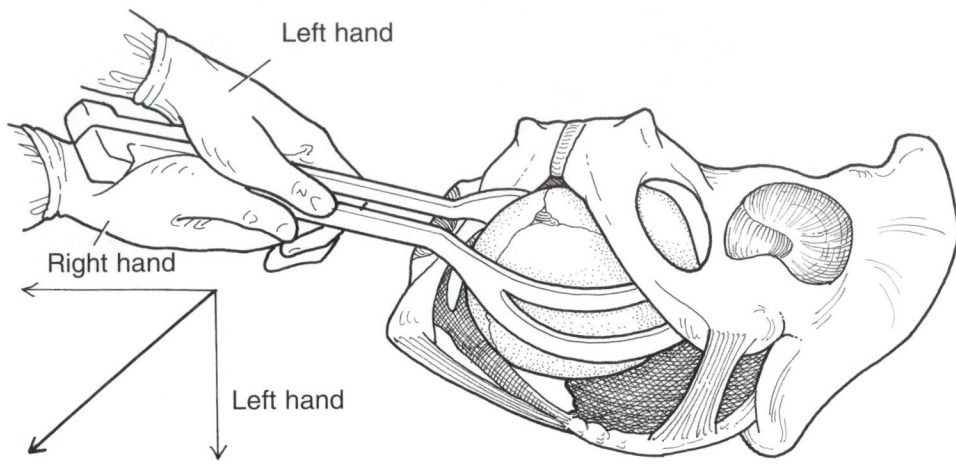

Figure 17-23 Vector of traction. Saxtorph–Pajot maneuver. Axis of traction is at a 45-degree angle downward from the horizontal in a low forceps or midforceps operation.

Left hand

Right hand

Left hand

to the parietal bones of the fetus. Traction should not be applied until the above steps have been verified in order to avoid injury to fetal soft tissue or bones.

Traction should be applied in a manner so that the force vector axis is parallel to the corresponding axis of the birth canal for the particular station of the biparietal diameter. When viewed from a sagittal section, the axis of the birth canal has an inverted **J** shape. For low forceps and midforceps procedures, the initial direction will be at a 45-degree angle downward from the horizontal plane, progressing to traction in the horizontal plane, and finally, at a slight upward angle as the vertex is crowning. The initial downward traction is accomplished by maintaining traction in the horizontal vector as downward traction is applied by the opposite hand to the shanks of the forceps (Saxtorph–Pajot maneuver Figure 17-23). Alternatively, axis traction devices may be attached to the forceps to aid in the application of force along the appropriate vector.

Once the largest portion of the biparietal diameter has passed under the symphysis pubis, the forceps may be disarticulated and the vertex delivered in the usual fashion with a modified Ritgen maneuver. Alternatively, the forceps may be left in place for traction and control of the head as it is delivered through the introitus. Care must be taken not to hyperextend the forceps toward the maternal abdomen, as this maneuver tends to drive the toes of the forceps blade into the posterior vaginal wall and perineal body, potentially creating or extending birth canal lacerations.

Vacuum-Assisted Delivery

The vacuum extractor has undergone several changes over the decades since it was originally developed to

assist delivery. The original device was the Malmström extractor, which was a rigid metal cup that was applied for 10 minutes prior to traction to allow formation of a chignon. A more malleable Silastic cup was introduced later and proved to be easier to apply and did not require chignon formation; therefore traction could be immediately applied. Current vacuum devices have smaller cups that are easier yet to apply and have less propensity to traumatize the vaginal mucosa.

The basic requirements for a vacuum-assisted delivery are the same as for forceps delivery, with the exception that surety of fetal head position is not required. The potential benefits of using the vacuum are (1) it occupies less space than forceps and, therefore, may require less anesthesia, (2) it is less likely to cause maternal genital-tract trauma, (3) it requires less training to use, and (4) it can be used to correct asynclitism (Figure 17-24). However, the use of vacuum does present several unique challenges. The vacuum is a pure traction instrument and cannot be used to exert rotational force without increasing the potential for fetal scalp laceration, cephalohematoma, and subgaleal bleeding.[60] Also, the operator should take care to apply suction only when the cup is verified to be applied to the vertex and vaginal mucosa is not pinched between the cup and the cranium. In general, vacuum-assisted operative deliveries should not be undertaken in cases in which forceps would not also be a viable option for treatment.

Vacuum versus Forceps

Once the decision is made to perform an operative delivery, the question of whether to use forceps or vacuum may be based on several considerations, as

| Normal | Anterior Asynclitism | Posterior Asynclitism |

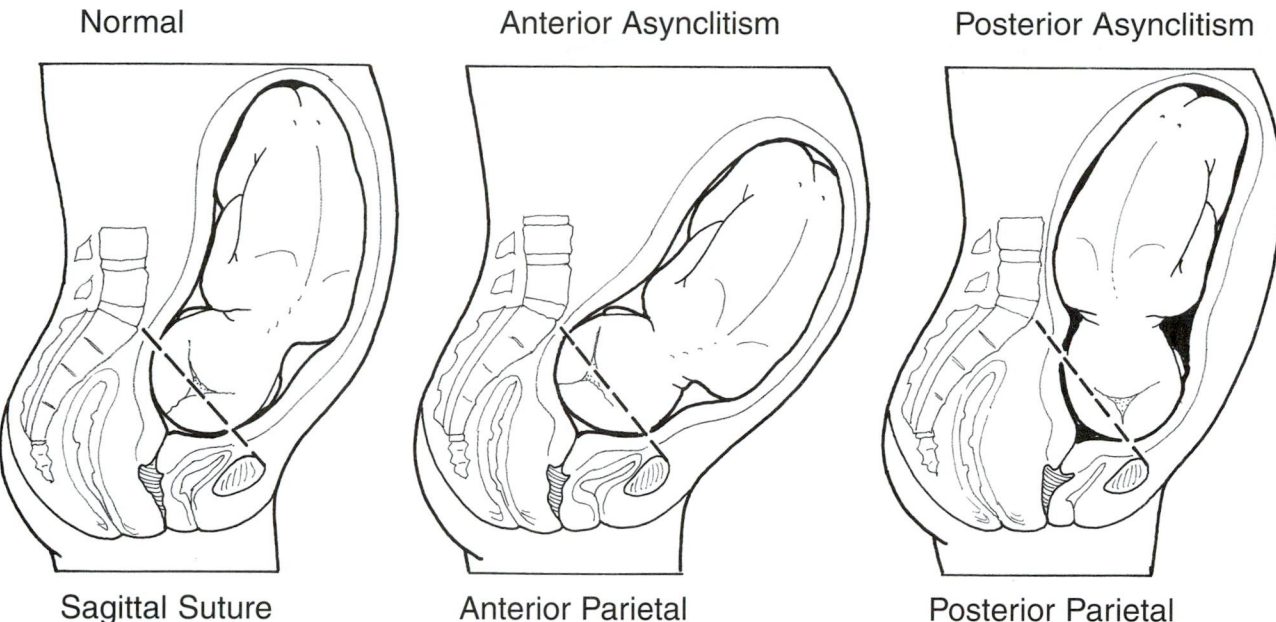

| Sagittal Suture | Anterior Parietal | Posterior Parietal |

Figure 17-24 Different forms of asynclitism. Note the location for the placement of the vacuum to correct for the asynclitism.

each method has its advantages and disadvantages.[61,62] Forceps are more likely to cause vaginal lacerations and facial bruising of the fetus. The vacuum extractor has a greater chance to fail because of a sudden loss of vacuum during traction, particularly when the head begins to crown. Of perhaps greatest importance in the decision to use either method in an operative delivery is the operator's experience with use of the instrument. While it is optimal to be facile with the use of both instruments, personal preference based on previous training and experience typically prevail in the decision to use a specific instrument. From the point of view of many patients, vacuum devices may be more appealing in comparison to forceps; however, education regarding the fundamental mechanics of forceps can usually overcome the misconception that some patients have of forceps functioning as pliers.

SHOULDER DYSTOCIA

Shoulder dystocia results from impaction of the anterior shoulder behind the symphysis pubis (Figure 17-25). Criteria used to define shoulder dystocia are easier to articulate than measure, as there is certainly a wide spectrum of difficulty encountered in delivery of the shoulders, and the defining point between mere assistance in delivery and "dystocia" is nebulous. Perhaps the most useful definition for shoulder dystocia is impaction of the shoulder after delivery of the fe-

tal vertex which requires specific maneuvers to relieve the impaction in order to effect delivery of the fetus. Defined as such, the incidence of shoulder dystocia is typically 0.5 to 2%.

Risk factors for shoulder dystocia include fetal macrosomia, diabetes mellitus, prolonged second-stage labor, and midpelvic operative delivery. However, the majority of shoulder dystocia cases occur in nondiabetic patients with fetuses weighing less than 4000 g.

As the frequency of shoulder dystocia increases in macrosomic fetuses, several investigators have performed decision analysis calculations to evaluate whether the incidence of shoulder dystocia could be decreased by managing these cases with elective cesarean delivery. One group of authors estimated that approximately 2345 such cesarean deliveries, at an expense of $4.9 million dollars, would have to be performed to prevent a single case of shoulder dystocia that resulted in permanent injury.[63] Therefore, the benefits of implementing a program of elective cesarean delivery for macrosomia are not well supported. Similarly, randomized trials of labor induction and expectant management in the nondiabetic patient with suspected or impending macrosomia have failed to demonstrate decreases in the abdominal or operative vaginal delivery rates or a decrease in the incidence of shoulder dystocia.[64,65] Thus, the implementation of protocols for cesarean delivery or induction of labor in an attempt to circumvent shoulder dystocia appear to be ineffective.

Fig. 17-25 Impaction of the anterior shoulder behind the pubic symphysis.

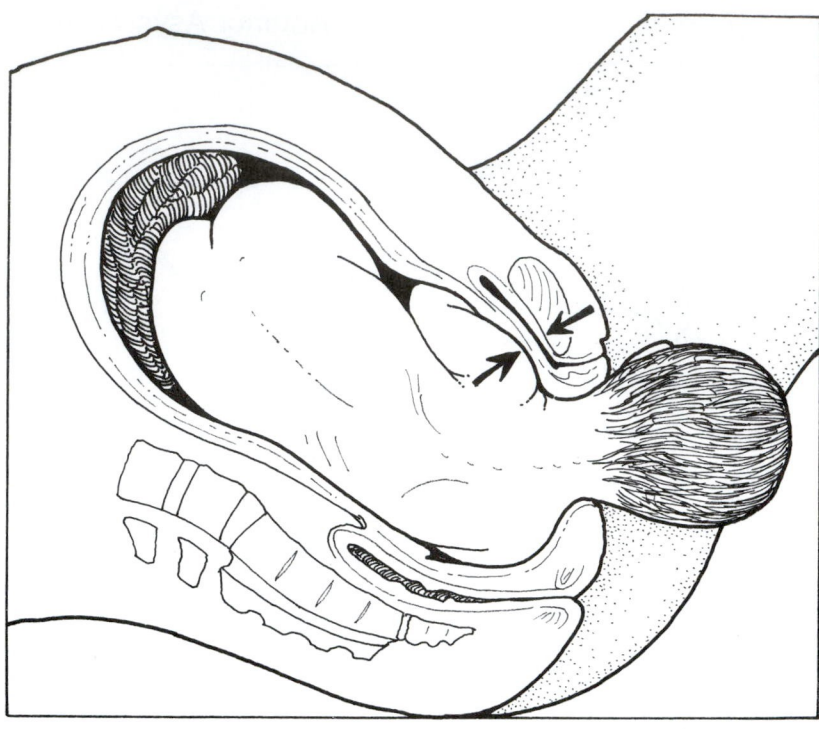

Given that the majority of deliveries complicated by shoulder dystocia cannot be prevented through the use of planned cesarean delivery, the key element in the effective management of shoulder dystocia is anticipation and preparation. Delivery room attendants should anticipate the potential for shoulder dystocia and discuss and rehearse their management plans ahead of time. Signs suggesting impending shoulder dystocia at the time of delivery include a turtle sign on delivery of the fetal vertex, retraction of the head against the inferior portion of the pubic symphysis, and failure of egress of amniotic fluid with delivery of the vertex.

If shoulder dystocia occurs, the following steps should be taken to facilitate disimpaction of the shoulder. There may be disagreement of the order in which each of the steps are undertaken; however, the most important factor in successful management of shoulder dystocia is that the practitioner has a clear plan of action for resolution of this emergency. By recognizing the potential for shoulder dystocia and rehearsing initial management steps, the delivery team may reduce the element of panic that can accompany this complication and lead to overzealous traction prior to disimpaction of the shoulder, setting the stage for nerve injury.

Following recognition of shoulder dystocia, the attendant should ensure that anesthetists and pediatricians are immediately notified by someone other than a needed member of the delivery team. Assistants should help the mother assume the McRoberts position with the hips hyperflexed and abducted (Figure 17-26). With the next contraction and maternal expulsive effort, suprapubic pressure should be applied by an assistant. If the shoulder is noted to descend under the symphysis, the delivery attendant may provide gentle traction to facilitate delivery. The attendant must make a concerted effort to refrain from applying excessive traction to the fetal head prior to relief of the impaction. The use of the McRobert maneuver has been demonstrated to achieve several effects that are likely useful in relieving the shoulder dystocia. Hyperflexion of the hips causes the anterior maternal pelvis to rotate cephalad, which brings the inlet directly perpendicular to the vector of maximal maternal expulsive forces while opening the pelvic inlet to its maximal dimensions and flattening the lumbosacrum. The McRobert maneuver with suprapubic pressure resolves up to 90% of shoulder dystocias.[66] If the McRoberts maneuver is unsuccessful, positioning the mother on all fours may result in disimpaction of the anterior shoulder.[67]

If these initial maneuvers are ineffective, episioproctotomy should be performed to eliminate the component of soft-tissue dystocia contributed by the perineal body. Rotation of the anterior shoulder to an oblique position can be attempted. If this maneuver is unsuccessful in effecting delivery, continued rota-

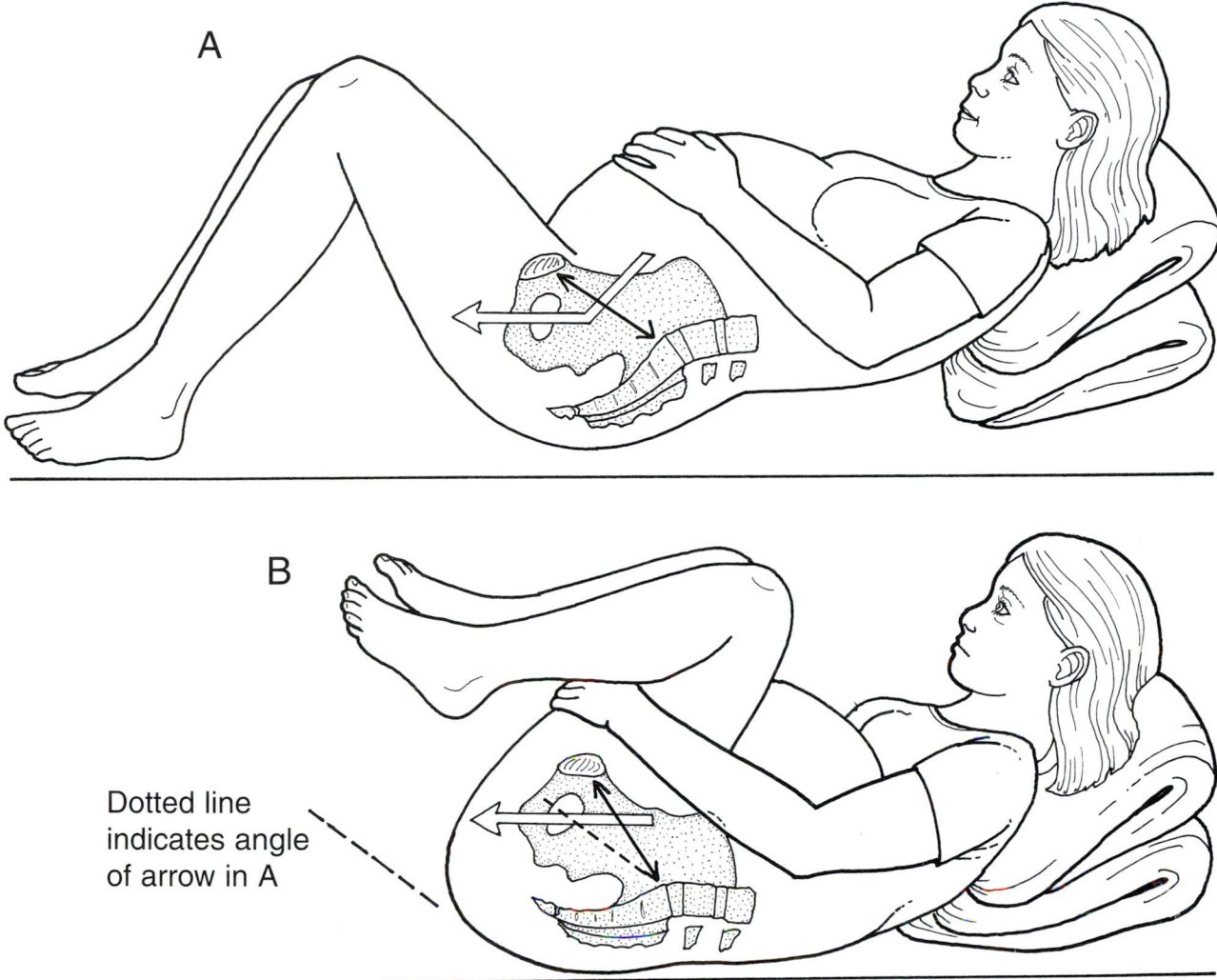

Dotted line
indicates angle
of arrow in A

Fig. 17-26 McRoberts maneuver. Hyperflexion of the maternal hips onto the abdomen and the resulting change in the pelvic orientation.

tion to a total of 180 degrees will bring the anterior shoulder to a posterior position, which may result in relief of the impaction. Continued rotation of the fetal trunk through 180-degree arcs combined with fundal pressure can result in descent and disimpaction of the shoulders, a manuever referred to as the Wood screw.[68] While the original description of this maneuver suggested that the attendant place several fingers on the anterior aspect of the posterior shoulder for rotation, this results in abduction of the fetal shoulders and an increase in the biacromial diameter. Therefore, Rubin's modification of this maneuver is recommended, in which the attendant's fingers are placed on the scapula to·effect rotation.[69] If the anterior shoulder remains impacted under the symphysis or the fetal trunk cannot be rotated, delivery of the posterior arm should be attempted (Figure 17-27). Intentional fracture of the fetal clavicle and

symphysiotomy are destructive maneuvers that are seldom practiced in developed countries but have been described as potential actions to facilitate release of the impacted shoulder. An alternative "last resort" popularized during the past decade is cephalic replacement, also known as the Zavanelli maneuver.[70] This maneuver is merely an effort to replicate the cardinal movements of labor in a reverse order while elevating the fetal head in the birth canal as preparations are being made for abdominal delivery. In the unusual situation in which the anterior shoulder is impacted under the symphysis and the posterior shoulder is impacted by the sacral promontory, cephalic replacement is often the only option and should be considered early. If this method fails, an abdominal incision should be performed, and the impacted shoulder should be disengaged from above. The remainder of the delivery can then be completed vaginally.[71]

A

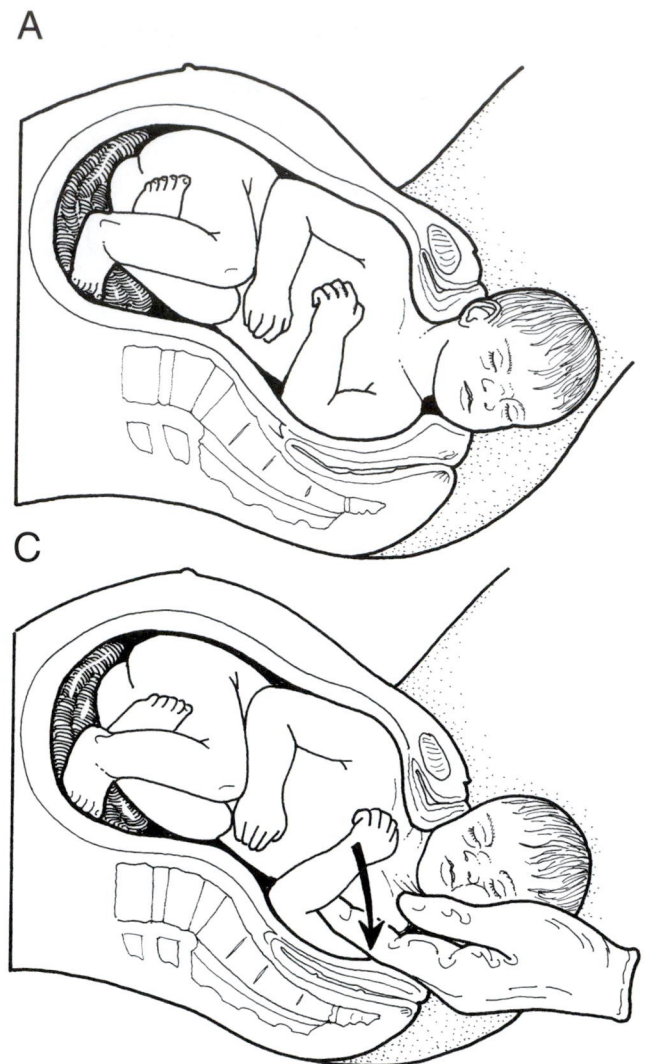

B

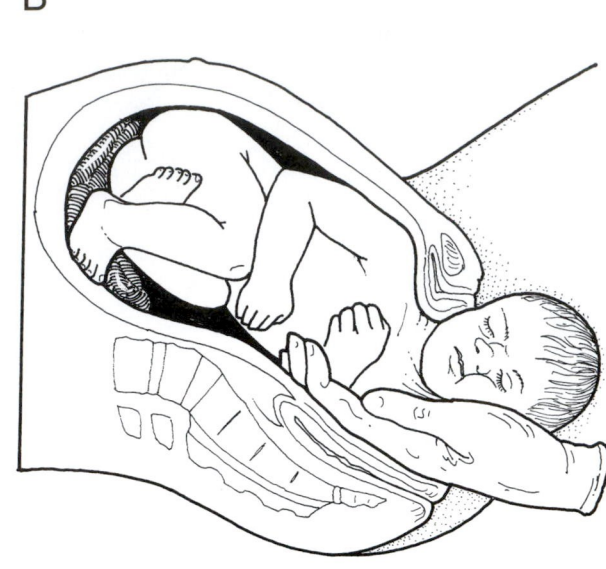

C

Figure 17-27 Sequence for delivery of the posterior arm to resolve shoulder dystocia. A. Shoulder dystocia. B. Placement of hand into posterior vagina. C. Sweep arm across chest and extension of arm to deliver shoulder.

The long-term sequelae from this obstetric emergency range from mild neurologic injury of the brachial plexus to severe neonatal acidosis and even fetal death. While the majority of infants delivered after shoulder dystocia do not have any apparent sequelae, some infants will suffer permanent disability, a situation associated with a high probability of medicolegal action. The incidence of brachial plexus injury following shoulder dystocia is approximately 10%, with over 90% of these resolving within 6 months of delivery.[72] If nerve dysfunction remains evident at 6 months of age, the deficit is likely to be permanent. Aside from brachial plexus injury, there is a significant increase in perinatal morbidity and mortality when shoulder dystocia occurs. Perinatal morbidity, often related to acute intrapartum hypoxia or delivery-related injuries occurs in up to 20% of neonates, and the perinatal mortality rate is increased 10-fold relative to

neonates delivered without shoulder dystocia. Thus, shoulder dystocia should be viewed as an often unpredictable, unpreventable complication of vaginal delivery that is associated with an approximate 1% risk of serious long-term disability. Appropriate contemporary management of this complication should be focused on anticipation and preparation for this event, with subsequent efforts directed at relieving the impaction as quickly as possible, but in a calm, orderly fashion, without excessive traction on the fetal neck prior to disimpaction of the anterior shoulder.

Shoulder Dystocia in the Diabetic Patient

The only subgroup of women who may benefit from elective cesarean delivery in order to prevent shoulder dystocia are women with diabetes. These women are more likely to have delivery complicated by shoulder dystocia, and their neonates are more likely to have long-term sequelae as a result. The fetus of a woman with diabetes has a greater propensity for truncal obesity, predisposing to impaction of the shoulders following delivery of the head. In addition, shoulder dystocia in the pregnant woman with diabetes is more likely to result in permanent neonatal sequelae such as brachial plexus injury or developmental disorders related to perinatal asphyxia. This increase in the risk for shoulder dystocia and resultant permanent injury have led some experts to advocate elective cesarean delivery when the fetus is anticipated to have macrosomia; however, the threshold fetal weight used to offer elective cesarean delivery remains controversial. Using data extracted from a large retrospective investigation, Langer and colleagues estimated that elective cesarean delivery of diabetic women with fetuses with a birth weight of more than 4250 g would prevent 76% of cases of shoulder dystocia in this population and increase the overall cesarean delivery rate by only 0.26%.[73] Unfortunately, this study assumes that the clinician is able to accurately predict the fetal weight based on ultrasonographic measurements. In fact, accurate prediction may be particularly difficult, especially at this extreme of fetal weight.

THIRD STAGE OF LABOR

The third stage of labor is designated as the period from expulsion of the fetus until delivery of the placenta. The average duration of the third stage is 8 minutes, and 95% of women complete this stage in 30 minutes. Intense uterine contractions following delivery of the fetus result in cleavage of the placenta from the decidua basalis and constriction of the spiral arteries as they course through the myometrium, a natural mechanism of hemostasis that is quite efficient.

The three common signs indicative of placental separation are a gush of blood from the introitus, lengthening of the umbilical cord, and the uterus appearing as a globular structure rising in the maternal abdomen. Efforts to facilitate the third stage by injecting uterotonic medications into the umbilical cord or allowing the blood to drain from the severed umbilical-cord remnant have not been demonstrated to be effective in reducing blood loss or reducing the duration of the third stage.

Disorders of the Third Stage of Labor

If separation does not spontaneously occur within 20 to 30 minutes, the practitioner should consider the possibility that the placenta is abnormally adherent, is separated and is held by a contracted lower uterine segment or cervix, or that this is a normal variant. Prolongation of the third stage should prompt manual exploration of the uterine cavity under the supervision of an experienced operator. The attendant should avoid excessive traction on the umbilical cord to minimize the risk for cord avulsion and uterine inversion. Manual exploration in a nonemergent situation should be performed under adequate anesthesia, typically regional anesthesia or intravenous sedation. The operator should put on a second set of gloves and a sterile sleeve, gently separate the labia and place the hand into the uterine cavity, using the umbilical cord to direct the examiner to the placenta. The placenta can then be gradually removed by identifying its plane with the uterus. The operator may facilitate removal of the placenta by placing the opposite hand on the abdomen and pushing the fundus toward the examining hand. Once the placenta has been removed, uterotonic agents should be administered and the extracted placenta examined to ensure complete removal. A second sweep of the cavity may be made with gauze placed over the hand to curette the uterine lining. Manual extraction does not appear to increase the risk for postpartum endometritis, and prophylactic administration of antibiotics is not necessary.[74,75]

Placenta Accreta

The absence of a normal layer of connective tissue (Nitabuch layer) between the placenta and the decidua basalis can result in invasion of chorionic villi beyond the superficial decidual layers into the decidua basalis. This is referred to as a placenta accreta, and normal separation of the placenta during the third stage does not occur (Figure 17-28). This potentially life-threatening condition occurs with an incidence of approximately 1 in 2000 to 1 in 3000 deliveries. Attempts at manual extraction are impaired by the inability to discern a normal plane of separation between a portion or all of the placenta with the uterine wall. Such efforts usually result in removal of only fragments of the placenta, with subsequent hemorrhage. Primary risk factors for placenta accreta include prior uterine curettage, prior uterine surgery, placenta previa, or endometritis.

Figure 17-28 Placenta acc-reta. Abnormal placentation versus normal implantation.

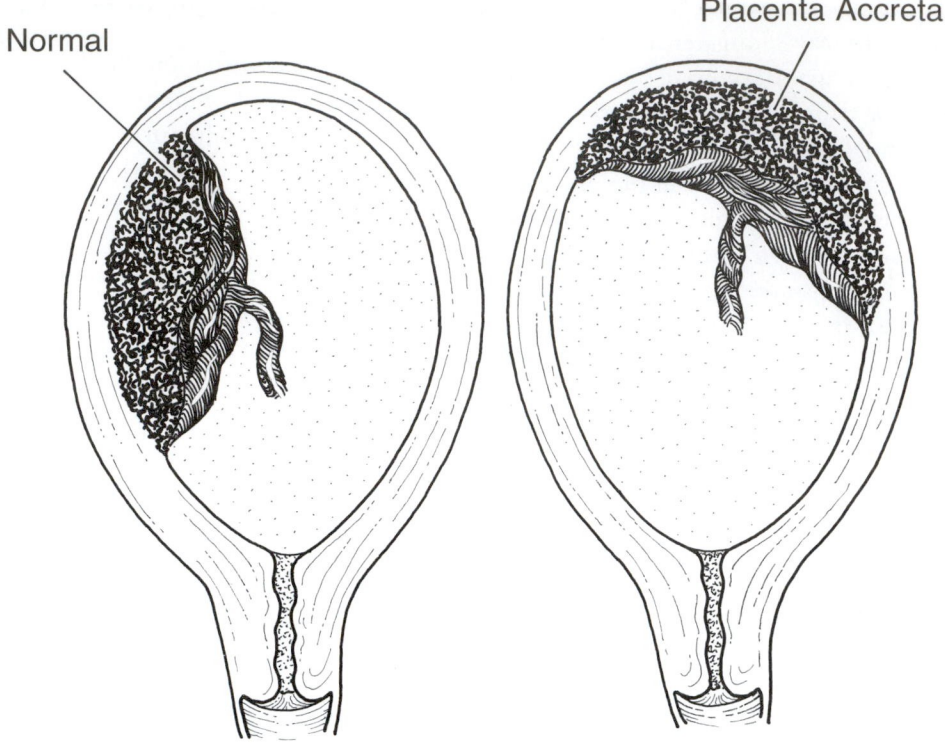

Normal

Placenta Accreta

The initial management of placenta accreta is critical to minimizing maternal morbidity and mortality. With a prolonged third stage, the practitioner should first recognize the possibility of placenta accreta, allowing the delivery room team to anticipate the potential needs for management of this disorder. If it is clear during attempted manual extraction that the placenta is firmly adherent to the uterus, immediate preparations should be made for the management of severe postpartum hemorrhage. Anesthesia, nursing, and blood bank personnel should be notified, and blood products should be available. Operating room personnel and equipment should be available as well. The patient should be informed of the situation and counseled for the possible need for emergency blood replacement and surgery, including uterine curettage, exploratory laparotomy, hypogastric or uterine artery ligation, and peripartum hysterectomy. After preparations have been made, the operator may proceed with extraction of the placenta and remove as much of the retained tissue as possible manually or by curettage. Ultrasound guidance may be helpful during uterine curettage to prevent perforation and to facilitate removal of the remaining placenta. Following placental removal, uterotonic medications such as $PGF_{2\alpha}$ or methergine can be used to aid hemostasis. If placental removal is successful and initial hemostasis is ade-

quate, the patient should be closely monitored for recurrent hemorrhage, which may occur in the first 12 to 24 hours postpartum.

Excessive bleeding following manual extraction and curettage should prompt reassessment of the patient's cardiovascular status, with fluid and blood product replacement as needed. While controversial, uterine packing has been advocated by some as a conservative means of treatment for postpartum hemorrhage. Advocates believe that adequate pressure can be applied to achieve compression of bleeding vessels, while opponents contend that packing only serves to distend the uterus, partially conceal hemorrhage, and interfere with the natural hemostatic method of myometrial constriction of uterine arterioles and venous spasm.[76,77] There are no prospective, randomized trials evaluating the effectiveness of uterine packing; however, case series have reported that up to 80% of women may avoid peripartum hysterectomy if this technique is used.[78] If uterine packing is attempted, care should be taken to tightly and completely pack the uterine cavity. This may be effective in helping to achieve hemostasis, and usually involves using several packs tied together to compress the actively bleeding endometrial bed. In addition, the packs should be counted closely and recorded to ensure none are retained following removal 12 to 24 hours

Chapter 18

Obstetr

and An

Christopher F. James

Five K

- **Curr**
  comb
  epidu
  signi
- **The**
  mort
  inabi
- **The**
  mort
  and
- **The**
  by u
  shou
  epid
- **"Mo**
  mort
  deliv

An obstetric anesthesi
strated a changing prac
rics in the United State
were approximately 15
obstetric care in 1992 b
Association's Guide to th
of this decrease occur
delivery units with fe
year.[1] More women are
with a twofold increase
sia from 1981 to 1992

later. Uterine packing may also slow hemorrhage to such a degree that the patient becomes a candidate for selective embolization by interventional radiographic techniques. These procedures typically require several hours to perform, so a patient with a significant amount of blood loss or who is hemodynamically unstable is not a candidate for embolization.

If the patient continues to bleed significantly, the only option available is to proceed with laparotomy for uterine and/or hypogastric artery ligation, specialized suture placement, or hysterectomy.[79] The decision-making process may hinge on consideration of factors such as age, parity, future fertility desires, and the clinical circumstances. Difficulties may arise when performing a postpartum hysterectomy due to the markedly dilated cervix and the potential to incite further intraoperative complications. In the patient who has suffered major postpartum hemorrhage and has a dilutional coagulopathy, it may be reasonable to perform a subtotal hysterectomy rather than risk further bleeding and extend the length of the operative procedure in an effort to perform a complete hysterectomy.

Uterine Inversion

Uterine inversion is a third-stage disorder that occurs in approximately 1 in 1500 to 1 in 2000 deliveries. This serious disorder can result in massive hemorrhage and maternal shock. Severe hypotension may occur before there is significant hemorrhage, possibly due to a parasympathetic response to extrusion of the uterus from the vagina. Fundal implantation of the placenta, excessive cord traction, and excessive use of uterine relaxing agents (such as magnesium sulfate) have all been implicated as causes of uterine inversion; however, uterine inversion may occur spontaneously, without the presence of any of the above factors.

There are several degrees of uterine inversion, ranging from partial to complete inversion with prolapse of the fundus through the cervix and introitus (Figure 17-29). Uterine inversion may also be temporally classified as acute (within 24 hours of delivery) or delayed (more than 24 hours after delivery).

The primary complications of uterine inversion are hemorrhage and hypovolemic shock. If uterine inversion occurs and the placenta remains attached to the uterus, it should be left in place until the uterus

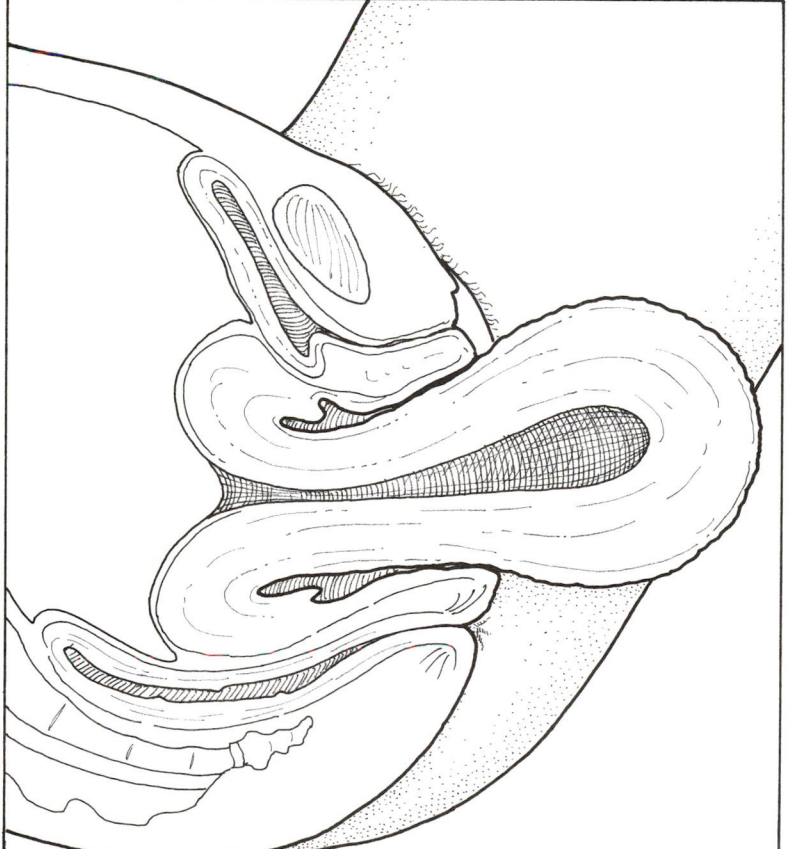

Fig. 17-29 Complete uterine inversion.

40. Secher NJ, Lange Al
    gaard JG. Induction
    amniotomy: a rando
    tablets and intraven
    Scand 1981;60:237.

41. O'Driscoll K, Jacks
    longed labor. BMJ 1

42. Friedman EA. Labo
    2nd ed. New York:

43. O'Driscoll K, Foley
    of labor as an altern
    Obstet Gynecol 19!

44. Frigoletto FD, Lieb
    Ringer S, Datta S. /
    labor. N Engl J Me

45. Caldwell WE, Mol
    female pelvis and tl
    classification. 1933;

46. Thurnau GR, Scat
    index: a method of
    in women attempti
    delivery. 1991;165:

47. Kopelman JN, Duf
    Computed tomogr
    the breech present

48. Baker ER, D'Altor
    cesarean hysterectc

49. Uldbjerg N, Ulms
    cervix in terms of
    Obstet Gynecol 1⁹

50. Koontz WL, Bishc
    of labor. Clin Obs

51. Caldeyro-Barcia R
    quantitative study
    the pregnant hum
    121:18.

52. Thorp JA, Hu Dl
    partum epidural a
    ized controlled pr
    1993;168:319.

53. Bowes WA, Bowe
    operation. Clin C

54. Bansal RK, Tan V
    there a benefit to
    natural experimei

55. Lede RL, Belizan
    siotomy justified?

56. Argentine Episioi
    versus selective e
    Lancet 1993;342:

57. Harrison RF, Bre
    EA. Is routine ep

58. Argentine Episio
    versus selective e
    Lancet 1993;342

59. American Colleg
    Operative vagina
    no. 196, August

obstetricians providing epidural analgesia, with anesthesiologists being more involved in the large hospitals and nurse-anesthetists in the small hospitals.

Anesthetic-related deaths make up approximately 4 to 7% of all maternal deaths and are superseded only by pulmonary embolism, hypertensive disorders, ectopic pregnancies, hemorrhage, and cerebrovascular accidents.[3] Although anesthetic-related mortality is decreasing overall, anesthetic deaths under general anesthesia have been steady, whereas there has been a significant decrease in deaths under regional anesthesia.[4]

Maternal physiologic effects of pain and stress of labor include an increase in catecholamine levels, with resultant increases in maternal blood pressure and decreases in uterine blood flow. Labor pain also leads to maternal hyperventilation, resulting in respiratory alkalosis, and may cause hypoventilation between contractions, resulting in maternal and fetal hypoxemia. Moreover, alkalosis will shift the oxyhemoglobin dissociation curve to the left, increasing maternal oxygen affinity and compromising the fetal transfer of oxygen. These complications have to be weighed against those associated with parenteral or neuraxial drugs. Gastrointestinal motility is decreased with pain, and this effect may be compounded by opioid administration. Of course, clinical implications of reduced gastrointestinal motility include the potential for pulmonary aspiration of gastric contents in pregnant patients who are undergoing general anesthesia or who are oversedated.

The management of pain in labor and delivery is a significant challenge for any health care provider. Labor pain is one of the most severe pain syndromes.[5] There is a wide variation in the degree of pain among laboring patients. In one survey, 50 to 70% of nulliparous patients described their labor pain as severe and intense.[5] It is not uncommon for multiparas to have less analgesic treatment than primaparas during labor and delivery; however, in a Scandinavian study, 50% of grand multiparous patients described their analgesia in labor as "insufficient," and a majority of them suffered intense pain during labor.[6] Pain can be caused by dilation of the cervix, distention and contraction of the uterus; distention of the perineum; pressure on pelvic organs, including the urinary bladder, urethra and rectum; and compression of the lumbosacral plexus. This pain is not only multifaceted, but its intensity increases with the progression of labor. Labor pain is referred from the 10th thoracic

to the 1st lumbar dermatome via afferent sensory nerves (C and A-delta fibers), subsequently entering the lumbar sympathetic chain. This visceral component is usually not well localized and is described as cramping, dull, and aching. In the late first stage and second stage of labor, the earlier visceral component of pain intensifies, with stronger and more frequent contractions. Moreover, during the later part of labor, there is also a somatic component of pain resulting from distention of the pelvic floor, perineum, and vagina by the presenting part of the fetus. These later somatic pain impulses are transmitted via the pudendal nerve or sacral 2nd through 4th nerve roots, and are localized and sharp in nature. Along with pain, labor is also compounded by anxiety, fear, expectations, motivations, and concerns of adverse fetal effects, along with diverse manifestations due to different sociocultural backgrounds.

Therefore, it is not surprising that there have been multiple methods for pain management in this setting. Nonpharmacologic techniques have included natural childbirth proposed by Dick-Read.[7] This approach was first described in the 1940s and was further popularized by Lamaze and his psychoprophylaxis technique of positive conditioning, education and concentration[7] (Table 18-1). These techniques, along with others, are the basis for the present-day prepared childbirth classes that are offered to most pregnant patients. Other nonpharmacologic techniques include hydrotherapy, massage and touch, temperature, and emotional support. More technical methods include acupuncture, biofeedback, hypnosis and transcutaneous electrical nerve stimulation (TENS). Although most of these techniques have very little scientific evidence of efficacy, in certain patient groups they can provide decreased anxiety, prompt less reliance on analgesics, and perhaps shorten labor and reduce the frequency of operative delivery. Pharmacologic techniques such as subcutaneous and intramuscular injections for labor analgesia are not used as frequently today due to their pain on administration. Intravenous administration includes intermittent bolus versus continuous infusion or patient-controlled analgesia (PCA).

Minor nerve blocks include bilateral sympathetic nerve blocks and paracervical blocks (Table 18-2). Although lumbar sympathetic blocks may enhance cervical dilation, they require multiple injections that may not be acceptable to patients. Paracervical blocks have also been used in labor; however, the high

TABLE 18-1
NONPHARMACOLOGIC AND SYSTEMIC
PHARMACOLOGIC ANALGESIA

Nonpharmacologic Analgesia	Effects/Complications
Nontechnical	
Prepared childbirth classes	Decreased anxiety/? Decreased pain
Emotional support	Decreased anxiety
Hydrotherapy	Decreased anxiety/relaxation
Massage and touch	Relaxation
Ambulation	? Shorten labor/? Increased rate of spontaneous delivery
Technical	
Acupuncture	Culture-specific
Biofeedback	Relaxation
Hypnosis	Requires antepartum and intrapartum specialist
Transcutaneous electrical nerve stimulation	Interference with fetal heart rate monitor
Pharmacologic Analgesia	
Opioids	Nausea, vomiting
	Dysphoria, drowsiness
	Neonatal respiratory depression
Subcutaneous/intramuscular	Painful administration
Intravenous	Fast onset
Intermittent bolus	Inconsistent analgesic effect
Continuous infusion	More consistently effective
	Overdose concerns
Patient-controlled analgesia	Greater patient satisfaction
Barbiturates	Sedation
Phenothiazines	Sedation
	Antiemetic effect
	Amnesia
Inhalation agents	Special apparatus required
	Environmental pollution—risk to health-care personnel
	Safety concerns
Nitrous oxide	Rapid onset
	Effective analgesia in <50% of cases
	Hyperventilation
	Hypoxia
	Drowsiness/dysphoria
Potent inhalation agents	Rarely used
	Loss of protective airway reflexes
	Pulmonary aspiration
	Amnesia

incidence of fetal bradycardia and repeated blocks for protracted labor have precluded the widespread acceptance of this technique. Major nerve blocks (neuraxial blocks) for labor include lumbar epidural, caudal epidural, spinal, and combined spinal-epidural techniques (see Table 18-2). Neuraxial analgesia offers superior pain relief with minimal systemic or hemodynamic effects if performed appropriately.

With the significant maternal hemodynamic changes that occur during gestation, labor, and the immediate postpartum period, the interaction of these maternal physiologic changes and the effects of neuraxial blocks can be either beneficial or detrimental. Maternal blood volume increases throughout gestation and peaks at approximately 40% above nonpregnant levels. This increase in blood volume is coupled with a 30 to 40% increase in cardiac output between 20 and 30 weeks of gestation.[8,9] During labor, cardiac output increases another 15 to 45% above prelabor values, with an additional 10 to 25% increase during uterine contractions and a further increase in the immediate postpartum period[9-12] (Figure 18-1). Patients with moderate cardiac reserve may tolerate pregnancy but may decompensate during labor or in the immediate postpartum period. Neuraxial analgesia can curtail the marked increase in cardiac output and potentially ameliorate this decompensation.[13] On the other hand, significant

Regional Block	Effects/Complications
Lumbar sympathetic block	Enhances cervical dilation
	Short-acting
	Requires multiple deep injections
	Accidental neuraxial block
	Maternal hypotension
Paracervical block	First stage of labor only
	Short-acting
	Fetal bradycardia
Epidural analgesia	Excellent analgesia
	Maternal hypotension
	Local anesthetic toxicity
	Accidental total spinal
	Contraindicated in presence of a coagulopathy
Intermittent bolus	Uneven anesthetic effect
Continuous infusion	Greater cumulative dose
Patient-controlled epidural analgesia	Patient satisfaction
	Dose-sparing
	Fewer top-up requirements
Spinal analgesia	Excellent analgesia
	Fast onset
	Short-acting
	Greater maternal mobility if opioids are used
	Uterine hypertonus
	Contraindicated in presence of coagulopathy
	High spinal block
	Headache
Combined spinal epidural analgesia	Flexibility
	Combined advantages of spinal and epidural
	Equipment concerns
Pudendal nerve block	Delivery only—minimal manipulation
	Intravascular injection
Saddle block (low spinal anesthesia)	Effective only for delivery
	Maternal hypotension
	Headache

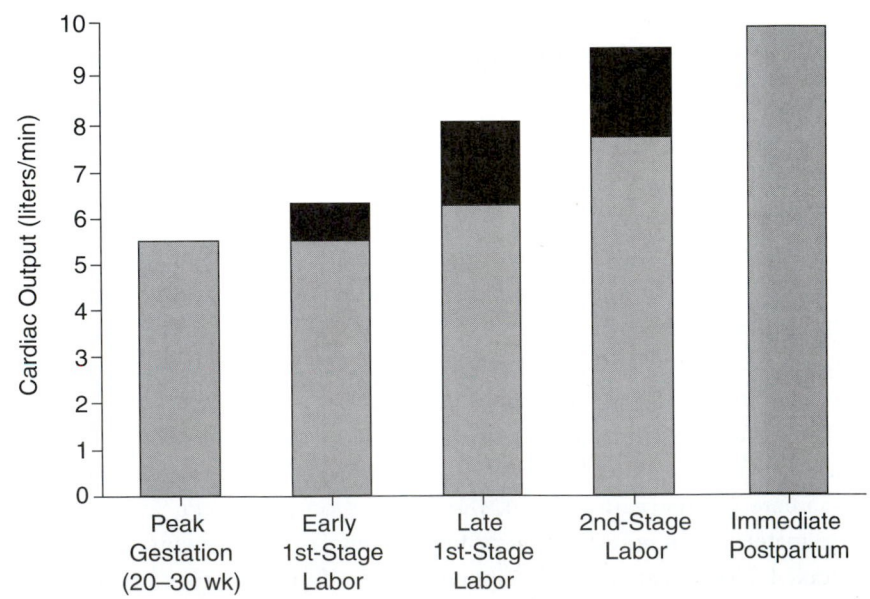

Figure 18-1 Cardiac output during pregnancy, labor, and delivery. Estimated values without regional anesthesia, because cardiac output may vary dramatically among individuals. Solid bars represent increases in cardiac output during contractions. *Reprinted, with permission, from James.*[11]

hypotension from a neuraxial block can also be detrimental in some of these patients. Another major physiologic disturbance that may have a significant interaction with neuraxial analgesia is aortocaval compression. Aortocaval compression occurs in 90% of near-term patients in the supine position; however, because of compensatory mechanisms, only about 10 to 15% of them manifest overt supine hypotensive syndrome.[14,15] With a neuraxial block, part of this compensatory mechanism is blocked, resulting in a high incidence of hypotension [see "Regional (Neuraxial) Analgesia, below].

Analgesia for vaginal delivery includes lumbar epidural analgesia with perineal "top-up" doses, saddle block (low spinal), and pudendal blocks. Low spinal blocks or pudendal blocks usually are reserved for difficult vaginal deliveries for patients who do not have a functioning epidural anesthetic. Anesthesia for cesarean delivery includes neuraxial anesthesia (epidural, spinal, or combined spinal–epidural), general anesthesia and, on rare occasion, local anesthesia. The benefits of regional anesthesia over general anesthesia are discussed below.

Most drugs cross the placenta, including the anesthetic agents. There are four main factors that determine placental drug transfer from mother to fetus. The characteristic of the drug—i.e., its molecular weight, lipid solubility, ionization, and configuration—are major factors, along with the maternal, placental, and fetal components. As part of the maternal component, the route of administration of a drug would determine the uptake and drug levels in the maternal circulation, rendering an intravenous dose of a drug substantially higher than an epidural dose, which in turn would be higher than a spinal dose. If the fetus is acidotic, the drugs that have crossed the placenta may be unable to circulate back to the maternal side due to the increased ionization in the fetus (see below). Because of the characteristics of nondepolarizing muscle relaxants, they do not cross the placenta very well and essentially have no effect on the fetus or neonate. Depolarizing muscle relaxants such as succinylcholine also have no appreciable effect because they are rapidly metabolized by maternal plasma pseudocholinesterase prior to crossing the placenta. However, in a patient with pseudocholinesterase deficiency, succinylcholine may not be metabolized, and, therefore, can cross the placenta and render the neonate weak or paralyzed.

SYSTEMIC MEDICATIONS

Opioids

All systemic medications used in labor for pain control and sedation cross the placenta and can cause either direct or indirect effects, resulting in fetal or neonatal depression, depending on the amount of drug, timing of administration related to delivery, and effects on placental perfusion. A classic example of timing is the use of meperidine in labor. Neonatal depression after meperidine administration occurs between 1 and 4 hours prior to delivery because maximal fetal tissue uptake of meperidine and its metabolite, normeperidine, occurs around 2 to 3 hours after administration to the mother.[16] Opioids are the mainstay for parenteral analgesia in the laboring patient and have usually been used as intermittent boluses because of concerns regarding the mother and the fetus. Concerns for the mother include nausea and vomiting, sedation, dysphoria, and potential respiratory depression. Intramuscular (IM) injections of morphine or meperidine have approximately a 10- to 20-minute onset with a duration of 2 to 3 hours, whereas an intravenous dose has a rapid onset of action (less than 5 minutes) and lasts about 1.5 to 2 hours.[17] The synthetic agonist–antagonist opioids nalbuphine and butorphanol have a purported ceiling effect for respiratory depression, with less nausea and vomiting; however, they can produce more sedation and dizziness.[18,19] Fentanyl, another synthetic opioid, has been shown to have fewer side effects than meperidine; its drawback is its short duration of action.

Besides the intermittent-bolus technique, a more recent adaptation in labor is the use of patient-controlled analgesia (PCA) with either fentanyl or nalbuphine.[20-22] Meperidine initially was the opioid of choice for PCA use. However, long-term use of meperidine in a continuous infusion or in PCA mode can lead to prolonged analgesic effects and potential seizure formation due to its active metabolite, normeperidine. The PCA technique with nalbuphine, fentanyl, or remifentanil would be appropriate for patients in moderate to severe pain who may have a contraindication for a regional anesthetic technique—e.g., a coagulopathy, or when anesthesia services are not provided. Obviously, sedation level and respiratory rate should be monitored. The mother and fetus should be closely monitored, as with a regional anesthetic technique. All sytemic administered opioids may cause a decrease in fetal heart rate (FHR) variability, and butorphanol and nalbuphine have been associated with a sinusoidal FHR pattern.[23]

The narcotic antagonist naloxone hydrochloride is used to reverse maternal and neonatal respiratory depression from narcotic agonists. The neonatal dose is 0.1 mg/kg, and it can be administered intravenously, intramuscularly, or subcutaneously.[24] The onset of action occurs within 2 minutes, and the analgesic effect persists for 20 to 30 minutes. A longer-acting oral narcotic antagonist, naltrexone, is now available. Oral naltrexone should be used to prevent the minor side effects over a prolonged period and not for acute reversal of respiratory depression. Moreover, the partial agonist–antagonists butorphanol and nalbuphine can be used to partially reverse opioid side effects without fully reversing the analgesia in cases in which respiratory depression is not the concern.

Phenothiazines

Phenothiazines often are used in conjunction with opioids because of their antiemetic and sedative effects. Phenothiazines do not appear to cause any appreciable neonatal respiratory depression. Promethazine is the most common phenothiazine used in labor. Other agents are not used because of their α-blocking properties, which can result in maternal hypotension.

Barbiturates

Barbiturates have been used for sedation in preterm labor and for management of anxiety. Barbiturates seldom lead to neonatal respiratory depression when given long before delivery. However, neonatal respiratory depression can occur when barbiturates are combined with opioids for labor analgesia or when large doses of thiopental ($\geq$6 mg/kg) are administered for induction of general anesthesia.[25]

Benzodiazepines and Dissociative Agents

Benzodiazepines and dissociative agents are seldom used in labor, as they can cause amnesia, which is not a desirable effect for most women in labor today. Concerns with benzodiazapines and the fetus include neonatal hypotonicity, hypoactivity, temperature deregulation, and respiratory depression.[26] Midazolam, unlike diazepam, is water-soluble, has a rapid onset, is shorter-acting, and has no active metabolites.

Thus, it has less of an adverse effect on the neonate. However, unlike phenothiazines and barbiturates, benzodiazepines have a specific antagonist, flumazenil, which can reverse the respiratory depression and sedative effects.[27] Flumazenil in large doses has been reported to cause seizure activity.[28] Ketamine is a phencyclidine derivative and is classified as a dissociative agent. It may be used for induction of anesthesia in cases of maternal hemorrhage or asthma at higher doses (1 mg/kg), and can be used as a sedative agent at lower doses (0.2 to 0.3 mg/kg) for difficult vaginal deliveries or postpartum procedures in patients without regional anesthesia. Possible adverse effects of ketamine include amnesia, hallucinations, increased salivation, hypertension, tachycardia, and increased uterine tone.[29]

Scopolamine

Scopolamine is an anticholinergic agent, with atropine being the prototype. During the middle of the 20th century, scopolamine was used in labor in combination with an opioid to cause heavy sedation or "twilight sleep" and amnesia. It also caused excitement and anxiety. Fetal effects included fetal tachycardia and loss of beat-to-beat variability. With changing practices and consumer concerns, scopolamine is seldom used today.

Inhalation Analgesia

Inhalation analgesia is seldom used for labor today in the United States. In an older survey in 1981, approximately 6% of centers used inhalation analgesia in labor[30] Intermittent nitrous oxide, given as a 50% mixture of nitrous oxide and oxygen, was the most common inhalation agent.[31] The advantage of nitrous oxide is its rapid uptake and excretion. However, adverse effects include hypoxia, dysphoria, drowsiness, nausea, and vomiting. Potent inhalation agents such as halothane, enflurane, isoflurane, desflurane, and sevoflurane have been sparingly used in this country during the second stage of labor and delivery.[32] Methoxyflurane was once a popular alternative in labor and delivery. It was administered via a vaporizer or whistle (Penthrane whistle). It had a great margin of safety in maintaining the patient's airway reflexes due to its marked lipid solubility. However, methoxyflurane is no longer used because of the risk of nephrotoxicity from one of its metabolites, inorganic fluoride. All the inhalation agents cause a dose-dependent decrease in uterine activity. Safety issues include loss of protective airway reflexes and environmental pollution. Loss of airway reflexes creates the potential for pulmonary aspiration and the risk is compounded if other systemic medications such as opioids are added to the inhalation agents. Moreover, with the changing practice of obstetrics in the United States today, an appropriate apparatus to administer these agents is difficult outside the operating room. In addition, with changing consumer attitudes and sophistication, maternal amnesia is unacceptable to most patients. Thus, for all these reasons, inhalation anesthesia in the United States is confined to cesarean delivery in the surgical suite.

REGIONAL ANALGESIA

Lumbar Sympathetic Block

Bilateral lumbar sympathetic blocks have been used for labor analgesia in the past, with some recent renewed interest. By blocking the lumbar sympathetic nerves, pain sensations from the uterus, cervix, and upper vagina are blocked. An advantage of this unopposed sympathetic block has been the enhancement of cervical dilation.[33] However, drawbacks of this technique may eclipse this advantage. The potential drawbacks include the relatively short duration of action (i.e., 2 to 3 hours even with the longer-acting local anesthetics, such as bupivacaine), inadequate pain relief for the second stage of labor, the potential technical difficulty of the procedure, and the lack of patient compliance for at least two deep injections. Moreover, due to the proximity of other structures besides the vertebral bodies, accidental epidural, intrathecal, and intravascular injections can occur. Also, with the potential spread of the local anesthetic, the splanchnic nerves and celiac plexus can be affected, resulting in maternal hypotension. Whether the "rediscovery" of this block for obstetrics becomes popular remains to be seen.

Regional (Neuraxial) Analgesia

Regional analgesia includes epidural, spinal, and the combined spinal–epidural technique. Initially, epidural analgesia was the only option for labor, and it included the lumbar and caudal approach. A caudal epidural is performed via the sacral hiatus and requires the patient to be either in the prone position with hips and knees flexed or in the lateral decubitus position. The perineum is easily numbed with this technique because of the proximity of the sacral nerves; however, to reach the T10 level for control of uterine contraction pain requires a significant volume of solution (15 to 20 ml). Because of the higher dose and the increased vascularity of the caudal epidural space, local anesthetic toxicity becomes a greater threat with this technique.[34] Because this technique relaxes the pelvic musculature, appropriate rotation of the fetal head to the occiput anterior position may be hampered, leading to more occiput posterior and transverse positions. Although rare, other problems with the caudal approach include the potential for traumatizing the fetal head or maternal rectum with the epidural needle.

The most common epidural technique is the lumbar approach, usually performed at the level of L2 to L5. With the lumbar, as opposed to the caudal, approach, the amount of solution required to block the appropriate nerve fibers (T10 to L1) is significantly less (6 to 10 ml) because of the proximity of the nerves and the smaller lumbar epidural space. Moreover, these sympathetic nerve fibers are smaller and more easily blocked, in contrast to the larger somatic nerves of S1 and S2. Obviously, the lumbar approach makes it more difficult to obtain perineal analgesia for the second stage of labor and for vaginal delivery. However, near the time of delivery, the combination of sitting the patient upright or positioning her in a semi-Fowler's position and increasing the volume of solution ("perineal dose") usually will suffice; otherwise, the obstetrician can supplement the epidural by performing a pudendal block or a local infiltration.

Epidural Intermittent Bolus

Prior to continuous epidural infusions, the intermittent bolus technique with local anesthetics was used. Today, single-injection epidural local anesthesia is used during initial epidural placement, for top-up doses to supplement a continuous infusion, or during the second stage of labor for perineal analgesia. A single-shot epidural bolus can also be given if delivery is imminent during placement. As the duration of any single-shot epidural local anesthetic is limited, i.e., 45 to 90 minutes, depending on the particular local anesthetic, sodium bicarbonate, epinephrine, and more commonly, opioids (e.g., fentanyl) are added to local anesthetics to enhance the onset and duration of action.[35-37]

The volume of local anesthetic solutions also plays a role in efficacy and duration. When comparing equipotent doses of a local anesthetic, solutions with greater volumes (i.e., 10 to 20 ml vs. 4 to 5 ml) offer superior pain relief and prolong the duration of action as compared with smaller volumes.[38] Alpha-2-adrenergic agonists, epinephrine and, more specifically, clonidine, have been added to the epidural local anesthetics to enhance labor analgesia. In one investigation, the combination of bupivacaine and clonidine provided a median duration of analgesia of 114 minutes as compared with 53 minutes with bupivacaine alone.[39] The analgesic effects of α_2-agonists appear to be secondary to effects on the α_2-adrenergic receptors in the dorsal horn of the spinal cord. Epidural clonidine also has a short duration of action, especially in labor, and requires a continuous infusion for prolonged relief. Advantages of clonidine include lack of nausea or pruritus as occurs with epidural opioids. However, it can cause mild maternal hypotension, maternal and fetal bradycardia, and sedation.[40] Sodium bicarbonate has also been added to local anesthetics to decrease time to onset of effective anesthesia.[41] Local anesthetics are more ionized at lower pH values, which restricts transfer across the dura mater. By increasing the pH of the solution, local anesthetics become more un-ionized and can cross membranes more readily. This property also is true for placental transfer and the concept of "ionic trapping" in an acidotic fetus. That is, the large un-ionized portion of the drug in a normal maternal pH environment will readily cross the placenta; however, once it reaches the acidotic fetus, the drug becomes ionized and remains "trapped."[42] Quicker-onset local anesthetics such as 2-chloroprocaine have been used for single top-up doses for impending delivery when rapid analgesia is required. However, if 2-chloroprocaine is used earlier in labor, the effectiveness and duration of subsequent epidural opioids or other local anesthetics can be significantly decreased.[36]

Local Anesthetic Toxicity

Intravascular injections can lead to local anesthetic toxicity. Local anesthetic toxicity is more prone to occur with the larger doses that are required for operative procedures such as cesarean delivery and is less likely to occur during labor unless larger doses are used. Local anesthetic toxicity affects the central nervous system (CNS) and the cardiovascular system. The CNS toxicity is biphasic and excitatory, followed

by a period of depression. Initial CNS symptoms include circumoral and tongue numbness, dizziness, and lightheadedness followed by tinnitus, difficulty in focusing, and restlessness. Further increases in local anesthetic levels result in slurred speech and muscle twitching, with eventual generalized tonic–clonic seizures. Higher drug levels may lead to unconsciousness and coma.

The cardiovascular toxicity is also biphasic, with an excitatory component manifested by hypertension and tachycardia. It is followed by hypotension, dysrhythmias, and cardiac arrest. Cardiovascular toxicity usually requires greater blood concentration of local anesthetic than the CNS toxicity, and the ratio of blood levels between cardiac and CNS is approximately 2.5 to 1 to 4.5 to 1, depending on the local anesthetic.[43] With the large separation of the two systems, the cardiac component usually does not occur at the same time as CNS toxicity. An exception to this rule is bupivacaine. There have been several reports of severe dysrhythmias—i.e., ventricular tachycardia and ventricular fibrillation—with bupivacaine without antecedent CNS effects. Moreover, laboratory studies have shown enhanced cardiotoxicity with bupivacaine in pregnant sheep versus nonpregnant ones.[44] These findings led to the ban of 0.75% bupivacaine in obstetrics in the mid-1980s and more than likely contributed to the declining maternal mortality rate with regional anesthesia since the mid-1980s. Physicians should note that high volumes of 0.5% bupivacaine can produce comparable serum levels as the 0.75% concentration of bupivacaine. Thus, bupivacaine or any other local anesthetic should be administered slowly, not exceeding 5 ml at a time. Bupivacaine is manufactured as a racemic mixture (dextro and levo). The S(−) enantiomer of bupivacaine is less cardiotoxic than the racemic mixture or R(−) enantiomer.[45] The S(−) enantiomer or L-bupivacaine has recently been released and will probably be competitive with the newer local anesthetic, ropivacaine.

Allergic Reactions

Allergic reactions to local anesthetics are extremely rare. There are two classes of local anesthetics, the amino-ester agents which are hydrolyzed by pseudocholinesterase—i.e., 2-chloroprocaine and tetracaine—and the amino-amide agents, which undergo hepatic metabolism—i.e., lidocaine, bupivacaine, mepivacaine, and ropivacaine. Allergic reactions are more commonly associated with the amino-esters and may be related to certain additives such as methylparaben. More likely, most of the reported reactions are not allergic reactions but, rather, are related to factors such as direct intravascular injections with epinephrine-containing solutions that lead to palpitations, restlessness, and tachycardia. Moreover, vasovagal reactions can occur with injections, which also may be construed as allergic reactions. True allergic reactions usually include an urticarial rash and wheezing. If an allergy to a particular local anesthetic exists, it is acceptable to use a local anesthetic from the other class.

Continuous Epidural Infusion

Continuous epidural analgesia was first described as early as the late 1950s and early 1960s and experienced a resurgence in the 1970s. However, it was not commonplace in obstetric suites until the 1980s. The emergence of this technique was refined with the advent of more reliable and manageable infusion pumps. It is more reliable because it avoids the fluctuations in pain relief seen with intermittent bolus injections and offers a greater margin of safety. This analogy can be made with continuous intravenous infusions versus intermittent boluses as well. The difference, however, is that an epidural injection may take about 20 minutes to be effective, similar to an intramuscular injection, as opposed to the more immediate nature of intravascular injections. An accidental single bolus injection of local anesthetic, especially at higher concentrations, into the intravascular or intrathecal space can be disastrous. The two most common causes of maternal morbidity and mortality from regional anesthesia are local anesthetic toxicity due to accidental epidural vein injection and a total spinal usually due to accidental spinal injection from an epidural dose (see below). In contrast, although rare, an epidural catheter could migrate into an epidural vein or the intrathecal space, which would lead to a gradual loss of analgesia (intravascular migration) or gradual increase in sensory and motor involvement (intrathecal migration). Although still a concern, there is a greater margin of safety with an errant catheter with a continuous infusion, especially with the lower concentrations of local anesthesia used today.

Bupivacaine, lidocaine, 2-chloroprocaine, and now ropivacaine have all been used for continuous epidural analgesia for labor. Various concentrations and volumes of local anesthetics have been used over the years; however, with the addition of opioids in the early 1980s, the concentration of local anesthetics has been decreasing. This trend has rendered the patient more mobile during labor, with a decreased incidence of motor blockade and more effective expulsion efforts during the second stage of labor. Older concentrations of bupivacaine typically ranged from 0.125% to 0.25%, as opposed to the present concentrations of as low as 0.03% to 0.10% (Table 18-3). Of course, the lower concentration local anesthetics require the addition of opioids—i.e., fentanyl or sufentanil— and α_2-adrenergic agents such as epinephrine or clonidine. These other neuraxial agents are added to minimize the side effects of local anesthetics, which include sensory and motor involvement and hemodynamic alterations, and the side effects of opioids, which include respiratory depression, nausea, and pruritus. These lower-concentration epidural infusions have allowed some patients to walk during labor,

---

TABLE 18-3
CONVENTIONAL VERSUS CURRENT NEURAXIAL ANALGESIA FOR LABOR

Older Classic Epidural		Newer Epidural "Lite"	
Technique (Dose)	Results	Technique (Dose)	Results
Continuous epidural Infusion (bupivacaine 0.125–0.25% infusion)	Pain-free Pruritus rare No sensation	Continuous epidural Infusion (bupivacaine 0.03–0.05% + fentanyl 1–2.5 μg/ml or sufentanil 0.2–0.4 μg/ml ± epinephrine or clonidine)	Pain-free Pruritus common Pressure sensation Functional
Intermittent epidural bolus (bupivacaine 0.25% or lidocaine 1–1.5%)	Weak-paralyzed immobile/bedridden Difficulty pushing	Spinal analgesia (fentanyl 25 μg or sufentanil 5–10 μg ± bupivacaine ≤2.5 mg or ropivacaine ≤3 mg)	mobile/sitting/walking Adequate pushing
		Combined spinal epidural (CSE) (spinal fentanyl or sufentanil as above with decreased epidural requirement)	

The efficacy of dosing a preexisting epidural for a postpartum tubal ligation has also been studied for cost effectiveness. Epidurals for labor that are subsequently used for postpartum tubal ligation have the greatest success rate if used within 4 hours of delivery.[179] The anesthesia and operating room times were the longest when the preexisting epidural catheter was used but not functioning, intermediate when the epidural was successful, and shortest when a spinal anesthetic was used in place of the epidural.

POSTPARTUM TUBAL LIGATION (PPTL)

A major controversy among anesthesiologists and obstetricians is the timing of postpartum tubal ligations. With the addition of pressures from various managed-care contracts, the timing of these procedures has become even more important. Of course, it is convenient and practical for the patient and the obstetrician to perform the PPTL soon after delivery. Moreover, the efficacy of using a preexisting epidural is improved if the procedure is performed within the first 4 hours after delivery.[180] However, other concerns include the safety of performing an elective procedure at certain times. Although 60% of postpartum patients undergoing PPTL were at risk for aspiration pneumonia, there was no difference in the incidence of at-risk criteria if the tubal ligation was performed 0 to 8 hours after delivery or 9 to 23 hours or 24 to 45 hours later.[181] Although some of the pregnancy factors contributing to an increased risk of aspiration and aspiration pneumonia are alleviated after delivery, residual hormonal and mechanical factors may continue for weeks in the postpartum period. Moreover, 36% of the postpartum patients had gastric contents with a pH <1.4.[182]

If there is a functioning epidural in place and no medical or obstetric complication is present, there is no reason to delay the procedure after delivery. Controversy does exist when there is no epidural in place for labor or when the labor epidural is not functioning. Despite the convenience of performing the PPTL after delivery, it is an elective procedure, and these patients by definition are still potentially at greater risk for aspiration. Although a regional block may appear safer than a general anesthetic, if a de novo neuraxial block is required, the risk for complications may be up to three times higher than dosing up a preexisting, functioning epidural.[172] Thus, the practice at our institution is to delay the procedure for either 6 to 8 hours or, more commonly, schedule it for the morning following delivery.

REFERENCES

1. Hawkins JL, Gibbs CP, Orleans M, Martin-Salvaj G, Beaty B. Obstetric Anesthesia Work Force Survey, 1981 versus 1992. Anesthesiology 1997;87:135.
2. Tsen LC, Pitner R, Camann WR. General anesthesia for cesarean section at a tertiary care hospital 1990–1995: indications and implications. Int J Obstet Anesth 1998; 7:147.
3. Berg CJ, Atrash HK, Koonin LM, Tucker M. Pregnancy-related mortality in the US, 1987–1990. Obstet Gynecol 1996;88:161.
4. Hawkins JL, Koonin LM, Palmer SK, Gibbs CP. Anesthetic-related deaths during obstetric delivery in the US: 1979–1990. Anesthesiology 1997;86:277.
5. Melzack R. The myth of painless childbirth. Pain 1984; 19:321.
6. Ranta P, Jouppila P, Jouppila R. The intensity of labor pain in grand multiparas. Acta Obstet Gynecol Scand 1996;75:250.
7. Dick-Read G. Childbirth without fear. New York: Harper, 1944.
8. Ueland K. Maternal cardiovascular dynamics. VII. Intrapartum blood volume changes. Am J Obstet Gynecol 1976;126:671.
9. Ueland K, Novy M, Peterson E, Metcalf J. Maternal cardiovascular dynamics. IV. The influence of gestational age on the maternal cardiovascular response to posture and exercise. Am J Obstet Gynecol 1969;104:156.
10. Robson SC, Dunlop W, Boys RJ, Hunter S. Cardiac output during labour. BMJ 1987;295:1169.
11. James CF, Banner T, Caton D. Cardiac output in women undergoing cesarean section with epidural or general anesthesia. Am J Obstet Gynecol 1989;160:1178.
12. James CF. Cardiac disease and hypertensive disorders in pregnancy. In: Civetta JM, Taylor RW, Kirby RR eds. Critical care. 3rd ed. Philadelphia: Lippincott-Raven, 1997:1389.
13. Ueland K, Hansen JM. Maternal cardiovascular dynamics. III. Labor and delivery under local and caudal analgesia. Am J Obstet Gynecol 1969;103:8.
14. Howard BK, Goodson JH, Mengert WF. Supine hypotension syndrome in late pregnancy. Obstet Gynecol 1953;1:371.
15. Bieniarz I, Crottogini JJ, Curachet E. Aortocaval compression by the uterus in late human pregnancy. Am J Obstet Gynecol 1968;100:203.
16. Shnider S, Moya F. Effects of meperidine on the newborn infant. Am J Obstet Gynecol 1964;89:1009.
17. Bonica JJ. Principles and practice of obstetric analgesia and anesthesia. Philadelphia: FA Davis, 1967:234.
18. Romagnoli A, Keats AS. Ceiling effect for respiratory depression by nalbuphine. Clin Pharmacol Ther 1980; 27:478.
19. Kallos T, Caruso FS. Respiratory effects of butrophanol and pethidine. Anaesthesia 1979;34:633.

20. Rosaeg OP, Kitts JB, Koren G, Byford LJ. Maternal and fetal effects of intravenous patient-controlled fentanyl analgesia during labour in a thrombocytopenic parturient. Can J Anaesth 1992;39:277.

21. Podlas J, Breland BD. Patient-controlled analgesia with nalbuphine during labor. Obstet Gynecol 1987;70:202.

22. Evans JM, Rosen M, MacCarthy J, Hoggs MIJ. Apparatus for patient-controlled administration of intravenous narcotics during labour. Lancet 1976;1:17.

23. Petrie RH, Yeh SY, Murata Y, et al. The effects of drugs on fetal heart rate variability. Am J Obstet Gynecol 1978;130:294.

24. American College of Obstetricians and Gynecologists. Obstetric Anesthesia and Analgesia. ACOG Technical Bulletin no. 225, July 1996.

25. Kosaka Y, Takahashi T, Mark LC. Intravenous thiobarbiturate anesthesia for cesarean section. Anesthesiology 1969; 31:489.

26. Cree JE, et al. Diazepam in labour: its metabolism and effect on the clinical condition and thermogenesis of the newborn. BMJ 1973;4:251.

27. Gross JB, et al. Flumazenil antagonism of midazolam-induced ventilatory depression. Anesthesiology 1991; 75:179.

28. Brogden RN, Goa KL. Flumazenil: a reapprasal of its pharmacologic properties and therapeutic efficacy as a benzodiapine antagonist. Drugs 1991;42:1061.

29. Akamatsu TJ, Bonica JJ, Rehmet R, et al. Experiences with the use of ketamine for parturition. I. Primary anesthesia for vaginal delivery. Anesth Analg 1974; 53:284.

30. Gibbs CP, et al. Obstetric anesthesia: a national survey. Anesthesiology 1986;65:298.

31. Rosen M. Recent advances in pain relief in childbirth: inhalation and systemic analgesia. Br J Anaesth 1971; 43:837.

32. Abboud TK, Gangolly J, Mosaad P, Crowell D. Isoflurane in obstetrics. Anesth Analg 1989;68:388.

33. Hunter CA. Uterine motility studies during labor: observations on bilateral sympathetic nerve blocks and abnormal first stage of labor. Am J Obstet Gynecol 1983; 85:681.

34. James CF. Local and regional anesthesia. In: Gravenstein N, ed. Manual of complications during anesthesia. Philadelphia: Lippincott, 1991:421.

35. McMorland GH, Douglas MJ, Jeffery WK, et al. Effect of pH-adjustment of bupivacaine on onset and duration of epidural analgesia in parturients. Can Anaesth Soc J 1986;33:537.

36. Grice SC, Eisennach JC, Dewan DM. Labor analgesia with epidural bupivacaine plus fentanyl: enhancement with epinephrine and inhibition with 2-chloroprocaine. Anesthesiology 1990;72:623.

37. Justins DM, Francis D, Houlton PG, et al. A controlled trial of extradural fentanyl in labor. Br J Anaesth 1982; 54:409.

38. Birnbach DJ, Johnson MD, Arcario T, et al. Effect of diluent volume on analgesia produced by epidural fentanyl. Anesthesiology 1987;67:A441 abstract.

39. O'Meara ME, Gin T. Comparison of 0.125% bupivacaine with 0.125% bupivacaine and clonidine as extradural analgesia in the first stage of labour. Br J Anaesth 1993; 71:651.

40. Eisenach J, Castro M, Dewan D, Rosen J. Epidural clonidine analgesia in obstetric sheep studies. Anesthesiology 1989;70:51.

41. DiFazio CA, Carron H, Grosslight KR, et al. Comparison of pH-adjusted lidocaine solutions for epidural anesthesia. Anesth Analg 1986;65:760.

42. Biehl D, Shnider SM, Levinson G, Callender K. Placental transfer of lidocaine: effects of fetal acidosis. Anesthesiology 1978;48:409.

43. DeJong RH, Ronfeld RA, DeRosa RA. Cardiovascular effects of convulsant and supraconvulsant doses of amide local anesthetics. Anesth Analg 1982;61:3.

44. Morishima HO, Pedersen H, Finster M. et al. Bupivacaine toxicity in pregnant and nonpregnant ewes. Anesthesiology 1985;63:134.

45. Aberg G. Toxicological and local anaesthetic effects of optically active isomers of two local anesthetic compounds. Pharmacol Toxicol 1972;31:273.

46. Santos AC, Arthur GR, Lehming EJ, Finster M. Comparative pharmacology of ropivacaine and bupivacaine in non-pregnant and pregnant ewes. Anesth Analg 1997; 85:87.

47. Feldman HS, Covino BG. Comparative motor-blocking effects of bupivacaine and ropivacaine, a new amino amide local anesthetic, in the rat and dog. Anesth Analg 1988;67:1047.

48. Standards and Guidelines for Professional Nursing Practice in the Care of Women and Newborns. 5th ed. Association of Women's Health, Obstetrics and Neonatal Nurses (AWHONN), pp. 32–33, Washington, DC.

49. Gambling DR, McMorland GH, Yu P, Lasxlo C. Comparison of patient-controlled epidural analgesia and conventional intermittent 'top-up' injections during labor. Anesth Analg 1990;70:256.

50. Ferrante FM, Lu L, Jamison SB, Datta S. Patient controlled epidural analgesia: demand dosing. Anesth Analg 1991;73:547.

51. Paech MJ. Patient-controlled epidural analgesia during labor: choice of solution. Int J Obstet Anesth 1993; 2:65.

52. Lambert DH, Hurley RJ, Hertwig L, Datta S. Role of needle gauge and tip configuration in the production of lumbar puncture headache. Reg Anesth 1997;22:66.

53. Cohen SE, Cherry CM, Holbrook RH, et al. Intrathecal sufentanil for labor analgesia-sensory changes, side effects, and fetal heart rate changes. Anesth Analg 1993; 77:1155.

54. Riley ET, Ratner EF, Cohen SE. Intrathecal sufentanil for labor analgesia: do sensory changes predict better analgesia and greater hypotension? Anesth Analg 1997; 84:346.

55. Abouleish E. Apnoea associated with the intrathecal administration of morphine in obstetrics. Br J Anaesth 1988;60:592.

56. Clarke VT, Smiley RM, Finster M. Uterine hyperactivity after intrathecal injection of fentanyl for analgesia during labor: a cause of fetal bradycardia? *Letter* Anesthesiology 1994;81:1083.

57. Nielsen PE, Erickson JR, Abouleish EI, et al. Fetal heart

rate changes after intrathecal sufentanil or epidural bupivacaine for labor analgesia: incidence and clinical significance. Anesth Analg 1996;83:742.

58. Palmer CM, Maciulla JE, Cork RC, Nogami WM,
Gossler K, Alves D. The incidence of fetal heart rate
changes after intrathecal fentanyl labor analgesia. Anesth
Analg 1999;88:577.

59. Segal S, Csavoy AN, Datta S. Placental tissue enhances
uterine relaxation by nitroglycerin. Anesth Analg 1998;
86:304.

60. Langevin P, Katovich M, James CF. Uterine smooth
muscle compliance: effect of nitroglycerine independent
of a contractile mediator. Anesthesiology 1996;85:A885
abstract.

61. Campbell DC, Banner R, Crone LA, Gore-Hickman W,
Yip RW. Addition of epinephrine to intrathecal bupivacaine and sufentanil for ambulatory labor analgesia. Anesthesiology 1997;86:525.

62. D'Angelo R, Evans E, Dean LA, Gaver R, Eisenach JC.
Spinal clonidine prolongs labor analgesia from spinal
sufentanil and bupivacaine. Anesth Analg 1999;88:573.

63. Carrie LES. Extradural, spinal or combined block for
obstetric surgical anaesthesia. Br J Anaesth 1990;65:225.

64. Norris MC, Greico WM, Borkowski M, et al. Complications of labor analgesia: epidural versus combined spinal
epidural techniques. Anesth Analg 1994;79:529.

65. Lyons G, MacDonald R. Miki B. Combined epidural/
spinal anaesthesia for caesarean section. Anaesthesia
1992;47:199.

66. Holmstrom B, Rawal N, Axelsson K, Nydahl P.-A. Risk
of catheter migration during combined spinal epidural
block: percutaneous epiduroscopy study. Anesth Analg
1995;80:747.

67. Robbins PM, Fernando R, Lim GH. Accidental intrathecal induction of an extradural catheter during combined
spinal epidural for cesarean section. Br J Anaesth 1995;
75:355.

68. Herman N, Molin J, Knape KG. No additional metal
particle formation using the needle-through-needle
combined epidural/spinal technique. Acta Anaesth Scand
1996;40:227.

69. Nageotte MP, Larson D, Rumney PJ, Sidhu M, Hollenbach K. Epidural analgesia compared with combined
spinal-epidural analgesia during labor in nulliparous
women. N Engl J Med 1997;337:1715.

70. Collis RE, Baxandall ID, Srikantharajah G, et al. Combined spinal epidural (CSE) analgesia: technique, management, and outcome of 300 mothers. Int J Obstet
Anesth 1994;3:75.

71. Breen TW, Shapiro T, Glass B, et al. Epidural anesthesia
for labor in an ambulatory patient. Anesth Analg 1993;
77:919.

72. Lieberman E, Lang JM, Frigoletto F, et al. Epidural analgesia, intrapartum fever, and neonatal sepsis evaluation.
Pediatrics 1997;99:415.

73. Camann WR, Hortvet LA, Hughes N, Bader AM, Datta
S. Maternal temperature regulation during extradural
analgesia for labour. Br J Anaesth 1991;67:565.

74. Fusi L, Maresh MJA, Steer PJ, Beard RW. Maternal
pyrexia associated with the use of epidural analgesia in
labour. Lancet 1989;1:1250.

75. Read MD, Hunt LP, Anderton JM, Lieberman BA.

Epidural block and the progress and outcome of labour.
J Obstet Gynecol 1983;4:35.

76. Moir DD, Willocks J. Management of incoordinate uterine action under continuous epidural analgesia. BMJ
1968;40:129.

77. Halpern SH, Leighton BL, Ohlsson A, Barrett JFR, Rice
A. Effect of epidermal vs. parenteral opioid analgesia on
the progress of labor. JAMA 1998;280(24):2105.

78. Schellenberg JC. Uterine activity during lumbar epidural
analgesia with bupivacaine. Am J Obstet Gynecol 1977;
127:26.

79. Gunther RE, Belville JW. Obstetrical caudal anesthesia.
II. A randomized study comparing 1% mepivacaine with
1% mepivacaine plus epinephrine. Anesthesiology 1972;
37:288.

80. Cheek TG, Samuels P, Miller F, Tomin M, Gutsche BB.
Normal saline i.v. load decreases uterine activity in active
labour. Br J Anaesth 1996;77:632.

81. Thorburn J, Moir DD. Extradural analgesia: the influence
of volume and concentration of bupivacaine on mode of
delivery, analgesia, efficacy, and motor block. Br J Anaesth
1981;53:933.

82. Chestnut DH, Vandewalker GE, Owen CL, et al. The influence of continuous epidural bupivacaine analgesia on
the second stage of labor and method of delivery in nulliparous women. Anesthesiology 1987;66:774.

83. Chestnut DH, Laszewski LJ, Pollack KL, et al. Continuous epidural infusion of 0.0625% bupivacaine-0.0002%
fentanyl during the second stage of labor. Anesthesiology
1990;72:613.

84. Rogers R, Gilson G, Kammerer-Doak D. Epidural analgesia and active management of labor: effects on length
of labor and mode of delivery. Obstet Gynecol 1999;
93:995.

85. Goodfellow CF, Hull MGR, Swaab DF, Dogertom J,
Buijs RM. Oxytocin deficiency at delivery with epidural
analgesia. Br J Obstet Gynaecol 1983;90:214.

86. Maresh M, Choong KH, Beard RW. Delayed pushing
with lumbar epidural analgesia in labor. Br J Obstet Gynaecol 1983;90:623.

87. Thorp JA, Parisi VM, Boylan PC, Johnson DA. The effect
of continuous epidural analgesia on cesarean section for
dystocia in nulliparous women. Am J Obstet Gynecol
1984;161:670.

88. Thorp JA, Eckert LO, Ang MS, Johnston DA, Peaceman
AM, Parisi VM. Epidural analgesia and cesarean section
for dystocia risk factors in nulliparas. Am J Perinatol
1991;8:402.

89. Thorp JA, Hu DH, Albin RM, et al. The effect of intrapartum epidural analgesia on nulliparous labor: a randomized, controlled, prospective trial. Am J Obstet Gynecol 1993;169:851.

90. Morton SC, Williams MS, Keeler EB, Gambone JC,
Kahn KL. Effect of epidural analgesia for labor on the
cesarean delivery rate. Obstet Gynecol 1994;83:1044.

91. Wuitchik M, Bakal D, Lipshitz J. The clinical significance
of pain and cognitive activity in latent labor. Obstet Gynecol 1989;73:35.

92. Ramin SM, Gambling DR, Lucas MJ, et al. Randomized
trial of epidural versus intravenous analgesia during
labor. Obstet Gynecol 1995;86:783.

93. Sharma SK, Sidawi JE, Ramin SM, Lucan MJ, Leveno

KJ, Cunningham FG. Cesarean delivery: a randomized trial of epidural versus patient-controlled meperidine analgesia during labor. Anesthesiology 1997;87:487.

94. Bofill JA, Vincent RD, Ross EL, et al. Nulliparous active labor, epidural analgesia and cesarean delivery for dystocia. Am J Obstet Gynecol 1997;177:1465.

95. Clark A, Carr D, Loyd G, Cook V, Spinnato J. The influence of epidural analgesia on cesarean section delivery rates: a randomized, prospective clinical trial. Am J Obstet Gynecol 1998;179:1527.

96. Gambling DR, Sharma SK, Ramin SM, et al. A randomized study of combined spinal–epidural analgesia versus intravenous meperidine during labor. Anesthesiology 1998;89:1336.

97. Chestnut DH, Vincent RD, McGrath JM, et al. Does early administration of epidural analgesia affect obstetric outcome in nulliparous women who are receiving intravenous oxytocin? Anesthesiology 1994;80:1193.

98. Chestnut DH, McGrath JM, Vincent RD, et al. Does early administration of epidural analgesia affect obstetric outcome in nulliparous women who are in spontaneous labor? Anesthesiology 1994;80:1201.

99. Roshanfekr D, Blakemore KJ, Lee J, Hueppchen NA, Witter FR. Station a onset of active labor in nulliparous patients and risk of cesarean delivery. Obstet Gynecol 1999;93:329.

100. Holt RO, Diehl SJ, Wright JW. Station and cervical dilation at epidural placement in predicting cesarean section risk. Obstet Gynecol 1999;93:281.

101. Gribble RK, Meier PR. Effect of epidural analgesia on the primary cesarean rate. Obstet Gynecol 1991;78:231.

102. Robson M, Boylan P, McParland P, et al. Epidural analgesia need not influence the spontaneous vaginal delivery rate. Am J Obstet Gynecol 1993;168:364. abstract.

103. Zhang J, Klebanoff MA, DerSimonian R. Epidural analgesia in association with duration of labor and mode of delivery: a quantitative review. Am J Obstet Gynecol 1999;180:970.

104. Flynn JM, Kelly J, Hollins G, Lynch PF. Ambulating in labour. BMJ 1978;2:591.

105. Chestnut DH. Does epidural analgesia during labor affect the incidence of cesarean delivery? Reg Anesth 1997;22:495.

106. May AE. The confidential enquiry into maternal deaths 1988–1990. Br J Anaesth 1994;73:129.

107. James CF. Maternal mortality. Semin Anesth 1992;11:76.

108. Hood DD, Dewan DM. Obstetric anesthesia. In: Brown DL, ed. Risk and outcome in anesthesia. Philadelphia: Lippincott, 1988:310.

109. Hogberg U. Maternal mortality—a worldwide problem. Int J Gynaecol Obstet 1985;23:463.

110. Cheney FW. The ASA Closed Claims Project: lessons learned. Annual Refresher Course. Atlanta, 1995.

111. Chadwick HS. An analysis of obstetric anesthesia cases from the American Society of Anesthesiologists Closed Claims Project database. Int J Obstet Anesth 1996;5:258.

112. Olsson GL, Hallen B, Hambraeus-Jonzon K. Aspiration during anaesthesia: a computer-aided study of 185,358 anaesthetics. Acta Anaesth Scand 1986;30:84.

113. Mendelson CL. Aspiration of stomach contents into lungs during obstetric anesthesia. Am J Obstet Gynecol 1946;52:191.

114. Lewis M, Crawford JS. Can one risk fasting the obstetric patient for less than 4 hours? Br J Anaesth 1987;59:312.

115. Carp H, Jayaram A, Stoll M. Ultrasound examination of the stomach contents of parturients. Anesth Analg 1992;74:683.

116. Colebatch HJH, Halmagyi DFJ. Reflex airway reaction to fluid aspiration. J Appl Physiol 1962;17:787.

117. Roberts RB, Shirley MS. Reducing the risk of acid aspiration during cesarean section. Anesth Analg 1974;53:859.

118. Gibbs CP, Schwartz DJ, Wynne JW, Hood CI, Kuck EJ. Antacid pulmonary aspiration in the dog. Anesthesiology 1979;51:380.

119. James CF, Modell JH, Gibbs CP, et al. Pulmonary aspiration: Effects of volume and pH in the rat. Anesth Analg 1984;63:665.

120. Wright PMC, Brown R, Lau M, Fisher DM. A phamacodynamic explanation for the rapid onset/offset of rapacuronium bromide. Anesthesiology 1999;90:16.

121. Sellick BA. Cricoid pressure to control regurgitation of stomach contents during induction of anesthesia. Lancet 1961;2:404.

122. Samsoon GLT, Young JRB. Difficult tracheal intubation: a retrospective study. Anaesthesia 1987;42:487.

123. Lyons G. Failed intubation. Anaesthesia 1985;40:759.

124. Lyons G, MacDonald R. Difficult intubation in obstetrics. Anaesthesia 1985;40:1016.

125. Cormack RS, Lehane J. Difficult tracheal intubation in obstetrics. Anaesthesia 1984;39:1105.

126. Hawthorne L, Wilkson R, Lyons G, Dresner M. Failed intubation revisited: 17-yr experience in a teaching maternity unit. Br J Anaesth 1996;76:680.

127. Archer GW, Marx GF. Arterial oxygen tension during apnoea in parturient women. Br J Anaesth 1974;46:358.

128. Mallampati SR, Gatt SP, Gugino LD, et al. A clinical sign to predict difficult tracheal intubation: a prospective study. Can Anaesth Soc J 1985;32:429.

129. Rocke DA, Murray WB, Rout CC, et al. Relative risk analysis of factors associated with difficult intubation in obstetric anesthesia. Anesthesiology 1992;77:67.

130. Farcon EL, Kim MH, Marx GF. Changing Mallampati score during labor. Can J Anaesth 1994;41:50.

131. Brain AIJ. The laryngeal mask—a new concept in airway management. Br J Anaesth 1983;55:801.

132. American Society of Anesthesiologists. Practice guidelines for management of the difficult airway. Anesthesiology 1993;78:597.

133. Barker P, Langton JA, Murphy PJ, et al. Regurgitation of gastric contents during general anesthesia using the laryngeal mask airway. Br J Anaesth 1992;69:314.

134. Hasham FM, Andrews PJD, Juneja MM, Ackerman WE. The laryngeal mask airway facilitates intubation at cesarean section: a case report of difficult intubation. Int J Obstet Anesth 1993;2:181.

135. Brain AIJ, Verghese C, Addy EV, Kapilla A. The intubating laryngeal mask. I. Development of a new device for intubation of the trachea. Br J Anaesth 1997;79:699.

136. Hood, DD, Dewan, DM. Anesthetic and obstetric outcome in morbidly obese parturients. Anesthesiology 1993;79:1210.

137. Brizgys RV, Dailey PA, Schnider SM, Kotelko DM, Levinson G. The incidence and neonatal effects of

maternal hypotension during epidural anesthesia for cesarean section. Anesthesiology 1987;67:782.

138. Clark RB, Thompson DS, Thompson CH. Prevention of spinal hypotension associated with cesarean section. Anesthesiology 1976;45:670.

139. Datta S, Kitzmiller JL, Naulty JS, et al. Acid-base status of diabetic mothers and their infants following spinal anesthesia for cesarean section. Anesth Analg 1982;61:662.

140. Ralston DH, Shnider SM, DeLorimier AA. Effects of equipotent ephedrine, metaraminol, mephentermine, and methoxamine on uterine blood flow in the pregnant ewe. Anesthesiology 1974;40:354.

141. Ramanathan S, Grant GJ. Vasopressor therapy for hypotension due to epidural anesthesia for cesarean section. Acta Anaesth Scand 1988;32:599.

142. Riley ET, Cohen SE, Rubenstein AJ, Flanagan B. Prevention of hypotension after spinal anesthesia for cesarean section: six percent hetastarch versus lactated Ringer's solution. Anesth Analg 1995;81:838.

143. Rout CC, Rocke DA, Levin J, Gouws E, Reddy D. A reevaluation of the role of crystalloid preload in the prevention of hypotension associated with spinal anesthesia for elective cesarean section. Anesthesiology 1993;79:262.

144. Jackson R, Reid JA, Thoburn J. Volume preloading is not essential to prevent spinal-induced hypotension at cesarean section. Br J Anaesth 1995;75:262.

145. Vandam LD, Dripps RD. Long-term follow-up of patients who received 10,098 spinal anesthetics. JAMA 1956;161:586.

146. Buettner J, Wresch K.-P., Klose R. Postdural puncture headache: comparison of 25-gauge Whitacre and Quincke needles. Reg Anesth 1993;18:166.

147. Vos PE, deBoer WA, Wurzer JAL, van Gijn J. Subdural hematoma after lumbar puncture: two case reports and review of the literature. Clin Neurol Neurosurg 1991; 93:127.

148. Miyazaki S, Fukushima H, Kamata K, Ishii S. Chronic subdural hematoma after lumbar-subarachnoid analgesia for a cesarean section. Surg Neurol 1983;19:459.

149. James CF. Labor analgesia in 1994. Adv Anesth 1995; 12:111.

150. Sechzer PH, Abel L. Post-spinal anesthesia headache treated with caffeine: evaluation with demand method. Part I. Curr Ther Res 1978;24:307.

151. Jarvis AP, Greenawalt LW, Fagraeus L. Intravenous caffeine for postdural puncture headache. Anesth Analg 1986;65:313.

152. Camann WR, Murray RS, Mushlin PS, et al. Effects of oral caffeine on postdural puncture headache: a double-blind, placebo-controlled trial. Anesth Analg 1990; 70:181.

153. Cheek TG, Banner R, Sauter J, et al. Prophylactic extradural blood patch is effective: a preliminary communication. Br J Anaesth 1988;61:340.

154. Colonna-Romano P, Shapiro BE. Unintentional dural puncture and prophylactic epidural blood patch in obstetrics. Anesth Analg 1989;69:522.

155. Trivedi NS, Eddi D, Shevde K. Headache prevention following accidental dural puncture in obstetric patients. J Clin Anesth 1993;5:42.

156. Carp H, Singh PJ, Vadhera R, Jayaram A. Effects of the serotonin-receptor agonist sumatriptan on postdural puncture headache: report of six cases. Anesth Analg 1994;79:180.

157. Breen TW, Ransil BJ, Groves PA, Oriol NE. Factors associated with back pain after childbirth. Anesthesiology 1994;81:29.

158. Macarthur A, Macarthur C, Weeks S. Epidural anaesthesia and low back pain after delivery: a prospective cohort study. BMJ 1995;311:1336.

159. Stevens RA, Urmey WF, Urquhart BL, Kao T.-C. Back pain after epidural anesthesia with chloroprocaine. Anesthesiology 1993;78:492.

160. Massey-Dawkins CJ. An analysis of the complications of extradural and caudal block. Anaesthesia 1969;24:554.

161. Scott DB, Tunstall ME. Serious complications associated with epidural/spinal blockade in obstetrics: a two-year prospective study. Int J Obstet Anesth 1995;4:133.

162. Ravindran RS, Bond VK, Tasch M, Gupta CD, Leurssen TG. Prolonged neural blockade following regional analgesia with 2-chloroprocaine. Anesth Analg 1980;59:446.

163. Reisner LS, Hochman BN, Plumer MH. Persistent neurologic deficit and adhesive arachnoiditis following intrathecal 2-chloroprocaine injection. Anesth Analg 1980;59:452.

164. Rigler ML, Drasner K, Krejcie TC, et al. Cauda equina syndrome after continuous spinal anesthesia. Anesth Analg 1991;72:275.

165. Schneider M, Ettlin T, Kaufmann M, et al. Transient neurologic toxicity after hyperbaric subarachnoid anesthesia with 5% lidocaine. Anesth Analg 1993;76:1154.

166. Beardsley D, Holman S, Gantt R, et al. Transient neurologic deficit after spinal anesthesia: local anesthetic maldistribution with pencil point needles? Anesth Analg 1995;81:314.

167. Pollock JE, Neal JM, Stephenson CA, Wiley CE. Prospective study of the incidence of transient radicular irritation in patients undergoing spinal anesthesia. Anesthesiology 1996;84:1361.

168. Tryba M. Epidural regional anesthesia and low molecular heparin: Pro (German). Anasth Intensivmed Notfallmed Schmerzther 1993;28:179.

169. Burrows RF, Kelton JG. Incidentally detected thrombocytopenia in healthy mothers and their infants. N Engl J Med 1988;319:142.

170. Beilin Y, Zahn J, Comerford M. Safe epidural analgesia in thirty parturients with platelet counts between 69,000 and 98,000 mm^3. Anesth Analg 1997;85:385.

171. Horlocker TT, Wedel DJ. Neuraxial block and low-molecular-weight heparin: balancing perioperative analgesia and thromboprophylaxis. Reg Anesth & Pain Med 1998;23(6) Suppl 2:164.

172. Dripps RD, Vandam LD. Long-term follow-up of patients who received 10,098 spinal anesthetics. JAMA 1954;156:1486.

173. Crawford JS. Some maternal complications of epidural analgesia for labour. Anaesthesia 1985;40:1219.

174. Scott DB, Hibbard BM. Serious non-fatal complications associated with extradural block in obstetric practice. Br J Anaesth 1990;64:537.

175. O'Connor RL, Sevarino FB. Cardiopulmonary arrest in the pregnant patient: a report of a successful resuscitation. J Clin Anesth 1994;6:66.

176. Ness TJ, Gebhart GF. Visceral pain: a review of experimental studies. Pain 1990;41:167.

177. Russell IF. Levels of anaesthesia and intraoperative pain at cesarean section under regional block. Int J Obstet Anesth 1995;4:71.

178. American College of Obstetrics and Gynecology Committee #231. Pain relief during labor. February, 2000.

179. Riley ET, Cohen SE, Macario A, Desai J, Ratner EF. Spinal versus epidural anesthesia for cesarean section: a comparison of time, efficiency, costs, charges and complications. Anesth Analg 1995;80:709.

180. Viscomi CM, Rathmess JP. Labor epidural catheter reactivation or spinal anesthesia for delayed postpartum tubal ligation: a cost comparison. J Clin Anesth 1995;7:380.

181. Vincent RD, Reid RW. Epidural anesthesia for postpartum tubal ligation using epidural catheters placed during labor. J Clin Anesth 1993;5:289.

182. James CF, Gibbs CP, Banner T. Postpartum perioperative risk of aspiration pneumonia. Anesthesiology 1984; 61:756.

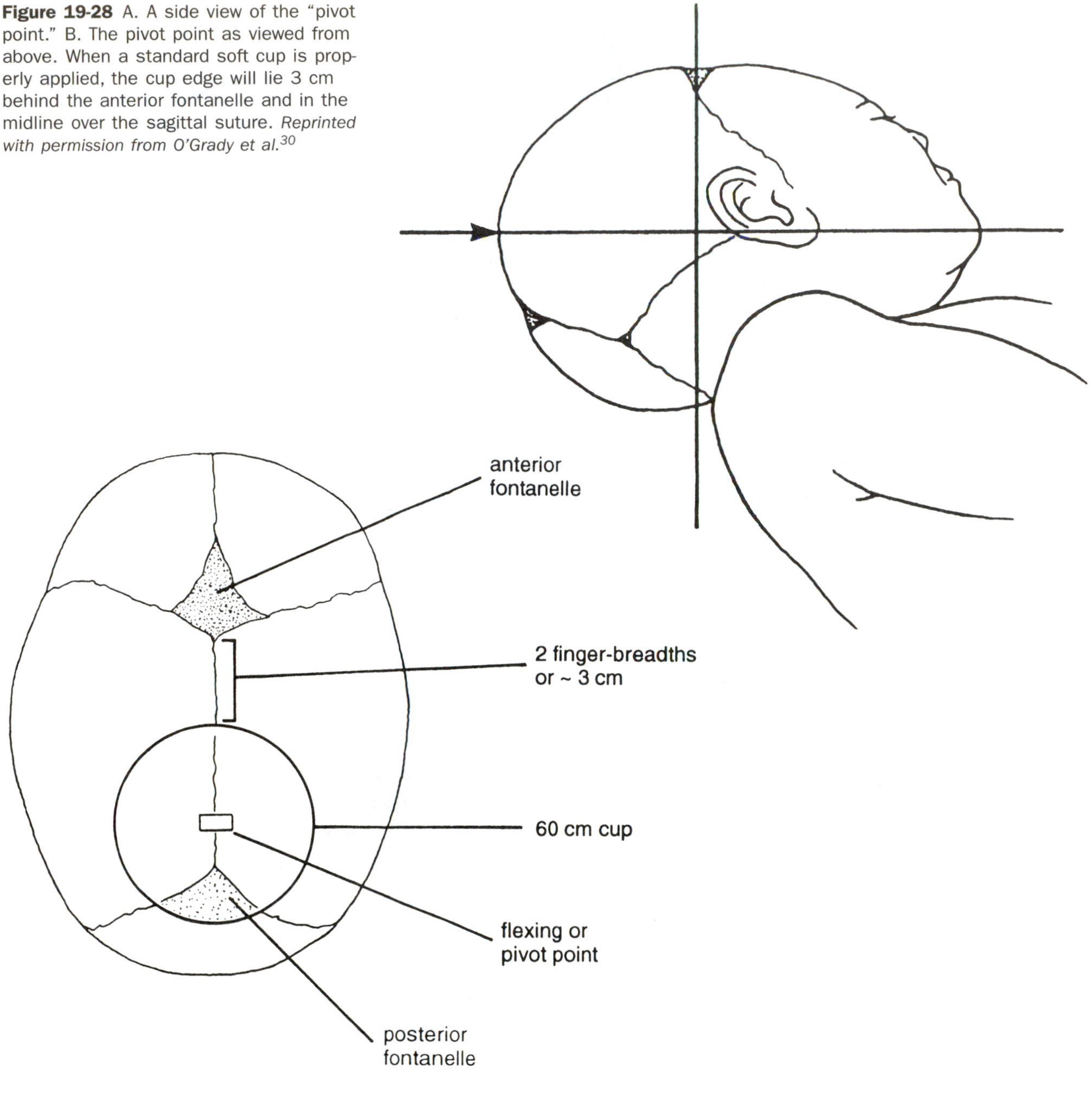

Figure 19-28 A. A side view of the "pivot point." B. The pivot point as viewed from above. When a standard soft cup is properly applied, the cup edge will lie 3 cm behind the anterior fontanelle and in the midline over the sagittal suture. *Reprinted with permission from O'Grady et al.*[30]

anterior
fontanelle

2 finger-breadths
or ~ 3 cm

60 cm cup

flexing or
pivot point

posterior
fontanelle

lack of consensus regarding the number of pulls required to effect delivery, the maximum number of cup detachments that can be tolerated, and the duration of time that the cup can safely be attached to the fetal head. It is generally recommended that no more than 3 cup dislodgments, 4 or 5 traction efforts, or 15 to 20 minutes of vacuum time be allowed on any one fetus.[37] Cosmetic scalp trauma has been reported to occur more frequently in vacuum applications exceeding 10 minutes.[44] Descent of the fetal head should begin with the first traction. Sjostedt,[45] in a study that is still widely quoted, reported that 93% of 433 women undergoing vacuum extraction with a Malmström-type

vacuum cup were delivered successfully using no more than four traction efforts. If descent does not occur with vacuum extraction, a forceps instrument should not be applied. Forceps trials following failed vacuum operations have been associated with an increased risk of life-threatening neonatal scalp injuries.[46]

What technique should be used when applying vacuum—continuous or intermittent? One study has shown no difference in maternal or fetal outcomes between the two techniques. Bofill et al.,[47] using the M-cup-type vacuum extractor, randomized 164 women to receive a continuous level of vacuum until the infant was completely delivered and instructed

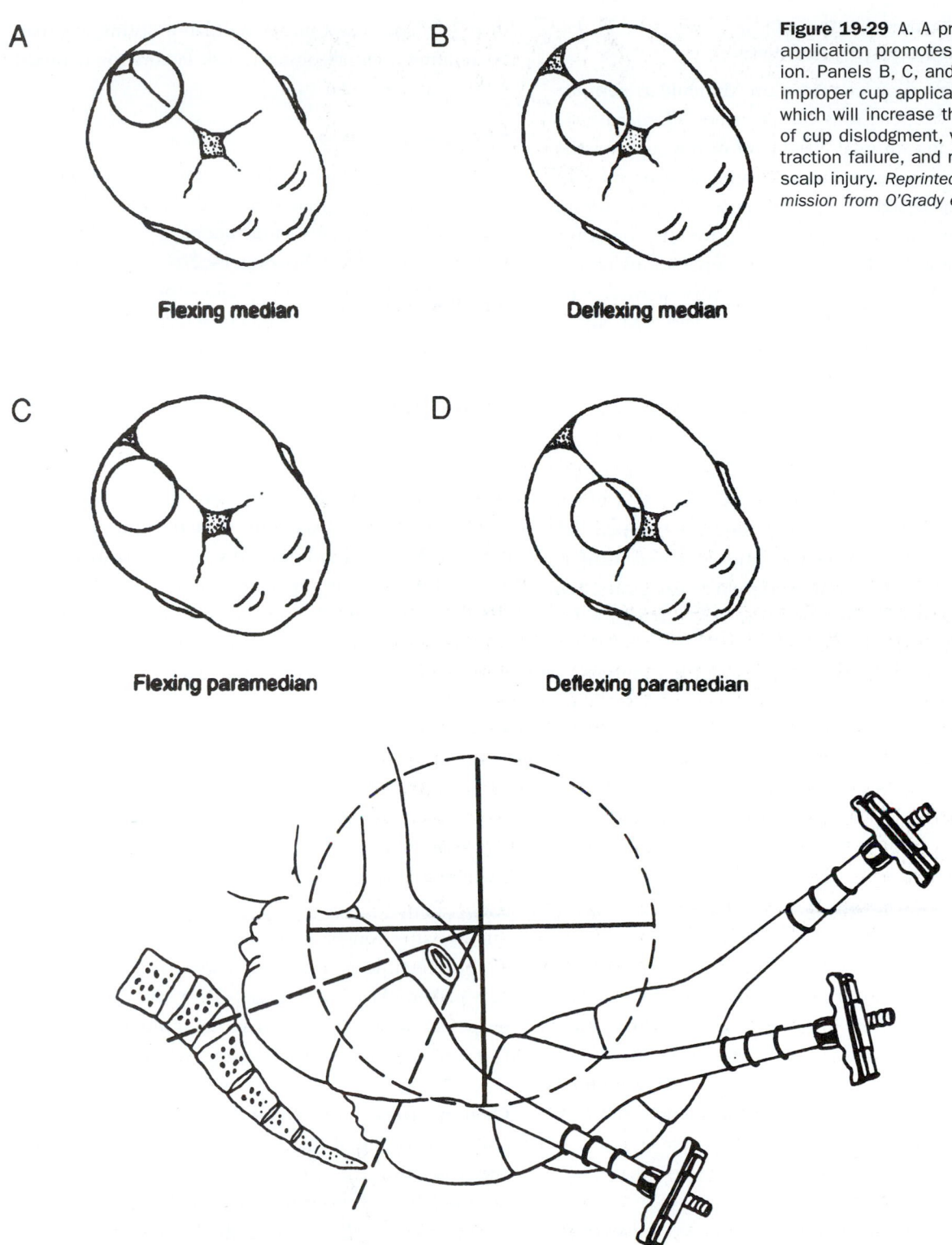

A

Flexing median

B

Deflexing median

C

Flexing paramedian

D

Deflexing paramedian

Figure 19-29 A. A proper cup application promotes cranial flexion. Panels B, C, and D show improper cup applications, all of which will increase the chance of cup dislodgment, vacuum extraction failure, and neonatal scalp injury. *Reprinted with permission from O'Grady et al.*[30]

Figure 19-30 The correct vector of traction with a vacuum-cup device changes as the fetal head descends through the pelvic curve. *Reprinted with permission from O'Grady et al.*[30]

the operator to actively prevent loss of station between contractions. One hundred fifty-eight women were randomized to an intermittent vacuum technique. The level of vacuum was decreased to 100 mm Hg between contractions, and the operator was instructed to make no effort to prevent fetal loss of station. The continuous vacuum technique did not effect delivery more quickly or reduce method failures, and the intermittent technique did not reduce the risk of neonatal injury.

In Occiput Posterior (OP) and Occiput Transverse (OT) Positions

Vacuum extraction can be more difficult to perform successfully in persistent OP positions. The fetal head is deflexed and optimal placement of the cup over the pivot point can be technically difficult using most of the soft-cup designs. Bofill[48] suggests that the use of the M-cup vacuum extractor allows the operator greater maneuverability for cup applications to the persistent OP fetus since the traction stem can be bent. He also states that application of the M-cup at the true pivot point of the fetal head may allow the fetus to "autorotate" to occiput anterior. Vacuum extraction can also be used instead of Kielland forceps for delivery of fetuses in a deep transverse arrest. Herabutya et al.[48] compared maternal and neonatal outcomes after a deep transverse arrest in 117 women delivered with Kielland forceps and 142 women delivered with the rigid vacuum cup. Maternal complications were more common in the forceps group, and cephalohematoma occurred more often in babies delivered by vacuum extraction.

If vacuum extraction is used to aid in the delivery of OP or OT presentations, torsion should not be applied to the vacuum cup in an attempt to rotate the fetal head. Cup torsion promotes cup displacement and scalp injury and thus causes the extraction procedure to be unsuccessful.[43]

Vacuum Complications

Maternal

Maternal complications following vacuum extraction are usually similar to those reported after a spontaneous vaginal delivery. Episiotomy extensions or soft tissue injuries—i.e., cervical, vaginal, or periurethral lacerations—may occur during the vacuum delivery process.[29,31,32,37,43]

Retinal Hemorrhages

Retinal hemorrhages are commonly seen in newborn infants. They can occur after a spontaneous delivery but are more common after an instrumental delivery, particularly vacuum extraction.[50] The clinical significance of retinal hemorrhages is unclear, as most of these lesions are transient and are associated with no long-term residual effects.[51] Williams et al.[52] noted that fetal distress, vacuum-assisted delivery, decreased birth weight for gestation, umbilical artery pH less than 7.20, and a second stage of labor lasting less than 30 minutes were all obstetric risk factors for neonatal retinal hemorrhage.

Fetal Cranial Injuries

In a 1979 report, Plauché[53] reviewed the world's literature up until that time and reported the type and the incidence of various neonatal cranial injuries that were detected following 14,276 vacuum extractions performed using the Malmström vacuum cup. These cranial injuries will be described below. No such large series has yet been reported after the use of soft-cup vacuum extraction devices, but one would surmise that a soft cup would cause fewer of these type injuries.

CHIGNON (100%) Some degree of chignon formation occurs with all vacuum extraction procedures. A chignon is an area of localized scalp edema that forms under the extractor cup when suction is applied and the fetal scalp is pulled up into the cup. A chignon is not serious and begins to regress in a few hours and is usually undetectable in a few days.[51,53]

SCALP ABRASIONS AND/OR LACERATIONS (12.6%) Scalp abrasions, lacerations, and ecchymoses have been noted with both metal- and soft-cup vacuum extraction. Usually these are minor, superficial injuries that rarely require suturing and can be treated with an antibacterial soap or ointment.[51,53] Cosmetic scalp trauma has been reported to occur more frequently after longer vacuum applications (exceeding 10 minutes), longer second stages, and paramedian cup placements.[44] Vesicular scalp rashes, mimicking herpes simplex infections, have been reported in 4 infants after vacuum delivery using a Mityvac cup.[54]

CEPHALOHEMATOMA (6%) A cephalohematoma is a collection of blood that lies beneath the pericranium and arises from the laceration of a subperiosteal vessel. On physical examination, a cephalohematoma is usually firm, well circumscribed, restricted to one cranial bone, and does not move with palpation of the scalp. Usually, these scalp lesions do not cause any serious neonatal problems. Neonatal hyperbilirubinemia may occur but rarely is so severe that phototherapy or a blood transfusion is required.[51,53]

Berkus et al.,[53] in a prospective study undertaken to determine the safety of the Silastic vacuum extractor, reported that the clinical diagnosis of a cephalohematoma often is not confirmed by a neo-natal cranial ultrasound examination. Only 3 of the 12 (25%) cephalohematomas clinically diagnosed after vacuum extraction in his study were later confirmed by neonatal cranial sonography. Cephalohematomas can occur after spontaneous delivery but have an increased incidence after instrumental delivery. Bofill et al.,[56] in a prospective, randomized, controlled trial of vacuum delivery in 322 women using a M-cup device, noted that the only predelivery factor found to predispose to neonatal cephalohematoma forma-tion was increasing asynclitism.

Life-Threatening Fetal Cranial Injuries

Subgaleal Hemorrhages (0.45%)

A subgaleal hematoma is a collection of blood be-tween the periosteum of the skull and the epicranial aponeurous. These hemorrhages can be life threaten-ing because of the large potential space in the scalp for blood to collect. Diffuse scalp swelling, extensive neonatal blood loss, hypotension, shock, and even convulsions may occur from these hemorrhages.[51] Plauché noted that fetal coagulopathies were associ-ated with almost half of the reported cases of sub-galeal hemorrhages.[53] Chadwick et al.[57] reviewed the records of 37 neonates admitted to the neonatal intensive-care unit over a 24-year period with the diagnosis of a subgaleal hematoma. All except one of these neonates had an instrumental delivery, and 89% had a vacuum extractor applied to their heads at some stage of the delivery process. Neonates who were de-livered by vacuum extraction and then developed a subgaleal hemorrhage were more likely to have had a failed vacuum procedure that was followed by a trial of forceps or had vacuum extractions that were diffi-cult, requiring several cup applications for prolonged periods. Treatment of subgaleal hemorrhage is support-ive and requires control of hemorrhage and restoration of blood volume.[51] If the neonate survives the acute event, long-term outcome is good for these infants, and long-term neurologic sequelae are uncommon.[57,58]

Intracranial Hemorrhage (0.35%)

Intracranial hemorrhage after vacuum extraction is a rare event and may be subarachnoid, subdural, or intraparenchymal. The prognosis after this event de-pends on the location of the bleeding. Infants with intracranial bleeding may present with symptoms such as depression, apnea, shock, or convulsions.[51,53] Risk

factors for this rare type of hemorrhage are difficult vacuum extractions requiring a prolonged time for delivery, nonreassuring fetal heart rate tracings, appli-cation of the vacuum cup at a high fetal station, or attempting a forceps delivery after the fetal head does not descend with vacuum extraction.[59]

Skull Fractures

The true incidence of skull fractures after vacuum extraction is unknown. Most cases probably go un-detected because cranial radiographs are not usually performed in asymptomatic neonates.[51,53] A skull fracture may be present in conjunction with a subgaleal or intracranial hemorrhage. Hickey and McKenna[60] reported a case of a term infant in whom a parietal bone skull fracture developed after delivery by vac-uum extraction using a Malmström cup placed in-correctly in a paramedian location. The authors sug-gested that the vacuum extractor can exert considerable traction force and may not always dislodge before causing serious head trauma.

Which Instrument Is Better to Use— Forceps or a Vacuum Extractor?

Johanson et al., in a 1993 study,[61] performed a meta-analysis of nine randomized controlled trials compar-ing maternal and neonatal outcomes with forceps de-livery versus vacuum extraction.[50,61-68] In analyzing the results of the meta-analysis, the authors found that delivery by forceps was associated with significantly more maternal perineal and vaginal trauma and with the need for regional/general anesthesia and delivery by cesarean. The vacuum extractor was found to be significantly more likely to fail at achieving a vaginal delivery and to cause neonatal injuries, such as cephalohematomas, retinal hemorrhages, jaundice, and low 5-minute Apgar scores. Thus, the above studies all found that using a forceps instrument to effect de-livery caused more maternal injuries, and performing an operative vaginal delivery by vacuum extraction caused more neonatal injuries.

Certain maternal injuries that are more common after a forceps delivery, such as third- or fourth-degree episiotomy extensions, damage the anal sphincter and may cause long-term anal incontinence and defeca-tory symptoms. Sultan et al.[69] studied primiparous women delivered by forceps (N = 26) and vacuum (N = 17) and compared them with 47 women who had spontaneous vaginal deliveries. Each patient in this study underwent anal endosonography, manometry, pudendal-nerve terminal motor latency testing, and perineometry. Defecatory symptoms were more common in women delivered by forceps [38% of forceps versus 12% of vacuum deliveries (p not significant), and 4% of controls ($p = 0.0003$)]. Anal sphincter defects identified by endosonography were more common in forceps deliveries [81% of forceps deliveries vs. 21% of vacuum extractions (p not significant) and 36% of control patients ($p = 0.0005$)]. Anal pressures were lower in women with sphincter defects, but pudendal-nerve terminal motor latency was not significantly altered by the type of delivery.

In a follow-up study, Sultan and colleagues[70] performed a retrospective analysis of obstetric variables in 50 women who had sustained a third-degree laceration at delivery and compared them with 88 matched controls delivered during the same period. Study and control patients underwent anal endosonography and manometry and pudendal-nerve terminal motor latency measurements. Factors found to be significantly associated with a third-degree laceration were forceps deliveries, nulliparity, and birth weight greater than 4000 g. If Sultan et al.'s data are confirmed by other large prospective investigations, findings from these studies should be used when the obstetrician is deciding which instrument to select for an operative vaginal delivery.

Most neonatal scalp injuries from vacuum extraction are not serious, but, in rare instances, a subgaleal hematoma or an intracranial hemorrhage may develop and can be fatal to the infant. As discussed previously in this chapter, Chadwick et al.[57] reported that difficult and prolonged vacuum extractions or failed vacuum procedures followed by a trial of forceps were significant obstetric risk factors for subgaleal hemorrhage. However, I am aware of several cases, through medicolegal case review or by discussions at national meetings, in which a subgaleal hematoma or an intracranial hemorrhage developed despite the fact that the vacuum procedure was performed correctly. Thus, these life-threatening neonatal scalp injuries from vacuum extraction may not all be preventable.

SUMMARY

The type of instrument any given operator will select for performing an operative vaginal delivery will depend on the clinical situation and his or her own training, skills, and personal biases. I recommend that every young obstetrician be trained during residency in the proper application and use of both obstetric forceps and vacuum extractors. With proper training, obstetricians can then continue to use both these instruments in their practices and select the best instrument for a given clinical situation. For example, a soft-cup vacuum extractor is the instrument of choice to perform an outlet or low operative vaginal delivery when a patient does not have adequate anesthesia. If the patient does have adequate anesthesia and needs an urgent delivery, obstetric forceps are more likely to succeed in achieving a prompt vaginal delivery. Forceps are the instrument of choice for delivering premature fetuses and fetuses with suspected coagulation defects.

REFERENCES

1. Kerr M. The obstetric forceps and the ventouse. In: Myerscough PR, ed. Munroe Kerr's operative obstetrics. 10th ed. New York: Bailliére Tindall, 1982:276.
2. O'Grady JP. Instrumental delivery. In: O'Grady JP, Gimovsky ML, eds. Operative obstetrics. Baltimore: Williams & Wilkins, 1995:176.
3. Yeomans E. Forceps delivery. In: Hankins GD, Clark SL, Cunningham FG, Gilstrap LC, eds. Operative obstetrics. Norwalk, CT: Appleton & Lange, 1995:129.
4. Burkman RT. Forceps and vacuum-assisted delivery. In: Repke JT, ed. Intrapartum obstetrics. New York: Churchill Livingstone, 1996:165.
5. Thompson JP. Forcep deliveries. Clin Perinatol 1995; 22:953.
6. Yeomans ER, Gilstrap LC. The role of forceps in modern obstetrics. Clin Obstet Gynecol 1994;37:785.
7. Healy DL, Laufe LE. Survey of obstetric forceps training in North America in 1981. Am J Obstet Gynecol 1985; 151:54.
8. Ramin SM, Little BB, Gilstrap LC. Survey of forceps delivery in North America in 1990. Obstet Gynecol 1993;81:307.
9. Bofill JA, Rust OA, Perry KG, et al. Forceps and vacuum delivery: a survey of North American residency programs. Obstet Gynecol 1996;88:622.
10. American College of Obstetricians and Gynecologists. Obstetric Forceps. ACOG Committee Opinion #59. February, 1988.
11. Hagadorn-Freathy AS, Yeomans ER, Hankins GD. Validation of the 1988 ACOG forceps classification system. Obstet Gynecol 1991;77:356.
12. American College of Obstetricians and Gynecologists. Forceps: new ACOG guidelines and definitions. Update vol. 15, issue 4. Washington, DC: ACOG, 1989.
13. Dennen PC. Prerequisites for forceps deliveries. In: Dennen PC, ed. Dennen's forceps deliveries. 3rd ed. Philadelphia: F.A. Davis, 1989:7.
14. Dennen PC. Special instruments: Kielland forceps. In:

Dennen PC, ed. Dennen's forceps deliveries. 3rd ed. Philadelphia: F.A. Davis, 1989:97.

15. Dennen PC. Special instruments: Piper forceps for the aftercoming head. In: Dennen PC, ed. Dennen's forceps deliveries. 3rd ed. Philadelphia: F.A. Davis, 1989:159.

16. Dennen PC. Special instruments: other. In: Dennen PC, ed. Dennen's forceps deliveries. 3rd ed. Philadelphia: F.A. Davis, 1989:169.

17. Dennen PC. Special instruments: Barton forceps. In: Dennen PC, ed. Dennen's forceps deliveries. 3rd ed. Philadelphia: F.A. Davis, 1989:135.

18. Megison JW. Save the Barton forceps. Obstet Gynecol 1993;82:313.

19. Dennen PC. Technique of application. In: Dennen PC, ed. Dennen's forceps deliveries. 3rd ed. Philadelphia: F.A. Davis, 1989:35.

20. Dennen PC. Traction. In: Dennen PC, ed. Dennen's forceps deliveries. 3rd ed. Philadelphia: F.A. Davis, 1989:53.

21. Phillips RD, Freeman M. The management of the persistent occiput posterior position. Obstet Gynecol 1974;43:171.

22. Dennen PC. Tranverse positions of the occiput. In: Dennen PC, ed. Dennen's forceps deliveries. 3rd ed. Philadelphia: F.A. Davis, 1989:67.

23. Yancey MK, Herpolsheimer A, Jordan GD, Benson WL, Brady K. Maternal and neonatal effects of outlet forceps delivery compared with spontaneous vaginal delivery in term pregnancies. Obstet Gynecol 1991;78:646.

24. Carmona F, Martínez-Román, Manau D, Cararach V, Iglesias X. Immediate maternal and neonatal effects of low-forceps delivery according to the new criteria of the American College of Obstetricians and Gynecologists compared with spontaneous vaginal delivery in term pregnancies. Am J Obstet Gynecol 1995;173:55.

25. Robertson PA, Laros RK, Zhao RL. Neonatal and maternal outcome in low-pelvic and midpelvic operative deliveries. Am J Obstet Gynecol 1990;162:1436.

26. Hankins GD, Rowe TF. Operative vaginal delivery—year 2000. Am J Obstet Gynecol 1996;175:275.

27. Rubin L, Coopland AT. Kielland's forceps. Can Med Assoc J 1970;103:505.

28. Revah A, Exra Y, Farine D, Ritchie K. Failed trial of vacuum or forceps—maternal and fetal outcome. Am J Obstet Gynecol 1997;176:200.

29. Hayashi RH. Vacuum delivery. In: Hankins GD, Clark SL, Cunningham FG, Gilstrap LC, eds. Operative obstetrics. Norwalk, CT: Appleton & Lange, 1995:173.

30. O'Grady JP, Gimosky ML, McIlhargie CJ. The history of the vacuum extractor. In: O'Grady JP, Gimosky ML, McIlhargie CJ, eds. Vacuum extraction in modern obstetric practice. New York: Parthenon, 1995:1.

31. Lucas MJ. The role of vacuum extraction in modern obstetrics. Clin Obstet Gynecol 1994;37:794.

32. Halme J, Ekbladh L. The vacuum extractor for obstetric delivery. Clin Obstet Gynecol 1982;25:167.

33. Paul R, Staisch K, Pine S. The new vacuum extractor. Obstet Gynecol 1973;41:800.

34. Maryniak G, Grank J. Clinical assessment of the Kobayashi vacuum extractor. Obstet Gynecol 1984;64:431.

35. Cohn M, Barclay C, Fraser R, et al. A multicentre randomized trial comparing delivery with a silicone rubber cup and rigid metal vacuum extractor cups. Br J Obstet Gynaecol 1989;96:545.

36. Hofmeyr GJ, Gobetz L, Sonnendecker EW, Turner MJ. New design rigid and soft vacuum extractor cups: a preliminary comparison of traction forces. Br J Obstet Gynecol 1990;97:681.

37. American College of Obstetricians and Gynecologists. Operative Vaginal Delivery. Technical Bulletin no. 196. August 1994.

38. Instruction Booklet for CMI vacuum delivery system. Redmond, OR: Columbia Medical & Surgical, Inc., 1994.

39. Witter F. Soft-cup vacuum extractors safely assist normal deliveries. Contemp Obstet Gynecol Technology Issue 1985; and Obstet Gynecol 1990.

40. Morales R, Adair CD, Sanchez-Ramos L, Gaudier FL. Vacuum extraction of preterm infants with birth weights of 1,500–2,499 grams. J Reprod Med 1995;40:127.

41. Thomas SJ, Morgan MA, Asrat T, Weeks JW. The risk of periventricular-intraventricular hemorrhage with vacuum extraction of neonates weighing 2000 grams or less. J Perinatol 1997;17:37.

42. Bird GC. The use of the vacuum extractor. Clin Obstet Gynecol 1982;9:641.

43. O'Grady JP, Gimosky ML, McIlhargie CJ. Vacuum extraction operations. In: O'Grady JP, Gimosky ML, McIlhargie CJ, eds. Vacuum extraction in modern obstetric practice. New York: Parthenon, 1995:57.

44. Teng FY, Sayre JW. Vacuum extraction: does duration predict scalp injury? Obstet Gynecol 1997;89:281.

45. Sjostedt JE. The vacuum extractor and forceps in obstetrics: a clinical study. Acta Obstet Gynecol Scand 1967;46:203.

46. O'Grady JP, Gimosky ML, McIlhargie CJ. Instruments, indications, and issues. In: O'Grady JP, Gimosky ML, McIlhargie CJ, eds. Vacuum extraction in modern obstetric practice. New York: Parthenon, 1995:13.

47. Bofill JA, Rust OA, Schorr SJ, Brown RC, Roberts WE, Morrison JC. A randomized trial of two vacuum extraction techniques. Obstet Gynecol 1997;89:758.

48. Bofill JA. The vacuum extraction to forceps in posterior presentation comparison. Am J Obstet Gynecol 1997;176:1398.

49. Herabutya Y, Prasertsawat PO, Boonrangsimant P. Kielland's forceps or ventouse—a comparison. Br J Obstet Gynaecol 1988;95:483.

50. Ehlers N, Jensen K, Hansen KB. Retinal haemorrhages in the newborn. Acta Ophthalmol 1974;52:73.

51. O'Grady JP, Gimosky ML, McIlhargie CJ. Complications and birth injuries. In: O'Grady JP, Gimosky ML, McIlhargie CJ, eds. Vacuum extraction in modern obstetric practice. New York: Parthenon, 1995:73.

52. Williams MC, Knuppel RA, O'Brien WF, Weiss A, Spellacy W, Pietrantoni M. Obstetric correlates of neonatal retinal hemorrhage. Obstet Gynecol 1993;81:688.

53. Plauché WC. Fetal cranial injuries related to delivery with the Malmström vacuum extractor. Obstet Gynecol 1979;53:750.

54. Hagadorn JI, Bogin FJ, Rasmussen CA. Vesicular neonatal rash at the site of vacuum application. Obstet Gynecol 1996;87:879.

55. Berkus MD, Ramamurthy RS, O'Conner PS, Brown K, Hayashi RH. Cohort study of silastic obstetric vacuum

cup deliveries: I. Safety of the instrument. Obstet Gynecol 1985;66:503.

56. Bofill JA, Rust OA, Devidas M, Roberts WE, Morrison JC, Martin JN. Neonatal cephalohematoma from vacuum extraction. J Reprod Med 1997;42:565.

57. Chadwick LM, Pemberton PJ, Kurinczuk JJ. Neonatal subgaleal haematoma: Associated risk factors, complications and outcome. J Paediatr Child Health 1996;32:228.

58. Benaron DA. Subgaleal hematoma causing hypovolemic shock during delivery after failed vacuum extraction: a case report. J Perinatol 1993;13:228.

59. Vacca A. Annotation: birth by vacuum extraction: Neonatal outcome. J Paediatr Child Health 1996;32:204.

60. Hickey K, McKenna P. Skull fracture caused by vacuum extraction. Obstet Gynecol 1996;88:671.

61. Johanson RB, Rice C, Arthur J, et al. A randomised prospective study comparing the new vacuum extractor policy with forceps delivery. Br J Obstet Gynaecol 1993; 100:524.

62. Dell DL, Sightler SE, Plauché WC. Soft cup vacuum extractor—a comparison of outlet delivery. Obstet Gynecol 1985;66:624.

63. Fall O, Ryden G, Finnstrom K, et al. Forceps or vacuum extraction? A comparison of effects on the newborn infant. Acta Obstet Gynecol Scand 1986;65:75.

64. Johanson R, Pusey J, Livera N, et al. North Staffordshire/Wigan assisted delivery trial. Br J Obstet 1989;96:537.

65. Lasbrey AH, Orchard CD, Crichton D, et al. A study of the relative merits and scope for vacuum extraction as opposed to forceps delivery. S Afr J Obstet Gynaecol 1964;2:1.

66. Loghis C. Comparison of assisted deliveries by forceps and silicone rubber cup vacuum extractor. Proceedings of the 13th World Congress on Gynaecology and Obstetrics (FIGO), Singapore, 1991. Abstract 64.

67. Vacca A, Grant A, Wyatt G. Portsmouth operative delivery trial—a comparison of vacuum extraction and forceps delivery. Br J Obstet Gynaecol 1983;90:1107.

68. Williams MC, Knuppel RA, Weiss A. A prospectively randomised comparison of forceps and vacuum assisted delivery. Am J Obstet Gynecol 1991;164:323.

69. Sultan AH, Kamm MA, Bartram CI, Hudson CN. Anal-sphincter trauma during instrumental delivery. Int J Gynecol Obstet 1993;43:263.

70. Sultan AH, Kamm MA, Hudson CN, Bartram CI. Third degree obstetric anal sphincter tears: risk factors and outcome of primary repair. BMJ 1994;308:887.

Chapter 20

Cesarean Delivery and Cesarean Hysterectomy

Patrick Duff

Five Key Points

- The most common indications for cesarean delivery in the United States are dystocia and repeat cesarean.

- The most common complication of cesarean delivery is endometritis.

- The principal advantage of the Pfannenstiel skin incision for cesarean delivery is enhanced wound strength. The principal disadvantage is decreased intraoperative exposure.

- For patients with a single prior low transverse cesarean, the probability of successful vaginal birth after cesarean is approximately 70%.

- The morbidity associated with cesarean hysterectomy is such that the procedure should be performed only when there is a clear indication both for cesarean delivery and hysterectomy.

In the eighth century B.C., the Roman ruler Numa Pompilius established a law requiring that postmortem abdominal delivery be performed whenever a woman died late in pregnancy. The purpose of the statute was twofold: to save the life of the fetus and to permit separate entombment of mother and fetus. This law, originally termed *lex regia*, was continued under the rule of the Roman emperors and became known as *lex caesarea*.[1]

Although isolated references to cesarean delivery appear in early scientific writings, the details of the operations are poorly documented. Not until 1500 was cesarean delivery performed on a living patient. In that year, Jacob Neufer, a German farmer, reportedly performed the operation on his wife. The woman survived and subsequently delivered two other children vaginally. This remarkable achievement was not described in the literature until 1591, and several historians question the authenticity of the report.[1]

In 1668, the French obstetrician, Francois Mauriceau, reviewed the European obstetric experience with cesarean delivery and concluded that the procedure almost invariably resulted in maternal death and, therefore, should be performed only in rare and desperate situations. Almost 160 years later, John Lambert Richmond (1830) became the first American physician to successfully perform a cesarean delivery.[2] His patient had been in labor for over 30 hours and was experiencing eclamptic convulsions when he took over her care from two midwives. Alarmed by the deterioration in the women's condition, Richmond, "feeling a deep and solemn sense of my responsibility, with only a case of common pocket instruments, about one o'clock at night ..." performed a cesarean. Despite making a classical uterine incision, Richmond was unable to extract the fetus.

> As soon as the gush of blood partially subsided, I commenced my efforts to remove the child, but it was uncommonly large. . . . Thinking the danger to the mother very great and believing . . . the child was dead from detachment of the placenta, and considering at all events that a childless mother was better than a motherless child, I determined to do all I could for the preservation of the mother. Accordingly I made a transverse incision across the back of the foetus . . . by which means I was enabled easily to extract it. . . . She commenced work in twenty-four days from the operation, and in the fifth week walked a mile and back the same day.[2]

Until the early 20th century, the maternal mortality rate associated with cesarean delivery was alarmingly high, ranging from 85 to 100%. For the 90 years ending 1876, French obstetricians were unable to report a single patient who survived the operation. The vast majority of deaths were the result of either exsanguination or overwhelming septicemia.[3] In the late 19th century, two major innovations greatly improved the safety of abdominal delivery. In 1876, Porro[4] performed the first cesarean hysterectomy in which both mother and child survived. Hysterectomy was recommended as a means of preventing the serious intraabdominal sepsis that resulted when an infected uterus was left in place. In 1882, Sanger described a technique for closure of the uterine wall with wire sutures.[5] Sanger had used this technique in only one operation and based his recommendation primarily on reports of 16 operations performed by American frontier surgeons such as William Polin, who in 1852 was the first American physician to close the uterus with silver wire.

The next major development in cesarean delivery was Frank's description in 1907 of the extraperitoneal operation.[6] Frank opened the peritoneal cavity just above the pubis and then sutured the parietal peritoneum to the visceral peritoneum at the point of the vesicouterine reflection. This maneuver sealed off the peritoneal cavity before the uterus was opened through a vertical incision. Two years later, Latzko[7] reported a major modification of the procedure that avoided entry into the peritoneal cavity, thereby preventing the peritoneal contamination that occurred once the uterus was opened.

In 1912, Krönig used a transperitoneal approach, dissected the bladder away from the lower uterine segment, and entered the uterus through a short vertical incision.[3] In the early 1920s, Beck[8] and DeLee and Cornell[9] popularized the vertical lower segment operation in the United States. In 1926, Munro Kerr[10] of Glasgow modified Krönig's technique and performed a transverse incision in the lower uterine segment. However, general acceptance of his procedure did not occur until 1949. The Kerr procedure now is the most popular type of cesarean delivery.

Several developments during the past 45 years have further enhanced the safety of cesarean delivery. Improvements in anesthetic techniques, blood-banking technology, and supportive medical care, particularly intravenous fluid therapy, have benefited all surgical patients. Surgical outcome for obstetric patients in particular has improved as our understanding of the pathophysiology and microbiology of postcesarean infection has increased.

INDICATIONS

A significant increase in the number of cesarean deliveries performed in the United States has occurred over the past 45 years. The average incidence of cesarean delivery rose from approximately 4% in 1950 to almost 20% in 2000. The increased incidence of operative deliveries has coincided with changes in obstetric practice, most notably: (1) widespread application of ultrasound and electronic fetal monitoring, (2) an intensified multidisciplinary approach to treatment of pregnant women with major medical illnesses, and (3) enhanced safety of the operation. The increase has coincided with a significant decrease in the perinatal mortality rate. However, this latter decline is due primarily to other changes in obstetric practice and only in part to the increased incidence of operative delivery.

Four indications account for most of the increase in the cesarean delivery rate: dystocia, repeat cesarean, breech presentation, and fetal distress.[11] Repeat cesarean now is the most common reason for abdominal delivery, accounting for almost one-third of procedures. Approximately 30% of cesareans are performed for dystocia. Third-trimester bleeding, malpresentation, and fetal distress each account for 10 to 15% of cesareans. Cesarean delivery has become the most commonly performed major operation in

American hospitals, and almost 1 million such procedures are now performed annually.

PERIOPERATIVE COMPLICATIONS

Maternal Mortality

In the 20th century, maternal mortality secondary to operative delivery has declined sharply.[11] For example, in 1970, maternal mortality was 113.8 per 100,000 operations. By 1978, mortality had decreased to 40.9 per 100,000. One report documented no maternal deaths in 10,231 cesarean deliveries performed during the 11-year period 1968 to 1978.[12]

The two leading causes of maternal death associated with cesarean delivery are hemorrhage and pulmonary embolism. Infection and complications of anesthesia are less common, but still important, causes of mortality. Despite major improvements in anesthetic and surgical techniques, cesarean delivery is associated with at least a two- to fourfold increased risk of maternal death as compared with vaginal delivery.[11]

Infection

Infection, specifically endometritis, is the single most common complication of cesarean delivery. On average, endometritis occurs in 15 to 20% of patients having an unscheduled cesarean delivery even when prophylactic antibiotics are administered. The incidence of endometritis is lower in women having a scheduled cesarean delivery before the onset of labor but still averages 5 to 10%. Approximately 5 to 10% of patients in whom endometritis develops have bacteremia, 3 to 5% have urinary-tract infections (UTIs), and 1 to 3% have wound infections.[13]

The principal risk factors for postcesarean infection are young age, low socioeconomic status, multiple vaginal examinations, extended duration of labor and ruptured membranes, and preexisting lower-genital-tract infection (e.g., group B streptococcal colonization, bacterial vaginosis). Variables such as type of anesthesia, duration of internal fetal monitoring, preoperative hematocrit, and level of experience of the surgeon have an inconsistent relationship with incidence of infection. The lowest incidence of infection occurs in middle and upper socioeconomic class, private patients undergoing scheduled abdominal delivery; the highest incidence occurs in indigent patients undergoing cesarean delivery after long labors with extended duration of ruptured membranes.[13]

Hemorrhage

The average blood loss during cesarean delivery is 1000 to 1100 cc. Placenta previa, abruptio placentae, severe preeclampsia, and multiple gestation predispose to excessive blood loss at abdominal delivery. In addition, surgical technique itself may influence intraoperative blood loss. For example, a classical uterine incision usually results in more blood loss than a low transverse or low vertical incision. When the lower uterine segment is poorly developed, as in a preterm gestation, lateral extension of the incision into the major uterine vessels may occur. Vertical extensions of the lower segment incision into the vagina or uterine fundus also may result in excessive intraoperative blood loss. Conversely, tubal ligation or incidental appendectomy generally do not increase the incidence of intraoperative hemorrhage.

The need for perioperative transfusion depends on several variables, the most important of which are the original indication for surgery, socioeconomic status of the patient, preoperative hematocrit, and the surgical skill of the obstetrician. Less than 5% of middle and upper socioeconomic class patients undergoing elective repeat or primary cesarean for arrest of progress in labor require transfusion. Conversely, the requirement for transfusion may be higher in indigent, anemic women undergoing emergency cesarean delivery.[11]

Urinary-Tract Injury

The incidence of bladder injury associated with primary and repeat cesarean is 0.19% and 0.60%, respectively. Injury typically occurs in patients who have had a prior cesarean delivery and who have extensive adhesions between the bladder and lower uterine segment or between the bladder and undersurface of the anterior abdominal wall. The most common site of injury is the lower posterior wall of the bladder. Primary intraoperative repair of the bladder defect usually results in healing without subsequent development of a vesicovaginal fistula.[14]

The incidence of ureteral injuries is about 0.09%. Most ureteral injuries occur when the ureter is ligated accidentally during efforts to control hemorrhage from the major uterine vessels. Ureteral injuries identified intraoperatively can be repaired primarily. When the ureter has been ligated, removal of the ligature is the only treatment necessary. If the ureter has been crushed by a clamp or actually severed, resection of the damaged tissue followed by ureteroureteral anastomosis or ureteroneocystostomy is necessary.[14]

OPERATIVE TECHNIQUE

Skin Incision

The peritoneal cavity may be entered through either a vertical or transverse skin incision (Figure 20-1). The vertical incision should be made in the midline, extending from a point approximately 2 cm above the pubic symphysis to just below the umbilicus. The principal advantages of the vertical incision are that it permits more rapid entry into the abdominal cavity and facilitates intraoperative exposure. The major disadvantages are its greater susceptibility to dehiscence and less attractive cosmesis.

The transverse or Pfannenstiel incision should extend transversely for approximately 15 cm (the length of an Allis clamp) at a point about 2 cm above the pubic symphysis.[15] The principal advantage of this incision is that it is less likely to result in dehiscence than the vertical incision. In addition, it affords a better cosmetic appearance. Disadvantages of the transverse incision include slower entry into the peritoneal cavity and decreased operative exposure, particularly when the procedure is performed under regional anesthesia.

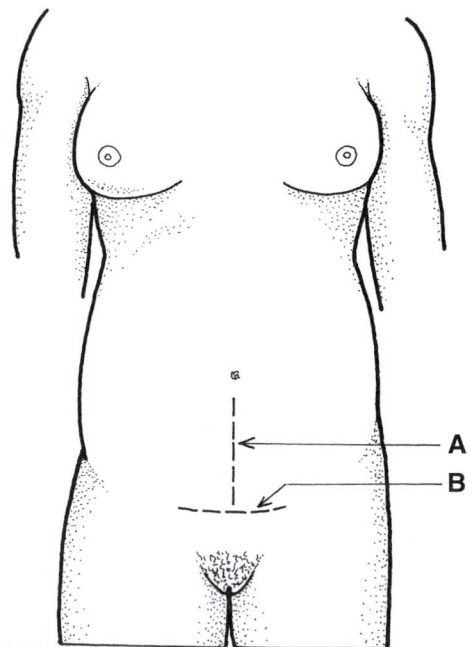

Figure 20-1 Skin incisions for cesarean delivery. A. Vertical midline incision. B. Transverse or Pfannenstiel incision.

UTERINE INCISION

Low Transverse Incision

The low transverse, or Kerr, incision is the procedure most frequently performed for cesarean delivery (Figure 20-2A). It generally is associated with less intraoperative blood loss than either the low vertical or classical incision. Its principal advantage is that it heals more securely than the vertical incisions and is less likely to dehisce during subsequent pregnancies.[9,10] Improved healing is a consequence of the fact that the lower-segment incision is made at a point in the uterus where there are relatively few myometrial fibers. Therefore, during the process of uterine involution, the incision is not subjected to contractile forces that disturb the integrity of the wound.

Low Vertical Uterine Incision

There are two principal indications for the low vertical, or Krönig, incision. It should be used for delivery of the very small preterm fetus, especially the fetus in footling breech presentation, when the lower uterine segment is poorly developed. In this circumstance, a transverse incision may result in exposure inadequate for atraumatic delivery of the fetus and in lateral extension of the incision resulting in laceration of the uterine artery and vein. The low vertical incision also is useful when cesarean hysterectomy is planned. In this instance, the vertical incision avoids the risk of laceration of the major uterine vessels prior to performance of the more extensive surgical procedure.

The initial steps of the low vertical procedure are the same as for the low transverse incision. After the plane between bladder and lower uterine segment has been developed, the bladder is retracted inferiorly. A vertical hysterotomy incision is made starting at the lowermost boundary of the lower uterine segment and extending upward for approximately 6 to 8 cm (Figure 20-2B). Ideally, this incision should be confined to the noncontractile lower segment, but, of necessity, it often extends into the thickened upper segment.

Classical Uterine Incision

The classical uterine incision is rarely indicated in modern obstetric practice. Its principal disadvantage is that it is much more likely than the low transverse

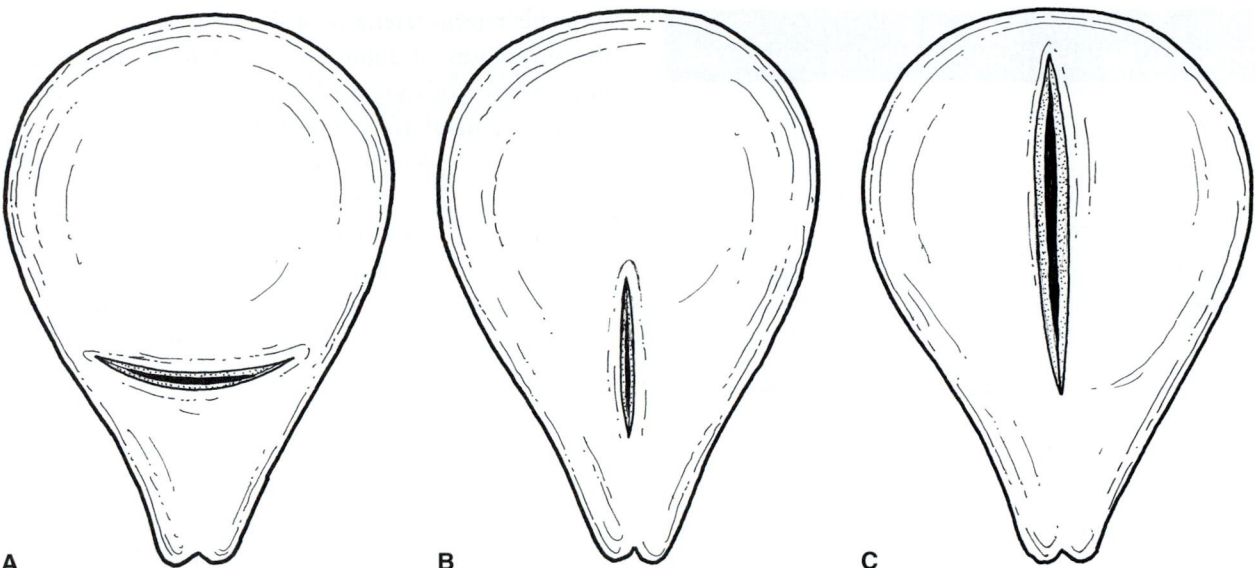

Figure 20-2 A. Low transverse uterine incision. B. Low vertical uterine incision. C. Classical uterine incision.

incision to dehisce in a subsequent pregnancy.[11,16] Disruption may even occur before the onset of labor. In addition, the classical incision usually results in increased intraoperative blood loss as compared with either the low transverse or low vertical incision.

The major advantage of the classical incision is that it provides complete access to the endometrial cavity. In selected clinical situations, such access may be necessary to accomplish safe delivery of the fetus (Table 20-1).

The classical incision should extend vertically from a point just above the bladder reflection to the superior portion of the uterine fundus (Figure 20-2C). The bladder does not need to be separated from the lower uterine segment.

**TABLE 20-1
SELECTED INDICATIONS FOR
CLASSICAL UTERINE INCISION**

Transverse lie with fetal back down
Fetal anomaly
  Severe hydrocephalus
  Large abdominal-wall defect
  Large sacrococcygeal teratoma
Premature twin gestation complicated by abnormal presentations
More than two fetuses
Extensive adhesions between bladder and lower uterine segment
Placenta previa combined with prominent varicosities of the
    lower uterine segment
Large leiomyoma obstructing access to the lower uterine
    segment

Extraperitoneal Cesarean Section

The extraperitoneal procedure was developed to decrease the risk of peritoneal contamination in patients who already had chorioamnionitis or who were at high risk for postoperative infection because of prolonged rupture of membranes.[6,7] In the preantibiotic era, the rationale for extraperitoneal cesarean delivery was clear. Maternal mortality rates were dramatically higher than at present, and sepsis was one of the two major causes of maternal death. With the advent of broad-spectrum antibiotics, the theoretical and practical advantages of the extraperitoneal procedure are questionable. In fact, in most clinical situations, extraperitoneal cesarean section, although not harmful, does not offer any significant advantage over the transperitoneal procedure and typically is more difficult and time-consuming to perform.[17]

UTERINE CLOSURE

Although there are differences of opinion with respect to the selection of suture for uterine closure, synthetic resorbable fibers such as polyglycolic acid (Dexon) and polyglactin (Vicryl), 0 gauge, appear to be the best choices. These materials have increased tensile strength and cause less inflammation as compared with chromic or plain gut suture. Improved manufacturing techniques, especially coating of the suture with polyglycolic or polyglactin polymer, have

TABLE 20-2
PRINCIPAL RISK FACTORS FOR WOUND DEHISCENCE

Wound infection
Obesity
Acute or chronic pulmonary disease
Postoperative ileus
Immunodeficiency disorders
Irradiation
Immunosuppressive therapy, i.e., systemic corticosteroids and
    chemotherapy
Ascites
Malnutrition

made these materials comparable to chromic suture in terms of ease of handling. Knot slippage is a possibility with the new synthetic materials, but this problem can be minimized by tying a minimum of four knots.

When the lower segment is well developed and reasonably thin, the endometrium and myometrium may be closed together as a single layer with a continuous suture. In one report, patients with single-layer closure actually had a lower frequency of post-cesarean endometritis as compared with patients with a double-layer closure.[18] If the patient has not labored and the lower segment is thicker and less well developed, a two-layer closure of the uterus may be necessary. In this case, the second layer should be reapproximated with a continuous horizontal or vertical imbricating suture. With classical uterine incisions, the myometrium is so thick that it always should be closed in a minimum of two layers.

Abdominal-Wall Closure

Closure of the visceral and parietal peritoneum is unnecessary. Peritoneal closure neither improves the

ultimate tensile strength of the wound nor prevents the formation of adhesions between the bowel and undersurface of the anterior abdominal wall.

As a general rule, multifilamented synthetic sutures such as polyglycolic acid or polyglactin polymers (0 gauge) are the preferred materials for closure of the fascia. In patients at increased risk for wound dehiscence (Table 20-2) either delayed resorbable monofilament polymers of polyglyconate (Maxon) or polydiaxonone (PDS) or a permanent monofilament suture such as nylon or polypropylene should be used for fascial closure.

The fascia may be closed with continuous or interrupted sutures. With a continuous suture, the individual needle bites should be placed at least 1.5 cm from the fascial edge, and the tissue should be coapted without excessive tension. Interrupted sutures are of most value in closure of a vertical incision in a patient who has other risk factors for wound dehiscence. In such circumstances, the sutures should be placed in a far-far (1.5 to 2.0 cm from the fascial edge), near-near (0.5 to 1.0 cm from the fascial edge) manner (Smead–Jones technique, Figure 20-3).

The subcutaneous layer need not be closed if it is less than 0.5 to 0.75 inch in thickness. If it exceeds this thickness, it should be loosely reapproximated with several interrupted sutures of 2-0 or 3-0 polyglycolic acid or polyglactin polymer. Del Valle et al.[19] have documented a decreased frequency of wound disruption, seroma, and hematoma when the subcutaneous layer was reapproximated as described.

The skin may be reapproximated with external sutures, surgical staples, or a continuous subcutaneous suture of 4-0 polyglycolic acid or polyglactin polymer. The latter two techniques produce the best cosmetic results. External sutures and staples should be

Figure 20-3 Smead–Jones technique for closure of the abdominal wound.

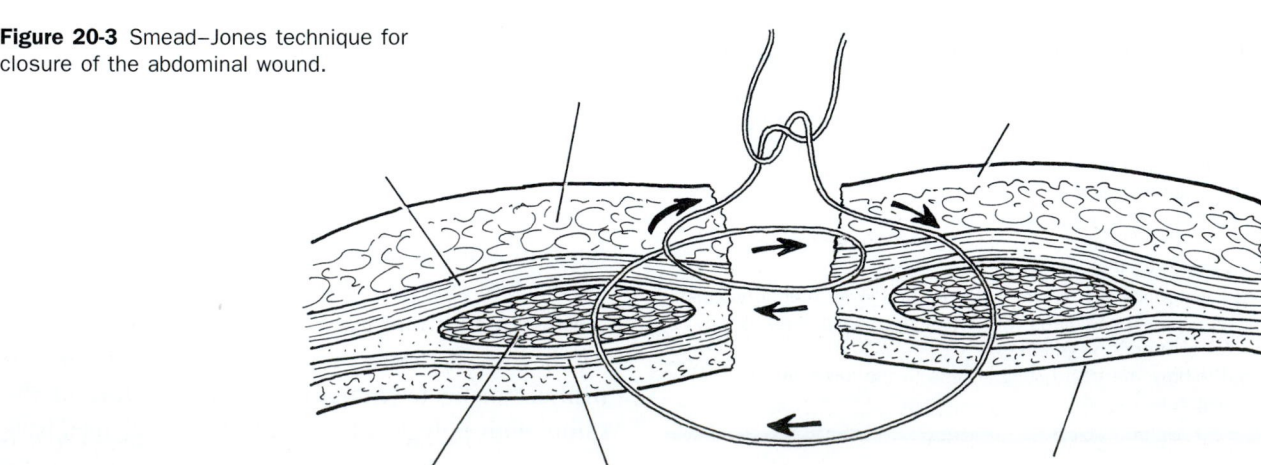

removed on approximately the third or fourth post-operative day, and steristrips should be applied to maintain coaptation of the skin edges.

ANESTHESIA FOR CESAREAN DELIVERY

Cesarean delivery can be performed under local anesthesia. This technique, however, does not provide optimal anesthesia and may require use of near-toxic doses of the local anesthetic agent. Therefore, in virtually all circumstances, regional or general anesthesia should be utilized for abdominal delivery. In the United States today, general, epidural, and spinal anesthesia are each used in about one-third of cases.[11]

The most frequent complications of spinal anesthesia are maternal hypotension and post spinal headache. Epidural anesthesia is more difficult to perform than subarachnoid block and, therefore, more frequently results in technical failure. However, it is less likely than subarachnoid block to cause maternal hypotension because it produces more gradual blockade of sympathetic vasomotor fibers. With either technique, systemic absorption of the local anesthetic agent may occur and lead to adverse effects such as seizures and cardiac arrest. Similarly, with either technique, unexpectedly high levels of blockade may occur, resulting in paralysis of the accessory muscles of respiration. Infection or prolonged neurologic injury are exceedingly rare complications of regional anesthesia.[11]

In situations in which general anesthesia is indicated for cesarean delivery, the patient must be intubated to minimize the risk of aspiration pneumonitis. Induction of general anesthesia usually is accomplished by administering thiopental intravenously (2 to 4 mg/kg of body weight). In the presence of hypotension, ketamine (1.0 mg/kg) may be preferred to thiopental because of its sympathomimetic properties. Succinylcholine (0.1 to 0.2%) usually is administered intravenously during the induction sequence to prevent laryngospasm during intubation. Nitrous oxide (50 to 75%) with oxygen then is given by inhalation to maintain a light level of anesthesia until the fetus is delivered. After delivery of the infant, the level of anesthesia can be deepened by administering intravenous narcotics and a short–acting benzodiazepine such as midazolam. If uterine relaxation is required, one of the nonflammable agents such as halothane, enflurane, or isoflurane should be administered. Adequate muscle relaxation can be maintained during delivery by administering a continuous intravenous infusion of succinylcholine or incremental doses of pancuronium.

ROUTINE POSTOPERATIVE CARE

Following surgery, the patient's bladder catheter should be left in place until sensation in the lower half of the body has returned. Early ambulation should be encouraged in an effort to reduce the risk of deep-vein thrombosis. Patients whose procedure was uncomplicated usually can advance quickly to a regular diet within 24 hours of surgery.[20,21] For the first 24 to 48 hours postoperatively, patients may require parenteral narcotics such as meperidine hydrochloride, 50 to 100 mg (25 mg IV or 50 to 100 mg IM) every 3 to 4 hours, for analgesia. Thereafter, oral agents such as acetaminophen (325 mg) plus codeine (30 mg) every 4 to 6 hours or ibuprofen (400 to 800 mg) every 6 to 8 hours provide adequate pain relief. Barring complications such as endometritis or wound infection, patients usually can be discharged from the hospital on the third postoperative day and occasionally as early as the second postoperative day.[22]

POSTMORTEM CESAREAN DELIVERY

Postmortem cesarean delivery rarely is performed except in unusual and tragic circumstances. In the small series of postmortem cesarean sections reported in the literature, neonatal survival has ranged from 0 to 40%.

Postmortem cesarean should be considered whenever maternal death is imminent and pregnancy has progressed to the point of fetal viability. In exceptional situations, it may even be appropriate to prolong maternal life for a short time after brain function has ceased in order to enhance the chances for the neonate's survival.[23]

In considering the possibility of postmortem cesarean delivery, the attending physician must be aware of the strict definition of brain death. All of the following criteria must be fulfilled before a patient is declared to be brain dead[23]:

• No response to painful stimuli.
• No muscular movement and no spontaneous breathing for 1 hour (or 3 minutes off the respirator).
• No reflexes, ocular movements, or blinking.
• Fixed and dilated pupils.
• Flat, isoelectric electroencephalogram during two separate recordings obtained 24 hours apart.
• Observations above must not have occurred as a result of barbiturate intoxication or hypothermia.

In ideal circumstances, the physician should discuss the procedure in advance with the patient's nearest relative. If this intervention is planned, a surgical instrument set should be kept at the bedside so that delivery can be completed as soon as possible after the declaration of maternal death. Cardiopulmonary support must be maintained in the interval between maternal death and delivery of the fetus.

TUBAL LIGATION AT THE TIME OF CESAREAN DELIVERY

Sterilization may be performed at the time of cesarean delivery by any of several accepted methods: Pomeroy, Parkland, Irving, or Uchida techniques. The failure rates of these techniques vary from about 1 in 200 with the first two to approximately 1 in 1000 with the latter two. In general, tubal ligation does not increase the morbidity associated with cesarean delivery. Counseling for permanent sterilization should be conducted well in advance of delivery. Prior to performing tubal ligation at the time of cesarean delivery, the surgeon should ascertain that the initial neonatal evaluation is normal and that no unusual neonatal complications are anticipated.

TRIAL OF LABOR AFTER PREVIOUS CESAREAN DELIVERY

In 1916, Edwin Cragin[24] presented a paper before the Eastern Medical Society of the City of New York in which he directed his associates' attention to the dangers associated with cesarean delivery, particularly the danger of maternal death due to overwhelming infection.

> Let me say, that it pays to be charitable toward any careful man who is unfortunate enough to have in his practice a case of puerperal infection. To criticize is easy, but alas! the tables may soon be turned and we may be the next unfortunate to spend anxious days and sleepless nights over a case of puerperal infection which came we know not how.

Cragin noted that most instances of severe infection occurred in situations in which cesarean delivery followed a long period of labor and an extended duration of ruptured membranes.

> If the woman has been a long time in labor with membranes ruptured many hours, the mortality of two to three percent rises to a mortality of ten to fifteen percent, and the operation ceases to be a conservative procedure and becomes one of considerable hazard. This emphasizes the importance of an early diagnosis in all cases with a positive indication

> for Caesarean Section so that the operation can be performed either just before or in the early stages of labor.

He cautioned, however, that cesarean delivery should be performed only in exceptional circumstances:

> (o)ne thing must always be borne in mind, viz., that no matter how carefully a uterine incision is sutured, we can never be certain that the cicatrized uterine wall will stand a subsequent pregnancy and labor without rupture. This means that the usual rule is, once a Caesarean always a Caesarean. . . . I believe that the extension of Caesarean section to conditions other than dystocia from contracted pelvis or tumors should be exceptional and infrequent.

Cragin's paper was presented at a time when cesarean delivery was not safe and when the vast majority of operations were performed through classical uterine incisions. For over 50 years, however, his dictum, "once a Caesarean always a Caesarean" was accepted without reservation by most American obstetricians. In spite of contrary rationale,[25] as late as 1984 more than 95% of women who previously had had cesarean deliveries were delivered by repeat cesarean section.[26]

In recent years, more than 30 reports describing trials of labor in patients with previous cesarean delivery have been published.[27] The principal findings of these studies may be summarized as follows.

- During a subsequent pregnancy, the classical incision is much more likely to dehisce than the low transverse incision. The incidence of disruption of the classical incision is 5 to 10%, as compared with 0.5 to 1.5% for the transverse incision. Disruption of the classical incision usually is a true rupture. It may occur prior to the onset of labor and be associated with potentially life-threatening maternal hemorrhage. Maternal and fetal mortality may be as high as 5% and 40 to 75%, respectively. The usual clinical manifestations of rupture are fetal distress, pain, shock, and cessation of labor.[27] Patients with a prior classical incision should not be allowed to labor. They should be delivered by repeat cesarean at approximately 37 weeks of gestation after documenting fetal lung maturity.

- The incidence of rupture of the low vertical incision has not been defined precisely but appears to be intermediate between the low transverse and classical incisions, depending on whether the vertical incision extended upward into the contractile segment of the uterus. If the low vertical incision is completely confined to the lower uterine segment, the frequency of disruption approximates that of a low transverse incision.[27]

- Disruption of the low transverse incision usually takes the form of a small dehiscence of the scar. It typically does not become apparent prior to the onset of labor, nor is it associated with major maternal blood loss. Only in rare circumstances does fetal mortality occur. Dehiscence of the lower uterine segment scar usually is asymptomatic but may present with fetal distress, mild to moderate abdominal pain, and loss of coordinated uterine activity.[27]

- The low transverse incision heals more rapidly and securely than the vertical incision because the former incision is not subjected to the same disruptive contractile forces as the latter.

- The majority of women who have had a prior cesarean delivery are acceptable candidates for subsequent trial of labor (vaginal birth after cesarean, VBAC). The principal contraindications to VBAC are prior classical incision, prior low transverse incision complicated by vertical extension into the thickened myometrium, and present indication for abdominal delivery such as placenta previa, abruptio placentae, malpresentation, or marked fetopelvic disproportion.

- In most investigations, the maternal morbidity and mortality associated with a management protocol that allows a trial of labor for selected patients is less than that associated with a policy that dictates elective repeat cesarean for all patients. In addition, such a protocol does not increase the frequency of perinatal morbidity or mortality.[27] In a large retrospective survey in Nova Scotia, McMahon et al.[28] observed no significant difference in the overall rate of maternal complications in women who elected to have a trial of labor as compared with those who had an elective repeat cesarean. Neonatal complications and perinatal mortality were similar in the two groups. "Major maternal complications" (need for hysterectomy, uterine rupture, operative injury) were twice as likely (odds ratio, 1.8) in the trial of labor group. However, the overall incidence of these "major complications" was quite low, 1.3%.

- More than one prior low transverse incision does not contraindicate a trial of labor. Patients with more than one prior low transverse cesarean do not have a disproportionately increased risk of uterine scar dehiscence.[29]

- At a minimum, at least half of women who are allowed a trial of labor will deliver vaginally. In most reports, the average frequency of successful VBAC is 60 to 70%, and, in selected series, 80 to 90% of patients have had successful trials of labor.[27,30,31]

- Unless markedly decreased pelvic capacity has been demonstrated conclusively, a prior diagnosis of cephalopelvic disproportion is not a contraindication to a trial of labor. Among women with a previous cesarean delivery for failure to progress or for cephalopelvic disproportion, approximately 50 to 60% will have a successful trial of labor. Of those delivering vaginally, 20 to 30% will have a larger infant than during the first delivery.[30,32]

- In women who have an unsuccessful trial of labor, the incidence of postcesarean infection is significantly higher than that in patients who undergo elective repeat cesarean delivery.[33]

- Regional anesthesia will not mask clinical manifestations of overt scar dehiscence and, therefore, is not contraindicated in women undergoing a trial of labor.

- Administration of oxytocin for induction or augmentation of labor in patients undergoing a trial of labor is not contraindicated, provided that uterine hyperstimulation is avoided.[34]

- In women delivering vaginally, small scar defects that are not bleeding do not need repair. If such defects are noted during repeat cesarean, they should be repaired as the uterine incision is closed. Only in exceptional circumstances will hysterectomy be necessary because of disruption of a transverse lower-segment scar.

Joseph et al.[35] have showed that, if women with a prior cesarean are allowed an open-ended choice between VBAC and repeat cesarean, only half opt for VBAC. The data presented above and the ethical principle of beneficence clearly support directed counseling in favor of VBAC. Repeat cesareans now account for more than one-third of all operative deliveries. At least half of these procedures could be avoided without significantly increasing the risk for either mother or fetus, resulting in major cost savings for patients and third-party payers. However, because rare, but very serious, complications can occur during trials of labor, the equally important ethical principle of autonomy ultimately should be decisive.[28,36] If the patient refuses to consent to VBAC, she should not be coerced into a procedure against her will. Table 20-3 outlines the criteria for VBAC, including the requirement for informed patient consent.

TABLE 20-3
CRITERIA FOR VAGINAL BIRTH AFTER CESAREAN

Prior low transverse incision or low vertical incision clearly confined to the noncontractile segment of the uterus
No recurring indication for cesarean delivery
No new indication for cesarean delivery
Appropriate ancillary support—anesthesia, blood bank, nursing staff
Informed consent of the patient

TIMING OF REPEAT CESAREAN DELIVERY

In patients who have had previous cesarean delivery and who are not candidates for a trial of labor, the timing of repeat cesarean is of critical importance. Unexpected delivery of a preterm infant is usually due to failure of the attending physician to satisfy rigid criteria for establishment of gestational age.

One way to avoid miscalculation of gestational age is to perform amniocentesis to document a mature surfactant profile prior to elective delivery. However, amniocentesis increases costs, and third–trimester amniocentesis may be associated with serious complications, including fetal and placental bleeding, rupture of membranes, infection, and initiation of labor. The usual incidence of such complications is less than 3%.[37]

Another method for avoiding elective prematurity is to delay repeat cesarean until the patient is in labor. One disadvantage of this policy is that patients with prior classical uterine incisions may experience dehiscence of their scar prior to labor. As noted, rupture of the classical incision may be associated with severe maternal hemorrhage and a high incidence of fetal mortality. Therefore, at least in this select group of patients, delivery should be performed on a scheduled basis prior to the onset of labor. Other disadvantages are: (1) the patient may go into labor during the night or weekend hours, when the surgical team is not immediately available, and (2) the patient may go into labor soon after eating a meal.

If the following strict criteria established by the American College of Obstetricians and Gynecologists are observed, elective repeat cesarean delivery can be performed without antecedent amniocentesis.[38]

- Fetal heart tones have been documented for 20 weeks by nonelectronic fetoscope or for 30 weeks by Doppler.
- 36 weeks have elapsed since a positive serum or urine human chorionic gonadotropin assay.

- An ultrasound measurement of the crown-to-rump length, obtained at 6 to 11 weeks, supports a gestational age ≥39 weeks.
- An ultrasound, obtained at 12 to 20 weeks, confirms the gestational age of ≥39 weeks determined by clinical history and physical examination.

PROPHYLACTIC ANTIBIOTICS FOR CESAREAN DELIVERY

Pathogenesis of Postcesarean Infection

Postoperative endometritis is a polymicrobial infection caused by bacteria normally present in the host's lower genital tract. The major microorganisms responsible for endometritis are aerobic gram-negative bacilli, principally *Escherichia coli*; anaerobic gram-negative bacilli, principally Bacteroides and Prevotella species; aerobic gram-positive such as, primarily group B streptococci and enterococci; and anaerobic gram-positive cocci, specifically Peptococci and Peptostreptococci species.[13,39]

The development of clinical infection is dependent on a complex balance between host defense mechanisms and bacterial virulence factors. Cesarean delivery alters this balance so as to predispose the patient to infection. During labor and abdominal delivery, the endometrium and peritoneal cavity inevitably are contaminated with large numbers of highly pathogenic aerobic and anaerobic bacteria. The serosanguineous fluid that collects in the abdomen after surgery and the injured uterine tissue at the site of the hysterotomy incision provide excellent culture media for microbial growth. The bacterial inoculum is particularly large when cesarean delivery is performed after multiple vaginal examinations and extended duration of labor and ruptured membranes.

Rationale for Prophylaxis

Antibiotic prophylaxis reduces the size of the bacterial inoculum and alters the characteristics of the culture medium at the operative site during the brief time that host defenses are impaired by the trauma of surgery.[40] The major objective in using prophylactic antibiotics is to reduce the incidence of postcesarean endometritis. This disorder causes the patient considerable discomfort and results in increased duration of hospitalization. In addition, it is the usual precursor for serious complications such as pelvic abscess, septic shock, and septic pelvic thrombophlebitis. A second objective of prophylaxis is to reduce the incidence of these life-threatening complications. The third objective is to reduce the incidence of major wound infections. Such disorders usually require a second surgical procedure to open and debride the incision and may lead to dehiscence and evisceration. Wound infection is even more likely than endometritis to result in marked prolongation of the patient's hospitalization.

Results of Clinical Trials

Since 1970, more than 20 reports of prophylactic antibiotics in cesarean delivery have been published in the American obstetric literature. The principal findings of these investigations may be summarized as follows.[39]

- Virtually without exception, all studies have shown a significant decrease in postcesarean endometritis in patients who received antibiotics. Even in patients who have elective repeat cesareans, antibiotic prophylaxis is of benefit if the base-line frequency of endometritis in untreated patients is in the range of 10%.[39]
- In very-high-risk, indigent patient populations, prophylactic antibiotics also may decrease the frequency of urinary-tract and wound infection.[39]
- Prophylactic antibiotics should be administered after the infant's umbilical cord is clamped.[33] Delay in administration until this point in the procedure does not compromise the efficacy of prophylaxis and avoids exposure of the neonate to antibiotics.
- Inexpensive antibiotics such as the first-generation cephalosporin, cefazolin, are as effective for prophylaxis as the more expensive, extended-spectrum cephalosporins and penicillins.[41]
- In patients who have an immediate hypersensitivity reaction to β-lactam antibiotics, a single dose of clindamycin (900 mg) plus gentamicin (80 mg) may be used for prophylaxis.
- In most patient populations, a single dose of antibiotic is as effective as two- and three-dose regimens. In no circumstance should more than three doses of antibiotic be administered as prophylaxis.[39,41] More extended courses of antibiotics represent actual treatment, not prophylaxis, and simply increase the expense of treatment and the risk of side effects.

- Serious adverse effects are unlikely when limited-spectrum agents are used for short courses of prophylaxis.

CESAREAN HYSTERECTOMY

Historical Evolution

In 1768, Joseph Cavallini described experimental cesarean hysterectomy in laboratory animals and suggested that there might be instances in which such a procedure would be necessary as a lifesaving measure for the gravid patient[42]:

All things having been duly weighed, I do not doubt that the uterus is not at all necessary to life, but whether it may be plucked out with impunity from the human body we cannot be certain without a further series of experiments of this kind which, perhaps, a more fortunate generation may obtain.

In speculative moments, I have sometimes felt inclined to persuade myself that the dangers of the Caesarean operation might be considerably diminished by removal of the uterus. Perhaps this method of operating may prove an eminent and valuable improvement.

Cavallini's investigations stimulated other scientists to investigate cesarean hysterectomy. In 1823, James Blundell published his study of cesarean hysterectomy in the rabbit model.[1] In 1869, Horatio Storer[43] performed the first subtotal hysterectomy in a living patient. Abdominal delivery was necessary because the patient's birth canal was obstructed by a large pelvic tumor, and removal of the uterus was performed because of life-threatening hemorrhage. Although the infant survived, the patient died on the third day after surgery.

In 1876, Eduardo Porro[4] reported the first cesarean hysterectomy in which both infant and mother survived. Porro's patient, Julia Cavallini, was a 25-year-old dwarf, and her pelvis was markedly distorted by rickets. After delivery of the infant, Porro performed a subtotal hysterectomy and unilateral salpingo-oophorectomy utilizing a snare called a "Cintrat's constrictor."

Despite the lack of blood products, intravenous fluids, and antibiotics, Julia Cavallini survived a turbulent 40-day hospitalization. The successful outcome in this case was due to Porro's adherence to surgical principles that are well recognized today but which certainly were not firmly established in 1876. He achieved hemostasis by use of the occluding snare. He irrigated the peritoneal cavity with carbolized sponges, drained the operative bed, and exteriorized the cervical stump in an effort to prevent infection. He closed the abdominal wound with wire to reduce the risk of dehiscence. Porro also personally attended the patient during the first 24 hours after surgery, feeding her "champagne and laudanum."

Porro's paper, "Dell' Amputazione Utero-ovarica come Complemento de Taglio Cesereo," stimulated a flurry of interest in cesarean hysterectomy. Within months of his report, Inzana and Previtali in Italy and Hegar in Germany presented single-case reports of cesarean hysterectomy. Although two of the three infants survived, all three mothers died in the immediate postoperative period. These fatalities are not surprising in view of the fact that one patient had osteosarcoma affecting the bones of the pelvis, one had eclampsia, and one had chorioamnionitis.[42,44]

Two years after publication of Porro's paper, Muller of Switzerland described a modification of Porro's technique. His patient had been in labor for 3 days, and chorioamnionitis had developed, resulting in fetal death. Muller's innovation was to remove the uterus from the peritoneal cavity and elevate it onto the abdominal wall before making the hysterotomy incision.[42,44]

In 1880, Robert P. Harris[45] of the United States reviewed the world literature and collected 50 cases of cesarean hysterectomy, reported from seven countries. The cumulative maternal mortality was 58%; fetal survival was 86%.

The first successful cesarean hysterectomy in the United States was performed by Richardson in 1881. His patient, like Porro's, was a young dwarf, 3 feet 10 inches tall. Richardson utilized Muller's technique of exteriorizing the uterus. Once the uterus was positioned on the abdominal wall, a wire snare was placed around the cervix at the level of the internal os and tightened to secure hemostasis. After delivery of the fetus, the uterus was amputated, and the cervical stump was cauterized with carbolic acid and placed back into the pelvis. Both mother and infant survived.[42,46]

One year later, the first cesarean hysterectomy was performed in Great Britain by Croom, Hart, and Caird.[40] In that same year, Wells,[47] also of Great Britain, completed the first total cesarean hysterectomy; all previous operations had been supracervical procedures. The indication for surgery in Wells's patient was invasive cervical carcinoma. The first two British patients died in the immediate postoperative period.

In 1884, Godson[48] performed the first cesarean hysterectomy in Great Britain that resulted in maternal survival. Additional modifications in Porro's operative technique were made by Tait[49] and Von Waerz and Weiss.[46] Each of these investigators directed special attention to management of the cervical stump after supracervical hysterectomy. Tait recommended exteriorization of the uterus, excision of the corpus, and suture of the cervical stump to the abdominal wall. Von Waerz and Weiss advocated leaving the cervical remnant within the pelvis and reapproximating the visceral peritoneum over the stump. Another modification in technique was suggested by several physicians, including Reymond and Cazalis in 1911, LeCoq in 1917, and Solieri and Rogers in 1922. These investigators described performance of hysterectomy before cesarean delivery and reported survivals in both mother and infant.[42,44,46]

Changing Indications

From its development in the mid-1800s until 1900, cesarean hysterectomy was performed exclusively as a lifesaving measure for the mother. In 1900, Reed outlined the following indications for the Porro procedure: (1) intrauterine fetal death in association with chorioamnionitis; (2) cervical cancer; (3) hemorrhage due to uterine atony; (4) uncontrolled hemorrhage due to placenta previa, placenta accreta, or abruptio placentae; and (5) ruptured uterus.[42,44,46]

In the early 1900s, some clinicians began to extend the indications for cesarean hysterectomy. Duncan and Targett[50] of Great Britain were among the first to suggest that subtotal hysterectomy be performed for sterilization at the time of indicated cesarean delivery. In 1922, J.W. Harris of Johns Hopkins reported 64 subtotal cesarean hysterectomies, of which 18 were performed for sterilization. He justified these elective procedures by citing an improved maternal mortality of 4.7% as compared with the 58% incidence reported earlier by Robert P. Harris.[42,44,46]

In 1935, Lash and Cummings listed the following indications for cesarean hysterectomy: intrauterine infection, acute blood loss, chronic renal disease, tuberculosis, and any case in which sterilization is indicated. Two years later, Wilson reported that 8.7% of all cesareans at the University of Rochester were accompanied by hysterectomy. He cited uterine leiomyoma, uncontrolled hemorrhage, intrauterine infection, and sterilization as acceptable indications for the procedure.[42,44,46]

In 1951, M.E. Davis[51] of the Chicago Lying-In Hospital advocated the extreme view that sterilization by cesarean hysterectomy was justified "in women near the end of their reproductive period, in whom the uterus no longer serves a useful function" and that "when reproduction is no longer desirable the uterus can be dispensed with, for, although it contributes little or nothing, the aging organ is subject to degeneration and serious disease." Addressing his contemporaries' concern with the psychological aspects of elective hysterectomy, Davis dismissed their fears by noting that "the complete removal of the uterus at delivery does not interfere with normal sex life, it actually improves it. . . . The roomy, plastic vagina, combined with the freedom from fear of conception results in ideal marital life."

Davis reported a series of 140 patients who underwent cesarean hysterectomy. Fifty-six percent of these procedures appear to have been performed solely for sterilization. Davis documented surprisingly low perioperative morbidity and an absence of maternal mortality.

In recent years, most authors have argued that the morbidity associated with cesarean hysterectomy is high enough that the procedure should be performed only when there is a clear indication both for cesarean delivery and hysterectomy.[52] In most instances, the procedure will be required on an emergency basis. Table 20-4 summarizes currently accepted nonemergency and emergency indications for cesarean hysterectomy.

TABLE 20-4
SELECTED INDICATIONS FOR CESAREAN HYSTERECTOMY IN MODERN OBSTETRIC PRACTICE

Nonemergency procedures
  Invasive cervical malignancy
  Prior cesarean and history of chronic pelvic pain not
    amenable to medical management
  Prior cesarean and large uterine leiomyoma
  Prior cesarean and severe endometriosis not responsive to
    medical management
  Prior cesarean and severe dysfunctional uterine bleeding not
    responsive to medical management
Emergency procedures
  Uncontrolled hemorrhage
  Uterine atony
  Placenta accreta, increta, or percreta
  Coagulopathy due to a condition such as abruptio placentae,
    severe preeclampsia, or amniotic fluid embolism
  Overwhelming infection
  Uterine rupture not amenable to surgical repair

Complications Associated with Cesarean Hysterectomy

Operative Mortality

The operative mortality in patients undergoing cesarean hysterectomy ranges from 0 to 10.1%, with a mean of 0.9%. In contrast, the operative mortality in patients undergoing cesarean delivery ranges from 0.07 to 0.11%, with a mean of 0.09%.[53] In patients having abdominal hysterectomy, operative mortality ranges from 0.10 to 0.24%, with a mean of 0.17%.[52]

Most deaths related to cesarean hysterectomy occur in indigent patients undergoing emergency operations. Acute hemorrhagic shock and pulmonary embolism are the leading causes of perioperative death. Most of the reported deaths occurred before the development of modern blood-banking procedures and anesthetic techniques and before the introduction of broad-spectrum antibiotics. Series from both public and private hospitals document several hundred elective and emergency procedures without a fatality. Nevertheless, when large series are considered cumulatively, the operative mortality associated with cesarean hysterectomy is five to eight times that associated with abdominal hysterectomy or cesarean delivery.[52]

Perioperative Hemorrhage

Many cesarean hysterectomies are performed because of life-threatening hemorrhage due to obstetric disorders such as placenta previa, placenta accreta, and abruptio placentae. Not surprisingly, therefore, 56 to 100% (mean, 75%) of patients undergoing emergency cesarean hysterectomy receive multiple blood transfusions, usually in the range of 2 to 3 units.[52]

Excessive blood loss also may occur during elective cesarean hysterectomy. Twelve to 66% of patients (mean, 40%) having elective operations receive transfusions, averaging 1 to 2 units. Even in this group of patients, the percentage of individuals requiring transfusions is approximately eight times that of patients having cesarean delivery[47] and three to four times that of women having abdominal hysterectomy.[54]

Perioperative hemorrhage is not always the result of an underlying obstetric disorder but often is due to technical difficulty with the surgical procedure itself. One to 13% of patients undergoing cesarean hysterectomy experience such extensive intraoperative blood loss that an unplanned surgical procedure such as adnexectomy, hypogastric artery ligation, or supracervical hysterectomy (rather than total hysterectomy) must be performed to control hemorrhage.

Approximately 2% (range, 0 to 6.3%) of patients require reexploration for control of postoperative hemorrhage. In these instances, bleeding usually has occurred from either the infundibulopelvic ligament or the uterine vascular pedicle. The incidence of reoperation for bleeding is well in excess of that reported in patients undergoing cesarean delivery or abdominal hysterectomy.[52,55]

Infection

Postoperative soft-tissue pelvic infection, abdominal-wound infection, and urinary-tract infection constitute the second most common group of complications associated with cesarean hysterectomy. The reported incidence of perioperative infection is difficult to assess for several reasons. Some authors have used an end point of standard febrile morbidity, which does not accurately reflect the true incidence of overt clinical infection. The sporadic, uncontrolled, and prolonged use of "prophylactic antibiotics" also has affected the reported incidence of infection. Finally, varying criteria are used for the diagnosis of pelvic infection. Many studies of cesarean hysterectomy were published before the pathophysiology of operative-site infection was well understood. Accordingly, many patients who were treated with antibiotics for fever of unexplained origin may have had pelvic cellulitis. Therefore, the true incidence of this disorder probably has been underreported.

With these caveats in mind, several general conclusions appear to be warranted. The most common perioperative infection is lower-urinary-tract infection, which occurs, on the average, in 5 to 10% of patients. Pelvic cellulitis is the second most common infection, occurring in 0.7 to 15% of patients, with a mean incidence of 6.1%. Wound infection is the third most frequent infection and occurs, on the average, in 4 to 5% of patients.[52] The highest reported incidence of pelvic abscess in patients having cesarean hysterectomy is 3.8% in a series of 1000 indigent patients.[56] Most investigators describe an incidence of abscess of less than 0.5%.

Urinary-Tract Injury

Injury to the urinary bladder occurs in 0.9 to 6.7% (mean, 3.5%) of patients undergoing cesarean hysterectomy. Most injuries occur in patients who have a history of prior cesarean and who have extensive adhesions between the bladder and lower uterine segment. Approximately 15% of bladder injuries result in vesicovaginal fistulas. Virtually every reported case of fistula developed because the original bladder injury was not recognized and repaired primarily.[52]

The reported incidence of ureteral injury varies from 0 to 1.8%, with a mean of 0.6%. Urinary-tract injury is 5 to 10 times more likely to occur during cesarean hysterectomy as compared with abdominal hysterectomy or cesarean delivery. Ureteral injury most commonly occurs at three anatomic sites. The ureter may be incorporated into the pedicle containing the infundibulopelvic ligament when adnexectomy is performed. It may be ligated or transected as the uterine vessels are clamped and incised. It also may be injured as it courses through the paracervical tissue and enters the bladder. Although ureteral injury is relatively rare, ureterovaginal fistulas develop in 33 to 40% of patients who sustain such injuries. If recognized promptly, most ureteral injuries may be managed by either reanastomosis or ureteroneocystostomy.[14,52,57]

Operative Technique

The reported operating time required for cesarean hysterectomy ranges from 65 to 132 minutes, with a mean of 100 minutes.[52] Important features of the operative technique are summarized in the following sections.

Skin Incision

When cesarean hysterectomy is performed for treatment of invasive cervical malignancy, the surgeon must have sufficient operative exposure to allow thorough exploration of the abdominal viscera and upper periaortic lymph nodes. Most oncologists prefer a vertical incision for this purpose. Alternatively, a transverse muscle-splitting (Maylard) or muscle-detaching (Cherney) incision may be used.

When surgery is performed because of an obstetric emergency, a vertical incision should be used, since it permits the most rapid abdominal entry and ensures maximal surgical exposure. When cesarean hysterectomy is performed for nonemergency indications, either a transverse incision or a vertical incision is acceptable. Operative exposure may be limited with the former incision, however, particularly when surgery is performed under regional anesthesia without muscle blockade.

Dissection of the Bladder

In order to reduce the risk of bladder injury, sharp dissection of individual adhesions should be employed if necessary to free the bladder from the underlying uterus. In the presence of adhesions, efforts to separate the bladder by blunt dissection may result in trauma to the posterior bladder wall. The surgeon should be particularly careful to avoid extension of the dissection laterally into the highly vascular bladder pillars. The dissection initially should be extended inferiorly only so far as is necessary to permit safe ligation of the uterine vascular pedicle. Fine-tip scissors are essential for this dissection.

Bladder injuries must be recognized and repaired immediately in order to prevent formation of a vesicovaginal fistula. A two-layer closure usually is adequate to repair the bladder defect. When bladder dissection has been difficult, bladder competency should be evaluated at the conclusion of the procedure by instilling marker media (such as sterile evaporated milk) through the urinary catheter. Although methylene blue has been used for this purpose, it may stain tissue, making subsequent identification of bladder defects and dissection planes more difficult.

Uterine Incision

A classical uterine incision should be performed for the selected obstetric indications noted previously. In other clinical situations, a low transverse or low vertical incision is acceptable.

The most serious complication associated with a transverse incision is extension into the uterine vessels and broad ligament, resulting in severe intraoperative hemorrhage. Lateral extension is particularly likely to occur in patients in whom the lower uterine segment is poorly developed. In contrast, a low vertical incision provides excellent access for delivery of the fetus and minimizes the risk of lateral extension of the incision into the broad ligament. It also facilitates exposure of the cervix and separation of the cervix from the vagina during removal of the uterus.

Identification of the Ureter

Ureteral injuries are largely preventable by employing meticulous surgical technique. Even when adnexectomy is not contemplated, the visceral peritoneum should be opened and the ureter should be identified as it courses along the medial leaf of the broad ligament. Dissection of the ureter is continued to the point where it passes below the uterine artery and vein so that the uterine vascular pedicle may be isolated without risk of injury to the adjacent ureter. Careful separation of the bladder from the lower uterine

segment also ensures that the ureters are displaced laterally away from the uterine vascular structures.

If radical cesarean hysterectomy is to be performed, the ureter must be dissected free from the paracervical tissue, and the point of insertion of the ureter into the bladder must be identified. In simple cesarean hysterectomy, this additional dissection is not necessary. However, the ureter should be palpated in the distal third of its course to ensure that it is lateral to the point where clamps and ligatures are applied to the cardinal ligaments, uterosacral ligaments, and upper vagina.

Isolation and Ligation of Vascular Pedicles

One to 13% (mean, 5.6%) of patients undergoing cesarean hysterectomy experience severe intraoperative hemorrhage because of uncontrolled bleeding from either the ovarian or uterine vascular pedicle. Unilateral or bilateral adnexectomy may be necessary to manage this complication.

During pregnancy, the ovarian and uterine vessels are dilated up to 10 times their normal caliber, and blood flow is increased severalfold above that of the nonpregnant state. Therefore, all vascular pedicles must be clearly identified and isolated and then securely clamped and ligated. The amount of tissue included in each pedicle should be minimized, and both leaves of the broad ligament should be incorporated into the pedicle to prevent retraction of vessels and bleeding from denuded peritoneal surfaces. Retrograde bleeding from the uterine side of pedicles may be prevented by clamping or ligating the proximal side of each pedicle.

Prevention of Perioperative Infection

No prospective, randomized, controlled investigations of prophylactic antibiotics in patients undergoing cesarean hysterectomy have been published. Therefore, conclusions about their value must be extrapolated from data reported for cesarean delivery. As noted previously, a limited course of prophylactic antibiotics is of value in decreasing the frequency of operative site infection after cesarean delivery and would seem to be a reasonable course of management in patients having cesarean hysterectomy.

Anesthesia for Cesarean Hysterectomy

Nonemergency, scheduled cesarean hysterectomies may be performed under either regional or general anesthesia. Most clinicians recommend endotracheal intubation and general anesthesia for emergency cesarean hysterectomy. Regional anesthetics usually require more time to administer and may exacerbate maternal hemodynamic dysfunction in the setting of an obstetric emergency.

The preferred agents for general anesthesia are those that produce the least depressive effect on the cardiovascular system of the mother and fetus. Inhalation gases that result in marked uterine relaxation, such as halothane and enflurane, should be avoided in patients with severe hemorrhage. The anesthetic regimen most commonly used for emergency cesarean hysterectomy is the same as the one outlined previously for emergency cesarean delivery.

REFERENCES

1. Trolle D. The history of cesarean section. Copenhagen: Reitzel Booksellers, 1982.
2. King AG. America's first cesarean section. Obstet Gynecol 1971;37:797.
3. Speert H. Obstetrics and gynecology in America: a history. Baltimore: Waverly Press, 1980.
4. Porro E. Dell'amputazione utero-ovarica come complemento de taglio cesareo. Milan: frat Rechiedei, 1876.
5. Eastman NJ. The role of frontier America in the development of cesarean section. Am J Obstet Gynecol 1932; 24:919.
6. Frank F. Suprasymphysial delivery and its relation to other operations in the presence of contracted pelvis. Arch Gynaekol 1907;81:46.
7. Latzko W. Der extraperitoneale Kaiserschnitt, seine Geschichte, seine Technik und seine Indikationen. Wien Klin Wochenschr 1909;22:477.
8. Beck AG. The advantages and disadvantages of the two flap low incision cesarean section, with a report of eighty-three cases done by fifteen operators. Am J Obstet Gynecol 1921;1:586.
9. DeLee JB, Cornell EL. Low cervical cesarean section (laparotrachelotomy). JAMA 1922;79:109.
10. Kerr JMM. The technic of cesarean section, with special reference to the lower uterine segment incision. Am J Obstet Gynecol 1926;12:729.
11. National Institute of Child Health and Human Development. Report of a Consensus Development Conference on Cesarean Childbirth. Bethesda, MD: National Institutes of Health, 1981, publication no. 82–2067.
12. Frigoletto FD Jr, Ryan KJ, Phillippe M. Maternal mortality rate associated with cesarean section: an appraisal. Am J Obstet Gynecol 1980;136:969
13. Duff P. Pathophysiology and arrangement of endomyometritis. Obstet Gynecol 1986;67:269.
14. Eisenkop SM, Richman R, Platt LD, Paul RH. Urinary tract injury during cesarean section. Obstet Gynecol 1982; 60:591.
15. Finan MA, Mastrogiannis DS, Spellacy WN. The "Allis" test for easy cesarean delivery. Am J Obstet Gynecol 1991; 164:772.
16. O'Sullivan MJ, Fumia F, Holsinger K, McLeod AGW. Vaginal delivery after cesarean section. Clin Perinatol 1981;8:131.
17. Wallace RL, Eglinton GS, Yonekura ML. Extraperitoneal cesarean section: a surgical form of infection prophylaxis? Am J Obstet Gynecol 1984;148:172.
18. Hauth JC, Owen J, Davis RO. Transverse uterine incision closure: one versus two layers. Am J Obstet Gynecol 1992; 167:1108.
19. Del Valle GO, Combs P, Qualls C, Curet LB. Does closure of Camper fascia reduce the incidence of post-cesarean superficial wound disruption? Obstet Gynecol 1992; 80:1013.
20. Soriano D, Dulitzki M, Keidar N, Barkai G, Mashiach S, Seidman DS. Early oral feeding against cesarean delivery. Obstet Gynecol 1996;87:1006.
21. Kramer RL, Van Someren JK, Qualls CR, Curet LB. Postoperative management of cesarean patients: the effect of immediate feeding on the incidence of ileus. Obstet Gynecol 1996;88:29.
22. Brooten D, Roncoli M, Finkler S, Arnold L, Cohen A, Mennuti M. A randomized trial of early hospital discharge and home follow-up of women having cesarean birth. Obstet Gynecol 1994;84:832.
23. Arthur RK. Postmortem cesarean section. Am J Obstet Gynecol 1978;132:175.
24. Cragin EB. Conservatism in obstetrics. NY Med J 1916; 104:1.
25. Pauerstein CJ. Once a section, always a trial of labor. Obstet Gynecol 1966;28:273.
26. Gleicher N. Cesarean section rates in the United States. The short-term failure of the National Consensus Development Conference in 1980. JAMA 1984;252:3273.
27. Lavin JP, Stephens RJ, Miodovnik M, Barden TP. Vaginal delivery in patients with a prior cesarean section. Obstet Gynecol 1982;59:135.
28. McMahon MJ, Lutter ER, Bowes WA, Olshan AF. Comparison of a trial of labor with an elective second cesarean section. N Engl J Med 1996;335:689.
29. Porreco RP, Meier PR. Trial of labor in patients with multiple previous cesarean sections. J Reprod Med 1983; 28:770.
30. Flamm BL, Goings JR, Liu Y, Wolde-Tsadik G. Elective repeat cesarean delivery versus TOL: a prospective multicenter study. Obstet Gynecol 1994;83:927.
31. Rosen MG, Dickinson JC. Vaginal birth after cesarean: a meta-analysis of indicators for success. Obstet Gynecol 1990;76:865.
32. Seitchik J, Rao VR. Cesarean delivery in nulliparous women for failed oxytocin-augmented labor: route of delivery in subsequent pregnancy. Am J Obstet 1982;143:393.
33. Merrill BS, Gibbs CE. Planned vaginal delivery following cesarean section. Obstet Gynecol 1978;52:50.
34. O'Connor RM. How safe is induction of labour following a previous cesarean section? J Obstet Gynaecol 1983;44:86.
35. Joseph GF, Stedman CM, Robichaux AG. Vaginal birth after cesarean section: the impact of patient resistance to a trial of labor. Am J Obstet Gynecol 1991;164:1441.

36. Scott JR. Mandatory trial of labor after cesarean delivery: an alternative viewpoint. Obstet Gynecol 1991;77:811.
37. Hayashi RH, Berry JL, Castillo MS. Use of ultrasound biparietal diameter in timing of repeat cesarean section. Obstet Gynecol 1981;57:325.
38. Fetal maturity assessment prior to elective repeat cesarean delivery. American College of Obstetricians and Gynecologists no. 98. September 1991.
39. Duff P. Prophylactic antibiotics for cesarean delivery: a simple cost-effective strategy for prevention of postoperative morbidity. Am J Obstet Gynecol 1987;157:794.
40. Ledger WJ, Gee C, Lewis WP. Guidelines for antibiotic prophylaxis in gynecology. Am J Obstet Gynecol 1975; 121:1038.
41. Carlson C, Duff P. Antibiotic prophylaxis for cesarean delivery: is an extended-spectrum agent necessary? Obstet Gynecol 1990;76:343.
42. Young JH. The history of cesarean section. London: Lewis, 1944.
43. Storer HR. Successful removal of the uterus and both ovaries by abdominal section; the tumor, fibrocystic, weighing thirty-seven pounds. Am J Med Sci 1866;51:110.
44. Riva HL. Indications and techniques for cesarean hysterectomy. Clin Obstet Gynecol 1969;12:618.
45. Harris RP. Results of the first fifty cases of "cesarean ovarohysterectomy," 1869–1880. Am J Med Sci 1880; 80:129.
46. Durfee RB. Evolution of cesarean hysterectomy. Clin Obstet Gynecol 1969;12:575.
47. Wells TS. Observations on recent improvements in the mode of removing uterine tumors. BMJ 1881;1:909.
48. Godson C: Porro's operation. BMJ 1884;1:142.
49. Tait L. Address on the surgical aspect of impacted labour. BMJ 1890;1:657.
50. Duncan W, Targett JH. Porro-Cesarean hysterectomy with retro-peritoneal treatment of the stump in a case of fibroids obstructing labour; with remarks upon the relative advantage of the modern Porro operation over the Sanger Cesarean in most other cases requiring abdominal section. Trans Obstet Soc Lond 1900;42:244.
51. Davis ME. Complete cesarean hysterectomy: a logical advance in modern obstetric surgery. Am J Obstet Gynecol 1951;62:838.
52. Park RC, Duff P. Role of cesarean hysterectomy in modern obstetric practice. Clin Obstet Gynecol 1980;23:601.
53. Amirikia H, Zarewych B, Evans TN. Cesarean section: a 15-year review of changing incidence, indications, and risks. Am J Obstet Gynecol 1981;140:81.
54. Dicker RC, Greenspan JR, Strauss LT, et al. Complications of abdominal and vaginal hysterectomy among women of reproductive age in the United States: the collaborative review of sterilization. Am J Obstet Gynecol 1982;144:841.
55. Ledger WJ, Child MA. The hospital care of patients undergoing hysterectomy: an analysis of 12,026 patients from the Professional Activity Study. Am J Obstet Gynecol 1973;117:423.
56. Barclay DL. Cesarean hysterectomy at the Charity Hospital in New Orleans—1000 consecutive operations. Clin Obstet Gynecol 1969;12:635.
57. Britton JJ. Sterilization by cesarean hysterectomy. Am J Obstet Gynecol 1980;137:837.

Chapter 21

Immediate Assessment and Resuscitation of the Neonate

Dean T. Theophilopoulos
David J. Burchfield

Five Key Points

- Several important physiological adaptations must occur for a normal transition from the intrauterine to the extrauterine environment.

- Several aspects of the maternal history are relevant to the immediate resuscitation of neonates.

- The obstetric provider must be able to identify an asphyxiated or distressed neonate who requires immediate resuscitation.

- Tissue hypoxia can be reversed by properly resuscitating asphyxiated or distressed neonates.

- Following resuscitation the neonate should be reassessed to determine if other problems are likely in the immediate neonatal period.

The first few minutes of a neonate's life may be the most critical and pivotal time for a favorable future. A neonate in distress who is not immediately and effectively resuscitated is at risk for long-term physical, mental, and emotional disabilities. The need for resuscitation in a typical delivery room is common and ranges from 0.4% in term neonates to over 70% in low-birth-weight neonates.[1] At delivery, the healthcare provider should be capable of performing an initial assessment of the neonate and be able to provide immediate resuscitation of the neonate in distress. This chapter will introduce the practitioner to the normal physiologic adaptations taking place at birth, an initial assessment of the neonate to identify if resuscitation is required, and key aspects of neonatal resuscitation that are aimed at preventing or reversing

tissue hypoxia. In addition, a secondary assessment of the neonate will be presented to identify potential problems that a neonate may experience during the early neonatal period.

NORMAL PHYSIOLOGIC ADAPTATION

Several physiological adaptations must occur for a normal transition from the intrauterine to the extrauterine environment.

LUNG LIQUID

The near-term fetus produces an estimated 5 ml/kg per hour of lung liquid that is important for normal prenatal lung growth and development.[2] The switch from placental to pulmonary gas exchange necessitates cessation of lung liquid production as well as rapid removal of this liquid, which is estimated to be 20 mL/kg near term.[3-5]

Lung liquid production is greatly attenuated in the days preceding normal labor; labor not only decreases formation, but also increases clearance of lung liquid. Lung water is reduced by 45% in animals allowed to labor compared to similar gestation animals delivered without labor.[6] The combination of decreased production and enhanced absorption of lung liquid with labor accounts for approximately 75% of lung liquid clearance prior to birth, with the remaining 25% requiring clearance after birth for a normal transition to pulmonary gas exchange.

Circulatory Changes

Due to the high pulmonary vascular resistance, low placental vascular resistance, and the intervening ductus arteriosus, only 10% of fetal cardiac output traverses the lungs. This low pulmonary blood flow in utero leads to a low left atrial filling pressure compared to right atrial pressure and allows for blood to flow across the foramen ovale from the right atrium to the left atrium. At birth, several events occur simultaneously to reverse this situation. With crying, the lungs are expanded, and mechanical obstruction to pulmonary flow is relieved. Establishment of a gas–liquid interface promotes pulmonary vasodilation and increased pulmonary blood flow. Clamping of the umbilical cord acutely removes the low-resistance placental circulation. Finally, with the increased pulmonary blood flow, left atrial pressure rises above right atrial pressure, causing the foramen ovale to close.

With the placenta serving as the organ of oxygen exchange, the fetal pO_2 is in the range of 25 to 30 torr, which is much lower compared to a normal neonate who has an extrauterine pO_2 of 50 to 80 torr. It is important to realize that the fetus has a lower pO_2, because at the moment of birth, prior to air-breathing, the neonate should have some degree of cyanosis, which rapidly resolves with pulmonary respiration.

PERTINENT RESUSCITATION HISTORY

At the time of delivery several pertinent questions should be asked regarding the maternal history, because the answers are relevant to the immediate resuscitation of the neonate.

Gestational Age

Special problems are associated with both preterm and postterm neonates, such as hyaline membrane disease in preterm neonates and meconium aspiration syndrome in postterm neonates. Equipment needs will vary, with the preterm neonates requiring smaller masks, laryngoscope blades, and endotracheal tubes.

Multiple Gestation Pregnancy

For multiple birth deliveries, each neonate will require a separate resuscitation team with its own equipment.

Meconium

When meconium is present in the amniotic fluid, a neonate may require intubation and tracheal suctioning immediately after birth. The equipment to intubate and aspirate meconium from the trachea must be ready when meconium is present in the amniotic fluid.

Emergent Conditions

Neonates born by emergent cesarean delivery because of maternal vaginal bleeding, prolapsed umbilical cord, or nonreassuring fetal heart rate tracing may have suffered intrauterine asphyxia.

Anesthesia

General anesthesia and narcotics administered to the mother may cross the placenta and cause respiratory depression, hypotonia, and decreased activity in neonates.

Magnesium Sulfate

Magnesium sulfate given to mothers for preterm labor or preeclampsia crosses the placenta and may cause respiratory depression, hypotonia, and decreased activity in neonates.

Congenital Anomalies

Certain congenital anomalies, such as congenital diaphragmatic hernia, abdominal wall defects, facial anomalies, hydrops fetalis, and myelomeningocele, require special interventions during resuscitation. These special circumstances will be discussed later in this chapter.

INITIAL ASSESSMENT

Following delivery, certain aspects of the neonatal physical examination are important to identify an asphyxiated or distressed neonate that may require immediate resuscitation. Abnormalities in a neonate's activity, tone, respirations, color, and/or perfusion usually signify that resuscitation will be required. The audible cry of a neonate is often the first reassuring sign that a neonate is doing well and is unlikely to require resuscitation. Spontaneous movement is another reassuring sign that the neonate will not require resuscitation. On the other hand, a silent neonate who is flaccid and hypotonic is worrisome and likely to require resuscitation.

Neonates that are hypoxic at birth undergo a well-defined sequence of events that is important to recognize. When a neonate is hypoxic, there is an initial period of rapid breathing followed by a period of apnea known as primary apnea. If the hypoxia continues, the neonate develops gasping respirations followed by another period of apnea known as secondary apnea. During primary apnea, a neonate may reestablish spontaneous respirations with minimal interventions such as tactile stimulation and administration of free-flow 100% oxygen. During secondary apnea, positive pressure ventilation (PPV) is required to reestablish spontaneous respirations. Furthermore, during secondary apnea, the longer the delay in initiating PPV, the longer it will take for a neonate to reestablish spontaneous respirations. The longer a neonate is in secondary apnea, the greater the chance for brain and other organ damage from hypoxia, hypercarbia, and acidosis. Because primary and secondary apnea are clinically indistinguishable, when faced with an apneic neonate at birth, one must assume that the neonate is experiencing secondary apnea and proceed with PPV if the neonate does not immediately respond to tactile stimulation.

Neonates with central cyanosis, which can be recognized by the appearance of cyanosis of the mucous membranes and entire body, are hypoxic and require supplemental oxygen. A dusky, mottled, or pale appearance of the skin with a prolonged capillary refill time, cool extremities, and weak pulses are signs of hypovolemia and indicate that a neonate requires volume expansion.

RESUSCITATION

Courses are available through the Neonatal Resuscitation Program (NRP) to train health-care providers in neonatal resuscitation. To date, over 430,000 health-care providers have been trained by the NRP.[7] Figure 21-1 is an overview of neonatal resuscitation. The different steps in neonatal resuscitation are aimed at preventing or reversing tissue hypoxia. In this section we will discuss important aspects of the various steps in neonatal resuscitation.

Adequate Preparation

To properly resuscitate a neonate, one must be adequately prepared. Proper preparation includes anticipating which neonates may require resuscitation, having appropriate and functioning equipment, and assuring that health-care providers capable of performing neonatal resuscitation are present for each delivery. Communication between the obstetrician and pediatrician regarding antepartum and intrapartum problems is very important and cannot be overemphasized. Health-care providers should frequently review the steps in neonatal resuscitation as well as practice their skills, because the more complex aspects of a resuscitation, such as intubation, chest compressions, and medications, are rarely required and are easily forgotten.

Initial Steps

During the initial part of a resuscitation, neonates should be thoroughly dried. The removal of wet linens following the drying of a neonate is a step that is often forgotten and results in increased heat loss, especially in preterm neonates. Neonates that have increased heat loss have increased metabolic demands and require more oxygen. Adequate positioning of a neonate with the neck slightly extended is important because it promotes a patent airway, whereas flexion or hyperextension of the neck leads to an obstructed airway. The mouth should be suctioned before the nose to prevent aspiration of oral secretions. Suctioning of the mouth is most effective when the head is turned to one side.

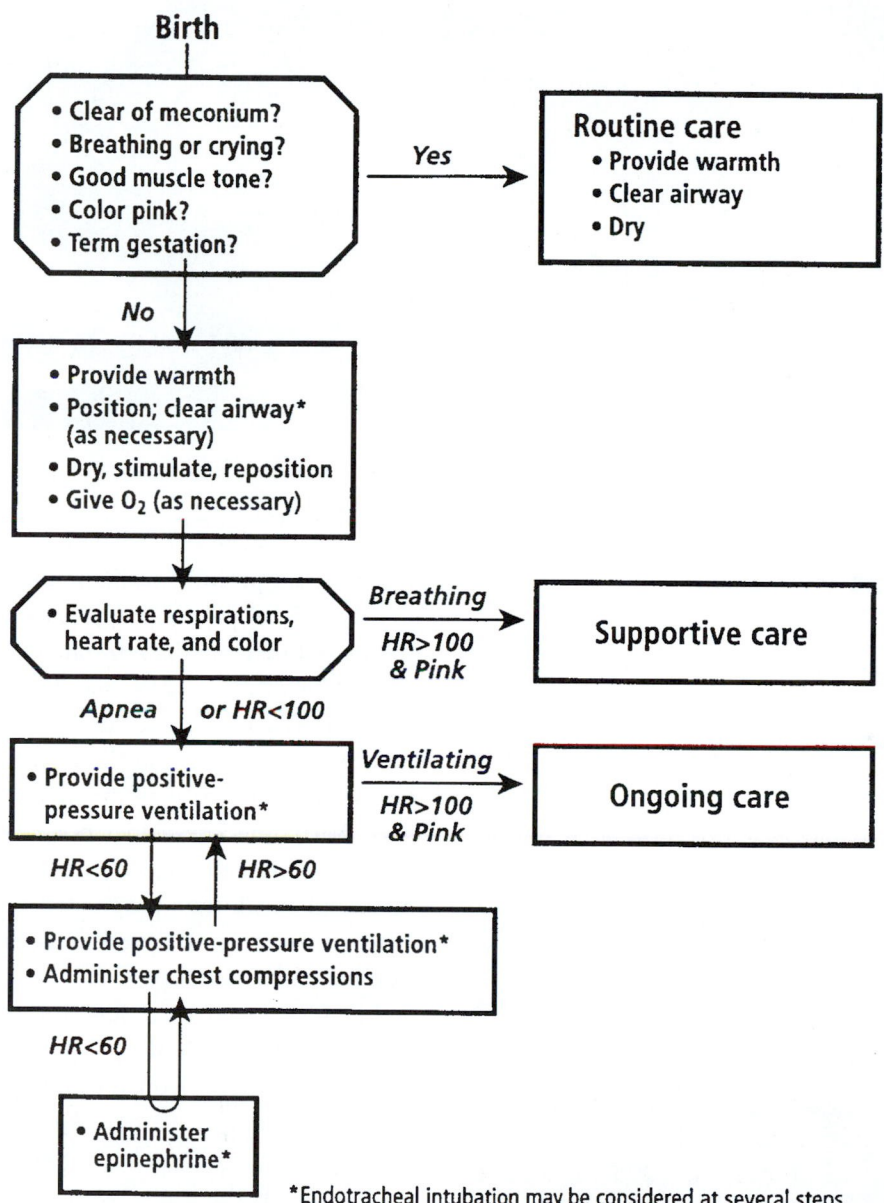

Birth

- Clear of meconium?
- Breathing or crying?
- Good muscle tone?
- Color pink?
- Term gestation?

Yes →

Routine care
- Provide warmth
- Clear airway
- Dry

No

- Provide warmth
- Position; clear airway*
  (as necessary)
- Dry, stimulate, reposition
- Give O₂ (as necessary)

- Evaluate respirations,
  heart rate, and color

Breathing
HR>100
& Pink →

Supportive care

Apnea | *or HR<100*

- Provide positive-
  pressure ventilation*

Ventilating
HR>100
& Pink →

Ongoing care

HR<60 | *HR>60*

- Provide positive-pressure ventilation*
- Administer chest compressions

HR<60

- Administer
  epinephrine*

*Endotracheal intubation may be considered at several steps.

Figure 21-1 Overview of neonatal resuscitation. *Used with permission of the American Academy of Pediatrics, Textbook of neonatal resuscitation, 1994 edition.*

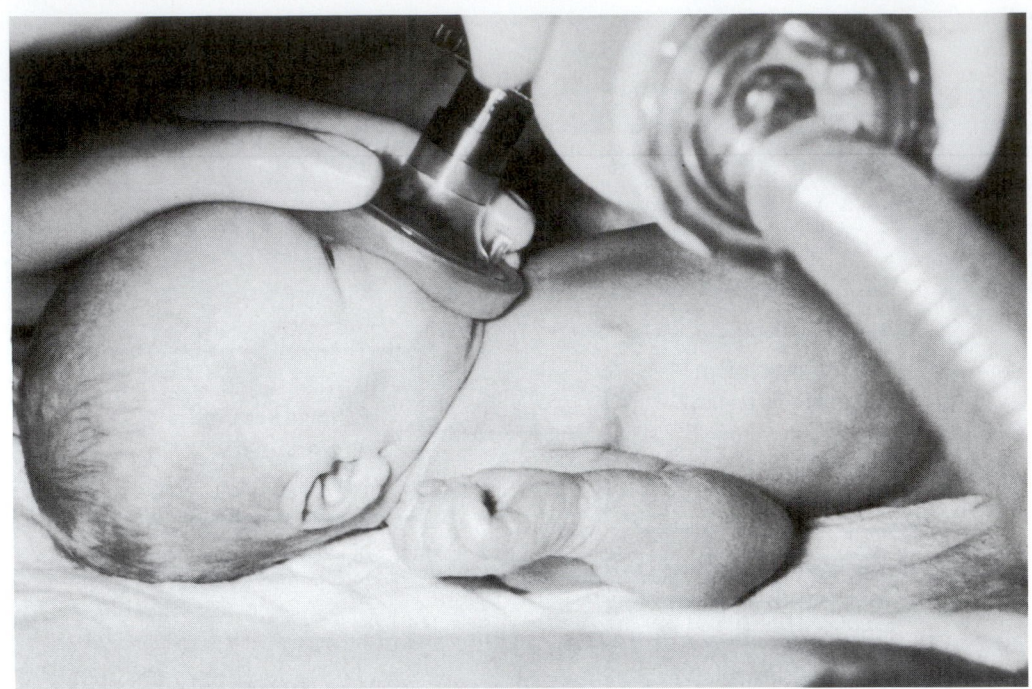

Figure 21-2 Improper PPV. Placement of the mask on the neonate's face has forced the neck into a flexed position, resulting in airway obstruction.

Positive Pressure Ventilation

Because of stress and anxiety that arises in practitioners during resuscitations, neonates are often ventilated at rates greater than the recommended 40 to 60 breaths per minute. While providing PPV by bag and mask, the neck should be kept in a slightly extended position, because there is a tendency to force the neck

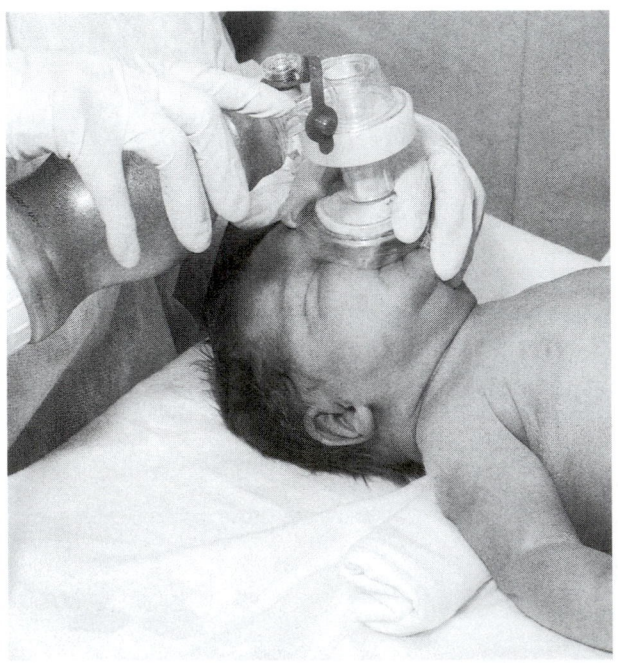

into a flexed position while holding the mask against the face. Examples of improperly and properly administered PPV are demonstrated in Figures 21-2 and 21-3. The obstetric provider should have an unobstructed view of the neonate's chest to observe it rise with each ventilation, so the resuscitation bag should be kept perpendicular to the neonate's chest, not parallel. When the chest does not rise while providing PPV, the following steps should be taken: reapply the mask and check for a proper seal, reposition the head while making sure the neck is slightly extended, suction secretions, ventilate with the mouth slightly open, and increase positive pressure. Too often during resuscitations not enough positive pressure is used to move a neonate's chest. Neonates often require more than the recommended 40 cm H_2O pressure for initial breaths after birth in order to remove lung liquid and establish a gas-fluid interface at the alveolus. When a neonate's condition worsens despite adequate PPV with bag and mask, intubation and bag-tube ventilation are required.

Figure 21-3 Proper PPV. Holding the mask on the face with the thumb and index finger in the form of the letter "C" and supporting the mandible in a slightly extended position with the third, fourth, and fifth fingers promotes airway patency. A blanket under the shoulders also facilitates airway patency.

Endotracheal Intubation

The key to intubation is visualization of the pharyngeal area landmarks, specifically the epiglottis, glottis, and false vocal cords. Because the vocal cords and glottis are located more anteriorly in preterm compared to term neonates, endotracheal intubation may be facilitated in preterm neonates by applying external cricoid pressure. While inserting the endotracheal tube, be sure that the view through the laryngoscope blade remains unobstructed. Some endotracheal tubes have a vocal cord guide, a black line near the distal end, that when placed at the level of the vocal cords places the tip of the endotracheal tube in a proper position between the vocal cords and carina. Once an endotracheal tube has been inserted, it should be held against the hard palate until taped securely to the upper lip. In extremely low-birth-weight neonates with noncompliant lungs, it is often difficult to initially confirm proper endotracheal tube placement by the normal routines of visualizing chest wall rise and absence of gastric distention with each ventilation and auscultating symmetric breath sounds over the chest. In this situation the obstetric provider must rely on visualizing the endotracheal tube in the trachea. During intubations, hypoxia can be minimized by providing free-flow 100% oxygen, limiting attempts to 20 seconds, and providing PPV before and between attempts. Table 21-1 lists proper laryngoscope blade sizes, endotracheal tube sizes, and depth of insertion of endotracheal tubes for neonates of different birth weights.

Heart Rate

During neonatal resuscitations, health-care providers often rush to evaluate the heart rate prior to evaluating respirations. This is a mistake that should be avoided, because the establishment of adequate respirations often results in resolution of bradycardia. For heart rate determination, the NRP recommends using a 6-second method where one listens to the heart beat or palpates the umbilical or brachial pulse for 6 seconds and multiplies this number by 10 for an approximation of the true 1-minute heart rate. In a recent study, we found that over 50% of health-care providers use a method other than the NRP's 6-second method for determining heart rates.[8] In this same study we demonstrated that the NRP's 6-second method for determining heart rates is difficult, often results in inaccuracies, and that a simple electronic timing device preset to 6 seconds improves accuracy of heart rate determination compared to when health-care providers use their own method or the NRP's 6-second method.[8]

Chest Compressions

Chest compressions should always be accompanied by PPV. Chest compressions should be performed over the lower third of the sternum, just below an imaginary line drawn between the nipples. While making sure the fingers remain in constant contact with the sternum, the sternum should be depressed $1/2$ to $3/4$ inch. Over a 2-second time interval, three chest compressions should be followed by one ventilation. This is easiest if the leader of the resuscitation coordinates chest compressions and ventilations by calling out "one, and two, and three, and breathe." Chest compressions should be discontinued whenever the heart rate is greater than 60 beats per minute.

Color

Acrocyanosis, which can be recognized by cyanosis of a neonate's hands and feet, is common after birth and does not require any intervention. A neonate with central cyanosis should receive free-flow 100%

	TABLE 21-1 APPROPRIATE LARYNGOSCOPE BLADE SIZES, ENDOTRACHEAL TUBE SIZES, AND DEPTH OF INSERTION OF ENDOTRACHEAL TUBES FOR NEONATES ACCORDING TO BIRTH WEIGHT		
Weight (kg)	Laryngoscope blade size	Endotracheal tube size	Depth of insertion (cm at upper lip)
<1.0	00-0	2.5	7
1.0–2.0	0	3.0	8
2.0–3.0	1	3.5	9
3.0–4.0	1	3.5–4.0	10

oxygen. If a neonate continues to have central cyanosis despite free-flow 100% oxygen, a trial of PPV should be given. When no longer needed during a resuscitation, free-flow 100% oxygen should be slowly discontinued.

MEDICATIONS

Medications are required infrequently during neonatal resuscitations. Nevertheless, because of the critical situations in which they are needed, health-care providers should be familiar with the most commonly used medications. Table 21-2 lists the most commonly used medications, their indications, proper dosages, and route, rate, and frequency of administration. Dosages for the various medications are based on birth weight, which is often not known in neonates requiring immediate resuscitation in the delivery room. Recent estimated fetal weights can be used, if available, or the obstetric provider may estimate the birth weight. Since gestational age is often known at the time of birth, one helpful method for estimating birth weights in neonates that are appropriate for gestational age is knowing that the 50th percentile birth weights for gestational ages of 27, 34, and 38 weeks are 1.0, 2.0, and 3.0 kg, respectively. In this section we will discuss key aspects regarding the medications used during neonatal resuscitations.

Epinephrine

Epinephrine enhances cerebral and myocardial blood flow by causing peripheral vasoconstriction. Epineph-rine is most frequently administered endotracheally, because intubation is often quicker and easier than obtaining vascular access. When administered endotracheally, epinephrine is more slowly absorbed, and thus 10-fold higher doses may be required to achieve the same effect as the intravenous dose.[9,10] The initial dose of endotracheal epinephrine should be 0.1 to 0.3 mg/kg. However, if a neonate does not respond to this dose, a 10-fold higher dose should be administered. To facilitate delivery of epinephrine endotracheally, the dose should be diluted with normal saline to a final volume of several milliliters.

Volume Expanders

Volume expanders increase tissue perfusion by increasing vascular volume. Normal saline, Ringer's lactate, whole blood, and 5% albumin are four types of volume expanders that are used in neonates. Because delays occur from the time volume expanders are requested during a resuscitation until the time that they are available, one should have volume expanders prepared prior to delivery if the maternal history suggests that a neonate may be volume depleted. Vaginal bleeding, bloody amniotic fluid, and a prolapsed umbilical cord are conditions that may be associated with neonatal hypovolemia.

Sodium Bicarbonate

Systemic acidosis compromises myocardial contractility, causes peripheral vasodilation resulting in hypotension, and decreases responsiveness to oxygen and

---

TABLE 21-2
MOST COMMONLY USED MEDICATIONS, THEIR INDICATIONS, PROPER DOSAGES, AND ROUTE, RATE AND FREQUENCY OF ADMINISTRATION

Medication	Indications	Dosage	Route	Rate	Frequency
Epinephrine (1:10,000)	1. HR < 80 despite 30 sec of adequate PPV and CC 2. HR = 0	0.1–0.3 ml/kg	ET IV	rapid	3–5 min
Volume expanders	Evidence or suspicion of acute blood loss with signs of hypovolemia	10 ml/kg	IV	5–10 min	Until signs of hypovolemia resolve
Sodium bicarbonate	Prolonged arrest that does not respond to other therapy	2 meq/kg	IV	Over at least 2 min	Avoid repeat doses if possible
Naloxone hydrochloride	Respiratory depression and a history of maternal narcotic administration within the past 4 hours	0.1 mg/kg	ET, IV preferred IM, SQ acceptable	Rapid	Dose may need to be repeated after 1–4 h

epinephrine.[11] In the presence of adequate ventilation, sodium bicarbonate corrects metabolic acidosis by raising the pH of blood as well as by providing some volume expansion resulting from the hypertonic solution of sodium. Effective ventilation must precede and accompany sodium bicarbonate administration. Although sodium bicarbonate administration increases arterial pH, it also transiently lowers intracellular pH.[12] When sodium bicarbonate is given, carbon dioxide is rapidly formed intravascularly and easily crosses cell membranes, thus lowering intracellular pH. With effective ventilation this effect may be minimized. Sodium bicarbonate should only be used during prolonged resuscitations where metabolic acidosis is likely to be present. Potential complications of sodium bicarbonate administration include hypernatremia and intraventricular hemorrhage, especially in preterm neonates. These complications may be avoided with proper dosage and rate of administration.

Naloxone Hydrochloride (Narcan)

Naloxone hydrochloride is a narcotic antagonist that reverses narcotic-induced respiratory depression. The intravenous and endotracheal routes of administration are preferred because of concerns with poor absorption when the drug is given via the intramuscular and subcutaneous routes. Neonates that receive naloxone hydrochloride in the delivery room subsequently should be monitored closely. Since the duration of action of narcotics often exceeds that of the antagonist, a second dose of naloxone hydrochloride occasionally may be needed. The average half-life of naloxone hydrochloride in preterm neonates is 70 minutes.[13] This drug should not be used in neonates born to narcotic-dependent mothers because it may precipitate an acute, life-threatening abstinence syndrome.

SPECIAL CIRCUMSTANCES

Meconium-Stained Amniotic Fluid

Passage of meconium in utero occurs in up to 10 to 15% of all pregnancies.[14,15] When meconium is present in the amniotic fluid, it may be aspirated into the lungs and cause atelectasis, airway obstruction, chemical pneumonitis, and meconium-aspiration syndrome. Because the presence of meconium in amniotic fluid is not always known before deliveries, the clinician should always be prepared to deal with this special circumstance. Meconium in the amniotic fluid is often described as "thin and watery" or "thick and particulate." Because of the more frequent use of amnioinfusions in the setting of meconium-stained fluid, amniotic fluid that was initially thick and particulate may later be thin and watery.

The most important step in managing neonates with meconium-stained amniotic fluid is performed by the obstetrician, who, following delivery of the head and prior to delivery of the shoulders, should suction the mouth, pharynx, and nose. Subsequent management of the neonate is controversial. The NRP recommends that for depressed neonates with thin or thick meconium the following steps be taken immediately after delivery: avoid stimulation, place under the radiant warmer, remove residual meconium from the hypopharynx by suctioning under direct vision, intubate, and suction meconium from the trachea with a meconium aspirator connected directly to the endotracheal tube. Reintubation and suctioning may be repeated as necessary and tolerated until no further meconium is suctioned from below the vocal cords. No attempts should be made to suction meconium from the trachea by passing a suction catheter through an endotracheal tube; suction catheters are too small to adequately remove meconium.

The major controversy is whether vigorous neonates with thick meconium require intubation. In a vigorous, crying neonate the risks of intubation may outweigh the risks of meconium in the airway. Studies have suggested that intrapartum pharyngeal suctioning prior to the first breath obviates the need for tracheal suctioning and that routine tracheal suctioning of vigorous neonates confers no benefit.[16-18] Once a neonate with meconium-stained fluid has been resuscitated and is stable, the stomach should be suctioned to prevent aspiration of meconium-containing gastric contents.

Congenital Diaphragmatic Hernia

Congenital diaphragmatic hernia (CDH) is characterized by the presence of abdominal organs in the thoracic cavity. Pulmonary development is often affected, resulting in pulmonary hypoplasia. Neonates with CDH should be intubated and given bag-tube ventilation. PPV with bag and mask should be avoided because air may enter the bowel and compromise lung expansion. Currently, over 50% of neonates with CDH are recognized prenatally so special care should be taken with these neonates. Unfortunately, in a sizeable minority of patients, the diagnosis is not known at the time of delivery. CDH should be suspected in any neonate with worsening respiratory distress and cyanosis despite adequate PPV with bag and mask, absent or diminished breath sounds or bowel sounds over one side of the chest, a scaphoid abdomen, an asymmetric chest, or auscultation of heart sounds over the right side of the chest. During the resuscitation, an orogastric tube should be placed to low intermittent suction, as soon as possible, to keep the stomach and bowel decompressed.

Abdominal Wall Defects

Neonates with abdominal wall defects, such as gastroschisis and omphalocele, who require assisted ventilation, should be intubated and provided bag-tube ventilation in order to prevent air from entering and distending the bowel. Surgical repair, which is performed as soon as possible after birth, is simplified when the bowel is not distended. Frequently meconium-stained amniotic fluid is present at the time of delivery. The amniotic fluid in these circumstances is most often discolored due to bile rather than meconium. Resuscitation of these neonates should also include careful handling of the bowel. A pediatric surgeon should be present at the delivery to assess the bowel and to ensure that the vascular supply to the bowel is not compromised. These neonates should be placed in a sterile isolation or "bowel" bag to decrease insensible water losses. If a "bowel" bag is not available, the bowel may be carefully covered with sterile, saline-soaked gauze. Neonates with gastroschisis should be positioned on their right side with the bowel slightly elevated on a blanket to help assure that the vascular supply to the bowel does not become compromised.

Facial Anomalies

Neonates with facial anomalies may present with respiratory distress in the delivery room and may be very difficult to ventilate with routine techniques. Neonates with Pierre-Robin sequence have a small jaw, which forces their tongues back against the posterior pharynx and obstructs their airways. Respiratory distress in a neonate with Pierre-Robin sequence

may improve and resolve by placing the neonate in a prone position that displaces the tongue anteriorly. Neonates that do not respond to prone positioning should have an oral airway inserted, which displaces the tongue anteriorly and relieves airway obstruction. If needed, bag and mask ventilation may be performed with the oral airway in place.

Choanal atresia is a congenital obstruction of the posterior nares caused by the persistence of a bony septum or a soft tissue membrane. Because neonates are obligate nasal breathers, those with choanal atresia present with severe respiratory distress and cyanosis in the delivery room that worsens when their mouth is closed and improves when they cry. The diagnosis is made by the inability to pass a suction catheter through the nose into the nasopharynx. The smallest available catheter should be inserted in a posterior and inferior direction into each nostril. Neonates with choanal atresia require an oral airway or intubation.

Hydrops Fetalis

Hydrops fetalis is a condition of excess fluid accumulation in a fetus that can manifest as anasarca, pleural effusions, ascites, and pericardial effusion. Because these fetuses suffer significant hypoxia in utero and are at increased risk for intrapartum asphyxia, they may be very difficult to resuscitate. These neonates frequently require assisted ventilation. During the resuscitation of a neonate with hydrops fetalis, the clinician should be prepared to perform thoracentesis, and possibly even paracentesis, if assisted ventilation is compromised, as well as pericardiocentesis if the cardiovascular system is compromised. Fluid aspirations are best accomplished by placing a 16-gauge angiocatheter into the body cavity and, after removing the needle, aspirating the catheter with a syringe.

Myelomeningocele

Neonates with myelomeningocele typically present at birth with a sac-covered mass of neural tissue over the lower spine. During resuscitation of these neonates, care should be taken not to disrupt the sac because it will lead to exposure of the underlying neural tissue and leakage of cerebrospinal fluid. These neonates should be resuscitated on their sides, and, following resuscitation, be kept in the prone position. The defect should be carefully covered in sterile, saline-soaked gauze. Because these neonates commonly have, or soon develop, a latex allergy, such products should be avoided.

SECONDARY ASSESSMENT

Immediately following resuscitation in the delivery room, each neonate should be reassessed to determine whether the neonate is able to go to the "well baby" nursery or requires more intensive observation. Aspects of the physical examination that can be used to identify neonates who require closer observation include abnormalities in activity, tone, respirations, color, and heart rate, as well as congenital anomalies and prematurity. Tachypnea, grunting, flaring, and retractions are signs that a neonate is in respiratory distress. Neonates commonly exhibit mild grunting and flaring after birth that usually resolve within 30 minutes. This mild grunting or flaring is often due to hypothermia and frequently resolves with drying and warming of the neonate. Underlying pathology usually causes a neonate's respiratory distress to worsen over the first few minutes of life. Tachycardia is an abnormal finding in neonates after birth and is most commonly due to hypovolemia or maternal fever.

During the secondary assessment one should identify potential problems that a neonate may be at risk for during the early neonatal period.

Risk for Sepsis

Risk factors for sepsis include prematurity, maternal fever or chorioamnionitis, maternal group B streptococcal colonization, a history of group B streptococcal infection in a previous sibling, prolonged rupture of membranes ($\geq$18 hours), and rupture of membranes at less than 37 weeks gestation and before the onset of labor. A neonate at risk for sepsis should receive an immediate evaluation and antibiotics, if indicated.

Hypothermia

Preterm neonates and neonates with intrauterine growth restriction (IUGR) are at risk for hypothermia and often require placement in an incubator or under a radiant warmer to maintain their temperature within the normal range.

Hypoglycemia

Preterm neonates, neonates with IUGR, large-for-gestational-age (LGA) neonates, and infants of diabetic mothers are at risk for hypoglycemia. Glucose levels in these neonates should be monitored closely, and feedings encouraged as soon as possible. These neonates may require intravenous glucose to maintain normoglycemia.

Feeding Difficulties

Neonates with conditions such as prematurity, neurologic abnormalities, tachypnea, cleft palate, and other facial anomalies may have difficulty feeding after birth. Preterm neonates do not develop a coordinated suck-and-swallow mechanism until approximately 34 weeks corrected gestational age, and until then may require orogastric feedings or parenteral nutrition. Neurologic disorders may affect a neonate's ability to suck and swallow, as well as to protect his or her airway. Tachypneic neonates should not be fed orally because of the risk of aspiration. Most neonates with a cleft palate tolerate oral feedings, but some have difficulties and may need a special nipple or feeding device such as a Haberman feeder.

Neonates at risk for any of the above-mentioned problems should not be allowed to stay in the delivery room for a prolonged period of time after birth and should be observed closely during the transition period.

REFERENCES

1. McDonald HM, Mulligan JC, Allen AC, et al. Neonatal asphyxia: Part I. Relationship of obstetrical and neonatal complications to neonatal mortality in 38,405 consecutive deliveries. J Pediatr 1980;96:898.
2. Adamson TM, Brodecky V, Lambert TF, et al. Lung liquid production and composition in the "in utero" foetal lamb. Aust J Exp Biol Med Sci 1975;53:65.
3. Humphreys PW, Normand ICS, Reynolds EOR, et al. Pulmonary lymph flow and the uptake of liquid from the lungs of the lamb at the start of breathing. J Physiol 1967;193:1.
4. Normand ICS, Reynolds EOR, Strang LB. Passage of macromolecules between alveolar and interstitial spaces in foetal and newly ventilated lungs of the lamb. J Physiol 1970;210:151.
5. Normand ICS, Oliver RE, Reynolds EOR, et al. Permeability of lung capillaries and alveoli to non-electrolytes in the foetal lamb. J Physiol 1971;219:303.
6. Bland RD, Hansen TN, Haberkern CM, et al. Lung fluid balance in lambs before and after birth. J Appl Physiol 1982;53:992.
7. Burchfield DJ. Medication use in neonatal resuscitation: epinephrine and sodium bicarbonate. Neonatal Pharmacol Quarter 1993;2:25.

8. Theophilopoulos DT, Burchfield DJ. Accuracy of different methods for heart rate determination during simulated neonatal resuscitations. J Perinatol 1998;18:65.

9. Burchfield DJ, Berkowitz ID, Berg RA, Goldberg RN. Medications in neonatal resuscitation. Ann Emerg Med 1993;22:435.

10. Emergency Cardiac Care Committee and Subcommittees, American Heart Association. Guidelines for cardiopulmonary resuscitation and emergency cardiac care, I: introduction. JAMA 1992;268:2172.

11. Preziosi MP, Roig JC, Hargrove N, Burchfield DJ. Metabolic acidemia with hypoxia attenuates the hemodynamic responses to epinephrine during resuscitation in lambs. Crit Care Med 1993;21:1901.

12. Graf H, Leach W, Arieff AI. Evidence for a detrimental effect of bicarbonate therapy in hypoxic lactic acidosis. Science 1985;227:754.

13. Stile LI, Fort M, Wurburger RJ, et al. The pharmacokinetics of naloxone in the premature newborn. Dev Pharmacol Ther 1987;10:454.

14. Gregory GA, Gooding CA, Phibbs RH, et al. Meconium aspiration in infants: a prospective study. J Pediatr 1974; 85:848.

15. Carson BS, Losey RW, Bowes WA, et al. Combined obstetric and pediatric approach to prevent meconium aspiration syndrome. Am J Obstet Gynecol 1976;126:712.

16. Dillard RG. Neonatal tracheal aspiration of meconium-stained infants. J Pediatr 1977;90:163.

17. Linder N, Aranda JV, Tsur M, et al. Need for endotracheal intubation and suction in meconium-stained neonates. J Pediatr 1988;112:613.

18. Cunningham AS. When to suction the meconium-stained newborn? Contemp Pediatr 1993;10:91.

Chapter 22
The Puerperium

Amy Boardman

Five Key Points

- In nonlactating women, the mean time to resumption of ovulation is 45 days. In lactating women, the mean interval varies from 3 to 6 months.

- The most common cause of delayed postpartum hemorrhage is subinvolution of the placental site.

- The principal medical benefit of breast-feeding is enhanced protection of the infant against respiratory and gastrointestinal infections.

- Puerperal mastitis is usually caused by staphylococcal and streptococcal bacteria. The condition can usually be treated with a short course of oral antibiotics. Women with breast abscesses should be hospitalized for intravenous antibiotics and surgical drainage.

- Postpartum mood disorders include postpartum blues, postpartum depression, and postpartum psychosis. The former condition can usually be treated by supportive therapy. The latter two conditions require more intensive medical treatment and psychological counseling.

The puerperium is defined as the interval immediately following delivery of the placenta until 6 weeks postpartum. During this period numerous changes occur that eventually lead to involution of the reproductive organs and resumption of normal menses in nonlactating women. This chapter will focus on normal and abnormal postpartum involution, management of the normal puerperium, lactation and complications of breast-feeding, contraception, and postpartum psychological reactions. For diagnosis and management of puerperal infections, the reader is referred to Chapter 5.

POSTPARTUM INVOLUTION

Uterus

The process of involution begins immediately after delivery of the placenta with intense myometrial contractions, which eventually restore the puerperal uterus to its normal proportions. These contractions initially control bleeding, and, by 24 hours postpartum, reduce the term, gravid uterus to a hard, globular mass of approximately the size of a 20-week uterus. At 1 week postpartum the uterine volume decreases by 50%. By 2 weeks after delivery, the uterus is no longer palpable on abdominal examination. Finally, the uterus resumes its nonpregnant weight of approximately 50 to 100 g by postpartum week 6.[1]

Immediately after delivery, the dramatic decrease in endometrial surface area leads to shearing off of the placenta at the decidual basalis. Within a few hours postpartum, an acute inflammatory cell infiltrate appears at the placental site and acts as an antibacterial barrier to early ascending infection.[2] After 10 days, a chronic plasma-cell and lymphocytic response replaces the acute inflammation and may persist for several months as the only evidence of a recent pregnancy. Further involution of the placental site occurs at 72 hours postpartum, as two distinct layers become apparent: first, a superficial layer eventually sloughed off as lochia; and second, an underlying layer of residual endometrial glands from which new endometrium regenerates. Restoration of the endometrium in areas other than the placental site occurs by postpartum day 16. Decidual necrosis begins within 24 hours of delivery, and any evidence of decidual reaction is usually gone by postpartum week 6.

Complete regeneration of the placental site takes longer than the remainder of the endometrium. Initial hemostasis is achieved primarily by compression of the blood vessels through contraction of uterine muscle, and to a lesser degree, by arterial smooth muscle. Blood vessels at the placental site undergo several changes during postpartum days 1 through 8: the veins develop thrombosis, hyalinization, and endophlebitis, while the arteries hyalinize, with evidence of obliterative fibrinoid endarteritis.[3] These vascular changes remain as the stigmata of the former placental site.

Lochia is defined as the normal postpartum uterine bleeding and conventionally has been subdivided into lochia rubra, serosa, and alba, based upon the evolving characteristics of the discharge. Lasting for several hours, the initial lochia rubra is the flow of bright red blood immediately after placental separation. Lochia rubra eventually changes into a reddish-brown color while it diminishes in flow over the next 3 to 4 days. When the discharge becomes more mucopurulent and somewhat malodorous in nature, it is then called lochia serosa. As the discharge tapers off, it becomes more yellow-white in color and lighter in flow. This discharge is called lochia alba.

The duration and character of lochia has not been well studied. Oppenhiemer et. al.[4] found a median duration of lochia of 4 weeks, although 13% of women

in this study experienced some lochial flow at 60 days postpartum. Primiparous women and those who delivered larger infants demonstrated a longer duration of lochia, which is due to slower regeneration of endometrium at the placental site. In another study of breast-feeding women, Visness and colleagues[5] found the median duration of lochia to be 27 days. Lochia was further characterized by intermittent spotting and bleeding. Neither breast-feeding nor oral contraceptive use appears to affect the duration of lochia.

Cervix

During pregnancy, the cervical epithelium increases in thickness and vascularity. The glands undergo hyperplasia and hypertrophy, consistent with the Arias–Stella reaction, while the stroma undergoes decidual change. After delivery of the placenta the cervix is essentially atonic, but within 2 to 3 days, the cervix appears normal, although still dilated 2 to 3 cm.[6] Colposcopic findings seen during the initial postpartum period include ulceration, laceration, and ecchymosis with regression of these changes and resolution of edema by postpartum day 4.[7]

Ovarian Function

Following delivery, the resumption of ovulation and normal menses depends on prior ovarian function and lactation status. In nonlactating women, after delivery of the placenta, serum estrogen and progesterone levels rapidly decline, allowing the gradual increase in secretion of the gonadotropins, follicle-stimulating hormone (FSH) and luteinizing hormone (LH), between 3 and 5 weeks postpartum. Prolactin falls to normal levels by the first postpartum week, thus permitting return of ovulation and fertility.[8] The mean time until ovulation is 45 days, with no evidence of ovulation prior to 25 days.[9] Normal menstruation usually resumes by 12 weeks postpartum in 70% of nonlactating women, with the first menstruation at 7 to 9 weeks.[10] These studies emphasize the need for initiation of contraception prior to the traditional 6-week postpartum evaluation.

Lactation induces anovulation and amenorrhea through the repeated nipple stimulation associated with breast-feeding.[11] FSH levels return to normal within 30 days after delivery, while LH levels remain suppressed at low-normal values. Thus, the release of LH from the pituitary is inhibited, while FSH

production is unaffected during breast-feeding. However, because of the inadequate LH signal, the follicles produce lower levels of estradiol. Although follicular growth and estradiol secretion eventually normalize, the follicles remain unruptured or atrophy due to the absence of a normal preovulatory LH surge.

Several studies have assessed the return of ovulation in breast-feeding women. In Scottish[12] and Mexican[13] studies of exclusively breast-feeding women (i.e., no supplemental feedings), ovulation did not occur in the first 3 months postpartum, while less than 20% of Australian women had ovulated by the 6th postpartum month of exclusive breast-feeding.[14] In a study of American women,[9] the average time to first ovulation was 27.2 weeks (range, 5 to 37 weeks) or approximately 6 months. Yet another study of exclusively breast-feeding women found that ovulation always occurred later than 8 weeks postpartum, with a range from 32 to 37 weeks, varying by the time interval from delivery to first postlochial bleeding.[15]

In conclusion, ovulation should not occur before 8 weeks postpartum and usually resumes between 3 and 6 months postpartum in women who breast-feed exclusively. However, the duration of anovulation depends on the frequency of breast-feeding, the duration of feeding episodes, and the proportion of supplemental feeds.[16] On average, ovarian suppression requires at least five feeds totaling at least 65 minutes of suckling a day.[17] Overall, the risk of ovulation within the first 6 months postpartum in exclusively breast-feeding women is approximately 2%.[18]

Thyroid Function

During pregnancy, thyroid volume increases by approximately 30%, with a compensatory rise in thyroxine (T_4) and triiodothyronine (T_3) levels and concomitant decreased triiodothyronine resin uptake (T^3RU). Thyroid volume reverts to normal gradually over a 12-week period. T_4 and T_3 levels and T^3RU normalize within 4 weeks postpartum.[19] During the puerperium, women are at increased risk for autoimmune thyroiditis followed by hypothyroidism.[20]

Cardiovascular System and Coagulation

The normal physiologic changes of pregnancy include a 35% increase in blood volume by the third trimester with an initial rise in plasma volume occurring during the first trimester. An additional 1200 ml of plasma accounts for the 50% increase in plasma volume seen by the third trimester.[21] Despite increases in red-cell mass, the overall increase in total blood volume causes a relative dilutional, or physiologic, anemia of pregnancy. Other changes in cardiovascular parameters consist of elevations of heart rate, stroke volume, and cardiac output. Most of the major circulatory alterations during pregnancy return to base-line, nonpregnant levels in the early postpartum period, usually by 6 to 8 weeks. However, the rate of return is variable and not well known.

For a singleton gestation the estimated blood loss for a spontaneous vaginal delivery, cesarean delivery, and cesarean delivery plus hysterectomy is 500 ml, 1000 ml, and 1500 ml, respectively.[22] This blood loss results in a 1000-ml decline in plasma volume immediately after delivery, but within 24 hours plasma volume increases by 900 to 1200 ml as extracellular fluid shifts intravascularly.[23] By postpartum day 3, total blood volume decreases by 16% of the antenatal peak value.[24] The rate at which red-cell volume returns to prepregnancy values is unknown, but it usually normalizes by 8 weeks postpartum.[25] For the first 30 to 60 minutes postpartum, heart rate, stroke volume, and cardiac output remain elevated or achieve higher values as compared with their pregnancy values. Cardiac-output values normalize by 8 to 10 weeks postpartum, but the rate at which normal values resume is unknown.[26]

During normal pregnancy, gradual changes in the coagulation and fibrinolytic systems occur in preparation for hemostasis following placental separation. Under the influence of rising circulatory estrogen, the liver increases synthesis of vitamin K–dependent coagulation factors, specifically fibrinogen, and factors VII, VIII, IX, and X. In contrast, levels of prothrombin (factor II) and factors V and XII remain unchanged, while the platelet count, factors XI and XIII levels, and other fibrinolytic factors decline slightly.[27,28] These parameters return to normal values within 3 weeks postpartum.[6] These changes contribute to the so-called hypercoagulable state of pregnancy. Additional features that increase the incidence of venous thromboembolic disease during pregnancy include increased venous stasis, vascular injury at the time of placental separation, cesarean delivery, and infection.[29] Because the hypercoagulable state persists for 2 weeks after delivery, hormonal contraception should be avoided during this time.[30]

Urinary Tract and Renal Function

Renal morphologic changes during pregnancy may last for several months and are manifested by dilated renal calices and ureters above the pelvic brim. The right collecting system is affected more than the left side.[31] The dilation is due to compression of the ureters by the adjacent vasculature, specifically, the iliac artery,[32] and to a lesser degree, by the gravid uterus. The enlargement of the collecting system has been confirmed by intravenous urography[33] as well as by ultrasonography.[34]

In contrast, renal function returns to nonpregnant basal levels within 6 to 8 weeks after delivery. Glomerular filtration rate, which increases 50% by early pregnancy, and creatinine clearance normalize by postpartum week 8.[35] Renal plasma flow, which increases 25% in the first trimester and reaches 200 to 250 ml/min by the third trimester, declines rapidly by postpartum day 5.[36]

Weight Loss

Most women will experience an immediate 10- to 13-lb weight loss following delivery of the infant, placenta, amniotic fluid, and normal blood loss.[37] Nearly 30% of women return to their prepregnancy weight by the 6th week postpartum. In a study by Schauberger et al.,[38] weight gain during pregnancy was considered the most critical determinant of weight loss postpartum: the more weight gained antepartum, the more weight lost postpartum. Most women required a longer interval to return to the range of their prepregnancy weight. Other factors that positively correlated with weight loss by the 6th month postpartum include smoking, primiparity, and early return to work outside the home. The mode of delivery, type of contraception used (including oral contraceptives), breast-feeding, and exercise, did not affect weight loss by 6 months postpartum.

Breast-feeding is often considered an important factor in postpartum weight loss because of the increased energy requirement of 750 to 1000 kcal/day for the production of breast milk.[38] However, in studies of well nourished breast-feeding women, the overall effect of breast-feeding on postpartum weight loss is negligible. Thus, the clinician should promote breastfeeding for its health benefits and not as a method for well-nourished women to compensate for excessive pregnancy weight gain or to increase postpartum weight loss.[39]

MANAGEMENT OF THE PUERPERIUM

According to the American Academy of Pediatrics (AAP) and the American College of Obstetricians and Gynecologists (ACOG),[40] the purpose of postpartum hospitalization is to identify both maternal and neonatal complications as well as to provide professional assistance when mothers are most likely to need support. Continuity of care is initiated during the intrapartum period, while the patient is in labor and delivery, and should be extended into the postpartum period through a multidisciplinary and collaborative approach. Comprehensive care begins immediately in the birthing room, LDR (labor-delivery-recovery), or designated recovery room. Following delivery, any of these areas should allow bonding of the family unit, observation for maternal complications, stabilization of the neonate within the first 6 hours, and initiation of breast-feeding, if desired.

Immediate Postpartum Care

If mothers have been given regional or general anesthesia, they are observed in LDRs or a postanesthesia care unit (PACU) following vaginal or cesarean delivery. During this time, close monitoring and recording of the patient's vital signs and clinical status is performed until the patient is discharged to the postpartum ward at the discretion of the physician, certified nurse midwife, or anesthesiologist. Postpartum sterilization can be performed immediately if the delivery was uncomplicated; anesthesia is continued (e.g., functional epidural in place); and necessary staffing is available.[40] Subsequent postpartum care is directed at teaching the mother how to care for herself and her baby.

Perineal Care

Many women have an episiotomy or vaginal or perineal laceration as a part of their delivery. Routine care for a midline first- or second-degree episiotomy or laceration involves cleansing the vulva from an anterior to perineal direction, application of ice packs to the perineum for 24 hours, and administration of oral analgesics, such as nonsteroidal antiinflammatory medication. Warm or cold sitz baths, as described by Droegmueller,[41] may also reduce perineal pain and discomfort.

Patients with a third- or fourth-degree laceration may experience significant perineal pain, edema, and ecchymoses. Narcotic analgesics may be required for additional pain relief. If marked periurethral edema or pain associated with voiding develops, intermittent catheterization or even placement of an indwelling catheter may be needed for the first 24 hours. Stool softeners should be administered in order to avoid straining and discomfort. Any patient with excessive perineal pain following delivery that is not relieved with analgesics should be examined to rule out the presence of an expanding vaginal or vulvar hematoma or early perineal cellulitis.

Hemorrhoids often develop in pregnant women; these may become exacerbated during delivery. Supportive treatment includes use of corticosteroid-containing foams or pads, witchhazel compresses, and local anesthetic sprays and compresses. In addition, stool softeners are helpful to avoid straining. A symptomatic, prolapsed, thrombosed hemorrhoid requires excision under local anesthesia. Such intervention usually provides prompt pain relief.

Bladder Care

Women should attempt to void as soon as possible after delivery. Voiding difficulties are common and arise from obstetrical trauma, regional anesthesia, vulvar and perineal edema and pain, and postdelivery diuresis leading to bladder overdistention.[40] Following a vaginal delivery, the bladder should be palpated frequently for the first 24 hours. If urinary retention develops, then either single catheterization or placement of an indwelling catheter is indicated.

Hospital Discharge

Over the past 30 years the average length of hospitalization for childbirth has decreased dramatically. The average length of stay following vaginal delivery is approximately 2 days shorter than it was 25 years ago.[42] ACOG and the American Academy of Pediatrics have defined early discharge as anything <48 hours postpartum for normal vaginal delivery. This trend arises from two nonmedical groups: first, the natural childbirth movement originating during the 1970s, and second, insurance companies attempting to reduce the expense of obstetric hospitalizations under the pressures of a managed-care environment.[42] Current evidence judging the safety and practicality of early postpartum discharge is equivocal; however, in selected, consenting patients, early discharge appears safe.[43] Nonetheless, current ACOG guidelines for postpartum discharge should be followed for the majority of patients.

Delayed Postpartum Hemorrhage

Early postpartum hemorrhage, described elsewhere, is defined as bleeding that occurs within the first 24 hours after delivery. Late, or delayed, postpartum hemorrhage occurs after the first 24 hours and within the first 6 weeks following delivery. Late postpartum hemorrhage is less common and is usually associated with less blood loss than early hemorrhage. Primary etiologies include subinvolution of the placental site, caused by retained placental tissue from a complete or partial cotyledon or succenturiate lobe, or less commonly, by endometritis.[44] Gestational trophoblastic neoplasia (GTN) also must be considered as part of the differential diagnosis.[45] Retained placental fragments usually undergo necrosis with subsequent fibrin deposition. If this tissue is not resorbed, it may eventually form a so-called placental polyp. If the eschar from that polyp sloughs, heavy, brisk bleeding may arise 1 to 2 weeks postpartum.[46] In a similar manner, the eschar from the normal placental site scar may cause a sudden, transient, brisk episode of uterine bleeding occurring during the same time interval.[47] While this bleeding may be profuse, it is usually self-limited and resolves in 1 to 2 hours.

Most patients with subinvolution present with persistent lochial discharge and irregular or excessive uterine bleeding during the puerperium. Bimanual examination demonstrates an enlarged, boggy, and sometimes tender uterus. Ultrasound evaluation is useful for detecting retained placental tissue.[48] In the absence of significant retained fragments documented on ultrasound, most cases will respond to conservative treatment with uterotonic agents, such as intravenous oxytocin, ergot alkaloids, or prostaglandins and antibiotics.[30] Ergonovine (Ergotrate) or methylergonovine maleate (Methergine) 0.2 mg orally every 3 to 4 hours for 24 to 48 hours may be effective.

Uterine curettage following late postpartum hemorrhage often does not remove identifiable placental tissue and may actually exacerbate bleeding by traumatizing the subinvoluted placental site.[46] Uterine curettage should be reserved for women with persistent heavy bleeding despite conservative measures or evidence of retained fragments on ultrasound. Informed consent for curettage should include the possibility of hysterectomy for control of bleeding.

Episiotomy and Pelvic-Floor Infections

Postpartum soft-tissue infections can be subdivided into a spectrum according to the depth of infection: simple episiotomy infection; superficial fascial infection; superficial fascial necrosis; and myonecrosis. The simple episiotomy wound infection is characterized by infection localized to the skin and superficial fascial edge adjacent to the episiotomy incision. Compared to deeper infections, edema and erythema are confined to the immediate area surrounding the episiotomy site. Bulla formation, skin necrosis, and systemic findings are absent.

Simple episiotomy infections should be opened, explored, and debrided under adequate anesthesia to exclude a hematoma or rectovaginal fistula. If extensive infection of the superficial fascial layer is present, antibiotics should be given that cover streptococci, staphylococci, Enterobacteriaceae, and anaerobic bacteria, including *Bacteroides fragilis*. Traditionally, the site is left open to heal by secondary intention,[49] but a more recent prospective, randomized study compared incision, curettage, and primary closure of episiotomy wound infections to "open" treatment and found no difference in outcome.[50]

A severe superficial fascial infection, or necrotizing fasciitis, typically involves necrosis of the superficial perineal fascial layers with further extension to the thighs, buttocks, and anterior abdominal wall along these fascial planes (Figure 22-1). This infection has an acute onset, a rapid course with prominent systemic manifestations, and a high fatality rate, ranging from 21 to 76%.[51,52] The superior layer of the superficial fascia (Camper fascia) is fibroadipose tissue and forms most of the labia majora. This fascia is recognized as subcutaneous fat on the anterior abdominal wall. The deep layer of the superficial fascia on the perineum (Colles fascia) is membranous and without adipose tissue, and extends onto the anterior abdominal wall as Scarpa fascia. Characteristically, the deep fascia of the urogenital diaphragm and levator ani are spared. Skin findings are variable. Initially, there may be cutaneous edema and erythema, with indistinct margins. Marked blue or brown discoloration occurs

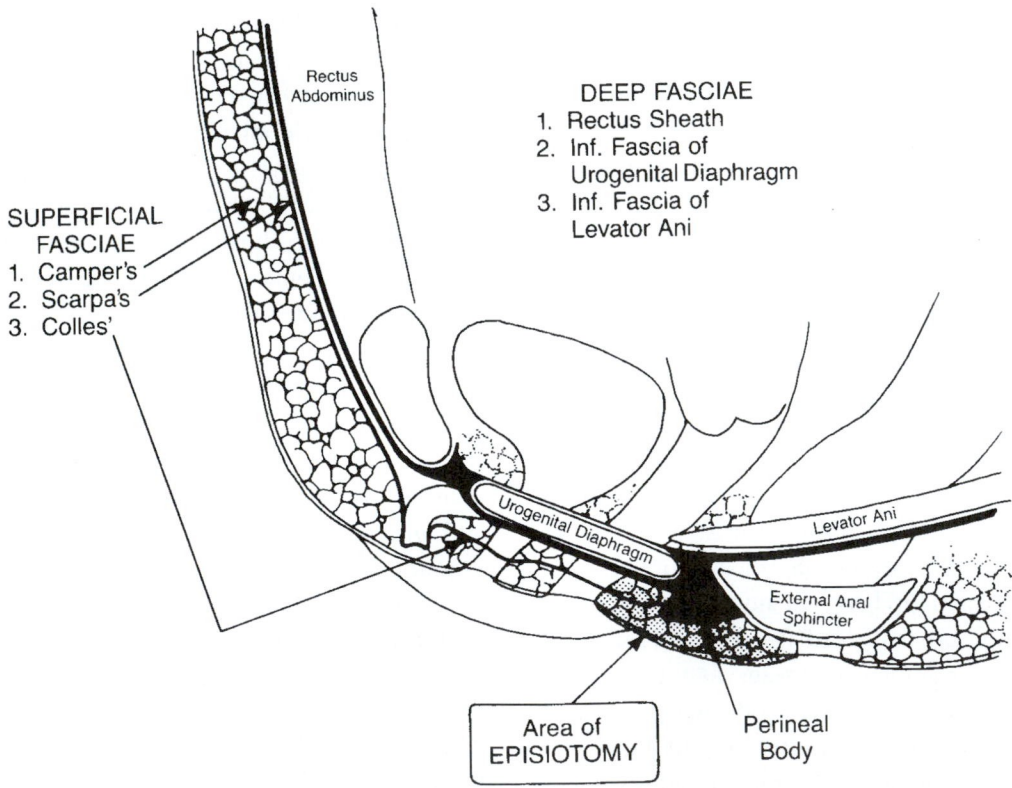

Figure 22-1 Diagrammatic representation of the fascial layers of the perineum (paramedian section), which may be involved by extension from an infected episiotomy. *Adapted from Isada NB, Grossman III JH. Perinatal infections. In: Gabbe SG, Niebyl JR, Simpson JL. eds. Obstetrics: normal and problem pregnancies. 2nd ed. New York: Churchhill Livingstone, 1991:1286.*

as the disease progresses; vesicles and bullae form; and the skin may become gangrenous. As the cutaneous nerves are affected, the lesion may become hypesthetic or even anesthetic. With delay in diagnosis, patients may progress to fulminant septic shock.

Specific pathogenic bacteria include group A, β-hemolytic streptococci and anaerobes. The most reliable method for culture requires a deep-tissue sample sent for immediate anaerobic and aerobic culture. Appropriate therapy requires rapid diagnosis and extensive surgical debridement in conjunction with appropriate antimicrobial therapy. Antibiotics alone are ineffective therapy. Surgical debridement is indicated if skin edema or erythema occurs beyond the immediate borders of the episiotomy, if severe systemic manifestations are present, or if the infection does not resolve after 24 to 48 hours of antibiotic treatment.[49] Surgical exploration that demonstrates separation of the skin from the underlying deep fascia and a bloodless incision of the superficial fascia are strong diagnostic signs of necrotizing fasciitis.

Myonecrosis is infection beneath the deep fascia that also involves the muscles. The most commonly associated microorganism is *Clostridia perfringens*. Clostridial infection may occur early in the postpartum period, and typically, the severity of the pain is disproportionate to the physical findings. Appropriate treatment for both myonecrosis and clostridial infections includes a combination of surgical resection and antibiotic therapy with high-dose penicillin. Hyperbaric oxygen should be considered only an adjunctive therapy, which does not replace adequate surgical debridement.

BREAST PHYSIOLOGY DURING PREGNANCY AND LACTATION

The hollow alveolus, or milk gland, forms the basic component of the breast and is lined by a single layer of milk-secreting epithelial cells. Each alveolus is encased in a interlacing shell of contractile myoepithelial fibers and an extensive outer capillary network. The breast is comprised of 15 to 20 pyramidal lobes of glandular tissue, which consist of multiple alveolar units. Each lobule drains into separate lactiferous ducts that empty into the lactiferous sinuses located under the areola. Fifteen to 20 lactiferous sinuses open onto the mammary papilla, or nipple. The lobes are defined and interconnected by the suspensory ligaments of Cooper, which are connective-tissue septa that attach

the breast to the skin and the deep layer of the superficial fascia.

Growth and development of this milk producing system depends on numerous hormonal factors that occur first during puberty and later during pregnancy. Estrogen is the major hormonal influence during puberty, while the combination of high levels of estrogen and progesterone, as well as prolactin, thyroxine, cortisol, insulin, and growth hormone, allow for the final differentiation of the alveolar epithelial cell into a mature milk-producing cell.[8] At only 3 to 4 weeks postconception, marked breast hyperplasia and hypertrophy occur. With increasing placental hormones, estrogen predominantly affects ductal epithelial growth while progesterone influences lobular or alveolar proliferation. Compared to the nonpregnant state, glandular elements predominate over the intervening stroma.[53]

Prior to pregnancy, serum prolactin levels are normally 10 to 25 ng/ml, and they progressively rise to peak levels at term of 200 to 400 ng/ml.[54] Although prolactin stimulates breast growth, only colostrum is produced until after delivery. The high levels of estrogen and progesterone inhibit full lactation by interfering with prolactin's action at the alveolar-cell prolactin receptor.[55,56] The hormonal trigger for the initiation of milk production is the rapid clearance of progesterone and estrogen from the maternal circulation after delivery that then allows prolactin to function at the receptor level.

Prolactin is the main hormone involved in milk production and is responsible for synthesis of casein, the primary protein, and lactose, the primary carbohydrate. In non–breast-feeding women prolactin clears at a much slower rate than the placental steroids, requiring seven days to reach normal levels after delivery. In breast-feeding women, serum prolactin levels decline approximately 50%—to 100 ng/ml.[8] Each episode of suckling transiently increases prolactin, which is important in initiating and maintaining milk production. During the first 2 to 3 months postpartum, basal prolactin levels are 40 to 50 ng/ml with a 10- to 20-fold rise after suckling. Thereafter, base-line prolactin levels remain elevated, with only a 2-fold increase in prolactin after suckling.[57]

Milk ejection from the breast does not result from a mechanically induced negative pressure caused by suckling.[8] Rather, suckling activates tactile sensors located in the areola and triggers an afferent sensory neural arc via thoracic nerve roots to the hypothalamus.

This stimulus causes the hypothalamic paraventricular and supraoptic nuclei to produce and transport oxytocin to the posterior pituitary. The pulsatile release of oxytocin into the maternal circulation then acts on the breast alveoli, causing tonic contraction of the myoepithelial cells and emptying of milk from the alveolar lumen. Milk contained within the lactiferous sinuses is ejected from openings in the nipple. This rapid release of milk is called a let-down. Eventually, the central nervous system response can be conditioned to respond to nontactile stimuli, such as the presence or cry of an infant. Conversely, anxiety, stress, pain, or fright can inhibit the normal milk ejection reflex.[58]

Suckling causes the release of both prolactin from the anterior pituitary and oxytocin from the posterior pituitary; both hormones are necessary for the maintenance of milk production.[59] Prolactin maintains the volume of secretion and the production of casein, lactose, and fatty acids, while oxytocin stimulates milk expression by contracting the myoepithelial cells and emptying the alveolar unit. Frequent emptying of the alveolar lumen is important for maintaining adequate milk production, as the amount of milk produced correlates with the amount removed by suckling. Suckling also suppresses the hypothalamic formation of prolactin-inhibiting factor (PIF), which is thought to be dopamine.[8] Dopamine is secreted by the basal hypothalamus into the portal system and is transmitted to the anterior pituitary, where it binds specifically to lactotrophs and inhibits prolactin secretion. If PIF, or dopamine, is absent, then prolactin is secreted.

Colostrum consists of desquamated epithelial cells and transudate and is the thick yellow liquid secreted by the breasts late in gestation and early after delivery. Colostrum contains more minerals and protein and less lactose and fat than mature breast milk. The primary protein of colostrum is globulin. Secretion of colostrum continues for approximately 5 days, with gradual conversion to mature milk over the next 4 weeks. Colostrum provides several host immunologic factors and antibodies, such as secretory immunoglobulin A (sIgA), which confer protection against enteric pathogens in the neonate. Other important components include complement, macrophages, lymphocytes, lactoferrin, lactoperoxidase, and lysozomes.[60]

Mature human milk consists of a suspension of fat and protein in a carbohydrate–mineral solution that is 88 to 95% water. Lactating women produce between 600 and 1000 ml of milk per day with peak volumes in the early morning hours and nadirs during the early evening hours.[61] Protein comprises less than 1% of mature milk, of which 60% is whey and the remainder casein.[62] The distribution of lactose and fat varies with the milk ejection reflex, maternal nutrition, and intake of fore or hind milk (i.e., fore milk occurs at the beginning of a nursing session and hind milk at the end). Peak fat content is present during the midpoint of the nursing interval.[63] Antibodies in breast milk and colostrum are poorly absorbed by the neonatal gut. Despite this fact, the predominant immunoglobulin in milk, sIgA, prevents bacterial adherence to epithelial-cell surfaces, thereby limiting tissue invasion and making breast-fed infants less prone to enteric infections.[64]

Management of Breast-feeding

Breast-feeding should begin with prenatal promotion. Health-care providers should avoid a neutral attitude toward breast-feeding, which may appear as tacit approval of bottle-feeding.[65] Ideally, the issue of breast-feeding should be addressed during prenatal care, and the more frequently this topic is approached, the more likely the mother is to breast-feed.[66] It is during the pregnancy itself that the health-care provider can promote the multiple long-term health benefits of breast-feeding (Table 22-1).

With rare exceptions, human milk is considered the preferred food for all infants. The American Academy of Pediatrics (AAP)[67] recommends that breast-feeding begin immediately after birth, within the first hour if possible, unless medically contraindicated. The newborn should remain with the mother during recovery, and procedures that could interfere with breast-feeding or traumatize the infant should be avoided. The mother should be assisted with proper latch-on technique for effective suckling: at least 2 inches of the areola should be in the baby's mouth to allow the tongue to stroke the areola over the collecting ductules against the hard palate. Once on the postpartum floor, the infant should room with the mother in order to facilitate both breast-feeding and maternal–infant bonding. The mother should nurse whenever the newborn shows signs of hunger, specifically, increased alertness, activity, rooting, or mouthing. Crying is actually considered a late indicator of hunger.

Since breast milk is digested more quickly than formula, the newborn should nurse 8 to 12 times in

TABLE 22-1 HEALTH BENEFITS OF BREAST-FEEDING	
Maternal	Decreased postpartum bleeding due to more rapid uterine involution and higher oxytocin levels Decreased menstrual loss due to lactational amenorrhea Delayed resumption of ovulation with child spacing Increased bone remineralization with decreased risk of postmenopausal hip fracture Decreased risk of ovarian and premenopausal breast carcinoma
Neonatal	Decreased incidence and severity of diarrhea Decreased incidence of lower-respiratory-tract infections, otitis media, bacteremia, bacterial meningitis, botulism, urinary tract infections, and necrotizing enterocolitis
Possible Neonatal	Protective effect against SIDS, IDDM, Crohn disease, ulcerative colitis, lymphoma, and allergic diseases Enhancement of cognitive function

SIDS = sudden infant death syndrome; IDDM = insulin-dependent diabetes mellitus.

Adapted from American Academy of Pediatrics. Breastfeeding and the use of human milk. Pediatrics 1997;100:1035.

24 hours until satiety, alternating 10 to 15 minutes on each breast. Because it takes approximately 7 to 10 days for the milk supply to be established, in the early weeks postpartum, nondemanding infants should be aroused to feed if an interval greater than 4 hours has elapsed since the previous nursing. Healthy, full-term, and most larger preterm infants should not be given any supplements unless medically indicated, including such agents as water, glucose water, or formula. Parents should avoid supplements and pacifiers if possible and only use them, if absolutely necessary, once breast-feeding has been well established. Intermittent bottle-feeding of a breast-fed infant may lessen the success of breast-feeding. Since breast-feeding follows a supply-and-demand pattern, any infant supplemented with water or formula will take less milk from the breast, and milk production will subsequently diminish. Furthermore, some infants may experience nipple confusion and have difficulty alternating between an artificial nipple and the breast.

An adequately nourished and hydrated newborn should take at least 8 feedings per day and sleep well between feedings. Appropriate output is monitored by the newborn's voiding and stooling patterns, as the neonate should urinate at least six times a day, form three to four stools a day by five to seven days of life, and gain weight over time. A normal neonate may actually feed 12 to 14 times a day and produce a small, moist stool with many of the feedings. The AAP recommends that all breast-feeding mothers be evaluated by a trained observer within 48 hours postpartum and then 2 to 3 days after discharge.[67] The recommended

ideal length of breast-feeding is at least 12 months, after that, for as long as mutually desired.

Feeding the Preterm Infant

Infants who weigh >1500 g at birth may be fed either breast milk or a regular 67 kcal/dl infant formula normally used for full-term infants.[40] Breast milk has many desirable features for preterm infants, including antibodies and triglycerides that are easy to absorb. In addition, breast milk lipases assist with fat digestion and supplement deficient pancreatic lipase levels in preterm infants. Despite these advantages, breast milk lacks the necessary protein, calcium, and phosphorus components for adequate nutrition of the preterm infant. Therefore, breast milk should be supplemented with various commercially available milk fortifiers.

Very-low-birth-weight infants (<1500 g) should be given a 67 to 80 kcal/dl formula specifically created for premature infants or breast milk supplemented with a commercial mixture. Formulas designed for premature infants contain easily digested and absorbed lipids with 15 to 50% medium-chain triglycerides as well as additional protein, easily absorbed carbohydrates (glucose polymers and lactose), and additional calcium and phosphorus to maintain bone remineralization at a faster rate than that achieved with the use of regular infant formulas or unfortified breast milk.[40]

Maternal Nutrition during Lactation

Postnatal dietary guidelines are similar to those established in pregnancy[68] (Table 22-2). The minimal

TABLE 22-2
RECOMMENDED DAILY DIETARY ALLOWANCES FOR ADOLESCENT AND ADULT PREGNANT AND LACTATING WOMEN

Nutrient	Pregnant	Lactating, First 6 Months
Energy (kcal)	+300	+500
Protein	60	65
Fat-soluble vitamins		
Vitamin A (μg retinol equivalents)	800	1300
Vitamin D (μg as cholecalciferol)	10	10
Vitamin E (mg α-tocopherol equivalents)	10	12
Vitamin K (μg)	65	65
Water-soluble vitamins		
Vitamin C (mg)	70	95
Thiamine (mg)	1.5	1.6
Riboflavin (mg)	1.6	1.8
Niacin (mg niacin equivalent)	17	20
Vitamin B_6 (mg)	2.2	2.1
Folate (μg)	400	280
Vitamin B_{12} (μg)	2.2	2.6
Minerals		
Calcium (mg)	1200	1200
Phosphorus (mg)	1200	1200
Magnesium (mg)	300	355
Iron (mg)	30	15
Zinc (mg)	15	19
Iodine (μg)	175	200
Selenium (μg)	65	75

Reprinted with permission from *Recommended Dietary Allowances*, 10th ed, © 1989 by the National Academy of Sciences. Published by National Academy Press, Washington, D.C., and adapted from Guidelines for Perinatal Care, 4th ed.

caloric requirement for adequate milk production for an average-sized woman is 1800 kcal/day, with an increased energy requirement of 750 to 1000 kcal/day.[38] New mothers should be adequately nourished with the intake of a balanced diet. Vitamin and mineral supplements are not necessary.[40] Only if the mother is at nutritional risk should a multivitamin supplement be given, such as calcium, vitamin B_{12}, or vitamin D. Iron supplements should be prescribed only if the mother is iron-deficient.

Contraindications to Breast-Feeding

According to the AAP,[68] breast-feeding is not in the best interest of the infant in certain situations. Infants with galactosemia cannot metabolize galactose and should not breast-feed. Mothers with active tuberculosis should breast-feed their infants only after they have received adequate treatment and are considered noninfectious.[40] If active maternal disease is present, the neonate should be isolated and given isoniazid prophylaxis. The infant may be reunited with the mother after 7 days of treatment. All antituberculous medications are acceptable during breast-feeding except streptomycin and pyrazinamide.

Certain viruses pose an infectious risk to the breast-fed infant. Cytomegalovirus (CMV) is excreted into human milk. Mothers with primary CMV infection should not breast-feed during the acute phase of the illness. Mothers with active hepatitis B infection should not breast-feed. However, mothers who are chronic carriers (test positive for hepatitis B surface antigen) may breast-feed provided that the neonate has received hepatitis B immune globulin and hepatitis B vaccine. Vertical transmission of hepatitis C infection through breast milk has not been clearly documented. In studies that evaluated breast-feeding in infants born to hepatitis C antibody–positive mothers, the average rate of infection was 4% for both breast-fed and formula-fed infants.[69] A history of herpes simplex virus (HSV) infection does not preclude breast-feeding. Mothers with active HSV may still breast-feed as long as no vesicles are located in the breast area and strict hand-washing techniques are followed.

In the United States, maternal human immunodeficiency virus (HIV) infection is considered a contraindication to breast-feeding.[70] For HIV-infected women in developing countries, breast-feeding offers

TABLE 22-3
DRUGS THAT ARE CONTRAINDICATED DURING BREAST-FEEDING

Drug	Reason for Concern, Reported Sign or Symptom in Infant, or Effect on Lactation
Bromocriptine	Suppresses lactation; may be hazardous to the mother
Cyclophosphamide	Possible immunosuppression, unknown effect on growth, association with carcinogenesis, neutropenia
Cyclosporine	Possible immunosuppression, unknown effect on growth, unknown association with carcinogenesis
Doxorubicin*	Possible immunosuppression; unknown effect on growth, unknown association with carcinogenesis
Ergotamine	Vomiting, diarrhea, convulsions with doses used for migraine medications
Lithium	One-third to one-half therapeutic blood concentration in infants
Methotrexate	Possible immunosuppression, unknown effect on growth, unknown association with carcinogenesis
Phenindione	Anticoagulant; increased prothrombin and partial thromboplastin time in one infant; not used in United States

*Drug is concentrated in human milk.

Reprinted with permission from American Academy of Pediatrics, Committee on Drugs. The transfer of drugs and other chemicals into human milk. Pediatrics 1994;93:137.

such high nutritional and health benefits that the mortality risks associated with not breast-feeding may outweigh the possible risk of HIV. However, in the United States, where formula is safe and available, HIV-infected women should be counseled not to breast-feed.[40] Unfortunately, no randomized controlled trials have accurately documented the incremental risk of HIV transmission through breast-feeding over that occurring during the antepartum and intrapartum periods.[70] Reports in various African populations have demonstrated a 3 to 12% risk of vertical transmission.[70] Furthermore, the controversial interpretation of results from one meta-analysis indicates that the incremental risk of transmission by breast-feeding from mothers with established infection antepartum is 14%, while the risk of vertical transmission approaches 29% in women who acquire primary infection during the postpartum period.[70]

Only a few medications require temporary cessation of breast-feeding; these include radioactive isotopes, antimetabolites, cancer chemotherapeutic agents, and a small number of other medications[68] (Tables 22-3 and 22-4).

Lactation Suppression

For women who choose not to breast-feed, lactation suppression is best achieved with supportive measures. Recommendations include the use of a comfortable, but tight breast binder or well-fitted brassiere, the application of cold packs to the breasts, and the administration of nonsteroidal antiinflammatory agents. Most signs and symptoms will resolve in 1 to 2 days as long as the breasts are not stimulated by nursing or pumping. Bromocriptine mesylate (Parlodel), a dopamine agonist and prolactin inhibitor, was used routinely during the 1980s for lactation suppression. When given in a dose of 2.5 mg orally twice daily for 14 days, bromocriptine prevented severe bilateral engorgement in 75 to 98% of women.[46] However, approximately 25% of women experienced rebound engorgement at the end of treatment. In 1989 the Maternal Health Advisory Committee of the Food

TABLE 22-4
RADIOACTIVE COMPOUNDS THAT REQUIRE TEMPORARY CESSATION OF BREAST-FEEDING

Radiolabeled Element	Recommended Time for Cessation of Breast-Feeding*
Copper-64 (^{64}Cu)	50 hr
Gallium-67 (^{67}Ga)	2 wk
Indium-111 (^{111}In)	Very small amount present at 20 hr
Iodine-123 (^{123}I)	36 hr
Iodine-125 (^{125}I)	12 days
Iodine-131 (^{131}I)	2–14 days
Radioactive sodium	96 hr
Technetium-99m (^{99m}Tc), ^{99m}Tc, Macroaggregates, ^{99m}TcO$_4$	15 hr to 3 days

*Duration of radioactivity in breast-milk

Reprinted with permission from American Academy of Pediatrics, Committee on Drugs. The transfer of drugs and other chemicals into human milk. Pediatrics 1994;93:137.

and Drug Administration recommended that bromocriptine no longer be used for lactation suppression because of case reports that bromocriptine had a small association with stroke, myocardial infarction, seizure activity, and psychiatric disturbances in puerperal women.[71] Despite limited evidence, the manufacturers voluntarily removed lactation suppression from the product labeling in 1994.[72]

Nipple Disorders

Nipple Discharge

A bloody nipple discharge during the second and third trimesters as well as during the postpartum period may occur due to the development of extensive ductal hyperplasia lined with a delicate capillary network. These capillaries can be easily injured, leading to a unilateral or bilateral sanguineous discharge. Cytologic evaluation of the discharge may be obscured by normal pregnancy-induced changes. The discharge is normally self-limited, and only observation and reassurance are necessary. However, if the discharge persists for longer than 2 months postpartum or is associated with a mass or other physical findings, further evaluation of the affected breast is indicated, including sonography, mammography, and possible exploration of the ductal system with a ductogram.

Depressed or Inverted Nipples

Approximately 10% of pregnant women have some type of nipple abnormality, which makes breast-feeding more difficult or even impossible.[73] Women with depressed nipples have lactiferous ducts that open directly into a depression at the center of the areola. If the depression is very deep, they are unable to nurse, but if the depression is more superficial, a breast pump can be used to evert the nipple and obtain milk. True inverted nipples are rare, affecting less than 1% of women.[74] Inverted nipples are clinically recognized by a ring of circular fibers that restrict the ability of the nipple to be everted even slightly. In order to prepare the breasts for nursing, daily attempts should be made to draw out the nipple with gentle traction using the mother's fingers. Use of breast shields or shells or a breast pump may also facilitate eversion of the nipples. If a woman's nipples are fibrous or inelastic, the infant may be unable to elongate the nipple in the mouth and use normal, peristaltic tongue motion to remove milk from the lactiferous sinuses, resulting in inefficient milk removal.[75]

Fissured or Cracked Nipples

Nipples can become cracked, blistered, ulcerated, and extremely sore. These conditions are commonly caused by poor breast-feeding technique, such as improper positioning, poor latch-on, or sucking problems. These skin breaks not only make nursing more painful, but they also may act as portals of entry for bacteria and yeast, possibly leading to mastitis. If such changes develop in a nursing mother, she should be evaluated by her healthcare provider or lactation specialist in order to identify any use of oils, soaps, ointments, or other self-medications and to assess her breast-feeding technique. Once poor technique is corrected, additional measures for comfort and support can be initiated. These measures include the use of topical agents, such as A&D Ointment, purified lanolin, or synthetic hydrocorticoid cream (Elocon), avoidance of soaps and other drying agents, allowing the breasts to air-dry, and the use of breast secretions for lubrication.[76] In cases of severe cracking, women may pump or manually express from the affected side and nurse from the unaffected side.

In women with persistently cracked nipples that do not respond to simple interventions, the most likely cause is a fungal infection of the breast ducts. The most common agent is *Candida albicans*, and this type of infection frequently follows antibiotic therapy. Women complain of sharp, shooting pain through the breasts. The nipple may appear normal despite the presence of severe pain. The infant should be treated with a nystatin oral suspension (Mycostatin), regardless of the presence or absence of oral thrush or diaper rash. Topical nystatin cream can also be applied to the nipples as well as all other artificial nipples and toys. A topical steroid cream or combined steroid–antifungal cream (Mycolog) may also provide relief. A course of oral fluconazole is also effective treatment, which eliminates the need for removing any topical agents from the nipples prior to nursing.[76]

Breast Disorders

Galactoceles

Galactoceles are simple, milk-filled cysts, which are usually associated with pregnancy or lactation. These cysts are caused by obstruction of the lactiferous ducts, with accumulation of milk in one or more breast lobules. A galactocele presents as a tender, fluctuant mass with pressure-type symptoms and is usually noted after discontinuation of breast-feeding. Palpation demonstrates a dominant, mobile, unilateral mass located in a subareolar position. The cyst may also assume a linear shape with a soft consistency. Evaluation includes aspiration, ultrasound, and possibly, mammography. Fine-needle aspiration can be both diagnostic and curative with the demonstration of grossly milky fluid; however, additional aspirations may be necessary. Ultrasonography demonstrates a hypoechoic, well-delineated mass with additional shadowing and compression. Although rarely indicated, mammography shows a characteristic appearance. Because of the partial fatty density of milk, mammography reveals a well-circumscribed, radiolucent mass with clean margins. The mammographic finding of a water–fat level within a mass is pathognomonic. Treatment is primarily supportive, with the use of ice packs and good breast support with a tight brassiere or breast binder. If the galactocele is recurrent, excision of the affected duct may be necessary to avoid infection and abscess formation. The histology of galactoceles appears as a dilated duct filled with proteinaceous material, showing cellular lactational change.

Fibroadenomas

Fibroadenomas are benign, well-demarcated, smooth, mobile breast nodules. The majority of these tumors are asymptomatic. During pregnancy, fibroadenomas may increase in size and show lactational histologic changes. For this reason, some authorities advocate their removal prior to pregnancy because of the risk of infarction during pregnancy and lactation.

Mammary Hamartomas

Mammary hamartomas are benign tumors that behave in a fashion similar to fibroadenomas. These tumors typically present during the postpartum period following breast involution. They form smooth, well-encapsulated masses that are usually asymptomatic. Excision is recommended if fine needle aspiration is inconclusive or the patient is symptomatic. Histologically, the specimen demonstrates fatty stromal and ductal tissue.

Breast Engorgement

Breast engorgement, or milk stasis, is an exaggerated response of the normal venous and lymphatic congestion associated with lactation. This condition does not result from overdistention of the lacteal system with milk. Breast engorgement most commonly occurs on postpartum day 2, with initiation of milk let-down, resulting in painful, distended, and nodular breasts. Engorged breasts are a common cause of puerperal fever and affect 13% of postpartum women.[77] Most temperature elevations are low-grade, ranging from 37.8 to 39°C, and of short duration, lasting from 4 to 16 hours. Supportive treatment includes the use of a breast binder or tight brassiere, application of ice to the breasts, and oral analgesics. The majority of cases resolve within 48 to 72 hours. For women who are breast-feeding, engorged breasts may make it difficult, and even impossible, for the nursing infant to latch on properly. In this situation, breast pumping or manual expression may be necessary for several days until nursing can be effectively resumed.

Puerperal Mastitis

By providing a lactose-rich environment for bacteria, milk stasis may allow the growth and possible ascent of the oropharyngeal flora from the nursing infant via the terminal nipple ducts. Such contamination of the alveolar–ductal complex ultimately may lead to a spectrum of complications, including noninfectious inflammation, acute mastitis, and even breast abscess. Puerperal mastitis affects approximately 2% of women postpartum.[78] Various risk factors include breast engorgement, hospital delivery, poor hygiene, inexperienced breast-feeding technique leading to cracked (fissured) nipples, and lowered maternal immunity due to fatigue, stress, or poor nutrition. Although most infections occur within the first 5 weeks postpartum, cases may present up to 10 months after delivery.[79]

In 1953 Gibberd classified mastitis into two basic types: epidemic, and nonepidemic, or sporadic.[80] In the past, acute mastitis was often epidemic and was associated with longer hospitalizations, lack of antibiotics, and nursery outbreaks of *Staphylococcus aureus* infection. Due to shorter hospital stays and institution of hospital infection-control policies, epidemic mastitis is uncommon today. Epidemic mastitis is the result of an acute adenitis and cellulitis within the lactiferous ducts, located between Cooper's ligaments and usually occurs in a hospital setting 1 to 2 days postpartum. Epidemic mastitis is more likely to lead to abscess formation. In comparison, the onset of sporadic mastitis occurs in the third to fourth postpartum week and usually arises during periods of sporadic nursing or weaning. Sporadic mastitis is characterized as a superficial cellulitis with extension into the periglandular connective tissue, clinically appearing as a V-shaped area located between the lobes of the breast. Sporadic mastitis rarely leads to breast abscess formation.

Women with mastitis typically present with a flu-like syndrome of malaise, fever, chills, and myalgias; localized symptoms develop 1 to 2 days later. The breast may become very hard and painful, and maternal temperatures may reach as high as 40°C following the onset of actual rigors. Clinical signs include tenderness, warmth, edema, erythema, and induration in a V-shaped, or fanned-out, distribution along the involved lobule of the breast. Unilateral involvement is most common, and often breast engorgement precedes inflammation.

The differential diagnosis includes breast engorgement versus an inflammatory breast carcinoma. Breast engorgement is usually bilateral, but mastitis can arise in this setting if the mother has recently discontinued breast-feeding. An inflammatory carcinoma should be considered if a woman has recurrent episodes of mastitis or does not respond to antimicrobial therapy. Knowledge of the antepartum breast examination is useful for differentiating mastitis from an inflammatory carcinoma. If the breasts were normal early in pregnancy, then it is much less likely for a neoplasm to arise de novo postpartum.[78] This form of breast carcinoma presents in a fashion similar to mastitis but with more diffuse erythema, warmth, and induration. Thickening, or peau d'orange, of the skin may be present due to lymphatic tumor infiltration. Satellite nodules and purplish discoloration may also be found.

The majority of culture isolates are *S. aureus*.[80] Other commonly identified organisms include *S. epidermidis*; groups A, B, and D streptococci; aerobic coliforms; and anaerobes. Most staphylococcal organisms are penicillin-sensitive, but methicillin-resistant strains can comprise up to 10% of isolates.[60] Epidemic mastitis can coincide with the appearance of a new strain of antibiotic-resistant *S. aureus* and usually occurs when the infant becomes infected after contact with colonized nursery personnel.[80]

Diagnosis is based primarily on clinical signs and symptoms. Prior to the initiation of antibiotics, milk should be expressed from the affected breast after discarding the first 2 to 3 ml, swabbed, and submitted to

TABLE 22-5
CLASSIFICATION OF NONEPIDEMIC MASTITIS

Milk stasis
  $<10^6$ leukocytes/ml milk
  $<10^3$ bacteria/ml milk
Noninfectious inflammation
  $>10^6$ leukocytes/ml milk
  $<10^3$ bacteria/ml milk
Infectious mastitis
  $>10^6$ leukocytes/ml milk
  $>10^3$ bacteria/ml milk

Adapted from Thomsen et al.[81]

the laboratory for Gram stain and culture. Although diagnosis is rarely based on culture results alone, identification of the organism and its antibiotic sensitivities not only guides treatment, but also provides useful information regarding hospital infection control policy and surveillance of nosocomial infections. If a woman presents with recurrent mastitis, culture of the infant's nasopharynx may be beneficial as well. Thomsen and co-workers[81] used milk leukocyte counts and quantitative bacterial cultures in order to differentiate between milk stasis, noninfectious inflammation, and infectious mastitis (Table 22-5). Blood cultures may be useful to define the duration of treatment, especially if epidemic mastitis with *S. aureus* infection is suspected. In general, mammography is not indicated in the evaluation of mastitis unless malignancy is strongly considered.[82]

Therapy should be initiated promptly, as delaying treatment over 24 hours can increase the incidence of abscess formation.[83] In cases of sporadic mastitis, the mother should continue emptying the breast either via pumping or breast-feeding.[79,81] Often it is easier to begin with the unaffected breast in order to initiate let-down and then switch to the contralateral breast. Abscess formation is more common if *S. aureus* is present.[84] If appropriate therapy is started before suppuration begins, the infection usually resolves within 48 hours. In order to proceed with outpatient therapy, the patient must be considered reliable and not acutely ill. An antistaphylococcal or a first-generation cephalosporin antibiotic is usually adequate, and therapy should be continued for at least 10 to 14 days to avoid recurrence[76] (Table 22-6). If a woman is penicillin-allergic, then erythromycin may be substituted, although staphylococcal coverage may be limited.

For those patients who appear more acutely ill, inpatient therapy with parenteral regimens is

TABLE 22-6
TREATMENT OF PUERPERAL MASTITIS

Antibiotic	Dose	Route	Interval (Hours)
Uncomplicated Acute Mastitis			
Penicillin	5 million units	Oral	6
Ampicillin	500 mg		
Oxacillin	500 mg		
Dicloxacillin	500 mg		
Erythromycin base	500 mg		
Clindamycin	500 mg		
Cephalexin	500 mg		
Cephradine	500 mg		
Breast Abscess			
Cefazolin or	1–2 g	Intravenous	8
Ampicillin or	1–2 g		6
Methicillin or	1–2 g		6–8
Nafcillin or	1–2 g		4
Oxacillin	1–2 g		4
and			
Clindamycin or	900 mg		8
Metronidazole	500 mg		12
MRSA Mastitis or Severe Penicillin Allergy			
Vancomycin	125 mg	Oral	6
	500 g	Intravenous	6

MRSA = methicillin resistant *S. aureus*.

Hager WD. Mastitis. In: Mead PB, Hager WD. eds. Infection protocols for obstetrics and gynecology. Montvale, NJ: Medical Economics, 1992:27.

recommended. Nafcillin, oxacillin, and cefazolin may be used with equal efficacy. If methicillin-resistant *S. aureus* is identified, then vancomycin should be administered. The parenteral antimicrobial regimen should be continued for at least 48 hours after the patient is afebrile, with subsequent completion of a 10 to 14 day course of oral antibiotics. In Thomsen's study, a good response was seen in 15% of women with no treatment, in 51% of women who emptied only the affected breast, and in 96% of women who both emptied their breasts and received oral antibiotics.[81] Additional supportive measures include the administration of analgesics, continued nursing using gentle pumping if necessary, and the application of moist heat to the affected breast. The milk of mothers with mastitis has a higher sodium and lower lactose, fat, and total protein content, and often the infant will reject the breast.[80] If the breast is persistently rejected, then inflammatory carcinoma should be considered as a cause.

Breast Abscess

The incidence of breast abscess is approximately 10% in patients with mastitis. Clinical suspicion may be apparent from failure to defervesce after 48 to 72 hours of antibiotics, presence of a palpable mass on examination, or spontaneous purulent drainage from the affected breast.[85] Most abscesses occur in inexperienced, young mothers not practicing proper hygiene. A second peak incidence occurs at the time of weaning, when the breasts are engorged and milk stasis occurs.[86]

When a breast abscess is diagnosed, nursing should be discontinued on the affected breast and parenteral antibiotics should be initiated, with the addition of adequate anaerobic coverage. If there is no improvement in 48 to 72 hours, the abscess should be incised and drained. If indicated, a biopsy should be obtained and sent for culture to exclude the possibility of an inflammatory carcinoma. Ultrasound-guided needle aspiration can be used instead of open drainage[87]; however, repeat aspirations may be necessary for effective resolution.[88]

In addition to surgical drainage, the breast must be kept empty of milk. Breast-feeding can continue on the unaffected side, but the infected breast should be emptied with gentle pumping. If the breast is too tender to pump, then either pumping or manual expression can be performed while the mother soaks in a warm bath with the breast suspended. The infant should not be allowed to nurse from the involved breast, especially if a staphylococcal infection is present, because pneumonia, lung abscesses, and even infant deaths have been reported.[89]

Postpartum Contraception and Prevention of Pregnancy

Each year 150 million pregnancies occur worldwide, 70% of them in developing countries. Of these, 50% are unplanned, and 50% of those are unwanted.[90] The postpartum period is an ideal time to initiate contraception and family planning. Reversible contraceptive measures include natural methods, barrier methods, and steroid contraceptive methods, such as combined oral contraceptives, progestin-only pills, injectable contraception, and subdermal implants. Irreversible methods include sterilization either by postpartum tubal ligation or vasectomy.

Contraception in Lactating and Nonlactating Women: Timing and Method Selection

The initial concern during the first 2 weeks postpartum is the increased risk of venous thromboembolic events due to the persistence of the hypercoagulable state that arises during pregnancy.[91] Administration of steroid contraceptives containing estrogen is not recommended until this interval has passed.[92] Once the hypercoagulable period has passed, lactation status then helps to determine the timing for the initiation of contraception.[93] The "Rule of Threes" serves as a useful guide for clinicians:[8]

• With full breast-feeding, contraception should begin in the third postpartum month
• With partial or no breast-feeding, contraception should begin in the third postpartum week

As an exception to these rules, women treated with dopamine agonists (e.g., bromocriptine) ovulate earlier, and, thus, contraception should be initiated by two weeks postpartum.[8]

Every contraceptive choice has advantages and disadvantages, and the risks and benefits of each one must be assessed in view of each woman's personal needs, beliefs, past experience, and lactation status.

Natural Methods

Lactational Amenorrhea Method

In addition to its many health and nutritional benefits for infants, breast-feeding can also provide the added advantage of contraception during the first postpartum months. Breast-feeding decreases fertility by inducing anovulation and amenorrhea. The lactational amenorrhea method (LAM) is based on this period of relative infertility that occurs in women who breast-feed.[11,94] Breast-feeding provides its greatest birth spacing effect when a mother "exclusively" or "nearly exclusively" breastfeeds and remains amenorrheic. When these two conditions are met, breast-feeding confers greater than 98% protection from pregnancy in the first 6 months postpartum[18,95] (Figure 22-2). However, only amenorrheic women who exclusively breast-feed at regular intervals, including nighttime, during the first 6 months, were considered to have contraceptive protection equivalent to that provided by combined oral contraceptives. Supplemental feedings increase the risk of ovulation and menses.[16] In a prospective study of 72 exclusively breast-feeding postpartum women, there was no evidence of ovulation before 8 weeks postpartum despite the fact that nearly 50% of these women experienced some amount of bleeding or spotting between 6 and 8 weeks postpartum.[15] Thus, the guidelines for LAM note that vaginal bleeding occurring in the first 56 days postpartum in fully or nearly fully breast-feeding women should be ignored when determining the return of menses.[18,94,96] Because ovulation has been

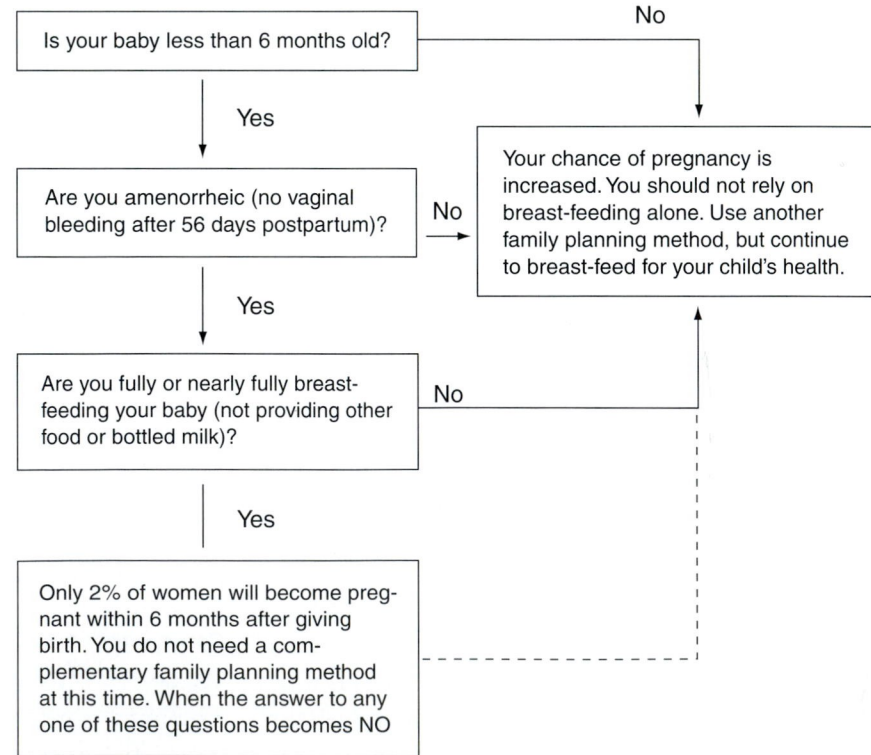

Figure 22-2 Lactational amenorrhea method and protection against pregnancy. Adapted from Kaunitz AM. Considering postpartum contraception and the role of lactation. Dialogues in contraception 1997;5:5; based on data from Labbok M, Cooney K, Coly S. Guidelines: Breastfeeding, family planning, and the lactational amenorrhea method—LAM. Washington, DC: Institute for Reproductive Health, 1994.

Is your baby less than 6 months old? — No
↓ Yes
Are you amenorrheic (no vaginal bleeding after 56 days postpartum)? — No
↓ Yes
Are you fully or nearly fully breast-feeding your baby (not providing other food or bottled milk)? — No
↓ Yes
Only 2% of women will become pregnant within 6 months after giving birth. You do not need a complementary family planning method at this time. When the answer to any one of these questions becomes NO

Your chance of pregnancy is increased. You should not rely on breast-feeding alone. Use another family planning method, but continue to breast-feed for your child's health.

documented to occur in fully breast-feeding women prior to 6 months,[9,15] it is wise to recommend a supplementary contraceptive method to fully breast-feeding women in the third postpartum month.[8]

Periodic Abstinence

Due to the many false positive and false negative interpretations of cervical mucus, periodic abstinence cannot be used with great reliability until the resumption of normal menses.[8]

Nonhormonal Methods

Barrier Methods

Barrier methods obviously have no impact on breast-feeding and include male and female condoms, diaphragms, cervical caps, and spermicides. Condoms are effective in preventing pregnancy if used correctly and consistently, but they do have a higher failure rate than other available methods (Table 22-7). Condoms also provide an approximately 50% reduction in the transmission of sexually transmitted infections and pelvic inflammatory disease.[8] Vaginal dryness can be a

TABLE 22-7
FAILURE RATES DURING THE FIRST YEAR OF USE IN THE UNITED STATES

Method	Women with Pregnancy	
	Ideal (%)	Typical (%)
No method	85.0	85.0
Combination pill	0.1	3.0
Progestin only	0.5	3.0
Intrauterine devices (IUDs)		3.0
Progesterone IUD	2.0	<2.0
Copper T 380A	0.8	<1.0
Norplant	0.2	0.2
Female sterilization	0.2	0.4
Male sterilization	0.1	0.15
Depo-Provera	0.3	0.3
Spermicides	3.0	21.0
Periodic abstinence		20.0
Calendar	9.0	
Ovulation method	3.0	
Symptothermal	2.0	
Post-ovulation	1.0	
Withdrawal	4.0	18.0
Cervical cap	6.0	18.0
Diaphragm and spermicides	6.0	18.0
Condom	2.0	12.0

IUD = Intrauterine device

Reprinted with permission from Trussell J, Hatcher RA, Cates W Jr, Stewart FH, Kost K. A guide to interpreting contraceptive efficacy studies. Obstet Gynecol 1990;76:558.

Adapted from Speroff L, Darney PD. A clinical guide for contraception. 2nd ed. Baltimore: Williams & Wilkins, 1996.

problem in lactating women due to relatively low serum estrogen levels, but the use of a water-based lubricant can reduce the degree of dyspareunia. Condoms should not be used with mineral oil- or petroleum-based products, which can break down the latex. Condoms should be used in conjunction with a spermicide that uses nonoxynol-9. Condoms are appropriate to use in the first 6 weeks postpartum.

Other barrier methods, such as the diaphragm and cervical cap, should be fitted after 6 weeks to allow for proper healing of the cervix and complete uterine involution. These devices should not be used if a woman is still having bleeding because they can become dislodged.[93] Diaphragms should be used in conjunction with a spermicide. Both the diaphragm and cervical cap may be difficult to fit in lactating women due to vaginal dryness. Additional lubrication may be necessary.

Intrauterine Devices (IUDs)

Only two IUDs are currently available in the United States: the Copper T 380A, (Paragard, Ortho Pharmaceutical Corp., Raritan, NJ) and the progesterone-releasing IUD, (Progestasert, Alza Corp., Palo Alto, CA). The copper-bearing IUD is effective for 10 years, making it the longest-acting, reversible contraceptive available.[8] The copper IUD prevents fertilization by incapacitating sperm in the uterine cavity and preventing them from reaching the fallopian tubes. All IUDs create a sterile foreign-body reaction that produces cytotoxic macrophages that reduce sperm survival. Few, if any, sperm reach the ovum in the fallopian tube.[97] If the spermicidal action fails, then the intrauterine inflammatory response will prevent implantation.[98] IUDs have no effect on ovulation,[99] and they do not act as abortifacients.[100] A major disadvantage of the copper-bearing IUD is its association with a higher incidence of dysmenorrhea and menorrhagia.

The progesterone-releasing IUD releases 65 μg of progesterone per day for 1 year, which results in thickening of the cervical mucus and decidualization of the endometrium. The progesterone-releasing IUD effectively inhibits implantation and interferes with sperm capacitation and survival, although fertilization rates are higher than with copper-bearing IUDs.[8] The progesterone-releasing IUD is associated with a 40 to 50% lower incidence of bleeding and cramping and may be useful in women with significant menorrhagia and dysmenorrhea.[8] Due to its limited duration of efficacy, the progesterone-releasing IUD must be replaced annually. After an IUD is removed, the normal uterine environment and fertility return rapidly.[101,102]

The typical failure rate during the first year of use for all IUDs is approximately 3%, with a 10% expulsion rate, and a 15% removal rate, primarily for pain and bleeding.[8] As duration of use and patient age increase, the failure rate and removals decrease. In some studies, the failure rate with the Copper T 380A is less than 1 per 100 women per year.[100,103] IUDs do not increase the risk of ectopic pregnancy and may offer some protection against it.[8] In a large WHO multicenter trial, IUD users were 50% less likely to have an ectopic pregnancy as compared with women not using contraception.[104] However, IUDs do not inhibit ovulation to the same degree as oral contraceptives. Thus, if pregnancy occurs in an IUD user, the pregnancy is more likely to be ectopic. The lowest ectopic pregnancy rates are seen with the copper-bearing IUDs, with slightly higher rates for progesterone-releasing IUDs. Finally, IUD-related infection is believed to be caused by endometrial contamination at the time of insertion; infection arising 3 to 4 months after insertion is probably due to a newly acquired sexually transmitted disease.[8]

Since IUDs do not affect lactation, they are an excellent contraceptive choice in breast-feeding women.[91] Insertion of IUDs in breast-feeding women as compared with non–breast-feeding women is less painful and the subsequent rate of removal for bleeding and pain is lower.[105] Compared with insertion after 8 weeks postpartum, copper-bearing IUDs can be safely inserted at 4 to 8 weeks postpartum with no increased postinsertion event rates, such as expulsion or perforation.[106] The Copper T 380A IUD can be inserted immediately postpartum, although some studies show a higher rate of expulsion than with insertion at least 6 weeks postpartum.[107]

Hormonal Methods

Combined Oral Contraceptives

Current oral contraceptives (OCs) contain 20, 30, or 35 μg of ethinyl estradiol with varying types and doses of 19-nortestosterone progestins. In nonlactating women oral contraceptives should be initiated during week two to three postpartum, or on the second or third Sunday.[93] Combined OCs should be avoided prior to this time because of the concern of the hypercoagulable state and risk for venous

thromboembolism. Since the earliest ovulation in lactating women does not occur before three weeks,[108] it is prudent to start OCs sooner to avoid selection of a dominant follicle and risk subsequent ovulation.[93] The easiest practice is to send women home with a pack of OCs to start in two to three weeks. Clinicians should be aware that the product labeling recommends deferring initiation of OCs until four weeks postpartum in the nonlactating woman.

Lactating women who regularly breast-feed at least every 4 hours, do not provide supplemental feeds, and avoid the use of pacifiers do not need to worry about pregnancy for 2 to 3 months.[109] If there is a concern, then women may initiate either OCs once their supply of breast milk is well established or use a progestin-only pill starting at 6 weeks until supplemental feedings begin. Some authorities recommend avoiding combination OCs in fully breast-feeding women because estrogen has been shown to decrease milk production as well as caloric and mineral content.[110] While the use of combination OCs can reduce the volume and duration of lactation,[111] there appears to be no effect on infant growth and development.[112] The authors speculated that either supplemental feedings or more prolonged intense suckling episodes compensated for the decreased milk volumes. Thus, OCs can be used in breast-feeding women once lactation is well established. Other less controversial options include nonhormonal methods, use of the progestin-only pill, or switching to combination OCs after weaning.

Progestin-Only Contraception

The progestin-only pills currently available in the United States include norethindrone 0.35 mg/day (Nor-QD, Syntex; and Micronor, Ortho) and norgestrel 0.075 mg/day (Ovrette, Wyeth-Ayerst). The progestin induces an atrophic endometrium, which impairs implantation, and also causes a thick, impermeable cervical mucus. The effect on inhibition of ovulation is less predictable.[8] Progestin-only pills can be used in both lactating and nonlactating women. Only small amounts of progestin are secreted into breast milk, which does not affect infant growth or development.[93] Progestin-only pills may provide a moderate increase in milk production and have been shown to be related to longer breast-feeding duration.[8]

Progestin-only pills can be used in non–breast-feeding women and should be started by at least the third postpartum week. Due to their lower efficacy, it is important to advise women to adhere to a strict schedule, taking one pill at the same time each day to provide adequate contraceptive protection. When pills are taken more than 24 hours apart, steroid levels diminish, as does their effect on cervical mucus. Women should use back-up contraception for at least 48 hours if they are more than 3 hours late after the last dose.[8] If given to breast-feeding women who are already hypoestrogenic, progestin-only pills may cause a higher incidence of breakthrough bleeding than combined oral contraceptives.

Injectable Contraception

Depomedroxyprogesterone acetate (DMPA, or Depo-Provera) is an aqueous suspension of low-solubility microcrystals and is given as a 150-mg intramuscular injection every 3 months. DMPA provides greater than 99% efficacy against pregnancy. DMPA has been used in developing countries for over 30 years but was not approved for use in the United States by the Food and Drug Administration until 1992. DMPA effectively inhibits ovulation for 14-week intervals and causes atrophic changes in the endometrium, making it less hospitable for implantation. Ideal failure rates approach 0.7 per 100 woman-years with typical use failure rates of 0.3 per 100 woman-years. The most common side effect is unpredictable bleeding and spotting. Additional side effects include headaches, bloating, mood changes, and weight gain.[92] Fifty percent of women are amenorrheic after 1 year of use, and 75% become amenorrheic with extended use. Long-term use is associated with reversible reduction in bone-mineral density, which may reflect the relative estrogen-lowering effect of DMPA.[93]

Women on DMPA may experience a delayed return to fertility unrelated to duration of use. In women attempting pregnancy after discontinuation of DMPA, 50% will become pregnant by 10 months after the last injection.[92] A small number of women may experience delayed ovulation until 18 months after the last injection. Noncontraceptive benefits of DMPA include a decreased risk of pelvic inflammatory disease, hematologic improvement in women with sickle-cell disease, and decreased seizure frequency in women with seizure disorders.[92] In large case–control trials there was no increased risk of breast, endometrial, ovarian, or cervical cancer. In fact DMPA provides even greater protection against endometrial cancer than oral contraceptives.[92]

Based on product labeling, DMPA may be administered to nonlactating women within the first 5 days and by the first 3 weeks postpartum. Women who are fully breast-feeding may wait until 6 weeks postpartum. When started immediately as opposed to 6 weeks postpartum, there was no decreased duration of lactation or infant weight gain noted in women given DMPA.[92] Immediate postpartum use of DMPA and implants, regardless of lactation status, appears safe and appropriate given the growing body of clinical evidence and lack of impact on the coagulation system.[93]

Contraceptive Implants

Levonorgestrel subdermal implants (Norplant) consist of six soft silastic capsules, each measures 34 by 2.4 mm and contains 36 mg of crystalline levonorgestrel. The initial daily release rate of 85 μg gradually declines to 30 μg by the fifth year of use.[92] Norplant was approved for use in the United States by the Food and Drug Administration in 1990. Norplant maintains one of the lowest failure rates for contraceptives, at 0.8 per 100 woman-years during 5 years of use, with rates rising to 2 per 100 by 6 years. Norplant works primarily by inhibiting ovulation; however, approximately one-third of users experience cyclic luteal activity during the first year and have normal menses.[8] The progesterone values are lower than those associated with normal ovulation, which in effect causes luteal insufficiency and impaired oocyte maturation, preventing fertility in users with ovulatory activity. An additional contraceptive action is alteration of cervical mucus.

Norplant can be inserted immediately postpartum, but it is usually inserted at 4 to 6 weeks. Small amounts of levonorgestrel are secreted into breast milk, but no effect has been observed on lactation and infant growth in women with implants inserted at 6 weeks postpartum.[92] Disadvantages include irregular, unpredictable bleeding, up-front expense, and potential difficulty in removal due to the fibrous capsules that develop around the rods.

Emergency Contraception

Women should be informed of the availability of emergency contraception in the event of unprotected intercourse or potential contraceptive failure, such as a broken condom. The most common estrogen–progestin regimen is two doses of a combination of 100 μg of ethinyl estradiol and 0.5 mg of levonorgestrel each, the first dose taken within 72 hours after intercourse and the second dose 12 hours later. Although the same hormones are present in some brands of oral contraceptives, this combination has been marketed under the brand name Preven and is available only through prescription. The mechanism of action is believed to be inhibition or delay of ovulation.[113] Since intervention occurs prior to implantation, this form of contraception does not act as an abortifacient. When administered within 72 hours after intercourse, the estrogen–progestin regimen is estimated to be 75 to 80% effective and is safe.[114] Significant side effects include nausea (50%) and vomiting (20%), but overall the regimen is well tolerated. An antiemetic can be prescribed to be taken 1 hour prior to the first dose. Women should expect their menses in 21 days: if menstruation does not occur, then medical evaluation and pregnancy testing should be performed. Other regimens include mifepristone, danazol, and insertion of a copper IUD within 5 days following intercourse.

Surgical Sterilization

Over 1 million voluntary sterilization procedures are performed annually (640,000 tubal ligations and 500,000 vasectomies).[92] Immediate postpartum procedures account for approximately one-third of all U.S. tubal sterilizations.[115] The most common type of procedure performed is the partial salpingectomy, or Pomeroy procedure, via a small infraumbilical incision.[115] Other surgical ligation techniques, such as the Irving or Uchida procedures, are usually performed at the time of cesarean delivery. Mechanical devices, such as surgical clips or silastic rings, can be used, but the edematous postpartum fallopian tubes require careful placement to decrease the likelihood of failure.[115]

All methods of sterilization are highly effective. The previously accepted failure rate of less than 1% was based on cumulative data from many small studies with different occlusion methods. However, data from the U.S. Collaborative Review of Sterilization (CREST) demonstrated a higher rate of method failure than previously recognized.[116] CREST is a prospective cohort study with over 10,000 women followed for up to 10 years. This study found that the risk of pregnancy persists for many years after the procedure and varies by method of tubal occlusion and patient's age. Young women were found to be at increased risk for failure, with an overall 10-year cumulative risk of

18.5 pregnancies per 1000 procedures performed. Of the 143 sterilization failures, the cumulative 10-year probabilities of pregnancy based on method used were: spring-loaded clip (36.5 per 1000); unipolar (7.5 per 1000); and postpartum partial salpingectomy (7.5 per 1000). When the cumulative risk of pregnancy was stratified based on age and method used, the highest failure rates were noted in women under 30 with a bipolar procedure (54.3 per 1000) and spring-loaded clip (52.1 per 1000). Interestingly, the CREST study found that the 10-year cumulative life-table probability of failure was 7.5 pregnancies per 1000 procedures for postpartum partial salpingectomy versus 20.1 per 1000 procedures for interval partial salpingectomy.[116] The authors concluded that the difference was due to chance or bias and could not be explained otherwise.

The risk of ectopic pregnancy was also found to be greater 2 or more years after the procedure than immediately after sterilization.[117] Thirty to 36% of all tubal sterilization failures resulted in ectopic pregnancy.[117,118] The 10-year cumulative probability of ectopic pregnancy for all methods of sterilization combined was 7.3 per 1000 procedures. The cumulative probability varied substantially according to the method used and the woman's age at the time of sterilization. Women under the age of 30 who underwent bipolar fulguration had a 27-fold higher risk of ectopic pregnancy (31.9 vs. 1.2 per 1000 procedures) than women under age 30 who underwent postpartum partial salpingectomy.[117] For women over the age of 30, no significant differences were detected in the probability of ectopic pregnancy among the different methods of tubal occlusion. The authors concluded that the primary effect of age on the risk of ectopic pregnancy is its effect on fecundity.

The major disadvantages of female sterilization include regret, surgical complications, and possible menstrual function changes. In an earlier report of the CREST data, 7% of women reported regret on at least one occasion following sterilization.[92] Risk factors include young age at the time of the procedure, (20- to 24-year-old women versus 30- to 34-year-old women), postpartum versus interval, low income, and longer time period elapsed since procedure—i.e., there was a higher rate of regret at 5 years after the procedure. These issues emphasize the importance of thorough presterilization counseling. Surgical complications are usually minor and occur in less than 1% of all procedures.[115] The mortality rate is 1 to 2 deaths per 100,000 procedures, which are most commonly the result of anesthetic complications.[92] Other specific complications include surgical trauma, burns, and wound infections. Menstrual function changes include an increase in menstrual flow and dysmenorrhea, although there is inconsistency between studies about whether the entity of posttubal syndrome exists.[92] One study found a threefold increased risk of hysterectomy in younger women following tubal sterilization, but there was no increased risk in older women.[92] A significant noncontraceptive benefit of tubal occlusion is the apparent protective effect against ovarian cancer.[92]

Vasectomy involves the occlusion of the vas deferens either by surgical ligation or thermocautery or electrocautery. The procedure is easily performed on an outpatient basis in approximately 20 minutes. Complications are uncommon and include vasovagal reaction, internal scrotal bleeding or hematoma, wound infection, and local anesthetic toxicity.[119] Vasectomy provides highly effective contraception, with a failure rate of 0.15% in the first year.[119] Disadvantages are few, with no long-term adverse effects.[8] Regret is expressed by 5 to 10% of men.[8,115] There are weak and conflicting epidemiologic data linking vasectomy to an increased risk of prostate cancer, which is an unlikely causal relationship.[119]

Postpartum Psychiatric Events

Although it has long been thought that pregnancy confers emotional well-being, the development of mood disorders during the postpartum period is one of the most common obstetrical complications, second in frequency only to cesarean delivery.[120,121] Up to 12.5% of all psychiatric hospital admissions of women occur during the puerperium,[122] and the Diagnostic and Statistical Manual of Mental Disorders, 4th ed. (DSM-IV) now includes the modifier for "postpartum onset" of mood disorders with symptoms starting within 4 weeks postpartum.[123] The three major subtypes of postpartum mood disorders include maternity blues, postpartum depression, and postpartum psychosis (Table 22-8).

Postpartum Blues

Postpartum, or maternity, blues are defined as depressed mood experienced shortly after birth.[124] The condition is manifested by mood lability, depressed affect, increased sensitivity to criticism, tearfulness, fatigue, irritability, poor concentration, and despondency. The onset of symptoms is usually within 1 to 5 days after delivery. The symptoms typically last from 2 to 3 days and usually resolve within 10 days of presentation.[120,121,125-127] This condition affects 50 to 80% of postpartum women.[124] Causes are unknown, but biologic correlates include low serum tryptophan levels, altered platelet monoamine oxidase activity, and increased serum-bound cortisol levels.[120,121,125-127] Because of the transient nature of the symptoms, little intervention by the health-care practitioner is needed other than reassurance and close follow-up. However, up to 20% of women with maternity blues will develop an episode of major depression within the first year postpartum.[124,128]

	Maternity Blues	Postpartum Depression	Postpartum Psychosis
Incidence	50–80%	10–20%	1–2/1000 deliveries
Symptoms	Insomnia, tearfulness, fatigue, irritability, poor concentration, depressed affect	Irritability, mood lability, evening exacerbation of symptoms, insomnia, phobias, anxiety, and obsessive worrying	Confusion, attention deficit, distractibility, and clouded sensorium
Onset	1–5 days	2 wk–12 mo	Acute, over 24–72 hr within 2 to 3 days after delivery
Resolution	10 days	3–14 mo	Variable
Cause	Unknown	Unknown	Unknown
Recurrence	High	50%	33–51%
Risk of suicide	None	Low, but still present	Moderate
Risk of infanticide	None	Low	4%
Treatment	Reassurance, time, and support	Antidepressants, psychotherapy, ECT	Antidepressants, psychotherapy, ECT; hospitalization often necessary

TABLE 22-8
POSTPARTUM MOOD DISORDERS

Adapted and reprinted with permission from Depressive disorders in women: diagnosis, treatment, and monitoring. APGO Monograph. Washington, DC: Association of Professors of Gynecology and Obstetrics, 1997.

Postpartum Depression

Postpartum depression (PPD) affects 10 to 22% of women and up to 26% of adolescent mothers.[120] Symptoms usually appear between 2 weeks and 12 months postpartum, and may last from 3 months to 14 months or longer.[120,121,125-127] For 60% of these women, the onset of PPD will represent their first episode of depression.[128] Compared with other non-puerperal depressive disorders, PPD is specifically characterized by increased levels of irritability, mood lability, evening exacerbation of symptoms, insomnia, phobias, anxiety, and obsessive worrying.[120,121,125-127]

Various risk factors can help identify women susceptible to depression during this period (Table 22-9).[129] The presence of prenatal depressive symptoms is the best predictor of PPD.[130] Other strong indicators include a personal or family history of depression, a prior episode of postpartum depression, and a history of depression predating the pregnancy. Postpartum depression will develop in up to 30% of women who have a history of depression prior to conception. Once an episode of PPD occurs, the risk of a subsequent episode in future pregnancies increases by 50%.[120,121,125-127] PPD is less likely than other depressive disorders to lead to suicide, but the risk is still present. Although the cause remains an enigma, large shifts in levels of serum and central nervous system estrogen, progesterone, cortisol, and β-endorphin may be contributory,[120,121,125-127] but no studies have definitively correlated specific neuroendocrine changes within the puerperal hypothalamic–pituitary axis and the development of postpartum depression.[131]

Any woman displaying features characteristic of PPD requires further clinical evaluation. It is also important for the physician to survey the patient's current psychosocial situation and to be wary of overlapping symptoms that could be caused by other clinical disorders. Thus, the work-up should include a directed history, medical review of systems, physical examination, and limited diagnostic testing as indicated, with a complete blood count to rule out significant anemia, measurement of electrolyte and glucose levels to rule out hypokalemia or hypoglycemia, ultrasensitive testing of thyroid-stimulating hormone levels to detect thyroid dysfunction, and urine drug screen to rule out substance abuse.

As clinicians, it is critical to elicit this type of history from our patients, as our society often anticipates that new mothers invariably experience only joy and happiness following delivery and that negative feelings are incompatible with motherhood. Accordingly, many women may feel embarrassed or ashamed about negative emotions and would be less likely to volunteer such information.[129] For this reason, psychometric testing has proven invaluable in screening for PPD. Various rating scales for early detection include a postpartum depression checklist and the Edinburgh Postnatal Depression Scale (EPDS). The PPD checklist is a physician-administered screen that helps to identify women for further evaluation of depressive symptoms.[132] The EPDS is a multilingual, self-rated measure that correlates well with physician-rated scales and diagnosis of depressive disorder.[133] Considered the most widely accepted scale, the EPDS is easily administered and scored, but it is not intended to replace a thorough history and further evaluation in making the diagnosis of PPD.

The initial treatment for PPD is supportive care and reassurance from family and health-care professionals. For women who do not respond to these simple measures, specific interventions include psychotherapy, pharmacotherapy, and electroconvulsive therapy (ECT). Controlled trials have shown that women with postpartum depression respond over time to interpersonal psychotherapy and nondirective counseling.[134] Antidepressants, such as tricyclic antidepressants (TCAs) and the newer, selective serotonin reuptake inhibitors (SSRIs), can also be used in the treatment of PPD. TCAs are effective in 60 to 70% of nonpuerperal patients,[135] but their disadvantages arise from the fact that they affect several neurotransmitter systems other than the ones involved in depressive disorders. While this class of drugs effectively blocks the reuptake of serotonin and norepinephrine, they

---

TABLE 22-9
RISK FACTORS FOR POSTPARTUM DEPRESSION

Personal or familial history of depression (especially postpartum depression)
Prior episode of postpartum depression (50% risk of recurrence with subsequent pregnancies)
History of depression prior to conception (up to 30% risk)
Anxiety and depression during pregnancy
Poor postpartum support
Stressful or adverse life events
Marital instability
Infants with health problems or disagreeable temperaments
Unwanted pregnancy

Reprinted with permission from Beck.[129]

also antagonize muscarinic–cholinergic, histaminergic, and α-noradrenergic receptors. Such blockades lead to the characteristic anticholinergic side effects of dry mouth, constipation, blurred vision, urinary retention, and cardiac arrhythmias; antihistaminic effect of sedation; and the anti-noradrenergic effect of orthostatic hypotension, reflex tachycardia, and dizziness.[136] Thus, patients may have to experience several adverse effects in order to derive therapeutic benefits. In addition, there is a potential for substantial weight gain, as well as a highly lethal risk if the medication is taken in overdose.[137,138] Onset of action usually takes 3 to 5 weeks before improvement is detected, and one study has shown that women may be less responsive to the medication than men.[139]

SSRIs, on the other hand, affect only the reuptake of serotonin, and therefore, have little to no effect on the other neurotransmitter systems. Although no more effective or faster acting than TCAs, SSRIs are generally better tolerated. Specifically, SSRIs are nonsedating and have no anticholinergic, hypotensive, or cardiac conduction effects. They are much safer in overdose.[138,140] They are, however, considered potentially lethal if given in combination with monoamine oxidase inhibitors.[137] The main side effects of SSRIs are nausea, which varies from 21% to 37%, depending upon the particular agent,[140] and sexual dysfunction, specifically with respect to achieving orgasm, which can occur in 10% to 30% of patients.[136] Both sertraline (Zoloft, Roerig, New York), an SSRI, and nortriptyline (Pamelor, Sandoz Pharmaceuticals, East Hanover, NJ), a TCA, have proven beneficial as single agents in the treatment of PPD.[141,142]

Combination treatment using behavioral therapy and antidepressant pharmacological therapy has also been studied in a randomized controlled trial of 61 non–breast-feeding women with postpartum depression. This investigation compared fluoxetine (Prozac, Lilly Research Laboratories, Indianapolis), a nonsedating, anxiolytic SSRI, versus placebo, and either one or six sessions of cognitive-behavioral counseling. Fluoxetine alone was found to be an effective treatment for PPD.[143] In addition, a course of six sessions of simple counseling derived from cognitive-behavioral therapy was found to be more effective than a single session. However, there was no advantage in receiving both therapies. Since many women with PPD are reluctant to take medication while breast-feeding, this study provides some reassurance that simple cognitive-behavioral therapy can be as effective as pharmacological therapy.

Transdermal estrogen has been found to have a beneficial effect in the treatment of PPD.[144] Unfortunately, further studies are needed to determine when, and in whom, to initiate this therapy, as well as duration of treatment. ECT is also beneficial in the treatment of PPD in cases of depression refractory to psychotherapy and pharmacotherapy and often provides rapid improvement for patients with vegetative depression or suicidal ideation.[145] Furthermore, ECT can be used safely in breast-feeding mothers without risk to the nursing infant.[146]

After a woman has been diagnosed with PPD, all treatment options should be reviewed with her, keeping in mind that few treatment studies for PPD have been conducted and that essentially no definitive treatment guidelines exist for clinicians to use. All antidepressants are lipid-soluble, and, therefore, are secreted into breast milk, but the concentration varies greatly depending on the individual agent. Furthermore, since there is a lack of data regarding the indirect effects of these medications on the breast-fed newborn, each situation needs to be individualized based on the patient's severity of symptoms and responsiveness to alternative interventions. Most of the information on SSRIs and breast-feeding is based on case reports, without the benefit of long term data on neurobehavioral effects and teratogenicity. The American Academy of Pediatrics does not specifically discourage breast-feeding in mothers on antidepressants.[147]

Breast milk is not only considered the optimal source of nutrients for infants, but the physical act of breast-feeding also provides enormous psychological fulfillment for the nursing mother. For some women, a prohibition against breast-feeding may place undue feelings of inadequacy, guilt, and failure upon them, which could potentially worsen their depression. As clinicians, we can only assist the patient in making an informed decision, balancing the risks versus the benefits of proceeding with or without pharmacotherapy for both the mother and infant. The patient's decision and the process of informed consent should be clearly documented in the medical record. In women who choose to breast-feed, the practice of timed feedings may reduce the infants' exposure to the medication. Specifically, the mother should take the medication just after she has breast-fed and just before the infant is expected to have a period of sleep.[147]

Postpartum Psychosis

The de novo development of postpartum psychosis is an extremely rare event that affects 1 to 2 mothers per 1000 live births.[148] The abrupt and unexpected onset of overt psychotic symptoms usually occurs over 24 to 72 hours within the first 2 to 3 days after delivery, but the risk for presentation persists for the first month postpartum. The majority of women affected typically have a history of bipolar disorder or unipolar depression with psychotic features. The cause is unknown, but may be related to low estrogen levels, which could precipitate psychosis through supersensitization of central dopamine receptors.[120,121,125-127]

Symptoms are often similar to those of organic brain syndrome, including confusion, attention deficit, distractability, and clouded sensorium. In addition, 50% of women with overt psychosis will also meet the diagnostic criteria for major depression, and the risk of a subsequent episode in future pregnancies increases by 33 to 51%. These women require psychiatric consultation. Often, hospitalization is necessary in the acute setting, but the overall prognosis is favorable, with the duration of illness usually lasting only 2 to 3 months. The risk of infanticide is considerably higher in this group of patients as compared with the other mood disorders, and any woman conveying neglect or threats of harm to her infant requires further evaluation and possible intervention.

REFERENCES

1. Hytten FE, Cheyne GA. The size and composition of the human pregnant uterus. J Obstet Gynaecol Br Commonw 1966;76:400.

2. Sharman A. Postpartum regeneration of the human endometrium. J Anat 1953;87:1.

3. Anderson WR, Davis J. Placental site involution. Am J Obstet Gynecol 1968;102:23.

4. Oppenheimer LW, Sherriff EA, Goodman JDS, Shah D, James CE. The duration of lochia. Br J Obstet Gynaecol 1986;93:754.

5. Visness CM, Kennedy KI, Ramos R. The duration and character of postpartum bleeding among breast-feeding women. Obstet Gynecol 1997;89:159.

6. Resnick R. The puerperium. In: Creasy RK, Resnick R, eds. Maternal fetal medicine: principles and practice. 3rd ed. Philadelphia: Saunders, 1994:140.

7. Coppleson M, Reid BL. A colposcopic study of the cervix during pregnancy and the puerperium. J Obstet Gynaecol Br Commonw 1966;73:575.

8. Speroff L, Darney PD. A clinical guide for contraception. 2nd ed. Baltimore: Williams & Wilkins, 1996.

9. Campbell OM, Gray RH. Characteristics and determinants of postpartum ovarian function in women in the United States. Am J Obstet Gynecol 1993;169:55.

10. Sharman A. Menstruation after childbirth. J Obstet Gynaecol Br Commonw 1951;58:440.

11. McNeilly AS. Suckling and the control of gonadotropin secretion. In: Knobil E, Neill JD, eds. The physiology of reproduction. 2nd ed. New York: Raven Press; 1994:1179.

12. Howie PW, McNeilly AS, Houston MJ, et al. Effect of supplementary food on suckling patterns and ovarian activity during lactation. BMJ 1981;283:757.

13. Rivera R, Kennedy K, Ortiz E, et al. Breast-feeding and the return to ovulation in Durango, Mexico. Fertil Steril 1988;49:780.

14. Lewis PR, Brown JB, Renfree MB, et al. The resumption of ovulation and menstruation in a well-nourished population of women breastfeeding for an extended period of time. Fertil Steril 1991;55:529.

15. Visness CM, Kennedy KI, Gross BA, et al. Fertility of fully breast-feeding women in the early postpartum period. Obstet Gynecol 1997;89:164.

16. Gray RH, Campbell OM, Apelo R, et al. Risk of ovulation during lactation. Lancet 1990;335:25.

17. McNeilly AS, Glasier A, Howie PW. Endocrine control of lactational infertility. In: Dobbing J, ed. Maternal nutrition and lactational infertility. New York: Vevey/Raven Press, 1985:1.

18. Kennedy KI, Rivera RR, McNeilly AS. Consensus statement of the use of breastfeeding as a family planning method. Contraception 1989;39:477.

19. Rasmusen NG, Hornnes PJ, Hegedus L. Ultrasonographically determined thyroid size in pregnancy and postpartum: the goitrogenic effect of pregnancy. Am J Obstet Gynecol 1989;160:1216.

20. Jausson R, Dahlberg PA, Winsa B, et al. The postpartum period constitutes an important risk for the development of clinical Graves disease in young women. Acta Endocrinol 1987;116:321.

21. Bowes WA Jr. Postpartum care. In: Gabbe SG, Niebyl JR, Simpson JL, Anderson GD, eds. Obstetrics: normal and problem pregnancies. New York: Churchill Livingstone, 1986:691.

22. Pritchard JA, Baldwin RM, Dickey JC, Wiggins KM. Blood volume changes in pregnancy and the puerperium. II. Red blood cell loss and changes in apparent blood volume during and following vaginal delivery, cesarean section, and cesarean section plus total hysterectomy. Am J Obstet Gynecol 1962;84:1271.

23. Lindesman R, Miller MM. Blood volume changes during the immediate postpartum period. Obstet Gynecol 1963;21:40.

24. Ueland K. Maternal cardiovascular dynamics. VIII. Intrapartum blood volumes changes. Am J Obstet Gynecol 1976;126:671.

25. Paintin DB. The size of the total red cell volume in pregnancy. J Obstet Gynaecol Br Commonw 1962;69:719.

26. Walters WAW, MacGregor WG, Hills M. Cardiac output at rest during pregnancy and the puerperium. Clin Sci 1966;30:1.

27. Hytten FE, Lind T. Volume and composition of the blood. In: Hytten FE, Lind T, eds. Diagnostic indices in pregnancy. Basel: Documenta Geigy, 1973:36.

28. Laros RK, Alger LS. Thromboembolism and pregnancy. Clin Obstet Gynecol 1979;22:871.

29. Barbour LA. Current concepts of anticoagulation therapy in pregnancy. Obstet Gynecol Clin North Am 1997; 24:499.

30. American College of Obstetricians and Gynecologists. Postpartum hemorrhage. ACOG Technical Bulletin no. 243. January 1998.

31. Baird D. The upper urinary tract in pregnancy and puerperium, with special reference to pyelitis of pregnancy. J Obstet Gynaecol Br Emp 1935;42:733.

32. Rubi RA, Sala NC. Ureteral function in pregnant women. III. Effect of different positions and of fetal delivery upon ureteral tonus. Am J Obstet Gynecol 1968;101:230.

33. Dure-Smith P. Pregnancy dilatation of the urinary tract: the iliac sign and its significance. Radiology 1970;96:545.

34. Peake SL, Roxburgh HB, Langlois SL. Ultrasonic assessment of hydronephrosis of pregnancy. Radiology 1983; 146:167.

35. Sims EAH, Krantz KE. Serial studies of renal function during pregnancy and the puerperium in normal women. J Clin Invest 1958;37:1764.

36. DeAlvarez RR. Renal glomerulotubular mechanism during normal pregnancy. Am J Obstet Gynecol 1958; 75:931.

37. Crowell DT. Weight change in the postpartum period: a review of the literature. J Nurse Midwifery 1995;40:418.

38. Schauberger CW, Rooney BL, Brimer LM. Factors that influence weight loss in the puerperium. Obstet Gynecol 1992;79:424.

39. Lederman SA. The effect of pregnancy weight gain on later obesity. Obstet Gynecol 1993;82:148.

40. Guidelines for perinatal care. 4th ed. Washington, DC: American Academy of Pediatrics and American College of Obstetricians and Gynecologists, 1997.

41. Droegmueller W. Cold sitz baths for relief of postpartum perineal pain. Clin Obstet Gynecol 1980;23:1039.

42. Braverman P, Egerter S, Pearl M, Marchi K, Miller C. Early discharge of newborns and mothers: a critical review of literature. Pediatrics 1995;96:716.

43. Grullon KE, Grimes DA. The safety of early postpartum discharge: a review and critique. Obstet Gynecol 1997; 90:860.

44. Khong TY, Khong TK. Delayed postpartum hemorrhage: a morphologic study of causes and their relation to other pregnancy disorders. Obstet Gynecol 1993;82:17.

45. Berkowitz RS, Goldstein DP. Gestational trophoblastic neoplasia. In: Berek JS, Hacker NF, eds. Practical gynecologic oncology. 2nd ed. Baltimore: Williams & Wilkins, 1994:457.

46. Cunningham FG, MacDonald PC, Gant NF, Leveno KJ, Gilstrap LC III. Other disorders of the puerperium. In: Cunningham FG, ed. Williams obstetrics. 19th ed. East Norwalk, CT: Appleton & Lange; 1993:643.

47. King PA, Duthie SJ, Dip V, et al. Secondary postpartum hemorrhage. Aust NZ J Obstet Gynaecol 1989;29:394.

48. Lee CY, Madrazo B, Drukker BH. Ultrasonic evaluation of the postpartum uterus in the management of postpartum bleeding. Obstet Gynecol 1981;58:227.

49. Shy KK, Eschenbach DA. Fatal perineal cellulitis from an episiotomy site. Obstet Gynecol 1979;54:292.

50. Christensen S, Anderson G, Detlefsen GU, Hansen PK. Treatment of episiotomy wound infections: incision and drainage versus incision, curettage and sutures under antibiotic cover—a randomized trial. Ugeskr Laeger 1994;156:4829.

51. Giuliano A, Lewis F, Hadley K, et al. Bacteriology of necrotizing fasciitis. Am J Surg 1977;134:52.

52. Stone HH, Martin JD. Synergistic necrotizing cellulitis. Ann Surg 1972;175:702.

53. Cotran RS, Kumar V, Robbins SL, eds. Robbins' pathologic basis of disease. Philadelphia: Saunders, 1989:1181.

54. Tyson JE, Hwang P, Guyda H, Friesen HG. Studies of prolactin secretion in human pregnancy. Am J Obstet Gynecol 1972;113:14.

55. Murphy LJ, Murphy LC, Stead B, Sutherland RL, Lazarus L. Modulation of lactogenic receptors by progestins in cultured human breast cancer cells. J Clin Endocrinol Metab 1985;62:280.

56. Simon WE, Pahnke VG, Holzel F. In vitro modulation of prolactin binding to human mammary carcinoma cells by steroid hormones and prolactin. J Clin Endocrinol Metab 1985;60:1243.

57. Battin DA, Marrs RP, Fleiss PM, Mishell DR Jr. Effect of suckling on serum prolactin, luteinizing hormone, follicle-stimulating hormone, and estradiol during prolonged lactation. Obstet Gynecol 1985;65:785.

58. McNeilly AS, Robinson, KA, Houston MJ, Howe PW. Release of oxytocin and prolactin in response to suckling. BMJ 1983;286:257.

59. Dawood MY, Khan-Dawood FS, Wahl RS, Fuchs F. Oxytocin release and plasma anterior pituitary and gonadal hormones in women during lactation. J Clin Endocrinol Metab 1981;52:678.

60. Ramin SM, Cunningham FG. The breast in pregnancy and lactation. In: Cunningham FG, ed. Williams obstetrics. East Norwalk, CT: Appleton & Lange; 1998(Suppl):1.

61. Jelliffe DB, Jelliffe EFP. The volume and composition of human milk in poorly nourished communities—a review. Am J Clin Nutrit 1978;31:492.

62. Murray L, Seger D. Drug therapy during pregnancy and lactation. Emerg Med Clin N Am 1994;12:129.

63. Sagraves R. Drugs in breast milk: a scientific explanation. J Pediatr Health Care 1997;11:230.

64. Cravioto A, Tello A, Villafan H, Ruiz J, del Vedovo S, Neeser JR. Inhibition of localized adhesion of enteropathogenic Esherichia coli to Hep-2 cells by immunoglobulin and oligosaccharide fractions of human colostrum and breast milk. J Infect Dis 1991;163:1247.

65. Graffy J. Breast-feeding: the general practitioner's role. Practitioner. 1992;236:322.

66. Hill P. Maternal attitudes and infant feeding among low-income mothers. J Hum Lact 1988;4:7.

67. American Academy of Pediatrics. Breastfeeding and the use of human milk. Pediatrics 1997;100:1035.

68. National Research Council, Subcommittee on the Tenth Edition on RDAs. Recommended dietary allowances. 10th ed. Washington, DC: National Academy Press, 1989.

69. CDC. Recommendations for prevention and control of hepatitis C virus (HCV) infection and HCV-related chronic disease. MMWR. 1998;47:9.

70. American Academy of Pediatrics. Human milk, breast-feeding, and transmission of human immunodeficiency virus in the United States. Pediatrics 1995;96:977.

71. Morgans D. Bromocriptine and postpartum lactation suppression. Br J Obstet Gynaecol 1995;102:851.

72. Food and Drug Administration. Bromocriptine indication withdrawal. FDA Med Bull 1994;24:2.

73. Alexander JM, Grant AM, Campbell MJ. Randomized controlled trial of breast shells and Hoffman's exercises for inverted and nonprotractile nipples. BMJ 1990; 304:1030.

74. DeCoopman JM. Breast-feeding management for healthcare professionals. 2nd ed. Wyandotte, MI: Resources for lactation professionals, 1995:51.

75. Shadigian E, Van Bonn P, Cook M. Management of breast-feeding. Female Patient 1998;23:47.

76. Lawrence RA. Breastfeeding: a guide for the medical profession. 4th ed. St Louis: Mosby-Year Book, 1994:215.

77. Almeida OD, Kitay DZ. Lactation suppression and puerperal fever. Am J Obstet Gynecol 1986;154:940.

78. Stehman FB. Infections and inflammations of the breast. In: Hindle WH, ed. Breast disease for gynecologists. Norwalk, CT: Appleton & Lange, 1990:151.

79. Niebyl JR, Spence MR, Parmley TH. Sporadic (nonepidemic) puerperal mastitis. J Reprod Med 1978;20:97.

80. Hager WD. Mastitis. In: Mead PB, Hager WD. eds. Infection protocols for obstetrics and gynecology. Montvale, NJ: Medical Economics, 1992;27.

81. Thomsen AC, Espersen T, Maigaard S. Course and treatment of milk stasis, noninfectious inflammation of the breast, and infectious mastitis in nursing women. Am J Obstet Gynecol 1984;149:492.

82. Hindle WH. Other benign breast problems. Clin Obstet Gnecol. 1994;37:916.

83. Devereux AP. Acute puerperal mastitis. Am J Obstet Gynecol. 1970;108:78.

84. Matheson I, Aursnes I, Horgen M, Aabo O, Melby K. Bacteriological findings and clinical symptoms in relation to clinical outcome in puerperal mastitis. Acta Obstet Gynecol Scand. 1988;67:723.

85. Hankins GDV, Clark SL, Cunningham FG, Gilstrap LC III. eds. Breast disease during pregnancy and lactation. In: Operative obstetrics. Norwalk, CT: Appleton & Lange, 1995:667.

86. Scott-Conner CEH, Schorr SJ. The diagnosis and management of breast problems during pregnancy and lactation. Am J Surg 1995;170:401.

87. Karstrup S, Solvin J, Nolsoe CP, Nilsson P, Khattar S, Loren I, et al. Acute puerperal breast abscesses: ultrasound-guided drainage. Radiology 1993;188:807.

88. Dixon JM. Repeated aspiration of breast abscesses in lactating women. BMJ 1988;297:1517.

89. Eschenbach DA. Acute postpartum infection. Emerg Med Clin North Am 1985;3:87.

90. Efficacy of lactational amenorrhea method as a family planning method (protocol for a Cochrane review). In: The Cochrane Library, Issue 4, 1998. Oxford: update Software.

91. WHO Task Force on Oral Contraceptives: Contraception during the postpartum period and during lactation: the effects on women's health. Int J Obstet Gynaecol 1987;25(Suppl):13.

92. American College of Obstetricians and Gynecologists: Hormonal contraception. ACOG Technical Bulletin no. 198. October 1994.

93. Kaunitz AM. Considering postpartum contraception and the role of lactation. Dialogues in Contraception 1997; 5:5.

94. Labbok M, Cooney K, Coly S. Guidelines: breastfeeding, family planning and the lactational amenorrhea method-LAM. Washington, DC: Institute for Reproductive Health, 1994.

95. Kennedy KI, Labbok MH, Van Look PFA. Consensus statement: lactational amenorrhea method for family planning. Int J Gynecol Obstet 1996;54:55.

96. Family Health International. Breastfeeding as a family planning method. Lancet 1988;2:1204.

97. Alvarez F, Guiloff E, Brache V, et al. New insights on the mode of action of intrauterine contraceptive devices in women. Fertil Steril 1988;49:768.

98. Sivin I. IUDs are contraceptives, not abortifacients: a comment on research and belief. Stud Fam Plann 1989; 20:355.

99. Ortiz ME, Croxatto HB. The mode of action of IUDs. Contraception 1987;36:37.

100. Sivin I, Diaz S, Pavez M, et al. Two-year comparative trial of the gyne T 380 slimline and gyne T 380 intra-uterine copper devices. Contraception 1991;44:481.

101. Vessey M, Meisler L, Flavel R, Yeates D. Outcome of pregnancy in women using different methods of contraception. Br J Obstet Gynaecol 1979;86:548.

102. Belhadj H, Sivin I, Diaz S, et al. Recovery of fertility after use of the levonorgestrel 20 mcg/day or copper T 380Ag intrauterine device. Contraception 1986;34:261.

103. Treiman K, Liskin L. Intrauterine devices, pop reports, Series B. Baltimore: Population Information Program, Johns Hopkins University, 1988.

104. WHO Special Programme of Research, Development and Research Training in Human Reproduction. Task Force on Intrauterine devices for Fertility Regulation, a multinational case-control study of ectopic pregnancy. Clin Reprod Fertil 1985;3:131.

105. Chi I-C, Farr G. Postpartum IUD contraception: a review of an international experience. Adv Contracept 1989;5:127.

106. Mishell DR Jr, Roy S. Copper intrauterine contraceptive device event rates following insertion 4 to 8 weeks postpartum. Am J Obstet Gynecol 1982;143:29.

107. Thiery M, Van Kets H, Van Der Pas H. Immediate post-placental IUD insertion: the expulsion problem. Contraception 1985;31:331.

108. Gray RH, Campbell OM, Zacur HA, Labbok MH, MacRae SL. Postpartum return of ovarian activity in nonbreastfeeding women monitored by urinary assays. J Clin Endocrinol Metab 1987;64:645.

109. Mishell DR Jr, Darney PD, Burkman RT, Sulak PJ. Practice guidelines for OC selection: update. Dialogues in Contraception 1997;5:7.

110. World Health Organization (WHO) Task Force on Oral Contraceptives, Special Programme of Research, Development, and Research Training in Human Reproduction. Effects of hormonal contraceptives on breast milk composition and infant growth. Stud Fam Plann 1988; 19:361.

111. Croxatto HB, Diaz S, Peralta O, et al. Fertility regulation in nursing women. IV. Long-term influence of a low-dose combined oral contraceptive initiated at day 30

postpartum upon lactation and infant growth. Contraception 1983;27:13.

112. WHO Special Programme of Research, Development and Research Training in Human Reproduction, Task Force on Oral Contraceptives. Effects of hormonal contraceptives on milk volume and infant growth. Contraception 1984;30:505.

113. Glasier A. Emergency postcoital contraception. N Engl J Med 1997;337:1058.

114. Trussell J, Ellertson C, Stewart F. The effectiveness of the Yupze regimen of emergency contraception. Fam Plann Perspect 1996;28:58.

115. Stewart GK, Carignan CS. Female and male sterilization. In: Hatcher RE, Trussel J, Stewart F, et al., ed. Contraceptive technology. 17th ed. New York: Arden Media, 1998:545.

116. Peterson HB, Xia Z, Hughes JM, et al. The risk of pregnancy after tubal sterilization: findings from the US collaborative review of sterilization. Am J Obstet Gynecol 1996;174:1161.

117. Peterson HB, Xia Z, Hughes JM, Wilcox LS, Ratliff Tylor L, Trussell J. The risk of ectopic pregnancy after tubal sterilization. N Engl J Med 1997;336:762.

118. Napolitano PG, Vu K, Rosa C. Pregnancy after failed tubal sterilization. J Reprod Med 1196;41:609.

119. Burkman RT. Contraceptive sterilization: trends, options, and surprising new data. Dialogues in Contraception 1997;5:5.

120. Stowe ZN, Nemeroff CB. Women at risk for postpartum onset major depression. Am J Obstet Gynecol 1995; 173:639.

121. Horowitz JA, Damato E, Solon L, Von Metzsch G, Gill V. Postpartum depression: issues in clinical assessment. J Perinatol 1995;15:268.

122. Duffy CL. Postpartum depression: identifying women at risk. Genesis 1983;11:21.

123. American Psychiatric Association. Diagnostic and statistical manual of mental disorders, 4th ed. Washington, DC: American Psychiatric Association, 1994:317.

124. O'Hara MW, Schlechte JA, Lewis DA, et al. Prospective study of postpartum blues: biologic and psychosocial factors. Arch Gen Psychiatry 1991;48:801.

125. Depression Guideline Panel. Depression in primary care. Vol. 1. Detection and diagnosis. Clinical practice guideline, no. 5. Rockville, MD: US Department of Health and Human Services, Public Health Service, Agency for Healthcare Policy and Research; April 1993. AHCPR publication no. 93-0550.

126. Weissman MM, Olfson M. Depression in women: implications for healthcare research. Science 1995;269:799.

127. Llewellyn AM, Stowe ZN, Nemeroff CB. Depression during pregnancy and the puerperium. J Clin Psychol 1997;58(Suppl 15):26.

128. Campbell SB, Cohn JF, Flanagan C, et al. Course and correlates of postpartum depression during the transition to parenthood. Dev Psychopathol 1992;4:29.

129. Beck CT. A checklist to identify women at risk for developing postpartum depression. J Obstet Gynecol Neonat Nurs 1998; 27:39.

130. O'Hara MW, Schlechte JA, Lewis DA, Varner MW. Controlled prospective study of postpartum mood disorders: psychological, environmental, and hormonal variables. J Abnorm Psychol 1991;100:63.

131. Depressive disorders in women: diagnosis, treatment, and monitoring. APGO Monograph. Washington, DC: Association of Professors of Gynecology and Obstetrics, 1997.

132. Stowe ZN, Landry JC, Porter MR. The use of depression rating scales in women with postpartum depression. In: New research program and abstracts of the 148th Annual Meeting of the American Psychiatric Association, May 23, 1995; Miami, Fla. Abstract NR309:138.

133. Cox JL, Holden JM, Sagovsky R, Detection of postnatal depression. Development of the 10-item Edinburgh Postnatal Depression Scale. Br J Psychiatry 1987;150:782.

134. Holden JM, Sagovsky R, Cox JL. Counselling in a general practice setting: controlled study of health visitors' intervention in treatment of postnatal depression. BMJ 1989;289:223.

135. Preskorn SH, Burke M. Somatic therapy for major depressive disorder: selection of an antidepressant. J Clin Psychiatry 1992;53(9, Suppl):5.

136. Zajecka JM. Special section: effexor. venlafaxine: a unique antidepressant medication. Innovations & Research 1994;3:7.

137. Richelson E. Pharmacology of antidepressants: characteristics of the ideal drug. Mayo Clin Proc 1994;69:1069.

138. Depression Guideline Panel. Depression in primary care, vol. 2. Treatment of major depression. Clinical Practice Guideline, no. 5. Rockville, MD: Department of Health and Human Services, Public Health Service, Agency for Healthcare Policy and Research; April 1993. AHCPR publication no. 93-0551.

139. Weissman MM, Olfson M. Depression in women: implications for healthcare research. Science 1995;269:799.

140. Rickels K, Schweizer E. Clinical overview of serotonin reuptake inhibitors. J Clin Psychiatry 1990;51(12, Suppl B):9.

141. Stowe ZN, Casarella J, Landry J, Nemeroft CB. Sertraline in the treatment of women with postpartum major depression. Depression 1995;3:49.

142. Wisner KL, Perel JM. Serum nortriptyline levels in nursing mothers and their infants. Am J Psychiatry 1991; 149:1234.

143. Appleby L, Warner R, Whitton A, et al. A controlled study of fluoxetine and cognitive-behavioural counselling in the treatment of postnatal depression. BMJ 1997; 314:932.

144. Gregoire AJP, Kumar R, Everitt AF, et al. Transdermal oestrogen for treatment of severe postnatal depression. Lancet 1996;347:930.

145. Repke JT, Berger NG. Electroconvulsive therapy in pregnancy. Obstet Gynecol 1984;63:39S.

146. Wisner KL, Perel JM. Psychopharmacologic agents and electroconvulsive therapy during pregnancy and the puerperium. In: Cohen RL, ed. Psychiatric consultation in childbirth settings: parent- and child-oriented approaches. New York: Plenum Medical, 1988:165.

147. Committee on Drugs. The transfer of drugs and other chemicals into human milk. Pediatrics. 1994;93:137.

148. Kendell RE, Chalmers JC, Platz CA. Epidemiology of puerperal psychoses. Br J Psychiatry 1987;150:662.

PART II

Gynecology/ Women's Health

SECTION 1
Women's Health Care Issues

Chapter 23

Cancer Screening

Frank W. Ling
Herbert Peterson

Five Key Points

- Cancer is either the first or second leading cause of death in all age groups of females in the United States.

- Breast cancer, cancer of the lung/bronchus, and colorectal cancer are the three leading causes of cancer and cancer deaths in women.

- The lack of proven effectiveness of a screening test does not mean that the test is ineffective, only that the quality of accumulated evidence in support of recommending the test is lacking.

- The U.S. Preventive Services Task Force provides one set of recommendations, with gradings rated A (good evidence to support) through E (good evidence to exclude).

- Other organizations also provide recommendations that may vary from those of the U.S. Preventive Services Task Force and/or each other. The clinician must individualize recommendations for each patient's unique circumstances.

As the second leading cause of death in the United States, cancer represents a major health concern for the nation. In 1994, cancer was the cause of over 500,000 deaths, approximately 23% of reported deaths.[1] The estimated number of cancer-related deaths by site for women is listed in Table 23-1.[2] Cancer remains either the leading or second-leading cause of death in females irrespective of age group. It is the leading cause of death in the 35 to 54 and 55 to 74 age group, while it is second only to accidents as the cause of death in the 1 to 14 and 15 to 34 age groups and second only to heart disease in the 75 and older patient population.[3]

Reducing the absolute number of deaths due to cancer requires intervention at many different levels, ranging from altering individual lifestyle choices to treating preinvasive disease to application of expensive, highly technologic methods in advanced cases. A critical component of promoting health and preventing morbidity and mortality related to cancer is the appropriate application of screening tests. Table 23-2 lists the estimated numbers of the most common new cancer cases in women in 1998.[4]

Cancer screening is the application of a test to detect whether or not an individual who has no signs or symptoms has the disease. In order to be an effective screening test, several criteria should be met. First, the disease should be an important health problem. Second, the disease should be detectable while it is still asymptomatic. Third, there should be acceptable methods available to treat the disease if present. Fourth, the natural history of the disease should be

Rank	Site	Number	Percent
	TABLE 23-1		
	CANCER DEATHS IN WOMEN, UNITED STATES, 1998		
1	Lung and bronchus	67,000	25
2	Breast	43,500	16
3	Colon and rectum	28,600	11
4	Pancreas	14,900	6
5	Ovary	14,500	5
6	Leukemia	12,600	4
7	Non-Hodgkin lymphoma	11,900	4
8	Endometrium	6,300	2
9	Brain and other nervous system	6,000	2
10	Stomach	5,600	2

Rank	Site	Number	Percent
	TABLE 23-2		
	NEW FEMALE CANCER CASES, UNITED STATES, 1998		
1	Breast	178,700	30
2	Lung and bronchus	80,100	13
3	Colon and rectum	67,000	11
4	Endometrium	36,100	6
5	Ovary	25,400	4
6	Non-Hodgkin lymphoma	24,300	4
7	Melanoma of skin	17,300	3
8	Pancreas	14,900	2
9	Urinary bladder	14,900	2
10	Cervix	13,700	2

known. Finally, the screening test must be safe and acceptable.

There are clear benefits derived from screening for cancer. Earlier detection of cancer improves prognosis, allows for less radical treatment, and ultimately provides for a savings in resources. In addition, there is reassurance for those whose screening results are negative. However, there are some disadvantages. There is a longer morbidity period, there is the potential for overtreatment of borderline cases, and the screening test itself may be a hazard to the patient. False positive and false negative tests results are also of concern; the former create possible morbidity resulting from the test itself or from teatment, while the latter generate false reassurance.

As described in the second edition of the *Guide to Clinical Preventive Services*, an effective screening test must be "able to detect the target condition earlier than without screening and with sufficient accuracy to avoid producing large numbers of false-positive and false-negative results." In addition, an effective screening test, when coupled with treatment of persons with early disease, "should improve the likelihood of favorable health outcomes (e.g., disease-specific morbidity or mortality) compared to treating patients when they present with signs or symptoms of the disease."[5]

Table 23-3 summarizes the categories to which scientific data are assigned in order to determine their relative value in reaching evidence-based recommendations. This scheme was adapted from that originally developed by the Canadian Task Force on the Periodic Health Examination. The recommendations provided by the U.S. Preventive Services Task Force are graded from A to E. Interventions that have been demonstrated effective or have proven benefits are given "A" (good evidence to support) or "B" (fair evidence to support) levels of recommendation. Those that have been proven ineffective or harmful have been assigned "D" (fair evidence to recommend exclusion from practice) or "E" (good evidence to exclude) recommendations.

In attempting to balance the uncertain benefit of a test with its potential harm, the Task Force acknowledged that there remains the possibility that further research in a particular field could result in a favorable benefit–harm relationship that would lead to a different level of recommendation.[6] A level C recommendation has been assigned to those tests for which there is insufficient evidence to demonstrate effectiveness or a lack thereof. As with so many areas of clinical practice, the lack of proven effectiveness does not mean that a test or maneuver is ineffective. Other factors such as potential harm to the patient,

	TABLE 23-3
	QUALITY OF EVIDENCE
I	Evidence derived from at least one properly performed randomized controlled trial
II-1	Evidence derived from controlled trials without randomization
II-2	Evidence derived from cohort or case-control studies
II-3	Evidence derived from multiple time-series with or without the intervention
III	Opinions of authorities, descriptive studies, expert committees

cost, burden of suffering, high-risk factors, patient preference, and legal requirements must all be considered.

BREAST CANCER

U.S. Preventive Services Task Force

1. 50 to 69 years old: screening every 1 to 2 years with mammography alone or mammography and annual clinical breast examination. A recommendation
2. 40 to 49 years old and over 70 years old: insufficient evidence for or against routine mammography or clinical breast examination, although other factors could affect recommendations in high-risk patients. C recommendation
3. Insufficient evidence for or against use of screening clinical examination alone or teaching of breast self-examination. C recommendation

Other Recommendations

1. Several other organizations such as the American Cancer Society (ACS), the American College of Obstetricians and Gynecologists (ACOG), and the American Medical Association (AMA) recommend screening with mammography every 1 to 2 years and annual clinical breast examination beginning at age 40. Beginning at 50 years of age, annual clinical examination as well as annual mammography have been recommended. More recently, age 40 has been the recommended age at which annual mammography and clinical examination are begun.
2. The ACS, ACOG, and the American Academy of Family Practice (AAFP) recommend routine teaching of breast self-examination.[7]

COLORECTAL CANCER

U.S. Preventive Services Task Force

1. 50 years old and older: screening with annual fecal occult blood testing or sigmoidoscopy (frequency not specified). B recommendation
2. Insufficient evidence to recommend routine screening with digital rectal examination, colonoscopy, and barium enema. C recommendation
3. Individuals at high risk for colon cancer should be referred for diagnosis and management.

Other Recommendations

1. ACS and ACOG recommend annual digital rectal examination beginning at age 40, annual fecal occult blood testing starting at age 50, and sigmoidoscopy every 3 to 5 years after age 50.
2. The American College of Radiology (ACR) recommends screening with barium enema as an alternative to sigmoidoscopy every 3 to 5 years.[8]

CERVICAL CANCER

U.S. Preventive Services Task Force

1. Pap tests for all women who have ever been sexually active and who have a cervix beginning at the age of first intercourse at least every 3 years. If sexual history is uncertain, begin at age 18. B recommendation
2. Insufficient evidence for upper-age-limit recommendation, although recommendations to discontinue over age 65 can be made on other grounds for patients with negative history. C recommendation
3. Insufficient evidence for routine screening using colposcopy or for screening for human papillomavirus infection. C recommendation

Other Recommendations

1. A consensus of the AMA, ACOG, ACS, AAFP, and others recommends annual Pap tests for all women who are or have been sexually active or who have reached age 18.
2. Pap testing at less frequent intervals after three or more normal annual smears at discretion of physician.[9]

LUNG CANCER

U.S. Preventive Services Task Force

1. Routine screening with chest radiography or sputum cytology is not recommended. D recommendation
2. Patients should be counseled against tobacco use.

Other Recommendations

No organization recommends routine screening of either the asymptomatic patients or smokers.[10]

OVARIAN CANCER

U.S. Preventive Services Task Force

1. Screening asymptomatic women with tumor markers, ultrasound, or pelvic examination is not recommended. D recommendation
2. Insufficient evidence for or against screening symptomatic women at increased risk. C recommendation

Other Recommendations

1. No organization recommends routine screening with ultrasound or serum tumor markers. Several, including ACOG, specifically recommend against such screening.
2. Careful family history-taking and annual pelvic examination recommended by many organizations.
3. National Institutes of Health (NIH) Consensus Conference recommended in patients with presumed hereditary cancer syndrome: annual pelvic examination, CA-125 measurements, and transvaginal ultrasound until childbearing completed or age 35. Prophylactic oophorectomy recommended at that time.[11]

SKIN CANCER

U.S. Preventive Services Task Force

1. Insufficient evidence to recommend for or against routine total-body examination. C recommendation
2. Consider referring patients at increased risk for malignant melanoma to skin cancer specialist.
3. Insufficient evidence to recommend periodic self-examination. C recommendation
4. Counseling of patients at increased risk for skin cancer to avoid sun exposure particularly between 10:00 a.m. and 3:00 p.m. and to wear protective clothing such as hats and shirts. B recommendation
5. Insufficient evidence to recommend for or against use of sunscreen to prevent skin cancer. C recommendation

Other Recommendations

1. ACS recommends monthly skin self-examination for all adults.

2. ACS recommends skin examination by physician every 2 to 3 years for those aged 20 to 39 and yearly for those aged 40 and over.
3. AAFP recommends complete skin evaluation for adolescents and adults with increased occupational or recreational sun exposure; also for a family or personal history of skin cancer or history of precursor lesion.
4. Several organizations recommend avoidance of both sun exposure and artificial tanning devices while recommending use of sunscreen.[12]

ORAL CANCER

U.S. Preventive Services Task Force

1. Insufficient evidence to recommend routine screening. C recommendation
2. Practitioners may choose to screen for lesions in patients who chew or smoke tobacco, older patients who drink regularly, and those with suspicious signs/symptoms.
3. Patients should be counseled regarding their use of tobacco and alcohol.
4. Persons with excessive sun exposure should be counseled to protect lips and skin from ultraviolet rays.

Other Recommendations

1. ACS recommends oral cavity examination every 3 years starting at age 20 and yearly starting at age 40.
2. National Cancer Institute recommends early detection through routine dental examinations.[13]

BLADDER CANCER

U.S. Preventive Services Task Force

1. Routine screening with urinalysis, cytology, or dipstick not recommended. D recommendation
2. Patients who smoke cigarettes should be counseled that this increases the risk for bladder cancer.

Other Recommendations

No major organization recommends routine screening in asymptomatic patients.[14]

THYROID CANCER

U.S. Preventive Services Task Force

1. Screening using ultrasound or neck palpation is not recommended. D recommendation
2. Insufficient evidence to recommend in patients with previous irradiation to head and neck, but palpation periodically justified based on factors such as patient preference or anxiety regarding cancer risk. C recommendation.

Other Recommendations

ACS recommends palpation every 3 years between the ages of 21 and 40 and annually for those over 40.[15]

REFERENCES

1. CA—a cancer journal for clinicians. New York: Lippincott-Raven, 1996;20.
2. Ibid., 11, 14.
3. Ibid., 18, 19.
4. Ibid., 11, 14.
5. Guide to clinical preventive services. 2nd ed. Report of the U.S. Preventive Task Force. Baltimore: Williams & Wilkins, 1996:xlii.
6. Ibid., li.
7. Ibid., 73–83.
8. Ibid., 89–99.
9. Ibid., 105–112.
10. Ibid., 135–138.
11. Ibid., 159–164.
12. Ibid., 144–148.
13. Ibid., 175–179.
14. Ibid., 181–185.
15. Ibid., 187–190

Chapter 24

Wellness Counseling/ Immunizations

Geeta Malik
Virginia W. Ward

Five Key Points

- Primary prevention is defined as preventing a disease process from manifesting, e.g., immunization.

- Secondary prevention is screening for asymptomatic diseases, e.g., Pap smears.

- Tertiary prevention is prevention of long-term sequelae in an established disease entity, e.g., prevention of nephropathy in a patient with diabetes.

- Exogenous obesity due to high caloric consumption/inadequate activity is second only to tobacco as a preventable cause of excess morbidity and mortality.

- In adult women, domestic violence is the most common cause of severe injury.

The bulk of medical education is focused on diagnosing and treating disease rather than preventing it. Fortunately, the medical community has begun to realize that physicians can play a vital role in preventing disease and improving quality of life by addressing issues of family history and personal habits with their patients. We seek to identify risk factors and provide counseling in the role of anticipatory guiders. This chapter seeks to address this new role in women's health care.

Three levels of prevention are commonly encountered in clinical practice. Our efforts should be directed toward primary prevention, which is defined as taking steps to prevent a disease from manifesting (e.g., childhood immunizations). The focus of wellness counseling in the United States has been secondary prevention, screening for asymptomatic disease (e.g., Pap smears). Tertiary prevention, which has been the more established role for physicians, involves preventing long-term sequelae in an already established disease entity (e.g., preventing nephropathy in a patient with diabetes).

This chapter will address both primary and secondary prevention, as it relates to wellness counseling, in the three distinct life stages during which women present to their obstetrician-gynecologist.

THE ADOLESCENT

Case 1

A 14-year-old white female presents to your office for the first time for evaluation of vaginal discharge.

Her medical history is insignificant. Patient lives with both parents and one sibling. She reports no tobacco, alcohol, or drug use. Her family history is noncontributory. Menarche occurred at 12 years of age. Her menses occur on the average of every 28 days; however, her last menstrual period was more than 8 weeks ago. The patient has had a 3-day history of white pruritic discharge; she denies any sexual activity. On physical examination, the patient appears nervous and distracted. She is a mildly obese white female. Her clothes have a strong odor of smoke. The examination is significant for an erythematous introitus and a thick vaginal discharge. The uterus is enlarged. Laboratory test results are positive for pseudohyphae on potassium hydroxide preparation and the test for human chorionic gonadotropin is positive.

Putting Prevention into Practice: Assessing the Adolescent Risk Factors

The situation presented in Case 1 is often how the adolescent first presents to the obstetrician-gynecologist for care. When patients present to us in crisis, preventive health is often pushed aside. One goal for those who care for adolescents is to develop a more proactive approach, identifying at-risk teens and providing counseling and education before high-risk behaviors are initiated. And when those high-risk behaviors—unprotected sex, obesity, and tobacco use—are identified at presentation, as in case 1, being willing to address those issues and to initiate secondary prevention.

Teenage Sexuality

Currently, 71% of teens report sexual activity. One million teenagers become pregnant annually. Teen pregnancy accounted for 13% of all U.S. births in 1991. Teen pregnancy is associated with more low-birth-weight infants—9% as compared with the national average of 4%. These babies carry a 1-month mortality rate 40 times higher than normal-sized infants and have a higher instance of morbidity as well. The teen mother is more likely to discontinue her education and thus find it difficult to care for her young child without the assistance of family or government aid. Sexually active teens comprise 3 million of the 12 million cases of sexually transmitted disease (STD) reported annually.[1] STDs, even when treatments exist, carry long-term sequelae for these young women, such as infertility, pelvic pain, higher ectopic pregnancy rates, neonatal morbidity, neurologic deficits, cervical cancer, and death. Most would agree that abstinence is the ideal for adolescents, but programs that promote abstinence only have failed to change teenage sexual activity.[2] Primary prevention should occur prior to the adolescent beginning intercourse, with the focus being on the rewards of delaying sexual activity and promoting safe sex. Information on contraception and STDs presented in an open and nonjudgmental manner has never been shown to promote sexual activity in teenagers and is fundamental to preventing the teenage pregnancy and STDs commonly seen in this age group. A discussion of sexuality with any teen should also address sexual orientation. Ten percent of teens are homosexual, and allowing them to discuss their particular issues with you in a nonjudgmental forum may provide them with support they have been unable to find elsewhere.

Maintenance of Healthy Weight

Obesity and weight-related conditions, are second only to smoking as the leading cause of death in the United States, and claim 300,000 people annually. The problem begins in childhood, where we have seen a 42% rise in obesity since 1980. By the time they reach their teen years, one of five teens is significantly overweight. Obesity appears to be the cause of 88 to 97% of cases of Type II diabetes, 57 to 70% of cases of coronary artery disease, 11% of cases of breast cancer, and 10% of cases of colon cancer diagnosed in the United States.[3] Hypertension and gallstones are more common in the obese, as are osteoarthritis and gout. Obesity raises cholesterol and triglyceride levels and lowers levels of high-density-lipoprotein cholesterol.

Obesity is defined by the American Heart Association as body weight that surpasses "desirable weight" by 20% and the excess body weight is due to fat rather than water, muscle, or bone. Desirable weight is gender-specific and based on height. Its two main causes are excess caloric consumption and inadequate exercise. New body mass index (BMI) measurements more accurately measured obesity by computing body fat:

$$BMI = $$
weight in kilograms $\div$ height in meters squared.

BMI in the range of 19 to 25 is healthy; between 25 to 28 a person may be at risk for cardiovascular

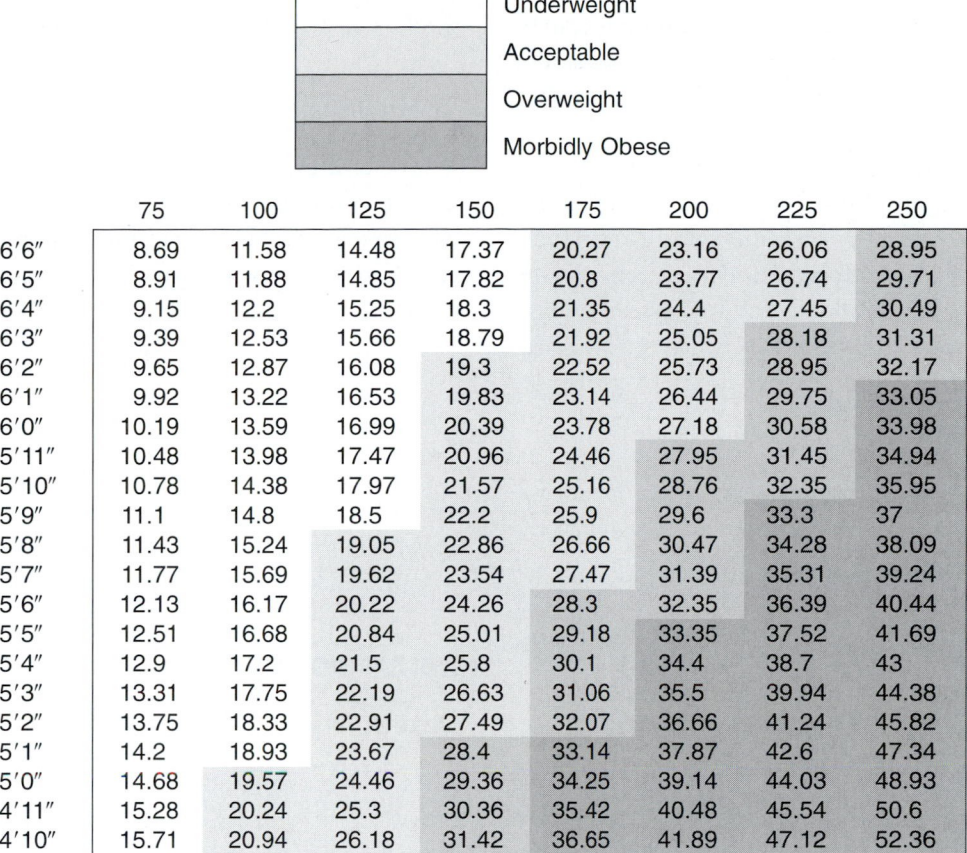

			Underweight
			Acceptable
			Overweight
			Morbidly Obese

	75	100	125	150	175	200	225	250
6'6"	8.69	11.58	14.48	17.37	20.27	23.16	26.06	28.95
6'5"	8.91	11.88	14.85	17.82	20.8	23.77	26.74	29.71
6'4"	9.15	12.2	15.25	18.3	21.35	24.4	27.45	30.49
6'3"	9.39	12.53	15.66	18.79	21.92	25.05	28.18	31.31
6'2"	9.65	12.87	16.08	19.3	22.52	25.73	28.95	32.17
6'1"	9.92	13.22	16.53	19.83	23.14	26.44	29.75	33.05
6'0"	10.19	13.59	16.99	20.39	23.78	27.18	30.58	33.98
5'11"	10.48	13.98	17.47	20.96	24.46	27.95	31.45	34.94
5'10"	10.78	14.38	17.97	21.57	25.16	28.76	32.35	35.95
5'9"	11.1	14.8	18.5	22.2	25.9	29.6	33.3	37
5'8"	11.43	15.24	19.05	22.86	26.66	30.47	34.28	38.09
5'7"	11.77	15.69	19.62	23.54	27.47	31.39	35.31	39.24
5'6"	12.13	16.17	20.22	24.26	28.3	32.35	36.39	40.44
5'5"	12.51	16.68	20.84	25.01	29.18	33.35	37.52	41.69
5'4"	12.9	17.2	21.5	25.8	30.1	34.4	38.7	43
5'3"	13.31	17.75	22.19	26.63	31.06	35.5	39.94	44.38
5'2"	13.75	18.33	22.91	27.49	32.07	36.66	41.24	45.82
5'1"	14.2	18.93	23.67	28.4	33.14	37.87	42.6	47.34
5'0"	14.68	19.57	24.46	29.36	34.25	39.14	44.03	48.93
4'11"	15.28	20.24	25.3	30.36	35.42	40.48	45.54	50.6
4'10"	15.71	20.94	26.18	31.42	36.65	41.89	47.12	52.36

Figure 24-1 Body Mass Index Chart [BMI = weight (kg) ÷ height (m^2)]

and other weight related disease according to the Mayo Clinic. The Centers for Disease Control and Prevention established 27.3 as its cutoff for defining obesity for women (Figure 24-1).

Obesity must be viewed in the same manner as other chronic diseases; rarely is the complete cure obtained, but the severity of the disease can be reduced. There are many practices adopted to reduce weight; behavior modification has been shown to produce the most sustained results. Patients should be warned to expect slow progress; it takes a deficit of 3500 calories to lose 1 lb. To lose 1 lb per week, one would have to consume 500 calories fewer each day. A weight loss of no more than 2 lb per week is now the recommended goal. Adding physical activity to a diet-modification regimen increases caloric expenditure. Programs such as Weight Watchers and Overeaters Anonymous provide information, encouragement, and support while stressing lifestyle changes in diet and exercise. The type of exercise chosen should be aerobic and should last 30 minutes, four to five times a week. A variety of nutritional supplements and meal

plans are available as well for those who wish to lose weight. Care must be taken to ensure they provide adequate nutrition. Patients may find it difficult to make the transition from these aids to "real meals" once the weight is shed.

There are also several pharmacologic options, both over-the-counter and prescription. Nonprescription drugs are usually noradrenergic agents chemically related to amphetamines, which serve as anorectics by affecting the appetite center. Scientific data have shown serious side effects as a result of use of some of the new prescription serotonergic agents, which affect the satiety center, and these drugs have been withdrawn from the market. Phentermine is still available, as are some newer agents such as orlistat (Xenical) and sibutramine (Meridia), but their use should be restricted to those who meet BMI criteria and should be used only in conjunction with diet modification and exercise. Weight is usually regained with discontinuation of medication.

When comparing weight-loss strategies, teen women tend to use more dysfunctional practices such as skipping meals, diuretics, laxatives, and induced vomiting. Fifteen percent of young women have markedly abnormal eating patterns and abuse diet aids and 5% have an eating disorder—either anorexia nervosa or bulimia.

Anorexia nervosa is a condition in which preoccupation with thinness leads to excessive and dangerous weight loss through extreme calorie restriction and excessive exercise. It affects 1% of teenage girls and claims the life of about 10% of those it affects. Those with bulimia experience cycles of bingeing and purging associated with feelings of guilt and shame. Up to 5% of United States college females are bulimic.[4]

It is the duty of the astute physician to screen for these disorders when these women present for visits. Clues on examinations that indicate young women with one of these disorders include rapidly fluctuating weight, secondary amenorrhea, dental problems, or lanugo.

Tobacco, Alcohol and Drug Use

The United States has enjoyed a 50% decrease in drug use over the past 15 years; our teens have not fared as well. Tobacco and marijuana use are on the rise and currently there are 9.5 million drinkers aged 12 to 20 years old. There is some encouraging news that teenage marijuana use is beginning to level off, especially among younger teens. Younger teens are also showing higher disapproval rates for drug use.

Our efforts at reducing teenage tobacco use should be directed to preventing smoking before it starts. Most adult smokers began smoking while they were teens. If we can prevent teens from lighting up in the first place, we can be more confident that they will remain tobacco-free. Today, 25% of Americans smoke, and while smoking is on the decline overall, adolescent tobacco use is rising—3000 adolescents become addicted each day.[5] Smoking remains the leading cause of preventable morbidity and mortality in the United States. Tobacco claims the lives of 400,000 annually from cancer, heart disease, stroke, and chronic obstructive pulmonary disease.[6] In preventing or stopping tobacco use in teens, we must make the benefit of abstention relevant to them. They may not appreciate the long-term consequences of their actions, but if you can show them how they will have more spending money, fresher breath and clothes, and an improved sports performance, they may be more likely to comply. Teaching them skills to recognize and

cope with situations in which they are more likely to smoke can help them stay away from tobacco.

Interventions in the Adolescent

The U.S. Preventive Services Task Force makes specific recommendations for interventions in the 11- to 24-year-olds (Table 24-1). In addition to those recommendations, we would add the following:

1. Teach breast self-examination and encourage monthly examinations.
2. Screen for scoliosis in the young adolescent.
3. Encourage routine use of sunscreens and discourage tanning and tanning bed use to prevent skin cancer in adulthood.
4. Moderation of noise/music volume to prevent noise-induced hearing loss in adulthood.

ADULT WOMEN

Case 2

A 28-year-old married African-American female presents to your office for a routine Pap smear. She is considering having a second child. Her medical history is insignificant. FH: strong (+) diabetes, (+) hypertension SH: (+) tobacco use and (+) alcohol on weekends, married × 3 yrs. ROS: G_1P_1. She is taking birth control pills and has normal menses. The physical examination is essentially normal except for the patient's morbid obesity.

Putting Prevention into Practice: Assessing the Adult Woman

Obstetrician-gynecologists are in an advantageous position to provide primary and secondary prevention through their access to women who are basically healthy but come in for an annual examination, i.e. to get their Pap smears. In Case 2, we have the opportunity to address both the obvious risk factors (obesity and tobacco) and the not-so-obvious risk factor (domestic violence) for this age group.

Maintenance of Healthy Weight

As discussed in the section on adolescence, obesity is now a national epidemic. Excessive weight that was tolerated in youth now begins to have an impact on your patient's current and future health. The patient may be pleased she has only gained 5 lb each year but

TABLE 24-1
U.S. PREVENTIVE SERVICES TASK FORCE RECOMMENDED INTERVENTIONS
IN YOUNG PEOPLE FROM 11 TO 24 YEARS OF AGE

Leading causes of death
    Motor vehicle-related and other unintentional injuries
    Homicide
    Suicide
    Malignant neoplasm
    Heart disease
Screening
    Height and weight
    Blood pressure
    Papanicolaou (Pap) test
    Chlamydia screen (sexually active females less than 20 years of age)
    Rubella serology or vaccination history (females more than 12 years of age)
    Assess for problem drinking
Counseling
    Injury prevention
        Lap/shoulder seat belts
        Bicycle/motorcycle/all-terrain-vehicle helmets
        Smoke detector
        Safe storage/removal of firearms from the home*
        Substance use
        Avoid tobacco use
        Avoid underage drinking and illicit drug use
        Avoid alcohol/drug use while driving, swimming, boating, etc.*
    Sexual behavior
        Prevention of sexually transmitted diseases: abstinence; avoiding high-risk behaviors;
            using condoms; female barriers with spermicide*
        Unintended pregnancy; contraception
    Diet and exercise
        Limit fat and cholesterol intake; maintain caloric balance; emphasize grains, fruits, and
            vegetables
        Adequate calcium intake (females)
        Regular physical activity*
    Dental health
        Regular visits to dental care provider*
        Floss, brush with fluoride toothpast daily
Immunizations
    Tetanus–diphtheria boosters (11 to 16 years of age)
    Hepatitis B (if not previously given)
    Measles–mumps–rubella (11 to 12 years of age, if booster not previously given)
    Varicella (11 to 12 years of age, if booster not previously given)
    Rubella (females at least 12 years of age, if not previously vaccinated)
    Chemoprophylaxis
    Multivitamin with folic acid (women planning or capable of pregnancy)
    Hormone prophylaxis (peri- and postmenopausal women)

*These interventions are suggested for low-risk patients in the general population.

Adapted from U.S. Preventive Services Task Force. Guide to clinical preventive services: report of the U.S. Preventive Services Task Force, 2nd ed. Baltimore: Williams & Wilkins, 1996.

over the next 20 years, if unchecked, will register 100 lb of additional weight. Forty-nine percent of American women over 25 years of age are obese. Sixty percent of all adult Americans are sedentary.[7] Exogenous obesity due to high calorie consumption and inadequate activity is second only to tobacco use in preventable causes of excess morbidity and mortality. All patients, particularly those with a strong family history for diabetes and hypertension, should be informed of the significant health risks that their excess weight present. Obese patients should receive nutritional counseling and a prescription to exercise (Tables 24-2 and 24-3).

Tobacco, Alcohol, and Drug Use

Substance abuse is highest in this age group, with 62 million smokers, 10 million marijuana users, and 2 million cocaine users.[8] Identifying and addressing a patient's use of these substances is the first step to stopping them.

TABLE 24-2
CONTRAINDICATIONS TO EXERCISE

Absolute Contraindications
Recent acute myocardial infarction
Unstable angina
Ventricular tachycardia and other dangerous
   dysrhythmias
Dissecting aortic aneurysm
Acute congestive heart failure
Severe aortic stenosis
Active or suspected myocarditis or pericarditis
Thrombophlebitis or intracardiac thrombi
Recent systemic or pulmonary embolus
Acute infection

Relative Contraindications
Untreated or uncontrolled severe hypertension
Moderate aortic stenosis
Severe subaortic senosis
Supraventricular dysrhythmias
Ventricular aneurysm
Frequent or complex ventricular ectopy
Cardiomyopathy
Uncontrolled metabolic disease (diabetes, thyroid disease, etc.) or electrolyte
   abnormality
Chronic or recurrent infectious disease (malaria, hepatitis, etc.)
Neuromuscular, musculoskeletal or rheumatoid diseases that are exacerbated
   by exercise
Complicated pregnancy

Adapted from British Columbia Ministry of Health and the Department of National Health and Welfare.
PAR-Q validation report.

TABLE 24-3
COMPONENTS OF AN EXERCISE PRESCRIPTION FOR CARDIORESPIRATORY FITNESS

Mode: Activities that exercise large muscle groups aerobically
Frequency: Three to five times per week
Duration: 20 to 60 minutes
Intensity: 55 to 90% of maximal heart rate; exercise intensity should be less vigorous initially for persons with a low level of fitness;
   maximal heart rate can be estimated by subtracting the age in years from 220.
Progress: Increase intensity and/or duration slowly over a number of weeks.

Derived from American College of Sports Medicine

Smokers in this age group have usually developed a physical dependence on nicotine. Assisting the patient in smoking cessation involves assessing nicotine dependence with the Fagerstrom test (Table 24-4) and recommending appropriate nicotine replacement (Table 24-5). Providing support and follow-up is important for the patient to be successful. Although 70%

of smokers want to stop smoking and 34% attempt to quit each year, only 2.5 succeed.[9]

Evaluating alcohol and drug use can be accomplished by a modified CAGE questionnaire designed by Rost and co-workers (Table 24-6). The questions are nonthreatening and may open the door to communication between the patient and physician. Once

TABLE 24-4
FAGERSTROM TEST FOR NICOTINE DEPENDENCE

Questions to Ask the Smoker	Scoring			
	0	1	2	3
1. How soon after you wake up do you smoke your first cigarette?	More than 1 hr	One-half to 1 hr	6 to 30 min	5 min or less
2. Do you find it difficult to refrain from smoking in places where it is forbidden (in church, at the library, in a movie theater)?	No	Yes		
3. Which cigarette would you hate to give up the most?	Any other	The first one in the morning		
4. How many cigarettes do you smoke per day?	Less than 10	11 to 20	21 to 30	More than 31
5. Do you smoke more frequently during the first hours after waking than during the rest of the day?	No	Yes		
6. Do you smoke if you are so ill that you are in bed most of the day?	No	Yes		

Note: Add the scores from the right-hand columns. A total score of 7 or greater indicates a high degree of dependence, possibly more severe withdrawal symptoms, greater difficulty quitting, and possibly the need for higher doses of nicotine supplements.

TABLE 24-5
FORMS OF NICOTINE REPLACEMENT

Dosage Form* Transdermal patches (hours worn per day)	Dosing Recommendations	Advantages Continuous delivery	Disadvantages Expense	Cost†
Habitrol (24)	21 mg per day for 4–6 wk, then 14 mg per day for 2–4 wk, then 7 mg per day for 2–4 wk	Fewer compliance problems than gum	Risk of skin irritation	7 mg: $109.50 for 24 patches 14 mg: $115.50 for 24 patches 21 mg: $121.50 for 24 patches
Nicoderm CQ (24)	21 mg per day for 4–6 wk, then 14 mg per day for 2–4 wk, then 7 mg per day for 2–4 wk	Less instruction time required	Risk of insomnia or nightmares	7 mg: $51.00 for 14 patches 14 mg: $55.00 for 14 patches 21 mg: $55.00 for 14 patches
Nicotrol (16)	15 mg per day for 4–12 wk	—	—	15 mg: $54.00 for 14 patches
Gum (nicotine polacrilex)		Useful on "as-needed" basis	Requires good dentition	Requires good dentition
Nicorette	2 mg per piece (maximum: 30 pieces per day); 4 mg per piece (maximum: 20 pieces per day)	Provides oral gratification	Risk of mouth irritation	$46.00 for 108 pieces; $26.50 for 48 pieces
Nicorette DS	4 mg per piece (maximum: 20 pieces per day)	—	Risk of developing dependence	$64.50 for 96 pieces

*Available over the counter or by prescription.
†Estimated cost to the pharmacist based on average wholesale prices, rounded to half-dollar amounts.

TABLE 24-6
CAGE QUESTIONNAIRE MODIFIED FOR SUBSTANCE ABUSE

1. Have you misused one of these substances more than five times in your life?
2. Have you ever found that you needed to increase your use of a substance in order to get the same effect?
3. Have you ever had emotional or psychological problems from using drugs—like feeling crazy or paranoid or uninterested in things.

Source: Rost K, Burnam MA, Smith GR. Development of screeners for depressive disorders and disorder history. Med Care 1993;31:189.

abuse or dependence is identified a multidisciplinary approach is needed to assist these patients through rehabilitation. Contacting local chapters of Alcoholics Anonymous and Narcotics Anonymous is a good starting point.

Domestic Violence

Domestic violence is the most common cause of serious injury in the adult woman. Two to four million women are assaulted by their partners each year.[10] Over a woman's lifetime she has a 54% cumulative exposure risk to domestic violence.[11] Domestic violence is not related to any set of socioeconomic or demographic factors. All women are at risk and should be screened, as was concurred by the 1992 statement

of the AMA, "Domestic Violence is sufficiently prevalent to justify screening of all women in medical and mental health settings."

The SAFE questions in Table 24-7 provide a screening tool to identify victims of domestic abuse. Once a patient has been identified as being at risk, our role becomes supportive. The National Domestic Violence Hotline (1-800-799-7233) has a database of support systems and emergency shelters for women who choose to extricate themselves from an abusive situation.

Interventions in the Adult Woman

The U.S. Preventive Services Task Force makes specific recommendations for interventions in the 25- to

TABLE 24-7 SAFE QUESTIONS	
Stress/Safety	What stress do you experience in your relationship?
	Do you feel safe in your relationship?
	Should I be concerned for your safety?
Afraid/Abused	Are there situations in your relationship in which you have felt afraid?
	Has your partner ever threatened or abused you or your children?
	Has your partner forced you to have sexual intercourse that you did not want?
Friends/Family	If you have been hurt, are your friends or family aware of it?
	Do you think you could tell them if it did happen?
	Would they be able to give you support?
Emergency Plan	Do you have a safe place to go and the resources you need in an emergency situation?
	If you are in danger now, would you like help in locating a shelter?
	Would you like to talk with social worker, a counselor or me to develop an emergency plan?

Source: Ashur ML. Asking about domestic violence: SAFE questions. JAMA 1993;269:2367.

64-year-old. A checklist in the patient's chart that includes these recommendations, will help to make sure each element is not overlooked during well visits (Table 24-8).

PERIMENOPAUSAL AND BEYOND

Case 3

A 53-year-old woman presents to your office for her annual examination according to your nurse's note. Thumbing through her chart you find her last visit was several years ago, as was her last mammogram. She also wants to talk to you about the hot flashes she has been experiencing. The patient works full-time and cares for her 75-year-old mother, who is incontinent and starting to wander. She smokes one pack of cigarettes per day, but is trying to quit. She is the divorced mother of three, and her last child has just left for college. Review of systems reveals shortness of breath with exertion. Her blood pressure is 153/92 mmHg. She has a flat affect, bilateral wheezes in her lungs, her vagina is dry, with atrophic mucosa, and rectal examination results are heme-positive.

Sexuality

As women approach this stage of life, sexuality remains an important issue to address. With advancing age, reported sexual frequency decreases and the sexual response does undergo changes, but both men and women can and do enjoy intercourse during their older years. In women, arousal may require more direct stimulation. Decreased lubrication and less ex-

pansion of the vaginal opening during excitement is also noted. In plateau phase, there is less vasocongestion and vaginal tenting. Orgasm has fewer uterine contractions, and clitoral tumescence resolves quicker than in younger women. Sexuality in the elderly has not been studied extensively, but one study of several California retirement communities showed that 50% of women reported sexual thoughts. Twenty-five percent of women respondents reported frequent sexual partners, though only 14% were married. Thirty percent had at least occasional intercourse. In order of decreasing frequency, sexual touching, masturbation, and intercourse were the most common behaviors reported. The average age of respondents was 86 years. As physicians, we must allow our patients to discuss sexual issues with us. Their sexuality should not be dismissed, and we should evaluate any sexual complaints as we would any other medical problem.[12]

It is important to counsel these patients regarding their preserved though diminished fertility until they undergo menopause, and they must still use contraception. Except in smokers, who should not use combined contraceptive pills after age 35, most forms of contraception can be safely used. Patients who may have been previously monogamous (divorcees, widows) need to be reminded about STD prevention before they begin to engage in sexual activity even after menopause.

Maintenance of Healthy Weight

Maintenance of healthy weight continues to be important for these women, as it is during this life stage that the complications of obesity such as coronary

TABLE 24-8 **U.S. PREVENTIVE SERVICES TASK FORCE RECOMMENDED INTERVENTIONS** **IN PEOPLE 25 TO 64 YEARS OF AGE**

Leading causes of death
  Malignant neoplasm
  Heart disease
  Motor vehicle–related and other unintentional injuries
  Human immunodeficiency virus infection
  Suicide and homicide
Screening
  Height and weight
  Blood pressure
  Total blood cholesterol levels (men, 35 to 64 years of age; women, 45 to 64 years of age)
  Papanicolaou (Pap) test
  Fecal occult blood test and/or sigmoidoscopy (at least 50 years of age)
  Mammography with or without clinical breast examination (women 50 to 69 years of age)
  Assess for problem drinking
  Rubella serology or vaccination history (women of childbearing age)
Counseling
  Substance use
  Tobacco cessation
  Avoid alcohol/drug use while driving, swimming, boating, etc.*
  Diet and exercise
  Limit fat and cholesterol intake; maintain caloric balance; emphasize grains, fruits and
    vegetables
  Adequate calcium intake (women)
  Regular physical activity*
  Injury prevention
  Lap/shoulder seat belts
  Bicycle/motorcycle/all-terrain-vehicle helmets*
  Smoke detector*
  Safe storage/removal of firearms from the home*
  Sexual behavior
  Prevention of sexually transmitted diseases: avoiding high-risk behaviors;* using condoms/
    female barriers with spermicide*
  Unintended pregnancy; contraception
  Dental health
  Regular visits to dental care provider*
  Floss, brush with fluoride toothpaste daily
Immunizations
  Tetanus-diptheria boosters
  Rubella (women of childbearing age; serology or history of vaccination)
  Hepatitis B (if not previously given)
Chemoprophylaxis
  Multivitamin with folic acid (women planning or capable of pregnancy)
  Discuss hormone prophylaxis (peri- and postmenopausal women)

*These interventions are suggested for low-risk patients in the general population.

Adapted from U.S. Preventive Services Task Force. Guide to clinical preventive services: report of the U.S. Preventive Services Task Force. 2nd ed. Baltimore: Williams & Wilkins, 1996.

artery disease (CAD), diabetes, and osteoarthritis begin to have an impact on quality of life. Truncal obesity appears to carry more of a risk for CAD than other forms and should be aggressively managed. As women age, their metabolism slows and lean body mass and bone density decrease. Regular exercise has been shown to reverse these changes. Exercise improves flexibility, agility, independence, and sense of well-being. Maintaining ideal body weight serves to decrease the risk of all–cause mortality and specifically,

myocardial infarction by 40 to 50%. Before embarking on an exercise program, patients should be screened for gait and balance disorders, visual deficits, and cardiopulmonary function. Exercise treadmill testing can assist in establishing fitness level and maximum heart rate (MHR) and ruling out coronary disease. Target heart rate (THR) can be calculated as:

$$THR = 0.7(MHR - RHR) + resting\ heart\ rate$$

MHR can also be estimated as $200 - age$.[13]

Fat intake should be no more than 30% of calories, and cholesterol should be limited to 300 mg daily. A low-sodium diet, including lean meats, low-fat dairy products, vegetables, fruit, and whole grains should be followed.[14]

Providers should also ensure that patients are getting adequate nutrition. Barriers to this include decreased mobility and sensory function, lack of transportation, financial constraints, and neglect. Unintentional weight loss should be evaluated and include an assessment for depression, thyroid dysfunction, medication side effects (interference with or loss of taste, anorexia), and cancer. Meal supplements such as Ensure, Meals-on-Wheels, and appetite stimulants have all been used with success.

Tobacco, Alcohol, and Drug Use

Continued counseling regarding alcohol consumption is important in this population. Up to 10% of women over age 65 years have an alcohol problem. Alcohol-related complications in the elderly include dementia, unintentional injury, and gastrointestinal bleeding.

Twenty percent of persons aged 65 to 74 smoke. While the prevalence of older male smokers has decreased, smoking in the older woman is on the rise. Cumulative risk from tobacco abuse increases with years and amount smoked. As stated before, smokers have higher rates of CAD, cerebrovascular disease (CVD), cancer, and respiratory disease. Risk reduction can be accomplished at any age. CAD mortality experiences a rapid decline within 1 to 2 years of cessation. Within 5 years, the risk compares with that of people who have never smoked. It may take 5 to 10 years for women to achieve cancer or COPD mortality reduction. Smoking status should be assessed at every visit and efforts should be taken to encourage patients to quit.[14]

General Considerations for the Older Patient

This life stage is often portrayed as a distressing one for women, although research has failed to bear this out. Freed from pregnancy concerns, these women may enjoy their sexual experiences more. With their children raised, women may have more time for educational, personal, and professional pursuits. Whether a woman experiences the often-spoken of "empty nest syndrome" appears to be more related to a woman's own sense of self-worth.

That is not to say that women do not experience difficulties during this time. Divorce, widowhood, or retirement can result in financial worries. Twenty percent of widows live in poverty.[15] These women now have to accept the changes of their aging bodies. Our role can be to reassure these patients that these changes are universal and normal. However, we should not miss an opportunity to intervene when we can. Every patient should be evaluated for hearing loss, which is the most common sensory loss; its prevalence increases with age. Hearing loss contributes to social isolation, increased safety risk, and risk for depression and psychosis. Hearing loss is thought to worsen cognitive losses in dementia. Those with cataracts should receive ophthalmologic referral and those with presbyopia will benefit from bifocals. Walkers, canes, and wheelchairs improve mobility for those with gait difficulties.

Dementia

When we see these patients in our office we should screen for dementia which affects 5 to 10% of those over age 65. After age 65, its incidence doubles every 5 years. Dementia is an impairment in cognitive function that affects memory, language, abstract thinking, arithmetic, and visuospatial function. Its onset is insidious and it is progressive. Alzheimer disease is the most common form, accounting for up to 90% of cases of dementia. It can be caused by CVD, infections, and metabolic, endocrine, and nutritional disorders. It is often misdiagnosed and unrecognized in its earlier stages and exposes our patients to undue safety risk. It is important not to interpret dementia as normal aging, delirium, or depression. Table 24-9 contains a list of symptoms that may constitute dementia. Any positive findings should prompt a focused history and physical, functional status assessment, and mental status examination.[16]

Elder Abuse

The physician of older women also needs to be ever vigilant for elder abuse. It can take the form of neglect, intimidation, violence, violation of their rights, or financial abuse. Older persons are at risk because of their relatively fragile, dependent, or impaired cognitive state. The U.S. House of Representatives Select Committee on Aging estimated in 1981 that 4% of the elderly are abuse victims. They found neglect to be the most common form, and the perpetrator was

TABLE 24-9
SYMPTOMS THAT MAY INDICATE DEMENTIA

Does the person have increased difficulty with any of the activities listed below?*

Learning and retaining new information: Is more repetitive; has trouble remembering recent conversations, events, appointments; frequently misplaces objects.

Handling complex tasks: Has trouble following a complex train of thought or performing tasks that require many steps, such as balancing a checkbook or cooking a meal.

Reasoning ability: Is unable to respond with a reasonable plan to problems at work or home, such as knowing what to do if the bathroom is flooded; shows uncharacteristic disregard for rules of social conduct.

Spatial ability and orientation: Has trouble driving, organizing objects around the house, finding his or her way around familiar places.

Language: Has increasing difficulty finding the words to express what he or she wants to say and following conversations.

Behavior: Appears more passive and less responsible; is more irritable than usual; is more suspicious than usual; misinterprets visual or auditory stimuli.

In addition to failing to arrive at the right time for appointments, the patient may have difficulty discussing current events in an area of interest and may show changes in behavior or dress. It may be helpful to follow up on areas of concern by asking the patient or family members relevant questions.

*Positive findings in any of these areas generally indicate the need for further assessment for the presence of dementia.

Source: Early Identification of Alzheimer's and Related Dementias Panel.[17]

most likely to be a family member. Being female, demented, or dependent on others for activities of daily living puts a person at greater risk. Abuse should be suspected in cases of weight loss, malnutrition, dehydration, trauma (especially recurrent), poor hygiene, or in medication overdose or noncompliance. The patient herself may be a barrier to diagnosis out of fear of retaliation, eviction from a facility, loyalty, or fear of loss of a familiar environment. The astute physician should recognize when caregivers have assumed too large a burden in caring for their elderly family member and offer assistance in the way of home health or resources such as Meals-on-Wheels to provide some respite.[17]

Immunizations

Immunization status is often an overlooked part of the clinic visit, yet underimmunization in the adult population remains a cause of needless morbidity and mortality. The National Center for Health Statistics found in 1995 that 41% of Americans older that 65 years received influenza vaccination and only 20% had received pneumococcal vaccine. Most influenza deaths occur in those over 65 years and it is estimated that an epidemic can claim 10,000 lives. The majority of the 40,000 pneumococcal deaths annually are also in the elderly or debilitated. Twenty to fifty percent of patients are behind in their tetanus immunizations. Practice teams that do not have effective means of educating their patients regarding immunizations and contacting them when

they are due will continue to have low immunization rates.[13,18]

Influenza is spread person-to-person or through objects, and occurs most often in the winter months. Because the offending virus mutates, the vaccine is reformulated annually. It is given yearly in the fall (mid-October to mid-November) and is recommended for all persons over age 65, health-care workers, institutionalized patients, and those with cardiac, respiratory, renal, metabolic, or immunosuppressive disease. Influenza complications include otitis media, sinusitis, and pneumonia. Protection does not occur until 2 weeks after immunization. It is not a live vaccine and therefore cannot cause influenza. Fever and a reaction at the injection site are reported side effects. Adults can receive either the whole or split virus vaccine. Those with sensitivity to eggs should not receive the vaccine.[18]

The elderly and those with debilitating illness are also more prone to severe pneumococcal illness, as are those who cannot mount a sufficient antibody response to polysaccharide antigens (HIV-positive, sickle cell disease, transplant and dialysis patients, asplenics). *Streptococcus pneumoniae* causes pneumonia, sepsis, and meningitis. All persons aged 65 and over should receive the vaccine because of their higher complication rate from infection. The available vaccines have antigens to the 23 bacteria that most commonly cause infection. Efficacy is estimated to be 57% and wanes with time. Revaccination is recommended only for those at highest risk (asplenics, dialysis, and transplant patients).

Tetanus can occur after puncture wounds, lacerations, or crush injuries. Mortality was one in four overall in one study of 110 cases but 50% for those over 80. While most children appear to be adequately immunized against *Clostridium tetani*, 49% of those over age 60 years do not have protective tetanus antibody. Boosters are recommended every 10 years. For adults not immunized in childhood, two doses, 1 month apart are recommended. For those with fewer than three previous doses, tetanus immune globulin is recommended at the time of penetrating injury.[19]

Interventions

The U.S. Preventive Services Task Force makes further specific recommendations for interventions in the age group over 65. Table 24-10 provides a complete summary.

SUMMARY

The physician has a new and developing role for the future care of his/her patients, to protect them from

---

TABLE 24-10
U.S. PREVENTIVE SERVICES TASK FORCE RECOMMENDED INTERVENTIONS IN PEOPLE 65 YEARS OF AGE AND OLDER

Leading causes of death
  Heart disease
  Malignant neoplasm
  Cerebrovascular disease
  Chronic obstructive pulmonary disease
  Pneumonia and influenze
Screening
  Height and weight
  Blood pressure
  Fecal occult blood test and/or sigmoidoscopy (at least 50 years of age)
  Mammography with or without clinical breast examination (women 50 to 69 years of age)
  Papanicolaou (Pap) test (less than 69 years of age)
  Vision screening
  Assess for hearing impairment
  Assess for problem drinking
Counseling
  Substance use
  Tobacco cessation
  Avoid alcohol/drug use while driving, swimming, boating, etc.*
  Diet and exercise
  Limit fat and cholesterol intake; maintain caloric balance; emphasize grains, fruits and
    vegetables
  Adequate calcium intake (women)
  Regular physical activity*
  Injury prevention
  Lap/shoulder seat belts
  Bicycle/motorcycle/all-terrain-vehicle helmets*
  Smoke detector*
  Safe storage/removal of firearms from the home*
  Hot water heater temperature less than 120 to 130°F*
  Cardiopulmonary resuscitation training for household
  Dental health
  Regular visits to dental care provider*
  Floss, brush with fluoride toothpast daily*
  Sexual behavior
  Prevention of sexually transmitted disease: avoid high-risk sexual behaviors*; use condoms*
Immunizations
  Pneumococcal vaccine
  Influenza
  Tetanus–diphtheria boosters
Chemoprophylaxis
  Discuss hormone prophylaxis (peri- and postmenopausal women)

*These interventions are suggested for low-risk patients in the general population.

Adapted from U.S. Preventive Services Task Force, Guide to clinical preventive services: report of the U.S. Preventive Services Task Force, 2d ed. Baltimore: Williams & Wilkins, 1996.

disease rather than solely treat disease. It is a complex and growing field of knowledge that takes considerable effort to incorporate into daily patient care. The benefits to our patients and the nation's health as a whole, make the effort this transition will require a worthwhile endeavor.

REFERENCES

1. Teenage Pregnancy: Facts You Should Know. Wilkes-Barre, PA: March of Dimes Birth Defects Foundation, May 1994.

2. Kantor L, Hoffner D. Comprehensive sexuality education: adolescents and abstinence. New York: Sexuality Information and Education Council of the United States, 1966.

3. Carek P, Sherer J, Carson D. Management of obesity: medical treatment options. Am Fam Physician 1997; 55:551.

4. The American Anorexia/Bulimia Association, Inc. 165 West 46th St., #1108, New York, NY 10036.

5. U.S. Department of Health and Human Services Fact Sheet. Substance abuse—a national challenge: prevention, treatment, and research at HSS. Washington, DC: Government Printing Office, December 20, 1997.

6. Smoking Cessation Guideline Panel. Smoking cessation: information for specialist. Am Fam Physician 1996; 53:2575.

7. Prevalence of sedentary lifestyle-behavioral risk factor surveillance system, United States, 1991. MMWR Morb Mortal Wkly Rep 1993;42:576.

8. National Institute on Drug Abuse. National household survey on drug abuse population estimates 1991.

9. Trends in cigarette smoking. New York: Epidemiology and Statistics, American Lung Association, December 1999.

10. American Medical Association Diagnostic and Treatment Guidelines on Domestic Violence. Arch Fam Med 1992;1:39 [Published erratum appears in Arch Fam Med 1992;1:287.]

11. Abbott J, Johnson R, Koziol-McLain J, Lowenstein SR. Domestic violence against women. incidence and prevalence in an emergency department population. JAMA 1995;273:1763.

12. Richardson J, Lazur A. Sexuality in the nursing home patient. Am Fam Physician 1995;51:121.

13. Malloy, et al. Common problems of the elderly. In: Taylor RB, ed. Family medicine: principles and practice. 4th ed. New York: Springer-Verlag, 1994.

14. Daly M, Taler G. Care of the elderly. In: Rakel RE, ed. Textbook of family practice. 5th ed. Philadelphia: Saunders, 1995.

15. Brummel-Smith K. Human development and aging. In: Taylor RB, ed. Family medicine: principles and practice. 4th ed. New York: Springer-Verlag, 1994.

16. Early Identification of Alzheimer's and Related Dementias Panel. Early identification of Alzheimer's disease and related dementias. Am Fam Physician 1997;55:1303.

17. Ham R. Elder abuse. In: Taylor RB, ed. Family medicine: principles and practice. 4th ed. New York: Springer-Verlag, 1994.

18. Zimmerman R, Clover R. Adult immunizations—a practical approach for clinicians: Part I. Am Fam Physician 1995;51:859.

Rockville, MD: National Institute on Drug Abuse, Division of Epidemiology and Prevention Research, Department of Health and Human Service,1991. DHHS publication no. (ADM)92-1887.

Chapter 25

Collaborative-Practice Models

Hal C. Lawrence
Susan F. Meade

Five Key Points

- **Definition of collaborative practice**
- **Identification of nonphysician collaborative providers**
- **Outline practice evaluation techniques**
- **Review of regulations regarding practice, billing, and physician oversight in collaborative practice.**
- **Evaluation of impact of your collaborative practice**

The delivery of health care by a team of professionals with different skills who work together to accomplish a common goal is a long-standing concept. Many obstetrician-gynecologists have worked with a multitude of nonphysician providers be these physician assistants, certified nurse-midwives, or nurse practitioners. Our changing health-care environment, with expansion of managed care, primary care, and health maintenance organizations, presents additional reasons to look at collaborative practice in the delivery of women's health care.

The American College of Obstetricians and Gynecologists has approved the following definition of collaborative practice:

Collaborative practice in the healthcare of women is a comprehensive, dynamic system of patient-centered healthcare delivered by a multidisciplinary team. The team consists of obstetrician/gynecologists and other healthcare professionals who function within their educational preparation and scope of practice. These team members work together utilizing mutually agreed upon guidelines and policies that define the individual and shared responsibility of each member. Although the responsibilities obstetrician/gynecologists place them in the role of ultimate authority because of their education and training, the contributions of each team member are valued and important to the quality of patient outcomes. The concept of a team guided by one of its own members and acceptance of shared responsibility for outcomes promotes shared accountability.

Using this definition, the obstetrician-gynecologist has the opportunity to evaluate his or her practice and determine whether collaborative practice would be beneficial. In these days of health-care reorganization and the need for the obstetrician-gynecologist to ensure access for women for primary, preventive health care, some physicians may find collaborative practice advantageous.

Collaborative practice offers the opportunity to:

- increase access to health care,
- facilitate continuity of care throughout the life span,
- improve patient satisfaction and compliance with treatment regiments and lifestyle modifications, and promote health and wellness,
- provide quality health-care services in a cost-effective manner, and
- optimize the individual expertise of all professionals.

This chapter will assist the obstetrician-gynecologist in understanding the different types of advanced-practice professionals and nonphysician providers;

their education and certification; how to evaluate one's practice; the three Rs (recruitment, regulation and reimbursement); and means of tracking the impact of the new collaborative practice.

TYPES OF NONPHYSICIAN PROVIDERS

Certified nurse-midwives, clinical nurse specialists, nurse practitioners, and physician assistants have different educational preparation and training. Understanding the differences among these types of providers may help identify the specific type of provider that would be most beneficial in meeting the goals of a particular practice.

Certified Nurse-Midwives

Certified nurse-midwives (CNMs) are registered nurses who have completed graduate-level education in midwifery. Nurse-midwifery education is based on theoretical preparation in sciences and clinical preparation with regard to judgment and skills needed to manage the care of women and newborns. Accreditation for certified nurse-midwives is through the Division of Accreditation of the American College of Nurse-Midwives. The Division of Accreditation also provides for periodic scheduled review of programs and monitors educational programs for nurse-midwives.

A student must demonstrate clinical and theoretical mastery of the program's curricular content prior to taking the National Certification Examination. CNMs are certified by the American College of Nurse-Midwives/American College of Nurse-Midwives Certification Council. Since 1971, national requirements for certification include graduation from an accredited program for nurse-midwifery and passing the examination administered by ACNM.

The practice of nurse-midwifery focuses particularly on pregnancy, childbirth, the postpartum period, and care of the newborn. Family planning and gynecologic care are also integral parts of the practice of nurse-midwifery. The CNM model of health care emphasizes health promotion, education, and disease prevention. Nurse-midwives practice in outpatient and inpatient clinical settings.

Clinical Nurse Specialists

Clinical nurse specialists (CNSs) are registered nurses who have completed formal education at a Master's level. Educational programs for nurses are accredited through the National League for Nursing. Length of the educational program varies depending whether an undergraduate degree is obtained in conjunction with the program. The courses in most CNS programs focus on the roles of clinician, educator, consultant, manager or administrator, and researcher. In some educational settings, the CNS student is allowed to select courses that focus on all of these roles as they would be applied in a specific setting or specialty. If the program is developed around a specialty area, the focus of some clinical courses may be determined by the specialty.

A wide range of physical and mental health problems may be handled by a clinical nurse specialist as these providers frequently work as educators, consultants, researchers, or managers. They generally work in inpatient settings and are certified by the Credentialing Unit of the American Nurse Association.

It is important to note that the term *clinical nurse specialist* is often used as a position or job title in some settings without a requirement for educational preparation at the Master's level. For the purpose of this document, the CNS designation applies only to those nurses who are prepared at the Master's level.

Nurse Practitioners

Nurse practitioners (NPs) are licensed, registered nurses with advanced education including both didactic and supervised clinical instruction in health maintenance and the diagnosis and treatment of illness. Completion of a nurse practitioner program may lead to a certificate or to a degree at the Master's level.

Certification is required to practice as a nurse practitioner in some states and is voluntary in others. Mandatory certification (which may be called "licensure" depending on the state's terminology) is based on completing an approved educational program, passing a National Certification Examination, or both. Voluntary credentialing is conferred by a nongovernmental agency and provides evidence of an individual's ability to apply advanced knowledge in a specialized setting. Nurse practitioners who specialize in women's health are certified by the National Certification Corporation for Obstetric/Gynecologic and Neonatal Nursing Specialties. Requirements for certification vary according to the specialty area and are determined by that certifying organization.

Nurse practitioners are qualified to provide a wide range of primary preventive health-care services, including obtaining medical, surgical, and psychosocial histories; performing physical examinations; and diagnosing and treating common illnesses and injuries. They are generally employed in primary-care outpatient clinics, health-maintenance organizations, specialty clinics, and schools. Nurse practitioners also function in subspecialty areas such as reproductive-endocrine-infertility, gyn-oncology, and high-risk obstetrics. An increasing number of nurse practitioners are being employed in inpatient settings.

Physician Assistants

Physician assistants (PAs) enter training from a variety of backgrounds and are educated to provide medical care under the direction and supervision of a physician or osteopath. Most of the physician-assistant training programs have been established within or with strong attachments to medical schools and require applicants to have at least 2 years of college education and experience in health care prior to entry. The educational program traditionally consists of a minimum of 2 years of classroom instruction and clinical rotations. Curriculum designed for most physician-assistant programs provides basic science, introduction to clinical sciences, and supervised clinical instruction. Completion of a physician-assistant program may lead to a certificate or to an Associate, Bachelor's, or Master's degree.

Most states require PAs to pass a National Certification Examination. The examination is given only to graduates of accredited PA programs and is developed by the National Board of Medical Examiners and administered by the National Commission on Certification of Physician Assistants (NCCPA). PAs must complete 100 hours of continuing medical education every 2 years and take a recertification examination every 6 years to maintain certification.

Physician assistants' duties include diagnostic and therapeutic procedures following a medical model of patient care. Typically, physician assistants work under a broad practice description that allows them to exercise clinical judgment while consulting a supervising physician as necessary as opposed to using detailed treatment protocols. Physician assistants practice in virtually all specialty areas, in outpatient and inpatient settings and as first or second assistants in surgery and provide preoperative and postoperative care.

PRACTICE EVALUATION

Understanding the physician's current practice structure and the desire to expand services or concentrate in a specific service area is essential before recruiting an advanced-practice professional to initiate collaborative practice. While many advanced-practice professionals are employed in educational formats, their primary role has been to expand clinical services. Therefore, identifying the area for practice focus or expansion is necessary. This identification will be influenced by multiple factors. Does the practice exist in an urban or rural environment? Is the population stable or changing? Is the population changing in any specific age group? If a new industry has come to town, bringing in new, younger individuals, obstetrics may be more of an issue. If the practice exists in a retirement area, gynecology and preventive health care will be more important.

The physician, in deciding the different services provided, must also clearly define the reporting responsibilities from the advanced-practice professional to the physician and the available supervision from the physician to the advanced-practice professional. Whether the advanced-practice professional will be purely office-based or hospital-based is an important issue to clarify early on. Hospital credentialing is an integral process for the advanced-practice professional to work with the physician in labor and delivery (certified nurse-midwife) or in the operating room (physician assistant). Many advanced-practice professionals are employed in making hospital rounds and would also require credentialing.

The level of care provided by the practice or desired to be provided is important. Does the obstetrician-gynecologist see himself or herself as a primary-care provider or as a specialist functioning for consultation? Does the hospital provide secondary or tertiary services?

Space requirements are important. Is there room in the current facility for an advanced-practice professional? The number of practice sites in which the practice delivers care must be considered. Will the advanced-practice professional practice in all these sites or will they be limited? Local regulations regarding physician oversight for the advanced-practice professional will be a determining factor in this decision. The reimbursement profile of your patient base is also important and will be addressed under the reimbursement section of the three Rs.

Once the focus of the practice has been identified, the provider needs to approach, realistically, what services the advanced-practice professional will provide. This answer is one that may change in the dynamics of collaborative practice, but its starting place must be defined. Visit types, such as new obstetrical patients, new gynecologic patients, returning obstetrical patients, annual physical examinations, contraceptive visits, and emergency work-ins all represent different opportunities in collaborative practice. Care must be taken on the obstetrical side that the advanced-practice professional does not greatly expand the obstetrical load of the practice, if that is not a desired outcome.

Once evaluation of facility and practice service goals has been completed, support staff (nurses, business offices, receptionists, billing) needs must be evaluated. Will this staff need to change? Are the staff prepared to work with a nonphysician provider?

Finally, the physician must clearly identify his or her personal goals. These goals must be kept in focus during the practice growth resulting from a collaborative format.

With the completion of the practice evaluation, it is recommended that the physician provider(s) seek out other physicians who have developed collaborative practices. Discussing with them the process and any pitfalls they have encountered may be helpful information in securing a successful outcome.

THE THREE Rs: RECRUITMENT, REGULATION, AND REIMBURSEMENT

Recruitment

The most important step in forming a collaborative practice is the recruitment of the correct nonphysician provider or advanced-practice professional. Not only do you need the right training for the identified responsibilities, equally important, you need the right person to fit in an ongoing practice. The same care given to recruiting a physician-partner should be given to recruiting a nonphysician provider. These individuals will be seen as integral parts of your practice by your patients. Your patients will expect the same level of interaction and education from these providers that they receive from you. Often the correct individual is more important than whether the individual is a nurse practitioner or a physician

assistant. Obviously, if you desire inpatient obstetrical care services, the certified nurse-midwife stands alone.

The following are suggestions for looking for qualified individuals:

- Place advertisements in the employment section of the local newspaper.
- Work with employment agencies, particularly those specializing in health-care personnel.
- Post a position announcement on bulletin boards in schools or universities with programs for certified nurse-midwives, nurse practitioners, or physician assistants.
- Send position notices to faculty in schools of nursing and physician assistant programs.
- Place advertisements in professional journals.
- Send position notices to professional associations and attend regional or national meetings for certified nurse-midwives, nurse practitioners, or physician assistants.

National organizations, such as the National Organization of Nurse Practitioner Faculty, the American College of Nurse-Midwives, and the National Physician Assistant Organization publish journals in which you could advertise.

Once a list of applicants has been identified, background evaluation and reference-checking are as important as they are for physicians recruitment. Speaking with an individual with whom this individual has previously worked is always helpful.

The interview is a critical part of the evaluation. Questions that may be construed as discriminatory—e.g., age, marital status, ethnic background—must be avoided. The advanced-practice nurse should be given the opportunity to meet with other office personnel. Understanding the strengths of the individual candidates and the services they will provide is an important component of the interview process.

The practice should carefully develop an employment agreement similar to a physician's contract that clearly delineates the nonphysician provider's job description and any restrictive covenants. Supervisory and reporting relationships must be clearly spelled out. A probationary period or "outclause" is an important component to have in the employment agreement. Refer to Guidelines for Implementing a Collaborative Practice, the American College of Obstetrician and Gynecologist, 1995, Appendix H, for an employment agreement checklist.[1]

After identifying the correct individual for the practice, it is important to establish a plan of integrating the advanced-practice professional into the practice and into the medical community, just as one would do with a new physician associate. Be sure the new member of the collaborative-practice team is introduced to all the office staff. Clarifying how the office staff will relate to the advanced practice professional is crucial to avoid conflict. If your collaborative practice is the first in your community, other physicians may be uncertain of the role of this individual. There is an opportunity and obligation to inform the community of how your collaborative practice will work. Physician colleagues may be concerned as to who will see a patient referred to your office. Clarify this in advance. Encouraging the advanced-practice professional to give educational programs to office staff and patients is a great way to ensure their success.

SCOPE OF NONPHYSICIAN PROVIDER PRACTICE

Legal authority, prescriptive authority, and reimbursement are important considerations in selecting a nonphysician provider for a practice. State laws and regulations play an important role in defining the scope of a nonphysician practice and must be consulted.

The guidelines included here are for general information. They are intended to provide a framework for considering important factors that apply to the various types of nonphysician providers. It is important to investigate laws and regulations for the state or jurisdiction in which a practice is located. This could involve inquiry regarding laws and regulations for more than one jurisdiction if the nonphysician provider's responsibilities will cross state or jurisdictional lines. Current pertinent statutes and recent regulations should be obtained from agencies that license or oversee nonphysician providers. Boards of nursing and medicine should be able to identify the agency responsible for specific types of nonphysician providers.

Statutes or regulations exist in most states to govern advanced-practice nursing. Typically, nurse practitioners, and in some states, certified nurse-midwives, are regulated under these statutes or regulations. Some states are becoming more involved in establishing requirements regarding regulation for clinical nurse specialists. There is much similarity regarding the scope of practice for nonphysician providers including

requirements for physician collaboration or supervision. However, the variations require individual state investigation into its particular regulations.

LEGAL AUTHORITY

The legal authority to practice as a nurse practitioner is granted solely by the board of nursing in most states or by a joint medical and nursing board in other states. Many states provide nurse practitioners with title protection (i.e., a license) for advanced-practice nursing. In other states, nurse practitioners practice under a broad nurse practice act that does not provide title protection for advanced-practice nursing. Nurse practitioners may be required to have written protocols, guidelines, or standardized procedures to outline their specific functions as nurses who practice in extended roles depending on the state's regulations.

Regulation of certified nurse-midwives can be by the board of nursing, the board of medicine, the department of public health, the board of midwifery or by joint medical and nursing boards, depending on state law. The scope of midwifery practice is well defined in most states. A state-by-state analysis of nurse-midwifery statutes and regulations can be obtained from the American College of Nurse-Midwives.

Generally, the practice of physician assistants is regulated under each state's medical practice act. State laws require physician assistants to work under the supervision of a doctor of medicine or osteopathy. Most states allow the physician to be in a different location as long as they are immediately available for consultation with the use of electronic communication.

PRESCRIPTIVE AUTHORITY

Most states allow nonphysician providers some level of prescriptive authority. Nurse practitioners are usually required to have some level of physician supervision or collaboration as a prerequisite for granting authority to prescribe medications. That authority may or may not include controlled substances. A few states grant nurse practitioners complete and independent authority to prescribe medications, including controlled substances. A number of states currently have no legislation covering prescriptive authority by nurse practitioners.

Although generalization is difficult, most states allow at least limited prescriptive authority to certified nurse-midwives. Other states allow broader authority. Some requirements may include development of a formulary or written practice guidelines to identify medications and circumstances under which medication would usually be prescribed. The prescriptive authority of certified nurse-midwives usually includes controlled substances due to management of labor and delivery.

Most states allow the physician to delegate prescriptive authority to physician assistants. This authority may include controlled substances. Prescription pads must include the name of the physician assistant and the supervising physician.

REIMBURSEMENT

Most states allow services provided by advanced-practice nurses and physician assistants to be eligible for third-party reimbursement. The Civilian Health and Medical Program of the Uniformed Services allows advanced-practice professionals to receive direct reimbursement for services provided to members of the uniformed services and their families. Direct reimbursement is also allowed to advanced-practice nurses for services provided to federal employees under the Federal Employee Health Benefit Plan. Payment levels for services provided by advanced-practice nurses under the Federal Employee Health Benefit Plan are determined by the individual health insurance plan. Traditionally, physician assistants have not sought direct reimbursement.

Medicare is a federal program that was established in 1966. A survey by the American College of Obstetricians and Gynecologists (ACOG), Department of Medical Economics, reveals that four-fifths of all obstetrician-gynecologists see Medicare patients. However, Medicare accounts for only 11% of the average obstetrician-gynecologist's practice. The Medicare program and its rules have undergone an evolution over time as it relates to physician assistants, nurse practitioners, and certified nurse-midwives. Under Medicare, services provided by employee-nonphysician providers under the on-site supervision by a physician are reimbursable to the physician at the physician rate, provided these services are an integral part of the diagnosis or treatment and would have been reimbursed if the physician had performed them. Under certain circumstances, Medicare reimburses physician assistants, nurse practitioners, and clinical nurse-specialists directly for services they are authorized to perform

under state law. The rate of reimbursement depends on the type of facility in which the services are rendered and whether the services are performed in a rural area. Medicare may directly reimburse certified nurse-midwives when the services rendered would be covered if performed by a physician. In this situation, the rate of reimbursement for the certified nurse-midwife does not vary with the type of facility or location in which the service is rendered. Certified nurse-midwife services provided outside the maternity cycle are included in Medicare coverage as of January 1, 1994.

Medicaid (Title 19) is a program jointly funded by states and the federal government to provide health care for the medically needy. In an ACOG survey, obstetrician-gynecologists who provided care for Medicaid participants noted that 23% of their patients were covered by Medicaid benefits. Most state Medicaid programs will reimburse for nurse practitioners, certified nurse-midwives, and physician assistant services with varying levels of reimbursement. Although states set their own reimbursement rates, they are required to set obstetric and pediatric reimbursement rates at a level that will ensure Medicaid patients access to care equal to that of privately insured patients. Some states have integrated managed-care concepts into their Medicaid programs that allow assigning enrollees to a primary care provider (PCP). The PCP is allowed a fixed number of patients. Some managed-care plans are recognizing physician assistants, certified nurse-midwives, and nurse practitioners as PCPs and are paneling them appropriately or increasing the number of enrollees that the physician may have. However, some plans have refused to recognize contributions of nonphysician providers.

There are approximately 1200 private insurance companies in the market and their coverage varies for nurse practitioners, certified nurse-midwives, and physician assistants. Under most fee-for-service and managed-care plans, insurance companies allow the nonphysician provider to bill "blind" using the physician's provider number.

Information about all types of reimbursement should be updated regularly since policies on reimbursement plans are always evolving.

PRACTICE REEVALUATION

With the institution of your collaborative practice, specific guidelines to enable assessment of the practice's effectiveness need to be instituted. The fact that advanced-practice professionals work within practice protocols facilitates this. These protocols identify the following areas:

- They specify the scope of supervision required for performance of specific procedures.
- They specify the circumstances or conditions that require the nonphysician to communicate immediately with the supervising obstetrician-gynecologist.
- They must be signed and dated by the obstetrician-gynecologist who approves the protocol.

By having this written documentation, it is easy to perform chart reviews that are provider- and procedure-specific. Documenting the appropriateness of the procedure, its outcome, and whether the reporting process was fulfilled are easily accomplished. This provides one way of evaluating the effectiveness of your collaborative practice.

Assessing changes in office efficiency represents another way to reevaluate the practice. Are appointment times more available? Are waiting times decreased? Are specific focus areas identified on your initial evaluation being addressed, with positive outcomes?

Evaluating these factors at a 6-month and 1-year interval is appropriate. The utilization of patient satisfaction questionnaires is an additional way to evaluate the impact of your collaborative practice. Patient acceptance is crucial. Their recognition of your concern regarding their care in your collaborative practice is, by itself, positive.

Looking at issues such as time with care providers, patients' perception about education regarding diet and preventive care, and patients' views regarding individualization of their care are all factors that lend themselves to inclusion in patient satisfaction surveys. In addition, these data may be beneficial in negotiating managed-care contracts. Specific issues relating to education, domestic violence screening, and value as perceived by the patients are easily incorporated into your patient satisfaction survey.

It is important to share the evaluation data between the physician and the nonphysician provider. This should be part of the nonphysician's review. Has your collaborative practice been viewed positively by the patients you serve?

The physician must look carefully at the expectations as defined in the initial evaluation. Are individual and professional goals being met? Has the practice and the collaborative structure been accepted by the patients and the community? Has expansion of the identified services been accomplished? Did the number of patients in the practice evolve in the direction desired by the physician? Has the collaborative-practice model been productive from an economic basis? The total practice revenue in a collaborative practice model must be looked at, not only the individual nonphysician provider's revenues. Surgical procedures identified by the nonphysician provider or new obstetrical patients brought into the practice usually are not identified as revenue by the nonphysician provider. This benefit accrues on the physician revenue side but was generated by the collaborative model. Likewise, the nonphysician provider may well have expanded the physician's time to perform surgical procedures or to have time away from the office. This needs to be calculated into the total economic impact. Has the physician leadership role evolved smoothly?

Using these tools, the physician is able to reevaluate the practice in a collaborative model. Most find this a positive evaluation.

SUMMARY

This chapter on collaborative practice should enable the reader to understand what a collaborative practice is, how to identify the different types of providers, and to evaluate one's own practice to see if a collaborative model will be useful. The reader should understand the recruitment processes to identify the correct advanced practice professional for their practice. The impact of state regulations and local credentialing requirements are identified. Reimbursement questions are highlighted for the reader.

The importance of reevaluating one's practice under a collaborative model must be stressed.

Currently there are many successful collaborative practices. Multiple, large, subspecialty groups such as the Ochsner Clinic in New Orleans uses this model with great success.

Three important factors must be remembered in the development of collaborative practice:

1. Time. It will take time for the collaborative practice to evolve and develop into its most positive structure.
2. Trust. Over the months to years, there needs to be a trust developed between the physician and nonphysician providers. This trust will portend ease in

communication and be readily identified by the patients. The care must be seamless.

3. Team. Team is the goal. As a team, a collaborative practice model can be incredibly strong and efficient. The "us" and "them" philosophy does not work. If the physician is unable or unwilling to be part of a team, collaborative practice will not be successful.

REFERENCES

1. Guidelines for Implementing a Collaborative Practice. Washington, DC: American College of Obstetricians and Gynecologists, 1995.

2. Collaborative Practice How to Get Started—060 Course Annual Clinical Meeting. Washington, DC: the American College of Obstetricians and Gynecologists, 1995.

3. Managed Care/Primary Care—Collaborative Practice: What Works in the Twenty-First Century. 060 Course Annual Clinical Meeting. Washington, DC: the American College of Obstetricians and Gynecologists, 1996.

4. Models of Collaborative Practice. Preparing for Maternity Care in the Twenty-First Century. Presentation Marriott Metro Center, Washington, DC, March 23–25, 1997.

5. Effective Collaborative Practice. 060 Course Annual Clinical Meeting. Washington, DC: American College of Obstetricians and Gynecologists, 1997.

Management of Chronic Medical Problems in Women's Health

TABLE 26-3 CLASSIFICATION OF BLOOD PRESSURE (NEW SYSTEM)			
Category	**Systolic**		**Diastolic**
Optimal	<120	and	<80
Normal	<130	and	<85
High-normal	130–139	or	85–89
Hypertension			
Stage 1	140–159	or	90–99
Stage 2	160–179	or	100–109
Stage 3	≥180	or	≥110

TABLE 26-4 CAUSES OF SECONDARY HYPERTENSION	
Primary aldosteronism	Renal artery occlusion/stenosis
Pheochromocytoma	Renal diseases
Cushing syndrome	Obstructive nephropathy
Drugs	Diabetic nephropathy
Oral contraceptives	Chronic pyelonephritis
Steroids	Polycystic disease
Vasopressor drugs	Interstitial nephropathy
Steroids	Glomerulonephritis
Coarctation of the aorta	

equal to 110 mm Hg. As with previous guidelines, the diagnosis is based on averaging two or more readings taken at each of two or more office visits after the initial screening (Table 26-3).

Hypertension is also stratified as either primary or secondary. Primary hypertension is any hypertension that cannot be attributed to an underlying cause. Secondary hypertension is related to an underlying condition. Any hypertension that appears refractory to normal treatment should be evaluated for secondary causes. Common diseases or entities that can cause secondary hypertension include renal disease, renal vascular disease, coarctation of the aorta, pheochromocytoma, and primary aldosteronism. Certain drugs, such as oral contraceptives, steroids, thyroid hormones, and vasopressor drugs, can also cause secondary hypertension (Table 26-4).

IMPACT OF HYPERTENSION

New data show a slight rise in the rate of stroke, increases in both end-stage renal disease and heart failure, and a leveling in the death rate for people with CHD. These statistics signal a need for a renewed effort by physicians and patients to prevent and treat hypertension. According to Centers for Disease Control and Prevention statistics,[3] as of 1993, almost 13,000 persons in the United States between the ages of 20 and 74 die each year from the effects of hypertension. The current death rate in the United States is 2 deaths per 100,000 population.

Over 50 million Americans (roughly 23% of the population) have high blood pressure. There are approximately 2 million new cases reported each year. Of those over the age of 65, about two-thirds have high blood pressure.[4] More than 10 million (more than 16%) visits to physicians in 1995 were for treatment of hypertension. Despite these visits, over 50%

of the patients with hypertension do not have their blood pressure adequately controlled.[5,6]

EVALUATION AND DIAGNOSIS

The diagnosis of hypertension requires more than one visit with the patient. The above definitions apply to an average of two or more readings, each of which are obtained at two or more separate office visits after the initial visit. The blood pressure should be taken the same way at each visit. The patient should be seated in a quiet area. It should be taken after the patient has rested for at least 2 to 3 minutes. The blood pressure cuff should be the correct size, covering about two-thirds of the upper arm. Too small a cuff can cause significant increases in the blood pressure measurement. The gauge should be correctly calibrated. Measurements should include both systolic and diastolic readings. Two or more readings should be obtained approximately 2 minutes apart. The measurements should be confirmed on two or more follow-up visits.

Sakuma[7] compared the reproducibility over time of blood pressure measured at health examinations (screening blood pressure) and blood pressure measured at home (home blood pressure). His results suggest that the reproducibility of home blood pressure over time is superior to that of screening blood pressure in the office. Blood pressure measurements obtained at home have a clinical significance for the diagnosis and treatment of hypertension and as a tool for evaluating the efficacy of antihypertensive drugs. Home blood pressure measurements also may be more useful than screening measurements in predicting future cardiac events.

The initial evaluation and work-up of hypertension begins with a thorough history and physical examination. This should include the patient's family

TABLE 26-5
LABORATORY EVALUATION OF HYPERTENSION

Routine
- Urinalysis including microscopic examination
- Chemistries
  - Creatinine
  - Glucose
  - Electrolytes
  - Lipids
  - Uric acid
- Chest x-ray examination
- Electrocardiography

Refractory (or diastolic pressure >115)
- Serum calcium
- Captopril test
- Urine for metanephrine
- Renal arteriography
- Plasma renin activity

TABLE 26-6
DRUGS OF CHOICE

Uncomplicated hypertension
- β-Blocker
- Diuretics

Special Considerations
- Diabetes mellitus (Type I) with proteinuria
  - Angiotensin-converting–enzyme inhibitors
- Congestive heart failure
  - Angiotensin-converting–enzyme inhibitors
  - Diuretics
- Isolated systolic hypertension
  - Diuretics
  - Dihydropyridine calcium-channel blockers (long-acting)
- History of myocardial infarction
  - β-Blockers
  - Angiotensin-converting–enzyme inhibitors

Note: Always start with a low dose and titrate upward, preferably a long-acting (once a day) drug. Consider low-dose combination therapy.

history as well as their own medical history. Laboratory studies are also useful in the initial work-up of newly diagnosed hypertension (Table 26-5). These should include urinalysis with microscopy and blood for glucose, uric acid, serum creatinine, electrolytes, and lipid profile. Chest x-ray films and electrocardiograms should also be obtained. These are useful for establishing a base line for comparison at follow-up visits as well as for evaluating end-organ damage from the hypertension. Special tests such as intravenous pyelography, renal arteriography, plasma renin, aldosterone, or catecholamine levels should be reserved for ruling out secondary causes.[8]

PREVENTION AND TREATMENT

Patients should be counseled about lifestyle modifications if they are at risk for hypertension.[9] Lifestyle modifications for preventing hypertension in patients who are at risk include smoking cessation, weight reduction, reducing daily sodium intake to less than 6 g of sodium chloride, moderate alcohol intake, exercising, increasing potassium intake from fresh fruits and vegetables, and ensuring adequate calcium and magnesium intake. Stress relief techniques are very helpful. This can be accomplished through community programs as well as patient education. Physicians should take advantage of any opportunity to encourage these lifestyle modifications.[10]

The ultimate goal of treatment is not simply to normalize blood pressure, but to decrease the morbidity and mortality associated with elevated blood pressure. The decision to treat hypertension should take into consideration overall risk for cardiovascular morbidity as well as the blood pressure. This includes risk factors such as diabetes mellitus, dyslipidemia, smoking, family history, age, and gender, as well as evidence of target organ damage and clinical cardiovascular disease. Antihypertensive therapy must be tailored to the individual patient. Risk of cardiovascular disease should influence blood pressure targets, and comorbid disorders should influence medication selection (Tables 26-6 and 26-7). Table 26-8 lists common antihypertensive agents.

TABLE 26-7
HYPERTENSIVE EMERGENCIES AND URGENCIES

Oral agents	
Captopril	25 mg orally, repeat as needed
Clonidine	0.1–0.2 mg orally, repeat every hour, up to 0.6 mg
Labetalol	200–400 mg orally, repeat every 2 to 3 hr
Intravenous medications	
Sodium nitroprusside	0.25–10 μg/kg/min (decrease within 10 min from maximum dose)
Nitroglycerin	5–100 μg intravenous drip
Diazoxide	50–150 mg intravenous bolus, or 15–30 mg/min intravenous drip
Hydralazine	10–20 mg intravenously or 10–40 mg intramuscularly
Enalapril	0.625–1.25 mg intravenously every 6 hr
Labetalol	20–80 mg intravenously every 10 min or 2 mg/min drip

TABLE 26-8
COMMON ANTIHYPERTENSIVE AGENTS

Drug	Iniftial Dose (mg/day)	Potentlal Adverse Reations
Diuretics		Weakness
Thiazides		Diabetes
Chlorthalidone	12.5	Gout
Hydrochlorothiazide	12.5	
Loop		Volume depletion
Bumetanide	0.5	
Furosemide	20	
Potassium-sparing		
Spironolactone	25	Menstrual irregularity
Triamterene	50	(Spironolactone)
Adrenergic inhibitors		Fatigue
β-blockers without ISA		Bronchospasm
Atenolol	25	Bradycardia/heart block
Metoprolol	50	Sleep disturbance
β-Blockers with ISA		Diabetes
Acebutolol	200	
α/β-Blockers		Headache/syncope
Labetalol	200	Orthostatic hypotension
α₁-Receptor blockers		Syncope
Prazosin	1.0	Orthostatic hypotension
ACE inhibitors		
Captopril	12.5	Angioedema
Enalapril	2.5	Renal failure
Calcium antagonists		
Nondihydropyridines		
Diltiazem	90	Bradycardia
Extended-release	180	Heart block
Verapamil	80	Constipation (Verapamil)
Long-acting	120	Headache (Diltiazem)
Dihydropyridines		Headache
Amiodipine	2.5	Dizziness
Felodipne	5.0	Edema/palpitations
Nifedipine	30	
Centrally acting α₂-agonists		Sedation
Clonidine	0.1	Dry mouth
Methyldopa	250	Orthostatic hypotension
		Liver toxicity/hemolytic anemia (methyldopa)
Peripherally acting adrenergic antagonists		
Guanethidine	10	Orthostatic hypotension
Reserpine	0.05	Dizziness (Reserpine)
Direct vasodilators		Palpitations
Hydralazine	10	Edema
Minoxidil	2.5	Hirsutism (Minoxidil)

ISA = intrinsic sympathomimetic activity

Source: Zoschnick LB. Management of hypertension in women. Female Patient 1996;21:77.

For example, a patient in Risk Group A with Stage 1 hypertension (140–159 mm Hg systolic and/or 90–99 mm Hg diastolic pressures) with no cardiovascular disease, organ damage, or other risk factors may be treated with lifestyle changes for 1 year before starting drugs if the patient is responding. By contrast, the earlier guidelines suggested that such patients should try lifestyle modifications for only 3 to 6 months before starting medications. Regardless of risk group, lifestyle modification is essential in all patients. Patients with risk factors should be consid-ered for antihypertensive therapy even with blood pressures below 140/90 mm Hg. Alternatively, before initiating drug therapy for patients with low risk-factor profiles, lifestyle modifications may be tested for 6 to 12 months for their effectiveness.

Weight reduction is an important step. Obesity, which is clearly associated with hypertension, is a growing public health concern in the United States and is becoming increasingly prevalent worldwide. Of particular note is that children are the most rapidly growing obese group in the United States. The

Nurses' Health Study demonstrated an exponential association of hypertension with weight gain in 85,000 women.[11] Furthermore, weight reduction clearly normalizes some elevated blood pressures. The Sodium Reduction and Weight Loss in Treatment of Old Persons (TONE) Trial demonstrated that 44 percent of patients randomized to a sodium-restricted, low-calorie diet were free of medications and cardiovascular events at 30 months as compared with only 16% who did not receive the same aggressive weight-loss and sodium-reduction counseling.[9] This occurred despite only an average 10-lb weight reduction over the 30 months of the study.

Decreased or moderated alcohol consumption improves blood pressure control.[1,2] Excessive alcohol intake is the most easily reversible cause of hypertension in the United States today. Eight percent of hypertension in men can be attributed to excessive alcohol consumption. Nevertheless, mild alcohol intake appears to be associated with reduced cardiovascular mortality (i.e, one drink/day). Absolute abstinence should not be encouraged in mild drinkers with hypertension. A general guideline would be to limit alcohol intake to no more than 1 oz of ethanol (i.e., 24 oz of beer, 10 oz of wine, or other drinks in an amount based on their ethanol content) per day for men and slightly less than 1 oz per day for women.

Increased physical activity also has a beneficial effect on hypertension. Endurance exercise training reduces systolic and diastolic blood pressures in approximately 75% of people who have essential hypertension. These reductions are approximately 10 mm Hg for both systolic and diastolic blood pressures. Exercise training at intensities of 40 to 70% of VO_{2max} appears to lower systolic blood pressure somewhat more and diastolic pressure to the same degree as higher-intensity training.[12] Additional benefits of endurance exercise training on other risk factors for coronary heart disease make such training an efficacious intervention for people who have mild to moderate elevations in blood pressure.

A healthy diet is an important part of this strategy. For the first time, the guidelines encourage the population-wide adoption of a specific diet. The diet was evaluated in a recent study, Dietary Approaches to Stop Hypertension (DASH). DASH found that eating a diet rich in fruits and vegetables that also includes low-fat dairy foods and a reduction in saturated and total fats significantly lowers blood pressure.[13] Patients should be advised to reduce daily sodium intake to no more than 2.4 g of sodium, or

6 g of sodium chloride, which is about 1 tsp of salt (reduce the intake of processed foods). Adequate dietary intake of potassium (90 mmol, or 3.5 g of potassium chloride) should be encouraged by including foods rich in potassium. Good sources of potassium include bananas, orange juice, potatoes, yogurt, prunes, and winter squash.

DRUG THERAPY

Drug therapy is needed when lifestyle modifications fail or when patients present with a systolic blood pressure greater than 130 mm Hg or diastolic pressure greater than 85 mm Hg and target-organ disease and/or diabetes. Based on several randomized controlled trials, the JNC VI treatment algorithm (Figure 26-1) recommends diuretics or β-blockers as the initial choice of therapy in cases of uncomplicated hypertension.[2,14,15] Despite this recommendation, calcium-channel blockers remain the most commonly prescribed antihypertensive medication today. Comparative data with agents other than β-blockers and diuretics are lacking. However, NHLBI studies are under way and more information will be available in coming years.

Patients with specific comorbid disease may gain particular benefit from medications other than diuretics and β-blockers (see Table 26-5). For example, angiotensin-converting–enzyme (ACE) inhibitors should be considered initial therapy in patients with renal disease or diabetes, especially Type 1 diabetes with proteinuria. Combination therapy with both diuretics and ACE inhibitors should be used in patients with congestive heart failure. β-Blockers should be

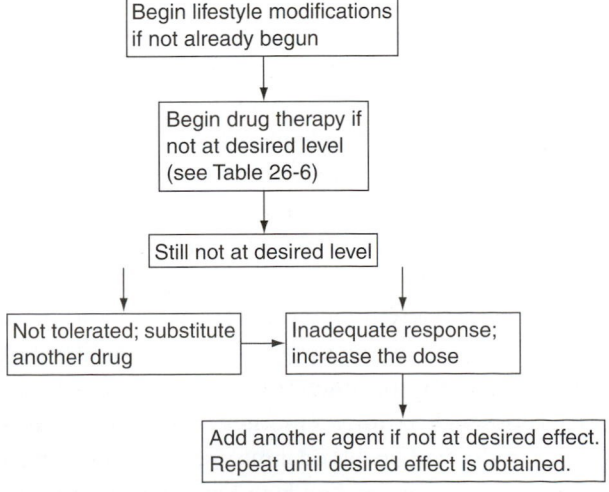

Figure 26-1 Treatment of hypertension.

considered in patients with a history of myocardial infarction. Myocardial infarction and left ventricular systolic dysfunction could benefit from ACE inhibitors. Elderly patients with isolated systolic hypertension have been shown to benefit from low-dose diuretics.[16,17] Studies have also shown that the use of long-acting dihydropyridine calcium-channel blockers in the elderly reduce morbidity and mortality from stroke by 42%. While survival data are less compelling, patients with prostatism may gain particular benefit from α-blockers, and patients with angina may benefit from either β-blockers or calcium-channel blockers.

When target blood pressure is not achieved with the initial agent, low-dose diuretics should almost always be considered as second-line additional therapy. The kidneys respond to antihypertensive medications with increased aldosterone and volume expansion. By countering this action, diuretics potentiate other therapies. Combination therapy with diuretics and ACE inhibitors, as well as diuretics and β-blockers, are available as a single pill.

Isolated systolic hypertension is most frequently encountered in the elderly.[14] When it is found in adolescents and young adults, it often is caused by hyperdynamic circulation and may be an indicator of future diastolic hypertension. Initially, lifestyle modifications should be attempted. Drug therapy should be considered for systolic pressures above 160 mm Hg.

Hypertensive emergencies require immediate blood pressure reduction, but not necessarily to normal ranges.[18] Examples of hypertensive emergencies include hypertensive encephalopathy, acute left ventricular failure with pulmonary edema, eclampsia or preeclampsia, intracranial hemorrhage, dissecting aortic aneurysm, unstable angina, and acute myocardial infarction. Hypertensive urgencies include malignant hypertension without severe symptoms or progressive target-organ damage. Calcium-channel blockers (especially short-acting nifedipine) are no longer recommended for treatment of urgencies or emergencies because of rapid and extreme drops in blood pressure. Several other medications that have proven to be safer to use in these situations (see Table 26-7) are available. Blood pressure should be reduced in a controlled manner over 30 minutes to several hours. Elevated blood pressure in the absence of target-organ damage often does not require emergency treatment. Too rapid a reduction in blood pressure can cause myocardial ischemia or cerebral hypoperfusion (watershed strokes).

LONG-TERM THERAPY

Patients on long-term therapy need continued follow-up care. With lifestyle modifications, patients often may be weaned from medications over the course of therapy. Patients with Stage 1 hypertension should be seen within 1 to 2 months of initiation of therapy to evaluate appropriate control. Comorbid conditions or the presence of target-organ damage may necessitate more frequent visits. Once blood pressure has stabilized, follow-up may be spaced out to every 3 to 6 months. Monitoring should include blood pressure monitoring and continued patient education.[1,2]

Good compliance requires ongoing patient education. Often planned programs or even group programs may help compliance. Always make sure patients understand the dosing regimen you have prescribed. Discussing treatment options and reasons with the patient will also improve compliance. Work to enhance family and/or social support for the patients. Try to answer the patient's questions (both asked and unasked). Individualize the regimen to better fit the patient's lifestyle and education level. Provide reinforcement for the patient as goals are met or surpassed. Take advantage of other community resources to help educate patients.

SPECIAL CONSIDERATIONS

Some of the drugs frequently encountered can cause or worsen hypertension. Oral contraceptives as well as estrogen-replacement therapy can cause hypertension. These medications are discussed in different sections of this book and will not be specifically dealt with here. Hypertension of pregnancy is a complicated topic that is covered in detail in other chapters.

TONE was the first multicenter clinical trial of sufficient size and duration to show that lifestyle modifications can be used to control high blood pressure in the elderly.[9] The patients selected to participate in TONE were 975 hypertensive men and women between the ages of 60 and 80 who were being treated with a single antihypertensive medication. The study included 585 overweight patients and 390 normal-weight patients. The overweight patients were randomized to one of four groups: sodium reduction, weight loss, combined weight loss and sodium reduction, or usual care. The normal-weight patients were assigned to either a sodium reduction or usual care group. At the end of the study, 30% of the participants were off their blood pressure medications. The study demonstrated that both weight loss and sodium restriction produced the best results as far as reducing the need for blood pressure medications. Sodium reduction lowered the need for antihypertensive medications by 31%, weight loss by 36%, and combination therapy by 53% as compared with usual care. Although TONE was not designed to look separately for effects on heart disease or stroke, the lowest rates of cardiovascular problems were seen in the groups receiving TONE interventions.

Hypertension in African-Americans as compared with Caucasians develops earlier in life, and the average blood pressures are much higher. As a result, African-Americans have an 80% higher rate of death from stroke, a 50% higher rate of death from heart disease, and a 320% higher rate of hypertension-related end-stage renal disease than the general population.[19] Lifestyle factors such as control of obesity and an awareness of an increased sensitivity to salt are particularly important for African-Americans who have a higher prevalence of risk factors for heart disease. Diuretics should be the first choice for this population.

Coexisting diseases can affect the choices of antihypertensive medications. For example, cardiovascular disease, coronary artery disease, congestive heart failure, and left ventricular hypertrophy can all influence choice of medications. These special considerations for combination therapy were discussed earlier in this chapter. Often the addition of an ACE inhibitor will be beneficial. Patients with vascular disease or angina may benefit from a calcium-channel blocker. Patients with renal disease or diabetes may delay further kidney damage with use of an ACE inhibitor. Patients with chronic obstructive pulmonary disease may not tolerate β-blockers well. If β-blockers must be used, consider the more cardioselective β-blockers. Patients with gout may not tolerate diuretics, which can worsen uric acid levels.

REFERENCES

1. The Fifth Annual Report of the Joint National Committee on Detection, Evaluation, and Treatment of High Blood Pressure. National Institutes of Health. National Heart, Lung, and Blood Institute. NIH publication no. 93-1088. January 1993.
2. The Sixth Annual Report of the Joint National Committee on Detection, Evaluation, and Treatment of High Blood Pressure. National Institutes of Health. National Heart, Lung, and Blood Institute. NIH publication no. 98-4080. November 1997.
3. Highlights of a new report from the National Center for Health Statistics (NCHS) Advance Report of Final Mortality Statistics, 1993 Monthly Vital Stat Rep 1996; 44(Suppl).
4. Kaplan NM. Southwestern Internal Medicine Conference: the promises and perils of treating the elderly hypertensive. Am J Med Sci 1993;3:305.
5. Lavrijssen ATJ, de Leeuw PW. Hypertension in the elderly: a brief overview. Neth J Cardiol 1993;1:16.
6. Hall WD, Ferario CM, Moore MA. Hypertension related morbidity and mortality in the Southeastern United States. Am J Med Sci 1997;313;195.
7. Sakoma M. Reproducibility of home blood pressure measurements over a 1-year period. Am J Hypertens, July 1997;10:7200-1.
8. Griner PF, Mayewski RJ, Mushlin AI, Greenland P. Selection and interpretation of diagnostic tests and procedures: principles and applications. Ann Intern Med 1981; 94(suppl):557.
9. Whelton PK, et al. Sodium reduction and weight loss in the treatment of hypertension in older persons: a randomized controlled trial of nonpharmacologic interventions in the elderly (TONE). JAMA 1998;279:839.
10. Bulpitt CJ, Fletcher AE. The measurement of quality of life in hypertensive patients—a practical approach. Br J Clin Pharmacol 1990;30:353.
11. Hu FB, Stampfer MJ, et al. Dietary fat intake and the risk of coronary heart disease in women. N Engl J Med 1997; 337:1491.
12. Koch GG. The use of nonparametric methods in the statistical analysis of the two period change over design. Biometrics 1972,28:577.
13. Sacks FM, et al. Rationale and design of the Dietary Approaches to Stop Hypertension trial (DASH): a multicenter controlled-feeding study of dietary patterns to lower blood pressure. Ann Epidemiol 1995;5:108.
14. Curb JD, Pressel SL, Cutler JA, et al. Effect of diuretic-based antihypertensive treatment on cardiovascular disease risk in older persons with isolated systolic hypertension. JAMA 1996;276:1886.
15. Nicholls MG. Age-related effects of diuretics in hypertensive subjects. J Cardiovasc Pharmacol 1998;12(Suppl):S51.
16. Holme I, Waaler T. Five-year mortality in the city of Bergen, Norway, according to age, sex, and blood pressure. Acta Med Scand 1976;200:229.
17. Agner E. Predictive value of arterial blood pressure in old age. Acta Med Scand 1983;214:285.
18. Kannel WB, Cupples A, D'Agostino RB, et al. Hypertension, anti-hypertensive treatment, and sudden coronary death: the Framingham Study. Hypertension 1988; (Suppl II):II-45.
19. Neutel JM, Smith DHG, Ram CVS, et al. Comparison of bisoprolol with atenolol for systemic hypertension in four population groups (young, old, black and nonblack) using ambulatory blood pressure monitoring. Am J Cardiol 1993;7:72.

Chapter 27

Diabetes Mellitus

Abbas E. Kitabchi
Michael Bryer-Ash

Five Key Points:

- Diabetes mellitus is a major cause of morbidity and mortality in our society and is a large and growing burden on our economy.

- Half of all Americans with type 2 diabetes are undiagnosed and approximately one-third will have one or more micro- or macrovascular complications when the diagnosis is finally made.

- Randomized controlled trials have established that intensive therapy to improve glycemic control prevents or delays progression of the major micro- and macrovascular diabetic complications.

- Two-thirds of all patients with diabetes die from vascular disease. Aggressive treatment of other associated cardiovascular risk factors is vitally important in persons with diabetes.

- The past 5 years have brought an explosion of new therapies for types 1 and 2 diabetes. Polypharmacy is now an important tool in achieving satisfactory glycemic control.

Human diabetes mellitus (DM) is a chronic disorder characterized by fasting hyperglycemia or plasma glucose levels that are above defined limits during oral glucose-tolerance testing (OGTT) or on random blood-glucose measurement as defined by established criteria.[1] DM is associated with abnormalities of protein, fat, and carbohydrate metabolism. There are approximately 16 million Americans with DM, of whom 1 million have type 1 and the remainder have type 2, representing approximately 6% of the total population. About 8 million of these individuals are undiagnosed or unaware of their DM.[2] In addition, there are approximately 20 million persons in the United States with a diagnosis of impaired glucose tolerance (IGT) who are at risk for developing DM.[3] Although these individuals may be asymptomatic for years before DM develops, some already have diabetic complications before the diagnosis is made.

The microvascular complications of DM are a major cause of morbidity.[4] DM is the leading cause of new cases of blindness in adults, and blindness is increased in DM about 20-fold as compared with nondiabetic subjects. Glaucoma and cataracts are increased by about 2- to 3-fold. Nephropathy occurs in 30% of patients with type 1 and 20% of those with type 2 DM, accounting for 30% of new cases of end-stage renal disease (ESRD) each year; the increased risk is about 25-fold over that for nondiabetic patients. Neuropathy is common in both type 1 and type 2 DM and is an important cause of morbidity (peripheral neuropathy, impotence, autonomic nervous dysfunction, anorgasmia, gastroparesis, etc.).

Coronary heart disease is four times more common in diabetic women than in nondiabetic women, and the risk for stroke is also increased fourfold. Peripheral vascular disease is present in 8% of patients at the time of diagnosis and in 45% after 20 years of DM. DM accounts for 40 to 50% of nontraumatic amputations and the 3-year survival of the other limb after contralateral amputation is 50%.[3]

The direct and indirect annual cost of DM in the United States in 1996 exceeded $98 billion.[5] There

TABLE 27-1	
ESTIMATED LIFETIME RISKS OF TYPE 1 DM	
Classification	**Risk (%)**
General population	
Background risk	0.2–0.3
DR3/4	2.4
Susceptible DR/DQ alleles	6–8.5
Family members	
Parents	3
Offspring	5
Siblings	6–8
Identical twins	30–50
HLA	
Identical	10–16
Haploidentical	2–9
Nonidentical	0–1

Derived from Eisenbarth GS, Ziegler AG, Coleman PA. Pathogenesis of insulin-dependent (type 1) diabetes mellitus. In: Kahn CR, Weir GC, eds. Joslin diabetes mellitus. Philadelphia: Lea & Febiger, 1994:216; and Bingley PJ, Gale EAM. Lessons from family studies. In: Harrison LC, Tait BD, eds. Clinical endocrinology and metabolism. London: Balliere-Tindall, 1991:261.

TABLE 27-2
POPULATION AT RISK FOR TYPE 2 DM

Persons with: classic signs and symptoms of diabetes (i.e., polyuria, polydipsia, polyphagia, and unexplained weight loss

Obesity (particularly upper-body adiposity) with body-mass index $\geq$30 kg/m^2 or $\geq$120% of ideal body weight

Primary relatives with history of type 2 DM

Susceptible ethnic groups (i.e., African-Americans, Hispanics and Native Americans, Asian-Americans)

Previous gestational DM or history of having a neonate weighing >9 lb

Having high-density lipoprotein cholesterol $\leq$35 mg/dl and/or TG $\geq$ 250 mg/dl

Previous impaired glucose tolerance or impaired fasting glucose

History of coronary artery or macrovascular disease and/or hypertension ($\geq$140/90 mm Hg)

Persons ingesting high doses of glucocorticoids

Derived from the Expert Committee on the Diagnosis and Classification of Diabetes Mellitus.[1]

are approximately 600,000 people who are diagnosed with DM each year; about half of these are older than 55, and the disease is diagnosed in more women than men (58% v: 42%, respectively). The annual incidence is 2.4 per 1000 people.

There has been an increase in the incidence of type 2 DM in this country during the past 35 years. Although the reason for this increase is not known, it is suggested that an increase in the age of the general population, a reduction in the mortality rate of people with DM, and better detection, as well as the increased severity of risk factors such as obesity and a sedentary lifestyle, have contributed to these increased rates.

Table 27-1 summarizes the lifetime risk for type 1 DM. The risk for DM of a primary family member of a patient with type 1 DM is increased 10-fold as compared with the general population.

The risk factors for type 2 DM are summarized in Table 27-2. It is important to point out that ethnicity and age have a contributory influence on DM 2.[6] For example, while the incidence of DM 2 in the Caucasian population is about 3%, the incidence in African-Americans is about 10%, in Hispanics about 12%, in Native American about 17%, and in Pima Indians about 35%. As an example, a 60-year-old Pima Indian woman has an approximately 60% chance of having type 2 DM. In addition, weight has a profound influence on the incidence of type 2 DM,[7] which rises steeply at greater than 140% of ideal body weight.

Having type 2 DM as well as its complications reduces life expectancy by approximately 5 to 10 years.[8] Table 27-3 demonstrates the approximate percentages of causes of death in persons with type 2 DM.

CLASSIFICATION AND DIAGNOSIS

DM classification and diagnostic criteria have gone through changes since 1979, when the National Institutes of Health Diabetes Data Group recommended two major classifications of DM with certain criteria. These were changed by the Expert Committee on the Diagnosis and Classification of Diabetes Mellitus and approved by the American Diabetes Association in 1997.[1] Table 27-4 depicts the new classifications of various forms of hyperglycemia, which recommend

TABLE 27-3
APPROXIMATE PERCENTAGE OF CAUSES OF DEATH IN TYPE 2 DM

Cause of Death	Percent of Deaths
Ischemic heart disease	40
Other heart disease	15
Metabolic decompensation of DM	13
Malignant neoplasm	13
Cerebrovascular disease	10
Pneumonia/influenza	4
All others	5
	100%

From Geiss et al.[8]

TABLE 27-4
CLASSIFICATION OF VARIOUS HYPERGLYCEMIAS

Diabetes mellitus
  Type 1
    a. Immune-mediated
    b. Idiopathic
  Type 2
  Individuals with insulin resistance who usually have
    relative rather than absolute insulin deficiency (obese or
    nonobese).
  Other Types
  Pancreatic disease and following pancreatic surgery, including
    tropical calcific DM
  Endocrinopathies (Cushing syndrome, acromegaly,
    glucagonoma, hyperaldosteronism, pheochromocytoma)
  Drug-induced
  Gestational (GDM)
  Maturity-onset DM of the young (MODY)
Impaired glucose tolerance (IGT)

Derived from the Expert Committee on the Diagnosis and Classification
of Diabetes Mellitus.[1]

that the older classification of insulin-dependent DM (IDDM) or juvenile-onset or ketosis-prone all be changed to the term *type 1 DM*, whereas the old terminology of noninsulin-dependent DM (NIDDM) adult-onset or ketosis-resistant DM all be changed to the term *type 2 DM*. Table 27-5 summarizes the new criteria for diagnosis of DM and IGT and furthermore, defines an additional term, *impaired fasting glucose*

TABLE 27-5
NEW CRITERIA FOR DIAGNOSIS OF DIABETES MELLITUS AND IMPAIRED GLUCOSE TOLERANCE

Diabetes mellitus
  Fasting plasma glucose ≥126 mg/dl on two separate
    occasions
  Casual blood glucose level ≥200 mg/dl with symptoms of
    DM (polyuria, polydipsia, unexplained weight loss)
  2-hr postprandial glucose ≥200 mg/dl on OGTT
Impaired glucose tolerance
  2-hr postprandial glucose ≥140<200 mg/dl on OGTT
Impaired fasting glucose (IFG)
  Fasting plasma glucose ≥110<126 mg/dl
Gestational DM (GDM)
  Following 100-g OGTT, plasma glucose reaching or exceeding
    any of the following two values: 95, 190, 165, 145 for
    fasting, 1 hr, 2 hr, 3 hr, respectively. Screen only high-risk
    subjects: (a) all women >25 years; (b) >120% of ideal
    body weight; (c) family history of DM; (d) ethnic groups at
    high risk; (e) previous GDM; (f) morbid obstetrical history
    or neonate birth >9 lb; (g) hypertension or hyperlipidemia
  Screen for DM in all individuals ≥45 years and if normal, re-
    peat at 3-year intervals. Screen at age <45 in high-risk
    individuals (see Table 27-2).

Derived from the Expert Committee on the Diagnosis and Classification
of Diabetes Mellitus.[1]

(IFG). The major differences between the old and new classifications are (a) fasting blood glucose (FBG) for diagnosis of DM is lowered from 140 to 126 mg/dl (on two separate occasions), (b) the number of abnormal blood glucose values required for diagnoses of DM and IGT from OGTT has now been changed from two to one, and (c) in gestational diabetes mellitus (GDM), although the earlier criteria have been retained, contrary to the previous recommendation, screening has been recommended only for those people who are older than age 25, or if under 25 years of age, are greater than 120% ideal body weight, have a family history of DM, or have any of the other risk factors described in Table 27-5. An additional important recommendation made by the Expert Committee is that individuals 45 years or older should be screened for type 2 DM and if normal, should undergo repeat screening every 3 years.

DIAGNOSTIC METHODS FOR DM

It is now well established that urine glucose testing is poorly related to blood-glucose levels.[9] Therefore, the use of urine glucose testing for diagnosis or follow-up of patients with DM is no longer an accepted procedure. As stated above and depicted in Table 27-5, the simplest method for diagnosis of DM is a fasting plasma glucose value of 126 mg/dl or higher on two separate occasions. Casual blood glucose of 200 mg/dl or higher with or without typical signs and symptoms of DM is also an accepted method. For individuals whose FBG >110<126 and who are at high risk for DM, 2-hour OGTT is the other method for diagnosis of DM. There are certain precautions as well as necessary preparations that need to be taken for satisfactory performance of the OGTT. These are summarized in Table 27-6.

Screening for GDM

As indicated in Table 27-5, the new guidelines recommend screening for DM during pregnancy only in certain groups. The standard procedure for screening during pregnancy is to administer a 50-g oral glucose load between the 24th and 28th week of gestation (without regard to time of day or time of last meal) to all pregnant women over age 25 (except those who are already known to have DM), and draw a 1-hour venous plasma glucose sample.[10] A value of ≥140 mg/dl (7.8mM) indicates the need for a full diagnostic OGTT (3 hours with preparation; see Table 27-6).

TABLE 27-6
PREPARATIONS AND PROCEDURES FOR PERFORMANCE OF OGTT

Administer only to otherwise healthy ambulatory subjects.

Allow at least 3 days of unrestricted diet and physical activity prior to the test. The diet should include 150 g of carbohydrate per day.

Subject should have fasted for 10 to 14 hours.

Test should be performed in the morning.

Administer 75 g of glucose orally for adults, 100 g for pregnant adults, and 1.75 g/kg of body weight for children, up to a maximum of 75 g.

Subject should remain seated and should not smoke nor use caffeine during the test.

Venous plasma glucose determinations are drawn fasting and every 30 minutes for 2 hours in nonpregnant adults.

Venous plasma glucose determinations are drawn every hour for 3 hours in pregnant adults.

Test should not be performed on subjects with previously diagnosed DM (by fasting or random blood glucose), as it may induce marked hyperglycemia.

Derived from Kitabchi AE, et al. Diabetes mellitus. In: Ling FW, Laube DW, Nolan TE, Smith RP, Stovall TG, eds. Primary care in gynecology. Baltimore: Williams & Wilkins, 1996:279.

Other Methods for Measurement of Glycemic Status

Although the only recognized and accepted methods for diagnosis of DM are the ones summarized in Table 27-5, there are other methods that provide useful information regarding glycemic status: intravenous glucose/tolerance tests (IVGTT) and glycated hemoglobin.[11]

Intravenous Glucose/Tolerance Test

The IVGTT, although less sensitive than the OGTT, may be a better index of glucose metabolism and clearance in individuals who have a compromised gastrointestinal (GI) tract, such as following GI surgery or in the presence of GI pathology.[12] In these situations, performance of an IVGTT and sampling of blood glucose at 2, 5, 10, 15, 20, 30, 40, 50, and 60 minutes after injection of 0.3g/kg of body weight of 50% dextrose in water ($D_{50}W$) and measuring the disappearance rate of glucose by the formula

$$K = (0.603/t\ 1/2) \times 100$$

where K = percent per minute glucose disappearance and where t 1/2 = time in minutes to reach half the initial peak, gives a fairly good separation between persons with and without DM. The nondiabetic individual has a K value of approximately 1.72% per minute and is above 1.3, but diabetic subjects have K

values of less than 1% per minute. Measurement of plasma insulin during IVGTT has been used to detect early pancreatic failure in family members of the patient with type 1 DM.[13] By measuring the early phase of insulin secretion (first 10 minutes) one can detect family members at high risk for type 1 DM. One caveat for performance of such a test is that the injected 50% dextrose (glucose), which is hypertonic, must be given into a major vein (antecubital) with precautions to prevent leakage of the $D_{50}W$ solution into the subcutaneous tissues.

Glycated Hemoglobin

Glycated (glycosylated) hemoglobin is the product of a ketoamine reaction between glucose and valine on the β-chain of hemoglobin in solution, which is the more stable form of this hemoglobin; it is abbreviated HbA_{1c}. In normal individuals this comprises 4 to 6% of total hemoglobin. HbA_{1c} is abnormally elevated in DM, as it depends on the concentration of glucose in the blood. As the half-life of HbA1 depends on the life span of red cells (120 days), HbA_{1c} values reflect the glycemic status over the past 8 to 10 weeks. In severely decompensated DM, HbA_{1c} is usually greater than 13%, indicating very poor control, whereas less than 7.5% indicates an acceptable range.[14] Measurement of HbA_{1c} as a diagnostic criterion for DM has not yet been accepted due to lack of adequate correlative data, but this may be forthcoming in the near future. Factors that can artificially lower HbA_{1c} include hemoglobinopathies (C, D, S), conditions with enhanced destruction of red cells (sickle-cell trait, hemolytic anemia, phlebotomies), and recent transfusion with nondiabetic blood. The conditions that cause falsely elevated HbA_{1c} are prehemoglobin A_{1c}, fetal hemoglobin(F) and uremia (carbamoylated hemoglobin), and high concentrations of alcohol or acetylsalicylic acid. Non−high−performance-liquid chromatography may be artificially altered by circulating lipids.[15]

Other Glycated Proteins

Increased glycation of protein such as serum protein can also occur with elevated plasma glucose in DM. Thus, serum albumin has a shorter half-life (17 to 20 days) than hemoglobin. In combination with glucose, this results in the production of fructosamine.[16] This compound provides an index of glycemia over a shorter duration (2 to 3 weeks), which may be useful in the treatment of patients with GDM or those unable to perform home blood-glucose monitoring.

PATHOPHYSIOLOGY OF TYPE 1 AND TYPE 2 DM

Table 27-7 summarizes the major characteristics of two types of DM. As can be seen from this table, type 1 DM is characterized by having onset in a younger age group and constitutes less than 10% of the diabetic population. This type has a strong autoimmune component, whereas type 2 DM has few indications of an autoimmune etiology, but has a strong familial association, with about an 80 to 85% prevalence of obesity. It is important to point out that metabolic ketoacidosis, although more frequent in type 1 DM, can infrequently occur in type 2 DM under extreme conditions with a greater incidence in certain ethnic groups (e.g., African-Americans).[17]

Type 1 DM

Type 1 DM is a metabolic disorder of autoimmune basis, characterized by insulinopenia, that is likely to be triggered by an environmental factor(s) such as a toxin or virus. It is important to note that other po-

tent risk factors, such as genetic susceptibility, impaired tissue and/or ineffective immunologic defenses can profoundly influence the development of DM.[18] The association of certain types of human leukocyte antigens (HLAs), abnormal immunologic responses, infection with pancreotropic viruses (mumps, rubella, Coxsackie B4, Epstein–Barr, hepatitis B and C, toxins), and excessive stress may all be contributing factors in bringing about the destruction of the β-cell that characterizes type 1 DM,[19,20] the hallmark of which is insulin deficiency. In type 1 DM an increased incidence of antibodies to various organs such as thyroid, adrenal glands, and gastric parietal cells has been observed.[21] Furthermore, antibodies to pancreatic islets have been detected by immunofluorescent techniques prior to diagnosis of overt disease, and some investigators have reported the presence of insulin antoantibodies in persons with newly diagnosed type 1 DM prior to therapy with insulin.[22]

The term HLA is used to describe the major histocompatibility complex (MHC) in humans, which consists of three classes of closely linked genes (I, II, and III) on the short arm of chromosome 6. Class II consists of DP, DQ, and DR loci. Certain HLA types (HLA-DR3 and HLA-DR4) are highly correlated with type 1 DM in Caucasians.[15] Although only 70% of persons with type 1DM have both DR3 and DR4,

---

TABLE 27-7
MAJOR CHARACTERISTICS OF TYPES 1 AND 2 DM

Features	Type 1 DM	Type 2 DM
Age at onset	Usually <40	Usually >40
Proportion of all DM	About 10%	About 90%
Seasonal trend	Fall and winter	None
Appearance of symptoms	Acute or subacute	Slow or subacute
Metabolic ketoacidosis	Frequent	Rare*
Obesity at onset	Uncommon	Common
β-cells	Decreased	Variable
Insulin	Decreased or absent	Variable
Inflammatory cells in islets	Present initially	Absent
Family history of DM	Uncommon	Common
Concordance in identical twins	30–50%	90–95%
HLA association	Yes	No
Islet-cell antibody (ICA)	Yes	Uncommon
Insulin autoantibodies (IAA)	Yes (in younger age)	No
"64K" GAD† antibodies	Yes	No
Treatment	Insulin and diet, Islet or Pancreas transplantation	Diet, weight reduction, exercise, OAA†, insulin

*Except in African-Americans.

†Glutamic acid decarboxylase (GAD).

†Oral antidiabetic agents.

Derived from Kitabchi AE, Fisher JN. In: Lomm R., ed. Current diagnosis. Philadelphia: Saunders, 1991:766.

about 95% express either one or the other of these alleles. These HLA types may vary with race, as African-Americans and Japanese may have different haplotypes.

Studies of HLA typing using refined DNA technology have shown the DR4 haplotype DQB10302 is the gene most associated with type 1 DM, whereas DQB10301 appears to increase incidence of DM in a subclass of the Caucasian population whereas DR1 is protective. In addition, some HLA types (such as DR4) may be more associated with the progression to diabetic complications, such as proliferative retinopathy or diabetic ketoacidosis.

Although the detailed mechanisms for the destruction of β-cells leading to type 1 DM are not known, certain factors appear to play important roles. Introduction of environmental pancreotropic virus into the pancreas leads to production of an antigen. The antigen is then processed by macrophages, which are antigen-presenting cells in whose membranes are located the major histocompatibility complex [MHC II (DR3, DR4, etc.)]. The appropriate antigen, consisting of a peptide that fits into the groove of the MHC class II molecule of the macrophage, must further fit into a receptor of the T lymphocyte for CD4 activation. Two cytokines, interleukin-1 and tumor necrosis factor-α (TNFα), are produced by macrophages, whereas lymphocytes produce interferon gamma (IFNγ), which collectively result in destruction of β-cells. When more than 90% of β cells are destroyed, the clinical condition of type 1 DM emerges. These events are summarized in Figure 27-1.[23] The onset of type 1 DM is usually preceded by the production of multiple antibodies, including islet-cell antibody (ICA), specific antibodies against a 64Kd antigen,[24] now identified as a sequence of the β-islet enzyme glutamic acid decarboxylase (GAD), and insulin autoantibody (IAA).[22]

Type 2 DM

Type 2 DM is a heterogeneous form of DM that usually occurs in individuals of older age (i.e., ≥40years). However, emerging data shows a 5- to 10-fold increase in the incidence of type 2 DM in children under age 18,[25,26] concometant with the rise in prevalence of obesity in this age group. In adults, it is 8 to 10 times more common than type 1 DM and accounts for greater overall morbidity. Genetic and environmental factors, aging, and adiposity play important roles,[27] but viral disease (except hepatitis B and C), HLA type and other immune factors apparently do not correlate with the disease. Analysis of identical twins with type 2 DM indicates approximately 90% concordance. By comparison, concordance in type 1 DM is about 25 to 50%. One sub-classification of type 2 DM is maturity-onset diabetes of the young (MODY), which seems to be transmitted as an autosomal dominant trait. MODY appears to be a rare condition that results in a less severe form of DM and, in certain families, is related to defects in the islet enzymes glucokinase and phosphofructokinase.[28]

Rates of insulin secretion and insulin levels in type 2 DM are variable depending on age, the duration of DM, dietary regimen, prior glycemic control, and adiposity. Thus, a newly discovered obese patient with type 2 DM and mild to moderate hyperglycemia

Figure 27-1 Pathogenesis of Type 1 DM.

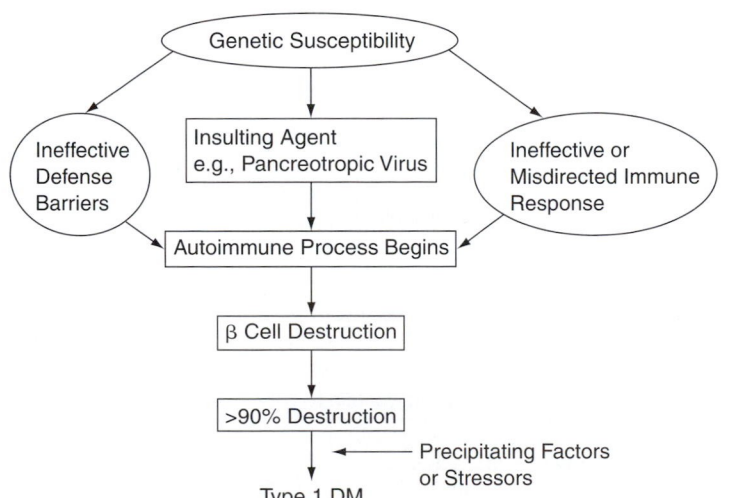

generally has a high basal insulin level (hyperinsulinemia) and fewer insulin receptors on insulin-responsive target tissues (i.e., muscle, fat, and liver cells). The high insulin level is due to a compensatory increase in phase 2 insulin secretion (as phase 1 insulin secretion in type 2 DM is decreased) to maintain near-normal fasting blood-glucose levels. With progression of the disease, even phase 2 insulin secretion is reduced, and the fasting plasma glucose gradually increases so that when the latter value ranges between 160 and 200 mg/dl, there is generally a significant reduction of overall insulin secretion and hence low C-peptide concentrations.[29]

Insulin Resistance in Type 2 DM

About 85% of patients with type 2 diabetes are obese (i.e. BMI >30 kg/m^2). These patients are insensitive to endogenous insulin, and the degree of insensitivity is positively correlated with the amount of fat tissue in the upper body (so-called apple-shaped or android habitus, as opposed to the increased lower body adiposity of the pear-shaped or gynoid habitus), producing a high waist-to-hip ratio. The major site of insulin resistance to glucose uptake in both obese and nonobese persons with type 2 DM is muscle.[27]

The insulin resistance that is the hallmark of type 2 DM may be the initial causative step as a result of either the genetic and/or environmental factors leading to compensatory increased insulin secretion to maintain fasting blood glucose near normal with abnormally elevated postprandial glucose levels (>140 but <200 mg/dl), which is defined as IGT (see Table 27-4). However, this postprandial hyperglycemia of IGT may have toxic effects on the pancreatic β cells.[28] Therefore, glucose toxicity,[30] insulin resistance, and genetic predisposition lead to a state of pancreatic exhaustion and frank DM.[31] These proposed etiopathological pathways are depicted in Figure 27-2.[32] The prediabetic state in such individuals is characterized by obesity, insulin resistance, IGT, hypertension, dyslipidemia, and hyperinsulinemia, which is collectively referred to as the dysmetabolic syndrome or syndrome X.[33]

CORRELATION OF CLINICAL CONDITIONS WITH METABOLIC AND BIOCHEMICAL ABNORMALITIES IN DM

As stated earlier, DM is a syndrome associated with abnormalities of carbohydrate, protein, and fat metabolism; therefore, alteration of their respective metabolic pathways brings about certain clinical manifestations

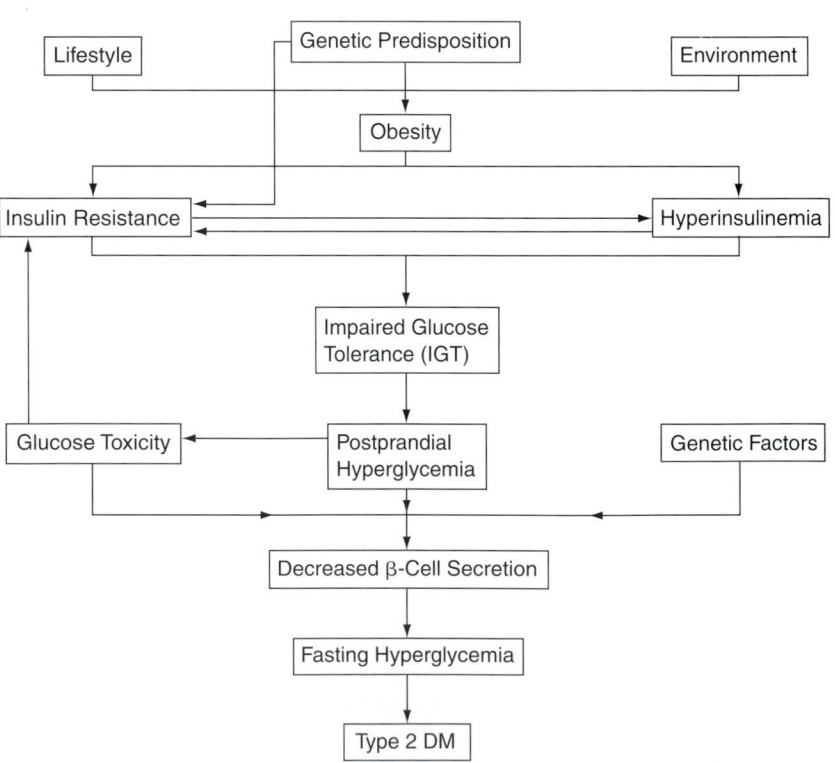

Figure 27-2 Hypothetical presentation for pathogenesis of obese type 2 DM, which could be preceded by insulin resistance, IGT, and glucose toxicity.

TABLE 27-8
CORRELATION OF CLINICAL CONDITIONS AND DIABETIC SYNDROMES WITH VARIOUS METABOLIC DEFECTS

Metabolic Defects	Chemical Abnormailities	Clinical Abnormalities
Carbohydrate metabolism		
1. Diminished uptake of glucose by tissues such as muscle, adipose, tissue, and liver	Hyperglycemia	Polyuria, polydipsia, polyphagia, fatigue, muscle weakness, pruritus
2. Overproduction of glucose (via glycogenolysis and gluconeogenesis by the liver)		Blurred vision
Diminished mental alertness, weight loss
Protein Metabolism		
1. Diminished uptake of amino acids and diminished synthesis of protein	Negative nitrogen balance
Elevated levels of branched-chain amino acids
Elevated blood urea nitrogen level	Loss of muscle mass
Weakness
2. Increased proteolysis	Elevated potassium level	Arrhythmia
Fat metabolism		
1. Increased lipolysis	Elevated plasma fatty acids
Elevated plasma glycerol level	Loss of adipose tissue
2. Decreased lipogenesis		Loss of adipose tissue
3. Increased production of triglycerides	Hypertriglyceridemia	Exudative xanthoma in skin lesions
Lipemia retinalis
Pancreatitis (abdominal pain)
4. Decreased removal of ketones and increased ketone production	Elevated plasma and urine ketones	Hyperventilation, metabolic acidosis abdominal pain, acetone on breath

Derived from Kitabchi and Fisher.[34]

characteristic of decompensated DM.[34] Table 27-8 shows the types of biochemical lesions that can lead to the presenting clinical features such as the polyuria, polyphagia, and polydipsia characteristic of uncontrolled DM, as well as further decompensation to diabetic ketoacidosis or hyperosmolarity, which may cause death if not treated promptly and correctly.

CLINICAL TRIALS OF INTENSIVE THERAPY OF PATIENTS WITH DM

For many years, controversies existed as to whether hyperglycemia per se could lead to microvascular (retinopathy, nephropathy, or neuropathy) or macro-

vascular (cardiovascular diseases, stroke, etc.) complications of DM. The important issue regarding microvascular complications was finally settled by 4 prospective randomized long-term studies.

The first major studies of this nature in type 1 DM were the NIH-sponsored Diabetes Control and Complications Trial (DCCT)[14] (conducted in 29 clinical centers in the United States and Canada) and the Swedish Diabetes Intervention Study (SDIS).[35] The Kumamoto Study,[36] which was conducted in Japan, and the UKPDS,[37,38] carried out in the United Kingdom, addressed similar issues in type 2 DM. Although the characteristics of type 1 and type 2 DM are different (Table 27-9), nevertheless, the results of these 4

TABLE 27-9
CHARACTERISTICS OF TYPE 1/DCCT VERSUS TYPE 2 DM PATIENTS

Features	Type 1 in DCCT	Typical Profile of Type 2 Patients
Age	27 years	40 years
Race	Caucasian >95%	Minority > Caucasian
Weight	Ideal body weight	Obese
Blood pressure	Normal	Hypertensive
Lipid profile	Normal HDL cholesterol
Low/normal total cholesterol
Low/normal total triglycerides	Low HDL cholesterol
Normal/high total cholesterol
High triglycerides
Blood insulin level	Insulinopenia	Hyperinsulinemia

HDL = high-density lipoprotein; LDL = low-density lipoprotein.
Derived from Kitabchi et al.[23]

TABLE 27-10
RELATIONSHIP OF GLYCEMIC CONTROL TO REDUCTION IN DIABETIC COMPLICATIONS

Outcome Parameters	Studies			
	SDIS[35]	DCCT[14]	Kumamoto[36]	UKPDS[37,38]
Type of DM	Type 1	Type 1	Type 2	Type 2
Number of Patients	102	1441	102	5102
Mean age (y)	30	27	49	53
Duration of follow-up (y)	7.5	6.5	6	10
Change in HbA$_{1c}$	−2.4	−1.9	−2.3	−0.9
Reduction in risk (%)				
Retinopathy	52	63	69	21
Nephropathy	89	54	70	33
Neuropathy	NS	60	—	—
Myocardial infarction	—	—	—	16
Any diabetes-related endpoint	—	—	—	25

studies clearly showed that reduction of hyperglycemia by intensive therapy does reduce the risk and incidence of microvascular complications in both type 1 and type 2 DM. Intensive therapy in the DCCT (characterized by three or more injections of insulin per day and self-monitoring of blood glucose (SMBG) 3 to 5 times per day by the patient, monthly outpatient visits with the goal of normalizing HbA$_{1c}$ and blood glucoses) versus conventional therapy (consisting of two or fewer insulin injections, one blood or urine test per day, and quarterly clinic visits) reduced the risk of progression of retinopathy by 63%, nephropathy by 39%, and neuropathy by 60%.[14] In the Kumamoto study of type 2 DM with a similar therapeutic protocol,[36] the risk of retinopathy was reduced by 69%, and nephropathy by 70% (Table 27-10). The UKPDS showed more modest beneficial reductions in these parameters (25 to 30%) but showed the important novel finding that control of blood pressure was equally as important in prevention of complications[39] as control of blood glucose. These studies also implied that the team approach to management of DM is extremely important to achieve a successful metabolic outcome. Therefore it has been recommended that physicians should work in cooperation with a team consisting of a diabetes educator, nutritionist, exercise physiologist, and behaviorist to bring about the desired outcome.[14]

MANAGEMENT OF DM

The goals of therapy in DM are to normalize metabolism, provide a state of well-being, and avoid the acute and chronic complications of DM. The recommended approach in achievement of these goals is initial evaluation of patients, education, meal planning and exercise, and therapy with pharmaceutical agents. These topics will be discussed under the separate headings of the various forms of DM.

Initial Evaluation of Patients with DM

Table 27-11 provides general management guidelines for patients recently diagnosed with DM. It is

TABLE 27-11
GENERAL GUIDELINES FOR MANAGEMENT OF DM

1. Establish diagnosis of DM and emphasize educational components. Do not perform OGTT if diagnosis of DM is already established.
2. Classify DM as type 1 or type 2, etc.
3. Inform patient of diagnosis and refer to DM education classes (to learn signs and symptoms, complications, SMBG, DM medications, sick days, etc.)
4. Place patient on American Diabetes Association diet with appropriate caloric, sodium, and lipid restrictions.
5. Identify and treat cardiac risk factors (blood pressure, lipids, etc.)
6. Determine status of kidney function (serum creatinine, 24-hour urine microalbumin), and reassess annually thereafter.
7. Evaluate for presence of neuropathy (refer to neurologist as necessary).
8. Establish extent of fundoscopic lesions (refer to ophthalmologist).
9. Check feet, pulses, and toenails at each visit.
10. Use SMBG for daily diabetic control and check urine only for ketones when blood sugar is >300 mg/dl.
11. Follow chronic glycemic control by HbA$_{1c}$ approximately every 3 months in the office, and perform complete physical examination annually.
12. Design exercise program for the patient with type 2 DM.

*At diagnosis if type 2 DM, at 5 years if type 1 DM.
Derived from Kitabchi et al.[23]

important to point out that if these patients had not been recently evaluated, they should have a complete history and physical examination with the following laboratory tests: complete blood count with differential, chemistry profile, fasting lipid profile, thyroid-stimulating hormone (and free thyroxine, if necessary), HbA$_{1c}$, and electrocardiography in adults.[40]

Since the diagnosis of DM in a previously unsuspecting individual may raise numerous social and emotional issues not only for the patient, but also for the family, it is important for the primary care physician to provide as much emotional support as possible and to approach the patient and family with compassion, empathy, and due consideration when first informing them of the diagnosis. This is particularly true in the case of children and young adults and their immediate families.[41]

Educational Program

As detailed in Table 27-12, the importance of an educational program is greater than mere itemization of various topics of discussion. It is necessary that, through the establishment of a one-on-one dialogue with the patient, a customized program of education commensurate with the work situation, family support network, educational background, psychological condi-

TABLE 27-13 METABOLIC GOALS IN DM		
	Normal Value	Goal Value for DM
Fasting blood glucose	70–110 mg/dl	80–120 mg/dl
Pregnant	69–90 mg/dl	69–90 mg/dl
Postprandial blood glucose (2 hr)	<140 mg/dl	<180 mg/dl
Pregnant (1 hr)	<140 mg/dl	≤130 mg/dl
Glycosylated hemoglobin (HbA$_{1c}$)	4–6%	<7%*
Total cholesterol	<200 mg/dl	<200 mg/dl
HDL cholesterol		
Men	>35 mg/dl	>35 mg/dl
Women	>45 mg/dl	>45 mg/dl
LDL cholesterol	<130 mg/dl	<100 mg/dl
Triglycerides	<150 mg/dl	<150 mg/dl
Body-mass index† (BMI) (weight [kg] ÷ height [m^2])	19–25	19–25

*In certain groups of patients.

†BMI >30 is defined as obese.

Derived from Kitabchi and Bryer-Ash.[30]

tion, physical ability, and presence or absence of various risk factors be considered and discussed in a frank and compassionate manner.[42] This is obviously a time-consuming and labor-intensive endeavor, which the primary care physician may not be able to accomplish alone. Therefore, as suggested by the results of the DCCT,[14] a team approach to education of patients is absolutely essential, with a minimum personnel requirement of a certified diabetes educator (CDE) and a nutritionist who can call on other individuals such as an exercise physiologist, social worker, podiatrist, and psychologist, under supervision of a knowledgeable physician, for further consultation. For any educational program to be effective, one must clearly establish metabolic goals for control of DM. Table 27-13 summarizes these goals for glucose, HbA$_{1c}$, lipids, and body weight. For patients with newly discovered DM, we ensure that the patient understands important aspects of self-management and emergency measures. Therefore, for such individuals we provide pretest and posttest questions to assess knowledge and the extent of retention of this knowledge after the educational program has been completed.

TABLE 27-12 EDUCATIONAL COMPONENT FOR DM TEACHING

1. Overview of DM
2. Establishment of metabolic goals (see Table 27-13)
3. Stress psychological adjustment
4. Family involvement and social support
5. Nutrition
6. Exercise
7. Work and recreational activities
8. Medications (oral antidiabetic versus insulin preparations)
9. Monitoring, keeping records, and proper use of results
10. Relationship of nutrition, exercise, and medication
11. Reduction of vascular risk factors (e.g., smoking)
12. Prevention, detection, and treatment of acute complications
13. Prevention, detection, and treatment of chronic complications
14. Foot, skin, and dental care
15. Benefits, risks, and management for improving glycemic control
16. Sick days
17. Various strategies for travel
18. Preconception care, pregnancy, and DM in pregnancy
19. Use of health care system and community resources
20. Provision of identification tag (i.e., MedicAlert) to be worn around the neck or wrist.

Derived from Kitabchi et al.[23]

Diet Management, Meal Planning, and Exercise

Establishment of Strategies

Since achievement of the desired outcome of self-management may necessitate changes in nutrition and

TABLE 27-17
CHARACTERISTICS OF HUMAN INSULINS AVAILABLE IN THE UNITED STATES

Action	Insulin Type	Onset	Peak Action	Duration
Ultrashort-acting	Lispro	5 minutes	45 minutes	3–4 hours
Short-acting	Regular, Velosulin	15–30 minutes	1–3 hours	5–6 hours
	Semilente	30–60 minutes	4–6 hours	12–16 hours
Intermediate-acting	Lente, NPH	1–3 hours	6–10 hours	16–20 hours
Long-acting	Ultralente	4–6 hours	8–20 hours	24–28 hours
	Glargine	1–2 hours	No peak	24–30 hours*
Mixture	(70/30, 50/50)	30 minutes	Biphasic	16–20 hours
	Lispro 75/25	5 minutes	Biphasic	16–20 hours

*Heinemann L et al. Diabetes Care 2000;23:644.
Derived from Kitabchi et al.[23]

achieve good metabolic control with only one injection of insulin per day, even if this contains two preparations (e.g., NPH and regular). Therefore, the physician must clarify to the patient at the outset that two or more injections per day or continuous insulin administration by insulin pump are necessary for optimal diabetic control and to achieve HbA$_{1c}$ values of less than 7%. Nevertheless, the emphasis should be on the achievement of satisfactory glycemic control itself and not merely on employment of a given number of daily insulin injections.

Availability of newer insulin delivery systems including subcutaneous insulin infusion (SCII, or the insulin pump) as well as insulin pens containing a cartridge for various insulin preparations, make administration of insulin more manageable for persons with sporadic meal schedules or activities.

As shown in Table 27-16, there are certain guidelines for treatment of type 1 DM that must be followed for successful treatment of such patients. Knowledge of these guidelines in the use of intensive insulin therapy, based on the results of the DCCT, clearly established a positive benefit:risk ratio for type 1 DM patients. However, it must be emphasized that, as was indicated in Table 27-9, the DCCT patients were young and relatively free of diabetic complications and also were older than 13 years of age. The better glycemic control, however, was achieved with a threefold greater incidence of severe hypoglycemia.[48] Therefore, intensive therapy in such patients must be carried out with caution and thorough education of the patient. In addition, such intensive therapy in selected groups of type 1 diabetic patients must be approached with care as the benefit:risk ratio of such intensive therapy with the accompanying higher incidence of hypoglycemia may be lower,

e.g. in the elderly.[49] We, therefore, recommend a cautious approach to the use of intensive therapy in the following groups of patients with type 1 DM: elderly patients, patients who live alone, children younger than 13 years of age, patients who have hypoglycemic unawareness, patients with a history of seizures and on medications for seizures, patients with advanced microvascular complications, and patients with major macrovascular complications.

Calculation of Insulin Dose

The dosage regimen that we propose for insulin is based on studies performed on rates of insulin secretion[50] and is consistent with the average dose used in the DCCT,[14] which ranged between 0.6 and 0.8 U/kg of body weight/day (higher in the adolescent group). Most nondiabetic, nonobese individuals (about 70 kg) secrete approximately 1 U of insulin per hour in the postabsorptive-fasting state (i.e., 24 U/day) as the basal rate of insulin production. In addition, approximately another 25 U are secreted during postprandial periods, which makes the total daily insulin secretion about 49 U or 0.7 U/kg/day in a 70-kg individual. It must be emphasized that calculations are oversimplifications, since endogenously secreted insulin is delivered directly to the liver in the portal system, while administered insulin is placed subcutaneously and bypasses the liver initially. As the basal insulin may be compared to intermediate-acting insulin and postprandial insulin response may resemble regular or Lispro insulin, we propose that in the initial empiric dosage calculations, 40 to 60% of the total dose should be given as regular or Lispro insulin and 40 to 60% be given as an intermediate-acting insulin. In individuals who are taking only two injections of insulin per day,

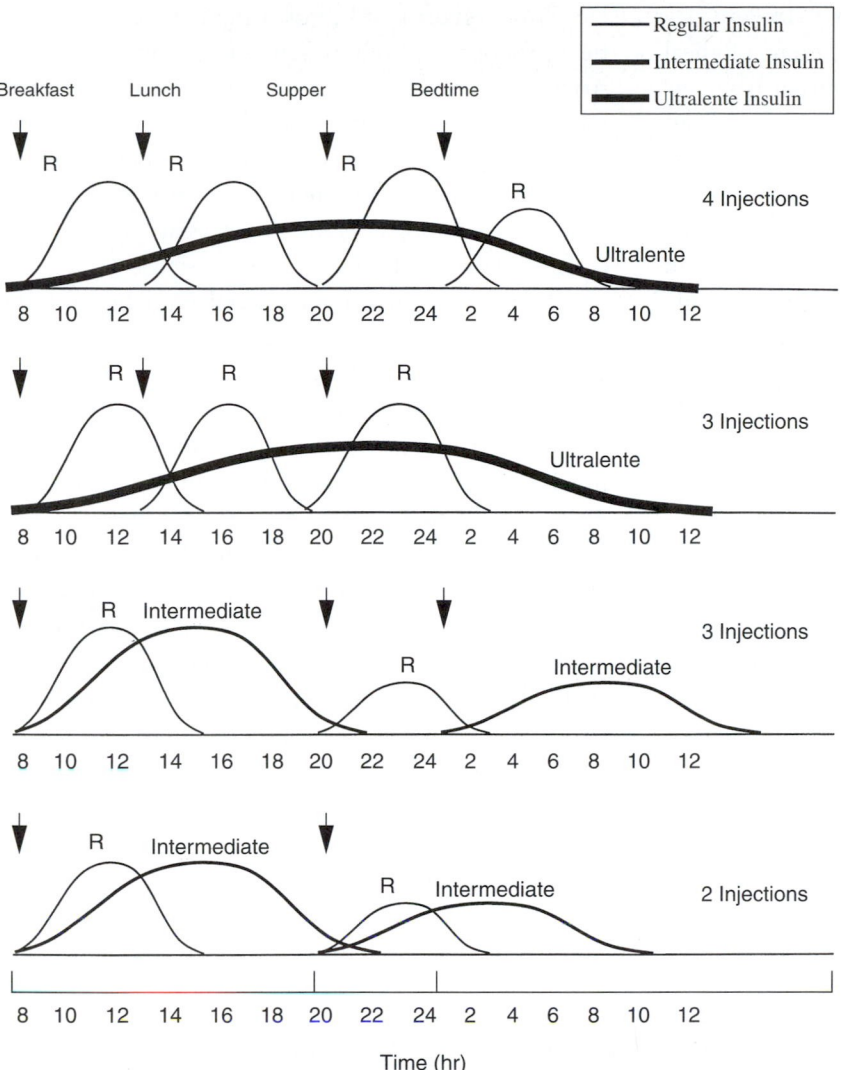

Regular Insulin
Intermediate Insulin
Ultralente Insulin

Figure 27-3 Hypothetical representation with peak and duration of action of various forms of insulin with different time schedule of subcutaneous injection.

two-thirds of the total dose (e.g., combined NPH plus regular) should be given before breakfast and one-third before supper. However, in some cases two injections may not provide optimal HbA$_{1c}$ values and, therefore, in certain patients evening NPH or Ultralente is given at bedtime, with the remaining dose of evening regular insulin being given before supper. Figure 27-3 provides a hypothetical representation of the duration of action of certain insulin preparations.

Occasionally, for people who desire a heavier lunch, a sliding-scale dose of regular or Lispro may be needed before lunch. As stated earlier, the availability of various convenient mechanical devices for blood-glucose monitoring and insulin injection pens makes determination of blood glucose and extra injections of insulin quite convenient and feasible. However, such intensive therapy for individuals with the conditions listed in the previous section, or with unpre-

dictable patterns of major physical exertion, must be approached with extreme caution, as there was a clear indication in the DCCT that intensive therapy resulted in a threefold increase in severe hypoglycemic events and that there is a strong correlation between lowering of HbA$_{1c}$ and the predicted incidence of severe hypoglycemia.[48]

Insulin Pump Therapy

Although the availability of insulin therapy by continuous subcutaneous insulin infusion (CSII) delivery systems has been a boon for certain individuals, these devices still continue to have some mechanical problems (in spite of the fact that manufacturers provide emergency replacement within 24 hours) and have a drawback in that they are open-loop systems, which necessitate patients to measure as many as seven to eight capillary blood glucose levels per day and develop dosing algorithms based on different physical activities, food intake, and varying diurnal basal insulin requirements. Therefore, it must be pointed out that the pump is not a panacea and should not provide a sense of false security that good control will automatically be forthcoming with its use,[51] but that only certain individuals with high motivation and commitment who are willing to measure multiple blood-glucose levels should attempt this under supervision of a diabetologist and with the support of a knowledgeable health-care provider. In such a situation, insulin pump therapy has proven to be very convenient, particularly in patients with brittle DM.

TREATMENT OF TYPE 2 DM

As outlined earlier, both modification of dietary patterns and exercise are essential parts of any program for control of DM. These components become even more important for patients with type 2 DM, since 85% of these individuals are overweight and more or less insulin-resistant.[8,27] Weight reduction can not only improve psychological well-being and improve the ability to exercise and thus improve cardiovascular fitness, but diet and exercise can also decrease insulin resistance[43,44] and improve dyslipidemia.[44] In

fact, in a certain number of patients who lose as little as 5% of their body weight and can maintain it by strict adherence to such a program, the use of pharmacologic agents may be significantly reduced or be unnecessary.[52] In the majority of the cases, however, supplementation of the dietary and exercise regimen with pharmacologic agents is necessary for optimal control of type 2 DM.

Table 27-18 provides a general guideline for the management of type 2 DM, without detailed discussion of the use of each drug.

As stated earlier, type 2 DM is a heterogeneous disease with strong familial associations where the incidence is further influenced by ethnicity, age, body weight, and physical activity.[21] Thus, whereas a few patients may respond positively to diet and exercise alone, in younger, lean patients sulfonylureas or a meglitinide may suffice, whereas in obese persons, an insulin-sensitivity modifier (e.g., metformin or a thiazolidinedione) may be indicated. A α-glucosidase inhibitor (e.g., acarbose or miglitol) may be adequate for patients with predominately postprandial hyperglycemia. Yet others may require insulin, and finally, in certain individuals a combination of two, three, or even four pharmaceutical agents may be required for optimal therapy.

Tables 27-19 and 27-20 provide a summary of the mechanism of action of various classes of oral

---

TABLE 27-18
GENERAL GUIDELINES FOR MANAGEMENT OF TYPE 2 DM

1. Place patient on an American Diabetes Association reducing diet, with three meals a day to achieve and maintain ideal body weight or to reduce weight by 7% in 6 months (if ≥120% of ideal body weight).
2. Encourage risk factor interventions (smoking, exercise, lipids, etc.). The exercise should be at least 100 kcal/day (1 mile of walking) for a total of 700 kcal/wk.
3. While on diet, check FBG and one 2-hr PPBG by finger stick daily for 2 months. If diet and exercise are effective, FBG will gradually decline during this period. If FBG does not decline or increases, consider use of oral antidiabetic agents (OAAs).
4. Patients with FBG >250 mg/dl or 2 HPPBG >300 mg/dl (after adequate dietary therapy) are suitable candidates for oral hypoglycemic agents (OHA).
5. While on OHA, check patient for FBG or 2 HPPBG every 2 months (with daily FBG and 2 HPPBG monitoring) at home; if 2HPPBG <200 mg/dl, omit OAA and place on diet and exercise alone and follow every 1–2 months. If BG values are unacceptable (2HPP >200 mg/dl) after sulfonylurea, add α-glucosidase inhibitor (acarbose or miglitol). If unsuccessful, place on combination OAAs. If still unsuccessful, add bedtime insulin.
6. Insulin dosage should be calculated on actual body weight (0.5–1.0 U/kg of body weight).
7. If total insulin requirement is less than 30 U/day, may try to give entire dose as NPH or Lente before a major meal and check for glycemic control (goal: FBG <140, 2HPP >200, HbA$_{1c}$ <7%, and no BG <60 mg/dl).
8. If the goal is not achieved by a single insulin injection, insulin may be given as a fixed combination of NPH and regular: 70/30 or 50/50 mixture, 1/2 hour before breakfast and 1/2 hour before supper or NPH and Lispro 75/25, 5 min before the meal.
9. Very obese patients may require more insulin/kg of body weight, and a greater percentage of total insulin as regular insulin than less obese patients with type 2 DM.
10. If the above regimen fails to control blood glucose or HbA$_{1c}$ (>8%), consider multiple regular or Lispro insulin injections before each meal with bedtime NPH or lente insulin and discontinue some or all oral agents.

Note: Refer insulin-resistant patients (requiring >200 U insulin/day) to an endocrinologist/diabetologist.

Derived from Kitabchi AE. Diabetes mellitus. In: Seltzer VL, Pearse WH, eds. Women's primary health care: office practice and procedures. New York: McGraw-Hill, 1995:541.

TABLE 27-19
AVAILABLE ORAL ANTIDIABETIC AGENTS

Generic Name	Brand Name	Daily Dosage (mg)	Duration of Action (hours)	Comments
First Generation Sulfonylureas				
Tolbutamide	Orinase	500–3000	6–12	Metabolized by liver to inactive product; excreted by kidneys; taken 2–3 times a day
Chlorpropamide	Diabinese	100–500	60	Metabolized by liver (~70%) to less active metabolites and excreted intact (~30%) by kidney; can potentiate anti-diuretic hormone action; taken once a day
Tolazamide	Tolinase	100–1000	12–24	Metabolized by liver to both active and inactive products; excreted by kidneys; taken 1–2 times a day
Second Generation Sulfonylureas				
Glipizide	Glucotrol	2.5–40	12–24	Metabolized by liver to inert products; excreted by kidneys; taken 1–2 times a day
	Glucotrol XL	5–20	24	Controlled-release preparation produces sustained plasma levels; taken once daily
Glyburide	Diabeta Micronase	1.5–20	16–24	Metabolized by liver to mostly inert products; excreted in bile and by kidneys; taken 1–2 times a day
	Glynase Pres Tab	0.75–12	12–24	Small particle size facilitates rapid absorption
Third Generation Sulfonylureas				
Glimepiride	Amaryl	1–8	24	Metabolized by liver; excreted 60% renal, 40% bile; lower incidence of hypoglycemia; taken once a day

antidiabetic agents, the preferred patient for treatment, as well as the expected change in fasting plasma glucose and HbA$_{1c}$. As stated, the effectiveness of these preparations is much enhanced by the use of these agents in combination.

ORAL ANTIDIABETIC AGENTS

In general antidiabetic agents are recommended alone or in combination in the patient who has not achieved the glycemic goal stated in Table 27-8 by

TABLE 27-20
OTHER ORAL ANTIDIABETIC AGENTS

Generic Name	Brand Name	Daily Dosage (mg)	Duration of Action (hours)	Comments
Meglitinides				
Repaglinide	Prandin	1.5–12	~1 hr	Taken only prior to meals. It is an insulin secretagogue, but is unrelated to sulfonylureas.
Biguanides				
Metformin	Glucophage	1000–2550	~5.5*	Not metabolized; excreted by kidneys; may be used alone or in combination with sulfonylureas or thiazolidinediones
α-Glucosidase Inhibitors				
Acarbose	Precose	25–150	8**	Slows absorption of polysaccharides and disaccharides from jejunum by inhibiting α-glucosidase; taken with first bite of meal, main action is on postprandial glucose
Miglitol	Glycet	25–300	8**	Slows absorption of polysaccharides and disaccharides from jejunum by inhibiting α-glucosidase; taken with first bite of meal, main action is on postprandial glucose
Thiazolidinediones				
Rosiglitazone	Avandia	4–8 mg	12	Decreases insulin resistance
Pioglitazone	Actos	15–45 mg	24	Decreases insulin resistance

*Plasma half-life

**Plasma half-life, which is unrelated to therapeutic effect, as this is mediated by unabsorbed drug.

diet and exercise alone, has no significant renal or hepatic disease, has a negative pregnancy test, and has no history of allergy to these drugs and in general has had DM for less than 10 years. Note that none of these oral agents is recommended (without the simultaneous use of insulin) in type 1 and C-peptide-negative diabetic subjects. Table 27-19 summarizes currently available oral sulfonylureas with their pharmacologic properties, mimimal–maximal dose, and any special comments. Table 27-20 summarizes features of other nonsulfonylurea compounds including α-glucosidase inhibitors, biguanides, thiazolidinediones, and the most recently available insulin secretagogue, which is not a sulfonylurea but is a meglitinide (repaglinide [Prandin]). A brief discussion of new preparations in each class follows.

Sulfonylureas

In general, sulfonylureas are insulin secretagogues, the mechanism of action of which entails binding to sulfonylurea receptors on the β-cell of the pancreatic islet to facilitate the intracellular influx of calcium and thence insulin secretion. They may also decrease hepatic insulin metabolism. They are effective in only 50 to 60% of patients and have a 3 to 5% annual failure rate.[53] Some sulfonylureas, such as chlorpropamide, glyburide, glimepiride, and extended-release preparations of glipizide may be used once a day; others such as tolbutamide, tolazamide, and standard-release glipizide, are usually used as twice-a-day preparations in relation to meals. From a mechanistic standpoint, glimepiride binds to the 65-kd component of the sulfonylurea receptor in the β-cell rather than the 140-kd element bound by other sulfonylureas. It also may exhibit insulinomimetic properties by improving the availability of glucose transporters (GLUT 4) in

insulin-sensitive tissues.[54] All sulfonylureas appear to be effective in combination with insulin as well as other antidiabetic agents such as biguanides, α-glucosidase inhibitors, or thiazolidinediones. Furthermore, certain drugs potentiate the hypoglycemic effects of sulfonylureas, including various sulfonamide preparations, dicumeral, oxyphenbutazone, and clofibrate.

Biguanides

The only biguanide preparation currently available in the United States is metformin (Glucophage®) which has been used in Europe, Canada, and much of the world for several decades. Its principal mechanism of action in improving hyperglycemia is by reduction of hepatic glucose production.[50,51] Since it has no effect on insulin secretion, it has minimal propensity to cause hypoglycemia. Furthermore, a certain number of obese diabetic patients appear to lose weight on this medication with reduction of peripheral insulin resistance.[57] Metformin may also have a modest action to reduce intestinal absorption of glucose. It is excreted unmetabolized by the kidney. The side effects of metformin are mainly GI-related. These are mild diarrhea, anorexia, nausea, and abdominal discomfort, which are dose-dependent and often transient. Lactic acidosis is a rare complication, and safety measures proposed for the use of metformin are detailed in Table 27-21 and should be closely followed. Effectiveness of metformin is enhanced in combination with sulfonylureas and thiazolidinediones.[56]

α-Glucosidase Inhibitors

Acarbose (Precose) and miglitol (Glyset) are α-glucosidase inhibitors that inhibit breakdown of complex carbohydrates (apart from lactose) and thus

---

TABLE 27-21
SAFETY MEASURES FOR THE USE OF METFORMIN

Do Not Prescribe in the Following Circumstances Due to Increased Risk of Lactic Acidosis	Withhold in Conditions Predisposed to Hypoxia or Renal Insufficiency
Serum creatinine ≥1.5 mg/dl in males and ≥1.4 in females	CV collapse
Creatinine clearance <75 ml/min or patients ≥80 years	Acute MI
CHF requiring therapeutic management	CHF requiring therapeutic agents
Moderate to marked respiratory dysfunction	Severe infection
Liver dysfunction	During and for at least 48 hours after use of iodinated contrast media
History of alcohol abuse/binge drinking	Following major surgical procedures
Acute or chronic metabolic acidosis	
Acutely ill hospitalized patients	
Prior history of lactic acidosis	

CHF = congestive heart failure; CV = cardiovascular; MI = myocardial infarction.

TABLE 27-22
PATIENT INSTRUCTIONS FOR ACARBOSE OR MIGLITOR

1. Suggested dosing schedule:
   - Step 1: Start with 25 mg at breakfast for 1 week.
   - Step 2: Take 25 mg with breakfast and dinner for 1 week.
   - Step 3: Take 25 mg with breakfast, lunch, and dinner for 1 week.
   - Step 4: Take 50 mg with breakfast and 25 mg with lunch and dinner for 1 week.
   - Step 5: Take 50 mg with breakfast and lunch and 25 mg with dinner for 1 week.
   - Step 6: Take 50 mg with breakfast, lunch, and dinner.
2. Do not go to a higher titration level if troublesome side effects occur. Stay at the same level or go to a lower step.
3. Take these drugs WITH THE FIRST BITE of each meal. They will not be as effective if taken before or after eating.
4. May increase to 100 mg t.i.d. if side effects are minimal at 50 mg t.i.d.

delay their intestinal absorption. They are, therefore, effective in reducing postprandial hyperglycemia, particularly in type 2 DM with HbA$_{1c}$ greater than 11 to 12%. These drugs are more effective in combination with sulfonylureas.[58,59] Since their principal side effect of flatulence is very much related to dosage, they should be titrated upwards very slowly as suggested in Table 27-22. They should not be used in patients with liver disease.

Thiazolidinediones

The thiazolidinediones comprise a class of antidiabetic agent, part of whose structure consists of α-tocopherol. The currently available thiazolidinediones are rosiglitazone (Avandia®) and pioglitazone (Actos®). They are peripheral insulin-sensitizers and are devoid of any effect on insulin secretion, and are ineffective in the absence of residual endogenous insulin secretion. They are effective adjuncts to insulin therapy and may markedly reduce or eliminate the need for insulin. Thiazolidinediones mimic insulin action by altering and modifying the glucose transport system to facilitate glucose metabolism. At the peripheral tissue, this reduces insulin resistance, the hallmark of type 2 DM, by enhancing proximal binding to and activating peroxisome proliferator activator receptor-γ (PPARγ), a superfamily of nuclear receptors.[60] These compounds may also improve insulin resistance in patients with IGT.[61] A comparative study indicated that biguanides and thiazolidinediones work via two distinctly different pathways in type 2 DM.[62]

Whereas biguanides exert a major effect to reduce hepatic glucose output, thiazolidinediones are most effective at enhancing peripheral glucose utilization.[62] The combined effect of the two classes of drugs is synergistic, and the combination thus may be an important therapeutic tool for obese patients with type 2 DM. The first thiazolidinedione on the market in 1997, troglitazone, was withdrawn in February 2000 after severe or fatal liver damage was found to be associated with its use and the safer rosiglitazone and proglitazone were available. Thiazolidinediones should be taken with meals, since food increases the secretion of bile acids and increases their absorption by 30 to 85%. The effect of the size of the meal on absorption is not known. Bioavailability of other drugs with thiazolidinediones is important; therefore, package inserts should be consulted for proper use of these drugs.

Due to the rare but severe side effects of troglitazone, which led to its withdrawal, safety guidelines have been established by the Food and Drug Administration (FDA) to guard against possible hepatic injury from the newer thiazolidinediones. Table 27-23 summarizes recent FDA guidelines for the use of these drugs. However, to date, after over a year of clinical availability, there have been no confirmed associations between the newer drugs and hepatic injury.

Meglitinides

The meglitinide drug repaglinide (Prandin) is an oral blood-glucose-lowering agent that is structurally

TABLE 27-23
THIAZOLIDINEDIONE SAFETY MEASURES

1. Due to withdrawal of troglitazone following approximately 150 reports of severe adverse liver effects, including over 50 deaths worldwide, the following recommendations are mandated by the FDA when using either of the currently available thiazolidinediones (rosiglitazone or priglitazone).
2. Recommend serum alanine aminotransferase (ALT, SGPT) levels be checked:
   a. At start of therapy
   b. Every 2 months for first 12 months
   c. Periodically thereafter
3. Perform liver-function tests at first symptoms suggestive of hepatic dysfunction.
4. Discontinue drug if patient has jaundice or if laboratory tests suggest liver injury or if ALT level is >3× upper limit of normal.
5. Do not start drug if initial ALT is >1.8× upper limit of normal.
6. Avoid in Class III or IV heart failure as fluid retention and edema may be exacerbated.

unrelated to sulfonylureas, but is a glucose-dependent insulin secretagogue. Its mechanism of action at the β-cell membrane is to close ATP-dependent K channels by binding at a characterizable site. This blockade depolarizes the β-cell membrane, thus opening calcium channels and stimulating insulin secretion. Unlike other insulin secretagogues, this compound needs to be taken with each meal in a dose of 0.5 mg to a maximum of 4 mg to be effective. It reduces fasting and postprandial blood glucose with an effective reduction of HbA_{1c} by about 1.7% (package insert, Novo Nordisk Pharmaceuticals). This drug is much more effective in combination with metformin or in conditions in which the latter is ineffective.

Comparative Effect of Various Oral Antidiabetic Agents

It is fortunate that we have at our disposal a large number of pharmacologic agents, each with its own special property, which can serve the particular needs of patients with type 2 DM. For example, while sulfonylureas in general can be used with more efficacy in less obese patients with type 2 DM, metformin and thiazolidinediones will be more effective in obese insulin-resistant patients,[56] while α-glucosidase inhibitors are best suited for individuals with postprandial hyperglycemia.[58,59] An important caveat for the use of any of the newer OAAs (especially metformin

and thiazolidinediones) is that consideration must be given to the safety guidelines for these drugs and to the contraindications to their use, which were presented in the previous tables under each heading. However, physicians are urged to read the drug insert for each preparation and to update themselves on any recent information on products that are relatively new on the market and whose long-term effects have not been studied in a large number of patients with type 2 DM. Table 27-24 provides a summary of various classes of OAAs, their mechanism of their action, and most suitable patients for treatment, as well as the average effect each class of compound has on fasting plasma glucose and HbA_{1c}. As stated, the effectiveness of these preparations is much enhanced by their use in combination.

The Use of Insulin with Oral Antidiabetic Agents

OAAs alone have been found to be ineffective in certain patients with type 2 DM, while other patients require large doses of insulin. Numerous investigators have evaluated the effect of insulin combined with OAAs, both to enhance the effectiveness of OAAs and to reduce insulin dosage. In the early 1980s, some studies indicated that a reduction of insulin dose could be achieved with OAA use,[63] while others proposed evening injection of insulin with some good results.[64,65] These were followed by data

TABLE 27-24
OAAS AND THEIR EFFICACY AS MONOTHERAPY

Oral Antidiabetic	Mechanism of Action	Preferred Patient Type	Reduction in FPG (mg/dl)	Reduction in HbA_{1c} (%)	Reduction in Postprandial Glucose (mg/dl)
Sulfonylureas	↑↑ Insulin secretion from β-cells	Insulinopenic, lean, young	60–70	1.5–2.0	92
Biguanides (Metformin)	↓↓ Hepatic glucose production ↑ Peripheral glucose utilization	Insulin resistant, overweight, dyslipidemic	59–78	1.5–2.0	83
α-glucosiase Inhibitors (acarbose, miglitol)	↓ Postprandial carbohydrate absorption	Postprandial hyperglycemia	20–30	0.5–1.0	40–50
Thiazolidinediones (rosiglitazone, pioglitazone)	↑↑ Peripheral glucose utilization ↓ Hepatic glucose production	Insulin-resistant, renal impairment, low HDL	62–75	1.5–1.6	N/A
Meglitinides (Repaglinide)	↑↑ Insulin secretion from β-cells	Insulinopenic, lean, young	61	1.7	104

NA = not applicable.

Source: Physician's Desk Reference, 54th edition, Sifton, DW, ed. Montvale, NJ: Medical Economics Company, 2000.

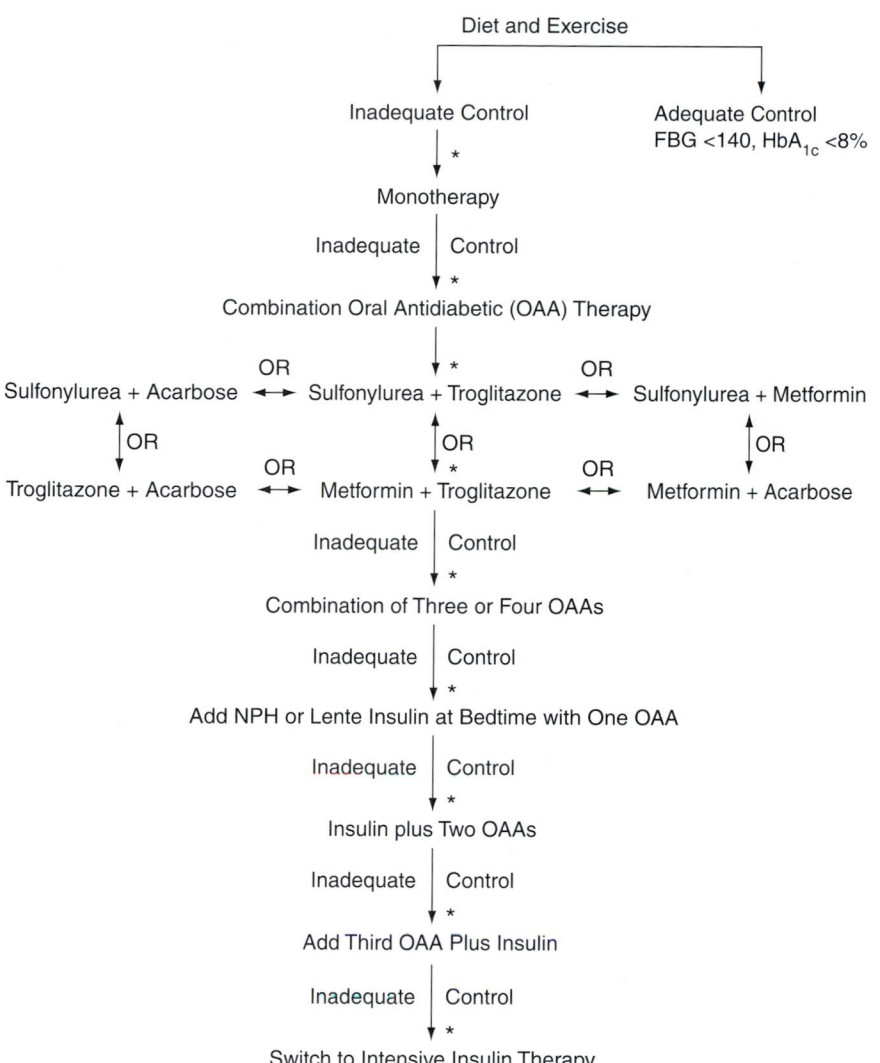

Figure 27-4 Management of type 2 DM (without acute complications or pregnancy). *Meal planning and exercise to be reviewed at each step.

showing similar salutary effects of other agents such as metformin in combination with insulin.[66] Therefore, in patients who cannot adhere to multiple insulin injections or in whom therapy with OAAs alone has failed, one or two daily injections may be tried in addition to the use of OAAs during the day. In addition to this simple regimen, the ADA guidelines provide certain protocols for combination of these agents (see below).

Algorithm for Management of Patients with Type 2 DM

Figure 27-4 provides a procedural algorithm for the use of OAAs alone or in combination. Failure of the combined drugs to attain therapeutic goals necessitates reevaluation of the patient in conjunction with counseling on diet and exercise and subsequent in-

clusion of insulin therapy along the guidelines stated in Figure 27-4.

Guidelines for Treatment of Acute Diabetic Emergencies

Because primary care physicians, at an ever-increasing rate, are involved with the care of moderately complicated cases of DM, it follows that they will also be dealing with the management of acute diabetic emergencies. These include insulin- or sulfonylurea-induced hypoglycemia, diabetic ketoacidosis (DKA), and the hyperglycemic hyperosmolar state (HHS). There are numerous review articles on the above topics,[67,68] but for the sake of brevity, we have prepared algorithms with diagnostic criteria for DKA and HHS and a step-by-step flow sheet for therapy of these conditions (Figures 27-5 and 27-6 respectively).

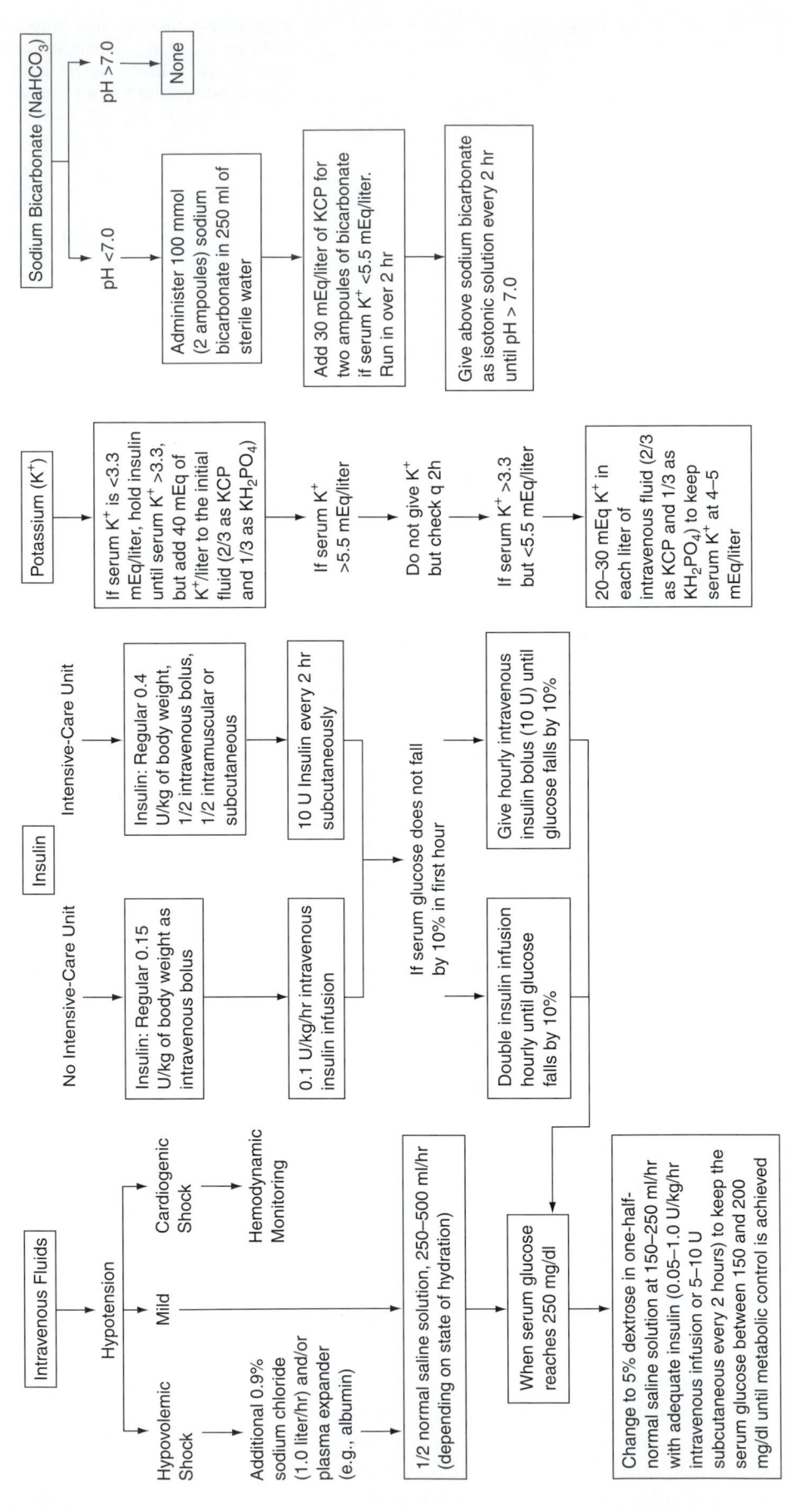

Figure 27-5 Proposed protocol for treatment of patients with DKA. Initial evaluation: After history and physical examination, obtain arterial blood gases, complete blood count with differential, urinalysis, blood glucose, blood urea nitrogen, electrolytes, chemistry profile and creatinine levels immediately as well as an electrocardiogram, chest x-ray films, and cultures as needed. Start intravenous fluid, 1.0 liter of 0.9% sodium chloride per hour initially. Diagnostic criteria: DKA: blood glucose >250 mg/dl, arterial pH <7.3, bicarbonate <15 mEq/liter, moderate ketonuria or ketonemia at 1:2 dilution. *Adapted from Kitabchi et al.*[6]

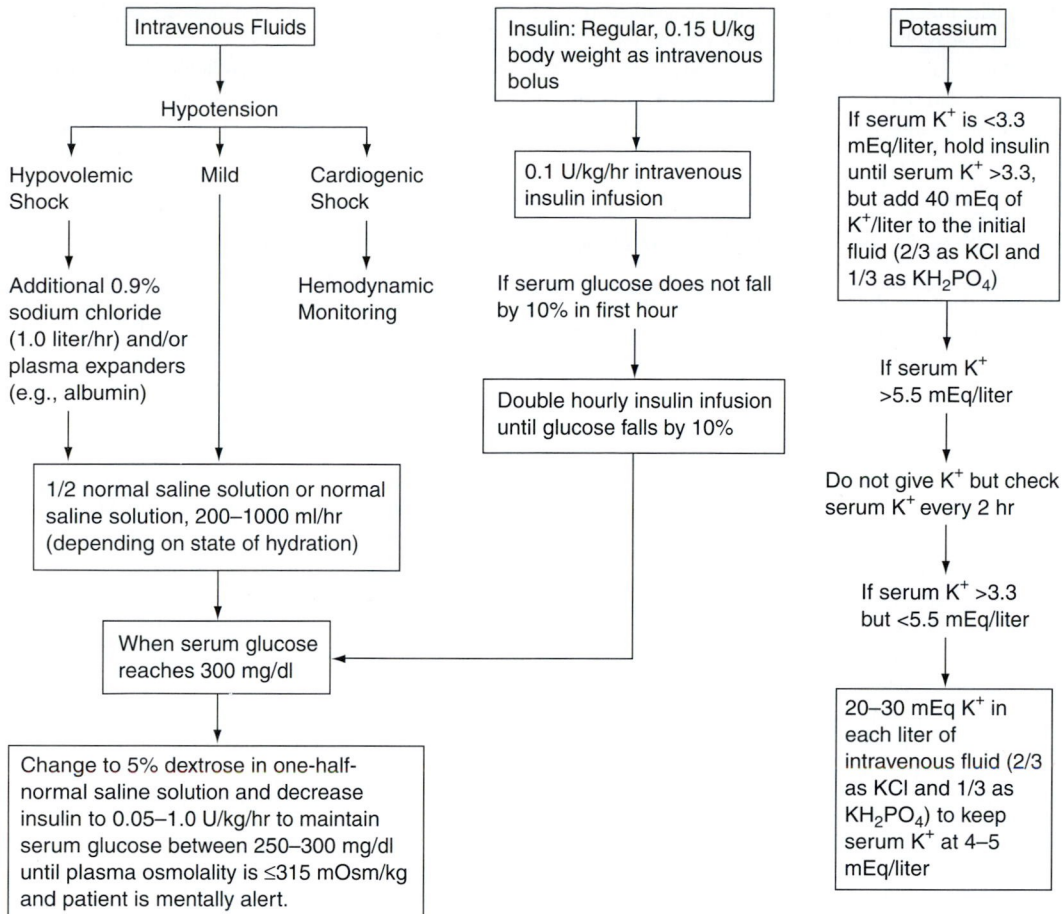

Figure 27-6 Proposed protocol for treatment of patients with HHS. Initial evaluation: After history and physical examination, obtain arterial blood gases, complete blood count with differential, urinalysis, blood glucose, blood urea nitrogen, electrolytes, chemistry profile and creatinine levels immediately. Electrocardiogram, chest x-ray films, and cultures as needed. Start intravenous fluid, 1.0 liter of 0.9% sodium chloride per hour initially. Diagnostic criteria: blood glucose >600 mg/dl, arterial pH >7.3, bicarbonate >15 mEq/liter, mild ketonemia (negative at 1:2 dilution) and effective serum osmolality >320 mOsm/kg. *Note: This protocol is for patients admitted with mental status change or severe dehydration who require admission to an intensive-care unit. For less severe cases see text for treatment guidelines. Adapted from Kitabchi et al.[6]*

REFERENCES

1. Expert Committee on the Diagnosis and Classification of Diabetes Mellitus. Report on the diagnosis and classification of diabetes mellitus. Diabetes Care 1997; 20:1183.
2. American Diabetes Association. Diabetes 1996 Vital Statistics. Alexandria, VA: American Diabetes Association, 1996.
3. National Institute of Diabetes and Digestive and Kidney Diseases. Diabetes statistics. Bethesda, MD: National Institute of Diabetes and Digestive and Kidney Diseases, 1995. NIH Publication no. H96-3926.
4. Klein R, Moss SE, Klein BEK, DeMets DL. Relation of ocular and systemic factors to survival in diabetes. Arch Intern Med 1989;21:296.
5. American Diabetes Association: Economic consequences of diabetes mellitus in the U.S. in 1996. Diabetes Care 1998;21;296.
6. Harris MI, Goldstein DE, Flegal KM, et al. Prevalence of diabetes, impaired fasting glucose and impaired glucose tolerance in U.S. adults: the Third National Health and Nutrition Examination Survey, 1988-1994. Diabetes Care 1998;21:518.
7. Golay A, Felber JP, Jequier E, DeFronzo RA, Ferrannini E. Metabolic basis of obesity and noninsulin-dependent diabetes mellitus. Diabetes Metab Rev 1988;4:515.
8. Geiss LS, Herman WH, Smith PH. Mortality in NIDDM. In: Harris MI, Cowie CC, Stern MP, et al. Diabetes in America. Bethesda, MD: NIDDK, 1995;236.
9. Morris LR, McGee JA, Kitabchi AE. Correlation between plasma and urine glucose in diabetes. Ann Intern Med 1981;94:469.

10. Ramus RM, Kitzmiller JL. Diagnosis and management of gestational diabetes mellitus. Diabetes Rev 1994;2:43.

11. Baynes JW, Bunn HF, Goldstein DE, Harris M, Martin DB, Peterson C. National Diabetes Data Group: report of the expert committee on glycosylated hemoglobin. Diabetes Care 1984;7:602.

12. Fajans SS. Classification and diagnosis of diabetes. In: Porte D Jr, Sherwin RS, eds. Ellenberg and Rifkin's Diabetes Mellitus, 5th ed. Stamford, CT: Appleton and Lange, 1997:357.

13. Vardi P, Crisa L, Jackson RA. Predictive value of intravenous glucose tolerance test insulin secretion less than or greater than the first percentile in islet cell antibody positive relatives of type 1 (insulin-dependent) diabetic patients. Diabetologia 1991;34:93.

14. The DCCT Research Group. The effect of intensive treatment of diabetes on the development and progression of long-term complications of insulin-dependent diabetes mellitus. N Engl J Med 1993;329:977.

15. Barker L, Koch DD, Wians FH Jr. Validation of the DCA 2000 hemoglobin A1c system. Clin Lab Sci 1995;8:331.

16. American Diabetes Association. Tests of glycemia in diabetes. Diabetes Care 1998;21(Supp 1):S69.

17. Umpierrez GE, Casals MMC, Gebhart SSP, Mixon PS, Clark WS, Phillips LS. Diabetic ketoacidosis in obese African-Americans. Diabetes 1995;44:790.

18. Lipton RB, Kocova M, LaPorte RE, et al. Autoimmunity and genetics contribute to the risk of insulin-dependent diabetes mellitus in families: islet cell antibodies and HLA-DQ heterodimers. Am J Epidemiol 1991;136:503.

19. Clements GB, Galbraith DN, Taylor KW. Coxsackie B virus infection and the onset of childhood diabetes. Lancet 1995;346:221.

20. Notkins AL. Virus-induced diabetes mellitus: brief review. Arch Virol 1977;54:1.

21. Goldstein RE, Drash A, Blizzard RM. Diabetes mellitus: the incidence of circulating antibodies against thyroid, gastric and adrenal tissue. J Pediatr 1970;77:304.

22. Palmer JP, Asplin CM, Clemons P, et al. Insulin antibodies in insulin-dependent diabetics before insulin treatment. Science 1983;222:1337.

23. Kitabchi AE, Murphy MB, Sherman AR, Lambeth H, Simons R. Diabetes mellitus. In: Ling FS, Laube DW, Nolan TE, Smith RP, Stovall TG, eds. Primary care in gynecology. Baltimore: Williams & Wilkins 1996:279.

24. Baekkeskov S, Aanstoot H, Christgau S, et al. Identification of the 64K autoantigen in insulin-dependent diabetes as the GABA-synthesizing enzyme glutamic acid decarboxylase. Nature 1990;347:151.

25. Pinhas-Hamiel O, Dolan LM, Daniels SR, Standiford D, Khoury PR, Zeitler P. Increased incidence of non-insulin dependent diabetes among adolescents. J Pediatr 1996; 128:608.

26. Scott CR, Smith JM, Cradock M, Pihoker C. Characteristics of youth-onset non-insulin-dependent diabetes mellitus and insulin-dependent mellitus at diagnosis. Pediatr 1997;100:84.

27. DeFronzo RA. Pathogenesis of type 2 diabetes: metabolic and molecular implications for identifying diabetes genes. Diabetes Rev 1997;5:177.

28. Froguel P, Zouali H, Vionnet N, et al. Familial hyperglycemia due to mutations in glucokinase: definition of a subtype of diabetes mellitus. N Engl J Med 1993; 328:697.

29. Chen Y-DI, Jeng C-Y, Hollenbeck CB, Wu M-S, Reaven GM. Relationship between plasma glucose and insulin concentration, glucose production and glucose disposal in normal subjects and patients with non-insulin-dependent diabetes. J Clin Invest 1988;82:21.

30. Leahy JL, Bonner-Weir S, Weir GC. β-cell dysfunction induced by chronic hyperglycemia: current ideas on mechanisms of impaired glucose-induced insulin secretion. Diabetes Care 1992;15:442.

31. Leahy JL. Natural history of β-cell dysfunction in NIDDM. Diabetes Care 1983;13:992.

32. Kitabchi AE, Bryer-Ash M. NIDDM: new aspects of management. Hosp Pract 1997;32:135.

33. Reaven GM. Banting Lecture: the role of insulin resistance in human disease. Diabetes 1988;37:595.

34. Kitabchi AE, Fisher JN. Diabetes mellitus. In: Glew R, ed. Clinical studies in medical biochemistry. 2nd ed. New York: Oxford Univesity Press, 1997:200.

35. Reichard P, Nilsson BY, Rosenqvist U. The effect of long-term intensified insulin treatment on the development of microvascular complications of diabetes mellitus. N Engl J Med 1993;329:977.

36. Ohkubo Y, Kishikawa H, Araki E, et al. Intensive insulin therapy prevents the progression of diabetic microvascular complications in Japanese patients with non-insulin-dependent diabetes mellitus: a randomized prospective 6-year study. Diabetes Res Clin Pract 1995;28:103.

37. UK Prospective Diabetes Study (UKPDS) Group. Intensive blood-glucose control with sulphonylureas or insulin compared with conventional treatment and risk of complications in patients with type 2 diabetes (UKPDS 33). Lancet 1998;352:837.

38. UK Prospective Diabetes Study (UKPDS) Group. Effect of intensive blood-glucose control with metformin on complications in overweight patients with type 2 diabetes (UKPDS 34). Lancet 1998;352:854.

39. UK Prospective Diabetes Study (UKPDS) Group. Tight blood pressure control and risk of macrovascular and microvascular complications in type 2 diabetes: UKPDS 38. BMJ 1998;317:703.

40. American Diabetes Association. Standards of medical care for patients with diabetes mellitus. Diabetes Care 1998; 21(Supp 1):S23.

41. Kovacs J, Brent D, Steinberg TF, Paulauskas S, Reid J. Children's self-report of psychologic adjustment and coping strategies during first year of insulin-dependent diabetes mellitus. Diabetes Care 1986;9:472.

42. American Diabetes Association. National standards for diabetes self-management education programs and American Diabetes Association review criteria. Diabetes Care 1998; 21(Supp 1):S95.

43. Bogardus C, Ravussin E, Robbins DC, Wolfe RR, Horton ES, Sims EA. Effects of physical training and diet therapy on carbohydrate metabolism in patients with glucose intolerance and non-insulin-dependent diabetes mellitus. Diabetes 1984;33:311.

44. Bjorntorp P, Fahlen M, Grimby G, et al. Carbohydrate and lipid metabolism in middle-aged physically well-trained men. Metabolism 1972;21:1037.

45. Edelman SV, Henry RR. Diagnosis and management of type 2 diabetes. Caddo, OK: Professional Communication, Inc., 1997.

46. Bittle J, Kitabchi AE. Obesity: an overview. In: Givens JR, ed. The hypothalamus. Chicago: Yearbook, 1984:73.

47. White JR, Campbell RK. Insulin analogues: new agents for improving glycemic control. Postgrad Med 1997;101:58.

48. The DCCT Research Group. Hypoglycemia in the Diabetes Control and Complications Trial. Diabetes 1997; 46:271.

49. Marker JC, Cryer PE, Clutter WE. Attenuated glucose recovery from hypoglycemia in the elderly. Diabetes 1992; 41:671.

50. Polonsky KS, Given BD, VanCauter E. Twenty-four hour profiles and pulsatile patterns of insulin secretion in normal and obese subjects. J Clin Invest 1988;81:442.

51. Kitabchi AE, Fisher JN, Matteri R, Murphy MB. The use of continuous insulin delivery systems in treatment of diabetes mellitus. In: Stollerman GH, ed. Advances in internal medicine, Chicago: 1983:449.

52. Vinik AI, Wing RR, Lauterio TJ. Nutritional management of the person with diabetes. In: Porte D, Sherwin RS, eds. Diabetes mellitus. 5th ed. Stamford, CT: Appleton & Lange 1997:609.

53. Lebovitz HE. Oral antidiabetic agents. In: Kahn CR, Weir GC, eds. Joslin's diabetes mellitus textbook. 13th ed. Philadelphia: Lea & Febiger, 1994:508.

54. Draeger E. Clinical profile of glimepiride. Diabetes Res Clin Pract 1995;28:138.

55. Stumvoll M, Nurjhan N, Perriello G, Dailey G, Gerich JE. Metabolic effects of metformin in non-insulin-dependent Diabetes Mellitus. N Engl J Med 1995;333:550.

56. DeFronzo RA, et al. Efficacy of metformin in patients with NIDDM. N Engl J Med 1995;333:541.

57. United Kingdom Prospective Diabetes Study Group. United Kingdom Prospective Diabetes Study Group Study 24: a 6 year randomized, controlled trial comparing sulfonylurea, insulin and metformin therapy in patients with newly diagnosed type 2 diabetes that could not be controlled with diet therapy. Ann Intern Med J 1998; 128:165.

58. Coniff RF, Shapiro JA, Seaton TB, Bray GA. Multicenter, placebo-controlled trial comparing acarbose (Bay g5421) with placebo, tolbutamide and tolbutamide plus acarbose in non-insulin-dependent diabetes mellitus. Am J Med 1995;98:443.

59. Chiasson JL, Josse RG, Hunt JA, et al. The efficacy of acarbose in the treatment of patents with non-insulin dependent diabetes mellitus. Ann Intern Med 1994; 121:928.

60. Saltiel AR, Olefsky JM. Thiazolidinediones in the treatment of insulin resistance and type II diabetes. Diabetes 1996;45:1661.

61. Nolan JJ, Ludvik B, Beerdsenp JM, Olefsky J. Improvement in glucose tolerance and insulin resistance in obese subjects treated with troglitazone. N Engl J Med 1994; 331:118.

62. Inzucchi SE, Maggs DG, Spollett GR, et al. Efficacy and metabolic effects of metformin and troglitazone in type II diabetes mellitus. N Engl J Med 1998;338:867.

63. Kitabchi AE, Soria AG, Radparvar A, Lawson-Grant V. Combined therapy of insulin and tolazamide decreases insulin requirement and serum triglycerides in obese patients with noninsulin-dependent diabetes mellitus. Am J Med Sci 1987;294:10.

64. Riddle M. New tactics for type II diabetes: regimens based on intermediate-acting insulin taken at bedtime. Lancet 1985;1:192.

65. Shank ML, Del Prato SD, DeFronzo RA. Bedtime insulin/daytime glipizide: effective therapy for sulfonylurea failures in NIDDM. Diabetes 1995;44:165.

66. Schwartz S, Raskin P, Fonseca V, Graveline JF. Effect of troglitazone in insulin-treated patients with type II diabetes mellitus. N Engl J Med 1998;338:861.

67. Kitabchi AE, Fisher JN, Murphy MB, Rumbak MJ. Diabetic ketoacidosis and the hyperglycemic hyperosmolar nonketotic state. In: Kahn CR and Weir G, eds. Joslin's Diabetes Mellitus textbook. 13th ed. Philadelphia: Lea and Febiger, 1994;738.

68. Kitabchi AE, Umpierrez GE, Murphy MB. Treatment of patients with diabetic ketoacidosis (DKA) or hyperglycemic hyperosmolar nonketotic state (HHNS). In: Rakel RES, ed. Conn's current therapy. Philadelphia: Saunders, 1999:555.

Chapter 28
Lipid Disorders

Thomas A. Hughes

Five Key Points

- **The goals of therapy are a low-density lipoprotein (LDL) cholesterol level <100 mg/dl; triglycerides <200 mg/day.**

- **Effects of diet therapy for hyperlipidemia are evident within 2 to 3 weeks and fully manifest within 6 weeks.**

- **The 3-hydroxy-3-methyl-glutaryl-coenzyme A (HMG-CoA) reductase inhibition should be the first-line pharmacologic therapy for elevated LDL cholesterol.**

- **An extremely ill patient should be taken off all lipid-lowering medications.**

- **Estrogen lowers LDL cholesterol and apolipoprotein B (apoB), whereas it raises high-density lipoprotein cholesterol, especially HDL_2 and apo A-I.**

Cholesterol is required by all cells to maintain normal membrane function; it is the substrate for steroid hormone synthesis in the gonads and adrenal glands. Triglyceride is the major energy source for most cells. Elevated concentrations of plasma cholesterol and triglyceride cause atherosclerosis and an increase in cardiovascular events such as myocardial infarction, stroke, and gangrene.[1-3] Reduction of these lipids has been shown to reduce cardiovascular events and decrease total mortality.[4-8] Severe elevations of triglyceride (>1000 mg/dl) can also cause pancreatitis.

LIPOPROTEIN STRUCTURE

Cholesterol and triglycerides are transported in the plasma in six different lipoprotein particles: chylomicrons (CM), chylomicron remnants (CM-R), very-low-density lipoproteins (VLDL), intermediate-density lipoproteins (IDL), low-density lipoproteins (LDL), and high-density lipoproteins (HDL). These particles differ in several ways: relative ratio of triglycerides (TG) to cholesterol ester (CE) in their core, size, buoyant density, and complement of apolipoproteins. An outer layer of phospholipids (PL) covers all lipoprotein particles, and separates the very hydrophobic core lipids (TG and CE) from the aqueous (polar) environment of the plasma. Almost all lipoproteins contain either apolipoprotein (apo) A-I (HDL) or apoB (all of the others). In general, the apoB-containing lipoproteins are atherogenic, while the apoA-I–containing lipoproteins are protective.

There are two varieties of apoB, apoB-100 (whole apoB or 100%), which is made in the liver, and apoB-48 (48% of B-100), which is made in the small intestine.[9] Each lipoprotein particle contains only one apoB molecule, and this apoB molecule is required for the particle's initial formation and secretion. In addition, apoB does not transfer from one particle to another. As a result, a measurement of apoB concentration provides an excellent measure of the number of apoB-containing particles present in the plasma. This is important because the number of lipoprotein particles corresponds fairly well with atherogenicity. ApoB-48 is an interesting molecule because it is derived from a very unusual cellular mechanism. The epithelial cells of the human small intestine contain an enzyme that specifically cleaves the messenger RNA (mRNA) of apoB-100, generating a message approximately half the length of apoB-100 mRNA. As a result, the intestine generates only apoB-48–containing particles. It is important to note that the deleted portion of apoB-100 contains the LDL receptor-binding region. Therefore, intestinally derived lipoproteins (CMs and CM-Rs) cannot bind to the LDL receptor via apoB.

Almost all HDL particles contain apoA-I but some also contain apoA-II.[10] This appears important because the particles that contain both apolipoproteins do not appear to be as protective as the "A-I alone" particles. There are patients who appear to have normal HDL levels but it is predominantly "A-I+A-II" HDL and is, therefore, largely ineffective in preventing atherosclerosis.[11] On the other hand, some patients with primarily "A-I alone" HDL may have relatively low total HDL cholesterol levels but still be at low risk for atherosclerosis.

All six major lipoprotein fractions contain an array of particles. For instance, as noted above, HDL can be subdivided into particles with and without apoA-II. In addition, there are five major discrete HDL particle sizes, which give them different densities. The most dense and least dense particles are "A-I alone" particles, while the three middle density particles also contain apoA-II. The numbers of apoA-I molecules in each of these particles range from two to five and the number of apoA-II molecules in each particle also varies. Therefore, the apoA-I concentration does not necessarily predict the number of HDL particles. However, the apoA-II:apoA-I ratio does reflect the relative amounts of "A-I+A-II" and "A-I alone" HDL particles. There are also several minor HDL subfractions.

Each of the apoB-containing lipoproteins consists of an array of particles that differ by the amount of lipid attached to each apoB molecule and the relative amount of TG versus CE in their cores. For example, small, dense LDL contains less total lipid per apoB and also has a core enriched with TG as compared with typical LDL. In general, a shift to the more dense particles within each lipoprotein subfraction is associated with an increased risk of atherosclerosis.[12] CMs, CM-Rs, VLDLs, and IDL are considered triglyceride-rich lipoproteins because their core lipid is 95 to 50% TG (respectively), while LDL and HDL are cholesterol-rich lipoproteins because their core lipid is approximately 80% CE. In pathological states, these ratios can be altered considerably.

Other apolipoproteins that are clinically important are discussed below.

ApoE is synthesized in the liver, macrophages, and brain. It acts as a general lipid scavenger and can bind to the LDL receptor as well as a specific apoE receptor(s).[13,14] This apolipoprotein is found in all lipoproteins except LDL and the denser subfractions of HDL. It is responsible for the hepatic clearance of CM-Rs and IDL (and possibly some HDL). There are three common isotypes of apoE: apoE2, apoE3, and apoE4, the most common being homozygous apoE3E3 (~60%). These isotypes are identified by isoelectric focusing gels and are caused by amino acid substitutions that add or subtract one negatively charged amino acid (arginine or lysine). The binding of apoE to its receptors is mediated through some of these charged amino acids, so these mutations can have a substantial impact on apoE/lipoprotein metabolism. ApoE2 generally binds poorly to the LDL receptor and is associated with increases in TG and reductions in LDL cholesterol, typically reducing the risk of cardiovascular disease (CVD). An extreme lipoprotein dysfunction is seen in a small percentage of patients homozygous for apoE2E2. In these patients β-VLDL or cholesterol-rich VLDL develops. This syndrome is designated type III Hyperlipidemia or Dysbetalipoproteinemia and is associated with an increased risk of CVD, especially peripheral vascular disease. Subjects who are heterozygous or homozygous for apoE4 tend to have high LDL cholesterol and low TG, an increased risk for coronary heart disease, and Alzheimer disease. ApoE2, on the other hand, appears to protect against Alzheimer disease.

ApoC-II is synthesized in the liver and is found on all lipoproteins except LDL. It readily transfers between lipoproteins and is required for activation of lipoprotein lipase. Its genetic absence causes severe hypertriglyceridemia in infancy, but this condition is very rare.[15]

ApoC-III is synthesized in the liver and has a lipoprotein distribution similar to apoC-II. It inhibits lipoprotein lipase activity (anti-apoC-II) and also prevents the premature clearance of triglyceride-rich lipoproteins from the plasma (i.e., prevents their removal before most of the triglyceride has been removed from the particle). High concentrations of apoC-III are atherogenic[16,17] and are probably partially responsible for the hypertriglyceridemia frequently seen in Type 2 Diabetes Mellitus[18-20] and renal insufficiency.[21,22]

LIPOPROTEIN PHYSIOLOGY

There are three major lipoprotein metabolic pathways (Figure 28-1):

1. Intestine $\Rightarrow$ Chylomicron $\Rightarrow$ Chylomicron Remnants $\Rightarrow$ Liver
2. Liver $\Rightarrow$ VLDL $\Rightarrow$ IDL $\Rightarrow$ LDL $\Rightarrow$ Liver
3. Intestine or Liver $\Rightarrow$ HDL $\Rightarrow$ Tissues $\Rightarrow$ "recycle"

Chylomicrons and VLDL have similar metabolic pathways (Figure 28-1). They are generated in their respective organs by first synthesizing apoB (apoB-48 for chylomicrons and apoB-100 for VLDL). The apoB then either associates with triglyceride (if it is available) or is degraded.[23] The amount of triglyceride associated with each apoB molecule depends on the relative abundance of TG. Therefore, after eating a high-fat meal both CMs and VLDL become larger because of the high concentration of TG in the cells. After secretion, CMs and VLDL will react with Lipoprotein Lipase (LPL) bound to endothelial cells of fat and muscle tissue, which cleaves the fatty acids from triglyceride. These fatty acids are then utilized for energy (muscle) or stored as triglyceride (fat).

As apoB-containing particles circulate, they accumulate cholesterol ester, transferred from HDL via cholesterol ester transfer proteins (CETPs).[24] At the same time, CETPs transfer some of their TG to HDL and LDL. As a result, CMs and VLDL become progressively smaller (from loss of TG) and more

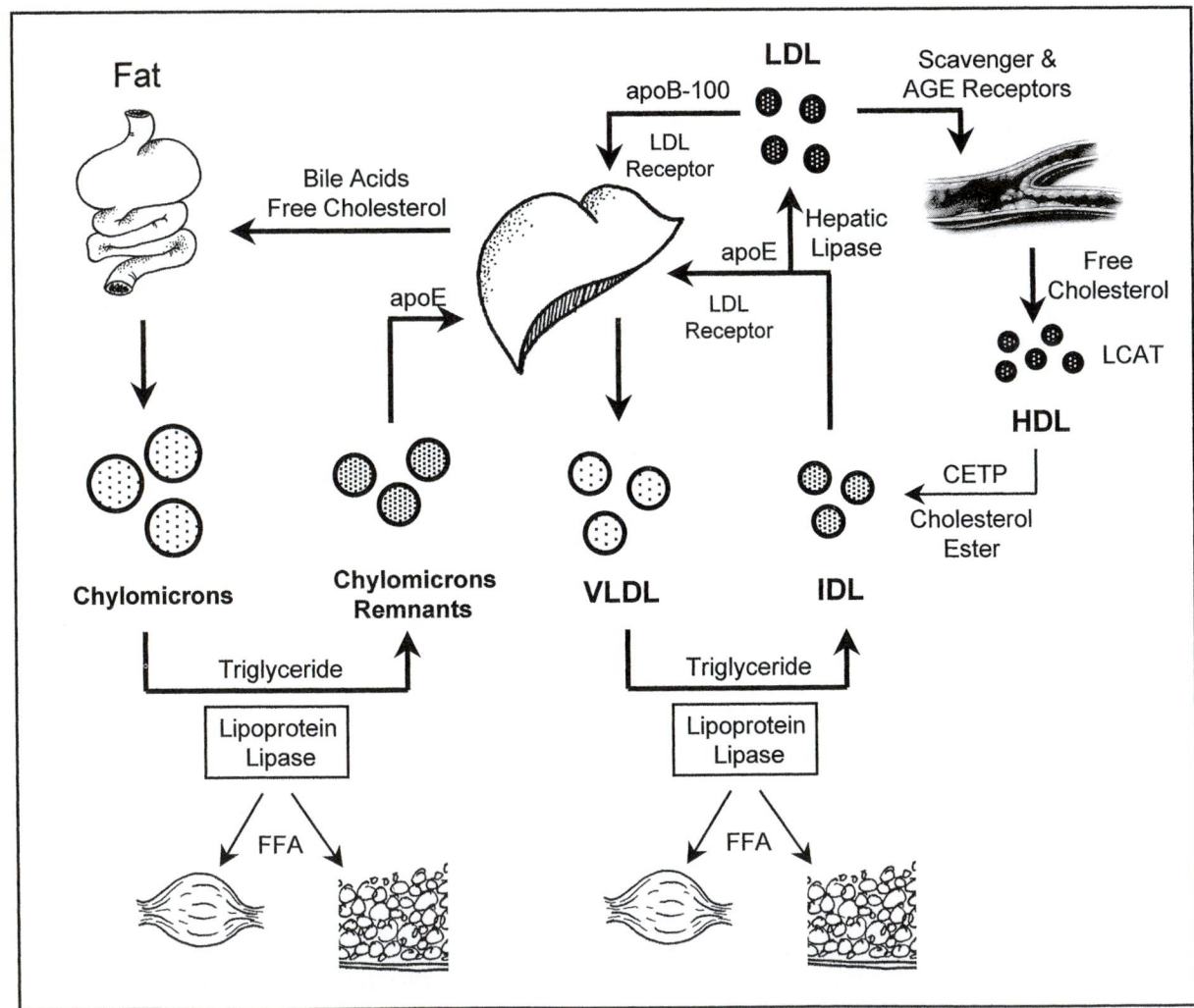

Figure 28-1 Lipoprotein metabolism.

CE-enriched. They also alter their apolipoprotein composition. As the particles shrink, they shed some of their surface phospholipids and apoCs, which HDL picks up. Lipoprotein Lipase activity also removes some apoCs. The loss of apoCs leaves space for apoE from HDL to attach to the particles. These alterations complete the transformation of CMs and VLDL to their remnant particles—CM-R and IDL, respectively. The apolipoprotein changes are critical for normal removal of these remnants by the liver. ApoC's block any binding of lipoproteins by hepatic receptors and, therefore, must be removed before clearance. In addition, apoB in CM-R and IDL are incapable of binding to any receptor because the receptor-binding region is missing in apoB-48 (CM-R), and is hidden in apoB-100 (IDL) until the particle shrinks to the size of LDL. Therefore, both CM-R and IDL must affix apoE before they can be removed by a variety of hepatic receptors,[25-30] including:

1. LDL receptor—Also called the B-E receptor since it binds both apolipoproteins.
2. LRP (LDL–receptor related protein)—This multifunctional receptor binds a variety of nonlipoproteins (α_2-macroglobulin, tissue-type plasminogen activator (t-PA), antithrombin III–thrombin, heparin cofactor II–thrombin, and α_1-antitrypsin–trypsin complexes), as well as apoE in IDL and CM-R.
3. Hepatic Lipase and Lipoprotein Lipase—These proteins can act as binding proteins for lipoproteins independent of their enzymatic function. These Lipase appear to work in conjunction with the LDL receptor and LRP to clear apoE-containing lipoproteins. Local delipidation by these enzymes also appears to increase lipoprotein particle uptake by the liver.

Normally, CM-R and IDL are cleared from the plasma in 12 to 18 hours. They deliver the cholesterol they have accumulated from HDL to the liver, where it can be excreted in the bile. However, in humans, a substantial number of the IDL particles are converted to LDL by an as-yet not fully understood pathway. This conversion removes much of the remaining triglyceride and all apolipoproteins except apoB-100. It involves Hepatic Lipase, occurs in the liver, and requires apoE3 or E4. The only known function of LDL (similar to IDL) is to deliver cholesterol transferred from HDL to the liver via the LDL receptor.[31-33] This activity appears to be maximal at LDL cholesterol (LDL-C) concentrations between 25 and 50 mg/dl. When LDL-C concentrations are above this level, LDL catabolism begins to be diverted to alternative tissues such as arteries.

HDL metabolism is very different from CM or VLDL/LDL metabolism. HDL begins as a small, disk-shaped particle containing primarily apoA-I ($\pm$apoA-II) and phospholipids (Figure 28-2). It is secreted from either the liver or small intestine. These particles collect "free" (nonesterified) cholesterol from the plasma membranes of tissues throughout the body. Cholesterol is vital to all nonplant tissues in order to maintain normal membrane function. However, most tissues synthesize more cholesterol than they require,[31-33] so the removal of their excess cholesterol by HDL is critical for maintenance of homeostasis. Free cholesterol is carried by lipoproteins interdigitated between the phospholipid molecules on their outer surface. This configuration is possible because of the slight polarity provided by its free −OH group. Because this type of transport provides rather limited carrying capacity, Lecithin: Cholesterol Acyltransferase (LCAT) esterifies free cholesterol to the much more hydrophobic cholesterol ester (CE), which is forced to move into the core of the particle. This process begins to convert the small disks to larger spheres, and opens up additional surface area for the adsorption of more cholesterol from overloaded tissues.[34]

Now that the cholesterol has been removed from the tissues and is essentially trapped in the interior of the HDL particle, some mechanism is required to deliver this cholesterol to the liver. This delivery is required because, despite the fact that almost every tissue can synthesize cholesterol, there is no tissue that can destroy it. Cholesterol must, therefore, be delivered to the liver where it can be excreted in the bile. This is accomplished by transferring the CE from HDL to the apoB-containing lipoproteins, which are normally rapidly removed from the circulation by the liver. Unlike the ready transfer of free cholesterol between the surfaces of all lipoproteins and cell membranes, CE will not transfer spontaneously because it is in the core of the particle. CE transfer requires a specific transport protein called "cholesterol ester transfer protein" (CETP). This protein can actually carry either TG or CE and moves them between various lipoprotein particles. Because of the presence of this protein, the longer lipoproteins remain in the circulation, the more closely their core compositions resemble each other. For example, LDL and HDL

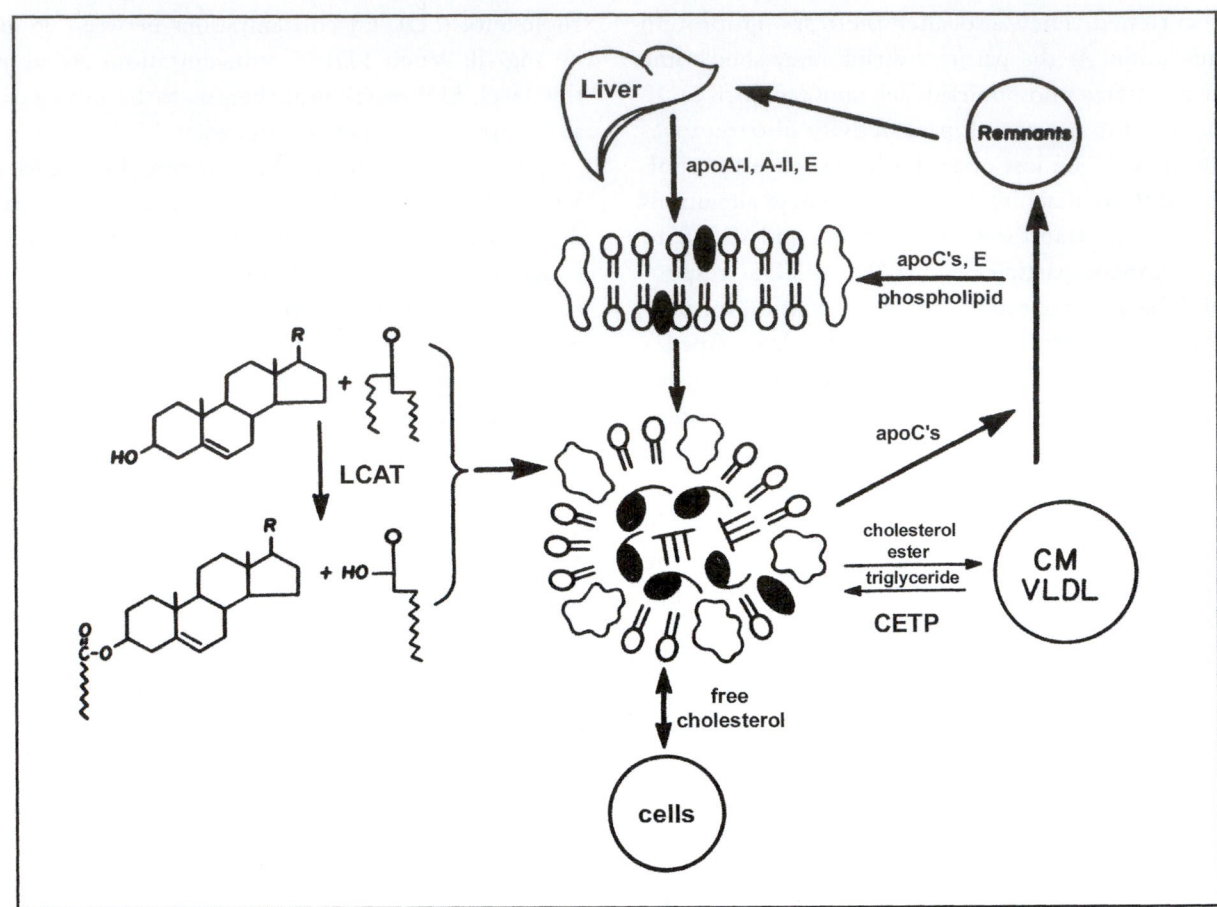

Figure 28-2 HDL metabolism

have very similar core compositions because they remain in the circulation for several days. As CE is removed from HDL, additional CE can be generated from free cholesterol and the HDL particle can accept more cholesterol from body tissues. This series of reactions, called "reverse cholesterol transport," allows HDL to be recycled as they fulfill their role in moving cholesterol from peripheral tissues to the liver.

CETP appears to be important in a number of common clinical syndromes. For example, CMs and VLDL remain TG-rich as long as they are cleared from the plasma fairly rapidly (hours). However, if these particles remain in the circulation for a prolonged period, such as in some patients homozygous for apoE2E2, they become cholesterol-rich and form β-VLDL (Type III Hyperlipidemia, or Dysbetalipoproteinemia). On the other hand, if there is an excess influx of triglyceride-rich lipoproteins in the circulation (such as in obesity, Type 2 Diabetes, renal insufficiency, etc.), TG is transferred to LDL and HDL and these particles become TG-enriched. TG-

enriched LDL and HDL are then converted to small, dense particles by Hepatic Lipase (discussed below). An inhibitor protein actually controls the activity of CETP. This inhibitor is present at modest levels in humans. Increased levels of this inhibitor reduce CETP activity and increase HDL-C concentration; typically levels of 70 to 90 mg/dl are seen. This increase in HDL is generally associated with reduced CVD. However, absence of CETP can lead to very high HDL-C concentrations (>100 mg/dl) and may actually be associated with an increase in CVD because of the severe deficiency in reverse cholesterol transport.

Hepatic Lipase (HL) is perhaps the most important enzyme involved in HDL metabolism. This enzyme removes both TG and phospholipid from lipoproteins and prefers to work on smaller lipoprotein particles, such as LDL, HDL, and IDL (as noted above). Hepatic Lipase appears to be the factor primarily responsible for eliminating HDL from the plasma. It does this by removing phospholipid from the outer surface of HDL. This allows apoA-I to detach from the particle.[35] Several tissues, including the kidney, rapidly remove this free apoA-I. Once apoA-I is lost from the plasma, it is not readily replaced and HDL concentrations fall. TG is also rapidly removed from HDL by Hepatic Lipase. Consequently, when HDL becomes TG-enriched because of an influx of VLDL or CMs, it is rapidly reduced in size by HL and apoA-I is lost.

In a similar fashion, when LDL becomes triglyceride-enriched in high-TG conditions, it is also attacked by Hepatic Lipase and small, dense LDL is formed.[36] This form of LDL appears to be more atherogenic than LDL of normal composition for several reasons.[37,38] First, it has a lower affinity for the LDL receptor than normal LDL, so it is cleared more slowly by the liver. Second, it penetrates the endothelial layer more easily, thus allowing it more ready access for plaque formation. Finally, it is more susceptible to oxidation and glycation, which are required before LDL can be taken up by macrophages to form foam cells.

Hepatic Lipase activity is hormonally regulated. Thyroid hormone, insulin, and androgens increase its activity while estrogens inhibit it. Hepatic Lipase is primarily responsible for the higher HDL-C concentrations seen in women and patients with hypothyroidism, and probably contributes significantly to the lower concentrations seen in insulin-resistant states and Type 2 Diabetes.

FAMILIAL HYPERLIPIDEMIAS

There are several familial hyperlipidemias that are relatively common and are major causes of CVD. Familial hypercholesterolemia[39,40] is caused by a genetic defect in the LDL receptor or apoB that reduces or abolishes binding of LDL (and other lipoproteins) to the LDL receptor. There are over 100 specific mutations identified with a variety of clinical presentations. These patients may have cholesterol deposits in their Achilles tendons (giving them "thick" ankles), which are rarely seen in other conditions. They may also have nodular xanthomas in the creases and/or on the extensor surfaces of their joints (similar to those seen in Familial Dysbetalipoproteinemia). Elevations of LDL-C are seen in utero. Heterozygotes typically have LDL-C levels between 300 and 800 mg/dl and begin having cardiac events in their 20s. This condition occurs in approximately 1 in 500 individuals.

Women with this disease do maintain some protection from CVD until menopause. Homozygotes have LDL-C >1000 mg/dl and frequently have cardiac events by the age of 5. Patients with this syndrome should be referred to a lipid specialist since intensive treatment will be required. All family members should be screened. Lifestyle changes (diet, alcohol, and exercise) have minimal impact on lipid concentrations.

Familial Combined Hyperlipidemia[41] is actually a syndrome since it represents a number of different mechanisms, most of which are poorly understood at present. The primary criterion for diagnosis is that different family members present with different lipid phenotypes—i.e., elevated cholesterol, elevated triglycerides, or both. These elevations may not be striking; levels of 240 to 300 mg/dl are common. HDL-C is typically reduced. An individual patient may also change phenotypes over time. The most frequent metabolic abnormality seen in this disorder is an overproduction of VLDL particles with a relatively normal composition. This disorder is typically identified by an increase in VLDL apoB with normal lipid to apoB ratios. VLDL size is, therefore, relatively normal. This increase in VLDL particle number will frequently lead to increases in the number of IDL and LDL particles, a very atherogenic situation. The hyperlipidemia will usually develop before the age of 30, although the low HDL may be evident at even earlier ages. Clinical CVD will frequently be present by the age of 40 and is often very malignant. Women appear to be at about the same risk as men, even before menopause, and therefore both should be aggressively treated. This syndrome is probably the most common cause of CVD in premenopausal women.

Familial Hypertriglyceridemia is a common cause for isolated hypertriglyceridemia (triglycerides: 150 to 600 mg/dl) and is characterized by an increased number of VLDL particles that are enlarged by extra triglyceride. These patients typically have low concentrations of LDL and HDL. The incidence of CVD is variable. Some families appear to be at high risk for CVD while others are not. Lipoprotein composition is not usually helpful in differentiating families at risk; therefore, a family history is critical in determining therapy. Insulin resistance is common in those patients with CVD and its presence is an indication for aggressive therapy.

Familial Dysbetalipoproteinemia is relatively rare (1 in 1000 to 5000 individuals) but common enough that many primary care providers will see these patients.

It is seen in individuals who are homozygous for apoE2E2 (described previously), and is characterized by the presence of large, cholesterol ester-rich VLDL (β-VLDL), formed by the delayed clearance of IDL. Both cholesterol and triglyceride plasma concentrations can vary from 150 to 1200 mg/dl, frequently with similar elevations. These patients may have orange cholesterol deposits in the creases of their hands (palmar xanthomas: only seen in this disease), as well as nodular xanthomas in the creases and on the extensor surfaces of their joints (similar to those seen in Familial Hypercholesterolemia). These patients are at increased risk for CVD, especially peripheral vascular disease. Lifestyle changes and many medical therapies can have a dramatic impact on their lipid levels.

THERAPEUTIC TARGETS

Normal human lipoprotein concentrations are LDL-C 30 to 60 mg/dl, triglycerides <140 mg/dl, and HDL-C >40 mg/dl in men and >50 mg/dl in women. "Normal" is defined as levels (a) that are not associated with disease (especially atherosclerosis) and (b) that are adequate to fulfill all known physiologic functions. "Acceptable" and/or "desirable" levels are currently defined by a number of committees based on a variety of factors, including cost-effectiveness analyses and levels shown to reduce cardiac events in clinical trials.[42] However, even the "normal" levels noted above may induce atherosclerosis if there is an abnormal lipoprotein present [i.e., β-VLDL or Lp(a)], or if the lipoproteins have been chemically altered, i.e., glycosylated and/or oxidized in diabetes). To date, clinical trials have shown that atherosclerosis will progress in approximately one-third of patients with venous bypass grafts at LDL-C concentrations of 95 mg/dl[43] and in native arteries at ~105 mg/dl.[44] In addition, teenagers with a LDL-C approximately 100 mg/dl usually have many fatty streaks in their arteries, which are the precursors of atheromatous plaques.

Risk factors for CVD are male sex, a family history of CVD, cigarette smoking, hypertension, estrogen deficiency in women, age >45 years, and HDL-C <35 in men and <45 in women (Table 28-1). Patients with Diabetes Mellitus should be treated as if they have known CVD.

Specific treatment goals are very controversial at this time. There is no question that a patient with known CVD of any kind or diabetes should maintain

---

TABLE 28-1
CARDIOVASCULAR RISK FACTORS

Positive risk factors:
  Age—Male ≥45 years; female ≥55 years or premature menopause without estrogen replacement
  Family history of premature CVD (definite myocardial infarction or sudden death before 55 years of age in father or other male first-degree relative, or before 65 years in mother or other first-degree relative)
  Current cigarette smoking
  Hypertension (blood pressure ≥135/85 mm Hg, or taking antihypertensive medication)
  Low HDL cholesterol (<35 mg/dl in men; <45 mg/dl in women)
  Diabetes mellitus
Negative risk factors:
  High HDL cholesterol (≥60 mg/dl)

Source: Grundy et al.[42]

LDL-C concentrations of <100 mg/dl. However, there is suggestive evidence that a more appropriate goal would be <70 mg/dl, especially if the HDL-C is <40 mg/dl in men or <50 mg/dl in women. Triglycerides should also be reduced to <150 mg/dl in these situations. Treatment goals for subjects without known CVD or diabetes are being debated at this time and are likely to change frequently in the near future. The risk of atherosclerosis can probably be almost eliminated if lipoprotein concentrations are maintained at the above "normal" levels (LDL-C <60 mg/dl and TG <140 mg/dl), even if their HDL is relatively low. The exceptions are patients with rare lipoprotein disorders that produce severely dysfunctional lipoproteins despite relatively normal concentrations, and possibly diabetes. It is generally agreed that everyone with an LDL-C >190 mg/dl and/or triglyceride >400 mg/dl should be treated. However, the type of therapy (lifestyle versus medications) and targets for therapy are controversial. Similarly, an LDL-C <100 mg/dl and/or TG <200 mg/dl in a patient with no other risk factors for CVD is generally not considered a candidate for medications (although diet and exercise could certainly be considered). Between these extremes, there is little agreement. The National Cholesterol Education Program (NCEP)[42] has proposed a set of minimum guidelines (Table 28-2). However, many experts believe that therapy should be much more aggressive, with everyone being treated to LDL-C <100 mg/dl and TG <200 mg/dl, and patients with one or two risk factors being treated to LDL <70 mg/dl and TG <150 mg/dl. Medications should be used if required

TABLE 28-2
TREATMENT DECISIONS BASED ON LDL CHOLESTEROL LEVEL (MG/DL)

Dietary Therapy			Drug Therapy		
Patient Category	Initiation Level	LDL Goal	Patient Category	Initiation Level	LDL Goal
No CVD, <2 Risk Factors	≥160	<160	No CVD, <2 Risk Factors	≥190	<160
No CVD, ≥2 Risk Factors	≥130	<130	No CVD, ≥2 Risk Factors	≥160	<130
With CVD	>100	≤100	With CVD	≥130	≤100

to achieve these targets. If NCEP minimum guidelines cannot be achieved in a specific patient, the patient should be referred to a lipid specialist (unless the patient is totally noncompliant with treatment).

DIET THERAPY FOR HYPERLIPIDEMIA

Dietary management must be adapted to the specific lipoprotein abnormality.

Severe Hypertriglyceridemia (TG >800 mg/dl)

Restriction of total fat to <20% of calories is extremely important. The only fat that should be allowed is fish fat or omega-3 fatty acids, which actually reduce triglycerides in these patients. Alcohol must also be eliminated since even a small amount can induce a substantial increase in triglycerides in just a few hours. If the patient has diabetes mellitus, the blood glucose level must be tightly controlled (<110 mg/dl). Restriction of dietary cholesterol is not required, but restriction of fructose and sucrose may be helpful. Substantial weight reduction will usually reduce triglycerides dramatically.

Mild to Moderate Hypertriglyceridemia (TG 150 to 800 mg/dl)

Restriction of fructose and sucrose is very important. It is important to remember that fruit has a high content of these sugars, therefore, only two to three servings of fruit per day should be allowed. Restriction of total fat does not appear to be helpful in these patients. However, reducing dietary fat should help them lose weight, which can produce a dramatic improvement in triglycerides. Alcohol should be highly restricted in these patients but cholesterol restriction will not alter their triglyceride concentrations. Controlling glucose by any means in diabetic patients will usually reduce triglycerides.

Hypercholesterolemia (LDL)

Fatty acid composition of food appears to be the most important dietary factor in determining LDL-C concentrations.[45-47] Myristate (saturated fatty acids with 14 carbons) and palmitate (saturated with 16 carbons) are the only common fatty acids that elevate LDL-C, with myristate being the more potent. Myristate is found in coconut, dairy fat, and some tropical oils. Palmitate is found in many tropical oils and animal fat. Stearate (saturated with 18 carbons) is found in animal fats and cocoa butter but does not increase LDL-C. Oleate (monounsaturated with 18 carbons) is found in most fat sources but is in particularly high concentration in olive oil. It appears to be neutral toward LDL but may cause a slight increase in HDL. Substituting oleate for myristate can reduce LDL and increase HDL, leading to an improvement in the LDL:HDL ratio. Linoleate (polyunsaturated with 18 carbons) is found in most vegetable oils and reduces both LDL and HDL concentrations to a similar degree. Therefore, there is little change in the LDL:HDL ratio. Cholesterol restriction has a variable response in patients because of individual variation in intestinal absorption. Probably a minority of patients will have a significant reduction in LDL-C by reducing dietary cholesterol to <150 mg/day. However, some patients may respond quite well to this change. The major source of dietary cholesterol is eggs (~250 mg/egg). Weight reduction will have a transient effect on LDL-C, but unless the weight loss is very large (>50 lb) the LDL will usually return to previous levels within several weeks of weight stabilization. HDL will also fall during weight reduction but it will usually increase to above initial levels with weight stabilization. Alcohol, fructose, and sucrose have little impact on LDL-C. However, alcohol will usually increase HDL-C a small amount.

The lipoprotein effects of all of these manipulations will become evident within 2 to 3 weeks and be fully manifest within 6 weeks, except for weight reduction. Lipoprotein composition will continue to change until 1 to 2 months after weight stabilization. In most instances, lipids should be rechecked within 4 to 6 weeks of starting a diet. If the target weight has been reached, the patient can be encouraged to continue. Otherwise, pharmacologic therapy should be instituted. If an excessive amount of time passes before rechecking lipid levels, many patients will have reverted to their previous diet and their success will have been missed. If no improvement is seen in 4 to 6 weeks, it is unlikely that continuing the regimen will produce significant reductions. Typical reductions seen with diet are 5 to 15% in LDL-C and 10 to 30% in triglycerides. Occasional, more dramatic improvements can be seen. If the therapeutic goal is significantly lower than these reductions would produce, then it is reasonable to institute dietary and pharmacologic therapy simultaneously.

LDL-C–LOWERING DRUGS

HMG-CoA Reductase Inhibitors[4-6,48-53]

Mechanism of Action

Inhibit cholesterol synthesis, primarily in the liver

Typical Response

LDL-C, −25 to −60%; TG, −10 to −40%; HDL-C, +5 to +10%. Also reduces apoB.

Complications

Approximately twofold increase versus placebo.

- Myositis (generalized muscle pains with creatine kinase level >3 times normal), rare (<1%); dose-related, increases with cyclosporin, niacin, or fibrate therapy.
- Rhabdomyolysis + acute renal failure (creatine kinase >10,000); very rare (<20 cases reported), almost always seen in ill patients on multiple medications
- Liver toxicity (transaminases >3 times normal), rare (<1% with usual doses); reversible when drug stopped; dose-related
- Cataracts—no increased risk
- Other—constipation, abdominal pain, myalgias, muscle cramps

Examples

Atorvastatin (Lipitor), 10 to 80 mg/day; Cerivastatin (Baycol), 0.2 to 0.3 mg/day; Fluvastatin (Lescol), 20 to 40 mg/day; Lovastatin (Mevacor), 10 to 80 mg/day;

Pravastatin (Pravachol), 20 to 40 mg/day; Simvastatin (Zocor), 5 to 80 mg/day.

Comparisons

Potency of maximum dosage—Fluvastatin/Cerivastatin < Pravastatin < Simvastatin/Lovastatin < Atorvastatin. Atorvastatin, cerivastatin, fluvastatin, pravastatin, and simvastatin are equally effective when the total dose is given once a day, in the evening, as compared with splitting the dosage to twice a day. Lovastatin, on the other hand, is slightly more effective when given as a split dose. Atorvastatin can be given any time of the day but all others are given in the evening. Pravastatin and fluvastatin are water-soluble and may be bound by bile-acid–sequestering agents (no data available). If side effects occur with one drug, another reductase inhibitor may not reproduce the same symptoms. *These agents should be the first-line pharmacologic therapy for elevated LDL-C.* Atorvastatin is the least expensive based on percent lowering of LDL-C.

Bile-Acid Sequestrants[54-56]

Mechanism of Action

Bind bile acids in the intestine, which reduces their reabsorption. This loss of bile acids stimulates hepatic synthesis of bile acids from cholesterol, which upregulates LDL receptors and lowers plasma LDL levels.

Typical Response

LDL-C, −20%; TG, +8%; HDL-C, +3%

Complications

- Constipation—frequent; should premix powder several hours before use and refrigerate; prescribe stool softeners very early
- Abdominal pain and bloating—frequent
- Gritty taste—mix with "pulpy" juices or soft foods (applesauce)
- Binds acidic drugs—warfarin, hydrochlorothiazide (HCTZ), propranolol, phenobarbital, thyroid, digoxin, tetracycline, penicillin G (and many more)
- May interfere with absorption of fat-soluble vitamins A, D, K

Examples

Cholestyramine (Questran Light), 1 to 6 packets or scoops/day; Colestipol (flavored Colestid), 1 to 6 packets or scoops/day.

Comparisons

Very similar responses. Some patients prefer the taste of one to the other. Patients must be prepared for gastrointestinal side effects. Both drugs should be given just before a meal, in divided doses.

Niacin (Nicotinic Acid, Not to Be Confused with Niacinamide)[56-58]

Mechanism of Action

Reduces VLDL secretion from the liver and increases Lipoprotein Lipase (LPL) activity. Reduces free fatty acid release from adiposites.

Typical Response

LDL-C, −20%; TG, −30%; HDL-C, +25%. Also lowers IDL-C, Lp(a), apoB, apoC-III, apoC-II, apoC-I, apoE, and increases apoA-I and HDL$_2$ (especially the "A-I alone" particle).

Complications

- Flushing, itching, urticaria—common: almost everyone will have some of these symptoms. Occurs 1 to 8 hours after dose and lasts a few seconds to an hour. Probable cause is direct degranulation of mast cells and vasodilatation. Treated by producing tolerance by starting with small, frequent doses and gradually increasing. Also prevented with antihistamines or prostaglandin inhibitors (aspirin). Sustained-release niacin reduces these symptoms. Most effective preventive measure is to take niacin with food.
- Orthostatic hypotension—rare but may be seen in patients with diabetes, probably an extreme manifestation of its typical vasodilatation.
- Glucose intolerance—common (~25%); usually seen with doses >2000 mg/day. Caused by increased insulin resistance in the muscle, not secondary to increases in counterregulatory hormones and apparently not related to changes in FFA. Lipids may be markedly improved despite increase in blood glucose.
- Transaminase elevations—common with sustained-release niacin but rare with crystalline niacin. May progress to severe jaundice, usually reversible.
- Dyspepsia—rare, but patients with a history of ulcers frequently have exacerbation of their peptic ulcer disease. Therefore, niacin should not used in these patients unless there is a very strong indication

and then it should only be used with appropriate preventive care.
- Gout—niacin frequently increases uric acid so patients should be monitored.
- Bronchitis—rare; niacin can induce an increase in mucus production in some patients.

Examples

Crystalline niacin, 500 to 4000 mg/day two to four times a day; Sustained-release N (Slo-Niacin), 250 to 1500 mg twice a day; Niaspan, 500 to 2000 mg at bedtime.

Comparisons

Some patients have very little triglyceride lowering with time-release niacin while their LDL effects are probably similar. However, there are marked individual variations in response so both formulations can be tried. Time-release niacin clearly produces more liver toxicity (Niaspan may be an exception) but also produces markedly fewer vasodilatory symptoms.

Neomycin

Mechanism of Action

Reduces intestinal cholesterol absorption by 45% and reduces LDL apoB synthesis.

Typical Response

LDL-C, −20%; TG, 0%; HDL-C, −10%. Also lowers Lp(a) 20%.

Complications:

- Nausea—10%
- Diarrhea—frequent; changes gut flora
- Neither ototoxicity nor nephrotoxicity has been seen.

Example

Neomycin, 500 mg three times a day or 1000 mg twice a day

Probucol[59]

Mechanism of Action

Enhances catabolic rate of LDL and enhances bile acid excretion. Prevents oxidation of LDL. Stimulates apoE secretion from macrophages and increases cholesterol ester transfer activity. Inhibits LPL activity.

Typical Response

LDL-C, -20%; TG, -5%; HDL-C, -30%. Also lowers apoB, apoA-I, and HDL_2; shrinks tendon xanthomas

Complications

• Diarrhea—10%

Example

Probucol (Lorelco), 500 mg twice a day.

TRIGLYCERIDE-LOWERING DRUGS

Fibric Acid Derivatives[60-63]

Mechanism of Action

Inhibit VLDL synthesis and stimulate LPL activity. Increase apoA-I and apoA-II synthesis.

Typical Response

LDL-C, $+10\%$; TG, -50%; HDL-C, $+10\%$. Also lowers VLDL and IDL while increasing apoA-I and HDL_3.

Complications

Nausea, diarrhea, dyspepsia—10% (will usually not improve with lower doses and will recur if the drug is restarted after discontinuation for even prolonged periods)

Examples

Gemfibrozil (Lopid), 600 mg twice a day; Clofibrate (Atromid-S), 500 mg twice a day.

Comparisons

Gemfibrozil appears to be more potent in lowering cholesterol.

Niacin (See Above)

Fish Oil (Omega-3 Fatty Acids)[64,65]

Mechanism of Action

Inhibits triglyceride, apoB, and VLDL synthesis. Increases LPL activity. Decreases platelet aggregation by inhibiting prostaglandin synthesis, and increases thrombolytic activity. Reduces blood pressure and inflammatory cell action.

Typical Response

LDL-C, $+10\%$; TG, -35%; HDL-C, $+5\%$. Also may increase HDL_2.

Complications

• Type 2 diabetes mellitus—Reduces insulin secretion; increases hepatic glucose production
• Prolonged bleeding time
• Flatulence, abdominal pain

Examples

EPA = eicosapentaenoic acid; DHA = docosahexaenoic acid (1-g capsules)

	EPA (mg)	DHA (mg)	Capsules/day
MaxEPA	180	110	3–15
SuperEPA	300	190	3–15
n-3 PUFA Caps	340	35	3–15
RES-Q1000	300	200	3–15
Sardine oil	300	0	3–15

Comparisons

Both EPA and DHA lower triglycerides similarly but DHA may have a more potent LDL-C lowering effect. Vitamin E (400 U) should be given with each dose of fish oil to prevent oxidation of these very unsaturated fatty acids.

DRUGS THAT INCREASE HDL

Niacin (See Above)

Fibric Acid Derivatives (See Above)

HMG-CoA Reductase Inhibitors (See Above)

Estrogen (See Below)

Dilantin, Phenobarbital

RECOMMENDATIONS

For the patient with only an elevated LDL-C level, a reductase inhibitor is the drug of choice. It is less expensive, more effective, and better tolerated than the sequestrants. It is also more effective and better tolerated than niacin. The reductase inhibitors are very similar in their effects but their maximum potencies are different. Atorvastatin is the most potent (lowers LDL by about 60% with 80 mg/day). It is also the least expensive in most situations if the degree of LDL-C lowering is considered.

If the patient has a relatively low HDL-C, then niacin should be given strong consideration, especially as a second drug. All lipid-lowering drugs provide some synergy so that it is usually better to use two or three drugs in moderate doses rather than pushing one drug to potentially toxic levels. Because of probucol's adverse effect on HDL, it should be reserved for patients with extremely high LDL-C (>400 mg/dl), while receiving two or more of the other medications. Reducing these extremely high LDL levels may offset the effects of reducing the HDL. The studies currently available have not been able to show a reduction in cardiac events with probucol monotherapy.

For patients with only an increase in triglycerides, either gemfibrozil or niacin can be used initially and the other added if adequate control is not achieved. Niacin is clearly less expensive but it is frequently difficult for patients to tolerate. On the other hand, patients with a borderline high LDL-C will usually not have an increase in LDL when treated with niacin, whereas LDL will frequently increase (occasionally into the abnormal range) with gemfibrozil therapy alone. If niacin is used, the crystalline form, or niaspan, should be tried first because it may be more effective in hypertriglyceridemia and has less hepatic toxicity. Whether fish oil is used before or after trying these drugs is a matter of personal preference. It is relatively expensive when given in therapeutic dosages (6 to 9 g/day), and many patients will not wish to take this many capsules. Fish oil can be obtained in the liquid form from some health food stores, and some patients may prefer this mode of treatment. Atorvastatin is slightly more effective in lowering triglycerides than the other HMG-CoA reductase inhibitors. In patients with moderate to severe hypertriglyceridemia (400 to 800 mg/dl), the maximum dosage of atorvastatin can reduce TG levels by over 40%.

For patients with significant elevations of both LDL and triglycerides, niacin and atorvastatin are probably the only single drugs that may potentially control both abnormalities. If one of these agents is not effective, then the other may be tried or a second drug added. An effective two-drug regimen for this problem is a reductase inhibitor plus gemfibrozil. This combination is not recommended in the *Physicians' Desk Reference* because of an increased risk of myositis. However, this risk is quite small (<5%) and rarely leads to rhabdomyolysis unless the patient is also on cyclosporin and/or is acutely ill. ANY PATIENT WHO IS SERIOUSLY ILL SHOULD BE TAKEN OFF OF ALL LIPID-LOWERING MEDICATIONS. Alternatively, gemfibrozil plus a sequestrant

or neomycin may be used. A reductase inhibitor plus niacin is also a very effective combination, but there is also a small increased risk of myositis with this combination.

The most effective drug for increasing HDL is niacin. However, since niacin increases HDL by a different mechanism than gemfibrozil, these two drugs can be relatively effective when used in combination. Dilantin (or phenobarbital) can also produce substantial elevations in HDL. However, the toxicity of dilantin and phenobarbital must be considered carefully. Estrogen therapy can cause substantial elevations of HDL in postmenopausal women, as well as have substantial direct antiatherogenic effects on the arterial wall (see below).

ANTIOXIDANT THERAPY[66-72]

There has been a substantial amount of evidence that indicates that LDL must be oxidized before it can be internalized by macrophages to form foam cells and, ultimately, arterial plaques. This required chemical step provides an additional mode of therapy for the prevention of atherosclerosis. Probucol is a very potent antioxidant, since this was the function for which it was originally designed. Unfortunately, probucol also substantially lowers HDL levels, and thus may have a detrimental effect on coronary disease. There are several other antioxidants currently being tested, including vitamin E (400 to 1200 U/day), vitamin C (250 to 1000 mg/day), and β-carotene. All have some clinical data that suggest that they prevent cardiac events and possibly some cancers.

ESTROGEN THERAPY[73-78]

Postmenopausal estrogen therapy has a major impact on cardiovascular disease in women. There have been more than 20 studies (case–control or cohort) that clearly demonstrate the substantial impact of estrogen therapy (typically reducing cardiovascular disease by about 50%). However, only one placebo-controlled, double-blind, prospective study has been reported that addresses this issue, and it included only 84 matched pairs of women. This study did demonstrate the expected 50% reduction in CVD. The "Women's Health Initiative," which is currently in progress, is designed to answer this question in a very large group of women. Unfortunately, these results may not be available until the year 2004. In the meantime, the current data must be used to decide whether to prescribe estrogen. Many lipid specialists believe that all women should receive this therapy unless they have a major contraindication.

There are several mechanisms by which estrogen therapy probably prevents atherosclerosis. (1) Estrogen lowers LDL and apoB while raising HDL, especially HDL$_2$, and apoA-I. These changes are usually only seen with oral estrogen therapy and are probably mediated through estrogen's effects on Hepatic Lipase (decrease) and Lipoprotein Lipase (increase) activities. Estrogen also increases the LDL receptor activity in the liver. (2) Estrogen inhibits smooth muscle proliferation and collagen synthesis, while increasing collagen degradation in the arterial wall. It also increases cholesterol efflux from foam cells, reduces fibrinogen and thromboxane, and increases prostacyclin and nitric oxide synthesis by endothelial cells. (3) Estrogen increases blood flow to the heart, brain, and kidney by stimulating nitric oxide production and has been shown to reduce angina. It also has calcium-channel-blocker activity. (4) Estrogen reduces insulin resistance and lowers insulin and glucose concentrations. (5) Estrogen prevents the accumulation of visceral fat, which is associated with hypertension, insulin resistance, hypertriglyceridemia, and low HDL. (6) Estrogen is a potent anti-oxidant and clearly inhibits LDL oxidation.

There are other reasons to use estrogen therapy. Estrogen clearly prevents bone resorption and prevents fractures. Estrogen prevents the vasomotor symptoms of menopause. It also appears that estrogen improves the reaction time in elderly women, allowing them to extend their arms to break their falls. This improved reaction time appears to lead to more wrist fractures but fewer hip fractures. Studies have also suggested that dementia may be slowed or prevented by estrogen therapy.

There are three major risks of estrogen therapy: (1) Endometrial cancer risk is increased by about 50%. It should be remembered that women have a 100-fold greater risk for cardiovascular disease than for endometrial cancer. Therefore, a 50% increase in risk actually accounts for very few cases as compared with CVD. In addition, mortality is not increased when endometrial cancer develops in women on estrogen-replacement therapy. This may be due to the occurrence of less-aggressive tumors or to better surveillance. Concomitant progestin or progesterone therapy reduces the endometrial cancer risk by about

80% versus no hormone therapy. Progestins can be given either by a low-dose, continuous regimen (2.5 to 5.0 mg/day) or cyclically, with higher doses (10 mg/day for 10 to 12 days every 2 to 3 months). However, progestins (but not progesterone) may blunt the beneficial lipid effects of estrogen. On the other hand, progestins will increase bone formation and may, therefore, reduce the risk of fractures even further. Some vaginal bleeding during the first 6 months of continuous estrogen–progestin therapy is common (about 60 to 70%). If this bleeding is not controlled with higher doses of progestin, an evaluation and possibly endometrial biopsy should be done. Annual endometrial biopsies should be recommended to women who have a uterus and who are receiving estrogen without progestin.

(2) Breast cancer incidence may be increased by as much as 10% with estrogen therapy, especially when high doses of Estradiol are given for long periods (>10 years). Few studies have implicated conjugated estrogens. There are as many (if not more) studies showing a reduction in breast cancer with estrogen therapy as an increase. In fact, the only controlled trial of estrogen therapy showed a substantial reduction in the incidence of breast cancer in the treated women, but this study only included 168 women. This remains a controversial issue. However, even if estrogen therapy does cause breast cancer, the relative incidence of atherosclerosis and breast cancer in postmenopausal women (10-fold difference) is such that breast cancer would develop in only one woman for every 20 women who would be saved from cardiovascular disease. There is no clinical evidence to date that indicates that there is a detrimental effect of estrogen in women with breast cancer even if they are receptor-positive.

(3) Thromboembolic events can occur with estrogen therapy. However, these are very rare when typical doses of estrogen (conjugated estrogens, 0.625 to 1.25 mg/day) are used, unless the patient has a hypercoagulable state, such as the presence of a lupus anticoagulant or an anticardiolipin antibody.

REFERENCES

1. Assmann G, Schulte H. Relation of high-density lipoprotein cholesterol and triglycerides to incidence of atherosclerotic coronary artery disease (the PROCAM experience). Am J Cardiol 1992;70:733.
2. Haheim LL, Holme I, Hjermann I, Leren P. The predictability of risk factors with respect to incidence and

mortality of myocardial infarction and total mortality—a 12-year follow-up of the Oslo Study, Norway. J Intern Med 1993;234:17.

3. Njolstad I, Arnesen E, Lundlarsen PG. Smoking, serum lipids, blood pressure, and sex differences in myocardial infarction: a 12-year follow-up of the Finnmark study. Circulation 1996;93:450.

4. Stark RM. Review of the major intervention trials of lowering coronary artery disease risk through cholesterol reduction. Am J Cardiol 1996;78:13.

5. Pedersen TR, Kjekshus J, Berg K, et al. Randomised trial of cholesterol lowering in 4444 patients with coronary heart disease: the Scandinavian Simvastatin Survival Study (4S). Lancet 1994;344:1383.

6. Jukema JW, Bruschke AVG, Vanboven AJ, et al. Effects of lipid lowering by pravastatin on progression and regression of coronary artery disease in symptomatic men with normal to moderately elevated serum cholesterol levels: the regression growth evaluation statin study (REGRESS). Circulation 1995;91:2528.

7. Shepherd J, Cobbe SM, Ford I, et al. Prevention of coronary heart disease with pravastatin in men with hypercholesterolemia. N Engl J Med 1995;333:1301.

8. Blankenhorn DH, Hodis HN. Arterial imaging and atherosclerosis reversal. Arterioscler Thromb 1994;14:177.

9. Patsch W, Gotto AM. Apolipoproteins: pathophysiology and clinical implications. Methods Enzymol 1996;263:3.

10. Fruchart JC, Degeteire C, Delfly B, Castro GR. Apolipoprotein A-I-containing particles and reverse cholesterol transport: evidence for connection between cholesterol efflux and atherosclerosis risk. Atherosclerosis 1994;110:S35.

11. Hughes TA, Moore MA, Joyce M, Go RCP, Segrest JP, Blackwell T. Sexual differences in lipoprotein composition in a family with dyslipidemic hypertension and premature atherosclerosis: deficiency of HDL-L and HDL-M "apoA-I alone" particle." J Lab Clin Med 1992;119:57.

12. Slyper AH. Low-density lipoprotein density and atherosclerosis—unraveling the connection. JAMA 1994; 272:305.

13. Dergunov AD, Rosseneu M. The significance of apolipoprotein E structure to the metabolism of plasma triglyceride-rich lipoproteins. Biol Chem Hoppe Seyler 1994;375:485.

14. Luc G, Fievet C, Arveiler D, et al. Apolipoproteins C-III and E in apoB- and non-apoB-containing lipoproteins in two populations at contrasting risk for myocardial infarction: the ECTIM study. J Lipid Res 1996;37:508.

15. Reina M, Brunzell JD, Deeb SS. Molecular basis of familial chylomicronemia—mutations in the lipoprotein lipase and apolipoprotein-C-II genes. J Lipid Res 1992;33:1823.

16. Alaupovic P, Mack WJ, KnightGibson C, Hodis HN. The role of triglyceride-rich lipoprotein families in the progression of atherosclerotic lesions as determined by sequential coronary angiography from a controlled clinical trial. Arterioscler Thromb Vasc Biol 1997;17:715.

17. Luc G, Fievet C, Arveiler D, et al. Apolipoproteins C-III and E in apoB- and non-apoB-containing lipoproteins in two populations at contrasting risk for myocardial infarction: the ECTIM study. J Lipid Res 1996;37:508.

18. Stewart MW, Laker MF, Alberti KGMM. The contribution of lipids to coronary heart disease in diabetes mellitus. J Intern Med 1994;236:41.

19. Alaupovic P, Bard JM, Tavella M, Shafer D. Identification of apoB-containing lipoprotein families in NIDDM. Diabetes 1992;41:18.

20. Manzato E, Zambon A, Lapolla A, et al. Lipoprotein abnormalities in well-treated type-II diabetic patients. Diabetes Care 1993;16:469.

21. Attman PO, Nyberg G, Williamolsson T, KnightGibson C, Alaupovic P. Dyslipoproteinemia in diabetic renal failure. Kidney Int 1992;42:1381.

22. Samuelsson O, Attman PO, KnightGibson C, et al. Effect of gemfibrozil on lipoprotein abnormalities in chronic renal insufficiency: a controlled study in human chronic renal disease. Nephron 1997;75:286.

23. Ginsberg HN. Role of lipid synthesis, chaperone proteins and proteasomes in the assembly and secretion of apoprotein B-containing lipoproteins from cultured liver cells. Clin Exp Pharmacol Physiol 1997;24:A29.

24. Murdoch SJ, Breckenridge WC. Influence of lipoprotein lipase and hepatic lipase on the transformation of VLDL and HDL during lipolysis of VLDL. Atherosclerosis 1995; 118:193.

25. Skottova N, Savonen R, Lookene A, Hultin M, Olivecrona G. Lipoprotein lipase enhances removal of chylomicrons and chylomicron remnants by the perfused rat liver. J Lipid Res 1995;36:1334.

26. Strickland DK, Kounnas MZ, Argraves WS. LDL receptor-related protein: a multiligand receptor for lipoprotein and proteinase catabolism. FASEB J 1995;9:890.

27. Kounnas MZ, Church FC, Argraves WS, Strickland DK. Cellular internalization and degradation of antithrombin III-thrombin, heparin cofactor II-thrombin, and alpha(1)-antitrypsin-trypsin complexes is mediated by the low density lipoprotein receptor-related protein. J Biol Chem 1996;271:6523.

28. deFaria E, Fong LG, Komaromy M, Cooper AD. Relative roles of the LDL receptor, the LDL receptor-like protein, and hepatic lipase in chylomicron remnant removal by the liver. J Lipid Res 1996;37:197.

29. Hardy MM, Feder J, Wolfe RA, Bu GJ. Low density lipoprotein receptor-related protein modulates the expression of tissue-type plasminogen activator in human colon fibroblasts. J Biol Chem 1997;272:6812.

30. Cooper AD. Hepatic uptake of chylomicron remnants. J Lipid Res 1997;38:2173.

31. Turley SD, Spady DK, Dietschy JM. Role of liver in the synthesis of cholesterol and the clearance of low density lipoproteins in the cynomolgus monkey. J Lipid Res 1995;36:67.

32. Osono Y, Woollett LA, Herz J, Dietschy JM. Role of the low density lipoprotein receptor in the flux of cholesterol through the plasma and across the tissues of the mouse. J Clin Invest 1995;95:1124.

33. Hill SA, McQueen J. Reverse cholesterol transport—a review of the process and its clinical implications. Clin Biochem 1997;30:517.

34. Dietschy JM. Theoretical considerations of what regulates low-density-lipoprotein and high-density-lipoprotein cholesterol. Am J Clin Nutr 1997;65:S1581.

35. Clay MA, Newnham HH, Forte TM, Barter PI. Cholesteryl

ester transfer protein and hepatic lipase activity promote shedding of apo A-I from HDL and subsequent formation of discoidal HDL. Biochim Biophys Acta 1992;1124(1):52.

36. Griffin BA, Freeman DJ, Tait GW, et al. Role of plasma triglyceride in the regulation of plasma low density lipoprotein (LDL) subfractions: relative contribution of small, dense LDL to coronary heart disease risk. Atherosclerosis 1994;106:241.

37. Raal FJ, Areias AJ, Joffe BI. Low density lipoproteins and atherosclerosis—quantity or quality? Redox Rep 1995; 1:171.

38. Gardner CD, Fortmann SP, Krauss RM. Association of small low-density lipoprotein particles with the incidence of coronary artery disease in men and women. JAMA 1996;276:875.

39. Shachter NS, Weinberger J. Mutations of the low-density-lipoprotein receptor gene and familial hypercholesterolemia. Trends Endocrinol Metab 1994;5:245.

40. Hegele RA. The genetic basis of atherosclerosis. Int J Clin Lab Res 1997;27:2.

41. Austin MA, Hokanson JE. Epidemiology of triglycerides, small dense low-density lipoprotein, and lipoprotein(A) as risk factors for coronary heart disease. Med Clin North Am 1994;78:99.

42. Grundy SM, Bilheimer D, Chait A, et al. Summary of the Second Report of the National Cholesterol Education Program (NCEP) Expert Panel on Detection, Evaluation, and Treatment of High Blood Cholesterol in Adults (Adult-Treatment-Panel-II). JAMA 1993;269:3015.

43. Post-CABG Trial Investigators. Impact of aggressive vs moderate lowering of LDL-C on atherosclerosis. N Engl J Med 1997;336:153.

44. Sacks FM, Pfeffer MA, Moye LA, et al. The effect of pravastatin on coronary events after myocardial infarction in patients with average cholesterol levels. N Engl J Med 1996;335:1001.

45. Woollett LA, Spady DK, Dietschy JM. Regulatory effects of the saturated fatty acids 6-0 through 18-0 on hepatic low density lipoprotein receptor activity in the hamster. J Clin Invest 1992;89:1133.

46. Daumerie CM, Woollett LA, Dietschy JM. Fatty acids regulate hepatic low density lipoprotein receptor activity through redistribution of intracellular cholesterol pools. Proc Natl Acad Sci U S A 1992;89:10797.

47. Horton JD, Cuthbert JA, Spady DK. Dietary fatty acids regulate hepatic low density lipoprotein (LDL) transport by altering LDL receptor protein and messenger RNA levels. J Clin Invest 1993;92:743.

48. Corsini A, Bernini F, Quarato P, et al. Non-lipid-related effects of 3-hydroxy-3-methylglutaryl coenzyme A reductase inhibitors. Cardiology 1996;87:458.

49. Elisaf M, Mikhailidis DP, Siamopoulos KC. Dyslipidaemia in patients with renal diseases. J Drug Dev Clin Pract 1996;7:331.

50. Lea AP, McTavish D. Atorvastatin: a review of its pharmacology and therapeutic potential in the management of hyperlipidaemias. Drugs 1997;53:828.

51. Hebert PR, Gaziano JM, Chan KS, Hennekens CH. Cholesterol lowering with statin drugs, risk of stroke, and total mortality: an overview of randomized trials. JAMA 1997; 278:313.

52. Playford DA, Watts GF. Management of lipid disorders in the elderly. Drugs Aging 1997;10:444.

53. Lennernas H, Fager G. Pharmacodynamics and pharmacokinetics of the HMG-CoA reductase inhibitors—similarities and differences. Clin Pharmacokinet 1997;32:403.

54. Heudebert GR, Vanruiswyk J, Hiatt J, Schectman G. Combination drug therapy for hypercholesterolemia—the trade-off between cost and simplicity. Arch Intern Med 1993;153:1828.

55. Lyons D, Webster J, Fowler G, Petrie JC. Colestipol at varying dosage intervals in the treatment of moderate hypercholesterolaemia. Br J Clin Pharmacol 1994;37:59.

56. Schectman G, Hiatt J. Dose-response characteristics of cholesterol-lowering drug therapies: implications for treatment. Ann Intern Med 1996;125:990.

57. Oster G, Borok GM, Menzin J, et al. Cholesterol-reduction intervention study (CRIS): a randomized trial to assess effectiveness and costs in clinical practice. Arch Intern Med 1996;156:731.

58. Schell WD, Myers JN. Regression of atherosclerosis: a review. Prog Cardiovasc Dis 1997;39:483.

59. Mao SJT, Yates MT, Jackson RL; Antioxidant activity and serum levels of probucol and probucol metabolites. Methods Enzymol 1994;234:505.

60. Schonfeld G. The effects of fibrates on lipoprotein and hemostatic coronary risk factors. Atherosclerosis 1994; 111:161.

61. Lozada A, Dujovne CA. Drug interactions with fibric acids. Pharmacol Ther 1994;63:163.

62. Spencer CM, Barradell LB. Gemfibrozil: a reappraisal of its pharmacological properties and place in the management of dyslipidaemia. Drugs 1996;51:982.

63. Farmer JA, Gotto AM. Choosing the right lipid-regulating agent: a guide to selection. Drugs 1996;52:649.

64. Schmidt EB, Kristensen SD, Decaterina R, Illingworth DR. The effects of n-3 fatty acids on plasma lipids and lipoproteins and other cardiovascular risk factors in patients with hyperlipidemia. Atherosclerosis 1993; 103:107.

65. Sassen LMA, Lamers JMJ, Verdouw PD. Fish oil and the prevention and regression of atherosclerosis. Cardiovasc Drugs Ther 1994;8:179.

66. Kappus H, Diplock AT. Tolerance and safety of vitamin-E—a toxicological position report. Free Radical Biol Med 1992;13:55.

67. Gey KF. Ten-year retrospective on the antioxidant hypothesis of arteriosclerosis: threshold plasma levels of antioxidant micronutrients related to minimum cardiovascular risk. J Nutr Biochem 1995;6:206.

68. Jha P, Flather M, Lonn E, Farkouh M, Yusuf S. The antioxidant vitamins and cardiovascular disease—a critical review of epidemiologic and clinical trial data. Ann Intern Med 1995;123:860.

69. Thakur ML, Srivastava US. Vitamin-E metabolism and its application. Nutr Res 1996;16:1767.

70. Reaven PD, Witztum JL. Oxidized low density lipoproteins in atherogenesis: role of dietary modification. Annu Rev Nutr 1996;16:51.

71. Weber P, Bendich A, Machlin LJ. Vitamin E and human health: rationale for determining recommended intake levels. Nutrition 1997;13:450.

72. Maxwell SRJ, Lip GYH. Free radicals and antioxidants in cardiovascular disease. Br J Clin Pharmacol 1997;44:307.

73. Zumoff B. Biological and endocrinological insights into the possible breast cancer risk from menopausal estrogen replacement therapy. Steroids 1993;58:196.

74. White MM, Zamudio S, Stevens T, et al. Estrogen, progesterone, and vascular reactivity: potential cellular mechanisms. Endocr Rev 1995;16:739.

75. Bluming AZ. Hormone replacement therapy—benefits and risks for the general postmenopausal female population and for women with a history of previously treated breast cancer. Semin Oncol 1993;20:662.

76. Samaan SA, Crawford MH. Estrogen and cardiovascular function after menopause. J Am Coll Cardiol 1995;26:1403.

77. Guetta V, Cannon RO. Cardiovascular effects of estrogen and lipid-lowering therapies in postmenopausal women. Circulation 1996;93:1928.

78. StClair RW. Effects of estrogens on macrophage foam cells: a potential target for the protective effects of estrogens on atherosclerosis. Curr Opin Lipidol 1997;8:281.

Chapter 29
Thyroid Diseases

Joseph N. Fisher

Five Key Points

- **Women have a much higher incidence of thyroid disorders than do men.**
- **Examination of the thyroid is often done in a cursory manner; therefore, significant pathology is overlooked.**
- **The single most useful test of thyroid function is a sensitive measurement of thyroid-stimulating hormone.**
- **A majority of thyroid disorders are autoimmune in nature.**
- **Thyroid nodules are common, thyroid cancer is not. So a rational plan must be made to distinguish the benign from the malignant nodule.**

Many surveys indicate that obstetricians and gynecologists are the primary physicians for a sizable majority of women. Thyroid disorders are more common in women than in men and account for a significant amount of morbidity. Therefore, the obstetrician-gynecologist should be well versed in the diagnosis and treatment of the more common thyroid diseases, especially those unique to women. The topics discussed in this chapter will include:

- Physical examination of the thyroid
- Basic thyroid physiology
- Tests of thyroid function
- Simple goiter
- Hypothyroidism
- Thyrotoxicosis
- Thyroid emergencies
- Thyroid nodules and thyroid cancer

PHYSICAL EXAMINATION

It is an unfortunate fact that examination of the thyroid is often neglected or performed in a cursory manner. While an obvious goiter will usually be noted, detection of a smaller thyroid gland will not, unless the examiner makes some effort to do so. Figure 29-1 illustrates the maneuvers suggested for scrutiny of the thyroid. It takes only a minute or two to accomplish and should be part of every physical examination. It should be noted that the normal thyroid gland is usually not palpable.

BASIC THYROID PHYSIOLOGY

The hypothalamic–pituitary–thyroid axis is illustrated in Figure 29-2. While intrathyroidal iodine concentration may exert an influence, the principal determinant of thyroid hormone secretion is thyroid-stimulating hormone (TSH). The synthesis and release of TSH in turn is modulated by the hypothalamic tripeptide thyrotropin-releasing hormone (TRH), and the set-point for the response of TSH to TRH is governed by the circulating levels of thyroxine (T_4) and triiodothyrinine (T_3), and ultimately by the amount of T_3 within the pituitary. Thyroid hormones

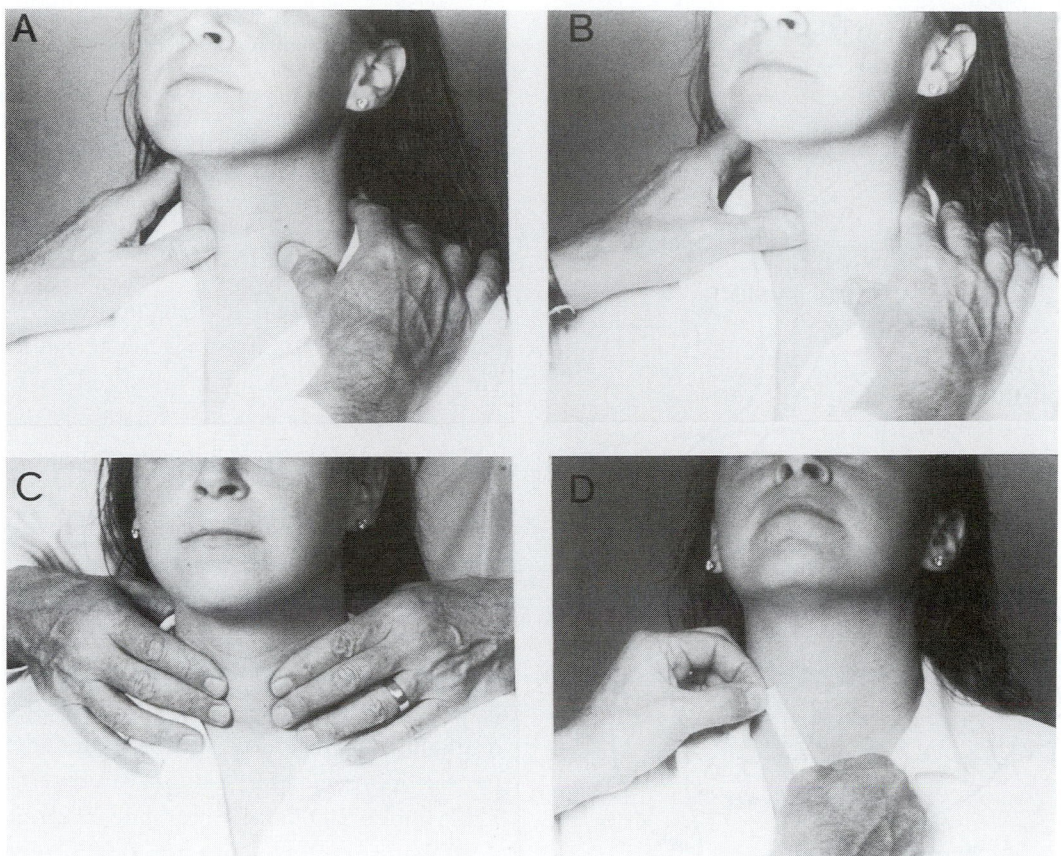

Figure 29-1 Examination of the thyroid. The subject is a young woman with a visible goiter due to autoimmune thyroiditis. A. The examiner's thumbs are palpating the anterior portion of both lobes. B. The examiner's left thumb has displaced the thyroid cartilage to the patient's left so that the left lobe of the thyroid can be more easily palpated. C. The examiner is palpating the gland from behind the patient. D. The examiner is measuring the gland by laying a ruler over the lobes.

circulate in the plasma bound to proteins, principally thyroxine-binding globulin (TBG), but also to albumin and thyroxine-binding prealbumin (transthyretin). In the euthyroid individual, about 75% of the circulating T_4 and 70% of T_3 are bound to TBG.

The equilibrium between T_4 and TBG can be expressed by the equation:

$$T_4 + TBG \rightleftharpoons T_4\,TBG$$

This equilibrium is shifted strongly to the right, with only about 0.03% of T_4 in the free or unbound form. The affinity of TBG for T_3 is lower, with the percentage of free T_3 approximately 0.3. Only the free hormones can be transported intracellularly and initiate metabolic events. When the amount of TBG is increased, as normally occurs with estrogen administration or during pregnancy, the equation is displaced to the right. The resulting decline in free hormone stimulates TSH release, which restores the absolute amount of free hormone, although at the expense of a larger amount of bound. Thus, the total T_4 (and to a lesser extent the total T_3) increases when the TBG is increased, but the free hormone and the metabolism are unchanged.

Thyroxine can be monoiodinated to either triiodothyronine or reverse triiodothyronine (rT_3) as noted in Figure 29-3. rT_3 is inactive, whereas T_3 is monodeiodinated more potent metabolically than T_4. Approximately 80% of circulating T_3 comes from the deiodination of T_4 by peripheral tissues. The enzyme 5′ deiodinase, which promotes that conversion, is inhibited by a number of conditions, including malnutrition, stress, acute and chronic illness, cirrhosis, and uremia, as well as high doses of glucocorticoids and propylthiouracil. Thus, the T_3 level is not always an accurate guide to thyroid function, especially hypothyroidism.

Many tissues in the body, including heart, kidney, brain, and liver, have receptors for thyroid hormones.

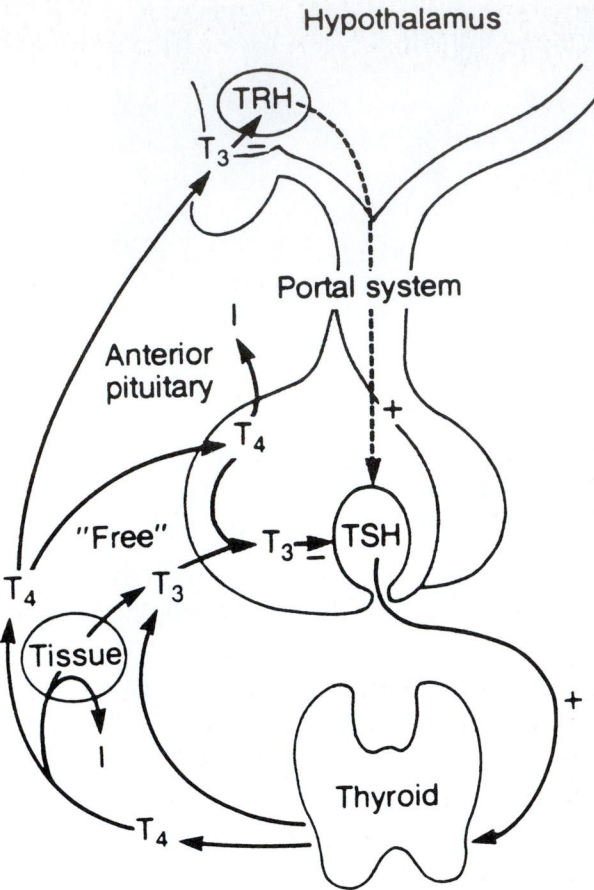

Hypothalamus

The putative mechanisms by which thyroid hormones effect calorigenesis, growth, and differentiation are reviewed elsewhere.[1]

TESTS OF THYROID FUNCTION

While quite a large number of tests and procedures are available for the diagnosis of thyroid disorders, in

Figure 29-2 The hypothalamic–pituitary–thyroid axis. Thyrotropin-releasing hormone produced in the hypothalamus reaches the anterior pituitary via the portal system, where it enables the secretion of thyroid-stimulating hormone. This response is modulated by triiodothyronine, which is produced in the thyroid by monodeiodination of thyroxine. *Source: Greenspan FS. The thyroid gland. In: Greenspan FS, Baxter JD, eds. Basic and clinical endocrinology. 4th ed. Norwalk, CT: Appleton & Lange, 1994:160.*

most instances only a few are needed. Tests that are readily available in most reference laboratories or nuclear medicine facilities are listed in Table 29-1. Perhaps the single most useful test is the sensitive TSH assay. This is true for at least three reasons. As noted in Figure 29-2, TSH is the central player in the negative-feedback control of the hypothalamic–pituitary–thyroid axis. Secondly, very small changes in thyroid function are amplified in TSH responses since arithmetic changes in thyroid hormone evoke logarithmic changes in TSH secretion.[2] Finally, unlike earlier assays, the newer supersensitive TSH assays can distinguish normal levels from low or suppressed values. Second-generation assays have a detection threshold of about 0.05 mU/liter, and the sensitivity of third-generation assays reaches 0.005 mU/liter. This becomes important in the separation of nonspecific TSH suppression from that seen in thyrotoxicosis.

In addition to the TSH measurement, a free thyroxine (FT$_4$) determination may serve to distinguish subclinical disease from frank hyperthyroidism or hypothyroidism or to identify the rare case of central (pituitary or hypothalamic) hypothyroidism. Indications for some of the other tests will be discussed in sections below, but a few brief comments are in order regarding the remaining serologic tests on the list.

Figure 29-3 Monodeiodination of the outer ring of T$_4$ produces the active hormone T$_3$, whereas inner-ring deiodination produces the metabolically inactive reverse T$_3$.

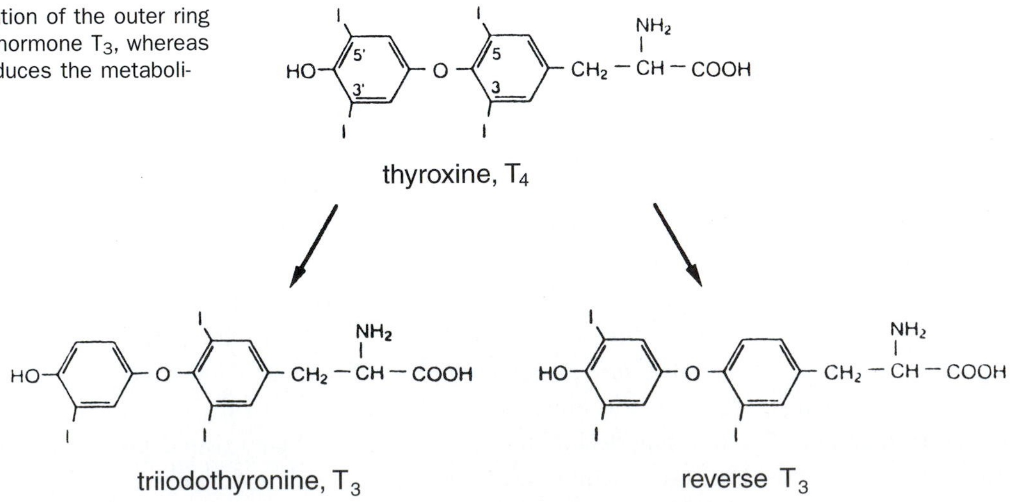

thyroxine, T$_4$

triiodothyronine, T$_3$

reverse T$_3$

TABLE 29-1 **TESTS OF THYROID FUNCTION**
Serologic tests
Total T_4 (T_4)
Total T_3 (T_3)
Free T_4 (FT_4)
Free T_3 (FT_3)
Resin T_3 uptake (RT_3U)
Free T_4 index (FT_4I)
TSH
TRH stimulation test
Antithyroid antibodies
Antithyroglobulin
Antimicrosomal (antithyroperoxidase)
Immunoglobulins of Graves' disease
Thyroid stimulating immunoglobulin (TSI)
TSH-binding inhibitory immunoglobulins (TBII)
Thyroid-binding globulin (TBG)
Nonserologic tests
Thyroid radioiodine uptake (RAIU)
Thyroid scintiscanning
Ultrasonography
Fine-needle thyroid aspiration

The resin T_3 uptake is perhaps the oldest test still in common use. It continues to confuse the uninitiated, who think it in some way measures the T_3 (tri-iodothyronine) level. Instead, it is an indirect measure of the binding sites available on TBG and other thyroxine-binding proteins. When the resin T_3 uptake is performed in conjunction with a total T_4 measurement, a calculation can be made that is called the free T_4 index, which approximates the measured free T_4. The measured free T_3 has become available in recent years, and occasionally may be useful when thyrotoxicosis is suspected and the TSH is suppressed but results of other tests are normal. The TRH stimulation test is rarely needed now that second- and third-generation sensitive TSH tests are widely accessible. Finally, antithyroglobulin and thyroperoxidase (TPO) antibodies are an indication of damage to the thyroid, as seen in Hashimoto's thyroiditis and Graves' disease, rather than the cause of these autoimmune disorders.

SIMPLE (NONTOXIC) GOITER

The term *simple goiter* has been applied to goiters that have no apparent cause, such as hypothyroidism or hyperthyroidism, thyroiditis, or neoplasm, and do not occur in regions of the world with iodine deficiency (endemic goiter). The cause of these goiters is probably multifactorial. The usual explanation is that an abnormality in the biosynthetic pathway of thyroxine

leads to an increase in TSH. That in turn would cause the thyroid gland to enlarge, reestablishing a eumetabolic state at the expense of goiter formation. Such a condition might arise as the result of exposure to a goitrogen, such as lithium. However, goiters develop in only a minority of patients who take lithium, and for that matter, even endemic goiter is not universal in iodine deficient regions, indicating that there are underlying genetic susceptibilities leading to goiter formation.[3] Furthermore, this concept is inconsistent with the observation that most patients with simple goiters do not by definition have an increase in TSH. Nevertheless, many such individuals will respond to thyroxine replacement with a shrinkage of the gland, particularly if the goiter has not been long-standing. Another possible explanation evokes the presence of antibodies that attach to receptors on thyroid cells and cause growth but do not stimulate production of thyroid hormones.[4]

In one follow-up of adolescents with simple goiter, after 20 years 60% were normal, 20% were unchanged, and thyroiditis or colloid goiters had developed in a few.[5]

Clinical Features

Patients are often unaware of goiters, which may be discovered only incidentally during a physical examination. When a goiter is sufficiently large it may produce symptoms of choking, dysphasia, a feeling of fullness in the neck, or rarely, interference with breathing due to compression of the trachea. Larger goiters may be of cosmetic concern. A report of sudden enlargement of a goiter, usually accompanied by pain, suggests hemorrhage into an adenoma.

Laboratory Tests

The serum TSH as well FT_4 and T_3 are normal in the patient with nontoxic goiter. The radioiodine uptake (RAIU) is usually within the normal range, but it might be increased in patients who are iodine-deficient or in whom there is a biosynthetic defect.

Therapy

While treatment should be directed at the underlying cause, one can rarely be discovered in patients with a nontoxic goiter. Iodine-deficiency goiter is seldom observed in the United States, as there is a plentiful supply of iodine in salt and other dietary sources. For that reason iodine solutions should not be given since they may produce either hypothyroidism[6] or thyrotoxicosis[7] in susceptible individuals. Adolescents and young adults with a nontoxic goiter will often have a decrease in the size of the gland when given replacement doses of levothyroxine. Multinodular goiters, which are more commonly seen in older individuals, will usually not response to suppressive therapy with thyroxine. In fact, since the multinodular goiter often develops areas of autonomous function, the TSH may already be at the lower end of normal, and exogenous thyroxine may produce thyrotoxicosis.[8]

Thyroidectomy is reserved for removal of malignancy or for patients in whom there are serious cosmetic concerns or who have objective symptoms that have been unrelieved by exogenous thyroxine. Surgical removal of the thyroid in part or in whole should be followed by thyroxine replacement therapy. This therapy should be monitored by use of a sensitive TSH assay and the dose adjusted to maintain the TSH at the lower end of the normal range. For older women in particular, this dose may be as little as 50 to 75 μg of thyroxine daily.

HYPOTHYROIDISM

An inadequate supply of thyroid hormone to the body is termed hypothyroidism. This may result from a variety of causes, including autoimmune thyroid disease, the destruction of the thyroid by surgery or radiation, goitrous hypothyroidism resulting from defective biosynthesis of thyroid hormone, pituitary insufficiency (secondary hypothyroidism), or hypothalamic disease (tertiary hypothyroidism). The latter two categories account for only about 5% of cases. Advanced hypothyroidism from any cause is termed myxedema.

Currently, the most common cause of primary hypothyroidism in the United States is that which commonly follows the use of radioactive iodine to treat thyrotoxicosis. A close second is that associated with chronic Hashimoto's thyroiditis. This autoimmune disease is more common in women than in men and may be associated with other autoimmune disorders such as Addison's disease, secondary ovarian failure, vitiligo, and even more rarely, idiopathic hypoparathyroidism, type 1 diabetes, and pernicious anemia. Furthermore, all of these disorders may be seen with greater frequency in the families of patients with autoimmune thyroid disease. Thyroid failure may also occur in patients who have received mantle radiation for lymphoma or Hodgkin's disease. A less common form of autoimmune disease involves antibodies that block the attachment of TSH to its receptors, producing thyroid failure without goiter.

Clinical Features

The signs and symptoms of myxedema are well known and readily discernible by a careful history and physical examination. The skin is cold, dry, and often pale or with a yellow tint due to carotinema. The voice may be hoarse and speech slow. Edema of the face and eyelids and decreased sweating may occur. A thickened tongue and coarse hair may be present. Reports of cold intolerance, memory impairment, constipation, fatigue, and weight gain should certainly lead to a suspicion of hypothyroidism. Unfortunately, for a number of reasons, the diagnosis is often missed for months or years. In the first place, it is only rarely that a patient becomes frankly myxedematous, with the classic features listed above. The condition tends to develop slowly, and particularly in older patients, the signs and symptoms may overlap with those of advancing age. The discovery of a goiter, a history of radioiodine treatment, or any of the above findings or symptoms should lead the physician to obtain a TSH. Cardiomegaly, which can be due either to cardiac failure or pericardial effusion, may be seen in more advanced cases. Galactorrhea may occur either due to the endogenous release of TRH in primary hypothyroidism or in association with a pituitary tumor. The recovery phase of the deep-tendon reflexes may be delayed. Anemia is common and may be due to iron deficiency from metrorrhagia, vitamin B_{12} deficiency secondary to an associated pernicious anemia, folic acid deficiency due to poor dietary intake, or a reduction in hemoglobin synthesis due to decreased oxygen consumption. The blood picture is unpredictable, therefore, and may range from normochromic to either microcytic or megaloblastic.

Diagnosis

Measurement of TSH is the single most useful diagnostic test. If the TSH is normal or low in a patient with suspicious findings, a FT_4 level should be obtained to exclude the 5% of patients with pituitary or hypothalamic disease. Detection of elevated antithyroglobulin and antimicrosomal (anti–TPO) antibodies will help to confirm the diagnosis of Hashimoto's thyroiditis. Cholesterol is often elevated in hypothyroidism and should decrease with thyroxine replacement. Since therapy for hypothyroidism is usually for a lifetime, the diagnosis should not rest on a single test. The sensitive TSH test should be used to monitor replacement therapy.

Synthetic levothyroxine is the treatment of choice. Brand name preparations should be used because generic forms of levothyroxine may have unpredictable results. Desiccated thyroid (USP) and synthetic combinations of levothyroxine and triiodothyronine should be avoided since the T_3 in those preparations may, in combination with the peripheral conversion of T_4 to T_3, result in transient thyrotoxic levels of T_3.[9] Excessive replacement should be avoided because it may cause symptoms such as anxiety and palpitations and, with chronic administration, result in excessive bone loss.[10]

THYROTOXICOSIS

The term *thyrotoxicosis* refers to the biochemical as well as the physiologic changes that take place when the body is presented with excessive quantities of thyroid hormones. As pointed out by Larsen et al.,[11] the term *thyrotoxicosis* is preferable to *hyperthyroidism*, as the latter term should be reserved for conditions in which thyrotoxicosis results from excessive production of hormone by the thyroid gland itself. Clinical manifestation of thyrotoxicosis may vary considerably depending on the cause, age of the patient, and severity of the disease. Table 29-2 lists the varieties of thyrotoxicosis discussed in this chapter.

TABLE 29-2
VARIETIES OF THYROTOXICOSIS

Associated with high RAIU
  Graves' disease
  Toxic multinodular goiter
  Toxic adenoma
  Trophoblastic tumors
  TSH hypersecretion
Associated with low RAIU
  Hashimoto's thyroiditis
  Subacute thyroiditis
  Postpartum thyroiditis (PPT)
  Drug-induced (amiodarone)
  Thyrotoxicosis factitia
  Struma ovarii

THYROTOXICOSIS ASSOCIATED WITH HIGH RAIU

Graves' Disease

The condition known as Graves' disease, or diffuse toxic goiter, also referred to as Basedow disease on the European continent, is in many ways the most important of thyroid diseases. As with other thyroid disorders, it is especially common in women, with an incidence 7- to 10-fold higher than in men. Graves' disease is the most common cause of thyrotoxicosis under the age of 40, and it may be seen in childhood and adolescence as well as occasionally in elderly patients.

Clinical Features

The characteristic features of the thyrotoxicosis of Graves' disease are a diffuse goiter, a predilection to infiltrative ophthalmopathy, and occasionally, infiltrative dermopathy. When the condition is fully developed it is easily recognized, even in the absence of exophthalmos. A patient may report palpatations and a forceful heartbeat (especially after exercise, but even at rest), tremor, and perhaps a change in handwriting, sleeplessness, emotional lability, and difficulty in concentrating, increased frequency of bowel movements, and occasionally, frank diarrhea, oligomenorrhea, loss of libido, excessive body heat and sweating, and weight loss despite a voracious appetite. Less often, weight gain is observed.[12] Although the patient may not have noticed a goiter unless it is large, it will usually be easily palpable. The goiter is characteristically smooth and nontender; a bruit may be heard over one or both lobes, and occasionally there will be a thrill to palpation. The skin is warm and often velvety, and the palms may be moist. Lid lag and poor convergence may be observed; if there is infiltrative ophthalmopathy, paresis may be noted, particularly of upward gaze. Tremor of the outstretched hands, along with characteristic nail changes (onycholysis) may be seen (Figure 29-4). Deep-tendon reflexes are usually brisk. In some cases there may be significant proximal muscle weakness. The hair is often extremely fine. The heartbeat is usually very forceful and rapid, and in older patients in particular, there may be accompanying auricular fibrillation. Such obvious features may not be present in the elderly, one-fifth of whom will not have a palpable goiter. Some elderly patients may present with "apathetic" or "masked" hyperthyroidism.[13] Thus, in elderly patients, as well as in

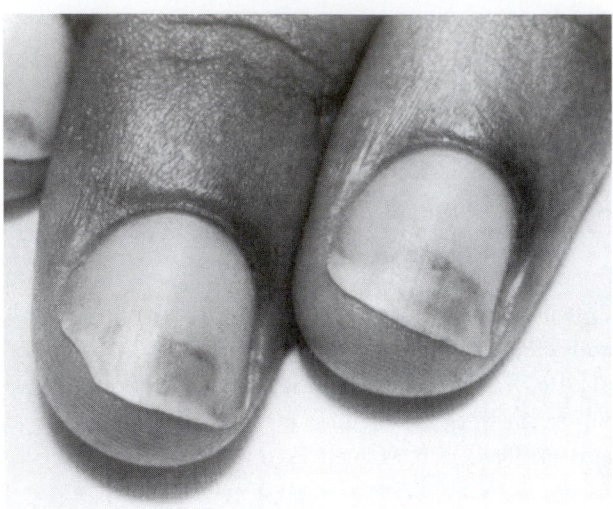

Figure 29-4 Onycholysis, or Plummer's nail, is a separation of the nail from its bed. Although nonspecific, it is often seen in thyroid disease, particularly hyperthyroidism.

younger patients who are severely ill, the classic signs of thyrotoxicosis may not be evident. In such patients the physician should be alert for tachyarrhythmias, congestive heart failure, weight loss, diarrhea, proximal muscle weakness, and change in mental status in making the diagnosis.[14] The cause of Graves' disease appears to be autoimmune due to immunoglobulins of the IgG class that attach to regions of the thyroid-cell plasma membrane, including the TSH receptor. This mimics the actions of TSH, resulting in increased vascularity and growth of the thyroid gland and hypersecretion of thyroid hormones, independent of TSH.

Diagnosis

In a patient with the classical clinical features of Graves' disease—thyrotoxicosis, diffuse goiter, and infiltrative ophthalmopathy—the diagnosis is obvious and laboratory studies are obtained for confirmation and to guide therapy. As noted, in severely ill or elderly patients, clinical findings may not be so obvious, and one must pay attention to subtle symptoms and signs in order to suspect the diagnosis and obtain appropriate laboratory tests. In most cases the serum T_4, T_3, FT_4, FT_3, and RT_3 uptake will be elevated and the TSH will be below the normal range. In severely ill patients the T_3 and FT_3 may be normal or even decreased because of diminished conversion of T_4 to T_3. Conversely, the T_3 may be elevated in the presence of a normal T_4 in the condition known as "T_3 toxicosis." The RAIU should be obtained if radio-

iodine therapy is planned, but it is not necessary as a diagnostic test unless thyrotoxicosis factitia, subacute thyroiditis, the syndrome of chronic thyroiditis with transient thyrotoxicosis or ectopic thyroid tissue (e.g., hydatidiform mole) is suspected. Routine laboratory tests may provide clues such as hypercalcemia (with an incidence near 25% in some reported series), low cholesterol or the reversal of previously documented hypercholesterolemia, and occasionally elevation of hepatocellular enzymes. The RAIU will be elevated above the normal range (5 to 35% in most nuclear medicine facilities), unless the patient has been exposed to a large amount of iodine (e.g. iodinated dyes, Lugol's solution, or supersaturated solution of potassium iodine [SSKI]). Measurement of autoantibodies (TSI or TBII) are expensive and usually unnecessary except perhaps in pregnant women with Graves' disease, in whom high levels should alert one to the possibility of neonatal thyrotoxicosis.[15]

Treatment

THIONAMIDE DRUGS. The thionamide drugs have been used to treat Graves' disease for half a century. Propylthiouracil (PTU) and methimazole (Tapazole) are the drugs employed in the United States, with each having some unique properties and theoretical advantages over the other. Both drugs appear to act by inhibiting the oxidation and organic binding of iodide in the thyroid. The initial dose of PTU is usually 100 to 200 mg every 8 hours but in very toxic patients, as much as 300 mg every 6 hours may be used for a brief time, especially since high doses of PTU, but not methimazole, block the conversion of T_4 to T_3 in the peripheral tissues. Such large doses are seldom continued beyond the first 7 to 10 days of therapy. Methimazole is ordinarily given in a dose of 5 to 20 mg every 8 hours initially, but because of its longer half-life in plasma (6 hours as compared with 1.5 hours for PTU), it may be given at less-frequent intervals, even once daily, especially after remission has been induced. Obviously, less-frequent dosing increases patient compliance.

In the past, PTU was said to be preferred in treating the pregnant woman with thyrotoxicosis since less of it was transferred across the placenta.[16] A more recent study, however, demonstrated that there was little reason to choose PTU over methimazole.[17] Treatment must be individualized in the pregnant patient with maternal FT_4 levels monitored as an index of fetal thyroid function in order to prevent fetal hypothyroidism.[18] A reason to choose methimazole over PTU is the retrospective discovery that, in patients treated with radioiodine following antithyroid drug therapy, the cure rate was considerably less for patients given PTU as compared with those treated with methimazole.[19] Both drugs have potential side effects, but serious complications are rare. Agranulocytosis (a granulocyte count below 500/mm^3) is reported to occur in approximately 0.1% of patients treated with methimazole and 0.4% of those treated with PTU. There is no clear relation to dose or duration of therapy, and it can occur at any age, although it occurs more commonly in patients over 40. Patients should be warned to discontinue treatment immediately if fever, sore throat, or sudden malaise develops, and to report for white-cell and differential-cell counts. Spontaneous recovery is observed in the great majority of patients after 2 to 3 weeks, but rare deaths have been reported.

It is of note that approximately 10% of untreated patients with Graves' disease have a white-cell count under 4000/mm^3 and a relative granulocytopenia, with true agranulocytosis being rare. Other rare complications of thionamide therapy include hepatitis, cholestatic jaundice, thrombocytopenia, aplastic anemia, and a lupus-like syndrome. Minor but more common side effects include skin rash, pruritus, urticaria, fever, arthralgias, and a bitter or abnormal taste.

Despite these considerations, most patients tolerate therapy with antithyroid drugs quite well. Treatment usually must be continued for a considerable period of time, with prospective studies indicating long-term remission rates from 62 to 82% in patients treated from 18 months to 2 years as compared with 31 to 42% in patients treated for only 6 months.[20,21] Relapse is most likely within 6 months after treatment is stopped, although it may occur years later. Long-term therapy appears to be safe if relapse occurs and the patient does not wish ablative therapy with radioiodine or surgery.[22] The studies of Hashizume and colleagues in Japan, who reported a striking reduction in both antibodies to TSH receptors and the frequency of recurrence of hyperthyroidism in patients administered thyroxine during antithyroid drug therapy,[23] have not been confirmed by other investigators.[24-26]

RADIOIODINE THERAPY. Radioiodine (RAI) has been used to treat thyrotoxicosis since the late 1940s. There is reduction in goiter size in virtually all

patients, and cure rates approach 100%. Most patients will respond adequately to a single dose, but some, particularly those with toxic multinodular goiter (see below), will require two or more doses. Most nuclear medicine physicians give a tracer dose of ^{131}I and bring the patient back for a 24-hour uptake measurement and calculation of the therapeutic dose. Some advocate giving a standard dose, usually around 10 mCi, without measurement of 24-hour uptake.[22] Patients are followed at 4- to 6-week intervals initially and then at increasingly longer intervals and are treated for hypothyroidism if the TSH rises above normal. It should be noted that the TSH usually remains suppressed for some time after other tests of thyroid function have returned to normal. Recurrence of hyperthyroidism is unusual once a euthyroid state is achieved.[27]

RAI therapy is contraindicated in pregnant and nursing women. A pregnancy test should be obtained prior to RAI treatment in all women of childbearing age. It is standard advice to recommend avoidance of pregnancy for a time, usually 6 months, after RAI therapy to allow any transient gonadal radiation effects to resolve. This advice is arbitrary, however, and not evidence-based. Many years of experience have demonstrated RAI therapy to be safe, with no increase in the risk of leukemia, thyroid cancer, or infertility; nor have there been any ill effects in the offspring of women previously treated with RAI. Permanent hypothyroidism is the principal side effect of RAI treatment, occurring in 50% or more of patients eventually. The incidence in the first year is dose-dependent, but thereafter continues to occur at a cumulative rate that approaches 3% per year. After radioiodine, patients should be followed indefinitely at approximately 1-year intervals with TSH measurement. Exacerbation of Graves' opthalmopathy following RAI treatment has been reported by some,[28] but not all,[29] observers. Use of corticosteroids to prevent progression of ophthalmopathy following radioiodine has been advocated.[29]

SUBTOTAL THYROIDECTOMY. Surgical treatment is reserved for patients unable or unwilling to be treated with medical therapy. Preoperative preparation is essential in order to avoid thyroid storm. Potassium iodide was a standard therapy in the past (it should not be used during pregnancy), but preparation for surgery with propranolol alone[31] or in combination with potassium iodide[32] is effective. Selection of a surgeon with experience is essential, but it is becoming increasingly difficult, since the demand for thyroid surgery has decreased recently. Recurrent laryngeal nerve damage, hypoparathyroidism, and other complications are possible; the incidence is inversely proportional to the skill of the surgeon.

Infiltrative Ophthalmopathy

Exophthalmos and periorbital edema are pathognomonic of Graves' disease, whereas lid lag and stare are manifestations of thyrotoxicosis from any cause. The latter are due to an increased sensitivity of the thyrotoxic patient to catecholamines and will respond to treatment by β-adrenergic blockade. Exophthalmos and other manifestations of infiltrative ophthalmopathy may follow a course independent of thyrotoxicosis, occurring years before or after therapy. Some 15% of patients recall that opthalmopathy began before symptoms of thyrotoxicosis, and about 40% recall it beginning at the same time.[33] Virtually all patients with Graves' disease will have some evidence of infiltrative ophthalmopathy, such as extraocular muscle enlargement or increased retro-orbital fat when examined by ultrasound or radiographic techniques,[34] but only about half will have clinically evident changes. Excessive tearing, irritation of the eyes, blurred or double vision, injected conjunctivae, and periorbital edema are among the symptoms and findings commonly seen. Eyelid retraction, chemosis of the conjuctivae, and limitation of ocular movement, especially upward gaze and abduction, may be observed. While exophthalmos itself is usually not painful, desiccation of the conjunctivae because of inability to fully close the eyelid during sleep is. For the latter, topical artificial tear solutions and ointments along with taping of the eyelids at night are beneficial. Chronic retraction due to infiltrative ophthalmopathy may necessitate tarsorrhaphy. Diplopia and strabismus may be treated by patching one eye or by placing a prism into the patient's glasses. Once the condition has been stable for a time, surgical correction of the condition may be attempted. If vision is threatened by increased intraocular pressure, high-dose glucocorticoid therapy is indicated and, if that fails, orbital decompression should be considered.[35] For patients who do not wish to undergo surgery or in whom operative management has failed, radiation treatment is available.[36] An experienced ophthalmologist should follow all patients with Graves' ophthalmopathy.

Toxic Multinodular Goiter

In time many simple nontoxic goiters become multinodular for reasons that are not altogether clear. Long-term exposure to a slight excess of TSH might lead to the development of anatomical and functional heterogeneity as well as to autonomous function. In that situation, one area, or usually several areas, of the gland becomes independent of TSH stimulation. This may remain clinically silent and undiagnosed unless the production of thyroid hormone is sufficient to suppress TSH and is picked up on routine thyroid testing. Eventually, frank hyperthyroidism may develop. Toxic multinodular goiter, in contrast to Graves' disease, usually occurs in patients over age 50. Like Graves' disease, it is far more common in women than in men. Infiltrative ophthalmopathy is not seen. Perhaps because of the older age group involved, cardiovascular abnormalities such as atrial fibrillation, tachycarda, and/or congestive heart failure may be presenting symptoms. Weakness and weight loss accompanied by anorexia rather than hyperphagia may suggest a malignancy.

Obstructive symptoms are more common than with Graves' because of the nature of the goiter and the fact that it often extends retrosternally. On palpation the gland is usually firm, with an irregular and sometimes asymmetrical enlargement, although as many as 20% of older patients with thyrotoxicosis may not have a distinct goiter.[11] A suppressed TSH may be the principal laboratory finding, along with a slight elevation of FT_4. The RAIU is usually of little help because thyrotoxicosis may be present in association with values that are within the normal range or only slightly elevated. It is of note that some healthy euthyroid elderly individuals can have a suppressed TSH,[37] so the diagnosis is sometimes difficult. In a retrospective analysis of persons 60 years of age or older who had a sensitive TSH measurement of less than 0.1 mU/ml, it was noted that there was a three-fold higher risk for auricular fibrillation over the next decade.[38]

Therapy

While RAI is the treatment of choice for toxic multinodular goiter, large doses and multiple treatments may be necessary to bring the patient into a euthyroid state. Even with successful treatment the goiter may fail to decrease in size. If obstructive symptoms are present, therefore, surgical removal may be the preferred approach, providing the patient's health permits it. In the presence of significant complicating illness, particularly cardiac disease, it is recommended that the patient be treated first with antithyroid drugs, followed by radioiodine after a euthyroid state is achieved. As noted previously, methimazole may be preferable to PTU in the patient who is eventually to be treated with RAI.[19] Once the patient is euthyroid, medication is withheld for approximately 4 to 7 days before administration of the radioisotope. A week to 10 days later, antithyroid drug therapy may be resumed if necessary and continued for another 2 or 3 months. If thyrotoxicosis recurs when medication is withdrawn, a second course of radioiodine should be administered. Multiple doses of radioiodine may be required in some patients.[39]

Uncommon or Rare Forms of Thyrotoxicosis

Occasionally, a single autonomous adenoma of the thyroid gland will produce sufficient thyroid hormone to cause symptomatic thyrotoxicosis. A toxic adenoma (Plummer's disease) is much less common than Graves' disease or toxic multinodular goiter. It tends to occur in a younger age group than the latter, though patients will often give a history of a longstanding nodule that has grown slowly over many years. In most, the pathogenesis appears to be a somatic point mutation in the TSH receptor gene, which leads to a constitutive activation of the TSH receptor.[40] On examination, there is usually a single nodule that is felt as a well-defined mass that moves freely on swallowing, is nontender, and is usually greater than 2.5 cm in diameter. Clinical manifestations of a toxic adenoma are usually milder than those seen in Graves' disease. There is no associated infiltrative ophthalmopathy or dermopathy.

Laboratory tests are as previously described except that thyroid autoantibodies will usually be negative. Early in the development of a toxic adenoma, a suppressed TSH may be the only abnormality noted. Once the TSH has been suppressed, a radioactive scan will demonstrate a "hot" nodule with partial or complete lack of uptake in the remaining thyroid gland. Treatment is either surgical or with radioiodine. Surgery is preferred for the younger patient, since exposure of the noninvolved thyroid to low doses of radioiodine could theoretically increase the risk of thyroid cancer later in the future.

Trophoblastic Tumors

Hydatidiform mole is said to occur in approximately 1 in 1500 pregnancies in the United States, with an occurrence 10 times more frequent in Asia and Latin America. Choriocarcinoma occurs in 1 in 40,000 pregnancies, about half in women with previously diagnosed hydatidiform moles.[41] A variant human chorionic gonadotropin (HCG) appears to be responsible for the hyperthyroidism observed in patients with a molar pregnancy. Prompt surgical removal of the mole in a thyrotoxic patient results in a rapid cure. Choriocarcinoma should be treated with chemotherapy by an experienced oncologist.

TSH Hypersecretion

A diffuse toxic goiter very rarely may be caused by hypersecretion of TSH. This can result from either a TSH-secreting pituitary adenoma or from a selective pituitary resistance to thyroid hormone. A normal or elevated serum TSH in the presence of thyrotoxic levels of total and free thyroid hormones would suggest one of these conditions. Surgical resection would be the treatment of choice for a TSH-producing adenoma.

THYROTOXICOSIS ASSOCIATED WITH LOW RAIU

While seldom used as a primary diagnostic tool, the RAIU is occasionally very useful in determining the correct cause of thyrotoxicosis. The treatment of conditions associated with a low RAIU is usually quite different from those of the conditions discussed above. Conditions associated with this finding include subacute thyroiditis, struma ovarii, factitious thyroid hormone ingestion, and very rarely, functioning thyroid cancer metastases. Iodine-induced hyperthyroidism, including that associated with amiodarone, may occur in susceptible individuals.[42]

Subacute Thyroiditis

This condition, which has been labeled with various names including giant-cell thyroiditis, granulomatous thyroiditis, and de Quervain's thyroiditis, has traditionally been thought to have a viral etiology, although that has been disputed.[43] The condition is far less common than Graves' disease or chronic lymphocytic thyroiditis and is rare at extremes of age, with a peak incidence in the fourth and fifth decades. As with other thyroid disorders, women are disproportionately affected. Multinuculated giant cells surrounding a central core of colloid are a characteristic histopathological feature.

Neck pain, which may be sudden or gradual in onset, is the usual presentation. Radiation of the pain to the jaw, ear, or occipital area and aggravation by head movement, swallowing, or pressure applied to the neck is commonly seen. Many patients have systemic symptoms, including fever, malaise, myalgia, and occasionally extreme lassitude.

Diagnosis

The gland is often exquisitely tender, and the patient will resist palpation. There is usually a slight to moderate enlargement of the gland, which may be asymmetrical, with one lobe more significantly involved than the other, at least initially. Acute otitis may be mimicked by radiation of pain to the ear. Acute suppurative thyroiditis must be excluded. Fine-needle thyroid aspiration may be of help in making the diagnosis.[44] A substantial number of patients will present with manifestations of thyrotoxicosis accompanied by elevated thyroid hormones and a suppressed TSH. RAIU is low because of the leakage of thyroid hormones into the blood due to inflammatory disease rather than to active production of thyroid hormone as in Graves' disease. The erythrocyte sedimentation rate is almost always increased, often to a very high level.

Treatment

When the condition is mild, aspirin or other nonsteroidal antiinflammatory drugs will be adequate. In the presence of severe neck pain, prednisone 40 mg/day will usually alleviate symptoms. Glucocorticoid therapy in a dose that alleviates symptoms should be given until the RAIU has returned to normal. At least partial relief of pain and tenderness of the neck should begin within 1 to 2 days after glucocorticoid therapy is begun. If pain is not resolved within 72 hours, the diagnosis should be questioned. Symptoms may recur if glucocorticoid therapy is withdrawn prematurely.

Painless Thyroiditis and Postpartum Thyroiditis

For the past couple of decades an entity has been recognized that consists of transient hyperthyroidism with a suppressed RAIU and a painless goiter. This has been labeled with many different names including "silent thyroiditis" to distinguish it from the painful subacute thyroiditis of de Quervain, lymphocytic thyroiditis with spontaneously resolving hyperthyroidism, subacute lymphocytic thyroiditis, painless lymphocytic thyroiditis, or painless thyroiditis (PT). When painless thyroiditis occurs during the postpartum period,\ it is called postpartum thyroiditis (PPT). It is histologically distinct from subacute thyroiditis with focal lymphocytic infiltration. With this inflammatory response there is damage of follicles, with release of thyroid hormone into the circulation resulting in elevation of serum T_4 and T_3 with suppression of TSH and the RAIU. Unless there are contraindications, the latter test should be done to exclude Graves' disease. The erythrocyte sedimentation rate is either normal or only slightly elevated in contrast to subacute thyroiditis. Antithyroglobulin antibodies are elevated in about one-fourth of patients and TPO in more than half. Thyrotoxicosis is usually mild and is self-limited, generally lasting only a few months. About 40% of patients will go through a euthyroid phase and then become hypothyroid. Again, this will spontaneously resolve after a couple of months, after which a majority of patients remain euthyroid.

PPT appears to have the same or at least a similar pathophysiology. By definition it occurs within a year after delivery, presumably as a result of a rebound of the maternal immune system, which had been suppressed during pregnancy. There is even a higher incidence of TPO antibodies (80 vs. 50%) in PPT as compared with PT.[45] In one review of 287 patients with PPT, 26% became hyperthyroid followed by the hypothyroid phase, 38% had hyperthyroidism alone, and 36% had hypothyroidism alone.[46] Thus, in that series at least, 64% of patients had hyperthyroidism.

Diagnosis

Transient thyrotoxicosis associated with PT and PPT is characterized by elevated circulating thyroid hormones in the presence of suppressed TSH and RAIU. The overall prevalence of silent thyroiditis as a cause of thyrotoxicosis has been estimated to vary between 5 and 20%.[47] The reported prevalence of PPT varies from 1.1% to 16.7%.[48] As noted, there is strong correlation between the presence of TPO antibodies and the subsequent development of PPT. The presence and the titer of thyroid autoantibodies can predict the likelihood of PPT. An incidence of PPT in women who had positive TPO autoantibodies during pregnancy has been reported as high as 33%. Furthermore, the women in whom PPT developed had higher titers of thyroid peroxidase and antithyroglobulin antibodies than did those in whom thyroiditis did not develop postpartum.[46,49]

Women with other autoimmune disorders would be expected to have an increased prevalence of PPT. One report, for example, indicated a prevalence of 10.5% of PPT in women with preexisting type 1 diabetes.[50] The recommendation has been made that all pregnant women should be screened for antithyroid antibodies in the first trimester of pregnancy, with determination of TSH at 3 and 6 months postpartum in antibody-positive subjects.[46]

Treatment

Most patients require no therapy, but β-agonist treatment may be helpful in the thyrotoxic phase. Thyroxine therapy is usually not necessary in the hypothyroid phase because that is ordinarily brief, but if symptoms occur it can be begun. It should be tapered within a year, however, in order to determine if thyroid function has spontaneously recovered.

Thyrotoxicosis Factitia

Self-administration of excessive quantities of thyroid hormone can lead to signs and symptoms that may be difficult to distinguish from some forms of spontaneous thyrotoxicosis. Individuals presenting in this fashion usually have some underlying psychiatric disease. Many are medical personnel who have easy excess to thyroid hormone or are patients for whom the drug has previously been prescribed. When confronted, they will usually deny having taken medication. Occasionally a patient may be unaware of having taken thyroid hormone, which had been given as part of an unscrupulous weight reduction program.

In the mid-1980s in the midwestern United States, an epidemic of thyrotoxicosis occurred that was traced to contamination of ground beef with bovine thyroid.[51] Recurrence of such an incident is unlikely, but should be kept in mind if more than one case of factitious thyrotoxicosis is encountered in a community.

Depending on the amount of hormone taken and the duration of exposure, the symptoms may vary from nervousness or insomnia to those of overt thyrotoxicosis. Although the thyroid should not be palpable, it could be in a patient with a nonsuppressible goiter. If thyroxine or desiccated thyroid has been ingested the total T_4 and FT_4 may be elevated, whereas they may be suppressed if triiodothyronine has been taken. In either case the T_3 should be elevated and the TSH and RAIU suppressed. Psychiatric referral may be indicated once the diagnosis has been established.

Struma Ovarii

Struma ovarii, an ovarian teratoma containing autonomous hyperfunctioning thyroid tissue, is a very rare cause of thyrotoxicosis. It could be easily confused with thyrotoxicosis factitia because of the finding of elevated thyroid hormones, a low RAIU, and absence of a goiter. The diagnosis may be confirmed by the detection of radioiodine uptake over the ovarian mass.[52] The treatment of choice is surgical resection, since these lesions are potentially malignant.[53]

THYROID EMERGENCIES

Thyroid storm and myxedema coma are rare but extremely dangerous conditions. Treatment must be initiated promptly based on clinical judgment since both are associated with a very high mortality rate, which will be increased if treatment is delayed pending laboratory confirmation.[54]

Thyroid Storm

Thyroid storm, or thyrotoxic crisis, is a serious, but uncommon complication of Graves' disease or, rarely, of toxic multinodular goiter. It is characterized by a severe, acute exacerbation of the usual signs and symptoms of hyperthyroidism. Cardinal features of thyroid storm are fever, marked tachycardia, and mental obtundation. Fever is usually quite high and may often be present without evidence of infection. There is marked tachycardia of either sinus or ectopic origin or as a result of atrial fibrillation. High-output congestive heart failure may be present. Pulse pressure is wide and, while blood pressure is usually well maintained, shock may occur terminally. Abdominal pain, nausea, vomiting, diarrhea, and occasionally mild jaundice may be observed. Most patients are extremely restless and hyperkinetic, but some may be apathetic, and confusion, delirium, psychosis, and convulsions may occur, progressing to stupor and coma. Untreated, the condition is invariably fatal. A number of precipitating causes may bring about thyroid storm in the undiagnosed or inadequately treated patient with thyrotoxicosis. These include infections, trauma, surgery, anesthesia, and severe nonthyroidal illness such as myocardial infarction and diabetic ketoacidosis.

Diagnosis

Circulating thyroid hormones will be in the thyrotoxic range, but treatment must be based on clinical judgment and not delayed pending laboratory confirmation. One study has suggested that FT_4 levels are disproportionately high in thyroid storm.[55]

Treatment

Patients should be placed in an intensive-care unit and therapy begun as soon as the diagnosis is suspected. Propylthiouracil 250 to 300 mg every 6 hours should be given by mouth or nasogastric tube. In the absence of cardiac insufficiency or bronchial spasm, a β-adrenergic drug should be given. Propranolol is the drug most commonly used, in a dose of 40 to 80 mg orally every 6 hours. If necessary, 2 mg can be given intravenously at a rate of 1 mg/min, but a shorter acting β-blocker such as labetaolol 20 mg by slow intravenous injection over a 2-minute period may be safer. Additional injections of 40 to 80 mg of labetaolol given at 10-minute intervals to a maximum of 300 mg can be administered until the pulse rate has been slowed to 100 beats per minute. Propylthiouracil (PTU) has the effect of inhibiting peripheral conversion of T_4 to T_3, and for that reason it is preferable to methimazole. Following a loading dose of PTU, which will prevent incorporation of iodine into glandular hormone stores, SSKI (5 drops every 6 hours) or sodium iodide intravenously (0.25 g/6 h) will acutely block the release of hormone from the thyroid gland. Iodide and PTU have been successfully administered per rectum when the oral route could not be used.[56] Digitalis is indicated for the control of auricular fibrillation, along with oxygen and diuretics for cardiac failure. High-dose intravenous glucocorticoids (cortisol 100 mg or dexamethasone 2 mg every 6 hours) have traditionally been given. Glucocorticoids, propranolol, and PTU, when given in high doses, will all tend to block the peripheral conversion of T_4 to T_3, which may hasten recovery. Precipitating causes such as infection or myocardial infarction should be sought in all patients. Clinical improvement is usually seen in 1 to 3 days, and total recovery ordinarily will occur within a week. Despite the advances in treatment, however, the mortality rate is still reported to be as high as 20%.[11]

Myxedema Coma

This condition, which occurs almost exclusively in elderly patients, is an acute deterioration of long-standing hypothyroidism. Coma, hypothermia, respiratory depression, and hypotension are frequent clinical features. It is most commonly seen in patients with primary hypothyroidism that has resulted from thyroidectomy, radioiodine therapy, or autoimmune thyroiditis, but it can complicate secondary (pituitary) or tertiary (hypothalamic) hypothyroidism. While it can be the result of neglected and progressive thyroid failure, it is usually precipitated by some definable cause, which in some cases is iatrogenic. Since drugs are slowly metabolized in the patient with hypothyroidism, anesthetic agents, opiates, barbiturates and psychotropic drugs may induce obtundation. Other precipitating causes include cold exposure, congestive heart failure, and myocardial infarction. The usual responses to infection such as fever and tachycardia may be obscured.

Diagnosis

Myxedema coma should be considered in the differential diagnosis of any elderly patient who presents in a coma. The more common situation, however, is for a patient who is already in a nursing home or hospital to go into myxedema coma as a result of one of the causes cited above. Hypothermia is nearly always seen, with temperatures as low as 74°F (23.3°C) having been reported.[11] While the typical findings of myxedema, including bradycardia, hypotension, pasty skin, puffy face, and delayed relaxation of deep-tendon reflexes are almost always present, they frequently are overlooked. Carbon dioxide retention due to alveolar hypoventilation may contribute to obtundation, as may dilutional hyponatremia from the syndrome of inappropriate antidiuretic hormone (SIADH). Brain-stem strokes or hypothermia from any cause may mimic the findings of myxedema coma. With a mortality rate as high as 80% when therapy is delayed or inadequate,[57] time is of the essence in the initiation of therapy.

Treatment

Administration of thyroid hormone and supportive therapy are the immediate goals of treatment. Because intestinal absorption may be unpredictable, levothyroxine should be given intravenously whenever possible. A loading dose of 500 μg of levothyroxine to replete the peripheral hormone pool is followed by daily doses of 50 to 100 μg intravenously thereafter. Cortisol should be given continuously via the intravenous route at a rate of approximately 100 mg/12 hr for the first few days. Saline and glucose may be required to alleviate hyponatremia and occasionally hypoglycemia. Respiratory function may require support with oxygen administration and even assisted ventilation. Internal warming by heated oxygen and/or gastric perfusion may be helpful, but external warming is to be avoided, as it may lead to vascular collapse. The patient should be covered with blankets to prevent further heat loss, and appropriate nursing care of the comatose patient should include prevention of aspiration, frequent turning to avoid pressure sores, urinary catheterization, and avoidance of fecal impaction. Precipitating causes, including infection or central nervous system or cardiac disease, should be sought. An increase in body temperature will usually begin to occur within 24 hours, and mental status will improve within a few days when treatment is successful.

THYROID NODULES AND THYROID CANCER

Thyroid nodules are very common. Indeed, ultrasound studies in normal volunteers have demonstrated nodular thyroid disease in over 60% of healthy adults.[58] The incidence of thyroid cancer recognized clinically, however, is only 4 cases per 100,000.[59] It is important, therefore, to formulate a plan for dealing with this very common problem in a manner that will avoid unnecessary operations, but at the same time will identify potentially malignant lesions.

Thyroid Nodules

As indicated, thyroid nodules are extremely common, whereas thyroid malignancy is relatively uncommon, and death from thyroid cancer quite rare. Obviously, surgical removal of all thyroid nodules is not only impractical, but undesirable. Therefore, a systematic approach is needed to identify the patient who should be referred for surgical removal of a nodule. A careful history and physical examination will help to identify women who are at greater risk for malignancy.

Age is one factor—patients <20 or >70 have a higher incidence of thyroid cancer in a palpable nodule. A history of irradiation to the head or neck during childhood is associated with an increased incidence of thyroid cancer (and nonmalignant nodular disease as well). A family history of thyroid cancer

suggests the possibility of medullary thyroid carcinoma. While a recent change in the size of the nodule is of concern, a sudden painful enlargement is likely due to hemorrhage into an adenoma. Hoarseness or dysphasia in the presence of a nodule should arouse suspicion. On physical examination, a firm irregular or hard nodule, fixation of the nodule on swallowing, the presence of tracheal deviation, or significant cervical lymphadenopathy all should alert the examiner to possible malignancy.

Several diagnostic studies are available to help separate benign from potentially malignant nodules. These include ultrasound, isotope scanning, and fine-needle aspiration. Although ultrasonography is an excellent way to determine the size and number of thyroid nodules, it is not of much value in distinguishing benign from malignant disease. It may be used to guide biopsy or to determine whether a nodule is changing in size over time. Historically, radionuclide scanning has been used to assess thyroid nodules for possible malignancy or autonomous function. The "hot" nodule that makes up perhaps 10% of scans is, for all practical purposes, nonmalignant. "Warm" and "cold" nodules may be malignant approximately 5 to 8% of the time. Isotopes commonly used for thyroid imaging include ^{131}I, ^{99m}Tc, and ^{123}I. While technetium scanning is rapid and convenient, it occasionally can be misleading since ^{99m}Tc scans may be "warm" or "hot," but the nodule will be "cold" on iodine scanning. Therefore, for a routine scanning, ^{123}I is recommended because it avoids the problem with technetium and also the excessive thyroidal radiation associated with ^{131}I. Magnetic resonance imaging and computed tomography are costly and have no role in the routine assessment of thyroid nodules. Fine-needle thyroid aspiration (FNA), on the other hand, is probably the most sensitive and cost-effective means of distinguishing benign from malignant thyroid nodules, and many authorities recommend this as the initial diagnostic approach rather than imaging studies.[60,61] In two reviews of FNA encompassing more than 27,000 patients, 69 to 72% were benign, 22 to 27% were nondiagnostic or suspicious, and only 4% were malignant. Of the suspicious group, up to 30% were ultimately found to be malignant. The sensitivity and specificity of FNA biopsy depends on the experience of the physician performing the biopsy and the cytopathologist interpreting the specimens. When both are skilled the diagnostic yield is in excess of 90%.

The treatment of benign solitary thyroid nodules and multinodular goiter (MNG) with TSH-suppressive

---

TABLE 29-3
CLASSIFICATION OF THYROID NEOPLASMS

Primary epithelial tumors
Tumors of follicular cells
    Benign: follicular adenoma
    Malignant: carcinoma
        Differentiated
            Papillary
            Follicular
        Poorly differentiated
            Insular
        Undifferentiated (anaplastic)
Tumors of C cells
    Medullary carcinoma
Primary nonepithelial tumors
Malignant lymphomas
Sarcomas
Secondary tumors

---

doses of thyroxine remains somewhat controversial. It seems reasonable in premenopausal women without cardiac contraindications to offer a 1-year trial of thyroxine. If the nodule or the MNG shows a significant decrease in size, then the treatment could be continued with a dose selected to suppress the TSH to the lower limit of the normal range.[62]

Thyroid Cancer

Cancers originating in the thyroid are almost always of epithelial origin and therefore, are carcinomas. Metastasis of a nonthyroidial cancer to the thyroid gland is extremely rare, but thyroid lymphoma may account for 1 to 2% of thyroid malignancies. A classification of thyroid neoplasms adapted from Larsen and colleagues[11] is seen in Table 29-3. This in turn was modified from guidelines published by the World Health Organization[63] and the Armed Forces

Institute of Pathology.[64] A staging system for thyroid cancer devised by the American Joint Committee on Cancer (AJCC)[65] is described in Table 29-4. This is based on three components: the extent of the tumor (T), and whether or not there are regional lymph-node metastases (N), or distant metastases (M).

Surgical therapy, often followed by radioiodine ablation, is the treatment of choice for differentiated thyroid cancer. The type and extent as well as the details of radioiodine and other medical therapies are beyond the scope of this chapter. Some general guidelines for diagnosis and treatment for thyroid cancer are summarized below.

Papillary Carcinoma

Papillary thyroid carcinoma (PTC) occurs most often between 30 and 50 years of age, although it may present in childhood as well as in the elderly. There is a distinct female predominance, with 60 to 80% of cases of PTC occurring in women. Most primary tumors average between 2 and 3 cm, and about one-third of patients have clinically evident lymphadenopathy upon presentation. Histologic evidence of lymph-node metastases is considerably higher; 35 to 50% of excised nodes are positive in adults and up to 90% in patients 17 years of age or younger.[66] More than 80% of patients with PTC present with Stage I or II tumor. Presentation with distant metastases and Stage IV disease (age 45 years or older with any T, any N, and M1) occurs in 3% or less of patients with PTC.

Follicular Carcinoma

Although follicular carcinoma (FTC) is thought to be more aggressive than papillary carcinoma, when

---

TABLE 29-4
AJCC STAGE GROUPINGS FOR THYROID CARCINOMA

| Stage | Papillary or Follicular | | Medullary (Any Age) | Undifferentiated (Any Age) |
	Age <45 yr	Age ≥45 yr		
I	M0	T1	T1	—
II	M1	T2–T3	T2–T4	—
III	—	T4 or N1	N1	—
IV	—	M1	M1	Any

T = size of primary thyroid tumor (T1 = ≤1 cm; T2 = >1 to ≤4 cm; T3 = >4 cm; T4 = extrathyroid invasion); N = regional nodal metastases (0 = absent; 1 = present); M = distant metastases (0 = absent; 1 = present).
Used with permission of the American Joint Committee on Cancer (AJCC®), Chicago, Illinois.[65]

patients with distant metastases at the time of diagnosis are excluded, follicular and papillary cancer mortality rates are similar (10% vs. 6%, P not significant).[67] The mean age in most studies of FTC is greater than 50 years, some 10 years older than the typical PTC. The Hürthle variant of FTC usually affects an even older group of patients, with an average median age around 60 years. For all FTC, women outnumber men by more than 2 to 1. A painless thyroid nodule is the usual presentation; clinical lymphadenopathy is rare (4 to 6%). The average size of FTC tumors is larger than those observed in PTC.

Poorly Differentiated (Insular) Carcinoma

This is an aggressive and often lethal carcinoma in which metastases to both regional nodes and distant sites are common. Controversy exists as to whether this is a morphologic variant of FTC or is a poorly differentiated variant of either PTC or FTC.

Undifferentiated (Anaplastic) Carcinoma

Anaplastic carcinoma usually occurs after the age of 60 and constitutes from 5 to 10% of all thyroid carcinomas. Women are at only a slightly greater risk than men (1.3:1 to 1.5:1). These are highly malignant tumors that rapidly invade locally and metastasize widely.

Medullary Thyroid Carcinoma

These tumors, which may account for as many as 10% of thyroid malignancies, most often occur after the age of 40 and are only slightly more common in women. Medullary thyroid carcinoma (MTC) resembles PTC in that it often invades the intraglandular lymphatics, spreading to other parts of the gland and to the pericapsular and regional lymph nodes. Unlike PTC it also frequently spreads via the bloodstream to lungs, bone, and liver. These tumors derive from the C cells of the thyroid rather than the follicular epithelium. The tumor may be sporadic, but about 20% are familial. The latter group commonly appears at a younger age and has a better prognosis. Both types secrete a biochemical marker, calcitonin, the early detection of which can lead not only to diagnosis, but to treatment and cure. It is now appreciated that the familial type may be diagnosed at a premalignant stage by calcitonin testing or by genetic identification of the *RET* proto-oncogene.[68]

Primary Malignant Lymphoma

It is important to differentiate thyroid lymphoma from an anaplastic carcinoma since the former has a relatively good prognosis. The risk of thyroid lymphoma is more than 60-fold higher in patients with Hashimoto's thyroiditis than in those with nodular goiters, although the incidence in patients with Hashimoto's thyroiditis is still only around 2%. The diagnosis can be made by FNA or open biopsy.

Treatment of Thyroid Carcinoma

Controversies exist regarding the extent of surgery and the use and amount of radioiodine in the treatment of differentiated thyroid carcinoma. Mazzaferri et al.[67] reported on more than 1300 patients with papillary and follicular cancer prospectively followed for up to 40 years. The survival rate was 76%, recurrence rate 30%, and cancer death rate 8% after 30 years. The most frequent recurrences were at the extremes of age (<20 and >55 years) but cancer mortality rates were lowest in patients younger than 40 years, increasing with each subsequent decade of life. Older age, larger tumors, greater mediastinal node involvement, and distant metastases were adverse prognostic factors. Factors reducing the likelihood of cancer death included female sex, operation more extensive than a lobectomy plus ^{131}I and thyroid hormone therapy. When ^{131}I treatment was given only to ablate normal thyroid gland remnants, the recurrence rate was less than one-third the rate after thyroid hormone alone, and no patient treated in that manner with ^{131}I had died of thyroid cancer over a follow-up period of thirty-five years.[67]

The treatment of medullary thyroid carcinoma is surgical; radioiodine has no role. Total thyroidectomy along with removal of nodes from the neck and upper mediastinum is required. Individuals with hereditary medullary thyroid carcinoma are treated in the same fashion, since prophylactic removal of all thyroid tissue and regional lymph nodes can be lifesaving if performed prior to distant metastatic spread.[69] Anaplastic thyroid carcinoma is rarely cured, and treatment is largely palliative. Patients with primary thyroid lymphoma are generally treated with chemotherapy and radiation.

REFERENCES

1. Brent GA. The molecular basis of thyroid hormone action. N Engl J Med 1994;331:847.

2. Spencer CA, LoPresti JS, Patel A, et al. Applications of a new chemiluminometric thyrotropin assay to subnormal measurement. J Clin Endocrinol Metab 1990;70:453.

3. Perez-Centeno C, Gonzalez-Sarmiento R, Mories MT, Corrales JJ, Miralles-Garcia JM. Thyroglobulin exon 10 gene point mutation in a patient with endemic goiter. Thyroid 1996;6:423.

4. Valente WA, Vitti P, Rotella CM, et al. Antibodies that promote thyroid growth: a distinct population of thyroid stimulating autoantibodies. N Engl J Med 1983;309:1028.

5. Rallison ML, Dobyns BM, Meikle AW, Bishop M, Lyon JL, Stevens W. Natural history of thyroid abnormalities: prevalence, incidence, and regression of thyroid diseases in adolescents and young adults. Am J Med 1991;91:363.

6. Silva JE. Effects of iodine and iodine-containing compounds on thyroid function. Med Clin North Am 1985; 69:881.

7. Fradkin JE, Wolff J. Iodine-induced thyrotoxicosis. Medicine (Baltimore) 1983;62:1.

8. Hurley DL, Gharib H. Evaluation and management of multinodular goiter. Otolaryngol Clin North Am 1996; 29:527.

9. Jackson IM, Cobb WE. Why does anyone still use desiccated thyroid USP? Am J Med 1978;64:284.

10. Ross DS, Neer MR, Ridgway EC, Daniels GH. Subclinical hyperthyroidism and reduced bone density as a possible result of prolonged suppression of the pituitary-thyroid axis with L-thyroxine. Am J Med 1987;82:1167.

11. Larsen PR, Davies TF, Hay ID. The thyroid gland. In: Wilson JD, Foster DW, Kronenberg HM, Larsen PR, eds. Williams textbook of endocrinology. 9th ed. Philadelphia: Saunders, 1998:389.

12. Jansson S, Berg G, Lindstedt G, Michanek A, Nystrom E. Overweight: a common problem among women treated for hyperthyroidism. Postgrad Med J 1993;69:107.

13. Nordyke RA, Gilbert FL, Harada ASM. Graves' disease: influence of age on clinical findings. Arch Intern Med 1988;148:626.

14. Isley WL. Thyroid dysfunction in the severely ill and elderly. Postgrad Med 1993;94:111.

15. Zakarijan M, McKenzie JM, Hoffman WH. Prediction and therapy of intrauterine and late-onset neonatal hyperthyroidism. J Clin Endocrinol Metab 1986;62:368.

16. Marchant B, Brownlie BEW, Hart DM, et al. The placental transfer of propylthiouracil, methimazole and carbimazole. J Clin Endocrinol Metab 1977;45:1187.

17. Momotani N, Noh J, Ishikawa N, Ito K. Effects of propylthiouracil and methimazole on fetal thyroid status in mothers with Graves' hyperthyroidism. J Clin Endocrinol Metab 1997;82:3633.

18. Momotami N, Noh J, Oyanagi H, Ishikawa N, Ito K. Antithyroid drug therapy for Graves' disease during pregnancy. N Engl J Med 1986;315:24.

19. Imesis RE, VanMiddlesworth L, Massie JD, Bush AJ, VanMiddlesworth NR. Pretreatment with propylthiouracil but not methimazole reduces the theraputic efficacy of iodine-131 in hyperthyroidism. J Clin Endocrinol Metab 1998;83:685.

20. Tamai H, Nakagawa T, Fukino O, et al. Thionamide therapy in Graves' disease: relation of relapse rate to duration of therapy. Ann Intern Med 1980;92:448.

21. Allannic H, Fauchet R, Orgiazzi J, et al. Antithyroid drugs and Graves' disease: a prospective randomized evaluation of the efficacy of treatment duration. J Clin Endocrinol Metab 1990;70:675.

22. Franklyn JA. The management of hyperthyroidism. N Engl J Med 1994;330:1731.

23. Hashizume K, Ichikawa K, Sakurai A, et al. Administration of thyroxine in treated Graves' disease. N Engl J Med 1991;324:947.

24. Reinwein D, Benker G, Lazarus JH, et al. A prospective randomized trial of antithyroid drug dose in Graves' disease therapy. J Clin Endocrinol Metab 1993;76:1516.

25. Tamai H, Hayaki I, Kawai K, et al. Lack of effect of thyroxine administration on elevated thyroid stimulating hormone receptor antibody levels in treated Graves' disease patients. J Clin Endocrinol Metab 1995;80:1481.

26. McIver B, Rae P, Beckett G, Wilkinson E, Gold A, Toft A. Lack of effect of thyroxine in patients with Graves' hyperthyroidism who are treated with an antithyroid drug. N Engl J Med 1996;334:220.

27. Goolden AWG, Stewart JSW. Long-term results from graded low-dose radioactive iodine therapy for thyrotoxicosis. Clin Endocrinol (Oxf) 1986;24:217.

28. Tallstedt L, Lundell G, Torring O, et al. Occurrence of ophthalmopathy after treatment for Graves' hyperthyroidism. N Engl J Med 1992;326:1733.

29. DeGroot LJ, Gorman CA, Pinchera A, et al. Theraputic controversies: radiation and Graves' opthalmopathy. J Clin Endocrinol Metab 1995;80:339.

30. Bartalena L, et al. Use of corticosteroids to prevent progression of Graves' ophthalmopathy after radioiodine therapy for hyperthyroidism. N Engl J Med 1989;321:1349.

31. Toft AD, Irvine WJ, Sinclair I, McIntosh D, Seth J, Cameron EHD. Thyroid function after surgical treatment of thyrotoxicosis: a report of 100 cases treated with propranolol before operation. N Engl J Med 1978;298:643.

32. Feek CM, Sawers JSA, Irvine WJ, Becket GJ, Ratcliffe WA, Toft AD. Combination of potassium iodide and propranolol in preparation of patients with Graves' disease for thyroid surgery. N Engl J Med 1980;302:883.

33. Marcocci C, Bartalena L, Bogazzi F, Panicucci M, Pinchera A. Studies on the occurrence of ophthalmopathy in Graves' disease. Acta Endocrinol (Copenh) 1989; 120:473.

34. Dallow RH, Momose KJ, Weber AL, et al. Comparison of ultrasonography, computerized tomography (EMI scan), and radiographic techniques in evaluation of exophthalmos. Trans Am Acad Opthalmol Otolaryngol 1976;81:305.

35. Lee AG, et al. Long term results of orbital decompression in thyroid eye disease. ORBIT 1995;14:59.

36. Kao SC, et al. Radiotherapy in the management of thyroid orbitopathy: computed tomography and clinical outcomes. Arch Opthalmol 1993;111:819.

37. Parla JV, Franklyn JA, Cross KW, Jones SC, Sheppard MC. Prevalence and follow-up of abnormal thyrotropin (TSH) concentrations in the elderly in the United Kingdom. Clin Endocrinol (Oxf) 1991;34:77.

38. Sawin CT, et al. Low serum thyrotropin concentrations as a risk factor for atrial fibrillation in older persons. N Engl J Med 1994;331:1249.

39. Cooper DS. Thyroid disorders. In: Cassel CK, Riesenberg

DE, Sorensen LB, Walsh JR, eds. Geriatric medicine. 2nd ed. New York: Springer-Verlag, 1990:239.

40. Salvatore D, Tu H, Harney JW. Type 2 iodothyronine deiodinase is highly expressed in human thyroid. J Clin Invest 1996;98:962.

41. Hershman JM. Trophoblastic tumors. In: Braverman LE. Utiger RD, eds. The thyroid. 7th ed. Philadelphia. Lippincott-Raven, 1996:573.

42. Newman CM, Price A, Davies DW, Gray TA, Weetman, AP. Amiodarone and the thyroid: a practical guide to the management of thyroid dysfunction induced by amiodarone therapy. Heart 1998;79:121.

43. Luotola K, Hyoty H, Salmi J, Miettinen A, Heiln H, Pasternack A. Evaluation of infectious etiology in subacute thyroiditis—lack of association with coxsackievirus infection. APMIS 1998;106:500.

44. Houghton DJ, Gray HW, MacKenzie K. The tender neck: thyroiditis or thyroid abcess? Clin Endocrinol (Oxf) 1998; 48:521.

45. Singer PA. Thyroiditis. Med Clin N Am 1991;75:61.

46. Stagnaro-Green A. Postpartum thyroiditis: prevalence, etiology, and clinical implications. Thyroid Today 1993; 16(4):1.

47. Klein I, Levy GS. Silent thyrotoxic thyroiditis. Ann Intern Med 1982;96:242.

48. Roti E, Emerson CH. Postpartum thyroiditis. J Clin Endocrinol Metab 1992;74:3.

49. Stagnaro-Green A, Roman SH, Cobin RH, el-Harazy H, Wallenstein S, Davies TF. A prospective study of lymphocyte-initiated immunosuppression in normal pregnancy: evidence of a T-cell etiology for postpartum thyroid dysfunction. J Clin Endocrinol Metab 1992;74:645.

50. Bech K, Hoier-Madsen M, Feldt-Rasmussen U, Jensen BM, Molsted-Pedersen L, Kuhl C. Thyroid function and autoimmune manifestations in insulin-dependent diabetes mellitus during and after pregnancy. Acta Endocrinol 1991;124:534.

51. Hedberg CW, Fishbein DB, Janssen RS, et al. An outbreak of thyrotoxicosis caused by the consumption of bovine thyroid gland in ground beef. N Engl J Med 1987; 316:993.

52. March DE, Desai AG, Park CH, et al. Struma ovarii: hyperthyroidism in a postmenopausal woman. J Nucl Med 1988;29:263.

53. Rosenblum NG, Livolsi VA, Edmonds PR, et al. Malignant struma ovarii. Gynecol/Oncol 1989;32:224.

54. Sacks HS. Thyroid storm and myxedema coma. In: Van-Middlesworth L, ed. The thyroid gland. Chicago. Yearbook, 1986:371.

55. Brooks MH, Waldstein SS. Free thyroxine concentrations in thyroid storm. Ann Intern Med 1980;93:694.

56. Yeung SC, Go R, Balasubramanyam A. Rectal administration of iodide and propylthiouracil in the treatment of thyroid storm. Thyroid 1995;5:403.

57. Hylander B, Rosenqvist U. Treatment of myxedema coma—factors associated with fatal outcome. Acta Endocrinol 1985;108:65.

58. Bruneton JN, Balu-Maestro C, Marcy PY, et al. Very high frequency (13 Mhz) ultrasonographic examination of the normal neck: detection of normal lymph nodes and thyroid nodules. J Ultrasound Med 1994;13:87.

59. Butler SJ, Young JL. Third national cancer survey incidence data. National Cancer Institute. Washington, DC: Department of Health, Education and Welfare, 1975:775.

60. Caruso D, Mazzaferri EL. Fine needle aspiration biopsy in the management of thyroid nodules. Endocrinologist 1991;1:194.

61. Gharib H, Goelner JR. Fine needle aspiration biopsy of the thyroid: an appraisal. Ann Intern Med 1993;118:282.

62. Zelmanovitz F, Genro S, Gross JL. Suppressive therapy with levothyroxine for solitary thyroid nodules: a double-blind controlled clinical study and cumulative meta-analysis. J Clin Endocrol Metab 1998;83:3881.

63. Hedinger C, Williams ED, Sobin LH. Histological typing of thyroid tumors. In: International histological classification of tumors. 2nd ed, No 11. World Health Organization. New York: Springer-Verlag 1988:1.

64. Rosai J, Carganio MI, Delellis RA. Tumors of the thyroid gland. Washington, DC: Armed Forces Institute of Pathology, 1992;1.

65. Fleming ID, Cooper JS, Henson DE, et al. AJCC Cancer Staging Manual 5th ed. American Joint Committee on Cancer. Philadelphia: Lippincott-Raven,1997;59.

66. Zimmerman D, Hay ID, Gough IR, et al. Papillary thyroid carcinoma in children and adults: long-term follow-up of 1,039 patients conservatively treated at one institution during three decades. Surgery 1988;104:1157.

67. Mazzaferri EL, Jhiang SM. Long-term impact of initial surgical and medical therapy on papillary and follicular thyroid cancer. Am J Med 1994:97:418.

68. Wohlik N, Cote GJ, Evans DB, et al. Applications of genetic screening information to the management of medullary thyroid carcinoma and multiple neoplasia type 2. Endocrinol Metab Clin N Am 1996;25:1.

69. Gagel RF, Tashjian AH Jr, Cummings T, et al. The clinical outcome of prospective screening for multiple endocrine neoplasia type 2a: an 18 year experience. N Engl J Med 1988;318:478.

Chapter 30
Mood Disorders

J. Sloan Manning
Beth Choby

Five Key Points

- Mood and anxiety disorders are common, debilitating, predominate in women, and serve as the chief stimulus to patient presentation or as a significant comorbidity in much of primary care to women.

- Most women receive care for mental illness in nonpsychiatric settings.

- Mental illness is a complex phenomenon, with heterogeneous biologic, psychological, and social underpinnings.

- Multiple psychiatric comorbidities are the rule, not the exception, in mental illness.

- Bipolar spectrum illness may be more common than previously realized.

BACKGROUND

Epidemiology

Primary care physicians frequently encounter patients with psychiatric disorders. Most of those patients experience depression and anxiety. Two-thirds of those who suffer never receive treatment. Generalist physicians treat about one-half of the remaining one-third. These patients are high users of medical resources. They are frequently stigmatized by practitioners and are often sources of frustration. The economic costs associated with depression and anxiety are estimated in the billions of dollars yearly just in lost productivity and absenteeism. The personal pain and disruptions in marriages, families, and relationships with significant others defy economic analysis. Recognition of such illnesses by primary care physicians may be poor and the treatment rendered often less than desirable as compared with that given in psychiatric

settings. This may lead to further deterioration of clinical status, refractory illness, and, unfortunately, death.

Women are disproportionately affected by mental illness, particularly depression and anxiety, for which the female:male ratio is about 2:1. According to epidemiologic data, as many as 25% of women ages 18 to 44 experience a diagnosable mental disorder in any given year. The reasons for this are not clear, but probably result from a combination of biologic differences and psychosocial issues. Primary care practitioners who are not prepared to recognize, diagnose, and manage mental distress and illness in women do them a disservice.

Vulnerability

In general, vulnerability (diathesis) to mental illness is inherited (primary vulnerability). The family histories

predisposition. In bipolar women there is often a predominance of depressive episodes before hypomania or mania are manifest. That these illnesses can occur during a normal period of tremendous personal and social upheaval should not be lost on physicians, since early onset illness is often predictive of chronic dysfunction and a high frequency of syndromal episodes. Aggressive screening and treatment may help reduce the severity of symptoms encountered and avoid negative psychological, social, and educational outcomes.

Women are not protected against mood disorders during pregnancy. High relapse rates have been documented for those electing to discontinue or change antidepressant treatment during pregnancy. Since approximately 50% of pregnancies are unintended, many women being treated for mood disorders will face decisions about the risks and benefits of continuing these medications. Antidepressant discontinuation prior to delivery increases the risk for postpartum depression. Women will have questions about the potential effects of antidepressants on breastfed infants. Medications should be considered when the benefits of treatment are felt to outweigh the risks of such treatment. Women should be appraised of relevant data and allowed to make an informed decision, realizing that no decision is devoid of risk.

Fortunately, the data for antidepressants on pregnancy outcomes is reassuring. The best safety data exists for TCAs and fluoxetine and suggest no increased risk for major congenital malformations resulting from first-trimester exposure. Substantial prospective safety data exists for fluoxetine in this regard. The preponderance of data also suggests no increase in perinatal complications for TCAs and fluoxetine. Data for other antidepressants is limited, but nonetheless reassuring.

All psychotropic medications are excreted in breast milk, but concentrations of such medications in breast milk vary greatly. Data on fluoxetine suggests no adverse effect on the infants of breastfeeding mothers nor adverse neurobehavioral outcomes for exposed infants. Significantly, the plasma of breastfed infants exposed to fluoxetine show no accumulation of the medication. Data for TCAs and other antidepressants is limited but similarly reassuring.

Postpartum depression is common, occurring in as many as 10% of women, and carries a high risk of recurrence. It is differentiated from "baby blues," a transient (1 to 2 weeks) period of depressed mood, which resolves spontaneously. Women at greatest risk of postpartum depression are those with previous histories of psychiatric illness. Postpartum psychosis, a severe form

of mood disturbance occurring uncommonly (<1%) is characterized by agitated states with overt psychotic symptoms. It is quite dangerous to mothers and their newborns. Many authorities consider postpartum psychosis a type of bipolar disorder. Lithium appears to be an effective preventive agent for women at risk.

Menopause may be a trigger for depressive or anxious episodes in women with known vulnerability, and women may experience depressive symptoms (fatigue, insomnia, difficulty concentrating) but the incidence of clinical depression per se does not seem to increase during menopause. Menopause can be a time of renewed personal growth for women freed from the responsibilities of child-rearing. So-called empty nest syndrome should be viewed as a euphemistic alias for depression and not a normal part of menopause. Estrogen replacement should not be considered first-line treatment for major depression associated with menopause, though some studies suggest that hormone replacement may be an effective antidepressant augmentation for some women. Minor disturbances of affect, particularly anxious mood associated with vasomotor instability and sleep disturbances, may respond to hormone replacement alone.

Chronic medical conditions may be associated with depressive and anxious illness. Notable among them are thyroid dysfunction, diabetes mellitus, rheumatoid arthritis, systemic lupus erythematosus, multiple sclerosis, stroke, cancer, and myocardial infarction. Any significant illness, chronic or acute, can trigger an episode of depression or anxiety. The mechanism may be one of uncovering latent vulnerability (e.g., major surgery) or de novo disturbances of neurologic integrity (stroke or multiple sclerosis). De novo disturbances of late onset (>50 years of age) in those without family histories may suggest an organic cause. It is important not to view chronic medical conditions simplistically, with demoralization leading to an "expected" disturbance in mood. The treatment of psychiatric illness comorbid with chronic medical conditions should combine appropriate psychiatric interventions with treatment optimization for the somatic condition.

Some medical treatments may exacerbate or uncover psychiatric illness. The list of offending medications includes steroids (including progestins and hormone replacements), antiestrogens, β-blockers, centrally acting antihypertensives (e.g., α-methyldopa), anticholinergics, antihistamines, bromocriptine, and gastrointestinal promotility agents (e.g., metoclopramide).

of depressed and anxious patients usually reveal affected relatives. Earlier conceptualizations of a reactive-endogenous dichotomy have not been borne out scientifically. Significant psychological stressors are strongly associated with an initial episode of major depression only. Subsequent episodes of major depression often appear in the absence of identifiable stressors. Since depressive disorders typically manifest a chronic pattern of waxing and waning symptoms with infrequent and sometimes brief remissions, much of the chaos and dysfunction seen in the lives of these patients may be secondary to the illness itself. For most, life events influence only the timing of syndromal episodes.

A vulnerability to mental illness may also be acquired. This often occurs when somatic illnesses such as stroke, multiple sclerosis, epilepsy, or closed head trauma damage brain structures of the limbic system. These widespread structures are both cortical and subcortical in location. A number of other somatic illnesses strongly associated with depression and anxiety may produce de novo disruptions in structural integrity or expose a primary diathesis by affecting normal neurophysiology. Among these illnesses are diabetes mellitus, acquired immunodeficiency syndrome (AIDS), multiple sclerosis, hypercortisolism, rheumatoid arthritis, and systemic lupus erythematosus.

CLINICAL PROCESS AS IT RELATES TO PRIMARY CARE PSYCHIATRY

The clinical process for the diagnosis and treatment of mental disorders is not unfamiliar to clinicians. It is the same process that is applicable to any somatic illness. We briefly review it here to highlight critical steps in the process and to familiarize physicians with the way that psychiatric illnesses fit known patterns of diagnosis and treatment. The basic steps of the clinical process are:

1. Recognition of dysfunction and screening for illness.
2. Assessment for pertinent comorbid conditions.
3. Application of diagnostic criteria.
4. Evaluation of the quality of the therapeutic alliance and a patient's readiness to proceed with treatment.
5. Selection of treatment(s) to be used.
6. Management of treatment(s) chosen to attain a robust, sustained response.

The remainder of this chapter will elaborate on depressive and anxious illness as it relates to this standard paradigm of practice.

RECOGNITION OF DYSFUNCTION

Common Symptoms

Alexithymia, a syndrome of difficulty verbalizing emotions, affects many depressed patients. Therefore, core depressive symptoms of sadness and anhedonia may be unreported, even on direct questioning. Initially, it may be more useful to screen for depression by focusing on nonspecific but common symptoms. These "trigger" symptoms should prompt more thorough questioning that would include inquiries about depressed mood and withdrawal or lack of interest in usual activities. Some common presenting symptoms are discussed below.

Abnormal Sleep Patterns

Either insomnia or hypersomnia (>10 hours of sleep per day) may be present. Any form of insomnia may be seen, and mixtures of initial insomnia (difficulty falling asleep), middle insomnia (frequent prolonged awakenings), and terminal insomnia (awakening early and unable to fall back to sleep) are not uncommon.

Fatigue

Fatigue, more precisely anergia, along with sleep problems, is the most common symptom of depression and anxiety. Anhedonia is often found mingled with the anergia. Is the patient tired or uninterested or both?

Pain

Not a DSM-IV symptom of depression, but often present and often overlooked by clinician and patient alike. Chronic, recurrent pain like headache, backache, or pelvic or abdominal pain is typical. The pain may be generalized and resemble a fibromyalgia syndrome.

Irritability

Outbursts of anger and impatience or even rage may be symptoms of irritability. Coping with small stresses becomes difficult. The patient may retreat or hide from identified stressors to remain comfortable or in control. This symptom is particularly likely to create interpersonal strife.

Anxiety ("Nerves")

Anxiety is usually present to some degree in depressive states, and it is often the acutely painful symptom complex that presents to the clinician. Many mild to moderate depressions may be compensated or normalized by patients until initial insomnia, restlessness, muscle tension, panic symptoms, or other manifestations of physiologic arousal arise. Anxiety disorders often predate depressive episodes. Generalized anxiety disorder and major depressive disorder may have similar biological underpinnings.

Euphemisms and Labels

Negative societal stigmata and the fact that depressed and anxious patients are heavy users of medical resources often result in clinicians and their staffs labeling patients or creating euphemisms to identify them. The terms *stressed out, crock, frequent flyer, supratentorial syndrome,* and *hypochondriac* are examples. The so-called worried well may not be so well after all, or we may use the term in a cavalier manner. Difficult patients and heavy users of telephone triage, urgent care, and on-call physicians are all good candidates for focused investigation.

Aliases and Specialty-Specific Pseudonyms

Because clinicians and patients may be unaware of psychiatric syndromes and unable or unwilling to make explicit diagnoses, depression and anxiety often carry a related somatic diagnosis. These diagnoses may be formal or informal. Clearly, the syndromes listed below are not always indications of psychiatric illness; however, their association with such is so strong that a diagnosis of depression or anxiety should be excluded in their assessment. In some, antidepressants are often primary or adjunctive treatments, regardless.

1. Migraine, tension, or mixed headache syndromes
2. Fibromyalgia, fibrositis, or idiopathic pain syndromes
3. Irritable-bowel syndrome, nonulcer dyspepsia, or other functional gastrointestinal complaints
4. "Hormone imbalance"
5. Hypoglycemia
6. Chronic dysequilibrium or tinnitus

Frequently Encountered Life Scenarios

A high suspicion of depression and anxiety is appropriate whenever patients present with psychosocial stressors. This is particularly true for situations with multiple stressors. To reiterate, stress is not the cause of depression and anxiety, but may trigger episodes of illness or escalate subsyndromal illness to syndromal levels. It is inappropriate for clinicians to decide how depressed or anxious a person should be, simply by reviewing a list of acute and chronic stressors. However, the presence of stressors can help identify patients for screening and are important contextual issues to be considered when planning well-rounded treatments that use medication, psychotherapy, or (preferably) both. Themes of discord, chaos, abuse, instability, change, or loss are common.

COMORBIDITY

When dysfunction or impairment is recognized clinically, the search for a cause and the foundation for management begins with a review of systems. It is this review that puts the identified symptoms in a clinical context and allows other illnesses, treatments, or situations to be assessed. The principal questions to be answered are:

1. Is the dysfunction secondary to a somatic condition or its treatment?
2. Is another somatic illness influencing a primary diathesis for mood/anxiety illness?
3. Is the dysfunction more properly seen as a consequence of another psychiatric syndrome?
4. To what extent does the psychosocial context of the illness contribute to its timing, severity, and duration or influence its management?

Somatic Issues

A number of somatic issues may affect the presentation of psychiatric disorders in women. These may be broadly divided into the areas of reproductive endocrinology and child-bearing, chronic medical conditions, and medical treatments.

Menarche is commonly associated with behavioral changes. For most women these aberrations will fall into a normal range of mood fluctuations, feelings of anxiety about self-image, individuation, and social role. However, women who have inherited strong predispositions for psychiatric disorders often have their first experience with syndromal illness in adolescence. This is particularly true for bipolar spectrum mood disorders and primary (early onset) dysthymia, with episodes often growing out of a temperamental

Psychiatric Comorbidity

Psychiatric comorbidity is the rule rather than the exception. Chief among other psychiatric conditions comorbid with depression and anxiety are substance-related disorders. All anxious and depressed patients should be screened carefully for substance use and abuse. This includes prescription and nonprescription products and the use of caffeine and herbal stimulants, including diet aids that contain ephedrine. A discussion of the diagnosis and treatment of chemical dependency is contained elsewhere in this textbook. Substance use may be the primary cause of the depressed or anxious mood, an attempt at self-treatment, or a parallel comorbidity. Aggressive management of comorbid anxiety and depression is associated with better outcomes in the treatment of alcoholism. Failure to eliminate substance abuse in depressed or anxious patients is associated with treatment failure.

Most patients with depression have significant anxiety. Conversely, most anxious patients have experienced depression, are currently depressed, or may be expected to become depressed during the course of their anxiety disorder. The genetic underpinnings of generalized anxiety disorder and major depression may be similar. Panic disorder, obsessive–compulsive disorder, and posttraumatic stress disorder (PTSD) are also commonly preceded by or complicated by mood disorders.

Anxiety/depression comorbidity has clinical significance. First, anxiety, as a pain state, is often more acute than the comorbid depression and may present more readily. Many patients tolerate mild to moderate depressed states by unloading life activities or relationships in the same way that discarding ballast may stabilize a sinking ship. Functioning often continues, albeit at a reduced level, and this impairment may be normalized. If anxiety is severe, however, its presence will often become a chief complaint because of restlessness, irritability, and initial insomnia. Therefore, anxious mood will prompt patient requests for intervention. Comorbid depression may then be hidden by the anxiety and ignored. Benzodiazepine anxiolytics and sedative hypnotics are commonly prescribed in these situations, but they do not represent the best treatments. Antidepressants are effective anxiolytics, with some allowance made for specific prescription based on the subtype of anxiety identified. All antidepressants may be expected to reduce symptoms of generalized anxiety in responders. If the presentation includes panic attacks, the antidepressant chosen should have antipanic activity. This excludes buspirone, bupropion, and trazodone, since these agents lack efficacy in panic disorder. If obsessive–compulsive disorder (OCD) is present, the antidepressant chosen should have efficacy in OCD. This situation excludes all antidepressants except the serotonin-specific reuptake inhibitors (SSRI) and the tricyclic antidepressant clomipramine. One can easily see why the SSRIs are now considered antidepressants of first choice by many clinicians—they are generally well tolerated and are broadly anxiolytic in generalized anxiety disorder, panic disorder, OCD, and PTSD, among other conditions.

There are two other psychiatric disorders commonly associated with anxious and depressed illness in women—somatization disorder and eating disorders. A pattern of physical complaints causing clinically significant distress that cannot be explained by a somatic illness or the effect of a treatment for such an illness defines somatization disorder. The prevalence of this disorder varies between 0.2 and 2% in general population studies but is more common in clinical populations. The symptoms are not intentionally feigned, but they are often presented in an exaggerated way or represent amplifications of expected symptoms from identifiable disorders. Descriptions of complaints are often vague. Histrionic, borderline, and antisocial personality disorders are more common in those with somatization disorder.

The diagnosis of somatization disorder is based on age of onset and the numbers of complaints and systems involved. Pain, gastrointestinal, sexual, and neurologic complaints must all be seen (Table 30-1). A strict application of the diagnostic criteria will help avoid overdiagnosis and the failure to consider treatable conditions. It is important to differentiate the anxious or depressed patient with somatic symptoms from those with somatization disorder. Somatic presentations for anxiety and depression are extremely common, and these symptoms improve with adequate treatment. Therefore, persons in whom somatization disorder is suspected should be adequately screened and treated for depression and anxiety.

The management of individuals with somatization disorder begins with strategies that limit a person's exposure to diagnostic and treatment interventions that might be costly and involve significant complications. A solid therapeutic alliance between the patient and a primary care physician is crucial.

TABLE 30-1
DIAGNOSTIC CRITERIA FOR 300.81 SOMATIZATION DISORDER

A. A history of many physical complaints beginning before age 30 years that occur over a period of several years and result in treatment being sought or significant impairment in social, occupational, or other important areas of functioning.

B. Each of the following criteria must have been met with individual symptoms occurring at any time during the course of the disturbance.

(1) Four pain symptoms. A history of pain related to at least four different sites or functions (e.g., head, abdomen, back, joints, extremities, chest, rectum, during menstruation, during sexual intercourse, or during urination).

(2) Two gastrointestinal symptoms. A history of at least two gastrointestinal symptoms other than pain (e.g., nausea, bloating, vomiting other than during pregnancy, diarrhea, or intolerance of several different foods).

(3) One sexual symptom. A history of at least one sexual or reproductive symptom other than pain (e.g., sexual indifference, erectile or ejaculatory dysfunction, irregular menses, excessive menstrual bleeding, vomiting throughout pregnancy).

(4) One pseudoneurologic symptom. A history of at least one symptom or deficit suggesting a neurological condition not limited to pain (conversion symptoms such as impaired coordination or balance, paralysis or localized weakness, difficulty swallowing or lump in throat, aphonia, urinary retention, hallucinations, loss of touch or pain sensation, double vision, blindness, deafness, seizures; dissociative symptoms such as amnesia; or loss of consciousness other than fainting).

C. Either (1) or (2):

(1) After appropriate investigation, each of the symptoms in criterion B cannot be fully explained by a known somatic condition or the direct effects of a substance (e.g., a drug of abuse, a medication).

(2) When there is a related somatic condition, the physical complaints or resulting social or occupational impairment are in excess of what would be expected from the history, physical examination, or laboratory findings.

D. The symptoms are not intentionally produced or feigned (as in factitious disorder or malingering).

Diagnostic and statistical manual of mental disorders, 4th ed. Washington DC: American Psychiatric Association, 1994.

Combinations of psychotherapy (aimed at stress management and understanding reactions to stress) and focused psychopharmacologic interventions (e.g., for significant depression) may also be used. Consultation is often helpful.

Eating disorders affect about 4% of adolescents and are 10 to 20 times more common in women than in men. Anorexia nervosa, a syndrome characterized by a refusal to maintain a minimal normal body weight for age combined with an intense preoccupation with weight, amenorrhea, and a disturbance of body image occurs in 0.2 to 0.8%. Among those affected, 85% are 13- to 20-year-olds. Bulimia nervosa affects 1 to 3% of young women. Bulimia is characterized by binge eating and efforts at compensation to prevent weight gain. Most bulimics maintain a normal weight. The syndrome often develops after a period of intense dieting. Compensation for bingeing comes in purging (self-induced vomiting, overuse of laxatives, diuretics, enemas) and nonpurging (fasting, excessive exercise) types. Self-induced vomiting (by gag reflex or ingestion of ipecac) is employed by 80 to 90% and may lead to dental erosion, electrolyte abnormalities, and cardiac or skeletal myopathies.

Mood disorders are extremely common in those with eating disorders. Substance abuse or dependence, typically stimulants or alcohol, occur in one-third. Psychotherapy combined with medication forms the basis for treatment. Fluoxetine has been approved by the Food and Drug Administration (FDA) for use in bulimia nervosa at a dose of 60 mg/day.

Psychosocial Context

Every illness occurs in a psychosocial context and, as such, is a biopsychosocial phenomenon. The particulars of that context help define illness apart from disorder. Psychosocial context is always important in depressive and anxious illnesses, because they are pervasive in their effects on the individual. Significant stressors may precipitate, accompany, or be secondary to depression and anxiety. Such contexts become factors in planning the assessment and treatment of patients. For those delivering primary care to women, several recurring contexts deserve special mention.

Spousal abuse may affect 1.8 million women in this country. All racial, religious, and socioeconomic backgrounds are affected. Pregnancy is a time of high risk for abuse, with 15 to 25% of women affected. Other risk factors include recent separation or divorce, age <30, and homelessness. About half of battered women grew up in homes with domestic violence. Abused women are frequently seen in ambulatory clinics and emergency rooms. Clinicians often miss important clues to an abusive situation. Patients will not often volunteer information on battering. However, clinicians will find that empathetic inquiries are appreciated by such women and may prevent further harm or death. Any suspicious injury or circumstance surrounding an injury should prompt direct questions about abuse after a male partner, relatives, or significant others have been invited out of the examination room. When abuse is suspected, a referral to an appropriate resource for battered women is indicated.

Divorce is common in this country, with about 50% of first marriages ending in legal separation. This often leaves women without adequate economic support and with sole or joint custody of their children. The result is tremendous stress from employment outside the home (often in more than one job) and the responsibility that comes with parenting alone added to the continued demands of household responsibilities. This may lead to sleep deprivation, poor nutrition, exhaustion, and ultimately, illness. Women facing this scenario often fail to make health maintenance visits with their primary care provider but present themselves in times of crisis. Clinicians have a role in helping patients identify when the demands of their lifestyle may be reaching critical levels and having a negative impact on their health.

Women typically outlive their spouses. During or after such a loss, there is a period of readjustment that often involves role change or conflict. Grief is a normal experience and may take months to resolve. Clinicians are often in a position to offer support and appropriate referrals to women in bereavement, screening for signs and symptoms of illness, since syndromal depression and anxiety may complicate grief, resulting in prolonged or worsened impairment.

DIAGNOSTIC FORMULATION

After the review of systems is complete, the patient's illness is compared to established criteria to formulate a working diagnosis. A reasoned working diagnosis facilitates communication with the patient and other clinicians, suggests areas of educational focus, and begins the consideration of various interventions.

Principles

Diagnoses are based on the presence of specific impairing symptom complexes. The current American standard of psychiatric diagnosis is the Diagnostic and Statistical Manual of Mental Disorders, 4th edition (DSM-IV). A primary care version of the DSM-IV

has been created (DSM-IV, PC). Symptom-driven diagnostic manuals are consensus statements offered as guidelines for clinicians. They form the basis for communication between clinicians. This chapter will supplement DSM-IV criteria with additional information to describe the clinical picture of the syndromes discussed.

Several types of evidence validate a diagnosis. These lines of evidence are:

1. Phenomenology (symptoms)—morbid and premorbid (temperamental)
2. Family pedigree
3. Longitudinal course
4. Treatment response
5. Biologic markers

Since no reliable, clinically useful biologic markers are available to assist in making psychiatric diagnoses, clinicians must focus on the first four types of evidence. An examination of each area will help in patient assessment. The most accurate diagnoses are made when experienced clinicians follow patients over time and make use of all available data.

Mood Disorders

Mood disorders fall into two spectra—unipolar (noncyclic) and bipolar (cyclic)—based on the absence or presence of a clinically significant period of expanded mood. Bipolar disorders may be more common in primary care than previously realized. Bipolar II disorder (nonmanic illness) is more common that bipolar I disorder (illness with mania). Hypomania, a brief and less severely impairing period of expanded mood, identifies the most common presentation of bipolarity (Figure 30-1). Hypomania characteristically appears and disappears abruptly. The DSM-IV requires a duration of 4 days for diagnosis, but 1- to 3-day durations are more typical. Hypomania may be triggered or exacerbated by sleep deprivation, antidepressants, and corticosteroids, or may be influenced in frequency and severity by menses and seasons of the year. The treatment of bipolar disorders with antidepressants alone may produce hypomania and mania, rapid cycling, or refractory depressions. A careful evaluation for these and other associated features of bipolarity in family pedigree, longitudinal course, premorbid temperament, and treatment response is essential to proper management. Bipolar disorders include bipolar I disorder, bipolar II disorder,

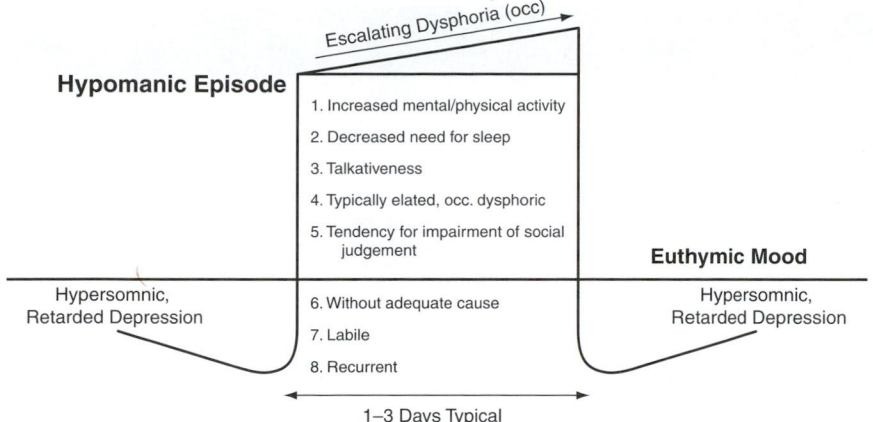

Figure 30-1 Hypomanic episode and euthymic mood. Elated mood may become mixed with depressive symptoms as the episode progresses. Hypersomnic, retarded depressions often precede and follow hypomanic expansions of mood. The base-line from which hypomanic episodes arise is typically one of chronic mixed anxious depressions. The shift from lethargy and depressed mood into productivity and elation is welcomed and perceived as normal. OCC = occasionally. From The Psychiatric Clinics of North America. Bipolarity: beyond classic mania, vol. 22. no. 3. September 1999. Saunders. Used with permission.

cyclothymic disorder, and bipolar disorder not otherwise specified (NOS) (Table 30-2).

Unipolar disorders include major depressive disorder, dysthymic disorder and depression not otherwise specified (minor depression). The prevalence of these disorders in primary care is 5 to 8%, 3 to 5%, and 8 to 11%, respectively. These figures are based on cross-sectional investigations and vary from study to study. Dysthymic disorder, in particular, may be underrepresented and better defined using the DSM-IV alternate criterion B that focuses on symptoms of

low self-esteem, pessimism, generalized loss of interest or pleasure, social withdrawal, chronic fatigue, feelings of guilt or brooding about the past, subjective feelings of irritability or excessive anger, decreased productivity, poor concentration/memory, or indecisiveness. Table 30-3 gives definitions of these disorders.

Minimally impairing symptoms clearly related to life stressors and lasting less than 6 months define adjustment disorders. Longitudinal observation and close questioning will differentiate these from minor

(Text continues on page 680.)

TABLE 30-2
BIPOLAR I AND II DISORDERS

Criteria for Bipolar I Disorder, Most Recent Episode Manic
A. The patient is currently (or most recently was) in a manic episode.
B. At least one previous major depressive episode, manic episode, or mixed episode has occurred.
C. The mood episodes listed in criteria A and B are not better accounted for by schizoaffective disorder and are not superimposed on schizophrenia, schizophreniform disorder, delusional disorder, or psychotic disorder not otherwise specified.

Criteria for Manic Episode
A. A distinct period of abnormally and persistently elevated, expansive, or irritable mood occurs that lasts at least 1 week (or any duration if hospitalization is necessary).
B. During the period of mood disturbance, three (or more) of the following symptoms have persisted (four if the mood is only irritable) and have been present to a substantial degree:
(1) Inflated self-esteem or grandiosity
(2) Decreased need for sleep (e.g., feels rested after only 3 hours of sleep)
(3) More talkative than usual or feels pressure to keep talking
(4) Flight of ideas or subjective experience that thoughts are racing
(5) Distractibility (i.e., attention too easily drawn to unimportant or irrelevant external stimuli)
(6) Increase in goal-directed activity (socially, at work or school, or sexually) or psychomotor agitation
(7) Excessive involvement in pleasurable activities that have a high potential for painful consequences (e.g., unrestrained buying sprees, sexual indiscretions, or foolish business investments)
C. The symptoms do not meet the criteria for a mixed episode.
D. The mood disturbance is sufficiently severe to cause marked impairment in occupational functioning or in usual social activities or relationships with others or to necessitate hospitalization to prevent harm to self or others, or psychotic features are present.
E. The symptoms are not due to the direct physiologic effects of a substance (e.g., a drug of abuse, a medication, or other treatment) or a somatic condition (e.g., hyperthyroidism).

Table continues on following page

TABLE 30-2 (CONTINUED)

Criteria for Mixed Episode

A. The criteria are met both for a manic episode and for a major depressive episode (except for duration) nearly every day during at least a 1-week period.

B. The mood disturbance is sufficiently severe to cause marked impairment in occupational functioning or in usual social activities or relationships with others, or to necessitate hospitalization to prevent harm to self or others, or there are psychotic features.

C. The symptoms are not due to the direct physiologic effects of a substance (e.g., a drug of abuse, a medication, or other treatment) or a somatic condition (e.g., hyperthyroidism).

Criteria That Distinguish Mania from Hypomania*

A. Meaningful conversation is difficult to maintain for any length of time.

B. Euphoric or ecstatic mood deteriorates to querulous belligerence.

C. Affective hallucinations, frank delusions of grandiose ability or identity, delusions of assistance or persecution, delusions of reference, or delusions of love are present.

D. Insight and judgment are lost to such a degree that frenzied expansive activity leads to serious social impairment.

Criteria for Bipolar II Disorder

A. One or more major depressive episodes.

B. At least one hypomanic episode is or has been present.

C. A manic episode or a mixed episode has never occurred.

D. The mood symptoms listed in criteria A and B are not better accounted for by schizoaffective disorder and are not superimposed on schizophrenia, schizophreniform disorder, delusional disorder, or psychotic disorder not otherwise specified.

E. The symptoms cause clinically significant distress or impairment in social, occupational, or other important areas of functioning.

Criteria for Hypomanic Episode

A. A distinct period of persistently elevated, expansive, or irritable mood occurs that lasts at least 4 days and is clearly different from the usual nondepressed mood.

B. During the period of mood disturbance, three (or more) of the following symptoms have persisted (four if the mood is only irritable) and have been present to a substantial degree:
   (1) Inflated self-esteem or grandiosity
   (2) Decreased need for sleep (e.g., feels rested after only 3 hours of sleep)
   (3) More talkative than usual or pressure to keep talking
   (4) Flight of ideas or subjective experience that thoughts are racing
   (5) Distractibility (i.e., attention too easily drawn to unimportant or irrelevant external stimuli)
   (6) Increase in goal-directed activity (socially, at work or school, or sexually) or psychomotor agitation
   (7) Excessive involvement in pleasurable activities that have a high potential for painful consequences (e.g., unrestrained buying sprees, sexual indiscretions, or foolish business investments)

C. The episode is associated with an unequivocal change in functioning that is uncharacteristic of the person when not symptomatic.

D. The disturbance in mood and the change in functioning are observable by others.

E. The episode is not severe enough to cause marked impairment in social or occupational functioning or to necessitate hospitalization, and there are no psychotic features.

F. The symptoms are not due to the direct physiologic effects of a substance (e.g., a drug of abuse, a medication, or other treatment) or a somatic condition (e.g., hyperthyroidism).

Criteria for Cyclothymic Disorder

A. For at least 2 years, numerous periods with hypomanic symptoms and numerous periods with depressive symptoms that do not meet criteria for a major depressive episode have been present in children and adolescents; the duration must be at least 1 year.

B. During the 2-year period (1 year in children and adolescents), the person has not been without the symptoms listed in criterion A for more than 2 months at a time.

C. No major depressive episode, manic episode, or mixed episode has been present during the first 2 years of the disturbance. After the initial 2 years (1 year in children and adolescents) of cyclothymic disorder, there may be superimposed manic or mixed episodes (in which case both bipolar I disorder and cyclothymic disorder may be diagnosed) or major depressive episodes (in which case bipolar II disorder and cyclothymic disorder may be diagnosed).

D. The symptoms listed in criterion A are not better accounted for by schizoaffective disorder and are not superimposed on schizophrenia, schizophreniform disorder, delusional disorder, or psychotic disorder not otherwise specified.

E. The symptoms are not due to the direct physiologic effects of a substance (e.g., a drug of abuse or a medication) or a somatic condition (e.g., hyperthyroidism).

F. The symptoms cause clinically significant distress or impairment in social, occupational, or other important areas of functioning.

*Diagnostic and statistical manual of mental disorders, 4th ed. Washington DC: American Psychiatric Association, 1994.
Adapted from Akiskal HS, Mallya G. Criteria for the "soft" bipolar spectrum: treatment implications. Psychopharmacol Bull 1987;23:68.

TABLE 30-3
CRITERIA FOR MAJOR DEPRESSIVE EPISODE

A. Five (or more) of the following symptoms have been present during the same 2-week period and represent a change from previous functioning; at least one of the symptoms is either (1) depressed mood or (2) loss of interest or pleasure.

Note: Do not include symptoms that are clearly due to a somatic condition, or mood-incongruent delusions or hallucinations.

(1) Depressed mood most of the day, nearly every day as indicated by either subjective report (e.g., feels sad or empty) or observation made by others (e.g., appears tearful). *Note:* In children and adolescents, can be irritable mood.
(2) Markedly diminished interest or pleasure in all, or almost all, activities most of the day, nearly every day (as indicated by either subjective account or observation made by others).
(3) Significant weight loss when not dieting, or weight gain (e.g., a change of more than 5% of body weight in a month), or decrease or increase in appetite nearly every day. *Note:* In children, consider failure to make expected weight gains.
(4) Insomnia or hypersomnia nearly every day.
(5) Psychomotor agitation or retardation nearly every clay (observable by others, not merely subjective feelings of restlessness or being slowed down)
(6) Fatigue or loss of energy nearly every day.
(7) Feelings of worthlessness or excessive or inappropriate guilt (which may be delusional) nearly every day (not merely self-reproach or guilt about being sick).
(8) Diminished ability to think or concentrate, or indecisiveness, nearly every day (either by subjective account or as observed by others).
(9) Recurrent thoughts of death (not just fear of dying), recurrent suicidal ideation without a specific plan, or a suicide attempt or a specific plan for committing suicide.

B. The symptoms do not meet criteria for a mixed episode.
C. The symptoms cause clinically significant distress or impairment in social, occupational, or other important areas of functioning.
D. The symptoms are not due to the direct physiologic effects of a substance (e.g., a drug of abuse, a medication) or a somatic condition (e.g., hypothyroidism).
E. The symptoms are not better accounted for by bereavement, i.e., after the loss of a loved one; the symptoms persist for longer than 2 months or are characterized by marked functional impairment, morbid preoccupation with worthlessness, suicidal ideation, psychotic symptoms, or psychomotor retardation.

Diagnostic Criteria for 300.4 Dysthymic Disorder

A. Depressed mood for most of the day, for more days than not, as indicated either by subjective account or observation by others, for at least 2 years. *Note:* In children and adolescents, mood can be irritable and duration must be at least 1 year.
B. Presence, while depressed, of two (or more) of the following:

(1) Poor appetite or overeating	(4) Low self-esteem
(2) Insomnia or hypersomnia	(5) Poor concentration or difficulty making decisions
(3) Low energy or fatigue	(6) Feelings of hopelessness

C. During the 2-year period (1 year for children or adolescents) of the disturbance, the person has never been without the symptoms in criteria A and B for more than 2 months at a time.
D. No major depressive episode has been present during the first 2 years of the disturbance (1 year for children and adolescents); i.e., the disturbance is not better accounted for by chronic major depressive disorder, or major depressive disorder, in partial remission.

Note: There may have been a previous major depressive episode provided there was a full remission (no significant signs or symptoms for 2 months) before development of the dysthymic disorder. In addition, after the initial 2 years (1 year in children or adolescents) of dysthymic disorder, there may be superimposed episodes of major depressive disorder, in which case both diagnoses may be given when the criteria are met for a major depressive episode.

E. There has never been a manic episode, a mixed episode, or a hypomanic episode, and criteria have never been met for cyclothymic disorder.
F. The disturbance does not occur exclusively during the course of a chronic psychotic disorder, such as schizophrenia or delusional disorder.
G. The symptoms are not due to the direct physiologic effects of a substance (e.g., a drug of abuse, a medication) or a somatic condition (e.g., hypothyroidism).
H. The symptoms cause clinically significant distress or impairment in social, occupational, or other important areas of functioning.

Specify if:
Early onset: before age 21 years
Late onset: age 21 years or older
Specify (for most recent 2 years of dysthymic disorder):
With atypical features

Depressive Disorder Not Otherwise Specified

The category of depressive disorder not otherwise specified includes disorders with depressive features that do not meet the criteria for major depressive disorder, dysthymic disorder, adjustment disorder with depressed mood, or adjustment disorder with mixed anxiety and depressed mood.

*Diagnostic and statistical manual of mental disorders, 4th ed. Washington DC: American Psychiatric Association, 1994.

TABLE 30-4
DIFFERENTIATION OF BIPOLAR ILLNESS FROM UNIPOLAR ILLNESS

Clinical Presentation	Bipolar Illness	Unipolar Illness
Age of onset in childhood or adolescence*	+	+/−
Family history of bipolar illness or lithium responsive first-degree relative	+	−
Loaded family pedigrees[†]	+	−
Atypical features	+	+/−
Premorbid affective temperament (dysthymic, hyperthymic, cyclothymic, irritable)[†]	+	−
Pharmacologic hypomania (antidepressants)	+	−
High frequency of episodes	+	−
Presence of mood lability and/or periods of energy-activity during depressed episodes	+	−
Mixed DSM-IV Axis II Cluster B/Cluster C Personality Disorders (e.g., Histrionic-Avoidant, Narcissistic-Dependent)	+	−

*Age of onset is significantly earlier for bipolar illness with recurrent depressions often predating hypomanic, manic, or mixed symptoms.

[†]Pedigree loading is defined as mood disorders affecting three or more persons in a generation.

[†]Affective temperaments are defined as early onset, enduring, but nonimpairing habitual traits. The dysthymic temperament manifests as a tendency to depressed mood, self-criticism, a guilt-ridden conscience, social avoidance, indecision, and a tendency to oversleep (≥9 hours). The hyperthymic temperament is just the opposite—a tendency to extroverted talkativeness, grandiose thinking, risk taking, impulsivity, and mild lapses of judgment combined with a decreased need for sleep (≤6 hours even on weekends). The cyclothymic temperament is a biphasic combination of both, where the individual manifests features of one for several days at a time before switching to the opposite phase. Cyclothymic temperament may manifest itself as romantic and geographic instability, uneven productivity, and odd working hours. The irritable temperament may be thought of as a concurrent blend of dysthymia and hyperthymia. Therefore, irritably tempered individuals tend to be restless, driven, and hypercritical or complaining.

Information on temperament adapted from Akiskal and Mallya.

depression and stress–related exacerbations of preexisting syndromal illness. The treatment of adjustment disorders is generally accomplished with support and various psychotherapies. Somatic (medication) intervention is appropriate, if a more severe illness emerges. Depressive symptoms represent attributable risk factors for major depression. Therefore, patients should be followed appropriately.

Bipolar disorders may be differentiated from unipolar disorders by associated historical factors and treatment response. These are summarized in Table 30-4. Atypical depressions, characterized by hypersomnia, hyperphagia, sensitivity to rejection by others, reversed diurnal variation (worse in evening), and reactivity of mood are listed as subtypes of major depression by DSM–IV. However, evidence suggests that many patients with atypical depression may eventually meet diagnostic criteria for a bipolar illness.

Bipolar illness is less likely than unipolar illness to respond to monotherapy with antidepressants, and the responses that do occur tend to be exaggerated, erratic, or problematic in some way. Sudden responses that begin within a few days to 2 weeks of beginning an antidepressant arouse suspicion. These abrupt recoveries are typically overly robust and short-lived. They may be reproducible with increases in the dose of antidepressant, but even then they are not sustained. Some bipolar patients will have responses to antidepressants that are punctuated by sudden drops into depression every few days or weeks. Such an uneven pattern resembles that of rapid cycling, which is a disruptive and refractory mood state. Others may respond to antidepressants with admixtures of agitation or dysphoric drivenness. This mixture of energy and depressed mood (mixed state) is often accompanied by increased suicidality (see Table 30-5).

Premenstrual dysphoric disorder (PMDD) is currently classified as a research diagnosis by the DSM-IV (Table 30-6). Though up to 75% of women will report minor premenstrual changes in mood, PMDD is thought to affect about 4 to 5% of women in their reproductive years. Its presence implies impairing symptoms of depression and anxiety during the late luteal phase of the menstrual cycle that abate at the onset of menses. About one-half of women who present with such complaints are actually experiencing a

---

TABLE 30-5
CLUES TO THE PRESENCE OF BIPOLARITY AND MIXED STATES

Detection of Subtle "Soft" Bipolar Disorders
Established bipolar family history, or lithium carbonate–responding first-degree relative, or both or loaded three-generational affective disorder pedigrees
Pharmacologically induced hypomania
History of mixed states
Spontaneous episodes of hypomania even when "adaptive"
Premorbid hyperthymic, cyclothymic, irritable, or dysthymic temperament
Periodic depression with abrupt onset and termination or seasonal pattern, especially with psychomotor retardation and hypersomnia
Psychotic depression in a teenager or young adult

Mixed States
Unrelenting dysphoria or irascibility
Severe agitation
Refractory anxiety
Unendurable sexual excitement
Intractable insomnia
Suicidal obsessions and impulses
"Histrionic" demeanor yet with genuine expressions of intense suffering

Adapted from Akiskal HS, Mallya G. Criteria for the "soft" bipolar spectrum: treatment implications. Psychopharmacol Bull 1987;23:68.

premenstrual exacerbation of a preexisting mood or anxiety disorder, and do not qualify for the diagnosis of premenstrual dysphoric disorder. The SSRI antidepressants are often effective in this disorder and may be administered intermittently or continuously with good results. Fluoxetine (Sarafem) is FDA approved for the treatment of PMDD. Both emotional and physical symptoms (bloating, breast tenderness, etc.) respond to SSRI treatment, often within 1 to 3 days.

Anxiety Disorders

As noted previously, anxiety and depression are frequently comorbid. It is useful to review specific diagnostic criteria for several of the anxiety disorders most commonly encountered. Anxiety disorders may have specific responses to psychopharmacologic interventions that overlap and compliment those of mood disorders. In general, anxious/depressive comorbidity identifies illness that is more chronic and associated with poorer outcomes. Important anxiety disorders include:

Generalized Anxiety Disorder

Generalized anxiety disorder is a syndrome of excessive worry lasting for more than 6 months by definition, but typically for years, often with an onset in young adulthood (Table 30-7). It often predates major depression and may be comorbid with dysthymic disorder or panic disorder. In fact, patients with generalized anxiety disorder who manifest significant shortness of breath, smothering sensations, or "air hunger" may be experiencing subsyndromal panic attacks. In this situation, antipanic interventions may be preferred treatments.

TABLE 30-6
RESEARCH CRITERIA FOR PREMENSTRUAL DYSPHORIC DISORDER

A. In most menstrual cycles during the past year, five (or more) of the following symptoms were present for most of the time during the last week of the luteal phase, began to remit within a few days after the onset of the follicular phase, and were absent in the week postmenses, with at least one of the symptoms being either (1), (2), (3), or (4):
  (1) Markedly depressed mood, feelings of hopelessness, or self-deprecating thoughts
  (2) Marked anxiety, tension, feelings of being "keyed up" or "on edge"
  (3) Marked affective lability (e.g., feeling suddenly sad or tearful or increased sensitivity to rejection)
  (4) Persistent and marked anger or irritability or increased interpersonal conflicts
  (5) Decreased interest in usual activities
  (6) Subjective sense of difficulty concentrating
  (7) Lethargy, easy fatigability, or marked lack of energy
  (8) Marked change in appetite, overeating, or specific food cravings
  (9) Hypersomnia or insomnia
  (10) Subjective sense of being overwhelmed or out of control
  (11) Other physical symptoms, such as breast tenderness or swelling, headaches, joint or muscle pain, a sensation of "bloating," weight gain
B. The disturbance markedly interferes with work or school or with usual social activities and relationships with others.
C. The disturbance is not merely an exacerbation of the symptoms of another disorder, such as major depressive disorder, panic disorder, dysthymic disorder, or a personality disorder (although it may be superimposed on any of these disorders).
D. Criteria A, B, and C must be confirmed by prospective daily ratings during at least two consecutive symptomatic cycles. (The diagnosis may be made provisionally prior to this confirmation.)

Diagnostic and statistical manual of mental disorders, 4th ed. Washington DC: American Psychiatric Association, 1994.

TABLE 30-7
DIAGNOSTIC CRITERIA FOR 300.02 GENERALIZED ANXIETY DISORDER

A. Excessive anxiety and worry (apprehensive expectation), occurring more days than not for at least 6 months, about a number of events or activities (such as work or school performance).

B. The person finds it difficult to control the worry.

C. The anxiety and worry are associated with three (or more) of the following six symptoms (with at least some symptoms present for more days than not for the past 6 months). *Note:* Only one item is required in children.
   (1) Restlessness or feeling keyed up or on edge
   (2) Being easily fatigued
   (3) Difficulty concentrating or mind going blank
   (4) Irritability
   (5) Muscle tension
   (6) Sleep disturbance (difficulty falling or staying asleep, or restless unsatisfying sleep)

D. The focus of the anxiety and worry is not confined to features of an axis I disorder, e.g., the anxiety or worry is not about having a panic attack (as in panic disorder), being embarrassed in public (as in social phobia), being contaminated (as in obsessive–compulsive disorder) being away from home or close relatives (as in separation anxiety disorder), gaining weight (as in anorexia nervosa), having multiple physical complaints (as in somatization disorder), or having a serious illness (as in hypochondriasis), and the anxiety and worry do not occur exclusively during posttraumatic stress disorder.

E. The anxiety, worry, or physical symptoms cause clinically significant distress or impairment in social, occupational. or other important areas of functioning.

F. The disturbance is not due to the direct physiologic effects of a substance (e.g.. a drug of abuse, a medication) or a somatic condition (e.g., hyperthyroidism) and does not occur exclusively during a mood disorder, a psychotic disorder, or a pervasive developmental disorder.

Diagnostic and statistical manual of mental disorders, 4th ed. Washington DC: American Psychiatric Association, 1994.

Panic Disorder

Panic disorder is characterized by attacks of intense anxiety, often associated with a fear of impending doom or death. Respiratory symptoms may be the most specific indicators of the syndrome. Panic attacks may trigger agoraphobia—an avoidance of places and situations where help is perceived by the patient to be unavailable or where significant embarrassment may occur (see Table 30-8).

Obsessive–Compulsive Disorder

Obsessive–compulsive disorder is characterized by either distressing, unwanted, obtrusive thoughts, ideas, or images (obsessions are typically related to contamination, safety, or order) or excessive, ritualistic behaviors performed to alleviate anxiety (compulsions are typically cleaning, counting, checking, ordering, saying certain words). The illness is sometimes known as the "doubting disease." In the United States obsessions are more common than compulsions. In Germany, the opposite situation exists (Table 30-9).

Posttraumatic Stress Disorder

Posttraumatic stress disorder is characterized by intrusive recollections of events involving the threat of death or severe harm to the one suffering from the disorder or others. Recollections may be stimulated by places, situations, or other cues related to the event.

Symptoms of physiologic arousal are prominent. A generalized numbness to surroundings and avoidance behaviors are also common (Table 30-10).

THERAPEUTIC ALLIANCE

The establishment of a therapeutic alliance is an essential task in the care of every patient. Patient and physician alike nurture the alliance, since both share accountability for the relationship. The goals of the alliance are shared decision-making and risk-taking and improved communication between patient and practitioner and adherence to the treatment plan. For the purposes of our discussion, the topic of therapeutic alliance has been placed after diagnostic formulation and before treatment selection, because treatment cannot proceed if there is no agreement as to the diagnosis and rationale of treatment. In reality, the therapeutic alliance begins the instant the patient steps into a practitioner's office and develops at every step in the clinical process. Several aspects of the therapeutic alliance are discussed below.

Empathy from the Clinician

Patients need some acknowledgment from their health-care provider that their distress is recognized and is considered legitimate. This should be no

TABLE 30-8
PANIC ATTACKS AND AGORAPHOBIA

Criteria for Panic Attack

Note: A panic attack is not a codable disorder.

A discrete period of intense fear or discomfort, in which four (or more) of the following symptoms developed abruptly and reached a peak within 10 minutes:

(1) Palpitations, pounding heart, or accelerated heart rate	(8) Feeling dizzy, unsteady, lightheaded, or faint
(2) Sweating	(9) Derealization (feelings of unreality) or depersonalization
(3) Trembling or shaking	(being detached from oneself)
(4) Sensations of shortness of breath or smothering	(10) Fear of losing control or going crazy
(5) Feeling of choking	(11) Fear of dying
(6) Chest pain or discomfort	(12) Paresthesias (numbness or tingling sensations)
(7) Nausea or abdominal distress	(13) Chills or hot flushes

Criteria for Agoraphobia

A. Anxiety about being in places or situations from which escape might be difficult (or embarrassing) or in which help may not be available in the event of having an unexpected or situationally predisposed panic attack or panic-like symptoms. Agoraphobic fears typically involve characteristic clusters of situations that include being outside the home alone, being in a crowd, standing in a line, being on a bridge, and traveling in a bus, train, or automobile.

Note: Consider the diagnosis of specific phobia if the avoidance is limited to one or only a few specific situations, or social phobia if the avoidance is limited to social situations.

B. The situations are avoided (e.g. travel is restricted) or else are endured with marked distress or with anxiety about having a panic attack or panic-like symptoms, or require the presence of a companion.

C. The anxiety or phobic avoidance is not better accounted for by another mental disorder, such as social phobia (e.g., avoidance limited to social situations because of fear of embarrassment), specific phobia (e.g., avoidance limited to a single situation like elevators), obsessive–compulsive disorder (e.g., avoidance of dirt in someone with an obsession about contamination), posttraumatic stress disorder (e.g., avoidance of stimuli associated with a severe stressor), or separation anxiety disorder (e.g., avoidance of leaving home or relatives).

Diagnostic and statistical manual of mental disorders, 4th ed. Washington DC: American Psychiatric Association, 1994.

TABLE 30-9
DIAGNOSTIC CRITERIA FOR 300.3 OBSESSIVE–COMPULSIVE DISORDER

A. Either obsessions or compulsions:

Obsessions as defined by (1), (2), (3), and (4)

(1) Recurrent and persistent thoughts, impulses, or images that are experienced, at some time during the disturbance, as intrusive and inappropriate and that cause marked anxiety or distress.

(2) The thoughts, impulses, or images are not simply excessive worries about real-life problems.

(3) The person attempts to ignore or suppress such thoughts, impulses, or images, or to neutralize them with some other thought or action.

(4) The person recognizes that the obsessional thoughts, impulses, or images are a product of his or her own mind (not imposed from without as in thought insertion)

Compulsions as defined by (1) and (2):

(1) Repetitive behaviors (e.g., hand-washing, ordering, checking) or mental acts (e.g., praying, counting, repeating words silently) that the person feels driven to perform in response to an obsession, or according to rules that must be applied rigidly.

(2) The behaviors or mental acts are aimed at preventing or reducing distress or preventing some dreaded event or situation; however, these behaviors or mental acts either are not connected in a realistic way with what they are designed to neutralize or prevent or are clearly excessive.

B. At some point during the course of the disorder, the person has recognized that the obsessions or compulsions are excessive or unreasonable. *Note:* This does not apply to children.

C. The obsessions or compulsions cause marked distress, are time-consuming (take more than 1 hour a day), or significantly interfere with the person's normal routine, occupational (or academic) functioning, or usual social activities or relationships.

D. If another axis I disorder is present, the content of the obsessions or compulsions is not restricted to it (e.g., preoccupation with food in the presence of an eating disorder; hair pulling in the presence of trichotillomania; concern with appearance in the presence of body dysmorphic disorder; preoccupation with drugs in the presence of a substance use disorder; preoccupation with having a serious illness in the presence of hypochondriasis; preoccupation with sexual urges or fantasies in the presence of a paraphilia; or guilty ruminations in the presence of major depressive disorder).

E. The disturbance is not due to the direct physiologic effects of a substance (e.g., a drug of abuse, a medication) or a somatic condition.

Diagnostic and statistical manual of mental disorders, 4th ed. Washington DC: American Psychiatric Association, 1994.

TABLE 30-10
DIAGNOSTIC CRITERIA FOR 309.81 POSTTRAUMATIC STRESS DISORDER

A. The person has been exposed to a traumatic event in which both of the following were present:
  (1) The person experienced, witnessed, or was confronted with an event or events that involved actual or threatened death or serious injury, or a threat to the physical integrity of self or others.
  (2) The person's response involved intense fear, helplessness, or horror. *Note:* In children, this may be expressed instead by disorganized or agitated behavior.
B. The traumatic event is persistently reexperienced in one (or more) of the following ways:
  (1) Recurrent and intrusive distressing recollections of the event, including images, thoughts, or perceptions. *Note:* In young children. repetitive play may occur in which themes or aspects of the trauma are expressed.
  (2) Recurrent distressing dreams of the event. *Note:* In children, there may be frightening dreams without recognizable content.
  (3) Acting or feeling as if the traumatic event were recurring (includes a sense of reliving the experience, illusions, hallucinations, and dissociative flashback episodes, including those that occur on awakening or when intoxicated). *Note:* In young children. trauma–specific reenactment may occur.
  (4) Intense psychological distress at exposure to internal or external cues that symbolize or resemble an aspect of the traumatic event.
  (5) Reactivity on exposure to internal or external cues that symbolize or resemble an aspect of the traumatic event.
C. Persistent avoidance of stimuli associated with the trauma and numbing of general responsiveness (not present before the trauma), as indicated by three (or more) of the following:
  (1) Efforts to avoid thoughts, feelings, or conversations associated with the trauma
  (2) Efforts to avoid activities, places, or people that arouse recollections of the trauma
  (3) Inability to recall an important aspect of the trauma
  (4) Markedly diminished interest or participation in significant activities
  (5) Feeling of detachment or estrangement from others
  (6) Restricted range of affect (e.g., unable to have loving feelings)
  (7) Sense of a foreshortened future (e.g., does not expect to have a career, marriage, children, or a normal life span)
D. Persistent symptoms of increased arousal (not present before the trauma), as indicated by two (or more) of the following:
  (1) Difficulty falling or staying asleep
  (2) Irritability or outbursts of anger
  (3) Difficulty concentrating
  (4) Hypervigilance
  (5) Exaggerated startle response
E. Duration of the disturbance (symptoms in criteria 13, C, and I) is more than 1 month.
F. The disturbance causes clinically significant distress or impairment in social, occupational, or other important areas of functioning.

Specify if:
  Acute: if duration of symptoms is less than 3 months
  Chronic: if duration of symptoms is 3 months or more
Specify if:
  With delayed onset: if onset of symptoms is at least 6 months after the stressor

Diagnostic and statistical manual of mental disorders, 4th ed. Washington DC: American Psychiatric Association, 1994.

problem for the anxious or depressed patient, since scientific evidence abounds to document the dysfunction experienced. Unfortunately, many clinicians still consider mental illness to be the result of personal weakness or project the attitude that they cannot be bothered with such matters.

Honesty from Both Clinician and Patient

Honesty leads to more and better communication with the patient. This results in a more accurate diagnosis and fewer misunderstandings about the nature of the illness and the rationale, potential risks, expected benefits of treatment, and treatment alternatives.

Assessment of a Patient's Health Beliefs and Readiness to Proceed

Patients, like clinicians, carry biases about the nature of mental illness and what constitutes acceptable treatment. Some patients may need several clinical encounters before a treatment contract can be negotiated.

Education to Improve Understanding of the Illness in Question

This is a critical and ongoing process that may include didactics at the bedside, written information, video presentations, interaction with community resources, or referral for outside consultation.

Shared Decision-Making

When clinicians assume a dominant role, patients may be left feeling powerless. For these patients, noncompliance is a common method of regaining control. Patients who share equally in making reasonable choices about their care will be more adherent, less likely to experience anger toward their caregivers, and less likely to take legal action in the event of a negative outcome.

Respect for Boundaries

Clinicians must respect the right of competent patients to make decisions about their health care, even when they strongly disagree about the rationale and potential effects of those decisions. Conversely, patients must respect the clinician's ethical mandate to act responsibly. There may be occasions when individual agendas or personal styles become burdensome to one party in the alliance. In these cases, an amicable parting with referral to a colleague is advisable before anger and resentment cloud clinical judgment.

SELECTION OF TREATMENT METHODS

Basis

The selection of treatment methods for the depressed and/or anxious patient involves consideration of three areas—acuity level, biologic underpinnings of the disorder(s) present, and the psychosocial context of the illness.

Acuity Level

Although many depressed and anxious patients can be treated adequately in an outpatient setting by a primary care physician, there are instances when consultation or referral is advised. The first such instance involves illness that contains significant suicidal ideation or plans. Women in general attempt suicide more often than men do. They typically choose less lethal means when making attempts, but the risk of death is still real. All depressed and anxious patients should be questioned about feelings of hopelessness, a sensitive measure of suicidality, whether they are experiencing thoughts of death, and whether suicide attempts have been made in the past. Patients deemed at risk should be immediately referred to appropriate care.

Clinicians differ in their interest in treating mentally distressed patients in their practices. Some clinicians who are otherwise interested do not have the time to properly assess and treat these individuals. There are also instances when the complexity of the psychopharmacology or the psychosocial support required for proper management may simply be beyond one's skills and scope of practice. Caregivers should always practice within the boundaries of their training, experience, and proven ability.

Biological Underpinnings

Psychiatric illness has biologic underpinnings that are often specific to treatment. Treatment must be targeted to address the disorders present. An effort should be made to use medications that are safe, effective, and well tolerated. Pertinent areas of consideration are discussed below.

SUBTYPE. Mood disorders are heterogeneous in cause and presentation. Recognized subtypes may suggest specific treatments.

Regardless of the various psychiatric disorders in an individual patient, the foundation of proper management in mood disorders is the differentiation of unipolar from bipolar conditions. Awareness of the historical (i.e., onset in childhood or adolescence, high frequency of episodes) and treatment responses that suggest bipolarity is crucial. Longitudinal assessment is often necessary. Many clinicians may be unfamiliar with the range of comorbidities that are possible. Panic attacks, obsessive–compulsive symptoms, social phobia, and substance-related disorders, among others, can all be the presenting manifestations of bipolar illness or may be comorbid with it. Bipolar disorders usually require mood stabilizers like lithium, valproate, or carbamazepine as the primary component of medical management. Antidepressants, benzodiazepines, antipsychotics, and the like can be added to mood stabilizers as indicated by comorbid findings and treatment response.

Likewise, symptom clusters may define subtypes and suggest effective therapy. For example, atypical depressions respond poorly to tricyclic antidepressants (TCAs). SSRIs and bupropion work better. Monoamine oxidase inhibitors (MAOIs) are also effective, but require dietary restrictions and avoidance of drug-drug interactions that may cause harm. Using sedating antidepressants to target insomnia has not correlated with improved antidepressant response.

PREVIOUS RESPONSE. Many patients will have had previous treatment experiences. Those experiences which produce significant, stable responses are good places to start when considering the treatment plan for the current episode of illness. However, clinicians should be careful when asking about past treatments. The severity of past episodes, symptom manifestations, and the quality of the response, reproducibility, and associated side effects should be evaluated.

COMORBIDITY. The coexistence of other disorders or conditions can be a useful guide to medical management. Examples include:

1. Medical comorbidity—Some somatic illnesses may be aggravated by certain psychopharmacologic interventions. For example, tricyclic antidepressants may worsen hyperglycemia in diabetes mellitus or induce dangerous arrhythmias in patients with coronary artery disease or recent myocardial infarction. Patients with chronic pain and depression or anxiety often find that their pain is more tolerable during antidepressant treatment. Bipolar patients with migraine headache may benefit from valproate's known effectiveness in migraine.
2. Anxiety disorders—Anxiety is usually responsive to antidepressant therapy with some allowance made for anxiety subtype in antidepressant selection (Table 30-11).
3. Pregnancy—Issues regarding antidepressant use during pregnancy and breastfeeding were discussed earlier.

Psychosocial context

As discussed earlier, psychosocial context is largely responsible for defining illness from a disorder. As pervasive illnesses with far-reaching implications, depression and anxiety often require intervention for this context. Important interventions to consider are discussed below.

SUPPORTIVE THERAPY. This is the encouragement, education, and human support that reside within the therapeutic alliance. In many cases, this may be the only psychotherapy needed. Despite misconceptions to the contrary, primary care providers can deliver supportive therapy within the time constraints of ambulatory practice. Stuart and Lieberman's *The Fifteen-Minute Hour* provides an excellent guideline for such interaction.

FORMAL PSYCHOTHERAPY. Two forms of psychotherapy deserve specific mention here. The first, cognitive therapy or rational-emotive therapy (RET) focuses on the irrational beliefs, thoughts, and feelings that often accompany depression. Cognitive therapy postulates that depressed feelings can often be reinforced by automatic negative thoughts that lack a rational basis. These thoughts are further reinforced by negative beliefs about self, the world, and the future. Patients are given techniques to combat these maladaptive patterns of thinking. Cognitive therapy is particularly useful in support of the chronically depressed patient. Interpersonal therapy (IPT) focuses on the transitions, role identity and conflict that can trigger depressed episodes. There is evidence for the usefulness of IPT as an effective maintenance therapy in recurrent depression.

SOCIAL WORK CONSULTATION. Social work services can be extremely helpful when legal or economic issues are prominent, or when community resources

---

TABLE 30-11
PSYCHOPHARMACOLOGIC INTERVENTIONS WITH SOMATIC OR ANXIETY DISORDER COMORBIDITY

Comorbid Condition	Possible Clinical Intervention
Diabetes mellitus	Avoid TCA or others associated with weight gain
Migraine headache requiring prophylaxis	TCA, SSRI, MAOI, valproate, lithium
Cluster headache requiring prophylaxis	Lithium, valproate
Tension headache requiring prophylaxis	TCA, SSRI, atypical antidepressants
Irritable-bowel syndrome	TCA, buspirone
Fibrositis/fibromyalgia	TCA, SSRI
Chronic pain/neuralgia	TCA, SSRI, atypical antidepressants, anticonvulsants
Coronary artery disease	Avoid TCA
Generalized anxiety disorder	TCA, SSRI, venlafaxine, buspirone
Panic disorder	TCA, SSRI, MAOI. Avoid bupropion, trazodone, buspirone
Obsessive–compulsive disorder	SSRI, clomipramine
Posttraumatic stress disorder	SSRI, MAOI

can be brought to bear in support of a distressed patient. Social workers are problem-solvers who often have expertise in psychotherapy. They make excellent partners in patient care.

MANAGEMENT OF TREATMENT

Therapeutic Goals

The goal of therapy is robust, sustained response and normalcy. While normalcy may be difficult to define for a particular individual, it implies an absence of symptoms and a level of functioning typified by productivity, flexibility, and resilience. This level of response is best achieved for most patients by combining biological and psychotherapeutic interventions, including lifestyle changes that are known to be beneficial to healthy emotional states. Regular exercise, adequate rest, proper diet, and avoidance of excessive alcohol and caffeine, among others, are important ancillary measures that will improve mental and general health.

Response rates to single antidepressants alone are approximately 60 to 70%. These figures are deceptive, however, when one considers that response in controlled trials is defined as a 50% improvement in the clinical scale used to track symptoms. For a moderately to severely depressed individual with a Hamilton Depression Rating Scale (HAM-D) of 30, this means a positive response for that person will be recorded if the final HAM-D score is 15. This suggests clinical improvement, of course, but a score of 15 still correlates with significant symptoms of depression and dysfunction. Clinical trials compare average improvement in depression for treated and placebo groups. It is easy to see that many individuals in trials of single antidepressants will not achieve full symptomatic remission. The rate of complete response to single antidepressants given at an adequate dose and duration is 40 to 60%.

Adequate treatment requires success in two areas. The first is in completeness of symptom remission. For most patients this correlates with a HAM-D score of less than 7. The second component is consistency of symptom relief. Some patients have responses that plateau or fade with time. Others will have a fragile response that leaves their mood vulnerable to external or internal stressors. This fragility has been referred to as reactivity, a term that may become perjorative, if reactivity becomes equated with character

defects or personality problems. Still others will cycle abruptly between improvement, hypomania or mania, and various levels of depressive or anxious symptoms. For many patients a rational polypharmacy will be necessary to fully control symptoms of depression and anxiety.

Psychopharmacology

Adequate dose and duration of therapy is the cornerstone of the medical therapy of depression and anxiety after an accurate working diagnosis is made. Within the boundaries of that diagnosis it is useful to select medications that are well tolerated and dosed conveniently. Several classes of agents deserve comment (Table 30-12) and are discussed below.

Tricyclic Antidepressants (TCAs)

TCAs are still effective, logical choices for well-chosen patients. The secondary amine members (nortriptyline, desipramine) are preferred due to better tolerability. The older members amitriptyline, imipramine, doxepin, or the heterocyclic trazodone are associated with higher side-effect profiles and generally are not good choices, unless the patient reports that a previous treatment with one of these agents was effective and well tolerated.

Serotonin-Specific Reuptake Inhibitors (SSRIs)

To date, these agents do not seem to differ significantly in spectra of activity. Minor differences in side-effect profiles may be seen, but are of limited significance as well. SSRIs are broad-spectrum antidepressant/anxiolytics that are well tolerated in most patients. Many consider them drugs of first choice in depression and anxiety treatment.

Aminoketones

Bupropion is the only available member. It is chemically unrelated to TCAs and SSRIs. It may have dopaminergic and noradrenergic activity. Bupropion is especially useful in atypical depressions, bipolar depression, smoking cessation, and in situations where sexual dysfunction as a side effect must be avoided.

Newer Tetracyclics

Mirtazapine is the only available member and is a potent $5-HT_2$ and $5-HT_3$ antagonist. It probably enhances central noradrenergic and serotonergic activity.

TABLE 30-12

PSYCHOPHARMACOLOGIC AGENTS USED IN THE TREATMENT OF DEPRESSION AND ANXIETY

Agent	Type	Starting Dose (mg/day)	Usual Total Daily Dose in Continuation Therapy (mg)	Typical Dose Titration	Comments
Nortriptyline	TCA	25	75–125	25 mg /3–5 days	Therapeutic window of plasma levels 50–150 ng/ml
Desipramine	TCA	25	100–200	25 mg/3–5 days	
Fluoxetine	SSRI	20	20–40	20 mg/4–6 weeks	Doses may be higher in OCD. Lower starting doses and slower titrations are advisable in panic disorder or in the presence of severe anxiety.
Sertraline	SSRI	50	100–200	50 mg/4–6 weeks	Doses may be higher in OCD. Lower starting doses and slower titrations are advisable in panic disorder or in the presence of severe anxiety.
Paroxetine	SSRI	20	20–40	20 mg/4–6 weeks	Doses may be higher in OCD. Lower starting doses and slower titrations are advisable in panic disorder or in the presence of severe anxiety.
Fluvoxamine	SSRI	50	100–300	50 mg/2–3 weeks	Doses may be higher in OCD. Lower starting doses and slower titrations are advisable in panic disorder or in the presence of severe anxiety.
Bupropion	Aminoketone	150 (sustained release)	300–400 (sustained release)	To 300 mg/day after 3–5 days	Added Norepinephrine reuptake inhibition at doses ≥ 225 mg/d
Venlafaxine	Novel	37.5 (extended release)	150–300 (extended release)	37.5 mg/1–2 weeks	
Nefazodone	Novel	200	300–600	50–100 mg/5–7 days	Rapid titration to 30 mg/day may reduce somnolence. 30 mg/day typical for generalized anxiety disorder.
Mirtazapine	Tetracyclic	15	15–45	15 mg/2 weeks	
Buspirone	Azapirone	15	30–60	10 mg/3–4 weeks	
Alprazolam	BZ	0.5 mg tid or 0.5 mg 1–3X per day prn	Variable, 3–5 mg for panic disorder, 0.25–1.5 mg in other situations	Rapid upward titration to therapeutic effect	Slow discontinuation of maintenance doses to avoid rebound symptoms and seizures.
Lorazepam	BZ	0.5 mg bid or bid prn	Variable, 4 mg for panic disorder, 0.5–1.0 mg in other situations	Same as above	Slow discontinuation of maintenance doses to avoid rebound symptoms and seizures.
Clonazepam	BZ	0.5 mg bid or bid prn	Variable, 2 mg for panic disorder, 0.5–1.5 mg in other situations	Same as above	Slow discontinuation of maintenance doses to avoid rebound symptoms and seizures.
Lithium	Novel	300	600–1500	300 mg/5–7 days	Usual therapeutic level is 0.6–1.0 mEq/liter.
Valproate	AED	250–500	500–1500 (10–15 mg/kg)	250 mg/3–5 days	Loading doses of 20 mg/kg/day often used in acute mania. Preferred over lithium in dysphoric (mixed) mania. Typical therapeutic level 50–100 μg/ml.
Carbamazepine	AED	200	400–1200	200 mg/–14 days	Plasma levels do not correlate with antimanic activity.

Novel Agents

Venlafaxine, nefazodone, and buspirone are examples. They are chemically unrelated. Venlafaxine and nefazodone are combined serotonin/noradrenergic reuptake inhibitors. Nefazodone is also a 5-HT$_2$ antagonist. Buspirone is an azapirone with 5-HT$_{1A}$ receptor affinity. It is an anxiolytic, indicated for generalized anxiety disorder, but has some antidepressant activity, particularly at higher doses (40 to 60 mg per day), and has been used to augment SSRI nonresponse.

Benzodiazepines (BZs)

A number of specific BZs are available. They are useful as adjuncts in the treatment of the anxious patient, but antidepressants are becoming first-line treatments for most anxiety disorders. Benzodiazepines are indicated for generalized anxiety disorder and several have antipanic activity and may be used alone or in combination with antidepressants in panic disorder patients. A few anxious or depressed patients may require extended treatment with combinations of antidepressants and benzodiazepines for best results.

Lithium

Lithium is a mood stabilizer that has significant antidepressant activity in many patients. It can be used to augment the effects of antidepressants.

Antiepileptic Drugs (AEDs)

Divalproex, carbamazepine, lamotrigine, and other anticonvulsants are being recognized as useful in the management of bipolar mood disorders and some anxiety disorders. They are considered mood stabilizers.

Follow-up and Length of Treatment

Patients just beginning treatment should be monitored frequently for tolerance, adherence, and efficacy. Weekly or biweekly office or phone visits will help strengthen the therapeutic alliance, and offer opportunities to demonstrate empathy, answer questions, reinforce rationale, and troubleshoot medication effects and needs. Since the clinical process is based on longitudinal assessment, the database should be reviewed regularly for masked or new problems. Evidence of substance abuse/dependency, and eating disorders, among others, is often hidden. The psychosocial context of the illness typically unfolds over time with careful history-taking. Any treatment plan is a work in progress, and changes are made when indicated.

Current guidelines recommend that an episode of depression or anxiety be treated for 6 to 9 months after symptoms resolve. For those with three or more previous major depressive episodes, maintenance therapy at acute antidepressant dosages may be recommended due to relapse rates that approach 100%. Remembering that most primary care patients with anxiety and depression are recurrently or chronically ill, many will benefit from maintenance treatment. Clinicians should inform patients of the risk of relapse and discuss the benefits and risks relative to the situation.

Factors that favor discontinuance (episodic treatment) are:

1. Cost savings
2. Avoidance of side effects, if any, including potential drug–drug interactions, and effects on a developing fetus.
3. Avoidance of long-term effects (if any arise from future study).
4. Less than a 100% risk of relapse for many patients, or relapse separated by long periods of time.

Factors that favor maintenance therapy are:

1. Risk of relapse is present for most patients and many will promptly relapse on discontinuance.
2. Insidious relapses are possible. This may interfere with the early reinstitution of treatment and result in dysfunction and negative consequences.
3. Avoidance of the impairment/disability commonly associated with illness.
4. Potential for refractory status on relapse.

Using Response Patterns as a Guide to Effective Management

Useful information can be obtained by observing one's response to medical treatment with antidepressants. Some patterns of response are common.

1. "Normal" response. Symptomatic improvement begins slowly 2 to 3 weeks after the drug dose reaches a therapeutic level. Continuation of treatment results in full remission of the illness in 6 to 12 weeks.
2. Plateau response. Symptomatic improvement begins on schedule, and may reach full remission levels, but after some weeks the patient experiences a partial relapse. This is not uncommon with TCAs and may occur with other antidepressants. Plateau may be a result of inadequate dose titration, tolerance to medication effects, or increasing

metabolism of the medication. Normally, only a dose increase is required to recover lost response. The body's ability to cause plateau is generally limited. There is usually a stable dose beyond which plateau does not recur.

3. Nonresponse. In this scenario, adequate doses of a particular antidepressant fail to induce symptom remission. Nonresponse can be complete or partial. Two types may be recognized: In stable nonresponse improvement is incomplete, but consistently so. No abrupt switches in activity or mood that may be indicative of bipolar illness are seen. In stable nonresponse a dose increase into the upper ranges of the recommended dosage of the antidepressant may be indicated, or more time for response may be needed. Switching to an antidepressant in a different class may overcome the problem. Augmentation strategies are often useful. In nonstable nonresponse the patient has better days and worse days, usually with a pattern of abrupt onset and termination. This pattern may suggest occult bipolar illness. De novo hypomania (or mania) may be seen. Augmentation with lithium may be a good strategy in this scenario, or a discontinuance of the antidepressant with a rebuilding of treatment on a foundation of mood stabilizers may be in order. Antidepressant-induced mixed states are a form of nonstable nonresponse.

Augmentation Strategies

When depression fails to respond adequately to an antidepressant trial, the clinician is faced with a therapeutic dilemma. A reassessment of the accuracy of the working diagnosis and consideration of confounding factors should precede changes in the treatment plan. Medical nonadherence, physical or emotional abuse, and unrecognized substance disorders, bipolar disorder, eating disorders, or obsessive–compulsive disorder are common causes of treatment failure. An unrecognized somatic condition like diabetes mellitus, hypothyroidism, or occult malignancy may also be present.

If the working diagnosis is confirmed and no complicating conditions are discovered, the decision in medical management centers on switching to another antidepressant (often, though in the case of SSRIs not necessarily, in another class) or augmenting the current antidepressant with another medication. Augmentation strategies are fairly new. Many clinicians prefer to try another antidepressant before

using augmentations. This is acceptable care in most instances. There are few data to suggest one strategy over the other. Since augmentation methods often work in days rather than weeks and obviate the need to discontinue one medication and reinstitute and titrate another, a strong case can be made for augmentation as a preferred initial strategy in refractory cases, especially if the patient already has a partial response to monotherapy. Consultation may be helpful in case selection.

Some commonly used augmentation strategies have been rigidly tested. Others are supported by open investigation only. Examples include:

1. Lithium. The best-studied and most effective augmentation strategy. Success rates range from 50 to 60%. Effective in unipolar and bipolar patients. Antidepressant augmentation may occur at lithium levels as low as 0.3 mEq/liter within days, but several weeks at levels of 0.7 mEq/liter or higher are necessary for an adequate trial.

2. Thyroid. Supported by controlled trials. Triiodothyronine (T_3) or levothyroxine (T_4) may be used. T_3 is preferred by many. T_3 doses start with 25 μg daily and titrated to 50 μg if needed. T_4 doses vary from 50 to 200 μg per day.

3. SSRI augmentation with TCA, trazodone, bupropion, or mirtazepine. Supported by open studies. For TCA, small doses are advisable because of cytochrome-P450 inhibition by most SSRIs. Bupropion may be useful for augmentation or to treat SSRI sexual dysfunction. Starting doses of 75 mg each morning may be advanced as tolerated.

4. SSRI augmentation with buspirone. Supported by open studies. Buspirone doses of 40 to 60 mg/day are used.

5. Psychotherapy. Often helpful with complex psychosocial contexts and chronic illness.

SUGGESTED READING

Akiskal HS. The prevalent clinical spectrum of bipolar disorders: beyond DSM-IV. J Clin Psychiatry 1996; 16(1 Suppl):4s.

American Psychiatric Association. Practice guideline for major depressive disorder in adults. Am J Psychiatry 1993; 150(4 Suppl):1.

Depression Guideline Panel. Depression in primary care. Vol. 1: Detection and diagnosis; Vol. 2: Treatment of major depression. Clinical Practice Guideline, no. 5. Rockville, MD: Department of Health and Human Services, Public Health Service, Agency for Health Care Policy and Research, 1993. AHCPR Publication no. 93-0550(1).

Diagnostic and statistical manual of mental disorders. 4th ed. Washington, DC: American Psychiatric Association, 1994.

Diagnostic and statistical manual of mental disorders. 4th ed. Primary care version (DSM-IV-PC). Washington, DC: American Psychiatric Association, 1995.

Goodwin FK, Jamison KR. Manic-depressive illness. New York: Oxford University Press, 1990.

Kessler RC. The prevalence of psychiatry comorbidity. In: Wetzler S, Sanderson WC, eds. Treatment strategies for patients with psychiatric comorbidity. New York: Wiley, 1997:23.

Kessler RC, McGonagle K, Zhao S, et al. Lifetime and 12-month prevalence of DSM-III-R psychiatric disorders in the United States: results from the National Comorbidity Survey. Arch Gen Psychiatry 1994;51:8.

Manning JS, Haykal RF, Akiskal HS. The role of bipolarity in depression in the family practice setting. In: Akiskal HS,

ed. Bipolarity: beyond classic mania. Psychiatr Clin North Am 1999;22:689.

Mental Health: A Report of the Surgeon General. Washington, DC: Department of Health and Human Services. Office of the Surgeon General, 1999.

Regier DA, Narrow WE, Rae DS, et al. The defacto mental and addictive disorders service system: epidemiologic catchment area prospective 1-year prevalence rates of disorders and services. Arch Gen Psychiatry 1993;50:85.

Savino M, Perugi G, Simonlini E, et al. Affective comorbidity in panic disorders: is there a bipolar connection? J Affect Disord 1993;28:155.

Stern TA, Herman JB, Slavin PL, eds. The MGH guide to psychiatry in primary care. New York: McGraw-Hill, 1998.

Stuart M, Lieberman J. The fifteen minute hour: applied psychotherapy for the primary care physician. New York: Praeger, 1986.

Chapter 31
Substance Abuse/Dependence

Verneeta L. Williams
James Franks

Five Key Points

- Alcoholism generally progresses from occasional relief drinking to constant relief drinking and ultimately to increased alcohol dependency.

- Fetal alcohol syndrome is the leading cause of mental retardation in the United States.

- Alcohol dependency and abuse affect all organ systems of the body.

- Acute alcohol withdrawal and long-term abstinence involve specific pharmacologic therapy as well as psychotherapy.

- Long-term abstinence from alcohol, sedatives, opiates, amphetamines, and caffeine-containing products requires a highly motivated patient and a multidisciplinary team.

ALCOHOLISM

Case Summary

B.C. started drinking alcohol as a child and increased her alcohol intake while in high school. She would drink alcohol "to get drunk" mostly on weekends while at parties because it made her emotionally free and happy. From her teen years into her 20s, the amount of alcohol consumed increased. Eventually, she married and continued to drink alcohol with her husband, mostly during the weekends. B.C. could control exactly when she drank; however, she could not control the quantity of alcohol consumed, i.e., when she drank, she never knew for sure if she would consume more than one drink per episode. B.C. had a low tolerance for alcohol. After consuming three glasses of wine, she would experience headaches and other symptoms of a hangover.

B.C. had a very strong family history of alcoholism, most prevalent in her mother. Subsequently, she attempted to stop drinking over a 2-week period. When it did not work, she began attending Adult Children of Alcoholics meetings. During a 4-year period, she continued to drink alcohol, but attempted to control how much and how often she drank. This also did not work.

B.C. and her husband were planning to have a family but were not initially successful. They were seriously considering in vitro fertilization when B.C. had a life-changing experience. She became intensely afraid of the injections that would be required during in vitro fertilization and this fear began to permeate into other areas in her life. She ultimately began attending Alcoholics Anonymous meetings as well as individual therapy. Today, B.C. is sober and living a victorious life with her son.

This case is one example of the prevalence of alcoholism in America. The alcoholic generally progresses from occasional relief drinking to constant

TABLE 31-1
TERMS AND CRITERIA FOR PATTERNS OF ALCOHOL USE

Term	Criterion
Moderate drinking (NIAAA)	Men: ≤2 drinks/day Women: ≤1 drink/day Over 65: ≤1 drink/day
At-risk drinking (NIAAA)	Men: >14 drinks/wk or >3 drinks/occasion Women: >7 drinks/wk or >3 drinks/occasion
Alcohol abuse (APA)	Maladaptive pattern of alcohol use leading to clinically significant impairment or distress, manifested within a 12-mo period by one or more of the following: failure to fulfill role obligations at work, school, or home; recurrent use in hazardous situations; legal problems related to alcohol; continued use despite alcohol-related social or interpersonal problems; symptoms have never met criteria for alcohol dependence

Alcohol dependence (APA)	Maladaptive pattern of alcohol use leading to clinically significant impairment or distress, manifested within a 12-mo period by three or more of the following:
	   Tolerance (either increasing amounts used or diminished effects with the same amount)
	   Withdrawal (withdrawal symptoms or use to relieve or avoid symptoms)
	   Use of larger amounts over a longer period than intended
	   Persistent desire or unsuccessful attempts to cut down or control use
	   Great deal of time spent obtaining or using or recovering from use
	   Important social, occupational, or recreational activities given up or reduced
	   Use despite knowledge of alcohol-related physical or psychological problems

Hazardous use (WHO)	Person at risk for adverse consequences
Harmful use (WHO)	Use resulting in physical or psychological harm

*NIAAA = National Institute on Alcohol Abuse and Alcoholism; APA = American Psychiatric Association; WHO = World Health Organization.

relief drinking to ultimately increased dependence on alcohol. The Diagnostic and Statistical Manual of Mental Disorders, 4th ed. (DSM-IV), distinguishes alcohol abuse from alcohol dependency (Table 31-1). The alcohol abuser uses alcohol for >12 months, resulting in detrimental effects in her life (i.e., work, family, and school). The definition of alcohol dependence includes tolerance and withdrawal symptoms and signs.

Alcohol is an equal opportunity employer. The primary care physician sees medical and surgical patients. Substantial numbers of patients have problems with alcohol at one time or another in their lives.[1] These alcohol problems may involve every organ system as well as produce various behavioral illnesses. Table 31-2 lists clinical manifestations and disorders associated with alcohol abuse.

Given the variety of medical and behavioral illnesses associated with alcohol use, it is important for the primary care physician to consider alcoholism in the differential diagnosis when evaluating a patient. Alcohol-associated illnesses generally have a gradually progressive pattern, with the patient often presenting early in the illness, during the mid-teen years. For example, a woman presenting in her teens with intermittent abdominal pain may be diagnosed with a behavioral disorder, while the same presentation during her 20s and 30s may be diagnosed as gastritis or peptic ulcer disease. Generally, as the alcoholic female patient continues to abuse alcohol, the health risks and environmental impact of her drinking increases.

Epidemiology

Within Western societies, 90% of people consume an alcoholic beverage at some time in their life.[2] "Data from the Epidemiologic Catchment Area (ECA) studies suggest that 13.8% of American Adults have abused or become dependent on alcohol at some

TABLE 31-2
CLINICAL MANIFESTATIONS AND DISORDERS ASSOCIATED WITH ALCOHOL ABUSE

Central nervous system—dementia, insomnia, peripheral neuropathy, cognitive, impairment
Cardiovascular—hypertension, vascular disease
Immunologic—recurrent infections, head and neck carcinomas
Hematologic—thrombocytopenia, anemia (megaloblastic)
Endocrine—amenorrhea, diminished fertility, anovulation, premature menopause
Nutritional—folate and thiamine deficiency, Wernicke–Korsakoff syndrome
Fetal—fetal alcohol syndrome
Gastrointestinal—carcinomas, pancreatitis, gastritis, esophageal varices, cirrhosis, malabsorption syndromes

point in their life."[3] The lifetime risk for alcoholism is 10% in men and 5% in women. There is a difference in alcohol consumption in specific populations. No single ethnic group is immune to alcoholism. Black Americans (both men and women) tend to begin heavy alcohol drinking later in life, but reportedly have more alcohol-related problems.[4] Native Americans have the highest rate of alcohol abuse, which is approximately 15% (varying from tribe to tribe).[4] Asian Americans reportedly have the lowest rate of alcoholism.[4] Women abuse alcohol but have a lower level of consumption than men. This is thought to be due to lower body fat and thus a lower volume of distribution as well as decreased activity of alcohol dehydrogenase.[1] Despite decreased alcohol intake in women, they are more often the recipients of the deleterious effects of alcohol abuse (i.e., spousal abuse, depression, divorce, separation, and violence).[5] Women also tend to have a later onset of alcohol abuse than men.[6]

Physiology/Mechanism of Action/Pharmacology

Typically, a standard drink equals 30 ml, or 1 fluid oz, of whiskey, 2 oz of fortified wine, 4 oz of table wine, or 10 to 12 oz of beer.[7] Each of these beverages has approximately 10 to 12 g of alcohol. Ethanol is metabolized in the liver to acetaldehyde by the enzyme alcohol dehydrogenase. Acetaldehyde is then metabolized to acetate by acetaldehyde dehydrogenase (which is one of the enzymes inhibited by disulfiram). Low amounts of alcohol are also directly excreted through urine, sweat, and the lungs.[8] Because alcohol is soluble in water and fat, one's blood alcohol level (BAL) is dependent on body weight, distribution of fat, and liver metabolism, which decreases with age and comorbid conditions. For example, 12 g of alcohol found in a standard drink will take approximately 1 hour to be metabolized and result in a BAL of 0.02 g/dl or 20 mg/dl if one drinks 1 drink per hour. In most states, a BAL of 80 mg/dl or 100 mg/dl defines legal intoxication.

Alcohol acts as a central nervous system (CNS) depressant. Alcohol potentiates the effects of other CNS depressants, including benzodiazepines and barbiturates. The resultant behaviors can be manifested as depression, mania, suicidal tendencies, anxiety, dementia, and psychosis. Behavioral changes can be observed with a BAL as low as 20 mg/dl and overdose and death can occur with a BAL of 300 to

400 mg/dl.[5] The mechanism of alcohol's effect on the CNS is only partially understood.[5] Liver metabolism of alcohol involves several oxidative processes in which the use of nicotinamide adenine dinucleotide (NAD) is one rate-limiting step. As cellular tolerance to alcohol develops (after daily use of alcohol over 1 to 2 weeks), larger amounts of cofactors and other enzymes are needed to metabolize ingested alcohol. Moreover, the liver's ability to metabolize alcohol can be maximized, resulting in direct passage of alcohol from the bloodstream to the brain.

Maternal–Fetal Effects of Alcoholism

As alcohol is metabolized to acetaldehyde and is distributed throughout a woman's bloodstream, it easily crosses the placenta and is directly toxic to the unborn fetus. It has been reported that placental distribution of alcohol is increased during the third trimester.[3] Alcohol not only has a direct toxic effect on the unborn fetus (through cardiovascular abnormalities and impaired growth), it can indirectly affect the delivery of nutrients and oxygen to the fetus.[3,9]

Fetal alcohol syndrome (FAS) is the leading cause of mental retardation in the United States. The overall incidence of FAS in the United States is 1 to 3 cases per 1000 live births. In contrast, the Native American population has a rate of 9.8 cases per 1000 live births.[9]

The severity of fetal abnormalities appears to be alcohol-dose–related. For example, about 10% of women who drink 1 to 2 oz of ethanol per day in the first trimester have infants with FAS, while approximately 50% of women who drink six ounces per day have infants with FAS (Table 31-3).

Other abnormalities such as strabismus, ear malformation, musculoskeletal defects (spina bifida), myopia,

---

TABLE 31-3
CRITERIA FOR FETAL ALCOHOL SYNDROME DIAGNOSIS

An infant with FAS must have one feature from each of the categories:

I.   Prenatal and postnatal growth retardation, with abnormally small-for-age weight, length, and head circumference continuing into adulthood.

II. CNS disorders, with signs of abnormal brain functioning, delays in behavioral development, and/or intellectual impairment.

III. At least two of the following abnormal craniofacial features—microcephaly, microphthalmia, short epicanthal folds, a hypoplastic absent philtrum, thin vermilion border, or flattened midface area renal abnormalities, undescended testicles, and hernias have also been associated with FAS.[9]

Factors associated with increased risk of an infant having FAS include persistent drinking throughout pregnancy, being African-American, multiparity, and the presence of alcohol related problems (as measured by the Michigan Alcohol Screening Test-MAST).[9] When the previously listed four characteristics were present, women had an 85% chance of having a baby with FAS versus a 2% chance if none of these risk factors were present.

For women who drink alcohol in smaller quantities throughout pregnancy, less severe behavioral and physical characteristics observed in the fetus are classified, by the American Medical Association, as fetal alcohol effects.[9] Researchers have observed various observations concerning the severity of fetal effects of alcohol use in association with the amount and duration and onset of alcohol use in pregnancy. (For example, binge drinking may place the fetus at greater risk for FAS than continuous intake of 1 to 2 drinks/day). However, the most important conclusion is that there is no safe level of alcohol intake that a fetus should be exposed to during pregnancy.

Alcohol is also transmitted in breast milk, where it reaches the same concentration as in the bloodstream.[9] Thus, with continuous breast-feeding, the infant will have a constant exposure to alcohol that can be clinically manifested as irritability, abnormal weight gain, and lethargy.

Pregnancy outcomes in women who drink alcohol are complicated by increased risk of spontaneous miscarriage and stillbirth. Obstetrical complications include an increased incidence of placenta previa, vaginal bleeding, and fetal distress. In addition, research shows that women in their second trimester who have 1 to 2 drinks per day have increasing obstetrical complications.[9]

Medical Complication of Alcoholism

Alcohol dependency and abuse affect all organ systems. In the central nervous system, heavy drinking can produce an alcoholic blackout, where an individual forgets part of what occurred while she was drinking.[2] These blackouts typically occur with acute alcohol intake. Sleep latency is also decreased with acute alcohol intake. Alcohol withdrawal symptoms can occur 24 to 48 hours after cessation of drinking and include elevations in blood pressure and pulse rate, nausea, vomiting, sweating, anxiety, and abnormal

sleeping patterns. The alcoholic typically resumes drinking, which ends the above symptoms. Alcoholic withdrawal seizures may occur 7 to 38 hours after cessation of alcohol drinking.[6] Alcohol withdrawal delirium, or delirium tremens, is defined as perceptual disturbances, clouded consciousness, and hallucinations, along with the usual signs and symptoms seen with alcohol withdrawal. Delirium tremens may develop within 2 to 3 days following the cessation of drinking, and may last for up to 4 or 5 weeks. The mortality associated with delirium tremens is less than 1%. Moreover, one-third of patients who experience alcohol withdrawal seizures go on to have delirium tremens.[6]

Chronic alcohol intake can also induce a peripheral neuropathy where distal extremities are affected, Wernicke encephalopathy (characterized by ophthalmoplegia, ataxia, and confusion), and Korsakoff syndrome (where the affected person has retrograde amnesia).[6] These problems are associated with thiamine and vitamin B deficiencies. Treatment of Wernicke encephalopathy with thiamine may reverse the symptoms. Other CNS-related problems with alcohol abuse include cerebellar degeneration and atrophy, alcoholic dementia, and psychiatric difficulties, including hallucinations (which are generally visual, occurring within 24 hours after cessation of drinking and lasting for minutes to days), paranoid delusions, anxiety, and depression.

Cardiovascular problems associated with alcohol abuse include hypertension and dilated cardiomyopathy. Prolonged use of alcohol can cause an increase in blood pressure that can ultimately lead to a dilated cardiomyopathy. The dilated cardiomyopathy can produce arrhythmias, mural thrombi, and mitral-valve regurgitation.

Gastrointestinal disorders related to alcohol abuse are not uncommon. Conditions such as peptic ulcer disease, esophagitis, gastritis with resultant pancreatitis, esophageal varices, an increase in carcinomas, and malabsorption diseases have all been identified.

Hematologic and endocrine disorders associated with chronic alcohol abuse include thrombocytopenia, megaloblastic anemia, amenorrhea, diminished fertility, anovulation, and premature menopause.

Laboratory Findings Associated with Alcoholism

Laboratory data serve as a useful adjunct to the history and physical examination when the physician is

TABLE 31-4
MICHIGAN ALCOHOLISM SCREENING TEST (MAST)

Points		Yes	No
	0. Do you enjoy a drink now and then?		
(2)	1. Do you feel you are a normal drinker? (By normal, we mean you drink less than or as much as most other people.)		
(2)	2. Have you ever awakened the morning after some drinking the night before and found that you could not remember a part of the evening?		
(1)	3. Does your wife, husband, a parent, or other near relative ever worry or complain about your drinking?		
(2)	4. Can you stop drinking without a struggle after one or two drinks?		
(1)	5. Do you ever feel guilty about your drinking?		
(2)	6. Do friends or relatives think you are a normal drinker?		
(0)	7. Do you ever try to limit your drinking to certain times of the day or to certain places?		
(2)	8. Have you ever attended a meeting of Alcoholics Anonymous?		
(1)	9. Have you gotten into physical fight when drinking?		
(2)	10. Has your drinking ever created problems between you and your wife, husband, a parent, or other relative?		
(2)	11. Has your wife, husband, or other family members ever gone to anyone for help about your drinking?		
(2)	12. Have you ever lost friends because of your drinking?		
(2)	13. Have you ever gotten into trouble at work or school because you were drinking?		
(2)	14. Have you ever lost a job because of drinking?		
(2)	15. Have you ever neglected your obligations, your family, or your work for two or more days in a row because you were drinking?		
(1)	16. Do you drink before noon fairly often?		
(2)	17. Have you ever been told you have liver trouble?		
(2)*	18. After heavy drinking have you ever had delirium tremens (DTs) or severe shaking, or heard voices or seen things that really weren't there?		
(5)	19. Have you ever gone to anyone for help about your drinking?		
(5)	20. Have you ever been in a hospital because of drinking?		
(2)	21. Have you ever been a patient in a psychiatric hospital or on a psychiatric ward of a general hospital where drinking was part of the problem that resulted in hospitalization?		
(2)	22. Have you ever been seen at a psychiatric or mental health clinic or gone to any doctor, social worker, or clergyman for help with any emotional problem, where drinking was part of the problem?		
(2)†	23. Have you ever been arrested for drunk driving, driving while intoxicated, or driving under the influence of alcoholic beverage? (If YES, how many times? _____)		
(2)†	24. Have you ever been arrested, or taken into custody, even for a few hours, because of other drunk behavior? (If YES, how many times? _____)		

*5 points for delirium tremens.

†2 points for each arrest.

Scoring system: In general. Five points or more would place that subject in an "alcoholic" category. Four points would suggest alcoholism, three points or less would indicate the subject was not alcoholic.

Programs using the above scoring system find it very sensitive at the 5-point level, and it tends to find more people alcoholics than anticipated. However, it is a screening test and should be sensitive at its lower levels.

Adapted from Selzer ML. The Michigan Alcoholism Screening Test: the quest for a new diagnostic instrument. Am J Psychiatry 1971;127:1653.

considering the diagnosis of alcohol abuse. In addition, abnormalities in laboratory data collected during routine physical examinations may prompt the physician to consider the diagnosis of alcoholism. Some laboratory findings associated with alcoholism include:

- γ-Glutamyl transferase (GGT) levels greater than 40 units

- Elevated aspartate transaminase levels with aspartate:alanine aminotransferase ratios greater than 3:1
- Uric acid levels greater than 7 mg/dl
- Triglyceride levels greater than 180 mg/dl
- Decreased white-cell count
- Decreased albumin, vitamin B_{12}, and folic acid levels
- Elevated lactate dehydrogenase levels

When a physician uses these laboratory tests along with history and physical examination information, the diagnosis of alcoholism can be confirmed.

Psychological Tests to Screen for Alcoholism

The physician can use psychological testing to aid in the screening and diagnosis of alcoholism. The Michigan Alcoholism Screening Test (MAST) was introduced in 1971 by Selzer. It has 25 questions that ask the patient specific items as they pertain to drinking alcohol and its effects (Table 31-4). The MAST is 90% sensitive. The CAGE questionnaire is also commonly used as a screening test for alcoholism. Similar in concept to the MAST, the CAGE asks four general questions concerning alcohol drinking (Table 31-5). Both the MAST and CAGE questionnaires can be used as screening tests along with history and physical information to help the physician diagnose alcoholism.

Treatment of Alcoholism

Treatment of acute alcohol withdrawal and long-term abstinence involve specific pharmacologic therapy as well as psychotherapy. The physician should approach alcoholism as a treatable disease. Successful treatment of alcoholism has been defined as "abstinence, or progressively longer periods of abstinence, with improved life functioning for the patient and his family."[10] Outpatient treatment of alcohol withdrawal should occur if the patient is medically stable, reliable, can follow up daily with a treatment regimen, can continue participation in the work force, and is highly motivated. Inpatient treatment and detoxification is also an option, and should be employed if the alcoholic fails to meet the above requirements or if a treatment program cannot be easily assembled. The patient's physician may need to consult with other health-care workers who have experience in treating the alcoholic and her family.

Acute alcohol withdrawal can be a medical emergency. Admission to the hospital for management of alcohol withdrawal should occur if there is hemodynamic instability, the presence of seizure activity, an associated traumatic event, protracted vomiting, or any signs of psychological instability (i.e., severe depression, hallucinations, or suicidal ideation).[10] Standard admission orders for treatment of alcohol withdrawal include frequent assessment of vital signs (every 4 hours), neurologic status, hydration, and

---

TABLE 31-5
CAGE SCREEN FOR DIAGNOSIS OF ALCOHOLISM

Have you ever:
C   thought you should CUT back on your drinking?
A   felt ANNOYED by people criticizing your drinking?
G   felt GUILTY or bad about your drinking?
E   had a morning EYE-OPENER to relieve hangover or nerves?

A score of 2 or 3 indicates a high index of suspicion of alcohol dependence, and a score of 4 is pathognomonic for dependence.

Adapted from Ewing JA. Detecting alcoholism: the CAGE questionnaire. JAMA 1984;252:1905.

---

seizure precautions. Medications that can be used to decrease the neurologic effects of alcohol withdrawal (i.e. tremors and anxiety) include chlordiazepoxide (50 to 100 mg initially and then 25 to 50 mg every 4 to 6 hours) and diazepam (5 to 10 mg initially, and then 5 to 10 mg every 4 to 6 hours). Diazepam is also used for the treatment of alcoholic seizures. In an outpatient setting, low-dose benzodiazepines and other anxiolytics can be used on an "as-needed" basis to help control CNS side effects of alcohol withdrawal (i.e., oxazepam, hydroxyzine, diphenhydramine). β-blockers and central α-agonist medications have also been used in conjunction with low-dose benzodiazepines to decrease the CNS irritability associated with withdrawal. Routine medications that should also be used include multivitamins, folic acid, repletion of magnesium, and thiamine.

Alcoholic rehabilitation involves intensive patient motivation and a multidisciplinary medical team approach. Alcoholics Anonymous (AA) can help the alcoholic recover and maintain long-term abstinence. AA was founded in 1935 by two chronic alcoholics. The basis of AA is a belief that alcoholics can achieve and maintain sobriety through daily discussions with other alcoholics of their drinking and its effects on their lives. There are 12 steps and traditions that serve to describe the purpose of AA (Tables 31-6 and 31-7). AA meetings occur throughout the world. A listing of meetings and their locations can be obtained from the National Council on Alcoholism. AA meetings are multiracial and nonprofessional, include both genders and all ages, and are nondenominational and apolitical. AA is a self-supporting entity without membership dues or financial investments. Participation in AA requires a motivated alcoholic who seeks help to become sober and remain abstinent throughout her life. Other groups exist that can be therapeutic to

cigarette smoke are distributed widely throughout the body and have interactions with nearly every organ system. Because of this, adverse effects can be seen globally, from the head (brain and CNS) to the toes (peripheral vascular disease).

Cancers directly and indirectly associated with smoking involve almost every major organ system in the body. Cigarette smoking has been implicated in cancer of the gastrointestinal tract including oral, esophageal, gastric, pancreatic, and colonic. Cancers of the respiratory tract (larynx and lung), central nervous system (brain), blood (leukemia), urinary system (kidney and bladder), and female reproductive tract (cervix and ovary) have also been associated with smoking. Female smokers have four times the risk of cervical cancer as nonsmokers.[11] Components of cigarette smoke have been found in the cervical mucus of smokers at levels 40 to 50 times those in the serum.[11] The risk of ovarian cancer is three times greater in the female smoker than in nonsmokers.[11]

Smoking has direct effects on the heart and cardiovascular system, and plays a major role in coronary artery disease. Nicotine increases the heart rate, raises systolic blood pressure, and causes vasoconstriction. Myocardial oxygen consumption increases. Nicotine also increases clotting and decreases the oxygen-carrying capacity of hemoglobin.[11] Carbon monoxide interferes with oxygen transport and use. Carbon monoxide displaces oxygen from hemoglobin and shifts the oxygen–hemoglobin dissociation curve to the left. Smokers have two to four times the risk of coronary artery disease as nonsmokers. In women, smoking can interact with oral contraceptives to increase the risk of stroke and premature myocardial infarction.[12]

Cigarette smoking is the main cause of chronic obstructive pulmonary disease and increases the incidence of asthma, bronchitis, pneumonia, and pulmonary infections. Ciliary activities of the respiratory epithelium and phagocytic activity of macrophages in the alveoli are inhibited by smoke, resulting in decreased clearance of foreign material and bacteria from the lungs.[12] Children of smokers have otitis media and upper respiratory tract infections more often.

Women who smoke have an increased incidence of infertility, spontaneous abortion, preterm labor, placenta previa, abruptio placentae, and premature rupture of membranes.[11] Infants of mothers who smoke during pregnancy weigh, on average, 170 g less than infants of mothers who do not smoke, and this

is probably a result of impaired uteroplacental circulation.[13] Fetal tobacco syndrome is fetal growth restriction in which the mother smokes five or more cigarettes a day throughout her pregnancy; there is no evidence of maternal hypertension; the infant has symmetrical growth restriction; and no other cause of intrauterine growth restriction can be found.[11] The incidence of fetal death, neonatal death, and sudden infant death syndrome is also increased. The long-term physical growth and intellectual development of the child may be adversely affected by smoking during pregnancy.[13]

Passive Smoking

It is estimated that about 15% of Americans are allergic to cigarette smoke.[11] Sidestream smoke is the smoke emitted into the air from the burning cigarette, while mainstream smoke is the smoke inhaled by the smoker. The majority of smoke from cigarettes diffuses into the air. The concentration of chemicals is initially greater in the sidestream smoke than the mainstream smoke because of a lower combustion temperature and lack of filtration through the cigarette.[11] It is only after the smoke mixes with air that the chemical concentration is lowered. Nonsmokers who are around smokers are exposed to the same chemicals as smokers but at lower concentrations. Nonsmokers exposed to smoke experience the harmful effects of smoking in these circumstances.

Spouses of smokers have increased lung and other cancers, increased coronary artery disease, and decreased pulmonary function. Passive smoke doubles to triples the incidence of lung cancer, cervical cancer, and myocardial infarction in female spouses of smokers as compared with female spouses of nonsmokers. It has been estimated that smoke in the home and workplace may be responsible for the deaths of more than 40,000 nonsmokers annually in the United States.[11]

Other Forms of Tobacco Use

Other forms of tobacco use include cigars, pipes, snuff, and chewing tobacco. There is increased morbidity and mortality associated with use of these tobacco products. Smokeless tobacco contains the same chemicals as cigarette tobacco, but some of them in much greater concentration.[11] Smokeless tobacco increases the incidence of oral and pharyngeal cancers and gum recession. While cigarette smoking increases user mortality by approximately 70%, cigar and pipe tobacco users experience about a 15 to 20% increase in mortality as compared with nonsmokers.[10] Cigar and pipe smoking is usually associated with less exposure to carbon monoxide and less lung tissue exposure to smoke.[10] Also, all of these tobacco products increase the risk of cardiovascular disease.

Benefits of Quitting

The benefits of quitting are numerous. Immediate benefits include the reduction in cardiovascular risk resulting from a decrease in nicotine and carbon monoxide levels. This results in decreased cardiac work and an increase in oxygenation. The risk of upper-respiratory-tract infections is also reduced. The reduction in cancer risk and the reduction in the rate of decline of pulmonary function occurs over a span of about 3 to 5 years.[10] Ten or more years after quitting, the death rates of persons who had smoked 20 or fewer cigarettes a day is approximately that of a nonsmoker.[13]

Withdrawal Symptoms

Nicotine, like many drugs, produces tolerance and dependence. Tolerance increases throughout the day and the effect of each cigarette decreases. Tolerance decreases throughout the night, resulting in the first cigarette of the day having the most effect.[12]

On quitting smoking, an abstinence syndrome usually occurs. The intensity varies greatly among individuals. The physiologic manifestations of the tobacco abstinence syndrome are inconsequential, consisting of a slight and gradual decline in heart rate and blood pressure.[10] About 80 to 90% of smokers experience the subjective aspects of the syndrome, starting within hours of quitting and peaking at 48 hours, and then diminishing over 2 to 5 weeks. Symptoms are the opposite of the pharmacologic effects. Symptoms include irritability, restlessness, sleep disturbances, difficulty in concentrating, impatience, anxiety dysphoria, gastrointestinal disturbances, hunger, weight gain, and cigarette craving.[10] Increased hunger and weight gain may persist for 10 to 12 weeks.[12] Cigarette craving may persist for months and may be experienced years later. Craving may be a learned phenomenon related to the powerful and persuasive associations rather than part of the abstinence

syndrome, since it is frequently experienced even in smokers not attempting to quit and not attempting to reduce their smoking.[10]

Treatment of Withdrawal

At present, the most widely used treatment for withdrawal is nicotine replacement. Nicotine replacement currently is available in the form of nicotine gum, transdermal nicotine patch, and nicotine nasal spray. Success in quitting smoking with nicotine replacement is enhanced when used in combination with strategies for behavior modification and support to enhance coping. Nicotine replacement will enhance the success of attempts to quit but will not induce or encourage an attempt to quit. Also, because smoking exposes the mother and fetus to many more toxins than nicotine alone, nicotine replacement can be used in pregnancy.

Nicotine gum is available in doses of 2 mg and 4 mg. Nicotine is absorbed through the buccal mucous membrane. The dose used is based on nicotine dependence. Nicotine blood levels are generally lower than those found in continued smoking. The gum should be placed in the mouth and chewed several times to elicit a peppery taste or a tingling feeling. The gum should then be placed between the gum and cheek to allow absorption. This should then be repeated every minute. The gum is not chewed like sweet gum and the juice swallowed. This will result in decreased absorption and an increase in its irritative effects, which include nausea, stomach upset, and sore throat. The gum should be discarded after 30 minutes. A steady blood level of nicotine should be maintained. This usually requires the use of one piece of gum an hour while awake. The advantages of nicotine gum are that the dosage can be adjusted to the individual and can be used in response to situational stimuli. A major disadvantage is that it requires a high level of compliance. The advantages and disadvantages of the nasal spray are the same, while they are the opposite for the patch.[10] The nicotine patch is available in several dosages and the dosage is gradually weaned over several weeks. The nasal spray delivers 0.5 mg of nicotine per spray and can be used up to five times an hour up to a total of 40 sprays a day.

Other medications used to reduce withdrawal symptoms include clonidine and bupropion. Clonidine is an α-adrenergic receptor agonist. It reduces symptoms, including irritability, anxiety, restlessness, hunger, and craving. It can be started at 100 μg twice a day and increased up to 400 μg a day. Clonidine should be used in conjunction with a behavioral modification program to achieve maximal benefit.

Bupropion is an antidepressant whose mechanism of action in smoking cessation is unknown at this time. It appears to ease withdrawal symptoms without working directly on depression. A study by Hurt and associates found that sustained-release bupropion at doses of 150 mg and 300 mg (150 mg twice a day) for 7 weeks more than doubled the smoking cessation rate over placebo at the end of the study, and nearly doubled the rate at one year post-treatment.[14]

Weight Gain

A reason frequently cited by smokers for not attempting to quit smoking or for relapsing is the fear of gaining weight. Physicians should address this early in the treatment program. Weight gain occurs because of a change in dietary habits and cessation of the metabolic effects of nicotine. Physicians should emphasize that the weight gained is medically insignificant in comparison to the benefits of smoking cessation. Weight gain averages 6 lb for men and 8 lb for women.[11] Physicians should give anticipatory guidance regarding weight control. Strategies could include daily weighings early in cessation, when weight control is most manageable; use of low-calorie snacks instead of high-calorie foods; initiation of an exercise program; and setting a limit on weight gain that will be tolerated for several months until smoking abstinence is well established.[10] Nicotine replacement may initially help to reduce weight gain in smoking cessation, but when it is stopped, weight is gained due to the cessation of nicotine's metabolic effects.

Treatment

The first and main idea that a physician should remember about smoking is that it is not simply an addiction to nicotine.[11] Smoking, or any substance abuse/dependence, involves the whole person. Social and psychological factors play significant roles. All these areas must be addressed in a treatment plan. There is not a single treatment that works for everyone.

The key to maintaining smoking cessation is behavior modification. Nicotine replacement and other medications are helpful in suppressing withdrawal symptoms in the acute period of days, weeks, and months, but long-term abstinence is achieved through behavior modification. The smoker is confronted with smoking stimuli in many aspects of her life, including the home, work, and social environments. The smoker must learn to confront these stimuli and develop habits and behaviors to deal with and overcome them. The physician can play a role in helping the patient to achieve these changes.

The first and most important change the physician can help to elicit is the motivation for the smoker to stop. Physicians should not underestimate the influence their advice to quit has on smokers.[10] Smokers cite physicians as the person most able to influence their decision to attempt to quit.[10] The main role physicians can play is to advise their patients to stop smoking and to help them to plan a course of action to stop and to maintain abstinence. Physicians can achieve increased smoking-cessation rates just by cautioning patients to quit at each office visit. Even greater cessation rates can be achieved if the physician adds reading or audiovisual material to advice.

Certain groups of patients are more susceptible to advice about quitting. Examples would include persons who have had a recent myocardial infarction or stroke and pregnant women. Some pregnant women have an increased willingness and desire to quit during pregnancy for the health of their babies. Unfortunately, a majority of those who quit during pregnancy return to smoking after delivery. This is a group in which a well-developed and structured abstinence maintenance program would be of enormous benefit in preventing relapse.

Physicians must tailor their quitting message and treatment regimens to the individual. Patients must be able to relate to what is being expressed to them. Emphasizing the long-term health hazards to teenagers, who feel they are invincible, does not work. Emphasizing the facts that smoking causes bad breath, yellows teeth, stinks up clothes, and decreases athletic endurance is more relevant and elicits a better response. Physicians should create or organize stop-smoking materials that pertain to their patient population. Materials given to patients should be individualized and personalized. They should be updated and revised frequently.

There are many brochures, pamphlets and guides available to physicians and patients to help in smoking cessation. Some of these include the American Academy of Family Physician's "Stop Smoking" program and guide, the American Cancer Society's "Smart Move!" guide, the National Cancer Institute's "Cleaning the Air" guide, and the American Heart Association's "Calling It Quits" guide. These are available through either local organization chapters or from the national organizations. Costs vary, and prices should be obtained from the providing organization.

Relapse is a frequent occurrence in smoking cessation. Most smokers will relapse on their first attempt. The physician and patient must be prepared to deal with this. When the patient presents to the physician after a relapse, the physician must not be critical. The physician should congratulate the smoker on the attempt and reassure her that relapses happen. The smoker should then be encouraged to attempt to quit again and the treatment plan resumed or a new plan formulated. The physician should not give up on the smoker, and the smoker should not give up on herself. Successful long-term cessation may take several attempts.

OTHER ABUSED SUBSTANCES

Amphetamines/Cocaine/Caffeine

Of the stimulant class of drugs of abuse, cocaine has been one of the most widely used and cheapest. There are different forms of cocaine available today. Cocaine extracted from its hydrochloride salt using ether (freebased cocaine); "crack," which is cocaine that is extracted using baking soda and water; the intravenous form; chewing the leaves, which is done by Peruvian Indians; and the natural pure alkaloid that is snorted or sniffed.

Other stimulants that are commonly abused include amphetamines and caffeine-containing products. One example of an amphetamine product includes methylphenidate (Ritalin), which is used in the treatment of attention-deficit disorder. The clinical effects of these stimulants result from stimulation of the sympathetic nervous system, causing any of the following:

- Cardiovascular: coronary artery spasm, myocardial infarction, hypertensive crisis, tachycardia
- Respiratory: sudden respiratory failure
- Endocrine: impotence, gynecomastia, menstrual irregularities, infertility
- Fetal: placental abruption, congenital malformations, withdrawal symptoms in the fetus

Psychological benefits of stimulant abuse include euphoria, increased energy, alertness, and confidence. These positive effects are seen with small amounts of stimulant abuse. However, when larger amounts are abused, anxiety, increased agitation, hallucinations, and seizures can occur. Withdrawal symptoms are commonly prevented by continuous and even increased stimulant abuse. The diagnosis of stimulant drug abuse is occasionally confirmed by clinical and laboratory information. Cocaine use can be detected from analysis of urine studies. Cocaine can be detected in adult urine for up to 36 hours after initial use, and maternal use within the past 6 to 9 days prior to delivery can be detected by testing the neonate's urine. Blood levels of cocaine can also be obtained; however, they can only detect recent ingestion and do not correlate with toxicity. Urine levels of amphetamines can also be detected. Some clinical tools that may be helpful in confirming stimulant use involve observing a patient's blood pressure and pulse rate, both of which may be elevated.

Opiates/Sedatives

Opioid abuse in the United States includes the use of heroin, morphine, meperidine, codeine, and methadone. Heroin can either be injected intramuscularly (skin-popping), injected intravenously, or inhaled (snorting, or sniffing).

Sedatives include benzodiazepines and barbiturates, which are commonly prescribed. As CNS depressants, these drugs have similar physiologic and psychological effects to alcohol. Benzodiazepines are appropriately used in certain clinical situations and should not be used in conjunction with other sedative medications. The margin of safety using benzodiazepines is greater than that of barbiturates, thus death from an overdose is less likely. In contrast to alcohol, benzodiazepines and barbiturates have less direct organ toxicity.

Intoxication with an opioid produces an initial euphoric effect, followed by a mellowed, relaxed state in which the participant can fall asleep. Other physical signs include pupillary constriction, decreased GI motility, slurred speech, and impaired memory. Long-term abuse of opioids can produce amenorrhea, and indirectly increase sexually transmitted diseases (STDs) and pelvic inflammatory disease (PID) secondary to the lifestyle choices of the drug abuser. The heroin abuser who is pregnant is at an increased risk for placental abruption, eclampsia, breech presentation, premature labor, premature of rupture membranes, and cesarean section. Use of benzodiazepine or barbiturates during pregnancy is associated with congenital birth defects that resemble those seen in fetal alcohol syndrome, neonatal respiratory depression, and decreased neonatal muscle tone. Neonatal withdrawal symptoms such as tremulousness, irritability, and sleep disturbances can be observed beginning 4 to 7 days after delivery, when there is chronic maternal abuse of benzodiazepines and barbiturates. It should be emphasized that barbiturate withdrawal can be lethal, while benzodiazepine withdrawal can cause CNS hyperactivity, insomnia, seizures, and delirium.

The main diagnosis of opiate and sedative abuse is based on history, clinical suspicion, and urine/serum analysis. It is important to remember that a detailed history may provide the primary care physician with the most useful diagnostic information. Both opiates and sedatives are categorized as psychoactive drugs, which have a depressant effect. Some clinical signs and symptoms of opiate and sedative use include decreased mental alertness, respiratory depression, decreased GI motility, and orthostatic hypotension.

TREATMENT FOR ABUSE OF OTHER SUBSTANCES

The treatment algorithm for withdrawal from abused substances can involve many different medical regimens and is usually a self-limited process. In contrast, the ability of the substance abuser to remain abstinent for the long term requires a long-term strategy to evaluate psychosocial and environmental issues surrounding addiction, in addition to using pharmacologic therapy.

Acute Withdrawal

Treatment of acute withdrawal from sedatives is similar to that of alcohol withdrawal. Long-acting benzodiazepines or barbiturates should be used to simulate the sedative effect while counteracting withdrawal symptoms. Detoxification can be achieved by estimating the total amount of sedative necessary to prevent withdrawal and decreasing dosage levels by 10% each day.[6] For example, a physician can estimate the total dose of benzodiazepines needed to initiate detoxification by history or by the pentobarbital challenge test (in which a 200-mg test dose of pentobarbital is given and the patient's physical condition is

rated on a quantitative scale). Diazepam is normally used (15 to 25 mg given four times a day).[6]

Treatment of opiate withdrawal can involve the use of methadone, a long-acting synthetic narcotic. Similar to benzodiazepines in action, methadone blocks withdrawal symptoms by providing cross-tolerance. The dose of methadone is eventually increased so that the patient is unable to experience any significant effects of narcotic intoxication.[14] The methadone-requiring patient is able to function safely in a working and home environment partly because she is not purchasing narcotics and because of the absence of withdrawal symptoms.[14] As with sedatives, detoxification from methadone can be achieved by decreasing dosage levels by 10% each day. Before complete discontinuation of methadone, clonidine (an α-adrenergic agonist) can be started at doses of 0.1 to 0.3 mg three times a day.[6] Researchers have shown that clonidine's effects are partly due to suppression of the autonomic nervous system as it relates to withdrawal. It should be noted that clonidine is not approved by the Food and Drug Administration (FDA) for opiate detoxification.[6]

Naltrexone is an opioid antagonist that is FDA-approved for use in opiate withdrawal and long-term abstinence. Naltrexone blocks opiate receptors, which helps to decrease the CNS effects of narcotic abuse. Naltrexone is usually given in doses of 25 to 50 mg daily. Research shows that naltrexone can also precipitate withdrawal symptoms in concurrent active narcotic users. Thus, the combination of clonidine and naltrexone may be more effective in maintaining abstinence for the long term.[6]

Treatment of acute withdrawal from amphetamines, cocaine, and caffeine-containing drugs involves securing a safe environment for detoxification and providing other supportive therapy from a multidisciplinary medical team. Because persons experiencing cocaine withdrawal can become dysphoric, anhedonic, and have a decreased appetite and weight loss, tricyclic antidepressant therapy can be used. Currently, research is inconclusive concerning the use of dopamine agonists (i.e., bromocriptine and amantadine), which are thought to enhance dopaminergic functioning, and thus decrease withdrawal symptoms.[6]

Maintenance of Abstinence

Similar to long-term abstinence from alcohol, long-term abstinence from sedatives, opiates, amphetamines, cocaine, and caffeine-containing drugs requires a highly motivated patient and multidisciplinary team. As with alcohol rehabilitation, the decision to enroll a patient in an inpatient or outpatient rehabilitation program depends on the patient's motivation, the presence of a supportive family network, the presence of comorbid medical conditions, and the presence of a multidisciplinary team preexisting within the community. Treatment groups such as Cocaine Anonymous and Narcotics Anonymous are available and should be used by the patient and physician.

SELECTED READING

Barker LR, Whitfield CL. Alcoholism. In: Barker LR, Burton JR, Zieve PD, eds. Principles of ambulatory medicine. 3rd ed. Baltimore: Williams & Wilkins, 1991:204.

Bigelow GE, Haines CS, Stitzer ML. Tobacco use and dependence. In: Barker LR, Burton JR, Zieve PD, eds. Principles of ambulatory medicine. 3rd ed. Baltimore: Williams & Wilkins, 1991:195.

Bigelow GE, Haines CS. Tobacco use and dependence. In: Barker LR, Burton JR, Zieve PD, eds. Principles of ambulatory medicine. 4th ed. Baltimore: Williams & Wilkins, 1995:212.

The Burton Goldberg Group. Addictions. In: Fife WA, ed. Alternative medicine: the definitive guide. New York: Futura, 1995:485.

Cross GM, Hoffman KJ. Alcoholism. In: Taylor RB, ed. Family medicine—principles and practice. 4th ed. New York: Springer-Verlag, 1994:451.

D'Lugoff B, Hawthorne J. Use and abuse of illicit drugs and substances. In: Barker LR, Burton JR, Zieve PD, eds. Principles of ambulatory medicine. 3rd ed. Baltimore: Williams & Wilkins, 1991:232.

Fingerhood MI, Barker LR. Alcoholism and associated problems In: Barker LR, Burton JR, Zieve PD, eds. Principles of ambulatory medicine. 4th ed. Baltimore: Williams & Wilkins, 1995:221.

Frances RJ, Franklin JE Jr. Alcohol and other psychoactive substance use disorders. In: Hales RE, Yudofsky SC, Talbott JA, eds. The American Psychiatric Press Textbook of Psychiatry. 2nd ed. Washington DC: American Psychiatric Association, 1994:355.

Gagné RJ. Care of the patient who misuses drugs. In: Taylor RB, ed. Family medicine—principles and practice. 4th ed. New York: Springer-Verlag, 1994:462.

Geller A. Common addictions. CIBA Clin Symp 1996;48:1.

Holbrook JH. Tobacco. In: Wilson JD, Braunwald E, Isselbacher KJ, et al., eds. Harrison's principles of internal medicine. 12th ed. New York: McGraw-Hill, 1991:2158.

Mendelson JH, Mello NK. Commonly abused drugs. In: Wilson JD, Braunwald E, Isselbacher KJ, et al., eds. Harrison's principles of internal medicine. 12th ed. New York: McGraw-Hill, 1991:2155.

Niswander KR, Arthur TE. Manual of obstetrics. 5th ed. Boston: Little Brown, 1996:27.

Rakel RE, Blum A. Nicotine addiction. In: Rakel RE, ed. Textbook of family practice. 5th ed. Philadelphia: Saunders, 1995:1549.

Rakel RE, ed. Textbook of family practice. 5th ed. Philadelphia: Saunders, 1995.

Schuckit MA, Rakel RE, Blum A, Sherin AM, Fawcett JA. Substance abuse. In: Rakel RE, ed. Rakel's textbook of medicine. 4th ed. Philadelphia: Saunders, 1990:1603.

Schuckit MA. Alcohol and alcoholism. In: Wilson JD, Braunwald E, Isselbacher KJ, et al., eds. Harrison's principles of internal medicine. 12th ed. New York: McGraw-Hill, 1991:2146.

Schuckit MA. Alcohol abuse. In: Rakel RE, ed. Rakel's textbook of family medicine. 5th ed. Philadelphia: Saunders, 1995:1537.

Schuckit MA, Segal DS. Opioid drug use. In: Wilson JD, Braunwald E, Isselbacher KJ, et al., eds. Harrison's principles of internal medicine. 12th ed. New York: McGraw-Hill, 1991:2151.

Sherin KM. Abuse of controlled substance. In Rakel RE, ed. Rakel's textbook of family medicine, 5th ed. Philadelphia: Saunders, 1995:1565.

Sullivan JT, D'Lugoff B. Illicit use and abuse of drugs and substances. In: Barker LR, Burton JR, Zieve PD, eds. Principles of ambulatory medicine. 4th ed. Baltimore: Williams & Wilkins, 1995:250.

U.S. Departments of Health and Human Services. Alcohol, tobacco, and other drugs may harm the unborn. Washington, DC: Department of Health and Human Services, Public Health Service, Substance Abuse and Mental Health Services Administration, 1994. DDHHS Publication no. (ADM)90-1711.

Wallach J. Interpretation of diagnostic tests. 6th ed. Boston: Little Brown, 1996:844.

REFERENCES

1. O'Connor PG, Schenfield RS. Patients with alcohol problems. N Engl J Med 1998;338:592.
2. Schuckit MA, Rakel RE, Blum A, Sherin AM, Fawcett JA. Substance abuse. In: Rakel RE, ed. Rakel's textbook of medicine. 4th ed. Philadelphia: Saunders, 1990:1603.
3. Prigerson HG, Frank E, Kasl SV, et al. Complicated grief and bereavement-related depression as distinct disorders: preliminary empirical validation in elderly bereaved spouses. J Am Psych 1995;152:22.
4. Cross GM, Hoffman KJ. Alcoholism. In: Taylor RB, et al., eds. Family medicine: principles and practice. 4th ed. New York: Springer-Verlag, 1994:451.
5. Schuckit MA, et al. Alcoholism and drug dependency. In: Harrison S, Tinsley R, eds. Harrison's principles of internal medicine. 12th ed. New York: McGraw-Hill, 1991: 2146.
6. Frances RJ, Franklin JE Jr. Alcohol and other psychoactive substance use disorders. In: Hales RE, Yudofsky SC, Talbott JA, eds. American Psychiatric Press textbook of psychiatry. 2nd ed. Washington DC: American Psychiatric Association, 1994:355.
7. Dufour MC. What is moderate drinking? Defining "drinks" and drinking levels. National Institute on Alcohol Abuse and Alcoholism, Bethesda, MD, Alcohol Res Health 1999;23:5.

8. Schuckit MA. Alcohol abuse. In: Rakel RE, ed. Rakel's textbook of family medicine. 5th ed. Philadelphia: Saunders, 1995:1537.

9. Cook P, et al. Alcohol, tobacco and other drugs may harm the unborn. Washington, DC: Department of Health & Human Services, Public Health Services, revised. 1994:15. DDHHS Publication no. (ADM)90-1711.

10. Bigelow GE, Haines CS, Stitzer ML. Tobacco use and dependence In: Barker LR, Burton JR, Zieve PD, eds. Principles of ambulatory medicine. 3rd ed. Baltimore: Williams & Wilkins, 1991:212.

11. Rakel RE, Blum A. Nicotine addiction. In: Rakel RE, ed. Textbook of family practice. 5th ed. Philadelphia: Saunders, 1995:1549.

12. Geller A. Common addictions. CIBA Clin Symp 1996; 48:1.

13. Holbrook JH. Tobacco. In: Wilson JD, Braunwald E, Isselbacher KJ, et al., eds. Harrison's principles of internal medicine. 12th ed. New York: McGraw-Hill, 1991:2158.

14. D'Lugoff B, Hawthorne J. Use and abuse of illicit drugs and substances. In: Barker LR, Burton JR, Zieve PD, eds. Principles of ambulatory medicine. 3rd ed. Baltimore: Williams & Wilkins, 1991:244.

15. Hurt RD, Sachs DPL, Glover ED, et al. A comparison of sustained-released bupropion and placebo for smoking cessation. N Eng J Med 1997;337:1195.

Chapter 32
Dermatologic Problems

Terri H. Henson
Robert A. Skinner, Jr.

Five Key Points

- Pregnant women are susceptible to the same common skin conditions as the general population; however, there are several dermatoses that are unique to pregnancy and must be considered when evaluating a pruritic eruption in a pregnant woman.

- Acne is one of the most common skin disorders treated by dermatologists and primary care providers alike. Treatment must be tailored to the individual based on multiple factors including morphology of the presenting lesions, skin type, and patient's desire for treatment.

- Topical medications, especially steroids, should be used cautiously in the vulvar area due to enhanced penetration, increased risk of irritancy, and local side effects.

- A biopsy should be considered when erosive or ulcerative vulvar lesions are refractory to treatment. Direct immunofluorescence testing can be very helpful in diseases such as lichen planus and the immunobullous disorders.

- Contact dermatitis of the vulva and vaginal introitus, which may be clinically subtle, can produce symptoms of vulvodynia. Consider patch testing in refractory cases.

Complaints involving the skin prompt many visits annually to both generalists and subspecialists. According to Fleischer et al., dermatologic problems account for 7.2% of all office visits to family physicians.[1] Because the problem is so visible, even psychiatrists and pathologists are caught at times by the anxious person who, at a family gathering or other social event, doesn't hesitate to expose the affected area to show the physician some "spot on my head," "rash on my stomach," or "this place on my arm." Patients and even some physicians erroneously believe that dermatologic diagnosis is easy and quick, requiring essentially no thought. However, like all other areas of medicine, the most important component of patient evaluation is the history and physical examination. This history is just as important to the dermatologist as to the internist (albeit usually shorter), and an appropriate physical examination is mandatory for accurate diagnosis. A proper skin examination requires that the patient be in a gown so that the skin surface may be visualized. (It's frequently as important to see where the rash is *not* as to see where it is.) Good lighting is essential and this is rarely the case outside an office setting.

The goal of this chapter is to present an overview of some common and a few uncommon dermatologic problems within the context of pregnancy and vulvar dermatoses.

PREGNANCY AND THE SKIN

Because of the complicated hormonal, immunologic, and vascular changes that occur during pregnancy, it is not surprising that there is a wide variety of associated skin changes. The effect of pregnancy on the skin can be categorized and will be dicussed as follows: physiologic skin changes, primary skin diseases acquired during or modified by pregnancy, and specific dermatoses considered unique to pregnancy.

Physiologic Skin Changes of Pregnancy

The cutaneous stigmata of pregnancy are sometimes pronounced and can be a source of distress to the patient. Due to the marked physiologic changes that occur, a number of skin manifestations may be seen (Table 32-1).

A variety of localized hyperpigmenting conditions may occur, most of which fade after delivery. However, melasma ("mask of pregnancy"), an irregular patchy macular hyperigmentation of sun-exposed areas, particularly the face (Figure 32-1), may persist beyond delivery in 30% of patients.[2] Melasma can also occur with oral-contraceptive use and is thought to be due to hormonal factors. Histologically, there is increased melanin in the basal-cell layer and sometimes deeper in the dermis within melanophages. This deeper (dermal) form is often refractory to treatment but the more superficial (epidermal) form may respond to treatment with combination creams containing hydroquinone 4%, tretinoin 0.05%, and hydrocortisone 1%. Long-term twice daily application is usually necessary for significant improvement to occur, and because ultraviolet-light considerably worsens melasma, photoprotection is mandatory.

Changes in the pattern of hair growth and shedding are often marked during pregnancy and the postpartum period. During pregnancy there is an increase in the number of hairs in the anagen (growing) phase of the hair cycle. After delivery (usually 1 to 5 months) these follicles are simultaneously shifted into the telogen (shedding) phase, which results in an apparent excessive loss of hair, which may be a source of anxiety for many women. Patients should be reassured

that these shedding hairs are being replaced by new hair. The shedding will resolve spontaneously and total baldness will not occur.

Striae distensae ("stretch marks"), which are almost universal in pregnancy, usually develop during the second and third trimester. The initial reddish-purple color eventually fades, but the atrophic lines are permanent. Reports have indicated that topical

TABLE 32-1
PHYSIOLOGIC SKIN CHANGES OF PREGNANCY

Hyperpigmentation
  Melasma
  Nipple, areolae, genital area
  Linea nigra
  Increase in size, number, and darkness of nevi
  Vulvar melanosis
Hair
  Increased growth
  Postpartum telogen effluvium
  Male pattern alopecia
Nails
  Brittle or softened
  Beau's lines (transverse grooving)
  Distal onycholysis
  Increased growth
Pruritus
Sweat glands
  Increased eccrine activity
  Decreased apocrine activity
  Increased sebaceous activity
Striae distensae
Skin tags (molluscum fibrosum gravidarum)
Vascular lesions
  Pyogenic granuloma of skin and mucosae
  Varicosities (anal, vulvar, and lower extremity)
  Palmar erythema
  Spider angioma

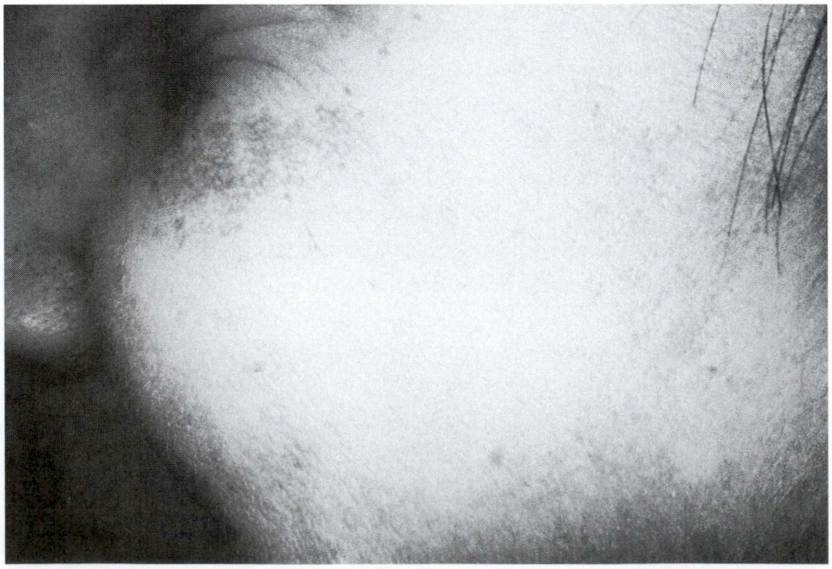

Figure 32-1 Close-up view of melasma. Note the reticulated brown patches on the cheek.

TABLE 32-2
EFFECT OF PREGNANCY ON SELECTED DERMATOLOGIC DISEASES

Acne	Variable, with approximately 50% improving
Atopic dermatitis (eczema)	Variable, with majority improving
Benign melanocytic nevi	Frequently increase in size, number, and darkness
Cutaneous T-cell lymphoma	May worsen
Discoid lupus erythematosus	Variable, frequently no effect
Erythema multiforme	Pregnancy may induce
Erythema nodosum	May be precipitated by or worsen during pregnancy
Fox-Fordyce disease	Majority improve
Hidradenitis suppurativa	Majority improve
Malignant melanoma	Controversial; may worsen prognosis if diagnosed during pregnancy
Neurofibromatosis	Cutaneous lesions may increase in size and number
Porphyria cutanea tarda	Most common porphyria; conflicting case reports regarding effect of pregnancy
Psoriasis	Variable; tendency to improve or remain unchanged during pregnancy; approximately 50% of patients deteriorate within 3 months postpartum

TABLE 32-3
SPECIFIC DERMATOSES OF PREGNANCY

Pemphigoid (herpes) gestationis
Impetigo herpetiformis (pustular psoriasis of pregnancy)
Polymorphic eruption of pregnancy (PEP)
Intrahepatic cholestasis of pregnancy
Prurigo of pregnancy
Pruritic folliculitis

tretinoin (Retin-A) 0.1% applied as early as possible (while still purpllish-red) can improve their appearance.[3] *Caution:* Although systemic absorption is negligible,[4] topical tretinoin should probably be avoided during pregnancy and nursing.

Primary Skin Diseases Acquired During or Modified by Pregnancy

Pregnant women are subject to the same skin diseases as the general population. However, pregnancy can modify many chronic dermatologic conditions and may actually induce some disorders, such as erythema multiforme and erythema nodosum. Some dermatoses are worsened; some are improved; but many are unpredictible. Table 32-2 lists some cutaneous diseases on which pregnancy is reported to have an impact.

Specific Dermatoses of Pregnancy

The specific dermatoses of pregnancy are a heterogenous group of distinct conditions considered unique to pregnancy and the puerperium (Table 32-3). They are not due to a preexisting disease, nor are they simply due to physiologic changes that occur during this time. The terminology over the past 20 years has been rather confusing, with overlap and redundancy of some of the reported entities. The following diseases have been well described and are considered distinct entities. With the exception of impetigo herpetiformis, these conditions all have in common severe pruritus. In addition to the specific dermatoses of pregnancy, the following differential diagnoses should be kept in mind whenever one is evaluating a pruritic skin disease in pregnancy: atopic dermatitis (eczema), contact dermatitis, drug reactions, insect bites, pityriasis rosea, scabies, and urticaria.

Pemphigold (Herpes) Gestationis

This rare immune-mediated blistering disease is considered by many to be identical to bullous pemphigoid. However, because of the unique clinical presentation, it continues to be described as a separate entity. It is an autoimmune vesiculobullous disorder in which there is antibody formation against a normal protein of the hemidesmosome complex, causing a cascade of proinflammatory events and ultimately subepidermal blister formation.

The clinical presentation of pemphigoid gestationis is dramatic. Patients present in the second or, more commonly, the third trimester with intensely pruritic vesicles and bullae on normal or erythematous skin (Figure 32-2). The blisters are frequently preceded (days to weeks) by a nonspecific urticarial or erythematous eruption. This prodromal eruption is often misdiagnosed unless there is a high index of clinical suspicion. Lesions tend to begin and predominate on the abdomen and usually involve the umbilicus, unlike PEP, which may resemble pemphigoid gestationis but tends to spare the umbilicus.

Diagnosis is based on the clinical appearance, routine histopathology, and most importantly, direct immunofluorescence. Routine hematoxylin and eosin staining of bullous lesions characteristically shows a subepidermal blister with eosinophils and neutrophils

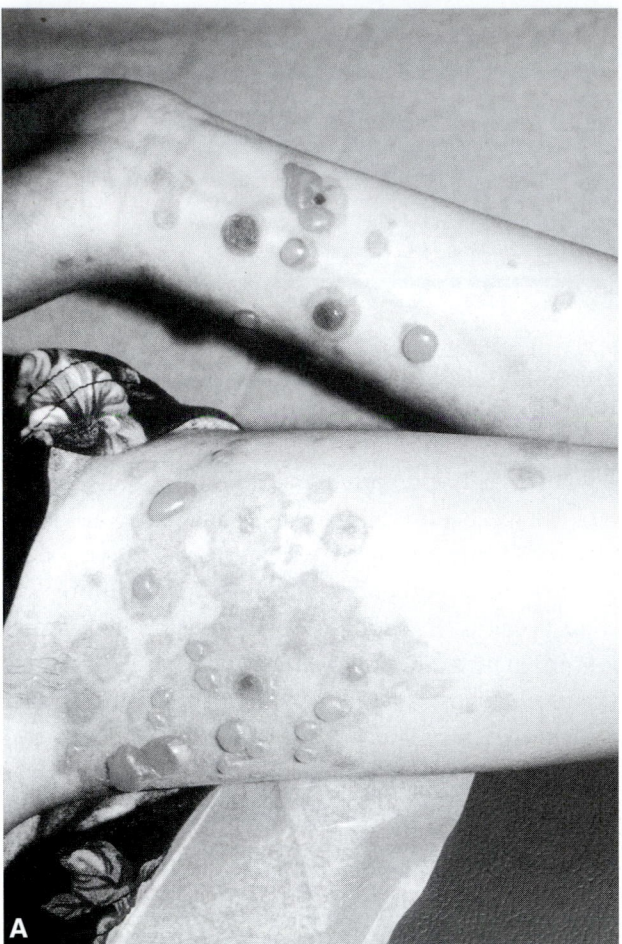 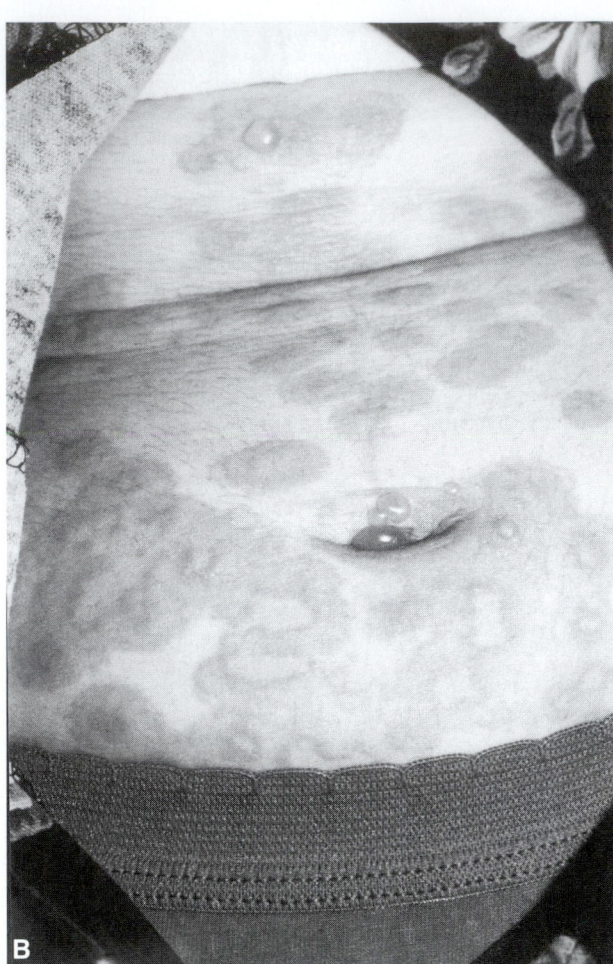

Figure 32-2 A and B. This patient with pemphigoid gestationis presented 3 days post-partum. Note the targetoid lesions and tense bullae on a background of urticaria. Umbilial lesions are very characteristic of this disease.

in the dermis, epidermis, and blister cavity. To accurately diagnose pemphigoid gestationis a second boispy for direct immunofluorescence is absolutely necessary. A punch biospy of perilesional skin is performed and transported in Michel's solution (*Note:* Formalin cannot be used as fixative for direct immunofluorescence.) Direct immunofluorescent staining of pemphigoid gestationis (which is positive in almost 100%) shows deposition of C3 alone or with IgG in a linear subepidermal pattern at the basement membrane zone. Complement-added indirect immunofluorescence, which detects circulating antibody, may be positive as well, but the titer does not correlate with disease activity or severity.

The course of pemphigoid gestationis is somewhat unpredictable. Patients often improve in the later part of pregnancy but most flare at or within days of delivery. Rarely, patients will actually present at or within days of delivery. Most women have complete clearance

after delivery (with or without treatment) but some experience exacerbations premenstrually and/or with the use of oral contraceptives. Pemphigoid gestationis tends to recur with subsequent pregnancies, often at an earlier time in gestation and with a more severe presentation. There is increased fetal morbidity (premature births), but not mortality, and because of transplacental IgG antibodies, infants may have similar skin lesions, which resolve spontaneously without treatment.

Therapy of pemphigoid gestationis is often difficult, especially during pregnancy. If the disease is localized (which is rare), supportive treatment and topical steroids may be beneficial.

In most cases, however, systemic steroids are required. Various immunosuppressive agents have been used after delivery with inconsistent and mostly disappointing results. Successful use of plasmapheresis has been reported in severe, refractory cases,[6] and Garvey et al. reported response to goserelin, a luteinizing-hormone—releasing hormone analogue in a patient with chronic, severe pemphigoid gestationis.

Impetigo Herpetiformis

Impetigo herpetiformis is an exceedingly rare skin disease (most dermatologists will never see it in a lifetime of practice). It is identical to pustular psoriasis, which is a true dermatolgic emergency. Patients, often without a prior history of psoriasis, present in the third trimester with sterile pustules on a background of bright erythema initially in flexural areas but quickly extending to the trunk and periumbilical area (Figure 32-3). It may be generalized and can involve mucous membranes. Patients are usually acutely ill with constitutional symptoms that may include fever, chills, nausea, vomiting, diarrhea, and changes in mental status. Diagnosis may be made clinically, but biopsy (with cultures) is advised to rule out infectious processes and pustular drug eruptions. Complications may be severe and include high-output congestive heart failure, renal failure, and fluid—electrolyte abnormalities, including hypocalcemia, which may be severe enough to induce tetany. Laboratory evaluation may reveal elevated erythrocyte sedimentation rate, leukocytosis, hypoalbuminemia, and hypocalcemia. Patients must also be monitored closely for the development of secondary infection and sepsis. There is increased fetal morbidity and increased maternal and fetal mortality. The disease may persist after delivery, but usually it will rapidly remit. Like pemphigoid gestationis, it usually recurs with subsequent pregnancies and is more severe. Exacerbation with oral contraceptive use is reported as well. Systemic steroids tapered slowly are the mainstay of treatment and in severe cases termination of pregnancy may be required.

Polymorphic Eruption of Pregnancy (PEP)

Also called pruritic urticarical papules and plaques of pregnancy (PUPPP), this relatively common disorder (1 in 240 pregnancies)[8] typically presents in the third trimester of a first pregnancy; however, there are reports of delayed onset within the first few days postpartum. These women present with a polymorphous eruption of intensely pruritic urticarial papules and plaques, vesicles, targetoid lesions, and polycyclic erythema. The lesions usually begin and predominate on the gravid abdomen, frequently within striae distensae. They may progress to involve the extremities as well. The umbilicus tends to be spared in PEP, in contrast to pemphigoid gestationis, which usually involves the umbilicus. Histology is nonspecific, but biopsy may be necessary to rule out pemphigoid gestationis. Direct immunofluorescence is always negative in PEP. Other common diseases to include in the differential diagnosis are erythema multiforme, drug eruptions, contact dermatitis, insect-bite reactions, scabies, and urticaria. Appropriate evaluation is necessary and may include (but is not limited to) biopsy, potassium hydroxide preparation for scabies, and patch testing. Infants are unaffected, and there is no increased maternal morbidity other than temporary discomfort. Treatment is symptomatic and consists of topical antipruritics such as calamine lotion, camphor and menthol lotions (Sarna), topical steroids, cool compresses, and diphenhydramine (Benadryl). In most cases, the disease resolves at or soon after delivery.

Until recently the cause of PEP was unknown, but a study by Aractingi et al.[9] found fetal DNA in lesional skin of women with PEP. Their findings suggest that "fetal cells can invade maternal skin during pregnancy and that their presence is associated with the development of unexplained skin disorders during pregnancy." These results using polymerase chain reaction analysis are exciting, although further investigation is necessary to determine the fetal cell type and to shed further light on the immunologic mechanisms involved.

Intrahepatic Cholestasis of Pregnancy (ICP)

ICP is a relatively uncommon disorder in which pregnant women manifest generalized pruritus secondary to intrahepatic cholestasis. Patients usually present in the third trimester with generalized itching, which tends to be worse at night. Physical examination may show excoriations and sometimes jaundice. The skin is otherwise completely normal. Generalized excoriations are common, often with marked sparing of the midback, an area not easily accessible to vigorous scratching. Laboratory abnormalities may include markedly elevated serum bile acids, mild to moderately elevated alkaline phosphatase and bilirubin, lipid abnormalities, and slightly elevated liver transaminases. However, there may be no laboratory evidence of cholestasis. There is associated fetal morbidity and mortality (increased incidence of perinatal complications and stillbirths). ICP resolves rapidly after delivery and tends to recur with subsequent pregnancies. Treatment is largely symptomatic (see section on PEP, above); cholestyramine and ultraviolet light may be

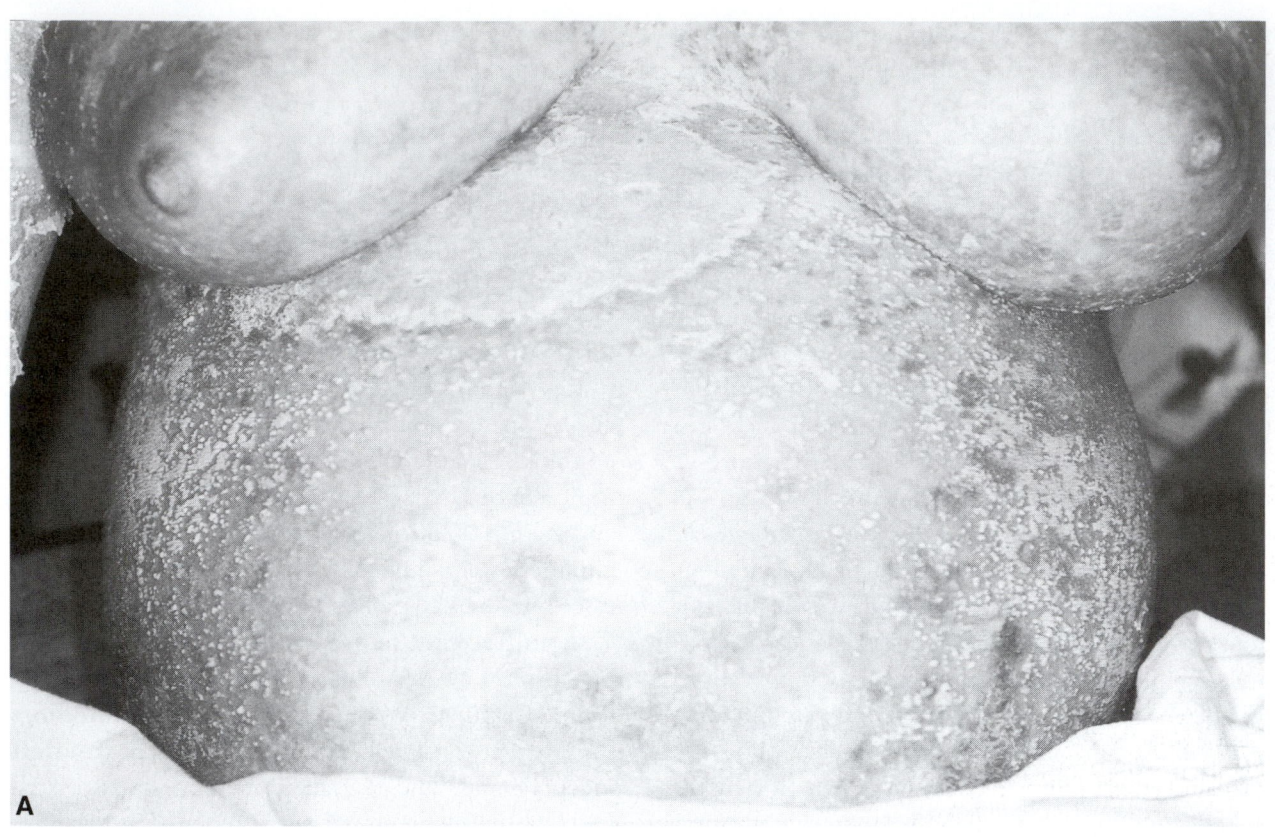

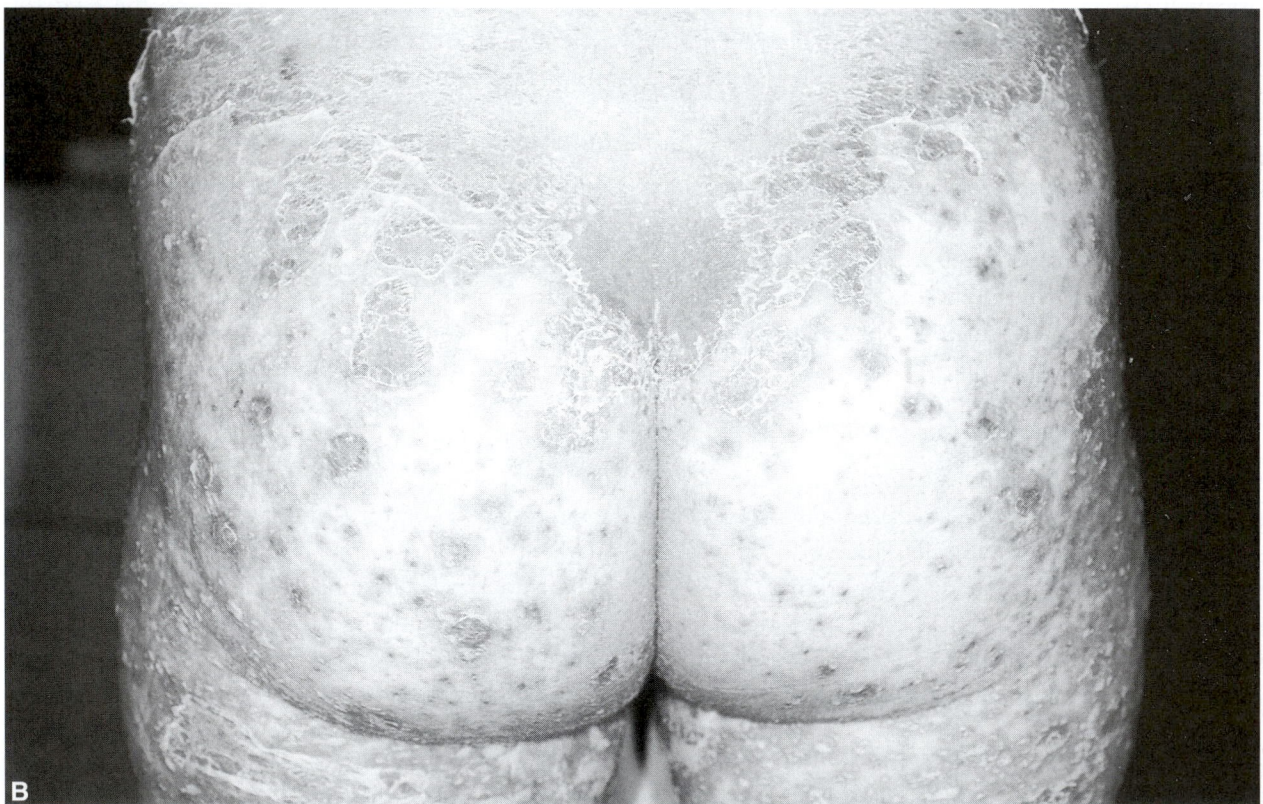

Figure 32-3 A, B, and C. Impetigo herpetiformis. Diffuse erythema studded with sterile pustules.

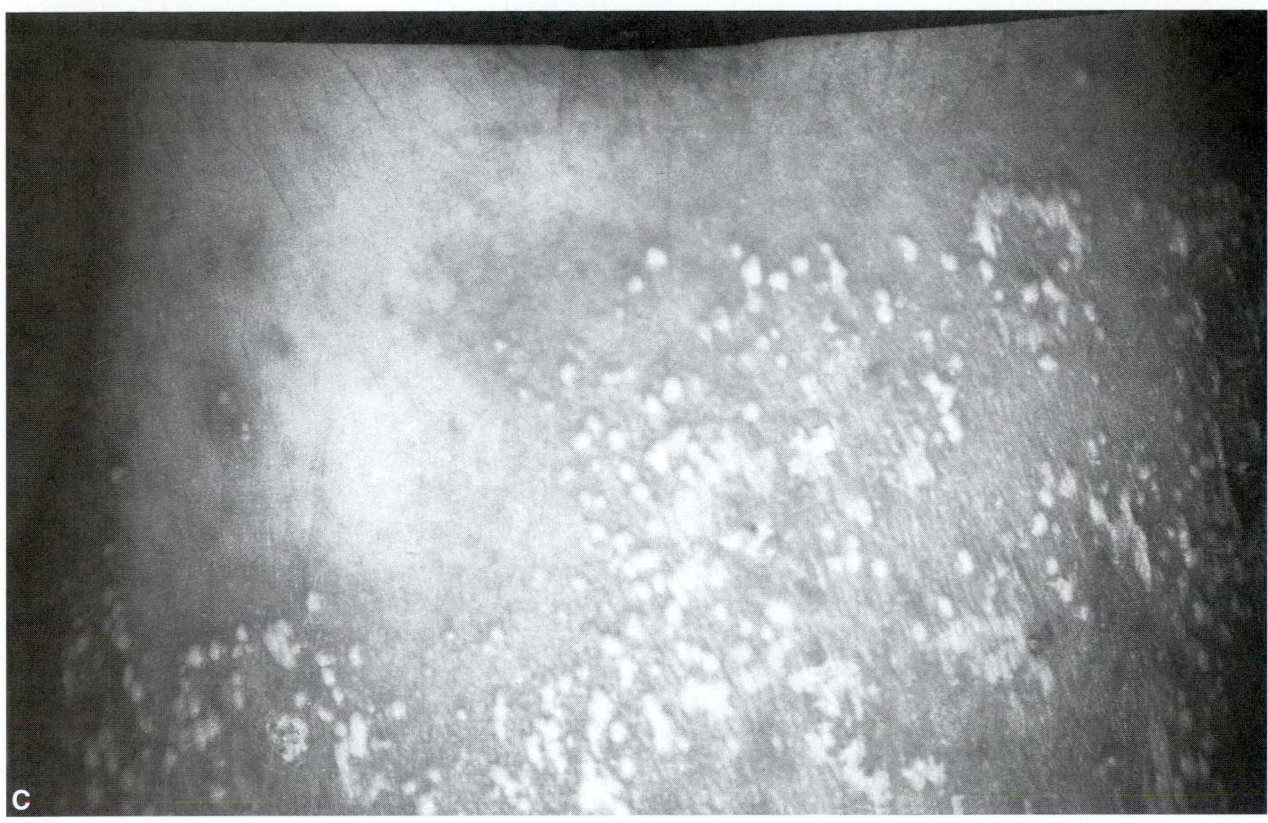

C

beneficial, and in prolonged ICP, vitamin K may be necessary.[10]

Prurigo of Pregnancy

This common, benign dermatosis of pregnancy presents earlier in gestation than the previously described disorders, usually between 25 and 30 weeks. The clinical appearance is characteristic, with extremely pruritic excoriated red or flesh-colored papules most commonly located on extensor surfaces of the trunk and extremities. There is no urticaria and no vesicle formation; this helps distinguish this condition from PEP. The histology of prurigo of pregnancy is nonspecific, and direct immunofluorescence is negative. It may recur with subsequent pregnancies. Treatment usually consists of oral antihistamines, midpotency topical steroids, and over-the-counter or prescription lotions containing α-hydroxy acids. Infants are unaffected, and other than maternal discomfort, there is no significant morbidity.

Pruritic Folliculitis

Patients present usually in the second or third trimester with pruritic monomorphous red follicular papules and pustules disseminated over the back and chest.

The clinical appearance strongly resembles steroid-induced acne. There is no adverse effect on baby or mother, and lesions usually resolve within several weeks of delivery.

A common skin problem that can mimic pruritic folliculitis is miliaria ("prickly heat"), which also manifests as variably pruritic red papules and pustules on the trunk and/or extremities in areas subject to sweating or occlusion. Treatment for miliaria requires keeping the area as cool and dry as possible using powders and loose clothing.

DERMATOSES EXACERBATED PREMENSTRUALLY

It is not uncommon for women to experience cyclical worsening of preexisting skin problems during the second half of the menstrual cycle. Many common dermatologic diseases are reported to worsen premenstrually and include such diverse diseases as acne, eczema, erythema multiforme, lichen planus, lupus, pruritis vulvae, psoriasis, rosacea, and urticaria.[11] Acne vulgaris is probably the most common of these and is the most common disorder treated by dermatologists.

Acne, a disorder of the sebaceous hair follicle, is found on the face, upper back, and chest. At puberty, the increase in circulating androgenic hormones causes enlargement of the sebaceous gland and, consequently, increased sebum production. There is concomitant hyperkeratinization of the follicular infundibulum (hair-follicle opening), which results in a follicular plug (microcomedo). *Propionibacterium acnes*, a lipophilic gram-positive anaerobic diphtheroid, native to the sebaceous hair follicle, begins to proliferate due to the increase in sebum, which is its natural substrate. This bacterium produces a lipase that converts triglycerides to free fatty acids, which are very irritating to the dermis. Because of the hyperkeratinization and plugging, the follicle dilates, the wall thins, and eventually ruptures, extruding sebum, keratin, bacteria, free fatty acids, and other debris into the dermis, causing a cascade of events leading to the development of inflammatory lesions such as papules, pustules, nodules, and cysts (Figure 32-4).

To treat acne effectively, one must attempt to address these mechanisms of pathogenesis. Treatment is also based on the clinical appearance of the lesions (Figure 32-5). There are essentially two clinical types of acne—comedonal and inflammatory—which, in most cases, coexist. Comedones are small, noninflammatory, open or closed papules (blackheads and whiteheads, respectively). Open comedones tend to resolve spontaneously but closed comedones can progress into the more inflammatory papules, pustules, nodules, and cysts, which can lead to permanent scarring.

For comedonal and mild inflammatory acne, topical keratolytics such as retinoids, benzoyl peroxide, salicylic acid, and α-hydroxy acids; topical antibiotics such as erythromycin and clindamycin; and astringents are often effective. For more inflammatory lesions, it is often necessary to add oral antibiotics and in the most severe types (nodulocystic), 13-*cis*-isotretinoin (Accutane) can be used. Extreme caution must be used, however, in females of reproductive age due to the teratogenicity of Accutane. A twenty-week course can cure acne in approximately 80% of cases; however, Accutane has significant side effects

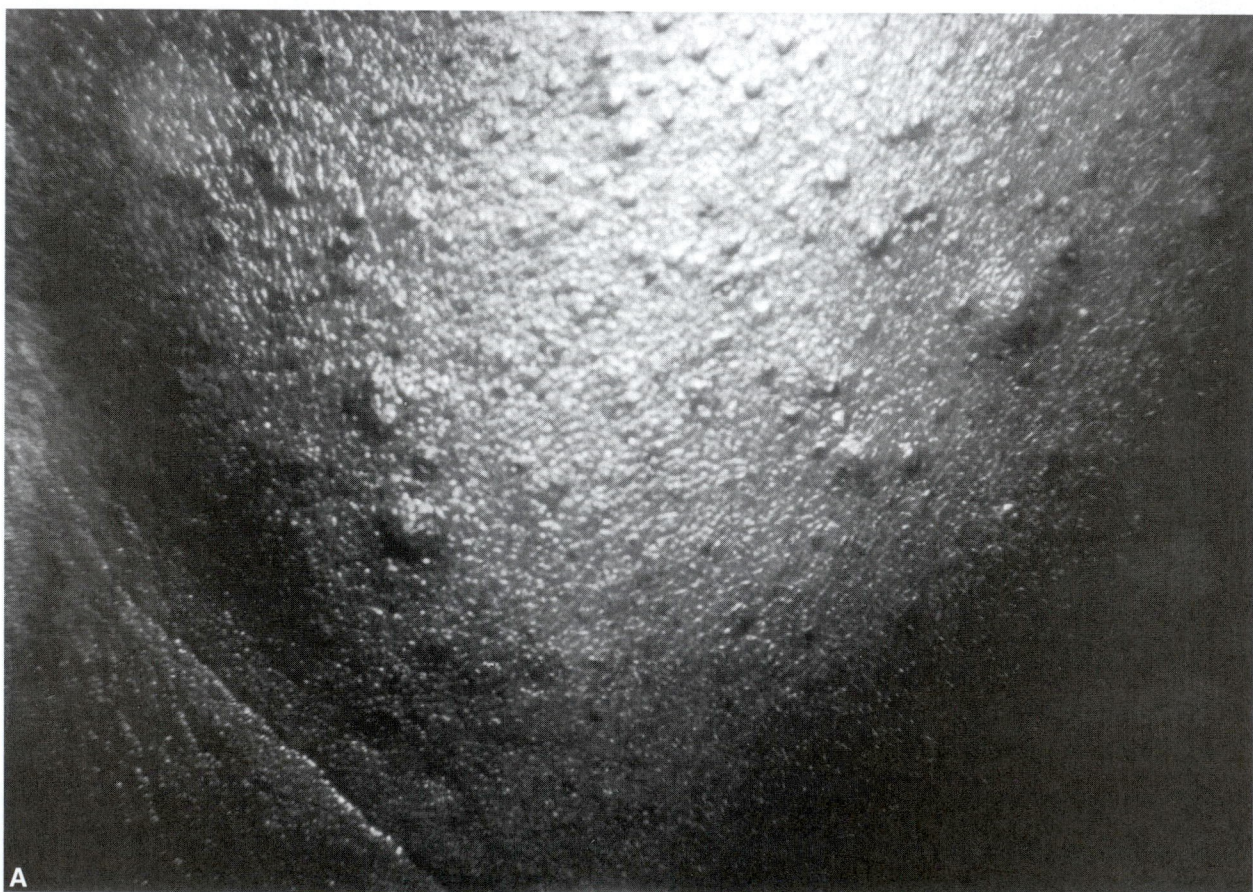

Figure 32-4 A. Noninflammatory comedonal acne. B. Papules and pustules of acne vulgaris. C. Severe inflammatory acne.

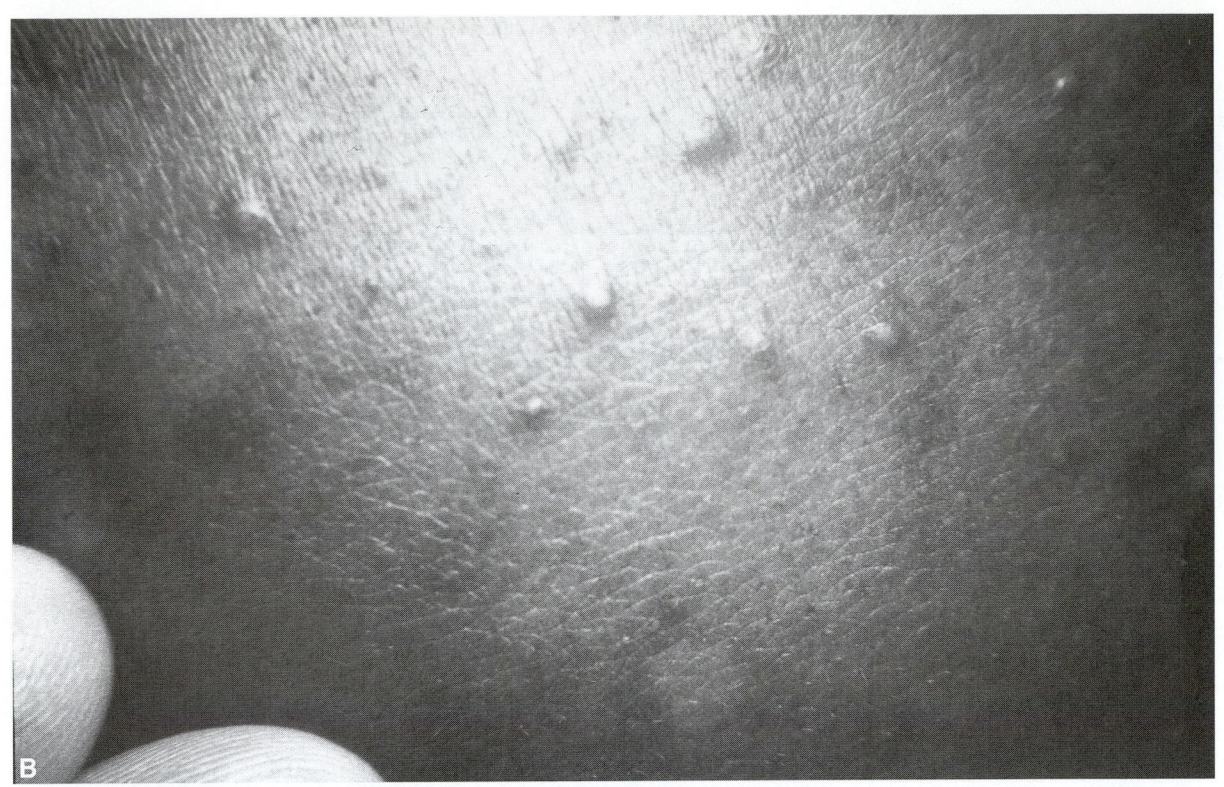

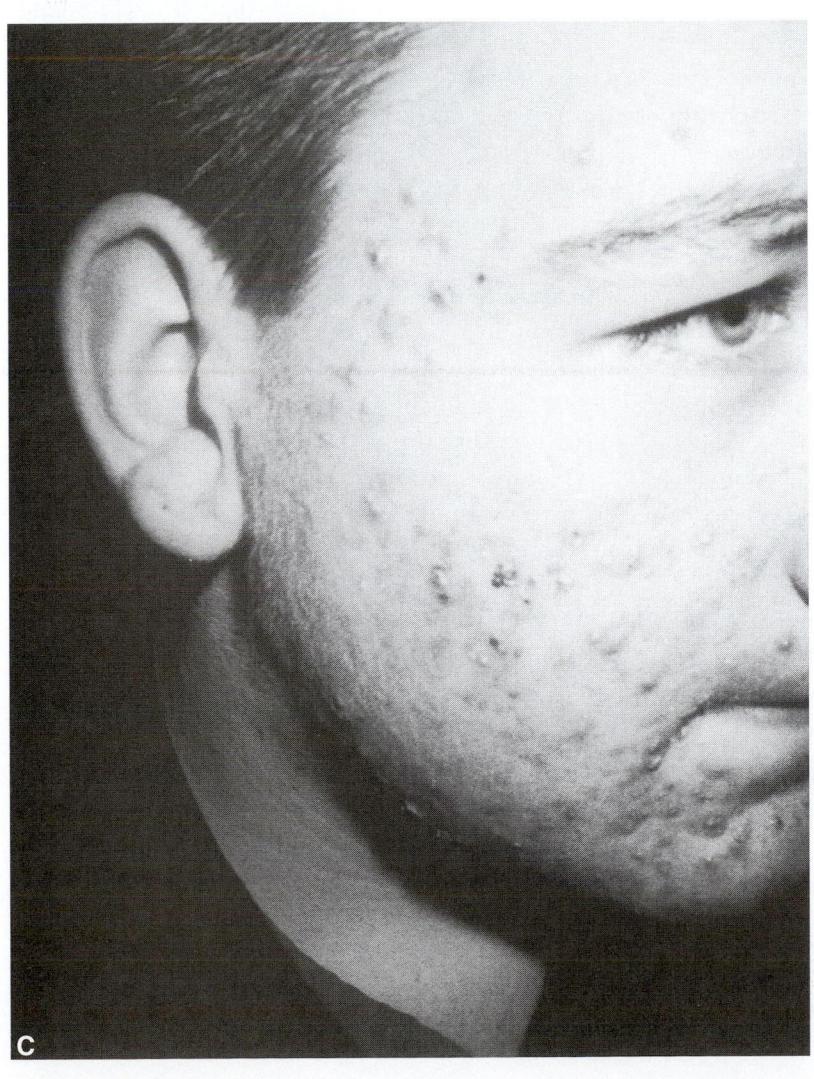

Figure 32-5 Treatment pyramid for acne vulgaris. Patients often require multiple agents aimed at different pathogenic mechanisms.

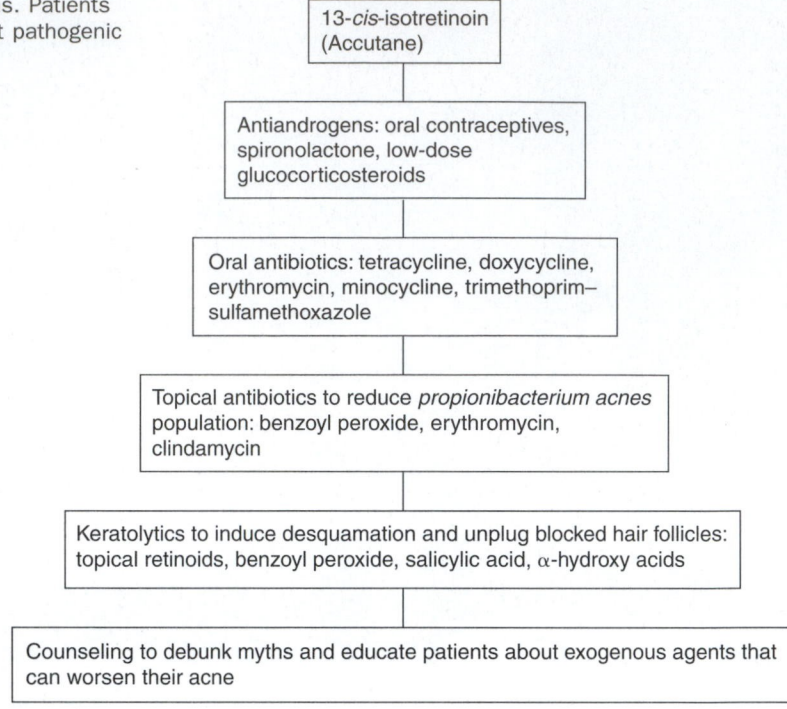

13-*cis*-isotretinoin (Accutane)

Antiandrogens: oral contraceptives, spironolactone, low-dose glucocorticosteroids

Oral antibiotics: tetracycline, doxycycline, erythromycin, minocycline, trimethoprim–sulfamethoxazole

Topical antibiotics to reduce *propionibacterium acnes* population: benzoyl peroxide, erythromycin, clindamycin

Keratolytics to induce desquamation and unplug blocked hair follicles: topical retinoids, benzoyl peroxide, salicylic acid, α-hydroxy acids

Counseling to debunk myths and educate patients about exogenous agents that can worsen their acne

and its use requires frequent laboratory monitoring. Isotretinoin should be reserved for severe refractory disease, and patients should probably be referred to someone familiar with its use.

When treating patients with acne, it is mandatory to discuss their use of hair care products, cosmetics, soaps, and any topical product they may be using, as these can contribute to or worsen their disease. It is also important to counsel patients regarding the pathogenesis of acne and dispel any myths they may believe regarding its development, such as foods, drinks, and poor hygiene. Patients should also be warned that any new acne regimen will take 8 to 10 weeks for maximum improvement. They should not expect results overnight.

For refractory disease in females that is exacerbated premenstrually, oral contraceptives containing low levels of progestin and ethinyl estradiol such as

Ortho-Tri-Cyclen can be beneficial. Spironolactone, with its antiandrogen activity, can also benefit this specific patient population.

It is important to remember that acne can be a sign of systemic disease, such as polycystic ovary disease, adrenal hyperplasia, virilizing tumors, and Cushing syndrome (see Table 32-4). Prolonged use of systemic steroids or topical steroids applied to the face can worsen preexisting disease or cause the development of new lesions. Other drugs, such as phenytoin, lithium, isoniazid, and halides can also contribute to the development or worsening of acne. It is important to have a high index of clinical suspicion and to examine the patient for other signs of virilization (Figure 32-6) when a systemic process is suspected.

Finally, it is important to realize that acne is not just a cosmetic disease. The severe forms can cause permanent scarring and can lead to serious psychosocial debilitation, especially in adolescents, whose self-esteem is often fragile. Residual postinflammatory pigmentary changes can be very distressing as well, especially in patients with dark skin. These changes may take months or even years to resolve, and can be as upsetting to the patient as the acne itself. Therefore, clinicians caring for these patients should be sensitive to their desire for treatment and willing to treat or refer to a dermatologist.

TABLE 32-4
SYSTEMIC CAUSES OF ACNE

Systemic steroids and other drugs*
Polycystic ovary disease
Cushing disease and syndrome
Adrenal hyperplasia
Adrenal tumors

---

*Adrenocorticotropic hormone, bromides, iodides, isoniazid, lithium, and phenytoin.

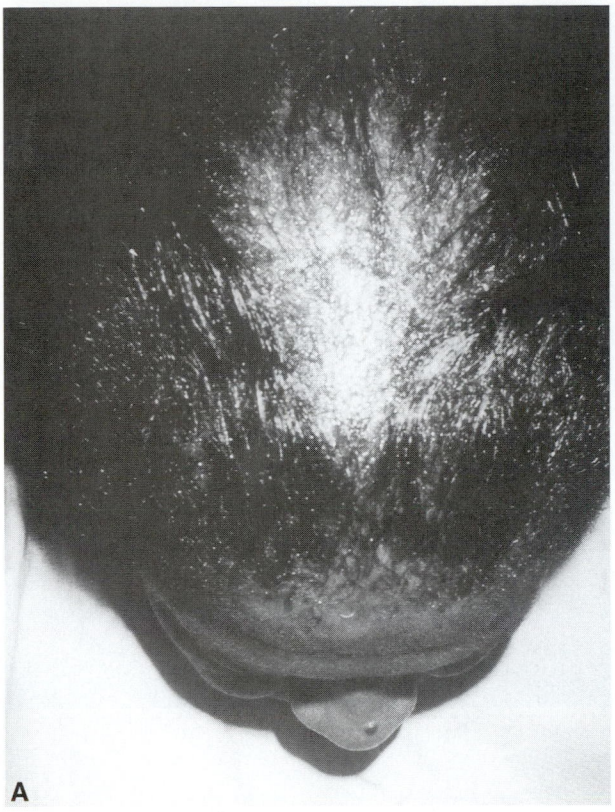

Figure 32-6 A and B. This constellation of androgenic alopecia, acne, and hirsuitism are suggestive of virilization.

VULVAR DISEASES

As mentioned earlier, the goal of this chapter is to present an overview of common dermatologic problems and their treatment in the context of pregnancy and vulvar dermatoses. The following discussion includes general principles of diagnosis and treatment, with special emphasis on the appearance and treatment of these diseases when they present in the vulvar area.

Infectious

This section on infectious diseases of the vulva will be limited to diseases that frequently present to and are treated by the dermatologist. A more detailed discussion of sexually transmitted diseases, including human papillomavirus, is included in elsewhere in this text.

Bacterial

PERIANAL STREPTOCOCCAL CELLULITIS Almost exclusively seen in children, this infection with β-hemolytic streptococci is probably introduced by fingers from other sites such as the oropharnyx.

Clinically, one sees pruritic perianal erythema resembling dermatitis. Patients may also complain of painful defecation, anal fissures, or blood-streaked stools. Cultures of the affected area show a moderate to heavy growth of β-hemolytic streptococci. Treatment consists of appropriate oral antibiotics.

ERYTHRASMA This relatively common form of axillary, vulvar, and toe-web intertrigo is caused by a gram-positive skin diphtheroid, *Corynebacterium minutissimum*. It characteristically presents as sharply demarcated brownish-red scaly intertriginous plaques that may or may not be pruritic. Because this bacteria produces a porphyrin byproduct, it will fluoresce coral red under long-wave UVA light, and a portable Wood's lamp (black light) can be a very useful diagnostic tool. Culture is difficult and not routinely done. Erythrasma can be treated effectively with oral or topical erythromycin.

IMPETIGO Impetigo is a superficial skin infection most commonly seen in children living in warm, humid climates, but it can occur in adults as well.

Figure 32-7 Honey-colored crust of impetigo.

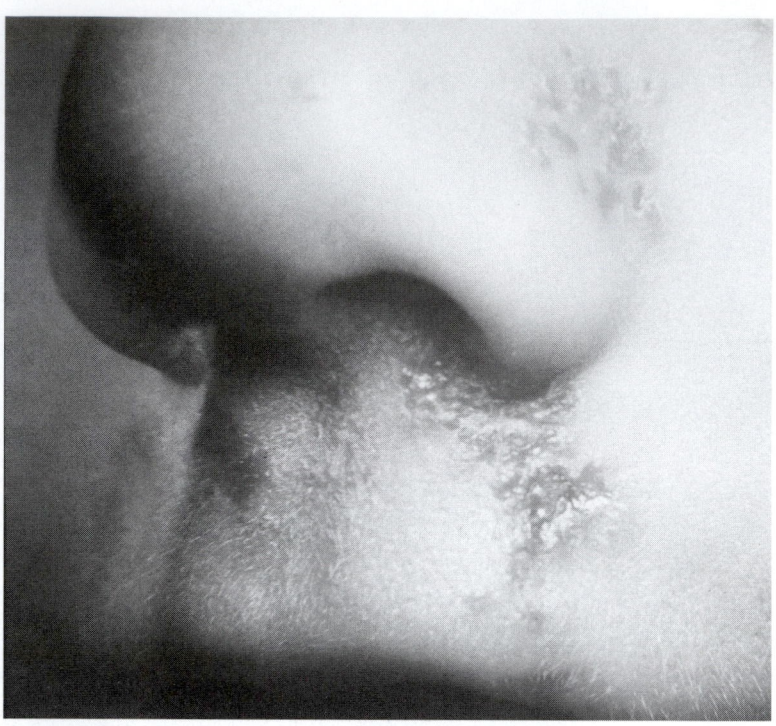

Any cutaneous surface may be affected, but areas that have been damaged by minor trauma (scratches, abrasions, insect bites) or primary skin diseases such as dermatitis, are more commonly involved. The classic nonbullous form begins as a papulovesicle or pustule on a base of erythema that rapidly ruptures and develops a honey-colored, varnish-like crust (Figure 32-7). Lesions may coalesce into large areas of involvement, and regional lymphadenopathy may be present, but systemic manifestations such as fever are rare. Bullous lesions can occur with certain toxin-producing strains of *Staphylococcus aureus* (phage group II, types 55 and 71). Culture of *Staph. aureus* or *Streptococcus pyogenes* from the lesion confirms the diagnosis. Treatment of localized infections can be accomplished with soaks and topical mupirocin (Bactroban), but widespread or bullous lesions are best treated with systemic antibiotics effective against penicillinase-producing *Staph. aureus*. For patients allergic to penicillin, erythromycin and clindamycin are alternatives. A rare but potentially life-threatening complication of impetigo is acute poststreptococcal glomerulonephritis, which occurs with certain nephritogenic strains of *Strep. pyogenes*.

FOLLICULITIS AND FURUNCULOSIS Bacterial folliculitis (superficial inflammation of hair follicles) and furunculosis (larger deep-seated nodules) are usually secondary to *Staph. aureus*. Any hair-bearing surface can be affected, but the scalp, buttocks, and extremities are more frequently involved. Crops of follicular papules and pustules (folliculitis) or tender, red, fluctuant nodules (furuncles) are seen, often with a halo of erythema. Pruritus is not uncommon. Precipitating factors include occlusion, friction, excessive sweating, and contact with oils. Treatment requires avoidance of these aggravating factors and antistaphylococcal therapy, which may be topical or systemic, depending on the extent of disease.

Pseudomonas folliculitis can occur after the use of contaminated swimming pools, hot tubs, or whirlpools. The eruption usually develops within 48 hours and consists of pruritic 2- to 10-mm red papules and pustules that tend to be most concentrated in areas occluded by tight swimsuits. Systemic infection is rare, and no specific treatment is necessary, as lesions will resolve spontaneously. Adequate disinfection of the water source is required.

TRICHOMYCOSIS This hair-shaft disorder is caused by several species of corynebacteria and characteristically consists of asymptomatic waxy, colorless to yellow-brown concretions on the axillary and/or pubic hair. Shaving of the affected area followed by twice-daily application of topical erythromycin is usually adequate treatment.

Color Plate

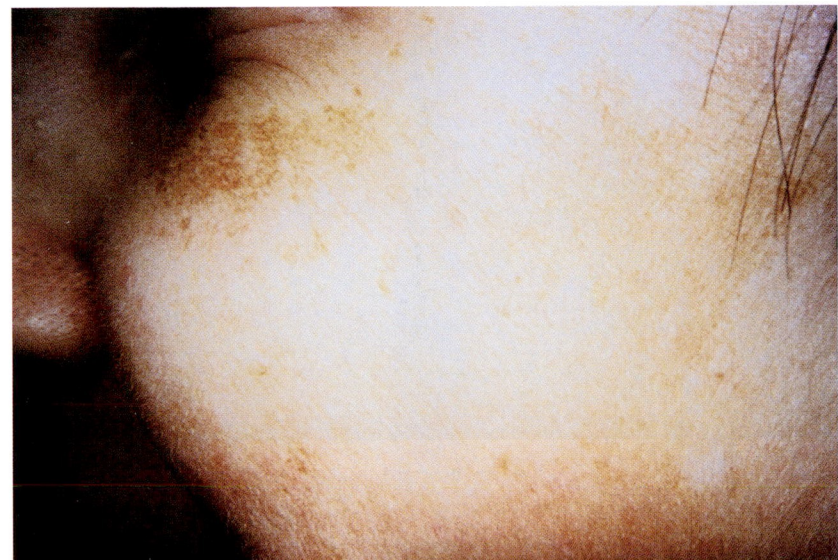

Figure 32-1 Close-up view of melasma. Note the reticulated brown patches on the cheek.

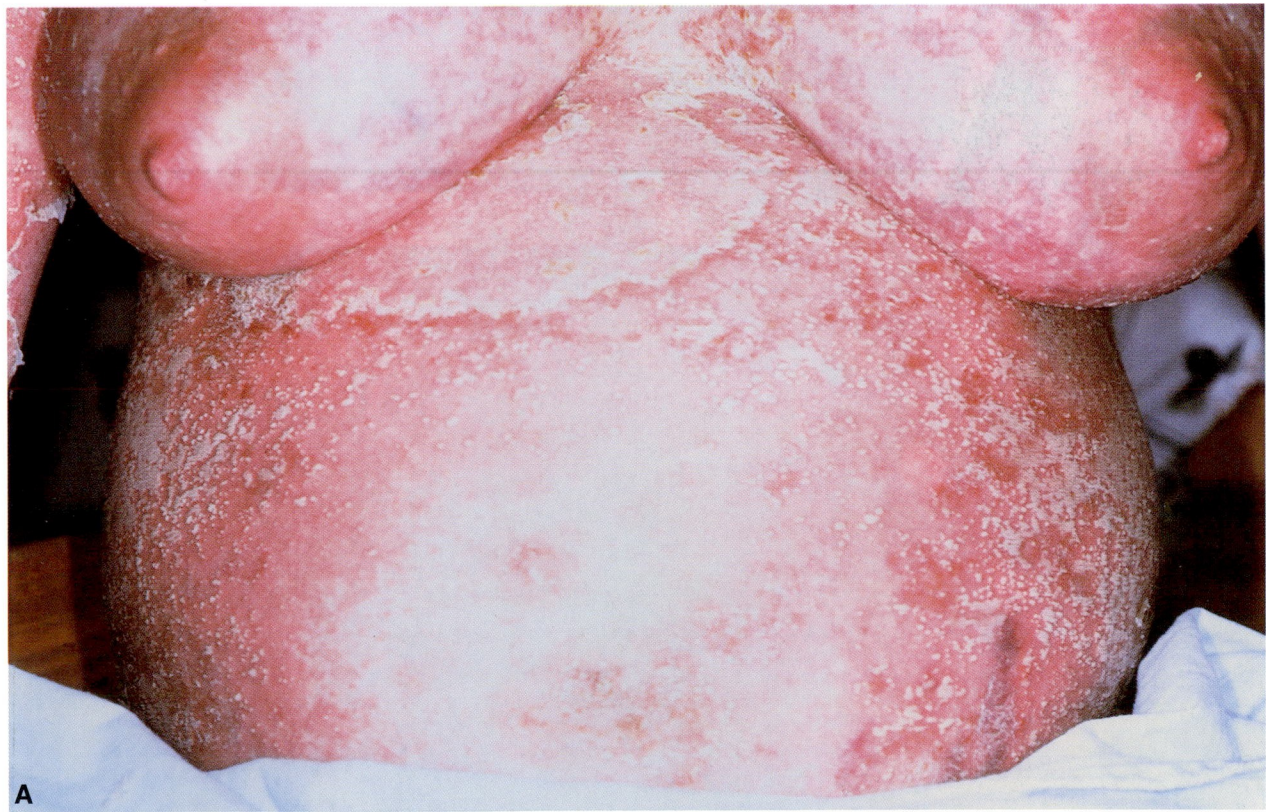

Figure 32-3 A. Impetigo herpetiformis. Diffuse erythema studded with sterile pustules.

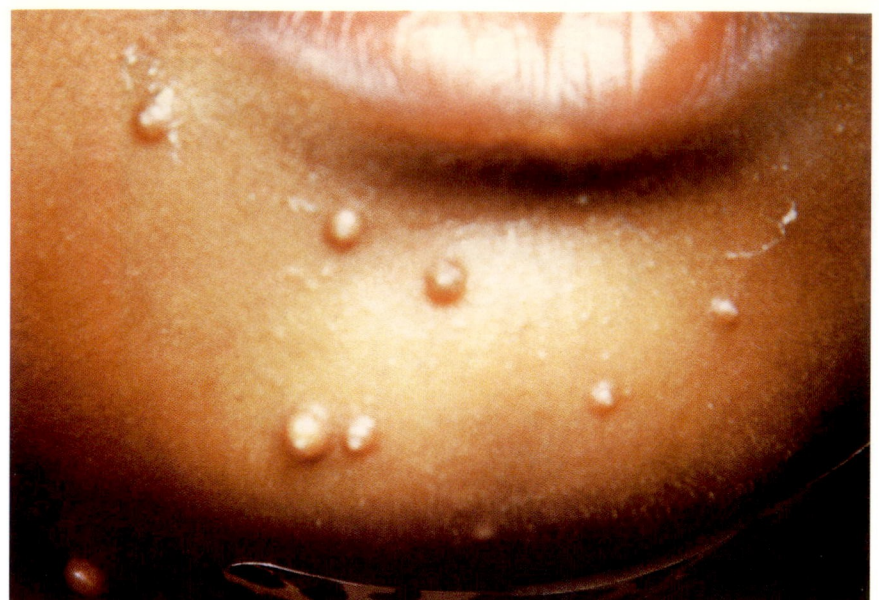

Figure 32-12 Molluscum contagiosum. Scattered flesh-colored and translucent dome-shaped papules, some of which are umbilicated.

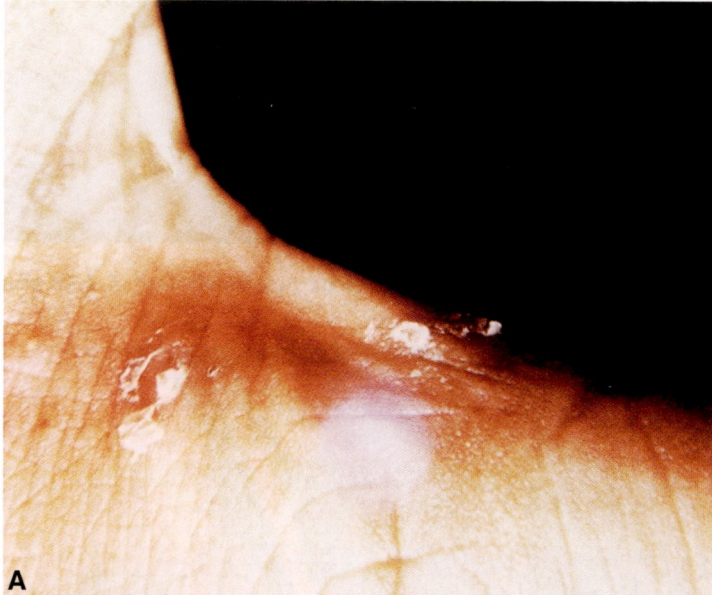

A

Figure 32-13 A. Interdigital scabies—subtle burrows and vesicles between fingers.

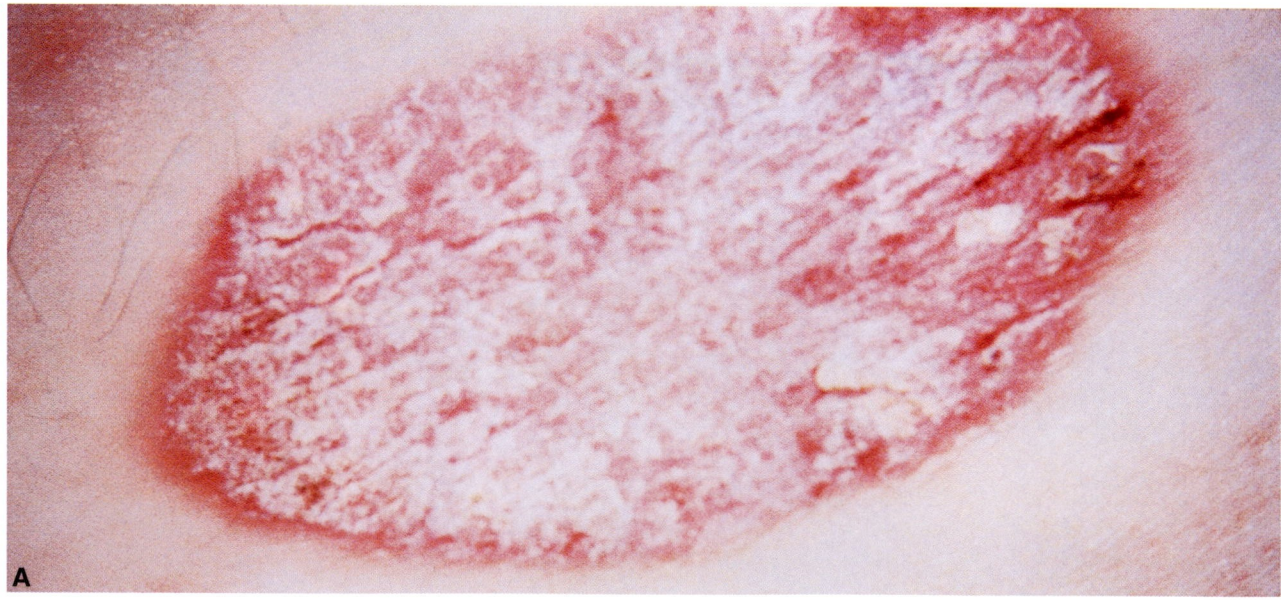

A

Figure 32-14 A. Classic plaque-type psoriasis. Sharply marginated erythematous plaques with overlying white micaceous scale.

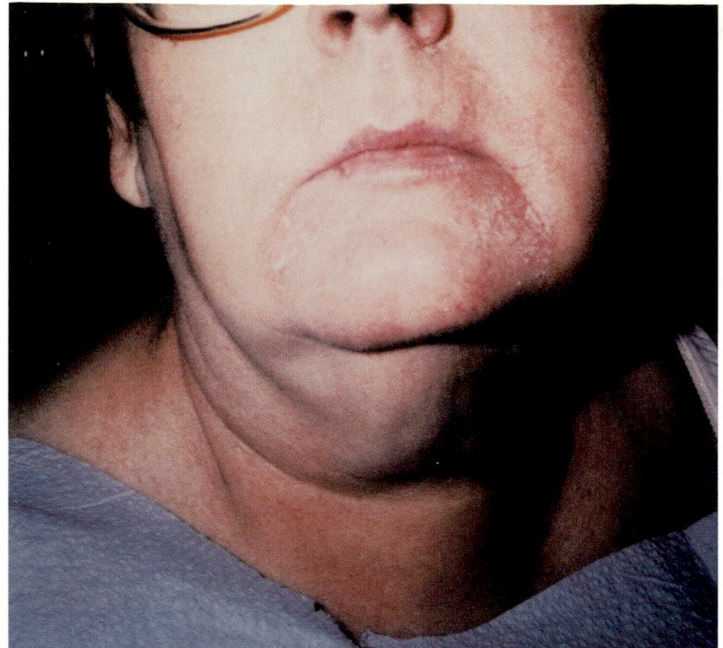

Figure 32-15 C. Seborrheic dermatitis.

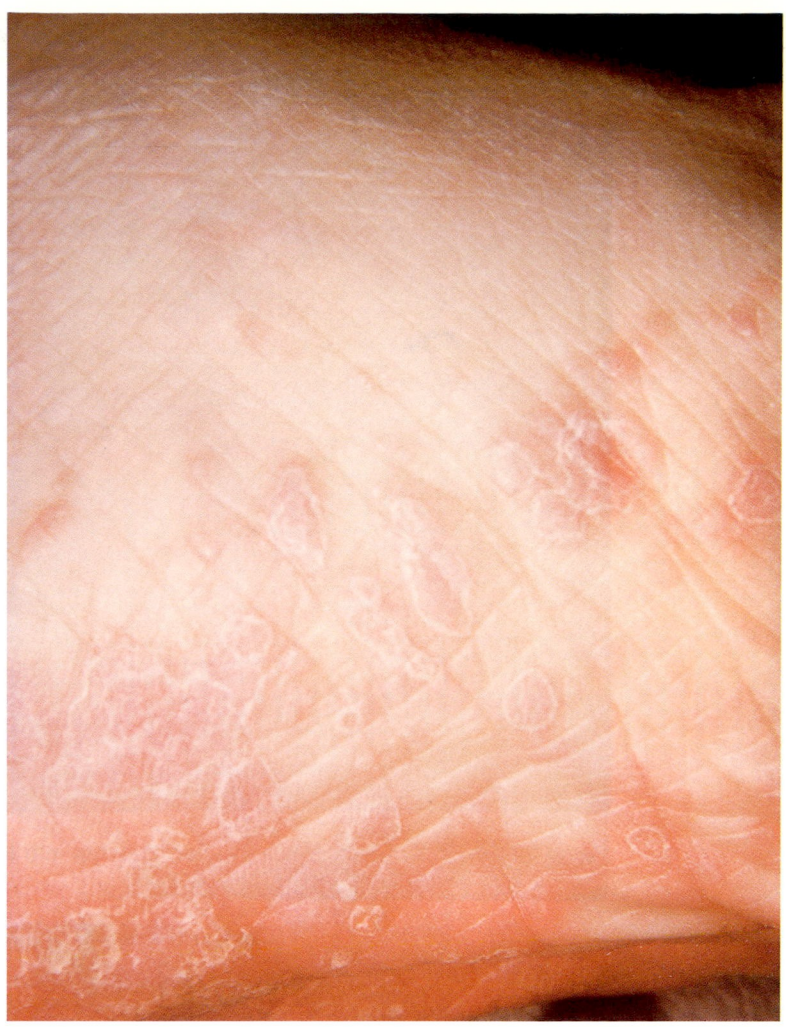

Figure 32-16 Polygonal purple pruritic papules of lichen planus. Note overlying Wickham striae.

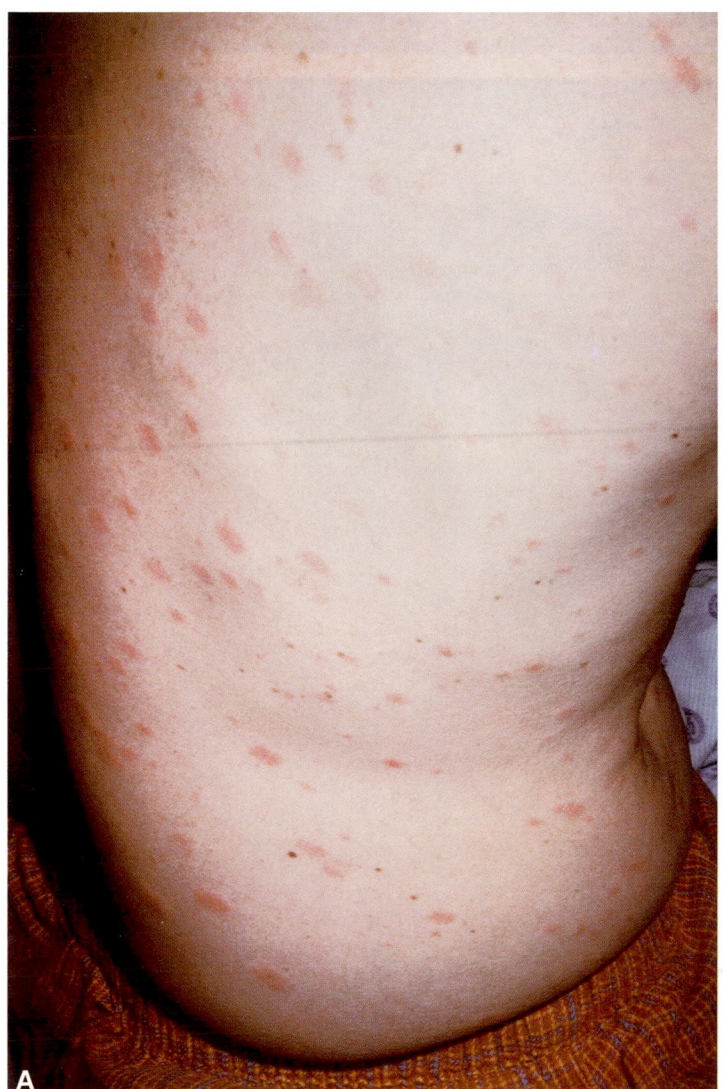

Figure 32-17 A. Pityriasis rosea. Pink oval lesions following skin cleavage lines of the lateral chest in a "Christmas tree" pattern.

5

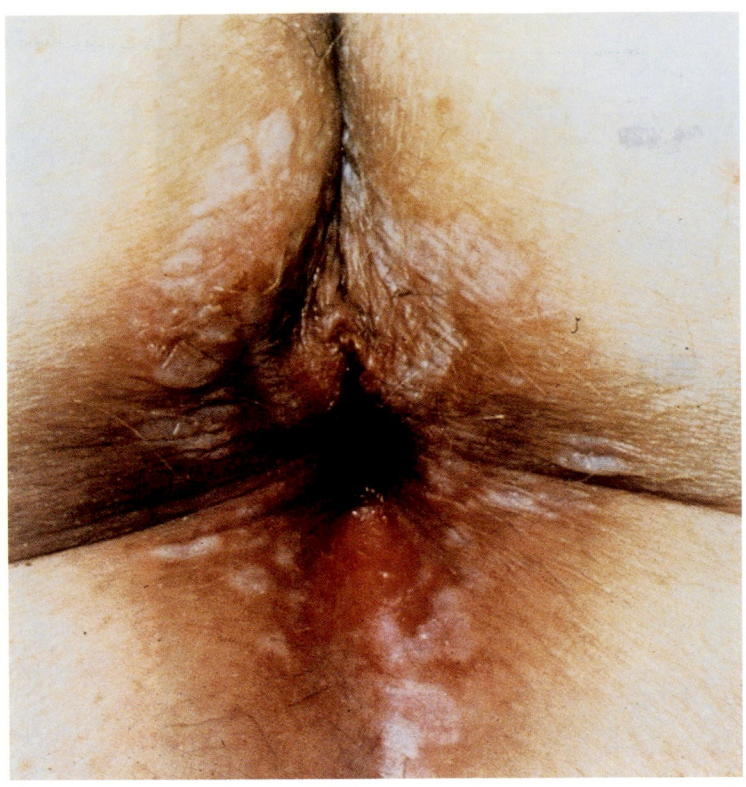

Figure 32-22 Perianal lichen sclerosis. Depigmented atrophic macules with characteristic "cigarette paper wrinkling."

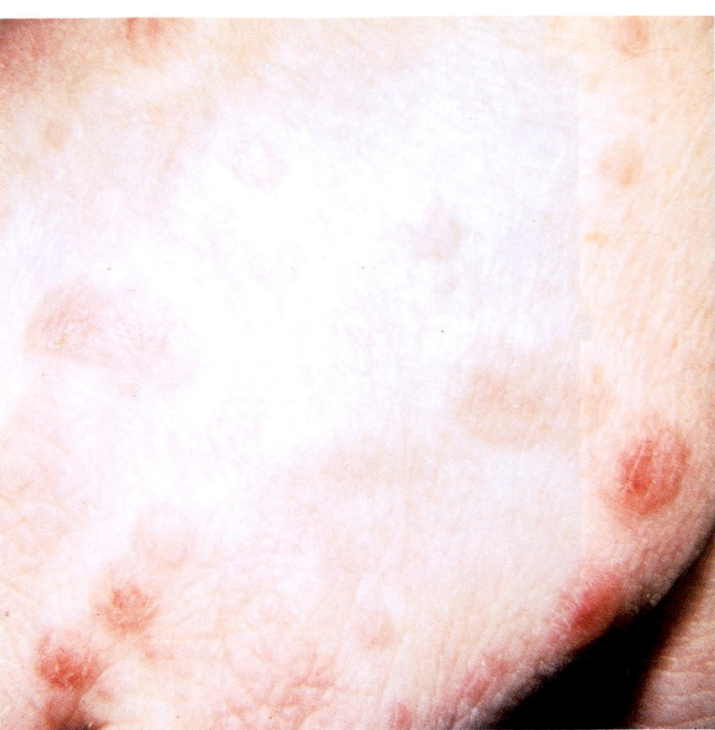

Figure 32-23 Close-up of target lesions of erythema multiforme on the dorsal hand.

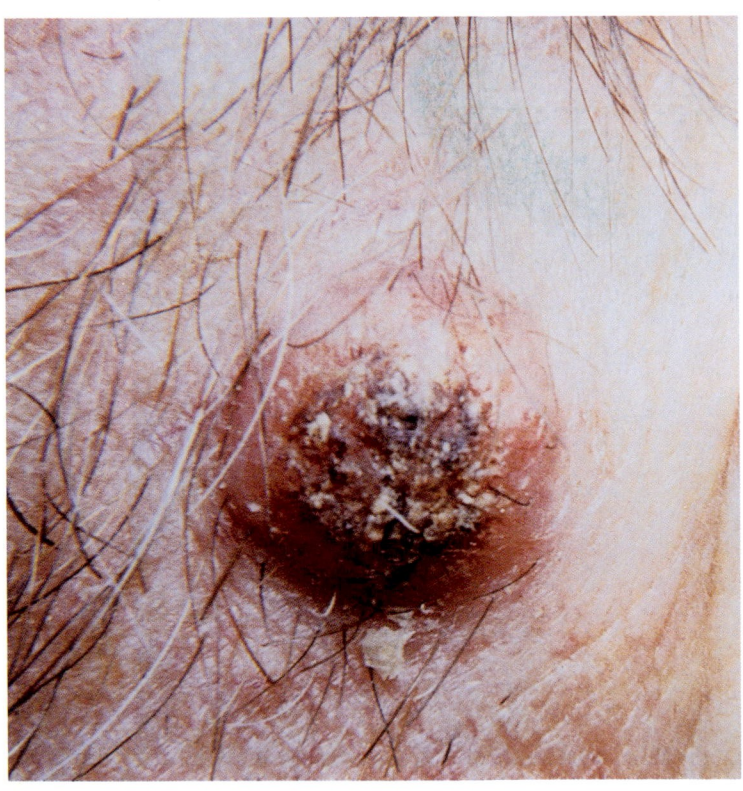

Figure 32-26 Preauricular squamous-cell carcinoma.

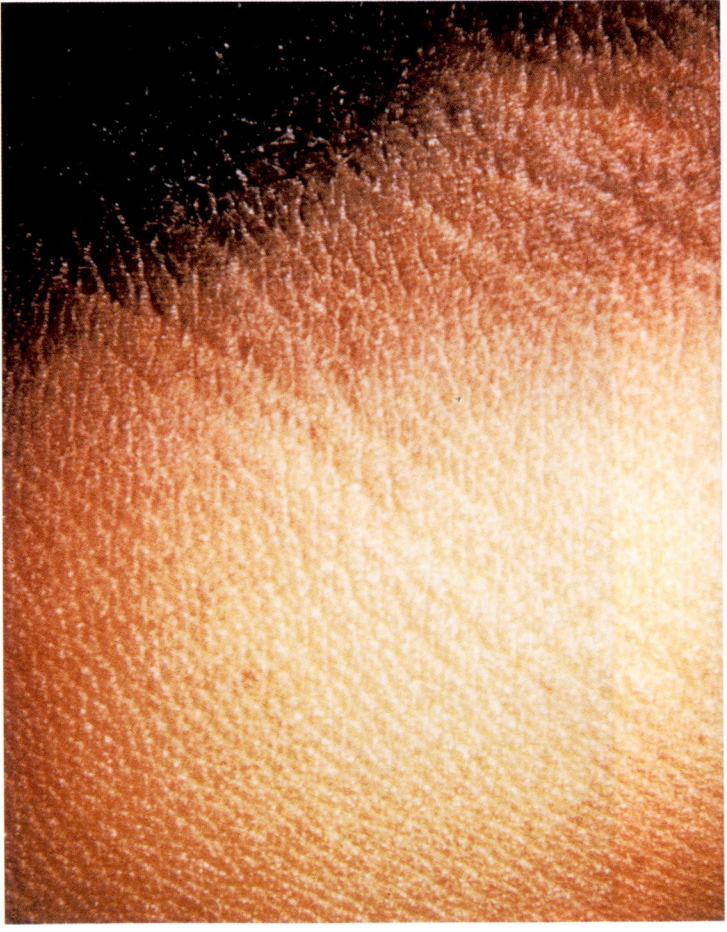

Figure 32-28 Close-up of acanthosis nigricans. Velvety, hyperpigmented, papillomatous skin of the neck.

Fungal

DERMATOPHYTOSIS (TINEA) Superficial fungal infections of the skin, hair, and nails are very common dermatologic problems and are caused by several species of dermatophyte, giving rise to a variety of clinical presentations. The classic clinical appearance is an inflammatory, variably pruritic annular plaque with a scaling red border (Figure 32-8); however, there is a clinical spectrum, and frequently at the time of presentation the appearance has been modified by the use of over-the-counter or prescription medication. Tinea incognito refers to tinea infections that have been masked by the use of topical steroids, which will reduce the erythema, pruritus, and scale, often leading to misdiagnosis by the unwary clinician. Tinea cruris usually involves the medial thighs, inguinal folds, and less often, the labia majora. The labia minora are rarely involved. Potassium hydroxide examination will reveal filamentous, septate, branching hyphae. If the potassium hydroxide examination is negative, fungal culture can provide accurate diagnosis. Localized skin infections can be treated twice daily with a topical antifungal such as terbenifine, an allylamine, or a variety of azoles, including ketoconazole, clotrimazole, econazole, and miconazole. More extensive cutaneous disease, and hair or nail disease, must be treated with systemic agents effective against dermatophytes.

Commonly used systemic drugs include terbenifine, itraconazole, and fluconazole. Griseofulvin is still the drug of choice for tinea capitis in children, but is not as effective in tinea corporis and is almost useless in onychomycosis. Because treatment of onychomycosis requires longer-term therapy with systemic agents that have potential side effects, mycologic diagnosis is required. This can be accomplished via potassium hydroxide preparation, fungal culture, or biopsy for histologic examination. A popular treatment regimen for onychomycosis is pulse therapy using itraconazole, 400 mg/day in single or divided doses for 7 days per month for 3 consecutive months. Proper patient selection is mandatory, however, because of potential side effects and drug interactions. Terbenifine has been approved by the Food and Drug Administration (FDA) only for daily dosing with 250 mg/day, and has the advantage of fewer drug interactions. Both of these agents are well tolerated, but physicians should be familiar with their side-effect profiles before prescribing them. Both itraconazole and terbenifine are keratophilic and are concentrated in the nail plate and although the clinical effect may be minimal after

---

| **TABLE 32-5** |
| **COMMON CAUSES OF INTERTRIGO** |

Irritant dermatitis due to friction, heat, and sweating
Candida
Seborrheic dermatitis
Psoriasis
Erythrasma

---

3 months, the antifungal effect persists even after discontinuation of the medication.

CANDIDA *Candida albicans* and *Candida glabrata* are common causes of intertrigo (dermatitis of flexural areas, such as the axillae, neck, diaper area, and inframammary areas). See Table 32-5 for other common causes of intertrigo. Local predisposing factors are moisture, heat, friction, and in the diaper area, incontinence of bowel and bladder. Predisposing systemic factors include diabetes mellitus, immunosuppresion, antibiotic use, topical steroids, and pregnancy. The classic presentation is erythematous patches or plaques, often pronounced in skin folds, with satellite papules or pustules (Figure 32-9). The eruption may be painful and/or pruritic, and erosions are sometimes present. Potassium hydroxide examination will show pseudohyphae and budding yeast. Culture is sometimes necessary if the potassium hydroxide examination is negative. Treatment consists of keeping the area as dry as possible and systemic or topical antifungals (topical nystatin or topical azoles), which can be combined with zinc oxide paste, which has a soothing as well as a drying effect.

Perleche (angular stomatitis) is due to candidiasis at the angles of the mouth due to chronic moisture caused by pooling of saliva. This may be secondary to ill-fitting dentures or the aging process, which causes a concavity in the area due to skin laxity.

Candida can also cause chronic paronychia in persons whose hands are frequently wet, such as housewives, bartenders, etc. It presents with pink edematous proximal and lateral nailfolds, with or without tenderness, and is frequently associated with horizontal banding of the nail plate. It is essential to keep the hands dry using gloves whenever possible. Topical therapy alone is sometimes effective, but systemic therapy is often necessary.

PITYROSPORUM *Pityrosporum ovale/orbiculare* is a biphasic lipophilic yeast that is commensal to the skin,

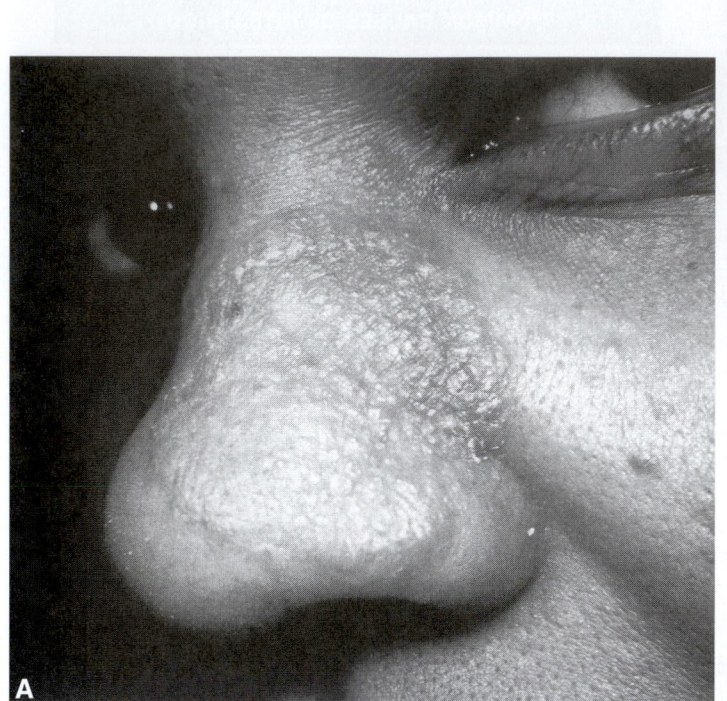

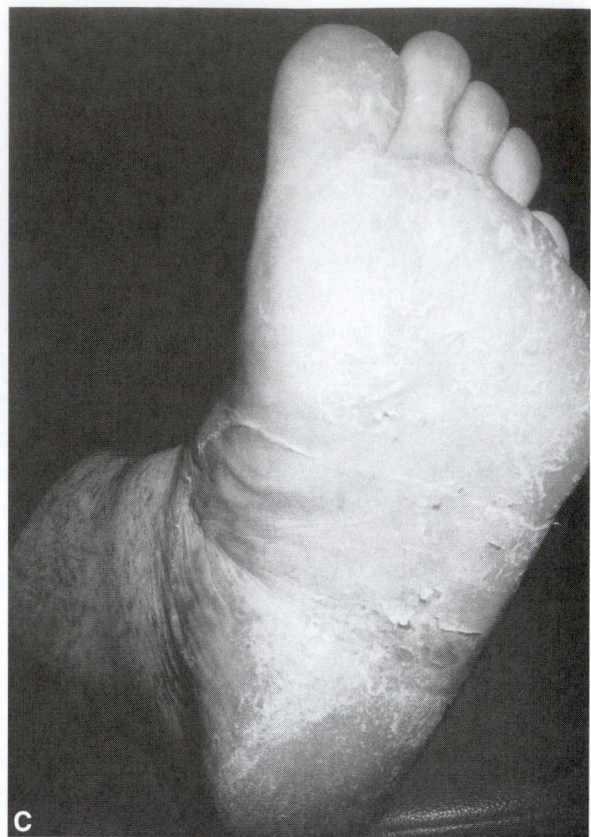

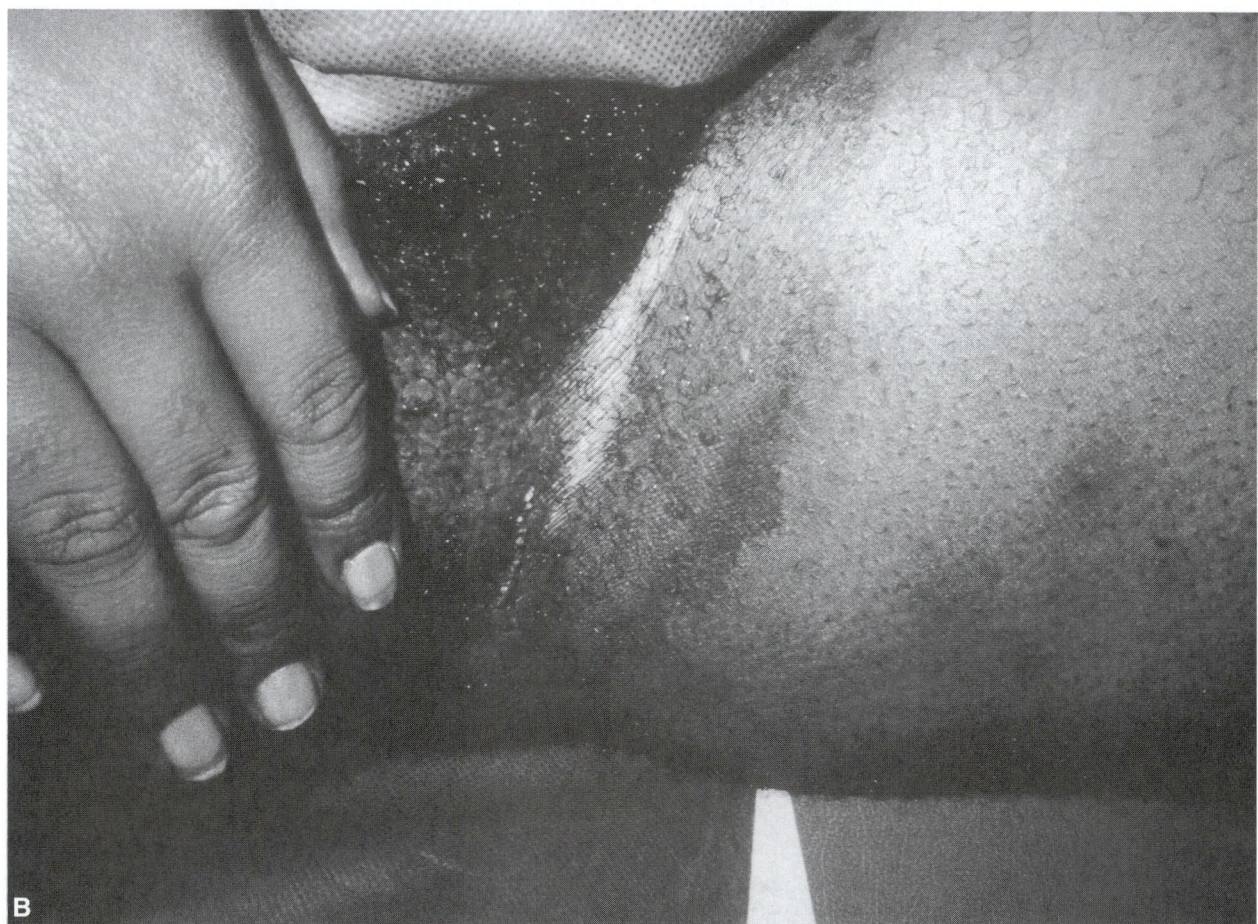

Figure 32-8 A. Characteristic annular scaling plaque of tinea facei. B. Tinea cruris.
C. Tinea pedis.

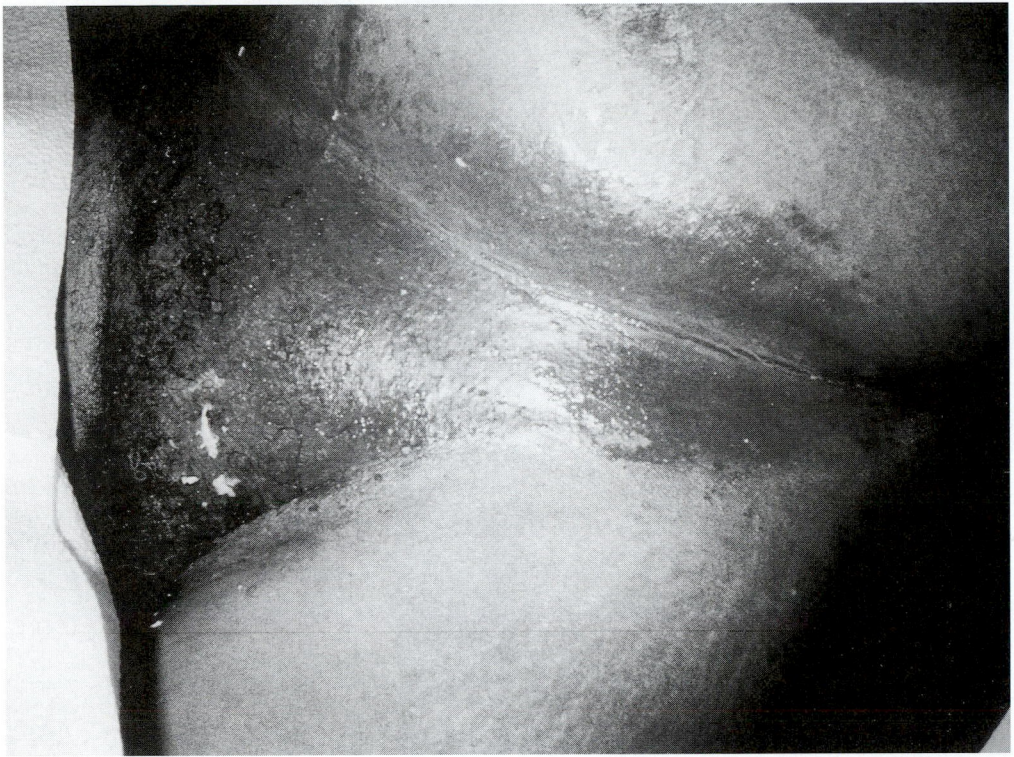

Figure 32-9 Bright erythema and satellite papules of intertriginous candidiasis.

colonizing the seborrheic areas (scalp, face, groin, upper back, and chest), which in certain situations (not clearly defined) becomes pathogenic, causing a variety of conditions such as seborrheic dermatitis, tinea versicolor, and in some individuals, pityrosporum folliculitis. Tinea versicolor presents with hypopigmented or hyperpigmented, mildly scaling patches, most commonly on the upper back, chest, and proximal extremities. Although uncommon, the vulvar area can be affected. The face is usually spared but can be involved. Potassium hydroxide examination of tinea versicolor shows short, fat, branching hyphae and grapelike clusters of spores with a "spaghetti and meatballs" appearance. Pityrosporum folliculitis usually presents as monomorphous follicular papules and pustules in the seborrheic areas. A variety of topical and systemic therapies is effective for both tinea versicolor and pityrosporum folliculitis and include selenium sulfide, propylene glycol, and topical azoles. A single dose or a short course of oral ketoconazole can be effective as well.

Viral

Many viruses can cause nonspecific exanthematous skin eruptions, but the number of viruses that can cause clinically specific skin lesions is limited. These include herpesvirus, human papillomavirus (HPV), and poxvirus, all of which are double-stranded DNA viruses. The section on herpes and HPV will be limited to nongenital lesions, as sexually transmitted diseases are described in more detail elsewhere in this text.

HERPES Two herpesviruses, varicella–zoster virus (VZV) and herpes simplex virus (HSV) have specific, clinically diagnostic skin lesions. Primary varicella (chickenpox) as well as varicella–zoster (shingles) and herpes simplex (Figure 32-10) all have similar primary lesions. VZV, in immunocompetent patients, is very characteristic, with clustered vesicles on an erythematous base in a unilateral or dermatomal distribution (see Figure 32-10). In primary varicella, the lesions are more numerous, much less clustered, and are disseminated over the entire body. Lesions are usually in many stages of development—i.e., papules (some of which may be umbilicated), vesicles, pustules, and crusted erosions. Mucosal involvement is not uncommon. Primary herpes simplex, unlike recurrent HSV, is often associated with constitutional symptoms such as fever, and tends to have larger numbers of lesions, which are more painful. Lesions of HSV are often less characteristic than those of VZV because their location on mucosal or modified

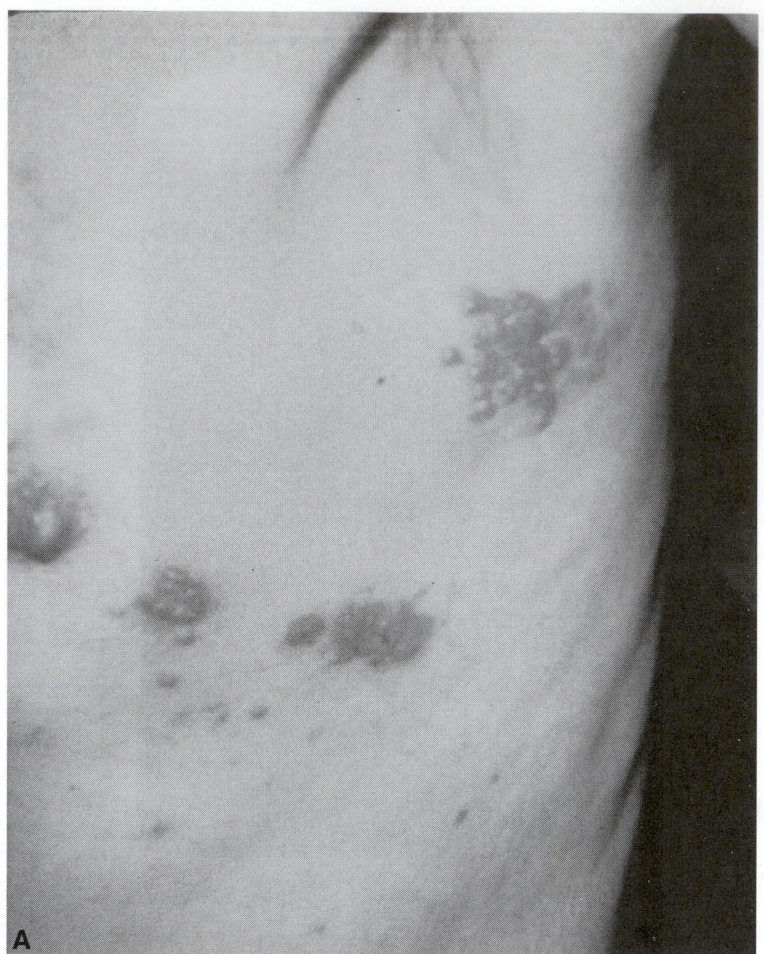

Figure 32-10 A. *Varicella zoster.* Clustered vesicles on an erythematous base in a dermatomal distribution. B. Close-up of herpetic vesicles.

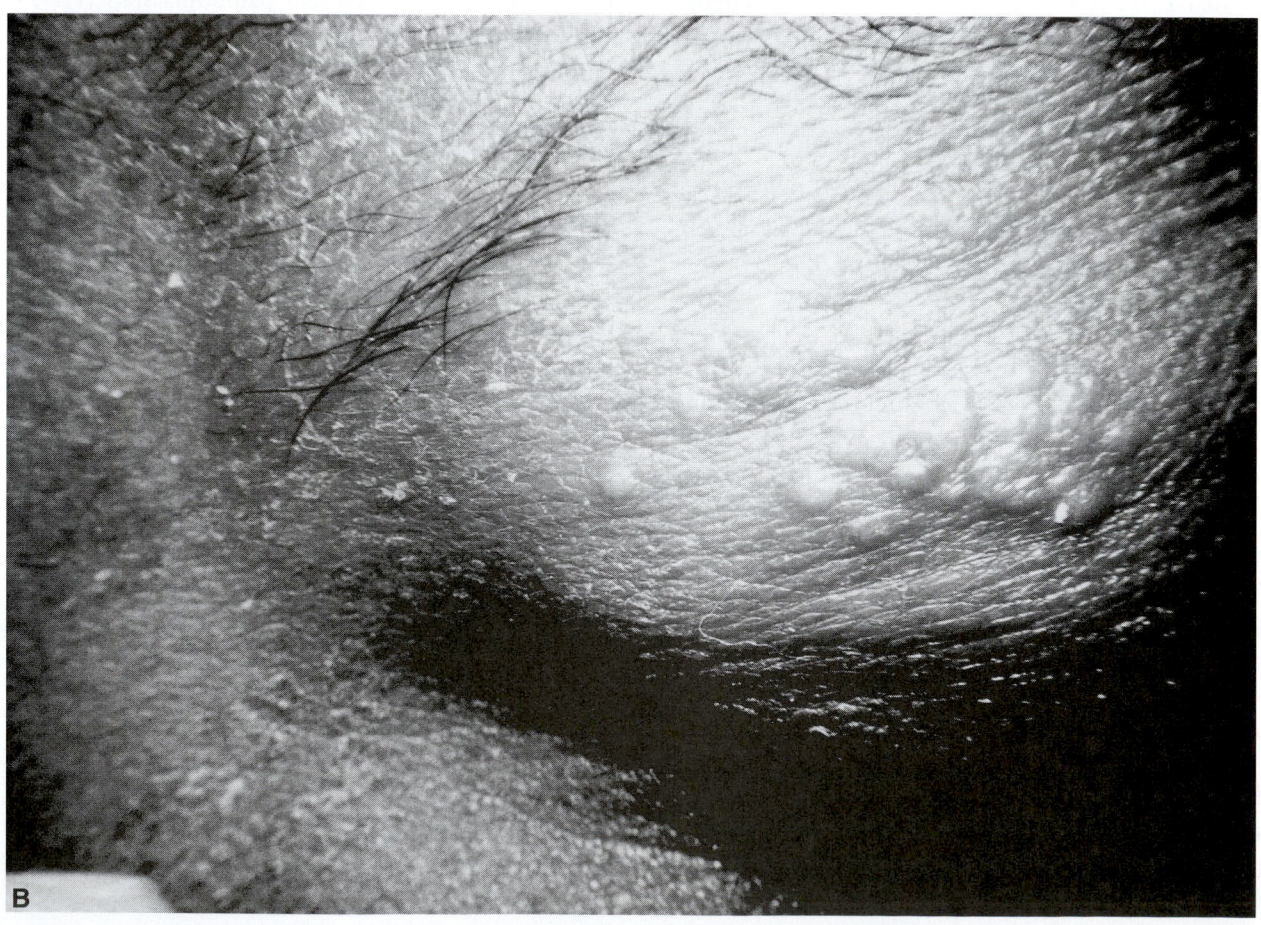

mucosal surfaces subjects them to trauma, and frequently at presentation there are few intact vesicles and only erosions or ulcers present. In immunosuppressed patients the lesions are rarely characteristic and may have been present for months, unlike non-immunosuppressed patients, in whom lesions heal spontaneously over several weeks. In a patient with human immunodeficiency virus, a nonhealing erosion or ulcer of the genitalia, buttocks, or perianal region is herpes simplex until proven otherwise.

HUMAN PAPILLOMAVIRUS HPV is an encapsulated double-stranded DNA virus that is anthropophilic and causes warts in genetically susceptible persons. Warts can occur on skin, modified mucosae of the lips and genitalia, and mucous membrane. Close to 100 HPV types have been described, and certain types are associated with specific clinical lesions. Some HPV types are oncogenic, it is believed, via the interaction between HPV E6 and E7 proteins and the host p53 tumor suppressor gene.

Plantar warts (Figure 32-11) on the sole of the foot are common in adolescents and young adults. They are often painful and can sometimes limit physical activity. These warts are associated with HPV-1. Verruca vulgaris (common wart) (see Figure 32-11) is due to HPV-2 and HPV-4. Verruca plana (flat warts) are usually seen in children and are notoriously difficult to treat. These are caused by HPV-3.

Numerous treatment methods have been employed to treat warts. Nothing works consistently in all patients. Destructive methods such as liquid nitrogen, curettage, electrodesiccation, and surgical excision, are most effective, but lesions will sometimes respond to topical keratolytics, such as salicylic acid and lactic acid, which are available over the counter and by prescription.

One must always consider the risk:benefit ratio when treating warts because inevitably they will spontaneously regress. Although the risk is low, scarring can occur with any destructive form of treatment, including liquid nitrogen, and one must keep in mind that these methods are painful and in young children can cause significant emotional distress.

MOLLUSCUM CONTAGIOSUM Molluscum contagiosum is caused by a large anthropophilic double-stranded DNA virus of the pox family. Its clinical appearance is very characteristic and consists of discrete, asymptomatic, translucent or pearly, dome-shaped papules, some of which may be umbilicated (Figure 32-12). The lesions may occur on any cutaneous surface. They usually range from 2 to 5 mm in size but, rarely, can become quite large. They may be limited in number or extensive, with hundreds of lesions present. Molluscum is extremely common in children and young adults, in whom it may be sexually transmitted. As the name implies, the virus is easily spread from person to person and from site to site on a given individual due to autoinoculation.

Other than cosmesis, the lesions are of no medical significance and in immunocompetent persons will spontaneously resolve without scarring over a period of months (up to several years). Effective therapy requires destruction of the lesions; this can be accomplished via cryosurgery, light curettage, or with chemicals such as cantharone or trichloroacetic acid. In immunosuppressed patients, especially those with human immunodeficiency virus (HIV), lesions tend to be numerous and have a predilection for the face. This can be cosmetically disfiguring and is very difficult, if not impossible, to treat. It is important to know that in HIV disease, infections such as cryptococcus and histoplasmosis can mimic molluscum when disseminated to the skin. Biopsy can easily distinguish these diseases, as the histology of molluscum is pathognomonic with large eosinophilic intracytoplasmic viral inclusions (molluscum bodies) within the epidermis.

Infestations

Two common human ectoparasites are pediculosis and scabies, both of which occur worldwide and respect no racial, sexual, age, or social boundaries.

Pediculosis

Infestation by the human louse is caused by *Pediculus humanus capitis* (head louse), *Pediculus humanus corporis* (body louse), or *Phthirus pubis* (pubic or crab louse). In the past, body lice were a major cause of disease, acting as a vector in the spread of rickettsial diseases such as typhus, relapsing fever, and trench fever; these diseases are still a problem in many underdeveloped countries, but are fortunately extremely rare in the United States.

Head lice (which do not transmit disease) are a growing problem in the United States. They are most common in children but can occur in adults as well. Transmission is via head-to-head contact and

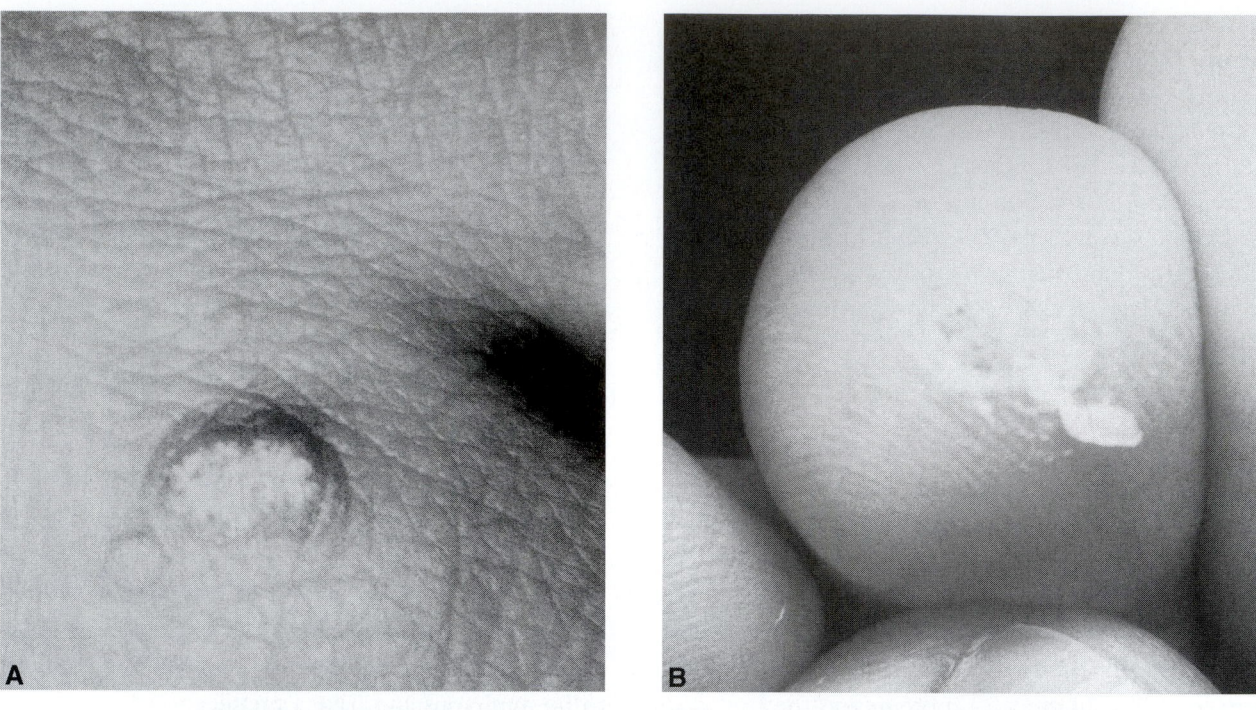

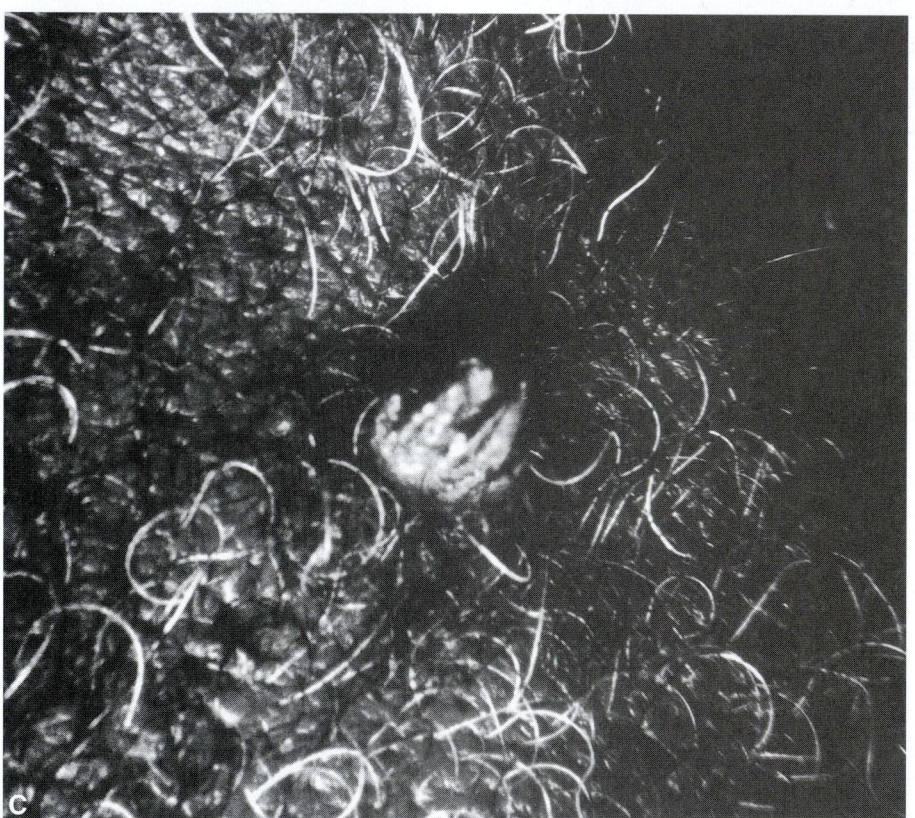

Figure 32-11 A. Common wart on the dorsal hand. B. Plantar wart with "black dots" representing thrombosed blood vessels. C. Filiform wart with typical frondlike projections.

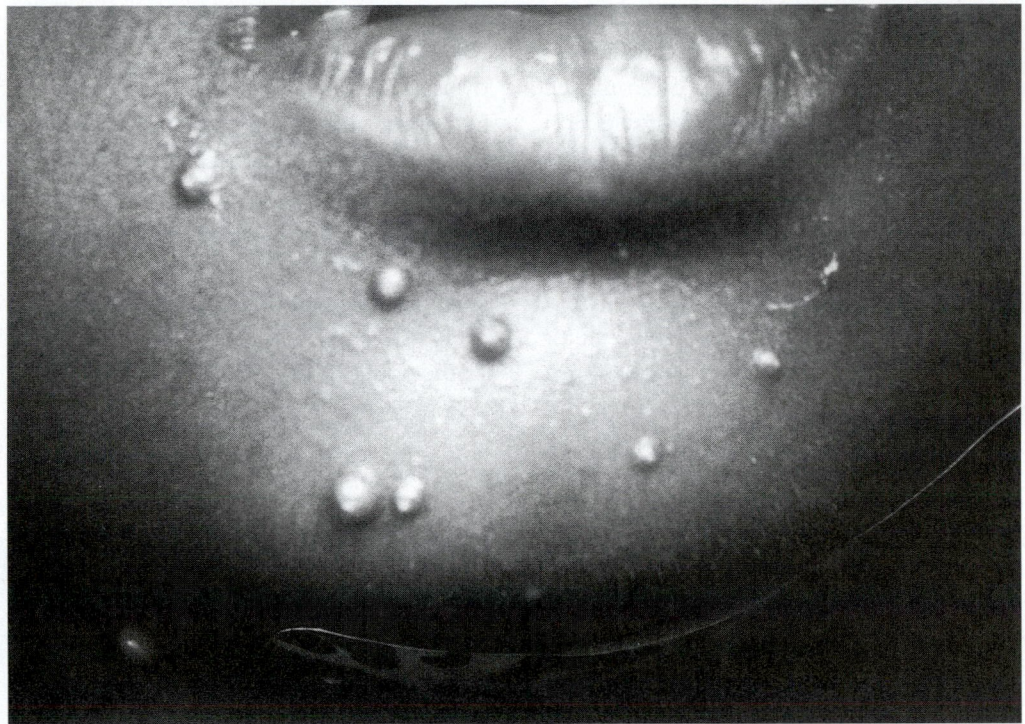

Figure 32-12 Molluscum contagiosum. Scattered flesh-colored and translucent dome-shaped papules, some of which are umbilicated.

fomites—i.e., shared brushes, combs, or hats). The main symptom is intense itching of the scalp. The scalp itself may be normal or show nonspecific erythema, scale, excoriations, or urticarial lesions. The posterior neck is frequently involved, and cervical lymphadenopathy is not uncommon. Secondary bacterial infection due to scratching is also a common occurence. The nits (eggs), which may be few in number or abundant, are firmly adherent to the hair shaft and plucking or cutting an affected hair and examining it microscopically shows a grayish-white ellipsoidal object on one side of the hair shaft. Adult lice are less frequently seen. The treatment of choice for head lice is a 1% permethrin cream rinse (Nix), available over the counter. Permethrin is a synthetic pyrethroid, which is ovicidal. Nits should be removed with a fine-toothed comb, and patients should probably be retreated with permethrin 1 week later. All close contacts should be treated simultaneously.

Body lice are seen mostly in persons with poor hygiene, such as the homeless. Transmission is via contaminated clothing or bed linens. The clinical picture is nonspecific, but numerous excoriations are usually present. Adult organisms are rarely seen on patients but numerous nits are usually found in the seams of clothing. Treatment is similar to that for scabies (see below) with special attention to proper laundering of contaminated clothing and bedding.

Epidemic in the United States, pubic (crab) lice, a common sexually transmitted disease, causes intense pruritus and sometimes sensations of crawling in the pubic area. Involvement of the thighs, trunk, axillae, eyelashes, and beard can occur as well. Sometimes small asymptomatic blue macules (maculae caerulae) are seen; these fade spontaneously. Diagnosis, again, is by microscopic examination of nits on the hair shaft. Treatment of sexual contacts, in addition to the patient, is essential. Other uninfested family members need not be treated. Therapy is the same as for head lice, but multiple treatments are usually required. For eyelashes, petrolatum applied three times daily for 3 days is usually adequate.

Scabies

Scabies, caused by the human itch mite, *Sarcoptes scabiei*, is a very common dermatologic problem. It is spread only via contact with infested persons. Patients present with intense, usually generalized, pruritus. As in many pruritic diseases, the itching of scabies is worse at night. There is often a history of multiple family members affected. Physical examination may be nonspecific, with excoriated red papules, nodules, or eczematous lesions. The classic primary lesion of scabies is a small (usually less than 1 cm) linear burrow (Figure 32-13), which is subtle and often missed by the unsuspecting physician. Areas of predilection include finger and toe-web spaces, genitalia, axillae, breasts in women, and palms and soles in children. It tends to spare the face and head in adults, but in children these areas may be involved. Diagnosis is confirmed with microscopic examination of a burrow using oil or potassium hydroxide to visualize the adult mite, eggs, or fecal material. Treatment consists of a topical antiparasitic such as Lindane (Kwell) or 5% permethrin (Elimite). The latter is favored because it

is less toxic and more efficacious. Either is applied to the entire body from the chin down and left on overnight for 8 to 12 hours and washed off with soap and water the following morning. Bed linens and clothing worn in the preceding 5 to 7 days must be washed in hot water. Treatment must include all family members and should be carried out simultaneously. Repeat application may be required 1 week later. The pruritus tends to persist for several weeks even if treatment is successful. Crusted (Norwegian) scabies occurs in immunosuppressed or debilitated patients and is very contagious due to the extremely high mite burden. These white, crusted lesions can be

Figure 32-13 A and B. Interdigital scabies—subtle burrows and vesicles between fingers.

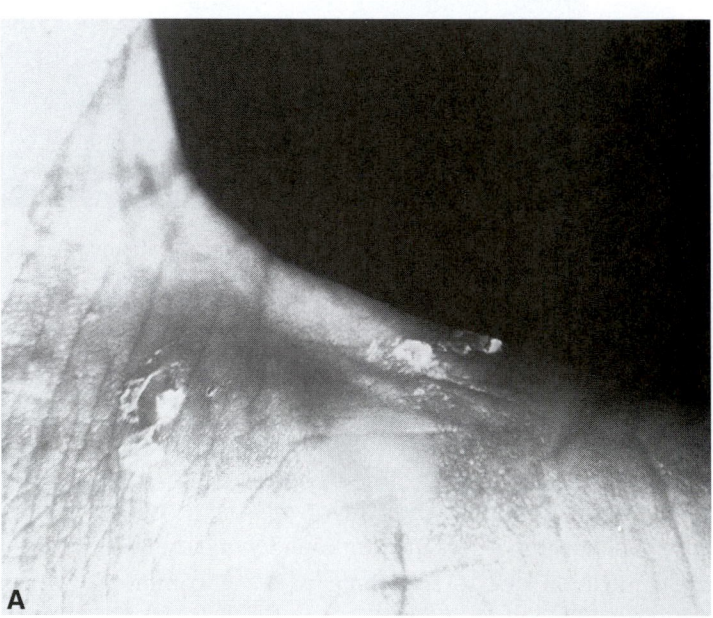

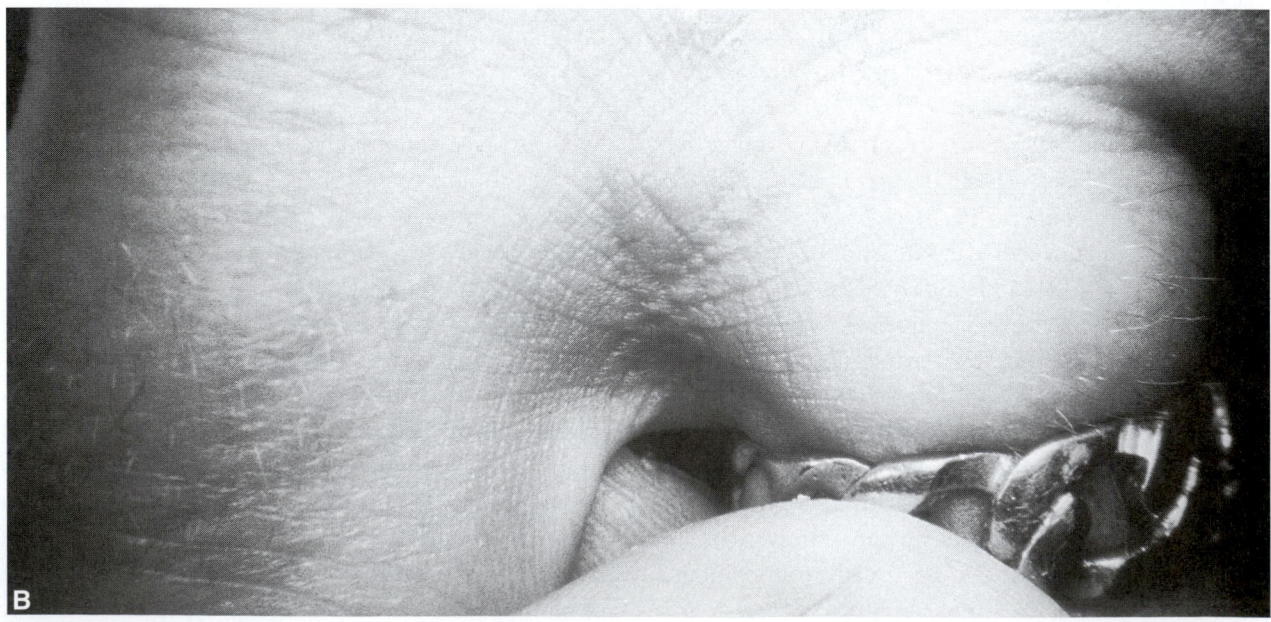

thick enough to mimic psoriasis or other papulosquamous skin diseases. Crusted scabies is more difficult to treat, and multiple treatments are usually required. Ivermectin (Stromectol), an antiparasitic used worldwide in the treatment of onchocerciasis and other endoparasites, may soon be approved for use in scabies. This single-dose oral agent should greatly enhance compliance.[12]

Papulosquamous Disorders

Papulosquamous disorders of the skin are those in which the primary lesion is a scaly papule or macule that may or may not coalesce into patches or plaques. Some have significant inflammation associated while others do not. The following discussion will be limited to common papulosquamous diseases that often present first to the primary care physician.

Psoriasis

Psoriasis is a common inflammatory skin disease (2% of the population) that can present at any age; however, most commonly the onset is in the second and third decades. The clinical spectrum is heterogeneous, from localized plaque psoriasis to severe, even life-threatening, exfoliative erythroderma and pustular forms. The variety of presentations can lead to misdiagnosis, but the classic picture of symmetric, red, sharply circumscribed plaques with white to silvery overlying scale located on extensor surfaces is easily recognized (Figure 32-14). Intertriginous psoriasis of the vulvar, gluteal, and axillary areas is easy to miss because the classic silver-white scale is usually absent due to friction and moisture, and the plaques tend to be smooth, red, and sometimes macerated (see Figure 32-14). When in such an intertriginous distribution, psoriasis can mimic seborrheic dermatitis, candidiasis, and dermatophyte infection, but the sharp margination and symmetry are clues that one is dealing with psoriasis.

With the exception of the less common severe forms (erythrodermic and pustular), which often are associated with fluid–electrolyte and thermoregulatory disturbances, there are few systemic complications, and the only extracutaneous manifestation of psoriasis is psoriatic arthritis, which also has varied presentations with a spectrum of severity. It is present in 7 to 21% of patients with cutaneous disease. Despite the rarity of systemic problems, psoriasis can be a debilitating disease both physically and psychosocially.

Treatment must be individualized, with special consideration for the patient's desire for treatment, as some who have severe disease are not particularly bothered, while others with mild or minimal disease may have significant psychological distress. Treatment is also based on the extent of involvement, age of the patient, location of lesions, and presence or absence of arthritis. Conventional therapies for mild to moderate plaque psoriasis include topical steroids, tar, anthralin, calcipotriene (Dovonex), and retinoids. The more extensive forms may respond to systemic antibiotics or ultraviolet light (UVB, psoralen and ultraviolet A [PUVA], combination UVB and UVA), which can be a relatively safe, very effective (although inconvenient) form of therapy. Methotrexate, systemic retinoids, and cyclosporine are also used to treat psoriasis. Although these agents can be very effective, they have significant and serious side effects. Proper patient selection and appropriate laboratory monitoring are absolutely mandatory. In treating intertriginous areas such as the vulva, one must exercise caution. Irritation can be especially problematic with some of the aforementioned topicals, and this area (because of enhanced absorption) is much more sensitive to the local and sometimes irreversible side effects of topical steroids—i.e, atrophy, striae, telangiectasia, ecchymoses, and steroid rebound dermatitis.

Seborrheic Dermatitis

This very common inflammatory skin disorder is due to pityrosporum, a yeast that is commensal to the skin. Scalp, ears, and the face, particularly the nasolabial folds, glabella, and brow and beard areas, are frequently involved and present with coarse white to yellow greasy scale overlying minimal to bright erythema (Figure 32-15). Pruritus is sometimes associated. Intertriginous areas including the vulva may be involved as well, and may be hard to differentiate from psoriasis. There is also histologic overlap with psoriasis, and some feel that pityrosporum may trigger psoriasis in susceptible individuals. Patients with mild facial seborrheic dermatitis commonly present to their physicians with "dry skin" and have been attempting to treat it with a variety of lotions and moisturizers. As this is a lipophilic organism, this only compounds the problem. Patients must be instructed to stop using these products. Mild seborrheic dermatitis may respond well to antiseborrheic shampoos (containing ketoconazole, zinc pyrithione, selenium

(Text continues on page 730.)

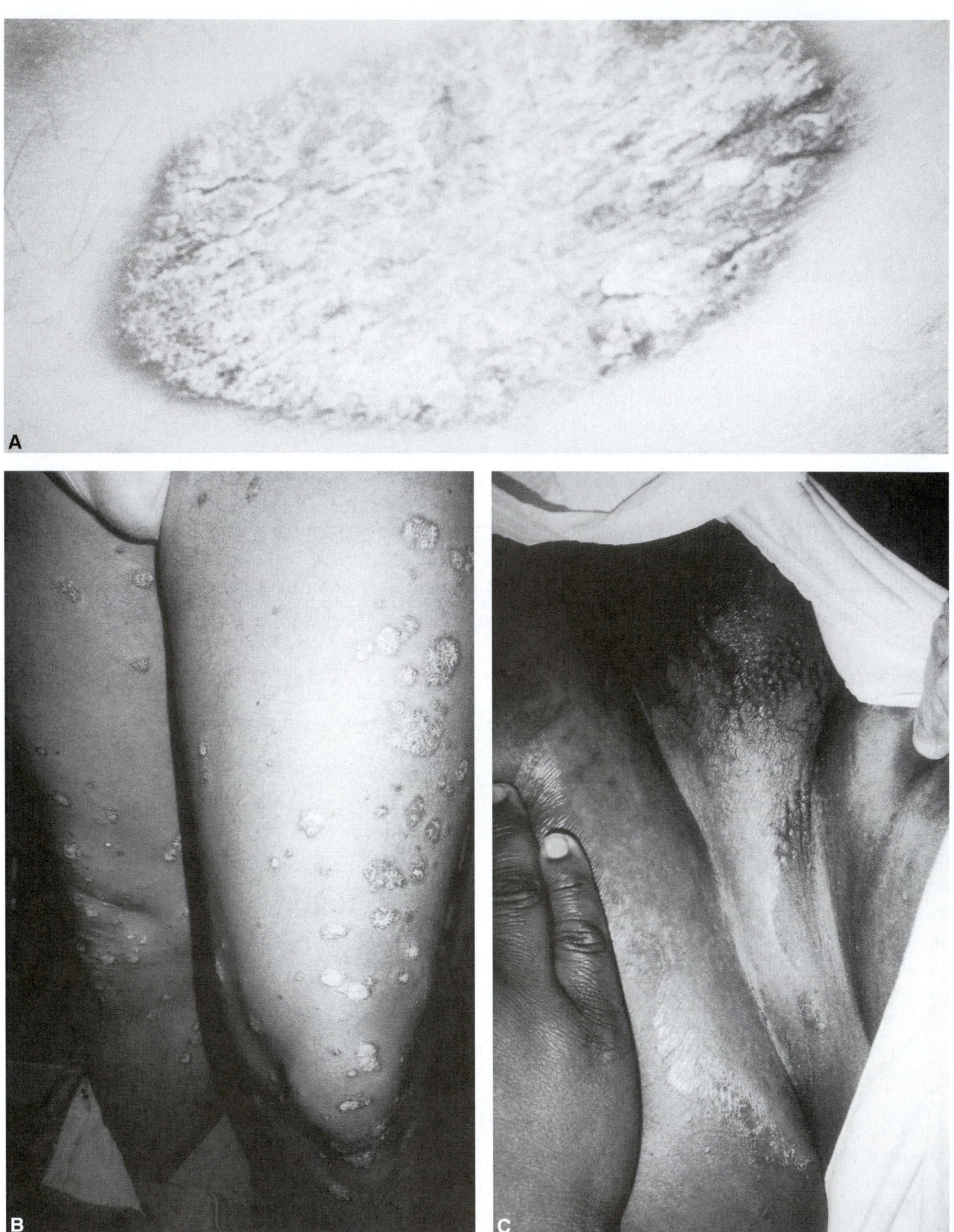

Figure 32-14 A and B. Classic plaque-type psoriasis. Sharply marginated erythematous plaques with overlying white micaceous scale. C. Intertriginous psoriasis. Note the sharp margination and lack of scale.

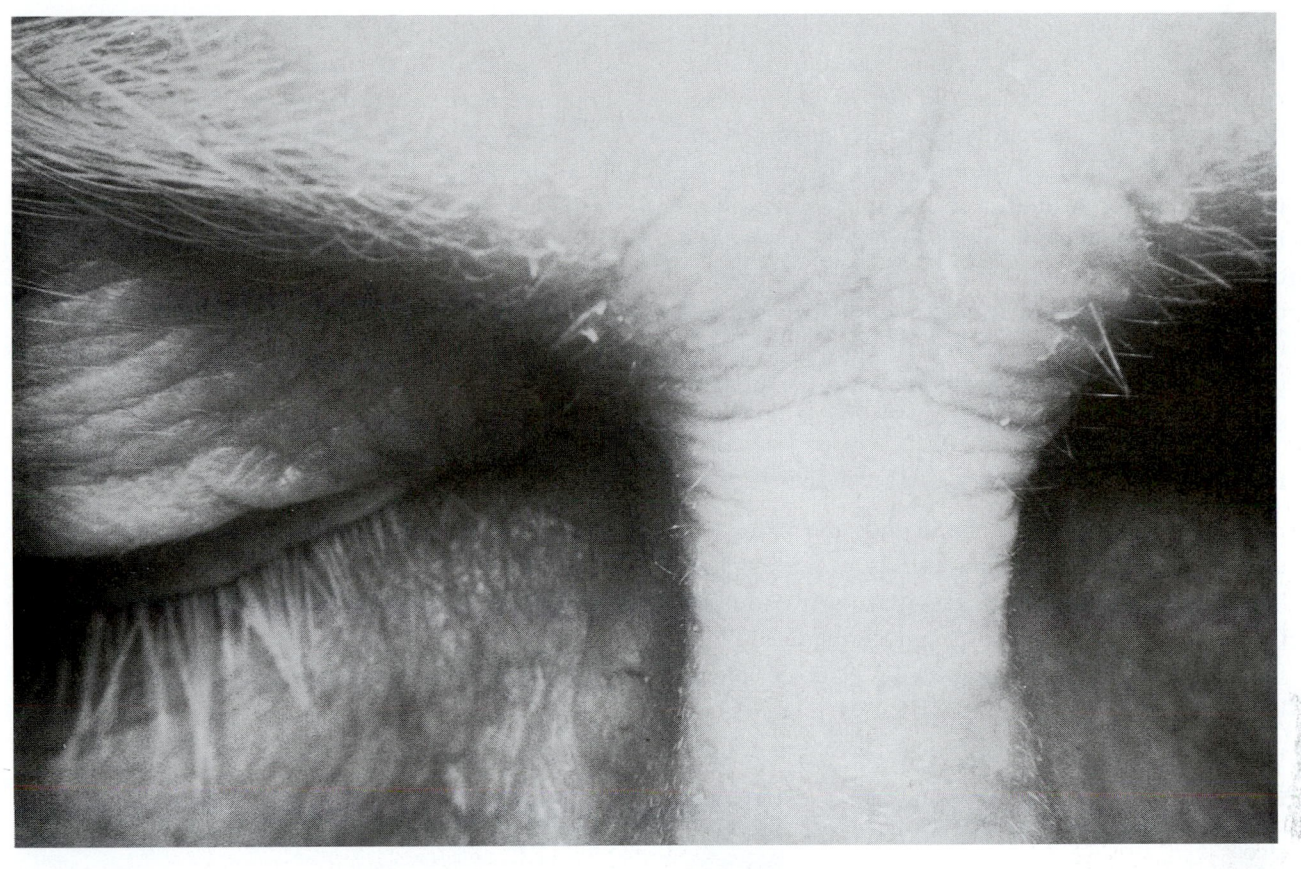

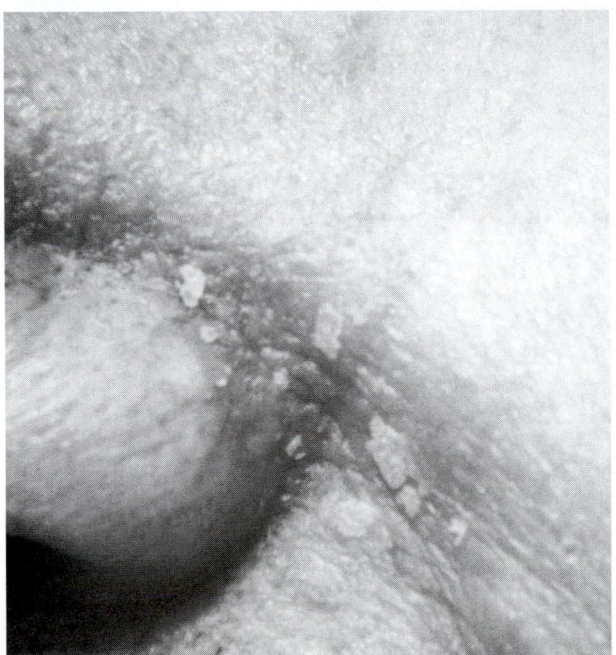

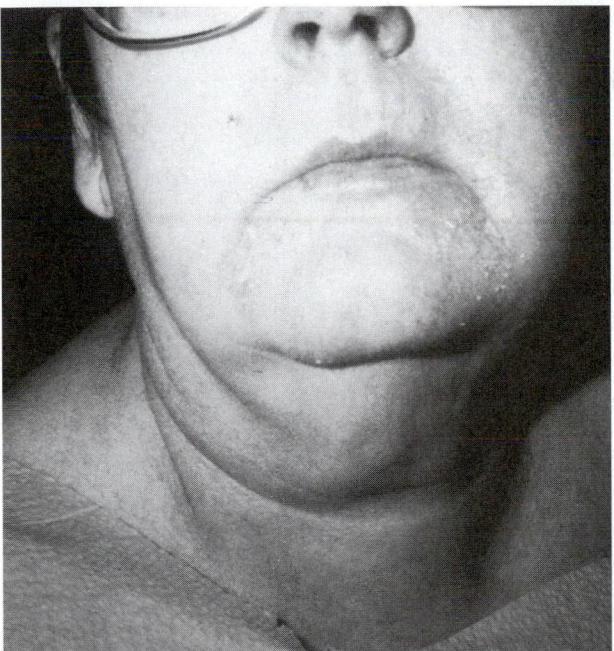

Figure 32-15 Seborrheic dermatitis.

sulfide, or tar), or topical ketoconzaole cream applied twice daily. For extensive or severe disease, oral keto-conazole is helpful. Short-term use of low-potency topical steroids can help control the erythema and pruritus but prolonged use may actually worsen the problem. Pityrosporum has no systemic complications in immunocompetent persons, but there have been cases of disseminated disease in severely immuno-compromised patients. It is also important to note that patients with HIV very commonly have refrac-tory seborrheic dermatitis, which may be the pre-senting sign of their disease.

Lichen Planus

A relatively common inflammatory dermatosis of unknown cause, lichen planus usually begins in adult-hood and is clinically characterized by the four Ps: intensely pruritic, polygonal, purple papules. These flat-topped papules may be discrete or coalesce into larger plaques (Figure 32-16). The surface has a char-acteristic lacy, white, reticulated scale (Wickham striae), which is often better visualized by placing a drop of mineral oil on the lesion. There is a predilec-tion for the volar wrists, forearms, dorsal hands, and ankles, but it can occur anywhere, including mucous membrane, hair follicles, and nails. Lesions can be lo-calized or, less commonly, disseminated. There is a clinical spectrum of mucosal disease from completely asymptomatic or intensely pruritic reticulated white patches to severe scarring erosive lesions. Lichen planus is a principal cause of desquamative vaginitis, and in the vulvar area it can cause significant mor-bidity. Long-standing erosive vulvar lichen planus can cause resorption of the labia minora.

There have been increased reports of lichen planus occuring in patients with hepatitis C, and the onset of lichen planus not infrequently precedes the diag-nosis of hepatitis. It is prudent in the right clinical setting to check the appropriate serology. Lichen planus–like lesions are also associated with certain

Figure 32-16 Polygonal purple pruritic papules of lichen planus. Note overlying Wickham striae.

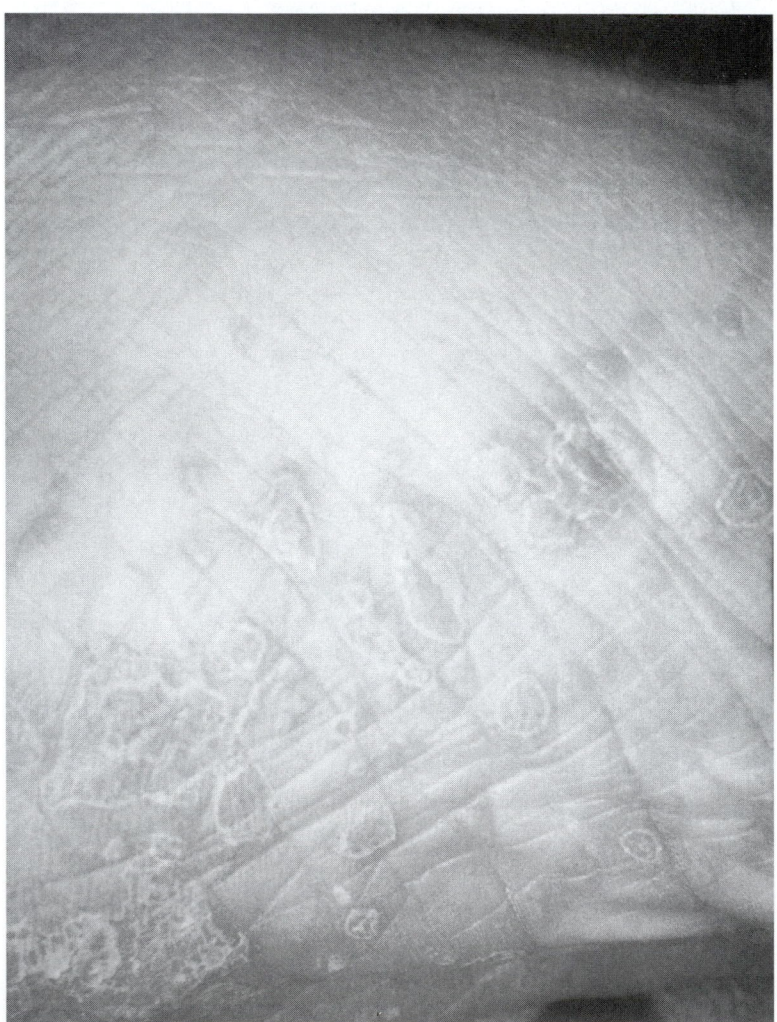

drugs, and histology can be helpful to distinguish idiopathic lichen planus from drug-induced lichen planus. Long-standing lesions of mucosal lichen planus (of the mouth and vulva) have eventuated in squamous-cell carcinoma; therefore, patients should be instructed to watch for change in mucosal lesions, and physicians should have a low threshold for biopsy.

Lichen planus has a characteristic histology showing acanthosis with a "saw-toothed" appearance of the rete ridges, hypergranulosis, absence of parakeratosis, and a bandlike mononuclear infiltrate at the dermal–epidermal junction.

Several distinct clinical variants of lichen planus may occur and often cause diagnostic uncertainty. These include such presentations as hypertrophic, annular, follicular, atrophic, bullous, and erosive lichen planus. Erosive lichen planus of the vulva will be discussed in more detail below.

Treatment may be difficult. Localized lesions often respond to ultrapotent topical or intralesional steroids. Erosive mucosal disease may require systemic steroids. Systemic retinoids and hydroxychloroquine are reportedly beneficial as well. For disseminated disease PUVA or UVB can be very effective, using the same protocols as for psoriasis therapy. Other agents that have been used include griseofulvin, dapsone, cyclosporine, cyclophosphamide, and metronidazole. The prognosis for typical acute lichen planus is good, with 85% clearing in 2 years. Recurrence is most common in those with extensive involvement.

Pityriasis Rosea

Pityriasis rosea does not often involve the genital area but is such a common papulosquamous disorder it will be included here. The cause is unknown, but it is thought to be viral because of seasonal associations and the rarity of recurrent episodes. It can be quite dramatic, with the sudden development of pink to red, round or oval papules and plaques usually with a peripheral collarette of scale (Figure 32-17); it tends to follow skin cleavage lines and on the back may have the characteristic "Christmas tree" pattern (see Figure 32-17). Pruritus may or may not be present, and there are no other associated symptoms. It is usually located on the trunk and proximal extremities, with sparing of the face, palms, and soles; however, atypical presentations sometimes occur. The herald patch, the first and largest lesion (2 to 10 cm) is usually present on the trunk, but it can occur anywhere. Within 3 to 14 days of the onset of the herald patch

the rash will generalize. Expectant management is best. If pruritus is present, soothing antipruritic preparations—calamine lotion, camphor, and menthol lotions—and sedating antihistamines may be helpful. For severe cases, UVB can be effective in relieving pruritus. Adolescents and young adults are most commonly affected but it can occur at any age. Because secondary syphilis can appear identical to pityriasis rosea, it is prudent to check a rapid plasma reagin in the right clinical setting. Pityriasis rosea is self-limited and usually lasts 6 to 10 weeks. If it persists beyond this time, biopsy may be necessary. One should also be aware that some drugs can induce pityriasis rosea–like eruptions (gold, angiotensin-converting–enzyme inhibitors, barbiturates, isoniazid, clonidine, non-steroidal antiinflammatory drugs, β-blockers, and metronidazole).

Dermatitis (Eczema)

Defined as "inflammation of the skin," this diagnosis is often very frustrating for physician and patient alike. The causes are numerous, and the clinical presentation is often nonspecific. The spectrum can range from subtle erythema to severe erosions, fissures, and excoriations. In acute dermatitis one can usually appreciate poorly marginated erythematous patches or plaques, papules, and sometimes scale, excoriations, blisters, or erosions. Pruritus, the primary symptom, is usually present and can be severe. Chronic vulvar dermatitis usually presents as lichenification, with or without pigmentary alteration. For practical purposes dermatitis can be divided into two main groups: endogenous and exogenous.

Atopic dermatitis is a classic example of an endogenous dermatitis. It is most common in children and typically begins between the ages of 6 and 12 months. It is an immunologically mediated skin disorder affecting the Th2 population of lymphocytes. There is often a family history of atopy and not infrequently, patients have coexisting asthma. Pruritus often begins first, followed by the skin eruption, and thus has often been called the "itch that rashes." Infants frequently present with facial and extensor involvement, while older children are more likely to have the classic flexural lesions. Lesions can be generalized, and in this situation are very difficult to treat. Genital lesions can occur and, more often than not, will have evidence of dermatitis at other sites. Treatment is aimed at reducing pruritus by avoidance of precipitating factors and through the use of antihistamines, emollients, and topical steroids; antibiotics

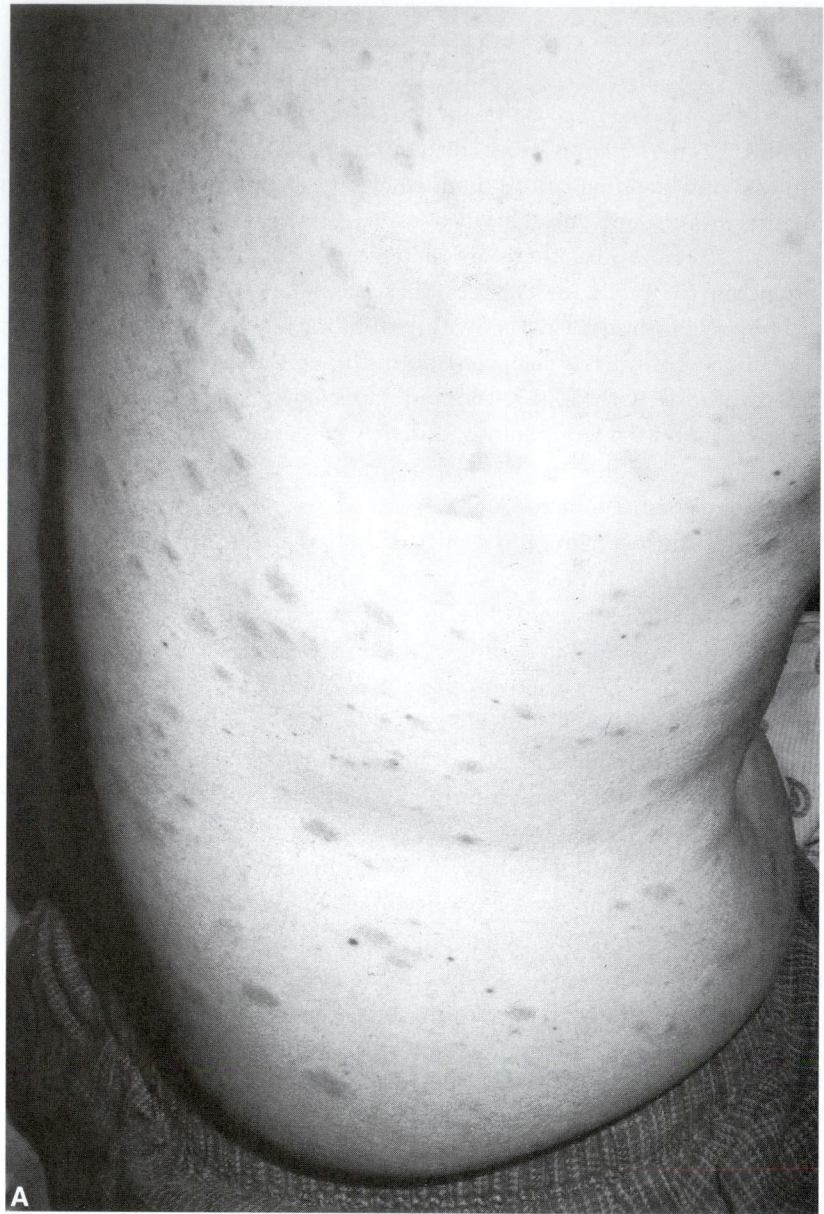

Figure 32-17 A. Pityriasis rosea. Pink oval lesions following skin cleavage lines of the lateral chest in a "Christmas tree" pattern. B. Collarette or "trailing scale" in pityriasis rosea.

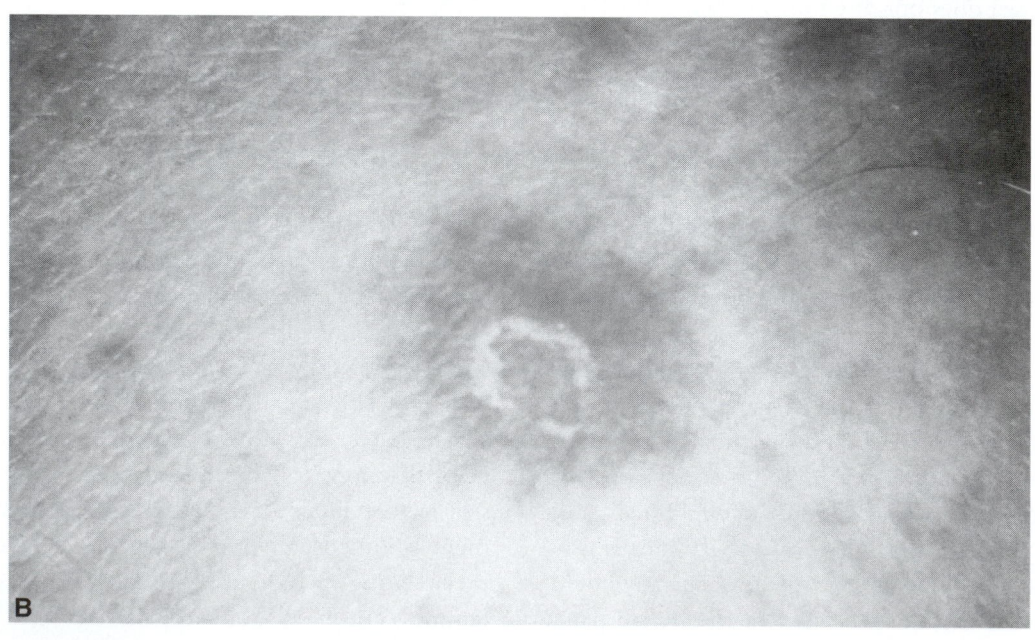

are often required, as colonization with staphylococcal species is a common occurence. In severe cases, UV light therapy can be very beneficial. Systemic steroids should be avoided, as the course is usually chronic, punctuated with exacerbations and remissions. Most children do outgrow their dermatitis by puberty but it is not uncommon for atopic dermatitis to recur in adulthood.

Exogenous dermatitis refers to dermatitis that is caused by an exogenous factor such as an irritant or allergen.

Irritant contact dermatitis should always be considered in patients with vulvar dermatitis in whom itching, burning, and discomfort are persistent and who fail to respond to appropriate therapy. Irritant contact is far more common than allergic contact dermatitis. Physical findings are variable and can range from minimal erythema to erosion and fissuring.[13] Commonly implicated irritants are soaps, alcohol, propylene glycol, deodorants, scented baths, bubble baths, and a variety of feminine hygiene products. Overzealous washing, even with a mild soap, can lead to irritation. Conversely, inadequate or infrequent cleansing can also be a problem because of the irritant effect of sweat, urine, and feces. Friction from tight clothing and self-medication using inappropriate medications are other causes of irritation. Treatment requires removal of all potential irritants, soothing agents such as zinc oxide paste, petrolatum (external genitalia only), loose-fitting clothing, and low-potency topical steroids for short duration (2 to 4 weeks).

Allergic contact dermatitis, a type IV delayed hypersensitivity reaction, is usually seen within 24 to 72 hours after exposure to the offending allergen. The natural course is 2 to 4 weeks, assuming that the patient is no longer exposed. When the allergen is not suspected and exposure continues, the course can be chronic and unremitting. The usual symptom is nonspecific itching, burning, and discomfort, and the physical findings are likewise nonspecific and range from subtle vulvar erythema to vesicles and erosions to chronic lichenification. Lack of response to or worsening with appropriate therapy can be a clinical clue. Patient and physician must play detective, and a detailed history is mandatory. Patch testing can be invaluable in many cases. One study of patch test data from patients referred from a "vulva clinic" revealed topical medications and their constituents as the responsible agent in the majority of cases.[14] This includes topical steroids, topical antibiotics, topical anesthetics, and preservatives used in these preparations. True allergic reactions to feminine hygiene sprays and deodorized sanitary napkins have been reported. Allergies to nickel, fragrances, adhesives, and rubber products (accelerators and vulcanizers) as well as latex itself can cause problems in the vulvar region. Rubber allergy can be especially problematic with the widespread use of condoms and diaphragms. Less common allergens that have been reported include propylene glycol in KY gel, chemical contraceptives, and semen.[13] Treatment is the same as for irritant dermatitis. Removal of the inciting agent is a prerequisite for the dermatitis to resolve. Bland, soothing topical preparations such as zinc oxide paste, emollients, and topical steroids are also beneficial.

LICHEN SIMPLEX CHRONICUS Any pruritic dermatosis that leads to chronic rubbing and scratching can result in lichen simplex chronicus. The physical findings are nonspecific, with pronounced lichenification being the most prominent feature. The chronic rubbing and scratching leads to thickening of the epidermis and uppermost dermis so that the normal skin lines are greatly accentuated. Frequently, there is associated postinflammatory hyperpigmentation or hypopigmentation. Pruritus vulvae is an example of lichen simplex chronicus. When involving the vulva, lichen simplex chronicus can be very challenging. The pruritus can be incapacitating and sleep cycles can be disturbed. Treatment is aimed at interrupting the itch–scratch cycle. The patient must be instructed not to rub or scratch; instead they can pat the area or use an ice cube for temporary relief. Sedating antihistamines are useful at night, as well as topical steroids, loose-fitting cotton underclothes, powders, and zinc oxide paste. Avoid precipitating irritants and allergens when applicable (most cases are idiopathic), and always consider unrecognized bacterial or yeast superinfection when patients do not respond to appropriate therapy.

Erosive and Ulcerative Disorders of the Vulva

Infectious

The differential diagnosis of infectious ulcerative vulvar diseases obviously includes the ulcerative sexually transmitted diseases (STDs) which will be covered in detail elsewhere in this text. In addition to STDs, other nonsexually transmitted infections can also present with erosions and ulcers. This would include varicella–zoster, candida, inflammatory vaginitis, and impetigo. Superficial cultures are usually diagnostic, but biopsy with tissue cultures is sometimes necessary for diagnosis. One caveat regarding ulcerative muco-cutaneous diseases in immunosuppressed populations (especially HIV): these diseases frequently lose their characteristic clinical features and any nonhealing erosion or ulcer of the perianal or genital region is herpes simplex until proven otherwise.

Noninfectious

The list of noninfectious mucocutaneous disorders which can present with erosions and/or ulcers is fairly extensive (Table 32-6). Some of these will be discussed in more detail in the following sections. The essential take-home message regarding erosive/ulcerative diseases is the following: BIOPSY. As the clinical features of many of these diseases are non-specific, biopsy is usually required for diagnosis. In addition, direct immunofluorescence is highly recom-mended to rule out immunobullous diseases such as bullous pemphigoid, pemphigus vulgaris, cicatricial pemphigoid, epidermolysis bullosa acquisita, and lin-ear IgA disease. A wedge or punch biopsy should be taken from the border of the lesion, and appropriate cultures should be performed as well.

APHTHOUS ULCERS (CANKER SORES) These com-mon lesions occur at any age, although tend to be most common in young adults. The cause is still un-known. Clinically, one sees painful recurrent, super-ficial ulcers, usually less than 1 cm, with an erythe-matous border. In the mouth they occur only on nonfixed mucosa in contradistinction to recurrent intraoral HSV, which are grouped and tend to occur more often on fixed mucosa, such as the hard palate and attached gingiva. In the genital area, aphthous ulcers occur more commonly within the vulvar vestibule. There are no associated systemic symptoms. If associated with systemic manifestations such as eye disease, arthritis, or central nervous system dysfunc-tion, one should suspect Behçet disease. The diagno-sis of aphthous ulcers is clinical and supported by a history of spontaneously healing ulcerations; but if lesions persist, or are clinically atypical, biopsy is necessary to exclude infectious or other inflammatory ulcers. Histology is nonspecific but can exclude other diseases. In addition to Behçet disease, recurrent or persistent aphthosis has been associated with other systemic diseases such as gluten-sensitive enteropathy, inflammatory bowel disease, iron-deficiency anemia, folate and vitamin B_{12} deficiency, systemic lupus erythematosus, and HIV. Typical aphthous ulcers re-solve spontaneously over 1 to 2 weeks. Symptomatic treatment with over-the-counter preparations such as benzocaine (Oragel), and prescription preparations containing viscous lidocaine and tetracycline may be helpful. Topical steroids early in the course may has-ten resolution. In severe cases, systemic antibiotics, colchicine, and dapsone are reportedly beneficial.

TRAUMATIC ULCERS Traumatic erosions/ulcers can be induced deliberately (factitial) or more commonly as a result of scratching. They may be superficial or deep and tend to be linear, geometric, or angular in nature. They may heal with hypopigmentation and scarring. In cases of psychogenic ulceration, there is

---

TABLE 32-6
NONINFECTIOUS MUCOCUTANEOUS DISEASES THAT CAN PRESENT WITH EROSIONS AND/OR ULCERS IN THE VULVAR AREA

Inflammatory	Malignant	Immunobullous
Aphthous ulcers	Vulvar intraepithelial neoplasia	Bullous pemphigoid
Contact dermatitis	Squamous-cell carcinoma	Cicatricial pemphigoid
Crohn disease	Extramammary Paget disease	Pemphigus vulgaris
Erythema multiforme	Leukemia	Linear IgA disease
Fixed drug eruption	Lymphoma	Epidermolysis bullosa
Hidradenitis suppuritiva		acquisita
Lichen planus		
Lichen sclerosis		
Necrolytic migratory erythema		
Pyoderma gangrenosum		
Trauma		
Zoon (plasma-cell) vulvitis		

no primary skin disorder, and lesions are confined to easy-to-reach areas of the body. Underlying psychiatric diseases include depression, anxiety, obsessive–compulsive disorder, and delusions of parasitosis.

Zoon's (plasma-cell) Vulvitis Zoon's (plasma-cell) vulvitis and balanitis present as asymptomatic, moist, shiny red, sharply demarcated plaques, which on biopsy show numerous plasma cells. The cause of this inflammatory disease is unknown but is thought by some to represent a variant of lichen planus. Reported treatments include intralesional interferon alfa, local excision, topical steroids, topical retinoids, and topical cyclosporine.

Pyoderma Gangrenosum Pyoderma gangrenosum is a chronic, painful, debilitating ulcerative skin disease that is idiopathic in 50% of cases. The remaining 50% are associated with systemic disease such as inflammatory bowel disease (ulcerative colitis more often than Crohn disease), rheumatoid arthritis, hepatitis, sarcoid, paraproteinemia and lymphoprolifera-

tive malignancies, and Behçet disease. The initial presentation is a painful deep nodule or pustule that rapidly ulcerates. Classically, the ulcer has undermined purplish borders (Figure 32-18) and heals with cribriform scarring. Pyoderma gangrenosum can occur at any site, including the genitalia. Although pathergy (development of new lesions at sites of skin trauma) is associated with pyoderma gangrenosum, biopsy is still indicated to rule out other causes of cutaneous ulcers (especially infection and malignancy). Treatment can be difficult, and high-dose systemic steroids are the mainstay.

Immunobullous Disorders Although there are several distinct autoimmune blistering diseases (Table 32-7), which have characteristic clinical, histopathologic, and immunofluorescent findings, the following discussion will be limited to the two prototypical immunobullous diseases: bullous pemphigoid and pemphigus vulgaris, both of which are characterized by antibody formation to specific structural proteins within the skin. It is unknown what triggers the

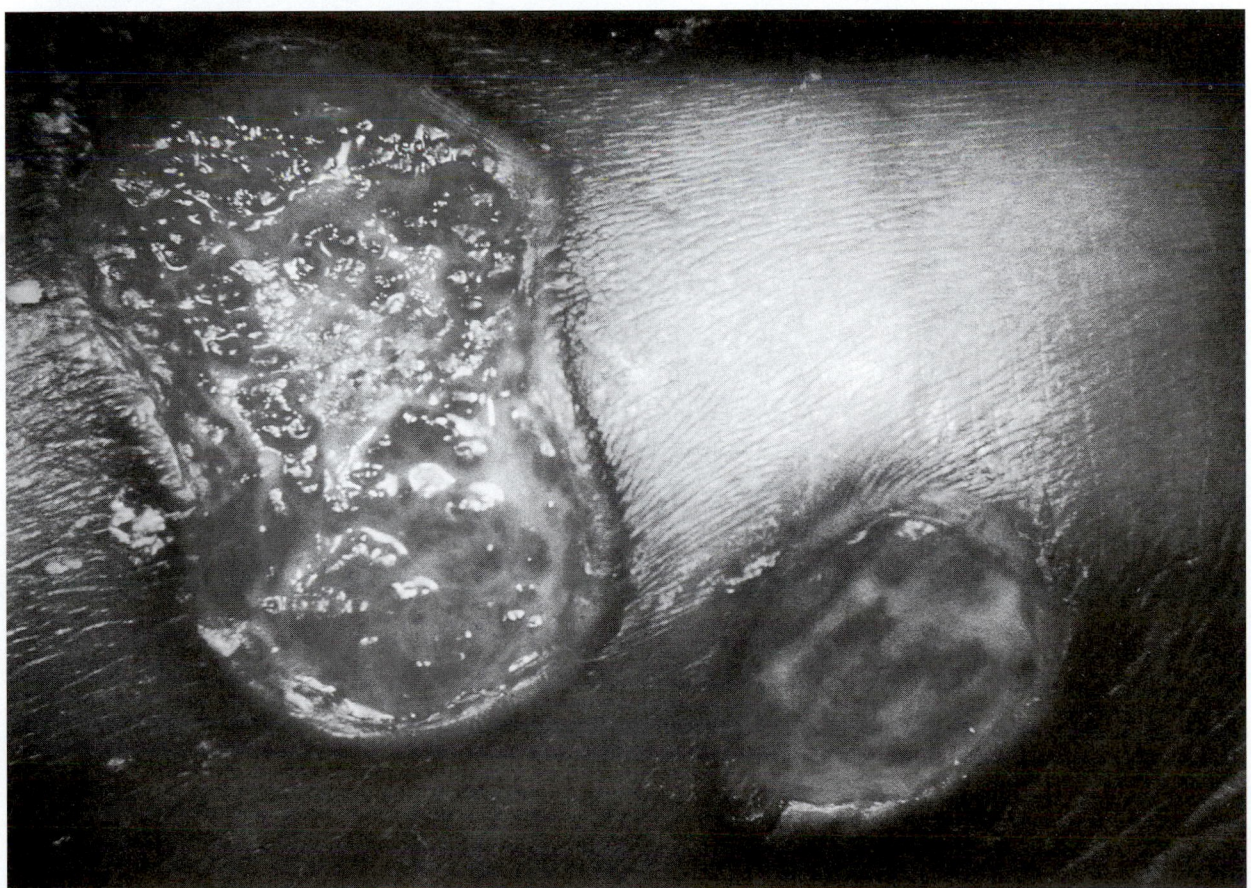

Figure 32-18 Pyoderma gangrenosum. Painful ulcers with a purple, undermined border.

TABLE 32-7
AUTOIMMUNE BLISTERING DISEASES

Pemphigoid
  Bullous pemphigoid
  Cicatricial pemphigoid
  Pemphigoid gestationis
Pemphigus
  Pemphigus vulgaris
  Pemphigus vegetans
  Pemphigus foliaceus
  Pemphigus erythematosus
Dermatitis herpetiformis
Linear IgA disease
Epidermolysis bullosa acquisita
Bullous lupus erythematosus

antibody formation but an inflammatory cascade is set in motion via the antigen–antibody complex that ultimately results in structural weakness that leads to blister formation.

Pemphigus vulgaris is a serious autoimmune blistering disease with significant morbidity and mortality. Prior to the availability of glucocorticosteroids, the mortality was approximately 100% (usually due to sepsis). Pathogenic autoantibody formation to a 130-kd cadherin-type protein, desmoglein III, a normal component of the epithelial desmosome, results in marked skin fragility, which clinically manifests as fragile, flaccid vesicles, bullae, and erosions, which are frequently crusted (Figure 32-19). Because of their

Figure 32-19 Erosions of pemphigus vulgaris.

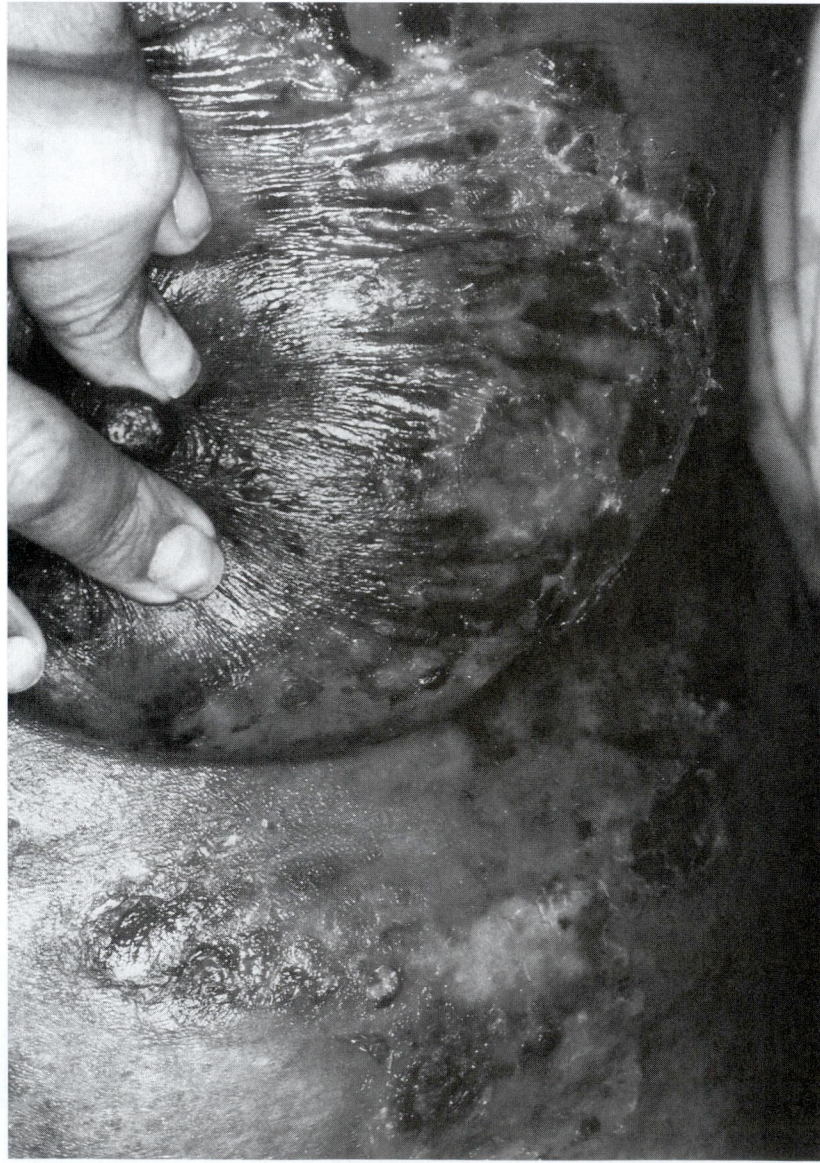

fragile nature, vesicles and bullae are not usually abundant, and erosions are the more prominent feature. The Nikolsky sign is positive—i.e., rubbing normal-appearing skin will induce a fresh blister. There is a predilection for mucosal surfaces (which may precede the cutaneous lesions by weeks to months). Lesions can occur on any cutaneous site; scalp, face, chest, axillae, and groin are common areas. These patients are usually ill and have constitutional symptoms. They must be monitored closely for associated fluid–electrolyte abnormalities and sepsis. Diagnosis is made by skin biopsy for hematoxylin and eosin staining and direct immunofluorescence. For the hematoxylin and eosin staining specimen, a new small intact blister is preferable, and for immunofluorescence, formalin cannot be used as a fixative; instead, Michels's solution, a nonformalin transport medium, should be substituted. On hematoxylin and eosin staining there is suprabasilar acantholysis, intraepidermal separation, and blister formation. Direct immunofluorescence is very characteristic with intercellular ("chicken wire") immunofluorescence within the epidermis due to deposition of C3 and IgG. Circulating antibodies to desmoglein III are present, and their titer correlates with disease activity and severity.

Treatment of pemphigus can be extremely difficult and usually requires aggressive management using high-dose steroids and steroid-sparing immunosuppressives such as gold, cyclophosphamide, azothiaprine, and methotrexate. Plasmapheresis has been used as well. Treatment in an intensive-care unit (preferably a burn unit) is often indicated when the disease is extensive.

More common than pemphigus vulgaris, bullous pemphigoid, unlike pemphigus, does not cause death; however, the morbidity can be significant. The presentation differs from pemphigus in that blisters are usually abundant and patients are not ill. The tense vesicles and bullae of bullous pemphigoid tend to be pruritic and may be present on normal or erythematous skin (Figure 32-20). There is no skin fragility, so the Nikolsky sign is negative. Lesions can occur anywhere, but there is a predilection for flexural areas. Although mucosal lesions do occur, they are much less common than in pemphigus. Some patients will have pruritic prebullous erythema or urticarial lesions weeks to months prior to onset of the bullae. Biopsy of lesional skin shows subepidermal separation and blister formation with eosinophils and sometimes neutrophils in the dermis, epidermis, and blister cavity.

Direct immunofluorescence of perilesional skin shows linear IgG and C3 at the basement membrane zone. In the majority of cases of bullous pemphigoid the antigen is a 230-kd intracellular component of the hemidesmosome. This differs from herpes gestationis (bullous pemphigoid of pregnancy), in which antibody formation is usually to a 180-kd extracellular component of the hemidesmosome complex. Circulating antibodies are usually present in bullous pemphigoid, but, unlike pemphigus vulgaris, do not correlate with disease activity or severity.

Cicatricial pemphigoid, a rare variant of bullous pemphigoid, is a scarring form that tends to affect primarily the mucosae of the mouth, eyes, and anogenital area. Complications of this disease are significant, and include blindness when the eyes are involved.

Treatment of bullous pemphigoid is challenging but, unlike pemphigus, it tends to be more responsive to a variety of agents, including systemic steroids, immunosuppressive agents, and combination tetracycline and nicotinamide. Localized disease sometimes responds to ultrapotent topical steroids.

EROSIVE LICHEN PLANUS Erosive lichen planus is a chronic, often debilitating mucosal disease. It is characterized by severe and extensive erosion and ulceration at affected mucosal sites. About 20 to 30% of patients with erosive mucosal disease will have cutaneous involvement as well.[15] Vaginal and vulvar symptoms include severe and unremitting pruritus, pain, burning, dyspareunia, and bleeding. Eroded areas may be surrounded by Wickham striae or classic papules of lichen planus, in which case the diagnosis is made easily. If these classic lesions of lichen planus are absent, biopsy of the erosion or ulcer is advisable, to rule out infectious or immunobullous diseases. A wedge or punch biopsy should be taken from the border of an erosion for hematoxylin and eosin staining and from perilesional skin for direct immunofluorescence.

Management of this chronic disease can be very challenging. Ultrapotent topical steroids in ointment or suppository form are the mainstay of treatment. Intralesional and systemic steroids are helpful, but erosions recur on tapering, and because of side effects are generally unsuitable for long-term use. Topical retinoids are reportedly helpful, but are very irritating when used in eroded mucosal sites; patient discomfort usually precludes their use. Systemic retinoids

(Text continues on page 740.)

have been reported to be beneficial in mucosal lichen planus, but extreme caution must be exercised in women of reproductive age. Topical cyclosporine is reportedly effective, but the cost is prohibitive for most patients.

Vitiligo

Vitiligo is an acquired idiopathic depigmenting condition of the skin and hair. The cause is unknown, and there is a family history in approximately 30% of patients.[16] In persons with dark skin, there can be significant social stigma. Vitiligo has been associated with autoimmune diseases such as diabetes mellitus, pernicious anemia, thyroid disease, Addison disease, and polyendocrinopathy with mucocutaneous candidiasis. Clinically, one sees sharply marginated, depigmented, irregularly shaped macules (Figure 32-21) and patches in a focal, segmental, or generalized pattern. This condition can occur at any age, but peak incidence is between ages 10 and 30. Biopsy of a fully developed lesion reveals an absence of melanocytes with otherwise normal-appearing skin. The course is unpredictable, and spontaneous repigmentation is the

exception rather than the rule. Treatment can be successful using topical steroids, topical or systemic PUVA, and in patients with stable, small areas of vitiligo, surgical therapy using punch grafts, minigrafts, suction blisters, autologous cultures, and autologous melanocyte grafts can be successful, as can micropigmentation (tattooing). In patients with extensive involvement, permanent depigmentation of remaining normal skin using irreversible bleaching agents is an option.

Hidradenitis Suppurativa

Hidradenitis suppurativa is a chronic, scarring disease of the apocrine-bearing skin of the groin, axillae, breasts, and buttocks. It is part of the follicular occlusion triad that also consists of dissecting cellulitis of the scalp and acne conglobata, all of which are caused primarily by occlusion of the follicular unit, which in the case of hidradenitis suppurativa leads to secondary inflammation of the apocrine glands. Clinically there are tender nodules, abcesses, and often fistulae with sinus-tract formation. Scarring is often pronounced. Hidradenitis is associated with obesity; weight loss may be beneficial in preventing progression of

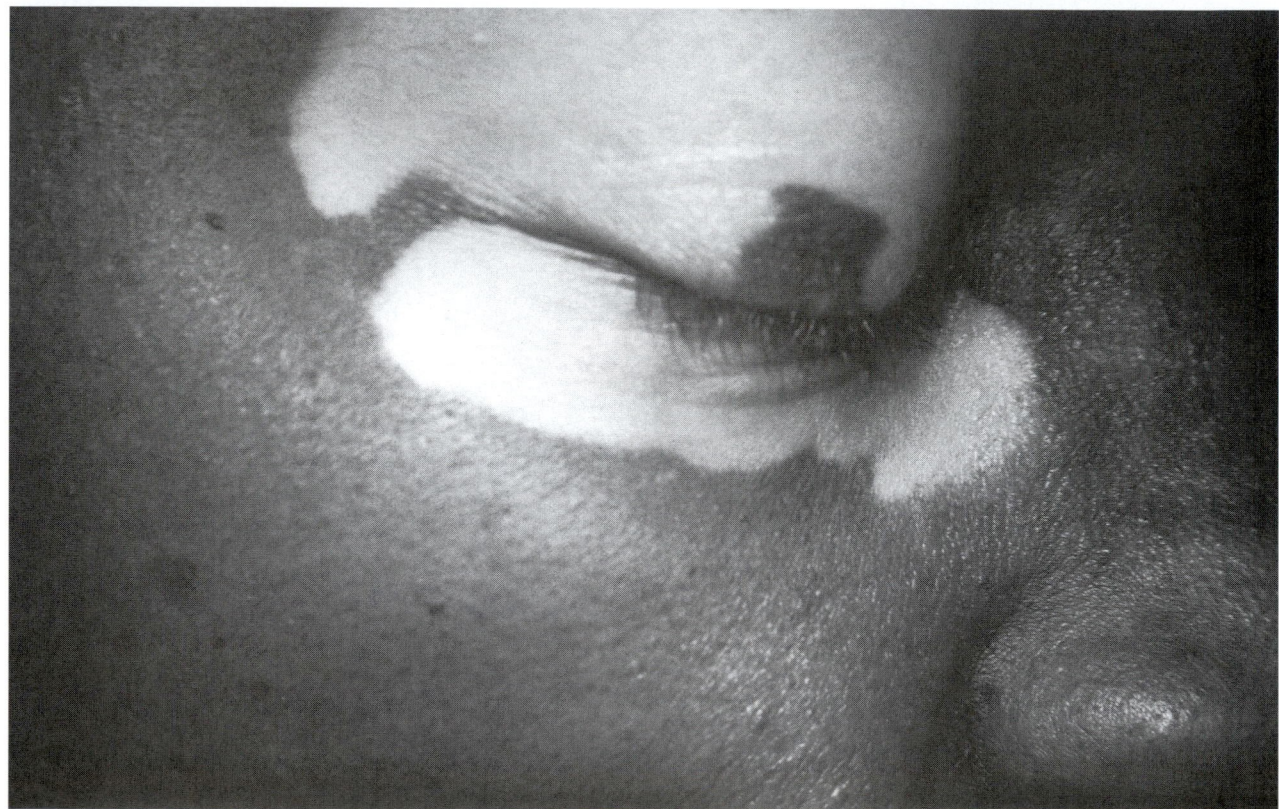

Figure 32-21 Vitiligo. Sharply demarcated patches completely devoid of pigment.

disease. As there is a clinical spectrum from mild to severe suppurative scarring disease, treatment must be individualized. Mild or early disease may respond to systemic antibiotics or high-dose isotretinoin (Accutane); intralesional and oral steroids can benefit severe pain and inflammation. Surgical treatment is the mainstay for severe hidradenitis suppurativa.

Fox–Fordyce Disease

This uncommon, but not rare, disorder of the apocrine gland is seen almost exclusively in women of reproductive age. Clinically, there are small, dome-shaped, flesh-colored, pruritic, follicular papules of the apocrine-bearing skin of the pubis and axillae. Onset is usually between the ages of 15 and 35. The course is chronic but improves considerably during pregnancy (especially the last trimester, when estrogens are highest), and regresses after menopause. Histologically, there is obstruction of the intraepidermal portion of the apocrine sweat duct. Hormonal factors are implicated, but no laboratory abnormalities have been identified. There is no cure, but some women respond well to oral contraceptives.

Lichen Sclerosis

Lichen sclerosis is a relatively common inflammatory dermatosis that can affect both sexes and any age group, although there is a bimodal peak of incidence in prepubertal girls and perimenopausal or postmenopausal women. There is a predilection for genital and perianal skin but there is no involvement of mucosal surfaces, so the vagina is spared. Extragenital cutaneous lesions, although less common, do occur. The clinical spectrum can range from minimally symptomatic disease to severe debilitating scarring disease, which has significant morbidity. The classic lesion is a well-demarcated atrophic hypopigmented or depigmented plaque. The surface may have a characteristic crinkled ("cigarette paper wrinkling") appearance (Figure 32-22), and, due to fragility, there may be purpura, bullae, or erosions. The labia minora, labia majora, clitoris, and perianal areas are often involved, giving a "figure eight" or "keyhole" distribution. Complications of severe disease are labial resorption, stenosis of the introitus, and burial of the clitoris. There is also an increased risk of squamous-cell carcinoma developing, especially in erosive lesions, and thickened, chronically rubbed areas. Patients

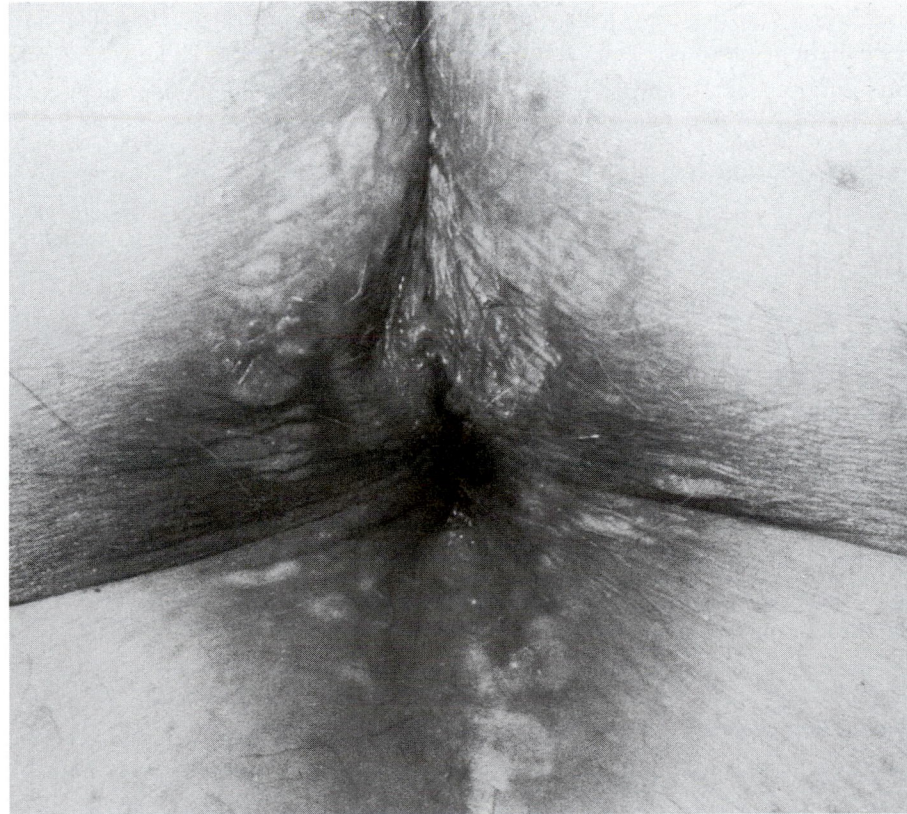

Figure 32-22 Perianal lichen sclerosis. Depigmented atrophic macules with characteristic "cigarette paper wrinkling."

should be informed of this risk and encouraged to examine themselves frequently. Physicians should have a high index of suspicion and a low threshold for biopsy. The diagnosis of lichen sclerosis is usually clinical, but biopsy may be necessary to differentiate lichen sclerosis from other hypopigmented lesions such as lichen planus, vitiligo, postinflammatory hypopigmentation, lichen simplex, and squamous-cell carcinoma. Lichen sclerosis has been associated with autoimmune diseases such as alopecia areata, vitiligo, thyroid disease, lichen planus, and morphea. The cause of lichen sclerosis is unknown, but it is thought by many to be autoimmune in nature because of its association with other autoimmune disorders. An association with *Borrelia burgdorferi* has been described as well.

The course is usually chronic, and ongoing topical therapy, which can be very helpful, is usually necessary to control disease. Potent or ultrapotent topical steroids in ointment vehicles are very beneficial but can increase the risk of secondary infection with bacteria or fungi; therefore, frequent follow-up is indicated to monitor infection and steroid-induced side effects. Other therapies reported to be helpful include topical testosterone and progesterone, topical and systemic retinoids, cryotherapy, aminobenzoate (Potaba), pulsed-dye laser, and surgical excision or ablation with the carbon dioxide laser. Surgery may be necessary to treat complications of lichen sclerosis such as introital stenosis and clitoral entrapment.

Genetic Skin Diseases with a Predilection for the Genital Region

Darier Disease

Darier disease is an uncommon, but not rare, papulosquamous disease of the skin, hair, and nails that is inherited in an autosomal dominant fashion. It usually presents in late childhood but can appear as late as the fourth decade. There is a predilection for the "seborrheic" areas of the face, scalp, central chest, retroauricular, sacral, and anogenital regions. Pruritus is variable and can be severe. The lesions are chronic and are exacerbated by heat, humidity, and UV radiation. Secondary infection with viruses, bacteria, and fungi is a frequent complication.

Hailey–Hailey Disease (Benign Familial Pemphigus)

Hailey–Hailey disease is an autosomal dominant genodermatosis that presents in the second or third decade, with recurrent nonscarring grouped vesicles, bullae, erosions, crusts, or papulosquamous lesions resembling tinea or candida. These lesions are found in the intertriginous areas of the neck, axillae, and groin. Malodorous, vegetating, pruritic plaques may be present. Secondary bacterial or yeast infection is common. The disease is chronic, with flares and remissions. Treatment is mostly supportive.

Epidermolysis Bullosa

Epidermolysis bullosa is a rare inherited blistering disease of the skin and mucosa. This genodermatosis is heterogeneous, with multiple subtypes that all have in common a genetic mutation that results in abnormal synthesis of an essential protein of the basement-membrane zone and, consequently, faulty adhesion of the epidermis to the dermis. This causes mechanical fragility, which is clinically manifest as vesiculobullous lesions and erosions, especially in areas subject to trauma. Some of the more severe subtypes are associated with dystrophic scarring and deformity. These often have systemic manifestations, and the onset is at birth or early infancy. Some of the less severe phenotypes (localized epidermolysis bullosa simplex) may not present until adolescence. Because the anogenital area is subject to trauma and friction (especially during infancy), it tends to be involved in the severe forms, and significant complications such as anal and vaginal stenosis are not uncommon. There is no available treatment at present other than supportive care. Genetic therapy may be available in the future.

White Sponge Nevus Syndrome

This autosomal dominant disorder is due to a genetic mutation causing abnormal mucosal keratins. Clinically, there are asymptomatic hyperkeratotic white plaques of the oral mucosa and genitalia. There is no available treatment.

Drug Eruptions

Erythema multiforme, Stevens–Johnson syndrome, and toxic epidermal necrolysis are probably a spectrum of disorders, each with their own clinical characteristics. They are immunologically mediated and can be triggered by a variety of antigenic stimuli such as drugs and infection with many different organisms.

Erythema multiforme can have a heterogeneous clinical presentation, but classic target lesions are usually present (Figure 32-23). Mucosal involvement, if

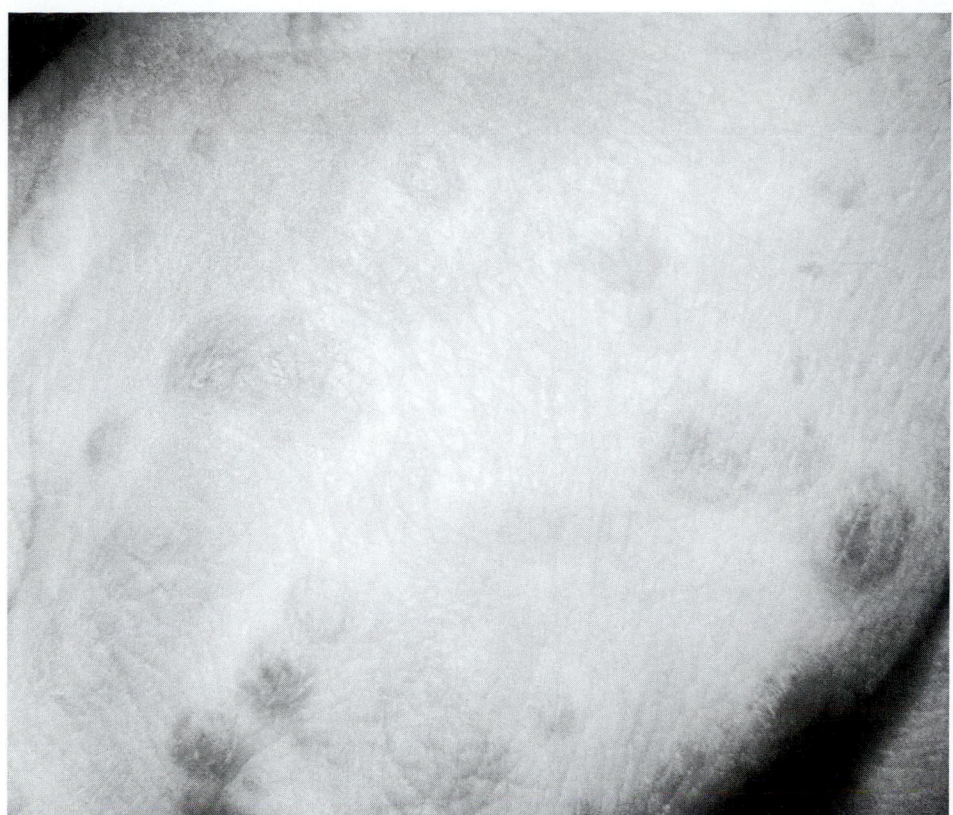

Figure 32-23 Close-up of target lesions of erythema multiforme on the dorsal hand.

present, tends to be minimal. The eruption is self-limited and will resolve without treatment. The inciting agent in erythema multiforme is more often infectious, with HSV and mycoplasma being especially common. Recurrent erythema multiforme is usually due to HSV, and prophylactic antiviral therapy may be warranted.

Stevens–Johnson syndrome is more severe, has more extensive) mucosal involvement (Figure 32-24), and has more associated morbidity, and rarely, mortality. Patients usually are ill and have constitutional symptoms such as fever and malaise; dehydration is not uncommon.

Toxic epidermal necrolysis (TEN) is the most severe of these disorders, with full-thickness epidermal necrosis resembling a second-degree burn. Stevens–Johnson syndrome and TEN are more often due to medications such as antibiotics, anticonvulsants, nonsteroidal antiinflammatory drugs, and allopurinol; however, there have been idiopathic cases reported. Treatment of severe Stevens–Johnson syndrome and TEN is controversial, with most recent studies advocating use of steroids ONLY if begun within the first 24 to 48 hours of rash onset. Supportive care in these cases in an intensive-care or burn unit is necessary.

These disorders have multisystem involvement and the mortality rate of TEN is very high, with death usually a result of sepsis.

Fixed Drug Eruption

A fixed drug eruption is a localized drug reaction characterized by a solitary (but sometimes multiple) lesion that occurs at the same site each time the patient is exposed to the offending drug. The classic appearance is a sharply marginated dusky red plaque, which may have a central bulla or erosion (Figure 32-25). Postinflammatory hyperpigmentation is usually present after healing. The genital skin is one of the most common sites for this type of drug reaction. Resolution occurs within weeks of stopping the drug. Medicines that commonly cause fixed drug eruptions are sulfonamides, tetracyclines, and phenolphthalein.

Miscellaneous Drug Eruptions

Other more common types of allergic drug reactions include exanthems and urticaria. Exanthems are pruritic, morbilliform (measleslike), symmetric erythematous eruptions sometimes associated with constitutional symptoms such as fever. Urticaria (hives) is characterized by pink-to-red transient wheals with

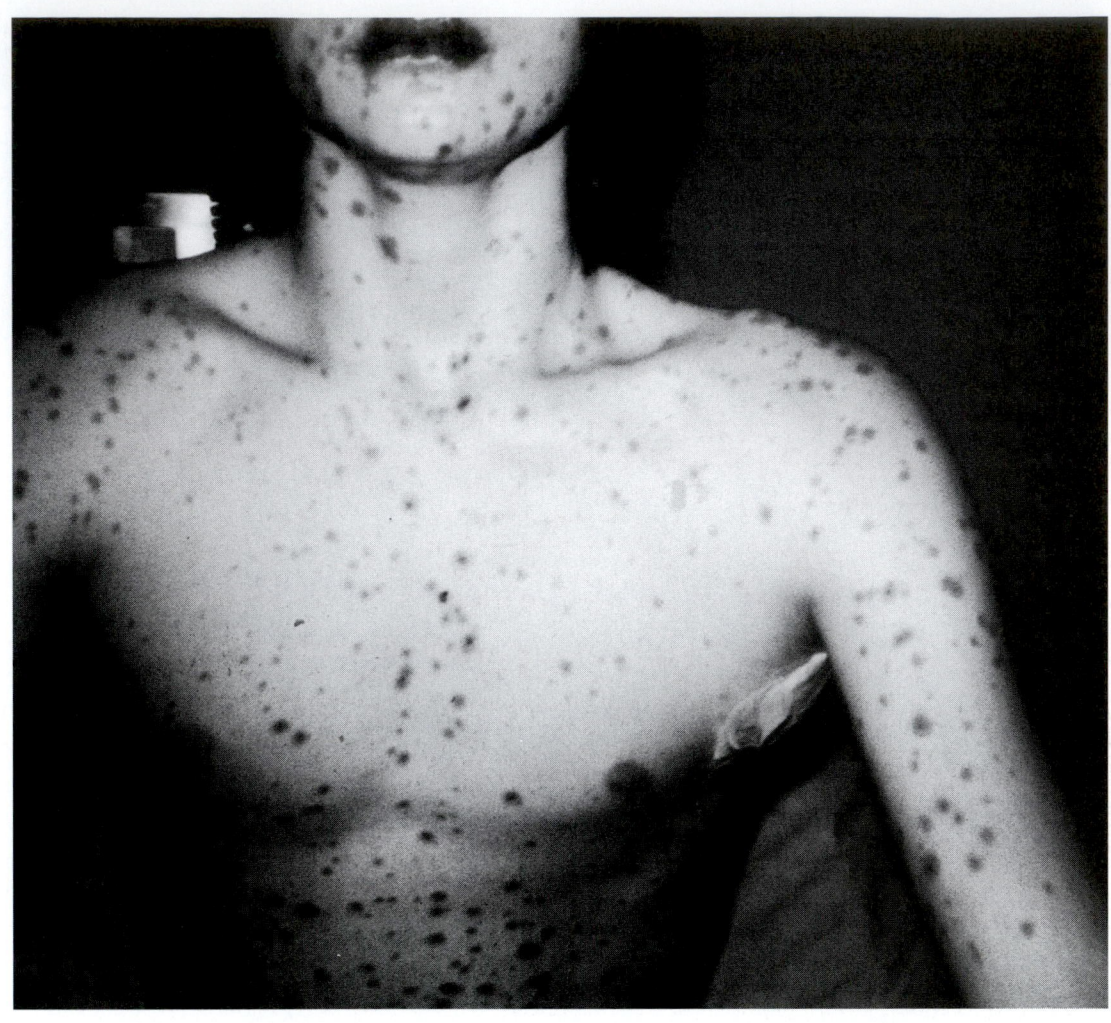

Figure 32-24 Stevens–Johnson syndrome. Polymorphous eruption with targetoid skin lesions and typical lip crusting.

Figure 32-25 Bullous fixed drug eruption in reaction to ibuprofen.

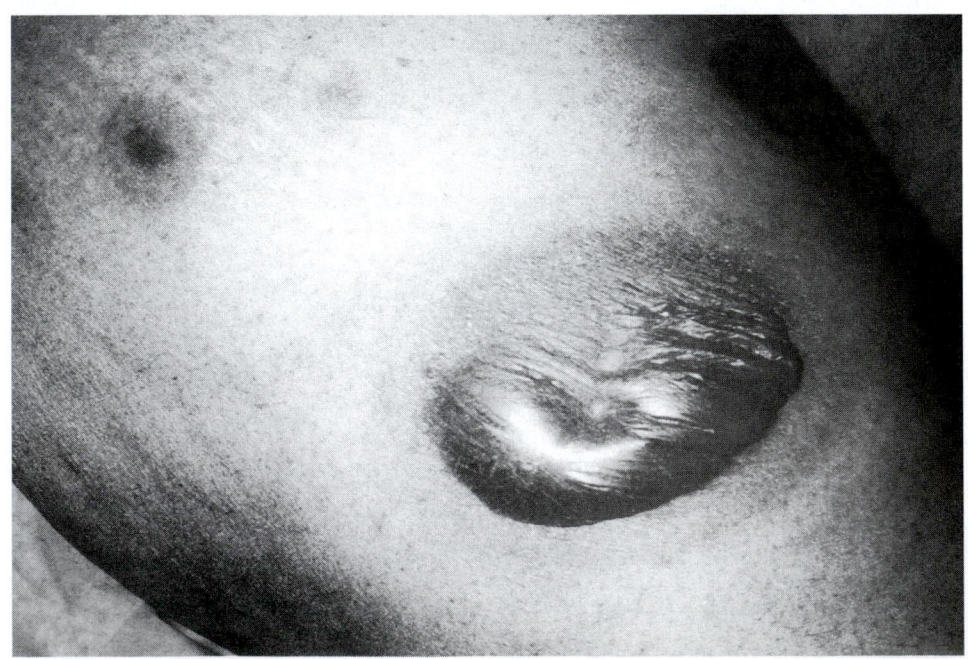

variable shape, arrangement, and distribution. They tend to change over hours and are extremely pruritic. Many drugs are capable of inducing exanthematous and urticarial eruptions, the more common of which are antibiotics and anticonvulsants. The time of onset of the rash in relation to the drug can be helpful in diagnosis. The rash can occur at any time between day 1 and 3 weeks after beginning the drug, with peak incidence occurring around day 9. In the case of penicillin, the reaction may not occur for 2 or more weeks after discontinuation of the drug. Treatment requires stopping the offending agent. Supportive measures such as topical and systemic antipruritics are beneficial.

Neoplastic Lesions of the Vulva

Table 32-8 outlines some of the more common benign tumors of the vulva. Malignant vulvar tumors are also discussed elsewhere in this textbook. It is important to note that the incidence of both melanoma and nonmelanoma skin cancer is rising dramatically in the United States, and, although these cancers occur much more often on sun-exposed skin, they can and do occur on the genitalia. Squamous-cell carcinoma (Figure 32-26) is the most common vulvar malignancy. Basal-cell carcinoma, which accounts for

TABLE 32-8 BENIGN TUMORS OF THE VULVA		
Solid	**Cystic**	**Vascular**
Skin tags	Bartholin cyst	Hemangiomas
Fibromas	Epidermal inclusion	Cherry angioma
Neurofibromas	cyst	Angiokeratoma
Syringoma	Pilonidal cyst and	Pyogenic granuloma
Hidradenoma	sinus	Endometriosis
papilliferum	Lymphangioma	
Lipoma		
Granular-cell tumor		

less than 5% of vulvar cancers,[17] has the same clinical appearance as basal-cell cancers on other skin sites. The classic lesion is a pearly, telangiectatic dome-shaped nodule (Figure 32-27), or an ulcer with a pearly, rolled border ("rodent ulcer"). However, basal-cell carcinoma has a variety of appearances, some of which are subtle. Biopsy is diagnostic, showing a basaloid proliferation with peripheral palisading and retraction artifact (clefting). Basal-cell carcinoma very rarely metastasizes, but if neglected can cause considerable local destruction.

Pigmented neoplasms are common on the vulva (see Table 32-9); the most common benign lesion is the lentigo. Vascular lesions, which can be dark in appearance, may simulate melanocytic lesions, but

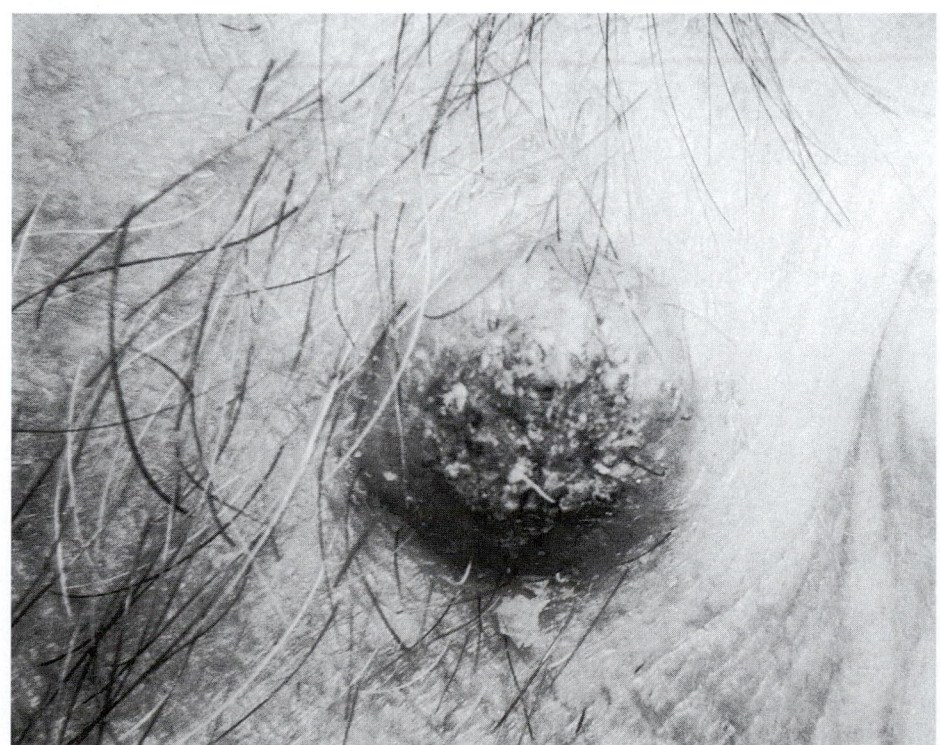

Figure 32-26 Preauricular squamous-cell carcinoma.

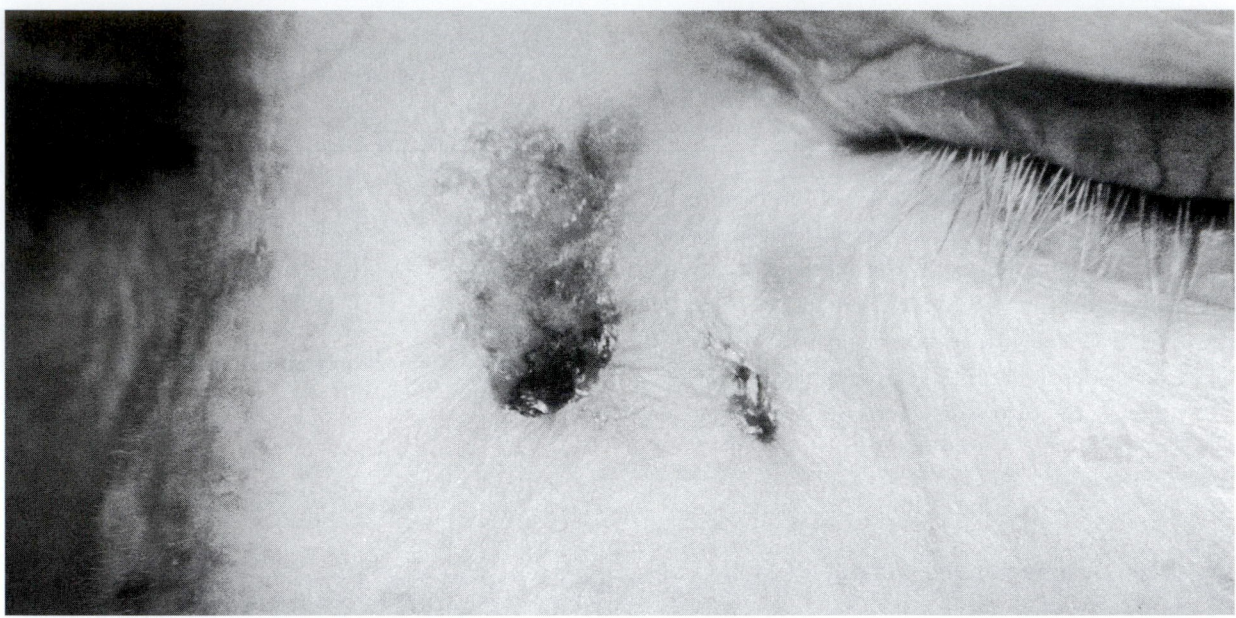

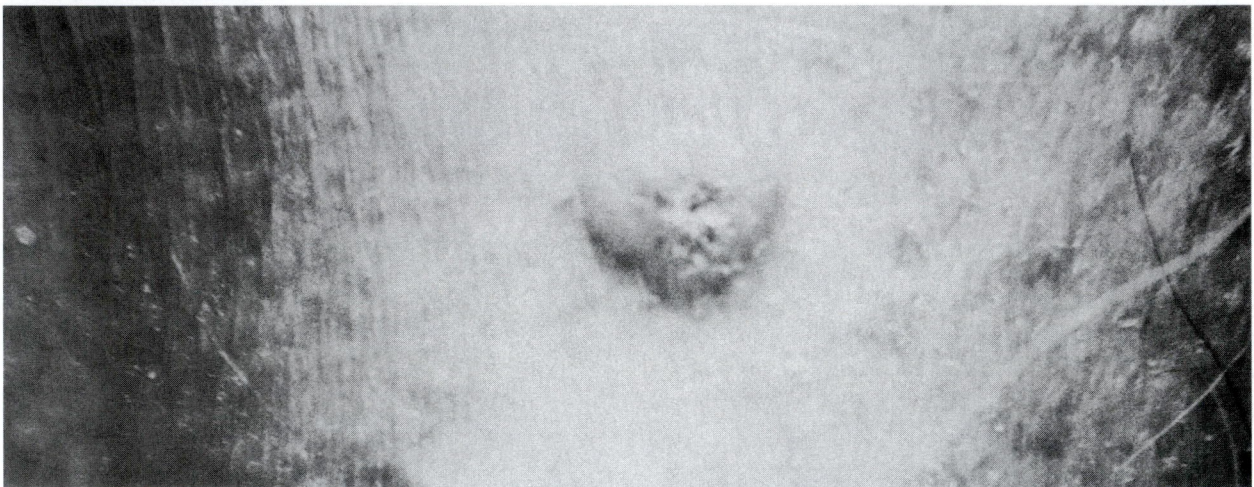

Figure 32-27 Pearly telangiectatic nodules of basal-cell carcinoma.

biopsy will easily differentiate these entities. In addition to melanoma, there are other malignancies that can be pigmented. These include basal- and squamous-cell carcinoma and extramammary Paget disease. Malignant melanoma of the vulva, which comprises 3% of all melanomas and is the second most common vulvar malignancy after squamous-cell carcinoma,[18] tends to be more advanced at the time of diagnosis than melanoma at other sites. Thin melanomas (less than 1 mm deep) have a good prognosis if they are detected early and completely excised; prognosis worsens with increased Breslow level, which is the depth of the tumor measured from the granular-cell layer of the epidermis to the base of the

tumor. Clinically, melanoma on the vulva resembles melanoma elsewhere on the body. There is asymmetry, border irregularity, color variegation, and the diameter is usually greater than 6 mm (ABCDs of malignant melanoma). Most are dark, but amelanotic melanomas are not uncommon on the vulva. Lesions are usually flat initially but become nodular as the atypical cells invade more deeply into the dermis; however, nodular melanoma can arise de novo and has a worse prognosis. Any pigmented lesion that raises suspicion for melanoma should be immediately biopsied. Ideally, an excisional biopsy should be performed but, if impractical at the time of presentation, an incisional biopsy (as large as possible) from the

TABLE 32-9
DARK LESIONS OF THE VULVA

Nonmelanocytic	Melanocytic
Freckles	Lentigines
Hemangioma	Compound, junctional, and
Angiokeratoma	intradermal nevi
Seborrheic keratoses	Blue nevi
Warts	Congenital nevi
Basal-cell carcinoma	Dysplastic nevi
Squamous-cell carcinoma	Malignant melanoma
Extramammary Paget disease	
Vulvar melanosis	
Postinflammatory	
hyperpigmentation	

worst, most nodular area can suffice. Assessment of depth is required in order to determine the width of margins as well as prognosis and staging.

Vulvar Manifestations of Systemic Diseases

The skin is sometimes a window to underlying systemic illness. Some diseases present with specific skin lesions such as sarcoidosis, lupus, neurofibromatosis, and others; but the majority of skin findings associated with systemic diseases are nonspecific. However, these nonspecific skin lesions can be very helpful diagnostic clues. Such examples include the association of generalized pruritus with lymphoma, acanthosis nigricans with adenocarcinoma of the stomach, pyoderma gangrenosum and erythema nodosum with inflammatory bowel disease, to mention just a few. This intriguing topic is very broad and most definitely beyond the scope of this chapter. Additional information can be found in standard dermatologic textbooks. The following paragraphs provide limited information on a few systemic diseases that have associated skin findings that are located on the vulva.

Chronic pruritus can be a symptom of iron-deficiency anemia, and although usually generalized, the pruritus can be localized to the anogenital region, often clinically manifest as lichen simplex chronicus. Other systemic causes of generalized pruritus include malignancy (especially lymphoproliferative malignancies) polycythemia vera, hepatic disease, renal disease, thyroid disease, medications, and psychiatric disorders.

Acanthosis nigricans presents as symmetric hyperpigmented velvety plaques of flexural areas of the neck (Figure 32-28), axillae, and groin, and has been associated with medications, obesity, carcinoma, endocrinopathies such as diabetes mellitus, Addison disease, polycystic ovary disease, hypogonadism, Cushing disease, and thyroid disease.

Generalized hyperpigmentation with accentuation in flexural areas and on mucosal surfaces may be seen in Addison disease.

Axillary freckling (Crowe sign), which is pathognomonic for neurofibromatosis (von Recklinghausen disease), can present in the anogenital region as well as the axillae.

Crohn disease can present with specific granulomatous lesions of the vulva or perianal area, or nonspecific lesions such as pyoderma gangrenosum, erythema nodosum, and aphthous ulcers.

A cardinal feature of Behçet disease, a multisystem inflammatory disorder, is the recurrent aphthouslike ulcers of the mouth and genitalia.

Erythema nodosum, a septal panniculitis, is an immunologic reaction pattern stimulated by multiple and diverse causes. Clinically, erythema nodosum presents as tender, red, poorly demarcated indurated nodules, most commonly seen on the anterior lower extremities. Fever, arthralgias, and malaise are sometimes present. Associated systemic diseases include group A streptococcus; granulomatous infections such as tuberculosis, histoplasmosis, and coccidioidomycosis; lymphogranuloma venereum; yersinia; drugs such as oral contraceptives and sulfonamides; sarcoidosis; inflammatory bowel disease; and Behçet disease. However, approximately 40 to 50% of cases are idiopathic and usually resolve spontaneously within 6 weeks. Treatment requires identifying and treating any underlying illness and supportive measures such as bed rest and nonsteroidal antiinflammatory drugs.

Zinc deficiency, which may be acquired or inherited (acrodermatitis enteropathica), can present with a variety of skin findings, such as eczematous patches or annular, vesiculobullous, pustular, or crusted erosive lesions of the hands, feet, scalp, and periorificial areas. Paronychia is common, as is alopecia, glossitis, oral erosions and perleche. The classic triad of zinc deficiency is dermatitis, diarrhea, and alopecia.

The skin findings of glucagonoma syndrome (necrolytic migratory erythema) associated with α-cell tumors of the pancreas can very much resemble the eruption of zinc deficiency. It also tends to be periorificial, but is more geographic because as old lesions heal, new ones appear, giving the appearance of migration. Biopsy of an early skin lesion can be

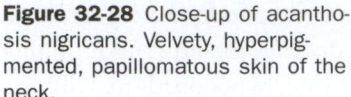

Figure 32-28 Close-up of acanthosis nigricans. Velvety, hyperpigmented, papillomatous skin of the neck.

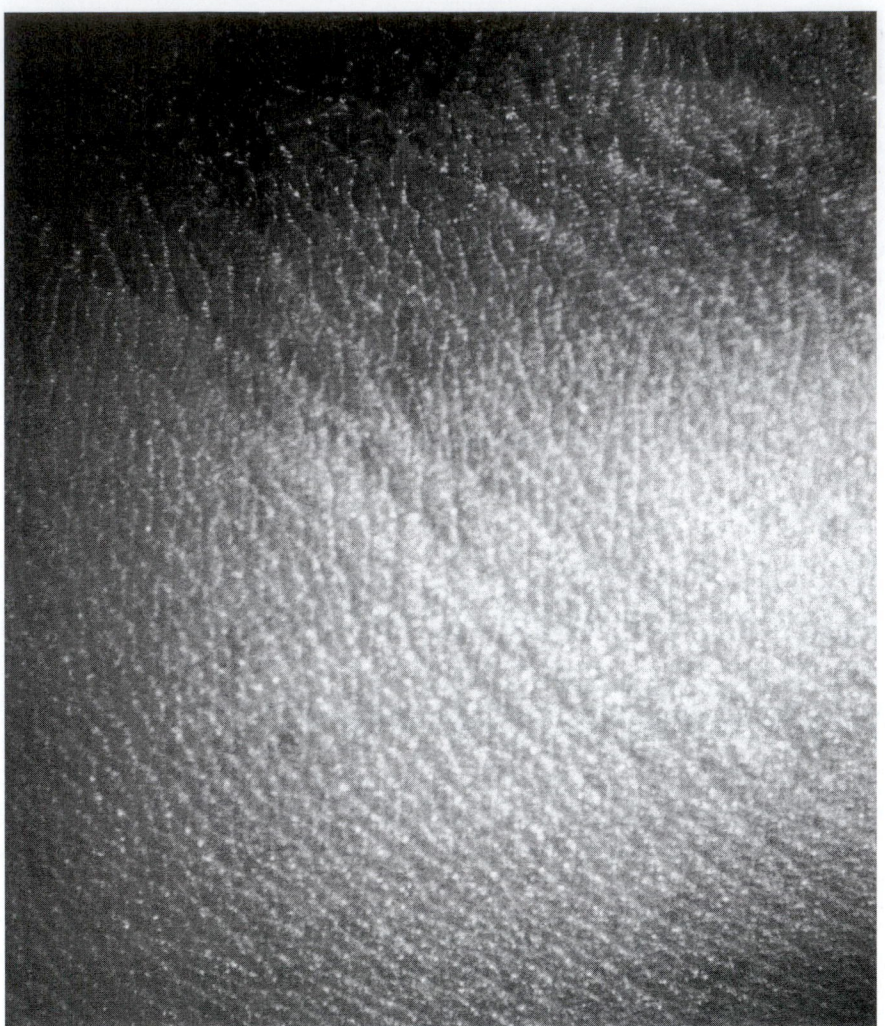

helpful if it shows the characteristic upper epidermal necrosis. Removal of the tumor can result in cure of the skin disease.

Vulvodynia from a Dermatologist's Perspective

The International Society of the Study of Vulvar Disease (ISSVD) defined vulvodynia as chronic vulvar discomfort with symptoms of burning, stinging, irritation or rawness.[19] McKay[20] has divided vulvodynia into five subsets: vulvar dermatoses, cyclic candidiasis, vulvar vestibulitis, squamous papillomatosis, and essential vulvodynia. The diagnosis of vulvodynia is based on a history of usually acute development of vulvar pain in a patient with good general health, unremarkable obstetric and gynecologic history, a normal gynecologic physical examination, and pain localized to the vaginal introitus (vestibule), which

can be reproduced by touching the vestibulum with a moist cotton-tipped swab.

Dermatologists treat the vulva as a skin structure and search the entire skin for a treatable skin disease (Table 32-10)[21] or infection (Table 32-11),[21] which may affect the vulva without being clinically obvious. Dermatologists mainly look for and treat vulvar dermatoses and cyclic candidiasis subsets of vulvodynia. Vulvodynia symptoms do not include pruritus, and pain precludes scratching, but chronic pruritic skin diseases or infection may produce the sensations of burning, stinging, irritation, or rawness. Most reports in the dermatologic literature have focused on dermatitis and urticaria as causes of vulvodynia.

Fischer et al.[22] found that of 144 adult patients with chronic vulvar symptoms, 64% were found to have dermatitis. Of patients with a histologic diagnosis of spongiotic dermatitis, 65% were found to be atopic and would be prone to the development of

---

TABLE 32-10
DERMATOSES IMPLICATED IN VULVODYNIA

Behçet syndrome
Benign familial pemphigus
Dermatitis herpetiformis
Dermatographism
Erythema multiforme
Estrogen deficiency (vulvar fragility, fourchette fissures)
Folate deficiency
Intraepithelial vulval neoplasia
Irritant and contact dermatitis
Lichen planus
Lichen sclerosis
Lichen simplex chronicus
Lupus erythematosus
Niacin deficiency (pellagra)
Pemphigoid
Pemphigus
Periorificial dermatitis (iatrogenic vulvodynia)
Psoriasis
Seborrheic dermatitis
Squamous-cell carcinoma
Tinea
Vulva papillomatosis

TABLE 32-11
INFECTIONS THAT MAY CAUSE
VULVAR PAIN/BURNING

Bacterial vaginosis
Cytolytic vaginosis
Desquamative inflammatory vaginitis
Genital herpes simplex
Genital warts
Genital zoster
Impetigo (rare in adults)
Intertrigo
Reiter syndrome
Syphilis (rare)
Vaginal lactobacillosis
Vulvovaginal candidiasis
Vulvovaginal trichomoniasis
Vulvovaginitis secondary to gonorrhea or chlamydia (rare)

---

irritation and dermatitis from topical irritant products and harsh soaps. Atopic dermatitis is diagnosed by a personal or family history of eczema, asthma, or hayfever and dermatitis of posterior neck and antecubital and popliteal fossae. If contact dermatitis is suspected by clinical appearance or skin biopsy, then a patch test is needed to discover the allergen causing the dermatitis. Brenan et al.[23] found that benzocaine was the most common allergen found in women with chronic vulvar symptoms and Lewis et al.[24] found medicaments or their constituents as the most common allergens. Successful treatment of dermatitis includes eliminating contact with allergens, avoiding irritants and harsh soaps in patients with atopic symptoms, using mild to moderate topical steroids, and treating superinfection, particularly candidiasis. Fischer et al.[22] reported that with a skin biopsy showing dermatitis and a positive candidal swab, the treatment of both dermatitis and candidiasis produced a 100% success rate.

Ricks et al.[25] reported successful treatment of vulvar vestibulitis with daily vulvar application of solid vegetable oil. Out of 47 patients, 15 had complete relief of symptoms after 14 months of oil use and an average of 5 years of symptoms. Thirty patients had partial relief of symptoms after 15.5 months with a 3-year average for symptoms. Several[26,27] reports have implicated the physical urticarias (local mast-cell activation due to an environmental factor), contact urticaria, and dermographism (increased wheal-and-flare response at the site of brisk stroking of the skin) as producing symptoms of vulvodynia. Urticarial lesions are pruritic, edematous, pink raised papules and plaques. Physical urticarias are suggested by a history of development of urticarial lesions when exposed to a definable environmental factor such as pressure, heat or cold. Contact urticaria is suggested by a clinical distribution of urticarial lesions that is consistent with contact. Dermographism is diagnosed by a history of development of linear whelts when the skin is scratched and demonstrated by production of linear whelts by briskly stroking the skin. Treatment of these conditions is oral antihistamines and an attempt to eliminate the cause of urticaria.

Isoprenosin,[28] flashlamp-excited dye laser,[29] amitriptyline,[30] psychological counseling,[31] oral calcium citrate combined with a low-oxalate diet,[32] and interferon alfa-2b[33] have been reported to alleviate the symptoms of vulvodynia.

RERENCES

1. Fleischer AB Jr, Feldman SR, McConnell RC. The most common dermatologic problems identified by family physicians. Fam Med 1997;29:648.
2. McKay M. Physiologic changes of pregnancy. In: Black MM, McKay M, Braude PR, eds. Obstetric and gynecologic dermatology. London: Mosby-Wolfe, 1995:19.
3. Kang S, Kwang JK, Griffiths C, et al. Topical tretinoin improves early stretch marks. Arch Dermatol 1996;132:519.
4. Shapiro L, Pastuszak A, Carto G, Koren G. Safety of first-trimester exposure to topical tretinoin: prospective cohort study. Lancet 1997;350:1143.

5. Jenkins RE, Black MM. Effect of pregnancy on other skin disorders. In: Black MM, McKay M, Braude PR, eds. Obstetric and gynecologic dermatology. London: Mosby-Wolfe, 1995:146.

6. Van de weil A, Hart HC, Flinterman J, et al. Plasma exchange in herpes gestationis. BMJ 1980;281:1041.

7. Garvey MP, Handfield-Jones SE, Black MM. Pemphigoid gestationis response to chemical oophorectomy with goserelin. Clin Exp Dermatol 1992;17:443.

8. Black MM, Mayou SC. Skin diseases in pregnancy. In: de Swiet M, ed. Medical disorders in obstetric practice. 2nd ed. Oxford: Blackwell Scientific, 1989:808.

9. Aractingi S, Berkane N, Bertheau P, et al. Fetal DNA in skin of polymorphic eruptions of pregnancy. Lancet 1998; 352:1898.

10. Reily CA. Liver diseases in pregnancy. In: Reece EA, Hobbins JC, Mahoney MJ, Petrie RH, eds. Medicine of the fetus and mother. Philadelphia: Lippincott, 1992:1077.

11. Stephens JM, Black MM. Perimenstrual skin eruptions. In: Black MM, McKay M, Braude PR, eds. Obstetric and gynecologic dermatology. London: Mosby-Wolfe, 1995:147.

12. Meinking TL, Taplin D, Hermida JL, et al. The treatment of scabies with ivermectin. N Engl J Med 1995;333:26.

13. Marren P, Wojnarowska F. Dermatitis of the vulva. Semin Dermatol 1996;15:36.

14. Marren P, Wojnarowska F, Powell S. Allergic contact dermatitis and vulvar dermatoses. Br J Dermatol 1992;126:52.

15. Marren P, Wojnarowska F. Erosive vulvovaginitis. In: Black MM, McKay M, Braude PR, eds. Obstetric and gynecologic dermatology. London: Mosby-Wolfe 1995:125.

16. Grimes PE. Diseases of hypopigmentation. In: Sams WM, Lynch PJ, eds. Principles and practice of dermatology. 2nd ed. New York: Churchill Livingstone, 1996:843

17. Monaghan JM, Horowitz IR, McKay M. Vulvar tumors. In: Black MM, McKay M, Braude PR, eds. Obstetric and gynecologic dermatology. London: Mosby-Wolfe, 1995: 147.

18. Lynch PJ, Edwards L. Genital dermatology. New York: Churchill Livingstone, 1994:163.

19. McKay M. Burning vulvar syndrome: report of the ISSVD task force. J Reprod Med 1984;29:457.

20. McKay M. Vulvodynia: a multifactorial clinical problem. Arch Dermatol 1989;125:256.

21. Mroozkowski, TF. Vulvodynia—a dermatovenereologist's perspective. Int J Dermatol August 1998;37:567.

22. Fischer G, Spurrett B, Fischer A. The chronically symptomatic vulva: aetiology and management. Br J Obstet Gynaecol 1995;102:773.

23. Brenan J, Dennerstein G, Sfameni S, et al. Evaluation of patch testing in patients with chronic vulvar symptoms. Aust J Dermatol 1996;37:40.

24. Lewis FM, Shah M, Gawkrodger DJ. Contact sensitivity in pruritus vulvae: patch test results and clinical outcome. Am J Contact Dermat 1997;8(3):137.

25. Ricks CM, Summers PR, Sharp HC. Topical oil application: a simple, safe remedy. Presented at the American College of Obstetricians and Gynecologists, San Francisco, 1995.

26. Lambiris A, Greaves MW. Urticaria: increasingly recognised but not adequately highlighted cause of dyspareunia and vulvodynia. Acta Derm Venereol 1997;77:160.

27. Perniciaro C, Bustamante AS, Gutierrez MM. Two cases of vulvodynia with unusual causes. Acta Derm Venereol 1993;73:227.

28. Sand Peterson C, Weisman K. Isoprenosine improves symptoms in young females with chronic vulvodynia. Acta Derm Venereol 1996;76:404.

29. Reid R, Omoto KH, Precop SL, et al. Flashlamp-excited dye laser therapy of idiopathic vulvodynia is safe and efficacious. Am J Obstet Gynecol 1995;172:1684.

30. McKay M. Dysesthetic ("essential") vulvodynia treatment with amitriptyline. J Reprod Med 1993;38:9.

31. Stewart DE, Reicher AE, Gerulath AH, Boydell KM. Vulvodynia and psychological distress. Obstet Gynecol 1994;84:587.

32. Solomon CC, Meimed MH, Heitler SM. Calcium citrate for vulvar vestibulitis. J Reprod Med 1991;36:879.

33. Larsen J, Peters K, Petersen CS, Damkjear K, Albrectsen J, Weisman K. Interferon alpha-2b treatment of symptomatic vulvodynia associated with koilocytosis. Acta Derm Venereol 1993;73:385.

Chapter 33

Approach to Anemia

Patricia Adams-Graves

Five Key Points

- Anemia is not a disease, but a sign of an underlying process that may be life-threating if ignored (e.g., colon cancer).

- Practitioners must first recognize anemia and become familiar with the normal values for hemoglobin, which are about 15% (2g/dl) lower for women as compared with men.

- Adaptive mechanisms to anemia are efficient during slowly developing and chronic anemias; therefore, practioners must not be eager to transfuse solely based on the hemoglobin or hematocrit values, but must base the decision on the clinical stability of the patient.

- Classification by expected patterns of anemia by mean corpuscular volume and red-cell distribution width, coupled with a meticulous history, physical examination, and laboratory evaluation, will help practitioners formulate a differential diagnosis and avoid the costly "shotgun" approach to diagnosing anemia.

- Erythropoietin is now available as an effective alternative for blood tranfusion for certain anemic states in which blood is contraindicated, as for Jehovah's Witnesses and for incompatible blood.

Anemia is not a disease, but a common, nonspecific sign of diverse underlying diseases. Therefore, obstetrician-gynecologists and other primary care providers should be sensitive to anemia. On recognition, a search for the underlying cause of anemia should be undertaken. A low hemoglobin concentration is often put aside to be dealt with after more urgent medical problems are under control. Even a minimal reduction in hemoglobin is usually a clue to a disease that may prove detrimental if not searched for (e.g., colon cancer).[1] Practitioners should think of anemia in a manner similar to symptons like fever, syncope, or abdominal pain, as an indicator of underlying disease rather than an entity in itself. Anemia should not only be recognized but included in the problem list during evaluation of patients with multiple medical problems. An understanding of the mechanisms of anemia will help practitioners to better evaluate anemia.

PATHOPHYSIOLOGY

General

Anemia should draw one's attention to a decrease in hemoglobin concentration. Anemia ultimately results in reduced oxygen-carrying capacity of the blood that does not match the body's metabolic needs.[2-6] Therefore, understanding the pathophysi-

---
**TABLE 33-1
PATHOGENETIC CLASSIFICATION OF ANEMIAS**

Impaired production
    Megaloblastic anemias
    Hypochromic anemias
    Aplastic and myelodysplastic anemias
    Myelophthisic anemias
Increased destruction (hemolytic anemias)
    Disorders of red-cell membranes
    Hemoglobinopathies
    Hemolytic anemias caused by red-cell infection
Altered erythropoiesis (secondary anemias)
    Anemia of chronic disease
        Chronic inflammation or infection
        Renal failure
        Collagen vascular diseases
        Liver disease
        Malignancy
        Endocrinopathy

---

ology of anemia will lead clinicians toward diagnosing specific diseases and then to implement the appropriate therapy.

Three basic pathogenic mechanisms of anemia include (1) those with decreased production or impaired release of red cells from the bone marrow, (2) those with increased destruction after release from the bone marrow, and (3) those associated with a variety of systemic disorders that alter normal erythropoiesis and secondarily result in anemia[2-6] (Table 33-1).

Physiologic Adaptation to Anemia

Under normal conditions, the body's hemoglobin concentration is maintaned within normal limits through a variety of regulatory and compensatory mechanisms. The ability of these adaptive mechanisms to maintain adequate oxygen delivery depends on whether the anemia developed rapidly (e.g., during states of acute blood loss and rapid hemolysis) or whether it developed slowly (e.g., with vitamin B_{12} deficiency and iron deficiency).[3,4] Other important factors include the degree of reduction in total blood volume, the degree of reduction of blood pH and partial pressure of oxygen (PaO_2) the integrity of the red cell (erythrocyte), hematopoietic cytokines,[7-10] the integrity of the bone marrow and its response to erythropoietin (a hormone secreted by the kidneys),[7,8] the capacity of the cardiopulmonary system to compensate for the anemia, and the general health of the patient.[2-12]

Rapidly Developing Anemia

Rapidly developing anemia, as with uncontrollable bleeding or the rapid red-cell destruction seen with brisk hemolysis, triggers immediate cardiopulmonary adaptation (e.g., tachycardia and hyperventilation) in an attempt to improve oxygen delivery to tissues and to avoid vascular collapse.[2-5,13] Although hyperventilation improves hemoglobin oxygen saturation, the sigmoidal oxygen-binding curve of intact hemoglobin in this setting is inefficient in unloading oxygen. During the process of unloading oxygen, the oxygen saturation of normal blood falls from 98% to about 74%, which minimally affects the PaO_2 of blood while unloading oxygen generously[4,14,15] (Figure 33-1). Cardiovasular adjustments include increase in blood flow by increasing stroke volume, heart rate (tachycardia), and redistribution of blood flow to areas most vulnerable to hypoxemia, such as the brain and heart. Centralization of blood flow during hypovolemia is responsible for anemia pallor by reducing skin perfusion. Uncontrollable hypovolemia and hypoxemia will ultimately lead to heart failure, tissue anoxia, and vascular collapse (hypovolemic shock).[2,4,5,13]

Slowly Developing Anemias

During slowly developing anemia (vitamin B_{12} deficiency, iron deficiency) or chronic hemolytic anemias (sickle-cell disease, hereditary spherocytosis) the normal physiologic cardiorespiratory and humoral feedback responses are well established to maintain oxygen delivery and to meet basic metabolic needs.[2-6] Therefore, otherwise healthy individuals and those with compensated chronic anemias may remain asymptomatic for a substantial amount of time, with hemoglobin values as low as 7.0 to 7.5 g/dl.[2-4,16] In contrast, individuals with diseased hearts or lungs may not be able to tolerate low hemoglobin concentrations and may become symptomatic of higher levels of hemoglobin.[13] Chronic, persistent cardiopulmonary adaptive mechanisms such as increased left ventricular filling pressure and increased heart rate (high-output dynamics) improve oxygen delivery and tissue perfusion but ultimately may lead to cardiomegaly and chronic congestive heart failure.[2,3,5,13,16] Persistent tissue hypoxia due to anemia stimulates more production of an erythrocyte metabolite in the Embden-Meyerof pathway of glycolysis, 2,3-diphosphoglycerate (DPG).[2-6,14,15] This

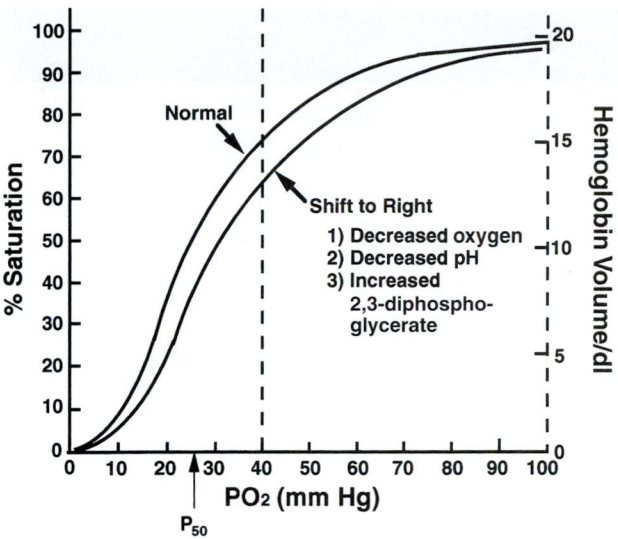

Figure 33-1 Normal oxygen binding curve for red-cell hemoglobin at 37°C and pH 7.4. P_{50} indicates the oxygen pressure that half saturates hemoglobin. The P_{50} of normal blood is 27 mm Hg. The right-shift curve results from chronic hypoxia due to anemia.

results in a sustained right shift of the hemoglobin dissociation curve, which leads to a new steady state for an ongoing increase in the unloading of hemoglobin-bound oxygen[14,15] (see Figure 33-1). Chronic hypoxia also results in an increase in aldosterone, a mineralocorticoid from the kidney, and an increase in pressor–antidiuretic hormone (ADH) from the posterior pituitary to promote sodium and free water retention, respectively.[13] Although this adaptive mechanism due to anemia partially corrects the plasma volume deficit, it is inefficent in restoring oxygen delivery and therefore results in perenal azotemia (decreased urinary output), orthostatic hypotension, and renal failure (shock kidney) if not corrected.[13] Moreover, a drop in PaO_2 (hypoxia) and pH (acidosis) due to anemia also triggers increased secretion of erythropoietin, a hormone from the renal tubules that stimulates bone marrow to increase the rate of erythropoiesis. Although the mechanism of erythropoietin production and release is unclear, erythropoietin, by increasing in vivo erythropoiesis, is the most efficent way to correct anemia and is now commercially available for clinical use for certain erythropoietin-sensitive anemias.[2,4,7-9,17,18] It is especially useful as an alternative to tranfusions in which blood therapy is contraindicated or undesirable because of religious beliefs, such as for Jehovah's Witnesses.[7-9,17-20]

APPROACH TO THE PATIENT

General Considerations

The main objective in evaluting patients with anemia is to make an appropriate diagnosis, including classifying and determining the cause, with the fewest laboratory studies and at the lowest possible cost.

It is imperative to obtain a meticulous history and to do a thorough physical examination. In general, some genetic anemias are common to certain ethnic groups (e.g., thalassemia in Italians, Asians, and Africans,[2-6,16]) whereas some acquired anemias (e.g., iron deficiency) are common in women of childbearing age with or without menorrhagia.[2,3,4,6,21,24] Certain lifestyle choices, such as the use of excessive alcohol and illegal drugs, sexual promiscuity, and poor or restricted eating habits can cause a variety of anemic states.[2,3,4,6,13,25] A mixed vitamin-B_{12} and iron-deficiency anemia resulting from malabsorption from a remote gastrointestinal surgery or ulcerative colitis might be obtained by history but would otherwise have gone unexplained.[4,25] Carefully obtained historical data will provide a guide for a differential diagnosis and later may lead to a specific cause of anemia (Table 33-2).

Recognition

Anemia is recognized in otherwise healthy individuals on the complete blood count (CBC) laboratory report and is based on a decrease in the number of red cells, hemoglobin concentration, or hematocrit per unit of blood below the level previously established by sampling large populations of men and women stratified by age, race, and residence (e.g., sea level)[6,25,26] (Table 33-3).

Medical History

Present Illness

In general, anemia is characterized by its underlying cause and whether it is genetic, acquired, or relative (selective increase in plasma volume)[2,3,4,16,23,24] (Table 33-4). The present illness can give clues to the presence, pace, and character of anemia prior to obtaining a CBC, including the onset of symptoms, rate of progession of symptoms, duration of symptoms, and any associated cardiopulmonary compensatory mechanisms present, such as the degree of weakness, shortness of breath, orthostatic hypotension, and palpitations.

TABLE 33-2
SYMPTOMS AND PHYSICAL SIGNS OF CLASSIC ANEMIA

	Symptoms	Physical Signs
Symptoms common to all anemias	Weakness, fatigue, lightheadedness, lassitude, shortness of breath (if severe)	Pallor, systolic flow murmur, tachycardia
Acute blood loss	Syncope or near syncope, headache; symptoms also referable to site of bleeding including hematemesis, melena, abdominal pain, back pain, crush injury, major lacerations, pain from fractures of long bones	Hypotension (with orthostatic changes), focal signs referrable to site of blood loss
Iron deficiency	Diminished work capacity, behavorial and learning disorders, palpitations, sicca; craving for clay (geophagia), etc.; cornstarch (amylophagia), or ice (pagophagia), etc.; dysphagia (thin membranous webs in the postcricoid area (Patterson–Kelly/Plummer–Vinson syndrome)	Koilonychia (nails dry, brittle, and ridged, with concave surface), angular stomatitis, glossitis, esophageal webs (if severe)
Vitamin B_{12} deficiency	Vertigo, tinnitus, palpitations, chest pain, paroxysmal nocturnal dyspnea, orthopnea, dependent edema, sore tongue, anorexia, weight loss, diarrhea, hypesthesia, parathesia, ataxia, poor fine motor coordination, diminished sphincter control, diminished proprioception, variable changes in mental status from irritability and forgetfulness to dementia or psychosis	Icterus, cardiomegaly, hepatosplenomegaly, low-grade fever, smooth beefy red tongue, hypesthesia, impaired proprioception, weakness, ataxia, abnormal Romberg test, poor fine motor coordination, diminished sphincter tone, hyperreflexia or hyporeflexia, Babinski sign abnormal, decreased memory, disorientation, confusion, psychosis
Folic acid deficiency	Vertigo, tinnitus, palpitations, chest pain, paroxysmal nocturnal dyspnea, orthopnea, dependent edema, anorexia, weight loss, diarrhea, psychosis, dementia, neurosis	Icterus, cardiomegaly, hepatosplenomegaly, glossitis, cheilosis, wasting, cachexia

Symptoms common to all anemias include weakness, tiredness, lightheadedness, and lassitude.[2,3,4,6,25] Table 33-2 lists symptoms of specific types of anemias.

Medications: Drug-induced Anemia

Identifying history of ingestion or injection of certain prescribed or nonprescribed medication is imperative when evaluating anemia.[2,3,4,6,25] For example, drugs such as phenytoin, commonly used for seizure disorders, can cause folate deficiency, resulting in the inhibition of DNA synthesis. Oral contraceptives can cause folate deficiency by impairing folate absorption or can increase urinary folate loss. Sulfasalazine used to treat inflammatory bowel disease may produce

TABLE 33-3
CRITERIA FOR ANEMIA IN ADULT WOMEN AND MEN

	Women	Men
Hemoglobin (g/dl)	<11.5	<13.5
Hematocrit (%)	<36	<40
Red cells ($\times 10^{12}$/liter)	<3.5	<4.0

Note: These values are at sea level from the hematology laboratory at The University of Tennessee William F. Bowld Hospital, Memphis. Normals may vary by location. Check values from your local laboratory or on the normal range included on the CBC report.

megaloblastosis (mean corpuscular volume [MCV] >100).[25] Knowing that these drugs cause macrocytic anemia may avoid an unnecessary evaluation for other causes of anemia. If possible, stopping or reducing the amount of the drug ingested by the patient can be curative. Therefore, all drugs in patients with anemia should be considered as the possible cause of their anemia (Table 33-5).

Family History

A family history is imperative in determining whether anemia is acquired or congenital. For example, a history of cholecystectomy, splenectomy, or jaundice in an otherwise asymptomatic patient and other asymptomatic family members may suggest a chronic hemolytic anemia such as hereditary spherocytosis, glucose-6-phosphate dehydrogenase (G6PD) deficiency, or sickle cell disease.[2,3,5,16]

Physical Findings

Physical examinations should be directed toward confirming a clinical suspicion of anemia. These exams should include looking for paleness in the oral

---

TABLE 33-4
ANEMIA CLASSIFICATION

Hereditary
  Hereditary membrane defects (spherocytosis, etc.)
  Red-cell enzyme defects (G6PD)
  Hemoglobinopathies
Acquired
  Vitamin deficiencies
  Anemia of chronic disease
  Splenomegaly
  Immune-mediated
  Mechanical trauma (TTP, HELP)
  Drugs (immune and nonimmune mechanisms)
  Infectious agents
Relative
  Pregnancy (selective increase in plasma volume)
  Splenomegaly (red-cell sequestration)

G6PD = glucose-6-phosphate dehydrogenase; TTP = thrombotic thrombocytopenic purpura; HELP = hemolysis, elevated liver enzymes, low platelet count.

mucosa and abnormalities of the tongue (e.g., beefy red tongue), as seen with vitamin-B$_{12}$ and folate-deficiency states, and angular cheliosis that is seen in both iron- and vitamin B$_{12}$–deficiency states.[2-4,6,25-29] Signs of severity include pale conjunctiva, poor capillary refill of the nail beds, systolic flow murmur, and signs of heart failure (S3 or S4 gallop).[2,3,4,13,16] The retina may show flame-shaped hemorrhages;

cerebral hypoxia can produce mental status changes as well as muscular weakness.[2-6,25] One may see difficulty with gait, position sense, and paresthesias due to vitamin B$_{12}$ deficiency.[2-4,6,27-29] Hypothyroidism may be identified by a delayed relaxation phase of deep tendon reflexes as a secondary cause of anemia (e.g., anemia of chronic disease).[13] Table 33-2 summarizes the numerous physical findings of common anemias.

Classification

Nearly all anemias can be categorized by their pathophysiology (Table 33-1) and/or by their morphology (Table 33-5).[5,25,29,30] Practitioners must have a working understanding of the red-cell indexes to appropriately classify anemia by morphologic features generated by automated cell analyzers.[4,25,26,31] The red-cell indexes address cell size, hemoglobin content, and hemoglobin concentration within red cells. The most important red-cell index for classification is the mean corpuscular volume (MCV).[4,25,26,30-34] It measures the red-cell volume or red-cell size in femtoliters (fl), with a normal range of 80 to 99 fl. The other indexes, such as the mean corpuscular hemoglobin (MCH) and the mean corpuscular hemoglobin concentration (MCHC), have little clinical usefulness in

---

TABLE 33-5
PHARMACOLOGIC AGENTS RESPONSIBLE FOR ANEMIA

Iron deficiency/acute blood loss	Inadequate or inactive folate	Megaloblastic anemia
Nonsteroidal/antiinflammatory drugs	Oral contraceptives	Inadequate or inactive vitamin B$_{12}$
Diclofenac sodium	Alcohol (chronic intake)	Azidothymidine (AZT)
Diflunisal	Diphenylhydantoin	Colchicine
Fenoprofen calcium	Isoniazid	Metformin
Flurbiprofen	Phenobarbital	Neomycin
Ibuprofen	Primidone	Nitrous oxide
Indomethacin	Sulfasalazine	p-Aminosalicylate
Ketoprofen	Dihydrofolate reductase inhibitors	Hemolytic Anemia
Mefenamic acid	Methotrexate	Cephalosporins
Meclofenamate sodium	Pyrimethamine	Dapsone
Phenylbutazone	Triamterene	Diflunisal
Piroxicam	Trimethoprim	Ibuprofen
Tolmetin sodium	Ribonucleotide reduction	Insulin
Aplastic anemia (pancytopenia)	Hydroxyurea	Penicillins
Azidothymidine (AZT)	Others	Quinine sulfate
Barbiturates	Phenothiazines	Sulfonamides
Cytotoxic agents (i.e., methotrexate,	Phenytoin	Thiazide diuretics
azathioprine, cyclophosphamide)	Quinacrine	
Valproic acid	Sulfonamides	
Dicumarol	Tegretol	
Furosemide	Thiazide diuretics	
Mephenytoin		

Note: Drugs that cause anemia may not be on this list, therefore, all drugs ingested or injected into patients with anemia should be considered to cause anemia.

TABLE 33-6
EXPECTED PATTERNS OF ANEMIA BY MCV AND RDW

MCV low, RDW normal	MCV low, RDW high	MCV normal, RDW normal	MCV normal, RDW high	MCV high, RDW normal	MCV high, RDW high
Heterozygous thalassemia	Iron deficiency	Normal	Mixed deficiency	Aplastic anemia	Folate deficiency
Chronic disease	Sickle β-thalassemia	Chronic disease (liver)	Early iron or folate deficiency	Myelodysplasia	B₁₂ deficiency
	Hemoglobin	Nonanemic hemoglobinopathy (AS, AC)	Anemic hemoglobinopathy (SS, SC)	Hypothyroidism	Immunohemolysis
	Red-cell fragments	Transfusion Chemotherapy	Myelofibrosis		Cold agglutinins
	Sideroblastic anemia	CLL, CML, hemorrhage hypothyroidism, hereditary spherocytosis	Sideroblastic anemia		CLL (high count)

AS = hemoglobin S-trait; AC = hemoglobin C-trait; SS = homozygous SS hemoglobinopathy; SC = double heterozygous SC hemoglobinopathy; CLL = chronic lymphocytic leukemia; CML = chronic myelogenous leukemia.

classifying anemias, except that an increased MCHC is seen in patients with hereditary spherocytosis.[4,25,26,30-34] The red-cell distribution width (RDW) measures the variance within the volume distribution of the red-cell population expressed as a percentage.[4,25,26,30-34] As such, it indicates the variation of red-cell sizes within the population of cells measured (anisocytosis). Normal RDW is 12 to 14%, and when increased can help in the differential diagnosis of anemia based on expected patterns of anemia by MCV and RDW (Table 33-6).

Bessman's Classification

The morphologic classification of anemia by Bessman[30] has been widely accepted as a guide to help health-care providers narrow diagnostic possibilities of the underlying cause. It is based on an orderly approach that classifies anemia first by the MCV or red-cell size, followed by a subclassification by the RDW. The MCV classifies anemia as microcytic (MCV, <80 fl), normocytic (MCV, 80 to 99 fl), and macrocytic (MCV, ≥100 fl). Each of the three categories is subclassified by the RDW. In the late 1960s and 1970s, Bessman conducted clinical studies that defined the utility of this new parameter.[30] There is no such thing as a low RDW; accordingly, increasingly high values for the RDW reflect greater degrees of anisocytosis (heterogenicity) per red-cell population. For example, a normal individual's RDW is around 12%, whereas a person with iron deficency has an RDW of about 15 to 16%, an abnormal value.[30-34] Increased RDW may reflect some type of vitamin deficiency or the presence of two or more

discrete cell populations. Examples of two discrete cell populations may be seen in patients recovering from iron deficiency or pernicious anemia (e.g., patients with iron deficiency have small cells mixed with newly produced large reticulocytes and normal cells). The Bessman trial suggested that the RDW can be used to substitute for peripheral blood smear assessment of anisocytosis.[30] However, when there are classification discrepancies, such as an increased RDW without anemia or normal indices associated with anemia, the peripheral smear should be viewed to identify any morphologic abnormalities that may otherwise have gone undetected.[2-6,26,31,33-35] Although Bessman's schema has met criticism from some who dispute its sensitivity and specificity,[32,33] it remains a useful classification tool that narrows the diagnostic possibilities for anemia. Clinicians now have a noninvasive guide to avoid the "shotgun" approach for determining the cause of anemia by using the fewest laboratory studies at the lowest possible cost and at the least discomfort to the patient.[30,34]

Reticulocyte Count

The reticulocyte count may be used for additional information to classify anemic states kinetically as either hypoproliferative or hyperproliferative. The absolute reticulocyte count provides a noninvasive means for evaluating whether the bone marrow is producing adequate red cells for the degree of anemia. In hypoproliferative anemic states, the reticulocyte count is often less than 2%. In hemolytic anemia or red-cell destruction after release from the bone marrow, the reticulocyte count is high, greater than 2%.

The definitive test to evaluate the bone marrow's ability to produce red cells appropriately and to evaluate the cause of unexplained anemia is a bone marrow aspiration and biospy.[2-5,4,6]

Peripheral Blood Smear

Careful examination of the blood smear remains one of the most important studies in the work-up of a patient with anemia.[2-6,25,35] It serves as a quality control in verifying the classification results generated by automated analyzers and may offer useful diagnostic information. When classification and subclassification of anemia are unclear by MCV and RDW, certain red-cell abnormalities of diagnostic value (e.g., spherocytes, fragments, sickle cells, target cells, hypochromic microcytes, oval macrocytes, and hypersegmented neutrophils) can be detected only by examining the blood smear (Figures 33-2, 33-3, 33-4, 33-5, 33-6, 33-7).

Special Groups with Anemia

Chronic Anemia

A concomitant anemia in individuals with chronically low hemoglobin concentrations (e.g., sickle-cell disease) is recognized by decreases in hemoglobin concentrations 10 to 15% (1 to 2 g) below base line in the absence of plasma volume increases. These individuals lack red-cell reserves and have maximized all adaptive mechanisms to maintain adequate oxygen delivery; therefore, symptoms occur sooner, and life-threatening anemias can develop very quickly.[16,36-44]

Anemia of Pregnancy

Appropriate evaluation of anemia of pregnancy is challenging, and requires a comprehensive focus on both the mother and fetus. Anemia is the most common hematologic complication of pregnancy and is associated with perinatal complications.[22-44] Although evaluation of anemia is no different from that in nonpregnant women, practitioners must distinguish the nonthreatening physiologic anemia of pregnancy (hemodilution or selective increased plasma volume over red-cell mass) from pathologic forms (absolute decrease in red-cell mass).[4,23,24,44] The most common pathologic anemia associated with pregnancy is iron-defiency anemia.[4,23,24,44] Folate deficiency is the most common cause of pathologic macrocytic anemia (MCV, >100) and is associated with neural-tube defects in the fetus.[2-4,23,24,44] Other anemias common to this group include sickle-cell trait and disease, the thalassemias, and G6PD deficiency.[16,23,24,39-44] Diagnostic criteria of pathologic anemia of pregnant women at the peak of hemodilution (~24 weeks of gestation) is a hemoglobin value than less than 10.5 g/dl or a 2 to 4 g/dl drop in hemoglobin concentration from base line, or a >25 to 30% drop in hematocrit in chronically anemic patients.[23,24,43,44] Therefore, a thorough history and physical examination during prenatal counseling and an appropriate

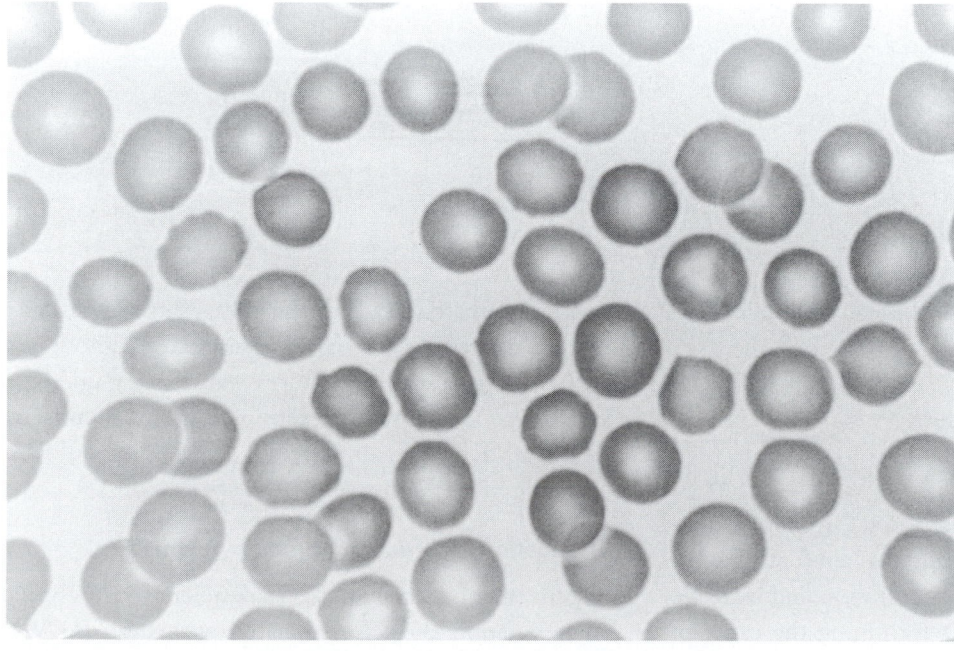

Figure 33-2 Normal peripheral blood smear. Normal erythrocytes. (Wright stain, ×1000).

Figure 33-3 Iron-deficiency anemia, peripheral blood. Marked hypochromia, microcytes, occasional oval cell. (Wright stain, ×1000).

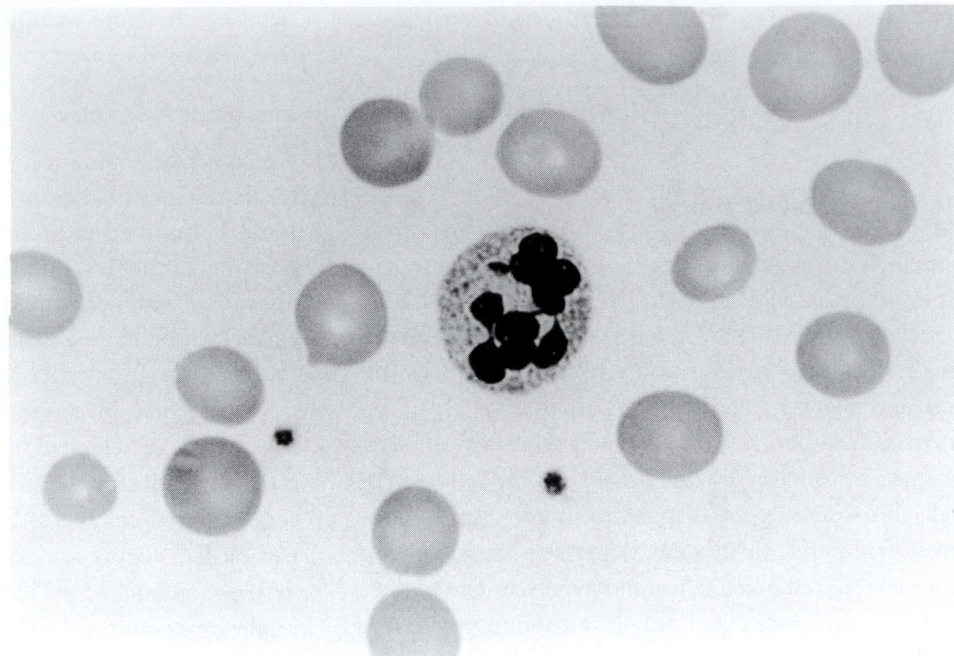

Figure 33-4 Vitamin B$_{12}$ deficiency, peripheral blood. Hypersegmented neutrophil (nine lobes) macrocytes, and oval macrocytes. (Wright stain, ×1000).

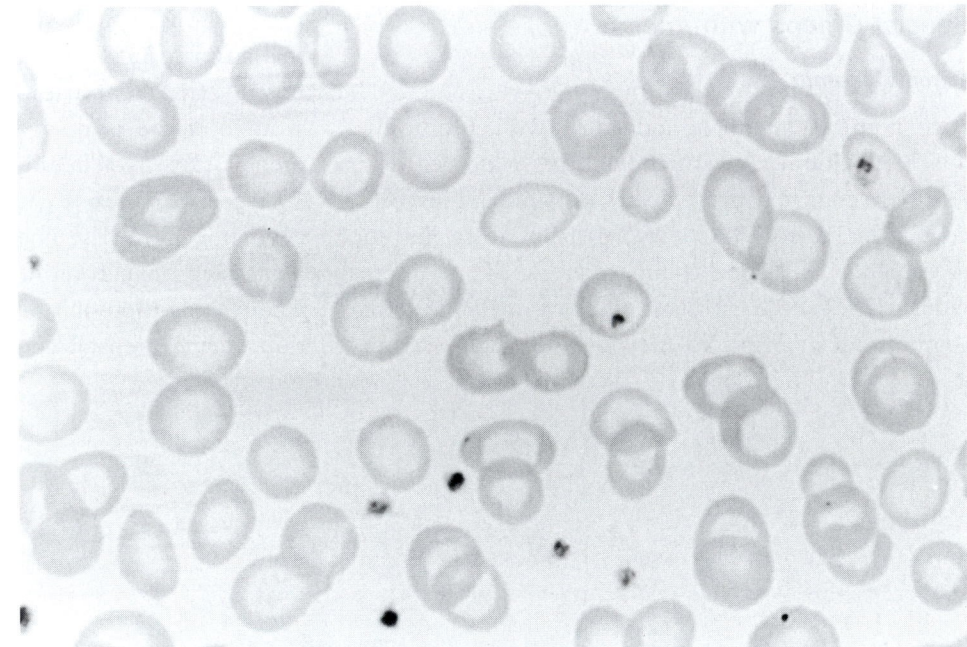

work-up for anemia can be clinically beneficial to both mother and baby.

Diagnosis of Anemia

General

The number of possible diagnoses for anemia goes beyond the scope of this chapter. Therefore, the approach to diagnosing the most common and treatable anemias will be addressed. Determining the cause of anemia ultimately leads to the therapy that will benefit the patient. An accurate differential diagnosis results from a careful laboratory evaluation guided by the history and physical examination for anemia; as such, the definitive underlying diagnosis should be determined in most cases.

Diagnostic Evaluation of Common Anemias

In general, most anemias due to deficiency states (iron, folate, vitamin B$_{12}$) are associated with high RDWs.

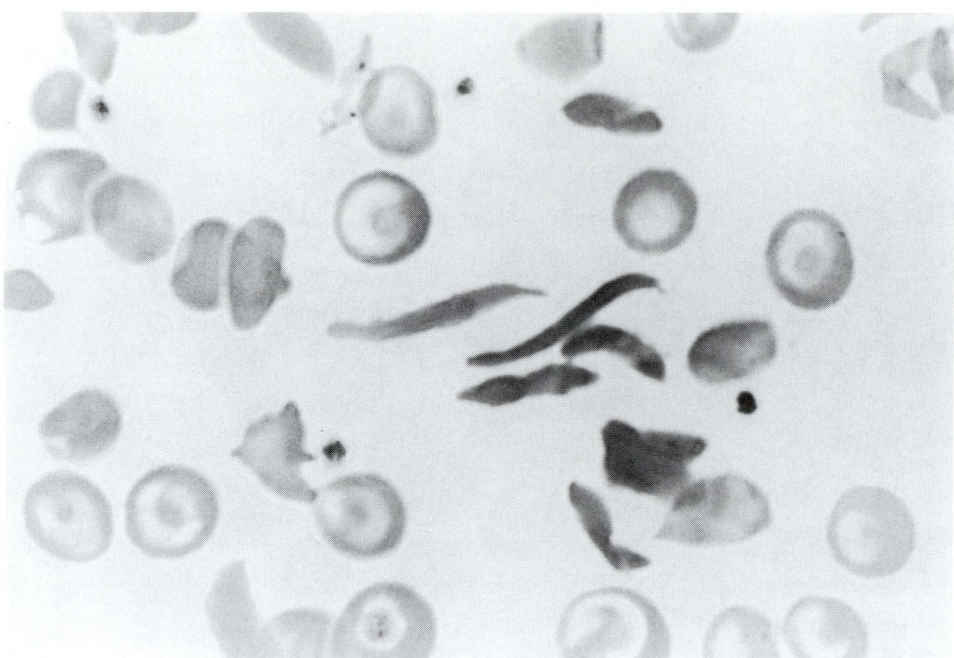

Figure 33-5 Sickle-cell anemia (hemoglobin SS), peripheral blood. Sickled red cells and target cells. (Wright stain, ×1000).

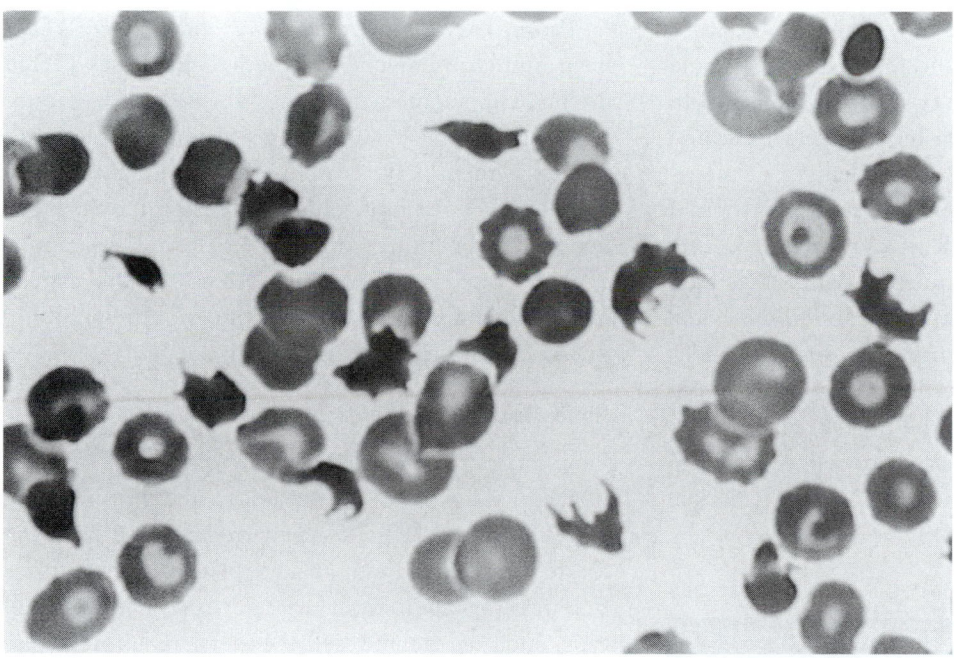

Figure 33-6 Thrombotic thrombocytopenic purpura, peripheral blood. Note membrane-injured erythrocytes, cell fragments, and thrombocytopenia. (Wright stain, ×1000).

For low-MCV, high-RDW anemias, it is appropriate to assume this is iron-deficiency anemia and iron studies should be done (Tables 33-7 and 33-8). A review of the peripheral-blood smear will be needed if routine studies are diagnostically uncertain. Sickle β-thalassemia is usually clinically obvious due to the lifelong sequelae associated with the disease. Nevertheless, individuals with low MCV anemias and high RDWs can also have concomitant iron deficiency, and this possibility should be evaluated. More than

likely, individuals with hemoglobinopathies have chronic iron overload (ferritin >250) due to receiving multiple blood transfusions and/or because empiric oral iron is administered merely because their MCV is low. Continued iron replacement therapy can potentially be harmful by causing cirrhosis of the liver, cardiomyopathy, or endocrinopathies directly associated with chronic iron overload.[2,3,4,6,45,46,50-52]

Anemia associated with high MCV and high RDW is commonly megaloblastic anemia secondary

Figure 33-7 Hereditary spherocytosis, peripheral blood. Note spherocytes in the center (small dense-staining erythrocytes). (Wright stain, ×1000).

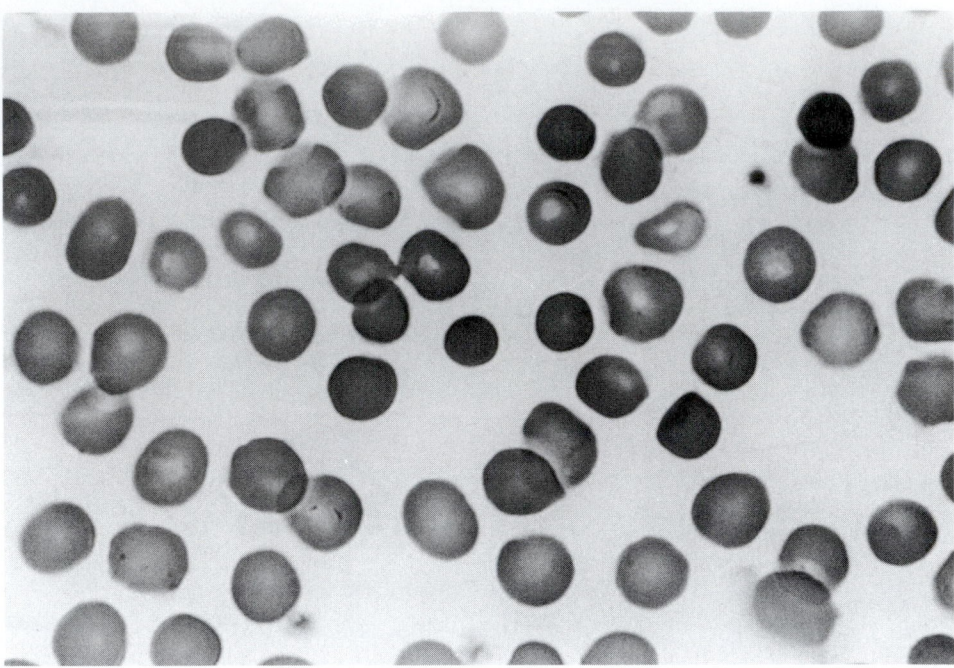

to vitamin B_{12} or folate deficiency (Table 33-9). Serologic studies of vitamin B_{12} and red-cell folate should make the diagnosis.[47] However, if these studies fail to diagnose anemia, a peripheral-blood-smear examination should look for morphologic changes of megaloblastic anemia such as hypersegmented neutrophils, giant platelets, and macrocytic erthyrocytes.

Anemia associated with normal MCV and high RDW is most commonly a mixed microcytic and macrocytic anemia (e.g., vitamin B_{12} or folate deficiency with iron deficiency). The MCV averages out in the blood-cell analyzer to the normal range; however, there are discrete populations of cells that are apparent by the consistent increased RDW (marked anisocytosis) (Table 33-10).

Patterns with a normal MCV and normal RDW have numerous diverse differential diagnoses (Table 33-11). The anemia of chronic disease is a diagnostic challenge.[2-4,6,10-12] Once the chronic underlying process is identified, a careful tracking of the hemoglobin and hematocrit values will determine the baseline values for future comparisons during evaluations of new concurrent anemias. Otherwise, the patient may be anemic for a lifetime if the associated chronic disease is not curable.

Bone Marrow Examination

Examination of the bone marrow is the gold standard in diagnosing many hematologic and nonhematologic disorders.[48] The bone marrow evaluation is indicated in patients with an unexplained excess or deficiency (cytopenia) of any peripheral-blood-cell type, such as the red cell. Modern technology has

---

TABLE 33-7
APPROACH TO ANEMIA WITH LOW MCV

RDW Normal	RDW High
Differential Diagnosis	
Heterozygous thalassemia	Iron deficiency
Chronic disease	Red-cell fragments
	Sideroblastic anemia
Laboratory Evaluation	
Iron studies (see Table 33-8)	
Serum ferritin for iron stores	
Hemoglobin electrophoresis and hemoglobin A_2 for thalassemia	
Review peripheral smear for fragments, targets	
If no diagnosis: +/− bone marrow aspirate for iron stores and ring sideroblast	

TABLE 33-8
EXPECTED PATTERNS FOR IRON STUDIES

	Normal	Iron Deficiency	Iron Overload	Chronic Inflammation
Serum iron	120 + 30	<40	120–280	20–50
Total iron binding concentration	330 + 30	300–480	<300	<260
% Saturation	35 + 10	16	40–100	10–25
Ferritin	100 + 60	<10*	>250	>150

*In age >65 the ferritin cut-off should be 45.

TABLE 33-9
APPROACH TO ANEMIA WITH HIGH MCV AND HIGH RDW

Differential diagnosis
  Folate deficiency
  Vitamin B_{12} deficiency
  Hemolysis
    Immunohemolysis
    DIC, TTP, HELP
    G6PD* deficiency
    Hemoglobinopathies
    Infection-related
    Drug-related
    Cold agglutinins
Laboratory evaluation
  Serum assays for vitamin B_{12}, folate
  Examination of the peripheral blood smear for evidence of microangiopathic changes of TTP** and DIC***, fragments, bite cells
  Urinary hemosiderin
  Direct and indirect Coombs test
  Reticulocyte count
  Serum lactic dehydrogenase and total bilirubin (elevated with hemolysis)
  Haptoglobin (low with intravascular hemolysis)
  Cold agglutinin titer
  Appropriate further tests as indicated by preliminary evaluation: Hemoglobin electrophoresis, G6PD screen (3 weeks later), bacterial cultures and examination of smear for malaria, babesiosis, bartonellosis.

*G6PD = glucose-6-phosphate dehydrogenase
**DIC = disseminated intravascular coagulation
***TTP = thrombotic thrombocytopenic purpura

precluded the frequent use of this study for the evaluation of anemia. It is very rare to diagnose folate, vitamin-B_{12}, and iron-deficiency anemias by bone marrow aspiration, due to the availability of red-cell indexes for classification, the quantitative

TABLE 33-10
APPROACH TO ANEMIA WITH NORMAL MCV AND HIGH RDW

Differential diagnosis
  Mixed deficiency (Vitamin B_{12} or folate with iron deficiency)
  Early iron deficiency
  Early folate deficiency
  Sickle cell disease (SS, SC, S-Thalassemia)
  Sideroblastic anemia
Laboratory evaluation
  Serum B_{12}, folate assays
  Iron studies (see Table 33-8)
  Hemoglobin electrophoresis
  Peripheral smear review for sickle cells, targets, hypersegmented neutrophils, macrocytes, microcytes, two discrete populations of cells
  Bone marrow for ringed sideroblast if all other studies negative

TABLE 33-11
APPROACH TO ANEMIA WLTH NORMAL MCV AND NORMAL RDW

Differential diagnosis
  Normal
  Chronic disease (uremia, HIV, liver failure, arthritis, lupus)
  Sickle cell trait (AS, AC)
  Hemorrhage
  Hypothyroidism
  Hereditary spherocytosis
Laboratory evaluation
  Search for chronic disease (renal failure, liver failure, arthritis), urea, creatinine, liver transaminases, sedimentation rate)
  If positive drug history do a drug screen
  Serial hematocrits for suspected bleeding
  TSH for hypothyroidism
  HIV testing
  Hemoglobin electrophoresis
  MCHC increased (suggest spherocytes)
  Peripheral smear review for spherocytes, sickle cells, C-crystals

serum assays for folate and vitamin B_{12}, ferritin as a measure of iron stores, and the widely accepted serum iron studies (Table 33-8). Although a bone marrow examination is less frequently used as a diagnostic tool for the cause of anemia, it is available for unexplained anemias associated with other abnormalities such as cytopenias, cellular excess, fever of unknown origin, and suspected malignancies.

THERAPY

Therapy for Common Anemias

Once it has been determined that a patient has a deficiency in iron, folate, or vitamin B_{12}, replacement therapy should be instituted without further delay.[2,3,4,6,49]

Iron Deficiency

The most common cause of iron-deficiency anemia is bleeding from the gastrointestinal tract (GI) or the uterus.[2-4,6,13,25,46,50-54] The most important factor in correcting iron-deficiency anemia is to localize and treat the underlying bleeding source, which will allow complete recovery of this anemic state.

Abnormal uterine bleeding is usually obvious and therefore is evaluated by taking a meticulous history for menorrhagia. Iron-replacement therapy may only partially correct this problem unless the bleeding is identified and controlled.

Dosing for iron deficiency in adults should provide between 150 and 200 mg of elemental iron daily (e.g., ferrous sulfate, 325 mg orally, three times daily). The iron may be taken orally in three divided doses per 24 hours 1 hour before meals for 4 to 6 months. That will allow iron stores to be replaced and hemoglobin concentration to return to normal.[2-4,6,25,49-53]

Side effects of oral iron therapy include GI upset, constipation, loose stools, and black-colored stools without melena. Iron overload may develop in individuals with ineffective erythropoiesis (e.g., sickle-cell disease or thalassemia).[2-4,6,16,21,45,52-54]

Most individuals with iron-deficiency anemia will fully recover after replacement therapy, especially if the underlying process is successfully treated. Correction of this anemia is gratifying, and symptons of anemia resolve within a few days.[2-4,6,37,54]

Folate-Deficiency Therapy

Folate is given orally, 1 to 5 mg daily, although 1 mg is usually enough in most cases. Pregnant women should be given 1 mg of folate per day to prevent neural-tube defects in the fetus.[2-4,6,23,24,44]

Vitamin B$_{12}$ Deficiency

A typical treatment schedule for vitamin B$_{12}$ deficiency due to malabsorption consists of 1000 μg intramuscular cobalamin (vitamin B$_{12}$) daily for 2 weeks, then weekly until the hemoglobin or hematocrit is normal, then monthly for life. Monthly maintenance injections may also be administered subcutaneously for patient comfort.[2-4,6,27-29,49] For dietary cobalamin deficiency and normal GI absorption, patients may decide to include vitamin B$_{12}$ in their diet, or oral cobalamin therapy should be adequate as an alternative to intramuscular injections.[2-4,6,49]

General Treatment for Severe Anemia

A standard low value of hemoglobin or hematocrit in itself has not been established to warrant the urgent administration of blood to a patient with anemia and therefore should be individualized based on clinical severity.[2-4,6,13] Although most patients will become symptomatic, with hemoglobin levels below 8.0 g/dl

or hematocrits below 25%, individuals with chronic anemia (base-line hemoglobin, 7.5 g/dl) may be asymptomatic until hemoglobin falls below 5.0 to 6.0 g/dl and below 16% for hematocrits.[13,16] Accordingly, clinically severe symptomatic anemia associated with shortness of breath, tachycardia, signs of heart failure (heart gallop), and extreme weakness warrants urgent intervention, regardless of the hemoglobin value, with supplemental oxygen, bed rest, and a blood transfusion.[16,39] Transfused blood complicates the ability to classify and diagnose anemia by altering the results of laboratory studies and is not an accurate reflection of the patient's condition. Therefore, it is imperative to first classify the anemia, collect appropriate pretransfusion diagnostic studies (e.g., iron studies or red-cell folate), and hold a few extra tubes (one purple-top for plasma and one red-top for serum) that can be sent for diagnostic studies after stabilizing the patient.

Erythropoietin

Erythropoietin (EPO) is now commercially available to be used as an alternative for blood for symptomatic anemias (Jehovah's Witnesses, incompatible blood). This hormone is very costly and has not been approved for use in all anemic states; however, for extenuating circumstances as previously described, second-payer sources may offer preapproval for its use on an individual basis. Dosing range is 50 to 150 units/kg of body weight three times per week. Some anemic states require higher doses, up to 300 units/kg three times per week. The dose should be adjusted individually by 25-unit increments or decrements three times per week every 2 weeks based on targeting the hematocrit between 25 and 35% or when symptoms of anemia resolve (e.g., chronic anemias may become asymptomatic at lower hematocrits). Hematocrits higher than 35% may cause hypertension or hyperviscosity in some individuals. Epoetin Alfa (Procrit) at 40,000 to 60,000 units given subcutaneously has shown to be effective in reducing preoperative blood transfusions in subsets of orthopedic surgical patients by increasing the pretreatment hemoglobin concentration.[55,56] Transfusion-dependent patients who respond to EPO therapy become transfusion-independent within 8 weeks. Others can be refractory to maximum-dose EPO therapy and remain severely anemic.[7-9,17-20,49]

CONCLUSION

Recognition of anemia based on classification by expected patterns of anemia by MCV and RDW, coupled with additional information from a meticulous history and physical, and laboratory evaluation should adequately diagnose most anemias. Failure to diagnose anemia should prompt clinicans to review a peripheral-blood smear or possibly do bone marrow studies to further aid in determining the diagnosis.

ACKNOWLEDGEMENTS

I wish to thank Ann Bell, M.S., S.H. (A.S.C.P.) for providing visuals aids, technical assistance, and guidance; Drs. Alvin M. Mauer, David Armbruster, and Marion Dugdale for sharing their knowledge and expertise; and Ms. Bobbie Clinton and Ms. Loretta Pitts for their patience and understanding as this manuscript was produced.

REFERENCES

1. Self KG, Conrady MM, Eichner ER. Failure to diagnose anemia in medical inpatients: is the traditional diagnosis of anemia a dying art? Am J Med 1986;81:786.
2. Jandl JH. Blood: textbook of hematology. 2nd ed. Boston: Little, Brown, 1996.
3. Wintrobe MM, Lukens JN, Lee GR. Wintrobe's clinical hematology. 9th ed. The approach to the patient with anemia. Philadelphia; Lea & Febiger, 1993:715.
4. Goyette RE. Hematology: a comprehensive guide to the diagnosis and treatment of blood disorders. Los Angeles: Practice Management Information Corporation (PMIC), 1997.
5. Jandl JH. Blood: pathophysiology. Boston: Blackwell Scientific, 1991.
6. Hoffman R. Hematology: basic principles and practice. New York: Churchhill Livingstone, 1991.
7. Facquin WC, Schneider TJ, Goldberg MA. Effect of inflammatory cytokines on hypoxia-induced erthropoietin production. Blood. 1992;79:1987.
8. Cash JM, Sears DA. The anemia of chronic disease: spectrum of associated diseases in a series of unselected hospitalized patients. Am J Med 1989;87:638.
9. Means RT, Krantz SB. Progress in understanding the pathogenesis of the anemia of chronic disease. Blood 1992;80:1639.
10. Baer AN, Dessypris EN, Krantz SB. The pathogenesis of anemia in rheumatoid arthritis: a clinical and laboratory analysis. Semin Arthritis Rheum 1990;19:209.
11. Lacombe C. Resistance to erythropoietin. N Engl J Med 1996;334:660.
12. Henry DH, Thatcher N. Patient selection and predicting reponse to recombinant human erythropoietin in anemic cancer patients. Semin Hematol 1996;33:2.
13. Wyngaarden JB, Smith LH Jr, Bennett JC. Cecil textbook of medicine. 19th ed. Philadelphia: Saunders, 1992.
14. Murray RK, Gragranner DK, Mayes PA, Rodwell VW. Harper's review of biochemistry. 24th ed. Stamford, CT: Appleton & Lange, 1996.
15. Martin DW, Mayes PA, Rodwell VW. Harper's review of biochemistry. 18th ed. Los Altos, CA: Lange Medical, 1981.
16. Embury SH, Hebbel RP, Mohandas N, Steinberg MH. Sickle cell disease: basic principles and clinical practice. New York: Raven Press, 1994.
17. Scott LL, Ramin SM, Richey M, Hanson J, Gilstrap LC. Erythropoietin use in pregnancy: two cases and a review of the literature. Am J Perinatol 1995:12;22.
18. Huch R, Huch A. Erythropoietin in obstetrics. Hematol Oncol Clin North Am 1994;8:1021.
19. Mann MC, Votto J, Kambe J, McNamee MJ. Management of the severely anemic patient who refuses transfusion: lessons learned during the care of a Jehovah's Witness. Ann Intern Med 1992;117:1042.
20. Kitchens CS. Are transfusions overrated? Surgical outcome of Jehovah's Witness. Am J Med 1993;94:117.
21. Viteri FE. Iron supplementation for the control of iron deficiency in populations at risk. Nutr Rev 1997;55:195.
22. Allen LH. Pregnancy and iron deficiency: unresolved issues. Nutrition Rev 1997;55:91.
23. Lops VR, Hunter LP, Dixon LR. Anemia in pregnancy. Am Fam Physician 1995;51:1189.
24. Williams MD, Whelby MS. Anemia in pregnancy. Med Clin North Am 1992;76:631.
25. Bick RL. Hematology: clinical and laboratory practice: clinical evaluation of the patient with anemia. St. Louis: Mosby, 1993:203.
26. Tilton RC. Clinical and laboratory medicine laboratory: diagnosis of erythroid disorders. St. Louis: Mosby, 1992.
27. Chanarin I, Deacon R, Lumb M, Perry J. Colobamin and folate: recent developments. J Clin Pathol 1992; 45:277.
28. Dickinson CJ. Does folic acid harm people with vitamin B_{12} deficiency? QJ Med 1995;88:357.
29. Clementz GL, Schade SG. The spectrum of vitamin B_{12} deficiency. Am Fam Physician 1990;41:150.
30. Bessman JD. Improved classification of anemia by MCV and RDW. Am J Clin Pathol 80;3:322.
31. Gulati GL, Hyun BH. The automated CBC—a current perspective. Hematol Oncol Clin North Am 1994;8:593.
32. Thompson WG, Meola T, Lipkin M, Freedman ML. Red cell distribution width, mean corpuscular volume, and transferrin saturation in the diagnosis of iron deficiency. Arch Intern Med 1988;148:2128.
33. Seward SJ, Safran C, Marton KI, Robinson SH. Does the mean corpuscular volume help physicians evaluate hospitalized patients with anemia? J Gen Intern Med 1990;5:187.
34. Savage RA. The red blood cell indices: yesterday, today, and tomorrow. Clin Lab Med 1993;13:773.
35. Gulati GL, Hyun BH. Blood smear examination. Hematol Oncol Clin North Am 1994;8:631.
36. Epstein FH, Young NS, Maciejewski J. The pathophysiology of acquired aplastic anemia. N Engl J Med 1997; 336:1365.

37. Snyder TE, Lee LP, Lynch S. Pregnancy-associated hypo-plastic anemia: a review. Obstet Gynecol Surv 1991; 46:264.

38. Pajor A, Kelemen E, Szakas Z, Lehoczky D. Pregnancy in idiopathic aplastic anemia (report of 10 patients). Eur J Obst Gynecol 1992;45:19.

39. Koshy K, Burd L, Wallace D, Moawad A, Baron J. Prophy-lactic red-cell transfusions in pregnant patients with sickle cell disease. N Engl J Med 1988;319:1447.

40. Koshy M, Burd L. Obstetric and gynecologic issues, sickle cell disease: basic principles and clinical practice. New York: Raven Press, 1994:689.

41. Koshy M, Burd L. Management of pregnancy in sickle cell syndromes. Hematol Oncol Clin North Am 1991; 5:585.

42. Mongomery KS. Caring for the pregnant woman with sickle cell disease. MCN 1996;21:224.

43. Adams S. Sickle cell disease in pregnancy: caring for the pregnant woman with sickle cell crisis. Pro Care Mother Child 1996;6:34.

44. Mani S, Duffy TP. Anemia of pregnancy. Clin Perinatol 1995;22:293.

45. Galloway R, McGuire J. Determinants of compliance with iron supplementation: supplies, side effects, or psychology? Soc Sci Med 1994;39:381.

46. Halliday CEW, Halliday JW, Powell LW. The clinical mani-festations of chronic iron overload. Baillere Clin Haematol 1989;2:403.

47. Colon-Otero G, Menke D, Hook C. A practical approach to the differential diagnosis and evaluation of the adult patient with macrocytic anemia. Med Clin North Am 1992;76:581.

48. Hyun BH, Stevenson AJ, Hanau CA. Fundamentals of bone marrow examination. Hematol Oncol Clin North Am 1994;8:651.

49. William WJ, Beutler E, Erslev AJ, Lichtman MA. Hema-tology. 5th ed. New York: McGraw-Hill, 1990.

50. Cook JD. Clinical evaluation of iron deficiency. Semin Hematol 1982;19:6.

51. Lanzkowsky P. Problems in diagnosis of iron deficiency anemia. Peditr Ann 1995;14:9:622.

52. Watson F. Routine iron supplementation—is it necessary? Mod Midwife 1997;7:22.

53. Engstrom JL, Sittler CP. Nurse-midwifery management of iron-deficiency anemia during pregnancy. Nurse-Midwifery 1999;39:20S.

54. Kumpf VJ. Parental iron supplementation. NCP 1996; 111:139.

55. Goldberg MA, McCutchen JW. A safety and efficacy comparison study of two dosing regimens of epoetin alfa in patients undergoing major orthopedic surgery. Am J Orthoped 1996;25:544.

56. Faris PM, Ritter MA. The effects of recombinant human erythropoietin on perioperative transfusion requirements in patients having a major orthopaedic operation. J Bone Joint Surg 1996;78-A:62.

Chapter 34

Respiratory Problems

Frank W. Ling
Roger P. Smith

Five Key Points

- Antibiotic use should be limited to cases in which a bacterial cause is strongly suspected.

- Adherence to guidelines for vaccinations against influenza and pneumococcal pneumonia should be strongly encouraged by clinicians.

- Effective medication to reduce the duration and severity of influenza is available.

- Use of throat culture and rapid strep test can aid in appropriate treatment of streptococcal pharyngitis.

- Individualized asthma management should include patient education, elimination of irritants, pharmacologic agents, and pulmonary function monitoring.

Respiratory problems are among the most commonly encountered in ambulatory medicine. For example, the National Ambulatory Medical Care Survey lists acute respiratory problems among the 10 most common reasons for office visits in the United States.[1,2] This chapter addresses the conditions that are not only common but also are manageable in a primary care outpatient setting.

SINUSITIS

Sinus infections develop in approximately 35 million people in the United States each year. A feeling of fullness and pressure in and over the involved sinuses is a result of accumulation of purulent material. Commonly, nasal congestion and a purulent, possibly blood-tinged discharge also are present. Associated symptoms include sore throat, malaise, and a low-grade fever. The sore throat is most likely caused by drainage of excess mucus down the back of the throat. Headaches, especially on waking in the morning, are common. The discomfort in these sinuses may be exacerbated by positional changes, or preceded by other events such as air travel, an upper respiratory infection, or seasonal allergies. Sinus infection may also occur as a secondary infection from a tooth abscess or from swimming in contaminated water. Sinus irritants include tobacco smoke, cold or damp weather, pollution, and structural abnormalities such as a deviated nasal septum. Table 34-1 lists clinical aspects of sinusitis as compared with the common cold and allergies.

The bacteria that usually cause sinusitis are normal inhabitants of the respiratory tract. When the body's defenses are compromised, or if normal sinus drainage is blocked, these bacteria can multiply to cause symptomatic infection. *Hemophilus influenzae* and Pneumococcus and Streptococcus species are the

TABLE 34-1
COMMON RESPIRATORY CONDITIONS

Symptom	Sinusitis	Common Cold	Allergy
Facial pain	Yes	Occasional	Occasional
Fever	Occasional	Occasional	No
Discharge	Thick, yellow/green	Thick, white	Clear, watery
Headache	Yes	Occasional	Occasional
Tooth pain	Occasional	No	No
Bad breath	Occasional	No	No
Cough	Yes	Yes	Occasional
Congestion	Yes	Yes	Occasional
Sneezing	No	Yes	Occasional
Duration	10–14 days	Less than 10 days	Variable

most common causative agents. Although less common, viral and fungal infections are also possible.

Sinusitis is most commonly diagnosed based on clinical signs and symptoms. In addition to the symptoms described above, tenderness over the involved sinuses or thickened/edematous mucosa may be found on examination. If sinus x-ray films are ordered, cloudiness and air–fluid levels can be seen. More sophisticated imaging such as computed tomography or magnetic resonance is not usually necessary in a primary care practice. Occasionally, a mildly elevated white-cell count is found. Cultures may be of greater help in the cases of patients who suffer from chronic sinusitis.

Generally, amoxicillin 500 mg three times a day or trimethoprim–sulfamethoxazole twice a day for 14 to 21 days is the prescribed treatment, with some data suggesting that treatment courses as brief as 3 days may be adequate.[3] Steam inhalation will aid in promoting drainage and provide a degree of comfort. If needed, alternative antibiotic therapy would include those with activity against β-lactamase-producing bacteria. In addition, antihistamines, analgesics and/or vasoconstrictors may help relieve congestion and the sense of fullness.[4] Use of nonprescription decongestant sprays for more than 5 days should be discouraged because of the potential of an induced rebound effect, causing the nasal passages to swell shut. Both alcohol and coffee should be avoided because they can cause swelling of the sinus membranes as well as dehydration.

COMMON COLD

The term *common cold* indicates by its name the frequency with which this condition is encountered in

modern medicine. It is estimated that two of every five Americans are afflicted each year, with some people having multiple episodes in 1 year. After an incubation period of 2 to 4 days, sneezing, runny nose, and malaise may last from 6 to 10 days, lasting sometimes upward of 3 weeks. Initially, the patient has a slight discomfort in the throat and nose, with scratchy eyes and a nonspecific sense of not feeling well. Sneezing and a clear, watery nasal discharge and nasal obstruction follow soon thereafter. After 2 to 3 days, the systemic symptoms begin to resolve, as the nasal discharge becomes thicker, cloudy, and yellowish in color. Local symptoms such as hoarseness, cough, or sore throat may last up to 7 to 10 days.

Contrary to common wisdom, a cold is not caused by a change in the weather, loss of sleep, going outside with wet hair, or fatigue. Although colds are, indeed, more prevalent in the winter, the risk for contracting a cold is due to exposure to the causative viruses through personal contact. As a result, situations that bring large numbers of people together increase the risk of contracting a cold. Examples would include the workplace, day-care centers, and schools. Droplets of infection are spread by sneezing, coughing, or by hand contact with the nose, eyes, or face.

The most common viral agents are the rhinoviruses, with over 100 serotypes having been associated with the common cold. Others include the coronaviruses, influenza types A, B, and C, parainfluenza virus, adenoviruses, and respiratory syncytial virus. No specific virus can be identified in up to 50% of cases. The common cold is highly contagious, as 75% of patients infected by the rhinovirus will have cold symptoms.

Table 34-1 summarizes some of the differences between the common cold and other common respiratory conditions. The diagnosis is made on clinical grounds, with laboratory and/or imaging studies indicated only if other conditions are strongly suspected. Viral isolation or culture is not practical. Other conditions that might be considered in the differential diagnosis include influenza, rubella, rubeola, group A β-hemolytic streptococcal infection, and mycoplasma pneumonia.

Treatment for the common cold includes supportive therapies: fluids, rest, humidification, and decongestants such as pseudoephedrine (Sudafed), phenylpropanolamine, and phenylephrine (Neo-Synephrine). Analgesics such as ibuprofen and naproxen treat general discomfort while also suppressing the cough reflex. In additional, cough suppressants (dextromethorphan and codeine), mucolytics such as guaifenesin, and antihistamines are helpful. Antihistamines such as chlorpheniramine (Chlor-Trimeton) and clemastine (Tavist) reduce nasal mucus secretions and suppress the sneeze reflex. Newer anithistamines, which have less of a tendency to cause sedation, include cetirzine (Zyrtec), fexofenadine (Allegra), and loratidine (Claritin). Short-term use of zinc lozenges (zinc gluconate 10 to 15 mg every 2 hours) can reduce the duration of subjective symptoms if begun early in the course of the disease.[5] Also, ipratropium bromide (Atrovent) appears to alleviate rhinorrhea and sneezing when sprayed into both nostrils three times per day.[6]

Although antibiotics are not appropriate in all cases initially, they should be considered if symptoms persist for 10 days or longer. At this point, the possibility that a secondary infection has occurred significantly increases, to 80% or more. Unfortunately, inappropriate prescribing of antibiotics for colds is common. In one survey, over 50% of patients diagnosed as having a cold were treated with antibiotics.[1] Purulent secretions in the history or on physical examination appear to influence the prescribing of antibiotics. Even though purulent secretions do not necessarily indicate a bacterial infection, nor do they suggest a antibiotic-susceptible organism as the causative agent, patients with this type of secretion were more likely to receive antibiotics.[7] Of note, factors in this study that increased the likelihood of antibiotic use were female patient and rural practice location. Empiric use of antibiotics such as erythromycin, amoxicillin, or sulfisoxazole–trimethoprim should be considered only if symptoms persist over 7 to 10 days.

Patient beliefs regarding the role of antibiotics in treatment of the common cold are a major factor in the inappropriate use of antibiotics. In a study of mostly white, suburban, educated patients, 50% believed that bacteria played a causal role. Over 85% believed that the upper respiratory infection would resolve on its own, but over 40% felt that antibiotics would be helpful. Interestingly, over 50% felt that too many patients took antibiotics for colds. Apparently patients, at least in this study, acknowledge the public health implications of the overuse of antibiotics, yet preferred to use them nevertheless.[8]

With the growing interest in disease prevention and complementary/alternative medicines, evaluation of other interventions will be forthcoming. One example of such an attempt is the report of the comparison of echinacea with placebo to prevent upper respiratory infections. It did not support the use of echinacea for this purpose, although it should be noted that other forms of echinacea are available and were not evaluated in this placebo-controlled trial.[9]

INFLUENZA

It is estimated that influenza is responsible for over 4 million excess respiratory illnesses each year as well as over 17 million excess bed and restricted activity days in the U.S. population over 20 years old. Up to 40,000 deaths and 200,000 hospitalizations annually are attributable to influenza.[10] The predominant viral strain may vary from year to year. As a result, the influenza vaccine, which is reformulated each year, includes antigens most recently detected from global viral surveillance. The inactivated influenza vaccine (killed-virus) containing antigens identical to circulating influenza A and B is 70 to 80% effective in preventing illness or reducing the severity of symptoms. The vaccine has also been shown to effectively prevent infection in health-care professionals, reducing work absences and febrile respiratory illnesses.[11] The benefits of immunizing health-care professionals is logically a lower risk of potential transmission of influenza to high-risk patients. Family contacts of high-risk patients should also be immunized yearly for this same reason.

Often it is necessary to differentiate influenza from a common cold. Table 34-2 summarizes some of the similarities and differences between the two conditions.

TABLE 34-2
COMMON COLD VERSUS INFLUENZA

Symptom	Cold	Flu
Fever	Occasional	Typical (up to 102–104°F) Lasts 3–4 days
Fatigue/ weakness	Mild	Up to 2–3 weeks
Extreme exhaustion	Rare	Common
Generalized aches	Slight	Common and severe
Headache	Occasional	Usual
Nasal congestion	Common	Occasional
Sneezing	Usual	Occasional
Cough	Mild/moderate	Common, possibly severe
Sore throat	Common	Occasional
Complications	Sinus congestion/ earache	Bronchitis/pneumonia Potentially life-threatening

Youth Risk Behavior Surveillance conducted by the Centers for Disease Control revealed that 73% of all deaths among those aged 10 to 24 were from motor vehicle crashes, other unintentional injuries, homicide, and suicide.[72] Sexually abused adolescents are more likely to have emotional problems, aggressive or criminal behaviors, addiction risk behaviors, and suicidal behaviors.

Characteristics that increase the risk of date rape include younger age at first date, early sexual activity, early age at menarche, and a past history of sexual abuse or prior sexual victimization. Adolescents may also believe myths regarding forced sex and its acceptability under certain dating circumstances. Risk factors include date-specific behaviors such as who paid for the date, who drove, and the type of dating activity. A high percentage of date rapes are associated with alcohol use. Adolescents may underestimate the effect of alcohol in diminishing their coping responses, their ability to ward off an attacker, and its ability to cause misinterpretation of usual dating cues as sexual invitations. The illicit drug flunitrazepam (Rohypnol) is also a risk factor for adolescents and young adults.[73] Adolescents with a history of physical abuse, sexual abuse, or rape are more likely to participate in HIV-risk behaviors such as having partners who use intravenous drugs.[74,75]

The pregnant adolescent is at higher risk for assault both during her pregnancy and postpartum. The abuse may not be from the father of the pregnancy but from a family member. An association has been demonstrated between sexual abuse and early coercive sexual experiences and teenage pregnancy.[76,77] A study of 100 pregnant women between the ages of 12 and 24 revealed that 32% of the subjects had a history of sexual abuse, 29% physical abuse, and 46% emotional abuse. A history of past abuse was significantly higher in girls who had been pregnant as compared with "never pregnant" girls. The past history of physical abuse accounted for the association in this study.[78] Pregnant teens were found to have a higher percentage not only of abuse during pregnancy as compared with adult women, but also a higher percentage of teens reported abuse during the year prior to pregnancy.[79]

The adolescent female may have many mental health and physical consequences of sexual or other types of abuse. The Guidelines for Adolescent Preventive Services recommends annual health visits for adolescents that include routine screening for any history of sexual abuse as well as other types of abuse and assault.[80]

CONCLUSIONS

The issues in this chapter focus on the aspects of secondary prevention of abuse. We have dealt with identification of abuse that has already occurred, prevention of consequences, and reduction of future abuse.

Primary prevention must be dealt with by society in its family units, schools, and public policy arenas. Physicians can have an important impact in this area. A study performed in New Zealand (similar socioeconomic culture to the United States) followed a large birth cohort for 21 years. Data were collected in the areas of socioeconomic resources, family relations, educational achievement, and problem behaviors. Partner abuse was measured at age 21. By the age of 3 some antecedents of later abuse could be identified. At each sequential 3-year evaluation, the correlations grew stronger. By the age of 15, there were strong correlations in all four areas, with the most consistent predictor being early problem behaviors.[81] This study suggests that we must begin prior to adolescence in order to prevent intimate partner violence. The challenge is not only to teach healthy relationships and conflict management in relationships, but also to model these behaviors. Excellent role-modeling programs have been developed for use in the schools. The teaching must begin at home. Only then will we have a major impact on the prevention of violence.

REFERENCES

1. Collins KS, Schoen C, Joseph S, Duchon L, Simantov E, Yellowitz M. Health concerns across a woman's lifespan: the Commonwealth Fund 1998 survey of women's health. May 1999. (Available at: http://www.cmwf.org/programs/women/ksc_whsurvey99_332.asp. Accessed October 7, 1999.)
2. Tjaden P, Thoennes N. Prevalence, incidence, and consequences of violence against women: findings from the National Violence Against Women Survey. Washington, DC: Department of Justice, National Institute of Justice, Centers for Disease Control and Prevention, November 1998. Publication no. NCJ 172837.
3. Pagelow MD. Marital rape. In: Van Hasselt VB, Morrison RL, Bellack AS, Hersen M, eds. Handbook of family violence. New York: Plenum Press, 1988:207.
4. Beebe DK. Emergency management of the adult female rape victim. Am Fam Pract 1991;43:2041.
5. Slaughter L, Brown CRV. Colposcopy to establish physical

and codeine), mucolytics such as guaifenesin, and antihistamines are helpful. Antihistamines such as chlorpheniramine (Chlor-Trimeton) and clemastine (Tavist) reduce nasal mucus secretions and suppress the sneeze reflex. Newer anithistamines, which have less of a tendency to cause sedation, include cetirzine (Zyrtec), fexofenadine (Allegra), and loratidine (Claritin). Short-term use of zinc lozenges (zinc gluconate 10 to 15 mg every 2 hours) can reduce the duration of subjective symptoms if begun early in the course of the disease.[5] Also, ipratropium bromide (Atrovent) appears to alleviate rhinorrhea and sneezing when sprayed into both nostrils three times per day.[6]

Although antibiotics are not appropriate in all cases initially, they should be considered if symptoms persist for 10 days or longer. At this point, the possibility that a secondary infection has occurred significantly increases, to 80% or more. Unfortunately, inappropriate prescribing of antibiotics for colds is common. In one survey, over 50% of patients diagnosed as having a cold were treated with antibiotics.[1] Purulent secretions in the history or on physical examination appear to influence the prescribing of antibiotics. Even though purulent secretions do not necessarily indicate a bacterial infection, nor do they suggest a antibiotic-susceptible organism as the causative agent, patients with this type of secretion were more likely to receive antibiotics.[7] Of note, factors in this study that increased the likelihood of antibiotic use were female patient and rural practice location. Empiric use of antibiotics such as erythromycin, amoxicillin, or sulfisoxazole–trimethoprim should be considered only if symptoms persist over 7 to 10 days.

Patient beliefs regarding the role of antibiotics in treatment of the common cold are a major factor in the inappropriate use of antibiotics. In a study of mostly white, suburban, educated patients, 50% believed that bacteria played a causal role. Over 85% believed that the upper respiratory infection would resolve on its own, but over 40% felt that antibiotics would be helpful. Interestingly, over 50% felt that too many patients took antibiotics for colds. Apparently patients, at least in this study, acknowledge the public health implications of the overuse of antibiotics, yet preferred to use them nevertheless.[8]

With the growing interest in disease prevention and complementary/alternative medicines, evaluation of other interventions will be forthcoming. One example of such an attempt is the report of the comparison of echinacea with placebo to prevent upper respiratory infections. It did not support the use of echinacea for this purpose, although it should be noted that other forms of echinacea are available and were not evaluated in this placebo-controlled trial.[9]

INFLUENZA

It is estimated that influenza is responsible for over 4 million excess respiratory illnesses each year as well as over 17 million excess bed and restricted activity days in the U.S. population over 20 years old. Up to 40,000 deaths and 200,000 hospitalizations annually are attributable to influenza.[10] The predominant viral strain may vary from year to year. As a result, the influenza vaccine, which is reformulated each year, includes antigens most recently detected from global viral surveillance. The inactivated influenza vaccine (killed-virus) containing antigens identical to circulating influenza A and B is 70 to 80% effective in preventing illness or reducing the severity of symptoms. The vaccine has also been shown to effectively prevent infection in health-care professionals, reducing work absences and febrile respiratory illnesses.[11] The benefits of immunizing health-care professionals is logically a lower risk of potential transmission of influenza to high-risk patients. Family contacts of high-risk patients should also be immunized yearly for this same reason.

Often it is necessary to differentiate influenza from a common cold. Table 34-2 summarizes some of the similarities and differences between the two conditions.

TABLE 34-2
COMMON COLD VERSUS INFLUENZA

Symptom	Cold	Flu
Fever	Occasional	Typical (up to 102–104°F) Lasts 3–4 days
Fatigue/ weakness	Mild	Up to 2–3 weeks
Extreme exhaustion	Rare	Common
Generalized aches	Slight	Common and severe
Headache	Occasional	Usual
Nasal congestion	Common	Occasional
Sneezing	Usual	Occasional
Cough	Mild/moderate	Common, possibly severe
Sore throat	Common	Occasional
Complications	Sinus congestion/ earache	Bronchitis/pneumonia Potentially life-threatening

The duration of symptoms in cases of Group A streptococcus does not help in making a diagnosis, as most patients become asymptomatic in 3 to 4 days even without therapy.

Other than cost, throat cultures are limited in their applicability by other factors. For example, the culture may be negative if the patient is partially treated with antibiotics. The culture could be taken improperly or the results misinterpreted. Results should not be expected for 24 to 48 hours.[18] There is an inherent false negative rate of 10%. Proper technique requires that the culture be taken directly from the tonsillar surface and/or the pharyngeal wall without touching the oropharynx or mouth. As an alternative to culture, the rapid strep test has become very popular. Although unable to identify small amounts of bacteria that could be potentially detected with traditional culture, the latex-agglutination test and enzyme immunoassay have a sensitivity of 80% and a specificity of 95%. When the test is positive, initiation of antibiotic therapy can prevent acute rheumatic fever as well as reduce the acute morbidity of the disease. A negative test, confirmed by a negative throat culture, can reassure both patient and clinician that the symptoms do not require antibiotics. The confirmatory culture is recommended for patients in whom the disease is strongly suspected on clinical grounds or who are considered at high risk because half of the patients with false negative rapid strep tests have a true infection.

Symptomatic treatment for pharyngitis of any cause includes salt-water gargles, acetaminophen, cool-mist humidification, and throat lozenges. Penicillin is the antibiotic of choice in the treatment of group A β-hemolytic streptococcal pharyngitis. The recommended dose is oral penicillin V 250 mg three times a day for 10 days. In cases in which patient compliance is a concern, 1.2 million units of benzathine G penicillin should be given intramuscularly. Alternative medications include erythromycin ethylsuccinate 300 to 400 mg three times a day, or cephalexin 250 mg three times a day for 10 days. Azithromycin is also an effective therapy.

A study designed to look at shorter duration of treatment of streptococcal pharyngitis found that a course of 3 days was no better than placebo in achieving relief of sore throat symptoms; however, 7 days of treatment might be as effective as 10 days.[19] Clinicians should be cognizant of the implications of the inappropriate use of antibiotics in the treatment of patients who present with simply a sore throat. Not only does this practice increase the incidence of antibiotic resistance, but it makes a medical condition of what otherwise would be a self-limiting condition. One study found that patients who received antibiotics for a sore throat were 30% more likely to return in the next year with a similar chief symptom. The increase in return visits went up 69% if the patient also received antibiotics in the previous year.[20]

ASTHMA

The prevalence of asthma in the U.S. adult population is estimated at 3 to 7%. The disease tends to present in childhood, during which time the incidence of wheezing is reported to be 10 to 15%. Asthma is a chronic inflammatory condition of the airways that leads to reversible airway obstruction and hyperresponsiveness. It is triggered by allergens, infections, and irritants, which results in the release of inflammatory mediators such as cytokines, histamine, and leukotrienes.[21] In addition to the underlying inflammation, the allergic response can be thought of as biphasic, i.e., a phenomenon that has an early and a late phase.

The early phase or acute asthmatic response occurs within the first 10 to 20 minutes, peaking within 30 minutes, and resolving within 1 to 3 hours. This early phase may not be easily identified. If an allergen is inhaled in low doses or the patient is using a β-adrenergic agonist, this early phase may be masked. In half of the patients in whom an early phase response is demonstrated bronchospasm that persists or recurs within 4 hours develops. This late-phase response may last up to 24 hours.

The most significant stimulus for asthma is exposure to inhaled allergens. Exposure to smoke, environmental pollutants, and household dust mites is commonly identified. Similarly, seasonal asthma is linked to pollen and molds in a predictable pattern. Viral respiratory diseases and exercise have been implicated, as have various medications such as aspirin, other nonsteroidal medications, and β-adrenergic blocking agents. The food additive monosodium glutamate has been associated with asthmatic symptoms termed the "Chinese restaurant syndrome." Medical conditions associated with asthma include gastroesophageal reflux and sinusitis.

Patients present with a classic triad of wheezing (inspiratory and/or expiratory), dyspnea, and cough.

Contrary to common thought, wheezing is not pathognomonic for asthma. The dyspnea tends to be on inspiration. The cough of asthma may be the sole presenting symptom and can be dry or productive.

The physical examination reveals end-expiratory wheezing in mild cases, with more extensive findings as the bronchospasm becomes more severe. The chest becomes more silent as airway obstruction worsens. Tachycardia and obvious use of accessory muscles of respiration are seen as the attack progresses.

In addition to the symptoms and physical findings, laboratory findings will support the presumptive clinical diagnosis. Measurement of arterial blood gases is only useful during the acute episode. Hypoxemia and respiratory alkalosis are frequently seen. Peak expiratory flow rate measurement is easily performed and correlates well with spirometry. It should be noted that pulmonary-function tests obtained between acute exacerbations may be normal. Ultimately, the diagnosis is not based on specific laboratory measurements, but on a recurrent clinical pattern of symptoms.

The management of asthma depends on four major components: (1) patient education; (2) control of environmental triggers; (3) measurement of pulmonary function; and (4) pharmacologic intervention. Successful asthma management may require close coordination with pulmonary specialists, including regular visits to ensure close supervision of all aspects of care.

β-Agonists are available in inhaled and oral forms. Inhaled short-acting agents are effective in relieving the bronchospasm of the early phase reaction. Because they are used on an as-needed basis, increasing use of these agents suggests a deterioration in the patient's status. Every patient with asthma should be encouraged to have ready access to an immediate-acting bronchodilator in case of acute respiratory problems. These medications can also be used prophylactically prior to exercising or exposure to cold air. Examples of short-acting β-agonists include albuterol (Proventil, Ventolin), pirbuterol (Maxair), bitolterol (Tornalate), metaproterenol (Alupent), and terbutaline (Brethaire). Each of these has an onset of action within 5 minutes and a duration of effectiveness approaching 3 to 6 hours. Salmeterol (Serevent) is the first agent in this class with a duration of action approaching 12 hours. It may be used twice a day for maintenance, 30 to 60 minutes prior to exercise for exercise-induced asthma, or at bedtime for nocturnal

asthma symptoms. When used for maintenance therapy, salmeterol should be used in combination with an antiinflammatory agent (see below).

The methylxanthine theophylline has mild bronchodilating and mild antiinflammatory effects. Its use reduces the need for β-agonists and also has a steroid-sparing effect. Theophylline protects against the late asthmatic response, but not the early response. The usual dose is 300 to 600 mg per day.

In addition to the β-agonists and methylxanthines, bronchodilators are a third class of anticholinergic agents. They are less effective than the β-agonists, but do cause some bronchodilation by inhibition of vagal cholinergic tone. They are commonly administered in conjunction with an inhaled β-agonist. Ipratropium (Atrovent) is administered at a dose of two to three puffs four times a day.

In addition to the bronchodilating agents listed above, the antiinflammatory agents comprise a second basis of pharmacologic management of asthma. The nonsteroidal antiinflammatory agents cromolyn (Intal) and nedocromil (Tilade) are considered first-line treatments for mild to moderate persistent asthma.[23] Cromolyn blocks early and late asthmatic responses and is useful for prophylaxis for exercise-induced asthma, although it is less efficacious than the inhaled steroid agents. Nedocromil also blocks both early and late asthma responses. Its primary drawback is an unusual bitter taste. Both agents are administered at a dose of 2 puffs four times a day.

Corticosteroids are available in both oral and inhaled forms. The oral medication is used to gain control of inflammation in patients who require a "steroid burst." It is considered last-line treatment in patients who suffer with severe persistent asthma. The inhaled corticosteroids are the most effective antiinflammatory agents and are considered primary therapy in persistent disease.[24] Adverse reactions are similar for all agents in this class. They include oral candidiasis, dysphonia, cough, and sore throat. Systemic adverse effects such as suppression of the hypothalamic–pituitary–adrenal axis, cataract formation, open-angle glaucoma, and bone demineralization occur with higher doses of inhaled steroids are used over a long period of administration, but are rare with normal doses used to treat asthma.[25] A useful comparison of the potencies of the steroids is: beclomethasone (Beclovent, Vanceril) is twice as potent as flunisolide (Aerobid) and triamcinolone (Azmacort); it is also about half as potent as fluticasone (Flovent).

Two antileukotriene agents have demonstrated efficacy in improving airway function and reducing asthma symptoms. Both are indicated as prophylaxis and treatment for chronic asthma. Zafirlukast (Accolate) is administered at a usual dose of 20 mg orally twice a day, while zileuton (Zyflo) has a usual dose of 600 mg orally four times a day. It is recommended that patients receiving zileuton have multiple liver-function tests during the first year of treatment.[26,27]

In summary, successful drug treatment of asthma is dependent on symptom severity, the side-effect profile of drugs, compliance, and individualized response. Inhaled corticosteroids are the most effective antiinflammatory agents and are considered first-line therapy. Short-acting bronchodilators are used on an as-needed basis for acute bronchospasm. The role of the antileukotriene agents continues to evolve.

LOWER RESPIRATORY INFECTIONS

Bronchitis can be considered a diagnosis of exclusion, after ruling out upper respiratory infection and pneumonia. It is an inflammatory condition of the tracheobronchial tree. It is most commonly seen several days after a viral syndrome, with the most commonly encountered infectious agents being those associated with the common cold and also *Mycoplasma pneumoniae*. Identification of the cause is rarely important. Patients present with cough, hoarseness, fever, and sputum production. The productive cough may last up to 3 weeks in 50% of cases and 4 weeks in 25%. Duration of symptoms is extended in smokers because of chronic airway changes. Bronchitis is more common than pneumonia and the absence of constitutional symptoms would favor the diagnosis of bronchitis.

The physical examination is aimed at ruling out pneumonia. Whereas bronchitis results in diffuse upper airway sounds with coarse rhonchi and rales, pneumonia presents with fine rales, decreased breath sounds, and egophony (E to A changes). Chest radiography is a useful diagnostic tool in cases of uncertainty. Because the cause is commonly viral, treatment is supportive in nature.

Antibiotics have been used with increasing frequency, particularly in patients with chronic bronchitis. If antibiotics are used, a wide range of options exists, including ampicillin, amoxicillin, erythromycin, azithromycin, tetracycline, and trimethoprim–sulfamethoxasole. In an attempt to limit the use of antibiotics to more appropriate cases, one investigation educated patients both in the office and at home regarding self-care and the appropriate use of antibiotics while their clinicians were given specific information regarding saying "no" to requests for antibiotics and a description of the patient education materials. As a result of the intervention, the use of antibiotics for acute bronchitis decreased from 74 to 48%.[28] Continued efforts such as this would seem appropriate in order to contain costs and reduce antibiotic resistance.

Pneumonia is classified into cases that are community acquired and those that are nosocomial. The differentiation is useful because of differences in cause, prognosis, and choice of antibiotics. Further differentiation of community-acquired pneumonia into typical and atypical is less useful because clinical aspects of the two overlap significantly.[29,30] Traditionally, typical pneumonia was described as presenting with classic symptoms of fever, dyspnea, and production of purulent sputum with physical findings suggestive of consolidation (rales, rhonchi, or bronchial breath sounds with dullness to percussion over the involved portion of the lung). In addition, findings on chest x-ray examination demonstrated alveolar infiltrates with a specific lobar distribution. In contrast, atypical pneumonia is most commonly described as not having significant sputum production, being associated with a long-term illness, and having an x-ray pattern that has diffuse and interstitial findings.

Table 34-3 lists the pathogens commonly found in community-acquired pneumonia, regardless of the typical–atypical differentiation. In most cases in the United States, *Mycoplasma pneumoniae, Chlamydia pneumoniae,* or various viral agents are probably the

---

TABLE 34-3
PATHOGENS ASSOCIATED WITH COMMUNITY-ACQUIRED PNEUMONIA

More common
  Streptococcus pneumoniae
  Chlamydia pneumoniae
  Mycoplasma pneumoniae
  Haemophilus influenzae
  Legionella species
  Viruses
Less common
  Gram-negative bacilli
  Staphylococcus aureus
  Pneumocystis carinii
  Mycobacterium tuberculosis

TABLE 34-4
INDICATIONS FOR HOSPITALIZATION OF PATIENTS WITH COMMUNITY-ACQUIRED PNEUMONIA

Age over 65
Altered mental status
Immunocompromised status
Unstable vital signs
Hypoxemia
Significant comorbid condition
Significant metabolic or hematologic derangement
Failure to respond to outpatient therapy

---

causative agent.[31] When a specific cause is identified, the most common single pathogen is *Streptococcus pneumoniae.*

Initial antibiotic therapy should be aimed at the most likely pathogens. In young, otherwise healthy patients, tetracycline or erythromycin are inexpensive first choices. For patients in whom significant gastrointestinal side effects develop, azithromycin (Zithormax) and clarithromycin (Biaxin) serve as alternatives. For patients over 60 and for patients with comorbid illness, trimethoprim–sulfamethoxazole is a recommended first-line therapy. Alternatives include a second-generation cephalosporin—e.g., cefuroxime (Ceftin, Zinacef), and cefprozil (Cefzil); a β-lactam/β-lactamase inhibitor—e.g., amoxicillin–clavulanate (Augmentin) and ampicillin–sulbactam (Unasyn); or erythromycin. Hospitalized patients with a community-acquired pneumonia may best be treated with a second- or third-generation cephalosporin or a β-lactam/β-lactamase inhibitor.[32] Table 34-4 lists indications for hospitalization of patients with community-acquired pneumonia.[33,34]

In general, since the specific causative agent is often difficult to determine in cases of community-acquired pneumonia, empiric therapy is appropriate, with the expectation that therapy will last for 10 to 14 days. Because of its long half-life, a course of 3 to 5 days of azithromycin is possible.[35] In hospitalized patients, once the fever has subsided and the patient's clinical condition has stabilized, parenteral antibiotics may be converted to oral agents with a comparable spectrum of coverage.[36]

Currently available pneumoccocal vaccines (Pneumovax 23 and Pnu-immune 23) include 23 capsular antigens, which represent 85 to 90% of the serotypes that cause pneumoccocal pneumonia. Pneumococcal vaccine may be given at the same time as the influenza vaccine, but by separate injection in the other arm. Approximately half the recipients have a transient local reaction at the injection site that lasts less than 48 hours. Candidates to be immunized include persons over 65 years of age, patients with chronic debilitating illnesses, inhabitants of special high-risk settings, and immunocompromised patients. Because antibody levels decrease after 5 to 10 years, it is recommended that patients over 65 who were less than 65 when immunized more than 5 years previously should be given another vaccination.[37]

REFERENCES

1. Schappert SM. National Ambulatory Medical Care Survey, 1991 summary. National Center for Health Statistics. Vital Health Stat 1994;13:116.
2. Adams GL, et al. Fundamentals of otolaryngology. 6th ed. Philadelphia: Saunders, 1989.
3. Williams JW Jr, Holleman DR, Samsa GP. Randomized control trial of three versus ten days of trimethoprim/sulfamethoxazole for acute maxillary sinusitis. JAMA 1995;273:1015.
4. Mossad SB, et al. Zinc gluconate lozenges for treating the common cold: a randomized, double-blind, placebo-controlled study. Ann Intern Med 1996;125:81.
5. Hayden FG, et al. Effectiveness and safety of intranasal ipratropium bromide in common colds: a randomized, double-blind, placebo-controlled trial. Ann Intern Med 1996;125:89.
6. Gonzales R, Steiner JF, Sande MA. Antibiotic prescribing for adults with colds, upper respiratory tract infections, and bronchitis by ambulatory care physicians. JAMA 1997;278:901.
7. Gonzales R, et al. The relation between purulent manifestations and antibiotic treatment of upper respiratory tract infections. J Gen Intern Med 1999;14:151.
8. Braun BL, et al. Patient beliefs about the characteristics, causes, and care of the common cold. J Fam Pract 2000;49:153.
9. Melchart D, et al. Echinacea root extracts for the prevention of upper respiratory tract infections. Arch Fam Med 1998;7:541.
10. Neuzil KM, Reed GW, Mitchell EF Jr, Griffin MR. Influenza-associated morbidity and mortality in young and middle-aged women. JAMA 1999;281:901.
11. Wilde JA, McMillan JA, Serwint J, et al. Effectiveness of influenza vaccine in health care professionals. JAMA 1999;281:908.
12. Glezen WP. Influenza control—unfinished business. JAMA 1999;281;944.
13. Hayden FG, et al. Use of the oral neuraminidase inhibitor oseltamivir in experimental human influenza: randomized controlled trials for prevention and treatment. JAMA 1999;282:1240.
14. Monto AS, Robinson DP, Herlocher ML, Hinson JM Jr, et al. Zanamivir in the prevention of influenza among healthy adults. JAMA 1999;282:31.

15. Hayden FG, et al. Use of the selective oral neuraminidase inhibitor oseltamivir to prevent influenza. N Engl J Med 1999;341:1336.

16. Komaroff AL, Pass TM, Aronson MD, et al. The prediction of streptococcal pharyngitis in adults. J Gen Intern Med 1986;1:1.

17. Poses RM, Cebul RD, Collins M, Fager SS. The accuracy of experienced physicians' probability estimates for patients with sore throats: implications for decision making. JAMA 1985;254:925.

18. Gerber MA. Comparison of throat cultures and rapid strep tests for diagnosis of streptococcal pharyngitis. Pediatr Infect Dis J 1989;8:820.

19. Zwart S, et al. Penicillin for acute sore throat: randomised double blind trial of seven days versus three days treatment or placebo in adults. BMJ 2000;320:150.

20. Little P, Gould C, Williamson I, et al. Reattendance and complications in a randomised trial of prescribing strategies for sore throats; medicalising effect of prescribing antibiotics. BMJ 1997;315:350.

21. National Asthma Education and Prevention Program. Expert Panel Report II (EPR II). Bethesda, MD: National Institutes of Health. February 1997.

22. Szefler SJ, Bender BG, Jusko WJ, et al. Evolving role of theophylline for treatment of chronic childhood asthma. J Pediatr 1995;127:176.

23. National Asthma Education and Prevention Program. Expert Panel Report II (EPR II). Bethesda, MD: National Institutes of Health. February 1997.

24. National Asthma Education and Prevention Program. Expert Panel Report. Bethesda, MD: National Institutes of Health. Publication no. 94-3042A. July 1994.

25. Garbe E, LeLorier J, Boivin J-F, Suissa S. Inhaled and nasal glucocorticoids and the risks of ocular hypertension or open angle glaucoma. JAMA 1997;277:722.

26. Accolate Product Monograph. Wilmington, DE: Zeneca Pharmaceuticals, 1996.

27. Zyflo Product Information Sheet. North Chicago, IL: Abbott Laboratories, 1996.

28. Gonzales R, et al. Decreasing antibiotic use in ambulatory practice: impact of a multi-dimensional intervention on the treatment of uncomplicated acute bronchitis in adults. JAMA 1999;281:1512.

29. Woodhead MA, MacFarlane JT. Comparative clinical laboratory features of *Legionella* with pneumococcal and mycoplasma pneumonias. Br J Dis Chest 1987;81:133.

30. Farr BM, Kaiser DL, Harrison BDW, Connolly CK. Prediction of microbial etiology at admission to hospital for pneumonia from the presenting clinical features. Thorax 1989;44:1031.

31. Rodnick JE, Gude JK. Diagnosis and antibiotic treatment of community-acquired pneumonia. West J Med 1991; 154:405.

32. American Thoracic Society Guidelines for the initial management of adults with community-acquired pneumonia: diagnosis, assessment of severity, and initial antimicrobial therapy. Am Rev Respir Dis 1993;148:1418.

33. Sue DY. Community-acquired pneumonia in adults. West J Med 1994;161:383.

34. File TM Jr, Tan JS, Plouffe JF. Community-acquired pneumonia: what's needed for accurate diagnosis. Postgrad Med 1996;99:95.

35. Pomilla PV, Brown RB. Outpatient treatment of community-acquired pneumonia in adults. Arch Intern Med 1994;154:1793.

36. Ramirez JA. Switch therapy in adult patients with pneumonia. Clin Pulmonary Med 1995;2:327.

37. Jackson LA, Benson P, Sneller V-P, et al. Safety of revaccination with pneumococcal polysaccharide vaccine. JAMA 1999;281:243.

Chapter 35

Sexual Assault and Intimate Partner Violence

Linn H. Parsons

Five Key Points

- One woman out of five will experience a sexual assault at some time in her life. Since at least of 80% of these are committed by an intimate partner, date, or acquaintance and occur under the age of 25, young women should be counseled on prevention of sexual assault.

- All women should be screened for a history of forced or unwanted sexual experiences and appropriate care offered to those responding in the affirmative.

- Physicians providing acute care to a sexual assault victim must be familiar with the complete medical evaluation (both physical and emotional concerns) and legal responsibilities necessary to protect the woman and the alleged assailant.

- Because survivors of intimate partner violence do not volunteer their history and the 1 in 5 women affected cannot be determined by race, social class, or other characteristics, ALL women must be screened for a history of abuse.

- Every physician caring for women needs to be familiar with the simple steps for intervention when a woman divulges a current or past history of partner violence: validation, documentation, safety assessment and plan, provision of appropriate resources, and referrals.

The prevalence of violence against women and the magnitude of its consequences make it imperative that all obstetricians and gynecologists incorporate concerns of interpersonal violence into their practices. The acute care of women experiencing violence includes not only medical care of direct injuries and prevention of potential medical sequelae, but also requires a knowledge of appropriate documentation, collection of legal evidence, and the ability to provide a link to community support services. The obstetrician-gynecologist needs knowledge regarding long-term consequences of a history of violence, including somatic symptoms and psychological sequelae, utilization of appropriate resources, and an awareness of the cost of providing health care to survivors. As health-care providers concerned for the well-being of female patients, the obstetrician-gynecologist is in a unique position to become involved in the community in dealing with the consequences of violence against women, including support of legislation for protection of women, and to take a public stand against abuse of women and children.

The aspects of violence against women that will be covered in this chapter are sexual assault, the adult consequences of sexual abuse, intimate partner violence, and special aspects of adolescent abuse. Definitions, prevalence, the potential consequences of each type of violence, and steps in the acute and long-term assistance of survivors will be discussed. Since a history of violence is not usually volunteered by women, recommendations for screening and identification of victims are included. Physical and sexual abuse of children, as well as assaults on men is beyond the scope of this chapter.

The 1998 National Survey on Women's Health by the Commonwealth Fund shows a continued alarming prevalence of violence against women. Of those women 18 and older surveyed, 16% reported a history of child abuse, 21% rape or sexual assault, and 31% domestic violence; 39% experienced violence in their lifetime. Unfortunately, only 8% reported that their physicians had discussed safety or violence at home with them.[1] The goal of this chapter is to assist the obstetrician-gynecologist in improving this response.

SEXUAL ASSAULT

Definitions

Sexual assault and rape are legal terms that will be defined differently in each state. Generally, a sexual assault is any sexual act performed by one person on another without their consent. While sexual intercourse is not required for a sexual assault, all states incorporate some level of sexual penetration in their law. Penetration may be of the vulva, vagina, mouth, or anus. Another critical element is the issue of consent. The alleged victim must be legally able to give consent and understand what consent means. Most states include in this definition those with physical or mental limitations that may prevent an understanding of the sexual event. Another component of the definition is the threat of force or use of force. An individual may also be coerced or intimidated into sexual activity by a person in a position of authority over her (e.g., supervisor or boss, provider of shelter or food). Submission or lack of physical trauma during a sexual assault does not imply consent.

Marital or partner rape is a sexual assault perpetrated by an intimate partner or spouse. Date rape is a sexual assault occurring when a woman voluntarily accompanies the perpetrator on a date. Alcohol or substance abuse may frequently be involved with date rape. In acquaintance rape, the perpetrator is a person known to the victim but not in an intimate or dating relationship. Acquaintance rape is a common type of sexual assault in adolescents. These three types of sexual assault are the most common and are less likely to be reported than stranger rape. Stranger rape, a sexual assault committed by an unknown perpetrator, accounts for only 15 to 20% of sexual assaults.

Prevalence

The 1996 National Institute of Justice and Centers for Disease Control and Prevention jointly sponsored the National Violence Against Women Survey.[2] For this survey, rape was defined as an event that occurred without the victim's consent, that involved the use or threat of force to penetrate the victim's vagina or anus by penis, tongue, fingers, or object or victim's mouth by penis. The definition included both attempted and completed rape. Of the 8000 women surveyed, 18% reported a completed or attempted rape at some point in their life. These women reported 22% of the assaults occurred at less than 12 years of age, 31% between 12 and 17 years, 29.4% between 18 and 24 years, and 16.6% at or after the age of 25 years. Eight percent of the women in the study reported rape by an intimate partner.

Although sexual assault is the most rapidly increasing violent crime in America, 90% of these crimes will go unreported. While most women fear sexual assault by a stranger, most sexual assaults are by an acquaintance or an intimate partner. Women are less likely to report an assault from someone they know. Women may choose not to report a crime for many reasons, such as feeling guilt or responsibility, embarrassment, fear of retribution, concern over potential medical evaluation and invasion of privacy, lack of faith in the legal system, or lack of knowledge of her legal rights. Studies of women experiencing intimate partner violence have found 25 to 50% of these women were sexually assaulted by their spouses. Marital rape is characterized by repeated victimization and more commonly associated with violence and physical injury.[3] Adolescent girls may also be concerned about confidentiality and parent notification, lack of financial resources and health insurance, and limited access to health care or lack of knowledge of health care resources. Date or acquaintance rape may not be viewed by the victim as a rape. Sexual assault by an acquaintance or intimate partner may have an even greater psychological impact than stranger rape because of the violation of trust.

Consequences of Sexual Assault

Rape trauma syndrome is a term used to describe the psychological aspects of rape.[4] The first phase is the acute phase or initial reaction and is characterized by disorganization. A woman feels shock and disbelief regarding the experience. She may appear subdued or controlled (appearing calm and composed) or she may display anger, fear, anxiety, and emotional instability. Physical shock or pallor, weak pulse, and shallow breathing may be present. This phase may last from 6 weeks to several months.

Phase two is a long-term process characterized by reorganization. The survivor must develop coping mechanisms in this phase. It will generally last for a few months to a year but may last indefinitely. During the adjustment stage, she may resume usual activities and deal with practical everyday life but may still experience daydreams or flashbacks regarding the assault. Counseling is helpful in expressing feelings and attaining closure to the experience. The second stage of this phase is integration. At this time a survivor may be depressed, focusing entirely on the rape, and having nightmares and flashbacks. The final stage is that of recovery, in which the woman returns to her base line level of functioning. Counseling is important in both phases.

Immediate consequences of rape involve both mental and physical health. Sexual assault victims are at risk for sexually transmitted infections, pregnancy, and physical injury. The reports of physical injuries are from 20 to 69%. Visual genital trauma occurs in about 20%. When colposcopy is added to the conventional rape examination, 87% of 131 women seen within 48 hours of an assault involving vaginal penetration had evidence of genital injuries. Injuries were most commonly at 3, 6 and 9 o'clock and consisted of lacerations, ecchymosis, and swelling.[5] Pregnant women are less likely to experience physical trauma.[6]

Postmenopausal women are more likely to experience genital trauma than premenopausal women.[73] Women less than 20 years old are more likely to suffer physical injury than those over 20 years of age.[8] Injury appears to be more common to the head, neck, and extremities than to the abdomen, chest, or back.

A population-based study of 4000 yielded a 5% risk of pregnancy per rape event. Only a small percentage of women received immediate medical attention after the assault and therefore did not have access to pregnancy prevention measures. In addition to lack of medical care after assault, women suffering from repeated sexual assault may be more likely to become pregnant and less likely to report their assault. This may occur in adolescent sexual abuse or intimate partner violence.[9]

It is difficult to estimate the risk of acquiring a sexually transmitted infection as a result of a sexual assault. First, it can be difficult to distinguish between a preexisting infection and one acquired during the assault. Second, most sexual assaults go unreported. Third, even for survivors reporting their assault initially, only a small percentage return for follow-up care. The Centers for Disease Control has estimated that an adult has a 6 to 10% risk of acquiring gonorrhea and 0 to 3% for acquiring syphilis. The risk of chlamydia is 4 to 17%.[10] A study by Jenny et al. found that in 204 women presenting within 72 hours of a sexual assault, 43% had at least one sexually transmitted infection: 6% gonorrhea, 10% chlamydia, 15% trichomonas, and 1% syphilis.[11]

The risk of human immunodeficiency virus (HIV) infection depends on the type of sexual exposure (vaginal, anal, or oral), the occurrence of trauma, the presence of other sexually transmitted infections, and exposure to sexual secretions and/or blood. The level of risk also depends on the HIV status of the assailant. More frequent assaults would be associated with a higher risk, such as in intimate partner violence. It is estimated that the risk of HIV transmission from a sexual assault involving anal or vaginal penetration and including ejaculation from a HIV-infected perpetrator is approximately 2 per 1000 contacts.[12] Certain populations of women will be at higher risk for acquiring HIV. One study of urban rape survivors showed rape to be most common among crack cocaine users, the homeless, sex workers, and women with a recent history of a sexually transmitted infection. Most of these urban survivors exhibited HIV risk behaviors. Unfortunately, while these women had a higher risk for HIV, they had a low perception of their risk.[13]

Extensive long-term consequences of sexual assault have been demonstrated. Mental health sequelae include sleep disturbances, eating disorders (both overeating and undereating), substance abuse, depression and suicide, anxiety disorders, phobias, and sexual dysfunction. Long-term physical sequelae commonly involve chronic pain, including pelvic and abdominal pain, headache, back pain, and temporomandibular joint pain. Vaginitis and concern over recurrent vaginal infections may be reported. Irritable bowel syndrome is more common in women with a history of sexual assault. Women with a history of sexual assault or abuse have a lowered perception of their health and a higher rate of use of medical services.[14,15]

The physician has two responsibilities in the acute care of a sexual assault victim: to provide a thorough medical evaluation and to fulfill the legal responsibilities. The physician's primary concern is the physical and emotional well-being of the alleged victim. In addition, there are legal steps required to protect the rights of both the victim and the alleged assailant and to fulfill state and local laws. Practitioners should be familiar with their local statutes. A conflict may seem to exist between these two responsibilities. The goal of a rape evaluation should be to minimize the physical and psychological trauma to the victim while maximizing the probability of collecting and preserving forensic evidence. The steps in acute care of the victim are summarized in Table 35-1.

The first step in the evaluation is to obtain informed consent. In addition to fulfilling a legal requirement, informed consent allows the woman to have a sense of control over the examination. She must feel safe during the medical encounter.

Major or life-threatening injuries should be addressed first. About 0.1% of assaulted women will die from asphyxiation, beating, lacerations, drowning, or gunshot wounds. The most common genital injuries will be of the posterior vaginal fornix and may result in bleeding significant enough to require surgical repair. Anal penetration may result in severe rectal injury. Intraperitoneal injury is less common but should be ruled out.

When acute injuries have been addressed and the patient is stable, a history is taken. The purpose of a medical history is to obtain information needed to guide the medical examination, to collect pertinent

---

TABLE 35-1
ACUTE CARE OF THE ALLEGED SEXUAL ASSAULT VICTIM

Medical
  Informed consent for examination
  Evaluate and treat physical injuries
  Obtain history: assault, medical, gynecologic
  Collect cultures, treat existing sexually transmitted infections, offer prophylactic antibiotics
  Offer emergency contraception
  Offer base-line hepatitis B and vaccination, syphilis testing
  Provide HIV counseling and offer testing
  ABO blood group
  Provide emotional support, mental health evaluation and referral
  Arrange medical follow-up
Legal
  Record patient's account of events
  Document injuries (consent for photos, body map)
  Collect and identify all physical evidence
  Local statues—report to authorities
  Maintain chain of evidence

---

physical evidence, and to assist in treating the victim. The history is not an investigative history. Any attempt to make a detailed history could provide subtle contradictions with police investigative history and cause problems with prosecution. The history should include whether there was actual or attempted oral, rectal, or vaginal penetration of the victim, oral contact with the perpetrator, ejaculation (if this is known by the victim), and penetration at any orifice with a foreign object or fingers.[16] She should also be questioned about activities following the assault that may have destroyed evidence such as bathing, douching, changing clothes, using tampons, brushing teeth, or having a bowel movement. A general medical history should be taken, including any chronic medical problems, medications used, allergies, and history of tetanus immunization. Previous mental health history will be important in providing assistance. Gynecologic history should include last menstrual period, contraceptive method, last episode of consensual intercourse, and history of sexually transmitted infections.

The general physical examination and the collection of physical evidence will be simultaneous (Table 35-2). States provide specific requirements for the collection of forensic evidence and a rape kit or step-by-step guidelines should be available in every facility caring for sexual assault victims. The victim should first undress over a large sheet of paper to collect any hair, debris, or other fibers. Any potential clothing

---

TABLE 35-2
PHYSICAL AND LABORATORY ASSESSMENT OF THE SEXUAL ASSAULT VICTIM

General
  Skin for cuts, bruises, abrasions, fingernail marks, bite marks
  Fingernail scrapings
  Woods lamp examination (in darkened room) for semen
  Hair combing
Oral cavity
  Search for injuries
  Collect specimens for saliva, semen of assailant, saliva of victim
  Culture for gonorrhea
Anogenital examination
  Pubic hair combing
  Colposcopic examination for injuries
  Vulvar and vaginal swabs for semen
  Vaginal swabs wet preparation
  Cervical cultures for gonorrhea and chlamydia
  Rectal swab for gonorrhea, semen
  Bimanual examination
Laboratory
  Hepatitis B
  HIV antigen/antibody (0 and 12 weeks, 6 months)
  Syphilis (0 and 12 weeks)
  Gonorrhea, chlamydia, wet preparation—as above, repeat after 2 weeks
  Pregnancy test

---

stains where there may be semen, blood, or other body fluids should be located and examined with a Woods lamp; dried semen will fluoresce under a Woods lamp in a darkened room. The outer clothing is placed in a collection bag along with the sheet of paper. Undergarments are similarly collected and placed in a container. Only the victim should handle her clothing. The victim's skin should be examined for any cuts, bruises, bite marks, abrasions, or fingernail scrapings. A body map can be used to document injuries. Photographs can be taken with informed consent. The mouth should also be examined for trauma and a saliva sample taken either with filter paper or directly into a small vial. This can later be used to look for secretion of ABO antigens. Culture of the oral cavity should be obtained for gonorrhea. If the assault has taken place within the past few hours, oral swabs can be taken for suspected semen. Areas of bite marks or kissing where the perpetrator may have deposited saliva are scraped to assist in discovering the assailant's blood type.

Controversy exists over the collection of hair evidence. Significant transfer of hair occurs in about 4% of assaults. The collection of hair by pulling pubic and

scalp hair can be very painful and humiliating for the victim. To compromise, hair can be obtained by combing both the pubic hair and head to collect any possible hairs from the assailant. If DNA identification of the victim is later necessary, hairs can be pulled at that time with her consent.[16]

A thorough anogenital examination is performed including a step-by-step explanation of the examination and the evidence collection. The use of a chaperone for the entire examination is necessary both for legal reasons and to provide support for the victim. The colposcope or a magnifying lens can be used on the anogenital area in order to increase detection of tears, abrasions, ecchymosis, and other trauma. Photographs or drawings should be used for documentation. Vulvar and vaginal swabs should be taken for suspected semen. Vaginal secretions can be aspirated and collected for later examination for evidence of seminal fluid. Vaginal swabs for saline and potassium hydroxide preparations should be examined for yeast, trichomonads, and bacterial vaginosis. Cultures of the cervix for chlamydia and gonorrhea should be collected. If anal penetration occurred, a rectal examination should be performed for injury, gonorrhea cultures taken, and a swab for semen collected. Injuries of the vagina, cervix, and rectum should be ruled out. A bimanual examination should be performed to identify any possible hematomas, other injuries, or preexisting gynecologic problems. Blood testing may be indicated by the state forensic protocol.

Another controversial area in evidence collection is examination for motile sperm. Seminal fluid can be examined for a prostatic antigen P30 and acid phosphatase. The ABO blood group antigens may be present in seminal plasma. Spermatozoa can be used for DNA profiling. Because individuals performing examinations of sexual assault victims may not be accustomed to identifying spermatozoa, an error can easily occur. Conflicting evidence regarding the presence, number, and motility of sperm reported in the emergency room and that determined by the forensic experts could undermine the case for the prosecution.[16]

The field of DNA profiling is expanding rapidly. Only small quantities of materials are needed for testing. Fresh material is not necessary for the analysis. Fluorescence in situ hybridization (FISH) has been used to detect nonsperm male cells, verifying sexual contact. This technique appears to be highly sensitive and specific in detection of male cells in cervical vaginal smears. Even in the absence of sperm or semen, male cells could be identified and DNA analysis performed. The use of FISH and its application in sexual assault is under investigation.[17]

State laws should be consulted regarding reporting of sexual assaults. Most states require the reporting of the assault prior to the forensic examination. Funds may be available for covering the costs of an examination. Some states allow anonymous reporting. A victim should be encouraged to report the crime. Since most physical evidence is gone after 72 hours, a forensic examination after this point may not be appropriate. Timely reporting is therefore critical in retrieving evidence and engaging the criminal justice system on behalf of the victim.

Evidence-collection kits are especially useful, not only in ensuring proper collection of all specimens, but also in maintaining the chain of evidence. If no collection kit is available, all specimens should be labeled with the victim's name, the examiner's name, the site of collection, the type of evidence, and the date and time of collection. Since wet specimens will decay rapidly, all specimens should be air-dried before packaging. The chain of evidence is maintained by handing a completed kit or other properly labeled sealed container to the law enforcement official.

The legal standard for documentation of chlamydia and gonorrhea is culture. Concern exists over false positive results with antigen testing. If cultures are not available, identification of an organism using antigen testing requires a second test using a different method on the same specimen in order to confirm the results.[18]

Any sexually transmitted infections found at the time of evaluation should be treated. Following evaluation, an empiric regimen for prophylaxis against chlamydia, gonorrhea, trichomonas, and bacterial vaginosis is recommended (Table 35-3). In patients requiring alternative regimens because of pregnancy or drug allergies, Centers for Diseases Control guidelines should be consulted for those details.[18] This regimen should also be effective against incubating syphilis. The efficacy of these regimens in preventing gonorrhea, bacterial vaginosis, or chlamydia genitourinary tract infections after sexual assault has not been studied. Possible benefits, toxicity, and side effects of medications must be considered in recommending treatment. Hepatitis B vaccination can be administered at the time of the initial evaluation. Follow-up dosages should then be given at 1 to 2 months

TABLE 35-3
PROPHYLAXIS AGAINST INFECTION

Empiric antimicrobial regimen
  Ceftriaxone 125 mg intramuscularly, one dose
    plus
  Metronidazole 2 g by mouth, one dose
    plus
  Azithromycin 1 g by mouth, one dose, or
  Doxycycline 100 mg by mouth, twice a day for 7 days
Hepatis B vaccination offered
HIV counseling, offer testing, prophylaxis only if HIV-positive
  assailant (use Centers for Disease Control guidelines)
In the case of injuries, tetanus booster, 0.5 ml intramuscularly
  if over 10 years since last booster

and at 4 to 6 months. The risk of acquiring hepatitis B from a sexual assault is unknown. Women should also be counseled regarding signs and symptoms of sexually transmitted infections and recommended to report for evaluation if any of these should occur. They should be advised to abstain from sexual intercourse until prophylactic treatment is completed.[18]

The recommendation to take zidovudine following a sexual assault is based on risk assessment of the exposure. Risk assessment includes the HIV status of the assailant; whether anal, vaginal, or oral penetration occurred; whether ejaculation occurred; the presence of physical injuries, including mucosal injuries; existence of sexually transmitted infection; and the number of assailants. Counseling at the time of the assault includes information regarding potential HIV transmission and helping survivors assess their risk for HIV and the utility of an HIV antibody test. This information may be overwhelming at an initial encounter at the time of an assault, but the lack of medical follow-up indicates that a discussion of this information should not be delayed. If the patient is unable to make a decision at this time, a serum sample can be frozen for later evaluation with consent. The effectiveness of zidovudine in preventing HIV infection after a known exposure remains unproven. Failures of zidovudine prophylaxis in health-care workers have been reported. In addition, the need to begin zidovudine within 4 hours of exposure and the cost of prophylaxis cause major problems in the setting of sexual assault.[12] If the patient decides to take zidovudine postexposure therapy, follow the Centers for Disease Control guidelines for occupational mucous membrane exposure to HIV.

In women susceptible to pregnancy, a pregnancy test is performed. If this test is negative, emergency

---

TABLE 35-4
EMERGENCY CONTRACEPTION

Yuzpe regimen
   Ethinyl estradiol 100 μg with levonorgestrel 0.5 mg within
      72 hours of the assault. Repeat in 12 hours. Antiemetic
      1 hour prior to each dose (e.g., Ovral 2 tablets stat,
      2 tablets in 12 hours. Nordette, LoOvral, or Levlen,
      4 tablets stat, then 4 tablets in 12 hours)
   PreVen
Levonorgestrel alone
   Levonorgestrel 0.75 mg stat and repeat in 12 hours (Plan B)

---

contraception should be offered (Table 35-4). The Yuzpe regimen uses 200 μg of ethinyl estradiol and 1.0 mg of levonorgestrel given in two divided doses 12 hours apart and is administered within 72 hours of unprotected intercourse. Provide an antiemetic to be taken 1 hour prior to each dose to reduce the nausea and vomiting. A product with levonorgestrel alone similarly uses two doses, each containing 0.75 mg of levonorgestrel. Significantly less nausea and vomiting occurs with levonorgestrel alone, with a similar pregnancy rate to the Yuzpe regimen.[19-21]

Follow-up Care

After the medical care is completed, give the patient a clear follow-up plan. Verbal as well as written instructions (including a list of tests performed) should be provided. A 24-hour emergency medical number and crisis line number should be given for problems or concerns. Arrange a mental health follow-up for 1 to 2 weeks after the event.

Assess the safety of the environment to which the woman will be returning. In the event of marital or acquaintance rape, ask the survivor if she is afraid of her assailant. Increased danger would be indicated if the behavior is repetitive, if the assailant has threatened or used weapons, if alcohol or drugs are involved, or if there is a threat to children in the house. Further information on danger assessment and safety planning are included in the section on "Intimate Partner Violence," below. In situations of marital rape, women may not be able to avoid intercourse or obtain partner treatment for sexually transmitted infections.

A 2-week follow-up appointment should be scheduled. If antibiotic prophylaxis against sexually transmitted infections was not used, follow-up cultures for gonorrhea and chlamydia and a wet preparation

examination are performed. The second hepatitis B vaccination shot will be due 1 month after the assault. A follow-up visit for 12 weeks will allow serologic testing for syphilis and HIV testing. Final HIV testing may be done at 6 months for patient reassurance.

In addition to providing follow-up medical care, the victim should be informed of the value of counseling following sexual assault. Women initially declining mental health services may be ready for this at the time of follow-up care. Refer the patient to mental health care providers who are trained to deal with sexual assault victims.

Screening

The reasons for routine screening for a history of sexual assault are quite simple. First, sexual victimization is a common occurrence, which has medical and mental health sequelae. Second, 90% of sexual victimizations are not reported and women with a history of victimization do not volunteer this history. Identification of a history of sexual assault requires use of nonjudgmental, sensitive questions asked in a private, safe environment.

Screening questions should exclude terms that may vary in their interpretation (examples: rape, assault, abuse, molestation). Questions that describe specific behaviors are much less open to interpretation and will yield more accurate results. Examples are: "Has anyone forced you to have intercourse or to participate in any other sexual activity that you did not want?"

If a woman discloses a history of sexual assault, the first step is to acknowledge the importance of this experience and to validate the assault as being a traumatic event that she did not deserve. Many women carry a burden of belief that the experience was caused by something they did and that they deserved the act. Next, determine the current status of the individual and whether the victimization is ongoing. Concerns over safety and ongoing violence are addressed in the section on "Intimate Partner Violence," below.

In a setting of ongoing sexual victimization, concerns over pregnancy and contraception, treatment of sexually transmitted infections, and other physical problems may be of concern to the woman. With a remote history of sexual victimization, she may still be concerned about sexually transmitted infections and an offer of screening can be helpful.

If the woman has never received counseling, the benefits of posttraumatic counseling should be discussed. Women often underestimate the impact of such a significant event on their physical and mental health. Knowledge of referral sources in the community who are specially trained in dealing with sexual assault and abuse is important.

Prevention

Primary prevention of sexual victimization will require society to exercise openness and frankness in dealing with sexual assault both of males and females. Children must be taught that it is inappropriate both to be touched and to have physical contact with another individual without requesting permission. Appropriate means of dealing with aggressive behavior in resolving conflict must be taught. Mixed messages received by adolescents and older women may confuse them, especially in the areas of acquaintance or date rape and marital rape. Adolescents are a population at great risk, and special issues regarding the care of the adolescent are covered in the section on "Special Issues for the Adolescent," below.

Practical issues in primary prevention include being cautious about alcohol and drug intake, not getting rides with strangers or individuals one knows only slightly, remaining alert to the environment, and avoiding situations of high risk. Since women assume that the greatest danger is from a stranger, we must educate women that the major risk is from people they know and from their intimate partners. Women will lower their guard because of trust and may actually feel guilty that caution indicates a lack of trust.

Secondary prevention includes both prevention of future sexual assault and reduction of the long-term sequelae of assault. A previous history of sexual victimization is a significant risk factor for future sexual assault.[22] Women found to have experienced a previous sexual assault should be advised of ways to prevent assault in the future. The obstetrician-gynecologist can address physical consequences that may occur because of sexual assault, screen for sexually transmitted infections, assist in pregnancy prevention, and be supportive of somatic complaints and problems that occur. Referral to counseling will help the survivor to move through the process of dealing with her sexual assault and to prevent and treat mental health sequelae associated with sexual assault, such as depression, anxiety disorders, panic attacks, the increased risk of substance use, and the initiation of risky sexual behaviors.

A sense of loss of control occurs for the sexual assault victim. Her obstetrician-gynecologist can assist her in the process of becoming a true survivor by using informed consent, asking permission to touch and proceed with a physical examination, and giving permission to stop the examination at any time if she is unable to continue. Compassion, confidentiality, and privacy are essential. Reduce self-blame by stating that it was not her fault and that assault is a very common problem in our society. She may also feel guilty if she did not resist the attacker. Emphasize that resistance sometimes leads to more severe injury and that her actions were necessary for her survival.

PROVIDING CARE TO ADULT SURVIVORS OF CHILDHOOD SEXUAL ABUSE

Studies show that one of every four women has had a nonconsensual sexual experience before the age of 14. Women presenting to the obstetrician-gynecologist as adults may have suffered from childhood or adolescent sexual victimization. About 75% of these experiences have never been reported, leaving women without the benefit of a counselor trained to help them recover from this experience. For women victimized prior to the age of 11, the perpetrator is most likely a relative, while for the young adolescent the perpetrator could be a relative or an acquaintance.

The family of origin for the victim of childhood sexual abuse may have contained diverse problems such as physical or sexual abuse of the mother, alcoholism, chronic illness in the mother, and serious mental health problems in the mother such as depression, suicide or suicide attempts, and psychosis.[23]

Finkelhor and Browne[24] have described four major outcomes of childhood sexual abuse that assist in understanding the sequelae and their categorization. The first is traumatic sexualization, which results in changes in attitudes and feelings toward the individual's sexuality. The results can be promiscuity, prostitution, and sexual dysfunction. Sarwer and Durlak studied 359 married adult women seeking sex therapy with their spouses.[25] They found that approximately 8 of 10 women with sexual dysfunction could be accurately identified with knowledge of their prior abuse. Sexual penetration was especially associated with adult sexual dysfunction. Specific problems identified were reduced libido, a disorder of orgasm, dyspareunia, and vaginismus.[25] A second major outcome is a sense of betrayal arising from a loss of trust. This may lead to difficulty in establishing intimate relationships in the future, feeling of vulnerability, anger, hostility, and depression. Next, a feeling of powerlessness or loss of control can lead to anxiety disorders, sleep disorders, phobias, and somatic complaints. Numerous chronic somatic complaints have been associated with childhood sexual abuse. Nonspecific symptoms such as sleep disorders, headaches, backache, and chronic pelvic and abdominal pain have been reported. Hot flashes or flushing of the skin, perspiration, exaggerated startle responses, restlessness, and rapid body movements may be associated with anxiety disorders or posttraumatic stress disorder.[23,26] The final category is that of stigmatization, in which the victim herself assumes the negative meanings associated with sexual assault. This might lead to guilt and shame, lowered self-esteem, and self-destructive behaviors. A wide range of self-destructive behaviors have been associated with childhood sexual abuse, including suicidal ideation and suicide attempts,[27] the use of psychoactive and illicit drugs, alcohol dependence,[28] and eating disorders (bulimia, anorexia, and obesity).[23] A national survey conducted in 1991 assessing substance abuse in women also found childhood sexual abuse associated with a significant risk of consensual sexual intercourse before the age of 15.[28] The severity of the consequences of childhood sexual abuse has been related to the duration of abuse, the use of force or threat or force, either oral or genital penetration, and father or stepfather as the abuser.[27,29]

The 1993 Commonwealth Fund Survey on Women's Health revealed a significant association between gynecologic problems and a previous history of childhood sexual abuse. Women with a history of childhood sexual abuse were also more likely to report having seen a physician for a gynecologic problem in the past 5 years, to rate their general health fair or poor, to report depression, and to have seriously considered suicide.[30] Robohm and Buttenheim[31] found that survivors of childhood sexual abuse were more likely to experience discomfort during a gynecologic examination including the time prior to the examination, the breast examination, and the pelvic examination. Survivors were also significantly more likely to become overwhelmed by emotion, have unwanted or intrusive thoughts, have a flashback or memory triggered, have body memories triggered,

or to feel detached from their body during the examination. Reddy and Wasserman[32] identified five behaviors during speculum insertion that indicated a higher level of anxiety during pelvic examination: holding hands or eyes covered or shut, hands on the shoulders, hands covering the pelvis, hands on the legs, and hands holding the table. Some women survivors will tightly close their eyes and silent tears will be the only sign of their distress. The gynecologist and his or her chaperone must stay tuned in to events at the head of the table in order to provide sensitive care.

Some studies have shown an increase in the cost of health care to women survivors of childhood abuse. Factors contributing to increased costs may be more operations and hospital admissions,[33] more primary care visits,[33,34] higher outpatient expenses, especially from mental health costs, and more frequent emergency room visits.[34]

The prevalence of childhood sexual abuse and its wide-reaching consequences, the increased frequency of somatic problems, including gynecologic concerns, and the increased difficulty with gynecologic examinations demonstrate the need for the obstetrician-gynecologist to incorporate routine screening into his or her practice. Questions such as "Has anyone ever forced you to have sexual activity or sexual intercourse that you did not wish to participate in?" can be included in a general screening for physical and sexual abuse, as discussed in the section on "Intimate Partner Violence," below.

INTIMATE PARTNER VIOLENCE

Epidemiology

The terms partner abuse, spouse abuse, and domestic violence are being replaced by a broader descriptive term, intimate partner violence. This violence is defined as a pattern of behavior designed to control a person with whom the abuser currently has or has had an intimate or romantic relationship. Estimates are that 25% or more of all women will at some time be in an abusive relationship. While it is difficult to know the true prevalence, women in the United States are more likely to be assaulted, injured, raped, or murdered by a current or former male partner than by anyone else. The victimization may be of three types: physical, sexual, emotional, or a combination of these.

Physical abuse includes a wide range of activities that threaten the physical well-being of the victim, such as verbal abuse, the threat of violence or use of weapons, throwing or breaking objects, pushing or shoving, and more serious behavior such as slapping, kicking, hitting, beating, or use of a weapon. Physical abuse is intentional and repetitive, increases in frequency and severity over time, and usually occurs in combination with one of the other two types of abuse.

Sexual abuse occurs in about 60% of physically abusive relationships. Activities include not only sexual intercourse but any type of sexual act or behavior unacceptable or undesirable to the abused woman. While forced intercourse is common, other activities may include forcing the partner to perform sexual acts with which she is uncomfortable or which make her feel degraded; assault to the genital area; the use of objects vaginally, orally, or anally; or the use of sexually degrading names. The risk of sexually transmitted infections and unwanted pregnancy accompanies sexual abuse.

Emotional or psychological abuse may be more difficult to identify. The threat of physical injury or threat of injury to her children; isolation from family and friends; withholding food, clothing, or money; ridicule and humiliation in public; control of finances; preventing access to health care; and any behaviors that intimidate her will result in loss of self-esteem and severe psychological consequences.

The face of a survivor of intimate partner violence may be the face of any woman. Intimate partner violence occurs in both heterosexual and same-sex relationships and to women in any socioeconomic group. Physical and sexual abuse has been documented in middle-class working women.[35] A survey of obstetricians and gynecologists examining attitudes and behaviors towards screening for domestic violence revealed that 20% of those responding to the survey had a personal history of violence.[36]

Characteristics of the Abusive Relationship

The basis of the abusive relationship is control. While an abuser may claim not to be in control, the abuser selects the tactics, their frequency, and severity. Abusers have been shown to have low self-esteem and feel unable to control the outside environment. Children in the house are also abused about 50% of the time. Yet, 100% of the time the children will be affected by witnessing abuse. There are myths that contribute to

the maintenance of the relationship. Women will feel responsible for the violence. They may have been raised in a house with family violence and therefore see violence as normal. Because of low self-esteem, a woman may believe that her own inadequacy and behaviors justify the violence. She may also believe that she can control the violence.

A second factor that may contribute to continuation of the relationship is the cycle of violence that characterizes the interaction. The first phase of the cycle is one of increasing tension, anger, arguing, and possible verbal abuse. In the second phase, the battering phase, verbal threats will increase, and physical and sexual abuse occur. Leaving the relationship in this dangerous phase can result in homicide for either partner. In the subsequent calm stage, the partner may apologize for his or her behavior, present gifts, and promise the behavior will never occur again. This hope may keep the abused woman in the relationship.

Twenty percent of women will leave an abusive relationship after the first episode of violence, 60% will eventually leave, and 20% will never leave. The two most common reasons for staying in an abusive relationship are lack of money and fear of retaliation. The time of leaving carries the greatest risk of homicide for the woman or her partner. Other reasons for staying include love, desire to maintain an intact household, children, the view that violence is normal, guilt, hope, powerlessness, depression, and feelings of worthlessness. Poverty is a significant problem for women and children who have left abusive relationships.

Consequences of Intimate Partner Violence (Table 35-5)

The first consequence of intimate partner violence is severe injury and death of women. About 4 million women each year are severely battered by their partners, and some of these women die.

Survivors of intimate partner violence may present with general somatic symptoms such as sleep disorders, nightmares, substance abuse (alcohol, tobacco, prescription and illegal drugs), eating disorders (anorexia, bulimia, overeating), repeated injuries, and apparent hostile, uncooperative, or noncompliant-appearing behaviors. Their partner may be present at all medical encounters and appear quite caring and protective. Frequent telephone calls to the office or frequent office visits with vague somatic symptoms

---

TABLE 35-5
CONSEQUENCES OF INTIMATE PARTNER VIOLENCE

Injury and death of victims
Medical sequelae
  Repeated injuries
  General symptoms (sleep disorders, eating disorders,
    noncompliance)
  Somatic symptoms (choking sensation, hyperventilation,
    pain, gastrointestinal symptoms)
  Gynecologic problems
  Sexually transmitted infections
Mental health sequelae
  Depression and suicide or suicide attempts
  Drug and alcohol use
Obstetric sequelae
  Maternal injury and mortality
  Late entry into prenatal care
  Substance abuse
  Unintended pregnancy
Access and health-care utilization problems
Increased health-care costs

---

may indicate a history of abuse. Women may present with symptoms such as a choking sensation, hyperventilation, asthma, allergic reactions, chest pain, gastrointestinal symptoms, and chronic or acute pain. Chronic abdominal and pelvic pain,[37,38] chronic headache,[39] functional bowel disease,[40] and fibromyalgia[40] may be associated with a history of intimate partner violence.

The 1993 Commonwealth Fund's National Survey of Women's Health included questions regarding gynecologic problems. Women with a history of spouse abuse (defined as currently married or cohabiting at the time of the survey) over the past 5 years reported a significantly higher occurrence of gynecologic diagnoses, sexually transmitted diseases, severe menstrual problems, and urinary-tract infections.[42,43]

Women with a history of intimate partner violence may have concerns over the presence of sexually transmitted infections. A study of African-American women in abusive relationships revealed a lower likelihood of using condoms and an increase in verbal abuse, emotional abuse, and threats of physical abuse when they discussed condom use with their partners.[44] A study of abused women living at shelters showed multiple risk factors for HIV, including illicit drug use, partners having sex with other partners, lack of condom use, and a prior sexually transmitted infection from their partner.[45] The Commonwealth Survey also found that women experiencing spouse abuse were more likely than other women

who were married or living with a male to report that their intimate partner had refused to wear a condom in the past year.[43]

The exposure to violence also leads to mental health consequences. Low self-esteem, depression, and anxiety diagnosed by a physician, depressive symptoms measured on a depression scale, and suicidal ideation have been found more commonly in women experiencing spouse abuse. These women were also more likely to have used illicit drugs and to have been counseled by a physician about substance abuse.[43]

A review of the prevalence of intimate partner violence in pregnancy showed that studies using detailed in person interviews or asking in a third trimester of pregnancy reported prevalence rates of 7.4 to 21.1%.[46] Women experiencing physical violence by their partner during the 12 months preceding delivery were more likely to have delayed entry into prenatal care than women not experiencing such violence.[47] The utilization of substances, including prescription drugs, alcohol, and illicit drugs have been associated with violence during pregnancy.[48,49] Maternal injury during pregnancy most often involves the abdomen, breasts, head, and neck. Injury is the most common cause of maternal mortality. A study in North Carolina revealed 51% of the maternal deaths from intentional injury were known or suspected of having experienced intimate partner violence.[50] Women with unwanted or mistimed (unintended) pregnancies are at increased risk for intimate partner violence as compared with women with intended pregnancies.[51] A qualitative study of the influence of abuse on pregnancy intention found intimate partner violence and unintended pregnancy were connected through the partner's control of contraception and pushing her to have a child. This study also found men's refusal to use condoms in an abusive relationship contributed to the partner's risk of acquiring sexually transmitted diseases, including HIV.[52] Two studies of women seeking pregnancy termination revealed a 39.5%[53] and 31.4%[54] prevalence of abuse in women seeking abortion. Women with a history of abuse were more likely to list relationship issues as the reason for pregnancy termination, were less likely to inform their partner of the pregnancy, and were less likely to have partner support for or involvement in the abortion decision.[53] The evidence is inconclusive regarding the association of intimate partner violence and obstetrical complications such as pregnancy loss, preterm labor, and low birth weight.

An excellent review by Petersen et al.[55] demonstrates the problems with the literature regarding abuse and pregnancy. Whether or not intimate partner violence is associated with obstetrical complications, the intimate partner violence in pregnancy will remain a major concern since many women are affected. Among women abused in pregnancy, one study found 87% had been physically abused prior to pregnancy. Abuse prior to pregnancy is the major risk factor for physical abuse during pregnancy.[56]

Health care access and utilization are influenced by intimate partner violence. Women with a history of physical or emotional abuse have more frequent telephone contacts with their health care provider, more physician visits, and more ongoing and acute prescriptions.[57] Women experiencing partner abuse are more likely to use the emergency room for their health care and less likely to have a regular doctor. While the Commonwealth Fund Survey found the mean number of physician visits in the past year did not differ between women who were abused and those who were not, a significantly greater percentage of abused women described themselves as having an unmet need for medical care in the past year.[58,59] Victims of intimate partner violence have been found to have more hospitalizations, more general clinic use, more mental health services, and more out-of-plan referrals in one health plan. Women with a history of intimate partner violence cost 92% more than a random sample of female enrollees.[60]

Access to medical care may be affected in an abusive relationship by many factors, including control of care by the abuser, lack of financial resources, lack of insurance, embarrassment or humiliation, and fear of retaliation. Two studies examining barriers that abused women encountered in the health care system found that women perceived health care providers to be disinterested or unsympathetic. The women felt humiliated and blamed for their abuse. Victims reported that their abuse was minimized, that they were given insufficient referrals and information, and that they were not identified as abused women. They also felt that the health-care system did not allow providers enough time to deal with their issues.[61,62]

Screening for Abuse

Although the previous section clearly indicates that women with certain medical presentations may be at higher risk for intimate partner violence, women

---

TABLE 35-6
STANDARDIZED ABUSE ASSESSMENT SCREEN

1. Within the last year, have you been hit, slapped, kicked, or otherwise physically hurt by someone? If yes, by whom?
   Number of times _____

2. Since you have been pregnant, have you been hit, slapped, kicked, or otherwise physically hurt by someone? If yes, by whom?
   Number of times _____

3. Has anyone ever forced you to have sexual activities? If yes, who?
   Number of times _____

---

cannot be identified by these factors alone. Women do not volunteer their history of abuse. Direct questions to screen for intimate partner violence are necessary. The standardized abuse assessment screen (Table 35-6) has been tested and shown to be more reliable than nursing or general social service interviews in the detection of abuse.[63-65] Repeated questioning on multiple prenatal visits yields a higher prevalence of abuse than single-event questioning.[46] The abuse assessment screen, developed in 1989 by the Nursing Research Consortium on Violence and Abuse, is not copyrighted and is available for use.[64] Questioning should take place in private, with no other family members or partner present. If a partner is constantly present, women can be screened by nursing staff in the restroom or the partner asked to leave for part of the visit. Two additional questions can be added to complete a five-question abuse assessment screen. First, "Within the last year, has anyone forced you to have sexual activities? Has anyone in the past forced you to have sexual activities? If so, who?" And second, "Are you afraid of your partner or anyone you listed above?"

If a patient has clearly obtained injuries such as a black eye or bruising but denies abuse, a statement such as, "I find that when I see women with injuries such as yours, they may have been caused by someone" may be helpful.

Annual screening can be done efficiently by the obstetrician-gynecologist. While asking about smoking, exercise, alcohol and drug use, or other screening questions, a simple question such as "Given the high incidence of violence against women, have you been hit or threatened since the last time I saw you?" is added.

Emotional abuse may be more subtle and difficult to identify. Extended questionnaires developed for this are cumbersome for use in an office. If a patient has difficulty making eye contact, appears to have low self-esteem, or has any of the problems identified under consequences of abuse, the following questions may be useful in identifying emotional abuse: Is your partner overly jealous or possessive? Does your partner insult or humiliate you especially in public or around friends? Has your partner threatened your children, other family members, friends, or pets? Does your partner keep you from working or going to school? Does your partner keep you from seeing your family or friends? Does your partner control the finances by not giving you money, taking your money or paycheck, or drinking or gambling away your money? Does your partner blame you for his problems or for any other household problems?

Potential barriers to screening and intervention for intimate partner violence have been identified.[36] Lack of education, discomfort dealing with psychosocial issues, and the perceived time required for screening and appropriate intervention were the most common barriers. Other barriers identified were the attitude that abuse is a problem only in lower socioeconomic women, provider frustration in being unable to resolve the victim's problems, and fear of offending patients. Extensive educational materials exist for dealing with domestic violence. An excellent reference for health providers is the book by Schornstein.[66] Confidence can also be gained by speaking with women with a history of abuse, speaking with mental health providers who deal with female victims, and visiting a local battered women's shelter. Time is certainly a major concern in today's medical environment. Training office personnel such as nurses and physician extenders about community resources, assistance with screening, and developing an office protocol will improve efficiency. Private patients are not offended by routine screening questions and nonabused women are grateful that their physicians are concerned.

Recommended Actions to Assist Survivors

The American College of Obstetricians and Gynecologists and the American Medical Association have devised specific recommendations for intervention in the area of intimate partner violence. These recommendations are listed in Table 35-7.[67,68]

TABLE 35-7
STEPS IN INTERVENTION—ACUTE EVENT

Validate that abuse is wrong.
Take a complete abuse history and document it.
Document the physical examination and any trauma (photographs, body map).
Perform safety or danger assessment.
Provide information on referral sources.
Provide emergency numbers and shelter information.
Assist in developing a safety or exit plan.
Inquire about child abuse.
Advise counseling and provide resources.
Inform her that you and your practice partners are available and concerned for her safety.

When the abuse assessment screening is positive, the first step is to verbalize that the abuse is wrong, this is a common problem, the abused woman is not alone in her victimization, and no one should have to live in such a situation. Women would prefer to be identified as "survivors" and not "victims."

The complete abuse history should be carefully documented in the chart using Table 35-8 (derived from Schornstein) as a guide.[66] Consent must be obtained for photographs. Because bruises can take 48 to 72 hours to develop, a return visit may be needed for documentation of some injuries. Schornstein states that a well-documented record will not only assist a survivor in obtaining a protection order or a criminal conviction, but it will also help keep a physician out of court.[66]

In addition to a physical examination for injuries, concerns regarding sexually transmitted infection and pregnancy should be addressed.

A safety or danger assessment is performed to assess the possibility of risk of homicide for either partner. Factors associated with an increased risk of homicide include a threat or an attempt to leave the relationship, an adolescent experiencing violence, the use of drugs or alcohol in the relationship, the presence of a gun in the house, sexual abuse, child abuse, suicide attempts or threats of suicide, and escalating violence with increased frequency or intensity. If any of these factors are present, women should be advised of your concern for their safety and their risk of death.

In addition to providing emergency numbers and shelter information, a nurse or physician extender can assist in the development of a safety plan. Women need to decide where they would go and how they

TABLE 35-8
DOCUMENTATION

Identify the patient by her full name, date of birth, and social security number on each page.

Provide the physician's full name and specialty.

Document all injuries (photographs, body map).

Document diagnosis and treatment, with date and time.

Record a brief statement from the patient regarding who caused the injuries and how (use abuser's name).

Record a brief statement of prior violence and cause of any prior injuries.

If an inconsistency appears in injury and stated cause, document this.

Record completely and accurately her statements. A trial could be a year away.

Use nonjudgmental terms such as "the patient states" or "the patient reports."

Write legibly—the report is useful only if it can be read.

Do not comment on areas outside your expertise.

Do not editorialize or interpret events or findings—record only facts.

would get there in an emergency. They should keep a suitcase containing a set of keys, money or bankbooks, identification, including Social Security card and driver's license, financial records such as car title, a change of clothes for herself and any children, and a special toy for each child with a friend or relative. After advising that the reporting of child abuse is mandatory in all states, inquire about child abuse.

Trained office staff can also provide information on referral sources, including legal resources, police, social services such as vocational rehabilitation, and support groups. Counseling should be offered, and the names and contact information for recommended providers given. Each patient should be informed that the physician and the practice are available if she has concerns or problems.

The presence of educational materials on intimate partner violence in the office will also designate the obstetrician-gynecologist as an individual concerned about abuse issues. Posters are available and along with emergency telephone numbers can be placed in every bathroom in the office.

For a women with a history of intimate partner violence who is no longer with her partner, assess for safety and determine if she is being stalked. If there is evidence of stalking, caution her regarding risk of homicide and refer to legal resources and the police. If the history of violence is remote and there appear to be no safety issues, an abuse history should still be documented. If she has never had counseling for the

abuse, provide recommended resources. Discuss her medical problems that may be related to the history of abuse.

With a protocol or plan in place, the well-prepared physician along with his or her staff can very effectively and efficiently assist present and past survivors of intimate partner violence. In order to provide appropriate treatment for somatic problems, recognize mental health concerns, avoid improper use of medications (antianxiety drugs, pain medications, antidepressants, and tranquilizers), and provide sensitive care, the identification of intimate partner violence must take place. It is clear that identification can take place only through routine screening. Women need their obstetrician-gynecologist to become an advocate for them in their struggle for survivorship.

SPECIAL ISSUES FOR THE ADOLESCENT

A multitude of factors combine to make the adolescent an especially high-risk population with regards to intimate partner violence and sexual assault. Women aged 16 to 24 years have the highest rate of rape, with the majority acquaintance or date rape. Many adolescents are unprepared for violent situations or behaviors they may encounter in a dating relationship. While date or acquaintance rape may occur during late night or early morning hours, the most common time is after school, when adolescents may be unsupervised. Verbal, physical, and sexual abuse as a child are all associated with an increased risk of subsequent date abuse.[69]

For the young adolescent, abuse is more likely to occur at home and to happen repeatedly, and the abuser is usually a family member. Girls usually do not tell anyone about the abuse. Twenty-four percent of girls in grades 5 to 8 and 29% of girls in grades 9 to 12 surveyed in the Commonwealth Fund in 1997 reported that they wanted to leave home because of violence or threat of violence at home. This study also showed that abused girls were twice as likely to have symptoms of depression, low self-confidence, and high stress. They were also more likely in grades 9 to 12 to smoke, drink, use drugs, and binge and purge. Girls with a history of physical or sexual abuse also reported more difficulty in accessing medical care.[70] In addition to finding substance abuse more common among adolescents with a history of sexual abuse, Hernandez also found substance abuse more likely in members of their immediate families.[71] The 1997

Youth Risk Behavior Surveillance conducted by the Centers for Disease Control revealed that 73% of all deaths among those aged 10 to 24 were from motor vehicle crashes, other unintentional injuries, homicide, and suicide.[72] Sexually abused adolescents are more likely to have emotional problems, aggressive or criminal behaviors, addiction risk behaviors, and suicidal behaviors.

Characteristics that increase the risk of date rape include younger age at first date, early sexual activity, early age at menarche, and a past history of sexual abuse or prior sexual victimization. Adolescents may also believe myths regarding forced sex and its acceptability under certain dating circumstances. Risk factors include date-specific behaviors such as who paid for the date, who drove, and the type of dating activity. A high percentage of date rapes are associated with alcohol use. Adolescents may underestimate the effect of alcohol in diminishing their coping responses, their ability to ward off an attacker, and its ability to cause misinterpretation of usual dating cues as sexual invitations. The illicit drug flunitrazepam (Rohypnol) is also a risk factor for adolescents and young adults.[73] Adolescents with a history of physical abuse, sexual abuse, or rape are more likely to participate in HIV-risk behaviors such as having partners who use intravenous drugs.[74,75]

The pregnant adolescent is at higher risk for assault both during her pregnancy and postpartum. The abuse may not be from the father of the pregnancy but from a family member. An association has been demonstrated between sexual abuse and early coercive sexual experiences and teenage pregnancy.[76,77] A study of 100 pregnant women between the ages of 12 and 24 revealed that 32% of the subjects had a history of sexual abuse, 29% physical abuse, and 46% emotional abuse. A history of past abuse was significantly higher in girls who had been pregnant as compared with "never pregnant" girls. The past history of physical abuse accounted for the association in this study.[78] Pregnant teens were found to have a higher percentage not only of abuse during pregnancy as compared with adult women, but also a higher percentage of teens reported abuse during the year prior to pregnancy.[79]

The adolescent female may have many mental health and physical consequences of sexual or other types of abuse. The Guidelines for Adolescent Preventive Services recommends annual health visits for adolescents that include routine screening for any history of sexual abuse as well as other types of abuse and assault.[80]

CONCLUSIONS

The issues in this chapter focus on the aspects of secondary prevention of abuse. We have dealt with identification of abuse that has already occurred, prevention of consequences, and reduction of future abuse.

Primary prevention must be dealt with by society in its family units, schools, and public policy arenas. Physicians can have an important impact in this area. A study performed in New Zealand (similar socioeconomic culture to the United States) followed a large birth cohort for 21 years. Data were collected in the areas of socioeconomic resources, family relations, educational achievement, and problem behaviors. Partner abuse was measured at age 21. By the age of 3 some antecedents of later abuse could be identified. At each sequential 3-year evaluation, the correlations grew stronger. By the age of 15, there were strong correlations in all four areas, with the most consistent predictor being early problem behaviors.[81] This study suggests that we must begin prior to adolescence in order to prevent intimate partner violence. The challenge is not only to teach healthy relationships and conflict management in relationships, but also to model these behaviors. Excellent role-modeling programs have been developed for use in the schools. The teaching must begin at home. Only then will we have a major impact on the prevention of violence.

REFERENCES

1. Collins KS, Schoen C, Joseph S, Duchon L, Simantov E, Yellowitz M. Health concerns across a woman's lifespan: the Commonwealth Fund 1998 survey of women's health. May 1999. (Available at: http://www.cmwf.org/programs/women/ksc_whsurvey99_332.asp. Accessed October 7, 1999.)
2. Tjaden P, Thoennes N. Prevalence, incidence, and consequences of violence against women: findings from the National Violence Against Women Survey. Washington, DC: Department of Justice, National Institute of Justice, Centers for Disease Control and Prevention, November 1998. Publication no. NCJ 172837.
3. Pagelow MD. Marital rape. In: Van Hasselt VB, Morrison RL, Bellack AS, Hersen M, eds. Handbook of family violence. New York: Plenum Press, 1988:207.
4. Beebe DK. Emergency management of the adult female rape victim. Am Fam Pract 1991;43:2041.
5. Slaughter L, Brown CRV. Colposcopy to establish physical

findings in rape victims. Am J Obstet Gynecol 1992; 166(Suppl):83.

6. Satin AJ, Hemsell DL, Stone IC Jr, Theriot S, Wendel GD Jr. Sexual assault in pregnancy. Obstet Gynecol 1991; 77:710.

7. Ramin SM, Satin AJ, Stone IC Jr, Wendel GD Jr. Sexual assault in postmenopausal women. Obstet Gynecol 1992; 80:860.

8. Peipert JF, Domagalski LR. Epidemiology of adolescent sexual assault. Obstet Gynecol 1994;84:867.

9. Holmes MM, Resnick HS, Kilpatrick DG, Best CL. Rape-related pregnancy: estimates and descriptive characteristics from a national sample of women. Am J Obstet Gynecol 1996;175:320.

10. Schwarcz SK, Whittington WL. Sexual assault and sexually transmitted diseases: detection and management in adults and children. Rev Infect Dis 1990;12(Suppl 6):S682.

11. Jenny C, Hooton TM, Bowers A, et al. Sexually transmitted diseases in victims of rape. N Engl J Med 1990; 322:713.

12. Gostin LO, Lazzarini Z, Alexander D, Brandt AM, Mayer KH, Silverman DC. HIV testing, counseling, and prophylaxis after sexual assault. JAMA 1994;271:1436.

13. Irwin KL, Edlin BR, Wong L, et al. Urban rape survivors: Characteristics and prevalence of human immunodeficiency virus and other sexually transmitted infections. Obstet Gynecol 1995;85:330.

14. Koss MP, Koss PG, Woodruff WJ. Deleterious effects of criminal victimization on women's health and medical utilization. Arch Intern Med 1991;151:342.

15. Koss MP, Heslet L. Somatic consequences of violence against women. Arch Fam Med 1992;1:53.

16. Young WW, Bracken AC, Goddard MA, Matheson S, New Hampshire Sexual Assault Medical Examination Protocol Project Committee. Sexual assault: review of a national model protocol for forensic and medical evaluation. Obstet Gynecol 1992;80:878.

17. Rao PN, Collins KA, Geisinger KR, et al. Identification of male epithelial cells in routine postcoital cervicovaginal smears using fluorescence in situ hybridization. Am J Clin Pathol 1995;104:32.

18. Center for Disease Control and Prevention. 1998 Guidelines for Treatment of Sexually Transmitted Diseases. MMWR 1998;47(No. RR-1):108.

19. ACOG Practice Patterns. Emergency Oral Contraception. Washington, DC: American College of Obstetricians and Gynecologists; December 1996, No. 3.

20. Fasoli M, Parazzini F, Cecchetti G, La Vecchita C. Postcoital contraception: An overview of published studies. Contraception 1989;39:459.

21. Lee SM, Dunn S, Evans F. Levonorgestrel versus the "Yuzpe" regimen. Can Fam Physician 1999;45:629.

22. Scott CS, Lefey HP, Hicks D. Potential risk factors for rape in three ethnic groups. Commun Ment Health J 1993;29:133.

23. Bachmann GA, Moeller TP, Benett J. Childhood sexual abuse and the consequences in adult women. Obstet Gynecol 1988;71:631.

24. Finkelhor D, Browne A. The traumatic impact of child sexual abuse. Am J Orthopsychiatry 1985;55:530.

25. Sarwer DB, Durlak JA. Childhood sexual abuse as a predictor of adult female sexual dysfunction: a study of couples seeking sex therapy. Child Abuse Negl 1996;20:963.

26. Lindberg FH, Distad LJ. Post-traumatic stress disorders in women who experienced childhood incest. Child Abuse Negl 1985;9:329.

27. Beitchman JH, Zucker KJ, Hood JE, daCosta GA, Akman D, Cassavia E. A review of the long-term effects of child sexual abuse. Child Abuse Negl 1992;16:101.

28. Wilsnack SC, Vogeltanz ND, Klassen AD, Harris TR. Childhood sexual abuse and women's substance abuse: national survey findings. J Stud Alcohol 1997;58:264.

29. Mullen PE, Martin JL, Anderson JC, Romans SE, Herbison GP. Childhood sexual abuse and mental health in adult life. Br J Psychiatry 1993;163:721.

30. Plichta SB. Violence and abuse: implications for women's health. In: Falik MM, Collins KS, eds. Women's health: the Commonwealth Fund Survey. Baltimore: John Hopkins University Press, 1996:237.

31. Robohm JS, Buttenheim M. The gynecological care experience of adult survivors of childhood sexual abuse: a preliminary investigation. Women Health 1996;24:59.

32. Reddy DM, Wasserman SA. Patient anxiety during gynecologic examinations. behavioral indications. J Reprod Med 1997;42:631.

33. Salmon P, Calderbank S. The relationship of childhood physical and sexual abuse to adult illness behavior. J Psychosom Res 1996;40:329.

34. Walker EA, Unutzer J, Rutter C, et al. Costs of health care use by women HMO members with a history of childhood abuse and neglect. Arch Gen Psychiatry 1999; 56:609.

35. Smikle CB, Satin AJ, Dellinger CL, Hankins GDV. Physical and sexual abuse: a middle-class concern? J Reprod Med 1995;40:347.

36. Parsons LH, Zaccaro D, Wells B, Stovall TG. Methods of and attitudes toward screening obstetrics and gynecology patients for domestic violence. Am J Obstet Gynecol 1995;173:381.

37. Rapkin AJ, Kames LD, Drake LL, Stampler FM, Nabboff BD. History of physical and sexual abuse in women with chronic pelvic pain. Obstet Gynecol 1990;76:92.

38. Walling MK, Reiter RC, O'Hara MW, Milburn AK, Lilly G, Vincent SD. Abuse history and chronic pain in women: I. Prevalences of sexual abuse and physical abuse. Obstet Gynecol 1994;84:193.

39. Domino JV, Haber JD. Prior physical and sexual abuse in women with chronic headache: clinical correlates. Headache 1987;27:310.

40. Drossman DA, Leserman J, Nachman G, et al. Sexual and physical abuse in women with functional or organic gastrointestinal disorders. Ann Intern Med 1990;113:828.

41. Walker EA, Keegan D, Gardner G, Sullivan M, Bernstein D, Katon WJ. Psychosocial factors in fibromyalgia compared with rheumatoid arthritis. II. Sexual, physical, and emotional abuse and neglect. Psychosom Med 1997; 59:572.

42. Plichta SB, Abraham C. Violence and gynecologic health in women <50 years old. Am J Obstet Gynecol 1996;174:903.

43. Falik MM, Collins KS, eds. Women's health: the Commonwealth Fund Survey. Baltimore: John Hopkins University Press, 1996.

44. Wingood GM, DiClemente RJ. The effects of an abusive primary partner on the condom use and sexual negotiation practices of African-American women. Am J Public Health 1997;87:1016.

45. Molina LD, Basinait-Smith C. Revisiting the intersection between domestic abuse and HIV risk. Am J Public Health 1998;88:1267.

46. Gazmararian JA, Lazorick S, Spitz AM, Ballard TJ, Saltzman LE, Marks JS. Prevalence of violence against pregnant women. JAMA 1996;275:1915.

47. Dietz PM, Gazmararian JA, Goodwin MM, Bruce FC, Johnson CH, Rochat RW. Delayed entry into prenatal care: effect of physical violence. Obstet Gynecol 1997; 90:221.

48. Amaro H, Fried LE, Cabral H, Zuckerman B. Violence during pregnancy and substance use. Am J Public Health 1990;80:575.

49. Campbell JC, Poland ML, Waller JB, Ager J. Correlates of battering during pregnancy. Res Nurs Health 1992; 15:219.

50. Parsons LH, Harper MA. An investigation of violent maternal deaths in North Carolina including a survey of the obstetric providers. Obstet Gynecol 1999;94:990.

51. Gazmararian JA, Adams MM, Saltzman LE, et al. The relationship between pregnancy intendedness and physical violence in mothers of newborns. Obstet Gynecol 1995; 85(6):1031.

52. Campbell JC, Pugh LC, Campbell D, Visscher M. The influence of abuse on pregnancy intention. Women's Health Issues 1995;5:214.

53. Glander SS, Moore ML, Michielutte R, Parsons LH. The prevalence of domestic violence among women seeking abortion. Obstet Gynecol 1998;91:1002.

54. Evins G, Chescheir N. Prevalence of domestic violence among women seeking abortion services. Women's Health Issues 1996;6:204.

55. Petersen R, Gazmararian JA, Spitz AM, et al. Violence and adverse pregnancy outcomes: a review of the literature and directions for future research. Am J Prev Med 1997; 13:366.

56. McFarlane J. Battering during pregnancy: tip of an iceberg revealed. Women Health 1989;15:69.

57. Sansone RA, Wiederman MW, Sansone LA. Health care utilization and history of trauma among women in a primary care setting. Violence Vict 1997;12:165.

58. Plichta SB, Weisman CS. Spouse or partner abuse, use of health services, and unmet need for medical care in U.S. woman. J Women's Health 1995;4:45.

59. Dearwater SR, Coben JH, Campbell JC, et al. Prevalence of intimate partner abuse in women treated at community hospital emergency departments. JAMA 1998;280:433.

60. Wisner CL, Gilmer TP, Saltzman LE, Zink TM. Intimate partner violence against women: do victims cost health plans more? J Fam Pract 1999;48:439.

61. Campbell JC, Pliska MJ, Taylor W, Sheridan D. Battered women's experiences in the emergency department. J Emerg Nurs 1994;20:280.

62. Gerbert B, Johnston K, Caspers N, Bleecker T, Woods A, Rosenbaum A. Experiences of battered women in health care settings: a qualitative study. Women Health 1996; 24:1.

63. Norton LB, Peipert JF, Zierler S, Lima B, Hume L. Battering in pregnancy: an assessment of two screening methods. Obstet Gynecol 1995;85:321.

64. McFarlane J, Parker B, Soeken K, Bullock L. Assessing for abuse in pregnancy: severity and frequency of injuries and associated entry into prenatal care. JAMA 1992;267:3176.

65. McFarlane J, Christoffel K, Bateman L, Miller V, Bullock L. Assessing for abuse: self-report versus nurse interview. Public Health Nurs 1991;8:245.

66. Schornstein SL. Domestic violence and health care: What every professional needs to know. Thousand Oaks, CA: Sage, 1997.

67. Council on Scientific Affairs of AMA. Violence against women: relevance for medical practitioners. JAMA 1992; 267:3184.

68. American College of Obstetricians and Gynecologists. Clinical Aspects of Domestic Violence for the Obstetrician/Gynecologist. Washington, DC, 1994.

69. Sappington AA, Pharr RE, Tunstall A, Rickert E. Relationships among child abuse, date abuse, and psychological problems. J Clin Psychol 1997;53:319.

70. Schoen C, Davis K, Collins KS, Greenberg L, Roches CD, Abrams M. The Commonwealth Fund Survey of the Health of Adolescent Girls. The Commonwealth Fund, New York, NY, November 1997.

71. Hernandez JT. Substance abuse among sexually abused adolescents and their families. J Adolesc Health 1992; 13:658.

72. Kann L, Kinchen SA, Williams BI, et al. Youth risk behavior surveillance—United States, 1997. State and local YRBSS coordinators. J School Health 1998;68:355.

73. Rickert VI, Wiemann C. Date rape among adolescents and young adults. J Pediatr Adolesc Gynecol 1998;11:167.

74. Cunningham RM, Stiffman AR, Doré P. The association of physical and sexual abuse with HIV risk behaviors in adolescence and young adulthood: implications for public health. Child Abuse Negl 1994;18:233.

75. Klein H, Chao BS. Sexual abuse during childhood and adolescence as predictors of HIV-related sexual risk during adulthood among female sexual partners of injection drug users. Violence Against Women 1995;1:55.

76. Boyer D, Fine D. Sexual abuse as a factor in adolescent pregnancy and child maltreatment. Fam Plann Perspect 1992;24:4.

77. Gershenson HP, Musick JS, Ruch-Ross HS, Magee V, Rubino KK, Rosenberg D. The prevalence of coercive sexual experience among teenage mothers. J Interpersonal Violence 1989;4:204.

78. Adams JA, East PL. Past physical abuse is significantly correlated with pregnancy as an adolescent. J Pediatr Adolesc Gynecol 1999;12:133.

79. Parker B, McFarlane J, Soeken K, Torres S, Campbell D. Physical and emotional abuse in pregnancy: a comparison of adult and teenage women. Nurs Res 1993;42:173.

80. American Medical Association. Guidelines for adolescent preventive services (GAPS), recommendations and rationale. Baltimore: Williams & Wilkins, 1994.

81. Magdol L, Moffitt TE, Caspi A, Silva PA. Developmental antecedents of partner abuse: a prospective–longitudinal study. J Abnorm Psychol 1998;107:375.

Chapter 36

Stress Management

Renate H. Rosenthal

Five Key Points

- Physical symptoms are often the first clue that emotional things are out of balance.
- Collectively, minor unremitting woes can create as much distress as some major calamities.
- We take better care of our cars than of ourselves.
- The authority vested in the medical profession can give patients the impetus to set limits on unreasonable demands.
- Stress management is not just a collection of techniques, but a way of life.

Stress is an inevitable part of the human experience. For purposes of this chapter, the word *stress* will be used to mean strain on personal endurance. Such strains can be due to acute trauma. More commonly, however, a whole host of normal events and challenges combine to cause an ongoing and, at times, overwhelming struggle to keep going.

Women who experienced or witnessed domestic violence, rape, or criminal assault may suffer from serious sequelae. Survivors of other disasters may show the same symptom constellation, collectively known as posttraumatic stress disorder.[1] Nightmares, flashbacks, severe anxiety, phobic avoidance, and depression are common in the wake of such episodes. In addition, there may be intense psychological distress surrounding cues that trigger recollections of the event. Memory may be affected, and there may be a marked desire to withdraw from social activities. There are persistent symptoms of increased autonomic arousal that were not present before the trauma. These include sleep disturbance, irritability and out-

bursts of anger, poor concentration, hypervigilance, and an exaggerated startle response. The patient may be unable to carry out the duties of everyday life, and psychiatric help may be required.

On the other hand, everyone is subject to benign stress. This condition is not, in and of itself, a psychiatric problem. However, if a person's endurance is challenged too severely, for too long a time, and to an extent that chronically exceeds available emotional and physical resources, symptoms appear. Patients may not even be fully aware that they are taxed beyond their limits. They come to the physician's office with a variety of physical problems and a general sense of malaise. Rarely is stress the actual chief complaint and often its impact is minimized or even denied at first.

Some sources of stress may be major life changes that would test anyone's coping skills: Death of a spouse or loved one; move to a new city that has required a major change in routine for the whole family; increase in responsibilities through promotion, job change, or "downsizing"; divorce, remarriage, with the challenge of being fair and understanding toward new stepchildren; empty nest; or financial woes. In addition, there are the inevitable daily hassles: Intricate logistics of juggling family schedules, babysitters, and careers. Add car trouble, a difficult boss, a chickenpox epidemic in the day-care center, manipulative officemates, a new neighbor who parties loudly all night long, a flea infestation afflicting the family pets, mice in the kitchen, squirrels in the attic, dead leaves in the gutters and nobody to clean them out, a backed-up toilet, and a sullen son or daughter with the mood swings and crises of puberty—none of these are, by themselves extraordinary events.

Nowadays, most women have complicated lives, trying to combine and juggle multiple roles. A constant sense of falling behind, of not living up to one's obligations, seems to be the norm. The financially secure "stay-at-home mom" is almost extinct. The notion of "having it all," career and family, has made way to women "doing it all," often as single parents and sole breadwinners, with minimal emotional support, in stressful and unrewarding jobs.

In his book *Drawing Life*,[2] David Gelernter, one of the survivors of the attacks of the "Unabomber," reflects on life and values in the latter part of the 20th century. In his musings about our society, he presents a very thought-provoking analysis of the consequences of the feminism of the 1960s. He refers to it as the Motherhood Revolution, which resulted in huge numbers of women joining the work force in the past 20 years or so. Far from having a fulfilling and challenging career with its financial and otherwise affirming rewards, "the average working mother sits at her desk in a big noisy room with a hundred other women at some insurance company in Peoria, and worries about her children. A generation ago she would have been at home taking care of them. Are we better off as a society now that she spends her day processing claims instead?"

As pressure mounts without constructive escape, a certain characteristic symptom picture emerges.

CLINICAL FEATURES

Physical Symptoms

Stress can bring out gynecologic and other physical symptoms that lack detectable organic causes, such as vague and shifting aches, exacerbation of premenstrual syndrome, pelvic pain, menstrual problems, and lack of libido. Musculoskeletal symptoms may include pain in the back, neck, and shoulders. Other manifestations of stress are: headaches, digestive trouble, shortness of breath, chest pain and tightness, numbness and tingling, sleep problems, lack of energy, chronic fatigue, and memory problems.

Psychological Symptoms

Psychological symptoms include anxiety, excessive worry, feeling of doom, heightened startle response, hypervigilance, irritability, impatience, forgetfulness, making mistakes, being accident-prone, argumentativeness and short fuse, bad temper, mood changes, emotional lability, tearfulness, crying spells, feeling easily hurt, and feeling seriously unappreciated, angry, or used. There also may be a decline in sense of humor, increased social withdrawal, brooding and rehashing problems, and an inability to "let go"—to shift focus to pleasant and constructive things. Often there is a defeatist attitude about making any positive changes.

DIAGNOSTIC CONSIDERATIONS

Stressed people run the gamut from well-adjusted individuals who have become overwhelmed to seriously ill psychiatric patients. The first order of business is to assess whether the patient satisfies the criteria for a psychiatric disorder. Many of the symptoms mentioned above also apply to panic and anxiety disorder, major depression, somatoform disorder, and substance abuse. Patients who fit those diagnostic criteria are discussed in more depth in Chapter 30. It is very important to keep these psychiatric illnesses clearly in mind as potential diagnoses before deciding that the patient is suffering mainly from "benign" stress. Many health-care dollars are wasted by failure to recognize readily treatable psychiatric problems early enough, by inadequate use of psychiatric drugs, and by reluctance to refer patients to psychiatic specialists who routinely and effectively deal with these disorders.

Psychiatric problems rarely emerge out of the blue. In predisposed patients, they can be triggered and compounded by overwhelmingly stressful circumstances. Medication may be the first line of treatment for these women, but the interventions outlined in this chapter can be combined with any psychiatric treatment.

Physical symptoms are often the first clue that things are out of balance. Patients may initially deny being stressed because they cannot point to some major recent tragedy or calamity and they have learned to accept their pressured lives as inevitable. However, the sheer cumulative amount of strains and daily hassles may keep tension and anxiety at an intolerably high level and may easily account for the symptoms at hand. A useful schematic is the stress turbine (Figure 36-1).

Collectively, minor unremitting woes can create as much tension and distress (or more) as some of the major problems that feed the "turbine" and keep the engine churning. The most significant and severe problems may be impossible to change, at least in the short run. For example, one may not be able to move on to a less stressful job or get out of a difficult marriage. Many of the minor issues, on the other hand, may lend themselves to creative solutions. Regardless of where the "flow" is reduced, the "turbine" will

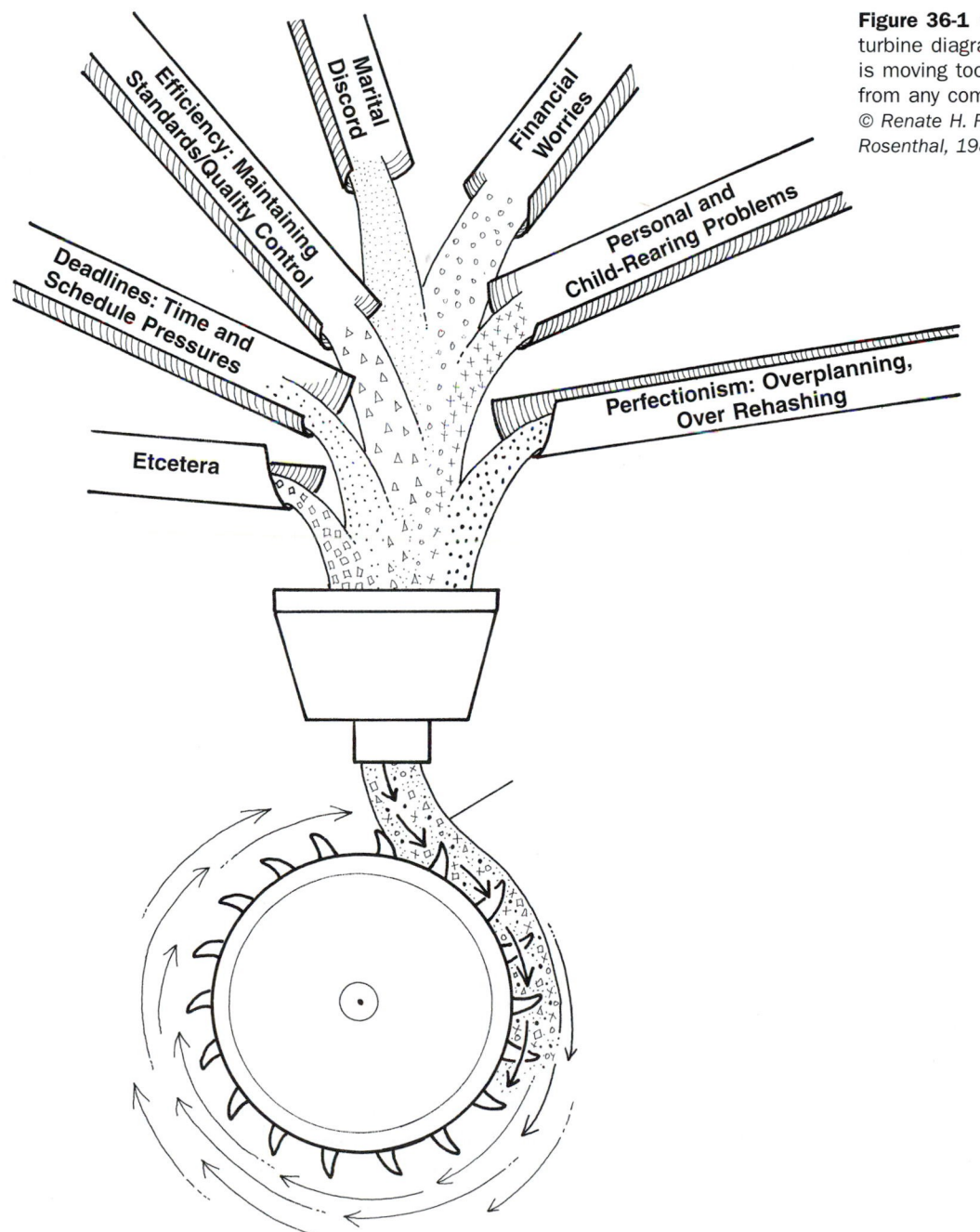

Figure 36-1 Combined flow stress turbine diagram. Once the turbine is moving too fast, reduce the flow from any combination of sources. © *Renate H. Rosenthal and Ted L. Rosenthal, 1981.*

turn at a slower speed when there is less stress feeding it. This reduction in "speed" will then permit some constructive escapes.

ASSESSMENT

As part of a good history and physical examination, questions about smoking, alcohol, drugs, and diet are routinely asked. However, in a busy office rarely is the time taken to learn about the texture of a patient's daily life. Very little is known about the pressures, problems, and daily hassles she has to face, about the challenges she has to meet. A few minutes of focused inquiry can yield a wealth of information. Ideally, all patients should have a chance to talk about themselves. Often the gynecologist is the only physician the woman sees on a regular basis, the only one to assess her physical and emotional well-being. In fact, unless she has other physical problems, her annual check-ups may be the only contact she has with the medical profession.

Many office appointments are precipitated by unstated emotional issues. Funds are wasted on tests and procedures and on prescriptions for low doses of antidepressants and anxiolytics when what is really needed is support, encouragement, guidance, and education about how to lead a more balanced existence.

Taking a Stress History

Patients with puzzling symptoms and those who seek care frequently should have the benefit of a psychosocial history to shed light on the context of the problem. This includes a thorough accounting of the pressures and changes that characterized the patient's life before she took ill. A good way to start is to ask: "Tell me what the last 18 months have been like for you. Have there been any major changes in your life? Any big challenges you have had to meet? What about the sheer amount of daily hassles and responsibilities?"

However, care must be taken to explain that inquiring about her life stress by no means implies that her physical complaints are not "real" or "in her head." She needs to be reassured that her symptoms will be carefully evaluated, no matter how much stress she has been under, and that even bona fide physical conditions are complicated and exacerbated by chronic stress.

Other important information includes personal and family history of abuse (physical, sexual, and emotional), of alcohol and drugs, and of psychiatric disorders. The latter is very important because it has major implications for the use of psychiatric medications. These concerns are discussed in more detail in Chapter 30.

Patients who were raised in abusive and emotionally unstable home situations are more likely in adulthood to have serious psychosocial problems. They often choose very troubled and abusive partners, and their lives may be chaotic. They are greatly overrepresented in the population of patients with chronic pain syndromes, depression, substance abuse, and somatization disorders.

Some patients are reluctant to admit to problems in their family of origin because they do not want to jump on the bandwagon of declaring themselves "victims" or they do not want to soil their own nest. It helps to explain that understanding and recognizing one's early problems is not the same as whining or feeling sorry for oneself, nor is the goal to pin blame on others for current problems. Rather, one needs to understand one's own background and upbringing so that one can allow for it and make good decisions as an adult.

Stressed people have lost the ability to balance work and play. Poverty or family troubles may have kept some from ever learning about sports, hobbies, or leisure interests. Others can easily point to fun activities they used to do and might enjoy again, but those have become very low priorities due to lack of time and energy. Stress management demands that the patient regain a balance of work and play.

INTERVENTIONS AND RECOMMENDATIONS

Patient Education—Setting the Stage

There is no substitute for fully educating patients about stress and about its effects and its management. They need to understand the conceptual framework that underlies the recommendations that are to follow so they do not mistakenly feel like their problems are being dismissed out of hand as "just stress." If a thorough assessment indicates that stress is a major problem, the subject can be introduced as follows:

It seems that you have been very stressed for a long time. Your symptoms are your body's way of telling you that things have gone too far, that you need to slow things down somehow and make time to take care of yourself. To get a better sense of balance in your life.

We take better care of our cars than of ourselves. For the car, we rotate the tires. We check the shock absorbers. We change the oil and flush out the cooling system. We use good gasoline.

Where are your shock absorbers? What happened to your personal maintenance schedule? What happened to the fuel you use to keep running?

At this juncture, patients typically admit they are stressed, start to enumerate their pressures, and insist that there are no changes that can be made in the situation.

It helps to then show the graphic of the stress turbine. A picture may be worth a thousand words:

This is how I think of your situation. There are so many things that contribute to keep your turbine running at top speed. We need to work on finding out which of these you can reduce or even eliminate for the sake of your physical and emotional health.[1]

People can develop all kinds of symptoms when they are very stressed. Again, this is not something that is "in your head"; it is a real problem. This is how the body tells a person that there are too many demands. The treatment is to reduce some of the stress, to help achieve more peace, to get things into a better balance. People tend to go on and on, to do what has to be done, to rise to the occasion, to carry on all duties and obligations until the body says "Too much! No more! Help!" This is a signal that things have gone too far, have gotten out of control, and that one needs to step back and look at what's going on.

"Stress" does not necessarily mean major disasters. Often it is the sheer number of demands—not any one of which would qualify as an extraordinary strain. Nevertheless, they can all add up to result in an overwhelming situation.

The bodily effects of stress—heightened anxiety, tension, sleep problems, and aches and pains—themselves become cause for worry. This further increases the speed of the "turbine." Recreation and leisure activities are the first thing to let go. This makes it even harder to unwind. Many people resort to alcohol or drugs as a shortcut to get some relief, which causes even more problems." This provides a good opportunity to inquire about substance use.

Once the stage has been set, the patient may decide to talk about her burdens. This can, in itself, be very therapeutic. Chances are she feels angry and overwhelmed, yet guilty about not being up to the task. Empathic, nonjudgmental listening may be the most effective intervention at this juncture.

Setting Priorities

The pressure in the stress turbine must be reduced to a more manageable level. This may include delegating tasks that can be done by others, setting firm limits on unreasonable demands, calling in favors from friends, and simplifying the daily routine. It is best to refrain from making too many specific suggestions. Rather, the physician can provide a road map of stress-management principles without getting involved in the details. The authority vested in the medical profession can give patients the backup they need to set necessary limits: "My doctor told me I have to slow down." "My doctor told me I need more rest." Many paths can lead to stress reduction. However, the common denominator is to reduce the flow into the turbine from any of the sources, and to achieve a better balance between work and play.

The better the patient's emotional health, the more responsive she will be to guidance. Some patients quickly find creative ways to help themselves once they understand just how overwhelmed they have become. They feel that they have a right to have their needs respected and are able to take the necessary steps. They do not have fundamental skill deficits in assertiveness or a deep-seated lack of self-esteem that keeps them from looking out for their own welfare. They just did not diagnose their own problem correctly to begin with. Now that they have learned what is wrong, they know how to ameliorate the problem, relieved that they are not medically ill.

Others, while agreeing that they are severely stressed, seem unable to envision how they could possibly simplify their lives. They remain highly dubious that stress could be at the root of their somatic complaints. Any suggestions are met with negativism and "yes—but" comments. There may be an almost masochistic insistence on being the listening ear and the leaning post for everyone else, on being the one who comes to the rescue of those in trouble when she has nothing left to give. Typically, these women have never learned how to nurture themselves, how to set appropriate limits. Although change occurs slowly, if at all, these patients benefit emotionally by having a chance to unburden themselves. Many are clinically depressed and in need of psychiatric and psychological help. They may accept medications, but resist the idea of getting some much-needed counseling; however, they can often be persuaded to get help for themselves once they understand the reasoning behind the referral. Being labeled as "crazy" or appearing to be of weak moral fiber is their greatest fear.

Time Management

Stressed people try to squeeze too many activities and chores into too short a time period. They add to their desperation by making themselves chronically run against the clock. They arrive wherever they go in a state of tension and emotional disarray.

Here are some rather simple techniques that may help the problem:

1. Set the alarm early enough to do what needs to get done in the morning. If you cannot decide the night before what to wear, allow time to make this decision in the morning. There are to be no last-minute "innovations," e.g., additions of chores and activities that delay departure, even if there are a few spare minutes. Problems need to be put on hold, and conversation must steer away from conflict unless it is a true emergency. Especially if two or more people have to leave home at the same time, this simple rule can prevent fights and acrimony and get the day off to a better start.
2. Allow enough time to drive safely or to meet your mode of transportation without getting down to the wire.
3. Do not routinely overschedule the day. Plan your lunch hour. If there is a good chance that there may not be a "lunch hour," take some wholesome food along to work, just in case. Fruit, cheese, raisins, and a bagel go a long way. Then you will not end up at the snack machine in desperation.
4. Keep a list handy and add to it when things that need to be done come to your mind. Do not try to rely on your memory alone. Prioritize the chores on the list and do them when you can, but do not try to squeeze them in without allowing sufficient time.
5. Allow yourself to take off a day now and then to catch up with chores and errands that cannot be done on the side.

Diaphragmatic Breathing

This relatively simple technique can enhance a patient's sense of well-being. Stressed people typically engage in very shallow breathing, punctuated by sighs and gasps. Many have tightness in the chest, a feeling of not getting enough air. Patients are instructed to take a deep breath, through the nose, using the muscles of the diaphragm rather than those of the rib cage, to hold it for about 5 seconds, and to slowly exhale through slightly pursed lips. Patients should take five such breaths, take a brief break, and practice this twice a day. They can learn to "spot-check" their breathing patterns throughout the day.

Watching a woman's breathing during the interview is very informative. Often sensitive topics provoke labored breathing and sighing. When asked, the patient will often admit to episodes of numbness, lightheadedness, feelings of derealization, and palpitations. In severe cases, this may lead to emergency room admissions for hyperventilation and panic attacks. Unfortunately, these spells are often misdiagnosed and dismissed as "just nerves." Some patients suffer for years, while they become more and more dysfunctional. Panic attacks are a readily treatable psychiatric disorder that requires proper diagnosis and close follow-up.

Relaxation Training

There are a whole host of relaxation techniques. Some patients may have had prior instruction in relaxation procedures, but are too stressed to practice the skill. Women already familiar with the Lamaze method through childbirth classes can be encouraged to refresh their memory and use what they learned there.

Another technique, known as guided imagery, involves deep breathing while visualizing a calm and peaceful scene. One of the secrets of managing stress is learning to distract onself, to shift one's mental focus from burdensome issues to pleasant and enjoyable things. This is not the same as engaging in denial. Rather, it is a refusal to unnecessarily rub one's nose in problems that one can do nothing about. Guided imagery provides a structured way of peaceful "daydreaming," combined with some deep-breathing exercises.

A good way to introduce the topic is as follows:

I would like for you to become good at shifting pictures in your head away from stressful things to calm and peaceful things. Stressed people become so caught up in their troubles that they need to make an extra effort to achieve a sense of mental calm. This is what this exercise is all about. It is a skill you can learn, and if you practice it and become good at it, you can take it with you wherever you go.

First I need to know what is really calm and peaceful for you. Try to think back to a time when you felt really calm, peaceful, carefree—when you had a sense of peace and joy. It could be a time long ago, a simpler time. Or it could be a vacation spot, a place where you felt far away from the cares of the world. Can you come up with such a place?

Most patients have no trouble with this. We hear about sunsets at the beach; a path through the woods; views from a mountain with a breeze blowing; floating on a raft in the swimming pool; sitting by the side of a lake on a warm summer evening; early morning in the back yard with bird songs and dewdrops and a fresh scent in the air.

The next step is to get the patient to elaborate on her image, to develop it into a three-dimensional scene. What season of the year? What time of day? What does the air smell like? What are the sounds? What is the temperature? Where is the sun? Where is the patient in the scene?

It is then necessary to add some elements that bring the scene alive. It is boring to focus on a static picture for any length of time. The scene needs movement and change: Clouds changing shape, a slight breeze that moves the leaves, wild birds in various activities and locations, ripples in the water, light reflecting from dewdrops and dancing in stippled shade.

Once the scene is complete, the patient is asked to settle comfortably into her chair, close her eyes, and take a deep breath through her nose:

Take a deep breath—hold it—and slowly exhale. When you are ready to do it again, take a deep breath—hold it—and slowly exhale. And again. . . .

Now, starting at the top of your head, relax your forehead. And your cheeks. And your jaws. And your upper arms. And your lower arms. And your hands, all the way down to your fingertips.

Relax your neck. Your shoulders. Your chest. Your back. All the way down to your waist. Relax your buttocks. Your stomach. Your thighs. Your calves. Your feet. All the way down to your toes.

Now, in your mind's eye, picture yourself in your peaceful place.

At this point, the therapist can elaborate on the patient's peaceful scene.

When you have the scene clearly in your mind, raise a finger of your left hand. Keep on imagining youself in the scene. You are calm and peaceful and nobody is making any demands on you.

After 3 or 4 minutes of this, the patient can be brought back to the present:

Now, I will count backward from ten, and when I get to three, I'll ask you to open your eyes. 10–9–8–7–6–5–4–3—open your eyes—2–1. Welcome back!"

The whole exercise takes no more than 10 minutes from start to finish. Most patients remark with surprise how far away they felt, and how refreshing it was to escape for a while. Imagery should be practiced daily, and the technique can be used to drift off to sleep.

This is a skill like any other skill. If you get good at this, you can use it when you find yourself getting uptight and anxious. For it to be beneficial, though, you have to already know what to do when you need it. So you need to practice it when you are feeling basically all right, to have the skill actually available to you when you first get tense.

As an aside, a number of medical students of the University of Tennessee College of Medicine learned this technique in their first semester as part of a stress-management class and reported using it throughout their medical school career with good results.

Deep muscular relaxation[3] is another popular technique. It consists of progressively tensing and relaxing muscle groups, until the whole body is relaxed. This procedure is useful for people who lack the ability to clearly visualize peaceful scenes. Unfortunately, most patients find this technique very boring. It requires more time and a physical setup where the patient can recline or lie down comfortably. Both guided imagery and deep muscular relaxation can be easily combined. Audiotaped relaxation instructions are available at "New Age" and health food stores. Also, some patients enjoy listening to recordings of peaceful nature sounds, for sale in record and CD outlets.

Biofeedback

Some people have a lot of trouble following any of the relaxation instructions. They may lack the ability to visualize peaceful scenes or the patience to tense and relax the various muscle groups for progressive relaxation. Mental imagery may impress them as esoteric hocus pocus. In rare cases, patients have fundamental religious objections to procedures and techniques that, to them, seem to be in conflict or competition with the power of prayer. Biofeedback offers an attractive alternative.

The patient is hooked up to recording equipment and receives direct feedback (auditory or visual) about changes in physiologic parameters, such as muscular tension or skin temperature. In addition to assisting in achieving a state of relaxation, biofeedback is a treatment option for tension and migraine headaches, Raynaud disease, and several other physical ailments.

Exercise and Movement

When stress mounts, recreational activities and physical exercise fall by the wayside. It is ironic that the activities that help patients the most to reduce tension and anxiety are the ones that are the most likley to be abandoned because there are not enough hours in the day. Stressed people may, indeed, have neither time nor energy to plan time-consuming exercise regimens. However, they may commit to going for regular short walks or to taking stairs instead of elevators. They might explore the idea of attending a weekly dance class. Dance and movement provide enjoyable stress relief and companionship. Except for ballroom dancing, a partner is not necessarily required, which makes it a pleasant diversion for single people. The patient's taste in music may dictate her choice of activity. There is tap, step dancing, American Square Dance, Scottish Ceilidh, English Morris and Country Dance, and Louisiana Zydeco, to mention just a few. The physical activity, combined with music and social companionship, is an excellent way to decompress. Rather than aiming for the "ideal" level of aerobic exercise and doing none of it, the patient should be encouraged to do what is enjoyable and practical.

T'ai Chi and Yoga

T'ai Chi, an ancient Chinese technique, is a "soft" martial art. It fosters a sense of balance, increases muscle tone and flexibility, and enhances concentration. The exercises, while simple, require full attention, effectively distracting the student from workday hassles and preoccupations. A main goal is the "harmonious merging of thought and action,"[4] providing respite from worry, anger, fear and fruitless ruminations. T'ai Chi is appropriate for people of all ages and can be recommended with confidence, not just as a calming technique, but as a way to enhance general well-being. Instructional books and videotapes are avail-

able; however, there is no substitute for a skilled teacher because the beginner needs extensive individualized guidance and support. Also, the social aspect of group interaction is therapeutic in itself.

Yoga is another avenue to increased physical and emotional well-being. It is more physically active and "athletic" than T'ai Chi and may be more appealing to people who lack the patience required for T'ai Chi.

Both Yoga and T'ai Chi are taught and practiced in many different styles. To find qualified instructors, one may need to shop around until one finds a person whose style and training inspire confidence. Some patients may say they have "tried" these disciplines and found them lacking. Chances are they did not have a congenial and well-trained instructor. It is a good idea to get names and telephone numbers of reputable Yoga and T'ai Chi institutes in the region so you can refer patients.

Nutrition

The higher the stress level, the more dismal the eating habits. Reducing caffeine and sugar intake, planning and procuring fresh nutritious meals, and staying away from alcohol are important aspects of a good stress-management program. Rather than eating on the run, viewing food as only fuel, patients need to place a higher value on making their meals a wholesome and restoring experience.

Contemporary society has bought into the idea that it is perfectly all right to eat in a rush and to settle for food that is neither tasty nor wholesome. A whole industry has sprung up around the concept that there is no such thing as a right or a wrong place to eat, drink, and munch, that sitting down to a meal is a rare luxury reserved for holidays. Mealtime at home should be a time of peace and a small celebration. Everything tastes better if the table looks nice and if the food is served attractively. Conversation should be pleasant and enjoyable. Controversial topics have no place at the dinner table.

Self-Care and Self-Nurturing

Many stress-prone people lack the skills to take good care of themselves. Often they were not well cared for and nurtured as children. Early attempts to assert their own needs and desires were labeled as "selfish" by punitive and controlling authority figures. In adult life, these people tend to neglect their own well-being for extended periods. They push on to the point of getting completely exhausted and threadbare, in the mistaken assumption that all of this can be undone during an anticipated vacation or holiday. More often than not, these yearned-for "escapes" prove to be not nearly as restorative as had been hoped and the grind begins anew.

Self-care skills can be learned. They involve paying attention to the small pleasures inherent in each day if the patient slows down enough to notice and enjoy them. A prerequisite is that the flow in the stress turbine be reduced to a manageable level. Then one can move from the mode of damage control to learning a new, slower, more conscious and more rewarding way of life.

A good way to start is to reduce clutter. In times of chronic stress, a person's environment is neglected to the point of utter chaos. A major clean-up, followed by discarding and giving away unwanted and unneeded items, may be the first step. Then, the aesthetics of the home deserve attention.

People should be encouraged to surround themselves with things they like and to arrange them in ways they find pleasing. One does not need to wait for special occasions to light candles, to scent the air, to put flowers on the table, to open the curtains and windows to let the sunshine in, to use nice soap for showers, to get the kind of toothbrush one likes. To keep fresh sheets on the bed and to play enjoyable music. People should work on making their home peaceful and inviting. The home should be a pleasant sanctuary rather than a dingy cave. It should look, feel, smell, and sound like a place one wants to come home to.

Intrusions and invasions of unnecessary stress into the home must be minimized. Unless firm boundaries are drawn, one is constantly invaded by unpleasant news and information that is neither needed nor wanted.

Radio and television are prime purveyors of bad news. There is no need to contaminate one's home by continuous blow-by-blow accounts of crime, wrongdoings, injustice, disasters, corruption, and impending doom. One is not enriched by inviting the flotsam and jetsam of the world into one's living room. Those who wish to reduce stress should keep

their television sets off unless there is a program they specifically and consciously wish to watch. Even educational programs can be disconcerting. Although it is sadly true that the environment is being degraded and that whole animal species are threatened with extinction, watching it happen in the living room does not help one's stress level.

The radio is easier to control, but even there, listening should be a conscious decision rather than a habit. Home computers and the World Wide Web have added a new dimension. Unsuspecting users can easily be seduced into wasting excessive time in front of the screen—time that might be used more wisely to enjoy nature and the outdoors, to move around, and to connect with friends.

Many people carry problems and gossip from work back into their homes where they get rehashed and rehearsed, invading what should be a safe and pleasant sanctuary from the outside world. Sometimes it takes some rather drastic steps to keep work-related stress at the office where it belongs. Self-discipline is required to ban intrusions from the home. Today's culture fosters the notion that one must be indispensable and always on call. Beepers, cell phones, call waiting, laptop computers—they all keep a person constantly yoked to whatever is happening. There is this constant nagging feeling that one may be missing out on something important by not being instantly available. Yet, anything that is truly important will still be around a few hours later, or even on the next day. Unwanted and inconveniently timed calls can be screened by an answering machine and returned later, if at all. Taking a leisurely bath, sitting down to a nice dinner with candles and flowers on the table, talking with loved ones, reading a good book—all these are important activities that nurture one's soul.

Therapeutic massage is a wonderful way to relieve stress. This is especially good for patients who do not have caring and supportive partners who might give them a good back rub at the end of the day. A good massage therapist should be on the same resource list as a good instructor for Yoga and T'ai Chi.

Some states license massage therapists as they do health-care providers. In addition, there is national certification. More information can be obtained from schools that teach therapeutic massage. However, word-of-mouth recommendations may be the best way to find a competent massage therapist.

CONCLUSION

Stressed people get buried in their multiple demands, unable to focus on what is truly important in life. The following saying may help keep things in perspective: "Walk around feeling like a leaf. Know you could tumble any second. Then decide what to do with your time."

Stress managment is not just a collection of techniques, but a way of life. It consists of a thorough assessment of the problems that stress the patient, followed by a conscious and considered effort toward a slower, less complex, and more meaningful and peaceful existence.

The philosophy of this chapter can be summed up in the famous Serenity Prayer:

God grant me the serenity to accept the things I cannot change, courage to change the things I can, and wisdom to know the difference.

SELECTED READINGS

Moore T. Care of the soul: a guide for cultivating depth and sacredness in everyday life. New York, Harper Perennial, 1992.

This book is not easy reading. The author draws on a wide array of sources, ranging from ancient philosophy to Jungian and contemporary psychological theory. The outcome is an interesting, thought-provoking and insightful book that addresses many of the value-questions raised in this chapter.

McQuiston JII. Always we begin again: the Benedictine way of living, Harrisburg, PA: Morehouse Publishing, 1996.

A little gem of a book, hip-pocket size, which outlines the directions for monastic life written by Benedict of Nursia in the 6th century in Italy. This is in no way a religious treatise. Rather, it provides the reader with a set of wise and extremely sensible "rules" and reflections that guide us toward a more balanced outlook on life.

Huff B. The tao of Pooh. New York, Penguin Books, 1983.

A delightful translation of the children's story of Winnie-the-Pooh, who was a master at managing his stress, into Taoist philosophy.

Rosenthal TL. To soothe the savage breast. Invited essay. Behav Res Ther 1993;21:439.

An exhaustive and scholarly review of stress-managment and calming techniques. It includes a comprehensive list of books and videotapes which can serve as enjoyable distractors from day-to-day hassles.

REFERENCES

1. American Psychiatric Association. Diagnostic and Statistical Manual of Mental Disorders, 4th ed. Primary Care Version. Washington, DC: American Psychiatric Association; 1994:47.
2. Gelernter D. Drawing life. New York: Free Press, 1997:97.
3. Benson H. The relaxation response. New York: Morrow, 1975.
4. Galante L. T'ai Chi: the supreme ultimate. York Beach, ME: S. Weiser, 1981.

Chapter 37
HIV/AIDS

Melissa Appleton
Robert E. Morrison
Rani Lewis

Five Key Points

- AIDS refers to the symptomatic evidence of immunocompromise caused by infection with the HIV virus.

- Medical therapy with highly active antiretroviral therapy (HAART) must be maintained appropriately (without missing doses) and indefinitely to avoid worsening disease.

- Treatment and management of HAART and of the multiple opportunistic infections to which these patients are susceptible is best performed with the assistance of an Infectious Disease or HIV specialist.

- Transmission of HIV virus to a fetus (vertical transmission) is decreased with the use of antiretroviral medications.

- Vertical transmission is possibly reduced with increased use of cesarean delivery.

Since physicians first noted a pattern of immunodeficiency and lymphadenopathy in gay men in 1981, human immunodeficiency virus (HIV) has spread rapidly around the globe. HIV-1, present in chimpanzees for centuries but not disease-causing, has probably been passed to humans on many occasions; but only in the past three decades have social conditions allowed an epidemic in humans.[1] Global travel, changing sexual mores, intravenous drug abuse, and undiagnosed contamination of the blood supply have contributed to the pandemic of HIV infection in the past 20 years. The HIV retrovirus was identified in 1983, and testing for the virus became available in 1985. Zidovudine (AZT), the first nucleoside reverse-transcriptase inhibitor available, was approved for use in 1987; although far from a perfect drug, it led to increased life expectancy and was an important advance in reducing vertical transmission and decreasing occupational spread. Protease inhibitors became available in September 1995, and the nonnucleoside reverse-transcriptase inhibitors later in June 1996. Also in 1996, the FDA approved the viral-load plasma viral RNA test. By 1997, triple combinations of dual nucleosides and protease inhibitors, so-called highly active antiretroviral therapy (HAART), were being employed in routine clinical practice, and more recently, even five or more drugs (MegaHAART) have been used. With these therapies, a sustained rise in CD4 and suppression of viral load have been observed in some patients for up to 5 years.[2]

BASIC SCIENCE OF HIV INFECTION

Although much has been learned regarding the pathogenesis and immune response to HIV as well as the clinical aspects and therapy of HIV-positive patients and those with the acquired immunodeficiency syndrome (AIDS), the remaining domain is a rapidly evolving field of study that requires a commitment to continued learning and practice. This chapter is designed to provide an initial overview of the topic, but those not willing to become expert should probably not care for these patients without consultation.

HIV-1 and the closely related HIV-2 are relatively large, 100 nm, enveloped RNA retroviruses of the lentivirus family. HIV-1 and HIV-2 are genetically related to retroviruses from other species of the animal kingdom. HIV-1 is the major cause of HIV infection worldwide; HIV-2 is closely related to the monkey AIDS virus, simian immunodeficiency virus (SIV). HIV-2 infection in humans appears to be less virulent, and to date, has been reported in West Africa, the United States, and Europe.[3] Mature HIV particles contain two copies of the HIV genome in single-stranded RNA wrapped in a tightly packed protein core (p24) surrounded by a lipid-containing envelope. The core also has been shown to contain partial, variably reverse-transcribed DNA chains as well as other proteins necessary for the early viral life cycle.[4,5]

A lipid envelope surrounds the core particle. The envelope contains imbedded glycoproteins (gp41 and gp120), which bind to specific receptors on T helper cells, macrophages, and monocytes. In addition, the binding and affinity of gp120 for CD4 is specific and very strong. Coreceptors, CCR-5 or CXCR-4, are chemotactic cytokine receptors that mediate the specific binding of virulent strains of HIV-1 into monocytes or T lymphocytes.[6-8]

On gaining entry into the cell, the viral RNA uncoats and becomes transcribed by reverse transcriptase into double-stranded proviral DNA. This may circularize or may, with viral integrase, become integrated into the host cellular DNA. Within the cell, the virus may then become latent until activated, with resultant viral production, budding, and cell death. Cellular activation is essential for the production and propagation of HIV.

Regardless of the route of infection, after transmission of HIV, the virus binds to CD4-positive cells of several kinds. Although the CD4-positive T lymphocyte is the principal cell type involved in infection, CD8 cells, human macrophages, monocytes, peripheral and follicular dendritic cells, oligodendroglia, microglia, astrocytes, retinal cells, renal cells, cardiac monocytes, trophoblastic cells, cervical cells, and rectal mucosal cells may be infected.

The virus usually enters the body by way of mucosal surfaces, such as the oropharynx, rectum, and genitalia. These tissues contain abundant Langerhans cells; dendritic cells, which communicate directly with the mucosal surface; and lymphocytes.

Based on experiments with SIV and macaque monkeys, it is believed that within a few days of intravaginal infection, virus spreads first to neighboring monocytes and lymphocytes and then to regional lymph nodes, with subsequent viremia and widespread lymphatic seeding.[9] Virus turnover and cell death occur very rapidly, with a viral half-life of about 6 hours and cell death within 2 days. During the primary viremia, the virus may reach titers of 10 billion particles per milliliter of blood. After the primary viremia, an initial drop in viral load occurs within 2 to 6 weeks, before the onset of detectable HIV antibodies, probably mediated by cellular cytotoxic T lymphocytes and by antibody-dependant cellular cytotoxicity. Events leading to cellular activation either by virus or cytokines may result in increases in viral load.[10,11]

During the acute HIV viral syndrome the relatively rapid rate of viral replication, and the naturally high variability of the genome, mediated by the imprecision of the reverse-transcriptase enzyme, may allow the virus to mutate into a new quasispecies in situ.[12] HIV virus has a mutation rate of 3×10^5 mutations per nucleotide per replication cycle (one mutation in every three 10,000-based paired genomes). Many mutated species are less lethal or less infectious. This is compensated for by the rapid rate of viral replication and by the recombinant sharing of RNA, which has been termed "primitive sexuality."[13] The heterogeneity and rapid viral turnover allow the virus to evolve into a more highly virulent syncytium-forming variant and to develop resistance to a host of antiviral agents while changing antigen coding so as to better evade immune surveillance in situ in a given patient.[14]

Since the virus also infects and destroys many of the very cells that would eliminate it, the resulting viral loads and T-cell counts may be viewed as a dynamic equilibrium between the ongoing competition between the virus and the host immune system. While initially the virus has the greatest affinity for macrophage–monocytes in the lymph nodes, after mutation to the more CD4-positive T-cell variant, the virus spreads more rapidly.

After resolution of the initial drop in CD4 cells, the CD4 and T-cell counts may rise, returning to near normal levels.[15,16] The virus seems to kill cells by multiple mechanisms, including programmed cell death, or apoptosis.[17] At all stages of infection, viral loads and replication are higher in the lymphoid organs than in the peripheral blood. Before the advent of HAART, the median time from infection to marked immunosuppression and opportunistic infection was up to 10 years; so the immune system would appear to have substantial reserve.

EPIDEMIOLOGY

HIV first became known in this country as a disease of homosexual white males, and that perception persists in some communities despite evidence to the contrary. Minority women now constitute the fastest-growing group of individuals with newly diagnosed HIV and AIDS. The disease is becoming increasingly spread by heterosexual means, with women showing a corresponding increase in infection rates. It is estimated that 6000 women with HIV give birth each year in the United States. Women now account for 20% of the cases of AIDS in the United States reported to the Centers for Disease Control and Prevention (CDC) and, depending on the geographical region, an even greater percentage of cases of HIV.[18]

The likelihood of sexual transmission of HIV is determined by the epidemiologic parameters of infectivity: duration of infection, rate of change of sex partners in the susceptible population, and the frequency of sexual activity. Infectivity depends on the viral load and the occurrences that increase viral numbers at the site of transfer—i.e., genital ulcerations, bleeding such as occurs during menstruation, tissue breaks or friable tissues, which occur in uncircumcised men or in females with cervical ectopy. Also, there is peak transmissibility soon after infection due to the high viral load found early in the epidemic curve. The principal means of transmitting HIV in the United States is through sexual contact, accounting for 76 to 85% of the over 28 million infections in humans. Other modes of transmission are via accidental needlestick, planned needle-sharing among intravenous drug users, mother-to-infant, and/or via transfusion of infected blood products. Rates of transmission can vary from as little as 1 in 1000 female-to-male episodes of sexual intercourse to up to 1 in 10 in some male-to-male sexual activities. Seroconversion following transfusion with HIV-infected material has been estimated to be as high as 1:1. In the absence of medical therapy, perinatal transmission (from mother to infant) has a prevalence rate of 22 to 25%.[19] With the use of oral AZT therapy antepartum, intravenous AZT intrapartum, and oral AZT elixir to neonates postpartum, the transmission rate decreases to 7.6%, a 67% reduction in transmission rate. The use of HAART and/or elective cesarean section further reduces the rate of transmission to ~2%. While antiretroviral therapy does not affect the detection of virus in cervical/vaginal specimens, the use of HAART has been estimated to yield an ~80% reduction in the rate of perinatal transmission.[19]

The prevalence of genital ulcer disease such as chancroid, syphilis, or herpes is associated with an increase in the relative risk of transmitting HIV in both men and women from 1.7 to 7. Concomitant infection with *Neiserria gonorrhoeae*, *Trichomonas vaginalis*, or *Chlamydia trachomatis* are associated with an increase of 60 to 340% in the prevalence of HIV infection, and a twofold increase in HIV transmission is associated with sexually transmitted diseases (STDs) with purulent cervical secretions. Cervical ectopy carries with it a 1.7- to 5-fold increased risk of infection.

PRIMARY INFECTION

More than 50% of patients with primary HIV infection will initially have nonspecific signs and symptoms, making an accurate diagnosis dependent upon a high index of suspicion on the part of the clinician. Patients with symptomatic infection tend to progress more rapidly and may particularly benefit from early potent antiretroviral treatment. Diagnosis of infection with HIV is made by enzyme-linked immunosorbent assay (ELISA), HIV-1 RNA quantitation, and p24 antigen testing. False positive and false negative results can occur, so diagnosis of HIV infection is only made after a positive ELISA is repeated, again found to be positive, and a Western blot test is performed for confirmation. The two ELISAs and Western blot can generally all be performed on a single blood sample; some physicians prefer to repeat an ELISA after a month for confirmation along with a Western blot if one of the initial tests is positive. With the requirement of serial positive tests, the false positive rate has been estimated at <1%.[20] The "primary HIV infection" portion of the syndrome occurs within 2 to 3 weeks after acquisition of the virus, is described as flu-like, and usually lasts an additional 2 to 3 weeks prior to spontaneously resolving.

Treatment of primary HIV-1 infection remains controversial; many experts recommend the early initiation of potent antiretroviral treatment, once the patient recognizes and accepts the need to continue this treatment indefinitely. The early hope of eradication of the virus by the use of potent therapy has been proven untenable at present; but early treatment may still benefit the patient by decreasing the rate of viral mutation, preserving immune function, and possibly reducing the risk of viral transmission. The drug combinations used in the treatment of primary infection are those used for established indications and have the same risks associated with their use.

Steady State

Generally, within 6 to 12 months of acquiring HIV, a steady-state level of viral replication will be reached that is predictive of the rate of progression to AIDS. The steady-state period extends from the time of the resolution of the primary infection to the development of clinical manifestations of AIDS. The length of the steady-state period will depend on the virulence of the infecting viral strain and the effectiveness of the host immune system. The "steady state" is most often a steady state of decline. While the majority of patients progress to AIDS in an average of 10 years after infection, about 5% progress to AIDS over a period of 15 to 20 years.[21,22] It has been theorized that these so-called long-term nonprogressors may have a less virulent strain of HIV, but it is generally believed that they may have a less susceptible immune system.

The absolute number of CD4 (helper) lymphocytes may drop below 200 mm³ during acute infection, but in most patients, the drop is less dramatic. A drop in CD4 cell counts of 200 to 300 cells in the first year after infection is common. CD4 cells decrease by an average of 60 to 75 cells/mm³/year in steady state in the untreated patient, and the average patient takes 10 years to progress to AIDS. A common laboratory marker for AIDS is an absolute CD4 count of <200 cells/mm³ or 14% of all lymphocytes. The

rate of progression to AIDS can be predicted by the level of viremia at steady state. The likelihood of AIDS developing within 3 years can be predicted by looking at both the viral load and the CD4-cell count. One explanation of the interaction of viral load and CD4-cell counts is to say that HIV might be thought of as a hill, with the viral load determining how steep the hill is and the CD4-cell count showing where the patient is on the slope.

Immunity wanes as the CD4-cell count decreases. During the CD4-cell count decrease from a normal level of 800 to 1200 to the AIDS-defining level of 200, the patient is often asymptomatic. The waning immunity makes the patient susceptible to common infections, such as mycobacterial tuberculosis, even prior to being classified as having AIDS. Sexually transmitted diseases such as syphilis, chancroid, herpes simplex virus (HSV), and human papillomavirus (HPV) may become more difficult to treat and often require higher doses of medications and longer courses of treatment. Shingles may appear in an otherwise healthy-appearing young person and should raise some concerns about HIV infection. The patient may present with chronic feelings of tiredness or other nonspecific symptoms. Again, a high index of suspicion on the part of the clinician may be required to make the diagnosis of HIV during this period.

AIDS

The transition from HIV to AIDS is frequently marked by nothing more than a decrease in the CD4-cell count to a level <200 cells/mm³. AIDS can be diagnosed at a higher CD4 level if an opportunistic infection (OI) is diagnosed. Most opportunistic infections, however, occur with a CD4-cell count less than 200 (Table 37-1). It is at this point also that systemic manifestations of HIV itself, such as dementia, wasting, and cytopenias begin to become more pronounced.

Studies have demonstrated that prompt and early treatment may help to prevent occupationally acquired HIV infection among health-care workers as well as vertical transmission from infected mothers to their children. Early recognition and treatment of primary infection with HAART may prevent the destructive polyclonal immune response. Although most people seroconvert within the first 6 to 12 weeks, the HIV ELISA antibody test may not become positive for up to 6 months or longer after primary

TABLE 37-1
CD4-CELL COUNT AT WHICH RISK FOR OI INCREASES

Cell Count	Opportunistic Infection
200 cells/mm^3	*Pneumocystic carinii* pneumonia
100 cells/mm^3	Coccidiodomycosis
	Histoplasma
	Cryptococcus
	Toxoplasma gondii
50 cells/mm^3	*Mycobacterium avium-intracellulare* complex
	Cytomegalovirus

infection. The viral RNA may not be detected until 3 to 6 weeks after infection, and the test results may be false negative, especially at lower titers. The earliest available test of infection is the HIV proviral DNA test; the use of this may demonstrate HIV-infected lymphocytes as early as 3 weeks after infection.

Although some patients with primary HIV infection are asymptomatic, symptoms have been described in as many as 50 to 90% of patients.[23,24] Individuals who have severe clinical symptoms at this time appear more likely to progress rapidly to AIDS than do those who experience asymptomatic primary infection.[25,26] The most common early signs and symptoms of HIV infection are fever, fatigue, and myalgias and/or arthralgias. Adenopathy, pharyngitis, diarrhea, headache, and a skin rash have also been reported in as many as 74% of patients. Nausea and vomiting, mucocutaneous ulcerations, and thrush have also been described. Neurologic involvement, including photophobia, meningitis, encephalitis, peripheral neuropathy, facial palsy, Guillian–Barre syndrome, brachial neuritis, radiculopathy, cognitive impairment, and psychosis have occurred.[27-30] A rash may occur, which has been described as erythematous, macular, mixed maculopapular, vesicular, or a pustular exanthem.[31,32] Histopathologic examination of a scraping from this rash may show a sparse lymphocytic infiltrate in the dermis surrounding the vessels of the superficial plexus.[31,32] Esophageal ulceration, candidiasis, vasculitis, nephritis, rhabdomylosis, acute renal failure, idiopathic pneumonitis, and aplastic anemia may occur but are less common.

During the primary infection, patients generally have a relatively homogeneous population of viral particles; in persons after long-term infection, a more diverse population of viruses and a greater likelihood that viruses have mutated to become resistant to antiviral agents may be present.[33,34] It therefore follows that treatment should be more effective during this phase of infection, and early treatment may have important beneficial effects on the immune system. However, in light of the many side effects of long-term HAART, controversy exists over the initiation of therapy during primary infection. The first regimen is considered the best chance of therapeutic effectiveness, regardless of when it is started.

Laboratory findings such as transient leukopenia and lymphopenia, CD8-cell lymphocytosis, a depletion of CD4 cells, and the development of atypical lymphocytes occur frequently. Thrombocytopenia, anemia, and elevation of hepatic enzymes may also occur.[35] The viral load is extremely variable during the primary HIV infection and may range from 20,000 copies to more than a million copies per milliliter. At this time, the individual is highly infectious. Mathematical models have predicted that from 56 to 92% of all HIV infections are transmitted during the period of acute infection.[36] The diagnosis of acute primary HIV infection should be based on a high index of suspicion and in individuals with high-risk behavior. In the absence of HIV antibodies, diagnosis may be confirmed by examination of proviral DNA or HIV RNA. It should be understood that with a low titer, the results of the quantitative HIV RNA test might be false positive. The HIV p24 antigen test may be positive but is less sensitive than the other tests of infection. Changes in the CD4 to CD8 ratio will eventually develop in all patients, and severe immunosuppression may develop in some. Cases of tuberculous meningitis, ocular cryptococcosis, *Pneumocystic carinii* pneumonia (PCP), prolonged cryptosporidiosis, esophageal candidiasis, and cytomegalovirus (CMV) colitis have been described in untreated primary infection. Investigators have related the duration and relative intensity of primary HIV infection with the subsequent course of HIV disease. The risk of AIDS developing within 3 years was eight times greater in subjects whose primary disease lasted longer than 14 days than in those who were asymptomatic.[37]

The likelihood of an opportunistic infection developing depends on the immunocompetence of the host and on the virulence and availability of the viral strain. As AIDS is diagnosed with severe immunosuppression, exposure to potential pathogens is required before disease can result. Opportunistic infection (i.e., with PCP, CMV, toxoplasmosis, and mycobacterial tuberculosis) may develop because of the interaction between the pathogen and host's depleted immune function. Superinfection with *Mycobacterium avium–intracellulare* (MAI), *Cryptococcus neoformans*, disseminated histoplasmosis, and cryptosporidiosis may be associated with latent reactivation of a previously sustained infection or newly obtained disease if the sufficiently immunocompromised host encounters the infectious agent.[38] More virulent organisms such as mycobacterial tuberculosis and *Streptococcus pneumoniae* may cause illness in patients with relative immunocompetence, as can latent varicella–zoster virus. Although Candida species can inhabit the gastrointestinal tract of many individuals, an overgrowth of oral candidiasis (frequently known as thrush) is itself an opportunistic infection and is an early clinical marker of immunosuppression, forewarning of the development of AIDS in many patients.[39] Age may be a confounding variable for the development of clinical disease.[40]

Clinical Findings

In the 1980s, generalized lymphadenopathy was seen in 50 to 70% of HIV-infected individuals and usually involved the posterior and anterior cervical, supraclavicular (best correlation), submandibular, occipital, axillary, epitrochlear, and femoral nodes. Marked generalized lymphadenopathy is not quite as common now, but some lymphadenopathy is still noted. Nodes may range in size from 0.5 to 2 cm. Localized or asymmetric nodes or rapid nodal enlargement suggests an infectious or malignant process. Peritracheal or hilar adenopathy is unusual, but abdominal imaging has revealed enlarged mesenteric and retroperitoneal nodes in HIV-infected persons. There is no correlation between the lymphadenopathy and rate of progression of immunodeficiency. Patients with HIV persisting in generalized lymphadenopathy may show follicular hyperplasia with loss of architecture and large germinal centers with viral replication occurring in the follicular and dendritic cells.[41] A node larger than 2 cm, rapidly enlarging, symptomatic, or suggestive of another entity such as Hodgkin disease, mycobacterial infection, lymphoma, Kaposi sarcoma, sarcoid, or secondary syphilis should be biopsied.

Early in HIV disease, immune thrombocytopenia may develop. Most cases are asymptomatic, with bleeding complications extremely rare. Platelet counts may remain low for years only to return to near normal in late-stage disease. On bone marrow examination, there will be increased megakaryocytes with erythroid hyperplasia. This destruction has been shown to occur peripherally. Chills, fever, weight loss, and thrombocytopenia with pancytopenia suggests opportunistic infections such as disseminated histoplasmosis, *Mycobacterium avium–intracellulare*, or lymphoma. Severe anemia may occur in patients with advanced HIV infection but also may be related to opportunistic infections or bone marrow suppression by drugs.[42] HIV-infected patients have been observed with parvovirus B19 infection causing pure red-cell aplasia with normal leukocyte counts.[43,44]

Fever, other than low-grade, is rarely due solely to HIV. A study of HIV infected outpatients with fever found that 83% had either opportunistic infections with PCP, MAI, related bacteremia, bacterial pneumonia, sinusitis, lymphoma, or drug reactions. Fever for longer than 2 weeks was most often associated with an AIDS-defining illness. Significant weight loss in the absence of opportunistic infections or malabsorption is highly unlikely.

Indications for Testing

There are six broad indications for offering HIV testing: signs and symptoms of acute HIV, signs and symptoms consistent with chronic HIV or AIDS, pregnancy, recognized risk factors, documentation of a patient's self-reported diagnosis of HIV, and persons requesting the test. The last group may include low-risk members of the "worried well" who should be gently discouraged if they repeatedly present for testing without identifiable risk factors on pretest counseling. This group may also be less willing to admit to a high-risk behavior, and should therefore not be assuaged too quickly.

The signs and symptoms of acute and chronic HIV are discussed elsewhere in this chapter, but of special concern in women are frequent and severe outbreaks of vaginal candidiasis and herpes. Pregnant women should be encouraged to be tested early in each pregnancy when possible or otherwise whenever they present for care. Recognized risk factors for HIV include other infections such as tuberculosis and STDs, intravenous drug abuse, unprotected sex (particularly men who have sex with men), multiple sexual partners, and occupational exposure. Documentation of a self-reported positive HIV test is important for medical and legal reasons. Some patients may have used home test kits of questionable efficacy or may have been incorrectly informed of a positive diagnosis in the past. In addition, there is a small subset of patients who falsely claim to be HIV-positive for secondary gain.

Pretest Counseling

The goals of pretest counseling are to obtain informed consent for testing; to educate the patient about HIV, its transmission, and tests employed; to address individual risk factors and risk reduction; and to address follow-up of the test results and follow-up care. The clinician should be aware of state laws governing informed consent. For example, is documentation of the patient's verbal consent sufficient or should consent be written? How is the positive test to be reported, and who will have access to the information? Too often only a brief attempt at obtaining informed consent is made, and patient education is neglected.

Posttest Counseling

Posttest counseling should be highly individualized. The test results should be conveyed in person, in a compassionate manner. For those who are seropositive, the importance of seeking treatment should be stressed and referrals made where necessary for medical care and case management. Often a patient will be too distraught to hear more than the positive result. However, an effort should be made to again discuss methods of transmission and ways to prevent spread of the virus to others. This visit also serves as a good time to address risk factors and ways to maintain a patient's seronegativity for those who have a negative test.

Available Tests

The most commonly used test is the HIV ELISA which, in low-risk groups, has a high rate of false positive results and always requires a confirmatory Western blot. The SUDS (single-use diagnostic systems) test for HIV has been licensed by the FDA for screening, but, like the ELISA, should be followed by a Western blot. Other somewhat less used tests are also available.

Initial Evaluation

The goals for the initial evaluation of persons with HIV are staging of the disease with CD4-cell counts/percentages and viral load, a thorough history-taking and physical examination, evaluation for other infections commonly associated with HIV, and continuation of the education process. Recommended laboratory studies are a Western blot for HIV (if this is not already documented); CD4-cell count and percentage of CD4 to CD8 lymphocytes; quantification of the viral load with the polymerase chain reaction (PCR) test; hepatitis B and C serologic tests; a complete blood count with differential; rapid plasma reagin (RPR) test; toxoplasma antibody; urinalysis; and a chemistry panel containing, at a minimum, electrolytes, blood urea nitrogen (BUN) and creatinine, liver-function tests, and total protein and albumin. In addition, a tuberculosis skin test/purified protein derivation (PPD) and chest radiography should be done. Laboratory abnormalities discovered should be further evaluated. In our referral clinic, the patient is also initially evaluated by a social worker, a nutritionist, and a nurse who takes a history, including a review of systems and risk factors.

The physical examination should look in particular for the following: wasting; skin disorders such as scalp or facial dermatitis, Kaposi sarcoma, bacillary angiomatosis, eosinophilic dermatitis, dermatophytoses; oral manifestations such as aphthous ulcers, thrush, oral hairy leukoplakia, and gingivitis; lymphadenopathy, thyromegaly, lung and heart abnormalities; hepatomegaly; splenomegaly; evidence of STDs, including pelvic and rectal examinations; and neurologic dysfunction.

After the initial evaluation and staging are complete, a decision regarding therapy should be reached with the patient. Treatment is generally indicated for any patient with symptomatic HIV and for an asymptomatic patient with a CD4-cell count less than $500/mm^3$ or a viral load greater than 10,000 on B-DNA test or greater than 20,000 on reverse transcription PCR (RT-PCR) (Roche). The treatment is chosen with the goal of suppressing the viral load to undetectable levels.

A pneumococcal vaccine is given early in the course of treatment, as is a course of hepatitis B vaccine if the patient does not show serologic evidence of prior infection. Tetanus–diphtheria vaccine is given if none has been received in the past 10 years. Influenza vaccine is given seasonally and is strongly encouraged. Persons with a positive PPD and a clear chest x-ray film with no evidence of active disease and no history of previous treatment should be started on a course of isoniazid for 9 months. Any active infection detected should be treated promptly and aggressively. Patients from areas where multidrug-resistant tuberculosis is endemic should be treated with the assistance of an infectious diseases specialist when possible.

The physician first treating a patient presumed to be HIV-positive must make certain of the diagnosis by personally viewing test results. These should be obtained, or if they are unable to be obtained, a new test should be performed and the positive ELISA and Western blot confirmation of the test should be documented. If the patient has other symptoms or signs of HIV, such as pharyngeal candidiasis, posterior cervical adenopathy, hairy leukoplakia, or Kaposi sarcoma, these may be viewed as a confirmatory test but should not replace personal viewing of the documentation of the HIV-positive ELISA and Western blot confirmation. Effort should be made to ascertain the most recent CD4-cell count if known and a viral load performed. The treating physician should ask the patient when they first found out that they were HIV-positive, where was the test was conducted, for what reason it was performed, where the patient obtained health care previously, and if the patient ever had a negative HIV test. In addition to the medical history, family history, and review of systems, careful attention should be addressed to any HIV-related illnesses, particularly the common OIs or weight loss (over 10% of body weight). Inquiry should be made about the patient's history of vaccination as well as of tuberculosis, PPD, and/or chest x-ray examination. A very careful gynecologic history should be taken, including history of pregnancies, premature births, miscarriages, abortions, number and outcome of pregnancies since diagnosed with HIV, and last menstrual period. Women should be asked about plans for pregnancy, what method of birth control has been used, and information regarding Pap smears. All patients should be asked about medications they are taking. A social history, including smoking and alcohol and illicit drug use, should be discussed. Sexual preference should be discussed, and safe-sex practices should be discussed. Inquiry should be made about the HIV status of the patient's partner as well as if any previous partners have tested positive.

A review of systems should include unexplained weight loss, night sweats or fevers, headaches, changes in appetite, difficulty thinking, any history of skin rash, sores in the mouth, painful swallowing, chest pain, cough, shortness of breath, abdominal pain, right-upper-quadrant pain, diarrhea, numbness, tingling or shooting pains in the legs or hands or feet, muscle weaknesses, or changes in vision or spots before the eyes. Keeping track of immunizations is a vital part of the history. Patients with stable disease should be followed every 3 to 4 months, with more frequent visits if laboratory values are changing rapidly or more opportunistic infections develop.

Treatment with Antiretroviral Agents

There are currently three classes of drugs available for the treatment of HIV and 18 drugs approved by the FDA. These drugs have multiple toxicities and drug interactions that can only be touched on here. The clinician is encouraged to exercise utmost caution in the use of these medications and to seek expert guidance.

Nucleoside Reverse-Transcriptase Inhibitors (NRTIs)

NRTIs act by competitively binding reverse transcriptase and lead to premature viral DNA chain termination.

Zidovudine (AZT, ZDV) was approved by the FDA in 1987 and is the oldest antiretroviral agent. It was initially given at higher doses than is given at present, which may contribute to its bad reputation among certain patient populations. The current dose is 300 mg orally every 12 hours for most indications, although higher doses may be used in the treatment of HIV dementia and the idiopathic thrombocytopenia associated with HIV. It has been associated with improving HIV dementia, as well as prolonging survival, lengthening the time of progression to AIDS, decreasing vertical transmission, and decreasing transmission after occupational exposure. Side effects are many and sometimes limit use of the drug. They include bone-marrow suppression, particularly anemia and neutropenia, headache, myopathy, nausea, vomiting, and fatigue. Caution should be used when this medication is given in conjunction with other drugs that have a suppressive effect on the bone marrow, such as ganciclovir or hydroxyurea. It is often used in combination with lamivudine as Combivir, which contains 300 mg zidovudine and 150 mg lamivudine and is taken every 12 hours.

Didanosine (ddI) is the second oldest antiretroviral agent. While effective, the major associated toxicities, including pancreatitis (5%), peripheral neuropathy (2 to 14%), and diarrhea, occasionally necessitate cessation of this medication. ddI is acid-labile, and therefore, the preparations are heavily buffered. This buffering can interfere with the absorption of medications, such as itraconazole and dapsone, which require acid for absorption, and medications such as tetracycline, which bind to the buffering agent. The usual adult dose is two 100-mg tablets dissolved in water and taken every 12 hours or two 200-mg tablets every 24 hours on an empty stomach. Other medications known to cause pancreatitis, such as pentamidine, should be used cautiously in a patient taking ddI.

The use of zalcitabine (ddc) has been severely limited because of its side effects and the availability of other, more potent, antiretroviral agents. The most common side effect is peripheral neuropathy, which occurs in up to 30% of patients. The other side effects include rash, esophageal ulcerations, and cardiomyopathy. The usual dose is 0.75 mg orally every 8 hours.

Stavudine (d4T) has modest antiretroviral activity but is generally well tolerated. The major side effect is peripheral neuropathy, and other medications with this side effect should be used cautiously in combination with stavudine; although it has generally been used without problems in combination with ddI. It should not be used in combination with ZDV because of antagonism of these medications when used in the same treatment regimen. The usual dose is 40 mg orally every 12 hours.

Lamivudine (3TC), also used in the treatment of hepatitis B, has rapid development of HIV resistance when used as a single agent, but the mutations responsible for the resistance cause the virus to regain sensitivity to ZDV. 3TC is well tolerated, with little systemic toxicity. It is given as 150 mg orally every 12 hours in the treatment of HIV, often as a component of Combivir.

Abacavir is the most potent of the current nucleoside analogs against HIV and is generally well tolerated. It may cause some gastrointestinal or central nervous system symptoms. The most important complication is the development of a hypersensitivity reaction in 3 to 5% of patients. This reaction, manifested as a rash plus systemic signs and symptoms such as fever, nausea, and vomiting, sore throat, cough, abdominal pain and arthralgias, may be deadly if the patient is rechallenged with the drug. The usual dose is 300 mg orally every 12 hours.

Nonnucleoside Reverse-Transcriptase Inhibitors (NNRTIs)

NNRTIs are effective agents without cross-resistance with NRTIs or protease inhibitors. However, they share cross-resistance as a group, with resistance to one generally conferring resistance to the others. There are multiple drug interactions associated with this class of drugs, only some of which are mentioned below.

Nevirapine shows good efficacy with sustained response when used in combination with other potent antiretroviral agents but rapidly develops resistance when used as a single agent. It induces cytochrome P-450 enzymes and its own metabolism, as well as decreases the plasma concentration of other medications such as protease inhibitors. Dosage adjustments are often indicated. The most common side effect is a morbilliform rash, although more severe rashes may be seen. The medication should be stopped and not restarted if the rash is severe or accompanied by constitutional symptoms. The usual dosage is 200 mg daily for 2 weeks; it is then increased to 200 mg twice a day.

Delavirdine is indicated in combination with NRTIs and seems to show synergy with this class of drugs. The most common side effect is a rash, which generally does not require discontinuation of the medication. There is cross-resistance with the other drugs in the NNRTI class but not with NRTIs or protease inhibitors. Drugs that induce cytochrome p3A (CYP3A) decrease delavirdine levels and should be avoided. Other drugs to be avoided with delavirdine include astemizole, cisapride, triazolam, alprazolan, and midazolam. The usual dose is 400 mg orally three times a day.

Efavirenz is a potent new NNRTI that can be used in place of a protease inhibitor in the initially prescribed antiretroviral combination. Side effects are common but not necessarily an indication to stop therapy. Vivid dreams noted by about 50% of patients are particularly common but resolve within a few weeks and can be modulated by 2 weeks of lorazepam, 0.5 mg orally at bedtime. A rash is also common in some instances but may be treated with antihistamines. Efavirenz is an inducer of CYP3A4. It should not be used with clarithromycin, astemizole, cisapride, midazolam, and triazolam. The usual dose is 600 mg at bedtime. Because of gross malformations seen in the offspring of pregnant cynomolgus monkeys given efavirenz, it is not currently recommended for use in pregnant women.

Protease Inhibitors

Protease inhibitors (PIs) prevent the cleavage of precursor proteins to mature proteins and enzymes. All may cause glucose intolerance, peripheral lipodystrophy manifested by fat wasting of the face and upper body, gynecomastia, and buffalo hump.

Ritonavir is a very potent antiretroviral drug. However, drug interactions, and until recently, the unpleasant taste of the liquid form, have kept the drug from wider usage. The formulation of the drug into capsules has helped palatability, as has the practice of taking ritonavir with chocolate beverages. Gastrointestinal side effects such as nausea, vomiting, and diarrhea are common but rarely cause discontinuation of therapy. Most important are the interactions with many medications used in the treatment of patients with HIV/AIDS as well as other medications. Ritonavir is frequently used in low doses as an "inducer" with other PIs. Ritonavir capsules should be kept refrigerated. The usual full dosage of capsules is 600 mg three times a day with food; lower doses are given when used as an inducer.

Saquinavir was the first PI to be approved by the FDA and is well tolerated. However, the first formulation (Invirase) had poor bioavailability due to metabolism by cytochrome P-450 enzymes. The new formulation (Fortovase) comes as soft gel capsules and addresses this problem, but ritonavir is often used in combination with saquinavir to increase the levels. Saquinavir has an attractive resistance profile that has little cross-resistance with the other PIs. Dosing must be carefully adjusted when given with drugs that affect the cytochrome P-450 enzymes, but the usual dose is 1200 mg orally three times a day with meals.

Indinavir is a potent PI with a prolonged antiretroviral effect when given in combination with nucleoside inhibitors. It is generally well tolerated, although the nephrolithiasis seen in 5 to 10% of patients is a potential problem. It is thought that this is caused by crystallization of the drug in the kidneys and might be prevented by the ingestion of large amounts of fluid. Resistance to indinavir may also mean resistance to the other PIs. It should not be used in conjunction with terfenadine, astemizole, cisapride, triazolam, or midazolam. The usual dose is 800 mg three times a day with 12 oz of fluid but without food. There are some concerns about this medication when used in pregnancy because of immature neonatal renal function, but this has not been fully established.

Nelfinavir is a potent drug and is one of the best tolerated of the PIs. The main side effect associated with usage is diarrhea, seen in up to 50% of cases, but this may be controlled with loperamide (Imodium) as needed and is rarely the cause of drug discontinuation. The diarrhea is rarely a problem when used in pregnant women, making this an effective therapy in this population. The recommended dosage is 750 mg orally (three pills) three times a day with or without food, but it is increasingly being used at 1250 mg orally (five pills) twice a day with or without food.

Amprenavir is the latest of the antiretroviral agents to be approved by the FDA. It is synergistic in combination with saquinavir, didanosine, zidovudine, and abacavir, and additive with indinavir and ritonavir. The most common side effect associated with amprenavir is rash in over 25%, with a severe rash such as Stevens–Johnson syndrome in 1%. Other side effects and drug interactions are common with the other PIs. The usual dosage is 1200 mg orally twice a day with or without food (avoid high-fat food).

Intensifiers

While not a classic antiretroviral drug, hydroxyurea is the most common intensifier of these therapies. It seems to work by increasing the activity of NRTIs, particularly the effect of didanosine. One side effect is bone-marrow suppression, and thus, the drug should be used cautiously, if at all, with other drugs known to suppress the bone marrow. The usual dose is 500 mg twice a day.

Ongoing Treatment

Physicians treating patients with HIV/AIDS should conceptualize their work in two frameworks. The first framework is that HIV/AIDS is a viral infection caused by a RNA retrovirus that uses reverse transcriptase and infects monocytes, macrophages, CD3 lymphocytes, skin cells, and neurons. The second framework addresses immune dysregulation and cell death. This, if left untreated, results in gradual and progressive depletion of immunocytes and depletion of CD4 cells and leads to the development of more frequent infections with common organisms such as staphylococcus and pneumococcus, predisposition to tuberculosis, and manifestations of herpes zoster. Immune dysregulation may result in a shift in immune response and in allergic reactions, rhinitis, sinusitis, asthma, and autoimmune disorders. As immune depletion continues, opportunistic infections such as PCP, cryptococcosis, disseminated fungal infections, candida esophagitis, toxoplasmosis, and bacterial pneumonias with common organisms such as the pneumococcus and uncommon organisms can occur.

The two frameworks are related by the amount of circulating virus. The higher the viral load, the more rapid progression of CD4-cell count loss. The average length of untreated HIV infections may be up to 10 years between the initial infection and the onset of opportunistic infections. With a viral load under 10,000, disease usually progresses very slowly. When the viral load is over 30,000, the disease progresses more rapidly, with the CD4-cell count falling over a period of 6 months to 2 years. From 10,000 to 30,000, the disease may progress in an intermediate fashion. A physician seeing a patient with HIV infection must address both the CD4-cell count and the viral load in order to provide appropriate care for the patient.

Viral Kinetics

Ho and colleagues[45] found that the CD4 cells survive an average of 6 hours after infection with rapid viral turnover. The CD4-cell count, therefore, represents a product of the infected immune system's ability to reconstitute and repair versus the ongoing viral productivity. Patients treated with PIs frequent develop viral loads that are undetectable in the serum. However, these patients are not "cured"; the virus can still be found in deep lymph nodes. If these patients were then to stop taking medications, they could easily regress from an undetectable viral load one day to as many as 10 billion virions the next day.[46] Montaner et al. have shown that missing as few as two or three doses over 52 weeks may result in suboptimal results.[46] Viral loads commonly range from a low of <40 (the current limit of detection using the ultrasensative PCR assay) to as high as 1 million virions per milliliter.

Current guidelines recommend beginning therapy with three drugs and changing at least two drugs or preferably all three drugs when either the viral load increases significantly, when the CD4-cell count falls significantly, or when the clinical condition deteriorates. It is no longer acceptable to treat with only two drugs, since all two-drug combinations are associated with deterioration in immune function. Monotherapy of any kind is contraindicated because it allows early emergence of resistance to whatever drug is used. The sole exception of this use is zidovudine in a pregnant woman if used prophylacticallly to decrease the risk of vertical transmission and not as a therapeutic regimen.

Patients should be seen every 3 to 4 months for assessment of their clinical course, viral load, and CD4-cell count. It is most beneficial to administer HAART early, before extensive immune damage has occurred. The patient's report of readiness to take the medication, appropriately, has been associated with improved compliance.

Treatment is based on the CD4 count, viral load, and the patient's clinical condition. The U.S. Public Health Service, CDC, and the IAS-USA recommend that individuals with a CD4-cell count below 500 or a viral load above 10,000 should be considered eligible for treatment. These recommendations apply to pregnant women already on therapy as well as patients with primary HIV infection. Antiretroviral therapy (ART) during pregnancy is best initiated with counseling regarding the limited number of placebo-controlled trials of ART in pregnant women. Use of ART drugs in pregnancy should be reported to the AntiRetroviral Pregnancy Registry (at 800-258-4263), which is collecting information in a retrospective and prospective fashion. Treatment involves using various antiretroviral chemotherapeutic agents to control viral load and render it as low as possible in combination with various prophylactic agents to prevent the development of opportunistic infections.

Combination Therapy

Triple therapy (HAART) generally includes the use of two nucleoside analogs and one PI. The use of protease-sparing regimens with two nucleosides and a nonnucleoside or three nucleosides has been attempted in a select population with low viral loads. Women of childbearing age are preferably placed on an AZT-containing regimen because of the effect of this drug in decreasing transmission to a fetus.

Resistance Testing

Genotypic and phenotypic testing to detect viral resistance to therapeutic agents has been suggested for use in determining new drug combinations when changing therapy for a failing combination. The decision to change therapy and the choice of a new regimen should be undertaken by a clinician with considerable experience and expertise in the care of persons with HIV infection. Less experienced clinicians should obtain consultation or refer the patient.

Treatment with HAART may result in a slow but incomplete recovery of the immune system. Opportunistic infections such as CMV retinopathy may improve and at times be arrested.

RECOGNIZING AND TREATING COMPLICATIONS OF HIV INFECTION

HIV is now recognized as a disease that can be treated as a chronic disease rather than in a standard infectious disease model of treating to cure. This involves using HAART to slow the progress of the disease, as well as the prophylactic or therapeutic management of opportunistic infections.

Pneumocystis carinii Pneumonia

The prevalence of PCP increased 1000-fold in the 1980s and early 1990s but has diminished in recent years due to prophylaxis and HAART. PCP was initially considered to be protozoan, however, it has been shown to share biologic properties with both protozoa and fungi. The pneumocystis organism contains several enzymes that may be used as drug targets. The principal pneumocystis drugs use the inhibition of pnemocystis dihydrofolate reductase (tetrahydrofolate). A combination of trimethoprim–sulfamethoxazole (TMP-SMX) has proven to be extremely efficacious clinically in this regard. Prevention is most commonly performed with TMP-SMX double strength orally three times a week or once daily if the CD4-cell count is <200 cells/mm^3 or ≤14%. Aerosolized pentamindine can be used for monthly treatments if specialized facilities are available. More recently, atovaquone, an antiprotozoal analogue of ubiquinone has been used as a second-line drug both for prophylaxis and for treatment of mild disease.

Patients presenting with unexplained pulmonary symptoms, productive cough, and/or chest pain and dyspnea should undergo chest x-ray examination. If there is an interstitial pattern present with scant sputum production and exercise oximetry reveals a ≥5% decrease in oxygen saturation, patients may be treated empirically for PCP. Patients who are hypoxic should have steroids added to their treatment regimen and additional diagnostic tests, such as induced sputums and/or bronchoscopy with bronchoalveolar lavage and/or lung transbronchial biopsy, should be performed to ascertain specific diagnosis. Patients may

not improve until 4 to 8 days after the initiation of therapy; although some patients respond within 24 hours. Many clinicians will switch to second-line therapy if the patient does not respond within 4 to 7 days.

Bacterial Infections

The incidence of infections with pneumococcus, *Haemophilus influenzae*, and salmonella are increased in patients with HIV, and apart from perhaps a greater propensity for bacteremia, do not present differently from these infections in a more general population. There is also an increase in *Staphylococcus aureus* infections, including otherwise unusual manifestations such as pyomyositis. Rare bacteria such as *Rhodococcus equi* may be seen.

As the patient becomes more immunosuppressed, *Mycobacterium tuberculosis* infections become more common. When the immune system is relatively more intact (e.g., a CD4-cell count ≥ than 500/mm^3), the typical apical infiltrate is frequently seen. With declining immunity, the infiltrate loses the typical pattern and may become more diffuse. A high index of suspicion is required to keep from spreading tuberculosis in the hospital setting. Many hospitals have a policy of putting every HIV-positive patient with an infiltrate and no other firm diagnosis into Acid Fast Bacillus (AFB) isolation. Treatment is for the standard 6 months when there is no drug resistance. Multidrug-resistant tuberculosis is almost impossible to eradicate in the immunocompromised patient.

Mycobacterium avium–intracellulare complex organisms often cause a disseminated infection in patients with CD4-cell counts less than 50/mm^3. It generally causes a nonspecific syndrome with fever, night sweats, weight loss, diarrhea, and cytopenias. Prophylaxis is generally instituted with clarithromycin 500 mg orally twice a day or azithromycin 1200 mg orally per week. Infection may be detected by bone-marrow smear and cultures, blood cultures, tissue cultures, or stool cultures. Treatment is often started empirically while cultures are pending and consists of a macrolide (azithromycin or clarithromycin) and ethambutol. Rifabutin is a potent addition to this regimen, but drug interactions may preclude its use.

An increase in the diagnosis of syphilis is frequently seen in geographic areas with high rates of HIV. The lesions of syphilis make acquisition of HIV during a sexual encounter more likely, and the immunodeficiency associated with HIV may make syphilis progress more rapidly or show unusual forms such as lues maligna. Diagnosis is generally made through serologic testing, although the organisms are occasionally seen on biopsy of tissues stained with silver stains. Treatment must be prolonged, and serologic titers should be followed carefully. Penicillin is the drug of choice.

Fungal Infections

Candida infections are ubiquitous in patients with HIV and AIDS. Manifestations range from persistent vaginal candidiasis to angular cheilitis of the mouth, thrush, and esophagitis. Clotrimazole and nystatin oral and topical preparations can be tried first for all of these except esophagitis, which requires systemic therapy, most frequently with fluconazole. Azole-resistant candida can appear after prolonged or intermittent treatment but usually responds to amphotericin B.

Cryptococcosis appears in about 5% of patients with AIDS. It is usually manifested by a central nervous system (CNS) infection of relatively gradual onset. Headache, stiff neck, fever, altered mental status, nausea, and vomiting may be seen. Diagnosis is made by lumbar puncture in the absence of papilledema. Cerebrospinal fluid will show cryptoccocal antigen and culture, but may have normal protein and cell counts. Occasionally, skin lesions are seen. Treatment depends on the severity of illness. For moderate illness, fluconazole may be used. For more severe illness, amphotericin B is indicated.

Histoplasmosis occurs in endemic areas in patients who have CD4-cell counts <100/mm^3 and is usually a reactivation of previous disease. The illness caused is difficult to distinguish from that caused by *Mycobacterium avium–intracellulare* complex and is diagnosed by bone marrow stains, cultures, and blood buffy coat cultures. Treatment depends on severity, with itraconazole being used in less severely ill patients, and amphotericin B for those who are seriously ill. Often treatment is initiated with amphotericin B and then switched to itraconazole after 2 weeks.

Blastomycosis may cause skin lesions or pneumonia. The pneumonia may be complicated by adult respiratory distress syndrome. Treatment is with amphotericin B or itraconazole. Coccidioidomycosis is more likely to be seen in endemic areas, where the CD4-cell count is <50/mm^3. It starts as a pulmonary infection and then may widely disseminate to skin, bone, and central nervous system. Treatment is with fluconazole or itraconazole.

Protozoan Infections

Protozoan infections, with the exception of toxoplasmosis, occur mostly in the intestines. *Crytosporidium parvum*, while self-limited in immunocompetent individuals, can be devastating in patients with a CD4-cell <100/mm^3. Diarrhea and cramping may be controlled symptomatically, but no treatment has been proven efficacious. Microsporidia can cause diarrhea and is treated with albendazole. *Giardia lamblia* causes the typical diarrheal and cramping syndrome and is usually treated with metronidazole or albendazole.

Toxoplasmosis in patients with AIDS is rarely primary but is instead a reactivation of latent infection. Although it can occasionally cause infection in other areas, it is the most common cause of mass lesions in the central nervous system of patients with AIDS. The frequency of toxoplasmosis is decreased in patients who have been taking TMP-SMX for PCP prophylaxis. It also may be decreasing with the use of HAART. It presents with fever, headache, and altered mentation progressing over a few days. Appearance on computed tomography (CT) is similar to that of CNS lymphoma, but there are usually more lesions with toxoplasmosis. Sometimes magnetic resonance imaging (MRI) is performed to look for lesions not seen with CT. Brain biopsy is helpful in extreme cases. Response to pyrimethamine plus either sulfadiazine or clindamycin leads to improvement in the majority of cases within 2 weeks. Maintenance therapy is continued lifelong after a 6-week induction course.

Viral Infections

Varicella–zoster virus (VZV) infection (chickenpox) is a member of the herpes family that rarely causes primary infection in the adult HIV population but can be disseminated and life-threatening when it does occur. Varicella–zoster immunoglobulin can be helpful in preventing infection in a susceptible individual if given within 96 hours of exposure. The licensed vaccine, however, is a live attenuated virus and should not be given to immunocompromised hosts.

More common in the patient with HIV/AIDS is localized recurrence of VZV, or shingles. It has a typical appearance but may rarely cause disseminated cutaneous and visceral disease. Care must be exercised when the ophthalmic branch of the trigeminal nerve is involved, as permanent visual loss may result. Immediate ophthalmologic consultation is indicated in this situation. Localized zoster may be treated with oral high-dose acyclovir or famciclovir, but if severe or disseminated disease is present, the patient should be hospitalized so that acyclovir can be administered intravenously. Acyclovir-resistant VZV is occasionally seen in patients with extensive acyclovir exposure for the treatment of HSV.

Cytomegalovirus (CMV) is the member of the herpes family that causes the most morbidity and mortality in AIDS patients. CMV retinitis, the most common manifestation of the virus, is usually seen at CD4-cell counts of $<50/mm^3$. Yearly ophthalmologic screening is instituted when CD4-cell counts drop below $100/mm^3$, and oral ganciclovir prophylaxis may also be instituted at this time. Visual symptoms such as floaters, blurry vision, or loss of vision are cause for immediate referral to an ophthalmologist. Lesions, consisting of exudates and hemorrhages, usually start peripherally but often progress rapidly toward the macula. Treatment is instituted immediately with intravenous ganciclovir at 5 mg/kg every 12 hours and continued at this dose until the disease has stabilized. At that point, gancyclovir, 6 mg/kg 5 days per week, may be continued indefinitely, although there have been studies showing that the partial immune reconstitution seen with effective antiretroviral treatment may allow secondary prophylaxis to be stopped in patients with stable disease who can be followed closely.[47] Cases failing to respond to ganciclovir may require the addition or substitution of foscarnet, 60 mg/kg every 8 hours or 90 mg/kg every 12 hours. CMV may also cause pneumonia, usually in conjunction with PCP and resolving with treatment of the PCP. Esophagitis, cholangitis, and colitis are sometimes due to CMV.

Another virus in the herpes family that is seen with HIV is Epstein−Barr virus (EBV). EBV is noted for its causative role in oral hairy leukoplakia and in some lymphomas, but antiviral treatment is rarely indicated with these complications. Viruses seen with HIV that are not members of the herpes family include the JC virus, which causes progressive multifocal leukoencephalopathy, and human T-cell lymphocytic virus type I (HTLV-I), which causes myelopathy. Genital human papillomavirus infections can be quite extensive and require surgical removal.

ORAL MANIFESTATIONS

HIV-positive individuals have an increased incidence of upper-respiratory-tract infections and allergies and experience sore throat either due to hypertonic postnasal drainage or streptococcal infection. Probably the most common opportunistic infection of HIV-positive individuals is candida pharyngitis (thrush), which may occur with characteristic cheesy plaques that can be removed with a tongue blade, leaving an erythematous base occurring on the tonsils, buccal mucosa, and soft palate. Thrush may also occur on the hard palate, hypopharynx, and posterior aspects and sides of the tongue. It may imitate hairy leukoplakia. Less commonly seen is atrophic candidiasis. Pseudomembranous candidiasis and angular kyelitis may occur. Patients who experience oral symptoms may have symptoms of dysphagia and indicate that food hangs up usually between the thyroid cartilage and the manubrium sternoid.

In individuals with <300 CD4 cells, oral hairy leukoplakia may occur. White lesions caused by the replication of EBV and keratinized cells of the epithelium are present on the tongue and buccal mucosa, showing the characteristic shaggy appearance on the sides of the tongue. These will not scrape off with a tongue blade and do not respond to antifungal therapy. Herpes simplex may cause painful oral ulcers, usually on the nonmovable surfaces of the buccal mucosa, hard palate, gums, and mucocutaneous surfaces. Aphthous stomatitis is manifested by several single or multiple painful ulcers often with exudate appearing throughout the oral cavity both on movable and nonmovable mucous membranes. Aphthous ulcers have been reported to respond to either thalidomide[48] or to the use of HAART. These occasionally respond to dexamethasone in orabase. Severe cases of oral candidiasis are best treated in HIV-positive people with systemic agents such as fluconazole 200 mg on the first day and 100 mg per day thereafter. Mild cases may also be treated with topical antifungal agents. After clearance of the lesions, many would advocate continued prophylaxis with fluconazole, although this has been subject to controversy and has not been shown to prolong life.

GASTROINTESTINAL MANIFESTATIONS

Reflux esophagitis, esophageal Kaposi sarcoma, lymphoma, carcinoma, and peptic ulcer disease also occur, as does CMV gastritis. Kaposi sarcoma of the stomach may occur with scant involvement. Right-upper-quadrant tenderness with acalculous cholecystis may occur, caused by a nonspecific bacterial sludge or cryptosporidium and cytomegalovirus.[49,50] Endoscopic sphincterotomy may relieve pain and obstruction. Colitis is common in HIV-positive individuals, caused by organisms such as salmonella, shigella, campylobacter, *Giardia lambia*, cryptosporidium, or isospori. Also, frequently in patients on antibiotics, *Clostridium difficile*–associated colitis may occur. CMV is a common viral cause of late-stage, painful diarrhea with fever, cramping, and tenesmus. Perforation of the colon has been described.[51]

RENAL MANIFESTATIONS

There is a specific HIV-related nephropathy. Patients have proteinuria and progressive renal failure. On ultrasound examination, large echogenic kidneys are seen; and on biopsy, focal, segmental sclerosing glomerular nephritis is seen. This disease may respond to high-dose steroid treatment or to angiotensin-converting–enzyme (ACE) inhibitors.

CUTANEOUS MANIFESTATIONS

Molluscum contagiosum, a cutaneous poxvirus infection, occurs more commonly in HIV-infected individuals through close sexual contact or other close contact.

Herpes lesions of the skin, especially the perirectal area, appear as giant, denuded, painful perirectal ulcers, which may be caused by acyclovir-resistant strains in patients previously treated with acyclovir. They may be diagnosed by typical appearance and location, viral culture, or positive Zanc preparation. Varicella–zoster virus often may reactivate with HIV infection, sometimes earlier, before the CD4-cell count has fallen but then may recur as the CD4-cell count continues to fall. In late HIV disease, it is 5 to 10% annually.[52-55] Chronic and multidermatomal herpes zoster may also be seen.

Seborrheic dermatitis occurs commonly. Other skin diseases that may occur are onychomycosis, bacterial folliculitis, eosinophilia folliculitis, xerosis, ichthymosus, staphylococcal skin infections, and warts. Kaposi sarcoma and bacillary angiomatosis have a characteristic appearance.

SEXUALLY TRANSMITTED DISEASES

Syphilis occurs more commonly in women with HIV infection and may increase the transmission and acquisition of HIV. Patients with HIV may have an accelerated form of neurologic syphilis in that progress to neurosyphilis occurs in months rather than years. Many physicians will proceed to lumbar puncture for HIV-positive patients with syphilis of unknown duration. Consideration must be given to lumbar puncture for patients not responding appropriately to penicillin therapy.

SPECIAL ISSUES IN WOMEN

Vaginal candidiasis occurs and recurs more frequently with severe symptoms in women with HIV even relatively early in the course of HIV infection. Women may self-medicate repeatedly prior to seeking treatment from a physician and may have a resistant strain upon presentation. Torulopsis glabrata can cause a persistent vaginitis that may respond to boric acid vaginal suppositories or second-generation topical antifungals. Physicians should be alert to the fact that women with persistent candidiasis may have underlying HIV.

STDs are well-known risk factors for the acquisition of HIV. HSV, syphilis, chancroid, and HPV are particularly virulent when they occur in women with HIV. Disorders associated with HPV are more common in women with HIV, becoming even more common as the immune system gets weaker. CDC recommendations suggest annual Pap smears after two normal smears 6 months apart. Reactive atypia calls for a repeat examination in 3 months. Colposcopy should be performed with ASCUS, AGCUS, SIL, or persistent inflammation that does not allow appropriate cytologic evaluation of the cervix.

Intrauterine contraceptive devices (IUDs) may increase the risk of acquisition of HIV in women. Women are generally counseled to encourage their partners to use latex condoms for contraception as well as to decrease the spread of potentially resistant virus between partners. The Depo form of progesterone is a good form of contraception, and is dosed every 3 months (can be done at the time of office visits).

PROPHYLAXIS FOR OPPORTUNISTIC INFECTIONS

Patients with CD4-cell counts <200 mm^3 are given prophylactic drugs to prevent PCP (trimethoprim–sulfamethoxazole, dapsone, or atovaquone). Those

If no focality or papilledema, but meningismus—obtain serum cryptococcal antigen and VDRL and strongly consider lumbar puncture

If focality—MRI or CT with contrast

A chronic, suspected primary headache with no physical findings does not require neuroimaging. Reasons for neuroimaging include abnormal neurologic signs, papilledema, visual field cut, fever, neck stiffness, nausea and vomiting with other suspicious findings, trauma, severe headache with exertion, "worst headache in my life," and increased severity over time.[31,40,41]

Treatment

Migraine

The goal of migraine headache therapy is to abort the acute attack and to prevent subsequent headaches. It is important to avoid narcotics if possible because of their addictive potential. Long-term analgesic and sedative use should also be avoided because of the rebound headaches with analgesics and the addictive potential of sedatives.

Some patients can achieve headache relief with use of simple analgesics such as acetaminophen, aspirin, or other nonsteroidal antiinflammatory drugs (NSAIDs). Some of these are available in suppository form. Improved efficacy can occur with an initial dose of 1000 mg orally for acetaminophen and aspirin and the maximum initial NSAID dose. Analgesics can also be given in combination with caffeine

and a barbiturate or in combination with codeine, but these medications carry significant addictive potential and should be limited to patients who have infrequent headaches.

Ergotamine tartrate and dihydroergotamine (DHE) are both effective agents for acute moderate to severe migraine treatment. See Table 38-5 for prescribing information. These drugs block neurovascular inflammation in the trigeminal vascular system and act as 5-hydroxytryptamine agonists. Both are vasoconstrictors. These agents are safe, but should not be used in uncontrolled hypertension, coronary or peripheral arterial disease, thyrotoxicosis, or sepsis.[42] Nausea is a side effect of the ergot alkaloids as well as a usual accompaniment to migraine. Concomitant administration of an antinausea agent such as metoclopramide or prochlorperazine facilitates the use of oral ergotamine in migraines. Use of ergotamine tartrate must not occur more than twice a week, and the total weekly dose should not exceed 10 mg to avoid physiologic dependence, which causes rebound headaches. The rectal suppository may be effective as a half dose, and refrigerating the suppository to permit hardening facilitates slicing it.[43] DHE may be given intravenously, intramuscularly, or subcutaneously. Repeat doses of intravenous DHE can be given in a hospital over 3 to 7 days up to 20 mg/wk to help break daily migraines, cluster headaches, or status migrainosus. Side effects of the ergot alkaloids include extremity ischemia, myocardial ischemia, and nausea. Side effects are rare if the drugs are used properly. All ergot alkaloids are relatively contraindicated in pregnancy (risk

TABLE 38-5
ERGOTAMINE PREPARATIONS*

Drug	Dose	Route	Dose per Attack	Maximum per Week
Ergotamine tartrate	2 mg	Sublingual	2 mg every 30 min up to 6 mg/24 hrs.	10 mg/week
Ergotamine tartrate/caffeine	1 mg/100 mg	Oral	2 mg initially and 1 mg every 30 min up to 6 mg/attack	10 mg/week
	2 mg/100 mg	Rectal	1/2 to 1 suppository initially; repeat as needed in 1 hour	2/day
Dihydroergotamine	1 mg (1 ml) intramuscularly, subcutaneously, or intravenously	1 mg hourly up to 3 mg intramuscularly or subcutaneously or 2 mg intravenously		6 mg/week
	0.5 mg intranasal	0.5 mg in each nostril; repeat in 15 min		6 mg/week

*Contraindicated in pregnancy (risk factor D, positive evidence of risk) and breast-feeding.

Comment: The use of ergotamine tartrate should be restricted to no more than two days per week except perimenstrually.

TABLE 38-6			
SELECTIVE 5-HYDROXYTRIPTAMINE RECEPTOR AGONISTS*			
Drug	**Dose**	**Route**	**Dose per Attack**
Sumatriptan	25–100 mg	Oral	25–100 mg initially; may give up to 100 mg additionally at 2 hr; do not exceed 300 mg/24 hr
	6 mg	Subcutaneous	6 mg initially; may repeat in 1 or more hours; do not exceed 12 mg per day
	5 mg, 20 mg	Intranasal	5, 10, or 20 mg. Repeat dose after 2 hours as needed; 40 mg/24 hr
Zolmitriptan	2.5 mg	Oral	2.5 mg initially; may repeat in 2 hr; do not exceed 10 mg/24 hr
Naratriptan	1–2.5 mg	Oral	1–2.5 mg initially; may repeat after 4 hr; do not exceed 5 mg/24 hr
Rizatriptan	5–10 mg	Oral	5–10 mg tablet or wafer (dissolves on tongue); may repeat in 2 hr; do not exceed 30 mg/24 hr

*Contraindicated in pregnancy (risk factor C, risk cannot be ruled out) and breast-feeding—minimal risk; can be decreased further by delaying feeding until 8 hours after dose.[44]

Comment: 5-HT agents should not be used if an ergotamine derivative was used within 24 hours. Limit use to ≤2 days/wk.

factor D, positive evidence of risk).[44] Ergotamine is also contraindicated during breast-feeding because of ergotism induced in infants.[45]

The newest group of drugs for abortive migraine therapy is the selective 5-hydroxytryptamine (5-HT) receptor agonists (Table 38-6). These include sumatriptan, zolmitriptan, naratriptan, rizatriptan, and others available outside the United States. Sumatriptan may be given subcutaneously, orally, or intranasally, while zolmitriptan, naratriptan, and rizatriptan are available orally. The 5-HT receptor agonists can relieve about 70% of migraines within 1 hour. In migraine with aura, one study suggests that subcutaneous dosing should be delayed until onset of headache to improve efficacy.[46] The dose may be repeated if the headache recurs, which is common.

From a practical standpoint, a fast-acting nonoral preparation such as intranasal or subcutaneous sumatriptan may be most useful in migraine with rapid onset of vomiting. Naratriptan may be helpful in avoiding triptan side effects since it has a low side-effect profile. DHE or naratriptan is also helpful in migraines that tend to recur because these drugs have a long half-life.[47]

In comparison with DHE, sumatriptan had slighter greater headache relief at 2 hours[48] but no difference at 4 hours. There was an increased risk of headache recurrence with sumatriptan. DHE nasal spray is less effective than subcutaneous sumatriptan.[49] For an acute attack, the patient should take 6 mg subcutaneously, 50 to 100 mg orally, or 20 mg intranasally of sumatriptan. The dose may be repeated once within 24 hours. Zolmitriptan, naratriptan, and rizatriptan appear to have similar efficacy. Naratriptan has a slower onset and longer duration of action. If one agent is

not effective, another may be tried.[50-53] Do not use the selective 5-HT receptor agonists within 24 hours of an ergot alkaloid. Side effects of the 5-HT agents are chest tightness, throat pain, paresthesias, nausea, and somnolence, but these are usually mild and self-limited; contraindications to use are ischemic heart disease and uncontrolled hypertension.[54] These agents are expensive. Caution is urged with use in postmenopausal women and women with cardiac risk factors.[52]

Other agents of proven efficacy in acute migraine treatment are butorphanol nasal spray, 1 mg, which can be repeated in 60 to 90 minutes and the sequence repeated in 3 to 4 hours if needed; metoclopramide, 10 mg intravenously; prochlorperazine, 25 mg suppository or 5 to 10 mg intravenously or intramuscularly; chlorpromazine, 0.1 mg/kg of body weight intravenously, which may be repeated every 15 minutes up to 3 doses; and meperidine, 50 to 100 mg intramuscularly or intravenously.[55-59]

Prophylaxis for migraine headaches (Table 38-7) should be considered when a patient has three or more severe attacks per month or if quality of life is impaired by the migraines. β-blocking agents, including propranolol, atenolol, timolol, metoprolol, and nadolol, have all been used successfully in migraine prevention. The mechanism of action in unknown. β-blockers must be used for at least 6 months to test efficacy. The usual starting dose for propranolol is 80 mg/day, which can be given conveniently as a once-a-day long-acting preparation. Dosage may be increased weekly by 40 to 60 mg/wk up to a target dose of 180 to 320 mg/day.[12] Efficacy is measured by a reduction in severity and frequency of headaches by 60 to 80%. Contraindications to β-blocker use are

TABLE 38-7
DRUGS FOR MIGRAINE PROPHYLAXIS

Drug Class	Drug	Initial Dose	Titration Interval	Titration Dose	Goal	Pregnancy Risk Factor*	Breast-Feeding
β-Blocker	Propranolol	80 mg/day	Weekly	40–60 mg/wk	180–320 mg/day	C	Permitted
	Atenolol	50 mg/day	Weekly	50 mg/wk	100 mg/day	D	Avoid
	Timolol	10 mg twice a day			10 mg twice a day	C	Permitted
	Metoprolol	50 mg twice a day	Weekly	50 mg twice a day	100 mg twice a day	C	Permitted
	Nadolol	80 mg/day	Weekly	80 mg	240 mg/day	C	Permitted
Tricyclic	Amitriptyline	25 mg at bedtime	2–7 days	25 mg	150 mg	D	Unknown, worrisome
	Desipramine	25 mg at bedtime	2–7 days	25 mg	150 mg	C	Unknown, worrisome
	Nortriptyline	25 mg at bedtime	2–7 days	25 mg	150 mg	D	Unknown worrisome
Antiepileptic	Valproate	250 mg/day	2 days	250 mg	Plasma level, 70–120 mg/liter (800–1500 mg/dl)	D	Permitted
Calcium-channel blocker	Verapamil	240 mg/day	1 week	120 mg	360 mg	C	Permitted
	Nimodipine	120 mg/day (divided dosages)			120 mg/day	C	Unknown
	Nifedipine (sustained release)	30 mg/day			30 mg/day	C	Permitted
NSAID	Naproxen	1100 mg/day (divided doses)			1100 mg/day	B	Permitted
	Tolfenamic acid	300 mg/day (divided doses)			300 mg/day	C	Permitted
	Aspirin	1300 mg/day (divided doses)			1300 mg/day	C	Use with caution

*B = no evidence of risk in humans; C = risk cannot be ruled out; D = positive evidence of risk.

asthma, chronic obstructive pulmonary disease, and congestive heart failure.

Tricyclic antidepressants also reduce severity and frequency of migraine attacks similarly to β-blockers. Agents used have included amitriptyline, desipramine, and nortriptyline. The usual starting dose for amitriptyline is 25 mg at bedtime, which can be increased by 25-mg increments every 2 to 3 days up to 150 mg at bedtime.[60] Efficacy is comparable to the β-blockers. Side effects are dry mouth, constipation, drowsiness, blurred vision, tachycardia, urinary retention, and postural hypotension. Amitriptyline should not be used in patients with underlying heart disease and generally should be avoided in postmenopausal patients because of anticholinergic side effects.

Sodium valproate reduces headache frequency by about 50 to 75%.[61-63] The starting dose is 250 mg/day, which is then increased every other day by 250 mg to achieve a plasma blood level of 70 to 120 mg/liter. Mean dose is 1087 mg/day. Another effective dose is 400 mg twice a day.[64] Nausea, dyspepsia, and fatigue are the primary side effects. There is risk of neural-tube defects if the drug is used during pregnancy.

Calcium-channel agents likely work by modulating neurotransmitters. The evidence for their efficacy is less well documented than for β-blockers. There is about a 50% reduction in headache frequency. Verapamil is used at a dose of 240 to 360 mg/day. Nimodipine and nifedipine have also been used. Side effects include constipation, dizziness, drowsiness, bradycardia, flushing, and congestive heart failure. Tolerance has been shown in some studies, necessitating an increase in dose.[65]

Other agents shown to have some efficacy in migraine prophylaxis are nonsteroidal antiinflammatory drugs (NSAIDs) such as naproxen[66] and aspirin.[67,68] Other NSAIDs such as ketoprofen, tolfenamic acid, and mefenamic acid are also effective.[69] Methysergide is effective[70] but has numerous side effects, including retroperitoneal fibrosis; there should be a medication-free period of 3 to 4 weeks after continuous use for 6 months.

Menstrual migraine can be managed acutely and from a preventive standpoint with the medications listed above. If associated with dysmenorrhea or menorrhagia, NSAIDs such as mefenamic acid, 500 mg 2 to 3 times a day for 5 to 7 days, with onset of menses may be helpful.[35] If treatment is not satisfactory, an estradiol continuous patch (Estraderm, 100 μg) provides a continuous estrogen level and can decrease migraines when applied several days before menses and during menses.[35,37] There is a relationship between oral contraceptives and stroke in migraine that is enhanced by smoking.[71,72] Caution should be exercised before prescribing oral contraceptives to migraineurs with risk factors for arterial disease, especially smoking. Previous stroke is a contraindication to use of estrogen contraception. Any woman with migraine and focal neurologic deficits should avoid estrogen-containing contraceptives.[35]

For the migraineur whose headaches require treatment during pregnancy, simple analgesics such as acetaminophen and caffeine may be used. Caffeine at a dose of <300 mg/day carries a B risk factor rating (no evidence of risk in humans). Aspirin should be avoided in late pregnancy because of bleeding risk to mother and fetus at birth. NSAIDs, also B drugs, cannot be used more than 48 hours during the third trimester because of decreased amniotic fluid volume, pulmonary hypertension, prolongation of labor, and prolongation of pregnancy.[37] Ergots must be avoided. The 5-HT$_1$ receptor antagonists carry a C risk factor rating (risk cannot be ruled out) and may be used with caution. β-Blockers and calcium-channel agents are risk factor C and can be used as preventives. Fluoxetine at doses ranging from 10 to 80 mg/day may be safely used with a risk factor B rating.[73]

Estrogen-replacement therapy at menopause can sometimes accelerate migraines. Use the lowest effective dose. Use continuous estrogen-replacement therapy if migraines are linked to estrogen withdrawal.

Cluster headaches can be treated similarly to migraines with ergotamines and sumatriptan. Inhalation of 100% oxygen is effective at 7 liters per minute for 15 minutes in patients under age 50.[74,75] Patients with chronic paroxysmal hemicrania respond well to indomethacin.

Prophylaxis is effective using verapamil at 80 to 240 mg three times a day,[76] prednisone at 20 to 40 mg/day tapered over 3 weeks,[77,78] lithium at 300 mg two to four times a day,[79,80] methysergide at 2 mg three to four times a day,[70,77] and divalproex sodium.[81]

While tension headache is the most common headache, most are of mild severity and are relieved by nonprescription analgesics. It is important to evaluate and treat for underlying depression as a cause of headache. Acetaminophen, aspirin, and other nonsteroidal agents are the primary form of therapy. Ibuprofen at 400 to 800 mg has been found to be more effective than aspirin at 650 mg or placebo.[82] Naproxen at 275 to 550 mg is similarly effective.[83,84] Tricyclic antidepressants (amitriptyline, doxepin, nortriptyline, desipramine, and imipramine) can be effective prophylactically.

Chronic daily headaches present a difficult challenge to the primary care physician. These headaches may have characteristics of both migraine and tension headaches, and there is often a history of migraines. Some call these transformed migraines, mixed headaches, or chronic daily headache. Analgesic dependency is common. Treatment requires withdrawal of the abused analgesic, which may include butalbital, caffeine, ergotamine, and/or codeine.[15] Intravenous DHE and hospitalization may be required.[85] The patient may then revert to her usual headache pattern (tension or migraine) and permit use of the usual prophylactic agent. Amitriptyline prophylaxis combined with analgesic withdrawal may also be helpful.[86] Analgesic rebound headaches have been successfully treated with a combination of dexamethasone, 4 mg intramuscularly daily for 2 weeks, and amitriptyline, 50 mg daily for 6 months, along with sumatriptan for acute headaches.[87] Addictive agents such as narcotics, barbiturates, ergotamine, and benzodiazepines must be avoided in long-term therapy.

DIZZINESS

Dizziness is one of the most common symptoms in a primary care medical practice, accounting for 8 million visits annually.[88] The majority of patients are female.[89] Among patients over 60 years old, 20% have had severe dizziness,[90] which increases their risk for falls. Dizziness is found in a variety of illnesses, including labyrinthine diseases, brain-stem problems, psychiatric illness, cardiovascular diseases, drug effects, and systemic illnesses. Including dizziness in a review of symptoms can generate many false positive responses and should be prefaced by "unusual" or "severe."

Pathophysiology

To better understand the diseases that cause vertigo it is important to review the anatomic and physiologic basis for balance. Within the temporal bone and adjacent to the cochlea is the vestibular system, consisting of three semicircular canals and the otolithic apparatus. This apparatus has two membranous sacs, the saccule and utricle. Endolymph fills the semicircular canals, and tiny hair cells within the canals detect angular and rotational movement as the endolymph moves across them. Endolymph continuously bathes both the cochlear and vestibular systems internally, and endolymph disorders may cause vertigo, hearing loss, and tinnitus. Linear motion and orientation to gravity are detected by hair cells embedded in the otolithic membrane. The cochlea and vestibular system share a common blood supply, and both are innervated by the eighth cranial nerve. Together they interconnect to produce the labyrinth. The vestibulo-ocular reflex provides for visual fixation during head movement. This reflex is produced by nerve connections between the vestibular nuclei and cranial nerves III, IV, and VI, which are responsible for eye movements. Unilateral peripheral vestibular injury generates nystagmus, which is a rhythmic repetitive movement of the eyes with fast and slow components. Nystagmus usually accompanies vestibular dysfunction. Absence of nystagmus on physical examination while the patient reports vertigo strongly suggests a nonvertiginous cause of dizziness.[91]

The vestibular labyrinth connects directly to the cerebellum and indirectly to the contralateral vestibular system, motor neurons of the spinal cord, and to the nuclei of the oculomotor system. Balance and spatial orientation also depend on proprioceptive nerves arising from tendons, joints, and muscles. Labyrinthine, brain-stem, and cerebellar lesions can all produce vertigo, and peripheral nervous system disease can cause imbalance.

Classification

Dizziness can be best grouped into four categories, depending on careful, nondirective questioning of the patient: true vertigo, in which a sensation of movement is experienced; presyncope, or faintness; disequilibrium characterized by staggering or sense of imbalance; and lightheadedness, often a feature of psychiatric or multisystem disease[92] (Table 38-8).

Presyncope has the same differential diagnosis as frank syncope and will be discussed in detail later. The most common causes of dizziness, accounting for more than 75% of final diagnoses are peripheral vestibular disorders, psychiatric disorders, and multiple sensory deficits.[93] Nearly half of patients may have more than one cause.[94]

Causes

Benign positional vertigo (BPV) is the most common type of vertigo and is characterized by transient vertigo associated with changes in head position. There is rarely nausea, if any. The posterior semicircular canal has free-floating particles (canaliths) heavier than the surrounding endolymph. These fall to the most dependent part of the canal on head movement. During their fall, the canaliths drag the endolymph and deflect the hair cells, leading to nystagmus and vertigo.[95] The condition is more common in the elderly but can occur as early as adolescence. Vertigo and nystagmus can be reproduced by rapid turning movements, bending over, and by the Dix–Hallpike (Nylan–Barany) maneuver, which is 50 to 78% sensitive in BPV[96,97] (Figure 38-1). This maneuver causes nystagmus, following a latency period of 5 to 30 seconds. The nystagmus is torsional, with the fast component directed down toward the undermost ear and the slow component upward.[95] Nystagmus parallels the sensation of vertigo.

Disabling positional vertigo may be caused by vascular compression of the vestibular nerve. In contrast to BPV, these patients have continuous vertigo when upright and an abnormal brain-stem auditory evoked response test (BAER).[98]

Acute labyrinthitis has sudden onset of hearing loss, vertigo, tinnitus, and usually nausea, with symptoms lasting for a few days up to 6 weeks. In contrast, vestibular neuronitis does not have hearing loss or tinnitus, but has persistent vertigo lasting for several weeks. A viral infection may be the inciting agent in both causes of vertigo.

An acoustic neuroma (technically, a vestibular schwannoma) usually presents with hearing loss and tinnitus. Vertigo is a symptom in fewer than 20% of patients.[99] Instead of vertigo, patients may complain of unsteadiness, particularly in the dark.[100] Brain-stem compression may occur from these cerebello-pontine-angle tumors, with accompanying numbness, weakness, ataxia, and corneal-reflex obliteration.

TABLE 38-8
DIFFERENTIAL DIAGNOSIS OF DIZZINESS

Vestibular disease (vertigo)
  Peripheral
    Acute and chronic otitis
    Acute labyrinthitis
    Anemia
    Benign positional vertigo
    Cerebellopontine-angle tumor
    Disabling positional vertigo
    Diabetes
    Hypotension
    Hypothyroidism
    Inflammatory labyrinthitis (syphilis, vasculitis)
    Internal auditory artery occlusion
    Meniere disease
    Motion sickness
    Otosclerosis
    Ototoxic drugs (salicylates, loop diuretics, quinidine, amino-
      glycosides, cisplatin)
    Perilymph fistula
    Phobic postural vertigo
    Posttraumatic vertigo
    Psychiatric
    Ramsay–Hunt syndrome
    Vestibular neuronitis
  Central
    Cerebellar hemorrhage/infarct
    Cerebellopontine angle tumor (acoustic neuroma, menin-
      gioma, etc.)
    Cranial neuropathy
    Demyelinating disease (multiple sclerosis, paraneoplastic
      syndromes, postinfections)
    Friedreich ataxia
    Intrinsic brain-stem lesions (tumor, arteriovenous malforma-
      tion, trauma)
    Migraine, complicated
    Other posterior fossa lesions
    Seizures
    Subclavian steal
    Vertebrobasilar insufficiency
Cardiac and vascular disease (syncope, near-syncope)
(see section on syncope for detailed listing)
  Anemia (severe)
  Autonomic insufficiency
  Arrhythmias
  Cardiomyopathy, hypertrophic
  Congestive heart failure
  Constrictive pericarditis
  Carotid-sinus hypersensitivity
  Neurocardiogenic (vasodepressor, vasovagal)
  Orthostatic hypotension
  Postprandial hypotension
  Pulmonary hypertension
  Situational
  Valvular heart disease

Disequilibrium (unsteadiness)
  Cataract surgery
  Cerebellar disease
  Cervical spondylosis
  Diabetes mellitus
  Drugs
  Motion sickness
  Multiple sclerosis
  Multiple sensory defects (eyesight, proprioception, motor)
  Nonfunctioning labyrinth
  Parkinson disease
  Posterior fossa tumors (preoperative and postoperatively)
  Proprioceptive deficits (vitamin B_{12}, tabes dorsalis, etc.)
Psychiatric disorders (lightheadedness)
  Anxiety
  Depression
  Hyperventilation
  Panic disorder
  Psychosis
  Somatization disorder
Systemic and metabolic disturbances (variable)
  Drugs (alcohol, analgesics, anticonvulsants, antihyperten-
    sives, anxiolytics, narcotics)
  Dysproteinemia
  Hypercapnia
  Hypoglycemia
  Hypoxia
  Hypocapnia
  Infections (meningitis, systemic infections)
  Leukemia
  Liver disease
  Paget disease
  Polycythemia
  Renal disease
  Respiratory infections
  Sarcoid
  Tuberculosis
  Toxins
  Vasculitis

Modified from Troost BT. Dizziness and vertigo in vertebrobasilar disease. Curr Concepts Cerebrovasc Dis 1979;11:301.

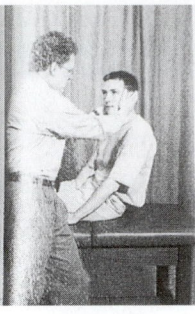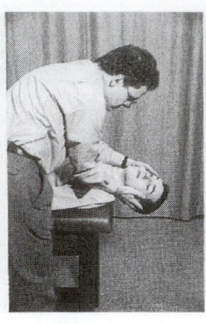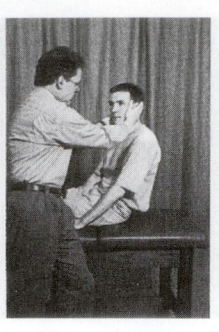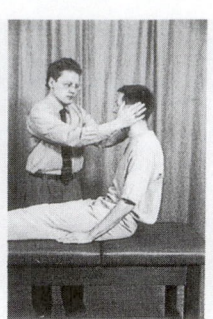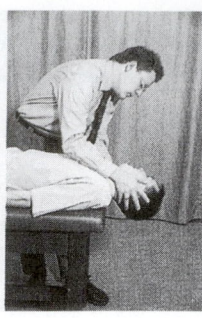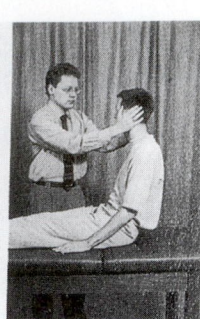

Figure 38-1 Dix–Hallpike positional maneuver for diagnosis of benign positional vertigo. Patients must be warned that transient vertigo may develop in any position. Patients are instructed to keep their eyes open throughout and to stare at the examiner's nose. In each position, observe the eyes closely for up to 30 seconds for development of nystagmus. This maneuver can be applied safely to patients with cervical spondylosis if the neck is not hyperextended. From left to right: Begin with patient sitting upright on a couch with the head turned 45 degrees to the left to test the left posterior canal. With the head in this position, lay the patient down rapidly until the head is dependent. Return the patient to the upright position. Approach the patient from the other side and rotate the head to the right to test the right posterior canal. Lay the patient down into the opposite head-hanging position. Return the patient to the upright position. *Reprinted with permission from Lampert T, Gretsy MA, Bronstein AM. Benign positional vertigo: recognition and treatment. BMJ 1995;311:489.*

Ototoxic drugs such as aminoglycosides, loop diuretics, aspirin, quinine, and cisplatin can cause vestibular toxicity. With aminoglycosides, disequilibrium usually occurs as the primary symptom. Vertigo is transient and positional. Severely ototoxic patients may have oscillopsia—i.e., objects in the visual field seem to jerk or wiggle.[101] Cinchonism is the labyrinthine dysfunction associated with cinchona alkaloid derivatives such as quinine and quinidine.

Meniere disease is categorized by the triad of vertigo, hearing loss, and tinnitus. The hearing loss is fluctuating, usually low frequency, and sensorineural. Vertigo is often severe and accompanied by nausea and vomiting. There is usually fullness in the involved ear. Poor endolymphatic drainage due to endolymphatic duct blockage may be the cause.[102]

Otologic syphilis can mimic Meniere disease in its presentation and can also cause sudden onset of deafness and vertigo. Phobic postural vertigo is a newly described cause of peripheral vertigo, with episodic vertigo or postural imbalance provoked by a perceptual stimulus or social situation.[103] It is unclear whether this is a psychiatric syndrome or a "space and motion" vestibulopathy with a psychiatric overlay.[104]

Vertebrobasilar insufficiency presents with brainstem symptoms and signs, including dysarthria, numbness, diplopia, or weakness along with vertigo. In 25% of patients with vertebrobasilar insufficiency, vertigo may be the presenting symptom, but additional neurologic clues almost invariably appear within 6 weeks. Cerebellar ischemia is more subtle, presenting with vertigo along with mild dysarthria, vertical nystagmus, focal dysmetria, headache, or mental status change.[105] Isolated vertigo due to vertebrobasilar insufficiency without other neurological signs or symptoms is uncommon. However, inferior cerebellar hemorrhage and infarction can present with vertigo, nystagmus, and postural instability alone and should be more strongly suspected in older patients with risk factors for stroke. Patients are often unable to walk without falling.[106] Internal auditory artery occlusion with sudden hearing loss and vertigo may occur with vasculitis, but rarely with atherosclerosis.[107]

Multiple sclerosis, a focal relapsing demyelinating disease affecting primarily women, is one of the most common causes of central vertigo. It can also present as disequilibrium. Weakness, numbness, unilateral visual impairment from optic neuritis, unsteadiness, and diplopia are the usual presenting symptoms, but vertigo can occur initially in 5% of patients.[108] Many research criteria for diagnosis have been published, all using two separate attacks at two separate times as the key finding. Supportive evidence comes from CSF examination with oligoclonal bands or elevated IgG, MRI with white matter lesions, and abnormal evoked potentials.[108,109]

Other common diseases causing disequilibrium include diabetes, Parkinson disease, cervical spondylosis, and vitamin B_{12} deficiency. Medications are also commonly associated either through side effects or withdrawal.[110] Younger patients with disequilibrium should be carefully evaluated for psychiatric causes, drug abuse, and vestibular causes.[111] Disequilibrium is a common symptom in the elderly and may be due to an abnormal visual vestibuloocular response[112] along with vascular, neuromuscular, and pharmacologic factors.[113]

Lightheadedness is the most common psychiatric description for dizziness, but psychiatric disease can occasionally produce disequilibrium, vertigo, or syncope. Persistent dizziness for a year or more is often psychiatric in nature. Vertigo preceding syncope is typically psychiatric, particularly if the patient is a young woman.[114] While a large number of psychiatric diagnoses can cause dizziness, the most common ones seen by the primary care physician are somatization disorder, panic disorder, and depression.

History

The history alone should diagnose about three-fourths of all cases of dizziness.[89] The physician should use open-ended questioning to obtain a careful description of exactly what the patient means by dizziness. If this is unsuccessful, then more specific questions about dizziness may be helpful—e.g., Is there a sensation of movement? (implying vertigo); Do you feel as if you're about to faint? (presyncope); Do you feel off balance when you stand or walk? (disequilibrium); and Are you lightheaded? (psychiatric). Disequilibrium typically is sensed by the patient as a problem in the feet or lower body rather than the head.

If vertigo is present, the history should focus on distinguishing central from peripheral vertigo. Central vertigo will have CNS symptoms (often brain-stem) such as dysarthria, dysphagia, headaches, focal numbness, focal weakness, or visual disturbance. Peripheral vertigo, caused by malfunction of the labyrinth, may have hearing loss, tinnitus, nausea and vomiting, recent viral illness, or head trauma. Trauma increases the possibility of a perilymph fistula, labyrinthine concussion, brain-stem injury, BPV, and cervical vertigo.[115] A disequilibrium description should encourage the physician to also ask about bowel and bladder dysfunction, exacerbation of symptoms in the dark, tremor, rigidity, and bradykinesia.

For the history relevant to presyncope and syncope, see the section on "Syncope," below.

Systemic and metabolic disturbances require a careful medication history; a past medical history, including chronic illnesses; and a review of systems to detect other symptoms. Substance abuse history and a careful psychiatric history focusing on symptoms of depression, somatization, and panic disorder should round out the history-taking.

Physical Examination

The examination for all forms of dizziness should start with the vital signs. Subclavian steal syndrome is suggested by a systolic blood pressure differential between arms of more than 20 mm Hg and at times the presence of a subclavian bruit. Orthostatic hypotension is detected by a 20-mm Hg drop in systolic pressure from supine to standing after a 2 minute lag. The pulse should be checked for irregularity. To check for nystagmus, have the patient look 45 degrees to the right, to the left, up, and down and note occurrence of nystagmus, both fast and slow components. Extremes of gaze generate spontaneous nystagmus in normal patients. Nystagmus due to peripheral vertigo typically is of short duration, has a few-second latency period, is increased on loss of visual fixation (with Frenzel glasses or by viewing one eye with an ophthalmoscope while uncovering and covering the other fixating eye), and is both positional and paroxysmal. The nystagmus increases when the gaze is shifted toward the fast phase and decreases when shifted away from this phase.[106] With central vertigo, nystagmus is often more severe than the vertigo, does not fatigue on repetition of the position change, and may be vertical (rather than rotatory or horizontal). Patients with acute cerebellar stroke are often unable to walk, in contrast to those with acute peripheral vertigo. Evaluate visual activity using newsprint or a Snelling chart. Exclude papilledema on funduscopic examination. Ears should be checked for the vesicles of Ramsay–Hunt syndrome. Removal of cerumen covering the tympanic membrane may resolve vertigo. Hearing acuity should be assessed. The tympanic membrane should be evaluated for otitis and cholesteatoma, which is desquamating keratin debris causing chronic otitis media and even perforation. The carotid arteries should be assessed for upstroke (diminished in aortic stenosis) and bruits. Also check for subclavian and vertebral bruits. A careful cardiac examination should be performed. A screening neurologic examination should be performed to include cranial nerves II to XII, mental status, deep tendon reflexes and Babinski sign, sensation (light touch, pinprick, and vibration), motor strength and tone, gait,

Romberg, and cerebellar testing (finger–nose and heel–shin).

There are specific tests that should be performed in vertigo, disequilibrium, and lightheadedness—Dix–Hallpike (see Figure 38-1), sudden right-angle turning, neck flexion and extension, and sitting and standing with eyes open and closed. Hyperventilation is neither sensitive nor specific for psychiatric dizziness and need not be performed. Benign positional vertigo may be precipitated by sudden turning, and cervical spondylosis can generate symptoms with neck movement. Removing all visual stimuli during sitting and standing may exacerbate disequilibrium.

If the patient's history does not distinguish between vertigo and presyncope, squatting for 30 seconds and then performing the Valsalva maneuver for 15 seconds can reproduce the symptoms in the case of presyncope.

In many, if not most cases of dizziness, no laboratory evaluation is required. This is particularly true of benign positional vertigo, acute labyrinthitis, vasovagal syncope, orthostatic hypotension from medications, and classic psychiatric syndromes. However, specific tests can yield a diagnosis in puzzling cases. Central vertigo should result in prompt referral to a neurologist, along with performance of an MRI. If seizure or migraine is suspected, then the primary care physician may elect to manage these. Persistent, undiagnosed peripheral vertigo should be evaluated with hematocrit, thyroid-stimulating hormone, fasting

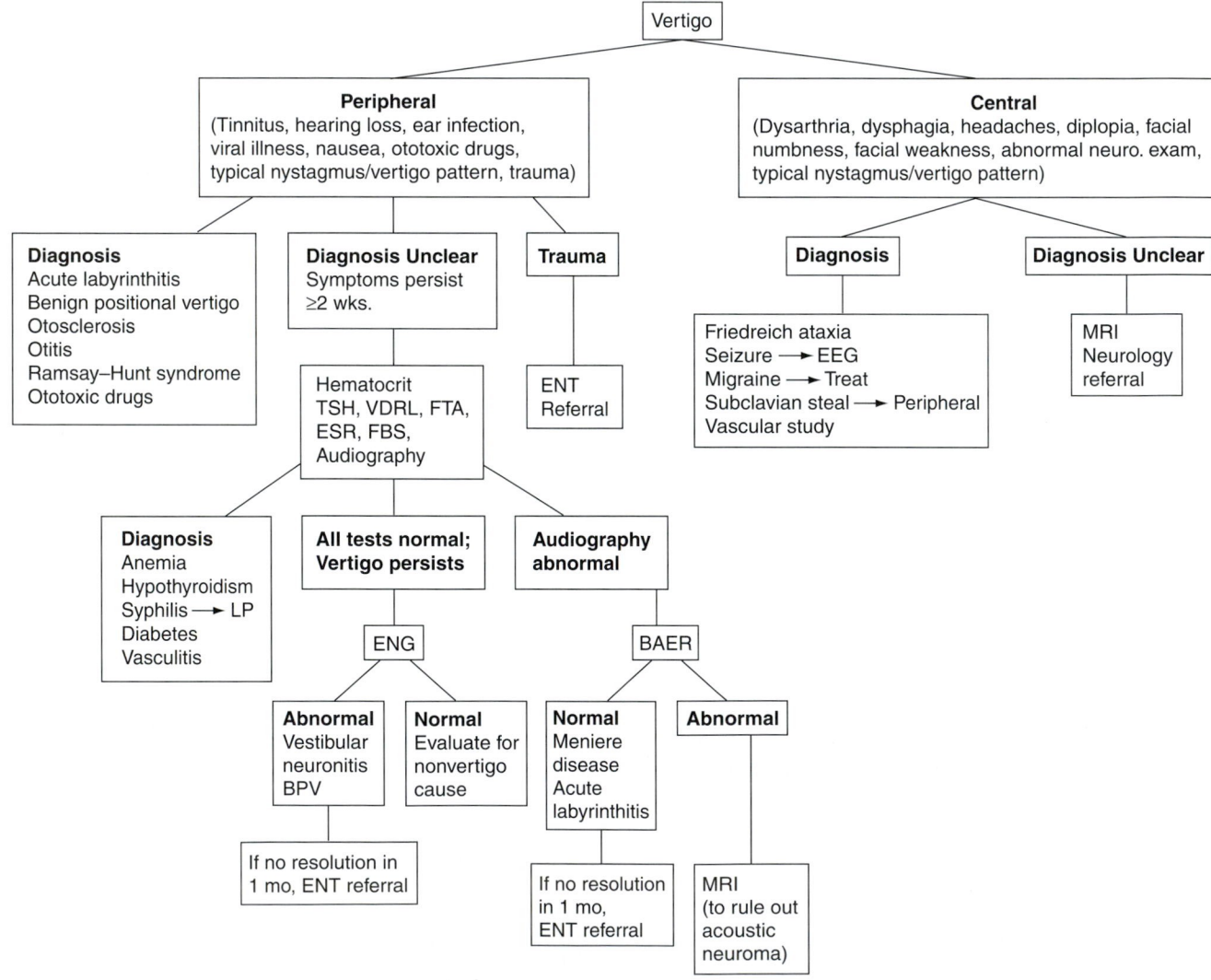

Figure 38-2 Evaluation of vertigo. TSH = thyroid-stimulating hormone; VDRL = Venereal Disease Research Laboratory; FTA = fluorescent treponemal antibody; ESR = erthrocyte sedimentation rate; FBS = fasting blood sugar; ENT = ear, nose, and throat; EEG = electrocardiography; LP = lumbar puncture; ENG = electronystagmyography.

blood sugar, treponemal and nontreponemal syphilis tests, and erythrocyte sedimentation rate to detect anemia, make the diagnoses of hypothyroidism and diabetes, and strongly suggest diagnoses of syphilis or vasculitis. Audiography should also be performed. If the audiogram is normal and vertigo persists, electronystagmography confirms the presence of true vertigo and limits the differential diagnosis largely to vestibular neuronitis and benign positional vertigo. If treatment with the Epley maneuver (see "Treatment") is unsuccessful, the patient should be referred to an ear, nose, and throat specialist. Abnormal results on audiography should be followed by brainstem auditory evoked response (BAER) testing, which is almost always abnormal in the presence of an acoustic neuroma.[116] If the BAER is abnormal, obtain an MRI to localize the acoustic neuroma. If normal, Meniere disease or acute labyrinthitis is likely. A patient with any peripheral vertigo that remains undiagnosed after 1 month should be referred to an otolaryngologist. See Figure 38-2 for a diagnostic algorithm of vertigo.

Treatment

General treatment of vertigo includes anticholinergic and antihistamine medications. Both have been shown in clinical trials to be effective (Table 38-9). Although benzodiazepines have been used in vertigo management, no trials have shown efficacy.[117] The scopolamine patch should be applied every 3 days to manage vertigo and motion sickness. Blurred vision and dry mouth are common side effects.

Benign positional vertigo is best treated through use of the canalith repositioning procedure, also known as the Epley maneuver (Figure 38-3). This maneuver directs debris out of the semicircular canal into the utricle. Premedication with an antiemetic may be advisable in severe BPV before treatment. Benign positional vertigo can be relieved 77% of the time with a single treatment and in another 20% after a second treatment.[118]

Treatment of Meniere disease is largely empiric. The acute vertiginous attacks may be treated with meclizine and the nausea with promethazine. Thiazide diuretics appear to help with the excessive production of endolymph. One regimen of hydrochlorothiazide, 25 mg twice a day, resulted in a reduction in both vertigo and hearing loss.[119] Endolymphatic surgery remains controversial. Consultation with an otolaryngologist may be beneficial.

Patients with BPV and vestibular neuronitis have an excellent prognosis, with almost all cases resolved at 1-year follow-up examination. Other vertiginous causes, psychiatric causes, and disequilibrium have a poorer prognosis.[94]

SYNCOPE

Up to 3.5% of women experience frank syncope,[120] with or without initial dizziness. Syncope, which is defined as transient loss of consciousness associated with postural tone loss,[121] has a narrower differential diagnosis than dizziness, encompassing valvular heart disease, arrhythmias, medications, orthostasis, vasovagal, and psychiatric causes.

Pathophysiology and Classification

Syncope usually occurs from a transient reduction in blood flow to the brain caused by hypotension. Reduction in cerebral blood flow may be caused by: (1) a decrease in systemic vascular resistance and/or

---

TABLE 38-9
DRUG TREATMENT OF VERTIGO

Drug Class	Drug	Dose	Side Effects	Comments
Antihistamine	Dimenhydrinate (Dramamine)	50 mg orally four times a day	Anticholinergic, drowsiness	Pregnancy B breast-feeding—unknown
	Meclizine (Antivert, Bonine)	12.5–50 mg orally four times a day	Anticholinergic, drowsiness	Pregnancy B breast-feeding—unknown
	Promethazine (Phenergan)	12.5–25 mg orally or rectally every 4–6 hr	Anticholinergic, sedation, extrapyramidal	Pregnancy C breast-feeding—unknown
Anticholinergic	Scopolamine (Transderm Scop)	1.5 mg every 3 days (transdermal)	Dry mouth, drowsiness, blurred vision	Pregnancy C breast-feeding—permitted

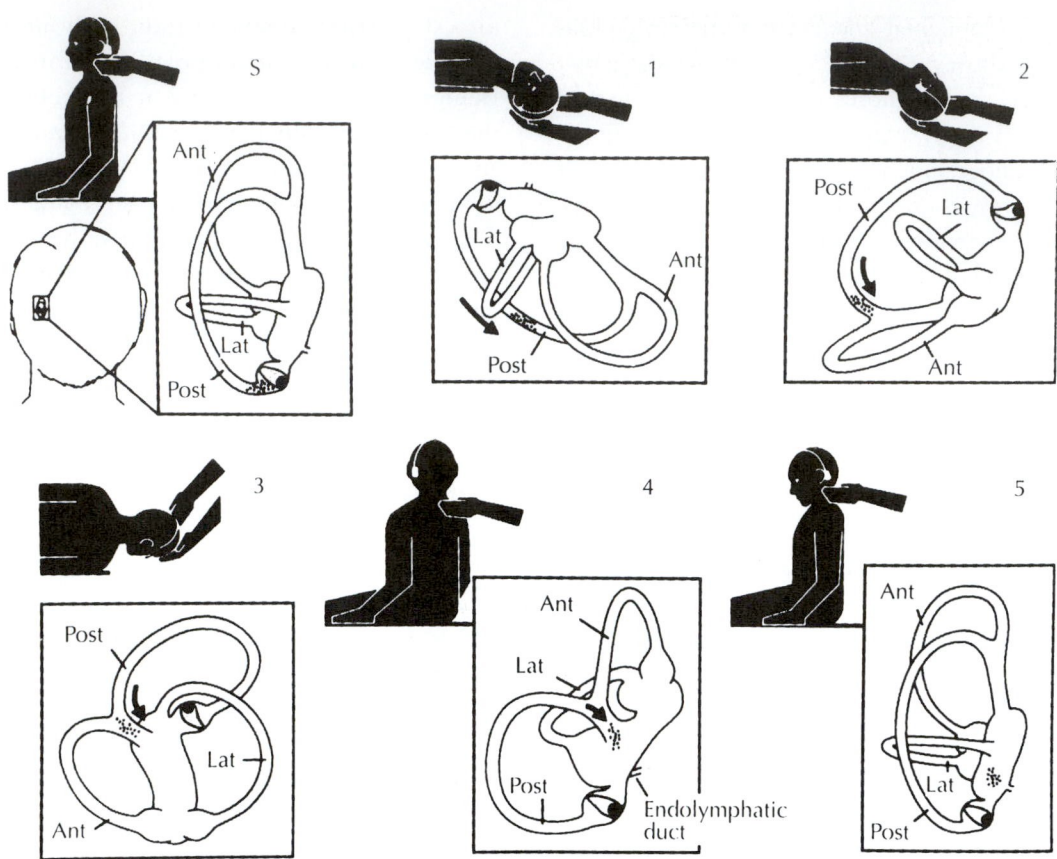

Figure 38-3 Illustration of canalith repositioning procedure, targeting the left posterior semicircular canal. General instructions: Pause at each position until induced nystagmus stops. If there is no nystagmus, pause until the latency plus duration period (in seconds) has passed. Repeat movements 1 through 5 until there is no nystagmus in any position. Position 5: Patient is seated with the operator behind and the oscillator is applied. (1) Head is placed over the end of the table 45 degrees to the left (canaliths gravitate to the center of the posterior semicircular canal). (2) While the head is tilted downward, it is rotated to a position 45 degrees to the right (canaliths reach the common crus). (3) Head and body are rotated until facing downward 135 degrees from the supine position (canaliths traverse the common crus). (4) While the head is turned to the right, the patient is brought to a sitting position (canaliths enter utricle). (5) Head is turned forward with chin lowered 20 degrees. The boxes illustrate the left labyrinth from the operator's viewpoint, showing gravitating canaliths. Semicircular canals are labeled. Ant = anterior; Lat = lateral; Post = posterior. *Reprinted with permission from Epley JM. The canalith repositioning procedure for treatment of benign positional vertigo. Otolaryngol Head Neck Surg 1992;107:399.*

venous return; (2) a decrease in cardiac output from obstruction of blood flow within the heart or pulmonary circulation or due to arrhythmias; or (3) cerebrovascular disease. Loss of consciousness may also occur from a reduction in cerebral metabolism due to hypoglycemia or hypoxemia and from seizures.[122]

A detailed list of causes of syncope is given in Table 38-10. From a pathophysiologic standpoint, the causes are neurally mediated from vasodilatation or bradycardia (vasovagal, neurocardiogenic, situational, and carotid sinus syncope), orthostatic and postprandial hypotension, neurologic (transient ischemic attacks and strokes, basilar migraine, seizures, and sub-

clavian steal), organic heart disease with decreased cardiac output (valvular heart disease, pulmonary embolism, pulmonary hypertension, ischemic heart disease, myxoma, pericardial tamponade, and aortic dissection), arrhythmias, psychiatric problems, and medications that may cause syncope by a variety of mechanisms. Roughly one-third of syncope remains undiagnosed, despite more sophisticated testing.[123]

Causes and Diagnostic Testing

The simple faint is not difficult to diagnose, with its attendant sweating, nausea, and precipitating event

TABLE 38-10
CAUSES OF SYNCOPE

Neurocardiogenic
    Vasovagal/vasodepressor
    Situational—cough, micturition, defecation, swallowing
Carotid-sinus syncope
Orthostatic and postprandial hypotension
Medications
Psychiatric
Neurologic—migraine, transient ischemic attack/stroke,
      seizure, subclavian steal
Cardiac
    Organic heart disease
      Aortic stenosis
      Hypertrophic cardiomyopathy
      Pulmonary embolism
      Pulmonary hypertension
      Myxoma
      Myocardial infarction
      Coronary spasm
      Tamponade
      Aortic dissection
    Arrhythmias
      Bradyarrhythmias
      Tachyarrhythmias
Metabolic
    Hypoglycemia
    Hypercapnia
    Hypoxemia
Undiagnosed

Modified with permission from Linzer M, Yang EH, Estes NA, Wang P, Vorperian VP, Kapoor WN. Diagnosing syncope. Part I. Value of history, physical examination, and electrocardiography. Clinical Efficacy Assessment Project of the American College of Physicians. Ann Intern Med 1997;126:989.

such as immobile position, stress, sight of blood, and fear. This is the most common cause of syncope. The term situational syncope is applied to syncope that is precipitated by coughing, micturition, defecation, or swallowing.

The broader category of vasodepressor or neurocardiogenic syncope can have a more subtle presentation. Along with psychiatric and alcohol-related causes, vasodepressor syncope is common in younger patients.[124] It should be suspected in unexplained, recurrent syncope with normal cardiac evaluation. Tilt-table testing is the key to diagnosis. Standardization of the procedure has now occurred.[125] The test is performed fasting with intravenous saline given prior to the procedure in an amount equal to 75 cc for each hour of the fasting period. The patient is placed on a tilt table for 20 minutes and then tilted upward to 60 to 80 degrees. A three-lead electrocardiogram is continuously recorded and beat-to-beat

blood pressure measured noninvasively. If after 45 minutes the test is nondiagnostic, pharmacologic provocation with isoproterenol at 1 μg/min is started with patient supine for 10 to 15 minutes and then tilted for 10 minutes. The dose can be increased twice to a maximum of 5 μg/min, repeating the tilt each time. A positive test occurs if syncopal or near-syncopal symptoms are reproduced by either hypotension and/or bradycardia.

Carotid-sinus syncope is a variant of vasodepressor syncope seen commonly in the elderly and in patients who report syncope with head turning or neck pressure. The key to diagnosis is carotid-sinus massage, which must not be done in the presence of carotid bruits, recent stroke or myocardial infarction, or history of ventricular tachycardia. The patient should have a continuously running cardiac monitor in place during the procedure and also an automatic blood-pressure measuring device. The carotid artery is massaged longitudinally for 5 seconds at the upper border of the thyroid cartilage. After a 1-minute respite, the procedure is repeated on the other side. Atropine should be readily available, though free-flowing intravenous administration is not a requirement. Carotid-sinus hypersensitivity syndrome is diagnosed by asystole >3 seconds (cardioinhibitory response), a drop in systolic blood pressure >50 mm Hg (vasodepressor response), or both (mixed response).[126]

Orthostatic and postprandial hypotension are common causes of syncope in the elderly. Orthostatic hypotension should be suspected in any elderly patient and in any patient on medications causing hypotension. A systolic blood pressure drop of 20 mm Hg or more from supine to standing is strongly supportive of the diagnosis.[127] The presence of orthostatic hypotension should not deter the physician from searching for other causes of syncope. Blood-pressure measurements may be more reproducible and diagnostic in the morning.[128] Postprandial hypotension may even be more common than orthostatic hypotension. It is seen in autonomic failure, diabetes, Parkinson disease, and during hemodialysis. It is more common in the elderly and may be associated with syncope, falls, dizziness, weakness, and stroke. Testing consists of blood-pressure measurements after a liquid meal with the patient seated.[129]

Medications associated with syncope typically cause vasodilation or bradycardia. They include β-blockers, angiotensin-converting–enzyme inhibitors, tricyclic antidepressants, centrally acting α_1-adrenergic agonists, vasodilators, α-adrenergic blockers, phenothiazines, barbiturates, and calcium-channel blockers.

Migraine and transient ischemic attacks are usually not difficult to diagnose as causes of syncope. Both transient ischemic attacks and strokes are almost always due to vertebrobasilar disease rather than carotid disease and will have concurrent symptoms such as vertigo, ataxia, and paresthesias.[130] Seizures are generally distinguished from syncope by their aura, sustained tonic–clonic movements, incontinence, and postictal phase. However, syncope induced by arrhythmias can cause brief tonic-clonic movements and up to 30 seconds of confusion ("convulsive syncope").[131]

Psychiatric disorders, particularly somatization disorder, depression, panic disorder, generalized anxiety, and alcohol/drug disorders appear to be related to syncope, particularly unexplained syncope.[132] Young patients who present with multiple episodes of syncope (e.g., five or more within a year) frequently have a psychiatric diagnosis.[121]

Cardiac causes of syncope include aortic stenosis, acute myocardial infarction, hypertrophic cardiomyopathy, pulmonic stenosis, pulmonary emboli, primary pulmonary hypertension, atrial myxoma, aortic dissection, pericardial tamponade, and both bradyarrhythmias and tachyarrhythmias. Exertional syncope mandates a careful search for valvular heart disease, coronary artery disease, arrhythmias, neurocardiogenic syncope, and if associated with arm movement, subclavian steal syndrome.

Electrocardiography is the first test performed to evaluate possible cardiac syncope and should be performed in any case of syncope without an obvious diagnosis. Complete heart block or a symptomatic arrhythmia may occasionally appear on the tracing and provide a diagnosis. More likely will be the presence of abnormalities that require further evaluation for arrhythmias such as Wolff–Parkinson–White (WPW) pattern, prolonged QT interval, nonsustained ventricular tachycardia, bundle-branch block, myocardial infarction, first-degree (or more severe) atrioventricular block, sinus bradycardia, or left ventricular hypertrophy.[123]

Echocardiography is a poorly studied method for the evaluation of cardiac syncope. However, it is useful in excluding an occult valvular lesion or an atrial myxoma, and evaluating an unexplained murmur. It should be done to detect unsuspected left ventricular hypertrophy, which can be an arrhythmia substrate. The echocardiogram is particularly important to order prior to treadmill testing to exclude hypertrophic cardiomyopathy and aortic stenosis as a cause of exercise-induced syncope. The echocardiogram is also useful in evaluating an elderly patient with risk factors for cardiac disease.[133]

Exercise stress testing should be performed in patients with exercise-related syncope or a likelihood of stable ischemic heart disease.[134] It should not be done in the setting of undiagnosed valvular heart disease, since sudden death during exercise can occur with severe aortic stenosis or hypertrophic cardiomyopathy.

Twenty-four-hour ambulatory cardiac monitoring (Holter) is useful in patients with symptoms suggesting an arrhythmia, such as brief loss of consciousness without warning and palpitations with syncope; known heart disease; an abnormal electrocardiogram; or unexplained recurrent syncope.[134] A loop monitor (event monitor), which is designed to be worn for a month, continuously records the patient's rhythm. The monitors store electrocardiogram rhythm strips for a programmable time period before and after the patient activates an event button. Following syncope, the previous electrocardiogram can be transmitted by telephone for analysis. Loop monitoring is particularly useful in frequent syncopal episodes with or without structural heart disease. However, loop monitors have a higher yield in the diagnosis of palpitations than of syncope.[135]

Significant arrhythmias detected by monitoring that require therapy are symptomatic tachyarrhythmia, symptomatic sinus-node dysfunction, symptomatic complete or second-degree atrioventricular block, asymptomatic complete heart block with rates <40 beats per minute (bpm) or asystole ≥3 seconds, bifascicular or trifascicular block with second-degree type II or third-degree atrioventricular block with or without symptoms, and possibly sinus-node dysfunction with heart rates <40 bpm and asymptomatic second-degree type II or complete heart block with heart rates >40 bpm.[136-138] If the patient has syncope or presyncope and a normal heart rhythm, then no further arrhythmia evaluation is required.

Electrophysiologic studies (EPS) are indicated for syncope associated with organic heart disease such as myocardial infarction or congestive heart failure without diagnostic findings on electrocardiographic or ambulatory monitoring.[139] EPS is also indicated for the following abnormalities on electrocardiographic or ambulatory monitoring: bundle-branch block, WPW, nonsustained ventricular tachycardia, sinus pauses, and atrioventricular block.[134,140]

The incidence of syncope may be increased during pregnancy. This may be caused by an increased number of arrhythmias[141] and by vena caval compression from a gravid uterus with reduction in cardiac output.[142] Further evaluation is merited if there is known heart disease; arrhythmias; exertional syncope; a murmur that is not a benign, flow murmur; or palpitations with syncope.[123]

Clinical Approach

History

To evaluate syncope, premonitory symptoms should be carefully explored, including exercise, chest pain, shortness of breath, arm movement (which can precipitate subclavian steal syndrome), sweating, yawning, nausea, aura, posture at time of syncope, blood loss, stressful situations, head-turning, cough, micturition, and defecation. If anyone witnessed the event, it is helpful to learn about tonic–clonic movements, the duration of syncope, and about a postsyncopal period of confusion. A cardiac and neurologic review of symptoms is also important. The frequency of syncope should be noted. Medications, substance abuse, and psychiatric symptoms round out the history.

Physical Examination

The physical examination should start with the vital signs. Both subclavian steal syndrome and orthostatic hypotension can be evaluated with bilateral arm blood pressures and supine and standing blood pressures as outlined earlier. A careful cardiac examination should be performed to detect an arrhythmia and to evaluate for organic heart disease. The murmur of hypertrophic cardiomyopathy may be exacerbated by the upright position or by the Valsalva maneuver. Pressing one hand gently on the abdomen during this maneuver and noting the tightening of abdominal musculature documents proper performance by the patient. Significant aortic stenosis is characterized by a slowly rising carotid pulse, a late peaking systolic murmur, a diminished S_2, and a delay in pulse transmission from the cardiac apex to carotids and from brachial to radial artery.[143] Patients with pulmonary hypertension often have a loud P_2 component of S_2,

a right ventricular lift, and tricuspid and/or pulmonic regurgitation murmurs. Atrial myxomas may have a low-pitched tumor plop in early to mid-diastole.

Hyperventilation using vigorous, open-mouthed breathing for 2 to 3 minutes is predictive of a psychiatric cause if syncope or near-syncope is produced.[144,145]

Laboratory Evaluation

The history and physical examination in the syncopal patient usually diagnoses vasovagal, situational, orthostatic, and postprandial hypotension and may strongly suggest the diagnoses of pulmonary embolus, myocardial infarction, subclavian steal syndrome, seizure, valvular heart disease, carotid-sinus syncope, and arrhythmia. Appropriate testing may include lung scan, cardiac enzymes, electrocardiography, peripheral vascular studies, electroencephalography, echocardiography, carotid-sinus massage, and Holter monitoring as indicated.

Unexplained syncope is a more difficult problem. The first step in evaluation is to determine if underlying heart disease is present. Exertional syncope, sudden syncope, cardiac symptoms, a history of ischemic heart disease or an abnormal electrocardiogram all point toward organic heart disease. These patients should be evaluated with an exercise treadmill test (ETT) (especially if there is exercise-induced syncope or a high likelihood of ischemic heart disease). In patients with exertional syncope, an echocardiogram should precede the ETT to exclude hypertrophic cardiomyopathy. Patients older than 60 have an increased risk for both carotid-sinus syncope and organic heart disease. Carotid-sinus massage may be done safely in elderly patients as long as no contraindications exist. If massage is negative, then organic heart disease may be excluded with stress testing and/or echocardiography. For patients in whom organic heart disease is suspected or who have symptoms suggestive of an arrhythmia, 24-hour Holter monitoring should be done next. The Holter monitoring may be diagnostic of the cause of syncope, may reveal nonsustained ventricular tachycardia or other arrhythmia suggesting a need for further study, or may show normal sinus rhythm in the face of syncope. The demonstration of syncope with a normal rhythm should prompt tilt testing and/or psychiatric evaluation if the syncope is recurrent. Electrophysiologic testing is the next step in the face of nondiagnostic but abnormal

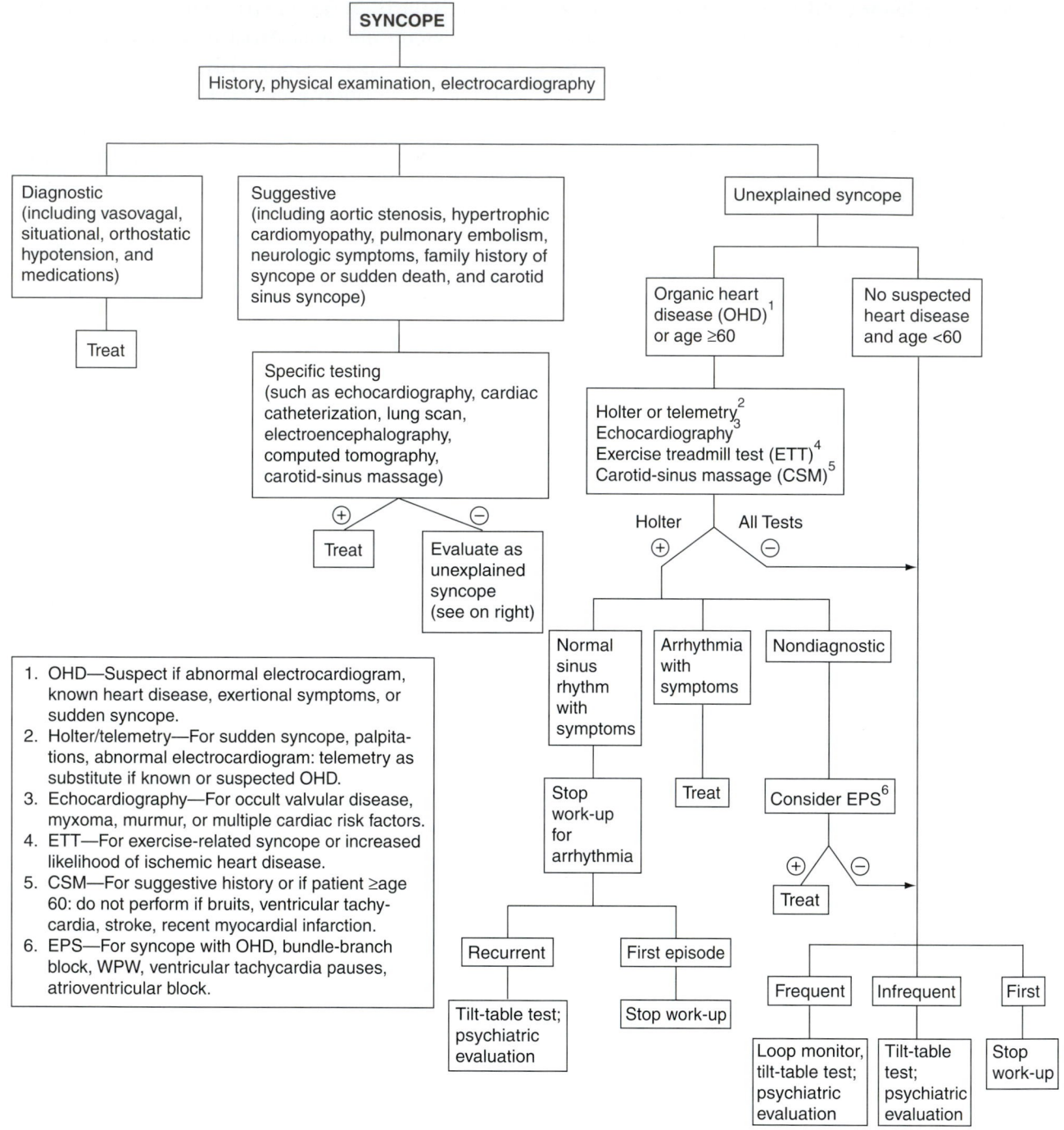

Figure 38-4 Evaluation of syncope. *Modified with permission from Linzer M, Yang EH, Estes NA, et al. Diagnosing syncope. Part I. Value of history, physical examination, and electrocardiography. Clinical Assessment Project of the American College of Physicians. Ann Intern Med 1997;126:989.*

symptoms on Holter monitoring as noted earlier.[134]

Patients in whom heart disease is ruled out or is clinically unsuspected should have work-up deferred unless syncope is recurrent. Work-up for recurrent syncope may include loop monitoring, tilt-table testing, and/or psychiatric evaluation. Loop monitoring is most effective in patients with frequent spells—one per week to one per 3 months.

Syncopal patients should be hospitalized for telemetry monitoring if they have known heart disease, chest pain, history of arrhythmias, or arrhythmogenic medications.[123,134]

See Figure 38-4 for an algorithmic approach to evaluation of syncope.

Treatment

The key to syncope treatment is identification of the underlying cause.

Postprandial hypotension can be managed by discontinuing medications that contribute to hypotension, lying down for up to 90 minutes after eating, drinking adequate fluids, reducing meal size and carbohydrate content, and possibly using medications such as caffeine, 250 mg or 2 cups of coffee preprandially; octreotide, 50 μg subcutaneously preprandially; fludrocortisone, from 0.1 to 1.0 mg daily; indomethacin, 25 to 50 mg twice a day, or midodrine, 2.5 to 10 mg twice a day.[129]

The treatment of orthostatic hypotension depends on the cause. Any offending medication should be stopped. Dehydration should be corrected. For orthostatic hypotension due to autonomic failure, nonpharmacologic measures such as elevation of the head of the bed at night and liberalization of salt and water intake may be helpful. Medications including fludrocortisone at 0.05 to 0.4 mg/day, midodrine at 2.5 to 10 mg three times a day, and recombinant human erythropoietin have all demonstrated efficacy.[146,147]

The management of neurocardiogenic syncope is based on a number of small trials, many with methodologic problems. Tilt-table testing, unfortunately, is less effective in predicting treatment efficacy than it is in diagnosis.[125] β-Blockers appear to be effective in managing neurocardiogenic syncope. Agents used have included metoprolol, 50 to 400 mg/day[148-150]; atenolol, 25 to 200 mg/day[150,151]; and propranolol, 40 to 160 mg/day.[150] Verapamil, scopolamine, and clonidine were less effective in more recent trials.[148,149,152] Fludrocortisone, disopyramide, mido-

drine, and serotonin reuptake inhibitors have also been used.[150,153-156] Pacemaker therapy may be considered in patients with cardioinhibitory vasovagal syncope unresponsive to β-blockers.[157-158] However, because of conflicting studies, the American College of Cardiology/American Heart Association guidelines note that the efficacy of a pacemaker in this situation is less well established.[138] Since many patients experience a decrease in their syncopal episodes following tilt-table testing and the condition is usually benign, long-term therapy is often not necessary. Patients with injury-causing syncope and no prodrome are the best candidates for empiric drug therapy.[159] Cardioinhibitory carotid sinus syncope is best managed with a dual-chamber pacemaker.[160,161]

REFERENCES

1. Lamberts H, Hofmans-Okkes I. Episode of care: a core concept in family practice. J Fam Pract 1996;42:161.
2. Silberstein SD, Merriam GR. Estrogens, progestins, and headache. Neurology 1991;41:786.
3. Stewart WF, Lipton RB, Celentano DD, Reed ML. Prevalence of migraine headache in the United States: relation to age, income, race, and other sociodemographic factors. JAMA 1992;267:64.
4. Rasmussen BK. Epidemiology of headache. Cephalalgia 1995;15:45.
5. Hainline B. Headache. Neurol Clin 1994;12:443.
6. Moskowitz MA. The neurobiology of vascular head pain. Ann Neurol 1984;16:157.
7. Lauritzen M. Pathophysiology of the migraine aura: the spreading depression theory. Brain 1994;117:199.
8. Headache Classification Committee of the International Headache Society. Classification and diagnostic criteria for headache disorders, cranial neuralgias, and facial pain. Cephalalgia 1988;8(Suppl 7):1.
9. Silberstein SD, Lipton RB. Overview of diagnosis and treatment of migraine. Neurology 1994;44(Suppl 7):S6.
10. Selby G, Lance JW. Observations on 500 cases of migraine and allied vascular headache. J Neurol Neurosurg Psychiatry 1960;23:23.
11. Lipton RB, Stewart W, Celentano DD, et al. Undiagnosed migraine: a comparison of symptom-based and self-reported physician diagnosis. Arch Intern Med 1992; 156:1.
12. Kumar KL, Cooney TG. Headaches. Med Clin North Am 1995;79:261.
13. Rasmussen BK, Jensen R, Schroll M, Olesen J. Epidemiology of headache in a general population—a prevalence study. J Clin Epidemiol 1991;44:1147.
14. Mathew NT. Transformed migraine. Cephalalgia 1993; 13(Suppl 12):78.
15. Mathew NT, Reuveni U, Perez F. Transformed or evolutive migraine. Headache 1987;27:102.
16. Mathew NT. Transformed migraine, analgesic rebound

and other chronic daily headaches. Neurol Clin 1997; 15:167.

17. Solomon S, Cappa KG. The headache of temporal arteritis. J Am Geriatr Soc 1987;35:163.

18. Weyand CM, Goronzy JJ. Polymyalgia rheumatica and giant cell arteritis. In: Koopman WJ, ed. Arthritis and allied conditions. Baltimore: Williams & Wilkins, 1997: 1610.

19. Forsyth PA, Posner JB. Headache in patients with brain tumors: a study of 111 patients. Neurology 1993;43:1678.

20. Juvela S. Minor leak before rupture of an intracranial aneurysm and subarachnoid hemorrhage of unknown etiology. Neurosurgery 1992;30:7.

21. Vermeulen M, Hasan D, Blijenberg BG, Hijdra A, van Gijn J. Xanthochromia after subarachnoid haemorrhage needs no revisitation. J Neurol Neurosurg Psychiatry 1989;52:826.

22. Garretson HD. Intracranial arteriovenous malformations. In: Wilkins RH, Rengachary SS, eds. Neurosurgery. New York: McGraw-Hill, 1996:2464.

23. American Academy of Neurology. Practice parameter: the utility of neuroimaging in the evaluation of headache in patients with normal neurologic examinations. Neurology 1994;44:1353.

24. Weiss NS. Relation of high blood pressure to headache, epistaxis, and selected other symptoms. N Engl J Med 1972;287:631.

25. Badran RHA, Weir RJ, McGuiness JB. Hypertension and headache. Scot Med J 1970;15:48.

26. Cooper WD, Glover DR, Hormbrey JM, Kimber GR. Headache and blood pressure: evidence of a close relationship. J Hum Hypertens 1989;3:41.

27. Giuseffi V, Wall M, Siegel PZ, Rojas PB. Symptoms and disease associations in idiopathic intracranial hypertension: a case control study. Neurology 1991;41:239.

28. Radhakrishnan K, Ahlskog JE, Garrity JA, Kurland LT. Idiopathic intracranial hypertension. Mayo Clin Proc 1994;69:169.

29. Durand ML, Calderwood SB, Weber DJ, et al. Acute bacterial meningitis in adults: a review of 493 episodes. N Engl J Med 1993;328:21.

30. Verghese A, Gallemore G. Kernig's and Brudzinski's signs revisited. Rev Infect Dis 1987;9:1187.

31. Bartlett JG 1998 medical management of HIV infection. Baltimore: Port City Press, 1998:274.

32. Epstein MT, Hockaday JM, Hockaday TD. Migraine and reproductive hormones throughout the menstrual cycle. Lancet 1975;1:543.

33. Somerville BW. The role of estradiol withdrawal in the etiology of menstrual migraine. Neurology 1972;22:355.

34. Fioroni L, Andrea GD, Alecci M, Canazi A, Faechinetti F. Platelet serotonin pathway in menstrual migraine. Cephalalgia 1996;6:427.

35. MacGregor EA. Menstruation, sex hormones, and migraine. Neurol Clin 1997;15:125.

36. Silberstein SD, Merriam G. Estrogens, progestins, and headache. Neurology 1991;41:786.

37. Silberstein SD. Migraine and women. Postgrad Med 1995;97:147.

38. Raskin NH. Headache. 2nd ed. New York: Churchill Livingstone, 1988:35.

39. Kudrow L. The relationship of headache frequency to hormone use in migraine. Headache 1975;15:36.

40. Gilman S. Imaging the brain. N Engl J Med 1998; 338:812.

41. Weingarten S, Kleinman M, Elperin L, Larson EB. The effectiveness of cerebral imaging in the diagnosis of chronic headache. Arch Intern Med 1992;152:2457.

42. Silberstein SD, Young WB. Safety and efficacy of ergotamine tartrate and dihydroergotamine in the treatment of migraine and status migrainosus. Neurology 1995; 45:577.

43. Capobianco DJ, Cheshire WP, Campbell JK. An overview of the diagnosis and pharmacologic treatment of migraine. Mayo Clin Proc 1996;71:1055.

44. Briggs GC, Freeman RK, Yaffe SJ. Drugs in pregnancy and lactation, 5th ed. Baltimore: Williams & Wilkins, 1998;389.

45. Committee on Drugs. American Academy of Pediatrics. The transfer of drugs and other chemicals into human milk. Pediatrics 1994;93:137.

46. Bates D, Ashford E, Dawson R, et al. Subcutaneous sumatriptan during the migraine aura. Neurology 1994; 44:1587.

47. Tepper SJ. Migraine: latest options for acute therapy. Consultant 1998;38:1163.

48. Winner P, Ricalde O, LeForce B, Saper J, Margul B. A double-blind study of subcutaneous dihydroergotamine vs subcutaneous sumatriptan in the treatment of acute migraine. Arch Neurol 1996;53:180.

49. Touchon J, Berlin L, Pilgrim AJ, Ashford E, Bes A. A comparison of subcutaneous samatriptan and dihydroergotamine nasal spray in the acute treatment of migraine. Neurology 1996;47:361.

50. Solomon GD, Cady RK, Klapper JA, Earl NL, Saper MD, Rumadan NM. Clinical efficacy and tolerability of 2.5 mg Zolmitriptan for the acute treatment of migraine. Neurology 1997;49:1219.

51. Ferrari MD. 311C90: increasing the options for therapy with effective acute antimigraine 5 HT$_{1B/1D}$ receptor agonists. Neurology 1997;48(Suppl 3):S21.

52. Zolmitriptan for migraine. Med Lett Drug Ther 1998; 40:27.

53. Mathew NT, Saper SR, Silberstein DS, et al. Migraine prophylaxis with divalproex. Arch Neurol 1995;52:287.

54. Pryse-Phillips WEM, Dodick DW, Edmeads JG, et al. Guidelines for the diagnosis and management of migraine in clinical practice. Can Med Assoc J 1997; 156:1273.

55. Gillis JC, Benefield P, Goa KL. Transnasal butorphanol: a review of its pharmacodynamic and pharmacokinetic properties and therapeutic potential in acute pain management. Drugs 1995;50:157.

56. Ellis GL, Delaney J, DeHart DA, Owens A. The efficacy of metoclopramide in the treatment of migraine headache. Ann Emerg Med 1993;22:191.

57. Lane PL. Comparative efficacy of chlorpromazine and meperidine with dimenhydrate in migraine headache. Ann Emerg Med 1989;18:360.

58. Jones J, Sklar D, Daugherty J, White W. Randomized double-blind trial of intravenous prochlorperazine for the treatment of acute headache. JAMA 1989;261:1174.

59. Thomas SH, Stone CK, Ray VG, Whitley TW. Intravenous versus rectal prochlorperazine in the treatment of benign vascular or tension headache: a randomized, prospective, double-blind trial. Ann Emerg Med 1994; 24:923.

60. Ziegler DK, Hurwitz A, Preskorn S, Hassanein R, Seim J. Propranolol and amitriptyline in prophylaxis of migraine. Arch Neurol 1993;50:825.

61. Jensen R, Brinck T, Olesen J. Sodium valproate has a prophylactic effect in migraine without aura—a triple-blind, placebo-controlled crossover study. Neurology 1994;44:647.

62. Kaniecki RG. A comparison of divalproex with propranolol and placebo for the prophylaxis of migraine without aura. Arch Neurol 1997;54:1141.

63. Mathew NT, Asgharnejad M, Peykamian M, Laurenza A. Naratriptan is effective and well tolerated in the acute treatment of migraine: results of a double-blind, placebo-controlled, crossover study: the Naratriptan S2WA 3003 study group. Neurology 1997;49:1485.

64. Hering R, Kuritzsky A. Sodium valproate in the prophylactic treatment of migraine: a double-blind study versus placebo. Cephalalgia 1992;121:81.

65. Jonsdottir M, Meyer JS, Rogers RL. Efficacy, side effects, and tolerance compared during headache treatment with three different calcium blockers. Headache 1987; 27:364.

66. Welch KM, Ellis DJ, Keenan PA. Successful migraine prophylaxis with naproxen sodium. Neurology 1985; 35:1304.

67. Grotemeyer KH, Scharafinski HW, Schlakc HP, Husstedt IW. Acetylsalicylic acid vs metoprolol in migraine prophylaxis—a double blind crossover study. Headache 1990;30:639.

68. Buring JE, Peto R, Hennekens CH. Low-dose aspirin for migraine prophylaxis. JAMA 1990;264:1711.

69. Welch KMA. Drug therapy of migraine. N Engl J Med 1993;329:1476.

70. Graham J. Methysergide for prevention of headaches. N Engl J Med 1964;270:67.

71. Lidegaard O. Oral contraception and risk of a cerebral thromboembolic attack: results of a case-control study. BMJ 1993;306:956.

72. Lidegaard O. Oral contraceptives, pregnancy and the risk of cerebral thromboembolism: the influence of diabetes, hypertension, migraine, and previous thrombotic disease. Br J Obstet Gynaecol 1995;102:153.

73. Silberstein SD. Migraine and pregnancy. Neurol Clin 1997;15:209.

74. Kudrow L. Response of cluster headache attacks to oxygen inhalation. Headache 1981;21:1.

75. Fogan L. Treatment of cluster headache: a double blind comparison of oxygen vs. air inhalation. Arch Neurol 1985;42:362.

76. Meyer JS, Hardenberg J. Clinical effectiveness of calcium entry blockers in prophylactic treatment of migraine and cluster headaches. Headache 1983;23:266.

77. Kudrow L. Comparative results of prednisone, methysergide, and lithium therapy in cluster headache. In: Green R, ed. Current concepts in migraine research. New York: Raven Press, 1978:159.

78. Kudrow L. Treatment of cluster headache. Headache Quarterly 1993;4(Suppl 2):42.

79. Kudrow L. Lithium prophylaxis for chronic cluster headache. Headache 1977;17:15.

80. Savoldi F, Bono G, Manzoni GC, Michieli G, Lanfranchi M, Nappi G. Lithium salts in cluster headache treatment. Cephalalgia 1983;3(Suppl 1):79.

81. Hering R, Kuritzky A. Sodium valproate in the prophylactic treatment of migraine: a double-blind study versus placebo. Cephalalgia 1992;12:81.

82. Diamond S. Ibuprofen versus aspirin and placebo in treatment of muscle contraction headache. Headache 1983;23:206.

83. Sargent JD, Peters K, Goldstein J, Madison DS, Solback P. Naproxen sodium for muscle contraction headache treatment. Headache 1988;28:180.

84. Miller DS, Talbot CA, Simpson W, Korey A. A comparison of naproxen sodium, acetaminophen and placebo in the treatment of muscle contraction headache. Headache 1987;27:392.

85. Silberstein SD, Schidman E, Hopkins M. Repetitive intravenous DHE in the refractory headache. Headache 1990;30:334.

86. Kudrow L. Paradoxical efects of analgesic use. Adv Neurol 1982;33:335.

87. Bonuccelli U, Nuti A, Lucetti C, Pavese N, Dell 'Agnello G, Muratoria A. Amitriptyline and dexamethasone combined treatment in drug-induced headache. Cephalalgia 1996;16:198.

88. Kroenke K, Mangelsdorff AD. Common symptoms in ambulatory care: incidence, evaluation, therapy, and outcome. Am J Med 1989;86:262.

89. Kroenke K, Lucas CA, Robenberg ML, et al. Causes of persistent dizziness: a prospective study of 100 patients in ambulatory care. Ann Intern Med 1992; 117:898.

90. Sloane P, Blazer D, George LK. Dizziness in a community elderly population. J Am Geriatr Soc 1989;37:101.

91. Harner SG. Peripheral labyrinthine causes of dizziness. Postgrad Med 1987;81:251.

92. Drachman DA, Hart CW. An approach to the dizzy patient. Neurology 1972;22:323.

93. McGee S. Dizzy patients—diagnosis and treatment. West J Med 1995;162:37.

94. Kroenke K, Lucas C, Rosenberg ML, Scherokman B, Herbers JE. One-year outcome for patients with a chief complaint of dizziness. J Gen Intern Med 1994;9:684.

95. Lempert T, Gresty MA, Bronstein AM. Benign positional vertigo: recognition and treatment. BMJ 1995;311:489.

96. Katsarkas A, Kirkham TH. Paroxysmal positional vertigo: a study of 255 cases. J Otolaryngol 1978;7:320.

97. Froehling DA, Silverstein MD, Mohr DN, Beatty CW, Offord KP, Ballard DJ. Benign positional vertigo: incidence and prognosis in a population-based study in Olmsted County, Minnesota. Mayo Clin Proc 1991; 66:596.

98. Jannetta PJ, Moller MB, Moller AR. Disabling positional vertigo. N Engl J Med 1984;310:1700.

99. Selesnick SH, Jackler RK, Pitts LW. The changing clinical presentation of acoustic neuromas in the MRI era. Laryngoscope 1993;103:431.

100. Ruckenstein MJ. A practical approach to dizziness. Postgrad Med 1995;97:70.

101. Black FO, Pesznecker SC. Vestibular ototoxicity. Otolaryngol Clin North Am 1993;26:713.

102. Gibson WP, Arenberg IK. Pathophysiologic theories in the etiology of Meniere's disease. Otolaryngol Clin North Am 1997;30:961.

103. Brandt T. Phobic postural vertigo. Neurology 1996; 46:1515.

104. Furman JM, Jacob RG. Psychiatric dizziness. Neurology 1997;47:1161.

105. Fisher CM. Vertigo in cerebrovascular disease. Arch Otolaryngol 1967;85:529.

106. Hotson JR, Baloh RW. Acute vestibular syndrome. N Engl J Med 1998;339:680.

107. Troost BT. Dizziness and vertigo in vertebrobasilar disease. Part II. Central causes and vertebrobasilar disease. Stroke 1980;11:413.

108. Rolak LA. The diagnosis of multiple sclerosis. Neurol Clin 1996;14:27.

109. Poser CM, Paty DW, Scheinberg L, et al. New diagnostic criteria for multiple sclerosis: guidelines for research protocols. Ann Neurol 1983;13:227.

110. Rosenstock HA. Sertraline withdrawal in two brothers: a case report. Int Clin Psychopharmol 1996;11:58.

111. Warner EA, Wallach PM, Adelman HM, Sahlin-Hughes K. Dizziness in primary care patients. J Gen Intern Med 1992;7:454.

112. Baloh RW, Jacobson KM, Socotch TM. The effect of aging on visual-vestibulocular responses. Exp Brain Res 1993;95:509.

113. Weindruch R, Korper SP, Hadley E. The prevalence of disequilibrium and related disorders in older persons. Ear Nose Throat J 1989;68:925.

114. Sloane PD. Clinical significance of a dizziness history in medical patients with syncope. Arch Intern Med 1991; 151:1625.

115. Fitzgerald DC. Head trauma: hearing loss and dizziness. J Trauma 1996;40: 488.

116. Hart RG, Gardner DP, Howieson J. Acoustic tumors: atypical features and recent diagnostic tests. Neurology 1983;33:211.

117. McClure JA, Willett JM. Lorazepam and diazepam in the treatment of benign paroxysmal vertigo. J Otolaryngol 1980;9:472.

118. Epley JM. The canalith repositioning procedure for treatment of benign positional vertigo. Otolaryngol Head Neck Surg 1992;107:399.

119. Klockhoff I, Lindblom U. Meniere's disease and hydrocholorothiazide—a critical analysis of symptoms and therapeutic effects. Acta Otolaryngol (Stockh) 1967;63:347.

120. Savage DD, Corwin L, McGee DL, Kannel WB, Wolf PA. Epidemiologic features of isolated syncope: the Framingham study. Stroke 1985;16:626.

121. Kapoor WN. Diagnostic evaluation of syncope. Am J Med 1991;90:91.

122. Kapoor WN. Workup and management of patients with syncope. Med Clin North Am 1995;79:1153.

123. Linzer M, Yang EH, Estes NA, Wang P, Vorperian VP, Kapoor WN. Diagnosing syncope. Part I. Value of history, physical examination, and electrocardiography: Clinical Efficacy Assessment Project of the American College of Physicians. Ann Intern Med 1997;126:989.

124. Day SC, Cook EF, Funkenstein H, Goldman L. Evaluation and outcome of emergency room patients with transient loss of consciousness. Am J Med 1982;73:15.

125. Benditt DG, Ferguson DW, Grubb BP, et al. Tilt table testing for assessing syncope: American College of Cardiology. J Am Coll Cardiol 1996;28:263.

126. McIntosh SJ, Lawson J, Kenny RA. Clinical characteristics of vasodepressor, cardioinhibitory, and mixed carotid sinus syndrome in the elderly. Am J Med 1993;95:203.

127. Atkins D, Hanusa B, Sefcik T, Kapoor WN. Syncope and orthostatic hypotension. Am J Med 1991;91:179.

128. Ward C, Kenny RA. Reproducibility of orthostatic hypotension in symptomatic elderly. Am J Med 1996; 100:418.

129. Jansen RW and Lipsitz LA. Postprandial hypotension: epidemiology, pathophysiology, and clinical management. Ann Intern Med 1995;122:286.

130. Davidson E, Rotenbeg Z, Fuchs J, Weinberger I, Agmon J. Transient ischemic attack-related syncope. Clin Cardiol 1991;14:141.

131. Aminoff MJ, Schienman MM, Griffin JC, Herre JM. Electrocerebral accompaniments of syncope associated with malignant ventricular arrhythmias. Ann Intern Med 1988;108:791.

132. Kapoor WN, Fortunato M, Hanusa BH, Schulberg HC. Psychiatric illnesses in patients with syncope. Am J Med 1995;99:505.

133. Fogoros RN. Cardiac arrhythmias: syncope and stroke. Neurol Clin 1993;11:375.

134. Linzer M, Yang EH, Estes NA, Wang P, Volperian VR, Kapoor WN. Diagnosing syncope. Part 2. Unexplained syncope: clinical efficacy assessment project of the American College of Physicians. Ann Intern Med 1997; 127:76.

135. Fogel RI, Evans JJ, Prystowsky EN. Utility and cost of event recorders in the diagnosis of palpitations, presyncope, and syncope. Am J Cardiol 1997;79:207.

136. Kusumoto FM, Goldschlager N. Cardiac pacing. N Engl J Med 1996;334:89.

137. Zimetbaum P, Kim KY, Ho KK, Zebede J, Josephson ME, Goldberger AL. Utility of patient-activated cardiac event recorders in general clinical practice. Am J Cardiol 1997;79:371.

138. Gregoratos G, Conill A, Epstein AE, et al. ACC/AHA guidelines for implantation of cardiac pacemakers and antiarrhythmic devices: a report of the American College of Cardiology/American Heart Association Task Force on Practice Guidelines (Committee on Pacemaker Implantation) J Am Coll Cardiol 1998;31:175.

139. Zipes DP, DiMarco JP, Gillette PC, et al. Guidelines for clinical intracardiac electrophysiological and catheter ablation procedures. J Am Coll Cardiol 1995;26:555.

140. Bachinsky WB, Linzer M. Weld L, Estes NAM. Usefulness of clinical characteristics in predicting the outcome of electrophysiologic studies in unexplained syncope. Am J Cardiol 1992;69:1044.

141. Kunzel W. Vena cava occlusion syndrome: cardiovascular parameters and uterine blood supply. Fortschr Med 1976;94:949.

142. Ikeda T, Ohbuchi H, Ikenoue T, Mori N. Maternal cerebral hemodynamics in the supine hypotensive syndrome. Obstet Gynecol 1992;79:27.

143. Etchells E, Bell C, Robb K. Does this patient have an abnormal systolic murmur? JAMA 1997;277:564.

144. Koenig D, Linzer M, Pontinen M, Divine GW. Syncope in young adults: evidence for a combined medical and psychiatric approach. J Intern Med 1992;232:169.

145. Hoefnagels WA, Padberg GW, Overweg J, Roos RA, van Dijk JG, Kamphuisen HA. Syncope or seizure? The diagnostic value of the EEG and hyperventilation test in transient loss of consciousness. J Neurol Neurosurg Psychiatry 1991;54:953.

146. Midodrine for orthostatic hypotension. Med Lett Drug Ther 1997;39:59.

147. Robertson D, Davis TL. Recent advances in the treatment of orthostatic hypotension. Neurology 1995; 45(Suppl 5):S26.

148. Jhamb DK, Singh B, Shada B, et al. Comparative study of the efficacy of metoprolol and verapamil in patients with syncope and positive head-up tilt test response. Am Heart J 1996;132:608.

149. Biffi M, Boriani G, Sabbatani P, et al. Malignant vasovagal syncope: a randomised trial of metoprolol and clonidine. Heart 1997;77:268.

150. Kapoor WN, Smith MA, Miller NL. Upright tilt testing in evaluating syncope: a comprehensive literature review. Am J Med 1994;97:78.

151. Mahanonda N, Bhuripanyo K, Kangkagate C, et al. Randomized, double-blind, placebo-controlled trial of oral atenolol in patients with unexplained syncope and positive upright tilt table test results. Am Heart J 1995; 130:1250.

152. Lee, TM, Su SF, Chen MF, Liau CS, Lee YT. Usefulness of transdermal scopolamine for vasovagal syncope. Am J Cardiol 1996;78:480.

153. Scott WA, Pongiglione G, Bromberg BI, et al. Randomized comparison of atenolol and fludrocortisone acetate in the treatment of pediatric neurally mediated syncope. Am J Cardiol 1995;76:400.

154. Grubb BP, Samoil D, Kosinski D, Kip K, Brewster P. Use of sertraline hydrochloride in the treatment of refractory neurocardiogenic syncope in children and adolescents. J Am Coll Cardiol 1994;24:490.

155. Ward CR, Gray JC, Gilroy JJ, Kenny RA. Midodrine: a role in the management of neurocardiogenic syncope. Heart 1998;79:45.

156. Grubb BP, Wolfe DA, Samoil D, Temesy-Armos P, Hahn H, Elliott L. Usefulness of fluoxetine hydrochloride for prevention of resistant upright tilt induced syncope. Pacing Clin Electrophysiol 1993;16:458.

157. Petersen ME, Chamberlain-Webber R, Fitzpatrick AP, Ingram A, Williams T, Sutton R. Permanent pacing for cardioinhibitory malignant vasovagal syndrome. Br Heart J 1994;71:274.

158. Benditt DG, Petersen M, Lurie KG, Gruff BP, Sutton R. Cardiac pacing for prevention of recurrent vasovagal syncope. Ann Intern Med 1995;122:204.

159. Barbey JT. Vasodepressor syncope-diagnosis and management. Cardiol Clin 1997;15:251.

160. Maloney JD, Jaeger FJ, Rizo-Patron C, Zhu DW. The role of pacing for the managment of neurally mediated syncope: carotid sinus syndrome and vasovagal syncope. Am Heart J 1994;127:1030.

161. McIntosh SJ, Lawson J, Bexton RS, Gold RG, Tynan MM, Kenny RA. A study comparing VVI and DDI pacing in elderly patients with carotid sinus syndrome. Heart 1997;77:553.

Chapter 39

Evaluation of Musculoskeletal Symptoms

Gurjit Kaeley
Laura Carbone

Five Key Points

- **A thorough history and physical examination is essential when evaluating a patient with a musculoskeletal condition.**

- **An inflammatory arthritis is characterized by morning stiffness and swelling within the joints.**

- **Nonarticular conditions, including fibromyalgia, bursitis, and tendonitis, are common causes of musculoskeletal complaints in a primary care office.**

- **In a patient presenting with pain in a single joint, it is critically important to examine the joint above and below the painful joint.**

- **In a patient presenting with a musculoskeletal symptom, order only those laboratory tests which are indicated by the history and physical examination.**

Musculoskeletal pain is a common symptom in primary care practice, and a systematic approach is needed to evaluate this pain. The history and physical examination are the most important aspects of the rheumatologic evaluation. Laboratory tests should be ordered only as guided by the history and physical examination.

In the following section, the initial approach to evaluation of arthritis will be discussed. Major rheumatic syndromes will then be discussed individually.

CLINICAL APPROACH TO THE EVALUATION OF ARTHRITIS

The important points to establish when obtaining a history of joint pain are the mode of onset, number and location of joints involved, and the characteristics of joint involvement. Articular pain may present abruptly or as gradual discomfort. When symptoms last more than 6 weeks, the condition is regarded as chronic. It is necessary to determine whether the joint involvement occurred simultaneously, in an additive fashion (pain persists in one or more joints and spreads to involve other joints), or in a migratory fashion (pain persists in one or more joints, then disappears in the initially involved joints and spreads to involve other joints).

The number and location of joints involved will also give a clue to the cause of the arthritis. Establishing whether the joint involvement is symmetric or asymmetric is also important. Inquiring about both peripheral joint involvement as well as specific questioning for axial complaints should be done.

Finally, it is important to establish whether the arthritis is inflammatory or noninflammatory. Historical clues to the presence of inflammatory arthritis include morning stiffness (usually more than 1 hour), joint swelling, and warmth.

A thorough review of systems should be done. Specific historical features of note include the presence of sicca symptoms; conjunctivitis or uveitis; alopecia; oral, nasal or vaginal ulcerations; weight loss; headaches; malar or discoid rashes; serositis; seizures; Raynauds phenomenon; morning stiffness; or diarrhea. On taking the social history, it is important to inquire about sexually transmitted diseases as well as intravenous drug use. A family history of arthritis and the nature of this arthritis should be sought. It is also desirable to establish whether the pain is articular or nonarticular.

The physical examination should be used to establish whether the pain arises from the joint (articular) or nonarticular structures, the extent and pattern of joint involvement, and involvement of other systems. The joint examination should proceed in an orderly manner, beginning with inspection, followed by palpation, then active and passive movement of the joints. On inspection, obvious abnormalities in alignment, swelling, and erythema over the joints should be noted. Palpation of the joint is used to confirm the presence of synovitis, effusion, or dactylitis. Next, using active and passive movement, the source of pain may be determined. Pain from articular structures arises during passive and active movements, while pain from nonarticular structures tends to occur during active movements only. If the active movement in the joint is incomplete, then passive movement should be used to determine the degree of limitation of the movement of the joint. The presence of crepitus may also be noted. A careful general examination should be done to uncover the extraarticular features of arthritis.

The laboratory evaluation should be thoughtfully guided by the history and physical examination, since no laboratory results are pathognomonic of rheumatic disease. Nonspecific laboratory results such as complete blood count, chemistry panel, and urinalysis are useful in determining multisystem involvement. The sedimentation rate and C-reactive protein (CRP) are nonspecific indicators of inflammation. Serologic tests should be ordered as indicated by the history and physical examination. Selected serologic tests are

TABLE 39-1 SELECTED SEROLOGIC TESTS	
Rheumatoid factor	High titer prognostic in rheumatoid arthritis. Also, positive in connective-tissue disease, cryoglobulinaemia, viral and parasitic infections, subacute bacterial endocarditis and hepatic disorders.
Fluorescent anti-nuclear antibodies	Positive in 2–5% of the general population, and over 90% of those with systemic lupus erythematosus (SLE), scleroderma, rheumatoid arthritis, drug-induced lupus and viral infections may also have a positive FANA.
Double-stranded DNA	Positive in 40% of patients with SLE. High titer increases risk for nephritis.
Anti-Sm (Smith)	Positive in 20% of patients with SLE.
Ribonucleoprotein	Positive in 30–40% of patients with SLE, 30% of those with systemic sclerosis. High titers may be indicative of mixed connective-tissue disease.
SS-A antibody	Positive in 35% of patients with SLE, and 55% of patients with Sjögren syndrome. Also associated with subcutaneous lupus, neonatal dermatitis, and congenital heart block.
SS-B antibody	Positive in 15% of patients with SLE, and 25–40% of those with Sjögrens syndrome. Also linked to neonatal dermatitis syndrome.
Antihistone	Associated with drug-induced lupus.
Scl-70	Positive in 20% of patients with systemic sclerosis.
Anticentromere	Positive in 40% of patients with limited scleroderma.
Cytoplasmic antineutrophil cytoplasmic antibody	Positive in most patients with Wegener's granulomatosis.
Perinuclear antineutrophil cytoplasmic antibody	Found in microscopic polyangitis, Churg–Strauss syndrome, Wegener's and inflammatory bowel disease.

shown in Table 39-1. Radiographs may be indicated in circumstances when infection, trauma, osteoarthritis, or crystalline arthropathy are suspected.

Arthrocentesis is central to the evaluation of monoarthritis and is a useful adjunct in cases in which infection and crystalline arthropathy are suspected. Aspirated fluid should be sent for cell count and differential, Gram stain and culture, as well as crystal examination. In addition, if there is sufficient synovial fluid, a portion should be directly inoculated into blood-culture bottles. Ideally, one should examine the synovial fluid for crystals promptly. Under plane polarized microscopy, gout crystals are needle-shaped and appear yellow parallel to the plane polarized light., (i.e., negatively birefringent). Calcium pyrophosphate crystals are rhomboid and positively birefringent—i.e., they appear blue parallel to the plane polarized light. The appearance of these crystals within macrophages is more specific.

POLYARTHRITIS

The initial assessment of polyarthritis will include the clinical evaluation as outlined above. Having established the nature of joint involvement, the flow diagram (Figure 39-1) may be used to generate a differential diagnosis.

In the following section the typical presentation of the common arthritides and connective-tissue diseases will be discussed.

Rheumatoid Arthritis

Rheumatoid arthritis is a symmetric polyarthritis involving the proximal interphalangeal joints, metacarpophalangeal joints, wrists, elbows, shoulders, hips, knees, ankles, and metatarsal phalangeal joints. It is more common in females. It may be associated with rheumatoid nodules, keratoconjunctivitis sicca, episcleritis, cutaneous vasculitis, pleural effusions, interstitial lung disease, and various hematologic abnormalities. Erosions at the articular surface may be seen on radiography. Diagnosis is based on clinical, laboratory, and radiographic findings. The 1987 American Rheumatism Association criteria for rheumatoid arthritis were designed to standardize clinical studies and may be used as an aid to memory (Table 39-2).

The Spondyloarthropathies

The spondyloarthropathies are a group of conditions of which ankylosing spondylitis is protypical. Other

TABLE 39-2 1987 AMERICAN RHEUMATISM ASSOCIATION CRITERIA FOR RHEUMATOID ARTHRITIS CLASSIFICATION*	
Criterion	**Definition**
Morning stiffness	Stiffness around joints that lasts more than an hour before maximal improvement
Arthritis of three or more joints	Minimum of three joint areas simultaneously swollen observed by physician (Possible joints: proximal interphalangeal, metacarpophalangeal, wrist, elbow, knee, ankle, or metatarsal phalangeal)
Arthritis of hand joints	At least one area swollen (wrist, MCP, or PIP)
Symmetric arthritis	Simultaneous joint involvement on both sides of the body
Rheumatoid nodules	Subcutaneous nodules observed over extensor surfaces
Serum rheumatoid factor	
Radiographic changes	Typical erosions or periarticular osteopenia on hand x-ray films.

*For the purposes of classification, the patient is said to have rheumatoid arthritis if four of seven criteria are present.

entities include reactive arthritis, Reiter syndrome, psoriatic arthritis, and arthritis associated with inflammatory bowel disease. The presentation includes an inflammatory oligoarthritis, with back pain and other associated features of the spondyloarthropathy. The back pain is usually inflammatory in nature, tends to be worse in the morning, and improves with exercise. Radiography may demonstrate sacroilitis, syndesmophyte formation, and calcification of the anterior longitudinal ligaments.

Reiter syndrome is associated with iritis, urethritis, and arthritis. Its dermatologic manifestations include circinate balanitis and keratoderma blenorrhagica.

Reactive arthritis occurs after urogenital or enteric infections from organisms such as chlamydia, shigella, yersinia, or salmonella. The arthritis presents 1 to 2 weeks after the infection and tends to be an asymmetric oligoarthritis that may be recurrent.

Psoriatic arthritis can present as a spondylitis, asymmetric oligoarthritis, arthritis mutilans, or symmetrical polyarthropathy indistinguishable from rheumatoid arthritis. The scalp and extensor areas, navel, and gluteal areas need to be inspected to detect the characteristic rash of psoriasis.

The spondyloarthropathy associated with inflammatory bowel disease presents as an inflammatory

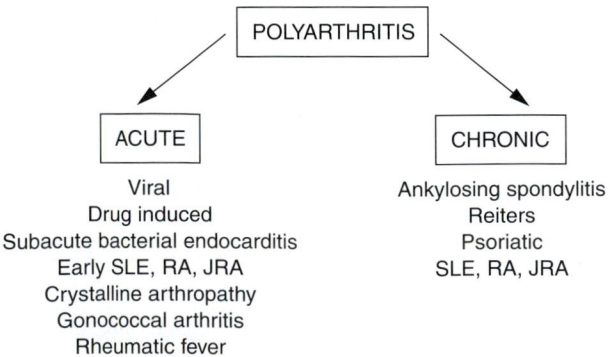

Figure 39-1 Flow diagram for evaluation of polyarthritis.

oligoarthritis. Enthesitis (inflammation of tendon attachments to bone) may be evident with heel pain or dactylitis. Extraarticular manifestations include erythema nodosum, iritis, and pyoderma gangrenosum.

Connective-Tissue Disorders

Systemic Lupus Erythematosus

Systemic lupus erythematosus (SLE) is a multisystem disease, predominantly of young females. In the United States it is more common in African-Americans and Hispanics. It may present with constitutional symptoms (fever, weight loss, night sweats), skin rash, polyarthralgia, or a nondeforming polyarthritis. Dermatologic manifestations include malar rash, discoid lesions, hair loss, mouth or nasal ulcers, urticaria, or cutaneous vasculitis. A history of photosensitivity or Raynaud phenomenon may also be elicited. Patients with serositis may present with pleuritis, pericarditis, or abdominal pain. Renal involvement may range from proteinuria to a nephritic sediment. Neurologic manifestations include neuropsychiatric disorders, seizures, headaches, cerebrovascular accidents, transverse myelitis, and neuropathy. Hematologic manifestations include leukopenia, hemolytic anemia, and thrombocytopenia. The patient may have various autoantibodies, including antinuclear antibody, anti-double-stranded DNA (anti-DNA) antibody, extractable nuclear antigens, and anticardiolipin antibodies. The 1982 revised criteria for lupus were designed for classification purposes (Table 39-3). However, they are useful as an aid to memory and underscore the fact that the diagnosis of SLE is not made solely on the

---

TABLE 39-3
1982 AMERICAN RHEUMATISM ASSOCIATION REVISED CRITIERIA FOR THE CLASSIFICATION OF SLE*

Malar rash
Discoid rash
Photosensitivity
Oral ulcers
Arthritis
Serositis
Renal disorder
Neurologic disorder
Hematologic disorder
Presence of anti-ds DNA, anti-Smith, Leprep, false positive VDRL
Antinuclear antibody

*For the purposes of classification, a patient with four or more criteria is deemed to have SLE.

TABLE 39-4
CLASSIFICATION OF SYSTEMIC SCLEROSIS

Type	Clinical Manifestations
Limited systemic sclerosis	Classified on the basis of skin thickening confined to neck, face, distal forearms, hands, and feet. Other features include Raynaud phenomenon, telangectasias, calcinosis, and esophageal involvement. Pulmonary hypertension may develop. These patients have a higher chance of having anticentromere antibody.
Diffuse systemic sclerosis	Classified on the basis of skin thickening involving proximal extremities and trunk. Raynaud phenomenon is common. Tendon friction rubs are specific to this disorder. Sclerodactaly, calcinosis, and digital pulp atrophy may also occur. Organ manifestations include pulmonary fibrosis and cardiac, intestinal, and renal involvement. 20% of these patients may have an anti-topoisomerase (anti-SCL70) antibody.

basis of positive results on the fluorescent antinuclear antibody (FANA) test.

Systemic Sclerosis

Systemic sclerosis is a condition of unknown cause in which fibrosis of skin and internal organs occurs. It is now classified into two forms—limited and diffuse (Table 39-4). The classification is dependent on the area of skin involvement. It is more common in middle-aged females. Patients may present with diffuse hand swelling or mild polyarthritis. Skin thickening, as well as changes in pigmentation, subsequently occur. Clinical manifestations are summarized in Table 39-4.

Infectious Causes of Polyarthritis

Viral

Acute infection with hepatitis A, B, or C, rubella, and parvovirus may all cause a polyarthritis. Chronic infection with hepatitis B may be associated with polyarteritis nodosa and mixed cryoglobulinaemia. Hepatitis C may lead to chronic infection. It has been associated with polyarthralgia, mixed cryoglobulinaemia, thyroiditis, sicca symptoms, glomerulonephritis and autoantibodies (FANA, rheumatoid factor, and cryoglobulins). Parvovirus infection may also cause an arthritis similar to rheumatoid arthritis, which usually resolves with time.

Gonococcal Arthritis

Arthritis may complicate 1 to 3% of cases of gonococcal infection. It is more common in women and presents with migratory polyarthralgia and tenosynovitis. The tenosynovitis commonly affects the hands, ankles, knees, and feet. A significant proportion of patients with disseminated gonococcal infection also have fever and dermatitis. Dermatitis may present as a maculopapular or a vesicular rash. Cultures of the throat, pustule, blood, cervix, and rectum are recommended. Recurrent gonococcal infection should prompt a search for early complement deficiencies.

Acute Rheumatic Fever

Acute rheumatic fever is a syndrome that occurs after a streptoccocal throat infection. It presents as a migratory polyarthritis and may be associated with carditis, chorea, erythema marginatum, or subcutaneous nodules. A similar clinical picture may be produced by subacute bacterial endocarditis, viral infection, gonococcal infection, or sarcoidosis.

Subacute Bacterial Endocarditis (SBE)

A subacute polyarthritis may complicate SBE. This is due to immune complex formation. Other manifestations of SBE include constitutional symptoms, splinter hemorrhages, Osler nodes, Janeway lesions, petechial hemorrhages, splenomegaly, and hematuria.

Sarcoidosis

Acute sarcoidosis may present with arthritis, usually of the lower extremities. In Caucasians a syndrome consisting of bilateral hilar adenopathy, erythema nodosum, and arthritis may occur (Lofgren syndrome). This is usually self-limiting and has a good prognosis. Ankle arthritis or periarthritis should prompt a search for sarcoidosis.

Polymyalgia Rheumatica

Polymyalgia rheumatica (PMR) is an inflammatory syndrome characterized by pain and stiffness of the upper and lower limb girdles that presents after the fifth decade of life and is commonly associated with a high sedimentation rate. Patients may present with constitutional symptoms as well as transient polyarthritis. A small subset of these patients may have giant-cell arteritis. Symptoms that suggest giant-cell arteritis include jaw claudication, headaches, scalp or temporal artery tenderness, or visual symptoms. Prompt biopsy of the temporal artery for diagnosis and treatment with high-dose corticosteroids are mandatory to prevent blindness.

Osteoarthritis

Osteoarthritis (OA) may affect a few joints or it may be generalized. Common joints involved include the hips, knees, distal interphalangeal, and first carpometacarpal joints. It presents with pain in the affected joints which is usually worse with exercise and toward the end of the day. Patients may report a gelling phenomenon with rest. Physical examination reveals crepitus on joint movement. In advanced cases, there may be pain on passive movement. Hand involvement may occur, with bony spurs forming in the proximal and distal interphalangeal joints, known respectively as Bouchard and Heberden nodes. Squaring of the first carpometacarpal joint may also be seen. Knee OA is characterized by pain and crepitus with passive motion. Evidence of meniscal or ligamentous damage or hypermobility may be elicited and indicates altered joint biomechanics. OA of the hip presents with pain and loss of motion. Loss of motion of internal rotation is usually most marked. Radiography reveals characteristic changes, including loss of joint space, subchondral cysts, and osteophyte formation, but does not always correlate to symptoms.

MONOARTHRITIS

Acute monoarthritis should be evaluated promptly, since infectious agents can destroy the joint rapidly. The differential diagnosis of acute monoarthritis is given in Table 39-5. However, the key differential diagnosis to consider are trauma, infection, and crystalline disease. A history of trauma is usually obvious.

Patients with infectious monoarthritis may present with fever. In addition, they may have factors contributing to relative immunosuppression. These include the use of immunosuppressive agents, renal failure, liver failure, rheumatoid arthritis, human immunodeficiency virus (HIV), and splenic dysfunction. Bacterial causes of monoarthritis may be divided into nongonococcal (Staphylococcus aureus most common) and gonoccocal. Aerobic gram–negative bacilli should be suspected if there is a concurrent urinary-tract infection (UTI), biliary-tract infection, or if the patient is immunocompromised. Intravenous drug abusers are

TABLE 39-5
DIFFERENTIAL DIAGNOSIS OF ACUTE MONOARTHRITIS

Trauma
Infection
Crystalline arthropathy
  Gout
  Pseudogout (calcium pyrophosphate)
Tumor
Osteoarthritis
Osteonecrosis

TABLE 39-6
SELECTED LABORATORY INVESTIGATIONS IN FIBROMYALGIA SYNDROME

Thyroid-stimulating hormone
Complete blood count with differential
Chemistry, including liver-function tests
Erythrocyte sedimentation rate
Urinalysis
Creatine kinase

more liable to be infected with aerobic gram-negative bacilli, anaerobes, and *Staph. aureus*. Prosthetic joints have a higher risk of infection with *Staph. epidermidis*. Mycobacterial and fungal infections may occur. Lyme disease and viral infections such as parvovirus and rubella may also present as a monoarthritis.

Monoarthritis may also be caused by crystalline disease. Gout commonly involves the lower extremities, and may present with podagra. Joint aspiration typically reveals intracellular negatively birefringent needle-shaped crystals. Hyperuricemia itself is not diagnostic of gout. Pseudogout occurs in middle-aged patients and may involve wrists, shoulders, or knees. Joint aspiration reveals rhomboid-shaped positively birefringent crystals under plane polarized microscopy.

Chronic monoarthritis not due to trauma, infection or crystalline arthropathy has frequently been found to be due to a spondyloarthropathy and less frequently rheumatoid arthritis.

Fibromyalgia Syndrome

Fibromyalgia is a common nonarticular condition that occurs predominantly in women. Its diagnosis is based on clinical findings and exclusion of other diseases. Treatment focuses on alleviating symptoms by promoting better sleep, aerobic exercise, and education.

Clinical Features

Fibromyalgia typically presents with chronic widespread pain. Exacerbating factors include cold or damp weather, unaccustomed exercise, lack of sleep, and psychological stressors. Fatigability and sleep disturbance are also common features. Patients typically describe nonrestful sleep and waking in the morning unrefreshed. Other somatic symptoms in patients with fibromyalgia include occipital and frontal headaches

and diffuse abdominal pain with variable bowel habits, as well as urinary frequency.

Pathophysiology

There are no distinct pathologic changes in this condition. There is an association of fibromyalgia with a sleep disturbance. In particular, stage IV non–rapid-eye-movement sleep is reduced.

Diagnosis

A history of widespread pain and the presence of 11 of 18 hyperanalgesic tender points are suggestive of fibromyalgia. The location of the tender points may include the occiput, trapezius, supraspinatus, gluteal, greater trochanter, lesser cervical, second rib, lateral epicondyle (2 cm distal to the epicandyle), and medial fat pad of the knee. Pain in these sites is elicited with digital palpation with force of 4 kg (just enough to blanch the fingernail).

A complete history and physical needs be done to exclude other medical disorders, and base-line investigations given in Table 39-6 may be conducted to assist in the work-up of these patients.

Treatment

First, the patient needs to be educated about fibromyalgia. This includes acknowledgment of the patient's suffering. In addition, the patient needs to be reassured that the pain does not indicate a serious inflammatory condition or carcinomatosis.

In clinical trials, the two interventions that have improved symptoms are improved sleep and a graded aerobic exercise program. It is worthwhile to counsel the patient on factors that may improve sleep (Table 39-7).

If the above interventions do not help sleep, a trial of tricyclic antidepressants may be warranted. Amytriptyline at a dose of 10 mg may be started and

TABLE 39-7
FACTORS THAT MAY IMPROVE SLEEP

Minimizing caffeine intake
Avoiding spicy and large meals prior to sleep
Scheduling a regular wakeup time
Avoidance of napping during the day
Ensuring that the bedroom is cool, dark and that distractions such as a television or a telephone are removed

gradually increased up to 100 mg daily. If the sedative or anticholinergic effects are intolerable, trazodone may be an alternative.

At the same time, the patient should be instructed in a gradual graded aerobic exercise program. It is important that the patient does not suddenly increase the exercise level since this may exacerbate symptoms. NSAIDs have a limited role in combination with the above modalities.

REGIONAL PAIN SYNDROMES

Shoulder Pain

Shoulder pain is one of the most common musculoskeletal symptoms in a primary care practice. The shoulder joint is a ball-and-socket joint that allows a large degree of movement. In order to perform clinical assessment of the shoulder joint, an understanding of its anatomy is critical. Figure 39-2 illustrates the anatomy of the shoulder joint.

Clinical Evaluation

The history of shoulder pain should include an inquiry about trauma and precipitating and alleviating factors of pain. Shoulder pain is often poorly localized, and it is difficult for patients to accurately pinpoint the source of pain. It is important to remember that shoulder pain can be referred from the cervical spine, thorax, breast, or abdomen, so examination of these sites is critical.

The shoulder joint should be examined with the patient undressed to the waist. Inspection, palpation, and special maneuvers (Table 39-8) may be used. Inspection of the shoulder should include a search for joint effusions (which usually present anteriorly), deformities of the scapula and clavicle, and ascertainment of muscle wasting.

Palpation should be done to elicit whether tenderness is present over the rotator-cuff tendon insertions, the bicipital groove, the subacromial bursa, and the acromiaclavicular and sternoclavicular joints.

Passive and active range of motion should be assessed. Active range of motion is conducted with the

Figure 39-2 Anatomy of the shoulder joint. *Reprinted with permission from Richards DB, Kibler WB. Sports-related shoulder rehabilitation: an overview of concepts. J Musculoskel Med 1997;14:46. © Charles Boyter, artist.*

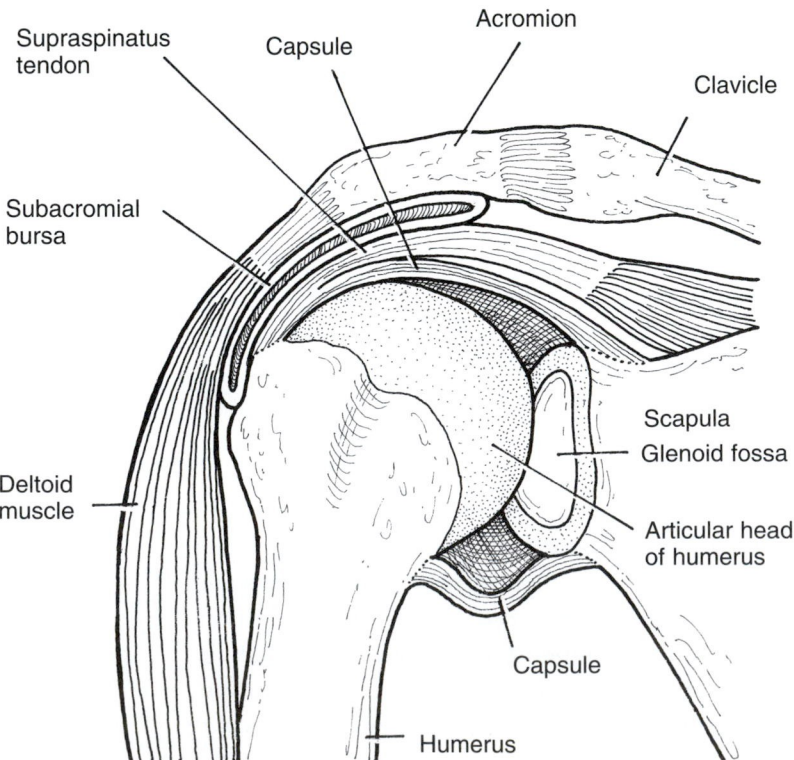

	TABLE 39-8 SPECIALIZED TESTS OF THE SHOULDER JOINT	
Test	**Procedure**	**Significance**
Rotator cuff pathology		
Drop arm test	Holding the arm abducted at 90 degrees	Severe pain or dropping of the arm suggests rotator-cuff tear
Impingement sign	Painful arc on abduction between 70 and 110 degrees	Rotator-cuff tendonitis (supraspinatus)
Bicipital tendon pathology		
Yergasson test	Resisting supination with the elbow flexed to 90 degrees elicits pain	Bicipital tendonitis
Speed test	Resisting shoulder flexion with the elbow extended elicits pain	Bicipital tendonitis

scapula fixed by the examiner. Extraarticular causes of shoulder pain usually primarily affect active range of motion; true shoulder-joint pathology (intraarticular) will affect both active and passive range of motion. The specialized tests shown in Table 39-8 may then be done if appropriate.

Shoulder pain may arise from articular or extraarticular structures.

Articular Causes of Shoulder Pain

The glenohumeral joint may be affected by various pathologies including OA, rheumatoid arthritis, crystalline arthritis, or avascular necrosis of the humeral head. A complete history is essential in evaluating the cause of glenohumeral involvement. Physical examination reveals decreased active and passive range of motion. Anteroposterior and lateral radiography should be done. Management depends on the cause of glenohumeral pathology.

Extraarticular Causes of Shoulder Pain

Rotator-Cuff Tendonitis

The rotator-cuff muscles consist of the supraspinatus, subscapularis, teres minor, and infraspinatus muscles. These muscles play an important role in stabilizing the shoulder joint during movement. The rotator cuff is subjected to stress when the arm is in an elevated position. Tendonitis may then be caused by repeated overhead activities such as throwing. The subacromial bursa may become secondarily inflamed. The supraspinatus muscle, which helps in stabilizing the shoulder joint during abduction, is usually involved in rotator-cuff tendonitis. Less commonly, the subscapularis, which controls internal rotation of the shoulder, or the teres minor and infraspinatus muscles, which control external rotation, may be involved.

Presentation

The presentation of rotator-cuff tendonitis depends on the age of the patient. In young patients, tendonitis may result from trauma or sudden throwing movements of the arm and present acutely. Middle-aged individuals may present with more gradual onset of symptoms. In the elderly there may be no history of antecedent trauma or activity. Patients may present with aching over the shoulder joint. In addition, they may report difficulty reaching behind their back or head.

Clinical examination of supraspinatus tendonitis reveals an arc of pain with active abduction of the arm from 70 to 110 degrees. Impingement signs may also be demonstrated. In subscapularis tendonitis, resisted internal rotation produces pain. Resisted external rotation of the shoulder causes pain in infraspinatus and teres minor tendonits.

The diagnosis is made on clinical grounds.

Management

Initial management of rotator-cuff tendonitis involves cessation of aggravating factors, use of physical therapy, and NSAIDs. Specific range-of-motion exercises such as Codman exercises are begun as soon as tolerated. If these initial therapeutic interventions do not help, a subdeltoid corticosteroid injection is usually given. In all patients, proper preparation for exercise and correct technique should be emphasized in order to prevent future injury.

Rotator-Cuff Tears

Rotator-cuff tears may present acutely or chronically. Acute presentations are usually after trauma and are easily recognized. However, a significant proportion of patients do not report a history of trauma. In this setting, there is usually a gradual degeneration of the rotator-cuff tendon that eventually results in rupture.

Presentation

Patients present with pain over the shoulder with a variable loss of function. The patient may report pain and weakness in abduction, flexion, and internal or external rotation of the shoulder. Physical examination may reveal features similar to rotator-cuff tendonitis, except that weakness is present. With larger tears the patient may be unable to maintain the arm in a horizontally abducted position (positive "drop-arm" sign).

The diagnosis may be confirmed by MRI or shoulder arthrography.

Management

Partial rotator-cuff tears are managed conservatively with physical therapy and strengthening. Acute tears in young patients should be referred for consideration for surgical repair. In older patients, a trial of physical therapy for 3 months may be attempted. With chronic tears, conservative therapy is usually recommended. Failure to achieve pain relief may be an indication for surgery.

Adhesive Capsulitis

The shoulder joint is one of the most complicated joints in the human body since it allows movement in virtually all planes. In order to permit this movement, the shoulder joint capsule has to be lax. Contracture of the shoulder capsule causes marked impairment of shoulder movement in all planes except forward flexion. Adhesive capsulitis refers to involvement and contracture of this capsule. The pathophysiology of this process is not entirely clear. However, capsulitis of the shoulder is common and has been associated with a variety of conditions, including diabetes mellitus, myocardial infarction, thyroid disease, pulmonary disease such as tuberculosis, cerebrovascular accident, and shoulder trauma.

Presentation

Adhesive capsulitis usually occurs after the age of 40 and is slightly more common in women. It is thought that there may be three phases of development and progression. The first phase is called the painful phase, and is characterized by the insidious onset of pain followed by stiffness. It may last for 3 to 8 months. The second phase is the adhesive phase, in which pain decreases but restriction of shoulder movement is more marked. This may last for 4 to 6 months. The final phase is the resolution phase. Pain further decreases and restriction of motion becomes dominant. Slow but gradual improvement of the range of motion usually occurs. Recovery may be incomplete and the whole condition may last for 1 to 3 years. Thirty to sixty percent of patients may have residual limitation of movement.

On examination, in contrast to rotator-cuff tendonitis there is a global limitation of active and passive movement. Disuse atrophy of the deltoid and rotator cuff muscles may also be noted. The diagnosis is established clinically. X-ray films may be obtained to exclude significant glenohumeral pathology and calcific tendonitis.

Management

Management of this condition is based on pain management as well as minimizing restriction of movement at the shoulder joint. Immobilization should be avoided if at all possible. NSAIDs may be prescribed for pain relief, and physical therapy is useful. Intraarticular injections should be used judiciously. These injections help reduce pain and increase range of motion but have not been shown to improve long-term outcome. In selected circumstances patients may be referred to an orthopedist for manipulation under anesthesia.

Elbow Pain

The elbow joint is a specialized hinge joint that allows complex precision movement of the upper extremity. Both flexion and extension (0 to 130 degrees) as well as supination and pronation (0 to 170 degrees) occur at this joint complex. The elbow joint is maintained at 7 degrees of valgus alignment (also known as the carrying angle). It is a common site of overuse injuries.

Clinical Evaluation

A thorough history and physical examination is essential. The onset and location of pain should be established. Pain at night or at rest is unusual and may suggest inflammation, infection, tumor, osteonecrosis, or nerve entrapment. Associated symptoms such as tingling or numbness over the forearm or the hand may suggest ulnar-nerve entrapment. It is important to remember that pain may be referred from the shoulder or the wrist, and one should examine these areas too.

Examination of the elbow joint should begin with inspection, which may reveal asymmetry, increased carrying angle, or ecchymoses. The elbow is then palpated for warmth or tenderness. Tenderness may be elicited over the condyles or over the radiocapitellum joints. Active and passive flexion, extension, supination, and pronation are observed. If trauma is suspected, the pulses and neurologic function of the forearm should also be tested. The common extensor origin at the lateral epicondyle may be stressed by resisted wrist extension (helpful in confirming lateral epicondylitis). Similarly, the flexor tendon origin at the medial epicondyle may be tested with resisted finger flexion (which is usually better than wrist flexion).

Radiography may be helpful for evaluation of articular problems. Standard anteroposterior and lateral views are usually sufficient.

Causes of Elbow Pain

Articular

Articular pain at the elbow may be caused by trauma, infection, or crystal arthropathy or may be part of an inflammatory arthropathy. A complete history may be helpful in further delineating the cause of elbow arthritis. The symtpoms may be bilateral. On physical examination, if there is active inflammation the joint may be warm and have synovial thickening and decreased range of motion. Further evaluation may involve radiography, joint aspiration, or specific laboratory tests if a systemic connective-tissue disorder is suspected (see Table 39-1).

Extraarticular

OLECRANON BURSITIS The elbow bursa is superficial and may be irritated with repeated trauma. It may also become infected with or without an overlying cellulitis. Olecranon bursitis may also occur secondary to crystalline arthropathy or a systemic arthropathy such as rheumatoid arthritis. The bursa is easily aspirated and the contents should be sent for Gramstain culture as well as crystal examination. If infection is suspected, antibiotics that have coverage for *Staph. aureus* should be begun.

LATERAL EPICONDYLITIS (TENNIS ELBOW) Lateral epicondylitis is a common condition, which may be associated with overuse syndromes.

Presentation Lateral epicondylitis presents with lateral elbow pain worsened by activities that involve repeated wrist supination and extension. Physical examination may reveal tenderness of the lateral epicondyle. In addition pain may be elicited at this site by resisted wrist extension and supination.

Management Treatment consists of modifying activities that may exacerbate the lateral epicondylitis. In addition to resting the forearm, ice may be applied and NSAIDs may be used. A splint is also is helpful in some patients. If these simple measures do not improve the symptoms, a local steroid injection may be used. Typically, 10 to 20 mg of methylprednisolone mixed with 1% lidocaine is used. The most tender area over the lateral epicondyle is identified and, using standard aseptic technique, injected. It is important to instruct in exercises to strengthen the forearm muscles to prevent recurrence. If the pain is resistant to the above measures, the diagnosis should be reevaluated. In some patients, entrapment of the posterior interosseous nerve may cause radiation of pain to the lateral epicondyle. Patients not responding to initial therapy should be referred to an orthopedist or rheumatologist.

MEDIAL EPICONDYLITIS (GOLFER'S ELBOW) Medial epicondylitis is much less common and has a similar presentation to lateral epicondylitis. On physical examination, tenderness may be elicited over the medial epicondyle at the common flexor tendon insertion. In addition, the pain may be worsened by resisted finger flexion and wrist pronation. Patients should be initially treated with rest or ice or both. Exercises to strengthen the flexor muscles of the forearm should be done to prevent recurrence. A local steroid injection may be helpful in refractory cases.

Wrist and Hand Pain

Pain at the wrist and hand is common and may originate from articular, extraarticular, and referred sources. In the following section, causes of hand pain will be briefly discussed.

de Quervain Tenosynovitis

de Quervain tenosynovitis refers to inflammation of the tendon sheaths of the abductor pollicis longus and extensor pollicis brevis. It usually occurs due to overuse and is most common in women between 30 and 50 years of age.

PRESENTATION Patients present with insidious onset of pain over the radial aspect of the wrist during pinch grip. The affected tendon sheaths may be tender or swollen. The Finkelstein test is used to distinguish de Quervain tendinitis from OA of the first carpometacarpal joint. (This test is conducted by folding the thumb into the palm, flexing the remaining fingers over the thumb, and gently deviating the wrist to the ulnar side. The involved tendons are stretched, in a de Quervain tendinitis, resulting in pain).

MANAGEMENT Treatment of de Quervain tendonitis consists of rest, heat therapy, NSAIDs and splinting. In more severe cases, local injection into the synovial sheath may be helpful. Surgical referral is indicated if symptoms persist for more than 6 months.

Trigger Finger (Stenosing Digital Tenosynovitis)

Trigger finger is a common repetitive strain injury of the hand. Tenosynovitis of the flexor tendons of the hand results in fibrosis and constriction localized to the first annular pulley that overlies the metacarpophalangeal joint and may, in addition, result in formation of a nodule. The constriction or tendon formation interferes with the normal excursion of the tendons, resulting in triggering or "catching" of the fingers.

Presentation

Patients report of pain over the flexor tendon of the finger. Intermittent locking of the digit in flexion may occur. Nodules over the tendons may be palpated.

Management

Modification of hand activities, local massage or heat treatment, and NSAIDs may be used. If simple measures do not help, a steroid injection of the affected flexor tendon sheath may be used effectively.

Hip Pain

Hip pain may be caused by articular or extraarticular structures or be referred from the spine or knee.

Clinical Evaluation

A detailed pain history is essential. It is especially important to inquire about trauma. Pain arising from the hip joint may radiate to the groin or buttock region and may be referred to the knee. In addition, pain from the spine and knee can be referred directly to the hip.

Physical examination of the hip joint should begin with observing the patient's gait. An antalgic gait occurs when walking is painful and the patient tries to relieve the pain by limping. A Trendelenburg gait occurs when there is weakness of the gluteus medius muscle or interference in its action as a hip abductor. The patient throws the body to the weak side to maintain balance. If there is bilateral gluteus medius weakness, a waddling gait may result. The patient should be examined for leg-length shortening (Table 39-9), and for contractures at the hip joint (Table 39-9). The inguinal area and trochanteric and ischial bursae should be palpated. Passive and active movements should then be examined. The lumbosacral spine should be examined as well as the neurovascular status of the lower limbs. Common clinical tests that may be used to examine the hip joint are given in Table 39-9.

Causes of Hip Pain

Articular

Inflammatory arthritis, osteoarthritis, and avascular necrosis are some of the more common causes of hip-joint pathology. Pain from the articular surface of the hip joint refers to the groin area. Physical examination may reveal limitation in joint movement or contractures. Assessment is aided by anteroposterior and lateral radiography of the hip joint. Therapy depends on the specific cause of hip joint pathology.

Extraarticular

TROCHANTERIC BURSITIS Trochanteric bursitis is one of the most common causes of hip pain. Most often it is induced by microtrauma, but it may also occur in conjunction with inflammatory arthritis. Microtrauma may occur to the trochanteric area if there is a change in the contralateral hip, spine curvature, and leg length, leading to alteration of gait. Jogging and other stressful activities may also cause microtrauma to the trochanteric area.

PRESENTATION Patients usually present with deep aching pain in the lateral aspect of the hip. They may also report of exacerbation by lying on it at night. Deep palpation elicits point tenderness over the area of the greater trochanter. Pain is reproduced with resisted abduction.

TABLE 39-9
COMMON CLINICAL TESTS THAT MAY BE USED TO EXAMINE THE HIP JOINT

Test	Procedure	Significance
Fabere test	Placement of the lateral malleolus of the tested leg onto the knee while patient is supine. Positive if there is pain or limitation of hip-joint motion.	Hip-joint pathology
Ober test	While patient is on the side, hip is abducted maximally, knee flexed to 90 degrees, and then released. Positive if thigh remains abducted.	Tight iliotibial band
Thomas test	While supine, one of the hip joints is flexed maximally. The degree of extension of the contralateral leg is observed. Positive if the contralateral leg cannot fully extend.	Hip-joint contracture
Trendelenburg test	Patient's pelvis is observed while bearing weight on one leg. Positive if pelvis on the unsupported side fails to elevate or descends.	Gluteus medius weakness or coxa vera on supported side.
True leg-length measurement	Distance between the anterior superior iliac spine and the medial malleolus.	Leg-length discrepancy
Femoral stretch test	With the patient prone, knee is flexed to 90 degrees and the hip joint extended. Positive if anterior thigh pain occurs.	Radicular pain

MANAGEMENT The acute phase of trochanteric bursitis may last for several days, followed by gradual resolution. Significant discomfort may persist in some patients. Treatment involves correction of identifiable underlying problems such as leg-length discrepancy as well as rest. Active athletes should be instructed to decrease activity. NSAIDs and physical methods such as ultrasound have had limited success. Injection of a mixture of lidocaine and long-acting corticosteroid may bring long-term relief. The injection is administered over the point of maximum tenderness just proximal to the periosteum in a fanlike fashion. Failure to resolve symptoms may be due to referred pain, a tight iliotibial band, or continued mechanical factors. Referral to a rheumatologist may be indicated for further evaluation.

Ischial Bursitis

The ischial bursa lies over the ischial tuberosity, and in the standing position has most of the gluteus maximus over it. In the sitting position with the leg extended, the gluteus medius muscle belly migrates, leaving the ischial tuberosity superficial, covered by the ischial bursa. Prolonged sitting or repeated trauma to this area may cause inflammation of the ischial bursa. This is sometimes termed the weaver's bottom.

PRESENTATION Patients may present with exquisite pain over the buttock area, which may radiate down the posterior thigh. Point tenderness over the ischial bursa may be elicited.

MANAGEMENT Therapy consists of use of cushions and in selected cases a local injection of corticosteroid mixed with lidocaine. The injection should be administered at the point of maximal tenderness, and care should be taken to avoid the sciatic nerve, which passes just lateral to the ischial bursa.

Referred Pain

Pain may be referred from the lumbar spine to the trochanteric region. In particular, mechanical problems at the T12–L1 junction can refer pain to the trochanteric region. Palpation of the lumbar spine may help differentiate this from hip-joint disorders. L2 to L4 nerve-root compression may cause referred pain to the inguinal area as well as to the anterior thigh region. The femoral stretch test (see Table 39-9) and neurologic examination may help in differentiating this from hip disease.

Pain from intraabdominal structures (such as retroperitoneal appendicitis, abscess, and pelvic inflammatory disease) may be referred to the inguinal and anterior thigh region. Ureteral stones and inguinal and femoral hernias may also be a cause of pain at the hip region. It is important to remember that aortic aneurysm or iliac-vessel narrowing may present with a pain at the buttock region with symptoms of claudication.

Knee Pain

The knee joint is a joint with complex movement whose integrity depends on its ligamentous support structures. Knee pathology may present with pain or mechanical loss of function. In the following section, selected causes of knee pain will be discussed.

Clinical Evaluation

There is a large number of causes of knee pain. Therefore, a logical history and physical examination are necessary. Initial assessment should include the mode and onset of knee pain, in addition to associated symptoms. Mechanical symptoms include locking, which refers to the inability of the patient to fully extend the knee. The patient may also report a "giving way" sensation of the knee, which is often secondary to reflex relaxation of the quadriceps following painful loading of the extensor mechanism. When trauma is involved, the mechanism of injury should be elicited. Twisting injuries may involve the menisci, while sudden deceleration of the leg may involve the anterior cruciate ligament, and a medial or lateral blow to the knee may involve the collateral ligaments. It is also important to note that knee pain may be referred from the hip or the lumbar spine.

The physical examination is used to localize the cause of pain as well as any deficiencies in the ligamentous structures of the knee. Inspection should start by watching the patient's gait and examining for quadriceps wasting and a knee effusion. The knees should then be palpated to detect warmth and effusion. If the knee effusion is small, a bulge test may be used to detect it. This is done by stabilizing the patella while gently messaging the fluid on either side of the patella while observing for a bulge on the opposite side. Larger amounts of the effusion can be confirmed by ballotting the patella. This is done by applying gentle pressure on the patella and feeling for its excursion. The joint margin and femoral and tibial condyles should be palpated for tenderness. Similarly, the superior and inferior margins of the patella and the insertion of the patellar tendon at the tibial tuberosity should be palpated. Active movements of the knees should the observed next, followed by passive examination. When placing the knee through passive range-of-motion exercises, the presence of crepitus should be noted. Provocative measures can then be applied to test the various ligaments. These measures and other common clinical tests are summarized in Table 39-10.

Some common causes of knee pain will be discussed below.

Causes of Knee Pain

Articular

The knee joint may be involved in systemic arthritis, infection, crystalline arthropathy, and osteoarthritis. These conditions may be evaluated clinically, with accompanying radiography and, if indicated, joint aspiration and laboratory testing. The knee is also frequently involved in injuries. These will be discussed later.

Extraarticular

BURSITIS

Prepatellar Bursitis Prepatellar bursitis, also known as housemaid's knee, is a common problem. It presents with a red fluctuant area over the front of the patella. It is usually caused by mechanical irritation, but infection or gout may also cause it. Most cases are self-limited and resolve with avoidance of kneeling. If sepsis is suspected, serial drainage and antibiotics may be indicated.

TABLE 39-10
COMMON CLINICAL TESTS USED TO EXAMINE THE KNEE JOINT

Test	Procedure	Significance
Anterior draw test	Place knee at 90 degrees and attempt to pull calf forward. Positive if there is laxity as compared with the contralateral side.	Anterior cruciate ligament tear
Posterior draw test	Place knee at 90 degrees and attempt to push tibia backward. Positive if there is laxity as compared with the contralateral side.	Posterior cruciate ligament tear
McMurray test	Palpation of the knee-joint margin with first internal and then external rotation of the knee while it is being extended from a flexed position. Positive if pain and click elicited.	Meniscal tear
Collateral ligament test	With the knee flexed at 15 degrees, apply valgus force to test medial collateral ligament and varus force to test lateral collateral ligament. Positive if laxity observed.	Medial or lateral collateral ligament tear
Patellar apprehension test	Apply a gentle lateral force to the patella while the patient tries to flex the knee from a fully extended position. Positive if discomfort or if the patella dislocates.	Patellar maltracking

Anserine Bursitis Inflammation of the pes anserinus bursa usually occurs in obese patients and presents with pain over the medial aspect of the upper tibia. Treatment is conservative at first, with NSAIDs and rest. The site may be injected with a local steroid injection if there is no improvement.

Patellar Tendonitis Tendonitis of the patellar tendon may occur due to overuse syndromes or sprain. It most commonly affects young athletes who participate in jumping, running, or climbing sports. It presents with pain over the inferior pole of the patella and is worsened by activity. Treatment includes rest and NSAIDs.

Osgood–Schlatter Disease Osgood–Schlatter disease is a traction apophysitis of the tibial tuberosity. It presents in a manner similar to that of patellar tendonitis. Patients are usually young athletes who present with pain over the tibial tuberosity that is worsened by activity. On physical examination the patient may have tenderness over the tibial tuberosity, which may be enlarged. Lateral radiography may reveal characteristic fragmentation of the tibial tubercle, and there may be a loose ossicle. This condition is treated by rest to allow time for the loose ossicle to fuse.

Chondromalacia Patellae Chondromalacia patellae refers to softening of the articular cartilage of the patella. It is a pathological diagnosis that requires arthroscopy. It is caused by overuse syndromes as well as patellar maltracking. The condition usually responds to quadriceps exercises and hamstring stretching.

Osteochondritis Ossicans This is a condition in which there is bony fragmentation of the lateral femoral condyles and the patella. It commonly occurs in the second decade, affecting boys more often than girls. It presents with aching pain after activity and there may be locking of the knee if there is a loose fragment. Physical examination may reveal quadriceps wasting, knee effusion, and tenderness over the lateral femoral condyles. Radiography is diagnostic, revealing fragmentation. Sunrise views of the patella and anteroposterior views of the knees are indicated. If there is no fragmentation, the patient is advised to avoid activities that may injure the knee. If fragmentation is present, the patient needs to be referred to an orthopedist. Isometric quadriceps exercises need to be prescribed to avoid quadriceps wasting.

Patellofemoral Disorders

The patella has a natural tendency to be shifted laterally. The lateral tendency is inhibited by fibers from the quadriceps medialis. Patellar dislocation or subluxation may be due to a variety of congenital abnormalities, which include joint laxity, patella alta, and persistent femoral anteversion.

Physical examination may reveal poor quadriceps tone as well as abnormalities such as patella alta or valgus of the knee, which predispose to subluxation. The apprehension test is positive in a large proportion of patients. Radiography may be performed to look for femoral tibial malalignment and patella alta, and skyline views of the patella may show an abnormal tilt. The initial management of recurrent subluxation is with quadriceps strengthening. If the symptoms are unabated and disabling, orthopedic referral for arthroscopy and lateral release may be indicated.

Knee Injuries

The knee is a common site for injuries. Initial evaluation and triage can be successfully conducted by the primary care physician. Highlights of the patient history that should be elicited should include the mechanism and site of injury and whether it involved contact. In addition, the patient should be questioned as to whether an audible pop was heard and if the knee joint is tender in any area. Inability to continue activities or bear weight is also important to establish. A history of prior injuries and ligamentous laxity may also be useful. The knees should be systematically examined as outlined above. Radiographic views that may be helpful include anteroposterior, lateral, and patellar tracking views. Orthopedic referral is indicated if the factors outlined in the Table 39-11 are found.

TABLE 39-11
FACTORS THAT MAY INDICATE ORTHOPEDIC REFERRAL FOR KNEE PAIN

Fracture

Extensor mechanism failure

Suspected Infection

Hemarthrosis (may suggest meniscal tear, osteochondral fracture, collateral ligament injury, and occurs in 70% of anterior cruciate ligament injuries)

Disabling lateral collateral ligament tears

Patellar dislocation (may be associated with osteochondral fracture)

Locking (may indicate fragments from meniscal tears or osteochondral fractures)

MENISCAL TEARS The menisci are semicircular cartilages that help in distributing weight over a large area as well as functioning as shock absorbers. In young patients, injury to the menisci may present as pain following a twisting injury. In older patients, the presentation is subacute and often presents as pain over the joint line. On physical examination a knee effusion may be palpated and the joint line may be tender. If there is locking, the McMurray test may be positive. The repair of the meniscal tear depends on the age of the patient, as well as the type and location of the tear.

LIGAMENTOUS INJURIES The ligaments of the knees may be sprained or torn. The resulting instability depends on the degree of compensation by the other structures and presence of associated injuries.

Medial Collateral-Ligament Injuries Medial collateral-ligament injuries may occur due to a valgus force and external rotation of the tibia. Such injuries may occur during sports such as skiing. The patient may report pain, tenderness, and swelling over the medial aspect of the joint. Physical examination may reveal a swelling and bruising over the course of the medial collateral ligament with a positive valgus stress test. Meniscal tears and anterior cruciate ligament injuries may also be present. Isolated medial collateral-ligament tears are treated nonoperatively with casting or bracing.

Lateral Collateral-Ligament Injuries Lateral collateral-ligament injuries occur with varus force applied to the flexed knee. These injuries are usually associated with damage to the lateral capsule, arcuate ligament, popliteus tendon, and anterior cruciate ligament. If the lateral collateral ligament ruptures, it usually occurs at the fibular styloid, which may compromise the peroneal nerve. Physical examination usually reveals tenderness and swelling at the lateral aspect of the knee joint with a positive varus stress test. Peroneal-nerve function should be tested. Isolated lateral collateral-ligament tears are often associated with little instability and are treated nonoperatively with casting or bracing.

Anterior Cruciate-Ligament Tears Anterior cruciate-ligament tears may occur if the flexed knee is subjected to a valgus and external rotational force or due to a hyperextension, internal rotational injury. The force may be small and the patient may report a popping sensation. Hemarthrosis usually accompanies this injury and is evident with knee swelling. However,

if the capsule of the knee is disrupted, blood tracks into the calf instead. (This may indicate serious knee disruption.) On physical examination the anterior draw sign is typically positive. Radiography may reveal a Segond fracture. This is seen as a chip off the lateral tibial spine and may be associated with a 60 to 70% chance of an anterior cruciate-ligament injury. Anterior cruciate-ligament injuries may also be associated with meniscal tears and osteochondral fractures. Orthopedic referral is warranted for evaluation of associated injuries. Anterior cruciate ligament repair is controversial and depends on the age and characteristics of the patient.

Posterior Cruciate-Ligament Tears Posterior cruciate-ligament tears usually occur in motor vehicle accidents when a posterior force is applied to a flexed knee. These injuries are much less common than anterior cruciate-ligament injuries. Physical examination reveals a positive posterior draw sign. Treatment is usually nonoperative.

Foot Pain

Foot pain is a common symptom in primary care practice. It usually occurs over the heel or the forefoot. Factors that might predispose to foot pain include sports activity, occupational activities that involve prolonged standing, and incorrect shoewear. If the pain is bilateral then rheumatic disease should be suspected.

Heel Pain—Plantar Fasciitis

Heel pain is commonly caused by plantar fasciitis. The plantar fascia plays an important role in maintaining the static and dynamic longitudinal arch. A large proportion of the force is concentrated at the medial calcaneal insertion of the plantar fascia. Repetitive stress by activities such as walking and jumping causes microtrauma and triggers chronic degenerative and reparative changes at this site, which may cause pain.

PRESENTATION Patients typically present with heel pain in the morning with the first few steps after getting out of bed or after an extended period of rest. On examination, tenderness is localized to the medial calcaneal insertion of the plantar fascia. Tenderness is worsened when the fascia is stretched (with foot dorsiflexion and toe extension). Radiography is seldom helpful.

DIFFERENTIAL DIAGNOSIS Painful compression of the first branch of the lateral plantar nerve may present with heel pain. However, the pain is typically greater at night, is stabbing in nature, and tends to radiate to the lateral aspect of the foot. Calcaneal stress fractures may also present with heel pain, especially after sporting activity involving jumping or running. The patient may recall the time of injury. There is usually exquisite point tenderness when the calcaneus is palpated bilaterally.

MANAGEMENT Initial management involves rest, minimizing time spent on the feet, and the use of heel pads. The patient is advised to stretch the plantar fascia, Achilles tendon, and hamstrings (this is important, since inelasticity in these areas may predispose to heel pain). NSAIDs may also be useful. In selected cases night splints may be indicated. This is usually in patients who have not responded to initial conservative therapy. Refractory cases may be referred to rheumatology or orthopedics.

Forefoot Pain—Morton Interdigital Neuroma

Morton interdigital neuroma is the most common cause of forefoot pain. This is caused by the entrapment of the interdigital nerve, commonly between the third and fourth metatarsals. A neuroma may be present. The most common causes of this condition are wearing tight-fitting shoes and, less frequently, mechanical foot problems.

Presentation

This condition typically occurs in middle-aged females who present with paroxysms of lancinating pain or dysthesia in the interdigital area. Patients typically are found to be wearing tight-fitting shoes and report worsening symptoms when walking on hard surfaces. Physical examination may reproduce the pain by compressing the metatarsals, and a neuroma may be palpated.

Management

The patient is instructed to wear wide-toe shoes and may also use soft metatarsal pads. If refractory, an orthopedic referral may be indicated.

Selected Nerve-Entrapment Syndromes

Peripheral nerves may become compressed and irritated at certain vulnerable anatomic sites. In addition, endocrinologic or systemic rheumatic disease may predispose to nerve entrapment. The initial evaluation is clinical by history and physical examination. If the clinical picture is uncharacteristic, electrophysiologic studies may be indicated to detect coexisting conditions such as radiculopathy or early polyneuropathy, or prior to surgery. In the following section, selected causes of nerve entrapment will be discussed.

Median-Nerve Entrapment

The most common site of median-nerve entrapment is at the carpal tunnel. Less commonly, the anterior interosseous branch of the median nerve may get trapped in the forearm.

CARPAL-TUNNEL SYNDROME This is the most common cause of entrapment neuropathy. It has a variety of causes, which are summarized in Table 39-12.

Presentation Patients typically present with parasthesia over the median-nerve distribution of the hand. These symptoms may be worse at night, and the patient may have to ease the symptoms by hanging the arm out of the bed. Some patients also may complain of dropping objects, or report sensory loss.

On examination Tinel or Phalen's sign (Table 39-13) may be positive. The median-nerve function is tested for both the motor and sensory components. Motor components are examined by testing opposition of the thumb to the little finger and by testing resisted thumb abduction. Sensory impairment should be tested over the second and third digits.

The patient may be referred for a nerve-conduction study if surgical referral is considered or if the diagnosis is unclear.

Management Initial management of carpal-tunnel syndrome involves avoiding precipitating activities and prescribing splints that place the wrist in a cock-up or neutral position. These should be worn as much

---

TABLE 39-12
CAUSES OF CARPAL-TUNNEL SYNDROME

Idiopathic
Cumulative trauma (e.g., use of keyboard, vibrating tools, etc.)
Endocrinologic disorders (e.g., diabetes mellitus, hypo-
 thyroidism, acromegaly)
Rheumatic disorders (e.g., rheumatoid arthritis, gout,
 osteoarthritis)
Pregnancy
Chronic renal failure
Amyloidosis

TABLE 39-13
CLINICAL TESTS USED TO DETECT CARPAL-TUNNEL SYNDROME

Test	Procedure
Tinel test	Percussion over base of hand. Positive test occurs with paresthesia over median-nerve distribution.
Phalen test	Hand held in acute passive flexion for about a minute. Positive if reproduction of paresthesia over median-nerve distribution.

---

as tolerated, particularly at night. Local steroid injection may be used by an experienced practitioner. Surgical referral is considered if the initial measures do not succeed, or if there is thenar muscle wasting, or if there is persistent sensory loss.

ANTERIOR INTEROSSEOUS-NERVE ENTRAPMENT
The anterior interosseous nerve is purely a motor branch of the median nerve. It may get trapped 5 to 8 cm distal to the lateral epicondyle. This may be due to trauma or to muscle hypertrophy. This nerve supplies flexor pollicis longus, flexor digitorum profundus of the index and middle fingers, as well as pronator quadratus.

Presentation The patient presents with forearm pain and may report difficulty using the index and middle fingers. On examination the patient is unable to make an O with the index and thumb. Electromyography and nerve-conduction studies may confirm the diagnosis.

Treatment of the patient initially involves resting the upper limb. NSAIDs may be used. If the symptoms do not resolve with 2 to 3 months, referral to an experienced hand surgeon may be indicated.

Ulnar-Nerve Entrapment

Ulnar-nerve entrapment at the elbow is the second most common cause of entrapment neuropathy. In addition, the ulnar nerve may get trapped at the wrist when it passes through the Guyon canal.

ULNAR-NERVE ENTRAPMENT AT THE ELBOW The ulnar nerve may get trapped at two sites. It may be trapped at the cubital tunnel between the medial epicondyle and the olecranon or under the aponeurotic band between the two heads of the flexor carpi ulnaris origin. Improper positioning during anesthesia or recurrent dislocation or fractures of the elbow predispose to ulnar-nerve entrapment.

Presentation Patients may present with pain, numbness, or tingling over the ulnar-nerve distribution. The symptoms may be made worse by elbow flexion. Athletes or artists may report a loss of fine control of the fingers. Physical examination may reveal weakness of finger abduction, thumb abduction, pinching of the thumb and forefinger, and if severe, power grip. There may be impaired sensation over the fifth digit. Usually there is no sensory impairment proximal to the wrist. In advanced cases, interosseous muscle wasting and claw-hand deformities may be noted. Radiography of the elbow may be helpful for detecting osteophytes. Electrodiagnostic studies may be helpful in confirming the diagnosis.

Management Nonsurgical therapy is indicated for patients with intermittent or mild neuropathy associated with an occupational cause. Patients are instructed to avoid repetitive flexion and extension of the elbow, to rest the elbow, and in some cases to use elbow splints in an extended position. Surgical referral is indicated for worse degrees of entrapment. However, the best surgical results appear to be in patients with mild signs and symptoms. In addition, a variety of ulnar-nerve palsy termed "tardy" palsy, which occurs after trauma, has a poor surgical outcome.

ULNAR NERVE ENTRAPMENT AT THE WRIST The ulnar nerve is infrequently trapped at the wrist. It passes through the Guyon canal, which does not contain any tendons. The causes of ulnar-nerve entrapment in the Guyon canal include repeated trauma to the palmar area (e.g., bicycling), ganglia, fractures, or falling on an outstretched hand.

Presentation Patients may present with pain at the wrist and may report sensory loss over the palmar aspect of the hand. Physical examination may reveal weakness in the hypothenar and thenar ulnar innervated muscles, with sparing of the dorsal hand from sensory abnormalities (because only the palmar branch is trapped). Electrodiagnostic studies may confirm the diagnosis.

Management Mild cases may be managed with avoidance of trauma with or without splints. In most cases this is sufficient. In refractory cases, surgical referral is indicated.

Radial-Nerve Entrapment Syndromes

The radial nerve may be compressed at level of the humerus, distal to the elbow or at the wrist.

RADIAL-NERVE COMPRESSION AT THE LEVEL OF THE HUMERUS High radial-nerve compression usually occurs before the division of the posterior interosseous nerve branch and the sensory branch. Compression may be caused by sleeping with the arm draped over the edge of a chair or other solid objects or by trauma. The patient may report weakness or paralysis of the wrist and finger extensors. Physical examination may confirm this weakness, and in addition, sensory loss over the radial nerve distribution over the dorsum of the hand may be detected. Patients with radial-nerve paresis due to compression tend to recover spontaneously.

POSTERIOR INTEROSSEOUS-NERVE SYNDROME The posterior interosseous nerve branch of the radial nerve may be compressed just distal to the elbow joint at the arcade of Frohse or at the entrance to the supinator muscle. Entrapment may occur due to ganglia or tumors, fibrous bands, or due to fractures or dislocation of the radius. Patients may present with a syndrome of resistant lateral epicondylitis and may note weakness of finger extensors, which may be confirmed on physical examination. Sensation is spared over the dorsum of the hand. Patients should be referred for consideration of surgical exploration with release of the extensor common tendon origin and for removal of any constricting vascular or fibrous bands.

SUPERFICIAL RADIAL-NERVE ENTRAPMENT The superficial radial sensory branch may be compressed at the wrist or in the forearm (where it is known as Wartenbergs syndrome). At the wrist, entrapment may be caused by laceration or blunt trauma as well as by wearing tight watch bands or handcuffs. When entrapment occurs at the forearm it may be associated with de Quervain disease (tenosynovitis of the extensor hallucis longus tendon) in 50% of the cases. The patient usually presents with sensory loss over the distribution of the radial nerve in the hand. The diagnosis is usually made on clinical grounds, and electrodiagnostic studies may be helpful in confirming the diagnosis and site of entrapment. Proximal superficial radial-nerve entrapment may be treated nonoperatively initially; however, surgical treatment may be indicated if it is nonresponsive.

Lateral Femoral-Cutaneous-Nerve Entrapment

Lateral femoral-cutaneous-nerve entrapment is also known as meralgia paresthetica. It refers to the entrapment of the lateral femoral cutaneous nerve as it passes underneath or through the inguinal ligament at the anterior iliac spine. It may occur in obese patients, or in patients who wear tight belts, corsets, or binders. Patients report dysthesia over the lateral aspect of the thigh. Therapy is nonsurgical, involving weight loss and avoidance of constricting belts about the abdomen. Resistant cases may respond to local nerve blocks or corticosteroid injection.

SELECTED READING

Baker DG, Schumacher HR. Acute monoarthritis. N Engl J Med 1993;329:1013.

Barth WF. Office evaluation of patients with musculosketal complaints. Am J Med 1997;102:1A.

Doherty M. Practical problems: fibromyalgia. Report Rheum Dis 1993;23:1.

Klippel JH, Dieppe PA. Rheumatology. 2nd ed. St. Louis: Mosby, 1998.

McGarvey W. Heel pain: "Front line" management of a "bottom line" problem. J Musculoskel Med 1998;15:14.

Nakano KK. Nerve entrapment syndromes. Curr Opin Rheumatol 1997;9:165.

Sack K. Monoarthritis: differential diagnosis. Am J Med 1997;102;1A:305.

Schenck RC, Rodriguez F. Office evaluation of the acutely injured knee. J Musculoskel Med 1992;9:17.

Schumacher R. Arthritis of recent onset: a guide to evaluation and initial therapy for primary care physicians. Postgrad Med 1995;97:52.

Shaffer B, O'Mara J. Common elbow problems: an algorithmic approach. J Musculoskel Med 1997;14:61.

Chapter 40

Gastrointestinal Disorders

R. James St. Hilaire
Charles Masbach II

Five Key Points

- **Acute gastrointestinal bleeding should not be overlooked and needs to be evaluated and treated expeditiously with the assistance of a specialist. Chronic gastrointestinal bleeding also should not be overlooked and an etiology must be determined.**

- **Adequate colonic screening is essential for the early diagnosis and therapy of all colonic neoplasia and the prevention of further neoplasic polyps and colon cancer.**

- **Hepatitis needs to be defined, screened for, vaccinated against and in some cases treated (B and C) to limit transmission, and long-term sequelae (cirrhosis, liver failure, and hepatocellular carcinoma). Remember, drugs often cause hepatitis.**

- **Irritable bowel syndrome is a major disease process with varying presentations that affects a high percentage of a primary care physician's patients, predominantly females. Look for red flags suggesting other disease and perform adequate screening. Multiple therapies exist and at present multiple new pharmacological therapies are in late phases of development.**

- **Peptic ulcer disease most often is the result of a bacterial infection, *Helicobacter pylori*, or as the result of NSAID ingestion.**

Within the past 30 years, gastroenterology has developed phenomenally, not only in diagnostic technology but also in the understanding of physiology, biochemistry, and pathophysiology of gastroenterologic disorders. An important example of this technology involves nonsurgical techniques for visualizing and treating gastrointestinal organ pathology. In addition, the critical role of the gastroenteric tract on other organ systems has been identified.

As primary care physicians, obstetricians and gynecologists will be caring for a larger number of patients with routine gastrointestinal (GI) disorders such as acid peptic disorders, heartburn, gastrointestinal reflux disease (GERD), abdominal pain, jaundice, constipation, diarrhea, chronic and acute GI bleeding, and irritable-bowel syndrome (IBS). In addition, appropriate screening of patients for colon polyps and carcinoma and other premalignant conditions is important, and certain GI disorders occur more frequently in pregnant patients—e.g., GERD, nausea and vomiting, abdominal pain, and anorectal or pelvic floor dysfunction.

A careful history is paramount in evaluating patients with potential gastrointestinal disorders and is therefore important to obstetricians and gynecologists. Specific emphasis and clarification of the cardinal symptoms can help to direct subsequent questioning, examination, evaluation, and testing. While physical examination and laboratory tests are important, the primacy of the history cannot be overstressed.

The symptoms and signs in addition to GI disorders that are most frequently encountered in a primary care practice are discussed in this chapter.

DYSPHAGIA

In dysphagia the patient describes an unpleasant sensation of food stopping or sticking behind the sternum or at the suprasternal notch soon after swallowing and before the food reaches the stomach. Dysphagia can occur with solids or both solids and liquids. Because this is a referred sensation, symptoms often do not localize the pathology. Dysphagia for solids alone, especially if progressive, is suggestive of an obstructing lesion such as a peptic stricture or malignancy. Peptic strictures are more common in patients who also have symptoms of chronic heartburn. GERD is the most common disorder of the esophagus and probably is one of the most prevalent clinical GI conditions originating from the gastrointestinal tract. This condition affects approximately 15% of the U.S. population. The prevalence of GERD increases with age, reaching 21% of patients who are ≥65 years of age as compared with 5% of patients under 65 years of age. The esophageal complications of GERD include Barrett's esophagus, esophageal ulcerations, and esophageal stricture, all of which can produce dysphagia. In addition to bleeding and perforation, GERD results from a complex interplay of several factors, including a dysfunctional lower esophageal sphincter and crural diaphragm, the inability of the esophagus to adequately clear refluxed material, the volume of gastric contents, the ability of the stomach to adequately empty, and the maintenance of the intrinsic resistance to injury of the esophageal epithelium.

Intermittent solid-food dysphagia, however, is more typical of patients with a ring or a web. Dysphagia for both solid and liquids suggests a motility disorder. Intermittent symptoms suggest spasm, while persistent symptoms suggest progressive motility disorders such as achalasia, the most common cause of motor-induced dysphagia. Achalasia of the esophageal body is slowly progressive and has a chronic course. Characteristics include partial or incomplete relaxation of the lower esophageal sphincter (LES), increased LES pressure, and decreased peristalsis of the body of the esophagus. Some patients have vigorous, sometimes extremely painful, tertiary contractions that may manifest as chest pain. This more often occurs early in the disease in younger patients. Patients commonly regurgitate, which can be provoked by changes in position or physical exercise. Therefore, aspiration has to be guarded against. In addition, foul breath occurs because of the pressure of stagnant food in the esophagus. Although patients have equal difficulty eating liquids and solids, by drinking small amounts and eating slowly, often the patient may be able to consume a full meal. Pain is frequently noted

if patients eat or drink rapidly, especially if the food is cold. Valsalva maneuvers or repeated swallowing can help pass material into the stomach. In approximately 5 to 10% of patients with achalasia, squamous-cell carcinoma of the esophagus is found as a complication. Patients with this disorder should be referred to a specialist for therapy, which includes balloon dilatation, treatment with botulinum toxin injections into the gastroesophageal sphincter, and surgery.

Other forms of solid and liquid dysphagia include carcinoma-induced achalasia, esophageal spasm, scleroderma, and fungal and viral esophagitis, in addition to esophageal ulcers, polyps, and foreign bodies. In oropharyngeal dysphagia (transfer dysphagia), patients describe difficulty in transferring food from their mouth into their upper esophagus. This difficulty initiating swallowing is often associated with aspiration, coughing, choking, and nasopharyngeal regurgitation. These symptoms are most often the result of a neurologic disorder. Often, other neurologic symptoms such as dysphonia, dysarthria, or nasal speech are associated with cough following deglutition. Upper esophageal dysfunction or a mechanical obstruction of the pharynx or upper esophagus may produce similar dysphagic symptoms. In addition to the anatomic and neurologic abnormalities, systemic muscular or neuromuscular disorders can result in this type of dysphagia.

Laboratory testing in patients with dysphagia should begin with barium esophagography, since it provides the best assessment of overall esophageal transport and also is more sensitive than esophagogastroduodenoscopy (EGD) in identifying both mild and moderate esophageal narrowing. Also, it outlines the anatomy for the endoscopist, such as the presence of a Zenker diverticulum, an endoscopic hazard, fistulae, lumen size, and other diverticula or pseudodiverticula, which could compromise endoscopic therapy. If no abnormality is noted in a patient with solid-food dysphagia, a bolus challenge should be done with a 12.5-mm barium tablet or marshmallow. If oropharyngeal dysfunction or aspiration is suspected, then a videotaped study should be performed or a modified barium swallow using barium of different consistencies with the head in different positions. Most information can be elucidated when this test is performed in consultation with a speech pathologist. More specialized testing of esophageal motility can be performed by a gastrointestinal specialist to help identify motor disorders.

In most cases an EGD is also necessary either for further diagnostic testing such as biopsies or for therapy such as dilatation of webs, rings or strictures, placement of esophageal stents, and injection of botulinum toxin.

HEARTBURN

Heartburn, the most prominent and classic symptom of GERD, is a substernal burning sensation that radiates toward the mouth. It may also be noted in the epigastrium, neck, throat, and occasionally into the back. It usually occurs postprandially, often after the consumption of spicy foods, citrus, fats, chocolate, and alcohol. In addition, recumbence and the act of bending over may further exacerbate the symptoms. It is often associated with the reflux of gastric acid or bile from the stomach into the esophagus because of decreased tone of the lower esophageal sphincter and/or increased abdominal pressure or an increased volume of gastric contents. Other symptoms with which it is associated include dysphagia, odynophagia, regurgitation, water brash, and belching.

ABDOMINAL PAIN

Abdominal pain, seemingly a single symptom, is in fact a group of symptoms. It is a very common human experience and is the most frequent reason that a patient consults a gastroenterologist and one of the most frequent reasons a patient consults a primary care physician. It is entirely a subjective experience that cannot be accounted for simply by the particular location of disease or tissue damage. A similar anatomical lesion can result in a widely different amounts and types of pain. It can also vary greatly in terms of location, character, and intensity. The physician's major tasks are to care for the patient in pain and to minimize suffering. Diagnosis is helped by a precise description of the location, quality, and characteristics of abdominal pain. Very often this symptom is very difficult for the patient to describe and therefore requires a clear and probing history-taking by the physician. The location of abdominal pain is generally divided into epigastric, periumbilical, and suprapubic, in addition to four quadrants. In addition to location, radiation of the discomfort is also important in determining the origin of the pain. The descriptive qualities of pain, such as burning, sharp, colicky, stabbing, aching, crampy, and throbbing help to further define the origin in addition to determining the presence of cyclicity or constancy of the pain. For example, ulcer pain is very frequently a burning pain often relieved by food, while the pain associated with

biliary disease is often colicky and is exacerbated by food. The pain associated with diarrhea and irritable-bowel syndrome is often described as crampy. Lastly, it is important to determine both temporal associations and causative associations in addition to those that result in pain relief.

GASTROINTESTINAL BLEEDING

Bleeding in the gastrointestinal tract can be segregated into acute and chronic and into upper gastrointestinal (UGI) bleeding and lower gastrointestinal (LGI) bleeding. Most acute GI bleeding involves the esophagus, stomach, or duodenum (75 to 80%). Acute UGI bleeding is subdivided into nonvariceal bleeding and variceal bleeding, while chronic UGI bleeding usually involves vascular or mucosal lesions in the esophagus, stomach, and duodenum.

Peptic ulcer disease (gastric and duodenal ulcers) is the most prevalent cause of acute UGI bleeding and requires immediate consultation with a gastroenterologist/endoscopist because endoscopy plays a pivotal role in the diagnosis and therapy of bleeding, especially in the acutely and rapidly bleeding patient. In addition, one should provide adequate vascular access, resuscitate, type and crossmatch for blood, do a complete physical examination looking for risk factors, and make sure the patient is well monitored in an acute-care hospital bed.

Acute UGI bleeding requires urgent evaluation, resuscitation, and reevaluation. Early determination of bleeding severity via the presence or absence of shock, tachycardia, pallor, orthostasis (>20 beats per minute and/or a drop in systolic blood pressure of ≥20 mm Hg), the presence of and frequency of melena, hematochezia, hematemesis (volume, frequency, bright red blood verses coffee grounds), and the presence of red blood in gastric contents (determined by nasogastric intubation) are all required. Of note, symptoms of abdominal cramps and lightheadedness suggest more rapid bleeding.

Other comorbid factors are very important in treating a bleeding patient (Table 40-1). These include age ≥70, concurrent major organ system disease, or hospitalization concurrent with the onset of bleeding. A careful medication history should be obtained (especially nonsteroidal antiinflammatory drugs [NSAIDs] and coumadin), in addition to a history of alcohol consumption, cirrhosis, chronic hepatitis, and atherosclerotic cardiovascular disease. Since the most common complications of an acute

TABLE 40-1
HIGH-RISK CRITERIA FOR SCREENING PATIENT WITH ACUTE UGI BLEEDING

History
  Age ≥70 yr
  Currently hospitalized
  Concurrent other major organ system disease
Symptoms
  Frequent melena
  Repeated hematemesis (large volume of fresh blood)
  Hematochezia
  Rapid development of orthostatic changes or syncope
  Abdominal cramps
Physical examination
  Blood pressure
    Hypotension (systolic <100 mm Hg)
    Othostasis (systolic drop ≥20 mm Hg)
  Heart rate
    Tachycardia >100 beats/min
    Orthostatic change >20 beats/min
  Pallor
  Bright red blood per nasogastric tube and on rectal
    examination
Transfusion requirements
  First 24 hr, >4 units
  With rebleeding event, >2 units
  Total 6–8 units

major UGI bleeding are myocardial ischemia events, the patient should be carefully assessed initially for ischemia, especially in elderly patients.

Important physical findings in the initial assessment of a patient with UGI bleeding include the presence of pallor, tachycardia (pulse rate >100 beats/min), orthostasis or "tilt" (≥20 mm Hg drop in systolic pressure) and an increase in pulse rate of ≥20 beats/min and hypotension (systolic pressure ≤100 mm Hg). Assessment for signs of chronic liver disease (splenomegaly, spider angiomata, palmar erythema, gynecomastia, small liver, ascites, caput medusae, testicular atrophy, muscle wasting, asterixis, and hepatic encephalopathy) is vital. A nasogastric tube should be placed and lavage and aspiration performed to establish the presence of blood and therefore confirm UGI bleeding. This is especially important in patients presenting with hematochezia without hematemesis. A rectal examination should *always* be performed to confirm the presence or absence of blood and whether it is melena (black) or red/maroon blood. The presence of bile after the initial clearing of the stomach suggests the absence of active bleeding in the proximal duodenum. Patients who have hematochezia usually have evidence of volume depletion by other parameters, if the bleeding source is from the upper tract. In addition, rapid resuscitation, evaluation, and treatment

of patients who have hematochezia and are vomiting up fresh blood is imperative because the mortality rate is high in these patients.

New-onset anemia or a drop in hemoglobin of ≥2 g/dl is indicative of significant bleeding or rebleeding. It is important to determine new acute bleeding from acute bleeding superimposed on chronic blood loss with a hematocrit and mean corpuscular volume (MCV) and red cell distribution width (RDW). However, it is important to remember that initial blood loss does not change the hematocrit, because the patient bleeds blood of the same hematocrit. A decrease in hematocrit is appreciated only after rehydration or reequilibration of fluid from the nonvascular compartment.

Profound anemia with a hemoglobin level <7.5 g/dl compromises the oxygen-carrying capacity of the blood; supplemental oxygen is beneficial to maximize available oxygen. Therefore, supplemental oxygen should be routinely provided in cases of hemodynamic instability, anemia, and advanced age and in patients with known ischemic disease. It is also important to immediately check the patient's coagulation status by obtaining a prothrombin time, an activated partial thromboplastin time, and a platelet count, in addition to obtaining a serum glucose, electrolytes, and calcium and drawing blood for a type and crossmatch for a minimum of four units of packed red cells.

Patient resuscitation should include placement of several large-bore (14-gauge) intravenous lines for volume replacement, and care should be directed at airway protection and protection from cardiac ischemia. Part of this initial evaluation and resuscitation should involve consultation with a gastrointestinal endoscopist and a surgeon so that endoscopy can be performed. It is important that this be done at the earliest time that the patient is stable if the bleeding is significant. If the bleeding is massive, central lines should be placed; in addition, an interventional radiologist should be consulted immediately in case endoscopy is impossible or yields no helpful results. Packed red cells are adequate to correct anemia. Fresh-frozen plasma is needed only to correct a coagulopathy or anticipated coagulopathy because of massive transfusion requirements or the presence of coagulopathy. Platelets are not usually needed unless the patient is thrombocytopenic (<20,000/μl).

Patients with significant UGI bleeding should be closely monitored in an acute-care setting with frequent monitoring of vital signs and repeat hematocrit determinations. Today, endoscopy is not only diagnostic but also allows for multiple therapeutic interventions that can affect the outcome of the bleeding. It is also useful in predicting rebleeding. Thus, it is important that early endoscopy be performed in the acutely bleeding patient. It is important to remember that H$_2$ receptor blockers and proton pump inhibitors do not decrease the chance of rebleeding of ulcers, varices, or Mallory-Weiss tears. However, early institution of these medications and/or antacid therapy aids in the early healing of many lesions.

The most common causes of UGI bleeding include duodenal ulcers, gastric ulcers, varices, Mallory–Weiss tears, gastritis, esophagitis, Dieulafoy lesions, acute hemorrhagic stress, gastritis, and tumors.

Chronic bleeding, on the other hand, is episodic, overt or occult, and mostly not associated with symptoms. Chronic bleeding from the esophagus, stomach, and duodenum is most commonly the result of persistent reflux esophagitis, a large hiatal hernia with ulcerations, large hypertrophic gastric polyps, watermelon stomach, portal hypertensive gastropathy, or angiodysplasia. If no other source is found, a RBC radionuclide scan should be performed. Because chronic bleeding is more insidious, it does not have to be evaluated as rapidly. However, a complete evaluation is still necessary and endoscopy is the most useful diagnostic method. If no source is found, evaluation of the small bowel should be performed.

RECTAL BLEEDING

Rectal bleeding or lower GI (LGI) bleeding, like UGI bleeding, can be separated into acute and chronic. Acute LGI bleeding initially is managed essentially the same way as acute UGI bleeding. First, assess the severity of bleeding and the cardiovascular status of the patient with a brief history and physical examination. As with UGI bleeding, determining the hemodynamic status of the patient is important. This is done by checking the vital signs and assessing the patient for shock or significant postural changes, which suggests a significant loss of blood volume. In addition, it is important to determine cardiovascular, clotting, respiratory, and renal status. It is also important to determine new acute bleeding from acute bleeding superimposed on chronic blood loss with a hematocrit and MCV. In addition, it is important to determine the presence of coagulopathy by checking a platelet count and clotting studies. Renal and hepatic function should also be determined. This is done while the patient is being resuscitated and stabilized.

Acute LGI bleeding presents with either bright red blood or maroon stool with or without clots. This depends on the coagulation status of the patient and the rate of bleeding. Some patients with slower right colonic or small intestinal bleeding can present with melena, as is found in UGI bleeding. It is important to document that the bleeding source is from the lower tract in case surgery should be necessary. Therefore, an endoscopist and a surgeon should be contacted early in the evaluation of the patient. If the patient is bleeding rapidly, it is important to rule out a UGI source with endoscopy. The lower tract needs to be evaluated with anoscopy and rigid sigmoidoscopy initially to determine the presence of low rectal or anal canal bleeding. Most often a rigid sigmoidoscope is used because the colon is unprepared and is difficult to visualize using a flexible sigmoidoscope. However, an initial evaluation can involve an enema followed by flexible sigmoidoscopy. If no source is found it is necessary to immediately prepare the patient for a colonoscopy with an electrolyte flush preparation (Golyte or Colyte). If there is a question regarding the level of the bleed, a radionuclide-red-cell study might be of value to separate a colon bleed from a small intestinal bleed. This detects active bleeding of 0.05 to 1.0 ml/min. If bleeding is more active (0.5 to 1.0 ml/min), selective angiography can be used to determine the site. There is little place at this time for colonic resection without preoperative imaging unless the extent of bleeding warrants emergency surgery. If bleeding is massive, emergency surgery either with or without intraoperative endoscopy may be necessary.

The most common cause of significant acute colorectal bleeding is diverticulosis, while the most common causes of chronic colorectal bleeding are hemorrhoids, neoplasms, diversion colitis, and angiodysplasia. Less common causes of acute bleeding include neoplasms, radiation, ischemic, ulcerative, and Crohn colitis, solitary rectal ulcer, varices, internal hemorrhoids, and Dieulafoy lesions. In addition, one has to consider small-bowel causes such as Meckel diverticula and aortoenteric fistulas.

Fecal occult blood testing best assesses chronic GI bleeding. These tests identify hemoglobin or altered hemoglobin in the stool. Ingestion of foods containing peroxidases (horseradish, cauliflower, turnips, melon, and broccoli) may result in a false positive test. Reducing agents such as ascorbic acid can reduce the sensitivity of these tests (Hemoccult II, HemoQuant, and Hemoccult SEMSA). All are not specific for human hemoglobin and therefore can be positive with red meat. Rehydration of the slides in the Hemoccult test increases the sensitivity but decreases the specificity. These tests are not affected by oral iron administration. The sensitivity of Hemoccult II tests for detecting asymptomatic colorectal cancer ranges from 45 to 89% and is less than 25% for colon polyps ≥1 cm. Of note, at least 50% of screened persons older than 40 years will be false positive or will have a UGI source of bleeding. Data suggest that annual fecal occult blood testing, with rehydration and colonoscopy in patients who test positive, has a 90% sensitivity in detecting colorectal cancers and is associated with a 33% decrease in 13-year cumulative mortality due to colorectal carcinoma. This was lost to a great degree by increasing the interval from 1 to 2 years. Colonoscopy is the best means of evaluating for chronic LGI bleeding. Not only is it effective in diagnosing mass lesions such as polyps and carcinomas, but it is also effective in diagnosing mucosal lesions not seen on high-quality air-contrast barium studies (angiodysplasia, vasculitis, Dieulafoy lesions). In addition, colonoscopy is effective in the treatment of many of these lesions.

DIARRHEA

One of the most common gastrointestinal problems in the world is diarrhea. It is a familiar affliction for physicians and patients alike, characterized clinically as the frequent passage of unformed stools. More precisely, it is the passage of >200 g of stool per 24 hours when consuming a standard Western diet or >400 g/day when consuming a diet in rural Africa, because of the increased consumption of absorbable fiber. Since measuring stool weight is difficult, a more pragmatic set of criteria is more useful clinically. These include an increase in the frequency of bowel movements mostly with an increase in the fluidity of the stool with or without the presence of abnormal constituents in stool. Normal stools are generally solid and brown. However, these features can depend on diet. Normal frequency can vary from one to three stools per day to two to three per week. In addition, blood, leukocytes, and oil are not usually present in normal stools.

Diarrhea can be either acute or chronic (Table 40-2). Chronicity is defined as diarrhea lasting >3 weeks. Since identifying a specific cause enhances the likelihood of a rapid response to therapy, a thorough

---

**TABLE 40-2
CAUSES OF DIARRHEA**

Acute Diarrhea	Chronic or Recurrent Diarrhea	
Viruses	Parasites	Malabsorption
Bacterial toxins	*Giardia lamblia*	Bile-salt malabsorption
Staphylococcus	*Entamoeba histolytica*	Lactase deficiency
Clostridium	Cryptosporidium	Pancreatic insufficiency
Bacteria	Inflammation	Sprue
Salmonella	Ulcerative colitis	Intestinal lymphoma
Shigella	Crohn disease	Whipple disease
Escherichia coli	Ischemic colitis	Other disaccharidase deficiencies
Yersinia	Microscopic colitis	Postsurgical
Vibrio parahemolyticus	Collagenous colitis	Postgastrectomy dumping syndrome
Vibrio cholerae	Drugs	Enterenteric fistuli
Parasites	Laxatives	Blind loops
Giardia lamblia	Antibiotics	Parasympathetic denervation
Entamoeba histolytica	Quinidine	Short-bowel syndrome
Cryptosporidia	Guanethidine	Other
Drugs	Caffeine	Cirrhosis
Laxatives	Alcohol	Diabetes mellitus
Antibiotics	Functional	Hyperthyroidism
Caffeine	Irritable-bowel syndrome	Scleroderma
Alcohol	Diverticulosis	Heavy-metal intoxication
Functional	Tumors	Other neurogenic diarrheas
Anxiety	Colonic carcinoma	Pellagra
Acute presentation of chronic diarrhea	Villous adenoma	Amyloidosis
	Islet-cell tumors	Addison's disease
	Carcinoid syndrome	
	Medullary carcinoma of thyroid	

TABLE 40-3
CLUES HELPFUL TO THE DIAGNOSIS OF ACUTE DIARRHEA

History	Possible Enteric Pathogens	Additional Tests
Bloody stools	Salmonella, Shigella, Campylobacter, Eschericia coli O157:H7, Clostridium difficile, amoeba	Stool for culture for enteric pathogens, ova and parasites, and C. difficile toxin
Recent antibiotic therapy, chemotherapy	C. difficile, Salmonella	Stool for C. difficile toxin, culture for enteric pathogens
Travel	E. coli O157:H7, Giardia lamblia, amebae, above listed organisms	Stool for ova and parasites and Giardia antigen
Several similarly affected family member of friends	Organisms causing food poisoning: Staphylococcus, Clostridium, Bacillus cereus, Salmonella	None usually required
Homosexual activities (male)	Herpesvirus, Chlamydia, Treponema pallidum, Shigella, Neisseria gonorrhoeae, amebae, Giardia lamblia	Sigmoidoscopy with rectal biopsy and stool specimen for ova and parasites, culture for gonococci, herpesvirus, and Chlamydia; serologic test for syphilis
Rectal pain, severe tenesmus	Campylobacter, Salmonella, Shigella, herpesvirus, Chlamydia	As above for homosexual activities
Severe or persistent abdominal pain	Campylobacter, Yersinia, Clostridium perfringens, Aeromonas	Notify laboratory for special culture
Hospitalization	C. difficile	Stool for C. difficile toxin
Participation or residence in day-care centers, mental institutions, nursing homes	Giardia lamblia, Salmonella, Shigella, C. difficile, rotavirus	Stool for culture for enteric pathogens, ova and parasites, Giardia antigen, and C. difficile toxin

Modified from Giannella RA. Gastrointestinal infections. In: Kelley WN, ed. Textbook of internal medicine. Philadelphia: Lippincott, 1991:554.

history and physical examination are essential. The severity and duration of symptoms directs the promptness and extent of the evaluation. Important factors (Table 40-3) in the history include travel, sexual preferences and activities, medications, type of water supply, whether diarrhea awakens patient from sleep, whether it is associated with blood in the stool, whether stools are foul-smelling or bulky (suggesting pancreatic insufficiency or malabsorption), and presence of steatorrhea. It is important to determine if the patient has any systemic disorder such as diabetes mellitus or thyroid disorders. In addition, it is important to check for a history of inflammatory-bowel disease, antibiotic use (pseudomembranous colitis), or use of other drugs (e.g., antacids, misoprostol, colchicine, conjugated estrogens, acute alcohol use, olsalazine). Evaluating the stool for fecal leukocytes or fecal fat also can provide important clues.

Understanding nutrient absorption in the gut is helpful in understanding the pathophysiology and complications found in malabsorption, maldigestion, and resultant diarrhea. Taken linearly, the duodenum absorbs calcium, magnesium, folate, monosaccharides, iron, and water-soluble vitamins, while the jejunum absorbs amino acids, monosaccharides, water-soluble vitamins, and fatty acids. Lastly, the ileum absorbs monosaccharides, amino acids, fatty acids, fat-soluble vitamins, vitamin B_{12}, and conjugated bile salts. It is important to remember that the distal small bowel has the capacity to adapt in order to absorb nutrients that are not absorbed in the proximal small bowel. The proximal small bowel cannot adapt to absorb bile salts or vitamin B_{12}, which are absorbed in the terminal ileum. The complexity of fat absorption makes it subject to malfunction at many stages, resulting in fat maldigestion and malabsorption and therefore steatorrhea. This can result in weight loss.

Diarrhea can be broken down into acute and chronic diarrhea, and each of these can be separated into four groups by mechanism:

- Osmotic diarrhea (increased amounts of osmotically active solutes)
- Secretory diarrhea (intestinal ion secretion or inhibition of normal active ion absorption)
- Exudative processes
- Intestinal-motility alterations

Osmotic diarrhea results when poorly absorbed water-soluble molecules remain in the intestinal lumen and therefore retain water or draw water into the intestinal lumen. Therefore, osmotic diarrhea follows the ingestion of osmotically active substances and stops with fasting. Stool volumes tend to be less than 1 liter per day, and there is an ion gap noted when measuring the stool electrolytes and osmolality (the stool osmolality is greater than the sum of the stool electrolyte concentrations). The stool pH can frequently be less than 7. This type of diarrhea subsides or is markedly reduced during fasting. Common causes of osmotic diarrhea (Table 40-4) include lactase deficiency, sorbitol in food (diet drinks, gum, etc), saline cathartics, and antacids. Lactose, a nonabsorbable 12-carbon sugar, is cleaved into two 6-carbon sugars, glucose, and galactose by lactase. When lactase is deficient, the lactose is not absorbable in the small bowel and therefore is fermented by colonic bacteria. This results in increased motility and a diarrheal stool with a low pH. This is the most common disaccharide deficiency. It is common in blacks, Eskimos, Orientals, and Middle Easterners and less common in societies where dairy farms are the rule. Diarrhea, abdominal cramps, and flatulence develop with the consumption of dairy products or other foods containing increased amounts of lactose. These symptoms are improved with a decrease in consumption of these products. The stool pH is very often <6. The diagnosis is made by withdrawal of lactose-containing foods, with a lactose-tolerance test, or by using a hydrogen breath test. The diagnosis is made using a lactose-tolerance test when the blood sugar increases <20 mg/100 ml after a lactose challenge. Lactose intolerance can occur in the clinical setting in which the intestinal mucosa is damaged—e.g., *Giardia lamblia* infestations. In addition, patients on weight-reduction diets who drink large amounts of diet drinks or chew sugarless gum may have an osmotic diarrhea from the sorbitol. Colon washouts used for preparation for colonoscopy also work as osmotic cathartics.

Secretory diarrhea is the result of abnormal fluid and electrolyte transport. An example of this type of diarrhea results when the intestine secretes more fluid than it absorbs. This results in a stool volume >1 liter per day, with a composition almost equivalent to extracellular fluid. Therefore, no ion gap is found and the diarrhea persists during fasting, although in some cases some decrease may occur because often there is also an osmotic component to the diarrhea. Because of the degree of the diarrhea, the patient often presents with hypokalemia. Common examples of secretory diarrhea include hormonal tumors; surreptitious laxative ingestion; bile acid diarrhea; bacterial-toxin—induced diarrhea; villous adenomas; and fatty acid diarrhea. The classic hormonal tumor resulting in a secretory diarrhea is Verner–Morrison syndrome (also called pancreatic cholera or WHDA [watery diarrhea, hypokalemia, and achlorhydria]). Patients with this disorder have massive diarrhea of 5 liters or more

---

TABLE 40-4
CAUSES OF OSMOTIC DIARRHEA

Ingestion of poorly absorbable solutes
  Magnesium sulfate
  Sodium sulfate
  Citrate-containing laxatives (magnesium citrate)
  Magnesium-containing antacids
  Mannitol
  Sorbitol
  Fructose (chewing gum, diet candy)
Maldigestion
  Disaccharidase deficiencies
  Lactose intolerance
  Sucrose intolerance
  Isomaltose intolerance
  Trehalose intolerance
  Gastrocolic fistula
  Jejunoileal bypass
  Short-bowel syndrome
  Postgastrectomy
  Postvagotomy states
  Chronic intestinal ischemia
  Lactulose therapy
Mucosal-transport defects
  Glucose–galactose malabsorption
  Chloridorrhea
  Congenital sodium diarrhea
  General malabsorption in diffuse disease of the small-bowel
    mucosa

---

per day, with associated dehydration and hypokalemia. It is often associated with other endocrine tumors, resulting in hypercalcemia and hyperglycemia in multiple endocrine neoplasia. The tumor is associated with non–β-cell tumors of the pancreas. Vasoactive intestinal peptide (VIP) is the most common mediator. However, prostaglandins, secretin, and calcitonin have also been implicated in secretory diarrhea. Treatment is surgical and/or therapy with octreotide. Secretory diarrhea can be caused by medullary carcinoma of the thyroid or Zollinger–Ellison syndrome. Patients with carcinoid syndrome can also have watery diarrhea syndrome. In these patients, dietary tryptophan is converted to serotonin, which causes diarrhea, abdominal cramps, and intestinal hypermotility in addition to histamine and other chemicals. Presence of carcinoid syndrome is indicative of hepatic metastases and is diagnosed by elevated urinary 5-hydroxyindoleacetic acid. Like WHDA, it is treated with octreotide.

Bile salt diarrhea, another cause of secretory diarrhea, is due to malabsorption of bile acids in the terminal ileum, resulting in their entering the colon thus stimulating secretion. The extent of this malabsorption determines the extent of symptoms and the mode of therapy. If the area of malabsorption is limited (e.g., limited resection), there are adequate bile salts in the proximal small bowel and adequate fat absorption resulting in no steatorrhea (fecal fat <20 g/24 hr). These patients can be effectively treated with cholestyramine. However, if there is extensive disease (e.g., extensive resection), then the bile salts are profoundly malabsorbed. The liver cannot compensate as it can with limited disease, and adequate micelles are not formed, resulting in fat malabsorption. Therefore, in this situation the malabsorbed fatty acids stimulate secretion in the colon. Thus, these patients must be treated with a low-fat diet and medium-chain triglycerides and not cholestyramine.

Laxative use is very common today, especially in persons over the age of 60. In fact, 15 to 30% regularly abuse laxatives. However with surreptitious laxative ingestion, diarrhea results; it is the commonest cause of watery diarrhea in referral centers. Patients often take the laxative to maintain a lower body weight. Proctosigmoidoscopy or colonoscopy reveals melanosis coli, and barium enemas often show a dilated, hypomotile colon lacking haustra. The laxatives that most commonly cause melanosis coli include anthracene derivatives such as senna, aloe, and cascara. Diagnosis is often made by history and stool phenolphthalein. If this is the problem, it is necessary to address the underlying psychological or emotional problems.

A classic example of toxin-induced secretory diarrhea is that caused by *Vibrio cholerae*. The toxin increases intracellular cAMP-mediated active ion secretion in the enterocyte, resulting in a profuse diarrhea. Onset is about 12 hours after exposure and is often associated with fever and dehydration due to the profuse diarrhea. This is a disease whose course can be shortened by therapy with tetracycline. It is important to remember that *few or no white cells are found in the stool of patients with toxigenic diarrhea*. Enterotoxigenic *Escherichia coli* results in traveler's diarrhea. The onset here is about 12 hours after ingestion and the disease is associated with fever. There are other bacterial infections of the gastroenteric tract that result in a secretory diarrhea but associated with tissue injury that can result in exudation and at times bleeding. These include *Campylobacter jejuni, Yersinia entercolitica*, Salmonella, Shigella, *Clostridium difficile, Staphylococcus aureus*, Aeromonas, and Plesiomonas. In addition to gut abnormalities, they can result in problems in distant organs.

Staphylococcus aureus toxin is found in egg products, cream, and mayonnaise when they have been at warm temperatures. It has a rapid onset, from 1 to 6 hours after ingestion, and lasts for 24 hours, and is not associated with fever, vomiting, or cramps. Only supportive therapy is necessary since it is a self-limiting disease.

Clostridium perfringens is a toxin that is ingested in precooked food such as beef and turkey. Heat-stable spores produce the toxin and are present, although the bacteria have been destroyed. Therefore, when the food is rewarmed the spores germinate, producing the toxin. Onset is 8 to 12 hours after ingestion and may be associated with fever. In this disease the diarrhea is worse than the vomiting and begins later. Like staphylococcal toxin disease, it lasts 24 hours and treatment is therefore supportive.

Bacillus cereus toxin is found in fried rice. There are two varieties of the diarrheal illness. One has a rapid onset, 1 to 6 hours after ingestion and is not associated with fever, and resembles the course of *Stap. aureus* toxin disease. The other has a much slower onset, 12 to 24 hours, is also not associated with fever but is associated with profuse diarrhea and resembles *Clostridium perfringens*–associated disease. Diagnosis is made by history and by isolating the organism from the contaminated food. Like most toxigenic diarrheas, treatment is supportive.

Most cases of *Clostridium difficile* diarrhea are associated with protein exotoxins A and B. A, an enterotoxin, triggers diarrhea, epithelial necrosis, and a characteristic inflammatory process, while B is a cytotoxin but does not by itself cause toxicity in animal models. The disease can range from mild diarrhea and little inflammation to severe colitis associated with pseudomembranes that adhere to necrotic colonic epithelium. This disorder occurs most commonly in elderly patients in hospitals or nursing homes, probably because of a combination of environmental contamination with the organism and the increased use of antibiotics. Other possible risk factors include surgery, nasogastric intubation, stay in an intensive-care unit, and lengthy hospital stays, in addition to use of antibiotics. Some patients have antibiotic-associated diarrhea but have no evidence of *C. difficile* infection. Virtually all antibiotics have been implicated except vancomycin. However, cephalosporins, ampicillin, amoxicillin, and clindamycin are most commonly implicated. Erythro-mycin, trimethoprim-sulfamethoxazole, and other penicillins are less commonly implicated. The typical clinical picture includes nonbloody diarrhea, lower abdominal cramps, leukocytosis, and low-grade fever (rarely high). However, severely ill patients manifest dehydration, hypotension, toxic megacolon, hypoproteinemia, and even colonic perforation. In these patients the diagnostic test of choice is a flexible sigmoidoscopy or colonscopy looking for classic findings. However, since the distal colon is involved in most patients, flexible sigmoidoscopy is usually sufficient. Referral for colonoscopy should be performed if flexible sigmoidoscopy is negative, since up to 30% of patients may have disease solely on the right. It is difficult to implicate *C. difficile* as the cause of antibiotic-associated diarrhea without identifying the cytotoxin. Therapy includes discontinuing the offending drug, if possible. If symptoms persist or are severe, the patient should be treated with metronidazole orally 250 mg four times daily for 7 to 14 days or oral vancomycin 125 mg four times daily for 7 to 14 days. In general, fever resolves in 24 hours with adequate therapy and diarrhea decreases within 4 to 5 days. If oral therapy is impossible, intravenous metronidazole is effective. Relapse rates are from 20 to 25% after successful therapy with either agent. Patients who relapse once have a higher incidence of relapsing additional times. About 5 to 10% have multiple relapses. Patients who have multiple relapses should be referred to a specialist for additional therapy.

Diarrhea as the result of exudation of serum proteins involves abnormal membrane permeability of the intestine. In addition, there can be exudation of blood or mucus into the bowel at sites of inflammation, ulceration, or infiltration. This type of diarrhea is frequently a small-volume and may be associated with blood and a high white-cell (WBC) count. Common examples include invasive bacterial pathogens such as Shigella and Salmonella and inflammatory-bowel disease.

Shigella causes a bloody diarrhea with fever and bacteremia and sometimes septicemia. It is diagnosed by clinical history, positive stool cultures, and blood cultures. It mostly can be treated with ampicillin. However, a resistant strain caused by plasmids is emerging; therefore, if no response is seen to ampicillin therapy, chloramphenicol might be considered. If no response to ampicillin is noted, it is beneficial to consult an infectious disease specialist.

Salmonella (mostly *Salmonella typhimurium* in the United States) from poultry is associated with fever but not bloody diarrhea. Diagnosis is based on positive stool cultures. It is important to note that therapy is supportive because antibiotics prolong the course of the disease and can result in the harboring of resistant organisms. In addition, antibiotics do not alter the course of the disease unless blood cultures are positive.

Vibrio parahaemolyticus may be ingested from undercooked shellfish, resulting in fever and bloody diarrhea. This disorder is common in Japan and is becoming more common in the United States. Diagnosis is based on positive stool cultures and, as with salmonella, antibiotics are of questionable value in treating the infection. However, of the antibiotics used, erythromycin is the most effective.

Staph. aureus enterocolitis is diagnosed on Gram staining of stool that is positive for a predominance of gram-positive cocci with a paucity of other organisms, while invasive *E. coli* is rare and presents as fever and bloody diarrhea in addition to profound toxicity.

Newer enteric pathogens include *Campylobacter jejuni*. These are gram-negative bacilli that result in the presence of blood and leukocytes in the stool, have an incubation period of 2 to 4 days before invading the small bowel, and may mimic granulomatous or idiopathic ulcerative colitis. Transmission is from infected water, poultry, unpasteurized milk, sick dogs, and infected children. In addition, because of explosive, frequent watery diarrhea due to the effect of many species that produce a cholera-type toxin, it can mimic a small-bowel secretory diarrhea. This diarrhea usually lasts from 3 to 5 days but may have a relapsing course. Treatment is often not needed, but if the illness is severe, the patient should be treated with erythromycin. Both hemolytic-uremic syndrome (HUS) and postinfectious arthritis are postdiarrheal illnesses associated with this infection.

Yersinia enterocolitica can result in diarrheal disorders that range from acute enteritis to chronic enteritis. It may cause enterocolities, ileitis, mesenteric adenitis, and septicemia. It appears to have its peak incidence in the winter. The acute form usually lasts from 1 to 3 weeks, as does shigella, and is characterized by fever, diarrhea, and leukocytosis, in addition to fecal leukocytosis. Chronic enteritis is found predominantly in children and is characterized by failure to thrive, hypoalbuminemia, hypokalemia, in addition to diarrhea. Bloody diarrhea is more apt to occur in children and adolescents, while joint pains more often occur in adults. Other features include right-lower-quadrant pain, tenderness, vomiting and nausea, and acute abdominal pain. These symptoms often mimic Crohn's disease and appendicitis. It is invasive and is transmitted by the fecal–oral route and via water and milk. In addition, extraintestinal manifestations are noteworthy. They include a nonsuppurative arthritis, ankylosing spondylitis in HLA27-positive patients, erythema nodosum, erythema multiforme, Graves disease, Hashimoto's disease, and liver abscesses and granulomata. A similar clinical picture is seen with *Yersinia pseudotuberculosis*. This disease is usually self-limited. However, if antibiotic therapy is required, trimethoprim–sulfamethoxazole or a fluoroquinone should be used. The bacteria also are sensitive to aminoglycosides but variably sensitive to tetracycline and chloramphenicol. Penicillin resistance is common because β-lactamases are frequently produced.

Campylobacter jejuni, motile microaerophilic gram-negative bacilli, are transmitted from animals, mostly poultry, to humans by infected water, contaminated food, and unpasteurized milk, or via sick dogs and infected children. These organisms are among the most common bacterial causes of diarrhea and can present as gastroenteritis, pseudoappendicitis, or colitis. After an incubation period of 2 to 4 days the infection results in 24 hours of constitutional symptoms and then diarrhea and abdominal cramps with blood and leukocytes in the stool after invasion of the small bowel; it may mimic either Crohn's or ulcerative colitis. In addition, it can mimic a small-bowel secretory diarrhea because many species produce a cholera-like toxin. This diarrhea lasts 3 days to more than week but may relapse. Carriage of the organism during the convalescent period for up to 5 weeks after the onset of the disease is common and is reduced with antibiotic therapy. Therapy with antibiotics—erythromycin or fluoroquinolones—is appropriate when the illness is severe. Newer macrolides such as azithromycin and clarithromycin also show excellent in vitro activity. However, this is generally not needed. Hemolytic–uremic syndrome and a postinfectious arthritis can occur as postdiarrheal illnesses.

A dangerous infection is enterohemorrhagic *Escherichia coli* O157:H7 infection that is transmitted in undercooked or raw ground beef from infected cattle, exposure to patients with bloody diarrhea, contaminated water supplies, and nonpreserved apple cider. It presents with nonbloody diarrhea, hemorrhagic colitis, and abdominal pain but with no fever. Large quantities of a Shiga-like toxin that is difficult to detect are instrumental in the disease. Infections with this organism may result in HUS and thrombotic thrombocytopenic purpura. The risk of HUS increases with older age and in children. It is gener-

ally believed that antibiotics are not indicated for active infections.

An extremely invasive organism that produces a necrotizing vasculitis associated with gangrene and shock is *Vibrio vulnificus*. It is isolated from shellfish, seawater, and zooplankton along the Gulf of Mexico, in addition to both coasts of the United States, most notably in warm seasons. It can result in two clinical syndromes. The first consists of a wound infection, cellulitis, fasciitis, or myositis. This occurs after exposure to seawater or after cleaning shellfish. The second clinical syndrome consists of septicemia following the ingestion of raw shellfish, most commonly oysters. Those who are at high risk for septicimia include patients with congestive heart failure, diabetes mellitus, renal failure, immunosuppressive states, or liver disease. Therapy involves treatment with tetracycline.

Entamoeba histolytica is the primary cause of dysentery. It may be complicated by fulminant colitis, toxic megacolon, bleeding, stricture formation, and perforation. Severe disease is most common in the elderly, the immunosuppressed, and the debilitated. It is usually acquired by ingesting cysts from fresh vegetables, contaminated water, and sexual practices that result in fecal–oral contamination. It is effectively treated with metronidazole, probably because the intestinal disease will not develop without the presence of bacteria. Three stool specimens should be examined via wet mount within 30 minutes of stool passage to look for motile trophozoites. A formalin–ethyl acetate concentration of the stool should be examined for cysts. It is important to avoid barium, bismuth, kaolin compounds, castor oil, hypertonic enemas, and magnesium hydroxide, because all will interfere with the ability to detect the parasite in the stool. A diagnostic test that is helpful is colonoscopy, which demonstrates colitis and scattered ulcers, which are most common in the cecum and ascending colon. If the patient still goes undiagnosed, serologic tests should be performed, such as indirect hemagglutination assay (IHA). It is positive in 90% of patients with amebic dysentery or amebic liver abcesses. However, it is important to remember that the IHA may remain positive for years after therapy for invasive amebiasis. Therapy for acute disease consists of oral metronidazole 750 mg three times daily for 10 days. This should be followed by a luminal-acting oral drug such as paromomycin 500 mg three times daily for 7 days or iodoquinol 650 mg three times daily for 20 days.

This will eliminate all cysts and therefore prevent possible relapse.

Other colitides include collagenous colitis, lymphocytic colitis, and drug-associated colitis (NSAIDs, gold, methyldopa, flucytosine, quinidine, and isotretinoin).

Lastly, motility disorders can result in diarrhea as the result of either rapid transit resulting in inadequate contact time for absorption or delayed transit resulting in bacterial overgrowth. Rapid transit can occur after gastrectomy, intestinal resection, and in metabolic disorders such as hyperthyroidism or carcinoid syndrome. However, delayed transit occurs with structural defects such as small-bowel diverticula, blind loops, or small-bowel strictures. It can also occur in myopathy such as scleroderma or visceral neuropathy such as diabetes mellitus. It is important to remember that, clinically, some cases of diarrhea are the result of more than one cause, such as malabsorption that often results in an osmotic and secretory diarrhea. In addition, many patients with irritable-bowel syndrome (IBS) present with diarrhea.

CONSTIPATION

One common gastrointestinal problem in the United States is constipation. It accounts for approximately 2.5 million physician visits per year and accounts for almost $500 million spent on over-the-counter (OTC) laxatives per year. It affects all ages and all educational and socioeconomic levels. It is more common in the elderly, with a dramatic increase in prevalence after age 65 years; women are affected two to three times more often then men.

The availability of OTC laxatives and their chronic and often inappropriate use can result in laxative dependency, produce damage to the bowel and its nervous system, and lead to many iatrogenic problems. Problems secondary to constipation add to the economic burden of this condition. Examples of this include the association with urinary-tract infections in women and pudendal nerve damage and fecal incontinence in middle-aged and older women. In young women, severe chronic constipation is associated with an increased incidence of unnecessary surgery, such as hysterectomy, ovarian cystectomy, and appendectomy. In the elderly, chronic constipation together with urinary incontinence is an important contributing factor in the removal of the aged from their homes and their placement in chronic-care facilities. However, while common, it is difficult to define. Patients who say that they are constipated may report bowel movements that are too infrequent; stools that are too hard; or defecation that feels incomplete, is painful, or requires them to strain or use laxatives in order to evacuate stool. These symptoms may or may not imply specific abnormalities in bowel function. Since stool frequency is the easiest to quantify, it is often used as the definition. However, difficulty arises because of the great variety in "normal" bowel frequency in the general population. This varies from two bowel movements per day to two bowel movements per week. Therefore, one must integrate the number of bowel movements with other signs and symptoms, such as stool firmness, ease of passage, excessive straining during defecation, discomfort during defecation, the feeling of incomplete evacuation, and the need for cathartics or digital means to facilitate evacuation. In addition, comparing the number of bowel movements with those that have been historically "normal" for the patient can also be used as a parameter of constipation, in addition to the age of onset. Onset in childhood suggests a congenital disorder such as Hirschsprung's disease. However, most cases are idiopathic.

When evaluating chronic constipation, the two objectives are to define the symptoms and identify possible causes. Stool frequency is most accurately measured by requesting that the patient keep a diary for several weeks. A stool frequency of <3 per week is one definition of constipation. Some patients define constipation as the need to strain in order to defecate as opposed to infrequent evacuation, or they feel that constipation is determined by one or more of the parameters mentioned above. Few of these are quantifiable or repeatable and therefore are subjective. Therefore, the determination of the presence of constipation requires both the objective parameter of number of bowel movements in conjunction with subjective symptoms. This is especially important if there has been a clear change in the patient's "normal" bowel habits. Thus, a complete, careful history is important, especially noting the patient's definition of constipation, the number of bowel movements that occur per week, and what other symptoms are associated with these bowel movements.

Once it is determined that chronic constipation is present, the patient should be screened for major causes by further history-taking, physical examination, and laboratory tests. Useful laboratory tests include thyroid-stimulating hormone (TSH), serum calcium, fasting blood glucose, electrolytes, and β-human

---

TABLE 40-5
CONDITIONS ASSOCIATED WITH CONSTIPATION

Disorders of the colon
  Irritable-bowel syndrome
  Chronic laxative use
  Inflammation
  Diverticulitis
  Crohn's disease
  Cancer
  Pelvic muscle injury
    Rectal prolapse
    Rectocele
  Pelvic-floor dysfunction
  Anal disease
    Anal stricture
    Incomplete anal relaxation
    Anismus
  Hirschsprung disease (hereditary)
  Neuromuscular disorders of colon
Endocrine and metabolic disorders
  Pregnancy
  Diabetes mellitus
  Hypothyroidism
  Hypokalemia
  Hypercalcemia
  Panhypopituitarism
  Pheochromocytoma
  Glucagonoma
  Porphyria
Neurologic
  Peripheral
  Neurofibromatosis
  Ganglioneuromatosis
  Stroke
  Spinal cord injury
  Multiple sclerosis
  Autonomic neuropathies
  Parkinson disease
  Shy–Drager syndrome
  Trauma to nervi erigentes
Other
  Immobility
  Psychiatric conditions
    Anorexia nervosa
    Bulimia
  Scleroderma and other infiltrating diseases
  Myotonic dystrophy
  Drugs (see Table 40-6)

---

chorionic gonadotropin if appropriate. Therefore, metabolic, systemic, neurologic, or drug causes can be ruled out (Tables 40-5 and 40-6). If there is a question as to the validity of the patient's symptoms or these tests are to validate a chronic problem, a better description of the type of constipation can be obtained by performing a sitz-marker (radiopaque marker) test. This test is performed by giving the patient 1 marker capsule per day for 3 days followed by an abdominal x-ray examination on day 4. The numbers of sitz markers and their locations in the colon

(right colon, descending colon, rectosigmoid colon) can be useful in determining if constipation is present and whether the cause is outflow obstruction, colonic spasm, or colonic hypotonia.

If the patient has occult blood in the stool or hematochezia it is important to rule out obstructive causes by referral to a colonoscopist to evaluate the patient for colon polyps, obstructive colon cancer, or other lower-tract lesions that might result in the presence of blood. If occult blood is not found then performing a flexible sigmoidoscopy and an air contrast barium enema is adequate. Endoscopy, however, provides little useful information on colonic and anorectal function. Once obstruction has been ruled out, a clinical trial of bowel training, an increased-fiber diet, and bulk laxatives should be implemented. However, this is not useful if the patient has megacolon or megarectum noted on the endoscopic and/or radiographic studies or if the patient appears to have colonic hypomotility.

TABLE 40-6
MEDICATIONS KNOWN TO CAUSE CONSTIPATION

Opiate-type pain medications
  Percodan
  Lortabs
  Codeine
  Percocet
  Demerol
  Street opiates
Cation-containing agents
  Iron supplements
  Antacids that contain aluminum or calcium
    Amphogel
    Basogel
  Sucralfate (aluminum)
  Barium sulfate (radiologic studies)
  Metallic intoxication
  Lead
  Mercury
  Arsenic
Anticholinergics
  Antispasmodic agents
  Antidepressants
  Antipsychotic agents
  Antiparkinson disease drugs
Neutrally active agents
  Antihypertension drugs
    Calcium-channel antagonists
      Linosopril
      Vasotec
      Capoten
    Clonidine
    Diuretics that cause potassium loss
    Ganglionic blockers
  Vinca alkaloids
  Anticonvulsants
  Nasal decongestants and antihistamines

Elderly patients often have constipation because of immobility, which can slow colonic transits; inability to respond to neuromuscular stimuli to defecate; and inadequate dietary and liquid intake, in addition to the effects of medications and depression or confusion. Patients may have neuromuscular disorders that may cause constipation as a result of muscle weakness or incoordination, dietary changes, use of medications with constipating effects or bowel dysfunction. Depression or social isolation often results in constipation. Therefore, dealing with bowel dysfunction is important in these patients because they often are fixated on bowel function.

Several types of underlying disorders result in constipation. Hypotonic constipation is characterized by delayed colonic transit in the colon proximal to the rectum as a result of diminished propulsive motor activity. Spastic constipation, as seen in irritable-bowel syndrome, is characterized by increased but nonpropulsive motility in the descending and sigmoid colon. It is thought that this causes retropulsion or a lack of propulsion of stool and segmenting of the colon, resulting in small, "meatball" stools associated with crampy abdominal pain. Outlet dysfunction results in stasis in the rectum, while transit is normal in the proximal colon. This can be determined by sitz marker testing. Further evaluation of functional-outlet obstruction, rectal spasm, paradoxical rectal contractions, or abnormal rectal angle can be performed by doing anorectal manometry and electromyography in conjunction with defecography looking for pelvic-floor dysfunction. There is often excessive discomfort and straining during defecation in patients presenting with this type of disorder.

Treatment usually involves supplementation with fiber, behavioral bowel training and biofeedback, non-irritative laxatives, and the use of prokinetic agents. Many patients respond to fiber intake of 20 to 30 g per day. This can include diet or high-fiber medications (bulk laxatives) and should be combined with an increase in fluid intake and increased ambulation. Fiber should be instituted slowly. However, fiber is contraindicated in patients with suspected obstructive lesions, megacolon, and megarectum. If this is unsuccessful, lactulose or sorbitol (15 to 30 ml per day in increasing doses) is added to result in a stool every day or every other day as well as use of the bathroom following meals. This uses the body's natural mechanisms of increased colonic motility following meals. Docusate salts are useful to soften hard stools. Stimulant laxatives should be avoided because their long-term use may result in abdominal cramps, fluid and electrolyte disturbances, malabsorption, and "cathartic colon."

Patients with chronic constipation refractory to the above therapies should be referred to a specialist for further evaluation and therapy.

GASTROESOPHAGEAL REFLUX DISEASE

Gastroesophageal reflux disease (GERD) is defined either by symptoms or tissue damage or by a combination of both. It is mostly the result of the movement of acidic gastric contents into the esophagus. However, it also can be the result of alkaline or bilious gastric contents into the esophagus. However, this is less frequent. Patients with GERD most typically present with postprandial symptoms of heartburn (83%) and regurgitation (70%). These symptoms are aggravated by bending over or lying down and are often relieved by over-the-counter histamine H_2-receptor antagonist (H_2RAs) and/or antacids. Other symptoms include dysphagia (37%), respiratory symptoms such as asthma, cough, wheezing, hoarseness (30%), abdominal pain (10%), chest pain (10%), nausea (8%), belching (7%), and bleeding (4%). In 50% of these patients, symptoms occur without evidence of esophageal erosions or ulcerations. GERD is perhaps the most common problem seen in medical practice. Approximately 10% of the U.S. population experiences daily episodes of heartburn, while 40% of the population has heartburn monthly. This results in approximately 40 million persons who use over-the-counter antacids or H_2-receptor antagonists at least twice weekly to relieve symptoms. In patients suffering from severe GERD the quality of life can be poor, significantly compromising daily living. This common clinical problem mostly is first seen by the primary care physician.

Many factors contribute to GERD. The esophagus is usually somewhat protected from gastric contents and acid by a competent lower esophageal sphincter (LES) with the aid of the crural diaphragm. Studies have revealed that some patients with GERD have low resting LES pressures and/or low sphincter pressures with increased intraabdominal pressure. An increased frequency of transient LES relaxation is noted in a larger number of patients with GERD. The acid that refluxes into the esophagus is usually promptly cleared. Delayed esophageal clearance is a result of a reduction in strength and frequency of esophageal peristaltic waves. In addition, gravity and salivary bicarbonate play a role in acid clearance. Hiatal hernias are thought to trap acid in the esophagus, delaying clearance. In addition, disordered gastric emptying can compromise a preexisting marginally functioning esophageal protective mechanism. Little is known about esophageal epithelial repair and cytoprotective mechanisms and factors such as epidermal growth factor. These may be important because up to 50% of patients with nonerosive esophagitis and a smaller proportion of patients with erosive esophagitis have an acid exposure time equal to that of normal healthy persons.

The natural history of GERD has not been clearly elucidated because few prospective studies have followed patients with reflux symptoms. In patients with grades I to III esophagitis, 46% have an isolated episode of GERD not requiring further therapy while 32% had recurrent episodes without progression in the esophagitis. Twenty-three percent of patients experience progressive disease, with half of these patients in the most severe group progressing to develop stricture and/or esophageal ulceration. Progression of GERD is frequently associated with progression in the severity of or a change in the type of symptoms. However, it is important to remember that severity of symptoms may not be a good measure of disease severity. Many patients who progress to Barrett's esophagus note a decrease in the severity of their symptoms, and the disease may progress in asymptomatic patients even with intensive therapy. The chronic nature of the disease is supported by the fact that at least 80% of patients have a relapse within 6 to 8 months of healing and cessation of therapy. Therefore, therapy is not curative, but helps to maintain the balance between esophageal cell damage and cytoprotection.

Chronic reflux disease can result in a condition in which the squamous lining of the esophagus is replaced by intestinal metaplasia or Barrett's epithelium. This indicates chronic, severe GERD and is a premalignant condition requiring regular endoscopic surveillance with biopsies to evaluate for dysplasia and cancer. The risk of cancer in Barrett's esophagus is thought to be approximately 1% per year. Some patients may progress to Barrett's esophagus or cancer without have symptoms of GERD.

Treatment should begin with elucidating activities or risk factors that induce or exacerbate symptoms. The patient should then be educated as to why these induce symptoms. It is the safest and least expensive way of reducing or alleviating symptoms and it empowers the patient to diminish the development of symptoms. Therefore, with mild to moderate GERD, simple continued lifelong lifestyle changes can improve symptoms no matter what other therapy might be instituted. These changes can enhance the effectiveness of pharmacotherapy. It is a very useful reminder to the patient to provide them with a list of these lifestyle changes. It is important to remember that very often when a patient is started on pharmacotherapy relief is obtained. This often results in the reduction or termination of lifestyle changes, resulting in the patient's perception that the medication's effectiveness stopped. However, it is not that the medication became ineffective but that the patient reinstituted behaviors that exacerbated symptoms.

Initial recommendations should include small rather than large meals; low-fat diet; and avoiding chocolate, mints, caffeine-containing beverages, carbonated beverages, highly acidic foods such as citrus and tomato products, and alcohol. Cigarette smoking should be avoided. It is also beneficial to chew gum or suck hard candies, as they stimulate alkaline saliva and also stimulate esophageal stripping motor activity. The patient should not lie down for 2 to 3 hours after meals and should sleep with the head of the bed elevated 5 to 6 inches (not three or four pillows). Weight loss is helpful, as is wearing loose-fitting clothing. Finally, the patient's medication list should be checked for drugs that have the potential to exacerbate reflux symptoms. Examples of these drugs include calcium-channel blockers, theophylline, cholinergic agents, and progesterone. These drugs relax the LES, which may permit or exacerbate reflux. The patient should understand the relationship between the use of these drugs and the development of symptoms, since very often the medications cannot be discontinued.

GERD occurs in nearly half of pregnant women. This is probably due to the lower LES pressure and altered motility resulting from pregnancy-induced hormonal changes. In addition, the increase in intra-abdominal pressure during pregnancy exacerbates symptoms. The symptoms are mostly mild and self-limiting during pregnancy and resolve after delivery. They often worsen as pregnancy progresses and are most pronounced during the third trimester. Therefore, GERD should be treated with lifestyle changes and with the use of prescription or OTC drugs without risk to the fetus. An example of these includes antacids and alginate since they are poorly absorbed or not absorbed. Metoclopramide and drugs that inhibit gastric secretion (ranitidine and cimetidine) should be reserved for severe cases and cases with severe esophagitis demonstrated by endoscopy. The fetal risk appears minimal especially if used during the last 3 months of gestation. If symptoms are severe, endoscopy is indicated to evaluate for esophagitis. It is important to remember in the pregnant patient that endoscopy should be performed if needed when essential to maternal diagnosis and therapy.

Initial evaluation of patients with suspected GERD should include a history and physical examination. Typical symptoms include heartburn (a burning pain behind the breastbone) and regurgitation (the spontaneous return of gastric contents into the esophagus or mouth). When both of these symptoms occur together, the diagnosis of GERD can be made with more than 90% certainty. These patients can be treated empirically without further diagnostic testing. Symptoms are likely to be exacerbated by large meals, high-fat meals, spicy foods, citrus products, cola drinks, coffee, tea, and beer and other alcoholic beverages. Often symptoms are worse at night, when the patient is supine. It is important to remember that while heartburn is highly specific for GERD, a heartburn-like symptom is often described in patients with achalasia, as the result of fermentation of undigested food in the esophagus resulting in inflammation. The presence of or the frequency of heartburn symptoms is not predictive of the severity of esophageal damage. Severe disease, including Barrett's esophagus and peptic strictures, can occur with infrequent or no heartburn. Also, many patients with daily heartburn show no endoscopic abnormalities. Only 50 to 60% of patients with heartburn who seek medical attention have erosive esophagitis on endoscopy. It is important to remember that patients with Barrett's esophagus, a premalignant condition, need to be screened and followed by a GI specialist. In addition, these patients need aggressive therapy.

Patients may present with symptoms that warrant early referral to a specialist for a diagnostic evaluation. These include dysphagia, odynophagia, early satiety, frequent vomiting, GI bleeding, or weight loss. In addition, patients who present with asthma, chronic cough, chronic hoarseness, nausea and vomiting, and unexplained chest pain should be referred for further diagnostic evaluation. It is important not to overlook atypical chest pain of cardiac origin.

In most cases, by the time a patient has seen the physician he or she has taken one or several OTC medications to relieve symptoms. Traditionally, the first medication chosen by the patient was an antacid either with or without alginic acid. They are either liquid or tablet formulations. Their mode of action involves neutralizing refluxate in the esophagus in addition to the stomach. The advantage is the rapidity of action; the disadvantage is the short duration of action because the medications are topically acting. The liquid formulation is not convenient for daytime use and therefore a tablet formulation was developed.

Several H₂RAs in a lower dosage form have been released for OTC use (Tagamet HB, 100mg; Pepcid AC, 10 mg; Axid AR, 75 mg; Zantac, 75 mg). When symptoms persist despite the use of OTC products and lifestyle changes, the primary care physician may next consider empiric prescription therapy or further diagnostic tests, depending on the initial history and physical examination. Because GERD is prevalent, heartburn is a quite specific manifestation of reflux, and because most patients with GERD do not have erosive disease, empiric therapy is frequently initiated on clinical suspicion alone. Many patients will have self-treated themselves with OTC therapy before seeking medical help. However, if no pharmacotherapy has been tried and the symptoms are mild, the physician should institute lifestyle changes with or without supplemental OTC therapy. If the patient does not achieve satisfactory relief, empiric prescription therapy should be instituted (H₂RA). Prokinetic agents seem to be more effective in patients with heartburn accompanied with bloating or fullness. If the patient experiences relief, a trial of therapy for 4 to 6 weeks should be tried. This should be followed by a trial off medications but with continued lifestyle changes. If the patient has no further symptoms or infrequent symptoms, episodic therapy is warranted. Otherwise continued long-term prescription therapy can be continued. However, if symptoms persist despite therapy, the drug therapy should be intensified either by increasing the dose of H₂RA alone or with a prokinetic agent or terminating that therapy and instituting therapy with a standard dose of a proton pump inhibitor (PPI) (Omeprazole-Prilosec 20 mg, Lansoprosole-Prevacid 30 mg, Pantoprazole-Protonix 40 mg, Rabeprazole-Aciphex 20 mg). Once satisfactory relief has been obtained it should be continued for 6 weeks and then tapered. If symptoms recur while on full dose or when tapering, the patient should be referred to an endoscopist for an esophagogastroduodenoscopy (EGD).

If the patient has symptoms suggestive of a serious non-GERD diagnosis or if she has atypical GERD symptoms suggestive of more severe disease, the patient should be referred to a specialist/

gastroenterologist endoscopist. This will help to further define the GERD and to rule out other serious non-GERD disorders such as malignancy, peptic ulcer disease, esophageal ulcers, or esophageal motility disorders. In addition, if the patient's symptoms worsen or change despite progressively increasing doses of pharmacotherapy, she should be referred to a specialist. In most cases EGD is warranted. At least half of these patients have either normal endoscopic findings or only mild to moderate esophagitis. Some consultants will perform 24-hour pH monitoring on these patients to confirm the presence of abnormal gastroesophageal reflux. If serious esophagitis is found, aggressive therapy should be instituted with continued lifestyle changes, PPI, and probably a prokinetic agent. If symptoms are persistent despite PPI, the dose should be increased, and if still refractory a prokinetic should be added with or without an evening dose of H_2-blocker. Refer patients with refractory illness to a GI specialist.

Reserve surgery for patients with chronic refractory illness who are dependent on PPIs for long-term symptom relief (young patients with severe disease) or some patients with chronic erosive esophagitis, Barrett esophagus, or recurrent reflux-induced esophageal strictures.

ACID PEPTIC DISEASE

Ulcers of the stomach or duodenum are thought to be the result of an imbalance between the digestive activity of pepsin and acid found in the gastric juice and other offensive factors and the mucosal defenses that resist mucosal digestion and promote repair. This delicate balance between offensive and defensive forces normally maintains mucosal integrity. Until recently the cause of most ulcer disease was thought to be idiopathic acid hypersecretion, and therapies were focused on controlling acid secretion or neutralizing acid. However, advances in the understanding of ulcer disease resulted in a reassessment of previous assumptions, especially following the discovery of the contribution of Helicobacter pylori. Major factors that alter this balance include H. pylori infection, NSAID use, pathologic hypersecretory states, genetics, the environment, and a disruption of mucosal defenses or a disruption in mucosal repair or repair mechanisms.

Acid peptic disease includes both gastric and duodenal ulcer disease and some forms of gastritis and duodenitis. In gastric ulcers, with normal or low acid secretion, the ulcers usually are found in areas of gastritis, mostly on the lesser curvature of the stomach at the junction between the antrum and the body. This is an area of the stomach where perfusion tends to be compromised because of the greater muscle mass. Diffuse mucosal injury allows back-diffusion of acid and ulcer formation even in a state of reduced acid secretion. The major defense mechanisms are mucus, bicarbonate secretion, mucosal blood flow, prostaglandin synthesis, and the presence and effectiveness of trophic factors. Regeneration restores injured mucosa to normal and is affected by blood flow and cytokines. Duodenal ulcers are more often found in states of normal to high acid secretion and occur most frequently in the duodenal bulb or in the pyloric channel. Duodenal ulcers that occur beyond the bulb are found in conditions of extreme acid secretion—e.g., Zollinger–Ellison syndrome (gastrinoma)—or as the result of exogenous influences—e.g., NSAIDs. H. pylori is known to play a major role in duodenal ulcer disease. It is found in islands of gastric metaplasia in the duodenum in a high percentage of patients with duodenal ulcers. Prepyloric ulcers very often behave like duodenal ulcers. Many of the mechanisms involved in ulcer formation in the stomach for gastric ulcers are operative in the evolution of duodenal ulcers.

Ulcers now can be classified into three groups based on causative factors: nonsteroidal antiinflammatory drugs (NSAIDS); Helicobacter pylori-related ulcers, and miscellaneous causes (5%). The miscellaneous causes include hypersecretory states (Zollinger–Ellison syndrome), idiopathic hypersecretion of acid, and duodenogastric reflux of gastric mucosal barrier-breaking substances such as bile salts. The most common cause of gastric ulcers is NSAIDS, while the most common cause of duodenal ulcer is H. pylori.

H. pylori is a fastidious gram-negative microaerophilic spiral bacillus that is found beneath and within the glycoprotein mucous coating of the gastric mucosa. It produces multiple enzymes and cytotoxins, such as urease and mucolytic proteases, that are important for survival and are pathogenic. These disrupt the protective gastric mucous barrier, damage the surface epithelial-cell layer, and make the mucosa more susceptible to acid-pepsin injury. H. pylori also elicits a local and systemic immune response that, through various cellular and humoral mediators, augments the inflammatory reaction initiated by the epithelial damage. Ingestion of the bacteria, which has several virulence factors, promotes colonization of the gastric mucosa. Urease is supposed to serve the function of protection from the acid environment by the cleavage of urea, resulting in carbon dioxide and ammonia. Unless treated, the organism survives in the mucous layer permanently. *H. pylori* can be thought of as a "slow bacteria" that causes a persistent gastric infection and chronic gastritis, although ingestion can cause acute symptoms. Following the acute infection, a chronic superficial gastritis evolves, and after many years or decades, chronic atrophic gastritis or gastric malignancy might develop.

In the early 1980s, Marshall recognized it as a cause of acute gastritis. In addition it was found to be a major risk factor for greater than 90% of duodenal ulcers and 70 to 80% of gastric ulcers. More recent data, however, demonstrate a higher percentage of duodenal ulcers associated with NSAIDs. There is, in addition, a potential role in the development of gastric adenocarcinoma and in gastric lymphoma (MALToma). *H. pylori* is present in 40 to 50% of the general population of the United States, with a prevalence related to older age. It is more prevalent in blacks, Hispanics, and poorer socioeconomic groups in addition to institutionalized patients. In underdeveloped countries, people are more frequently infected at a younger age than in developed countries. Therefore, as many as 50% of the children are infected by the age of 10 in many countries. A fecal–oral route of transmission has been postulated, and *H. pylori* has been isolated from human stool. This has resulted in the development of a diagnostic test, *H. pylori* fecal antigen. There is clustering of the infections within families, and a higher than expected prevalence of *H. pylori* is found in institutionalized patients and gastroenterologists. Transmission of the infection by endoscopic procedures and biopsies has been reported. Following eradication of the organism, a reinfection rate of 1% per year or less occurs.

Tests of *H. pylori* infection include serologic tests, C13 or C14 breath test, biopsy urease test, histologic tests, and biopsy and culture, which is seldom used (see Table 40-6).

There are three types of active chronic gastritis: Type A, associated with a supposed immunologic mechanism and pernicious anemia; Type B, found in association with *H. pylori* infection; and Type C, chemical injury gastritis found in association with NSAIDs, aspirin, bile salts, and alcohol. Therefore, *H. pylori*–induced gastritis is in fact the basic disease, while the development of both duodenal and gastric ulcers or malignancy is a complication of gastritis. Traditionally, these disorders have been thought of separately rather than as part of a continuum. The most important link between *H. pylori*–induced gastritis and the development of duodenal ulcers is the presence of gastric metaplasia in the duodenal bulb. Some data support the contention that infection of this gastric metaplasia with *H. pylori* is required to cause the development of duodenitis and duodenal ulcers. *H. pylori* is found in 90 to 95% of patients with duodenal ulcers and in about 70 to 90% of patients with gastric ulcers. The role of *H. pylori* as a causative agent is more convincing because it is present in most patients with ulcers and its eradication reduces the rate of recurrence of duodenal ulcers. The recurrence rate decreases by 50 to 80% after 1 year to <5% following eradication of *H. pylori*. The mechanism is not exactly clear. Further data link *H. pylori* to noncardiac gastric adenocarcinoma. It is postulated that *H. pylori* gastritis progresses to atrophic gastritis and, in the presence of other risk factors, evolves into gastric adenocarcinoma. However, this appears to be a rare but real occurrence. It is thought that between 35 and 89% of cancers would not occur if *H. pylori* were not present. Meta-analyses and animal model studies strongly suggest a causal relationship. In addition, primary B-cell lymphoma (MALToma) has been found associated with *H. pylori* with an odds ratio of 4.0. Regression of low-grade MALToma has been reported following eradication of *H. pylori*.

The prevalence of peptic ulcer disease (PUD) varies depending on several factors. These factors include population, geographic area, era, social and dietary habits, and traditions of the individual populations. In the United States, the annual incidence of PUD was 1.6% in the 1980s, with a lifetime incidence for men ranging from 11 to 13.5% and for women ranging from 7.7 to 11%. The incidence has been increasing for older women. This increasing incidence is probably due to the increased use of NSAIDs. There is a decreasing incidence for younger men because of a decrease in cigarette smoking. In the United States, duodenal ulcer is four times more common than gastric ulcer, a disorder that is rare before the age of 40 and has a peak incidence at ages 55 to 65. It is interesting that hospitalization rates for uncomplicated duodenal ulcers have been declining more rapidly than for gastric ulcers. However, hospitalization rates for complicated duodenal ulcers have remained constant despite the development of more potent treatments for PUD. The hospitalization rate for complicated gastric ulcers, on the other hand, has increased. Mortality rates have remained low except for patients >65 years of age. This might be because of the increased use of NSAIDs in this age group. However, with the recent development of cyclo-oxygenase-2 (COX-2) inhibitors, these figures should decrease in the future.

The principal risk factors for gastric ulcers are NSAIDs, *H. pylori* infection, and cigarette smoking. Other factors include altered antral motility and pyloric sphincter abnormalities. These lead to an increased reflux of duodenal contents (bile salts and lysolecithin), perhaps by stimulating gastrin release. Alcohol breaks down the mucosal barrier but is not a risk factor for either gastric or duodenal ulcer disease. Also, there is no definite evidence that stress, corticosteroids, or caffeine cause chronic gastric ulceration.

The principal risk factors for duodenal ulcer are acid hypersecretion, *H. pylori* infections, NSAIDs, cigarette smoking (which delays healing), and genetics. Other factors include altered duodenal bicarbonate secretion and the presence of other diseases, such as cirrhosis, renal failure, and chronic pulmonary disease. However, most people with *H. pylori* infections never have duodenal or gastric ulcers. Therefore, additional mechanisms must be involved. Diseases associated with duodenal ulcers include Zollinger–Ellison syndrome (gastrinoma), systemic mastocytosis, multiple endocrine neoplasia type 1 (MEN-1), chronic pulmonary disease, chronic renal failure, hypercalcemia, renal stones, and α_1-antitrypsin deficiency. Suggested associated diseases include Crohn's disease, hyperparathyroidism without MEN-1, coronary artery disease, polycythemia rubra vera, and chronic pancreatitis.

While acute stress can result in gastritis, the type of gastritis implicated is different from that associated with peptic ulcer disease. No associations have been established with chronic stress. Steroids do not appear to be associated with ulcer disease when administered alone. Therefore, no prophylaxis is needed for patients on oral steroids unless they are concurrently taking NSAIDs. In addition, there is no causal relationship between alcohol intake and the development of peptic ulcer disease. However, there is a causal role for ethanol in the development of gastritis.

The natural history of gastric ulcers is that 65 to 70% heal in 12 weeks with placebo therapy. However, the rate of recurrence on placebo is from 55 to 89%. Most of these ulcers recur at the same location; repeated recurrences do occur but not more than two to three times.

The symptoms of PUD include epigastric pain, nausea, vomiting, anorexia, weight loss, bloating, and belching. The pain is most often burning or gnawing in quality, epigastric, and at times radiating to the midback. It occurs at night in up to 80% of patients and if it wakens a patient at night it tends to be early in the morning rather than early in the night. The pain of ulcer disease is often relieved by meals, antacids, and acid suppression therapies and brought on by fasting, alcohol, coffee, or fatty meals (duodenal ulcer). At times, the pain is made worse with meals; this occurs more often with gastric ulcers.

It is important to note that up to 3% of adults undergoing voluntary endoscopy have clinically silent ulcers. Also, approximately 20% of complicated ulcers (i.e., bleeding) present without heralding symptoms. This occurs more frequently in elderly patients and patients taking NSAIDs. This is a very important fact to remember clinically when evaluating patients who are taking NSAIDs (the dissociation of symptoms and pathology).

Physical findings are few unless there are associated diseases or the presence of complications such as perforation or bleeding. The most common physical finding is epigastric tenderness. In addition, physical examination may reveal evidence of diseases or complications associated with ulcer disease such as cirrhosis, respiratory disease, or cardiovascular disorders. Complications of ulcers include bleeding, perforation, obstruction, and weight loss.

Diagnosis can be made radiographically or endoscopically. The advantage of an endoscopic diagnosis is that it allows for biopsies to rule out malignancy (in gastric ulcers) and to evaluate for the presence of *H. pylori* in addition to the histologic characterization of the ulcer. All gastric ulcers should be examined endoscopically and biopsied and should be restudied to confirm healing at approximately 8 to 12 weeks. In addition, endoscopy and biopsy are indicated if there is a radiologically diagnosed gastric ulcer, especially if it is a large ulcer (>2.5 cm) or one that does not appear to be typically benign. The same is *not* true for duodenal ulcers or pyloric-channel ulcers because most prepyloric and pyloric-channel ulcers behave like duodenal ulcers.

Further evaluation of patients with diagnosed peptic ulcers includes a complete history and physical examination, including a rectal examination and test for occult blood in stool. A complete history of associated medical problems, a complete drug history, surgical history, and family history for ulcer disease, malignancies, renal stones, or MEN are also needed. Laboratory tests should include an *H. pylori* serology (if endoscopy is not being performed), a serum calcium measurement, renal- and hepatic-function tests, a complete blood count, and urinalysis.

Therapy of patients with PUD involves multiple components. First, if the patient has a duodenal ulcer or a gastric ulcer with evidence of *H. pylori* he or she should be treated for the bacterium (Table 40-7). This can be diagnosed using serology with history, urea breath test, Clo test with EGD, or EGD with histopathology. Second, the patient should be treated with an acid-suppressing medication to promote ulcer healing. Third, the patient should discontinue behaviors that are detrimental to healing—e.g., smoking and NSAID use. Fourth, if the patient has a gastric ulcer it should be biopsied to rule out a malignant cause. Therefore, referral to an endoscopist for endoscopy and biopsy is imperative for a gastric ulcer. In addition, a UGI, or preferably endoscopy, should be performed to confirm healing at 8 to 12 weeks. If the ulcer were bleeding, it might be prudent to treat the patient with a 6- to 12-month course of chronic acid suppressive therapy to ensure healing. However, suppressive therapy (H$_2$-blockers and proton pump inhibitors) does not decrease the incidence of rebleeding. Lastly, it is useful to confirm eradication of the *H. pylori*. The urea breath test is an easy, accurate, and inexpensive means of confirming eradication, especially in patients in whom compliance is an issue or when an inadequate clinical response was noted. The stool *H. pylori* antigen might also prove useful.

Since treatment of *H. pylori* very significantly reduces ulcer recurrence, patients with gastric ulcers and *H. pylori* and all patients with duodenal ulcers or a history of ulcer disease who have not been treated should receive treatment for *H. pylori*. There is good evidence for the efficacy of 14-day triple-drug regimens that include a PPI or ranitidine bismuth citrate (RBC). Whether it will be possible to shorten these regimens to 7 to 10 days is actively being investigated. Because of the importance of eradicating *H. pylori* infection in patients with ulcer disease, it is important that optimal therapy be used and that the patient adhere to the regimen. All of the regimens have some unwanted side effects; therefore, the patient should be warned of the possible effects and encouraged to take the whole treatment course. See Table 40-7 for therapeutic regimens. Currently, routine posttreatment testing is recommended only in patients with a history of ulcer complications, gastric mucosal-associated lymphoid tissue (MALT) lymphoma, or early gastric cancer. Patients with recurrent symptoms after treat-

---

TABLE 40-7
THERAPEUTIC REGIMENS FOR
HELICOBACTER PYLORI **INFECTION**

PPI (omeprazole 20 mg or lansoprazole 30 mg) + amoxicillin 1 g + clarithromycin 500 mg (each drug given twice a day for 14 days)

PPI (omeprazole 20 mg or lansoprazole 30 mg) + metronidazole 500 mg + clarithromycin 500 mg (each drug given twice a day for 14 days)

RBC 400 mg + clarithromycin 500 mg + amoxicillin 1 g OR metronidazole 500 mg OR tetracycline 500 mg (each drug given twice a day for 14 days)

Bismuth subsalicylate 525 mg four times a day + metronidazole 500 mg three times a day + tetracycline 500 mg four times a day + PPI (omeprazole 20 mg or lansoprazole 30 mg) (each drug given in the dosage and frequency indicated daily for 14 days)

Bismuth subsalicylate 525 mg four times a day + metronidazole 250 mg four times a day + tetracycline 500 mg four times a day + H$_2$-receptor blocker (each drug given in the dosage and frequency indicated daily for 14 days, in addition the H$_2$-receptor blocker continued for an additional 14 days)

---

ment of *H. pylori* infection will also need further evaluation, including testing for *H. pylori*. Serologic tests should *not* be used since antibody titers decrease very slowly and inconsistently precluding its use for confirming irradication. However, if there were a question about the adequacy of the therapy or compliance, then a test such as the urea breath test is indicated. It is better to perform the C13 urea test on children and women of childbearing age.

Proton pump inhibitors (PPI) are more effective in suppressing acid production. However, they do not decrease the recurrence of bleeding from ulcers but do result in more rapid healing of duodenal ulcers. These drugs are most beneficial in refractory or recurrent ulcers and in patients with hypersecretory states such as Zollinger–Ellison syndrome. At present there are four drugs available (omeprazole 20 mg, pantoprazole 40 mg, lansoprazole 30 mg, and rabeprazole 20 mg). Pantoprazole is available in an intravenous formulation.

Approximately 20% of peptic ulcers fail to heal after 4 weeks of therapy. Ulcers are categorized as refractory if healing is not noted after 8 to 12 weeks of therapy. This is found in approximately 5% of ulcers. It is important to note that symptoms may persist after healing. Therefore, documentation of gastric ulcer healing is necessary. If the ulcer is not healed after 8 to 12 weeks of therapy check for *H. pylori* and consider retreatment in addition to excluding Zollinger–Ellison syndrome by getting a serum gastrin. At this time increase the dose or potency of the medication (i.e., switch to a more potent medication [PPI] if treating with H$_2$-blockers).

Intractability of ulcer disease or recurrent bleeding are the most common indications for surgical therapy. However, with *H. pylori* therapy and with the introduction of PPIs a decrease has occurred in the need for surgical management. It appears that 15% of patients with severe symptoms require surgical treatment. Hemorrhage occurs in 15 to 20% of patients with ulcers and is most common in elderly persons taking NSAIDs. More than 50% of patients treated medically hemorrhage again in 10 to 15 years. Less-common complications requiring surgery include perforation (pyloroduodenal more frequent than gastric) and gastric-outlet obstruction (2% of ulcer patients). Duodenal ulcers cause 90% of cases of gastric-outlet obstruction in adults. Of these, only 25 to 35% respond to medical treatment and therefore require surgical treatment. Multiple operations are available for treatment of PUD, but they will not be discussed here.

Complications of surgery for peptic ulcer disease include recurrent ulcer at anastomosis, gastric antrum retention, dumping syndrome, diarrhea, gastrocolic fistula or gastrojejunocolic fistula, afferent-loop syndrome, blind-loop syndrome, alkaline reflux gastritis, anemia, and susceptibility to infections. Dumping syndrome can present early with diaphoresis, tachycardia, hypotension, giddiness, abdominal cramps, and diarrhea. In addition, it can present late. The symptoms of late dumping include faintness, sweating, and coldness as the result of hypoglycemia. Dumping can be treated with multiple small meals low in carbohydrates.

Today, NSAIDs are commonly used for a variety of conditions. In fact, approximately 3 million people take NSAIDs daily and 100 million prescriptions are dispensed each year in the United States alone. Both ulcer and ulcer complication rates have increased dramatically in patients taking these medications. The incidence of ulcers in patients taking NSAIDs is three times that in patients not taking NSAIDs. In patients taking long-term NSAID therapy the prevalence of PUD is 15 to 30%, with a ratio of three gastric ulcers to two duodenal ulcers. NSAIDs are the most frequently reported cause of serious gastrointestinal side effects, leading to 2000 to 10,000 deaths and more than 25,000 hospitalizations in the United States each year from NSAID-induced ulcers and ulcer complications. In addition, patients taking NSAIDs have a risk of a bleeding gastric ulcer that is 10 to 20 times higher and a risk of a bleeding duodenal ulcer that is 5 to 15 times higher than patients not taking NSAIDs. Elderly females have the highest risk of bleeding gastric ulcers, possibly related to NSAIDs. In addition, patients who take long-term prophylactic doses of aspirin also have more ulcers and more bleeding ulcers. Thus, although NSAIDs gastrointestinal injury may be dose-dependent, even an aspirin every other day can be ulcerogenic. In patients requiring long-term NSAID therapy, the use of a COX-2 inhibitor or concomitant therapy with misoprostol is indicated.

NSAIDs inhibit gastroduodenal prostaglandin synthesis. This results in a decreased secretion of mucus and bicarbonate in addition to a reduced mucosal blood flow. Therefore, NSAID-induced ulcers are ischemic in nature and are most often located in the prepyloric area or in the antrum. It is important to remember that there is a different dose–response relationship for analgesia and antiinflammatory properties of NSAIDs. Thus, the maximum analgesic effect is well below the effective antiinflammatory dose. Since the inflammatory properties of NSAIDs predispose to ulceration, newer NSAIDs have been sold in dosages that have marked antiinflammatory activity without an equivalent increase in analgesia. Therefore, the use of these drugs may subject the patient to an increased risk for ulcers without providing increased analgesia. The use of NSAIDs at the lowest effective dose is therefore important. Of note, in the elderly the risk of PUD with NSAID use is maximal during the first month of treatment. Patients with a previous history of PUD are at highest risk. H$_2$-receptor antagonists and sucralfate are ineffective in preventing gastric ulcers and for reducing the incidence of NSAID-induced mucosal erosions. However, the use of the synthetic prostaglandin misoprostol does decrease the incidence of NSAID-induced gastric ulcers.

At present there are two COX-2 specific antagonists that are approved for clinical use. These medications are not only effective for pain relief but appear to result in a substantial decrease in ulcerogenesis. Multiple more potent COX-2 inhibitors are being clinically evaluated.

BILIARY-TRACT DISEASE

Cholesterol gallstones and associated clinical symptoms develop more frequently in women than in men. In the United States 35% of women and 20% of men have gallstones at some time during their life. Most are asymptomatic and therefore unaware of their gallstones. Death is rare, ~5000 per year, while cholecystectomy is very common, 500,000 to 700,000 patients per year. The increased incidence in females begins at menarche, is related to the number of pregnancies, and then tapers off after menopause. This suggests that female sex hormones may be important causative factors. In addition, women exhibit increased saturation of bile with cholesterol and have a smaller bile acid pool. Both pregnancy and the use of oral contraceptives increase the concentration and total output of cholesterol in both hepatic and gallbladder bile. In addition, there is no change or an effective decrease in bile acids secreted into bile and enterohepatic cycling of bile acids during pregnancy. This, along with the increased concentration of cholesterol, predisposes precipitation of cholesterol in bile, resulting in the formation of gallstones. Other factors predisposing the formation of gallstones during pregnancy include an increase in the residual volume of the gallbladder and a reduction in the contractility and rate of emptying of the gallbladder. As a result of this, biliary sludge develops in approximately one-third of pregnant women and progresses to ultrasonographically demonstrable gallstones in 10 to 12% of patients at delivery. During pregnancy, biliary colic does not appear to be found in patients with biliary sludge or with normal gallbladders. However, colic does occur in one-third of patients with existing stones, but these can mostly be managed conservatively. After delivery, approximately one-third of stones disappear, while biliary sludge disappears in virtually all patients. It appears that estrogens may accelerate the development of symptoms in patients with preexisting gallstones. Therefore, pregnancy not only predisposes to the formation of gallstones but also enhances the development of symptoms.

The two most common types of gallstones include cholesterol and pigment stones. Cholesterol stones are primarily made of cholesterol in addition to calcium, pigment, and glycoproteins. Pigment stones, however, are of two types: black and brown. The black pigment stones are formed under sterile conditions and consist of large amounts of calcium bilirubinate, carbonate, phosphate, and palmitate, in addition to small amounts of cholesterol. Brown stones, conversely, are formed in the biliary tree, are associated with infection, and are a result of bile stasis. They are composed of calcium salts, lipids degraded by bacteria, and small amounts of bilirubin and cholesterol. Cholesterol stones are radiolucent and constitute 85% of gallstones.

The pathogenesis of cholesterol gallstones depends on abnormalities of hepatic and gallbladder function that result in bile that is supersaturated with cholesterol. Supersaturated lithogenic bile may result either from enhanced cholesterol secretion (as occurs in obesity, pregnancy, or fasting) or from decreased bile acid secretion (as occurs in certain ethnic groups such as North American Indians or in association with distal small-bowel disease). Enhanced cholesterol secretion is more common. Hypomotility of the gallbladder also is involved in gallstone formation. This leads to incomplete emptying of the gallbladder and therefore an accumulation of gallstones forming along with mucin, providing a gel matrix for the development of gallstones. Because prostaglandins appear to regulate mucin secretion, prostaglandin inhibitors appear to inhibit mucus hypersecretion and therefore may interfere with gallstone nucleation. Hypomotility, as seen in diabetes mellitus, pregnancy, fasting, and total parenteral nutrition (TPN), may in part account for the increased incidence of gallstones in these populations. The normal gallbladder absorbs cholesterol and acidifies and concentrates bile. These functions decrease stone formation. Therefore, an inflamed or dysfunctional gallbladder can lead to conditions that allow for the formation of stones. Cholesterol-supersaturated bile leads not only to decreased gallbladder motility but also to an induction of the production of mucin. Both of these predispose to the formation of gallstones.

Hemolytic disorders, especially hemoglobinopathies, may lead to the formation of calculi composed of unconjugated bilirubin in the gallbladder or in the biliary tree. These black pigment gallstones also can occur in patients with cirrhosis, alcoholism, pancreatitis, or on TPN. These stones, which occur mostly in the gallbladder, consist mainly of the calcium salt of polymerized unconjugated bilirubin. Calcium is important in the formation of these stones. It is present as calcium bilirubinate, calcium carbonate, and calcium phosphate. While unconjugated bilirubin is soluble in healthy individuals, excess calcium or excess unconjugated bilirubin in bile leads to bilirubin precipitation.

Bile-duct obstruction due to biliary strictures or impacted gallstones can lead to biliary infection. This infected condition can lead to brown pigment gallstones as a complication. These stones, which consist primarily of calcium bilirubinate, calcium palmitate, mucin, bacterial glycoproteins, and biliary epithelium, in addition to cholesterol, form primarily in the bile duct and are frequently associated with bouts of cholangitis. Three major factors are important in the pathogenesis of brown pigment stones. These include lecithin hydroxylation to free fatty acids and their calcium salts, the reduction in cholesterol and bilirubin solubilizers resulting in precipitation, and bacterial β-glucuronidase conversion of soluble conjugated bilirubin to insoluble unconjugated bilirubin, which is then precipitated as calcium bilirubinate.

The prevalence of gallstones varies among different ethnic and racial groups. Black Africans have a prevalence of 3 to 5% and in some tribal groups, gallstones are almost unheard of, while in North Americans and Europeans the prevalence is from 10 to 20%. However, the prevalence in North American Indians is 60%.

Other risk factors have been identified, including female sex, increasing age, and pregnancy. Pregnancy appears to predispose to gallstones because of an increase in estrogens. Therefore, estrogen-containing oral contraceptives increase the risk of gallstones in women of childbearing age, as do estrogens given to postmenopausal women. However, transdermal estrogens do not appear to have this effect. The increased progesterone found in pregnancy causes decreased motility of the gallbladder. Because of both of these hormonal changes, biliary sludge can be detected during the third trimester in almost 50% of pregnant females. This is especially notable in multiparous females. However, this resolves in most women during the postpartum period. However, approximately 10% of patients go on to have small asymptomatic stones.

Other risk factors include hypertriglyceridemia, obesity, crash weight-reduction programs, and some lipid-lowering drugs, such as clofibrate and gemfibrozil. These drugs promote biliary cholesterol excretion. Cholestyramine also increases the risk of stones. Hypomotility of the gallbladder can occur with the fasting during TPN. This results in the development of biliary sludge or gallstones in 50% of these patients. Co-administration of cholecystokinin with TPN markedly reduces this finding. Gallbladder hypomotility can also result from autonomic dysfunction as found in patients with diabetes, spinal cord injury, or primary autonomic dysfunction.

Gallstone formation and dissolution is a dynamic process. Therefore, small (<5 mm) cholesterol stones may disappear spontaneously. Most patients with gallstones are asymptomatic; therefore, no therapy is indicated or advocated. However, each year symptoms develop in about 2 to 4% of patients with silent gallstones. The risk of complications from gallstones is approximately 0.1% per year. These complications include common-bile-duct obstruction, pancreatitis, cholangitis, and acute cholecystitis. However, subsequent severe symptoms or complications requiring hospitalization develop in approximately 66% of symptomatic patients. Mild recurrent symptoms occur at a rate of 6 to 10%, while severe complications, as mentioned above, occur at a rate of 1 to 3% per year. In addition, it appears that patients with gallstones have an increased risk of gallbladder carcinoma, as 75% of patients with gallbladder carcinoma have gallstones. The benefit of prophylactic cholecystectomy in high-risk patients (North American Indians) is unclear, even when a calcified gallbladder wall is found.

Cholelithiasis is found in 90% of patients with acute cholecystitis. No stones are found in the remaining 10%. Acute cholecystitis is due to inflammation of the gallbladder wall and stasis of bile flow due to obstruction of the cystic duct, ischemia, or de novo infection. Secondary bacterial infection often occurs; however, bacteria are not thought to be causative of the initial process. However, bacteria do appear to be causative in immunoincompetent or high-risk patients (diabetes, systemic lupus erythematosus, polyarteritis nodosa) in whom acalculous cholecystitis develops.

Gallstones either can form in the bile duct or can migrate from the gallbladder. Most of the stones found in the common bile duct are cholesterol stones, and 95% of patients with common-duct stones also have cholelithiasis. Duct stones can be asymptomatic or can result in obstruction, biliary colic, jaundice, pancreatitis, cholangitis, or gallstone ileus. Acute pancreatitis is associated with gallstones in 30 to 50% of cases. This occurs especially from ages 50 to 70 years and occurs in women two times as often as in men. Infection in the biliary tree, cholangitis, most often occurs as the result of biliary obstruction as the result of an impacted stone at a bile-duct stricture or at the papilla. This can also occur with neoplasms of the biliary tree, inflammatory disease such as primary sclerosing cholangitis, parasitic infections with Ascaris or *Chlonorchis sinensis*, as a result of congenital disorders such as Caroli disease or choledochal cysts, and with papillary stenosis or chronic pancreatitis.

The presentation of gallstones usually includes episodic biliary colic. The pain is usually epigastric or in the right upper quadrant and often radiates to the right subscapular region. It is severe and is not relieved by position, passage of flatus, or most home-based remedies. Therefore, the patient is restless.

Dyspepsia, nausea, bloating, diarrhea, and fatty-food intolerance have been found not to correlate with the presence of gallstones. However, if the cystic duct is obstructed by a stone, acute cholecystitis frequently occurs; if the common duct is obstructed, jaundice and cholangitis may occur. Most patients with cholangitis present with a subtle onset and do not present with fully manifest Charcot classic triad (fever, chills, right upper abdominal pain and jaundice). The stone can migrate into the ampullary region and result in acute pancreatitis. This may necessitate emergency endoscopic retrograde cholangiopancreatography (ERCP), papillotomy and drainage. In addition, acalculous cholecystitis can occur. This is found most frequently postoperatively and in diabetic patients, patients receiving corticosteroids, patients in the ICU, and patients with burns. If acalulous cholecystitis is not promptly diagnosed and treated, it can progress to gallbladder necrosis, bile peritonitis, and death.

Diagnosis of patients with gallstones is best made using ultrasonography. Computed tomography (CT) is less sensitive and more expensive. The thickness of the gallbladder wall can be misleading when evaluating the patient for cholecystitis. Hypoalbuminemia, ascites, pregnancy, acute hepatitis, and vasculitis can result in an apparent gallbladder wall thickening >2 mm. HIDA is useful to rule out acute or rule in the diagnosis if acute cholecystitis is suspected. Visualization of the common bile duct with no visualization of the gallbladder is highly suggestive of acute cholecystitis, while visualization of the gallbladder virtually rules out the diagnosis. False positive tests (nonvisualization of the gallbladder) can occur in a fasting patient or in patients with severe liver disease or pancreatitis. The presence of radionuclide in the small intestine in a HIDA scan virtually rules out complete bile-duct obstruction.

Patients with symptomatic gallstones and patients with acute cholecystitis are most often treated surgically. Laparoscopic cholecystectomy has revolutionized the management of symptomatic gallstones and in most uncomplicated cases has replaced open cholecystectomy. The advantages include decreased hospital stay, ease of recovery, rapid return to work, and minimal scarring and general patient satisfaction. Laparoscopic cholecystectomy requires conversion to an open procedure in approximately 5% of patients. This is primarily due to technical factors such as obesity, adhesions, or aberrant anatomy. However, bile-duct injury is more frequent with laparoscopic cholecystectomy, occurring with a frequency of 0.5%. This

problem is more common during the learning curve of the procedure. If the gallstones are asymptomatic then watchful waiting is the most prudent approach. In patients with decompensated liver disease, surgical mortality is prohibitive and even ERCP with sphincterotomy is very dangerous. The usual approach in dealing with symptomatic cholelithiasis has been first to clear the duct with ERCP and sphincterotomy if required, followed by laparoscopic cholecystectomy. However, many centers are now performing ERCP only in patients with abdominal cholestatic liver tests before surgery. Another alternative is an open cholecystectomy with common-bile-duct exploration. In patients with high medical risks and acute gallbladder disease, medical alternatives include percutaneous cholecystolithotomy or percutaneous cholecystostomy. Surgical alternatives include a surgical cholecystostomy. This is followed later by surgical removal of the gallbladder.

There are several nonsurgical treatments of gallstones. These include dissolution therapy with ursodeoxycholic acid for patients with pure cholesterol gallstones, lithotripsy (extracorporeal shock-wave lithotripsy [ESWL]), and infusion dissolution therapy. These methods are seldom used; therefore, if this therapy is considered, referral to a specialty center is advisable. The presence of stones in the bile ducts is best treated with ERCP and sphincterotomy.

In patients with acute cholecystitis, initial management should include intravenous fluids to correct dehydration and electrolyte imbalance and the administration of antibiotics. The combination of an aminoglycoside and ampicillin with or without a third antibiotic with good anaerobic coverage should be administered if the disease is severe. Surgery should be performed after the patient is stabilized. High-risk patients with serious cardiovascular or pulmonary disorders should be treated relative to the severity of their biliary-tract disease. For example, if gangrene, overwhelming sepsis, or perforation is suspected, a percutaneous or surgical cholecystostomy is indicated, followed by more definitive therapy if the patient's condition improves.

Following a cholecystectomy, 25 to 30% of patients can have nausea, vomiting, dyspepsia, or abdominal pain. Recurrent symptoms are more common if no stones were found at surgery. The pain is often postprandial, sharp, and stabbing in nature, associated with bloating, dyspepsia, and intolerance to fatty food, with flatulence. The symptom complex is often referred to as postcholecystectomy syndrome. It requires careful evaluation by a gastroenterologist or surgeon to rule out other organic disease of the gastrointestinal tract. It is important to note that abnormalities on liver-function tests are unusual in this syndrome. Their occurrence suggests the presence of a retained common bile duct or cystic duct stones. In addition, patients may also have postprandial diarrhea. This is treated effectively with bile-salt–binding resins.

PANCREATIC DISEASE

Pancreatitis is separated into acute and chronic types. Both present with abdominal pain. Patients with acute pancreatitis have pain that reaches a peak in intensity quite rapidly and may be quite severe and refractory to narcotics. The pain, which often radiates to the back and even the lower abdomen and commonly is associated with vomiting and nausea, may persist for from one to several days. Chronic pancreatitis, however, presents with a more varied constellation of symptoms. Patients more often have severe epigastric pain that can persist for from hours to months without apparent relief and frequently recurs or is exacerbated by food. In 10 to 20% of patients, the pain is very mild or absent and the patient may present only with a feeling of fullness or bloating most notable in the upper abdomen. If the disease is severe and associated with a significant amount of pancreatic parenchymal destruction the patient may have steatorrhea, but patients rarely pass more than two to five bulky steatorrheic stools per day. Chronic pancreatitis can make carcinoma of the pancreas difficult to diagnose because of the similarity of symptoms and because parenchymal changes of the gland can obscure small masses.

The pathophysiology of acute pancreatitis is not well understood. It appears to involve a cascade of events leading to and including the activation of digestive enzymes synthesized in the pancreas. After activation, these enzymes result in autodigestion of the pancreas. After acute pancreatitis occurs, the enzymes, including other toxic materials, can be extravasated into peripancreatic spaces and tissues and into the circulation. This is thought to lead to the systemic complications found in severe disease.

Acute pancreatitis is most frequently caused by alcohol and biliary calculi. Other causes include hyperlipidemia (serum triglycerides >1000 mg/dl), hypercalcemia, ampullary obstruction (tumor, Ascaris, periampullary duodenal diverticula, sphincter of Oddi

dysfunction), pancreatic ductal obstruction (tumor, stricture, stone), anatomic abnormalities (pancreas divisum), and hereditary pancreatitis. In addition, several medications have been shown to be causative (azathioprine, valproic acid, pentamidine, sulfonamides, and a significant number of other drugs). Blunt penetrating or surgical trauma to the pancreas, including the trauma caused by endoscopic retrograde cholangiopancreatography (ERCP) and sphincter of Oddi manometry, have all been shown causative. Finally, vascular disease and infectious agents and toxins such as parasites (Ascaris), viruses (mumps and cytomegalovirus), and bacteria (mycoplasma and others) have all been shown to result in acute pancreatitis. However, in up to 30% of diagnosed cases no cause can be found. It is important to keep in mind that some patients with idiopathic pancreatitis have been shown to have microliths in their bile.

Since the course can vary from benign to severe, it is important for the clinician to quickly determine the disease severity and therefore adjust his management and need for referral appropriately. Two scales of severity have been developed: Ranson's 11 prognostic signs, which are assessed within the first 48 hours, or measurement of the Acute Physiology and Chronic Health Evaluation II (APACHE II) points daily for the first two days (Table 40-8).

Using Ranson's criteria, if there are fewer than three positive signs, mortality is essentially zero; if there are three to five signs, mortality is from 10 to 20%; and with more than six signs there is a greater than 60% mortality. One problem with this scale is that it requires a full 48 hours of observation to complete the measurements, often a critical time. However, the APACHE-II score allows for earlier evaluation. An APACHE-II score >7 during the first 48 hours helps predict a severe attack of acute pancreatitis. On admission, the accuracy of the score in predictive severity is approximately 75%. However, after 48 hours the accuracy of the Ranson and APACHE-II scores are 70 to 80%. The most important indicator of severity is the presence of organ failure (shock, pulmonary failure, renal failure, and gastrointestinal bleeding). The second most important indicator of severity is local complications (necrosis, pseudocyst formation, and abscess formation). Dynamic CT scanning is useful in determining the presence and extent of necrosis in addition to the presence of periglandular involvement. If necrosis is present after 5 days of illness and associated with fever and an elevated

TABLE 40-8
SEVERITY OF ACUTE PANCREATITIS

RANSON'S CRITERIA
  Admission
    Age >55 years
    Leukocyte count >16,000/μl
    Plasma glucose >200 mg/dl
    Serum lactate dehydrogenase >350 U/liter
    Serum aspartate aminotransferase >250 U/liter
  Initial 48 hours
    Hematocrit decrease of >10%
    Blood urea nitrogen increase >5 mg/dl
    Serum calcium <8 mg/dl
    PO$_2$ <60 mm Hg
    Base deficit >4 meq/liter
    Fluid sequestration >6 liters
APACHE-II*
  Physiologic variables (points depend on variance from normal)
    Temperature
    Heart rate
    Mean arterial blood pressure
    Hematocrit
    White cells
    Serum sodium
    Serum potassium
    Serum bicarbonate
    Creatinine
  Oxygenation (points depend on variance from normal)
    FiO$_2$
    Arterial pH
  Age points (set scale)
  Chronic health points (set scale)

*APACHE-II = total APACHE-II physiologic score + age points + chronic health points

white-cell count, fine-needle aspiration (FNA) should be done for Gram stain and culture. It is also useful in severe cases with protracted pain or fever.

Therapy involves appropriate fluid replacement and close monitoring. Patients with severe disease should be monitored in the intensive-care unit (ICU) and should be treated by a team including a gastroenterologist, a surgeon, a radiologist, and critical-care personnel. Aggressive fluid management in addition to treatment of complications is important in severe cases. Antibiotics are usually administered in these severely ill patients even though their value is uncertain. If organ failure has developed after 5 days a dynamic contrast-enhanced CT scan should be performed. If there is evidence of interstitial disease, a successful outcome is almost inevitable. If necrotizing pancreatitis is present, improvement can occur with aggressive medical treatment in an ICU; however, no clinical improvement can be the course. If leukocytosis and a fever are present, CT-guided fine-needle aspiration of the pancreas with Gram stain and culture

is useful for determining the presence of infection and guiding antibiotic therapy. If the patient continues to deteriorate despite maximal therapy and an infected pancreas is confirmed, surgical debridement should be done. If no bacteria are found, aggressive medical therapy should be continued to attempt to reverse the process. However, surgical debridement of sterile necrosis may be necessary.

Other complications of acute pancreatitis include pancreatic pseudocysts and pancreatic abscesses. Asymptomatic pseudocysts should be left undisturbed. However, when symptomatic, pseudocysts should be decompressed. In the presence of fever, leukocytosis, or other signs of toxicity a guided percutaneous aspiration with Gram stain and culture can differentiate infected from noninfected cysts. Decompression can be performed surgically, radiographically, or endoscopically.

The prognosis of acute pancreatitis is good with interstitial pancreatitis. With sterile necrosis the mortality is 10%; with infected necrosis the mortality increases to 30%. However, the prognosis largely depends on the presence of systemic complications.

Patients with recurrent bouts of acute pancreatitis should be referred to a specialist. Mostly in these cases alcohol, gallstones, hyperlipidemia, hypercalcemia, and other obvious causes have been ruled out by a careful history-taking and appropriate laboratory tests. Searching for a cause by the specialist often requires specialized testing such as ERCP and endoscopic ultrasound to rule out more uncommon causes.

In chronic pancreatitis, clinical features are often dominated by abdominal pain, and if severe, signs and symptoms of diabetes mellitus or evidence of steatorrhea with associated weight loss are often noted. The pain, which often radiates to the back, tends to be chronic and is both intrapancreatic and extrapancreatic. It involves pancreatic inflammation, neural inflammation, increased pancreatic pressure, and stenosis of the common bile duct and at times stenosis of the duodenum. Chronic pancreatitis is usually established by evaluating pancreatic structure. The most commonly used and least sensitive is the flat abdominal x-ray examination, while CT and ultrasound are more sensitive because they visualize pancreatic calcification more often. The most sensitive test is the ERCP because it also assesses pancreatic ductal anatomy. Tests of pancreatic function rarely play a role in diagnosis. Approximately 70% of cases of chronic pancreatitis are caused by alcohol, while

20% are idiopathic. The remaining 10% have a variety of other causes. Therapy involves controlling pain, controlling inflammation, treating steatorrhea, and attempting to relieve causes of pain such as perineural inflammation (celiac plexus block and cutaneous stimulators) and increased intrapancreatic pressure (decrease the duct by decreasing secretion with proton-pump inhibitors (PPIs), oral pancreatic enzyme supplements and ocetreotide; in addition to stents and surgery). All the above therapies are limited in their effectiveness. It is therefore important for the patient to refrain from alcohol consumption, use narcotics sparingly and only by one physician, and be treated with a PPI or H$_2$RB and pancreatic enzyme supplements. An operation should be performed only if there is a chance of improvement such as dilated pancreatic ducts. The steatorrhea is best treated with pancreatic enzyme supplementation before and after meals in addition to a PPI or an H$_2$-blocker. In refractory cases the patient should reduce dietary fat to 50 g per day and should substitute medium-chain triglycerides for dietary fat. If the bile duct is stenosed, a biliary stent can be installed to assess effectiveness. Surgical bypass has been shown to be effective. If a duodenal obstruction is the cause of the pain, a gastrojejunostomy can be performed.

Tumors of the pancreas include cystic tumors such as serous cystadenomas, mucinous cystadenomas, or cystadenocarcinomas and cystic islet-cell tumors. It is important to distinguish pseudocysts from cystic neoplasms because of the difference in prognosis and therapy. However, ductal adenocarcimas account for >90% of pancreatic exocrine tumors with a predominance for men (1.4/1) and blacks (1.4/1). Contributing factors include age, gender, occupation (exposure to carcinogens), cigarette smoking, and possibly a high-fat diet. In addition, patients with long-standing diabetes and pancreatitis may be predisposed to adenocarcinoma.

Carcinoma of the pancreas is the fourth leading cancer in adults and has a grim prognosis: <20% are alive beyond 1 year and only 3% are alive beyond 5 years. More than 85% of tumors have spread beyond the glands at the time of diagnosis, most commonly to the liver, peritoneum, and lungs. Tumor markers such as CA 19-9 are usually normal early in the disease and have only a moderate specificity. Diagnosis is most often made with CT or ultrasound. ERCP may be helpful in diagnosis. Dynamic contrast-enhanced CT with thin cuts through the pancreas should be the first test performed to determine if the tumor is resectable. The patient should be cared for by a specialist. Angiography can show vascular involvement. If CT and angiography suggest resectability then laparoscopy should be performed to look for seeding of tumor. In addition, endoscopic ultrasound has been shown to be useful in evaluating the gland and metastases. Surgery for resectable carcinoma of the head of the pancreas usually involves a Whipple operation. If resection cannot be done, gastrojejunostomy should be performed in addition to biliary diversion or biliary stenting for impending obstructive symptoms. Nonoperative palliation includes relief of jaundice, management of pain, and a combination of chemotherapy and radiotherapy.

COLON POLYPS AND COLON CANCER

Colorectal carcinoma is the second most common cancer in the United States. In 1995 there were an estimated 140,000 cases of colorectal cancer in the United States, accounting for 55,000 deaths. The lifetime risk of being diagnosed with colorectal cancer in the United States is 5.9% in women and 6.1% in men, and the incidence rates increase with age, being uncommon among those younger than age 40. However, the rates of disease rise rapidly after age 50. Screening is most cost effective among those at higher risk, more specifically those at age 50 or older. However, in 1992, only 9% of people over 50 had undergone a proctoscopy and 25% had undergone a fecal occult blood examination in the previous 3 years. This was only a 3 to 4% increase from 1987.

Colorectal cancer is now thought to be a preventable disease. While it is common in the United States, Western Europe, Australia, and New Zealand, it is realtively uncommon in Asia, South America, and Africa. When these peoples immigrate to high-incidence areas, their risk of disease rises promptly. This often occurs within a single generation, suggesting the importance of environmental factors in the development of colon cancer and colon polyps. Therefore, if these factors can be identified it would be possible to prevent or significantly diminish the incidence of this common malignancy. Pathologic, genetic, and epidemiologic studies indicate that most colorectal cancers arise from previously benign neoplastic polyps—the adenoma–carcinoma sequence or relationship. Removal of these premalignant polyps decreases the incidence of colorectal carcinoma. More than 70% of all polyps detected by colonoscopy are these adenomas. In addition, autopsy and screening studies suggest that 20 to 30% of seniors in Western countries have one or more adenomas in their colon or rectum. Thus, it is especially important for primary care physicians to understand screening for colorectal polyps and cancer and institute a screening program consisting of fecal occult blood and endoscopic and

radiographic screening at regular intervals (Table 40-9) as part of their program of continuing total patient care.

There are multiple types of polyps found in the colon, which can be divided into two groups in terms of further screening: those with malignant risk and

---

TABLE 40-9
CURRENT GUIDELINES FOR SCREENING AND SURVEILLANCE FOR EARLY DETECTION OF COLORECTAL POLYPS AND CANCER*

Risk category	Recommendation[†]	Age to Start	Interval
		Average Risk	
All persons 50 yr or older who are not in categories	One of the following: FOBT plus flexible sigmoido-scopy[†] or TCE[§]	Age 50	FOBT every year and flexible sigmoidoscopy every 5 yr; colonoscopy every 10 yr or DCBE every 5–10 yr
		Moderate Risk	
People with single, small (<1 cm) adenomatous polyp	Refer to gastroenterologist for colonoscopy	At time of initial polyp diagnosis	TCE within 3 yr after initial polyp removal, if normal, as per average-risk recommendations
Persons with large (≥1 cm) or multiple adenomatous polyps of any size	Refer to gastroenterologist for colonoscopy	At time of initial polyp diagnosis	TCE within 3 yr after initial polyp removal; if normal, TCE every 5 yr
Personal history of curative-intent resection of colorectal cancer	TCE, colonoscopy preferred	Within 1 yr after resection	If normal, TCE in 3 yr; if still normal, TCE every 5 yr
Colorectal cancer or adeno-matous polyps in first-degree relatives younger than 60 yr or in two or more first-degree relatives of any age	TCE, colonoscopy preferred	Age 40 or 5–10 yr before the youngest case in the family, whichever is earlier	Every 5 yr
Colorectal cancer in other relative (not included above)	As per average-risk recom-mendations (see above); may consider beginning screening before age 50 yr	As per average-risk recom-mendations (see above); may consider beginning screening before age 50 yr	As per average-risk recommenda-tions (see above); may consider beginning screening before age 50 yr
		High Risk	
Family history of familial adenomatous polyposis	Early surveillance with endo-scopy, counseling to con-sider genetic testing and referral to a specialty center	Puberty	If genetic test positive or polyposis confirmed, consider colectomy; otherwise endoscopy every 1–2 yr
Family history of hereditary nonpolyposis colon cancer	Colonoscopy and counseling to consider genetic testing	Age 21	If genetic test positive or if patient has had genetic testing, colonos-copy every 2 yr until age 40, then every year
Inflammatory-bowel disease	Colonoscopies with biopsies for dysplasia	8 yr after the start of pan-colitis; 12–15 yr after the start of left-sided colitis	Every 1–2 yr

DCBE = double-contrast barium enema; FOBT = fecal occult blood testing; TCE = total colon examination.

*Approximatley 70 to 80% of cases are in average-risk individuals, approximately 15 to 20% are in moder-ate-risk individuals, and 5 to 10% are in high-risk individuals.

[†]Digital rectal examination should be done at the time of each sigmoidoscopy, colonoscopy or DCBE or during examination (by specialist or primary care physician) preceding the tests.

[†]Annual FOBT has been shown to reduce the mortality from colorectal cancer, so it is preferable to not screening; however, the ACS recommends that annual FOBT be accompanied by flexible sigmoidoscopy to further reduce the risk of colorectal cancer mortality.

[§]TCE includes either colonoscopy or DCBE. The procedure performed should depend on the medical condi-tion of the patient and the quality of the medical examinations available in the specific community. A flexi-ble sigmoidoscopy should also be performed when the rectosigmoid colon is not well visualized by DCBE. A DCBE should be performed when the entire colon has not been adequately evaluated by colonoscopy. Assumes that a preoperative TCE was done.

those with no malignant risk. The polyps with malignant risk include in progressive order of risk: tubular adenoma (2 to 3%), tubulovillous adenomas and villous adenomas (15 to 25%), while the polyps with no malignant risk include hyperplastic polyps, inflammatory polyps, hamartomas, and lymphoid aggregates. Seventy-five percent of adenomas are tubular adenomas, 10 to 25% are tubulovillous adenomas, and only 5% are of the highest-risk variety—villous adenomas. The likelihood of detecting a nidus of invasive carcinoma in these polyps is directly proportional to its size. Only 2 to 3% of polyps found at colonoscopy are larger than 3 cm, with a higher chance of containing carcinoma. Therefore, since there is quite persuasive evidence that colorectal carcinoma proceeds through a discontinuous process from normal mucosa to benign adenoma and finally to carcinoma, detection and removal of the polyps provides a secondary means for preventing colorectal carcinoma. This was supported by the prospective National Polyp Study where colonoscopic polypectomy and post polypectomy surveillance reduced the incidence of colorectal cancer by 76 to 90%. *Therefore the risk of cancer in any adenomatous polyp depends on a size >1 cm and the presence of villous elements. If a biopsy of the polyp shows an adenomatous polyp, perform colonoscopy.*

The epidemiologic data support that the incidence of colon polyps and colon cancer is affected by environmental factors. This suggests that modifying some of these environmental factors can be prevetive. Several dietary habits have been implicated as incidence risk factors, including excessive fat consumption and inadequate intake of vegetables, dietary fiber, and fruit. Some evidence suggests that fiber may not be protective in female patients. However, adequate exercise, maintenance of a normal body weight; avoidance of excessive alcohol or tobacco consumption; and consumption of antioxidants (vitamins A, E, and C) and folate, calcium, and selenium; and postmenopausal hormone replacement all might be protective. Epidemiologic studies suggest that NSAIDS may reduce the risk of colorectal cancer and colon polyps. Other studies have demonstrated that sulindac (an NSAID) reduces the number and size of colon adenomas in patients with familial adenomatous polyposis but does not cause regression of sporadic colonic polyps. Therefore, there are not sufficient data to support routine use of these agents outside of controlled clinical trials.

Today, unlike previously, most polyps are initially detected by flexible sigmoidoscopy or a primary colonoscopy performed as a part of a cancer-screening program or to evaluate symptoms. This is due to the realization that colonoscopy is the most accurate method of detecting polyps and in addition provides an immediate method of treating and diagnosing premalignant and malignant lesions, respectively. Experienced endoscopists can now examine the entire colon safely, in more than 95% of cases, using light intravenous sedation. In addition, most polyps can be removed safely and completely using electrocautery techniques at the initial examination. Serious complications such as bleeding or perforation requiring surgery occur in approximately 0.1 to 0.2% of patients. Comparative studies reveal that the accuracy of colonoscopy is superior to barium enema in the diagnosis of polyps. However, when a barium enema is ordered to screen for or diagnose polyps in the colon a double-contrast (air-contrast) technique should be requested because it increases the accuracy for detecting small filling defects. When an air-contrast barium enema is used to investigate a patient for colonic neoplasia, a proctosigmoidoscopy should also be performed. This should be done to evaluate the rectosigmoid, an area not always seen clearly in a barium enema, and the area of the colon where polyps are most likely to be found. While the cost of a colonoscopy far exceeds that of a flexible sigmoidoscopy and barium enema by 30 to 50%, 30 to 40% of patients undergoing a barium enema examination to detect polyps will have findings that subsequently require a colonoscopy. Therefore, the average cost and cost effectiveness of the two methods are approximately the same. Thus, colonoscopy is being performed more frequently as the primary test to evaluate the colon for polyps and/or cancer.

Screening as suggested by the American College of Gastroenterology is stratified based on risk. Approximately 70 to 80% of patients are at average risk, approximately 15 to 20% are at moderate risk, and 5 to 10% are at high risk. All patients 50 years or older who have no other risk factors as listed in Table 40-10 (average risk) should have fecal occult blood tests (FOBT) every year and flexible sigmoidoscopy every 5 years in conjunction with an air-contrast barium enema examination every 5 to 10 years. Another option is colonoscopy every 10 years since more polyps and cancers are being found out of the reach of a flexible sigmoidoscope. If an adenoma is found on flexible sigmoidoscopy, the patient should be referred to a colonoscopist to perform a colonoscopy

TABLE 40-10
RISK FACTORS FOR COLORECTAL CANCER

Strong risk factors
  Advanced age
  Country of birth
  Familial polyposis
  Gardner syndrome
  Hereditary nonpolyposis colorectal cancer
  Long-standing ulcerative colitis
Moderate risk factors
  High red-meat diet
  Previous adenoma
  Pelvic irradiation
Modest risk factors
  High-fat diet
  Alcohol
  Cigarette smoking
  Obesity
  Tall stature
  Cholecystectomy
  High sucrose consumption
Modest protective factors
  High vegetable/fruit diet
  High-fiber diet
  High folate/methionine intake
  High calcium intake
  Postmenopausal hormone-replacement therapy
Moderate protective factors
  High physical activity
  Aspirin
  NSAIDs

to screen the remainder of the colon and remove the adenoma. If a fecal occult blood test is positive, the patient should undergo endoscopic evaluation of the colon to determine the cause of the occult blood. It is important to remember that when performing fecal occult blood screening that a number of factors can affect the test. The consumption of red meats and peroxidase-containing foods (melon, uncooked broccoli, horseradish, cauliflower, and turnips) can result in false positive tests, and vitamin C may decrease the sensitivity of the test. However, *all positive tests have to be assumed true positives. Therefore, if a patient has a positive fecal occult blood test, she needs to be evaluated.* The sensitivity of the FOBT for the detection of small and medium-sized polyps is low; however, a significant fraction of larger, clinically significant polyps are detectable using FOBT. Since there is a higher risk of invasive carcinoma in these larger polyps, therefore FOBT screening is useful for finding carcinomas and polyps that have a higher risk of developing carcinoma. Some data suggest that annual FOBT, combined with rehydration and colonoscopy in patients who screen positive for occult blood, has a 90% sen-

sitivity in detecting colorectal cancers and is associated with a decrease of 33% in 13-year cumulative mortality from colorectal cancer. Flexible sigmoidoscopy is useful because it accurately detects 50 to 60% of all colorectal polyps because that percentage of polyps is located in the left colon in the viewing range of the flexible sigmoidoscope. A small polyp detected during a routine flexible sigmoidoscopy should be biopsied to determine whether it is an adenoma, which requires referral for colonoscopy, resection, and follow-up. The incidence of synchronous adenomas in patients with one confirmed adenoma is 30 to 50%. However, if it is a hyperplastic polyp, no further follow-up is required unless the patient has a clinical history suggesting a familial predisposition to right-sided lesions or if the patient has right-sided symptoms. A patient with an abnormality on barium enema should be referred for colonoscopy for biopsy and removal. Most polyps can be completely removed by electrocautery during colonoscopy. However, it is important to individualize the treatment of each patient with consideration to age, the presence of comorbidity, and the size of the lesion. A significant number of outcome studies have supported the contention that the risk of residual carcinoma following a colonoscopic resection of a malignant polyp is appreciably lower than the risk of surgical resection if the endoscopist is confident that the resection was complete, the cancer did not invade the margin of the electrocautery resection, the tumor was well differentiated, and there was no evidence of lymphatic or vascular invasion. The incidence of residual or nodal cancer in cases with favorable prognostic criteria was 0.3% and 1.5% for pedunculated and sessile malignant polyps, respectively. With one or more unfavorable criteria, the incidence of nodal metastases increases to 8.5% for pedunculated polyps and 14.4% for sessile polyps. Patients with a sessile polyp and these favorable prognostic criteria need a follow-up colonoscopy in 2 to 3 months to check the site for residual polyp tissue. However, if the polyp was pedunculated and cleanly excised, the subsequent follow-up surveillance is identical to that recommended for patients with nonmalignant adenomas. In good-risk patients, surgical referral and resection including lymph nodes should be performed if any of the above criteria are lacking. See Table 40-9 for the definitions and recommendations for screening and surveillance of moderate- and high-risk patients and for patients who have had adenomatous polyps removed.

IRRITABLE-BOWEL SYNDROME

Irritable-bowel syndrome is one of over 20 functional gastrointestinal disorders characterized by chronic or recurrent symptoms not explained by structural or biochemical abnormalities. They occur throughout the gastrointestinal tract from the pharynx and esophagus to the anorectum and also include the stomach, biliary tree, and small and large intestine. It appears that these disorders are involved with abnormalities in motility and/or the afferent sensitivity modulated by the central nervous system. Disorders of the esophagus include globus sensation or globus hystericus—a chronic or intermittent feeling of a lump in the throat that is not present during meals and that is not associated with dysphagia. In fact, it does not interfere with swallowing and may be relieved by deglutition. It is not associated with a known physiologic abnormality of deglutition. Patients are more commonly female and more often below 50 years of age, making up 18% of a normal gynecologic practice and 34% of patients with irritable-bowel syndrome. However, in patients older than 50 years of age, globus occurs in an equal proportion of males and females. A large proportion of patients does not seek medical assistance for this problem. It is widely believed that stress and anxiety are contributing factors in the genesis of globus. Globus tends to be difficult to treat. It is often recurrent, probably due in part to the multiple causative factors involved in symptom production. Because of the strong association between globus and emotional distress, a psychological assessment should be obtained for all patients. In addition, evaluations for GERD and esophageal motility disorders are often helpful to rule out these disorders. Supportive therapy is essential. A trial of antidepressant therapy can produce substantial and rapid improvement in patients with globus. However, this is based only on case studies.

Rumination syndrome is the chronic or recurrent regurgitation of recently ingested food into the mouth, associated with the rechewing of the food in the absence of nausea and vomiting. This is an uncommon problem but is more frequently found in infants and institutionalized adults and children with emotional and intellectual deficits. There are three subgroups of this disorder: emotionally deprived patients, mentally retarded patients, and persons in whom the behavior develops as a maladaptive habit that worsens with stress. In addition, in some persons rumination is associated with bulimia. The diagnosis is based on identifying the typical clinical features and excluding other medical or psychiatric disease. Patients with this disorder should be referred to a specialist to be evaluated for a primary structural or motility disorder of the esophagus. Since this disorder appears to be a learned maladaptive habit, behavioral modification and biofeedback techniques are recommended as therapeutic approaches, although PPIs have been shown to be of some value.

Functional chest pain of presumed esophageal origin is a midline chest pain with or without dysphagia in the absence of achalasia, esophagitis, pathologic reflux, or cardiac disease. A complete evaluation by a specialist is warranted if this diagnosis is suspected. However, it is important that cardiac disease be ruled out. Beyond a complete history and physical examination to eliminate systemic illnesses and musculoskeletal pain, initial evaluation should include electrocardiography, treadmill stress test, barium swallow, and a trail of antireflux therapy. If no diagnosis or an inadequate result is obtained with the empiric therapy, the patient should be referred to a gastrointestinal specialist for further evaluation, which often will include a 24-hour pH study, endoscopy, and esophageal motility studies. If the cardiac evaluation is unremarkable, it is often beneficial to reassure the patient that she or he does not have a dangerous cardiac illness. It is often useful to have the patient participate in psychometric testing, (Minnesota Multiphasic Personality Inventory [MMPI]).

Functional heartburn is characterized by a burning retrosternal discomfort that occurs in the absence of pathologic gastroesophageal reflux or esophagitis. Evaluation should include investigations to exclude GERD, esophagitis, hiatal hernia, and esophageal diverticula, and a cardiac cause of the symptoms. If these are excluded, a referral to a specialist is warranted to evaluate for an esophageal motility disorder. A trial of tricyclic antidepressants may be helpful despite known effects of lowering the LES pressure.

Functional dysphagia is the sense of solid or liquid foods sticking or passing abnormally in the absence of achalasia or other structural or motility disorder with a recognized pathophysiologic basis. Evaluation is similar to that of functional heartburn and functional chest pain.

Gastroduodenal functional disorders include functional dyspepsia and aerophagia. Functional dyspepsia is defined as pain or discomfort centered in the upper abdomen with no clinical, biochemical, endoscopic, or ultrasonic evidence of known organic disease to explain the symptoms. While controversy still does exist regarding subclassification, the Rome committees defined two subgroups. The first is ulcer-like dyspepsia, in which the patient experiences epigastric pain, not severe in nature and relieved by food or antacid agents. In addition, the pain is mostly focal and does not radiate. The second subgroup is dysmotility-like dyspepsia, possibly associated with gastric dysmotility in which pain is not a dominant symptom, but the patient reports early satiety, postprandial fullness, and nausea, often aggravated by food.

In evaluating these patients, it is most important to address the symptoms of greatest concern to them. It is important to rule out organic abnormalities. Patients with recent onset of symptoms and who have a normal physical examination and routine laboratory tests may be given 2 to 3 weeks of empiric H_2-receptor-blocker therapy. If no resolution of symptoms is noted, a full evaluation should be undertaken. It is important to remember that the diagnosis of a functional gastrointestinal disorder presupposes that no structural, metabolic, or infectious disorder is the cause. Careful attention should be paid to the type of symptoms. If the primary symptom is pain or discomfort, referral for endoscopy is warranted to rule out inflammation, ulceration, malignancy, *Helicobacter pylori* infection, gastric-outlet obstruction, and gastric retention. Also, *H. pylori* can be ruled out with a carbon-radiolabeled urea breath test or *H. pylori* serologic tests (remember that antibody titers stay elevated for a substantial amount of time following therapy). Ultrasonography should also be done to exclude both biliary and pancreatic disorders. If indicated by the symptoms, barium studies of the small bowel and/or colon are also warranted. A careful history and physical examination, in addition to blood tests, can be very rewarding and save expensive testing. It is also important to remember that some patients with these symptoms have subtle abnormalities in the central nervous system that might be contributory.

Some patients with pain with and without nausea have pylorospasm or spasm of the antral smooth muscle. These patients often respond to therapy with anticholinergic drugs. However, these drugs should be used sparingly in patients with suspected gastroparesis because they also decrease motility.

If the patient's symptoms include significant nausea with or without vomiting or bloating, and especially if retained food is found on endoscopy, a gastric emptying test should be performed. In addition,

a trial of a prokinetic drug (metaclopramide) should be initiated along with an H_2-receptor blocker. In addition, since stress decreases gut motility, improved stress management is thought to be helpful. Patients who are refractory to this type of therapy would be referred to a gastroenterologist, especially one with a special interest in gastrointestinal motility.

A greater understanding of GI motility has evolved and many disorders once thought to be functional have a physiologic defect. In addition, many new and novel medications that may be beneficial in therapy are in the process of development. Lastly, the patient should be monitored for clinical changes that might either suggest improvement or a different diagnosis.

Aerophagia is characterized by air swallowing with repetitive belching. It is often exacerbated by stress and can be associated with GERD, peptic ulcer disease, or gallbladder disease. Therefore, it is important to rule out these disorders. In addition, a great number of patients with aerophagia are very anxious. This learned behavior involves relaxing the upper esophageal sphincter, resulting in the swallowing of large amounts of air, which after a while becomes difficult to control. Mostly the patient presents with symptoms of uncontrollable belching. This can be so severe that it can be socially compromising. However, closely observing the patient during history-taking often reveals air swallowing or air-gulping behavior. It is again important to rule out other causes for these symptoms. The most successful therapy is behavior modification.

Biliary functional disorders include gallbladder dysfunction, which is characterized by recurrent moderate to severe pain in the epigastrium or right upper quadrant lasting 20 or more minutes and associated with pain after meals, nausea, vomiting, and evidence of abnormal gallbladder functioning. These patients are best evaluated with a good history, an abdominal ultrasound, and if no stones, sludge, mass, or dilated ducts are present, a radionuclide gallbladder ejection fraction test should be performed. At this time, the patient should be referred to a specialist for other hepatobiliary testing and therapy. Sphincter of Oddi dysfunction is also included in this group. It is characterized by a similar pain but in the absence of a gallbladder and at times it is associated with transient elevations of liver chemistries, a dilated common bile duct with delayed drainage, and the absence of structural abnormalities (i.e., biliary stricture, papillary stricture, or gallstones) to explain the symptoms. Sphincter of Oddi manometry is another diagnostic test used to establish the diagnosis. In certain subgroups of patients, endoscopic sphincterotomy relieves the symptoms, while in other subgroups it is not an effective therapy. Nitrates also can very transiently relieve symptoms is some cases.

Bowel-function gastrointestinal disorders include irritable-bowel syndrom, functional abdominal bloating, functional constipation, functional diarrhea, and functional abdominal pain. These occur chronically or recurrently at times of life stress, changes in diet, menses, or emotional tension. It is important that the presence of organic GI disease that can produce similar symptoms be ruled out. The most common and clinically important disorder is irritable-bowel syndrome (IBS), also called functional bowel disease, spastic colitis, and spastic colon. Approximately 28% of the population have this syndrome. It can present in several forms. The first form involves cyclic diarrhea and constipation with or without crampy abdominal pain often brought on or made worse by eating (especially salads, spicy food, or stress). However, IBS can also present in a pure constipation form, a pure diarrhea form, and an abdominal pain form. Diarrhea or constipation can exist with or without abdominal pain. Historically, IBS was a diagnosis of exclusion. If the patient had the symptoms and no organic disease was found the diagnosis was IBS. However, this very often required many tests to exclude organic disease. A number of physiologic factors were found to be associated with this disorder. However, the difficulty in testing these made them impractical. Finally, the Manning symptom criteria were developed and a few years later the Rome symptom criteria were developed. Using the Rome I symptom criteria studies with follow-up extending to 3 years resulted in the same diagnosis in up to 97% of cases. In 1999 these criteria evolved into the Rome II criteria (Table 40-11).

Multiple nonmutually exclusive hypotheses have been postulated to explain the cause of symptoms in IBS. First, patients have an underlying disorder of gastrointestinal motility. Second, emotional tension and psychological factors lead to the gastrointestinal symptoms and health-seeking behaviors. Third, these patients have enhanced visceral perception or an excessive response to a normal signal from the gastrointestinal tract, and other pathophysiologic factors such as luminal irritants and postinfectious neuromodulation may be operative.

While previous studies suggested an association between abnormal motility with IBS at rest, more re-

---

TABLE 40-11
ROME II CRITERIA* FOR IRRITABLE-BOWEL SYNDROME

At least 12 weeks or more, which need not be consecutive, in the preceding 12 months of abdominal discomfort or pain that has two of three features:

1. Relieved with defecation, and/or
2. Onset associated with a change in frequency of stool, and/or
3. Onset associated with a change in consistency of stool

Symptoms that cumulatively support the diagnosis of irritable-bowel syndrome:

a. Abnormal stool frequency (may be defined as more than three bowel movements per day and less than three bowel movements per week)
b. Abnormal stool form (lumpy/hard or loose/watery stool)
c. Abnormal stool passage (straining, urgency, or feeling of incomplete evacuation)
d. Passage of mucus
e. Bloating or feeling of abdominal distention

*In the absence of structural or metabolic abnormalities to explain the symptoms.
Modified from Thompson et al. GUT 1999;45(Suppl II):43.

---

cent evidence has not supported abnormal motility at rest. Previous studies have also supported an exaggerated response to physical and neurohumoral stimuli.

Patients with IBS with more psychopathology seek medical advice more frequently. In addition, patients who seek health care for IBS at a tertiary-care center are more likely to report a history of sexual, physical, or verbal abuse than patients diagnosed with organic disease. The current data suggest that psychological overlay and personality traits are not related to the development of motility disorders but are related to whether patients consult a physician for their symptoms. Data do support the contention that patients with IBS have a reduced threshold to discomfort induced by rectal or colonic distention. This decreased threshold to discomfort is not noted in nongastrointestinal locations in their bodies, resulting in their focusing on gastrointestinal discomfort.

The diagnosis of IBS is based on three steps: first, identification of a symptom complex compatible with IBS (Rome II Criteria); second, the presence of a frequent association of symptoms with factors that activate gut motility; and lastly, a limited screen of organic causes of symptoms. Therefore, prudence in the use of studies to exclude organic disorders is important. The tests should be based on the presenting symptoms and how that relates to the total clinical picture. It is also important to include long-standing symptoms, psychological issues, and the results of previous evaluations.

A basic evaluation should include a personal inventory, a complete blood count, basic chemistry screening, liver-function tests, thyroid-stimulating hormone, stool for ova and parasites, occult blood, and sedimentation rate. A flexible sigmoidoscopy with biopsy is very useful in patients with diarrhea and/or pain, especially if it is left lower quadrant pain. If the patient has diarrhea, a laxative screen, and stool for white cells is useful. It is important to remember that organic disease can occur concurrently in patients with IBS. Therefore, if the patient presents with an appropriate history or if the patient is ≥50 years of age, a colonoscopy or flexible sigmoidoscopy and ACBE should be considered instead of a flexible sigmoidoscopy alone. A complete history is very important, including travel, all medications (especially magnesium-containing antacids, PPIs, colchicine, misoprostol, quinidine, antihypertensives, narcotics, and anticholinergics), foods and drink, relationship of symptoms to life events, sexual history, and a psychological profile. *There are several red flags to watch for: blood per rectum, positive occult blood in the stool, weight loss, anemia, fever, elevated white-cell count, abnormal results on liver-function tests, persistent diarrhea, severe constipation, nocturnal symptoms of pain and abnormal bowel function, family history of GI cancer, inflammatory bowel disease or celiac disease, and new onset of symptoms in patients over 50 years of age.* In patients with these signs or symptoms it is important to rule out alternative or coexisting disease.

Current management components of IBS include education, reassurance, dietary modification, fiber, symptomatic treatment, psychological/behavioral options, and giving the patient realistic goals.

It is very important to build a bond of reassurance with the patient from the first visit. The general approach involves reassurance, listening, clear instruction, behavior modification, and making specific dietary changes (excluding caffeine and lactose-, fructose-, and sorbitol-containing foods, in addition to drugs that might affect the gut). It is important to reassure the patient that there is no serious organic disease or alarming symptoms. In addition, it is important to give the patient realistic goals for improvement. Start with lifestyle changes such as bowel training, dietary changes, and minimal medication unless the patient is having severe pain. There has been a 70% placebo effect in some trials with patients

with IBS. Drug therapy should be tailored to the patient's symptoms. Currently, many of the pharmacologic agents available for the treatment of IBS target only one symptom. Therefore, patients may need to take more than one medication in order to get their symptoms under control. Antispasmodic drugs (anticholinergics) tend to be useful in patients with pain. In addition, antidepressants can be helpful because of their central nervous system effects in addition to the anticholinergic effects. Therefore, these and SSRIs are predominantly used for patients with severe or intractable pain. Bulk agents and fiber also can be very useful for patients with cyclic constipation and diarrhea or pure constipation. Also, in patients with constipation, osmotic laxatives and stimulant laxatives should be tried. However, these may exacerbate abdominal pain and bloating. Several prokinetic drugs are in development that may prove useful for these patients in the future. However, it is important to see the patient frequently initially and establish a trusting relationship. It is important to understand that these patients most often have real symptoms and to explain to the patient how the symptoms occur and what is happening. At each visit reinforce all improvements, however small, and help to establish future goals based on current improvement. Some patients appear obsessed with abdominal symptoms. In these patients, relatively small doses of a tricyclic antidepressant may induce remission even if you cannot determine whether depression is present. Modulating the enteric nervous system appears to be effective in patients with IBS. In addition, antidiarrheals are useful for patients with diarrhea-symptom IBS. If idiopathic bile-salt malabsorption is suspected, or if patient has had a cholecystectomy, cholestyramine may be helpful.

In patients with long-term symptoms with minimal improvement or with severe maladaptive behavior, psychotherapy might be beneficial and should be used in this small group of patients.

It important to remember that pelvic-floor dysfunction may present with symptoms consistent with constipation-predominant IBS. Symptoms such as a sense of incomplete evacuation in addition to secondary abdominal pain result from the failure of orderly muscular coordination that normally enables rectal evacuation. These patients, identified by history, physical examination, and clinical and radiologic tests, can improve markedly by biofeedback and pelvic exercises. It is important to remember that no pharmacologic therapy is useful in treating these patients, and diagnosis and treatment of pelvic-floor dysfunction is the key to at least partial relief. However, patients may have concomitant disease.

INFLAMMATORY-BOWEL DISEASE

The term *idiopathic inflammatory-bowel disease* refers to both Crohn's disease and chronic ulcerative colitis. The cause of both disorders is unknown. It is important to rule out other causes, especially infections, before making the diagnosis of idiopathic inflammatory-bowel disease. Ulcerative colitis (UC) involves mucosal inflammation only in the colon and is a continuous inflammatory process from the anal verge proximal. The more extensive the disease, the more proximal the involvement. More than 95% of patients have rectal involvement, and patients usually present with frequent bloody diarrhea with tenesmus and little abdominal pain. Unlike Crohn's disease, UC does not form fistulas and perianal disease is uncommon.

Crohn's disease, on the other hand, involves segmental transmural inflammation and thickening of the gastroenteric tract which can occur anyplace from the esophagus through the anus, sparing the rectum in 50% of the patients. This segmental and transmural inflammation results in strictures of the intestine and is associated with episodes of partial or complete bowel obstruction. Early in the disease, apthoid uclers are often observed, while deep linear and serpiginous ulceration are often noted in more advanced disease. This may result in a cobblestone appearance. It presents with fewer bowel movements and less bleeding and is more commonly associated with abdominal pain. In addition, it is associated with intestinal fistula and fistula to other organs in addition to perianal disease. The spectrum of findings includes right lower quadrant pain with or without a palpable mass and diarrhea. This diarrhea may result from mucosal inflammation, partial bowel obstruction, malabsorption, bacterial overgrowth, transit through fistulas, and bile salt diarrhea due to a diseased terminal ileum.

Systemic findings include fever, weight loss, growth retardation in children and nutritional deficiencies. Patients may have anemia resulting from chronic blood loss, chronic disease, or deficiencies in folate, vitamin B_{12}, or iron. Some patients have solely ileal or small-bowel disease, other patients have granulomatous colitis, and some have both. Patients with colitis have more diarrhea, often with blood. The disease can involve almost any site in the gastrointestinal tract. Thus,

patients with Crohn's disease are more varied in their clinical presentation than patients with ulcerative colitis. The colon alone is involved in 30% of patients, the small intestine in 40%, and both small intestine and colon in 30% of patients. The diagnosis of Crohn's disease is based on clinical history and characteristic findings on colonoscopy, biopsy, and barium radiography. CT and magnetic resonance imaging have become more useful in recent years, as have indium-11-labeled granulocyte scans. However, none of these methods is as sensitive as colonoscopy in detecting mild disease.

The peak incidence of inflammatory-bowel disease (IBD) is between the ages of 15 and 35 years, but it may be present at any age. In <10% of patients the onset is after the age of 60 years. In fact, the onset of ulcerative colitis in a patient older than 60 years of age may be characterized by a severe initial attack that carries a high mortality rate. However, older patients who survive the initial attack and patients with Crohn's disease have a mostly favorable prognosis with age-specific mortality rates no higher than that of the general population. Relapse rates after medical or surgical therapies tend to be lower in older as compared with younger patients. They are more likely to have distal disease, while older patients with Crohn's disease are more likely to have colonic involvement than younger patients. Smoking is associated with a worse course in Crohn's disease while it decreases the risk of ulcerative colitis. In fact, relapses or the initial onset of UC often correlate with discontinuation of smoking. In nonsmokers, the use of oral contraceptives may increase the risk of Crohn's disease.

Extraintestinal manifestations of IBD include axial arthritis (spine and sacroiliac joints), whose activity is independent of the bowel disease, while peripheral oligoarticular arthritis tends to parallel the activity of the bowel disease. Other manifestations include uveitis and episcleritis. Erythema nodosum is most often associated with Crohn's disease and generally parallels the activity of the bowel disease. Patients with terminal ileal disease have an increased incidence of calcium oxalate kidney stones. Pyoderma gangrenosum pursues an independent course in 50% of the cases and is mostly associated with UC. Approximately 2.5 to 7.5% of patients with pancolitis have primary sclerosing cholangitis. This can progress to cholangiocarcinoma.

Patients with IBD should be referred to a gastroenterologist for specialist care.

Patients with long-standing ulcerative colitis have an increased risk of colon cancer and therefore need to have surveillance colonoscopy. In patients with pancolitis, the risk of cancer begins to increase after 8 years. Subsequently, the incidence of cancer ranges from 0.5 to 1% per year. A lower risk is found in patients with left-sided disease. Patients with pancolitis for 10 years or more or left-sided colitis for 15 years or more should be referred to a gastroenterologist for yearly surveillance colonoscopy. Patients are screened with colonoscopy, looking for dysplasia or carcinoma. There is a 20 to 40% chance of discovering carcinoma in a colon in which dysplasia is found. Therefore, colectomy is indicated in these patients.

An increased risk (5.6-fold) of colon cancer has been noted in patients with Crohn's disease, especially Crohn's colitis. This risk may be equivalent to that seen with UC risks after being adjusted for the less extensive involvement of the colon in Crohn's colitis. However, the value of surveillance colonoscopy has not been shown as of yet.

5-Aminosalicylic acid (5-ASA) and 5-ASA derivatives are the mainstay of therapy of IBD. Sulfasalazine, 5-ASA linked to sulfapyridine, is cleaved to the two constituent drugs by bacteria in the colon. The 5-ASA acts topically on inflamed colonic mucosa and is most effective on mildly to moderately severe ulcerative colitis and in Crohn's colitis. In addition to its role in treating active disease it is also effective in reducing the frequency and severity of relapses of UC. However, much more controversy exists about the efficacy of the drug in preventing relapses or postsurgical recurrence of Crohn's disease. One problem is that side effects occur in up to 50% of patients receiving the drug and it has to be discontinued in up to 20% of patients. Side effects, which are dose-dependent, include nausea, vomiting, anorexia, and headache. Idiosyncratic reactions include rash, dermatitis, neutropenia, pancreatitis, hepatitis, fever, and pneumonitis. In addition, sulfasalazine has been reported to cause reversible abnormalities of sperm structure and function in addition to infertility. Concentrations of the drug are sufficiently low and albumin-binding bilirubin-displacing kinetics are sufficiently weak to allow for complete safety in pregnancy and breast-feeding. No case of kernicterus has ever been attributed to sulfasalazine and no teratogenicity or adverse effects in pregnancy have been documented. Several newer preparations permit delivery of the 5-ASA moiety to the small bowel and colon without the need for sulfapyridine. These are olsalazine (Dipentum), two 5-ASA molecules held together by a diazo linkage, mesalamine (Asacol),

5-ASA coated with acrylic resin such that the drug is released in alkaline pH (terminal ileum and colon), and mesalamine (Pentasa), 5-ASA microsphere coated so that the drug is slowly released throughout the intestinal tract. Some data support the contention that Pentasa is more effective for patients with small bowel, especially ileal disease. 5-ASA formulations have been shown to be useful as maintenance treatment of Crohn's disease, especially in patients with ileal disease or previous resection, at dose of *at least* 2 g per day. 5-ASA can also be administered as enemas or suppositories for proctitis or left-sided disease.

The next group of drugs that play a role in IBD are steroids. Corticosteroids play an important role in the treatment of moderate to severe UC or Crohn's colitis. Their limitations lie in the significant toxicity associated with long-term use. They can be administered as an enema for proctitis or distal colitis. Long-term administration can result in adrenal suppression and systemic toxicity. In addition, it is difficult to wean patients from steroids, especially if they have been on the drug for a long time. Another drug, which is not available in the United States, is bude-sonide, which is more potent but has fewer side effects in clinical trials.

Metronidazole is a useful drug to treat colonic and perineal Crohn's disease in addition to pouchitis. Effective doses are from 10 to 20 mg/kg per day. It is useful for fistulas, perianal disease, complex perineal abscesses, and preventing recurrence. It is important to remember that at high doses, patients may experience paresthesias, which at times can become disabling, a metallic taste, and a disulfiram-like effect in patients who drink alcohol. In addition, the possibility of teratogenicity has to be considered. It appears to reduce the frequency and severity of recurrences of Crohn's disease after ileal resection. Some data suggest that ciprofloxacin may also be useful in both ileocolonic and perineal Crohn's disease.

Immunomodulatory and prednisone-sparing drugs are the next line of therapy. These include azathiprine and its metabolite 6-mercaptopurine. These drugs are an important adjunct to conventional therapy for IBD. Both are useful in treating fistulas in Crohn's disease, in treating patients who have relapses on other conventional medical therapies or surgery, and in decreasing or eliminating corticosteroid requirements. They prevent relapses both in patients with UC and Crohn's disease and do not appear to lead to an increased risk of malignancy. It is important to remember that there is a delay period of from 2 to 8 months before a therapeutic effect is noted. The therapeutic dose for 6-mercaptopurine is 1.5 mg/kg per day and 2.5 mg/kg per day for azathioprine. A starting dose of 50 mg per day of azathioprine is often used. Side effects include pancreatitis (~3% of patients), bone marrow suppression (~2%), and lymphoma (one case in a study of 400 patients). Therefore, symptoms and complete blood counts should be assessed regularly.

Other agents such as cyclosporine and methotrexate are beneficial in severe and refractory Crohn's disease and UC. However, a specialist should care for patients with severe disease requiring these therapies, including azathioprine. It is important to follow cyclosporine levels, renal function, blood pressure, and signs of neurotoxicity in patients receiving cyclosporine. Patients receiving methotrexate may have nausea, anorexia, diarrhea, stomatitis, cytopenia, hypersensitivity pneumonitis, and hepatotoxicity. Therefore, regular tests of hepatic inflammation should be performed.

New therapies, especially anti-tumor necrosis factor (TNF-α) (infleximide) have been introduced and have been found to be effective in patients who do not respond to conventional therapy, who are intolerant to or dependent on steroids, or who have fistulas not responsive to conventional therapy. Patients with disease of this severity should be cared for by a gastroenterologist if possible. Experts have suggested that early therapy with drugs of this type might minimize the complications from the disease and from other therapies, such as steroids. However, this is not the standard at present.

The role of bowel rest and diet therapy in IBD management is controversial. However, tube feedings and total parenteral nutrition may be indicated in patients with malnutrition, short-bowel syndrome, fistulas, or growth failure or as an adjunct to surgery. Elemental and polymeric diets used as primary therapy in patients with mild to moderately severe Crohn's disease have been shown in some studies to be equivalent in efficacy to steroid therapy. However, due to lack of palatability of the diets there is poor long-term compliance. These therapies have no role in primary therapy of UC.

Surgical therapy is therapy of necessity in IBD. The principal indications are intractable disease, obstruction, or cancer prophylaxis. With UC, ileoanal anastomosis after a proctocolectomy is the surgical treatment of choice, regardless of the extent of the disease. However, it is not appropriate for patients with Crohn's disease because of the frequency of recurrence and the frequency of perianal and perineal disease, despite rectal sparing. Surgery is required in most patients with Crohn's disease for intractability and failure of medical therapy, intestinal obstruction, symptomatic fistulas, abscesses, or cancer. In some patients with strictures a strictureplasty rather than resection permits preservation of bowel length when the stricture is fibrotic and not inflamed. In Crohn's disease with colonic involvement, a conventional proctocolectomy is preferred, especially in the elderly. In other cases, an ileoanal anastomosis is done with the construction of an ileal pouch. These patients often have 6 to 8 bowel movements per day. However, some fecal incontinence at night does occur, and in 20% of patients it occurs during the daytime. Approximately 2% of patients require excision of the pouch and an ileostomy. The most frequent complication in ileal pouches is pouchitis, characterized by tenesmus, bloody diarrhea, and inflammation seen on endoscopy. It is best treated with metronidazole 250 to 500 mg three times per day for 7 to 14 days or other antibiotics. Topical or oral aminosalicylate drugs or corticosteroids may also be beneficial.

The frequency and severity of recurrent flares is variable in patients with UC. Within 10 years of diagnosis, most patients have at least one relapse, and colectomy is ultimately required in 25% of patients. In patients with pancolitis, up to 30% of patients require a colectomy for uncontrolled disease within the first 3 years after diagnosis. Since Crohn's disease is a chronic recurrent disease, nearly all patients have a recurrence within the first 10 years after diagnosis. In addition, 30% require some surgical intervention within the first year after diagnosis. After that time, surgery is required at a rate of 5% per year. Subclinical recurrence after surgery is invariable.

LIVER TESTS

Understanding tests used in the diagnosis and management of liver disorders is important in that abnormalities in tests in the various groups have different implications and help define for the clinician the nature of the hepatic abnormality. In general, the tests can be divided into three groups: (1) tests of liver function or functional hepatic mass, (2) tests of hepatocellular injury; and (3) tests of hepatobiliary injury. Some tests overlap the different groups.

The tests of liver function involve synthesis and secretion, excretion, and drug metabolism and detoxification. These include serum albumin, serum cholesterol, prothrombin time, serum ammonia, serum bilirubin, and the rate of metabolism of various drugs by cytochrome P-450 enzymes (still in research phase). While the liver secretes other plasma proteins, albumin is secreted in the greatest quantities and is the most important. It is a nonglycosolated protein that is predominantly used for the binding and transport of poorly soluble substances in the body. It has a half-life of 22 days and therefore is most useful in assessing the liver's long-term function, assuming adequate nutrition. Serum albumin can be decreased in patients with a normal liver who are consuming insufficient nutrients and in conditions resulting in a significant protein loss such as nephrotic syndrome and protein-losing enteropathies such as Cronkite Canada syndrome or Ménétrier's disease.

In acute liver disease, especially fulminant hepatic failure, measurement of proteins with much shorter half-lives such as prealbumin, prothrombin, and factor V are of much greater prognostic value than albumin. While extracellular plasma albumin content is unaltered during normal pregnancy, serum albumin concentrations decrease at times, resulting in levels 60% of normal nonpregnant levels. This appears be due to hemodilution. Albumin losses can occur as a result of proteinuria in cases of preeclampsia and eclampsia. Therefore, in pregnancy it can be difficult to use low serum albumin levels as an assessment of chronic liver disease.

Some of the other proteins that the liver synthesizes include several of the coagulation factors: fibrinogen (factor I), prothrombin (factor II), and factors V, VII, IX, X, and XII. Therefore, a prolonged prothrombin time may indicate acute or chronic liver dysfunction or a decrease in hepatic mass, in addition to a malabsorption of clotting factors or the use of medications. Improvement of prothrombin time after the parenteral administration of 10 mg of vitamin K differentiates vitamin K deficiency states from hepatic dysfunction. While the prothrombin time does not correlate well with the severity of chronic liver disease, it is useful in gauging the severity of acute hepatocellular dysfunction. For example, in fulminant hepatic failure, factors II, V, and VII are affected earliest because these proteins have very short half-lives.

The liver synthesizes the majority of the body's cholesterol, which is then released into the bloodstream or excreted into the bile. Therefore, patients with disorders of impaired bile secretion, such as primary biliary cirrhosis, often have a high serum cholesterol, while patients with severe liver dysfunction or a significant decrease in functioning hepatic mass have low serum cholesterol. However, it is important to remember that elevated serum cholesterol is often the result of a disorder of lipoprotein metabolism. Pregnant patients, especially at the end of the first trimester, can have serum cholesterol levels up to two times normal nonpregnant levels. Thus, elevated serum cholesterol levels do not provide specific evidence of liver dysfunction during pregnancy. In reality, serum cholesterol is most useful in supporting severe liver dysfunction when serum levels are decreased.

Serum bilirubin is also an important test of hepatic function since the liver hepatocyte plays a major role in the metabolism (conjugation) and excretion of this organic anion, a breakdown product of hemoglobin. A normal serum bilirubin is 0.2 to 1 mg/dl. Some women normally manifest a modest rise in bilirubin during pregnancy (Table 40-12). Bilirubin is transported to the liver as unconjugated bilirubin, which on reaching the hepatocyte, separates from the albumin carrier protein and is transported across the cell membrane, where glucuronyl transferase converts it

TABLE 40-12
LIVER LABORATORY TESTS IN A NORMAL PREGNANCY

Nonpregnant		Pregnant Trimester (Mean Value)		
Test	Normal range	First	Second	Third
Albumin (g/liter)	42–56	43	40	39
Alkaline phosphatase (IU/liter)	17–68	29	35	71
Alanine aminotransferase (IU/liter)	2–30	7	8	8
Aspartate aminotransferase (IU/liter)	1–37	5	7	7
γ-Glutamyl transpeptidase	2–38	8	7	7
Total bilirubin (μmol/liter)	2–20	5	4	3
5' Nucleotidase (IU/liter)	3–14	4	5	6
Total bile acids (μmol/liter)	0.5–13	2	2	2

to conjugated bilirubin. The conjugated bilirubin is actively secreted by the biliary canaliculi into the biliary ducts, eventually reaching the intestinal tract. Elevated serum bilirubin levels often reflect either one or both of the following conditions: increased production due to hemolysis or decreased hepatic clearance due to a decreased functional hepatic mass (a result of hepatocyte function). In addition, bile clearance can also be affected by macrobiliary or microbiliary duct obstruction.

Serum ammonia, also a test of hepatocellular function, is much more useful when evaluating trends in ammonia level. Many situations can result in spurious singular values. The liver converts ammonia into urea via the Krebs urea cycle and then the urea is excreted in urine. Decreased hepatocellular function, as in hepatic insufficiency, results in hyperammonemia and a reduction in blood urea nitrogen. There is a correlation between elevated blood ammonia and hepatic encephalopathy but not with the ammonia level and the severity of the encephalopathy. Elevated blood ammonia is also associated with ureterosigmoidostomy, strenuous muscular activity, infections with the ammonia-producing bacteria *Escherichia coli* and patients with a deficiency in urea-cycle enzymes.

Therefore, the three major tests of hepatocellular function or functional hepatic mass (true liver-function tests) used clinically are serum albumin, prothrombin time, and serum bilirubin. Serum cholesterol is a useful adjunct test, as is serum ammonia. There are many other tests used in the research setting that are not useful for the primary care physician.

The second group of tests assesses hepatocellular injury. These include the aminotransferases: aspartate aminotransferase (AST) and alanine aminotransferase (ALT), which are involved in hepatocyte energy processing. Both of these enzymes are cytosolic and leak into the bloodstream when the hepatocyte is injured. AST is also found in the mitochondria. Alcohol, a mitochondria toxin, causes AST to be elevated more than ALT. Rarely is either aminotransferase raised by more than five times normal in patients with alcoholic hepatitis. These findings are unusual in acute viral hepatitis and therefore can be useful in differential diagnosis. Another disorder in which the AST tends to be raised more than ALT is acetaminophen hepatotoxicity. However, in that condition the levels are frequently more significantly elevated. Since hepatotoxicity occurs at lower doses of acetaminophen in heavy drinkers, acetaminophen hepatotoxicity can often be missed and therefore not treated early. There-

fore, if acetaminophen hepatotoxicity is suspected treat with *N*-acetylcysteine. Serum levels of acetaminophen may be below the nomogram in these cases. The nomogram was developed for acetaminophen overdose in the average patient when the consumption of the drug is significantly greater. Certain disorders result in very rapid rise and fall of ALT and AST, such as an ischemic or hypotensive event and acute extrahepatic biliary obstruction. A third test, γ–glutamyl transpeptidase (GGT), is also affected by hepatocellular injury. In addition, it is elevated in cholestatic disorders. Certain drugs, which induce P-450 enzymes also, result in an elevation in GGT. Examples of these include alcohol and phenytoin.

Therefore, the tests in the second group assess acute or ongoing damage to the hepatocyte and do not measure hepatic function. Tests of hepatocellular injury are useful in determining the extent of ongoing injury to the hepatocyte or the extent of an acute insult to the liver. Thus, transaminases are useful to follow the progress of acute and chronic hepatitis of all types, toxic injury, ischemic injury, traumatic injury, or other inflammatory injury.

The other final group of tests assesses biliary-tree cellular injury and/or cholestasis. Alkaline phosphatase (AP) is an enzyme with an unknown function. Isoenzymes of alkaline phosphatase are found in many tissues of the body including the liver, bone, placenta, and intestine. The AP found in the bile-duct epithelium is isoenzyme 1 and is secreted into bile. Direct bilirubin is a potent inducer of this secretory process. Therefore, an increased hepatic AP is a function of an enzyme-induced secretory process rather than duct obstruction to the flow of the enzyme from the hepatocyte with spillage into the blood. AP is elevated with extrahepatic and intrahepatic duct obstruction in addition to canalicular obstruction. It is also elevated in conditions resulting in duct or canalicular damage, in conditions involving macroscopic and microscopic space-occupying lesions of the liver, physiologic bone growth during puberty, and following fractures or associated with disorders of bone turnover. In addition, serum AP concentrations increase during pregnancy, increasing gradually during the first two trimesters and then more significantly during the last trimester, during which levels may be four times the upper limit of normal found in nonpregnant females. However, this is mostly due to an increase in concentrations of placental AP. Of note, estrogen therapy in nonpregnant patients may be accompanied by an increase in serum AP level. The pregnancy-induced elevated levels of AP usually return to normal within 2 to 3 months following delivery. A decrease in AP before delivery has been associated with fetal death. This is thought to result from placental dysfunction. Raised levels of AP can be corroborated to be of liver origin by checking for elevations of biliary-tract enzymes such as GGT or 5′ nucleotidase or by obtaining AP isoenzymes (heat-stable AP and heat-labile AP). Elevation of these enzymes associated with an elevation in AP suggests that the elevated AP is of hepatic origin. However, both of these enzymes also can be elevated during pregnancy; however, GGT activity decreases slightly during late pregnancy. In addition, GGT can be elevated by certain medications and by the consumption of alcohol. Disorders of cholestasis can result in the obstruction of the normal excretion and transport of bilirubin via the biliary ducts to the small intestine. This results in an elevation of the serum bilirubin. In most of these disorders, a significant proportion of the bilirubin is conjugated or direct bilirubin. However, this is not a necessary finding, because hemolysis or hepatocellular dysfunction may be present at the same time.

Of note, total and free bilirubin concentrations are lower in pregnancy than in nonpregnant controls during all three trimesters. This can confuse the situation of mild cholestasis during pregnancy. Fasting serum bile acids or serum cholylglycine (a bile acid) usually remain within normal limits during normal pregnancy; therefore, this laboratory test remains a specific test for the diagnosis of cholestasis during pregnancy.

Thus, assessing for biliary-duct disease, obstruction, or other causes of cholestasis involves the use of tests from the cholestatic group of tests with the caveat that bilirubin and GGT are also included in the liver-function test and hepatocellular groups, respectively.

HEPATITIS

Hepatitis, or inflammation of the hepatic parenchyma, is manifested by an elevation in parenchymal enzymes. It can be an acute self-limiting process or a chronic process. Infections, especially viral (A, B, C, D, E, G, cytomegalovirus, herpes simplex [Table 40-13]), are the most common causes, but hepatitis can have many other causes, such as toxic (alcohol and drug),

TABLE 40-13
VIRUSES CAUSING HEPATITIS

	HAV	HBV	HCV	HDV	HEV	HGV
Viral properties						
Size (mm)	27	42	~55	~36	~32	?
Nucleic acid	RNA	DNA	RNA	RNA	RNA	
Classification	Picornavirus	Hepadnavirus	Flavivirus-like	Calicivirus or Alphavirus-like	Flavivirus	
Incubation (days)	15–45	30–180	15–160	21–140	14–63	?
Transmission						
Fecal–oral	+++	−			+++	
Percutaneous	Rare	+++	+++	+++	−	++
Sexual	?	++	Unusual	++	+−	?
Perinatal		+++	Unusual			?
Clinical features						
Severity	Usually mild	Moderate	Mild	Possibly severe	Usually	Mild
Prognosis	Generally good	Worse with age, debility	Good		Good	
Chronic infection	No	1–2%: up to 90% neonates	80–90%	Common	No	Yes
Carrier state	No	Yes	Yes	Yes	No	Yes
Fulminant hepatitis	0.1%	1%	Rare	Up to 20% in superinfection	1–2% (10–20% in pregnancy)	?
Hepatoma	No	Yes	Yes	?	No	?
Prophylaxis	IG, vaccine	HBIG, vaccine	None	None (HBV vaccine for susceptible persons)	None	None

HAV = hepatitis A virus; HBIG = hepatitis B immune globulin; HBV = hepatitis B virus; HVC = hepatitis C virus; HDV = hepatitis D (delta) virus; HEV = hepatitis E virus; HGV = hepatitis G virus; IG = immune globulin; ++ = sometimes; +++ = often; ? = possibly; − = not.

autoimmune, genetic (Wilson disease, hemochromatosis), and ischemic. The most common forms of viral hepatitis are A, B, and C. The clinical features are quite similar. While the onset is more abrupt with hepatitis A, it is more insidious with hepatitis B and C. An influenza-like prodrome precedes the development of jaundice. However, anicteric disease can be common. The development of nausea, anorexia, a distaste for cigarettes in smokers, and altered bowel habits occur frequently during this prodrome period and during the early phase of icterus. In general, the onset of improvement usually begins after 1 to 2 weeks of jaundice. Once this occurs it tends to be progressive in hepatitis A and B, resulting in recovery within 3 to 4 months in the majority of patients. However in hepatitis B, the illness can be prolonged (6 to 12 months) with a resultant benign outcome.

During pregnancy, the clinical manifestations of acute viral hepatitis do not differ from those found in nonpregnant women and men. In addition, laboratory data are also similar to those found in nonpregnant individuals. Acute hepatitis has little adverse maternal effect in Western Europe and the United States except in cases of fulminant hepatic failure. However, there appears to be an increased risk in the underdeveloped world, possibly due to poor nutrition and an increased incidence of hepatitis E. However, in late pregnancy acute hepatitis can result in premature labor but without adverse fetal effect. Lastly, acute viral hepatitis is associated with a greater but small increased rate of fetal loss in well-nourished mothers.

In addition to hepatitis there are many other liver disorders that can occur either caused by or contingent with pregnancy. It is important to realize this possibility so that these patients can be followed by the appropriate specialist in addition to the patient's obstetrician/gynecologist (Table 40-14).

Hepatitis A

Hepatitis A virus (HAV) is caused by an RNA virus and accounts for from 20 to 25% of all acute hepatitis. It is transmitted primarily by the fecal–oral route either by person-to-person spread or by consumption of contaminated food or water. However, percutaneous transmission has been reported. It is unclear whether sexual intercourse not involving fecal–oral contamination is a mode of transmission. The incubation period is from 15 to 50 days. Because of its predominant mode of spread, it is more common in underdeveloped and overcrowded areas with poor sanitation. In the developed world, epidemics of hepatitis A are found in the military, associated with day-care centers, or associated with food handlers. In addition, epidemics can be caused by the ingestion of shellfish caught from areas near sewage effluent pipes. The acute disease is mostly mild and rarely fulminant; however, it may be severe in patients >60 years of age. It often has a subclinical course in children, while adults are more ill and more often have a disease associated with jaundice. Fecal shedding is maximal approximately 2 weeks before and 1 week after the

---

TABLE 40-14
HEPATIC DISORDERS DURING PREGNANCY

Hepatic disorders as a result of pregnancy
  Preeclampsia
  Eclampsia
  Hyperemesis gravidarum
  Acute fatty liver of pregnancy
  HELLP
  Hepatic infarction
  Hepatic rupture
  Intrahepatic cholestasis of pregnancy
  Tetracycline-induced fatty liver
  Budd–Chiari syndrome
Intercurrent hepatic disorders during pregnancy
  Acute hepatitis
    A
    B
    C
    D (delta)
    E
    Herpes simplex
    Cytomegalovirus
    Drug
    Autoimmune
  Fulminant hepatic failure
    Infectious
    Toxic
    Drug
    Ischemic
    Other
  Acute cholecystitis
  Acute cholangitis
  Biliary-tract calculus disease
  Other biliary-tract disorders
Pregnancy in patient with preexisting liver disease
  Chronic hepatitis
    Infectious
    Autoimmune
    Wilson disease
    α_1-antitrypsin deficiency
  Cirrhosis with or without portal hypertension
  Primary biliary cirrhosis
  Sclerosing cholangitis
  Hepatobiliary tumors
  Pregnancy following liver transplantation

onset of the illness. Since the virus is usually cleared from the feces soon after the onset of jaundice, isolation of jaundiced patients after that time usually does not prevent the spread of the illness. It is notable that during the period of fecal shedding the virus is present in the serum and saliva at low levels. The most frequent risk factors for HAV in the United States are household or sexual contacts with an infected person (24%), day-care attendance or employment (15%), international travel (6%), and food- or water-borne outbreaks (5%). Therefore, immune globulin a dose of 0.02 ml/kg intramuscularly should be given to institutional possible contacts or household contacts of the infected patient. In addition, immune globulin should be given to those exposed to a possibly infected food source. This passive immunization may be effective when administered as late as 2 weeks after exposure. However, passive immunization may inhibit the induction of endogenous anti-HAV. Therefore, these patients most likely will be susceptible to future exposure to HAV. Maternal–fetal transmission of HAV is uncommon. However, transmission may occur if acute hepatitis is present in late pregnancy. Immune globulin at a dose of 0.5 ml at birth is optional in this case.

Since a vaccine has been developed, it should be given to high-risk individuals. Persons likely to benefit from this vaccine include military recruits, persons working or residing in institutional settings, travelers to endemic regions, patients who participate in high-risk behavior for fecal–oral contamination, and patients with chronic liver disease who would be at greater risk of an unfavorable outcome if they contacted the disease. Protective antibody levels are usually detectable within 14 to 21 days after the first injection. It most probably will be given to a broad spectrum of people early in life in the future in the hope of eliminating the disease.

The prognosis of the disease is excellent, and neither chronic liver disease nor chronic hepatitis develops from HAV infections. Serologic tests are useful in the diagnosis of the disease. IgM anti-HAV is present during the acute disease and generally persists from 2 to 6 months. This is overlapped by the development of an IgG anti-HAV that persists and confers lifelong immunity. However, several cases of reinfection have been reported, but these are very rare. Acute hepatitis A rarely is characterized by very significant cholestatsis (bilirubin >20 mg/dl) and may be mistaken for biliary obstruction. Direct infection of the biliary epithelium lining the intrahepatic and extrahepatic bile ducts and gallbladder by HAV infection is thought to be the cause. Sufficient therapy with strict hand washing is important.

Hepatitis B

Hepatitis B virus (HBV), a DNA virus, consists of a surface and a core. The core consists of a core and e protein or antigen. Antibodies to these components are useful in the diagnosis, prognosis, and characterization of this disease. Worldwide, it is estimated that 300 to 400 million persons are carriers of HBV, resulting in an average hepatitis B surface antigen seroprevalence of 5%. However, in the United States, 1.2 million carriers are estimated from a seroprevalence of 0.1 to 0.5%. Thus, there are approximately 300,000 new infections annually in the United States.

The United States, Canada, Australia, and Western and Northern Europe have the lowest prevalence rates. However, within these areas certain groups participate in high-risk behavior such as intravenous drug abuse and homosexual acts. In the United States, African Americans have a higher seroprevalence than do whites. The risk is highest (70 to 80%) in infants born to mothers with active viral replication (positive e antigen and/or positive HBV-DNA) as compared with those who are chronic carriers without viral replication (10 to 20%). Children not infected at birth are still at high risk for acquiring HBV infection in endemic areas.

Hepatitis B is spread parentally, by sexual contact, by homosexual practices, by having multiple sex partners (homosexuals and heterosexuals), by being a sex partner of an infected patient, or by vertical transmission from mother to child during childbirth. Therefore, the groups at high risk for this disease include intravenous-drug users, health-care workers, and persons with multiple sexual contacts. Also, household contacts of infected patients are at increased risk. Most infections in adults are subclinical, while most symptomatic infections resolve within 6 months.

HBV causes liver injury mediated by a cellular immune response rather than any direct cytopathic effect. Therefore, after entry into the hepatocyte cytoplasm the virus is encoded and the nucleocapsid core transported to the nucleus, where the viral genome undergoes completion of it double-stranding by DNA polymerase. This forms covalently circular DNA, which serves as the template for four major RNA transcripts. These are packaged in the cytoplasm and

Figure 40-1 Time sequence of serologic markers in acute HBV infection, with recovery. anti-HBc = hepatitis B core antibody; HBsAg = hepatitis B surface antigen; anti-HBs = hepatitis B surface antibody; HBeAg = hepatitis B e antigen.

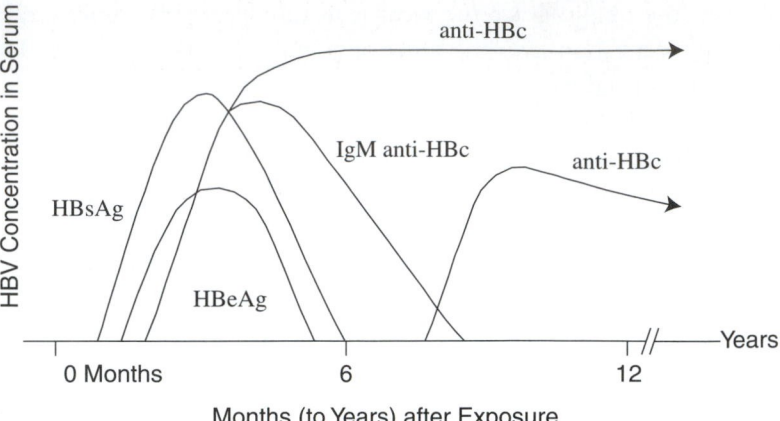

then transported out of the cell. This is followed by a recycling back into the nucleus. Core material is processed and transported out of the hepatocyte and is then spread throughout the liver. The core antigen on the hepatocyte is recognized by the HLA cells, therefore attracting cytotoxic T lymphocytes. The nature and extent of the immune recognition and response defines whether the HBV infection is terminated at that time or becomes a chronic infection.

The three antigens HBsAg, HBcAg, and HBeAg induce specific antibody responses that can be assessed by serology (Fig. 40-1). In acute, self-limited disease, HBsAg, HBeAg, and anti-HBcAg can be identified by serologic testing from 2 to 4 weeks before clinical hepatitis symptoms begin. In addition, HBV-DNA and DNA polymerase are elevated before the onset of symptoms. Initially, IgM and IgG anti-HBc are present; however, IgM anti-HBc generally declines to undetectable levels during the first 6 months while the IgG anti-HBc remains elevated permanently. HBV-DNA, HBeAg, and DNA polymerase are the first markers to be lost. This often occurs be-

fore the onset of symptoms. HBsAg disappears, with recovery from the disease being followed by the rise of anti-HBs and anti-HBe 2 weeks to 6 months later. This signifies the end of the disease. The period between these two events is referred to as the window period. During this period anti-HBc may be the only serologic evidence of the disease. Therefore, in a case of suspected hepatitis B it is important to repeat the serologic tests later to confirm the diagnosis. (See Tables 40-15, 40-16, and 40-17).

When symptoms occur during acute hepatitis B they are usually more severe than in patients suffering from acute hepatitis A or C, and the primary symptom of jaundice usually resolves within 4 weeks. HBV is not a cytopathic virus and the hepatocellular damage is due to the host's immune response to the viral-infected cells and accounts for the symptoms. Some patients have preicteric symptoms similar to "serum sickness," which includes urticaria and arthralgias that may be related to the presence of immune complexes. These complexes can result in glomerulonephritis and polyarteritis. Therefore, symptomatic

---

TABLE 40-15
SUMMARY OF HEPATITIS B MARKERS

Marker	Characteristics
HBsAg	First serologic marker to appear; disappears with clinical improvement; presence with anti-HBc IgM indicates acute infection; persistence beyond 6 months indicates chronic infection (and infectivity).
anti-HBc	Indicates current or previous infection; together with a negative HBsAg, indicates recovery; must determine the anti-HBc IgM status to definitively diagnose an acute infection; persists indefinitely.
anti-HBc IgM	Indicates acute disease, converts to anti-HBc IgG after acute
HBeAg	Present during acute infection, may persist for up to 6 months; helps distinguish acute from chronic infection; simultaneous presence with HBsAg confirms acute infection. Indicates active replication of the virus; highly infectious; may be detectable in acute or chronic HBV infection.
anti-HBs	Indicates recovery and/or immunity; detectable after HBsAg disappears and recovery is complete; indicates immunity after inoculation with hepatitis B vaccine or may be passively acquired from HBIG.

TABLE 40-16
MOST COMMON PATTERNS OF HEPATITIS B VIRUS SEROLOGY

HBsAg	Anti-HBs	Anti-HBc	HBeAg	Anti-Hbe	Interpretation
+	−	IgM	+	−	Acute HBV infection, high infectivity
+	−	IgG	+	−	Chronic HBV infection, high infectivity
+	−	IgG	−	+	Late-acute or chronic HBV infection, low infectivity
+	+	+	+ −	+ −	HBSAg of one subtype and heterotypic anti-HBs (common)
					Process of seroconversion from HbsAg to anti-HBs (rare)
−	−	IgM	+ −	+ −	Acute HBV infection; anti-HBC window
−	−	IgG	−	+ −	Low-level HbsAg carrier; remote past infection
−	+	IgG	−	+ −	Recovery from HBV infection
−	+	−	−	−	Immunization with HBsAg (after vaccination); remote past infection(?)
					False (+)

From Dienstag JL, Wands JR, Isselbacher KJ. Acute hepatitis. In: Wilson JD, Braunwald E, Isselbacher KJ, Petersdorf RG, Martin JB, Fauci AS, Root RK, eds. Harrison's principles of internal medicine. 12th ed. New York, McGraw-Hill, 1991:1322.

patients are more likely to clear the virus than patients with subclinical disease and symptomatic patients are less likely to become carriers. Thus, 90% of children who are more likely to have a subclinical disease are more likely not to clear the virus after 6 months, while 10% of adults, who are more likely to have symptomatic disease, are not likely to clear the virus. In addition, the patients who recover from fulminant hepatitis B rarely become carriers.

Various proportions of acutely infected persons become carriers. A carrier is defined as having (+) HBsAg for more than 6 months. Two major forms of chronic HBV have been described: those with active viral replication and those without active viral repli-

TABLE 40-17
HEPATITIS B SEROLOGY INTERPRETATION

Test	Results	Interpretation	Recommendation
HBsAg	Neg	Susceptible to infection (never	Consider vaccination especially
Anti-HBc	Neg	exposed to virus)	if high-risk patient
HBsAg	Pos	Acute or chronic infection	Further evaluation
Anti-HBc	Pos or Neg		
HBsAG	Neg	Multiple interpretations*	Consider vaccination especially
Anti-HBc	Pos		if high-risk patient
HBsAg (For further evaluation consider)	Pos	Carrier with chronic infection (HBsAG [+] for ≥6 mos),	Further evaluation Refer for possible therapy
Anti-HBc	Pos		
Anti-HBs	Neg		
HBeAg (last 2 not part of screening)	Pos	Highly infectious	
HBsAg	Pos	Carrier with chronic infection	Further evaluation
Anti-HBc	Pos	(HBsAG [+] for ≥6 mos),	
Anti-HBs	Neg	less infectious	
HBeAg (last 2 not part of screening)	Neg		

*An individual positive of Anti-HBc and negative for anti-HBs (four possible interpretations):
1. Patient recovering from acute HBV infection, with loss of HBsAg, but anti-HBs has not appeared (often called the serological window);
2. Immune to HBV, but anti-HBs never appeared for has fallen below detection levels;
3. Chronic HBV infection, with low levels of HBsAG that are undetectable in serum; or
4. False positive anti-HBc, with susceptibility to HBV infection.

cation. The chronic carrier state is defined by the absence of viral replication (HbsAg-positive and e-antigen-negative and/or HBV-DNA-negative). Chronic HBV infection with active viral replication is seen in 40 to 70% of adults who are chronic hepatitis B surface antigen carriers. This state is defined by the presence of HBV-DNA with or without the presence of e antigen. The probability of cirrhosis developing in these patients in 5 years is 15 to 20%. The frequency of the carrier state ranges from <5% in acutely infected immunocompetent adults to >90% in infected newborns. In addition, anti-HBc is found in high titers in the carrier state. In addition, HBeAg is found in the highly infectious replicative phases or anti-HBe in the less infectious nonreplicative phase. HBsAg is absent in the majority of carriers. Of note, patients who are HBeAg-positive have a high HBV-DNA that correlates with ongoing replication and indicates infectivity. In the absence of cirrhosis with marginal hepatocellular function and psychiatric dysfunction, the hepatitis B carrier should be referred to a gastroenterologist/hepatologist to be evaluated for possible therapy. Variants do exist that are unable to synthesize and secrete HBeAg. These variants may have high HBV-DNA levels but have a negative HBeAg. Patients with chronic hepatitis B with normal transminases in addition to normal histology are carriers with a good prognosis. Patients who are chronic carriers of HBsAg with elevated transaminases and evidence of ongoing liver disease or cirrhosis have a worse prognosis. These patients have an increased risk for hepatocellular carcinoma and should be screened regularly (every 6 months) with high-quality ultrasound and α-fetoprotein levels.

Since safe and effective vaccines have been available since 1983 for protection against hepatitis B, it is important that all persons in high-risk groups be vaccinated against hepatitis B. The American Liver Foundation recommends vaccination for these groups: health-care workers, emergency workers, pregnant women, international travelers, military personnel, morticians and embalmers, patients and staff of institutions for the mentally handicapped, intravenous-drug users who are not already positive, and ethnic groups with a high rate of hepatitis B, including Chinese, Koreans, Indochinese, Filipinos, Alaskan Eskimos, and Haitians. Persons who participate in promiscuous sex (prostitutes and hustlers) in addition to sexually active homosexual males would benefit from being vaccinated. Universal childhood vaccination is currently being advocated by many. In addition children aged 11 years and older who have not been previously immunized should receive vaccine.

The normal vaccine schedule is at 0, 1, and 6 months. For more rapid protection, a schedule of 0, 1, and 2 months has been shown to be as effective. Booster doses are not currently recommended for the majority of patients.

No treatment is considered necessary for acute hepatitis B except for supportive therapy, unless the disease is very severe and results in acute fulminant hepatic failure. For patients with asymptomatic chronic HbsAg carrier states no treatment is currently available. However, with chronic hepatitis B with active viral replication (e-antigen-positive and/or HBV-DNA-positive with chronic hepatitis features on liver biopsy and elevated transaminases), the patient should be referred to a specialist for further treatment.

Hepatitis C

Hepatitis C virus (HCV), a single-stranded RNA virus, causes most cases of posttransfusion hepatitis for transfusions prior to the development of hepatitis C screening assays (~1989). Of the six genotypes of the virus, ~70% of HCV in the United States are types 1a or 1b.

Acute HCV is now rarely seen, since posttransfusion cases have largely disappeared. However, cases are seen following acute needle sticks or other parenteral exposures. The incubation period is 7 weeks (range, 3 to 20 weeks). The symptoms include malaise, right upper quadrant discomfort, nausea, and jaundice. The ALT levels begin to rise prior to the onset of symptoms. The AST and ALT values are usually less than 1000 U per liter (mostly lower than hepatitis A or B). Clinical illness lasts from 2 to 12 weeks. Fulminant hepatic failure is rare. Diagnosis is confirmed by finding HCV-RNA, which is detectable within 1 to 2 weeks of infection. However, anti-HCV does not appear for several weeks or months. Acute HCV is thought to resolve completely in only 15% of cases. Chronic infection develops in 85% of cases, with persistence of HCV-RNA and often with elevated ALT resulting in the evolution to chronic hepatitis by biopsy. At present it is believed that 20 to 30% of adults with chronic infection will have cirrhosis after the first 20 to 25 years. Excessive use of alcohol, being male, or being older than 50 years at the time of infection suggests a higher rate of cirrhosis.

Chronic infection is often discovered during the evaluation of asymptomatic chronically elevated AST or ALT, screening for blood donation, or as part of a routine physical or insurance examination. Seventy-five percent of patients are asymptomatic. The most common symptoms include nonspecific chronic fatigue, weakness, right upper quadrant discomfort, and less often, itching, anorexia, weight loss, and jaundice.

Several nonhepatic diseases are associated with chronic HCV. These include clinical depression, essential mixed cryoglobulinemia, arthritis, Mooren corneal ulcers, glomerulonephritis, Sjögren syndrome, lichen planus, thyroiditis, peripheral-nerve vasculitis, and porphyria cutanea tarda.

The most common presentation of hepatitis C is an asymptomatic elevation of AST and ALT, of which <10% present with icterus and >90% are anicteric. The major mode of transmission is by the percutaneous spread of infected serum. Therefore, patients at risk include those with a history of blood transfusions, parenteral drug abuse, tattoos, piercing, scarification, acupuncture, and needle-stick exposure. Sexual transmission is still unclear. Thirty percent to 40% of patients with HCV have no identifiable risk factors.

While most cases of transfusion-related hepatitis can be accounted for by HCV, <5% of all cases of hepatitis C are transfusion-related while 50% are the result of intravenous-drug use at some time in the patient's life. Maternal–fetal transmission of hepatitis C virus is uncommon, as evaluated by HCV-RNA—approximately 6% of infants born to mothers positive for anti-HCV. Infection occurred only if the mother was HCV-RNA-positive. In addition, the likelihood of infection correlated directly with the titer of HCV-RNA in the mother's serum, requiring more than 10^6 genome-equivalents per milliliter of serum. Sexual transmission has been difficult to either prove or disprove. Studies have shown no evidence of sexual transmission to as many as 27% of sexual partners of patients with HCV. Both sexual and perinatal transmission may be more common when the person is infected with both HCV and human immunodeficiency virus. Hepatitis C antibody may be detectable in the blood of infants of mothers with hepatitis C. This appears to be maternal–fetal transfer of the antibody, while maternal–fetal transfer of the virus needs to be checked with HCV-RNA. Since anti-HCV appears later in the course of the disease, initial presumptive diagnosis is based on a characteristic clinical and biochemical course in addition to risk factors for

HCV. In addition, ruling out other causes that have early markers helps with the diagnosis. HCV-RNA can be measured using polymerase chain reaction (PCR) with a high degree of sensitivity and specificity. It is important to remember that anti-HCV may be false positive if the serum specimens undergo prolonged storage. The correlation between symptoms and degree of hepatic inflammation is poor and the chronic disease is characterized by the fluctuations in liver transaminases. A high percentage of cases of acute hepatitis C evolve into chronic disease (50 to 90%). At least 20% progress to cirrhosis after about 20 years. These patients have an increased risk of hepatocellular carcinoma developing. Some of the complications noted to occur with hepatitis C include membranoproliferative glomerulonephritis, cryoglobulinemia, vasculitis, urticaria, erythema nodosum, lymphocytic sialadenitis, neuropathy, idiopathic pulmonary fibrosis, and autoimmune thyroiditis. Also, HCV might play a role in causing liver disease in nongenetic porphyria cutanea tarda and α_1-antitrypsin deficiency. Patients with chronic HCV infection may also have other autoantibodies such as fluorescent antinuclear antibody and anti-smooth muscle antibodies (ASMA), but in low titers.

The recommendations for prevention of HCV summarized by the Centers for Disease Control include the following:

- Avoid excess alcohol intake.
- Receive hepatitis A vaccine if not immune.
- Avoid donation of blood or semen.
- Avoid sharing razor blades or other articles with which blood-to-blood transfer might occur, and keep cuts and sores covered to prevent spread.
- There is no need to change current sexual practices and no need for mandatory use of condoms in individuals with a long-term steady sexual partner.
- There is no need to avoid pregnancy or breast-feeding.
- There is no need to avoid routine daily contact with other individuals in school or place of work; patients with chronic HCV infection should not be excluded from these settings.
- Health-care workers should maintain universal precautions.

Standard immune globulin has no place in treating HVC following a blood transfusion or needle stick. Persons who are acutely exposed should be tested for the presence of HCV-RNA; if they become positive, treatment with an interferon-based regimen is recommended to reduce the probability of chronic infection. These patients should seek the expertise of a specialist as therapies are constantly changing. However, immune globulin is optional therapy—0.5 ml immune serum globulin at birth for neonates of either acutely or chronically infected mothers. However, efficacy is questionable. No effective vaccine is available at this time.

The 1997 NIH Consensus Conference recommends treatment for patients with chronic HCV with associated evidence of portal or bridging fibrosis, detectable HCV-RNA, and elevated ALT values. These individuals were felt to be at the highest risk for cirrhosis. For all other patients, treatment should be offered on an individualized basis.

Interferon appears to be effective in normalizing aminotransferase levels in 40 to 50% of patients treated with 3 million units subcutaneously three times weekly for 6 months. However, 50% of these relapse after 6 months. Therefore, it would be advisable to refer patients with HCV to a specialist with expertise in treating hepatitis C or who has ongoing clinical trials for hepatitis C therapy. The combination of interferon and ribavirin has been used with better success. *Patients with hepatitis C should be referred to a specialist for the consideration of therapy.*

Hepatitis D (Delta)

Delta agent or HDV, an RNA virus, endemic around the Mediterranean region, requires the helper functions of the DNA virus, HBV, in order to cause an infection. Therefore, HDV is not found without the presence of HBV infection. An infection with HDV can coinfect with an acute infection with HBV or more commonly superinfect with a chronic HBV infection that results in a more severe hepatitis than with HBV alone. This results in a more rapid progression to cirrhosis and often results in fulminant hepatic failure. Spontaneous improvement is uncommon. Interferon at a dosage of 5 million units per day or 9 million units three times per week has been effective in resulting in a biochemical improvement in 50%. However, fewer patients show histologic improvements. Unfortunately, relapse rates can be up to 90% following discontinuation of therapy. Therefore, a gastroenterologist or hepatologist should treat these patients. Transmission varies. In North America and Western Europe HDV spread is predominantly via the percutaneous routes, intravenous-drug users, and hemophiliacs requiring many blood transfusions.

However, in the Mediterranean, transmission usually occurs by a nonpercutaneous route, such as intimate contact.

The diagnosis is based on the clinical picture, the fact that the patient is infected with HBV and detection of anti-HDV. This antibody is found in the blood transiently and in low titers in coinfected patients; but in superinfected patients the titers tend to be high and sustained. The only preventive measure available today is vaccination of patients at high risk for HDV with vaccine for HBV to prevent hepatitis B and therefore HDV infections.

Hepatitis E

Hepatitis E, another RNA virus, is (as hepatitis A) transmitted enterically. It tends to be found in the Indian subcontinent, Southeast Asia, Africa, and Mexico. The source of the infection is contaminated water after the rainy season. The disease, which is frequently cholestatic, is most commonly seen in persons from ages 15 to 40 years. However, subclinical disease may occur in children. Therefore, in the West it is most commonly seen in travelers from those regions. It resembles hepatitis A clinically. However, it is important to note that there is a high risk (mortality rate of 10 to 20%) of fulminant hepatitis in women who acquire hepatitis E during the third trimester. Hepatitis E does not result in a chronic infection or in chronic hepatitis. At present, an antibody test is available. IgM tends to be found during the acute phase followed by a rise in IgG. The titers of both diminish with time.

Herpes Simplex Virus Hepatitis

Herpes simply virus hepatitis (either Type I or II), although rare in healthy adults, is relatively more common in pregnant females. Approximately half of reported cases occurred in association with pregnancy, with a 50% mortality rate. Presentation generally begins with a 4- to 14-day history of systemic virus-like symptoms and fever in addition to right upper quadrant pain. Laboratory tests are characterized by an increased prothrombin time, a low bilirubin level (typically less than 3 mg/dl), and very high aminotransferase levels (>1000 units). If herpes simplex virus hepatitis is suspected, a gastroenterologist or hepatologist should be consulted. Liver biopsy is often diagnostic. In addition, vaginal, cervical, throat, and liver cultures are often positive. Aggressive evaluation and treatment of pregnant women is important since therapy with agents such as acyclovir has been successful in saving both mother and fetus. Pregnant females who exhibit fever, a viral syndrome, and significantly elevated aminotransferase values with associated moderately elevated or low serum bilirubin should be evaluated aggressively by a specialist (gastroenterologist or hepatologist) followed by immediate institution of antiviral therapy. Infants born to infected women should be closely observed and treated as needed.

Other

Many gastrointestinal diseases occur in obstetric patients either coincident or as a result of or exacerbated by pregnancy. As a result of this, very often medications would be helpful or are necessary. Table 40-18 is a listing of commonly used gastrointestinal drugs and their purported safety during pregnancy.

REFERENCES

Banerjee S, LaMont JT. Treatment of gastrointestinal infections. Gastroenterology 2000;118:S48.

Boland CR, Sinicrope FA, Brenner DE, Caethers JM. Colorectal cancer prevention and treatment. Gastroenterology 2000;118:S115.

Bond J. Practice guidelines: Polyp guideline: diagnosis, treatment and surveillance for patients with colorectal polyps. Am J Gastroenterology 2000;95:3053.

Davis GL. Current therapy for chronic hepatitis C. Gastroenterology 2000;118:S104.

Graham DY. Therapy of helicobacter pylori: Current status and issues. Gastroenterology 2000;118:S2.Killenberg PG. Extrahepatic manifestations of chronic hepatitis C. Seminars in Gastrointestinal Disease 2000;11:62.

Klinkenberg-Knol EC, Nelis F, Dent J, et al. Long-term omeprazole treatment in resistant gastroesophageal reflux disease: Efficacy, safety, and influence on gastric mucosa. Gastroenterology 2000;118:661.

Muir AJ. The natural history of hepatitis C viral infection. Seminars in Gastrointestinal Disease 2000;11:54.

Pandolfino JE, Howden CW, Kahrilas PJ. Motility-modifying agents and management of disorders of gastrointestinal motility. Gastroenterology 2000;118:S32.

Sands BE. Therapy of inflammatory bowel disease. Gastroenterology 2000;118:S68.

Shamoun DK, Anania FA. Which patients with hepatitis C virus should be treated? Seminars in Gastrointestinal Disease 2000;11:84.

Thompson WO, Longstreth GF, Drossman DA, Heaton KW, Jivine EJ, Mueller-Lissner SA. C. Functional bowel disorders. D. Functional Abdominal Pain. In: Drossman DA,

Thompson WG, Whitehead WE, Corazziari E, eds. Rome II: functional gastrointestinal disorders: Diagnosis, pathophysiology, and treatment. 2nd ed. McLean, VA: Degnon Associates, Inc., 2000.

Wolfe MM, Sachs G. Acid suppression: optimizing therapy for gastroduodenal ulcer healing, gastroesophageal reflux disease, and stress-related erosive syndrome. Gastroenterology 2000;118:S9.

TABLE 40-18
SAFETY OF GASTROINTESTINAL DRUGS DURING PREGNANCY

Disease/Drug	Safe*	Questionable Safety†	Unsafe‡
Gastroesophageal reflux			
Antacids§		X	
Sucralfate§	X		
Cimetidine§		X	
Ranitidine§	X		
Famotidine		X	
Nizatidine			X
Omeprazole§		X	
Metaclopramide§			X
Cisapride			X
Nausea and vomiting			
Meclizine			X
Promethazine		X	
Metaclopramide	X		
Pyridoxine	X		
Ondansetron		X	
Constipation			
Bulking agents (psyllium)	X		
Stool softeners (docusate)	X		
Lubricants (mineral oil)			X
Hyperosmotics (sorbitol, lactulose)	X		
Saline laxatives			
Milk of magnesia (low-dose)	X		
Glycerin suppositories	X		
Stimulants			
Senna			X
Biacondyl	X		
Phenolphthalein		X	
Castor oil		X	
Diarrhea			
Kaolin with pectate	X		
Loperamide		X	
Diphenoxylate/atropine			X
Bismuth subsalicylate			X
Gallstone			
Chenodeoxycholic acid			X
Urosodeoxycholic acid		X	

*Nonabsorbable, nonsytemic drugs, prospecive trials show safety.

†Not teratogenic in animals, human data are limited.

‡Teratogenic in animals or adverse human data.

§Safe in late third trimester of pregnancy.

Torbey CF, Richter JE. Gastrointestinal motility disorders in pregnancy. Semin Gastrointest Dis 1995;6:203.

Chapter 41

Chronic Fatigue Syndrome

Nancy S. Fuller
Robert E. Morrison

Five Key Points

- Fatigue is a very common symptom in patients presenting to primary care physicians, with many possible causes.

- Chronic fatigue syndrome is a relatively uncommon but debilitating cause of fatigue that most often affects women of childbearing age.

- Fatigue, constitutional symptoms, cognitive dysfunction, and exercise intolerance are the most frequently reported symptoms of chronic fatigue syndrome.

- Currently, there are no reliably reproducible laboratory tests that correlate with a diagnosis of chronic fatigue syndrome.

- Support and reassurance are the cornerstones of therapy for patients with chronic fatigue syndrome.

Fatigue is frequently reported by patients seeking medical attention from physicians, with as many as 25% of people seeking care from a primary care clinic citing fatigue as a major problem.[1] There are many identifiable diseases and syndromes that can cause patients to come to the primary care physician with fatigue: infections such as human immunodeficiency virus (HIV) and hepatitis B and C, autoimmune disorders, malignancy, psychiatric problems, diabetes, hypothyroidism, drug abuse, multiple sclerosis, myasthenia gravis, and chronic cardiac, pulmonary, or hepatic illness. For hundreds of year, however, there have been patients whose fatigue could not be categorized into any known disease process described in the medical literature and did not fit the medical model framework. In 1850, Sir Richard Manningham described a syndrome of "dullness, great lassitude, and weariness all over the body," which he called febricula or small continued fever. Austin Flint called this disorder nervous exhaustion, and George Beard coined the term *neurasthenia*. In 1871, Da Costa described chronic fatigue in veterans of the Civil War. The disease has been attributed to chronic brucellosis and premorbid personality traits leading to a higher frequency of prolonged recovery after acute illness. Straus has meticulously catalogued the multiple descriptions of the syndrome and its many considered causes throughout the history of medicine to recent times.[2] Interest was rekindled in 1987 after reports of an outbreak of chronic fatigue in Incline Village, Nevada.[3] The term *chronic fatigue syndrome* was coined by a group of experts gathered together by the Centers for Disease Control and Prevention (CDC) in 1988 and was chosen to reflect the most common symptom. Initially, chronic mononucleosis or chronic Epstein–Barr viremia were commonly used to describe chronic fatigue syndrome, and some patients may still use these terms; but these are incorrect and inappropriate labels.

Chronic fatigue syndrome, also known as chronic fatigue immune dysfunction syndrome, or CFIDS, is an illness characterized by debilitating fatigue of at least 6-month's duration resulting in at least 50% reduction in normal, preillness capabilities. It is associated with flulike symptoms, such as pharyngitis, adenopathy, low-grade fever, myalgia, arthralgias, headaches, difficulty concentrating, and exercise intolerance.[4] Fifty to 70% of patients meet criteria for the diagnosis of depression. Although a premorbid or concomitant diagnosis of depression was initially thought to be an exclusionary feature when diagnosing chronic fatigue syndrome, this was later changed.[5] Komaroff et al. have suggested adding a weight loss of at least 10% of body weight and anorexia to the case definition as well.[6] Cognitive dysfunction is very common and is one of the most debilitating symptoms. Patients report an inability to concentrate, marked forgetfulness, and difficulty with information-processing.

The incidence of chronic fatigue syndrome, as estimated by an ongoing CDC surveillance system, ranges between 4 and 8.6 cases per 100,000 adults in the United States.[4] Most cases are sporadic, but occasionally case clusters occur or close contacts become ill with chronic fatigue syndrome at about the same time. However, there are no published data to indicate that chronic fatigue syndrome is contagious through close or intimate contact. Chronic fatigue syndrome has been found in many countries, but most cases have been reported from the United States, Canada, United Kingdom, Australia, New Zealand, Spain, and France. There is a female : male ratio of 2 : 1, making chronic fatigue syndrome of special interest to obstetricians and gynecologists. Ninety percent of patients are between the ages of 20 and 50, but it has been reported in both children and the elderly. Initial reports from Nevada seem to reflect a tendency toward victims with higher education and middle-class status.[3] The term *yuppie flu* was coined to describe this phenomenon, but this socioeconomic grouping was possibly artifactual.[7] In 1988 the CDC first published a set of criteria by which the syndrome was defined for purposes of research, and this was updated in 1992 and 1994 (Table 41-1).

Because of the nonspecific nature of these complaints, the current lack of any specific laboratory markers, and the lack of knowledge of the pathophysiology of chronic fatigue syndrome, it has been slow to gain acceptance as a "real disease" in the

TABLE 41-1
1994 REVISED DIAGNOSTIC CRITERIA FOR CHRONIC FATIGUE SYNDROME*

Clinically evaluated, unexplained, persistent, or relapsing fatigue for at least 6 months that:
is of new or definite onset,
is not the result of ongoing exertion,
is not substantially alleviated by rest, and
results in substantial reduction in previous levels of occupational, educational, social, or personal activities.
Four or more of the following concurrent symptoms on a persistent or recurrent basis during 6 or more consecutive months of illness, none of which may predate the fatigue:
self-reported impairment in short-term memory or concentration that is severe enough to cause substantial reduction in previous levels of occupational, educational, social, or personal activities
sore throat
tender cervical or axillary lymph nodes
muscle pain
multiple joint pain without joint swelling or redness
headaches of a new type, pattern, or severity
unrefreshing sleep
postexertional malaise lasting more than 24 hours

*Both criteria are required conditions for a diagnosis of chronic fatigue syndrome.

After Fukuda K, Gantz N. Management strategies for chronic fatigue syndrome. Fed Pract. 1995;July:12.

medical world. Acceptance of chronic fatigue syndrome as a somatic disease is complicated by the fact that a large percentage of patients meet the diagnostic criteria for depression. Chronic fatigue syndrome accounts for probably less than 5% of all patients who present with fatigue; but because of the high percentage of patients who report fatigue and the marked functional impairment shown by patients with chronic fatigue syndrome, all primary care physicians will see in their practices patients who meet this case definition.

In patients who meet the case definition of chronic fatigue syndrome, no reproducible laboratory abnormalities have been found. Blood chemistries, complete blood count, and erythrocyte sedimentation rate are all typically within normal limits. Immunologic abnormalities cited in various studies have remained unconfirmed and are often contradictory and have not been shown to correlate with symptoms. These include depressed natural-killer cells, modest increases in the number of activated lymphocytes, and slight elevation of circulating immune complexes. None are specific for chronic fatigue syndrome or abnormal in all patients with chronic fatigue syndrome.[8] Causative agents have been widely sought. Infectious agents considered include Brucella, Epstein–Barr virus, herpesvirus type 6, coxsackieviruses, and retroviruses. One study identified viral RNA suggestive of a retrovirus, but despite intense efforts, this study has not been duplicated.[9] Controlled studies have found no evidence of consistent elevation of antibodies to viruses, although reactivation of dormant viruses is found in some patients. Patients with chronic fatigue syndrome do not get an AIDS-like illness or immunosuppression. Various researchers have described low cellular magnesium levels, low carnitine levels, and subtle cardiomyopathy as possible causes of chronic fatigue syndrome; but none of these theories has been validated.[10,11]

Changes in the central nervous system, specifically the limbic system, have been described by several researchers.[12] In a review of patients from a large cohort in Nevada in the 1980s, whose description stimulated the current interest in chronic fatigue syndrome, more than 75% of the patients with chronic fatigue syndrome tested by magnetic resonance imaging (MRI) showed unidentified bright spots (UBOs) as compared with 21% of controls.[13] Single-photon-emission computed tomography (SPECT), which evaluates cerebral blood flow, had abnormal results in a significant number of patients with chronic fatigue syndrome, although the findings are nonspecific and displayed a significant overlap with SPECT scans of patients with primary depression.[14] Demitrack and associates studied a small number of patients who displayed hypothalamic–pituitary–adrenal axis dysfunction with hypothalamic hypocorticolism as compared with controls, and significantly, opposite to findings typically associated with major depression.[15] A small study found neurally mediated hypotension in a population of patients with chronic fatigue syndrome, and 9 of 23 reported resolution of symptoms with fludrocortisone treatment.[16] A case–control study looking at possible triggers or associations found only a higher likelihood of regular exercise in the year preceding development of chronic fatigue syndrome.[17] A larger number of potential cofactors and triggers, including history of allergies; depression; sleep disorders; fibromyalgia; irritable bowel syndrome; drug and/or sexual abuse; life stresses; consumption of raw milk or meat, vitamins, or food supplements; cigarette smoking; travel; or exposure to animals were not associated with a statistically significant increase in the development of chronic fatigue syndrome.[17] These reports, like much of the literature on chronic fatigue

---

TABLE 41-2
SOME CONDITIONS THAT CAN EXPLAIN CHRONIC FATIGUE

Hypothyroidism
Sleep apnea
Narcolepsy
Unresolved hepatitis B or C
Alcohol or substance abuse
Severe obesity
Medication site effects
Systemic lupus erythematosus
Multiple sclerosis
Major depressive disorder
Anorexia nervosa
Bulimia
Schizophrenia
Bipolar disorder
Dementia

From National Institute of Allergy and Infectious Diseases. Chronic fatigue syndrome: information for physicians. Washington, DC: Government Printing Office, 1997. Publication no. 97-484.

---

syndrome, should be regarded as exploratory. Although the studies reported above generally represent controlled, blinded research, many of the published reports do not reflect the application of optimal statistical methods or a rigorous experimental design.

In evaluating patients with fatigue, a careful history should be taken to exclude diseases known to be associated with fatigue and to include criteria associated with the case definition of chronic fatigue syndrome (Table 41-2). Special reference should be made to the onset of symptoms. Was there a flu-like illness or was the onset gradual and insidious? A majority of patients report onset of symptoms following an acute illness; however, this is not definitive. A substantial number of patients report a more gradual onset without an inciting event. The character of the fatigue is important. Is the fatigue present on awakening (nonrestorative sleep)? Is the fatigue brought on by exertion? Does it progress throughout the day, and is it accompanied by weakness? The fatigue in chronic fatigue syndrome is typically present throughout the day, including on awakening, and is worsened with exercise and not improved by rest. It is different from the fatigue associated with sleepiness or sleep disorders such as sleep apnea.

Careful attention to the patient's description of fatigue is essential in differentiating chronic fatigue syndrome from very treatable sleep disorders. Constitutional symptoms associated with fatigue can be significant. Has the patient had fever, chills, or night sweats? Is there significant weight loss or anorexia?

TABLE 41-3
DRUGS COMMONLY ASSOCIATED WITH FATIGUE

Antihypertensives
  β-Blockers, e.g., propranolol
  α-Blockers, e.g., α-methyldopa
  Reserpine
Antihistamines
Antispasmodics, e.g., hyoscyamine sulfate
Muscle relaxants, e.g., carisoprodol
Antidepressants, e.g., amitriptyline
Anxiolytics, e.g., hypnotics, diazepam
Steroids
Anticonvulsants

These may indeed be seen in chronic fatigue syndrome but would direct the physician to look more closely for infectious diseases or malignancy and to periodically reevaluate the patient after a diagnosis of chronic fatigue syndrome is made. Cognitive dysfunction is important. Has the patient had difficulty with thought processes or noted confusion? These are key symptoms in chronic fatigue syndrome and are reported by nearly all patients. Headaches, myalgias, arthralgias, and painful subjective adenopathy are common in patients with chronic fatigue syndrome, although a description of arthritis should cause the physician to ask careful questions pertinent to the diagnosis of connective-tissue diseases. If anhedonia is present, depression is more likely to be the primary diagnosis rather than a related finding. Recent travel, insect bites, and tick exposure, and skin rashes should be discussed, as this may point to other diagnoses for consideration. Many prescription and over-the-counter medications, including antihypertensives, antihistamines, and antidepressants, have fatigue or somnolence as side effects (Table 41-3). Ascertaining a detailed medical history, family history, and social habits is essential, including inquiring about the use of illicit drugs and alcohol and caffeine consumption. In addition to medical conditions that may cause fatigue, severe obesity, acute or recent alcohol or substance abuse, and severe mental illness are conditions that exclude the diagnosis of chronic fatigue syndrome.

A careful physical examination is required to evaluate the patient for other causes of fatigue. Specific physical findings such as nonexudative pharyngitis, tender lymphadenopathy, skin rashes, muscle tenderness (often in tender point areas such as seen with fibromyalgia), and orthostatic hypotension are seen in various combinations in a large number of patients with chronic fatigue syndrome. The Romberg test and tandem gait should be tested and may be abnormal in up to 20% of patients with chronic fatigue syndrome. However, peripheral neuropathy or other neurologic sensory motor deficits are not seen in chronic fatigue syndrome.

Laboratory tests should include a complete blood count with differential, erythrocyte sedimentation rate, serum electrolytes, glucose, blood urea nitrogen and creatinine, calcium, phosphorus, total bilirubin, aspartate and alanine aminotransferases, alkaline phosphatase, creatine kinase, urinalysis, fluorescent antinuclear antibodies, thyroid-stimulating hormone, HIV antibodies, a purified protein derivative with controls, and chest radiography. There is no value in obtaining viral titers, immune function studies, MRI unless otherwise indicated, or other tests being described in research articles. These are very expensive, not validated, and will not change the treatment of the patient. A National Institutes of Health consensus panel on chronic fatigue syndrome specifically recommended against obtaining exotic laboratory tests.[4]

Once a diagnosis of chronic fatigue syndrome is made, the physician's main role is to provide the patient with caring, support, and acknowledgment that their fatigue is real, as the patient's perception of the physician's attitude toward chronic fatigue syndrome is important (Table 41-4). It is also important to stress that patients tend to improve over time, that continued downward progression of the syndrome is unlikely, and that no one dies from chronic fatigue syndrome.[18] Efforts should be made to decrease secondary gain with reassurance and encouragement of

TABLE 41-4
ELEMENTS OF TREATMENT OF PATIENTS WITH CHRONIC FATIGUE SYNDROME

Establish therapeutic alliance with patient
Dispel misinformation about the disease
Use a medical team approach
Prescribe symptomatic treatments
Urge stress reduction
Introduce slowly graduated exercise
Suggest rehabilitation therapy to develop energy-conservation techniques
Schedule regular follow-up visits
Give emotional support

From National Institute of Allergy and Infectious Diseases. Chronic fatigue syndrome: information for physicians. Washington, DC: Government Printing Office, 1997. Publication no. 97-484.

normal functioning and activities. However, patients should be advised not to engage in extremely strenuous activities, but to progressively increase their activities and maintain follow-up. Deconditioning is a major problem in chronic fatigue syndrome and tends to increase fatigue and decrease exercise tolerance. A study of a controlled trial of exercise versus relaxation showed a marked trend of improvement in function both in short- and long-term follow-up.[19] Being available to the patient for reassurance and caring is important. Cognitive behavioral therapy, which also incorporates psychological interest in with reconditioning, was also helpful.[20] Medical treatment of chronic fatigue syndrome has been frustrating, as very few controlled clinical trials have been published and anecdotal reports abound. Symptom-specific treatment may be helpful. Since chronic fatigue syndrome is closely related to fibromyalgia, many patients may benefit from the use of low-dose tricyclic antidepressants, such as amitriptyline, which help with the sleep disturbance commonly seen with these disorders. Small doses of serotonin reuptake inhibitors have also been shown to be helpful in some patients, starting with lower doses than are typically used in depression. One controlled Scottish study showed some improvement in chronic fatigue syndrome patients who took omega-3 and omega-6 fish oils, and these are readily available in health food stores.[21] Some patients with chronic fatigue syndrome may try other nutritional supplements recommended by chronic fatigue syndrome support groups and the lay literature, but no valid scientific data are available to support their use. Trials, some scientifically sound and others not, have been conducted to test the use of acyclovir, immunoglobulins, interferon alfa, liver extract, magnesium sulfate, and transfer factor. None showed any significant benefit over placebo. Pdy (1)-Poly(C12c) (Ampligen) is an immune-mediated molecule that has been shown to improve function in patients with chronic fatigue syndrome but cannot universally be recommended because of problems with side effects.[4] Because of the study showing neurally mediated hypotension in chronic fatigue syndrome, tilt table testing and a trial of treatment directed toward correcting the abnormal response may be considered, although the trial was small and as yet unconfirmed.

If patients present claiming a disability, remember that disability is a lack of ability to perform. Careful evaluation of signs and symptoms that would indicate disability, such as weakness or psychological disorders,

should be documented with comparisons to premorbid abilities. Altered mental abilities should be evaluated by careful psychometric testing. It is important to remain as objective as possible in determining disability.

Chronic fatigue syndrome is a recurring, debilitating illness complicated by the fact that its diagnosis is based largely on subjective complaints. No reproducibly reliable diagnostic tests are currently available. Care must be taken to exclude potentially treatable causes of fatigue, to intermittently rethink the diagnosis of chronic fatigue syndrome, and to consider any new problems distinctly rather than to assume that all future complaints arise from chronic fatigue syndrome. Eventually, new information regarding diagnosis and treatment of chronic fatigue syndrome may help physicians and their patients who struggle with it. For now, support and reassurance remain the cornerstones of therapy.

REFERENCES

1. Cathebras PJ, Robbins JM, Kirmayer LJ, Hayton BC. Fatigue in primary care: prevalence, psychiatric comorbidity, illness behavior, and outcome. J Gen Intern Med. 1992; 7:276.
2. Straus SE. History of chronic fatigue syndrome. Rev Infect Dis 1991;13(Suppl 1):S2.
3. Holmes GP, Kaplan JE, Stewart JA, et al. A cluster of patients with a chronic mononucleosis-like syndrome: is Epstein–Barr virus the cause? JAMA 1987;257:2297.
4. Fukuda K, Straus SE, Hickie I, et al. The chronic fatigue syndrome: a comprehensive approach to its definition and study. Ann Intern Med 1994;121:953.
5. Schluederberg A, Straus SE, Peterson P, et al. Chronic fatigue syndrome research: definition and medical outcome assessment. Ann Intern Med 1992;117:325.
6. Komaroff AL, Fagioli LR, Geiger AM, et al. An examination of the working case definition of chronic fatigue syndrome. Am J Med 1996;100:56.
7. Shafran SD. The chronic fatigue syndrome. Am J Med 1991;90:730.
8. Mawle AC, Nisenbaum R, Dobbins JG, et al. Seroepidemiology of chronic fatigue syndrome: a case-control study. Clin Infect Dis 1995;21:1386.
9. Khan AS, Heneine WM, Chapman LE, et al. Assessment of a retrovirus sequence and other possible risk factors for the chronic fatigue syndrome in adults. Ann Intern Med 1993;118:241.
10. Cox I, Campbell M, Dowson D. Red blood cell magnesium and chronic fatigue syndrome. Lancet 1991;337:757.
11. Plioplys A, Plioplys S. Meeting the frustrations of chronic fatigue syndrome. Hosp Pract 1997;June 15:147.
12. Goldstein J. Chronic fatigue syndrome: limbic encephalopathy in a dysfunctional neuroimmune network. CFIDS Chronicle 1991;3:19.

13. Buchwald D, Cheney PR, Peterson DL, et al. A chronic illness characterized by fatigue, neurological and immunologic disorders, and active herpes virus type 6 infection. Ann Intern Med 1992;116:103.

14. Schwartz R, Komaroff A, Garada B, et al. SPECT imaging of the brain: comparison of findings in patients with chronic fatigue syndrome, AIDS dementia complex, and major unipolar depression. AJR Am J Roentgenol 1994; 162:943.

15. Demitrack M, Gold PW, Chrousas GP, et al. Evidence for impaired activation of the hypothalamic-pituitary-adrenal axis in patients with chronic fatigue syndrome. J Clin Endocrinol Metab 1991;73:1224.

16. Bou-Holagah I, Rowe PC, Kan J, et al. The relationship between neurally mediated hypotension and the chronic fatigue syndrome. JAMA 1995;274:961.

17. MacDonald KL, Osterholm MT, LeDell KH, et al. A case-control study to assess possible triggers and cofactors in chronic fatigue syndrome. Am J Med 1996;100:548.

18. Gold D, Bowden R, Sixbey J, et al. Chronic fatigue—a prospective clinical and virologic study. JAMA 1990; 264:48.

19. Fulcher K, White P. Randomized controlled trial of graded exercise in patients with the chronic fatigue syndrome. BMJ 1997;314:1647.

20. Deale A, Chalder T, Marks I, Wessely S. Cognitive behavior therapy for chronic fatigue syndrome: a randomized controlled trial. Am J Psychiatry 1997;154:408.

21. Behan PO, Behan WMH, Horrobin D. Effect of high doses of essential fatty acids on the postviral fatigue syndrome. Acta Neurol Scand 1990;82:209.

Chapter 42

Contraception/Family Planning

Christine W. Jordan
Andrew M. Kaunitz

Five Key Points

- **In healthy, nonsmoking women, use of combination oral contraceptives does not increase the risk of heart attack or stroke.**

- **Use of combination oral contraceptives is associated with important noncontraceptive benefits, including prevention of ovarian and endometrial carcinoma.**

- **Use of progestin-only contraceptives, including Depo-Provera, "minipills," and implants is appropriate in lactating and other women in whom contraceptive doses of estrogen should be avoided.**

- **The copper T IUD is as effective as sterilization and does not cause infertility.**

- **The copper T IUD prevents pregnancy through a spermicidal action which prevents fertilization; the risk of ectopic pregnancy is lower than in women using no contraception.**

Half of all pregnancies in the United States are unintended. In addition, some 1.4 million induced abortions are performed annually in the United States. These sobering observations underscore the important role obstetrician-gynecologists can play in encouraging their patients to use effective methods of contraception. Unfortunately, no single method is ideal for all patients. Clinicians must therefore consider such factors as overall effectiveness, patient compliance, and side effects as they help their patients to make prudent contraceptive choices. Hormonal and intrauterine methods represent approaches to fertility regulation more cost effective than female sterilization.

This chapter reviews oral, injectable, implantable, intrauterine, barrier, and periodic abstinence contraception, focusing on approaches that help candidates select appropriate methods and on management measures that maximize contraceptive efficacy and patient

satisfaction. Placement of contraceptive implants and intrauterine devices (IUDs), as with any minor surgical procedure, is best learned through directly supervised training. The manufacturers of implants and IUDs have prepared useful teaching videos. In addition, package labeling for these methods includes illustrations detailing insertion techniques.

Among women in the United States of reproductive age, approximately 64% utilized some form of contraception in 1995 (Figure 42-1). The most popular method, used by 27.7% of women practicing contraception, was female sterilization. The next most common method chosen by American women was combination oral contraceptives (OCs), used by 26.9%. Nearly as many women used condoms for contraception, with approximately 21% choosing that method. Three percent reported using medroxyprogesterone acetate injections (DMPA), while 1.3% and 0.8%, respectively, reported using implants and IUDs.

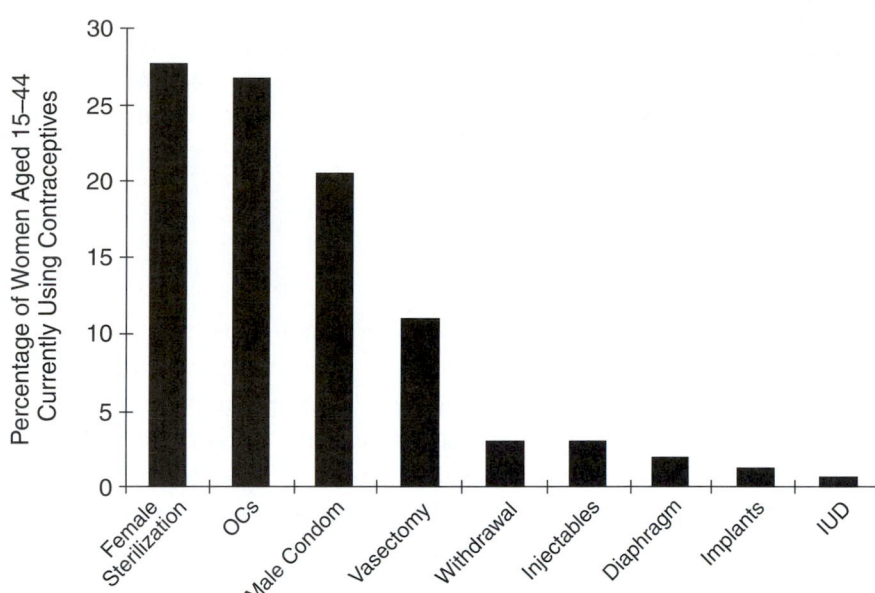

Contraception Use in the United States, 1995.

Figure 42-1 Contraceptive Use in the United States: 1995, Percentage of Women Ages 15–44 Currently Using Contraceptives. *Adapted from Piccinino LJ, Mosher WD. Trends in contraceptive use in the United States: 1982–1995. Fam Plan Persp 1998;30:4.*

Lowest expected and typical first-year contraceptive failure are listed in Table 42-1.

ORAL CONTRACEPTIVES

Since they first were marketed in the 1960s, the dose of sex steroids in combination OCs has dramatically declined. The highest-dose formulations now available contain 50 μg of ethinyl estradiol, while the majority of OCs currently prescribed contain 30 or 35 μg. Formulations with 20 μg of estrogen represent the OCs with the lowest estrogen combination currently available. Monophasic OCs contain a constant dose of both estrogen and progestin in each of the 21 active tablets. Phasic OCs alter the progestin and/or estrogen dose during the administration of the

TABLE 42-1
FIRST-YEAR CONTRACEPTIVE FAILURE AND CONTINUATION RATES

Method	Percent of Women with Pregnancy		% Continuing Use after 1 Year
	Lowest Expected	Typical	
No method	85	85	
Spermicides	6	21	43
Periodic abstinence	1–9	20	67
Withdrawal	4	19	
Cervical cap			
Parous	26	26	45
Nulliparous	9	18	58
Diaphragm	6	18	58
Condom			
Female (Reality)	5	21	56
Male	3	12	63
Combination OCs	0.1	3	72
Progestin-only OCs	0.5	3	72
Progesterone T IUD	1.5	2	81
Copper T 380A IUD	0.6	0.8	78
Depo-Provera	0.3	0.3	70
Norplant (6 capsules)	0.09	0.09	85
Female sterilization	0.4	0.4	100
Male sterilization	0.1	0.15	100

Adapted from Hatcher R et al.[1]

TABLE 42-2
CLINICAL SETTINGS IN WHICH PROGESTIN-ONLY CONTRACEPTIVES CAN BE USED

Smokers older than age 35
Vascular disease associated with diabetes or lupus
Coronary artery disease
Congestive heart failure
Cerebrovascular disease
Complicated migraine headaches (migraine with focal neurologic phenomena, migraines that intensify during combination OC use)
Increased risk of thromboembolism
Diabetes
Lipid disorders including hypertriglyceridemia
Postpartum (partial breast-feeding or nonbreast-feeding beginning within 3 weeks postpartum)
Fully breast-feeding (begin 6 weeks postpartum)
When combination OCs cause persistent estrogen-related side effects

---

21 active tablets in an effort to minimize total steroid dose, as well as metabolic and side effects, while maintaining contraceptive efficacy.

Progestin-only OCs ("minipills," or POPs) do not contain estrogen, with all of the 28 tablets in each pack containing hormone. Because POPs contain progestins in even lower doses than combination OCs, many clinicians feel that they are less effective. Nevertheless, the documented rates of failure for POPs are comparable to those of combination OCs, in women who are meticulous about taking the pill at the same time every day. POPs are well suited for use by lactating women and those of older reproductive age who have cardiovascular risk factors, two relatively less fertile groups, for whom contraceptive doses of estrogen are contraindicated (Table 42-2).

Mechanism of Action

Combination OCs prevent ovulation by inhibiting gonadotropin secretion. The progestin suppresses secretion of luteinizing hormone (LH), while the estrogen component suppresses secretion of follicle-stimulating hormone (FSH), preventing selection of a dominant follicle. The estrogen component also stabilizes the endometrium, thereby minimizing breakthrough bleeding. The progestin component also thickens the cervical mucus, preventing sperm from entering the endometrial cavity.

The substantially lower progestin doses of POPs blunt, but do not totally eliminate, midcycle LH peaks, with ovulation sometimes occurring in POP users.

The effects of the POP on cervical mucus last about 20 hours, making meticulous pill-taking of paramount importance to ensure high contraceptive efficacy. When a woman takes her POP more than 3 hours late, a backup method of contraception, such as condoms or a spermicide, should be used for the next 48 hours.

Initiation and Use

When OCs are initiated either on the first day of menses or the first Sunday after menses starts, there is no need for backup contraception. Associating pill-taking with a daily ritual, such as tooth brushing, may enhance compliance. If one or two tablets are missed, the patient should take one tablet as soon as possible. Then, one tablet should be taken twice a day until all the missed tablets are taken. If three or more tablets have been missed, a backup form of contraception should be used until the current pack is completed. With the progestin-only pills, backup contraception should be used for 48 hours if a pill is taken 3 or more hours late.

Side Effects

As with all hormonal contraceptives, OC side effects represent the major cause of non-compliance and discontinuation. Because breast tenderness and nausea are common estrogen-related side effects, clinicians can consider prescribing 20-μg estrogen OCs when these side effects persist for more than several months. Breakthrough bleeding occurs in up to one-third of women during their first 3 months of OC use, subsequently becoming less common. Rates of breakthrough bleeding are higher among women using 20-μg estrogen than those using 30- or 35-μg formulations. The new onset of intermenstrual bleeding after 3 months of OC use should alert clinicians to noniatrogenic causes, such as cervical infection or neoplasia. Once these conditions are excluded, oral estrogen (e.g. 1.25 mg of conjugated estrogen, esterified estrogen, or estropipate; or 1 to 2 mg of estradiol) can be taken with each active OC tablet to minimize breakthrough bleeding caused by progestin-induced changes.

Amenorrhea due to progestin-induced endometrial changes may result after long-term OC use. In this setting, patient anxiety may occur due to fear of possible pregnancy. Oral estrogen supplementation can be used as described above for breakthrough bleeding. Concerns that combination OCs cause weight gain are unfounded.

Health Risks

The estrogen component of combination OCs increases hepatic production of serum clotting factors, particularly factors VII and X and fibrinogen. With use of OCs formulated with less than 50 μg of ethinyl estradiol, the risk of venous thromboembolism (VTE) is three to four times that in nonusers. Accordingly, women with a history of thromboembolism should not use combination OCs. To place this risk in perspective, pregnancy is associated with a VTE risk six times higher than that in nonpregnant, non-OC-using women. Epidemiologic data do not suggest that VTE risk is lower with 20-μg estrogen formulations as compared with those with 30 to 35 μg. Although initial data suggested that VTE risk was higher with OCs containing the newer progestin desogestrel, subsequent studies have not confirmed such differential risk.

Combination OC use, even in the long term, does not cause atherosclerosis. Likewise, the risk of myocardial infarction or stroke does not appear to be increased among healthy, nonsmoking women using OCs formulated with less than 50 μg of estrogen. Because OC use and smoking synergistically increase the risk of myocardial infarction, women aged 35 and older who smoke should not use combination OCs.

Fears regarding breast cancer prevent many women from using OCs. A massive reanalysis has clarified associations between OC use and breast cancer. Ten or more years after discontinuing OCs, breast cancer risk is the same in ever-users and never-users of OCs. A modestly increased breast cancer risk noted in current and recent OC users may reflect increased screening in this population of women.

Although the use of OCs may increase the risk of cervical adenocarcinoma, well-controlled modern studies have not found an increased risk of the more common squamous-cell cervical cancer among OC users. Likewise, OC use has not been noted to have an impact on the natural history of cervical human papillomavirus infection. As with all sexually active women, regular cytologic screening is appropriate in women using hormonal contraception. A history of cervical intraepithelial neoplasia does not contraindicate OC use.

TABLE 42-3
HEPATIC ENZYME-INDUCING MEDICATIONS THAT MAY IMPAIR EFFICACY OF POPS AND IMPLANTS

Carbamazepine
Felbamate
Phenobarbital
Phenytoin
Primidone
Rifampin
Topiramate

Concomitant Medications

Certain anticonvulsants, as well as the antibiotic rifampin, may reduce the efficacy of OCS (particularly POPs) (Table 42-3). The anticonvulsant valproic acid and the antibiotics doxycycline, tetracycline, and metronidazole do not appear to reduce OC efficacy.

Noncontraceptive Benefits and Therapeutic Uses

Prevention of endometrial and ovarian cancer represents the most important noncontraceptive benefit of OC use. Because this protection persists for at least two decades after discontinuing pills, OC users in their late 30s and 40s can reduce their risk of being diagnosed with these malignancies during those decades of life when they would otherwise experience their highest lifetime risk of these cancers. OC noncontraceptive and therapeutic benefits are listed in Tables 42-4 and 42-5.

TABLE 42-4
ORAL CONTRACEPTIVE HEALTH BENEFITS

Prevention of
  Endometrial cancer
  Ovarian cancer
  Ovulatory pain
  Functional ovarian cysts
  Ectopic pregnancy
  Pelvic inflammatory disease
  Loss of bone mineral density
  Severe rheumatoid arthritis
Menstrual improvement
  Regular cycles
  Less flow
  Less dysmenorrhea

TABLE 42-5
THERAPEUTIC USES* OF ORAL CONTRACEPTIVES

Hypothalamic amenorrhea
Premature ovarian failure
Functional ovarian cysts
Chronic anovulation
Hirsutism
Acne†
Endometriosis
Control of bleeding in women with blood dyscrasias
Menorrhagia/dysmenorrhea (including when associated with
    uterine leiomyomata)

*Use of OCs for indications other than contraception represents off-label
use not approved by the FDA.
†Triphasic norgestimate/ethinyl estradiol (Tri-cyclen) approved for the
treatment of acne.

Postcoital or Emergency Contraception (EC)

About half of the unintended pregnancies in the United States occur in women not using contraception. Emergency contraception (EC) (commonly referred to as the "morning after" pill or postcoital contraception) is a method of preventing pregnancy after unprotected sexual intercourse. Many physicians are not familiar with EC; this has limited the use of this approach to fertility regulation. Many hormones have been used since this method was introduced in the 1960s, including synthetic or conjugated estrogens, antiprogestins, danazol, mifepristone, and progestins. EC is thought to be about 75% effective in preventing pregnancy. Emergency contraception prevents pregnancy by interfering with ovulation, causing corpus luteum dysfunction, or altering the endometrium to prevent implantation. No increased risk of fetal malformation has been noted in offspring born after use of the estrogen/progestin (EC) regimen described below.

The best studied and most commonly used EC method in the United States consists of 0.1 mg of ethinyl estradiol and 4.0 mg of DL-norgestrel taken within 72 hours of unprotected intercourse, with a second dose taken 12 hours later. In addition to a dedicated product (Preven), various approaches to prescribing the estrogen/progestin EC exist, and are listed in Table 42-6. The most common side effect of EC is nausea and vomiting. Use of an antiemetic taken 1 hour before each dose may reduce this side effect. Use of POPs can provide effective EC without estrogen-induced nausea. However, this approach uses twenty 75-μg norgestrel tablets (Ovrette), with this dose then repeated in 12 hours. A new dedicated progestin-only emergency contraceptive formulation (Plan B) facilitates use of this approach.

Progestin-Only Contraceptives

Because injectable, implantable, and progestin-only OCs contain no estrogen, they can be used by women who are not appropriate candidates for combination OCs (see Table 42-2).

INJECTABLE CONTRACEPTION

Medroxyprogesterone acetate (DMPA) is marketed in the United States as Depo-Provera, a 150-mg solution of aqueous microcrystals administered by deep intramuscular injection every 3 months. A monthly contraceptive injection combining 25 mg of medroxyprogesterone acetate with 5 mg of estradiol

TABLE 42-6
ORAL CONTRACEPTIVES FOR EMERGENCY CONTRACEPTION

Formulation	Brand Name	Tablets per Dose/Color	Doses Required	Time of First Dose
Norgestrel 0.50 mg + ethinyl estradiol 50 μg	Ovral	2/white		
Norgestrel 0.30 mg + ethinyl estradiol 30 μg	Lo-Ovral	4/white	2	Within 72 hr of unprotected sex.* Second dose 12 hr later
Levonorgestrel 0.15 mg + ethinyl estradiol 30 μg	Levlen, or Nordette	4/light-orange 4/light-orange		
Levonorgestrel 0.125 mg + ethinyl estradiol 30 μg	Tri-Levlen, or Triphasil	4/yellow 4/yellow		
Norgestrel 0.075 mg	Ovrette	20	2	Within 48 hr of unprotected sex.* Second dose 12 hr later.

*The patient may wish to time her first dose so as not to have to wake up during the night to take the second dose.

cypionate (Lunelle) was approved by the Federal Drug Administration in October 2000.

Mechanism of Action

DMPA provides highly effective contraception by blocking the LH surge and preventing ovulation.

Initiation and Use

When DMPA is initiated within 5 days of the onset of menses, there is no need for backup contraception. Following initial or subsequent injections, ovulation does not occur for at least 14 weeks, allowing a 2-week grace period when 3-month injection intervals are followed. For women more than 2 weeks late for their reinjection, pregnancy should be ruled out prior to reinjection, and backup contraception used for 1 week subsequently. Clinicians should note that Depo-Provera package labeling states that pregnancy should be excluded in women more than 1 week late for reinjection. Fortunately, contraceptive doses of DMPA inadvertently administered during pregnancy do not appear to result in increased risk of congenital anomalies.

Side Effects

Menstrual changes occur in all women using DMPA. Episodes of unpredictable, irregular bleeding and spotting lasting 7 or more days commonly occur in the first months of use. With increasing duration of use, the frequency and duration of these episodes decrease, and amenorrhea becomes common. After four injections of DMPA, half of women report amenorrhea, with this proportion increasing to over three-fourths with longer use. Based on unrealistic expectations of immediate amenorrhea, users may prematurely discontinue their contraceptive injections after experiencing unpredictable spotting and bleeding. Candid counseling prior to the first injection, as well as supportive follow-up measures, can enhance continuation of injectable contraceptives. If reassurance is not sufficient to encourage women experiencing menstrual changes to continue DMPA, persistent, irregular bleeding can be treated with continuous daily oral estrogen supplementation (as described above for OC breakthrough bleeding). After the discontinuation of supplemental estrogen, however, the bleeding may return. Side effects sometimes caused by DMPA

include alopecia, reduced libido, and possibly weight gain.

Return to Fertility

Return to fertility can be delayed after discontinuing DMPA. Within 10 months of the last injection, half of women who have discontinued DMPA to become pregnant will have conceived. However, fertility does not return in some women for up to 18 months after the last injection, underscoring that DMPA is not an appropriate choice for women who may wish to conceive in the next 1 or 2 years.

Health Risks

Use of DMPA is associated with modest suppression of ovarian estradiol production. Some, but not all studies, have noted lower bone mineral density in users. This reduction in bone mineral density reverses after drug discontinuation. Also, levels of high-density lipoproteins have been found to be lower in DMPA users. World Health Organization studies have found that use of DMPA does not have an impact on the risk of cervical or ovarian cancer, and it profoundly reduces endometrial cancer risk. DMPA's impact on breast cancer risk appears similar of that of OCs.

Noncontraceptive Benefits and Therapeutic Uses

Noncontraceptive benefits and therapeutic uses of DMPA are listed in Tables 42-7 and 42-8. Concomitant

---

TABLE 42-7
THERAPEUTIC USES* OF
MEDROXYPROGESTERONE ACETATE

Menorrhagia/dysmenorrhea (including when associated with uterine leiomyomata)
Premenstrual syndrome
Pain in women with endometriosis
Seizures refractory to conventional anticonvulsants
Painful crises in women with hemoglobinopathy
Menstrual hygiene problems in handicapped women
Vasomotor symptoms in menopausal women
Pelvic pain/dyspareunia of ovarian origin, posthysterectomy
Ovulatory pain
Endometrial hyperplasia
Metastatic endometrial cancer
Metastatic breast cancer

---

*Use of DMPA for indications other than contraception or endometrial cancer represents off-label use not approved by the FDA.

TABLE 42-8
HEALTH BENEFITS OF
MEDROXYPROGESTERONE ACETATE

Prevention of
  Iron deficiency anemia
  Pelvic inflammatory disease
  Ectopic pregnancy
  Endometrial cancer
  Hysterectomy in women with uterine leiomyomata

use of liver-enzyme–inducing medications (see Table 42-3) does not impair the effectiveness of DMPA. In addition, DMPA has intrinsic anticonvulsant properties. Therefore, some experts feel that DMPA should be considered the contraceptive of choice for women with seizure disorders.

CONTRACEPTIVE IMPLANTS

The Norplant subdermal contraceptive system consists of six 34-by-2.4-mm silastic tubes that contain 36 mg each of crystalline levonorgestrel. The six implants release a total of 85 μg per day initially, with the levels dropping to 30 μg per day by the fifth year of use. Annual pregnancy rates with subdermal implants are 0.8/100 woman-years during the 5-year period of use. Although package labeling indicates that Norplant is approved for 5 years of use, high efficacy persists for a total of 7 years. The risk of congenital anomalies does not appear to be increased among offspring born to women who have conceived with implants in place.

Mechanism of Action

Circulating progestin levels are sufficient to prevent ovulation in most women using implants. However, approximately one-third of implant users do experience cyclic luteal activity in the first year, with this luteal activity becoming more frequent in subsequent years. This luteal activity is associated with regular withdrawal bleeding episodes. In these ovulatory implant users, fertilization is prevented by progestin-induced luteal insufficiency, impaired oocyte maturation, and progestin-induced hostile cervical mucus. Implant users with cyclic menses are at higher risk of pregnancy and should be counseled about the importance of pregnancy testing if their regular menses abruptly cease.

Medications that induce hepatic enzymes can decrease implant efficacy (see Table 42-3). Some physicians have successfully placed two sets of implants (12 total implants) in women taking concomitant hepatic enzyme inducers. A two-implant levonorgestrel system that provides at least 3 years of contraception has been approved by the FDA but is not currently marketed in the United States.

Initiation and Use

Insertion of the implants within 7 days of the onset of menses avoids the need for backup contraception. Insertion and removal of implants are minor office procedures performed under local anesthesia. Removal takes longer and is associated with more discomfort than insertion. Appropriate insertion technique facilitates removal. Because serum progestin levels fall rapidly after removal, fertility returns within days or weeks of removal. This observation underscores that women having their implants removed need to initiate an alternative method of contraception immediately if they wish to avoid conceiving.

Side Effects

Irregular bleeding represents the most common side effect leading to implant discontinuation, and can be treated with estrogen supplementation, as with DMPA. Headache (nonmigraine) represents the most common nonmenstrual side effect leading to implant discontinuation. Some women using implants have reported hair loss, a side effect that appears to diminish during implant use.

Health Risks

No epidemiologic data assessing risk of reproductive tract cancers in implant users have been published. Functional ovarian cysts arising from persistent dominant follicles develop in some implant users, but rarely require surgical intervention.

Noncontraceptive Benefits and Therapeutic Uses

Amenorrhea occurs in 5 to 10% of women using implants. Some users report improvement in symptoms of dysmenorrhea or premenstrual syndrome.

INTRAUTERINE DEVICES

IUDs offer users convenient, highly effective, and safe contraception. Low use of IUDs among U.S. women likely reflects myths that IUDs act as abortifacients and cause pelvic inflammatory disease, infertility, and ectopic pregnancies. By educating women and dispelling myths, obstetrician-gynecologists can encourage appropriate candidates to take advantage of this underused contraceptive.

The two IUDs currently available in the United States are the Copper T 380A (Paragard) and the progesterone-releasing IUD (Progestasert). The Copper T is a polyethylene device covered with 380 mm^2 of copper. Two white monofilament threads are tied to the device's bulbous stem. The progesterone-releasing IUD (Progestasert) is a T-shaped ethylene/vinyl acetate copolymer device whose stem is filled with 38 mg of progesterone, which is released at a rate of 65 μg per day. Two blue-black monofilament strings are attached to the stem base. Barium sulfate is incorporated into the frames of these IUDs, making them radiopaque.

Mechanism of Action

IUDs prevent fertilization by creating a sterile, inflammatory foreign-body response in the endometrial cavity that is hostile to sperm. Copper causes local prostaglandin production and inhibits endometrial enzymes, intensifying the spermicidal impact of the copper IUDs. The copper T 380A (Paragard) is approved for 10 years of use, with first-year failure rates of 0.5 to 0.8 per 100 woman-years, and a cumulative 10-year failure rate of 2.1/100 woman-years. Recent data suggest that this IUD remains effective for at least 12 years.

The progesterone releasing IUD (Progestasert) not only inhibits sperm survival, but may also prevent implantation by creating an atrophic decidualized endometrium. The progesterone-releasing IUD also thickens the cervical mucus, preventing sperm entry into the endometrium. Approved for 1 year of use, the first-year failure rate has been reported to be 1.5 per 100 woman-years.

Initiation and Use

Many obstetrician-gynecologists feel that optimal timing of IUD placement is during menses, when insertional bleeding will be masked, discomfort may be minimized secondary to increased cervical dilatation, and pregnancy is ruled out. However, insertion may be performed at any time during the cycle as long as pregnancy can be reliably excluded. Although uterine perforation can occur at the time of IUD insertion, this complication rarely occurs with the copper or progesterone T. Skilled clinicians who pay attention to uterine anatomy during the preinsertional bimanual examination have perforation rates of approximately 1 per 1000 insertions. Appropriate attention to sterile technique and patient selection (i.e., avoiding insertion in patients with genital infections) precludes the necessity for prophylactic antibiotics, although some practitioners give a single dose of 200 mg of doxycycline or 1 g of azithromycin 1 hour prior to insertion.

Expulsion rates are approximately 5% in the first year of copper IUD use. Vaginal discharge, cramping, a lengthening string, or plastic protruding from the cervix are signs that suggest partial expulsion. In this setting, barrier backup contraception should be used until the patient can be evaluated. Partially expelled IUDs should be removed. A new device can be inserted after infection and pregnancy are ruled out.

Side Effects

Copper IUDs increase both menstrual flow and cramping. Careful screening of candidates to avoid insertion in women with preexisting menorrhagia and/or dysmenorrhea will reduce patient discontinuation due to these problems. Use of nonsteroidal antiinflammatory drugs is appropriate for women who use copper IUDs and experience dysmenorrhea. Because the progesterone T reduces menstrual flow and cramps, women with underlying heavy flow or dysmenorrhea may be good candidates for (even benefit from) the progesterone-releasing IUD. A multiyear levonorgestrel-releasing IUD (Mirena) may soon become available in the United States.

Health Risks

In contrast to barrier and hormonal contraception, IUDs do not prevent sexually transmitted diseases or PID. Selection of mutually monogamous candidates with no evidence of genital-tract infection, as well as good insertion technique, should result in little if any increased risk of pelvic infection following IUD insertion. Because use of copper IUDs reduces the overall risk of ectopic pregnancy, a history of ectopic pregnancy is a contraindication only to use of the progesterone-releasing IUD. Conditions no longer considered contraindications to IUD use include nulliparity, diabetes mellitus, valvular heart disease, treated cervical dysplasia, anovulatory cycles, lactation, and corticosteroid use without immunocompromise.

Uncomplicated vaginitis or cervicitis encountered in IUD users should be treated as in any other patient. Simple endometritis can be treated with doxycycline and metronidazole (or ampicillin/clavulanic acid) for 14 days without IUD removal if the patient responds appropriately. The occurrence of PID requires removal of the IUD after initiation of antibiotics. Actinomyces has been found on Pap smears in up to one-third of women with plastic IUDs and in almost 1% of copper IUD users with long duration of use. In women with Actinomyces with either uterine tenderness or an associated pelvic mass, appropriate treatment includes removal of the device along with a 1-month course of oral penicillin.

Clinicians diagnosing contraceptive failure in an IUD user should promptly determine the implantation site, due to the high probability of ectopic pregnancy. The risk of spontaneous abortion is increased if an IUD remains in place with an intrauterine pregnancy. If the string is visible, the IUD should be gently removed, regardless of the woman's pregnancy intentions. Once the IUD is removed, the increased risk of abortion resolves. If the string is not visible, some experts recommend sonographically guided removal by a clinician skilled in such procedures. If the IUD cannot be retrieved, the risk for congenital anomalies has not been shown to be increased, but the risk of preterm labor or intrauterine infection is heightened.

Noncontraceptive Benefits and Therapeutic Uses

Insertion of a copper-bearing IUD within 7 days after unprotected intercourse, or within 5 days after ovulation, is an alternative to the more commonly employed hormonal approaches to emergency contraception, with the added advantage of continued contraception for the next 10 years.

The progesterone-releasing IUD decreases menstrual blood loss by about 50% and reduces dysmenorrhea.

BARRIER AND SPERMICIDAL METHODS

Paralleling increased awareness of HIV and other STDs, the use of condoms among U.S. couples has become more common. Barrier methods can be relatively effective when used consistently and correctly. Younger age, lower socioeconomic class, and less education correlate with higher barrier and spermicide failure rates. Vaginal foams, jellies, suppositories, creams, and films containing the spermicidal detergent nonoxynol-9 kill or immobilize sperm on contact. Combining these spermicidal methods with barriers may increase contraceptive efficacy. Many couples perceive spermicides as messy or having an unpleasant flavor.

Initiation and Use

Diaphragms and spermicides used alone require proper placement prior to penile–vaginal contact, with additional spermicide placed with each subsequent sex act. Diaphragms should be left in place for at least 6 hours after sexual relations. Arcing-spring diaphragms are the most commonly used diaphragms, and can be used by women with pelvic relaxation or an anterior cervix associated with a posterior uterus. Flat-spring diaphragms are also available.

In contrast with diaphragms, cavity rim cervical caps have the advantage of allowing longer use, up to 36 hours at a time, not requiring concomitant spermicide use with each coitus, and maintaining appropriate placement in women with pelvic relaxation by means of the suction that is created. Failure rates with the cap are higher in parous women than nulliparas, with rates as high as 20% reported among parous women consistently using this device. Diaphragms and cervical caps are available in different sizes, must be professionally fitted, and require users who are knowledgeable about and comfortable with their genital anatomy. Male and female condoms can be used effectively without spermicides.

Side Effects

Vaginal pain or ulceration is rare with a properly fitted diaphragm or cervical cap. Diaphragm users should be reevaluated for correct fit annually, after any 10-lb or greater weight change, after an abortion, and post partum.

Health Risks

Urinary-tract infections are approximately twice as common among women using diaphragms as among those using OCs. Some individuals are allergic to latex condoms, diaphragms, or cervical caps.

Noncontraceptive Benefits and Therapeutic Uses

Use of barriers and spermicides reduces the transmission of bacterial and viral sexually transmitted diseases.

PERIODIC ABSTINENCE

The rhythm or calendar method, cervical mucus method, and symptothermal method are approaches to contraception that rely on observation of signs and symptoms of the "fertile" period during the menstrual cycle. Accordingly, women with irregular menses, vaginitis, or cervicitis are not appropriate candidates for the use of periodic abstinence. Periodic abstinence is the only method of contraception allowed by some religions. However, the need to abstain from sex for many days each menstrual cycle, as well as the method's high failure rate, limits this approach to fertility regulation.

CONCLUSION

Hormonal and intrauterine contraception offer women safe, effective, and reversible contraception. Barrier and spermicide methods are, in many cases, readily accessible and offer women protection against STDs. By individualizing counseling and recommendations based on relevant behavioral and medical considerations, obstetrician-gynecologists can maximize their patients' success with contraceptives.

REFERENCES

1. Henshaw SK. Unintended pregnancy in the United States. Fam Plan Persp 1998;30:24.

2. Piccinino LJ, Mosher WD. Trends in contraceptive use in the United States: 1982–1995. Fam Plan Persp 1998;30:4.

3. American College of Obstetricians and Gynecologists. Hormonal contraception. ACOG Technical Bulletin no. 198. October 1994.

4. Speroff L, Darney P. A clinical guide for contraception, 2nd ed. Baltimore, Williams & Wilkins, 1996.

5. Hatcher RA, Stewart F, Trussel J, et al. Contraceptive technology. 16th rev. ed. New York: Irvington, 1996.

6. Kaunitz AM, Illions EH, Jones JL, Sang, LA. Contraception: a clinical review for the internist. Med Clin N Am Office Gynecol 1995;79:1377.

7. Carr BR, Ory H. Estrogen and progestin components of oral contraceptives: relationship to vascular disease. Contraception 1997;55:267.

8. Redmond GP, Olson WH, Lippman JS, Kafrissen ME, Jones M, Jonizzo JC. Norgestimate and ethinyl estradiol in the treatment of acne vulgaris: a randomized, placebo-controlled trial. Obstet Gynecol 1997;89:615.

9. Collaborative Group on Hormonal Factors in Breast Cancer. Breast cancer and hormonal contraceptives: collaborative reanalysis of individual data on 53,297 women with breast cancer and 100,239 women without breast cancer from 54 epidemiologic studies. Lancet 1996;347:1713.

10. Kaunitz AM, Benrubi GI. The good news about hormonal contraception and gynecologic cancer. Female Patient 1998;January 23:43.

11. Grimes DA, Mishell DR, Speroff L. Contraceptive choices for women with medical problems. Am J Obstet Gynecol 1993;168:1974.

12. American College of Obstetricians and Gynecologists. The use of hormonal contraception in women with coexisting medical conditions. ACOG Practice Bulletin no. 18. July 2000.

13. American College of Obstetricians and Gynecologists. Emergency oral contraception. ACOG Practice Patterns. December 1996.

14. Kaunitz AM. Revisiting progestin-only OCs. Contemp Obstet Gynecol 1997;42:91.

15. Kaunitz, AM, Jordan CW. Two long-acting hormonal contraceptive options. Contemp Obstet Gynecol 1997;42:27.

16. Kaunitz AM, Mishell DR. Depot medroxyprogesterone acetate (DMPA) contraception in the United States: the first three years. J Reprod Med 1996;41(Suppl):379.

17. Kaunitz AM. Reappearance of the intrauterine device: a "user-friendly" contraceptive. Int J Fertil 1997;42(2):120.

18. United Nations Development Programme; United Nations Population Fund, World Health Organization; World Bank, Special Programme of Research, Development and Research Training in Human Reproduction. Long-term reversible contraception. Twelve years of experience with the TCu380A and TCu220C. Contraception 1997;56:341.

Chapter 43

Sexually Transmissible Infections

Roger P. Smith

Five Key Points

- The prevalence of sexually transmitted disease is increasing.
- All sexually active patients are potentially at risk.
- Treatment of sexually transmitted infections must be tailored to the infection, site, and special needs of the patient.
- Because of the lifetime implications of the diagnosis of "PID," the use of the diagnosis should be limited to those who meet diagnostic criteria.
- Screening for HIV infections should become as routine as screening for other sexually transmitted infections.

Changing behavior patterns and the emergence of fatal sexually transmitted diseases have made a familiarity with the area of sexually transmissible infections imperative. It is essential to be alert to the possibility of sexually transmitted disease in all patients, to perform diagnostic evaluations, and to promptly institute appropriate treatments. This is no longer a condemnation of the patient's lifestyle or personal choices, but rather a simple fact of today's life, and we must watch for and educate our patients about the risks involved in today's sexually open society.

Sexually transmitted diseases can run the gamut from the acquired immunodeficiency syndrome (AIDS) to vaginitis. They can be anything from a minor inconvenience to infections that cause loss of fertility or create long-term disability to life-threatening illness. Over 85% of sexually transmitted infections occur in people aged 15 to 29, often with lifelong

consequences. While many of these diseases can be acquired through nonsexual means, sexual transmission represents the major route by which they spread.

The prevalence of sexually transmitted disease has increased. Far from the success of declining rates reported a few years ago, we must now deal with a new upsurge of infections. In the United States there are approximately 13 million cases of sexually transmitted diseases annually, excluding human immunodeficiency virus (HIV) infections. This country has seen an increase of approximately 75% in the number of cases of syphilis reported in recent years. Steady or increased rates of gonococcal infections, herpes vulvitis, and other sexually transmitted diseases are the rule. Women have the fastest-growing rate of HIV infection in the United States. In 1994, AIDS was the third leading cause of death for women between the ages of 25 and 44, and it is anticipated that, at the current

TABLE 43-1
MINOR SEXUALLY TRANSMITTED DISEASES

Disease	Causative Agent	Main Symptom	Diagnosis	Treatment
Chancroid	*Hemophilus ducreyi*	Painful soft chancres, adenopathy	Clinical, smears, culture	Erythromycin 500 mg four times a day for 10 days
Granuloma inguinale	*Calymmatobacterium granulomatis*	Raised, red lesions	Clinical, smears	Tetracycline 500 mg every 6 hr for 3 wk
Lymphogranuloma venereum (LGV)	*Chlamydia trachomatis*	Vesicle, progressing to bubo	Clinical, complement-fixation test	Tetracycline 500 mg every 6 hr
Molluscum contagiosum	Molluscum contagiosum (DNA virus)	Raised papule with waxy core	Clinical, inclusion bodies	Dessication, cryotherapy, curettage
Parasites	Pediculosis pubis, scabies	Itching	Inspection	Lindane 1%
Enteric infections	*Neisseria gonorrhoeae, Chlamydia trachomatis,* Shigella species, Salmonella, protozoa	Diarrhea	Culture	Based on agent
Vaginitis (sexually transmitted)*	Trichomonas	Odor, irritation	Microscopic examination of secretions	Metronidazole 500 mg twice a day for 7 days

*Debate persists about the sexual transmission of bacterial vaginosis.

Reprinted with permission from Sexually transmitted disease. In Beckman CRB, Ling FW, Barzansky BM, et al., eds. Obstetrics and gynecology. 2nd ed. Baltimore: Williams & Wilkins, 1995:309.

rate of spread, by the time statistics for the year 2000 are available it will rank second behind heart disease as an overall cause of death for women.

The most common sexually transmissible infections may be conveniently divided into bacterial and viral types: The bacterial infections are *Chlamydia trachomatis, Neisseria gonorrhoeae* (GC), and syphilis, while the viral infections include herpes genitalis, human papillomavirus (HPV), and HIV, which causes AIDS. A number of so-called minor sexually transmissible infections exists, including chancroid, granuloma inguinale, lymphogranuloma venereum, and others (Table 43-1). Because of the predilection of these infections to cause vulvar lesions, they will be addressed in detail in Chapter 60.

EVALUATING THE PATIENT

A detailed sexual history must be obtained from all patients; it is invaluable for any patient in whom a sexually transmitted disease is either likely or suspected. Most sexually transmitted infections require skin-to-skin contact or the exchange of body fluids for transmission. Nonsexual activities that meet these criteria may also put the patient at risk.

All patients who are (or might be) sexually active should be examined for the possibility of sexually transmitted disease. The inguinal region should be inspected for rashes, lesions, and adenopathy. The vulva should be inspected for lesions, ulcerations, or abnormal discharge and palpated for thickening or swelling. The Bartholin glands, Skene ducts, and urethra cannot be overlooked. In patients with urinary symptoms, the urethra should be gently "milked" to express any discharge. The vagina and cervix must be inspected for lesions and abnormal discharges using a warmed speculum. When suspicion, risk, or prevalence is high, cultures for gonorrhea, Chlamydia, or other infections should be obtained. Lastly, the perineum and perianal areas must be evaluated for signs of sexually transmitted diseases. Cultures of the rectum for gonorrhea should be obtained in patients who engage in anal intercourse. The oral cavity, as well as cervical and other lymph nodes, must also be evaluated. The findings obtained by this process, combined with the patient's history, will generally make the establishment of the proper diagnosis much easier. Because 20 to 50% of patients with a sexually transmitted disease have more than one coexisting infection, when one venereal disease is found, others must be suspected. When a sexually transmitted disease is diagnosed or suspected, all sexual partners of the patient within the preceding 30 days should be evaluated.

period both before recurrent episodes and after lesions have healed, patients should be instructed to avoid intercourse from the first prodrome to until after all lesions have completely reepithelialized.

The diagnosis of herpes genitalis is made on the basis of suspicion and clinical findings. The lesions of herpes infections should be easily distinguishable from the ulcers found in chancroid, syphilis, or granuloma inguinale by their character and extreme tenderness. The diagnosis of herpetic infection may be confirmed by viral cultures of material swabbed from the lesions. This is the most sensitive method of diagnosis and allows confirmation in as little as 48 hours. Scrapings from the base of vesicles may be stained using immunofluorescence techniques to detect the presence of viral particles. Immunofluorescence evaluation is faster than culture techniques and carries approximately 65 to 80% agreement with culture. Smears of vesicular material may also be treated with Wright stain to visualize giant multinucleated cells with characteristic eosinophilic intranuclear inclusions. Rapid diagnostic kits are available, but current experience suggests that these kits are associated with poor sensitivity and specificity in clinical application.

When treating initial infections, the lesions should be kept clean and dry. Sitz baths, followed by drying with a heat lamp or warm hair dryer, work well for this purpose. Occasionally, the use of a topical anesthetic, such as 2% lidocaine jelly, may be required. If secondary infections occur, therapy with a local antibacterial cream (such as Neosporin) may be of help. Acyclovir ointment (5%, applied locally every 3 hours, begun within 48 hours of onset) has been recommended to decrease the duration of symptoms and viral shedding. This therapy has not been shown to decrease the likelihood of recurrence, and the decrease in symptom duration is often minimal. For patients who have frequent recurrences, oral acyclovir (200 mg three times a day increased to five times a day with lesions) is effective in decreasing both frequency and severity of flare-ups, but it should be limited to a duration of six months or less.

For pregnant patients with active herpes infections, cesarean delivery may be considered. Vaginal delivery is associated with roughly a 50% chance that the baby will acquire the infection. In infants, this infection is associated with significant morbidity and an almost 80% mortality rate. When there has been prolonged rupture of the amniotic membranes, infection may have already taken place, blunting the value of cesarean delivery.

Human Papillomavirus

Human papillomavirus (HPV) infection is the most common viral sexually transmitted disease in the United States, responsible for almost as many cases of sexually transmitted disease as N. gonorrhoeae. This DNA virus is found in 2.5 to 4% of women. The highest prevalence of HPV infections is among women aged 16 to 25, with the most common presentation of symptomatic infection being genital warts (condylomata acuminata). Long-term complications of HPV infection, most notably cervical cancer, may take years to develop. Subtypes 16, 18, 31, 33, 35, and others have been associated with the development of cervical neoplasia. Roughly 90% of patients with cervical squamous-cell carcinoma have evidence of HPV DNA in their cervical tissues.

This virus is easily spread. The virus is hardy, and may resist even drying, making transmission and auto-inoculation common. Fifty percent of sexual partners of women with HPV have visible lesions, and 25% have subclinical infections. The usual incubation period from infection to clinical manifestation is 3 months, but may vary from 1 to 6 months. Active viral replication in condylomata may last 6 to 9 months. The use of condoms has not been shown to reduce the spread of HPV, but should still be encouraged to reduce the spread of other sexually transmitted infections.

Clinical signs develop in approximately 30% of patients infected by HPV. Infection by HPV causes soft, fleshy growths on the vulva, vagina, cervix, urethral meatus, perineum, anus, and the tongue or oral cavity. These distinctive lesions may be single or multiple and generally cause few symptoms by their presence. They are often accompanied by Trichomonas infection or bacterial vaginosis. HPV is spread by direct skin-to-skin contact, making symmetrical lesions across the midline common. The diagnosis of condylomata acuminata is made based on physical examination, but may be confirmed through biopsy of the warts. While cytologic changes typical of HPV are often found on Pap smears, Pap smears of the cervix will diagnose the virus in only about 5% of patients.

Because the condylomata lata of syphilis may be confused with venereal warts, some care must be taken in making the diagnosis in patients at high risk for both infections. Venereal warts are usually characterized by their narrower base and more heaped-up appearance.

The treatment of small, uncomplicated venereal warts is generally by cytolytic topical agents, such as podophyllin (podophyllum resin), bichloroacetic or trichloroacetic acid (TCA), or physical ablative methods such as laser, cryotherapy, or electrodesiccation. Solutions must be carefully applied to the warts, protecting the adjacent skin, and allowed to remain for 30 to 60 minutes. Treatment may be repeated every 7 to 10 days as needed. Podophyllin should not be used during pregnancy. If lesions persist or recur, cryosurgery, electrodesiccation, surgical excision, or laser vaporization may be required. If cryotherapy is chosen, three to six treatments are often required, but cure rates are higher than for podophyllin and comparable to laser ablation (60 to 80%). Even with laser ablation, recurrence rates are reported to vary from 25 to 100%. Treatment with 5-fluorouracil cream is often used as an adjunct for cervical or vaginal lesions. Therapy with autologous vaccine, dinitrochlorobenzene, and interferon have been advocated but have yet to gain a significant place in clinical practice.

Lesions will be more resistant to therapy during pregnancy in patients with diabetes or in patients with immunosuppression. In patients with extensive vaginal or vulvar lesions cesarean delivery may be needed to avoid extensive lacerations and problems suturing tissues with these lesions. Cesarean delivery also decreases the possibility of transmission to the infant, which can cause subsequent development of laryngeal papillomata.

Any patient with a history of condyloma should have at least yearly Pap smear evaluations of the cervix. The sexual partners of patients with HPV should also be screened for the development of genital warts.

Human Immunodeficiency Virus and Acquired Immunodeficiency Syndrome

As of the end of 1998, an estimated 33.4 million people worldwide—32.2 million adults and 1.2 million children younger than 15 years—were living with HIV or AIDS. Approximately 43% of these adults are women. AIDS has become the number one killer of Americans aged 25 to 44. In the United States, 665,357 cases of AIDS had been reported to the Centers for Disease Control and Prevention (CDC) as of June 30, 1998. Of these, 553,048 (83%) were males aged 13 or older, 104,028 (16%) were females aged

13 or older, and 8280 (1%) were children under age 13. In New York City, it is estimated that 1 in every 30 adults is infected with HIV. In the United States, there is one AIDS-related death every 15 minutes, and someone is infected with HIV every 13 minutes. Though transmission of the human immunodeficiency virus may occur via blood transfusion, pregnancy, or the drug-associated use of contaminated needles, sexual transmission has become a major mode of spread, making HIV infection and AIDS sexually transmitted diseases.

Women have the fastest-growing rate of HIV infection in the United States. From 1985 to 1997, the proportion of AIDS cases in United States women reported each year increased from 7 to 22 percent. The American Academy of Pediatrics estimates that the number of HIV-infected teenagers in the United States doubles every 14 months. While HIV affects a disproportionate number of black and Hispanic women (77%), any sexually active woman is potentially at risk. Among women diagnosed with AIDS in the United States in 1997, most acquired HIV infection through sexual contact with a man with or at risk for HIV infection (38%) or through injection-drug use (32%). Heterosexual transmission accounts for an increasing proportion of AIDS cases in the United States. From 1991 to 1996, the estimated proportion of adult AIDS cases in the United States attributed to heterosexual contact each year grew from 8.5% to 17.5%.

The generally accepted prevalence of HIV infections is between 1.6 and 1.7 per 1000 live births, though this rate varies regionally (e.g., 3.4 per 1000 births in the Northeast) and is rising annually. Because the risk of transmission of AIDS to a fetus is high despite prophylactic therapies (30 to 50%), and the fact that maternal AIDS often worsens during pregnancy, pregnancy should be postponed until more is known or effective therapies become available.

Incubation from infection to clinical symptoms ranges from 5 days to 3 months, with an average of 2 to 4 weeks. In 90% of patients, infection by HIV produces only nonspecific symptoms, often mimicking mononucleosis. Febrile pharyngitis is most common, with fever, sweats, lethargy, arthralgia, myalgia, headache, photophobia, and lymphadenopathy seen soon after infection. These symptoms may last up to 2 weeks. Following the initial infection, the patient enters a carrier state during which symptoms are absent but viral shedding occurs. Immune dysfunction generally becomes apparent roughly 10 years after the initial infection. The development of immunocompromise is rare before 3 years after infection, and less than 35% of patients will have symptoms of AIDS before 5 years.

The diagnosis of HIV infection is made on the basis of serum screening tests (enzyme immunoassay), confirmed through repeated testing and the use of Western blot or immunofluorescence assays. Intermediate Western blot results may be obtained due to incomplete antibody response to HIV in serum or nonspecific reaction in sera from uninfected persons. Recent infection may not be reflected by these tests, which require antibody formation. False positive Western blot tests are uncommon—on the order of less than 1 in 130,000.

Current Centers for Disease Control and Prevention (CDC) guidelines suggest that aggressive screening be offered to all women who are at risk and all women who are pregnant. The latter is especially important because trials show that vertical transmission to the fetus may be reduced by as much as two-thirds if early treatment is instituted.

Once the diagnosis of HIV infection is made, base-line diagnostic testing will be essential for the eventual treatment of these patients. Current recommendations for base-line diagnostic tests for these patients is outlined in Table 43-3.

The results of long-term therapy for HIV infection or AIDS is not available, and the development of improved treatment options is incomplete. Therapy with antimetabolites such as zidovudine (Retrovir) or

combination multidrug therapy have been successful in delaying the progress of HIV infection for some patients. The treatment of both HIV infection and AIDS is continually evolving, the details of which lay beyond the scope of this discussion. For the foreseeable future, prevention is the only meaningful intervention available.

OTHER ISSUES

Enteric Infections and Hepatitis B

It is important to remember that enteric infections and vaginitis may also be a part of the spectrum of sexually transmitted diseases (STDs). They should be considered in patients with other STDs and, conversely, should suggest the possibility of STDs when found themselves. In patients who engage in anal intercourse, proctitis caused by *N. gonorrhoeae, C. trachomatis,* herpes, and syphilis may all arise. Fecal–oral contamination may lead to infection with Shigella species, Salmonella, or protozoa. Suspicion, anoscopy or proctoscopy, and laboratory evaluations may all be indispensable in establishing the diagnosis.

Though seldom grouped with "sexually transmitted diseases," hepatitis B is an STD that affects about 23,000 patients annually, 37% of which are women. It is estimated that 19,000 infected pregnant women deliver each year, with a vertical transmission rate of up to 90%, leading to a chronic carrier state for the baby. Most prevalent among Asians, this STD can have a great impact if not suspected and diagnosed in a timely way.

Parasites

Phthirus humanus (pubic or crab lice) and *Sarcoptes scabiei* (scabies or itch mite) are parasitic insects that may be transferred through sexual activity or through contact with contaminated clothing or bedding. Infestations by both agents occur most frequently in pubic hair, though spread to other hairy areas can take place. Scabies infections are not confined to hairy areas, but may be found in any area of the body. The bites of these insects produce intense itching; with scabies, the itching is greatest at night. Close inspection of the affected area will generally reveal nits, feces, burrows, or the insects themselves. These organisms are treated with local cleansing and topical applications of Lindane 1% (Kwell). Other family

---

TABLE 43-3
BASE-LINE DIAGNOSTIC TESTS FOR
HIV-POSITIVE PATIENTS

Laboratory
 CD4 and T-cell count and percentage
 Complete blood count, with differential white-cell count
 Electrolytes
 Glucose-6-phosphate dehydrogenase
 Hepatitis B screen
 Liver- and renal-function tests
 Platelet count
 VDRL or RPR
Other tests
 Cervical culture for gonorrhea and chlamydia
 Pap smear
 Tuberculin skin test with control (Candida, mumps, tetanus)

Compiled from American Medical Association Advisory Group on HIV Early Intervention. HIV early intervention: physician guidelines. 2nd ed. Chicago: American Medical Association, 1994:8.

members should be treated and the home disinfected at the same time.

Pelvic Inflammatory Disease (PID)

PID represents the most serious infection in women aged 16 to 25. Eighty-five percent of cases of this ascending infection are associated with sexually active women of menstrual age. The remaining 15% of cases follow instrumentation such as endometrial biopsy, hysterosalpingography, placement of an intrauterine contraceptive device, or the like. In roughly one-third of cases, the causative organism is *N. gonorrhoeae* by itself; one-third involve infection with *N. gonorrhoeae* and additional "mixed" infections with other organisms; the final third of infections is due to mixed aerobic and anaerobic bacteria. Chlamydia is involved in roughly 20% of cases, with this rate rising to roughly 40% among hospitalized patients. Death from pelvic infections or their complications (for women 15 to 45) is reported to be 0.29 in 100,000.

Even though PID is an ascending infection, acute pelvic infections develop in only about 15% of women with cervical *N. gonorrhoeae* infections. *N. gonorrhoeae* infection of the fallopian tubes, adnexa, or pelvic peritoneum cause symptoms of pain and tenderness, the development of fever or chills, and an elevated white-cell count. Peritoneal involvement may spread to include perihepatitis (FitzHugh–Curtis syndrome). Infection of the upper genital tract by Chlamydia causes a milder form of salpingitis with more insidious symptoms. Once a chlamydial infection is established, it may remain active for many months, furthering the tubal damage. Characteristics of these two similar, but different, infections are summarized in Table 43-4.

PID results in ectopic pregnancy, tubal factor infertility, and chronic abdominal pain in a high percentage of patients. Women with documented salpingitis have a fourfold increase in their rate of ectopic pregnancy, and the risk of infertility roughly doubles with each subsequent episode, culminating in a 40% rate of infertility after only three episodes.

Vaginitis

Sexual activity is a major route of spread for some forms of vaginitis. This is well established in the case of trichomonas infection and is debated in the case of bacterial vaginosis. The coexistence of vaginal infections and other more serious sexually transmitted diseases dictates that appropriate additional screening should be considered for these patients.

SELECTED READINGS

Albrecht H. Redefining AIDS: towards a modification of the current AIDS case definition. Clin Infect Dis 1997; 24:64.

American College of Obstetricians and Gynecologists. Genital human papillomavirus infections. ACOG Technical Bulletin no. 193. June 1994.

American Medical Association Advisory Group on HIV Early Intervention. HIV early intervention: physician guidelines. 2nd ed. Chicago: American Medical Association, 1994:8.

Anastos K, Denenberg R, Solomon L. Human immunodeficiency virus infection in women. Med Clin N Am 1997;81:533.

Bauer HM, Ting Y, Greer CE, et al. Genital human papillomavirus infection in female university students as determined by a PCR-based method. JAMA 1991;265:472.

Berry MC, Dajani AS. Resurgence of congenital syphilis. Infect Dis Clin N Am 1992;6:19.

Black CM. Current methods of laboratory diagnosis of Chlamydia trachomatis infections. Clin Microbiol Rev 1997;10:160.

Cates W Jr. A risk-assessment tool for integrated reproductive health services. Fam Plann Perspect 1997;29:41.

Centers for Disease Control and Prevention (CDC). HIV/AIDS Surv Rep 1998;10:1.

Centers for Disease Control and Prevention. 1993 sexually transmitted diseases treatment guidelines. MMWR 1993; 42(RR-14):1.

Centers for Disease Control and Prevention. Antibiotic-resistant strains of *Neisseria gonorrhoeae*: policy guidelines for detection, management, and control. MMWR 1987; 36(5 suppl):1s.

Centers for Disease Control and Prevention. Decreased susceptibility of *Neisseria gonorrhoeae* to fluoroquinolones—Ohio and Hawaii, 1992–1994. MMWR 1994;43:325.

Centers for Disease Control and Prevention. Recommendations for the prevention and management of *Chlamydia trachomatis* infections, 1993. MMWR 1993;42(RR-12):1.

Centers for Disease Control and Prevention. Sexually transmitted disease surveillance, 1992. Atlanta: Division of STD/HIV Prevention, 1993:10.

TABLE 43-4 COMPARATIVE SYMPTOMS OF GONORRHEA AND CHLAMYDIA INFECTIONS		
	Gonorrhea	**Chlamydia**
Onset	Rapid	Slow
Location	General	Mucosa
Inflammatory response	Strong	Mild
Impact	Cytotoxic	Immunologic

Reprinted with permission from Smith RP. Gynecology in primary care. Baltimore: Williams & Wilkins, 1996:561.

Centers for Disease Control and Prevention. Sexually transmitted diseases: treatment guidelines. MMWR 1989; 38:31.

Centers for Disease Control and Prevention. Update: AIDS among women—United States, 1994. MMWR 1994; 44:881.

Centers for Disease Control and Prevention. Update: barrier protection against HIV infection and other sexually transmitted diseases. MMWR 1993;42:589.

Centers for Diseases Control and Prevention. HIV/AIDS Surv Rep 1997;9(2):1.

Coates TJ, Feldman MD. An overview of HIV prevention in the United States. J Acquir Immune Defic Syndr Hum Retrovirol 1997;14(Suppl 2):S13.

Cohn JA. Recent advances. HIV infection—I. BMJ 1997; 314:487.

Crombleholme W, Landers D, Ohm-Smith M, et al. Sulbactam/ampicillin versus metronidazole/gentamicin in the treatment of severe pelvic infections. Drugs 1986; 31(Suppl 2):11.

Dodson MG, Faro S, Gentry LO. Treatment of acute pelvic inflammatory disease with aztreonam, a new monocyclic ß-lactam antibiotic, and clindamycin. Obstet Gynecol 1986;67:657.

Dodson MG. Antibiotic regimens for treating acute pelvic inflammatory disease: an evaluation. J Reprod Med 1994; 39:285.

Douglas GC, King BF. Maternal-fetal transmission of human immunodeficiency virus: a review of possible routes and cellular mechanism of infection. Clin Infect Dis 1992; 15:678.

Droegemueller WR. Infections of the upper genital tract. In: Mishell DR, Stenchever MA, Droegemueller WR, Herbst AL, eds. Comprehensive gynecology. 3rd ed. St Louis: Mosby, 1997:601.

El-Zaatari MM, Martens MG, Anderson GD. Incidence of the prozone phenomenon in syphilis serology. Obstet Gynecol 1994;84:609.

Ellen JM, Irwin CE Jr. Primary care management of adolescent sexual behavior. Curr Opin Pediatr 1996;8:442.

Fiumara NJ. Treatment of primary and secondary syphilis: serological response. JAMA 1980;243:2500.

Gazzard B. What we know so far. AIDS 1996;10(Suppl 1):S3.

Gibbs RS, Amstey MS, Sweet RL, Mead PB, Sever JL. Management of genital herpes infection in pregnancy. Obstet Gynecol 1988;71:779.

Hammerschlag MR, Golden NH, Oh MK, et al. Single dose of azithromycin for the treatment of genital chlamydial infections in adolescents. J Pediatr 1993;122:961.

Hankins C. Sexual transmission of HIV to women in industrialized countries. World Health Statistics Quarterly—Rapport Trimestriel de Statistiques Sanitaires Mondiales 1996;49:106.

Heath CC, Sulik SM. Contraception and preconception counseling. Prim Care Clin Office Pract 1997;24:123.

Jacobson LJ. Differential diagnosis of acute pelvic inflammatory disease. Am J Obstet Gynecol 1980;138:1006.

Jha PK, Beral V, Peto J, et al. Antibodies to human papillomavirus and to other genital infectious agents and invasive cervical cancer risk. Lancet 1993;341:1116.

John GC, Kreiss J. Mother-to-child transmission of human immunodeficiency virus type 1. Epidemiol Rev 1996; 18:149.

Koutsky LA, Stevens CE, Holmes KK, et al. Underdiagnosis of genital herpes by current clinical and viral-isolation procedures. N Engl J Med 1992;326:1533.

Landers DV, Sweet RL. Sexually transmitted infection. In: Glass RH, ed. Office gynecology. Baltimore: Williams & Wilkins, 1993;1.

Lange JM. Changing therapy in HIV. AIDS 1996;10(Suppl 1):S27.

Larsen S, Hunter E, Kraus S, eds. A manual of tests for syphilis. Washington, DC: American Public Health Association, 1990:1.

Lewis JE, Malow RM, Ireland SJ. HIV/AIDS risk in heterosexual college students: a review of a decade of literature. J Am Coll Health 1997;45:147.

Martin DH, Mroczkowski TF, Dalu ZA, et al. A controlled trial of a single dose of azithromycin for the treatment of chlamydial urethritis and cervicitis: the Azithromycin for Chlamydial Infections Study Group. N Engl J Med 1992; 327:921.

Marx R, Aral SO, Rolfs RT, Sterk CE, Kahn JG. Crack, sex, and STD. Sex Transm Dis 1991;18:92.

Matson SC, Pomeranz AJ, Kamps KA. Early detection and treatment of sexually transmitted disease in pregnant adolescents of low socioeconomic status. Clin Pediatr 1993; 32:609.

Miller KE. Women's health: sexually transmitted diseases. Prim Care Clin Office Pract 1997;24:179.

Morrison J, Alp NJ. Vertical transmission of human immunodeficiency virus. QJ Med 1997;90:5.

Mulhall BP. Sex and travel: studies of sexual behaviour, disease and health promotion in international travellers—a global review. Int J STD AIDS 1996;7:455.

National Institute of Allergy and Infectious Diseases. Clinical alert: important therapeutic information on the benefit of zidovudine (AZT) for the prevention of the transmission of HIV from mother to infant. Bethesda: NIAID, 1994.

Opal SM. Infectious disease challenges in the 1990's. Med Health RI 1996;79(3):100.

Pastorek JG II, Cole C, Aldridge KE, et al. Aztreonam plus clindamycin as therapy for pelvic infections in women. Am J Med 1985;78(Suppl 2A):47.

Pearlman MD, McNeeley SG. A review of the microbiology, immunology and clinical implications of Chlamydia trachomatis infections. Obstet Gynecol Surv 1992;47:448.

Perry CM, Faulds D. Valaciclovir: a review of its antiviral activity, pharmacokinetic properties and therapeutic efficacy in herpesvirus infections. Drugs 1996;52:754.

Phillips RS, Hanff PA, Wertheimer A, Aronson MD. Gonorrhea in women seen for routine gynecologic care: criteria for testing. Am J Med 1988;85:177.

Richman DD. New strategies to combat HIV drug resistance. Hosp Pract 1996;31:47, 53.

Romanowski B, Sutherland R, Fick GH, Mooney D, Love EJ. Serologic response to treatment of infectious syphilis. Ann Intern Med 1991;114:1005.

Royce RA, Sena A, Cates W Jr, Cohen MS. Sexual transmission of HIV. N Engl J Med 1997;336:1072.

Searight HR, McLaren AL. Behavioral and psychiatric aspects of HIV infection. Am Fam Physician 1997;55:1227, 1241.

Selwyn PA, Schoenbaum EE, Davenny K, et al. Prospective study of human immunodeficiency virus infection and pregnancy outcomes in intravenous drug users. JAMA 1989;261:1289.

Sloand EM. Viral risks associated with blood transfusion. Photochem Photobiol 1997;65:428.

Smith RP. Gynecology in primary care. Baltimore: Williams & Wilkins, 1996:549.

Sweet RL, Roy S, Faro S, et al. Piperacillin and taxobactam versus clindamycin and gentamicin in the treatment of hospitalized women with pelvic infection. Obstet Gynecol 1994;83:280.

Tapp A, Wise B, Cardozo L. Efficacy and safety of piperacillin/tazobactam in gynecologic infections. J Antimicrob Chemother 1993;Suppl B:61.

Waller SC. A meta-analysis of condom effectiveness in reducing sexually transmitted HIV. Soc Sci Med 1993;36:1635.

Washington AE, Cates W, Zaidi AA. Hospitalization for pelvic inflammatory disease. JAMA 1984;25:2529.

Weiss SH. Risks and issues for the health care worker in the human immunodeficiency virus era. Med Clin N Am 1997;81:555.

White JC. HIV risk assessment and prevention in lesbians and women who have sex with women: practical information for clinicians. Health Care Women Int 1997;18:127.

Chapter 44

Breast Disorders

James A. Hall

Five Key Points

- The diagnostic triad for breast disorders consists of physical examination, mammography, and fine-needle aspiration.

- Mammography is the only way to discover early breast cancer in a preclinical stage.

- Fine-needle aspiration can immediately differentiate cystic from solid masses and provide cells for cytology if the mass is solid.

- Breast preservation treatment (lumpectomy, axillary-node dissection, radiation therapy) offers the same opportunity for survival as mastectomy in most breast cancers.

- Estrogen use is not associated with a clinically significant increased risk of breast cancer.

Breast cancer is the most common malignancy found among women in the United States and is second only to lung cancer for cancer deaths. Approximately 185,000 new cases are diagnosed annually. Breast cancer is the number one cause of all deaths for women in their 40s. Breast cancer will develop in one in eight women living beyond 90 years. While there is no known prevention, early diagnosis offers an excellent opportunity for cure. Unfortunately the mortality from advanced breast cancer has not changed in the past 50 years. The average obstetrician-gynecologist will discover more breast cancers than all other malignancies combined. While the fear of breast cancer is the primary motivating factor bringing most women to the doctor with reported breast complaints, benign causes are far more common than malignancy. However, every report of a breast complaint deserves a full and prompt evaluation.

ANATOMY

The breasts are modified sebaceous glands within the superficial fascia of the anterior chest wall. The adult female breast is approximately 80% fat and connective tissue with glandular tissue making up the remaining 20%. The axillary tail of Spence is the lateral projection of the breast extending in the upper-outer direction toward the axilla. The breast is composed of 15 to 20 lobes arranged in a radial fashion extending from the nipple. Each lobe has one terminal excretory duct or collecting duct. The collecting ducts are 2 mm in diameter and converge into subareolar lactiferous sinuses that are 5 to 8 mm in diameter. Five to ten major milk ducts drain to the outside thru the nipple. The anatomical relationship of each lobe to its own terminal duct is important when evaluating multiduct and single-duct nipple discharge. Each lobe consists of 20 to

40 lobules. A lobule consists of 10 to 100 alveoli which are the secretory units of the breast. Cooper ligaments extend from the skin to the pectoralis major muscle fascia. Tumor growth may shorten these ligaments and cause skin retraction. The nipple is located over the fourth intercostal space and contains sebaceous and apocrine sweat glands as well as sensory nerve endings. The areola is the circular pigment tissue around the nipple. It contains the gland's of Montgomery which are sebaceous and capable of secreting milk. Morgagni tubercules are elevations on the surface of the areola formed by the openings of the Montgomery gland duct. Accessory breast tissue or nipples may occur along the breast line running from the axilla to the groin. This tissue may be functional or rudimentary.

The vascular supply to the breast is from the internal mammary artery and lateral thoracic artery. The internal mammary artery mainly supplies the medial and central part of the breast, while the lateral thoracic artery supplies the upper–outer quadrant. Approximately 75% of lymphatic drainage is to axillary nodes, with the remaining 25% going to internal mammary nodes and skin lymphatics. Axillary nodes are divided into three anatomical levels. Level I nodes are lateral to the pectoralis minor muscle. Level II nodes are beneath the pectoralis minor. Level III nodes are medial to the pectoralis minor muscle. Interpectoral nodes (Rotter nodes) are found between the pectoralis major and minor muscles. Lymphatic drainage proceeds sequentially from levels I to III and skip metastasis of cancer to a higher node level without involving lower node levels is rare. The axilla contains 30 to 60 lymph nodes. Internal mammary nodes are found in the intercostal spaces in the parasternal region. They are found close to the internal mammary vessels in the extrapleural fat. Lymphatic drainage proceeds from the internal mammary nodes to the intercostal glands located posteriorly along the vertebral column as well as subpectoral and subdiaphragmatic areas. While lymphatic metastasis usually proceeds in physiologic pathways, tumor may spread through any of the lymph-node groups in any direction. Unusual drainage paths may be explained by tumor blocking lymphatic routes, causing alternative routing and the direct spread of tumor into various organs.

RISK FACTORS FOR CANCER

The presence or absence of risk factors should not influence the diagnostic evaluation. Each breast

TABLE 44-1 CHANCES OF BREAST CANCER DEVELOPING IN WOMEN BORN IN 1990		
Age	**Risk**	
25	1:19,608	
30	1:2,525	
35	1:622	
40	1:217	0.5%
45	1:93	1%
50	1:50	2%
55	1:33	3%
60	1:24	4%
65	1:17	5%
70	1:14	6%
75	1:11	
80	1:10	10%
85	1:9	
95 and over	1:8	

Reprinted with permission from Cady B. Diseases of the breast. In: Current therapy. Philadelphia: Saunders, 1995:979.

complaint should be evaluated on its own merit. An abnormal mammogram is no more or less likely to be malignant because the patient has risk factors for breast cancer. Gender and age are the risk factors of most clinical significance. Less than 1% of breast cancers occur in men and risk increases with age. Table 44-1 shows that breast cancer is rare before the age of 35 and increases to one in eight women at the age of 95. A summary of clinically significant risk factors is shown in Table 44-2. The relative risk from having a first-degree premenopausal relative (mother or sister) with unilateral breast cancer is 1.8 and from bilateral cancer 8.8. The relative risk from a postmenopausal first-degree relative with unilateral breast cancer is 1.2 and bilateral cancer 4.0. Having a mother and sister with breast cancer raises the relative risk to

TABLE 44-2 CLINICALLY SIGNIFICANT RISK FACTORS FOR BREAST CANCER
Age
Female gender
Family history in first-degree relative
Personal history of breast cancer
Obesity
Personal history of endometrial or ovarian cancer
History of significant radiation
Immunological compromise
High-fat diet
Personal history of lobular carcinoma-in-situ of the breast
Proliferative fibrocystic changes, especially atypical hyperplasia
Birth of first child after age 34
Nulliparity

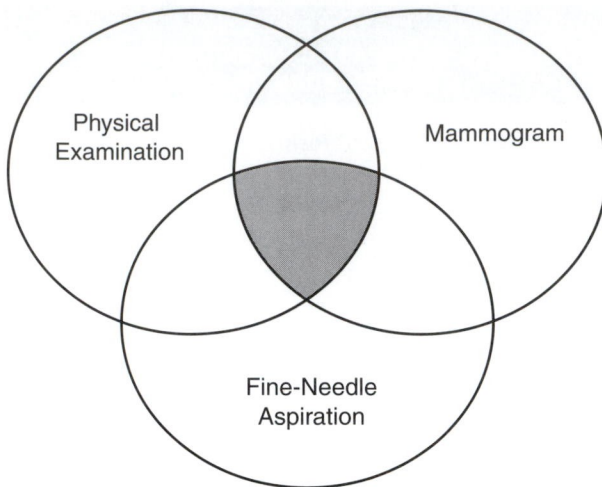

Figure 44-1 Diagnostic triad. Shaded area represents concordance of results from all the diagnostic tests.

14. It is imperative to remember that less than 30% of women over the age of 50 with breast cancer have any risk factor other than age or gender.

DIAGNOSTIC TRIAD

The diagnostic triad consists of physical examination, mammography, and fine-needle aspiration. Concordance of results for these three methods will allow the practitioner to reach the correct diagnosis in almost every case. Lack of concordance of all three parts of the triad leaves the diagnosis in doubt and demands further evaluation (Figure 44-1).

PHYSICAL EXAMINATION

Clinical breast examination is an important part of the evaluation of breast pain or annual patient visit. A proper breast examination needs to be done with the patient disrobed in both the sitting and supine position. It is important to ask the patient if she has any concerns and use this opportunity to stress self-breast examination. Most patients are effective examiners of their breasts. Self-examination should not be complicated but should be merely a search for significant change in structure from month to month. The ideal time is the week following menses and while bathing. Although mammography is superior in discovery of small, nonpalpable tumors, self-examination may shorten the lead time for diagnosis if a patient's only breast evaluation is during routine physician visits. A true breast mass is three-dimensional and distinct. Ill-defined thickened areas should not be equated

with a mass, and recording such observations on the chart may prove to be a medical/legal problem. Any charted drawings must be fully explained in the chart or later review may presume a mass was noted but not investigated properly. All abnormalities and masses must be fully investigated until a definite diagnosis is reached. It is permissible to have a patient with a questionable mass return in a month for a follow-up visit: however there is no reason to delay the investigation of a true breast mass until after a later menstrual cycle. A mass less than 1 cm can rarely be palpated and large, dense breasts may make a mass nonpalpable until it is several centimeters in diameter. A clinically suspicious mass requires a tissue diagnosis no matter how benign it appears on other testing methods.

MAMMOGRAPHY

Mammography offers the best opportunity for early diagnosis of breast cancer. Patients should be encouraged to follow screening protocols. Screening mammography should begin annually at age 40 and continue as long as the patient leads a productive life. Patients with a first-degree relative affected with breast cancer should begin screening mammograms 10 years before the age of diagnosis of their relative. Diagnostic mammography is done for investigation of a specific problem and should be done when indicated, irrespective of the time of the last screening mammogram. Mammography will discover approximately 90% of breast cancers. Those missed are usually either smaller than imaging is capable of detecting or larger palpable masses that do not contrast with surrounding tissues. Clinical examination is a necessary adjunct to mammography to rule out a palpable mass not visible mammographically. Mammography cannot make a definitive diagnosis and can never rule out the presence of breast cancer.

The average breast cancer doubling time results in a 6-year time period between its beginning and reaching a size of approximately 1 cm. Breast cancers less than 1 cm rarely metastasize but are also nonpalpable. At least 50% of cancers 2 cm in size have metastasized by the time of diagnosis. Therefore the goal is to discover breast cancer at its premetastatic size. This can be done only with screening mammogram programs. The mammographic window (Figure 44-2) is the time related to size in the life of a breast cancer that it is discoverable only with mammography. With better imaging techniques, the ability to

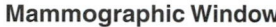

Mammographic Window

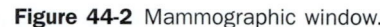

Figure 44-2 Mammographic window.

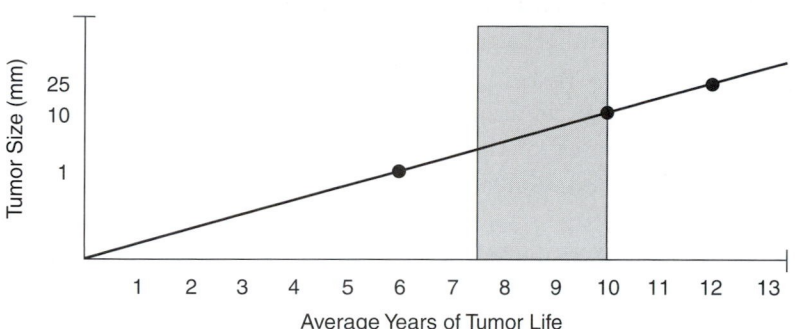

find smaller tumors is improving and the mammographic window is expanding. Mammography remains the most effective way of discovering early breast cancer. Various trials of screening programs have shown a 30 to 50% decrease in breast cancer mortality (Table 44-3).

Direct signs of cancer include microcalcifications and a spiculated or ill-defined mass. Indirect signs include a single dilated duct, architectural distortion, focal asymmetric density, or a developing density (Table 44-4).

It is important that the primary care physician communicate with the radiologist so there is no confusion concerning the report. A clear, concise report with an easily understood conclusion should be required of the mammographic facility. The Breast Imaging Reporting and Data System (BI-RADS) is a systematic reporting system that resulted from a collaborative effort of several professional societies with the hope of providing a clear, concise reporting system. The BI-RADS system is available from the American College of Radiology and its use is encouraged. Physicians should review difficult or confusing mammograms with the radiologist to lessen the chance of a misunderstanding regarding the report or recommendations. Mammographic centers should be

able to provide statistics regarding the frequency of patients called back for extra views, percentage of films read as abnormal, and percentage of abnormal films recommended for biopsy that ultimately proved to be benign or malignant.

Ultrasound is an adjunct to mammography and has a limited role in breast screening. Breast ultrasound may be performed in the office with a 7.5-MHz transducer but only after adequate training and credentialling. The primary use of ultrasound is to evaluate a target lesion to determine if it is cystic or solid. Because intracystic carcinoma is rare, the identification of a cystic lesion by ultrasound may eliminate the need for biopsy. This is most valuable in nonpalpable masses discovered mammographically, as palpable masses can be needle-aspirated without imaging studies. It is not possible to differentiate malignant from benign based on the ultrasound appearance of a solid mass. Cystic lesions may be observed, while solid masses need a tissue diagnosis. Strict criteria for identification of a cyst include round or oval mass with well-circumscribed margins, horizontal orientation that may flatten with compression, enhanced-through transmission of sound with back-wall enhancement, and no internal echoes (Table 44-5). Ultrasound may be used to guide needle aspiration of

---

TABLE 44-3
REDUCED BREAST CANCER MORTALITY FROM MAMMOGRAPHY SCREENING PROGRAMS

Study	Schedule	Reduced Mortality
HIP	Annual × 4 years	30%
Verbec	Biannual × 4 years	33%
Colette	1, 12, 18, and 24 months	50%
Tabar	Biannual, age 40–49; every 33 months after age 50	31%

Reprinted with permission from DiSaia PJ, Creasman WT. Breast disease. In: DiSaia PJ, Creasman WT, eds. Clinical gynecologic oncology. St. Louis: Mosby, 1997:382.

TABLE 44-4
MAMMOGRAPHIC SIGNS OF MALIGNANCY

Direct signs
  Abnormal clustered microcalcifications
  Spiculated or ill-defined mass
Indirect signs
  Single dilated duct
  Architectural distortion
  Focal asymmetric density
  Developing density

TABLE 44-5
ULTRASOUND EVIDENCE OF BREAST CYST

Round or oval mass with well-circumscribed margins
Horizontal orientation that may flatten with compression
No internal echoes
Enhanced through-transmission with back-wall enhancement of
  sound

nonpalpable cysts if there is uncertainty about the sonar appearance or the patient requests aspiration. Ultrasound may also be used to guide needle aspiration or core biopsy of solid breast masses.

FINE-NEEDLE ASPIRATION

Fine-needle aspiration (FNA) may be carried out for cystic or solid lesions. There is nothing more gratifying to the patient than to immediately discover that her mass is a cyst and is not malignant. Strict criteria must be followed when aspirating breast cysts to confirm benign status. The mass must completely resolve, the fluid must be nonbloody, and the mass must not recur. The color of the fluid is not significant as long as it is not bloody. Cytology is not indicated on nonbloody fluid and may be confusing as benign cells from cysts may appear cytologically abnormal. Nontraumatic bloody fluid necessitates biopsy of the mass. Surgical removal is indicated if the mass recurs more than twice after aspiration to rule out rare cystic carcinoma. Patients are asked to return 1 to 3 months after cyst aspiration to evaluate for recurrence. Equipment needed for cyst aspiration is a 10-cc syringe and 22-gauge needle. Local anesthesia is not necessary and pain is minimized by stretching the skin with two fingers over the mass prior to needle insertion. Care must be taken to observe the depth of the mass to prevent needle puncture into the pleural cavity.

Needle aspiration is also performed to evaluate solid masses and can be done immediately in the office on discovery. The value of diagnostic mammography for evaluation of a breast mass is more for investigation of the remainder of both breasts rather than the mass itself, as it can be evaluated immediately with fine-needle aspiration cytology. Equipment needed for needle aspiration includes a 10-cc syringe, 22-gauge needle, glass slide, and cytology fixative. The technique involves stabilizing the mass between two fingers and stretching the skin. Local anesthesia is not needed. Attempts are made to stabilize the mass

over a rib for protection of the pleural cavity. It is important to estimate the depth of the mass in relation to the length of the needle. Even a deep lesion will be close to the skin when the patient is supine and pressure is applied over the mass. Overzealous needle insertion risks pneumothorax. Once the needle is into the mass, negative pressure in the syringe is created by pulling back on the plunger. The needle is then moved several strokes in bayonet fashion with care to keep the needle in the mass. Negative pressure is released prior to removing the needle from the mass. The tissue aspirate is found within the hub of the needle and is expelled onto a glass slide and promptly spread and fixed. It is important that a cytologist be chosen who has expertise in breast cytology. Pressure is applied after FNA to minimize the chance of hematoma (Figure 44-3).

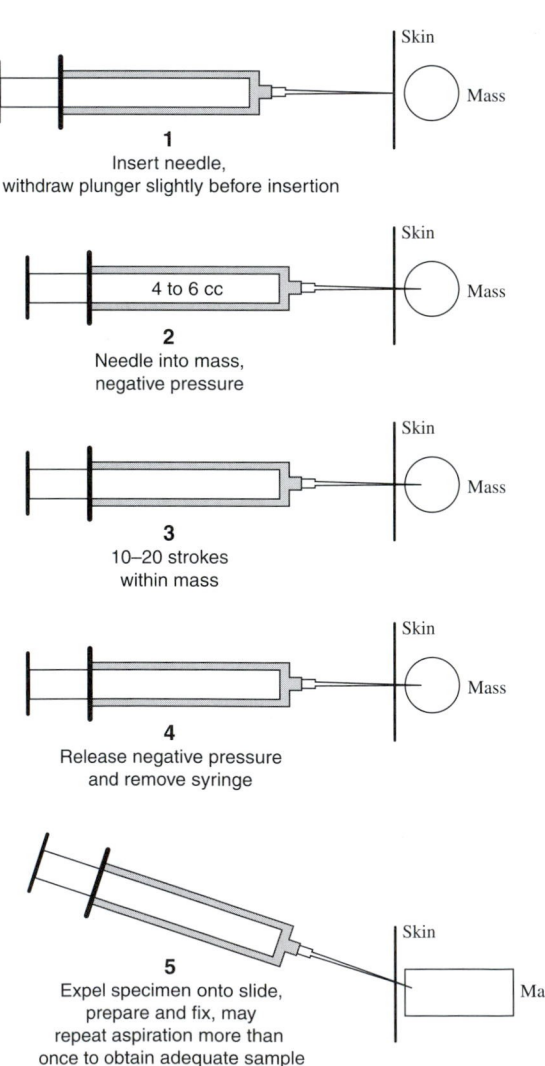

1
Insert needle,
withdraw plunger slightly before insertion

2
Needle into mass,
negative pressure

3
10–20 strokes
within mass

4
Release negative pressure
and remove syringe

5
Expel specimen onto slide,
prepare and fix, may
repeat aspiration more than
once to obtain adequate sample

Figure 44-3 Fine-needle aspiration cytology: solid breast mass.

False positive results with cytology are rare, and false negative rates are less than 10%. Hazards to a reliable diagnosis with FNA result from attempts to aspirate an ill-defined or nonexistent mass. Blood in the syringe may also make interpretation difficult. Prompt fixation is necessary to avoid air-drying of the specimen. The cytology aspirate must contain an adequate amount of ductal cells, and the report should comment about specimen adequacy. Absence of ductal cells prohibits any conclusion being drawn from the cytology specimen. Fine-needle-aspiration cytology (FNAC) cannot differentiate between atypical ductal cells, carcinoma in situ, or invasive cancer. Tissue diagnosis is required in these situations. A clinically suspicious mass should be biopsied even if the FNAC report is benign. A traumatic FNA with hematoma formation may require delaying mammographic investigation. Some radiologists prefer that FNA be delayed until after the mammogram is obtained.

Reliance on the diagnostic triad of physical examination, mammography, and FNAC will provide the clinician with an invaluable diagnostic tool for evaluation of breast complaints. Biopsy must always be done if there is not concordance of results. None of the individual components of the diagnostic triad stand alone, but together they provide an excellent method for office diagnosis of the majority of breast abnormalities. Algorithms for diagnostic evaluation of palpable and nonpalpable abnormalities are shown in Figures 44-4 and 44-5.

BENIGN BREAST CONDITIONS

Nipple Discharge

Although breast cancer rarely presents with nipple discharge, most women fear that it indicates malignancy. History and physical examination, combined

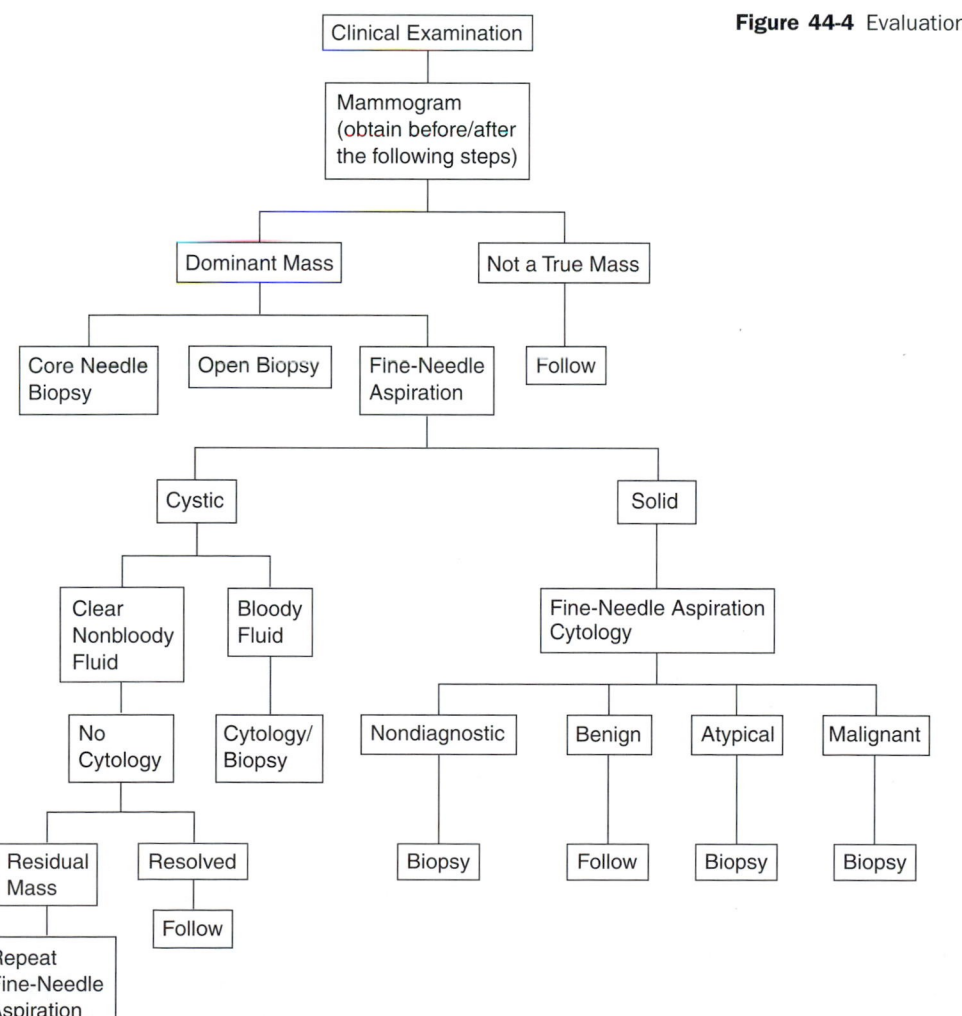

Figure 44-4 Evaluation of a palpable breast mass.

Figure 44-5 Evaluation of an abnormal mammogram.

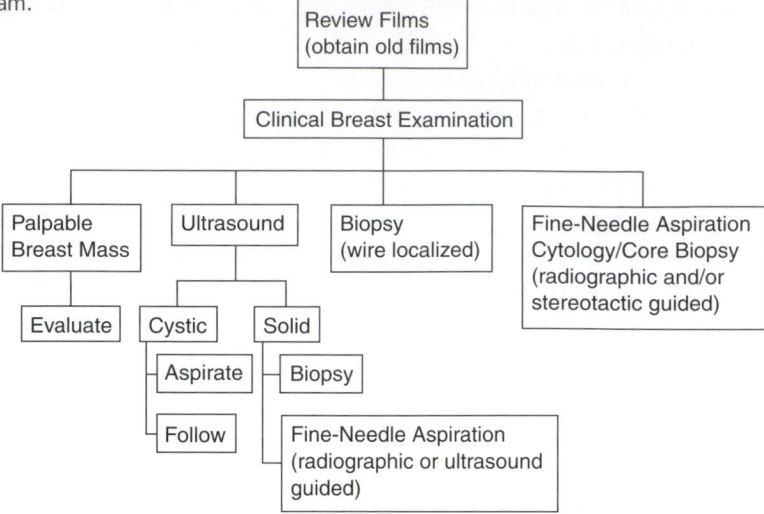

with knowledge of breast anatomy, will usually lead the clinician to the correct diagnosis. The anatomical relationship of isolated breast lobes with their own unique terminal duct communicating with the nipple is essential to understand the difference between galactorrhea and pathologic nipple discharge. An algorithm for diagnostic possibilities is shown in Figure 44-6.

Galactorrhea

Galactorrhea or hormonal nipple discharge is defined as milky secretion of fluid from the breast that is nonphysiologic and that is not related to pregnancy or nursing. Galactorrhea is present in 10% of women and can be elicited in 80% with manipulation. History nearly always reveals that it is induced, bilateral, and seen from multiple duct openings at the nipple. It is nonbloody. The color may be milky or various shades of green, gray, or brown. Although there are many causes, the ultimate cause of hormonal galactorrhea is an increased release of prolactin. Estrogen sources such as birth control pills can lead to galactorrhea by hypothalamic suppression, resulting in lowered production of prolactin-inhibiting factor (PIF), with a resulting rise in serum prolactin. Reduction of PIF may also result from hypothalamic neoplasm, cervical spine lesions, emotional stress, breast suckling, or chest-wall stimulation by trauma, surgery, or herpes zoster. Many drugs inhibit hypothalamic production of PIF or act directly on the pituitary. Phenothiazines, reserpine derivatives, opiates, diazepams, butyrophenones, methyldopa, and tricyclic antidepressants may

all stimulate galactorrhea. Phenothiazine-stimulated prolactin levels will not exceed 100 ng/ml. Hypothyroidism can stimulate galactorrhea, as excess hypothalamic thyroid-releasing hormone mimics prolactin-releasing hormone. Hyperprolactinemia can result from nonpituitary sources such as lung and renal tumors, as well as uterine leiomyomata. Renal disease with a lowered glomerular filtration rate may elevate prolactin levels. The pituitary gland itself may produce excess prolactin due to hyperfunction, tumor (adenoma) or empty sella syndrome. Treatment options are based on the patient's tolerance to the galactorrhea, prolactin level, and presence or absence of pituitary tumor. Simple measures such as changing medications or avoiding breast stimulation may produce dramatic results. Patients with elevated prolactin levels and no obvious cause should be imaged with magnetic resonance imaging (MRI) to rule out pituitary tumor. Patients with elevated prolactin levels but normal imaging studies are offered dopamine agonist medication (bromocriptine) or observation. Pituitary adenomas are divided into micro and macro groups, with 1 cm as the dividing line. Dopamine agonists are recommended, and surgery is reserved for rapidly growing adenomas or macroadenomas that do not respond to medical management.

Pathologic Nipple Discharge

Pathologic nipple discharge results from an abnormality within the breast. It is nearly always spontaneous, unilateral, and exists from a single duct opening at the nipple. The fluid is either serous, bloody, or

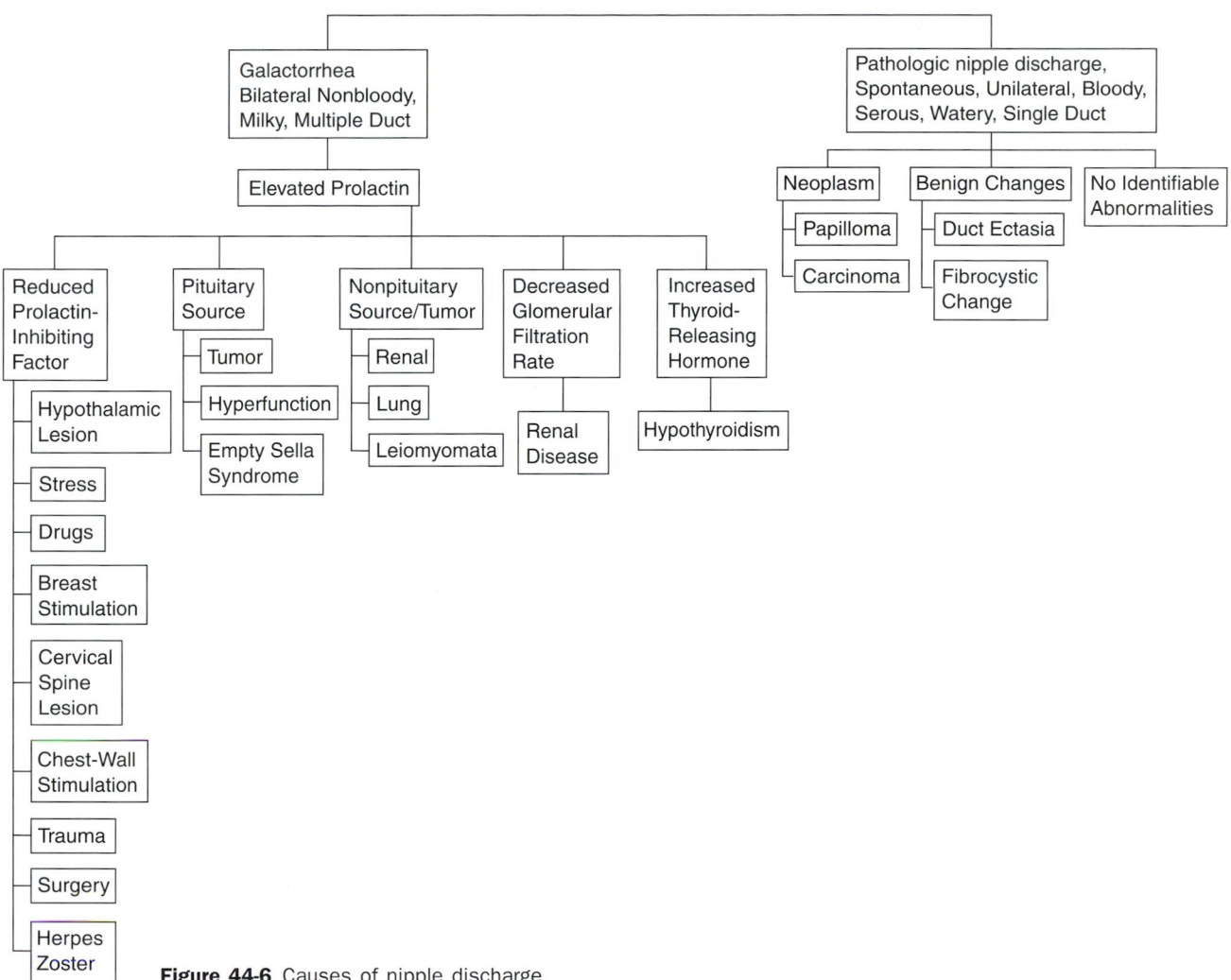

Figure 44-6 Causes of nipple discharge.

watery. While most pathologic nipple discharge is from trauma or benign disorders such as intraductal papilloma, it is imperative that the possibility of carcinoma be investigated. Guaiac testing of the discharge can be used to determine if the fluid is bloody. Galactography has limited value, but it may help in the case of a ductal tumor in a peripheral area of the breast. Cytology of the nipple discharge has no value. Evaluation consists of history, physical examination, and mammography. Nearly all papillomas are in the terminal ducts under the nipple–areola complex. The site of the papilloma can usually be elicited by sequential pressure around the areola. One will see discharge expressed from the nipple when the abnormal area is compressed. The duct in this area can then be excised under local anesthesia for histologic examination. Care must be taken not to interrupt a significant number of terminal ducts if the patient plans on breast-feeding in the future. Duct ectasia (see section

on "Duct Ectasia," below) may also cause nipple discharge. A palpable mass or mammogaphic abnormality should be evaluated as outlined previously. An algorithm for diagnostic evaluation of galactorrhea is shown in Figure 44-7.

Mastalgia

Breast tenderness is commonly reported. There is no universal agreement as to the cause of mastalgia and even less agreement as to what is effective treatment. Reports about caffeine-induced mastalgia are not scientifically validated, although some patients believe that caffiene reduction is helpful. The evaluation of mastalgia requires a careful history and physical examination. The cause may not originate in the breast but from the chest wall or muscular discomfort. Mammography is indicated if a neoplasm is suspected. While breast cancer is usually painless, the presence of

Figure 44-7 Diagnostic evaluation of nipple discharge.

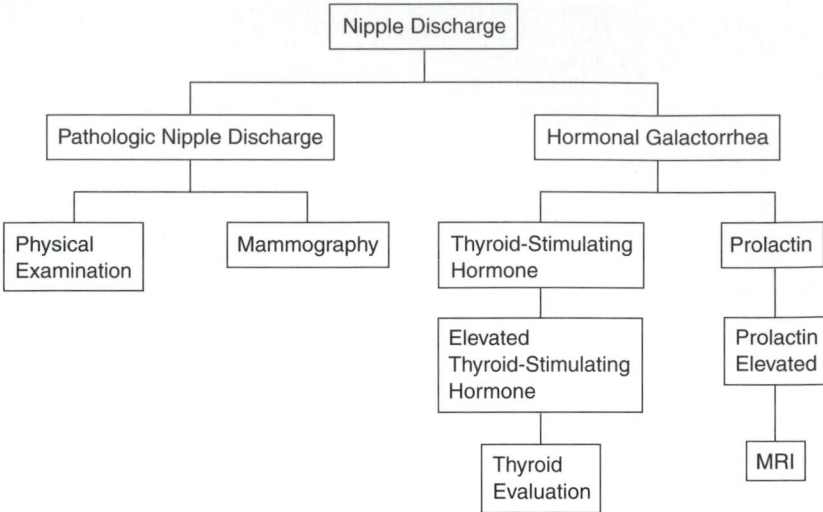

tenderness cannot be used to exclude malignancy. A palpable mass or mammographic abnormality should be appropriately investigated. When neoplasm is not suspected, the patient is offered various treatment options. The majority of patients are relieved there is no tumor, and reassurance often produces dramatic relief. Local measures include a well-fitting support bra without an underwire apparatus. Salt restriction during the luteal phase may be helpful. Medical management may be directed through the use of nonsteroidal analgesics or evening primrose oil tablets. Low-dose therapy of danocrine, 200 to 400 mg per day, may produce excellent results without androgen

side effects. Doses as low as 50 mg per day may be beneficial. Danocrine therapy is continued for 3 to 6 months, and care must be taken to ensure that the patient does not become pregnant. Low-dose birth control pills or bromocriptine may also be helpful. Tamoxifen taken 10 to 20 mg per day may be helpful because of its antiestrogen effect. Menopausal patients may experience mastalgia from estrogen-replacement therapy; lowering the dose is usually effective. Newer estrogens such as raloxifen (a selective estrogen-receptor modulator) that do not bind to breast tissue rarely cause mastalgia. An algorithm for evaluation and treatment of mastalgia is shown in Figure 44-8.

Fibrocystic Changes

Fibrocystic change is a nonspecific term used to describe lumpy or painful breasts. It is not a disease and should not be labeled as such. Fibrocystic changes are normal but exaggerated responses of breast tissue to female hormones. Classic symptoms are premenopausal cyclic engorgement, with increased density of the breast. The malignant risk of fibrocystic changes has been heavily debated. Studies have shown that it is the degree of ductal epithelial proliferation or hyperplasia that predicts malignant potential. Table 44-6 shows the cancer risk of various benign breast conditions, including proliferative changes. Reports of dietary methylxanthine elimination and administration of vitamin E have not demonstrated uniformly beneficial effects, although individual patients may report reduction of symptoms.

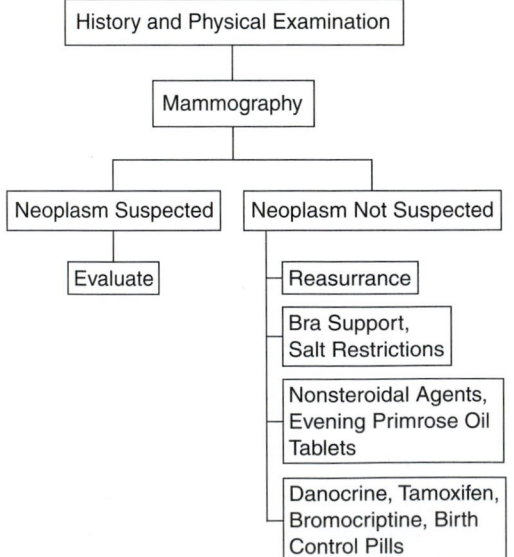

Figure 44-8 Mastalgia.

TABLE 44-6
CANCER RISK OF BENIGN BREAST CONDITIONS

No increased risk
  Adenosis
  Apocrine metaplasia
  Cysts
  Duct ectasia
  Fat necrosis
  Fibroadenoma
  Fibrosis
  Mastitis
  Mild hyperplasia
  Trauma
Slightly increased risk (1.5 to 2× risk)
  Moderate or florid hyperplasia
  Papilloma
Moderately increased risk (3 to 5× risk)
  Atypical hyperplasia: ductal or lobular

Duct Ectasia

Duct ectasia usually presents with multiduct nipple discharge with subareolar pain, itching, or burning. Swelling or a mass may be palpated under the areola. Duct ectasia results from periducteal inflammation which leads to fibrosis and dilatation of the duct. Rupture may occur, resulting in inflammation and fat necrosis. Excision of the involved duct is required for treatment and to rule out carcinoma.

Mastitis

Mastitis is usually an obstetric condition but can also be found in the nonpregnant woman. Treatment consists of antibiotics specific for Staphylococcus species and drainage of any abscess cavity. Drainage may be successful with serial needle aspirations and careful follow-up. Incision and drainage should be performed if there is not rapid improvement. Breast-feeding may continue, although any sores on the nipple must be allowed to heal. Inflammatory carcinoma should be considered in any patient with mastitis that does not rapidly improve.

Fat Necrosis

Fat necrosis originates from trauma, although the patient may not know when the injury took place. A tight bra, especially the underwire style, may lead to fat necrosis. The patient presents with a tender, ill-defined mass that may be more of a ridge. Mammography may suggest malignant changes with microcal-

cifications and a stellate mass. Fat necrosis has no malignant potential, although biopsy may be required to rule out carcinoma.

Fibroadenoma

Fibroadenoma is the most common breast neoplasm. They are benign and do not increase the patient's risk for subsequent cancer. Fibroadenomas are firm, rubbery nodules and often present in adolescents and women in their 20s. They are painless and do not change size in relationship to the menstrual cycle. Twenty percent of patients with fibroadenoma will have more than one. Approximately one-third of fibroadenomas will regress in size or disappear when followed over a long period. Nonpalpable fibroadenomas may be discovered mammographically and have a classic ovoid homogeneous appearance, with smooth margins surrounded by a halo. Serial mammography is appropriate as long as the appearance remains consistent with benign fibroadenoma. Palpable fibroadenoma may be diagnosed accurately with FNAC. Fibroadenoma may be observed or removed at the patient's request as Hindle and Alonzo have shown that expectant management of fibroadenoma is appropriate if the diagnostic triad has been satisfied.[3] Enlarging or giant fibroadenoma should be excised. Removal is done under local anesthesia with a small cosmetically placed incision. They are easily shelled out and there is no need to take wide margins.

Phylloides Tumor

Cystosarcoma phylloides are slow-growing fibro-epithelial tumors with hypercellular connective tissue. They are rare and account for only 2.5% of all fibro-epithelial tumors. While 25% are malignant, only 10% metastasize. They grow rapidly and most commonly present in women in their 50s. Treatment is excision with wide margins.

Adenoma

An adenoma of the breast is a well-circumscribed nodular tumor with benign epithelial elements and scant stroma. Tubular adenomas are mobile rubbery nodules that resemble fibroadenoma except that they lack a conspicuous stroma. Lactating adenomas are discrete mobile masses that arise during pregnancy or the postpartum period. Microscopically they have lactational changes similar to normal breast tissue.

Sclerosing Lesions

Sclerosing lesions have been called a variety of names but are more correctly included with the benign fibrocystic changes. Their gross and mammographic appearance mimics carcinoma. They are typically 1 cm or less in size and are firm, with central retraction. Their malignant potential relates to the degree of proliferation of the epithelial component. Surgical excision is the treatment of choice.

Invasive Breast Cancer

The United States has one of the highest rates of breast cancer incidence and mortality. Attempts have failed to discover the cause of breast cancer. The long latent period (average, 6 years) before a breast cancer becomes clinically evident makes epidemiologic research difficult. Five to ten percent of breast cancers are thought to occur as a result of genetic inheritance and mutation involving tumor-suppressive genes. The *BRCA1* gene is located on chromosome 17 and *BRCA2* gene on chromosome 13. Both express as autosomal dominant. Eighty-five percent of patients who carry a mutation to *BRCA1* and *BRCA2* will develop breast cancer. Accepted clinical guidelines for testing and recommendations for those with the mutations are lacking. The high cost of genetic testing, multiple mutations, and possible varying penetrance of the mutation make clinical recommendations unclear. If testing is to be performed, it is most appropriate in high-risk familes. It is not known what effect carrying the *BRCA1* and *BRCA2* mutations will have on a patient's ability to obtain health, life, or disability insurance. Present recommendations for those with the mutation range from intense screening to prophylactic mastectomy.

Patients with invasive breast carcinoma should undergo metastatic evaluation prior to any definitive cancer operation. Extensive local treatment to the breast will have little advantage if the patient already has distant disease. Breast cancer is potentially systemic at the time of diagnosis. Removal of axillary lymph nodes is for staging purposes only and does not improve the patient's chance of survival. Skip metastasis from lower- to higher-level axillary nodes is rare; thus, sampling of lower-level nodes (levels I

TABLE 44-7 FIVE-YEAR BREAST CANCER SURVIVAL RATES ACCORDING TO SIZE OF TUMOR AND AXILLARY NODE INVOLVEMENT			
	Axillary-Node Involvement		
Tumor Size	*Negative*	*1–3 Positive*	*4 or More Positive*
<0.5 cm	99.2%	95.3%	59.0%
0.5–0.9	98.3%	94.0%	54.2%
1.0–1.9	95.8%	86.6%	67.2%
2.0–2.9	92.3%	83.4%	63.4%
3.0–3.9	86.2%	79.0%	56.9%
4.0–4.9	84.6%	69.8%	52.6%
>5.0	82.2%	73.0%	45.5%

Reprinted with permission from Carter CL, Allen C, Henson DE. Reduction of tumor size, lymph node status, and survival in 24,740 breast cancer cases. Cancer 1989;63:181.

and II) is adequate. The internal mammary nodes are not sampled. Removal of the first axillary node in the drainage route from the breast may accurately predict the nodal status of the remainder of the axillary nodes. This first node has been named the sentinel node and is discovered by injection of the tumor bed with a dye or radioisotope. However, until sentinel-node removal stands the test of time, the standard of care remains an axillary dissection of levels I and II when node sampling is indicated. The presence of breast cancer in axillary lymph nodes only indicates that the cancer has the capacity to metastasize and has already done so. Survival rates worsen inversely with the number of involved nodes. The absence of spread into axillary lymphatics does not guarantee lack of distant disease, as there are alternate lymphatic routes and hemotogenous pathways. Distant metastases are usually found in lung, liver, and bone. Autopsy studies confirm that breast cancer has the capacity to spread into virtually any body site. Table 44-7 shows survival rates in relation to tumor size and lymph-node status.

Metastatic evaluation involves a complete physical examination as well as mammography to evaluatate the remainder of the ipsilateral and contralateral breast. Chest x-ray films and liver enzyme measurements are indicated. Imaging studies of bone structures are obtained if there is suspicion of metastasis. Serum tumor markers (CA 27.29) are obtained and followed on a serial basis. Estrogen and progesterone receptors are obtained for prognostic value only. Large tumor size and negative estrogen receptors remain the most predictive of all indicators for metastatic potential. DNA

**TABLE 44-8
CONTRAINDICATIONS TO BREAST-
PRESERVATION SURGERY**

Patient preference
Diffuse or multifocal disease with unobtainable clear margins
Medical contraindications to radiation therapy or prior breast
  radiation
Suspected poor cosmetic results from large ratio of tumor to
  breast size
Active pregnancy (radiation contraindicated)

flow cytometry will give prognostic information about the tumor's biological behavior.

Extensive radical surgery was once the standard of care for breast cancer. It was assumed that breast cancer spread in a logical stepwise fashion first through the axillary lymph nodes. Axillary nodes were thought to provide a barrier to distant spread. We now know that this is incorrect and that local control will not prevent distant disease. Through extensive investigative trials, it is now agreed that breast-preservation surgery (lumpectomy and axillary-node dissection with postoperative radiotherapy) offers the patient equal opportunity for survival as compared with mastectomy. Critical factors mandatory for breast-preservation surgery to be appropriate treatment are obtaining clear tumor margins (hopefully, 1 cm) and the absence of known multicentric disease. The patient must be involved in the decision whether to proceed with lumpectomy or mastectomy. Cosmesis and patient convenience are taken into account. Table 44-8 shows the contraindications to a breast-preservation procedure.

Postcancer adverse psychological sequelae are more closely related to the withdrawal of estrogen and fear of cancer than the choice of operation. Radiation therapy (XRT) is indicated after lumpectomy to eliminate microscopic undetectable multicentric disease. Early trials of lumpectomy without radiotherapy resulted in a 30% local recurrance rate. XRT reduces the local recurrence rates to 5%. With early detection of breast cancer, nearly all patients will be candidates for breast preservation.

Breast cancer occurs in 1 in 3000 pregnancies. The diagnostic evaluation should not differ from that for the nonpregnant woman. FNA and biopsy should be performed when indicated. Pregnancy is no longer thought to convey a worse prognosis as compared with nonpregnant patients stage for stage.

Unfortunately, most cancers in pregnant women are diagnosed at a more advanced stage than their nonpregnant counterparts. There are no conclusive data to suggest that subsequent pregnancies alter survival rates; therefore, there is no contraindication to future pregnancy.

Ductal Carcinoma in Situ

Ductal carcinoma in situ (DCIS) is found in increasing numbers as a result of mammographic screening programs. DCIS is a preinvasive lesion with a 20 to 40% risk of later development of infiltrating carcinoma. Axillary-lymph-node involvement is rare. It is imperative that extensive histologic examination be carried out to exclude the presence of an invasive component. DCIS is often multifocal and can be demonstrated mammographically. Simple mastectomy (removal of the breast without axillary-lymph-node dissection) has been the historical treatment of choice, with a cure rate of nearly 100%. Breast preservation is appropriate for those with localized disease and clear tumor margins. XRT is usually recommended after lumpectomy and has been shown to reduce the rate of local recurrence. Axillary-lymph-node dissection is not indicated.

Lobular Carcinoma in Situ

Lobular carcinoma in situ (LCIS) has no characteristic mammographic signs and is nonpalpable. It is diagnosed at biopsy for associated indications. Invasive disease is found in approximately 5% of patients. LCIS is viewed more as a marker of increased risk for future invasive disease than cancer itself. Patients with LCIS have a 30% lifetime risk (1% per year) of later development of invasive cancer, which is usually ductal, and the risk is equal in both breasts. Treatment options include bilateral simple mastectomy or no further surgery and careful follow-up. The patient must be involved in the decision for treatment. Factors relating to the patient's age and risk tolerance are important. Most patients will do well with no further surgery and reliance on close suveillance. LCIS is not radiosensitive and thus XRT has no role.

Paget Disease of the Nipple

Paget disease of the nipple is DCIS of the nipple–areola complex. Invasive changes may also be found.

Biopsy is mandatory for any suspicious lesion of the nipple or areola. A careful mammographic search should be carried out for other abnormal areas and palpable nodules should be excluded. Because the location involves the nipple–areola complex, most patients will be treated with mastectomy to ensure clear margins and a satisfactory cosmetic result. XRT is indicated if mastectomy was not performed. Axillary node dissection is not recommended for in situ disease.

Inflammatory Carcinoma

Inflammatory carcinoma is invasive ductal carcinoma with spread of malignant cells into dermal lymphatics. The classic appearance of mastitis may delay diagnosis. Mammography is indicated and may discover a mass difficult to feel due to skin thickening and induration of the breast. Biopsy of a mass or the skin will provide the diagnosis. Inflammatory carcinoma is considered systemic at the time of diagnosis, and historical survival rates were less than 5%. Aggressive chemotherapy has improved the chances for survival. Lumpectomy offers adequate local control, and mastectomy is rarely indicated. Axillary-node dissection is not recommended, as the disease is already known to be metastatic. Postlumpectomy radiation therapy will help with local control. An algorithm for treatment options for breast cancer is shown in Figure 44-9.

BREAST BIOPSY

Open breast biopsy is indicated either for a palpable mass or a mamographic abnormality. Biopsy for a palpable mass is indicated if the diagnostic triad fails to make a diagnosis. Biopsy is an outpatient procedure nearly always done under local anesthesia. Excellent cosmetic results can be obtained by making curvilinear incisions along Langer's lines. Circumareolar incisions are best and allow adequate exposure for most breast masses. With a tunneling technique, the incision can be placed in a more cosmetically acceptable location and does not have to be directly over the mass. It is imperative that the incision be placed in a location that does not compromise potential future cancer surgery. Meticulous hemostasis is obtained through the use of cautery. Deep sutures are avoided, if possible, to reduce induration and dimpling of the skin. Wound closure is with subcutaneous absorbable suture, and a pressure dressing is applied after surgery.

Cancer surgery can safely be deferred, pending pathological investigation, counseling, and metastatic evaluation. Complications are rare and include hematoma and infection. Most hematomas resolve without drainage. Except when the mass is known to be benign by FNAC, it is recommended to try to obtain a wide margin of tissue around the mass. This may eliminate the need for reoperation of the primary site if cancer is discovered and the margins were clear. The specimen should have the margins marked with ink and evaluated by pathology. Frozen-section diagnosis will not alter immediate management and only increases the cost. Hormone receptors and DNA flow cytomety studies can be obtained from fresh tissue or paraffin tissue block. Approximately 25% of biopsies for a palpable mass will be malignant.

Breast biopsies are more commonly performed for nonpalpable mammographic abnormalities than for palpable masses. This is a result of mammographic screening programs and the ability to evaluate a palpable mass with the diagnostic triad. The abnormal area is localized preoperatively with image-guided wire placement, and the patient taken to surgery for open biopsy. An alternative option is stereotactic image-guided core needle biopsy. Specimen radiography or a postbiopsy mammogram is obtained to confirm removal of the abnormal area. Wire localization with open biopsy has proven to be an accurate method to remove abnormal mammographic areas. We have failed to remove the abnormal area in only 4 (99.4% success rate) out of 611 patients from 1980 through 1999. Image-guided core biopsy techniques are accurate in skilled hands: although as many as 10 to 20% of patients will need open biopsy to establish a diagnosis due to sampling errors or the inability to rule out invasive cancer when the cored tissue reveals atypical hyperplasia or in situ disease. Reports indicate that 20 to 30% of all biopsies done for abnormal mammography will reveal cancer (Table 44-9). The

TABLE 44-9
PERCENT OF ABNORMAL MAMMOGRAPHIC AREAS CONFIRMED MALIGNANT AT OPEN BIOPSY

Series	Percent Malignant
Hall 1980–1993[17]	14
Hall 1993–1996	21
University of Kentucky 1981–1989[18]	19
University of Kentucky 1990[18]	31
Multiple series[18]	25

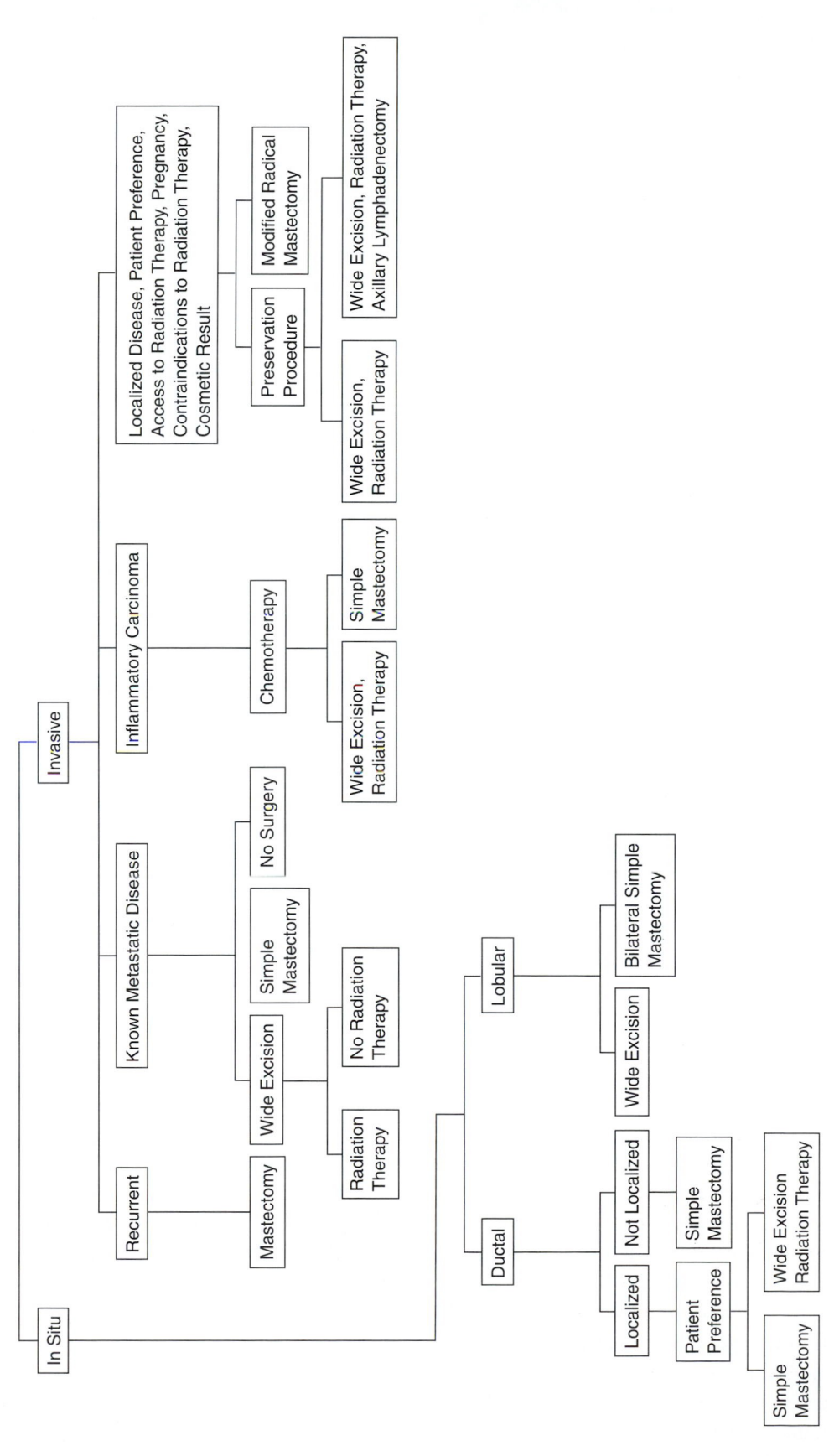

Figure 44-9 Surgical treatment of breast cancer.

TABLE 44-10 YIELD RATE OF CANCER FOR SPECIFIC MAMMOGRAPHIC ABNORMALITY		
Asymmetric density		
Hall[5]	2%	
Bauer[7]	6.6%	
McCreery[8]	6%	
Abnormal calcifications		
Hall[5]	22%	
Baute[9]	31%	
Bauer[7]	15.8%	
McCreery[8]	29%	
Mass		
Hall[5]	11%	
Baute[9]	36%	
Bauer[7]	9.7%	(63% spiculated)
McCreery[8]	3%	(45% spiculated)
Mass with calcium		
Hall[5]	21%	
Baute[9]	54%	
McCreery[8]	20%	

Reprinted with permission from Hall JA, Hall BR, Murphy DC, et al. Mammographic abnormalities and the detection of carcinoma of the breast. Am J Obstet Gynecol 1993;168:1677.

highest yield of cancer for mammographic abnormality is a spiculated mass with asymmetric density the lowest (Table 44-10). Nonpalpable occult breast cancers discovered mammographically should have a cure rate over 90%.

LONG-TERM FOLLOW-UP OF PATIENTS WITH BREAST CANCER

Patients will return to their primary care physician for integration of breast cancer treatment with other health-care concerns. Teamwork and coordination of all health care providers is essential. Psychological issues relating to body image, fear of cancer and death, and sexuality should be addressed. Side effects of chemotherapy and estrogen withdrawal are important considerations. Support groups are invaluable to some patients. Most want to return to a normal lifestyle and should be encouraged to do so. Emotional well-being may be more adversely affected by estrogen deprivation than by the disease itself. Long-term concerns relate to cancer recurrence, menopausal symptoms, contraception, and pregnancy. Some patients may question the advisability of prophylactic mastectomy of the contralateral side. This is generally discouraged in favor of careful surveillance. Neither subcutaneous mastectomy or simple mastectomy guarantees removal of all breast tissue or total prophylaxis.

Opinions vary about how extensive should be the testing carried out for recurrence. While early discovery of recurrence may not affect overall survival, it may lengthen the survival time as well as the quality of life. Searching for local recurrence, new primary disease in the contralateral breast, or distant metastases is appropriate. Mammographic screening is recommended every 6 months on the affected side for 3 years after treatment and annually on the contralateral side. After 3 years, the screening interval goes to annually bilaterally. Testing for metastatic disease includes annual chest x-ray examination, serum antigen CA 27.29, liver chemistries, and biannual physical examination. Pregnancy is not contraindicated after treatment and has not been proven to worsen the chance of survival. Estrogen is offered to all women with estrogen deficiency, and its use has not been shown to adversely affect survival rates. Selected estrogen-receptor modulators such as raloxifene may offer an advantage to those concerned about the safety of estrogen use, as they are antagonistic to uterine and breast tissue while maintaining positive estrogen benefits elsewhere. The known benefits of estrogen regarding prevention of osteoporosis, cardiovascular disease, and dementia must be made available to the patient. Tradition has held that estrogen is not to be used in patients who have had breast cancer; however, this belief lacks scientific validation. Wile and DiSaia's literature review[10] concluded that there is no evidence that estrogen usage is detrimental to surviving breast cancer. The American College of Obstetricians and Gynecologists states, "There are no data that support an increased risk of breast cancer recurrence or reduced survival rate after administration or reinstitution of ERT."[11]

Tamoxifen has antiestrogen activity to breast tissue but also acts as a weak estrogen systemically. The exact mechanism for tamoxifen's reduction on recurrence rates is not known. There are also data to suggest that tamoxifen may reduce breast cancer risk as much as 40%. Tamoxifen is generally recommended for patients with estrogen-receptor–positive tumors and is continued for 5 years. The risk of tamoxifen inducing endometrial cancer is the same as taking unopposed estrogen. Periodic transvaginal ultrasonography or endometrial biopsies have not been shown to lower mortality from tamoxifen-induced endometrial carinoma. Patients on tamoxifen are followed routinely with no special testing but are encouraged to report immediately any vaginal bleeding.

Concurrent use of progesterone with tamoxifen is not routinely recommended. Oral contraceptives, Depo-Provera, sterilization, or barrier methods are available for contraception depending on the patient's needs, desires, and risk tolerance.

ESTROGEN AND RISK OF BREAST CANCER

Opinions vary about whether estrogen increases the risk of breast cancer. Unfortunately, no prospective study answers this question. Available data are retrospective, and conclusions are expressed in terms of relative risk. Although a relative risk greater than 1.0 may be mathematically correct, the association between the risk factor and the event is considered weak until the relative risk reaches 2, or even perhaps 3, to 1.

Colditz et al.[12] reported results from the Nurses Health Study based on 60,000 women with 18 years follow-up, showing a possible 50% (relative risk, 1.46) increased risk of breast cancer after 5 to 10 years of estrogen use. The risk returned to base line 5 years after discontinuation of estrogen. It is important to note that there was a 40% decrease in the risk of overall mortality for current hormone users, with the primary benefit for women with cardiovascular risk factors. Progesterone had no effect on breast cancer risk.

Several studies report a different conclusion from the Nurses Health Study. Dupont and Page's[13] meta-analysis of 28 studies provides strong evidence that menopausal therapy of 0.625 mg/day of conjugated estrogens does not increase the risk of breast cancer. Nachtigall et al.[14] reported that 22 year administration of estrogen and progesterone did not increase the incidence of breast cancer in a small group of continuously hospitalized postmenopausal women. Stanford et al.[15] reported in 1995 that use of estrogen and progesterone was not associated with any increased risk of breast cancer in either current or long term (8 or more years) users. Newcomb et al.[16] also reported in 1995 there was no increased risk in estrogen users either current or long term of over 15 years. Figure 44-10 shows the relative risk estimate and 95% confidence intervals of estrogen use and breast-cancer risk from several studies. A significant clinical association between a risk factor and a disease requires a relative risk and its 95% confidence limits of at least 2:1. There appears to be no conclusive evidence of significant increased risk of breast cancer from estrogen usage.

Users of estrogen at the time of diagnosis also appear to have a better prognosis or at least no worse than nonhormone users. Willis et al.[20] reported a 16% reduction of risk of mortality among estrogen users and Strickland et al.[21] concluded that estrogen-replacement therapy did not compromise survival in women in whom breast cancer subsequently developed. Studies by Bergvist[22] and Gambrell[23] and their colleagues report a reduction in breast cancer mortality in current users of estrogen from 10 to 24% as compared with nonusers. Available evidence also fails

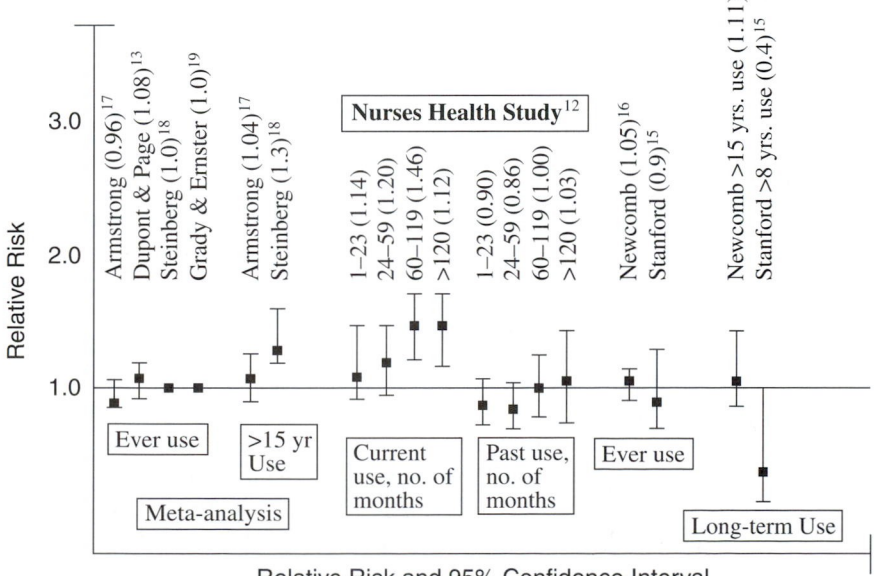

Figure 44-10 Estrogen and breast cancer risk.

to show an association between oral contraceptive use and breast cancer risk. Thomas[24] reviewed 15 case–control and 5 cohort studies and found no overall increased risk of breast cancer in users of birth control pills. There are no conclusive studies regarding risk for testosterone use but data suggest no increased risk. Depo-medroxyprogesterone acetate use has not been shown to increase the risk of breast cancer.

In conclusion, review of the literature suggests there is no conclusive clinically significant association linking estrogen use to breast cancer. Estrogen use at the time of diagnosis does not worsen the chance of survival and may actually improve the prognosis. Administration of estrogen after diagnosis has not been shown to reduce survival rates. The risk:benefit ratio heavily favors estrogen use, as overall mortality is significantly decreased and improved quality of life issues are well known.

REFERENCES

1. Cady B. Diseases of the breast. Current therapy. Philadelphia: Saunders, 1995:979.
2. DiSaia PJ, Creasman WT. Breast disease. In: DiSaia PJ, Creasman WT, eds. Clinical gynecologic oncology. St. Louis: Mosby, 1997:382.
3. Hindle WH, Alonzo LJ. Conservative management of breast fibroadenomas. Am J Obstet Gynecol 1991;164:1647.
4. Carter CL, Allen C, Henson DE. Reduction of tumor size, lymph node status, and survival in 24,740 breast cancer cases. Cancer 1989;63:181.
5. Hall JA, Hall BR, Murphy DC, et al. Mammographic abnormalities and the detection of carcinoma of the breast. Am J Obstet Gynecol 1993;168:1677.
6. Stelling CB. Preoperative mammographic localization of nonpalpable breast lesions. In: Powell DE, Stelling CB, eds. The diagnosis and detection of breast disease. St. Louis: Mosby, 1994:118.
7. Bauer TL, Pandelidis SM, Rhoads JE, Owens RS. Mammographically detected carcinoma of the breast. Surg Gynecol Obstet 1991;173:482.
8. McCreery BR, Frenkle G, Frost DB. An analysis of the results of mammographically guided biopsies of the breast. Surg Gynecol Obstet 1991;172:223.
9. Baute PB, Thibodeau M, Newstead G. Improving the yield of biopsy for nonpalpable lesions of the breast. Surg Gynecol Obstet 1992;174:93.
10. Wile AG, DiSaia PJ. Hormones and breast cancer. Am J Surg 1989;157:438.
11. American College of Obstetricians and Gynecologists. Estrogen replacement therapy in women with previously treated breast cancer. ACOG Committee Opinion no. 135. April 1994.
12. Colditz GA, Hankinson SE, Hunter DJ, et al. The use of estrogens and progestins and the risk of breast cancer in postmenopausal women. N Engl J Med. 1995;332:1589.
13. Dupont WD, Page DL. Menopausal estrogen replacement therapy and breast cancer. Arch Intern Med 1991;151:67.
14. Nachtigall MJ, Smilen SW, Nachtigall RD, et al. Incidence of breast cancer in a 22 year study of women receiving estrogen-progestin replacement therapy. Obstet Gynecol 1992;80:827.
15. Stanford JL, Weiss NS, Voight LF, et al. Combined estrogen and progestin hormone replacement therapy in relation to risk of breast cancer in middle-aged women. JAMA 1995;274:137.
16. Newcomb PA, Longnecker MP, Storer BE, et al. Long-term hormone replacement therapy and risk of breast cancer in postmenopausal women. Am J Epidemiol 1995;142:788.
17. Armstrong BK. Oestrogen therapy in menopause—boon or bane? Med J Aust 1988;148:213.
18. Steinberg KK, Thacker SB, Smith SJ, et al. A meta-analysis of the effect of estrogen replacement therapy on the risk of breast cancer. JAMA 1991;265:1985.
19. Grady D, Ernster V. Does postmenopausal hormonal therapy cause breast cancer? Am J Epidemiol 1991;134:1396.
20. Willis DB, Calle EE, Miracle-McMahil HL, et al. Estrogen replacement therapy and the risk of fatal breast cancer in a prospective cohort of postmenopausal U.S. women. Cancer Causes Control 1996;7:449.
21. Strickland DM, Gambrell RD, Butzin CA, et al. The relationship between breast cancer survival and prior postmenopausal estrogen use. Obstet Gynecol 1992;80:400.
22. Bergvist L, Adami HO, Persson I, et al. Prognosis after breast cancer diagnosis in women exposed to estrogen and estrogen-progesterone replacement therapy. Am J Epidemiol 1989;130:221.
23. Gambrell RD. Proposal to decrease the risk and improve the prognosis of breast cancer. Am J Obstet Gynecol 1984;150:119.
24. Thomas DB. Update on breast cancer and oral contraceptives: the contraceptive report. Monograph 1991;2:3.

Chapter 45
Sexual Counseling

Charles R.B. Beckmann

Five Key Points

- 50% of couples, 60% of women, and 40% men of experience sexual dysfunction at some time.

- Three questions will discover most sexual issues and problems: "Are you sexually active?" "Are you satisfied with your sexual activity?" "Do you have any sexual problems or questions?"

- Sustained and sufficient sexual stimulation is requisite to initiate the human sexual response; problems with either component are common and sometimes represent easily correctable causes of sexual dysfunction.

- Any gynecologic or medical disorder that causes pain, that alters physical appearance in an undesirable manner or anatomy or function in a manner not conducive to sexuality, or that alters a woman's view of herself and/or her sexuality may cause or contribute to sexual dysfunction.

- Gynecologists appropriately treat a number of the simpler sexual issues when they demonstrate a nonjudgmental, empathetic attitude, and a willingness to truly listen, combined with sufficient knowledge and skill to make a correct diagnosis. The PLISSIT model is a simple yet effective model for such management.

SEXUAL ISSUES AND THE ROLE OF THE GYNECOLOGIST

In the 21st century, there will be great diversity in the kinds of gynecologic practice. Some gynecologists will function strictly as specialists and others as primary care generalists, while still others will have practice patterns in between. In all cases, gynecologists will encounter concerns about sexual issues. How they respond will depend in part on the nature of their practice, in part on financial issues such as provided coverage and ability to bill for services, and always on their knowledge and skill in dealing with

these issues. The goal of this chapter is to present basic information about sexual issues and problems and a general approach to them. It is aimed at general gynecologists, who will identify and treat a number of simpler sexual problems and refer the remainder to sex therapists, psychologists and psychiatrists, and other mental health specialists. Physicians who wish to provide a full range of sexual counseling and therapy as part of their practice should acquire additional training.

Sexual issues are common. Up to 50% of couples, 60% of women, and 40% of men experience sexual dysfunction at some time; one-third of women have difficulty reaching orgasm and 1 in 10 never do; 40% of teens aged 13 to 19 are sexually active, before they have the maturity to deal with this powerful life experience; emotional and physical discomfort with sex, to the level of dysfunction, is common. Yet patients are reticent to discuss these matters with their physicians and physicians are hesitant to raise such discussion. Why? Two reasons: First, a simple lack of knowledge and skill about such issues. It is difficult and uncomfortable to deal with problems when ill-prepared to do so. Second, confused and uncomfortable attitudes and feelings about sexuality are common in society and inculcated in physicians as members of it.

Society places great emphasis on sex and sexuality in the media, the sale of products and services, and entertainment, yet simultaneously children are raised in family environments in which parents rarely discuss their sexuality or sexuality in general between themselves or with their children. Children eventually recognize their parents as sexual beings, but their sexuality is rarely acknowledged or discussed; children observe confusing, often violent or aberrant sexuality about them, but it is never explained. Children learn from other children, whose information base is lacking and emotional growth insufficient for understanding. Young people hear the paradox, "sex is dirty," and then, "save it for someone you love." The situation is aptly described as "unreal" and secrecy-ridden, and the resultant confusion and discomfort of patients and physicians, who grew up in this environment, is understandable. The situation is exacerbated by the number of men and women who have suffered sexual abuse as children or adults and who suffer the emotional and physical sequelae thereof. Physicians must be comfortable with and understand their own sexuality and any sexual issues they may have in order to be able to effectively help their patients. This may in some cases involve professional help, but often may be facilitated by quiet introspection. Table 45-1 provides a list of questions that may prove helpful when thinking about these issues. The level of discomfort noted while considering these questions may be a clue about how much work is needed in this area.

PHYSIOLOGY AND PSYCHOLOGY OF THE HUMAN SEXUAL RESPONSE

The human sexual response is functionally volitional (unlike the cycle-dependent estrus of lower animals) and deeply related to emotions and the type and timing of physical events, albeit based in a reasonably well-defined sequence of physiologic events. The human sexual response for women as described initially by Masters and Johnson[1] remains a useful paradigm to understand sexual function and issues. It describes the sexual response in four stages (Table 45-2 and Figures 45-1 to 45-4) although it is understood to be a continuum of events rather than four discrete, circumscribed ones.

TABLE 45-1
SELF-EVALUATION QUESTIONS IN SEXUALITY

What were Mom and Dad like with their sexuality, demonstration of affection, nudity, and verbal expressions about sex?

Were Mom and Dad sexual with each other? In your presence? How did what they did, or did not do, make you feel?

What did Mom or Dad or other adults say to you about sex and sexuality? About making or having babies? Where did you get your information about these topics?

Were you religious? If so, what was said about sex/sexuality? How about now?

How "girlish" or "boyish" were you as a child? Were you comfortable then? Now?

What was puberty like for you (menstruation, wet dreams, body changes, and emotions)? Who did you talk to about these matters? Were you comfortable with these changes, or uneasy? Why?

What was dating like for you? Successful, unsuccessful, why? What about your first sexual experience?

How satisfying have been/are your significant heterosexual or homosexual relationships? Can you talk to your partner easily? About sex? About fantasies you have? About what you like and dislike? Is your relationship comfortable, or uncomfortable, or both, and why? What about masturbation?

What are your theories about sexual identity (heterosexuality, bisexuality, homosexuality, asexuality, and so forth)?

TABLE 45-2
SEXUAL RESPONSE CYCLE IN THE FEMALE

Phase	Sex-Organ Response	General-Body Response
Excitement	Vaginal lubrication	Nipple erection
	Thickening of vaginal walls and labia	Sex-tension flush
	Expansion of inner vagina	
	Elevation of cervix and corpus	
	Tumescence of clitoris	
Plateau	Orgasmic platform in outer vagina	Sex-tension flush
	Full expansion of inner vagina	Carpopedal spasm
	Secretion of mucus by Bartholin gland	Generalized skeletal muscle tension
	Withdrawal of clitoris	Hyperventilation
		Tachycardia
Orgasm	Contractions of uterus from fundus toward lower uterine segment	Specific skeletal muscle contractions
	Contractions of orgasmic platform at 0.8-sec intervals	Hyperventilation
	External rectal sphincter contractions at 0.8-sec intervals	Tachycardia
	External urethral sphincter contractions at irregular intervals	
Resolution	Ready return to orgasm with retarded loss of pelvic vasocongestion	Sweating reaction
	Return of normal color and orgasmic platform in primary (rapid) stage	Hyperventilation
	Loss of clitoral tumescence and return to position	Tachycardia

Reprinted with permission from Masters and Johnson.[1]

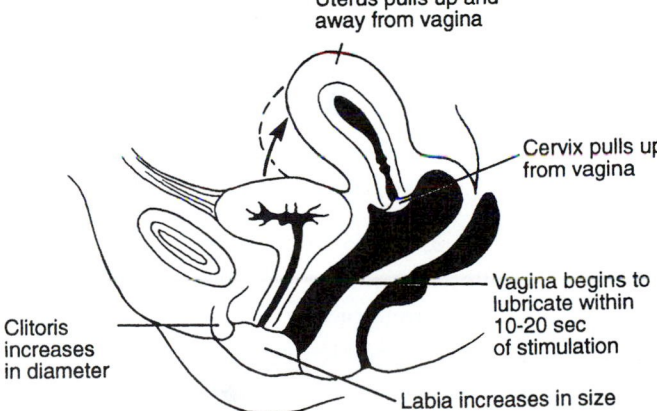

Uterus pulls up and away from vagina

Cervix pulls up from vagina

Vagina begins to lubricate within 10-20 sec of stimulation

Labia increases in size

Clitoris increases in diameter

Figure 45-1 Excitement stage of female sexual response. *Reprinted with permission from Masters and Johnson, p. 571.*[1]

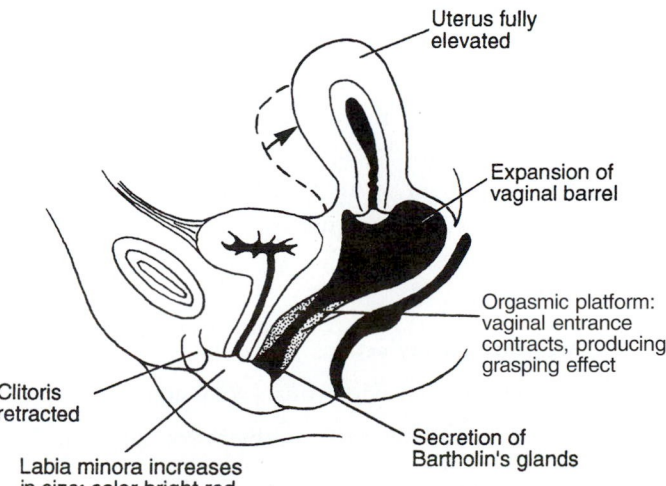

Uterus fully elevated

Expansion of vaginal barrel

Orgasmic platform: vaginal entrance contracts, producing grasping effect

Secretion of Bartholin's glands

Clitoris retracted

Labia minora increases in size: color bright red

Figure 45-2 Plateau stage of female sexual response. *Reprinted with permission from Masters and Johnson, p. 571.*[1]

Figure 45-3 Orgasm stage of female sexual response. *Reprinted with permission from Masters and Johnson, p. 571.*[1]

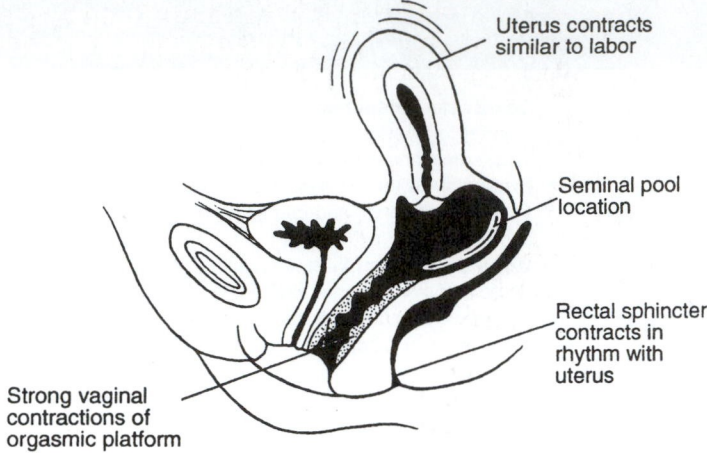

Uterus contracts similar to labor

Seminal pool location

Rectal sphincter contracts in rhythm with uterus

Strong vaginal contractions of orgasmic platform

Figure 45-4 Resolution stage of female sexual response. *Reprinted with permission from Masters and Johnson, p. 572.*[1]

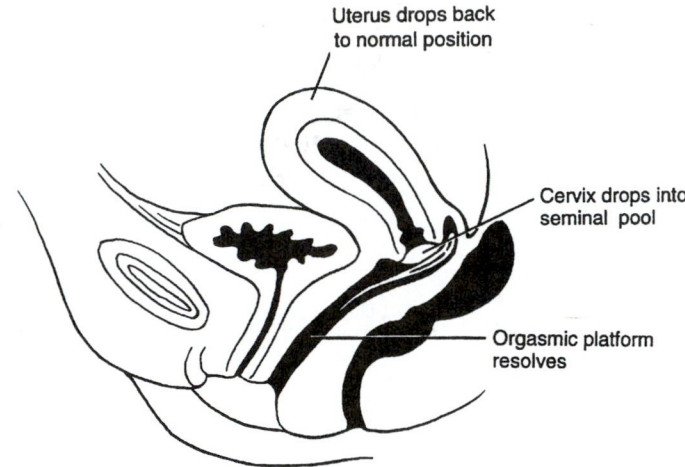

Uterus drops back to normal position

Cervix drops into seminal pool

Orgasmic platform resolves

Sustained and sufficient sexual stimulation is requisite to initiate the human sexual response. *Sustained sexual stimulation* means stimulation that occurs over a long enough time to effect arousal. *Sufficient sexual stimulation* might also be called *effective sexual stimulation*, and means stimulation that is correct and comfortable so as to initiate and sustain the sexual response. Problems with either stimulation component are common and sometimes represent easily correctible causes of sexual dysfunction. The quality and duration of foreplay is the most obvious example of an issue involving sustained and sufficient stimulation, although other issues such as timing and environment are often germane.

RECOGNITION AND DIAGNOSIS OF SEXUAL PROBLEMS

History Taking and the Professional Relationship

Sexual issues requiring attention may be discovered in two ways: reported directly as a complaint or revealed as part of the review of systems. In either case, adequate, comfortable, honest communication is requisite. The cornerstone of an effective history-taking is a physician comfortable with and knowledgeable about sexuality and sexual issues who wants to know about the patient's concerns and to help with them. Attention to other communication issues is helpful: a communication style characterized by warmth, supportiveness, active listening, professionalism, and a nonjudgmental attitude; a private, comfortable physical environment; realistic and defined time limits, which avoid frustration for patient and physician; and careful choice of terms to establish commonality of level and sexual words used.

Three questions will discover most sexual issues and problems:

"Are you sexually active?"

"Are you satisfied with your sexual activity?"

"Do you have any sexual problems or questions?"

When a response to any of these three questions reveals an issue or problem, the history-taking process is in many ways just like that for any other medical problem: onset, description, duration, and so forth. This paradigm is familiar and comfortable for patient and physician and should facilitate the effort. Given the emotions often associated with these issues (embarrassment, shame, guilt, anger, frustration, anxiety), the value of active listening techniques cannot be overemphasized. Issues and problems may be presented as seemingly trivial or unfounded complaints ("vaginal odor" in a young woman with physiologic secretions, pelvic pain where no organic cause is present) because the patient is at that time unable or unwilling to openly express her real concern. Careful, thoughtful listening is needed to recognize the actual problem.

In the course of history-taking, the elements of the general sexual history should be elicited. These may include the age at and nature of the first sexual experience and first intercourse (if not the same event), number and kind of lifetime partners and quality of these relationships, and present sexual life including partner(s), type, frequency, and satisfaction with sexual practices and forms of expression. Causes of or factors contributing to a sexual issue may be found in the "medical and emotional" review of systems and review of medications and drugs used, which should be carefully done in the light of an expressed or discovered sexual issue.

Physical Examination and Laboratory Evaluation

The complete general physical examination, and especially the abdominopelvic/gynecologic examinations with the usual laboratory evaluations, are the basis of the physical examination associated with sexual issues. As appropriate, the patient's state of sexual development (Tanner stage) should be noted. Examinations specific to possible causes of dysfunction or discomfort should be performed as discussed below. Routine laboratory evaluation may include a Pap smear, gonorrhea and Chlamydia cultures, and a wet preparation with pH determination, depending on the patient's symptoms or lack thereof.

SEXUAL PROBLEMS AND THEIR MANAGEMENT

Gynecologic Problems

Any gynecologic disorder that causes pain; alters physical appearance, anatomy, or function in a manner not conducive to sexuality; or alters a woman's view of herself may contribute to sexual dysfunction. For example, estrogen-deficiency–associated lack of lubrication may cause dyspareunia; women who have had a hysterectomy may falsely believe part or all of their sexual responsiveness has also been removed, a response that may be averted by effective preoperative counseling; malignancy and its treatment require sensitive discussion with a woman and her partner, as sexuality and interpersonal relations may be strained by the disease or its perceived effects; infertility and its treatment may create sexual problems for one or both partners, depending on the nature of the infertility issue and its specific therapy. A careful review by the gynecologist may ameliorate or eliminate sexual problems if addressed in a timely fashion.

Pain

DYSPAREUNIA. Painful intercourse is experienced by about 15 to 20% of women at some time in their lives, but is recurrent, severe, and leads to significant sexual dysfunction in about 2%. It should be evaluated because of its effect on sexual function and because it may be evidence of significant organic pathology. Two classifications are used: primary and secondary, insertional and deep-thrust. Primary dyspareunia is manifest at the first coitus and may involve anatomic conditions such as vaginal agenesis, duplication, septation, or hymenal stenosis. Secondary dyspareunia is manifest in women with previously comfortable coitus. Insertional dyspareunia is manifest with penetration and may be mild or so severe as to prevent intromission, and is localized to the vulva, perineum, and outer vagina. Deep-thrust dyspareunia arises during deep thrusting, is often dependent on the type and position of coitus, and may involve abdominal, pelvic, or vaginal pain. The causes of the dyspareunias are noted in Table 45-3, and their therapy is dependent on accurate diagnosis of the cause. History-taking is the important diagnostic maneuver, including location and description of the pain, what situations or actions preceded and/or cause the pain, frequency and duration of pain, how the pain has changed over time, if it has changed, how the pain has affected sexual and emotional health, and any solutions that have been attempted and their results.

VAGINISIMUS. Vaginisimus is insertional dyspareunia characterized by intense, involuntary painful vaginal muscle spasms in the pelvic floor and vaginal wall, causing functional narrowing of the vaginal vault. It

TABLE 45-3
CAUSES OF DYSPAREUNIA

Insertional
Vulvar
  Dystrophy
  Lichen sclerosis
  Vestibulitis
  Vulvitis
    Atrophic
    Chemical
    Infectious (chancroid, herpes, yeast, lymphogranuloma
      venereum)
    Vulvodynia
Vaginal
  Episiotomy/colporrhapy repair problems
  Inadequate lubrication
    Abuse
    Arousal disorder
    Insufficient foreplay
    Medication
  Trauma scarring
  Vaginismus
  Vaginitis
Other
  Congenital abnormality (duplication, agenesis, septum)
  Cystitis
  Gastrointestinal
    Diverticula
    Hemorrhoids
  Genitourinary
    Urethral diverticula
    Urethral stenosis
    Urethral syndrome
    Urethritis (bacterial, Chlamydia)
  Hymen—intact, stenosis
  Pelvic floor muscle spasm

Deep Thrust
Gynecologic
  Adhesions, abdominopelvic (chronic pelvic inflammatory dis-
    ease, surgery, endometriosis)
  Pelvic relaxation (cystocele, urethrocele, rectocele, entero-
    cele)
  Pelvic tumors (benign, malignant; uterus or adnexae; cystic
    or solid)
  Retained ovary syndrome
  Uterine
    Adenomyosis
    Malposition, especially retroversion/retroflexion
Gastrointestinal
  Chronic constipation
  Diverticular disease
  Inflammatory bowel disease
  Irritable-bowel syndrome
Urologic
  Chronic cystitis
  Detrusor dyssnergia
  Interstitial cystitis
  Urethral syndrome
Other
  Hernias (abdominal, femoral)
  Low back pain syndromes (low back strain; displaced/
    herniated disk)

may be so intense as to prevent intromission, and may be in response to the introduction of anything (tampon, finger, etc.) into the vagina. These women are anatomically normal, so that vaginisimus is often described as a phobic or hysterical reaction. These patients may remain orgasmic or have an orgasmic disorder as well.

At speculum or digital examination, about 25% of women with vaginisimus will not demonstrate spasm, so diagnosis is based on history. For the other 75%, gradual insertion of a digit so as to minimize or perhaps avoid spasm is a first and often therapeutic step. Two other physical "exercises" are therapeutic. First, the examiner and then patient inserts a finger(s) and the patient is asked to tighten the muscles as if to stop a urine stream. The patient learns to tighten and then relax these vaginal muscles. The goal is to learn to voluntarily relax the spastic muscles. The second exercise is the sequential insertion by patient and/or

partner of larger dilators (fingers, dilator sets, etc.) with the goal of learning to allow progressively larger objects in the vagina without spasm. As progress is made, patient-controlled penile insertion ensues and, as patient and partner gain confidence and skill that intromission without spasm is possible, attention can turn to resumption of intercourse and pleasure. Counseling completes the therapy. Simple counseling such as reassurance of anatomic normality, etc., is easily done by the gynecologist but referral may be indicated if there are associated sexual dysfunctions, psychiatric issues, or a history of sexual abuse.

Pregnancy and Infertility

Successful expression of sexuality during pregnancy may be complicated by fear of intercourse-associated injury to the pregnancy, pain, or difficulty with sex due to changes in anatomy. Progressive loss of sexual interest and expressiveness is common as pregnancy progresses, and orgasmic potential may decline as well. The frequency of intercourse is reported to drop by an average of 50%, the reason expressed being discomfort in about one-half of cases and fear of harm and lack of interest in the remaining cases. Fear of injury to the pregnancy may often be eliminated by simple provision of information that intercourse is not dangerous in normal pregnancy and confirmation that only bleeding and ruptured membranes actually preclude coitus. Fear of pain and anatomic problems may also be dealt with by counseling about techniques such as side-to-side and female-superior positions and mutual masturbation. Nursing mothers often have heightened sexual interest but a couple may have difficulty with vaginal intercourse due to the dryness of the vagina associated with nursing. The use of lubricants usually corrects this problem.

In cases of infertility, emotions are extremely strained, making sexual dysfunction particularly difficult for patient and partner, as well as the physician. Depending on the cause of the infertility and the requisite infertility therapy, unprecedented pressures may be placed on the couple's sexual relationship, especially if sexual performance is required. Sensitive discussion with special emphasis on active listening is the most important. Consultation with the infertility specialist and/or a sexual counselor may be required.

Hysterectomy

"Without a uterus I can't have an orgasm." "My partner will know I don't have a uterus and it won't feel right to him." "I'm not really a woman without a uterus." These are the kinds of issues ensuing from hysterectomy. Empathetic counseling can usually ameliorate these issues, with special emphasis on prehysterectomy counseling. Careful attention to cultural issues is important, as attitudes may vary significantly among various groups.

Menopause

Menopause is not directly associated with decreased sexuality, but physical changes associated with estrogen deficiency (lack of vaginal lubrication, loss of muscle tone, and pelvic relaxation) or aging in general may interfere with sexual expression. Counseling should be directed at affirmation that sexuality and sexual expression is appropriate in later years and attention should be given to hormone-replacement therapy and evaluation of general gynecologic health.

Urologic Problems

Treatment of male sexual dysfunction is directed primarily toward erectile dysfunction and impotence. Medical therapies include testosterone replacement in documented primary hypogonadism, bromocriptine and pergolide mesylate in hyperprolactinemia, the α_2-adrenergic antagonist yohimbine, which may decrease outward penile blood flow and erectile dysfunction in diabetics, and intracavernous injection of papaverine and phentolamine, in combination, or multidrug injection combinations, which also include prostaglandin E_1 and atropine. The first of a number of drug treatments for impotence has been released. Treatment with the drug Viagra (sildenafil citrate; 50 mg orally 1 hour before coitus) has been reported highly successful, although the experience with this drug and others like it is still quite limited. It acts by activating guanylate cyclase, leading to increased penile levels of cyclic guanosine monophosphate, increased blood flow to the corpus cavernosum, and increased likelihood of and quality of erection given sufficient sustained stimulation. Its use in patients using medications based on organic nitrates in any form is contraindicated due to potentiation of the vasodilatory effect of circulating nitric oxide, which results in the risk of significant hypotension. Surgical therapies, including the insertion of permanently tumescent or inflatable penile implants, are effective in some situations. Premature ejaculation, another common male problem, is discussed in the section on orgasmic disorders.

Chronic Illness and Medications

A multitude of medications have been associated with sexual dysfunction in males and females—e.g., drugs that block central dopamine action and may affect libido, opiates that may exert antiandrogenic effects, and medications that alter hemodynamics may affect erectile function. Medications that alter sympathetic tone may divert blood from penile erectile tissues and contribute to retrograde or absent ejaculation. A partial list of such medications is presented in Table 45-4.

Sexual dysfunction may be associated with a medical condition, and may be worsened by the medications specific for it, e.g., hypertension and antihypertensives. Mental disorders, especially depression, are often associated with altered libido and sexual

TABLE 45-4
MEDICATIONS AND DRUGS THAT AFFECT SEXUALITY AND SEXUAL FUNCTION IN MEN AND WOMEN

Medication	Used For	Effect
Acetazolamide (Diamox)	Glaucoma	Decreased desire, potency
Alcohol	In excess, a substance of abuse	In small amounts, may stimulate sexual interest by disinhibition; in larger amounts, interferes by general depression and psychomotor skill dysfunction; in chronic overuse (alcoholism), may affect liver function and metabolism of other drugs as well as estrogen, an antagonist of testosterone
α-Methyl dopa (Aldomet)	Hypertension	Erectile dysfunction; some effect on libido and orgasm
Alprazolam (Xanax)	Anxiety	Orgasmic inhibition, delayed or absent ejaculation; see also Benzodiazepines
Amiloride (Midamor)	Hypertension (adjunctive therapy with thiazide or other kaliuretic-diuretics)	Decreased desire; impotence
Amitriptyline (Elavil, Limbitrol)	Depression	Loss of desire; impotence; ejaculatory dysfunction
Amphetamines	Substances of abuse	Impotence, delayed ejaculation, anorgasmia
Amyl nitrate	Substance of abuse	Intense and prolonged orgasms in male and female; chronic use: decreased libido
Atenolol	Hypertension	Erectile dysfunction
Barbiturates	Anxiety, seizure disorders	Low doses: increased libido; higher doses: central nervous system depression, decreased libido and sexual performance
Benzodiazepines (lorazepam [Ativan], chlordiazepoxide [Librium], diazepam [Valium])	Anxiety	Low doses: increased libido; higher doses (especially if mixed with alcohol): central nervous system depression, decreased libido and sexual performance
Carbamazepine (Tegretol)	Seizures	Impotence
Chloral hydrate	Anxiety	see Sedatives
Chlorathlidone (Hygroton)	Hypertension	Decreased desire; impotence
Chlorpromazine (Thorazine)	Psychosis; nausea of pregnancy	Decreased desire; impotence, no ejaculation, priapism
Cimetidine (H_2-receptor antagonist) (Tagamet)	Peptic ulcer	Decreased libido, erectile dysfunction, gynecomastia, probably antiandrogenic effect; anorgasmia
Clomipramine (Anafranil)	Obsessive–compulsive disorders	Decreased libido; impotence; retarded ejaculation; anorgasmia
Clonidine (Catapres)	Hypertension	Erectile dysfunction; some effect on libido
Cocaine	Substance of abuse	Low doses: enhanced sexual desire; higher dose: arousal dysfunction, ejaculatory dysfunction, anorgasmia; chronic use: loss of sexual interest and performance ability, hyperprolactinemia; priapism
Digoxin	Heart failure, atrial fibrillation, paroxysmal atrial tachycardia	Decreased libido; impotence
Disulfiram (Antabuse)	Alcohol abuse	Impotence
Doxepin (Sinequan)	Psychoneurotic patients with anxiety or depression	Decreased libido
Famotidine (Pepcid, Mylanta)	Heartburn	Impotence
Hallucinogens	Substances of abuse	Low doses: may enhance libido; higher doses: severe depression of libido
Haloperidol (Haldol)	Psychosis, Tourette disorder, combative behavior	Impotence; painful ejaculation
Hydralizine (Apresoline)	Hypertension	Impotence; priapism
Indomethacin (Indocin)	Rheumatoid arthritis; osteoporosis; bursitis; gouty arthritis; ankylosing spondylitis	Decreased libido; impotence
Lithium	Manic–depressive illness	Decreased libido; impotence
Lorazepam (Ativan)	Preanesthesia; anxiety	Decreased libido
Marijuana	Substance of abuse	Decreased libido with chronic use
Methaqualone (Quaalude)	Anxiety; easily a substance of abuse	see Sedatives
Methyldopa	Hypertension	Erectile dysfunction
Metoclopramide (Reglan)	Gastroesophageal reflux, diabetic gastroparesis, antiemesis	Decreased libido and erectile dysfunction

TABLE 45-4 CONTINUED

Medication	Used For	Effect
Metoprolol (Lopressor)	Hypertension; angina pectoris; myocardial infarction	Impotence
Monoamine oxidase inhibitors	Depression	Decreased libido, anorgasmia, retrograde ejaculation, erectile dysfunction; bethanecol (Urocholine) may ameliorate symptoms in some men and women
Naproxen (Naprosyn)	Pain	Impotence, no ejaculation
Nefazodone (Serzone)	Depression	An SSRI and blocks norepinephrine uptake; same but probably less effect than pure SSRIs
Nifedipine	Hypertension	Erectile dysfunction
Nortriptyline (Aventyl; Pamelor)	Endogenous depression	Impotence, decreased libido
Opioids	Substances of abuse	Sexual dysfunction: erection lubrication, orgasm, ejaculation; chronic use: decreased libido
Paroxetine (Paxil)	Depression; obsessive–compulsive disorder; panic disorder	Decreased libido, delayed or no orgasm
Phenothiazines	Psychosis	Decreased libido, erectile and ejaculatory discomfort
Phenoxybenzamine (Dibenzyline)	Hypertension	Priapism; retrograde ejaculation; inhibited emission
Phenytoin (Dilantin)	Seizures	Decreased libido; impotence; priapism
Prazosin (Minipress)	Hypertension	Impotence, priapism
Propranolol (Inderal)	Hypertension, angina, mitral-valve prolapse	Decreased libido; erectile dysfunction; impotence
Sedatives	Anxiety	As a class, in low doses may increase sexual interest by disinhibition; in higher doses or when mixed with alcohol, general inhibition of sexual interest and function
Selective serotonin-reuptake inhibitors (SSRI) (fluoxetine [Prozac], sertraline [Zoloft], paroxtine [Paxil], venlaxafine [Effexor])	Depression	Orgasmic inhibition (antihistamine cyproheptadine taken one hour before sex may block much of this effect)
Sertraline (Zoloft)	Depression, obsessive–compulsive disorder, panic disorder	Decreased libido; retarded or no orgasm
Spironolactone (Aldactone)	Hypertension	Impotence, decreased libido
Spironolactone	Hypertension	Decreased libido, impotence, gynecomastia
Testosterone	Testosterone deficiency syndromes	Priapism
Thiazide diuretics	Hypertension	Erectile dysfunction
Thiothixene (Navane)	Psychosis	Spontaneous ejaculation; impotence; priapism
Thorazine	Psychosis, especially the schizophrenias	Erectile dysfunction, decreased libido, anorgasmia, impotence, and priapism; separating from aspects of primary disorder often difficult
Trazodone (Desyrel)	Depression	Priapism, clitoral priapism; increased libido; anorgasmia; retrograde or absent ejaculation
Tricyclic antidepressants	Depression	Decreased libido, anorgasmia, retrograde ejaculation, erectile dysfunction
Trifluoperazine (Stelazine)	Psychosis; acute nongeneralized nonpsychotic anxiety; behavioral symptoms of intellectually challenged individuals	Painful or spontaneous ejaculation

interest, and again, specific medications such as selective serotonin-reuptake inhibitors (SSRIs) may have an additional adverse effect on sexuality. Caution must be taken in ascribing sexual dysfunction to a medication rather than a chronic disease process. A partial list of such disorders is presented in Table 45-5.

Sexual Dysfunctions

Arousal and Orgasmic Disorders

Arousal disorders involve difficulty or inability to become sexually excited, while orgasmic disorders include problems with orgasm, as well as the inability

TABLE 45-5
MEDICAL CONDITIONS ASSOCIATED WITH SEXUAL PROBLEMS

Diabetes	Strongly associated with impotence, probably related to atherosclerotic changes or autonomic neuropathy
Hypertension/cardiovascular disease/atherosclerosis	Impotence probably related to neurovascular/atherosclerotic changes, often worsened by side effects of antihypertensive medications
Smoking	May exacerbate existing erectile dysfunction
Depression	Decreased libido, sexual interest, performance; altered interpersonal relationships; medical therapy may exacerbate
Hyperprolactinemia of any cause	Impotence
Thyroid dysfunction (hyper- or hypo-)	Impotence
Hypotestosteronemia of any cause	Erectile dysfunction and decreased libido in male; decreased libido and orgasmic dysfunction in female
Multiple sclerosis	Musculoskeletal dysfunction
Spinal-cord injury	Neurologic dysfunction specific to level of injury
Stroke	Neurologic and mental function specific to lesion(s)
Carcinoma	Organic dysfunction specific to lesion; emotional dysfunction/depression

to attain orgasm. The diagnosis is primarily by history, where differentiation of physical from emotional causes is based on whether or not successful masturbation is possible. If it is, physical causes are unlikely as compared with emotional ones. In either case, confusion with desire disorder is common, as the initial commentary from the patient may be focused on lack of desire. When an arousal or orgasmic disorder is long-standing, frustration and tolerance may wane and manifest as lack of desire. Patients with arousal or orgasmic disorders, however, are interested in having satisfactory sex.

Arousal and orgasmic disorders arise in association with specific diseases (see Table 45-5) and the use of some medications (see Table 45-4), as the result of specific sexual disorders (female arousal disorder, female orgasmic disorder, male erectile disorder or impotence, and male orgasmic disorders, including premature ejaculation), and as the result of inadequate sexual stimulation. They also arise in association with interpersonal and intrapersonal issues such as anxiety and shame, which in turn are often associated with commonly held sexual myths and misinformation.

Adequate sexual stimulation involves a mixture of physical stimulation, mental imagery (including fantasy), and positive emotion extended over a sufficient time. Identification of such factors and brief counseling often suffices as therapy, although referral for specialized sex therapy is usually required after identification of the problem, given the specialized skills and length of treatment often required. Counseling, which is appropriate for the general gynecologist, often involves "debunking" commonly held sexual myths and misinformation—e.g., practices such as fantasy, oral or manual sex, etc., are wrong or unhealthy; men should always be able to "perform"; women should respond like men with respect to arousal and orgasm. Performance anxiety (fear of not being able to perform adequately) may be a significant problem, with difficulty getting sexually aroused a common result. Significant ongoing interpersonal conflict (money, authority, child care, jobs and relationship roles, etc.) may also cause or contribute to these problems, and require identification and resolution.

PREMATURE EJACULATION. Some general gynecologists may choose to initiate treatment for a couple in which the male suffers premature ejaculation. The most simple and usually effective method is based on making the male aware of impending ejaculation, leading to control of the process—the "stop and start method." First, in the male supine position and progressing toward the male superior position, the male is stimulated to near ejaculation whereupon his partner uses thumb and forefinger to squeeze the penis just below the glans, impeding ejaculation. Alternatively, the male learns to know when ejaculation is about to happen and to alter his thrusting speed to avoid ejaculation until desired. If such initial therapy fails, however, referral is recommended, as other unidentified problems may be present.

Disorders of Desire

Disorders of desire may present as chief complaints or embedded in other sexual problems, such as depression, relationship changes or loss, or marital conflict. Two disorders are defined: hypoactive sexual desire disorder (HSDD)—deficiency or absence of sexual fantasies or desire for sexual activity that causes distress not related to a medical condition or medication; and sexual aversion disorder (SAD)—aversion to or avoidance of genital sexual contact, causing distress or interpersonal difficulty not related to a medical condition.

HSDD usually presents as a troublesome relationship issue, both partners feeling that there is a lack or deficiency of desire of one partner relative to the other. This lack may be a real sexual function problem, or may represent a significant difference in sexual desire between two normal persons with markedly different levels of sexual desire. Absent sexual desire is relatively uncommon, as often sexual relationships are never initiated so that motivating conflict does not ensue. SAD is also relatively uncommon; it manifests as a powerful adverse somatic response to sexual activity—e.g., nausea and emesis, headache, abdominopelvic pain, and panic.

Finally, mention should be made of hyperactive sexual desire, a condition usually misapplied to higher than normal but not pathological sexual desire. Terms such as promiscuous, compulsive, nymphomania, and the like are applied. Evaluation and possibly treatment in these situations is probably best reserved for cases in which the level of sexual activity is disturbing to the individual or interferes with her partner relationship or when it leads to dangerous self-destructive behaviors such as unsafe sex in high-risk situations.

All of these disorders of desire are complex situations requiring considerable time and expertise for correct diagnosis and treatment. The role of the gynecologist is, most appropriately, identification of an issue, complete gynecologic evaluation to correct "organic problems" or to identify ones to be dealt with as part of sex therapy, evaluation of medications, and referral to a sex therapist or mental health professional.

Paraphilias

Paraphilias are intense sexual experiences outside those generally considered normal (*para*, meaning "beside" and *philia*, meaning "love"). *Perversion* is often used as a synonym, appropriately so if used to indicate a sexual practice outside that considered normal in a given society and associated with secretiveness and guilt, as opposed to a moral judgment.

Paraphilias have similar basic characteristics:

Intense, recurrent for more than 6 months, involving fantasy, urges, or behaviors

Focus on a specific object (examples: animals, nonhuman things, children, individuals who are humiliated or suffer, the dead, etc.)

Resulting clinical distress and/or psychosocial dysfunction.

There are eight basic paraphilias as noted in Table 45-6. The role of the general gynecologist is rarely

---

TABLE 45-6
THE PARAPHILIAS

Pedophilia	The most dangerous of paraphilias, as it involves the victimization of children who are the focus of sexual acts. More pedophiles are focused on girls than boys, but those who focus on boys are more resistant to mental health or legal interventions. This behavior is criminal and must be reported when discovered.
Voyeurism	Surreptitious observation of others unclothed or engaged in sex, often with masturbation during or after the observational episode.
Exhibitionism	Exposure of genitals in anticipation of the shocked response of the observer, often combined with masturbation. More often younger males rather than older males or females.
Fetishism	Sexual focus, often with masturbation, on an object symbolic of a person, such as underclothes, leather or rubber clothing, and statues, etc. Vibrators and other sex devices made for sexual arousal are not fetish objects.
Frotteurism	Rubbing against a stranger in a public place to obtain sexual gratification.
Masochism	Sexual excitement resulting from one's own humiliation, suffering, or pain. Physical practices ranging from spanking and light bondage to extreme and dangerous practices such as coitus-associated asphyxiation. Fantasy practices include rape, torture, slavery, etc. Usually starting in early life, masochism often continues, competing with and often overcoming normal sexual and interpersonal relationships.
Sadism	A spectrum of behaviors from fantasy of dominance to physical attack of another, nonconsenting person, including murder and rape. Often combined with masochism, including fascination with urination ("golden showers") and feces.
Transvestic fetishism	A male (often a transsexual) wearing female clothing to elicit sexual stimulation, often associated with masturbation.

TABLE 45-7
THE PLISSIT MODEL

Permission	Given the confused attitudes and feelings often associated with sexuality, many patients need permission to think about and work on sexual issues; permission to feel better. Permission is granted as long as the goals are realistic and will add to the quality of life if achieved and cause no harm and involve no danger or coercion. Permission alone often is quite therapeutic.
Limited Information	Fear and concern based on lack of knowledge or reliance on sexual myth is often the issue in a sexual problem. Provision of information is often all that is required. For example: anal intercourse is not abnormal and is safe with certain precautions; sex when pregnant is generally safe, but often requires trying new positions and methods of expression; not achieving orgasm at every sexual encounter does not mean one is inadequate or abnormal
Specific Suggestions	Simple suggestions specific to the patient's issue, but not obvious to the patient; these often focus on increased communication about the identified issue. For example: helping a couple understand the physiology of lubrication, hence the value of foreplay and proper position.
Intensive Therapy	Where intensive therapy starts and specific suggestions end depends on the knowledge and skill and scope of practice of the gynecologist; psychotherapy, marital/couple therapy, surrogate therapy, and the like are almost always beyond those without extended training in the area.

---

more than identification of a paraphilia and the establishment of a physician–patient relationship of sufficient strength and trust to facilitate referral to a sex therapist/mental health specialist.

MANAGEMENT BY THE GYNECOLOGIST: EMPATHY AND THE PLISSIT MODEL

Gynecologists appropriately treat a number of the simpler sexual issues when they demonstrate a non-judgmental, empathetic attitude and a willingness to truly listen, combined with sufficient knowledge and skill to make the correct diagnosis. The Permission, Limited Information, Specific Suggestions, and Intensive Therapy (PLISSIT) model is a simple yet effective paradigm for management by the gynecologist (Table 45-7).

REFERENCES

1. Masters W, Johnson V. Human sexual response. Boston: Little, Brown, 1966.

SELECTED READINGS

American College of Obstetricians and Gynecologists. Sexual dysfunction. ACOG Technical Bulletin no. 211. September 1995.

Annon JS. The behavioral treatment of sexual problems. Honolulu: Enabling Systems, 1974.

Barbach LG. For yourself. New York: Doubleday, 1990.

Comfort A. The new joy of sex. New York: Crown Publishers, 1993.

Frank E, Anderson C, Rubinstein D. Frequency of sexual dysfunction in "normal couples." N Engl J Med 1978; 299:111.

Kritzinger S. Women's experience of sex. New York: Putnam, 1983.

LaHaye TF, LaHaye B. The act of marriage—the beauty of sexual love. Grand Rapids, MI: Zondervan, 1998.

Plouffe L. Screening for sexual problems through a simple questionnaire. Am J Obstet Gynecol 1985;151;166.

Renshaw DC. Seven weeks to better sex. New York: Random House, 1995.

Solberg DA, Butler J, Wagner NN. Sexual behavior in pregnancy. N Engl J Med 1973;288:1098.

Chapter 46

Hirsutism

Stephen R. Lincoln

Five Key Points

- A limited number of disorders result in hirsutism and the most common are idiopathic, polycystic ovarian syndrome and stromal hyperthecosis.

- Adult onset or nonclassical congenital adrenal hyperplasia may account for up to 5% of hirsutism patients.

- Androgen-producing tumors are a rare cause of hirsutism, recognized by rapid onset of symptoms, followed by virilization.

- Long-term medical treatment of hirsutism includes the use of oral contraceptives and spironolactone.

- New therapies may include long-acting gonadotropin-releasing hormone analogs with estrogen progesterone educt therapy.

Excessive facial and body hair in locations where hair is not commonly found in women is defined as *hirsutism*.[1] Hirsutism may result from a hyperandrogenic state that signifies metabolic alterations allowing activation and stimulation of hair follicles in male pattern locations. *Virilization* is a more severe state of hyperandrogenism resulting in masculinization of the female, as well as hirsutism[2] (Table 46-1). Although hirsutism may cause cosmetic disfigurement, it rarely is associated with a life-threatening disease. Virilization, on the other hand, may represent a potentially malignant androgen-producing neoplasm and deserves a more extensive evaluation.

A brief review of the physiology and endocrinology of hair growth is followed by a management plan for the patient with hirsutism. The differential diagnosis, laboratory investigation, and treatment of hirsutism are presented for the clinician faced with the patient with hirsutism.

HAIR FOLLICLE GROWTH AND DEVELOPMENT

Hair follicles begin developing in utero at 8 to 10 weeks of gestation. The total endowment of hair follicles is determined by birth and can never increase. The number of follicles varies by ethnic origin (for example, Italians tend to have more hair than do Asians), but interestingly do not vary by gender. Hair follicles

TABLE 46-1
SIGNS OF ANDROGEN EXCESS

Hirsutism	Virilization
Facial hair	Clitoromegaly
Intermammary hair	Amenorrhea
Male escutcheon	Deepening of the voice
Hair on back	Decreased breast size
Abdominal hair	Increased muscle mass
Hair on upper legs	Temporal balding

begin as nests of columnar epithelium invaginating into the underlying dermis, where the hair follicle root bulb is derived. The epithelial column hollows out to form the hair canal, arrector pili attach, and sebaceous glands arrive to form the pilosebaceous apparatus.

Hair growth occurs in cycles and is a result of three phases. The anagen phase is initiated with shedding of the old hair within the follicle, followed by stimulation and growth of the new follicle. Once the growth phase is complete, the hair follicle enters the catagen, or rapid involution, phase and the shaft ceases to grow, the root moves upward within the follicle, and the hair bulb shrivels. After the catagen phase, hair follicles enter the telogen, or resting, phase until a new cycle begins.

Hair follicles on the head have a very long growing (anagen) phase (2 to 3 years) and short resting (telogen) phase, resulting in this hair constantly growing in length and shedding.[3] However, hair follicles on the thigh or forearm have a short anagen phase and long telogen phase, resulting in short stable hair.[4] This is important clinically, as it may take 6 to 12 months for medical treatment for hirsutism to have any visual effect.

ENDOCRINOLOGY OF HAIR GROWTH

Sexual hair refers to the hair follicles that respond to the sex steroids. Locations of sexual hair follicles include the pubic area, axillae, lower abdomen, thighs, legs, arms, chests, and face. Androgens predominantly initiate and stimulate hair growth, as well as increase the diameter and pigmentation of individual hairs. In contrast, the estrogens retard initiation and stimulation of hair growth. In addition, estrogens may increase the synchrony of growth phases, leading to periods of exclusively growth or shedding. This synchrony may lead to clinical perceived increased growth or shedding in high estrogen states (e.g., pregnancy). Once the high estrogen state is removed, the synchrony disappears. The effects of progestins are controversial and they probably have minimal effects on hair growth (Table 46-2).

TABLE 46-2 EFFECT OF STEROIDS ON HAIR GROWTH	
Androgens	Initiate and stimulate growth
Estrogens	Synchronize growth stages and may retard androgen effects
Progestins	Minimal

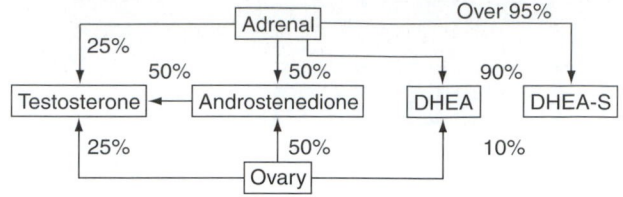

Figure 46-1 Androgen production.

ANDROGEN PRODUCTION

Hair follicles responsive to sex steroids remain dormant until puberty when rises in androgens begin stimulation and growth of pubertal hair. When levels reach the "adult female" range, hair growth occurs in the pubic region, axillae, and extremities in female areas. If levels rise to the "adult male" range, hair growth occurs on the face, chest, and back, and male pattern escutcheon occurs. Androgen production in the female occurs from two sources, the adrenal glands and the ovaries. The most important androgens include testosterone, dihydrotestosterone (DHT), androstenedione, dehydroepiandrosterone (DHEA), and dehydroepiandrosterone sulfate (DHEA-S). Figure 46-1 reviews the contributions of the androgens from adrenal and ovarian sources.

Approximately 25% of circulating testosterone in normal women is secreted directly by the ovary and another 25% directly from the adrenal glands. The remaining 50% of testosterone arises from peripheral conversion of androstenedione, which in turn is secreted equally from the adrenals and ovaries. The adrenal glands also secrete the vast majority of the less androgenic steroids DHEA and DHEA-S. At target sites for androgen activities (e.g., hair follicles), testosterone is converted to DHT by the enzyme 5α-reductase. Both testosterone and DHT interact with the androgen receptor, stimulating androgen response, but DHT has a higher binding affinity and hence is more potent.

Circulating testosterone is bound to protein carriers for transport and only a small fraction is free and active. The majority of testosterone molecules are bound to the protein sex-hormone–binding globulin (SHBG), while the remaining molecules are bound to albumin. In normal women, only 1% of circulating testosterone is free, whereas hirsute women may have higher levels of the unbound fraction. The protein SHBG is synthesized in the liver, and small changes in SHBG can greatly increase free testosterone. The balance of SHGB depends on levels of other steroids

TABLE 46-3
DIAGNOSIS OF HIRSUTISM

Cause	Testosterone	DHEA-S	17α-Hydroxy-progesterone	Virilized	Comments
Idiopathic	Normal	Normal	Normal	No	Tissue sensitivity increased
Polycystic ovary syndrome	Normal to slightly increased	Normal to slightly increased	Normal	No	Luteinizing hormone/follicle-stimulating hormone increased
Stromal hyperthecosis	Slightly increased	Normal to slightly increased	Normal	Occasionally	Normal luteinizing hormone/follicle-stimulating hormone
Congenital adrenal hyperplasia	Normal	Normal to slightly increased	>200 μg/dl	No	ACTH test
Cushing syndrome	Normal	Normal	Normal	No	Dexamethasone suppression test
Ovarian tumor	>200 ng/dl	Normal	Normal	Yes	Rapid progression
Adrenal tumor	Normal	>700 μg/dl	Normal	Yes	Rapid progression

that have action on or are metabolized by the liver. The production of SHBG is increased in states of excessive estrogens or thyroid hormones and decreased by excessive androgens or decreased thyroid hormones. Hypothyroidism, for example, can result in hirsutism due to decreased SHBG, where the total concentration of testosterone remains constant.[5,6]

EVALUATION OF THE HIRSUTE PATIENT

Only a limited number of disorders result in hirsutism. Hirsutism in pregnancy will be considered separately at the conclusion of the chapter; intersex disorders (undermasculinized XY patient or virilized XX patient) are an extremely rare form best referred to a subspecialist. If a female patient has normal pelvic anatomy on examination, is not pregnant, and is not taking androgen medications (e.g., danazol, anabolic steroids, etc.); the differential diagnosis of hirsutism is summarized in Table 46-3.

Evaluation of the hirsute patient focuses on ruling out the rare but serious pathologic conditions resulting in androgen excess. Testosterone or DHEA-S will be elevated in neoplasms of the ovary or adrenal respectively. Elevations of 17α-hydroprogesterone (17OHP) will be found in congenital adrenal hyperplasia. If menstrual irregularities are present, thyroid, pituitary, and gonadotropin evaluations are indicated. When Cushing syndrome is suspected, a screening test (i.e., dexamethasone suppression) is indicated. Table 46-4 summarizes the initial laboratory assessment of the hirsute patient.

The initial history and physical examination will often lead to the cause of hirsutism. Particularly important is the presence of rapidly developing hirsutism

followed by virilization, which suggest neoplasm. Assessment of the quantity of hirsutism can include the use of the Ferriman–Gallwey system to document the location and extent of disease.[7] Photographs may also be used to record data for comparison after treatment. Microscopic measurement of hair follicle diameter is another method to observe progression or regression of hirsutism.

DIFFERENTIAL DIAGNOSIS OF HIRSUTISM

Idiopathic hirsutism (also called constitutional or familial) is the most common nonpathologic cause of hirsutism and may represent over 50% of patients. It is characterized by normal laboratory evaluations, regular menstrual cycles, and an absence of virilization. Idiopathic hirsutism is frequently familial and found more commonly in women of Mediterranean ancestry. The hirsutism is slow growing (measured in years) and may be viewed as an increased tissue sensitivity to normal levels of androgen. Increased 5α-reductase activity has been found in this group of women.[8]

TABLE 46-4
INITIAL LABORATORY ASSESSMENT

Testosterone
Dehydroepiandrosterone sulfate
17α-Hydroxyprogesterone
Menstrual irregularities
    Prolactin
    Thyroid-stimulating hormone
    Follicle-stimulating hormone
    Luteinizing hormone
Suspect Cushing syndrome
    Dexamethasone suppression test

The important consideration is that idiopathic hirsutism is a diagnosis of exclusion, and other pathologic causes must be ruled out.

Polycystic ovary syndrome (PCO) is the most common pathologic cause of hirsutism. The triad of obesity, hirsutism, and oligo-ovulation is the hallmark of PCO, but it is important to remember that not all three signs are always present. The unifying features of the group includes mild androgen excess and an increased luteinizing hormone (LH) to follicle-stimulating hormone (FSH) ratio. The cause of PCO continues to be an enigma for researchers, and various theories have been proposed. It is helpful to consider PCO as an end point of several mechanisms that cause a steady state of anovulation. Interruption of the cyclicity of the hypothalamic–pituitary axis can occur, resulting in the steady state of low or weak estrogens from the periphery (extraglandular production by adipose tissue).

Menstrual irregularities in hirsute patients with PCO often begin soon after menarche. Virilization is rarely present and basic laboratory evaluation is essentially normal. However, slight elevations of testosterone (100 to 150 ng/dl), or DHEA-S (400 to 600 μg/dl) may occur and the LH:FSH ratio is usually $\geq 2:1$ (normal, 1:1). Not all patients need gonadotropins measured, but sometimes levels are helpful to confirm the diagnosis. Ultrasonography is not helpful in the diagnosis of PCO. The often-described necklace-like pattern of follicular cysts within the ovaries of PCO patients can be found in 25% of women with normal ovulation.[9,10]

Central mechanisms of the hypothalamic–pituitary tract resulting in excess LH production will lead to excess androgen production from the ovaries, causing chronic anovulation and androgen excess.[11] Increased insulin resistance has also been shown to modulate PCO syndrome in some patients by virtue of the hyperinsulinemic state, resulting in activation of insulin-like growth factor 1 (IGF-1) receptors, which leads to stimulation of the theca cells of the ovarian stroma to produce excess androgens. In addition, hyperinsulinemia has been shown to decrease production of SHBG, resulting in increased unbound testosterone.[12] Other causes of the PCO syndrome probably exist and have been described, but clinical management for hirsutism remains consistent regardless of the cause.

Stromal hyperthecosis can be viewed as a severe extreme of PCO, but certain different characteristics exist. The history is consistent with PCO, including menstrual irregularities and androgen excess, but progressive signs of virilization may begin to occur with hirsutism. Mild degrees of temporal balding, decreased breast size, and clitoromegaly may occur, as well as weight gain and increased muscle mass. Virilization signs should alert the physician to the possibility of a neoplasm, but stromal hyperthecosis has a slow but relentless progression whereas neoplasms present with a rapid history of virilization.

Laboratory values reveal testosterone approaching tumor levels (200 ng/dl), with minimal elevation of DHEA-S. Retrograde ovarian vein catheterization has shown that elevated testosterone arises from the ovary, and ovarian biopsy will reveal nests of luteinized theca cells. In contrast to PCO, the gonadotropin ratio is frequently close to equal (LH:FSH).[13,14]

Late-onset (also known as nonclassical or adult-onset) congenital adrenal hyperplasia (CAH) may be present in 1 to 10% of hirsute patients.[15,16] Incidence varies according to ethnic populations studied, and late-onset CAH is most common in Alaskan Yupik Eskimos, Ashkenazi Jews, and Hispanics. The syndrome arises when inadequate production of enzymes required for cortical secretion by the adrenal signals a compensatory increase of adrenocorticotrophic hormone (ACTH) by the pituitary. The pituitary "recognizes" a decreased cortisol production and drives the adrenal by increased ACTH production to maintain adequate cortisol levels. However, precursors to cortisol may build up at the stage of partial enzyme deficiency (Figure 46-2) and the excess precursors are shunted into androgen production. The excess androgens lead to hirsutism.

The most common enzyme defect in late-onset CAH is 21-hydroxylase deficiency and others include 11β-hydroxylase and the rare 3β-hydroxysteroid dehydrogenase deficiency. The enzyme defects are inherited and the gene (located on chromosome 6) responsible for 21-hydroxylase has been described, including various nucleotide inversions, deletions, and mutations. The variable defects result in a range of clinical presentations, and some hirsute women formerly thought to have PCO have been found to have late-onset CAH.

Diagnosis is made by finding elevated precursor levels of 17α-hydroxyprogesterone (>200 ng/dl) in a screening test. The 17α-hydroxyprogesterone (17OHP) screen must be drawn in the follicular phase to avoid false positive results (17OHP rises due to corpus luteum production in the secretory phase) and in the

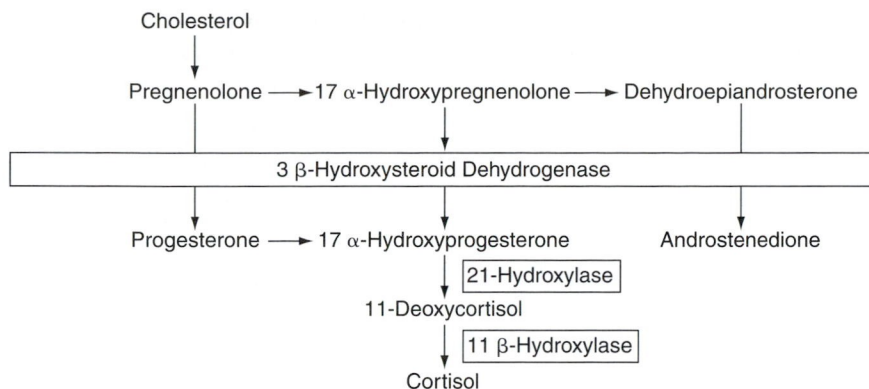

Figure 46-2 Steroidogenesis pathway and congenital adrenal hyperplasia enzyme defects.

early morning to avoid false negative results (circadian decrease of 17OHP that parallels cortisol and ACTH). If the screening level is elevated, the ACTH stimulation test is performed to confirm the diagnosis. Synthetic ACTH (cosyntropin, 250 μg) is given intravenously and 17OHP is measured at time zero (x-axis) and at 1 hour (y-axis).[17,18] Levels of 17OHP greater than 1000 ng/dl make the diagnosis and usually are greater than 1500 ng/dl.

Cushing syndrome is another rare cause of hirsutism. Cushing syndrome is a state of excess cortisol production and can arise from several sources. Pituitary ACTH-producing adenoma (Cushing disease), ectopic ACTH production by tumor (lung or kidney), or autonomous oversecretion of cortisol by the adrenal (adrenal tumor) all lead to a cushingoid state. The overproduction of cortisol by the adrenal is accompanied by overproduction of androgens, resulting in hirsutism. Characteristics include hirsutism of a fine lanugo type, centripital obesity, pigmented abdominal striae, dorsal neck fat pads, peripheral muscle wasting, moon facies, hypertension, hypokalemia, and ecchymosis.[19]

Laboratory diagnosis begins with initial screening, but not all hirsute patients require testing. When clinical suspicion arises, the dexamethasone overnight suppression test (1 mg dexamethasone at 11:00 p.m. followed by 8:00 a.m. cortisol level) or the 24-hour urinary free cortisol level can be used for screening. Levels of serum cortisol <5 μg/dl (dexamethasone test) or urinary free cortisol, 10 to 90 μg (urine test), rule out Cushing syndrome. If the screening test is abnormal, more extensive testing, including extended low- and high-dose suppression, serum ACTH levels, and possibly radiographic studies are required to confirm Cushing syndrome and define the cause of cortisol excess.

Androgen-producing tumors are the most uncommon, but potentially lethal, cause of hirsutism. The clinical history of rapidly progressing hirsutism followed by virilization can take place in only a few months. As androgen levels rise, masculinizing and defeminizing signs occur, such as deepening of the voice, decreased breast size, increased muscle mass, menstrual irregularity, and clitoromegaly. Base-line measurements of testosterone (<200 ng/dl) and DHEA-S (<700 μg/dl) effectively rule out an androgen-producing tumor as a cause of hirsutism.[20,21] Androgen-secreting ovarian tumors are usually palpable (80%) on bimanual examination and include Sertoli–Leydig-cell tumors, granulosa-cell tumors, gynandroblastomas, and Brenner tumors. Adenomas and carcinomas of the adrenal gland can secrete large amounts of DHEA-S and other androgens that lead to rapid progression. Metastasis of both ovarian and adrenal tumors can frequently occur before detection.

SPECIAL CIRCUMSTANCES OF HIRSUTISM IN PREGNANCY

Hirsutism is common in pregnancy and often is associated with the synchrony of hair growth phases cause by high levels of estrogens. When virilization occurs with hirsutism, clinical suspicion for a luteoma of pregnancy should arise. A luteoma is not a true ovarian neoplasm, but represents an exaggerated response of ovarian stroma to human chorionic gonadotropin (HCG). Solid luteomas (unilateral in approximately 45% of cases) are associated with normal pregnancy and androgen excess.[22] Luteomas may rarely cause virilization of a female fetus, and surgical evaluation of the mother should be considered in the second trimester.[23,24] True androgen-secreting tumors of the ovary are rare, as neoplasms inhibit ovulation.

Theca luteal cysts may arise in pregnancy and the condition is referred to as hyper reactio luteinalis. Multiple theca luteal cysts arise, usually due to high levels of HCG, are almost always bilateral, and may be associated with trophoblastic disease. Virilized female fetuses have not been reported with theca luteal cysts and the cysts regress post partum.[25] Surgery is rarely required except in extreme cases of rupture or torsion. The clinician should be cognizant of the cross reactivity of the HCG molecule with thyroid stimulating hormone and possible hyperthyroid states.

TREATMENT OF HIRSUTISM

Hirsutism is not a specific disease but a sign of a spectrum of conditions. The cause of hirsutism should be ascertained and treatment should focus on the condition that results in hirsutism. Serious pathologic causes of hirsutism are rare and require specialized care. Androgen-producing neoplasms of the adrenal or ovary require surgical exploration and often adjuvant chemotherapy. Cushing syndrome requires precise localization of the excess ACTH and treatment involves removal of the source. Late-onset congenital adrenal hyperplasia requires replacement doses of the delinquent corticosteroids (usually prednisone or dexamethasone).

Treatment of the remaining causes of hirsutism (idiopathic, PCO, and stromal hyperthecosis) can be considered together. Medical treatment is aimed at reducing the amount of androgens produced (usually at the ovary) and decreasing the synthesis and actions of androgens at their peripheral sites. It is important to remember that new hair follicles will no longer be stimulated with medical therapy, but previously established hair follicles are not affected. Only mechanical removal will show initial visible improvement, and this is temporary. It often requires 6 months to a year before medical therapy shows visible results, and mechanical removal may be required more than once before results take effect. Mechanical therapies include shaving, tweezing, waxing, or depilatories. Permanent removal can be accomplished only with electrolysis.

MEDICAL THERAPY

Oral contraceptives (OCs) have been a mainstay in the treatment of hirsutism and function by suppression of ovarian steroidogenesis and inhibition of the LH surge. Patients with PCO also benefit from the induction of regular menses and protection from the effects of continuous estrogen on the uterine endometrium. There is no clinically apparent distinction between low-dose, high-dose, or multiphasic combination of OCs and the treatment of hirsutism. New formulations of OCs include less-androgenic progestins (gestodene, norgestimate, and desogestrel) and are associated with increases in SHBG and decreases in free testosterone levels in laboratory studies, but these effects remain to be verified clinically.

Spironolactone is the other mainstay of medical treatment,[26,27] and often is used in conjunction with OCs for maximal effect. Spironolactone is a diuretic found to have significant antiandrogen actions. It competes with androgens at the androgen receptor in the hair follicle and also reduces 5α-reductase activity. Spironolactone is most effective at doses of 200 mg daily in divided doses (100 mg twice a day) and may be reduced after 3 to 6 months of therapy. Side effects can occur and include diuresis in the beginning stages of treatment, fatigue, and occasionally dysfunctional bleeding. Spironolactone is a potassium-sparing diuretic, and hyperkalemia may also occur.

Flutamide is a new nonsteroidal antiandrogen showing promising results in the treatment of hirsutism.[28,29] Like spironolactone, flutamide directly inhibits hair growth and may have fewer side effects than spironolactone. Doses of 250 mg three times a day have been shown to be effective.[30] Both flutamide and spironolactone have not been approved for use in pregnancy and if a patient is not taking OCs, other methods of contraception should be employed.

Finasteride, another new agent being considered for the treatment of hirsutism, is a competitive inhibitor of 5α-reductase, the enzyme responsible for intracellular conversion of testosterone to dehydrotestosterone. Originally approved for treatment of benign prostatic hyperplasia, finasteride has been shown to effectively treat idiopathic hirsutism with a daily dose of 5 mg.[31-33]

Long-acting gonadotropin-releasing hormone analogs (GnRH-A) also show promise as a new treatment for hirsutism. The reversible "medical menopause" effectively inhibits pituitary LH secretion and may be extremely effective in the treatment of hirsutism. However, long-term treatment (>6 months) is not recommended due to adverse effects of osteoporosis and lipid profiles in the estrogen-deprived patient who is taking GnRH-A. GnRH-A treatment combined with estrogen and progesterone add-back therapy has shown excellent results in alleviating these side effects. The add-back therapy can be given as oral contraceptives[34] or conjugated estrogens (0.625 mg/day) and medroxyprogesterone acetate (10 mg for 12 days/month).[35] However, before recommending GnRH-A with add-back therapy, its costs and alternatives should be considered.[35,36]

Cyproterone acetate is a potent progesterone and antiandrogen agent that has been use worldwide for hirsutism,[37] but is not available in the United States. Significant side effects, including decreased libido and mental depression will probably preclude its use here as it has not been shown to be more effective than spironolactone.

REFERENCES

1. Rittmaster RS. Hyperandrogenism—what is normal? N Engl J Med 1992;327:194.
2. Rittmaster RS. Evaluation and treatment of hirsutism. Infertil Reprod Med Clin N Am 1991;2:511.
3. Kligman AM. The human hair cycle. J Invest Dermatol 1959;33:307.
4. Seago SV, Ebling FJG. The hair cycle on the human arm and upper thigh. Br J Dermatol 1985;113:9.
5. Perloff WH. Hirsutism: a manifestation of juvenile hypothyroidism. JAMA 1955;157:651.
6. Stern SR, Kelnar CJH. Hypertrichosis due to hypothyroidism. Dis Child 1985;60:763.
7. Ferriman D, Gallwey JD. Clinical assessment of body hair growth in women. J Clin Endocrinol Metab 1961; 21:1440.
8. Serafini P, Lobo RA. Increased 5a reductase activity in idiopathic hirsutism. Fertil Steril 1985;43:74.
9. Polson DW, Wadsworth J, Adams J, Franks S. Polycystic ovaries: a common finding in normal women. Lancet 1988;2:870.
10. Clayton RN, Ogden V, Hodgkinson J, et al. How common are polycystic ovaries in normal women and what is their significance for the fertility of the population? Clin Endocrinol 1992;37:127.
11. Burger CW, Korsen T, van Kessel H, van Dop PA, Caron JM, Schoemaker J. Pulsatile luteinizing hormone patterns in the follicular phase of the menstrual cycle, polycystic ovarian disease (PCOD) and non-PCOD secondary amenorrhea. J Clin Endocrinol Metab 1985;61:1126.
12. Bergh C, Cartlsson B, Olsson J-H, Selleskog U, Hillensjo T. Regulation of androgen production in cultured human thecal cells by insulin-like growth factor I and insulin. Fertil Steril 1993;59:323.
13. Judd HL, Scully RE, Herbst AL, Yen SSC, Ingersol FM, Kliman B. Familial hyperthecosis: comparison of endocrinologic and histologic findings with polycystic ovarian disease. Am J Obstet Gynecol 1973;117:979.
14. Nagamani M, Lingold JC, Gomez LG, Barza JR. Clinical and hormonal studies in hyperthecosis of the ovaries. Fertil Steril 1981;36:326.
15. Kuttenn F, Couillin P, Girard F, et al. Late-onset adrenal hyperplasia in hirsutism. N Engl J Med 1985;313:224.
16. Benjamin F, Deutsch S, Saperstein H, Seltzer BVL. Prevalence of and markers for the attenuated form of congenital adrenal hyperplasia and hyperprolactinemia masquerading as polycystic ovarian disease. Fertil Steril 1986;46:215.
17. New MI, Lorenzeu F, Leiner AJ, et al. Genotyping steroid 21-hydroxylase deficiency: hormonal reference data. J Clin Endocrinol Metab 1983;57:320.
18. Azziz R, Zacur H. 21-hydroxylase deficiency in female hyperandrogenism: screening and diagnosis. J Clin Endocrinol Metab 1989;69:577.
19. Kamilaris TC, Chrousos GP. Adrenal diseases. In: Moore WT, Eastman RC, eds. Diagnostic endocrinology. Philadelphia: Decker; 1990:79.
20. Lobo RA. Ovarian hyperandrogenism and androgen-producing tumors. Endocrinol Metab Clin N Am 1991; 20:773.
21. Meldrum DR, Abraham GE. Peripheral and ovarian venous concentrations of various steroid hormones in virilizing ovarian tumors. Obstet Gynecol 1979;53:36.
22. Garcia-Bunuel R, Bered JS, Woodruff JD. Luteomas of pregnancy. Obstet Gynecol 1975;45:407.
23. Grumbach MM, Ducharme JR. The effects of androgens on fetal sexual development: androgen-induced female pseudohermaphroidism. Fertil Steril 1960;11:157.
24. Jewelwicz R, Perkins RP, Dyrenfurth I, Vande Wiele RL. Luteomas of pregnancy: a cause for maternal virilization. Am J Obstet Gynecol 1971;109:24.
25. Bradshaw KD, Santos-Ramos R, Rawlins SC, MacDonald PC, Parker CR Jr. Endocrine studies in pregnancy complicated by ovarian theca lutein cysts and hyperreactio luteinalis. Obstet Gynecol 1986;67:66S.
26. Schapiro G, Evron S. A novel use of spironolactone treatment of hirsutism. J Clin Endocrinol Metab 1988;51:363.
27. Tremblay RR. Treatment of hirsutism with spironolactone. J Clin Endocrinol Metab 1980;15:363.
28. Erenus M, Gurbuz O, Durmusoglu F, Pekin S. Comparison of the efficacy of spironolactone versus flutamide in the treatment of hirsutism. Fertil Steril 1994;61:613.
29. Cusan L, Dupont A, Gomez JL, Tembley RR, Labrie F. Comparison of flutamide and spironolactone in the treatment of hirsutism: a randomized controlled trial. Fertil Steril 1994;61:281.
30. Marcondes JAM, Minnani SL, Luthold WW, Wachenberg BL, Samojlik E, Kirschner MA. Treatment of hirsutism in women with flutamide. Fertil Steril 1992;57:543.
31. Moghetti P, Castello R, Magnani CM, et al. Clinical and hormonal effects of the 5α-reductase inhibitor finasteride in idiopathic hirsutism. J Clin Endocrinol Metab 1994; 79:1115.
32. Wong IL, Morris RS, Chang L, Spahn M, Stanczyk FZ, Lobo R. A prospective randomized trial comparing finasteride to spironolactone in the treatment of hirsute women. J Clin Endocrinol Metab 1995;80:233.
33. Ciotta L, Cianci A, Calogero AE, et al. Clinical and endocrine effects of finasteride, a 5α-reductase inhibitor, in women with idiopathic hirsutism. Fertil Steril 1995; 64:299.
34. Heriner JS, Greendale GA, Kawakami AK, et al. Comparison of a gonadotropin-releasing hormone agonist and a

low dose oral contraceptive given alone or together in the treatment of hirsutism. J Clin Endocrinol Metab 1995; 80:3412.

35. Azziz R, Ochoa TM, Bradley EL Jr, Potter HD, Boots LR. Leuprolide and estrogen versus oral contraceptive pills for the treatment of hirsutism: a prospective randomized study. J Clin Endocrinol Metab 1995;80:3406.

36. Rittmaster R. Editorial: Gonadotropin-releasing hormone (GnRH) agonists and estrogen/progestin replacement for the treatment of hirsutism: evaluating the results. J Clin Endocrinol Metab 1995;80:3403.

37. O'Brien RC, Cooper ME, Murray RML, Seeman E, Thomas AK, Jerums G. Comparison of sequential cyproterone acetate/estrogen versus spironolactone/oral contraceptives in the treatment of hirsutism. J Clin Endocrinol Metab 1991;72:1008.

Chapter 47

Abnormal and Dysfunctional Uterine Bleeding

Edward J. Stanford

Five Key Points

- **Abnormal and dysfunctional uterine bleeding (DUB) may affect women throughout their entire lives: childhood, adolescence, reproductive years, perimenopause, and menopause.**

- **A careful work-up, a comprehensive examination, and good clinical judgment are essential in treating DUB.**

- **Consider changes in anatomy, physiology, and the potential for systemic disease when evaluating and treating DUB.**

- **Understand the complex mechanisms that control the normal menstrual cycle.**

- **Treatment of DUB may be medical, surgical, or both and should be directed at the underlying pathophysiology.**

INTRODUCTION

Dysfunctional uterine bleeding (DUB) is one of the most common diagnostic problems encountered by the gynecologist and primary care physicians. This is primarily due to the potential for abnormal bleeding patterns seen throughout a woman's life from early menarche through her perimenopausal and postmenopausal years. Most patients who seek care for DUB notice a change in their otherwise normal cycle length, duration, or amount of bleeding. They may notice heavier flow, larger clots, spotting between cycles, increased dysmenorrhea, or an increase in the use of sanitary products. Excessive bleeding may cause economic hardship, may interfere with work and physical activity, or may lead to sexual dysfunction. Likewise, amenorrhea or infrequent menses may concern the patient sufficiently to seek medical care.

The term dysfunctional uterine bleeding does not necessarily identify the underlying cause and is therefore a diagnosis of exclusion—i.e., the diagnosis of DUB is generally reserved for those patients in whom organic causes of abnormal bleeding have been excluded. The presence of an abnormal bleeding history necessarily mandates that the physician rule out the many possible causes. Advances in imaging techniques and less invasive surgical treatments have generally led to an overall improvement in the treatment of DUB.

DUB is traditionally discussed in terms of endocrinologic causes and organic causes. To fully understand DUB, it is important to have a comprehensive understanding of normal menstrual patterns seen in women during the different phases of their reproductive life. When a physician is faced with medical disorders that are as variable as DUB, it is prudent to consider to what extent to pursue a work-up. Considerations of cost and comfort are very real concerns in health care today and should be taken seriously when approaching the patient presenting with DUB.

DEFINITIONS

The "normal" menstrual cycle requires a balance of hormonal stimulation and withdrawal with associated endometrial growth and shedding. It is generally agreed that the normal menstrual cycle is between 24 and 35 days[1,2] although a slightly broader range of 28±7 days is traditionally taught, indicating a normal range of 21 to 35 days. The clinician should consider initiating appropriate work-up when the menstrual cycles occur less frequently than every 35 days, more frequently than every 24 days, or if the patient notices a difference in her usual pattern of frequency or flow. Treloar et al.[3] reported a prospective, 30-year study of 275,947 menstrual cycles in Caucasian women attending the University of Minnesota. The most consistent cycle interval was in women aged 20 to 40 years, with a median duration at age 20 of 28.9±2.75 days and at age 40, 26.8±2 days. Cycle length varied by 1 to 2 days each month, with only 50% falling in the 28-day lunar cycle (26 to 30 days). The length or duration of the average menstrual period is 3 to 7 days.

DUB can be defined as alterations in the interval between menstrual cycles or the duration of menstrual flow (Table 47-1). Abnormal intervals are defined as: oligomenorrhea—frequency of menstrual flow is greater than 35 days; amenorrhea—no menstrual flow for at least 6 months; and polymenorrhea—frequency less than 24 days. When the duration of menstrual flow is prolonged (greater than 7 days) it is referred

to as menorrhagia or hypermenorrhea. Intermenstrual bleeding or bleeding at a time other than the menstrual cycle is termed metrorrhagia.

Quantifying uterine blood loss is difficult and not clinically practical in the office setting. Loss of more than 80 ml per cycle is accepted as the objective definition for menorrhagia; however, the risk of developing iron-deficiency anemia becomes significant when the monthly blood loss exceeds 60 ml per cycle. Due to variations in hygienic practices, a patient's pad or tampon count does not correlate with objectively measured menstrual blood loss.[5] A more practical approach is to inquire whether there has been a change in the patient's usual duration or whether the cycles are heavier, with an increased passage of blood or blood clots requiring the use of more sanitary products. Most of the patient's menstrual blood loss will occur early in the menstruation phase, with 70% of the blood loss occurring by day 2 and 90% by day 3.[6,7]

MENSTRUAL CYCLE REGULATION

A general overview of the complex mechanisms involved in regulating menstrual cycles is important to understanding abnormal uterine bleeding. The menstrual cycle can be viewed in terms of the ovarian cycle and the endometrial cycle. The ovarian cycle is divided into three phases: the follicular phase, ovulation, and the luteal phase. The endometrial cycle is discussed in terms of the proliferative and secretory phases.

Normal, regular menstrual cycles require maturation of the hypothalamic–pituitary–ovarian axis and estrogen feedback mechanism. In the absence of pregnancy, there is a fall in luteal-phase steroids and in a compound called inhibin. Low levels of estrogen and progesterone stimulate the pulsatile release of gonadotropin releasing hormone (GnRH) from the hypothalamus. GnRH, a decapeptide, travels to the anterior pituitary, stimulating the release of follicle-stimulating hormone (FSH) and luteinizing hormone (LH) in a pulsatile manner from gonadotropic cells. Follicle development appears to be independent of gonadotropin stimulation. However, it does rely on a rise in FSH toward the end of the preceding cycle to promote the growth of a dominant follicle through the different stages of follicle maturation. Although the growth of the follicle is initiated during the luteal phase of the preceding cycle the follicular phase, by

---

TABLE 47-1
DEFINITIONS OF DYSFUNCTIONAL UTERINE BLEEDING

Amenorrhea	No menstrual flow for at least 6 months
Oligomenorrhea	Frequency greater than 35 days
Polymenorrhea	Frequency less than 24 days
Menorrhagia	Excessive bleeding or duration of menstrual flow greater than 7 days; (also hypermenorrhea) at regular intervals
Metrorrhagia	Intermenstrual bleeding between regular cycles
Menometrorrhagia	Prolonged uterine bleeding with frequent or intermenstrual bleeding

definition, begins with the onset of menses and extends to the LH surge.

FSH propagates an increase in its own receptors on the granulosa cells. As the follicle develops, FSH initiates estrogen production in granulosa cells, converting them from an androgenic to an estrogenic microenvironment. Failure in the conversion to an estrogenic microenvironment will result in an atretic follicle. The hypothalamus becomes increasingly more sensitive to the rising estradiol level until there is a large release of GnRH leading to the LH surge. There is a surge in estradiol levels at approximately 14 to 24 hours, followed by a surge in LH levels. Ovulation occurs approximately 36 hours after the onset of the LH surge and 10 to 12 hours after the LH peak. The luteal phase follows ovulation and lasts until the onset of the next menstrual cycle. After ovulation, the corpus luteum is formed. During the luteal phase, progesterone levels rise and reach a peak approximately 8 to 9 days after ovulation. Capillary growth and penetration into the granulosa layer can result in a hemorrhagic corpus luteum. The length of the normal luteal phase is 11 to 17 days.[6] In the absence of pregnancy, the corpus luteum will begin its demise 9 to 11 days following ovulation.[7] As the corpus luteum declines, FSH levels begin to increase as estradiol, progesterone, and inhibin levels decrease. Inhibin levels decline as the luteolytic mechanisms within the corpus luteum affect steroid production allowing FSH to increase. Approximately 2 days prior to menses, FSH levels begin to rise and the cycle of selecting a dominant follicle repeats.

The dominant follicle continues to develop as estrogen inhibits FSH production. LH is not usually present in the follicular fluid until approximately midcycle, when LH increases or surges, during which granulosa cells begin to acquire LH receptors. In a FSH-stimulated estrogenic environment, LH induces formation of its own receptors necessary to respond to the LH surge. A sustained increase in estradiol precedes the LH surge. Ovulation requires a complex interaction of a GnRH surge, sustained estradiol levels for at least 36 hours, an LH surge, and a smaller FSH surge.

In the hypothalamus, several neurotransmitter compounds stimulate or inhibit GnRH release. Norepinephrine (NE), γ-aminobutyric acid (GABA), and acetylcholine (ACh) stimulate GnRH release. Dopamine, serotonin, and melatonin inhibit release. Following ovulation, progesterone levels increase and LH, FSH, and estrogen levels drop.

At the endometrial level, increasing estradiol levels stimulate proliferation of epithelial and stromal cells. Progesterone receptors are synthesized under the influence of estrogen on the epithelial cells. This phase is referred to as the proliferative phase. During the luteal phase, there is an increase in progesterone and estradiol levels and a decrease in LH and FSH levels. The endometrium undergoes secretory changes reflecting the increase in progesterone. In the early secretory phase, glycogen vacuoles are formed in the glandular epithelium. In the midsecretory phase, the endometrium demonstrates three distinct layers. Endometrial growth stops, probably under the influence of progesterone since there is adequate estrogen to continue promoting proliferation, and the endometrium becomes stable. If fertilization does not occur, the corpus luteum involutes, estrogen and progesterone levels drop, and menses ensues. With menses the endometrium becomes edematous, with constriction and necrosis of blood vessels resulting in sloughing. Initially, stromal autolysis inhibits coagulation. Thrombin is generated by the action of tissue thromboplastin through the extrinsic coagulation pathway. Menstrual bleeding slows as the spiral arterioles vasoconstrict and the endometrium begins to regenerate. Prostaglandins (PGs) are released locally in the endometrium and play a role in regulating menstruation. Their actions help regulate menstrual flow by inducing uterine contractions (PGE_2, PGF_2), causing vasoconstriction (PGF_2, thromboxane A_2 [TXA_2]) or vasodilation (PGE_2, PGI_2).

In terms of the endometrial cycle, the proliferative phase corresponds with the estrogen effect on the endometrium prior to ovulation, causing endometrial proliferation. This is a period of reepithelialization, or regrowth, of the uterine lining. The secretory phase follows ovulation, during which the endometrium is prepared for implantation. The histologic changes in the endometrium are predictable and can be reliably dated from endometrial biopsy samples, with particular accuracy in the luteal phase.[8] The innermost layer, the stratum basalis, is refractory to the effects of progesterone and maintains a proliferative pattern throughout the menstrual cycle. At menstruation, the functional zone, consisting of the outer layer (stratum compactum) and the middle layer (stratum spongiosum), sloughs. During the follicular phase, endometrial-layer changes are not consistent or ordered enough to be dated. The maturing endometrium can be reliably dated in the luteal phase. Prior to menses, the spiral arterioles vasoconstrict under the influence of prostaglandins. The cessation of menstrual flow is influenced predominantly by the action of prostaglandins. TXA_2, derived from platelet membranes is a vasoconstrictor and promotes platelet aggregation. Prostaglandin I_2 opposes TXA_2 in a delicate balance to achieve hemostasis. Prostaglandins E_2 and $F_{2\alpha}$ stimulate platelet activity and uterine muscle contraction. $PGF_{2\alpha}$ is a potent vasoconstrictor. In patients with menorrhagia, there is an increase in arachidonic acid in the endometrium (a precursor to prostaglandin production)[9] and increased PGE_2, PGD_2 with lower levels of $PGF_2\alpha$ and TXA_2.[10]

The first day of the menstrual cycle is often considered day 0 of the menstrual cycle. Many however, will report the LH peak as day 0, with the days before the peak minus days and the days after, plus days.[11] The critical event in the regulation of the menstrual cycle is whether ovulation has occurred. According to Bates et al.,[12] a reasonable approach is for the clinician to ask whether FSH, LH, estradiol, or progesterone is elevated or suppressed when evaluating patients for disorders of ovulation. Premenstrually, all are suppressed and the patient is anovulatory. In anovulatory patients during their reproductive years (typically, polycystic ovary patients), estrogen is elevated, with positive feedback to the pituitary stimulating LH secretion. In the menopausal patient, FSH is elevated and estradiol is suppressed due to ovarian failure, resulting in anovulation.

MENORRHAGIA

Menorrhagia is excessive menstrual blood loss. By definition, menorrhagia indicates heavy flow (greater than 80 ml) or flow lasting longer than 7 days, but occurring at regular, predictable intervals. In clinical terms, for the practitioner caring for patients with DUB, menorrhagia is menstrual bleeding that is heavier as compared with the patient's previous history, duration of flow that has increased (i.e., 5 days to 9 days), or menstrual blood loss leading to anemia or somatic symptoms such as chronic fatigue. Since quantifying menstrual blood loss is not clinically practical, the clinician should rely on a careful clinical history, menstrual cycle diaries, and sound clinical judgment.

Under most circumstances, medical therapy should be the first-line therapy for menorrhagia. Endome-

---

TABLE 47-2
ETIOLOGIES OF ABNORMAL UTERINE BLEEDING

Organic
  Systemic disease
    Blood dyscrasias
    Hepatic disease
    Renal disease
    Obesity
    Iatrogenic
  Mechanical or gross lesion disease
    Uterine leiomyomas
    Uterine or cervical polyps
    Infection
    Intrauterine contraceptive device
    Estrogen-producing tumor of the ovary
    Pregnancy (abortion or ectopic pregnancy)
    Uterine or cervical neoplasia
Endocrinologic
  Gross endocrinopathy
    Thyroid dysfunction
    Diabetes mellitus
    Adrenal disease
    Prolactin disorders
  Dysfunction of the reproductive hormones
    Anovulation
    Inadequate corpus luteum
    Polycystic ovarian syndrome

---

trial sampling should be performed for patients with menorrhagia who are over age 35, are not responding to medical therapy, and are at high risk for adenocarcinoma (obese, unopposed estrogen use). Work-up may uncover a treatable cause such as endometrial polyps, leiomyoma, or endometritis (see Tables 47-2 and 47-3 and Figure 47-1). Prior to proceeding with work-up, the patient should be counseled with informed consent. Also, consider the impact to the patient and the cost-effectiveness of the planned therapy. In acute situations in which bleeding may be life-threatening, aggressive management may be required. High-dose estrogen therapy can stop bleeding in most who present acutely (Table 47-4).

Reproductive Years

The causes of abnormal uterine bleeding in the reproductive years can be attributed to the organic and endocrinologic causes referred to in Table 47-2. The most common causes are anovulation, polycystic ovary syndrome, and obesity. Work-up and treatment require a complete history and physical examination to ensure that more serious causes are not overlooked.

TABLE 47-3
ABNORMAL UTERINE BLEEDING WORK-UP

Comprehensive history
    Attention to menstrual history
Complete physical examination
    Rule out systemic illness
Laboratory studies
Complete blood count (rule out thrombocytopenia, iron-
    deficiency anemia)
Quantitative human chorionic gonadotropin
    Thyroid function studies (thyroid-stimulating hormone)
    Gonadotropin levels (FSH, LH)
    Prolactin
Consider
    Renal and liver function studies
    Progesterone level (midluteal)
Coagulation studies (prothrombin time, partial thromboplastin
    time, bleeding time, clotting factors)
Serum androgens (testosterone, dehydroepiandrosterone
    sulfate)
Adrenal function testing (serum cortisol, 17-hydroxyproges-
    terone)
Ultrasonography (early pregnancy, ectopic, uterine pathology)
Endometrial sampling
Hysteroscopy with or without sampling
Computed tomography or magnetic resonance imaging

Perimenopausal

DUB is quite common in the perimenopausal period. Most women are concerned about their general health during this period of their life and visit their physicians more regularly and are usually aware of their increased risk of female cancers and that menopause may be approaching. This may be heightened by the onset of irregular uterine bleeding. In past years, perimenopausal DUB was a common indication for hysterectomy.[14] In some instances, despite advances in therapeutic options, this trend may be continuing. Fortunately, newer therapeutic approaches and stricter guidelines for hysterectomy have made it less likely that DUB in the perimenopausal period will lead to a major surgery.

TABLE 47-4
TREATMENT OF ACUTE UTERINE BLEEDING

Conjugated estrogen, 25 mg intravenously every 4 hours, fol-
    lowed by combined oral contraceptives.[13]
Combined oral contraceptives, 1 tablet every 4 hours for 5 to
    7 days or until bleeding stops

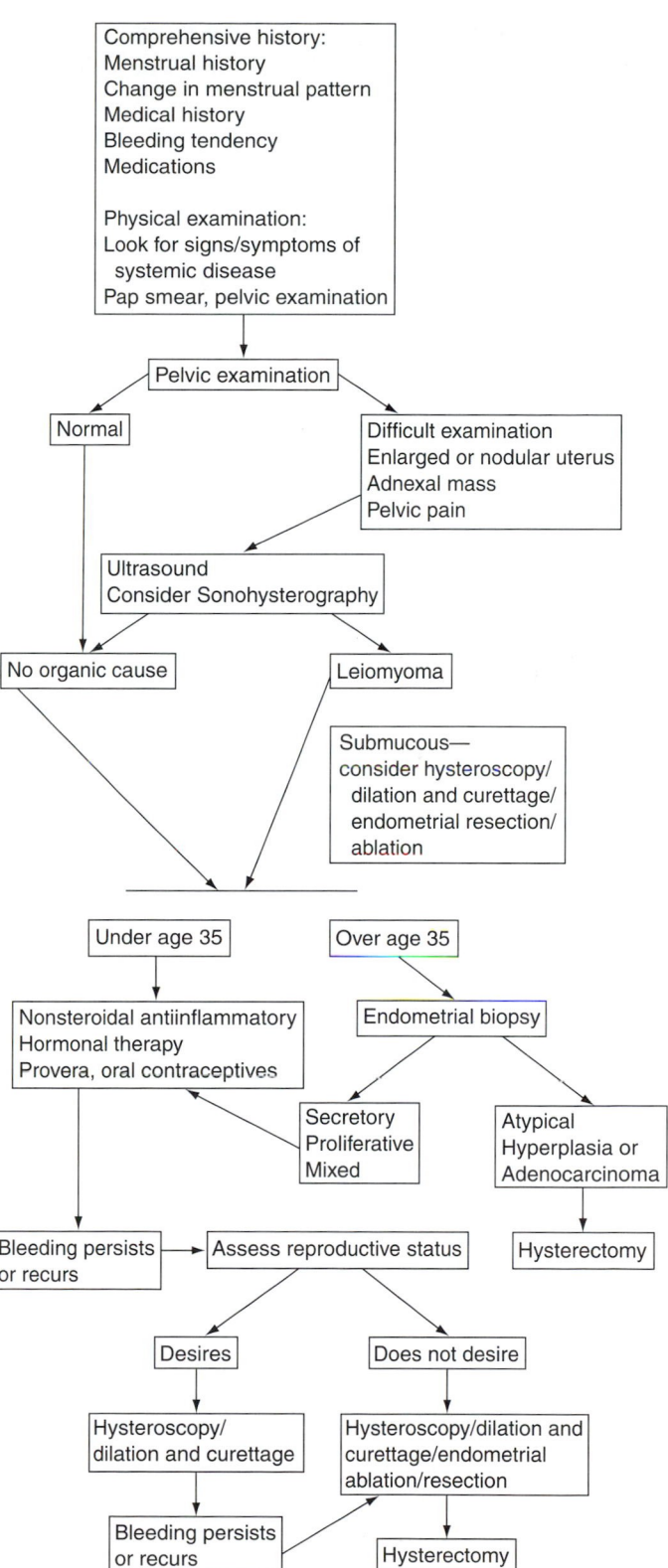

Figure 47-1 Menorrhagia.

In the perimenopausal period, the ovary gradually becomes less sensitive to FSH and LH. The follicular and luteal phases shorten.[15,16] Ultimately, the frequency between cycles lengthens and the patient becomes anovulatory. Anovulation occurs in a fashion similar to that of adolescent DUB in that there is estrogen stimulation but insufficient amounts to cause an LH surge. FSH levels slowly elevate and estradiol secretion decreases.[17] Inhibin also plays a role during this decline in ovarian function. As the population of follicles declines, the amount of estradiol also declines. The onset of this occurs in the late perimenopausal period as inhibin levels begin to decrease.

Initially, medical therapy should be considered in all women with DUB, including perimenopausal patients. As estrogen levels drop, estrogen-replacement therapy (ERT) should be considered if there are no contraindications. Work-up should be complete, to rule out more common, organic causes in this age group such as endometrial polyps, uterine fibroids, and endometrial hyperplasia (see Tables 47–2 and 47–3). Initially, the clinician may wish to start the patient on cyclic progestins. Breakthrough or failure of treatment may lead to hysteroscopy and possibly endometrial surgery.

If the patient is started on hormone replacement, it is not uncommon for her to experience breakthrough bleeding and require additional estrogen. For this reason, the clinician may wish to initiate hormone replacement with low-dose combined oral contraceptives containing 20 μg of estrogen in lieu of lower-dose regimens. As the patient approaches menopause, decreasing the estrogen dose may be better tolerated.

POSTMENOPAUSAL BLEEDING

Menopause occurs when ovarian function fails and menstruation ceases. The average age at which menopause occurs is 51. We are, in essence, treating a new disorder manifested by the longer lives women are living. At the turn of the last century, most women did not live to the onset of menopause. Now, women are living for decades after the onset of menopause. Factors that can influence the age at menopause include cigarette smoking, chemotherapy, pelvic irradiation, and hysterectomy. Cigarette smoking appears to cause menopause to occur 1 to 2 years prematurely.[18] During the perimenopausal period, estrogen levels fall, along with a fall in androgen levels and the androgen precur-

sors dehydroepiandrosterone and dehydroepiandrosterone sulfate. In the late perimenopausal period, there is a rise in FSH followed by a slow, steady decline in the menopausal period over several years. These hormonal changes bring about physical changes, some of which are readily apparent, such as irregular menstrual bleeding, insomnia, hot flushes, and urogenital atrophy.

Patients who present with postmenopausal bleeding should be carefully examined to uncover the source of bleeding. A common rule of thumb is that postmenopausal uterine bleeding should be considered endometrial carcinoma until proven otherwise. This conservative approach should be balanced by the knowledge that atrophic changes are the most common source of postmenopausal genital bleeding. Prior to initiating any form of therapy, work-up should include a thorough physical examination, including pelvic and rectal examinations, a Pap smear, and an endometrial biopsy. Severe atrophy or cervical stenosis may not allow the physician to examine the patient completely or to obtain an endometrial sample. Under these circumstances, a short course of estrogen therapy (4 to 8 weeks) may allow future evaluation. Usually, once the work-up has been initiated, the patient can be started on a course of combined estrogen and progesterone therapy or cycled with progestin therapy for 10 days per month for 2 to 3 months. This will usually control bleeding. If the work-up is negative for adenomatous hyperplasia or adenocarcinoma but the patient continues to have bleeding, hysteroscopy and fractional dilation and curettage (D&C) are indicated. When starting treatment, the patient should be warned about the possibility of breast tenderness, which can be pronounced.

Hormone replacement can be continuous or cyclic. Using either method, patients who are started on hormone-replacement therapy may resume bleeding or spotting. Many patients elect to discontinue treatment, often without informing their physician; therefore, the patient should be reassured that some bleeding is normal when initiating hormone-replacement therapy. With continuous therapy, work-up can wait 2 to 3 cycles. However, any heavy or persistent bleeding or spotting necessitates further evaluation.

CHILDHOOD AND ADOLESCENT DUB

Prepubertal children may occasionally present with vaginal bleeding. Inspection of the vagina and vulva is important to rule out a foreign body or lesions. In young girls, the examination may be difficult because of fear. The child's parents may be able to calm the young patient, allowing an examination. It is not uncommon to require sedation in order to fully examine the vagina and perform a rectovaginal examination to palpate the pelvic organs. A flexible hysteroscope (4 mm) is ideal for vaginoscopy under sedation, particularly when warmed saline is gently flushed. Naturally, trauma to the genitalia should prompt a full history to rule out the possibility of sexual abuse. Vulvovaginal infections usually do not cause bleeding. However, the associated pruritus may cause the child to scratch, leaving open wounds. A wet mount and potassium hydroxide (KOH) preparation is important to rule out bacterial or yeast vaginitis, trichomonads, or parasites. A Gram stain and cultures should be considered. Additional treatment with topical hydrocortisone to control itching and topical estrogen cream to promote healing may speed recovery and relieve discomfort.

If a vulvar lesion is encountered, a biopsy should be taken. If human papillomavirus (HPV) is encountered, sexual abuse should be considered. However, the three modes of transmission reported for HPV include sexual contact, close nonsexual contact, and contact at the time of delivery.[19] Colposcopy is generally of limited use in this situation.[20] Other potential causes of vaginal bleeding in childhood include urethral prolapse, lichen sclerosis, foreign body, and genital tumors. Urethral prolapse is treated conservatively with local application of estrogen cream unless urinary obstruction and retention are noted. Lichen sclerosis may affect this age group and usually produces the characteristic white lesions. Bleeding may occur if local irritation has led to scratching and tissue excoriation. Foreign-body insertion is relatively common and may result in vaginal infection and bleeding.

Genital tumors may present with vaginal bleeding. Vulvar carcinoma is exceedingly uncommon. Benign tumors such as cavernous hemangiomas may produce serious hemorrhage, and surgical removal should be considered. The most common malignant genital tumor is sarcoma botryoides (vulvar embryonal carcinoma). Treatment for sarcoma botryoides is usually started with chemotherapy (cyclophosphamide, vincristine, dactinomycin). After a course of treatment, surgical removal may be attempted. Other tumors to suspect are endodermal carcinoma, mesonephric carcinoma, and clear-cell adenocarcinoma.[21]

Childhood and early adolescent vaginal bleeding may also be associated with exogenous or endogenous estrogen production. Granulosa-cell tumors may produce large amounts of estrogen and cause isosexual precocious puberty. Symptoms and findings may include abdominal pain, enlargement of abdominal girth, uterine bleeding, endometrial hyperplasia, breast enlargement, or ovarian enlargement.[22] Exogenous sources may include accidental ingestion and exposure to creams or patches containing estrogen.

Prior to maturation of the hypothalmic–pituitary–ovarian axis, adolescent females may experience abnormal menstrual cycles. These are the prototypical examples of DUB. The feedback mechanism is not matured and anovulation may not occur due to the absence of the LH surge. There is estrogen stimulus without sufficient progesterone, resulting in irregular bleeding patterns. Basically, the endometrium proliferates under the influence of unopposed estrogens until the endometrium can no longer maintain its integrity and breaks down. The patient may have regular monthly bleeding, although patterns of DUB include missed periods or intermenstrual bleeding, and bleeding may be heavier or longer.

Occasionally, bleeding disorders cause abnormal bleeding. If the medical history shows evidence of easy bruising, a family history of bleeding dyscrasia, gingival bleeding, or frequent epistaxis, the patient should be screened for von Willebrand disease and idiopathic thrombocytopenia purpura (ITP). Obtain a complete blood count with platelets, prothrombin time, and partial thromboplastin time, and consider obtaining a bleeding time.

Treatment for adolescent DUB not related to an underlying medical condition is essentially the same as in adults. Oral contraceptives or intermittent progestins are both effective. Emergency treatment of symptomatic uterine hemorrhage may include D&C (rule out pregnancy and abortion), intravenous fluid replacement, parenteral conjugated estrogens, or rarely, transfusion.

POLYCYSTIC OVARY SYNDROME

Polycystic ovary syndrome is generally referred to as PCO, indicating simply polycystic ovaries. This syndrome is associated with anovulation and may be manifested as hirsutism, obesity, and infertility. Most patients present with symptoms suggesting anovulation, with irregular menstrual cycles or oligomenorrhea.

Other signs of PCO may be present, such as oily skin or acne, change in hair thickness, or difficulty conceiving. Work-up should include a physical examination, laboratory evaluation of LH, FSH, and thyroid levels, and a pelvic ultrasound. An LH:FSH ratio of greater than 2:1 is suggestive of PCO. Ultrasound of the ovaries reveals multiple small cortical cysts. Further evaluation, such as serum testosterone levels, may be indicated based on initial findings. Treatment depends on whether the patient desires to become pregnant immediately. If pregnancy is not desired, combined oral contraceptives are very effective in restoring normal menstrual patterns and improving androgenic signs. If the patient desires conception, induced ovulation with clomiphene citrate is an appropriate therapy to consider initially.

LEIOMYOMA

Uterine leiomyomata are the most common organic cause of increased menstrual bleeding.[23] Although, the pathogenesis of leiomyoma formation is incompletely understood, it is estimated that 20% of all women over age 35 have leiomyomas.[24] Leiomyomata do not have to be palpable to cause abnormal bleeding. Those associated with menorrhagia tend to be either submucous or intramyometrial in location. Bleeding occurs, in theory, due to abnormal contractility or enlargement of the endometrial surface area adjacent to the leiomyoma and abnormal venous drainage in myomatous uteri.[25] Doppler ultrasound is not routinely used clinically but reduced mean uterine artery resistance indexes may be seen in women with uterine myomas, indicating abnormal vascularization.[26]

Treatment naturally depends on location, size, and symptoms. Hysterectomy has been a mainstay of treatment for symptomatic leiomyomata since it definitively cures the patient. Traditionally, hysterectomy has been recommended when the uterine size is equivalent to a 12-week gestation. Operating before the uterus grows larger avoids a higher prevalence of blood transfusion, ureteral injury, or silent ureteral obstruction and decreases the risk of missing leiomyosarcoma. The literature does not support this teaching in asymptomatic patients. Alternative treatments should be considered and offered to the patient, although she may elect definitive hysterectomy. Alternatives include treatment with GnRH agonists to shrink the leiomyomata; myomectomy, which may require laparoscopy or laparotomy for intramural or subserosal leiomyoma; or endometrial resection if submucosal. Newer treatment options requiring further follow-up research include bipolar electrocautery and cryosurgery. The risk of regrowth of leiomyomata in the 10 years following myomectomy is 20%.[27] When obtaining informed consent, the patient should consider that myomectomy may be palliative, there may be more significant blood loss as compared with hysterectomy, and the incidence of postoperative fever and adhesion formation may be higher.

ADENOMYOSIS

Adenomyosis is characterized by the presence of ectopic endometrial glands and stroma within the myometrium. The depth of invasion correlates with the heaviness of bleeding.[28] Pathologists will usually report adenomyosis when ectopic endometrial tissue is seen to extend more than two low-power microscopic fields deeper than the basalis layer into the myometrium. Magnetic resonance imaging (MRI) and ultrasound can be used to diagnose adenomyosis in patients in whom this condition is suspected.[29] However, diagnosis usually requires myometrial tissue, most commonly obtained at hysterectomy. Adenomyosis is a diffuse process but appears to involve primarily the posterior wall.[30] Failure to control bleeding after endometrial ablation may be due to deeply invading adenomyosis.[31] Endometrial resection specimens and, less commonly, ultrasound-guided needle biopsy, mainly of the posterior uterine wall, may yield sufficient tissue for pathologic diagnosis of adenomyosis. Patients with adenomyosis typically have uterine enlargement (usually less than 12-weeks-gestational size); globular, soft, and tender uterus; dyspareunia; menorrhagia; or dysmenorrhea. Many patients treated with hysterectomy for menorrhagia not controlled by medication will have adenomyosis as the final pathologic diagnosis. Unfortunately, it is difficult to be sure that adenomyosis is not merely a co-finding since it is also found in asymptomatic women treated with hysterectomy. When a patient does not respond to medical therapy for menorrhagia and work-up does not reveal other pelvic pathology, surgical therapy may be suggested to the patient. Hysterectomy may be indicated; however, physicians who perform endometrial resection or ablation may wish to offer this outpatient surgical approach instead of hysterectomy.

ENDOMETRIAL POLYPS

Endometrial polyps can arise anywhere in the endometrium. It is not uncommon to find endometrial polyps when performing an annual cervical smear. Removal with ring forceps is usually sufficient. Occasionally, the patient with an endometrial polyp may present with abnormal uterine bleeding in the form of postcoital bleeding or intermenstrual bleeding. They are more easily appreciated when the polyp prolapses or extends through the endocervical os. When the uppermost portion of the polyp cannot be seen or retrieved, hysteroscopy may be warranted to investigate further and remove the polyp or polyps in their entirety. In perimenopausal and menopausal patients, it is essential to rule out endometrial hyperplasia and adenocarcinoma.

PREMATURE OVARIAN FAILURE

Premature ovarian failure is rare. By definition, premature ovarian failure is the cessation of menses prior to the age of 35 years, associated elevated gonadotropin levels (FSH >40 IU/liter), and decreased estrogen levels.

SYSTEMIC ILLNESSES

Systemic illnesses are not a common cause of DUB, although the clinician must consider them in the work-up of each patient.

Bleeding Disorders

Idiopathic thrombocytopenia purpura; von Willebrand disease; prothrombin deficiency; factors II, V, VII, and XI deficiencies; disseminated intravascular coagulopathy (DIC); and acute leukemias can present or have as part of their symptoms dysfunctional menstrual bleeding patterns. Most commonly, menorrhagia and metrorrhagia are reported and the work-up does not reveal a mechanical cause such as polyps or leiomyomata. Patients with leukemia may present with easy bruising. Up to 20% of adolescents presenting with severe menorrhagia may have blood dyscrasias.[32]

Weight Loss/Anorexia Nervosa

Severe fluctuations in body weight affect ovarian function and menstruation as demonstrated by the well-known documentation of Dutch women in World War II.[33] Patients suffering anorexia nervosa or other forms of severe weight loss usually become amenorrheic. FSH, LH, thyroid-stimulating hormone (TSH), and estradiol levels decrease. Testosterone levels may be elevated. Basal levels of serum growth hormone and serum cortisol levels increase. The responses of gonadotropin increase to GnRH stimulation and TSH to thyrotropin-releasing hormone (TRH) stimulation are depressed, signaling hypothalamic hypofunction. Weight gain and reestablishment of body mass corrects the hormonal imbalances.

Very active women who engage in strenous physical activity may decrease their body mass sufficiently to develop dysfunctional menstrual patterns such as oligomenorrhea or amenorrhea.[34] Long-distance runners, dancers, and gymnasts are prone to exercise-induced amenorrhea. Adolescent swimmers are prone to delayed menarche. In contrast to runners and dancers, who tend to be hypoestrogenic, swimmers in whom postmenarchal amenorrhea develops have normal estrogen, normal FSH, elevated LH, increased dehydroepiandrosterone sulfate (DHEA-S), and androstenedione, and normal testosterone, suggesting a different mechanism.

Liver Disease

Patients with liver disease such as alcoholic cirrhosis can present with DUB due to impaired metabolism of estrogens and decreased production of fibrinogen and coagulation factors.[35] Patients with liver dysfunction may present initially or later in their disease with amenorrhea, oligomenorrhea, or metrorrhagia. Patients with chronic cirrhosis, whether alcoholic or nonalcoholic, may have higher levels of estradiol, progesterone, and testosterone due to impaired clearance, with higher levels of estrone due to peripheral conversion of elevated androgen precursors.[36,37] Liver-transplant recipients, even those with abnormal liver-function studies, frequently resume normal menstrual function.[38]

Renal Disease

DUB or amenorrhea commonly develops in patients with renal insufficiency, but a pattern is not predictable. Patients on dialysis tend to have amenorrhea and to undergo menopause at an earlier age, although many will continue to have regular menses. The duration of the menstrual cycle lasts essentially the same number of days. Bleeding is reported as being heavier as compared with before dialysis.[39] Heparin is administered with each dialysis session, and many patients take oral anticoagulants. Amenorrhea may occur when serum creatinine levels reach 5 mg/dl or greater and often persists despite hemodialysis. The use of recombinant human erythropoietin may be a factor in delayed amenorrhea. Renal-transplant patients often resume normal menses[40] and ovulatory cycles.[41] Patients with uremia behave similarly to patients with PCO, with elevated LH levels due to poor renal clearance.[42] Hyperprolactinemia develops in about 50% of patients on dialysis and does not respond to levodopa or dopamine suppressors.[43]

Hyperprolactinemia

Prolactin is secreted from the anterior pituitary and is under the inhibitory control of dopamine released into the portal circulation from the hypothalamus. TRH, vasoactive intestinal peptide (VIP), and GnRH affect prolactin secretion. The chief role of prolactin is lactogenesis; therefore, galactorrhea is a possible result of elevated prolactin levels in the nonlactating female. Hyperprolactinemia can lead to amenorrhea due to central anovulatory dysfunction. As prolactin levels increase, GnRH suppression leads to inadequate luteal phase, anovulation, and possibly amenorrhea. Work-up should proceed from establishing a prolactin level. In patients with levels greater than 100 ng/ml, computed tomography (CT) of the sella turcica may reveal a microadenoma. Treatment with the dopamine receptor agonist bromocriptine (2.5 to 10 mg daily) is usually effective in restoring menstrual cycles. Patients whose disease does not respond to bromocriptine may be candidates for newer dopamine agonists depending on availability in the United States.[44]

Thyroid Disease

Patients with DUB should be screened for thyroid disorders. Hypothyroidism is associated with increased estradiol secondary to conversion of androstenedione to testosterone and peripheral aromatization of testosterone to estradiol.[45] Approximately 20% of patients with subclinical forms of hypothyroidism will report heavy periods.[46] Thyrotropin replacement usually corrects the menstrual disorder. Oligomenorrhea or amenorrhea may develop with hyperthyroid patients. In these patients, testosterone, androstenedione, estrone, and LH levels are elevated, leading to anovulatory DUB.

TABLE 47-5
AUTOIMMUNE DISORDERS ASSOCIATED WITH PREMATURE OVARIAN FAILURE

Addison disease (idiopathic)
Autoimmune thrombocytopenic purpura
Diabetes mellitus (juvenile-onset type)
Hyperthyroidism (Hashimoto thyroiditis, Graves disease)
Hypoparathyroidism
Myasthenia gravis
Pernicious anemia
Rheumatoid arthritis
Systemic lupus erythematosus

Reprinted with permission from Steinkampf.[48]

Diabetes

Ovarian function is normal in most women with diabetes, although premature ovarian failure is reported with type 1 diabetes. The relationship between polycystic ovary syndrome and diabetes is well known. Oligomenorrhea and amenorrhea is seen in approximately 30% of women with diabetes who are receiving treatment.[47]

Autoimmune Disorders

Amenorrhea and premature ovarian failure are not uncommonly seen in women with autoimmune disease (Table 47-5). Adrenal failure (Addison disease) is associated with autoimmune-related premature ovarian failure.[49] Amenorrhea, virilization, and androgen hypersecretion are well documented in 21-hydroxylase deficiency.

Cushing Syndrome

Cushing syndrome, in which there is an excess of glucocorticoid production, is associated with amenorrhea and other glucocorticoid-mediated changes such as hirsutism and striae. The disorder is 10 times more prevalent in women. FSH, LH, and sex hormone–binding globulin levels are depressed, while testosterone and estrogen (from peripheral conversion) are increased. GnRH agonists will cause an increase in FSH but not LH in the patients.[50]

Cancer/Chemotherapy

Every patient who presents with abnormal uterine bleeding should be evaluated for cervical lesions, with a physical inspection of the cervix and a Pap smear to rule out cervical cancer. Suspicious lesions should be

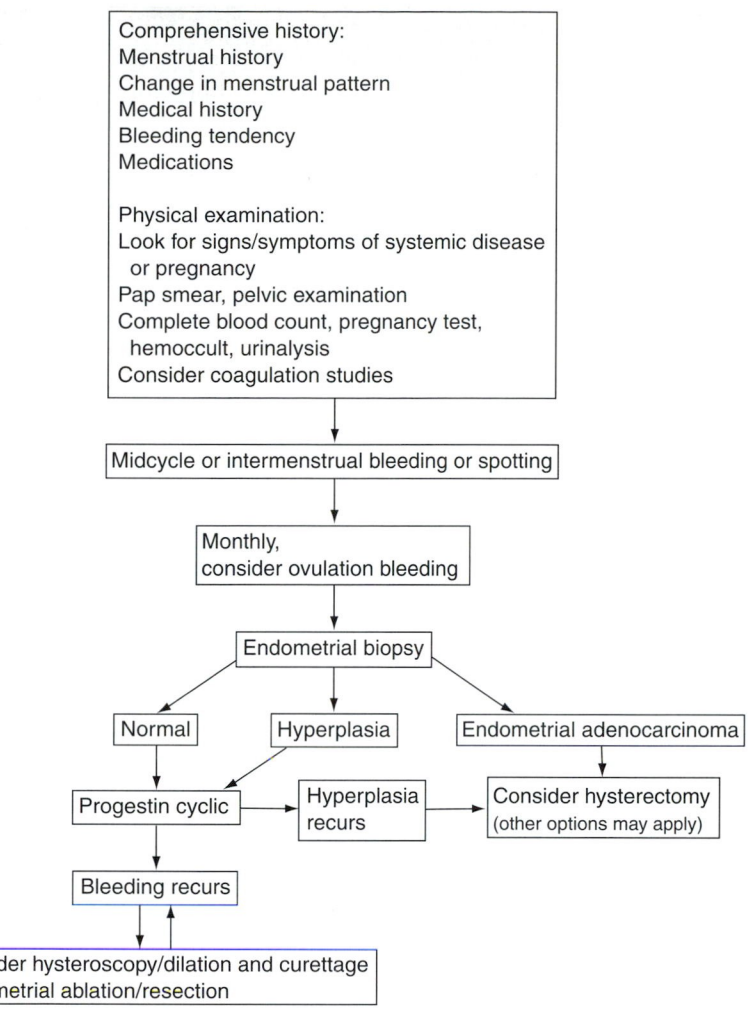

Figure 47-2 Metrorrhagia.

biopsied and submitted for pathologic diagnosis. Similarly, consider endometrial biopsy and hysteroscopy for patients with menorrhagia or metrorrhagia (Figure 47-2).

Rarely, granulosa-cell tumors, which produce excess estrogen, may be encountered when a patient presents with DUB. Arrhenoblastomas or lipoid-cell tumors may produce sufficient androgen and estrogen to cause DUB.[51]

Exposure to alkylating chemotherapeutic agents such as chlorambucil, cyclophosphamide, nitrogen mustard, busulfan, and melphalan can cause sterility and amenorrhea due to their effects on the ovary. Also, exposure to pelvic irradiation can lead to ovarian failure.

Thalassemia Major

Patients with β-thalassemia major have been shown to have lower estradiol, FSH, and LH levels.[52] Menstrual patterns are not predictable.

TRAUMA

Transient amenorrhea may develop in patients who suffer severe trauma. Patients with spinal-cord injuries appear to proceed to menarche without delay, and about one-third have transient postinjury amenorrhea. Most show some evidence of central neurotransmitter changes when tested.[53] Studies of women in the intensive-care unit and after follow-up for trauma are limited.

LACTATION

Lactation is the most common form of contraception and is used to prevent pregnancies more often than all other forms of contraception.[54] Local release of β-endorphins depresses GnRH secretion, decreases FSH and LH secretion, and inhibits dopamine production, causing increased prolactin secretion. DUB may develop in the form of oligomenorrhea or amenorrhea.

ORAL CONTRACEPTIVES

Breakthrough bleeding is a common problem with all forms of hormonal contraception and is a cause for the patient to discontinue use. Approximately 10 to 30% of oral contraceptive users report breakthrough bleeding during the first few months of use. No additional treatment is usually required during these initial months other than considering additional contraceptive prevention. It is important to counsel the patient prior to initiating oral contraceptives and to reassure the patient should bleeding occur. If bleeding continues beyond the first three cycles, it is likely due to progestin-induced decidualization, in which the endometrium is prone to breakdown. Having the patient take supplemental estrogen (2 mg of estradiol or 1.25 mg of conjugated estrogens daily for 7 days) may control bleeding. Late-cycle bleeding usually requires no additional therapy. The patient can be instructed to stop her pills, undergo a withdrawal bleed, and resume a new packet in 7 days. Instruct the patient to use additional contraception if applicable.

Medroxyprogesterone acetate (Depo-Provera) injections are an effective and convenient form of contraception. Unfortunately, bleeding occurs in up to 70% in the first year and is a principal reason for patients to discontinue this method.[55] Bleeding can be treated with nonsteroidal antiinflammatory drugs or in the same manner as breakthrough bleeding on oral contraceptives, with a 7-day course of supplemental estrogen. Reassuring the patient is appropriate since amenorrhea will develop in most during the first year of therapy.

INTRAUTERINE CONTRACEPTIVE DEVICES

Patients with intrauterine devices (IUDs) often report abnormal bleeding, mainly menorrhagia with associated dysmenorrhea. Most likely the cause of their excess bleeding is a mass effect, in which the myometrium does not adequately contract around the IUD. Other possible explanations include local endometrial inflammation and local effects on clotting mechanisms.

WORK-UP

History and Physical Examination

The work-up for DUB is no different from any other medical condition in that it should include a complete history and physical examination. A comprehensive health questionnaire with an emphasis on the patient's menstrual history, particularly as it relates to a change in the patient's previous cycles, is quite helpful. Patients who present to the office or are referred for specialty consultation deserve a complete physical examination looking for signs of systemic disorders since they often present with dysfunctional menstrual patterns.

Laboratory Analysis

Before proceeding to laboratory evaluations, the practitioner should consider the cost, discomfort, and efficacy of the planned work-up. A review of the literature does not reveal any studies to address the most cost-effective approach to evaluating DUB in its many possible scenarios. The rule of thumb is to be prudent.

The majority of patients will have abnormal bleeding due to anovulation. If the physical examination does not reveal any systemic illness, structural abnormality, or pregnancy, laboratory analysis for hyperprolactinemia, hypothyroidism, or anemia may be in order. Suspicion of an underlying systemic disease or uterine abnormality may lead more directly to a focused work-up (e.g., ultrasound, liver-function studies, etc.).

Endometrial Sampling

Although endometrial hyperplasia and adenocarcinoma may occur at any age, it is reasonable to treat women under the age of 35 at low risk for endometrial carcinoma empirically with combined oral contraceptives or cyclic progestins. For patients in whom initial therapy fails, those at high risk, those with midcycle heavy bleeding (metrorrhagia), or patients over age 35, the physician should consider performing endometrial sampling prior to initiating treatment. Some suggest that all women over age 35 with DUB should undergo endometrial biopsy to rule out endometrial cancer or hyperplasia.[56] A biopsy showing proliferative endometrium or mixed proliferative and secretory endometrium obtained at or near the beginning of menses is consistent with anovulation.

Ultrasound/Sonohysterography

Ultrasound imaging of the uterus and pelvic structures has become a common diagnostic study for patients with DUB. Scanning images can be obtained transabdominally (3.5 to 5 MHz probe) or transvaginally (5 to 8 MHz probe). During the reproductive years the uterus measures ≤10 cm in length, ≤5 cm in width, and ≤4 cm in height. Postmenopausally, the uterus measures <9 cm in length, while many years after menopause the uterus may measure 5 to 6 cm.[57] The endometrium is easily visualized with transvaginal scanning. The endometrial echogram is considered abnormal relative to the phase of the menstrual cycle. Other abnormal findings include focal or bulbous thickening or disruption of the endometrial echogram and focal or diffuse heterogeneity of the endometrial echotexture. In the proliferative phase the endometrium measures between 4 and 8 mm in premenopausal women[58] and has a characteristic triple-lined or five-layer appearance. In the secretory phase, the endometrium thickens to 7 to 14 mm with a less distinctive appearance. Measurements greater than 8 mm in the proliferative phase and >15 mm in the secretory phase should be considered abnormal in menstruating women. Postmenopausally, the endometrium becomes atrophic and measures usually less than 6 mm. In the Nordic trial,[59] a cutoff of ≤4 mm yielded 96% sensitivity and 69% specificity for endometrial pathology.

Tamoxifen stimulates the uterus and endometrium, and a potential complication of tamoxifen therapy includes endometrial hyperplasia and adenocarcinoma. Sonographically, the endometrial cavity may appear normal or may have a mixed echogenic or "Swiss-cheese" appearance. Any patient taking tamoxifen who has bleeding or endometrial thickness ≥6 mm should undergo endometrial sampling and hysteroscopic evaluation.

Sonohysteroscopy is an ultrasonographic technique in which sterile saline is introduced into the uterine cavity to improve visualization. The technique is useful in the preoperative evaluation of abnormal uterine bleeding by providing a detailed transvaginal ultrasound image of the endometrial lining and uterine wall. Common endometrial abnormalities that are seen easily with this method and that are amenable to endometrial surgery are endometrial polyps and submucous fibroids.

TREATMENTS

Prostaglandin Synthase Inhibitors

Prostaglandin synthase inhibitors can significantly reduce menstrual blood loss and reduce symptoms of dysmenorrhea in the absence of other causes, such as uterine myomata or bleeding disorders. The agents inhibit the production of cyclooxygenase in endometrial tissue,[60] resulting in reduced levels and altered ratios of the platelet-aggregating vasoconstrictor TXA_2 and the antiaggregating vasodilator prostacyclin.[61] Ovulatory menorrhagia may respond favorably to prostaglandin synthase-inhibitors. Contraindications include hepatic or renal disease, bronchospastic pulmonary disease, or allergy to aspirin.

Hormonal Therapy

Hormonal therapy using combined oral contraceptives reduces menstrual blood flow over time and is the preferred treatment in chronic menorrhagia. Alternatively, empiric treatment with progestins can be initiated in most patients. Patients in whom initial treatment fails or who are at high risk for endometrial hyperplasia or those over age 35 should be investigated with endometrial sampling. Progestins can be effective given alone or when given prior to initiating combined oral contraceptives. Medroxyprogesterone acetate 10 mg/day for 10 days per month given during the luteal phase, micronized oral progesterone 200 mg/day for 10 days per month, 100 to 400 mg of progesterone in oil, or 150 to 300 mg medroxyprogesterone acetate are effective in inhibiting endometrial proliferation and, with cyclic withdrawal, results in what some consider a medical curettage.

Intrauterine Devices

After treating DUB with medical therapy, one option is to place a progestin-releasing IUD. The Progestasert IUD has been shown to produce a 65% decrease in menstrual blood loss over 12 months.[62] The levonorgestrel-releasing IUD may reduce menstrual blood flow 97% at 12 months.[63]

Antifibrinolytic Agents

The antifibrinolytic agents tranexamic acid and ε-aminocaproic acid are effective in treating menorrhagia. These are not used commonly in the clinical setting, although they have been shown to reduce ovulatory menorrhagia in up to 50% of cases. Side effects such as nausea, dizziness, diarrhea, and intracranial thrombosis limit their use.

Ergot Derivatives

When considering the current and contemporary treatments of DUB, ergot derivatives have a limited clinical role. Their use should be abandoned in the treatment of menorrhagia.

Dilation and Curettage

Dilation and curettage (D&C) should be reserved for patients in whom medical therapy has failed or for those in whom hysteroscopy is being performed. D&C provides only temporary relief when used alone.[64] A D&C may not detect a causative factor.[65] The goal of a D&C in DUB is to detect a cause such as endometrial hyperplasia and endometrial carcinoma and to control bleeding. In 60% of hysterectomy specimens obtained immediately after curettage, less than half of the endometrial lining is sampled and the cause of DUB is frequently missed.[66] Control of menorrhagia with a D&C is short-term, and often bleeding is slowed only during the first menstrual cycle after the procedure. [66,67]

As compared with D&C, endometrial sampling is clearly superior when considering cost, convenience, adequacy of sampling, complications, safety, and diagnostic accuracy.[68] Several types of sampling devices exist. Most devices are 3 to 4 mm and are small enough not to require dilation prior to the procedure. A D&C costs approximately 10 times more than outpatient endometrial biopsy.[69] Acceptability is high for the procedure, with severe pain being reported by 5 to 7% when the Pipelle device was used. As compared with hysterectomy specimens, the Pipelle specimen was in agreement in 96%, with 97.5% sensitivity in patients with known endometrial adenocarcinoma.[70,71] Samples are obtained in over 90% of patients, and the specimen is adequate for pathologic diagnosis.[72]

To increase the specificity and sensitivity of diagnosing endometrial adenocarcinoma, transvaginal ultrasonography and endometrial biopsy (EB) can be used in conjunction. It has been shown in postmenopausal women that when the full endometrial thickness (double layer) is ≤5 mm, the endometrial mucosa is atrophic.[73] When the endometrial thickness is ≥6 mm, pathology is more likely to be diagnosed.[74] Using a 5-mm cutoff, endometrial adenocarcinoma has been diagnosed by Pipelle EB. Transvaginal ultra-

sonography and EB used together reportedly increases the sensitivity and specificity of diagnosing endometrial adenocarcinoma to 100%.[75]

Hysteroscopy/Endometrial Surgery

Hysteroscopy is endoscopy of the uterine cavity; the main indication for hysteroscopy is abnormal uterine bleeding.[76,77] Advantages of hysteroscopy are that it is an outpatient diagnostic and therapeutic procedure, it is well tolerated by patients, the patient returns quickly to work and normal activities, and it can be performed in the office or surgical suite depending on the indications and suspected findings. As a diagnostic tool, it has essentially replaced the "blind" D&C.[78] Compared to D&C in a hospital surgical setting, outpatient diagnostic hysteroscopy is better tolerated and significantly reduces time, expense, and postoperative disability.[79] Motashaw and Dave demonstrated in patients with DUB, normal endometrium (33%), endometrial hyperplasia (23%), endo-metrial polyps (21.5%), submucous fibroids (11.3%), synechiae (5.7%), endometrial atrophy (1.6%), and adenocarcinoma (1.35%).[80] However, hysteroscopy is not a first-line diagnostic procedure for most patients. It is reasonable to perform endometrial sampling on all women with DUB over the age of 35, any patient with metrorrhagia, any patient with postmenopausal bleeding (PMB), whether or not she is receiving hormone-replacement therapy, and any patient in whom medical therapy fails and who has persistent or recurrent DUB. Hormonal treatment can be safely initiated if the biopsy results are negative and there are no contraindications. Other indications for diagnostic hysteroscopy include to evaluate an abnormal hysterogram, to search for intrauterine adhesions, or to locate an occult IUD.[81] Adenomatous hyperplasia and small endometrial polyps may be difficult to distinguish from lush polypoid secretory endometrium[82]; therefore, it is recommended that endometrial sampling be performed regardless of the hysteroscopic findings.

In the menopausal patient, bleeding while on hormone-replacement therapy is a primary reason for discontinuing treatment. A reasonable and cost-effective approach to patients with postmenopausal bleeding who are on hormone-replacement therapy is to perform an endometrial biopsy initially. If biopsy results are normal, showing proliferative or atrophic endometrium, the treatment options include cyclic medroxyprogesterone, altering the dose or sequence of hormone replacement, or no therapy. Recurrent or persistent PMB warrants hysteroscopic evaluation and directed sampling. In both perimenopausal and postmenopausal patients with DUB, abnormal pathology may be seen in as many as 48% of patients.[83]

Operative hysteroscopy is performed for abnormal uterine bleeding to remove endocervical polyps, submucous myomata, or to resect or ablate the endometrium. Endometrial ablation or resection is becoming more commonly used to treat abnormal bleeding, in lieu of hysterectomy. It is particularly suited to patients who are not candidates for hysterectomy or who desire a minimally invasive, conservative procedure. Hysteroscopy is generally contraindicated for patients with upper-genital-tract infection, submucous myomata >10 cm, endometrial hyperplasia, or adenocarcinoma. According to Neuwirth,[84] indications for hysteroscopic myomectomy in symptomatic patients are to preserve fertility, to resect submucous myomata measuring ≤4-by-4 cm (absent submucous myomata on the opposing surface of the uterine cavity), and for abnormal uterine bleeding caused by submucous myomata in a patient who does not wish an abdominal operation. As compared with endometrial ablation, success appears to be higher for endometrial resection in controlling DUB. Amenorrhea after endometrial ablation is approximately 50%.[85,86]

Diagnostic and operative hysteroscopy requires a distention medium to provide visualization of the expanded uterine cavity. The cervix is placed under traction and the endocervix is dilated gently. An appropriate distention fluid is run into the uterine cavity. Diagnostic hysteroscopy can be easily performed by instilling lactated Ringer's or saline through intravenous tubing through the inlet port of the hysteroscope. Operative procedures require the fluid to be injected under pressure; however, the pressure should not exceed the mean arterial blood pressure of the patient. Potential complications of hysteroscopy include fluid overload, cervical laceration, and uterine perforation. Too much fluid instilled intravenously through open vascular channels in the uterus can cause noncardiogenic pulmonary edema or cerebral edema. To avoid the complication of fluid overload, the amount of distention medium instilled should be compared carefully to the amount of fluid retrieved.

Should the surgeon note that the fluid balance is negative by greater than 500 cc, he or she should consider finishing the surgery as soon as possible. A negative fluid balance of greater than 800 cc should alert the surgeon to stop the procedure or finish the endometrial procedure at another time.

Endometrial surgeries are becoming more commonly used in patients who do not desire further childbearing. In many, when medical therapy has not produced optimal results, diagnostic hysteroscopy with endometrial ablation or resection is a good alternative. The indications for endometrial surgery are evolving. Currently, candidates include patients with persistent postmenopausal bleeding, menorrhagia or metrorrhagia not responsive to medical therapy, endometrial polyps, and submucosal leiomyomata. Patients with obesity or disease who are poor candidates for hysterectomy may be appropriate candidates for endometrial surgery. Prior to endometrial surgery, work-up to exclude endometrial hyperplasia and adenocarcinoma is mandatory.

The indications for hysteroscopic endometrial surgery include DUB unresponsive to other treatments and, in some patients, postmenopausal bleeding. Patients who desire endometrial resection or ablation should have completed childbearing. Pregnancy has been reported following ablation[87] but so far not following endometrial resection. Patients with dysmenorrhea, pelvic pain, and premenstrual syndrome may show short-term improvement from endometrial surgery, but these are not primary indications for ablation or resection.[88]

Historically, various methods to destroy the endometrium and thus produce endometrial scarring (Asherman syndrome) have been attempted. Agents used have included methyl-cyanoacrylate, paraformaldehyde, quinacrine, liquid nitrogen, super-heated steam, and intracavitary radium.[89] Currently, electrosurgery and neodymium:yttrium–aluminum–garnet laser are used most commonly for ablation and resection. Newer techniques such as the ThermaChoice Balloon System may prove effective in performing endometrial ablation in an office setting. Amenorrhea is the desired effect in performing endometrial resection or ablation. Patients should be counseled that some will have recurrent bleeding in the form of spotting, light flow, or perhaps a recurrence of heavy flow. Regrowth and bleeding occur unless the stratum basalis of the endometrium is destroyed. Hormonal

TABLE 47-6
HYSTEROSCOPIC DISTENTION MEDIA

Diagnostic
  Carbon dioxide
  Saline
  Lactated Ringer's
  Hyskon
Operative
  Glycine, 1.5–2.2%
  Sorbitol, 5%
  Mannitol, 5%

TABLE 47-7
INDICATIONS FOR ENDOMETRIAL BIOPSY

DUB, age >35
Metrorrhagia
Postmenopausal bleeding
Failed medical therapy

therapy, repeat endometrial surgery, or hysterectomy may be indicated.

Preoperatively, it may be beneficial to thin the endometrium with progestins or GnRH agonists, particularly to facilitate endometrial destruction. Laminaria can be placed the day prior to endometrial surgery in patients who have cervical stenosis. Postoperatively, the patient should be counseled that she might have a discharge for several weeks. Following ablation, spontaneous menses may be seen 4 to 6 weeks postprocedure.

Distention mediums include carbon dioxide, saline, lactacted Ringer's solution, and Hyskon for diagnostic procedures and glycine 1.5 to 2.2 %, sorbitol 5%, and mannitol 5% for operative procedures (Table 47-6). Saline and Ringer's solution contain electrolytes and are not indicated in electrosurgical procedures. Glycine is an electrolyte-free, nonhemolytic solution ideal for electrosurgical and laser procedures. It is metabolized to serine and glyoxalic acid. Fluid overload with glycine can cause hyponatremia, hypokalemia, pulmonary edema, and encephalopathy. In patients undergoing urologic procedures, encephalopathy with hyperammonemia has been reported. Nausea or vertigo may develop and if not treated may cause death.[90] Sorbitol is metabolized to carbon dioxide and water and may cause hyperglycemia. Hyskon is a viscous electrolyte-free solution of 32% dextran. It can be used for diagnostic and operative procedures, but it is known to damage equipment if not completely cleaned after use and, due to the high viscosity, requires high pressure to flow. Dilutional hyponatremia, pulmonary edema, anaphylaxis, acute respiratory distress syndome, and disseminated intravascular coagulopathy have been reported with the use of Hyskon.

Endometrial surgery, either endometrial resection or ablation, is indicated in patients with menorrhagia,

metrorrhagia, endometrial polyps, submucous leiomyomata, or bleeding not responding to medical therapy if they desire to preserve the uterus, or are a poor surgical risk for hysterectomy (Table 47-7). In the past, when patients with DUB did not respond to medical therapy, they often underwent dilation and curettage (sometimes on multiple occasions) or hysterectomy. Currently, if one or more courses of medical treatment fails, hysteroscopy and endometrial sampling should be considered. Prior to surgery, work-up with ultrasound or sonohysterography may reveal endometrial pathology such as endometrial polyps or submucous leiomyomata. Operative hysteroscopy can then be performed for these patients (Table 47-8).

In unusual cases, the surgeon may uncover atypical endometrial hyperplasia or adenocarcinoma not previously detected with endometrial sampling. Other possible pitfalls include creation of a false passage with dilation, uterine perforation, and excess fluid absorption.

Although operative hysteroscopy is very effective, this treatment will fail in a percentage of patients and repeat hysteroscopy or hysterectomy will be required. Unger and Meeks,[91] in a small sample of 42 patients, reported a 34% hysterectomy rate within 5 years of

TABLE 47-8
INDICATIONS FOR HYSTEROSCOPY

DUB not responding to medical therapy
Postmenopausal bleeding
Multiple D&Cs
Acute anemia with heavy menstrual flow
Insufficient tissue on prior endometrial biopsy
Inability to perform endometrial biopsy
Thickened endometrial stripe
  >15 mm in the follicular phase
  >4 mm in postmenopausal bleeding
Ultrasound reveals intracavitary lesion
Abnormal hysterogram
Uterine synechiae
Occult IUD

endometrial ablation. Others report lower failure rates with endometrial resection and those in whom it fails usually have myoma or deep adenomyosis.[92] Reasons to repeat hysteroscopy or perform hysterectomy include pelvic pain, fibroids, persistent bleeding, and endomyometritis.

Hysterectomy

By age 60, more than one-third of American women will have had a hysterectomy.[93] It is estimated that more than 85% of hysterectomies are elective in the sense that there is almost always at least one other reasonable alternative to the procedure.[94] Hysterectomy is reserved for patients in whom no treatment has proved effective or in whom there is evidence of malignancy, adenomyosis, leiomyomata, endometrial hyperplasia, severe adhesive disease, infection, or endometriosis. The decision to remove the uterus should be one decided by the patient after she understands all of the options available.

Complications of hysterectomy vary depending on the type of hysterectomy performed. The Collaborative Review of Sterilization (CREST) is thus far the most reliable study regarding complications of hysterectomy.[95] Harris[96] provides an excellent review of the complications of hysterectomy. Postoperative fever occurs in 32.3% after abdominal hysterectomy (AH) and 15.3% after vaginal hysterectomy (VH). As many as 50% of these postoperative fevers may have no identifiable source.[97] Patients treated with laparoscopic hysterectomy (LH) have a lower incidence of unexplained fever, perhaps due to early discharge and early ambulation. Pelvic infection is seen in 9% after AH, 3.9% after VH, and 1.4% after LH. Urinary-tract infections and pneumonia are the most common nonoperative-site infections. With shorter times for indwelling urinary catheters, the incidence should be less than 1 to 2% after hysterectomy. The risk of pneumonia is higher in patients with a history of alcoholism, underlying pulmonary disease, and in the elderly. Intraoperative hemorrhage is reported in 0.2% for AH and 0.7% for VH. Transfusion rates are lower than in the past because of more conservative use of blood products. Transfusions and postoperative hemorrhage rates should be less than 1 to 2% for all forms of hysterectomy. Injuries occurring from surgery can include bladder, bowel, and ureters and should be discussed as part of the consent process.

Prophylaxis against thromboembolic disease is current practice for patients undergoing hysterectomy. Compression stockings, intermittent compression devices, or low-dose heparin may be employed, particularly in patients with high risk. Patients at high risk for thromboembolism include those with malignancy, history of deep-vein thrombosis, lower-extremity edema, large varicose veins, obesity, prior radiation therapy, prolonged operative times, intraoperative hypotension, or increased blood loss.

Wound dehiscence occurs most often in patients who are obese, in those who suffer from diabetes, and in the elderly. Delayed recognition of bowel perforation may occur and may not be seen during hospitalization. Prolonged ileus may also occur, resulting in longer hospital treatment. Damage to the pelvic floor's complex neurovascular system may cause postoperative dysfunction of the urinary system[98] (incontinence, retention, frequency, and dysuria) and intestinal tract (constipation, decreased rectal sensation, increased rectal volume, and decreased sigmoid motility).[99] Although some patients may report decreased vaginal lubrication, sensation, orgasm, and libido after hysterectomy, in patients studied prior to and following elective hysterectomy, there is no increased incidence of psychosexual dysfunction[100] except that related to decreased estrogen associated with oophorectomy. Detailed preoperative questioning and counseling are imperative for elective hysterectomy. When necessary, psychometric testing should be considered.

REFERENCES

1. Landgren BM, Unden A, Diczfalusy E. Hormonal profile of the cycle in 68 normally menstruating women. Acta Endocrinol 1980;94:89.
2. Johannison E, Landgren BM, Rohr HP, et al. Endometrial morphology and peripheral hormone levels in women with regular menstrual cycles. Fertil Steril 1987; 48:401.
3. Treloar AE, Boynton RE, Behn BG, Brown BV. Variations of the human menstrual cycle through reproductive life. Int J Fertil 1970;12:77.
4. Hallberg L, Hogdahl A, Nilsson L, Rybo G. Menstrual blood loss—a population study. Acta Obstet Gynecol Scand 1966;45:320.
5. Fraser IS, McCarron G, Markham R. A preliminary study of factors influencing perception of menstrual blood loss volume. Am J Obstet Gynecol 1984;149:788.
6. Lenton EA, Langren B, Sexton L. Normal variation in the length of the luteal phase of the menstrual cycle:

identification of the short luteal phase. Br J Obstet Gynaecol 1984;91:685.

7. Speroff L, Glass RH, Kase NG, eds. Clinical Gynecologic Endocrinology and Infertility. 5th ed. Baltimore: Williams & Wilkins, 1994.

8. Noyes RW, Hertig AW, Rock J. Dating the endometrial biopsy. Fertil Steril 1950;1:3.

9. Downing I, Hutchon DJ, Poyser NL. Uptake of (3H)-arachidonic acid by human endometrium: differences between normal and menorrhagic tissue. Prostaglandins 1983;26:55.

10. Cameron IT, Kelley RW, Baird DT. Prostaglandins in the human uterus: an interaction between endometrium and myometrium. Prostaglandins Leukotrienes Med 1985; 17:329.

11. Vermesh M, Kletzky OA, Davajan V, Israel R. Monitoring techniques to predict and detect ovulation. Fertil Steril 1987;47:259.

12. Bates GW, Garza DE, Garza MM. Clinical manifestations of hormonal changes in the menstrual cycle. Obstet Gynecol Clin North Am 1990;17;299.

13. DeVore GR, Owens O, Kase N. Use of intravenous Premarin in the treatment of dysfunctional uterine bleeding: a double-blind, randomized control study. Obstet Gynecol 1982;59:285.

14. Pokras R, Hunagel V. Hysterectomy in the United States, 1965-1984. Am J Public Health 1988;78:852.

15. Lenton EA, Landgren B-M, Sexton L, et al. Normal variation in the length of the follicular phase of the menstrual cycle: effect of chronological age. Br J Obstet Gynaecol 1984;91:681.

16. Lenton EA, Landgren B-M, Sexton L. Normal variation in the length of the luteal phase of the menstrual cycle: identification of the short luteal phase. Br J Obstet Gynaecol 1984;91:685.

17. Jutras ML, Cowan BD. Abnormal bleeding in the climacteric. Obstet Gynecol Clinics North Am 1990;17:409.

18. Hammond CB. Menopause and hormone replacement therapy: An overview. Obstet Gynecol Feb 1996: 87(Suppl 2);2S.

19. DeJong AR, Weiss JC, Brent RL. Condyloma acuminata in children. Am J Dis Child 1982;136:704.

20. Muram D, Elias S. Child sexual abuse—genital findings in prepubertal girls. II. Comparison of colposcopic and unaided examination. Am J Obstet Gynecol 1989;160:333.

21. Huffman JW, Dewhurst CJ, Capraro VJ. The gynecology of childhood and adolescence. 2nd ed. Philadelphia: Saunders, 1981.

22. Anikwue C, Danwood MY, Kramer E. Granulosa and theca cell tumors. Obstet Gynecol 1978;51:214.

23. VenEijkeren MA Christiaens GCML, Sixm JJ, Haspels AA. Menorrhagia: a review. Obstet Gynecol Surv 1989; 4406:421.

24. Buttram VC Jr, Reiter RC. Uterine leiomyomata: etiology, symptomatology, and management. Fertil Steril 1981;36:433.

25. West CP, Lumsden MA. Fibroids and menorrhagia. Ballieres Clin Obstet Gynaecol 1989;3:357.

26. Weiner Z, Beck D, Rottem S, et al. Uterine artery flow velocity wave forms and color flow imaging in women with perimenopausal bleeding and postmenopausal bleeding: correlation to endometrial histopathology. Acta Obstet Gynecol Scand 1993;72:162.

27. Candiani GB, Fedele L, Parazzini F, Villa L. Risk of recurrence after myomectomy. Br J Obstet Gynaecol 1991;98:385.

28. McCausland AM. Hysteroscopic myometrial biopsy: its use in diagnosing adenomyosis and its clinical application. Am J Obstet Gynecol 1992;166:1619.

29. Ascher SM, Arnold LL, Patt RH. Adenomyosis: prospective comparison of MR imaging and transvaginal sonography. Radiology 1994;190:803.

30. Novak ER, Woodruff BS Adenomyosis uteri. In: Novak ER, Woodruff BS, eds. Novak's gynecologic and obstetric pathology. Philadelphia: Saunders, 1979:443.

31. McCausland AM, McCausland VM. Depth of endometrial penetration in adenomyosis helps determine outcome of rollerball ablation. Am J Obstet Gynecol 1996; 174:1786.

32. Claessens EA, Cowell CA. Acute adolescent menorrhagia. Am J Obstet Gynecol 1981;139:277.

33. Smith CA. The effect of wartime starvation in Holland upon pregnancy and its product. Am J Obstet Gynecol 1947;53:599.

34. Cooper GS, Sandler DP, Whelan EA, Smith KR. Association of physical and behavioral characteristics with menstrual cycle patterns in women age 29-31 years. Epidemiology 1996;7:624.

35. Green P, Rubin L. Amenorrhea as a manifestation of chronic liver disease. Am J Obstet Gynecol 1959;78:141.

36. Valimaki M, Pelkonen R, Salaspuro M, et al. Sex hormones in amenorrheic women with alcoholic liver disease. J Clin Endocrinol Metab 1984;59.

37. Shaaban MM, Ghaneimag SA, Hammad WA, et al. Sex steroids in women with liver cirrhosis. Int J Gynaecol Obstet 1980;18:181.

38. Mass K, Quint EH, Punch MR, Merion RM. Gynecological and reproductive function after liver transplantation. Transplantation 1996;62:476.

39. Holley JL, Schmidt RJ, Bender FH, Dumler F, Schiff M. Gynecologic and reproductive issues in women on dialysis. Am J Kidney Dis 1997;29:685.

40. Alper MM, Garner PR. Premature ovarian failure: its relationship to autoimmune disease. Obstet Gynecol 1985;66:27.

41. Mantouvalos H, Metallinos C, Makrygiannakis A, et al. Sex hormones in women on hemodialysis. Int J Gynaecol Obstet 1984;22:367.

42. DeKretser DM, Atkins RC, Paulsen CA. Role of the kidney in the metabolism of luteinizing hormone. J Endocrinol 1973;58:425.

43. Lim VS, Kathpalia SC, Frohman LA. Hyperprolactinemia and impaired pituitary response to suppression and stimulation in chronic renal failure: reversal after transplantation. J Clin Endocrinol Metab 1979;48:101.

44. Razzaq R, O'Halloran DJ, Beardwell CG, Shalet SM. The effects of CV205-502 in patients with hyperprolactinemia intolerant and/or resistant to bromocriptine. Horm Res 1993;39:218.

45. Yen SSC. Chronic anovulation caused by peripheral en-

docrine disorder. In: Yen SSC, Jaffe RB, eds. Reproductive endocrinology. 2nd ed. Philadelphia: Saunders, 1986: 482.

46. Wilansky DL, Greisman B. Early hypothyroidism in patients with menorrhagia. Am J Obstet Gynecol 1989; 160:673.

47. Djursing H. Hypothalamic-pituitary-gonadal function in insulin treated diabetic women with and without amenorrhea. Dan Med Bull 1987;34:139.

48. Steinkampf MP. Systemic illness and menstrual dysfunction. Obstet Gynecol Clin North Am 1990;17:316.

49. Turkington RW, Lebovitz HE. Extra-adrenal endocrine deficiencies in Addison's disease. Am J Med 1967;43:449.

50. Boccuzzi G, Angeli A, Bisbocci D, et al. Effect of synthetic luteinizing hormone releasing hormone (LH-RH) on the release of gonadotropins in Cushing's disease. J Clin Endocrinol Metab 1975;40:892.

51. Long CA, Gast MJ. Menorrhagia. Obstet Gynecol Clin North Am 1990;17:343.

52. De Sanctis V, Vullo C, Katz M, et al. Hypothalamic-pituitary-gonadal axis in thalassemic patients with secondary amenorrhea. Obstet Gynecol 1988;72:643.

53. Huang TS, Wang YH, Lai JS, Chang CC, Lien IN. The hypothalamus-pituitary-ovary and hypothalamus-pituitary-thyroid axes in spinal cord-injured women. Metabolism 1996;45:718.

54. Short RV. Lactational infertility in family planning. Ann Med 1993;25:175.

55. Cromer BA, Smith RD, Blair JM, Dwyer J, Brown R. A prospective study of adolescents who choose among levonorgestrel implant (Norplant), medroxyprogesterone acetate (Depo-Provera), or the combined oral contraceptive pill as contraception. Pediatrics 1994;94:687.

56. Bayer SR, DeCherney AH. Clinical manifestations and treatment of dysfunctional uterine bleeding. JAMA 1993;269:1823.

57. Hall DR, Yoder IC. Ultrasound evaluation of the uterus. In: Callen PW, ed. Ultrasonography in obstetrics and gynecology. 3rd ed. Philadelphia: Saunders, 1994:586.

58. Fleischer AC, Gordon AN, Entman SS, et al. Transvaginal sonography (TVS) of the endometrium: current and potential applications. Crit Rev Diagn Imag 1990; 30:85.

59. Lerner JP, Timor-Tritsch IE, Monteagudo A. Use of transvaginal sonography in the evaluation of endometrial hyperplasia and carcinoma. Obstet Gynecol Surv 1996; 51:718.

60. Chan WY. Prostaglandins and nonsteroidal anti-inflammatory drugs in dysmenorrhea. Ann Rev Pharmacol Toxicol 1983;23:131.

61. Smith JB. The prostanoids in hemostasis and thrombosis. Am J Pathol 1980;99:743.

62. Bergkvist A, Rybo G. Treatment of menorrhagia with intrauterine release of progesterone. Br J Obstet Gynecol 1983;90:255.

63. Andersson JK, Rybo G. Levonorgestrel-releasing intrauterine device in the treatment of menorrhagia. Br J Obstet Gynaecol 1990;97:690.

64. Nilsson L, Rybo G. Treatment of menorrhagia. Am J Obstet Gynecol 1991;110:713.

65. Siegler AM. Hysteroscopy. In: Osofsky HJ, ed. Advances in clinical obstetrics and gynecology. Vol. 2. Baltimore: Williams & Wilkins, 1984:158.

66. Stock RJ, Kanbour A. Prehysterectomy curettage. Obstet Gynecol 1975;45:537.

67. Haynes PJ, Hodgson H, Anderson ABX, Turnbull AC. Measurement of menstrual blood loss in patients complaining of menorrhagia. Br J Obstet Gynecol 1977; 84:763.

68. Grimes DA. Diagnostic dilation and curettage: a reappraisal. Am J Obstet Gynecol 1982;142:1.

69. Lutz MH, Underwood PB Jr, Kreutner A, Mitchell KS. Vacuum aspiration: an efficient outpatient screening technique for endometrial disease. South Med J 1977; 70:393.

70. Stovall TG, Ling FW, Morgan PL. A prospective, randomized comparison of the Pipelle endometrial sampling device with the Novak curette. Am J Obstet Gynecol 1991;165:1287.

71. Stovall TG, Photopulos GJ, Poston WM, Ling FW, Sandles LG. Pipelle endometrial sampling in patients with known endometrial carcinoma. Obstet Gynecol 1991; 77:954.

72. Check JH, Chase JS, Nowroozi K, Wu CH, Chern R. Clinical evaluation of the pipelle endometrial suction curette for timed endometrial biopsies. J Reprod Med 1989;34:218.

73. Nasri MN, Shepherd JH, Setchell ME, Lowe DG, Chard T. The role of the vaginal scan in measurement of endometrial thickness in postmenopausal women. Br J Obstet Gynecol 1991;98:470.

74. Goldstein S, Nachtigall M, Snyder J, Nachtigall L. Endometrial assessment by vaginal ultrasonography before endometrial sampling in patients with postmenopausal bleeding. Am J Obstet Gynecol 1990; 163:119.

75. Goldchmit R, Katz Z, Blickstien I, Caspi B, Dgani R. The accuracy of endometrial pipelle sampler with and without sonographic measurements of endometrial thickness. Obstet Gynecol 1993;82:727.

76. Barbot J. Hysteroscopy for abnormal bleeding. In: Baggish MS, Barbot J, Valle RF, eds. Diagnostic and therapeutic hysteroscopy: a text and atlas. St. Louis: Mosby Year Book, 1989:147.

77. Nagele F, O'Connor H, Davies A, Badawy A, Mohamed H, Magos A. 2500 outpatient diagnostic hysteroscopies. Obstet Gynecol 1996:88;87.

78. Brooks PG, Serden SP. Hysteroscopic findings after unsuccessful dilation and curettage for abnormal uterine bleeding. Am J Obstet Gynecol 1988:158;1354.

79. Gimpleson RJ. Office hysteroscopy. Clin Obstet Gynecol. 1992;35:270.

80. Motashaw ND, Dave S. Diagnostic and therapeutic hysteroscopy in the management of abnormal uterine bleeding. J Reprod Med 1990:35;616.

81. Siegler AM. Office hysteroscopy. Obstet Gynecol Clin North Am 1995;22:457.

82. Valle RF. Hysteroscopic evaluation of patients with abnormal uterine bleeding. Surg Gynecol Obstet 1981; 153:521.

83. Downes E, Al-Azzawi F. The predictive value of outpatient hysteroscopy in a menopause clinic. Br J Obstet Gynaecol 1993:100;1148.

84. Neuwirth RS. Hysteroscopic submucous myomectomy. Obstet Gynecol Clin North Am 1995;22:541.

85. Townsend E, Richart RM, Paskowitz RAN, et al. "Rollerball" coagulation of the endometrium. Am J Obstet Gynecol 1990;76:310.

86. DeCherney AH, Diamond MP, Lavy G, Polan ML. Endometrial ablation for intractable uterine bleeding: hysteroscopic resection. Obstet Gynecol 1987;70:668.

87. Goldberg, JM. Intrauterine pregnancy following endometrial ablation. Obstet Gynecol 1994;83:836.

88 O'Connor H, Magos, A. Endometrial resection for the treatment of menorrhagia. N Engl J Med 1996;335:151.

89. Ke RW. Endometrial ablation: an alternative to hysterectomy. Clin Obstet and Gynecol 1997;40:914.

90. Hoakstra PT, Kahnoski R, McCamish MA, et al. Transurethral resection syndrome—a new perspective: encephalopathy with associated hyperammonemia. J Urol 1983;130:704.

91. Unger JB, Meeks GR. Hysterectomy after endometrial ablation. Am J Obstet Gynecol 1996;175:1432.

92. Salat-Baroux J, Hamou J, Antoine JM. Hysteroscopic resection of the endometrium: an alternative to hysterectomy? Bull Acad Natl Med 1996;180:2139.

93. Carlson KJ, Miller BA, Fowler FJ. The Maine women's health study. 1. Outcomes of nonsurgical management of leiomyomas, abnormal bleeding, and chronic pelvic pain. Obstet Gynecol 1994;83:556.

94. Gambone JC, Reiter RC. Hysterectomy: improving the patient's decision-making process. Clin Obstet Gynecol 1997;40:868.

95. Dicker RC, Greenspan JR, Strauss LT, et al. Complications of abdominal and vaginal hysterectomy among women of reproductive age in the United States: the collaborative review of sterilization. Am J Obstet Gynecol 1982;144:841.

96. Harris WJ. Complications of hysterectomy. Clin Obstet Gynecol 1997;40:928.

97. Hemsell DL, Reisch J, Nobles B, et al. Prevention of major infection after elective abdominal hysterectomy: Individual determination required. Am J Obstet Gynecol 1983;147:520.

98. Hanley HG. The late urological complications of total hysterectomy. Br J Urol 1969;41:682.

99. Varma JS. Autonomic influences on colorectal motility and pelvic surgery. World J Surg 1992;16:811.

100. Bachmann GA. Psychosexual aspects of hysterectomy. Women's Health Issues 1990;1:41.

Chapter 48
Hyperprolactinemia

Debra A. Minjarez
Khaled Zeitoun
William H. Kutteh

Five Key Points

- Hyperprolactinemia frequently presents with disruption of the menstrual cycle and/or galactorrhea due to disruption of gonadotropin-releasing hormone secretion.
- Evaluation should include prolactin, thyroid-stimulating hormone, and pituitary imaging with computed tomography or magnetic resonance imaging.
- Dopamine agonist is the treatment of choice for both microadenomas and macroadenomas of the pituitary.
- Cabergoline, a recently approved dopamine agonist, has a better efficacy and side-effect profile than bromocriptine.
- Hypoestrogenism associated with hyperprolactinemia is a potential cause of osteopenia in premenopausal women.

Hyperprolactinemia is a common endocrine disorder encountered in young women of reproductive age. The clinical presentation is often manifested by menstrual irregularities, secondary amenorrhea, galactorrhea, infertility, and decreased libido.[1] The purpose of this chapter is to review the pathophysiologic causes, diagnosis, and treatment of hyperprolactinemia. The ultimate goal for physicians is to restore normal menstrual function for patients desiring fertility, symptomatic control of galactorrhea, and prevention of the severe consequences associated with hypoestrogenism.

PROLACTIN

Hyperprolactinemia is the most common endocrine disorder of the hypothalamic–pituitary axis. Hyperprolactinemia is diagnosed by an elevated plasma prolactin >20 ng/ml. A single gene on chromosome 6 encodes this 197 to 199 amino acid protein.[2] A transcription factor, Pit-1, is important for the transcription of prolactin as well as pituitary differentiation. There are at least five known isoforms of prolactin. The predominant form is a nonglycosylated monomer form (little prolactin) of 23 kD, which has the most bioactivity.[3] Dimeric and polymeric forms (45 to 160 kD) also exist but their significance is unclear.[3]

Prolactin is secreted by the lactotroph cells of the anterior pituitary in a pulsatile fashion of 13 to 14 peaks per day at 90-minute intervals.[4] Peak levels occur between 3 A.M. and 5 A.M., with a modest increase in the afternoon. Prolactin is also produced in decidualized endometrium, myometrium, and leiomyomata.[5] The mechanism regulating secretion of prolactin in these tissues is under a different mechanism than the lactotroph cells of the pituitary and beyond the scope of this chapter.

Secretion of prolactin by the pituitary is predominantly regulated by inhibitory control via dopamine produced in the arcuate and ventromedial nuclei of the hypothalamus. Dopamine binds to D2 receptors on lactotroph cells, inhibiting adenylate cyclase and thus inhibiting synthesis and release of prolactin.[6] In hyperprolactinemia, dopamine is increased within the central nervous system; however, for reasons poorly understood, it is unable to inhibit prolactin secretion. These high levels of dopamine eventually inhibit gonadotropin-releasing hormone (GnRH) pulsatility either directly or through increased endorphins, resulting in menstrual dysfunction.[7]

γ-Aminobutyric acid (GABA) and cholinergic pathways also inhibit prolactin release while estrogen, thyrotropin-releasing hormone (TRH), serotonin, and endogenous opiates stimulate prolactin secretion.[8] The physiologic significance of these other inhibitory and stimulatory factors is unknown.

Prolactin action is mediated via the prolactin receptor in multiple tissues including the breast, liver, kidney, gonads, and brain. The prolactin receptor belongs to the superfamily of cytokine/growth hormone/prolactin receptors. Members of this family are associated with cytoplasmic tyrosine kinases of the Jak family (Janus kinases).[9] Signaling activation occurs as a result of the dimerization of the receptor on binding to prolactin. Phosphorylation and/or dephosphorylation by Jak will then affect the activity of intracellular and plasma membrane proteins.

The main function of prolactin is the initiation and maintenance of lactation.[10] Prolactin, in conjunction with estrogen and insulin-like growth factor 1, causes proliferation of the breast ducts and stroma in preparation for lactation. During pregnancy, the high circulatory levels of estradiol inhibit lactation. After delivery, the immediate decrease in estrogen allows prolactin to initiate lactation. Prolactin levels then remain elevated above basal levels. These levels increase to a maximum within 10 to 30 minutes after nursing begins and decline within 30 to 120 minutes.[11]

CAUSES OF HYPERPROLACTINEMIA

Multiple physiologic, pharmacologic and pathologic entities are known to affect prolactin secretion (Table 48-1). TRH, psychotropic medications, stress, nipple stimulation, sleep, protein-rich diets (especially tryptophan-rich meals), and tumors are the most

---

**TABLE 48-1
CAUSES OF HYPERPROLACTINEMIA**

Physiologic
Stress
Diet
Nipple stimulation
Exercise
Intercourse
Hypoglycemia

Pharmacologic
Anesthetics
Dopamine-depleting
  Methyldopa
  Monoamine oxidose inhibitors (MOA)
  Reserpine
Receptor-blocking
  Estrogen
  Oral contraceptives
  Phenothiazines
Inhibition of dopamine release
  Opiates
Antihypertensives
  Verapamil
Antihistamines
  Cimetidine

Pathologic
Hypothalamic tumors
  Craniopharyngioma
  Germinoma
  Metastatic carcinoma
  Hamartoma
Infiltrative disease
  Sarcoid
  Histiocytosis X
  Leukemia
  Infection
  Tuberculosis
  Encephalitis
Pituitary disease
  Prolactinoma
  Acromegaly
Cushing disease
  Pituitary-stalk compression
  Empty-sella syndrome
  Mixed tumors
Hypothyroidism (TRH)
Renal failure
Cirrhosis
Head trauma
Chest wall lesions/surgical incisions
Bronchogenic carcinoma (mostly small cell undifferentiated)

Other
Pregnancy

well known causes.[1] The most important causes to consider are adenomas and hypothyroidism.

Adenomas are derived from three cell types—basophil, acidophil, and chromophobe. The basophil is a rare tumor associated with the secretion of adrenocorticotropic hormone (ACTH). Acidophilic adenomas secrete growth hormone and/or prolactin. Chromophobe adenomas account for the majority of pituitary adenomas and sometimes secrete prolactin, growth hormone, and/or ACTH.[12]

Asymptomatic pituitary adenomas have been demonstrated in about 10% of the normal adult population, and occult adenomas are estimated to occur in up to 27% of the general population at autopsy.[13] They can vary in size and occasionally encroach on the walls of the sella turcica. Tumors <10 mm are classified as microadenomas and those >10 mm as macroadenomas.

Other mixed-cell tumors may increase prolactin secretion.[14] If a tumor is >10 mm, with a prolactin level less than 200 ng/ml, the standard evaluation should include growth hormone, ACTH, and urinary free cortisol. These other tumors increase prolactin secretion by pituitary stalk compression or interference with dopamine transport from the hypothalamus to the anterior pituitary. This is important to recognize, as treatment will usually reduce prolactin levels but shrinkage of the tumor will not occur and patients will continue to report persistent or worsening central nervous system (CNS) symptoms.

There are other CNS lesions in addition to adenomas that cause increased prolactin secretion. Craniopharyngiomas, sarcoidosis, metastatic tumors, and Hodgkin tumor infiltration may also eliminate dopaminergic inhibition of prolactin secretion.[15] The prolactin levels with these tumors are usually less than 100 ng/ml.

Empty-sella syndrome can also mimic a pituitary tumor. It is caused by a congenital weakness in the sella diaphragm that enables cerebrospinal fluid to extend into the pituitary fossa. The increased pressure can interrupt normal portal blood flow, lowering the concentration of dopamine in the anterior pituitary.[16]

TRH plays an important role in controlling prolactin secretion. Increased TRH stimulates prolactin release and may affect dopamine action. Patients with primary hypothyroidism can present with galactorrhea and menstrual irregularities.[17] In addition to an elevated prolactin level, radiologic studies may reveal an enlarged pituitary secondary to a hyperplastic response to TRH. Treatment of hypothyroidism will result in complete resolution of symptoms and normalization of prolactin levels.

An increasingly common cause for hyperprolactinemia is pharmacologic. Many prescription and over-the-counter medications interfere with the synthesis, metabolism, reuptake, or receptor binding of dopamine.[18] The most frequently encountered medications are the neuroleptics, such as phenothiazine, thioxanthines, and butyrophenones. Other drugs include antihistamines, antidepressants, antihypertensives, and antiemetics. One study revealed that prolactin levels increase immediately after the initiation of haloperidol and plateau between 30 and 50 ng/ml.[19] Other studies have demonstrated that with long-term therapy, 30% of patients who initially had an elevated prolactin, will have levels return to baseline.[20] Some clinicians advise discontinuation of potentially causative medications followed by a repeat measurement of the prolactin level. However, in some cases it is not possible to discontinue medications, such as antipsychotics, because of the risk to patients. Alternative medications may be an option; however, these are also often associated with hyperprolactinemia. Limited studies have investigated the use of bromocriptine in patients treated with psychiatric medication who were followed closely. Understandably there is concern for worsening psychiatric symptoms, as bromocriptine may interfere with the pharmacologic mechanisms of certain medications. Ultimately, the clinician must decide which course of action to follow in these difficult cases.

Any disease state that alters the metabolism of prolactin or metabolic clearance, such as cirrhosis of the liver and renal failure, are associated with elevated prolactin levels. Other conditions such as chest-wall lesions, surgical incisions, trauma, herpes zoster, and spinal-cord disease are also known to increase prolactin levels. The mechanism is poorly understood but thought to be secondary to activation of the afferent loop involved in the initiation of lactation.

In the past, transient hyperprolactinemia was thought to be the cause of infertility by disrupting normal luteal function.[21] These patients would present with high normal prolactin levels, which would increase during the menstrual cycle. Therapy was thought to improve pregnancy rates; however, controlled studies have demonstrated no benefit.

CLINICAL PRESENTATION

Hyperprolactinemia classically presents with galactorrhea and/or menstrual cycle disturbances. Galactorrhea is characterized by the presence of a clear or white nipple discharge that occurs spontaneously or after nipple stimulation and is not associated with the peripartum period.[22]

In general, as prolactin levels increase, luteal dysfunction will occur first, followed by oligomenorrhea and finally amenorrhea. The higher the prolactin level, the more severe the symptoms. Hyperprolactinemia is found in 30% of women with amenorrhea, 60% of women with galactorrhea, and 75% with both amenorrhea and galactorrhea.[23] The clinical manifestation of symptoms in women allows for earlier diagnosis and intervention.

Regardless of the pathologic cause for hyperprolactinemia, hypogonadotropic hypogonadism will eventually develop in most patients. Patients will present not only with amenorrhea and galactorrhea, but also with reports of hypoestrogenism, including vaginal dryness, pruritus, and rarely, hot flushes. The long-term consequences of hypoestrogenism and hyperprolactinemia are decreased bone density.[24] In women with hyperprolactinemia and amenorrhea, bone mineral content is decreased more than women with amenorrhea alone.[25] Furthermore, men with hyperprolactinemia also display lower bone density; thus it appears that prolactin may have a direct effect on bone.[26]

In men, hyperprolactinemia is often present for many years without symptoms being reported. Men will present with symptoms of decreased libido and/or erectile dysfunction related to complete or partial hypogonadism. Galactorrhea in men is not commonly encountered, however it has been reported to occur in 14 to 33% of cases.[27] At the time of evaluation, a higher proportion of men will be diagnosed with macroadenomas, which is thought to be due to the duration of the disease before presentation. However, the exact mechanism is unknown.

Both men and women will frequently present with headache and visual disturbances. The headaches are described as variable in intensity and nonspecific in character. The most common visual abnormality is bitemporal hemianopsia secondary to compression of the optic chiasm.[28] Other visual symptoms include decreased visual acuity, blurred vision and scotomata. If the tumor extends laterally into the cavernous sinus,

oculomotor function will be impaired due to impingement of cranial nerves III, IV, VI, and V. Large tumors extending into the temporal lobe may present with seizure activity.

EVALUATION

With careful history-taking, physical examination, and diagnostic work-up one can virtually exclude other causes of amenorrhea and/or galactorrhea. The history should focus on duration of amenorrhea or galactorrhea, exacerbation factors such as breast stimulation, and use of medications including both prescription and over-the-counter. Questions should be directed to elicit symptoms of headaches or visual disturbances.

On physical examination, practitioners should note the size and consistency of the thyroid, the presence of galactorrhea with microscopic evaluation for the presence of fat globules, and hypoestrogenic effects such as vaginal ruggation, color, and cervical mucus.

Laboratory evaluation should include a human chorionic gonadotropin (HCG) level to exclude pregnancy and TSH in addition to a prolactin level (Figure 48-1). If a prolactin is elevated and physiologic factors are suspected, a fasting prolactin level should be measured between 9 A.M. and 11 A.M. If TSH levels are increased, the patient is hypothyroid. Elevated TRH may stimulate prolactin secretion.

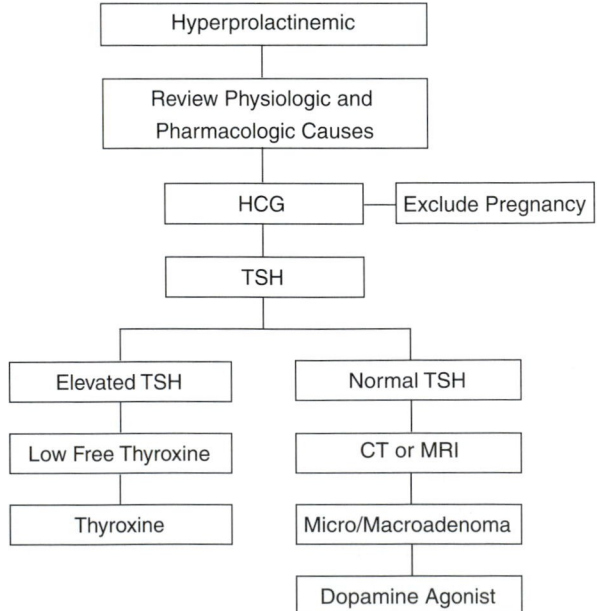

Figure 48-1 Evaluation of hyperprolactinemia.

Once TSH levels are normalized, reevaluate prolactin and determine if additional therapy with dopamine agonists is required. If results reveal a normal TSH with an elevated prolactin, patients should be referred for a CT or MRI.

An MRI yields higher contrast resolution and is safer than CT due to the lack of ionizing radiation to the ocular system. Although MRI is less helpful than CT in the evaluation of bone erosion, it is far better for the evaluation of any extrasellar expansion and involvement of the hypothalamus, blood vessels, sinuses and optic chiasm. MRI also allows for better resolution of microadenomas less than 1 cm, with a specificity of 90 to 100%; however, the sensitivity remains unknown.[29] One must keep in mind that despite the higher resolution in identifying microadenomas, MRI is more costly, and identification of such microadenomas will not affect treatment. Thus, in some cases, selective CT scans may be appropriate. Historically, lateral cone views were used to diagnose prolactinomas. Due to the variation in normal bony morphology and of inability to diagnose soft tumors, these x-ray examinations have now been replaced with MRI and CT.[30]

In approximately one-third of cases microadenomas are not visualized by CT or MRI. In one-third of these cases, idiopathic hyperprolactinemia will resolve spontaneously and 10-15% will eventually develop evidence of a microadenoma.[31] Thus, further diagnostic imaging for these patients may be tailored to the prolactin levels.

Assessment of visual fields yields little information when medical management is initiated unless surgical intervention is considered or patients have failed medical therapy.[32] It is recommended that visual-field testing be used in patients with symptoms of visual disturbances, if imaging studies confirm the presence of a macroadenoma, and/or if medical treatment is unsuccessful.

TREATMENT

There is general consensus that medical therapy is first choice in treating patients with prolactinomas.[33] There is also a role for observation in selected patients. Patients with significant extension of the tumor into either the third ventricle or the cavernous sinus require surgical intervention. The objectives of treatment are to reduce tumor size, correct visual or cranial-nerve abnormalities, restore normal menstrual function, alleviate galactorrhea, and/or treat the associated hypoestrogenism.

In 1971, the introduction of bromocriptine (Parlodel), a semisynthetic ergot alkaloid dopamine agonist, allowed for conservative management of hyperprolactinemia.[34] Numerous studies have shown that bromocriptine has a dramatic effect in reducing prolactin levels, shrinking the tumor and rapidly improving symptoms by binding to D2 receptors, inhibiting prolactin synthesis and secretion, and producing cellular necrosis. The response to bromocriptine is thus dependent on the number and affinity of tumor dopamine receptors.

Bromocriptine has been shown in multiple studies to be effective in restoring menses in 80% of patients and eliminating galactorrhea in 57 to 100%.[35] After a single dose, peak plasma levels are attained in 2 to 3 hours and remain detectable for 8 to 12 hours. The short half-life of bromocriptine, 3.5 hours, requires its administration twice daily.[36] The drug is metabolized in the liver and excreted in the feces. Due to hepatic metabolism, bromocriptine should be used only with extreme caution in patients with cirrhosis and ascites.

The usual starting dose is 2.5 mg/day, increasing by 2.5 mg weekly until prolactin normalizes. The majority of patients will respond to a regimen of 2.5 mg twice a day; however, a maximum dose of 10 mg/day can be used. Ten percent of patients are non-compliant with this regimen because of side effects.[37] The most common symptoms are nausea, dizziness, and orthostatic hypotension, which frequently occur at the initiation of treatment. To avoid these symptoms patients are encouraged to take their medication before bedtime with a small amount of food. In certain cases, it may be necessary to begin treatment with 1.25 mg (half a tablet) at bedtime and increasing the dose every 3 days over a 1- to 2-week period. Less common side effects are headache, nasal congestion, abdominal cramping, constipation, and hypertension. Studies looking at intravaginal administration of bromocriptine have shown that side effects are diminished and prolactin levels remain suppressed.[38]

Resistance to bromocriptine develops in 5 to 18% of treated patients, usually resulting from poor patient compliance.[39] There are reported cases of receptor defects causing resistance to dopamine agonists. In these cases, new medical methods are successful in treating resistant hyperprolactinemia.[40]

Cabergoline (Dostinex) is a synthetic ergoline with high specificity and affinity for the dopamine receptor.[41] It has received FDA approval for the treatment of hyperprolactinemia in the United States. It is a potent and long-acting inhibitor of prolactin secretion. A single dose of cabergoline rapidly lowers prolactin within 3 hours of drug administration and suppression has been documented to persist for at least 14 days.

Studies have shown that cabergoline is better tolerated than bromocriptine and easier dosing allows for greater patient compliance.[42] The initial recommended dosage is 0.5 to 1.0 mg twice weekly. An initial dose of 0.5 mg once weekly is suggested, increasing in increments of 0.5 mg/week until a therapeutic response is seen. The recommended maximum dose is 1.0 mg twice weekly but clinical studies have reported benefit at 3.0 mg weekly.

The side effects of cabergoline are similar to bromocriptine, with the most commonly reported being nausea, vomiting, headaches, and dizziness. Orthostatic hypotension occurs in up to 50% of patients but are rarely symptomatic.[43] Multiple studies have shown that the overall incidence of adverse symptoms and discontinuation of the drug is significantly lower for cabergoline than bromocriptine.[44] Eighty percent of patients who do not tolerate bromocriptine do well with cabergoline.[45]

Both bromocriptine and cabergoline have been shown to reduce tumor size and restore menstrual function. Bromocriptine was investigated with regard to its ability to reduce tumor size in eight studies. Sixty-nine percent of patients had at least a 25% reduction in tumor size, 12% had less than a 25% reduction, and 19% had no reduction.[46-50] In comparison, cabergoline was investigated in six studies, with 70% of patients having at least a 25% reduction and 13% having less than 25% reduction. In these studies, 16% of patients had no change.[51,52] In the treatment of women with hyperprolactinemic amenorrhea, cabergoline 0.5 mg to 1 mg twice weekly was significantly more effective than bromocriptine 2.5 mg to 5.0 mg twice daily in restoring ovulation and menses.[53]

Other dopamine agonists include pergolide, quinagolide, metergoline, and lisuride.[54] All these agonists act by directly binding to and stimulating D2 receptors. Pergolide is currently available in the United States for the treatment of Parkinson disease but not approved for the treatment of hyperprolactinemia. Quinagolide, metergoline, and lisuride are available only in certain European markets. Studies overseas have confirmed that both these agents have similar efficacy to bromocriptine in the treatment of hyperprolactinemia; however, overall, cabergoline is superior to bromocriptine.

In summary, both bromocriptine and cabergoline reduce prolactin levels, reduce tumor size and restore ovulatory function. Because of the side-effect profiles and patient compliance with cabergoline it will undoubtedly become first-line therapy. The initial cost of cabergoline is greater than bromocriptine[55]; however, improved patient compliance and the potential of once-a-week dosing may decrease unnecessary physician visits and laboratory costs.

There is no consensus for long-term therapy, but in general it is recommended that therapy continue for 2 years in microadenomas and idiopathic hyperprolactinemia and 4 years with macroadenomas. The natural course of the disease is well documented. In patients with idiopathic hyperprolactinemia followed for over 10 years few have evidence of a pituitary tumor.[56] These patients respond well to medical therapy, with restoration of prolactin levels even after treatment is halted. In patients with microadenomas the tumor is generally stable, with minimal enlargement, and in some cases spontaneous resolution has been documented. After a 1- to 2-year period of treatment for microadenomas, prolactin levels remain normal for several years after discontinuation of medication.[57] However, patients should continue to be monitored periodically and re-evaluated with the reappearance of symptoms.

The history of macroadenomas is less clear. Treatment is warranted to prevent worsening side effects and expansion into the optic chiasm, which may impair vision. In the majority of patients treated for 4.9 years, prolactin levels remain low or normal after withdrawal of medication.[58] Thus, in both microadenomas and macroadenomas, withdrawal of medication is an acceptable alternative as long as patients are monitored for recurrence of symptoms.

In patients with asymptomatic microadenomas or idiopathic prolactinemia, observation is also an acceptable alternative to medical treatment once the MRI returns as normal. One of the health risks of hyperprolactinemia-induced amenorrhea is osteoporosis.[59] The use of cyclic estrogen with provera or oral contraceptives is sufficient to prevent further decrease in bone mineral density. Patients should be monitored annually and repeat imaging performed if prolactin levels increase or symptoms occur. At this point treatment should initiated.

Over 20 years ago, one treatment option was transcranial surgery. Complications were common and mortality approached 10%, with rates closely associated to tumor size and surgeon experience.[60] Total or partial hypophysectomy through the transphenoidal route is now the preferred surgical method. There is less trauma and fewer complications but a higher recurrence rate. Immediately after surgery, prolactin levels are restored to base line in 70% of microadenomas and 30% of macroadenomas.[61] Unfortunately, recurrence occurs between 17% and 50% for microadenomas and between 20% and 80% for macroadenomas requiring medical treatment.[62]

Radiation therapy is reserved for patients for whom medical and surgical treatment fails. The effect is minimal and may take several years before prolactin levels are normalized. Published literature shows a cure rate of only 10% in patients using radiation alone and 30% in patients treated with radiation and bromocriptine.[63] The major consequence of radiotherapy is pituitary insufficiency requiring lifelong treatment.

PREGNANCY

The major issues to consider in a pregnancy are the effect of pregnancy on tumor size and the effect of treatment on the fetus. Enlargement of a pituitary tumor occurs from the stimulatory effect of estrogen on the lactotroph cells. Reviewing data, the risk of clinical enlargement of a microadenoma is 1.6 to 5.5%, but it is 15.5 to 35.7% for macroadenomas.[64] Before conception, it is recommended that patients receive at least 3 months of therapy. The risk of expansion in patients previously treated with bromocriptine is <10%.[65] Once pregnancy is achieved, medical therapy is discontinued and patients monitored carefully. If any symptoms develop during pregnancy, treatment is restarted. In pregnancy, prolactin cannot be used as a marker for tumor enlargement as prolactin from placental sources during pregnancy may rise to peak levels of 150 to 200 ng/ml.[66]

The safety of bromocriptine in utero has been well established. There is no increased incidence of congenital anomalies, spontaneous abortions or multiple pregnancies and no adverse effects on postnatal development.[67] Fewer data are available on cabergoline and pregnancy. Limited studies have shown no increase in congenital anomalies; however, due to its long half-life, it is currently recommended that women seeking pregnancy should discontinue cabergoline therapy 1 month before intended conception.[68] As such, therapeutic abortion is not warranted if pregnancy ocurrs during cabergoline treatment.[34]

In a non-breast-feeding woman, prolactin levels will return to base line within a week. For women who wish to breast-feed, lactation does not increase the risk for tumor progression[68,69] and some patients have displayed a spontaneous regression of the tumor possibly through infarction.[71]

CONCLUSION

Hyperprolactinemia is a relatively common disorder that most clinicians will encounter. Women will most frequently present with amenorrhea and/or galactorrhea. A comprehensive history and physical evaluation combined with the appropriate laboratory and imaging studies will identify the cause in the majority of cases. The optimal treatment for these patients is with dopamine agonists and observation in certain cases. In patients who do not desire fertility, estrogen-replacement therapy is essential to prevent further loss of bone mineral density. The approval of a new dopamine agonist will no doubt increase patient compliance and improve symptoms. Ultimately, the clinician must tailor diagnosis and treatment for each individual patient.

REFERENCES

1. Billier BM, et al. Guidelines for the diagnosis and treatment of hyperprolactinemia. J Reprod Med 1999;44(12Suppl):1075.
2. Mehta AE, Tolis G. Prolactin update. Pathobiolog Annu 1981;11:337.
3. Sarapura V, Schlaff WD. Recent advances in the understanding of the pathophysiology and treatment of hyperprolactinemia. Curr Opin Obstet Gynecol 1993;5:360.
4. Lewis V. Hyperprolactinemia. In: Cowan BD, Seifer DB, eds. Clinical reproductive medicine. Philadelphia: Lippincott-Raven, 1997:85.
5. Jones EE. Hyperprolactinemia and female infertility. J Reprod Med 1989;34:117.
6. Chang RJ, Knockenhauer ES, Slayer S, et al. Anovulation of CNS origin. In: Carr BR, Blackwell RE, eds. Textbook of reproductive medicine. 2nd ed. Norwalk, CT: Appleton & Lange, 1998:289.
7. Quigley MM, Haney AF. Evaluation of hyperprolactinemia: clinical profiles. Clin Obstet Gynecol 1980;23:337.
8. Blackwell RE. Diagnosis and management of prolactinomas. Fertil Steril 1985;43:5.
9. Ciccarelli E, Camanni F. Diagnosis and drug therapy of prolactinoma. Drugs 1996;51:954.

10. Fraser WM, Blackard WG. Medical conditions that affect the breast and lactation. Clin Obstet Gynecol 1975;18:51.

11. Sakiyama R, Quan M. Galactorrhea and hyperprolactinemia. Obstet Gynecol Surv 1983;38:689.

12. Keye WR, Chang J, Jaffe RB. Prolactin secretin pituitary adenomas in women with amenorrhea or galactorrhea. Obstet Gynecol Surv 1977;32:727.

13. Burrow GH, Wortzman G, Rewcastle NB, et al. Micro-adenomas of the pituitary and abnormal selected tomo-grams in an unselected autopsy series. N Engl J Med 1981;304:156.

14. Abboud CF, Laws ER. Clinical endocrinological approach to hypothalamic-pituitary disease. J Neurosurg 1979; 51:271.

15. Malarkey WB. Prolactin and the diagnosis of pituitary tumors. Ann Rev Med 1979;30:249.

16. Dollar JR, Blackwell RE. Diagnosis and management of prolactinomas. Cancer Metast Rev 1986;5:125.

17. Katz E, Adashi EY. Hyperprolactinemic disorders. Clin Obstet Gynecol 1990;33:622.

18. Ohaman R, Axelsson R. Prolactin response to neuro-leptics: clinical and theoretical implications. J Neural Transm Suppl 1980;17:1.

19. Spitzer M, Sajjad R, and Benjamin F. Pattern of develop-ment of hyperprolactinemia after initiation of haloperidol therapy. Obstet Gynecol 1997;91:693.

20. Conner P, Fried G. Hyperprolactinemia, etiology, diagnosis and treatment alternatives. Acta Obstet Gynecol Scand 1998;77:249.

21. Franks S. Use of bromocriptine in hyperprolactinaemic anovulation and related disorders. Drugs 1979;17:337.

22. Fiorica JV. Nipple discharge: contemporary management of breast disease. I. Benign disease. Obstet Gynecol Clin N Am 1994:453.

23. Yazigi RA, Quintero CH, Salameh WA. Prolactin disor-ders. Fertil Steril 1997;67:215.

24. Sanfilippo JS. Implications of not treating hyperprolactine-mia. J Reprod Med 1999;44(12 Suppl):1111.

25. Schlechte JA, Sherman B, Martin R. Bone density in amenorrheic women with and without hyperprolactine-mia. J Clin Endocrinol Metab 1983;56:1120.

26. Greenspan SL, Neer RM, Ridgway EC, et al. Osteoporo-sis in men with hyperprolactinemic hypogonadism. Ann Intern Med 1986;104:777.

27. Thorner MO, Vance ML, Laws ER, et al. The anterior pituitary. In: Wilson JD, Foster DW, Kronenberg HM, Larsen PR, eds. Williams textbook of endocrinology. 9th ed. Philadelphia: Saunders, 1998;751.

28. Newman SA. Advances in diagnosis and treatment of pituitary tumors. Intern Opthalmol Clin 1986;26:285.

29. Kulkarni MV, Lee KF, McArdle CB, et al. MR imaging of pituitary microadenomas: technical considerations and CT correlation. Am J Neuroradiol 1988;9:5.

30. Wolpert SM, Molitch ME, Goldman JA, et al. Size, shape and appearance of the normal female pituitary gland. AJR 1984;143:377.

31. Molitch ME, Thorner MO, Wilson C. Therapeutic contro-versy: management of prolactinomas. J Clin Endocrinol Metab 1997;82:996.

32. Dollar JR, Blackwell RE. Diagnosis and management of prolactinomas. Cancer Metast Rev 1986;5:125.

33. Molitch ME. Management of prolactinomas during preg-nancy. J Reprod Med 1999;44(12 Suppl):1121.

34. Kinch RA. The use of bromocriptine in obstetrics and gynecology. Fertil Steril 1980;33:463.

35. Moriondo P, Travaglini P, Nissim M, et al. Bromocriptine treatment of microprolactinomas: evidence of stable pro-lactin decrease after drug withdrawal. J Clin Endocrinol Metab 1985;60:764.

36. Breckwoldt M, Crosignani PG, et al. A new treatment for hyperprolactinemic disorders. Presented at the 11th annual meeting of the European Society of Human Reproduc-tion and Embryology, June 30, 1995, Hamburg.

37. Robinson AG, Nelson PB. Prolactinomas in women: cur-rent therapies. Ann Intern Med 1983;99:115.

38. Motta T, Vincentiliis S, Marchini M, et al. Vaginal caber-goline in the treatment of hyperprolactinemic patients intolerant to oral dopaminergics. Fertil Steril 1996; 65:440.

39. Soule SG, Powell M, Jacobs HS. Prolactinomas resistant to dopamine agonists: insights into pathogenesis and therapy. Curr Opin Obstet Gynecol 1994;6:393.

40. Colao A, Di Sarno A, Sarnacchiaro F, et al. Prolactinoma resistant to standard dopamine agonists respond to chronic cabergoline treatment. J Clin Endocrinol Metab 1997; 82:876.

41. Ferrari C, Piscitelli G, Crosignani PG. Cabergoline: a new drug for the treatment of hyperprolactinemia. Hum Reprod 1995;10:1647.

42. Webster J. A comparative review of the tolerability profiles of dopamine agonists in the treatment of hyperprolactine-mia and inhibition of lactation. Drug Safety 1990;14:228.

43. Ciccarelli E, Giusti M, Miola C, et al. Effectiveness and tolerability of long-term treatment with cabergoline, a new long-lasting ergoline derivative, in hyperprolactine-mic patients. J Clin Endocrinol Metab 1989;69:725.

44. Webster J. Dopamine agonist therapy in hyperprolactine-mia. J Reprod Med 1999;44(Suppl):1105.

45. Biller BMK, Molitch ME, Vance ML, et al. Treatment of prolactin-secreting macroadenomas with the once-weekly dopmine agonist cabergoline. J Clin Endocrinol Metab 1996;81:2338.

46. Gen M, Uozumi T, Ohta M, et al. Necrotic changes in prolactinomas after long term administration of bromocriptine. J Clin Endocrinol 1984;59:463.

47. Thorner MO, Perryman RL, Rogol AD, et al. Rapid changes of prolactinoma volume after withdrawal and re-institution of bromocriptine. J Clin Endocrinol Metab 1981;53:480.

48. Bassetti M, Spada A, Pezzo G, et al. Bromocriptine treat-ment reduces the cell size in human prolactinomas: a morphometric study. J Clin Endocrinol Metab 1984; 58:268.

49. Hallenga B, Saiger W, Ludecke DK. Necroses of prolactin-secreting pituitary adenomas under treatment with dopamine agonists: light microscropical and morphometric studies. Exp Clin Endocrinol 1988;92:259.

50. Vanít Verlaat JW, Croughs RJM. Withdrawal of bromo-criptine after long-term therapy for macroprolactinomas: effect on plasma prolactin and tumour size. Clin En-docrinol 1991;34:175.

51. Jeffcoate WJ, Pound N, Sturrock NDC, et al. Long-term

follow-up of patients with hyperprolactinemia. Clin En-docrinol 1996;45:299.

52. Webster J, Piscitelli G, Polli A, et al. Dose-dependent suppression of serum prolactin by cabergoline in hyper-prolactinemia: a placebo controlled, double-blind, multi-centre study. Clin Endocrinol 1992;37:534.

53. Webster J, Piscitelli G, Polli A, et al. A comparison of cabergoline and bromocriptine in the treatment of hyper-prolactinemic amenorrhea. N Engl J Med 1994;331:904.

54. Crosignani PG, Ferrari C. Dopaminergic treatments for hyperprolactinaemia. Clin Obstet Gynecol 1990;4:441.

55. Faber K. A pragmatic approach to evaluating, managing hyperprolactinemia. Obstet Gynecol Manage 1998; June:66.

56. Martin TL, Kim M, Malarkey WB. The natural history of idiopathic hyperprolactinemia. J Clin Endocrinol Metab 1985;60:855.

57. Sisam DA, Sheehan JP, Sheeler LR. The natural history of untreated microprolactinomas. Fertil Steril 1987;48:67.

58. March CM, Kletzky OA, Davajan V, et al. Longitudinal evaluation of patients with untreated prolactin-secreting pituitary adenomas. Am J Obstet Gynecol 1981;139:835.

59. Klibanski A, Neer RM, Beitins IZ, et al. Decreased bone density in hyperprolactinemic women. N Engl J Med 1980;303:1511.

60. Guiot G. Transphenoidal approach in surgical treatment of pituitary adenomas: general principles and indications in nonfunctioning adenomas. In: Kohler PO, Ross GT, eds. Diagnosis and treatment of pituitary tumors. New York: American Elsevier, 1973:159.

61. Carr BR. Disorder of the ovaries and female reproductive tract. In: Wilson JD, Foster DW, Kronenberg HM, Larsen PR, eds. Williams textbook of endocrinology. 9th ed. Philadelphia: Saunders, 1998;751.

62. Bevans JS, Adams CB, Burke CW, et al. Factors in the outcome of transphenoidal surgery for prolactinoma and non-functioning pituitary tumor including pre-operative bromocriptine therapy. Clin Endocrinol 1987;26:541.

63. Frantz AG, Cogon PH, Chang CH, et al. Long-term eval-uation of the results of transphenoidal surgery and radio-therapy in patients with prolactinoma. In: Crosignan PG, Rubin BL, eds. Endocrinology of human infertility: new aspects. New York: Grune & Stratton, 1981:161.

64. Molitch ME. Pregnancy and the hyperprolactinemic woman. N Engl J Med 1985;312:1364.

65. Lamberts SWJ, Klijn JG, de Lange SA, et al. The inci-dence of complications during pregnancy after treatment of hyperprolactinemia with bromocriptine in patients with radiologically evident pituitary tumors. Fertil Steril 1979;31:614.

66. Noel GL, Suh HD, Frantz AG. Prolactin release during nursing and breast stimulation in postpartum subjects. J Clin Endocrinol Metab 1974;38:413.

67. Krupp P, Turklj I. Surveillance of parlodel (Bromocriptine) in pregnancy and offspring. In: Jacobs HS, Harrison RF, et al., eds. Prolactinomas and pregnancy. Lancaster, PA: MTP Press, 1983:45.

68. Prager D, Braunstein GD. Pituitary disorders during preg-nancy. Endocrinol Metab Clin North Am 1995;24:1.

69. Webster J. A comparative review of the tolerability profiles of dopamine agonists in the treatment of hyperprolactine-mia and inhibition of lactation. Drug Safety 1990;14:228.

70. Rains C, Bryson H, Fitton A. Cabergoline: a review of its pharmacological properties and therapeutic potential in the treatment of hyperprolactinemia and inhibition of lactation. Drugs 1995;49:255.

71. Kutteh WH, Carr BR, Le SQ. Long-term follow up after a severe haemorrhage within a prolactin-producing ade-noma resulting in successful pregnancies. J Obstet Gy-naecol 1997;17:1158.

Chapter 49

Premenstrual Syndrome

Candace S. Brown
Frank W. Ling

Five Key Points

- Premenstrual syndrome is a recurring cyclical disorder involving emotional and physical symptoms during the luteal phase of the menstrual cycle.

- Premenstrual syndrome is diagnosed with prospective charting of symptoms and should be differentiated from other disorders that can be exacerbated premenstrually.

- Mild premenstrual symptoms are best treated with lifestyle changes, such as a healthy diet, sodium and caffeine restriction, exercise, and stress reduction.

- Moderately severe premenstrual mood symptoms are most effectively treated by selective serotoninergic reuptake inhibitors.

- Moderately severe premenstrual physical symptoms respond to low-dose oral contraceptives, nonsteroidal antiinflammatory drugs, and diuretics.

Premenstrual syndrome (PMS) is a recurring cyclical disorder involving behavioral, emotional, and physical symptoms during the luteal phase of the menstrual cycle. Behavioral and emotional symptoms include irritability, mood swings, depression, hostility, and social withdrawal, whereas physical symptoms include bloating, breast tenderness, myalgias, headache, and fatigue. Up to 70 to 80% of women experience some premenstrual symptoms, with 2 to 10% reporting disabling, incapacitating symptoms resulting in work or social impairment.[1]

Theories about the cause of PMS include progesterone deficiency, estrogen excess, increased activity of aldosterone or of the renin-angiotensin system, vitamin B_6 deficiency, and serotonin deficiency. Current research suggests that PMS is most likely of multifactorial origin, with involvement of neurohormones and neurotransmitters.[2] Although the underlying cause remains unclear, significant progress has been made in symptomatic treatment.

The *International Statistical Classification of Diseases and Related Health Problems* (10th rev.) (ICD-10) includes PMS as a genitourinary system disorder.[3] It is defined as a condition in which there is mild psychological discomfort and physical symptoms of bloating and weight gain, breast tenderness and swelling, swelling of hands and feet, various aches and pains, poor concentration, sleep disturbance, and change in appetite. Only one of these symptoms is required for this diagnosis, although the symptoms

---

TABLE 49-1
DSM-IV CRITERIA FOR PREMENSTRUAL DYSPHORIC DISORDER

On prospective evaluation of patient symptom charting for 2 to 3 menstrual cycles, 5 (or more) of the following symptoms are present during the last week of the luteal phase and are absent postmenstrual. At least 1 of the symptoms must be 1, 2, 3, or 4.

1. Markedly depressed mood, feelings of hopelessness, or self-deprecating thoughts
2. Marked anxiety, tension, feeling of being "keyed up" or "on edge"
3. Marked affective lability (e.g., feeling suddenly sad or fearful or increased sensitivity to rejection)
4. Persistent and marked anger or irritability or increase in interpersonal conflicts
5. Decreased interest in usual activities (e.g., work, school, friends, hobbies)
6. Subjective sense of difficulty in concentrating
7. Lethargy, easy fatigability, or marked lack of energy
8. Marked change in appetite, overeating, or specific food cravings
9. Hypersomnia or insomnia
10. A subjective sense of being overwhelmed or out of control
11. Other physical symptoms, such as breast tenderness or swelling, headaches, joint or muscle pain, a sensation of bloating, weight gain

The disturbance *must* markedly interfere with work or school or with usual social activities and relations with others (e.g., avoidance of social activities, decreased productivity and efficiency at work or school).

Adapted with permission from the American Psychiatric Association.[5]

TABLE 49-2
SYMPTOMS OF PREMENSTRUAL DYSPHORIC DISORDER (PMDD) AND MAJOR DEPRESSIVE DISORDER (MDD)

Found in MDD and PMDD	Found in PMDD
Depressed mood	Anxiety and tension
Decreased interest	Affective lability
Difficulty concentrating	Marked anger/irritability
Fatigue	Sense of being overwhelmed
Changes in appetite	Physical symptoms: breast pain,
Changes in sleep	bloating, headache

Adapted with permission from Yonkers.[6]

DIAGNOSIS

Diagnosis is determined by results of a thorough interview, physical examination, routine laboratory tests, and use of prospective daily diaries. Optimally, the initial interview should be scheduled for two sessions, including one during the premenstrual period in order to obtain a direct observation of any possible symptoms, and another session during the midfollicular phase, when no symptoms are expected. If only a single session is possible, a premenstrual visit is preferred for direct observation.

The interview should contain a psychological history, which includes questions about postpartum depression, oral contraceptive use, and alcohol and substance use, since studies have shown an increased incidence in women with PMS as compared with controls.[7] A family history should be obtained because almost 50% of women with PMS have a family history of either a mood disorder or alcoholism.[8] The presence of relationship conflicts, work problems, parenting, and health concerns should be determined, since these factors often contribute to the severity of PMS.

A complete physical and gynecologic examination should be conducted to rule out underlying medical disorders that may mimic PMS. Laboratory tests should include a complete blood count (CBC), fasting blood sugar, thyroid studies, liver-function tests, and creatinine. The incidence of perimenopausal symptoms is also high in this population, and determining the serum follicle-stimulating hormone (FSH) level may be helpful in establishing the latter diagnosis in women over 40. Laboratory studies should be conducted 1 to 7 days prior to menses or when symptoms are most severe.

must be restricted to the luteal phase of the menstrual cycle, reach a peak shortly before menstruation, and cease with the menstrual flow or soon after.

A severe form of PMS, characterized predominantly by mood symptoms, has been defined in the third and fourth editions of the *Diagnostic and Statistical Manual of Mental Disorders*. In the third edition (DSM-III-R),[4] the disorder was termed late luteal phase dysphoric disorder (LLPDD) and was placed in the appendix as a condition in need of further study. In the fourth edition (DSM-IV),[5] the name of the disorder was simplified to premenstrual dysphoric disorder (PMDD). Table 49-1 lists the DSM-IV criteria for PMDD. PMDD was placed under the mood disorders section because of its symptom similarity with major depressive disorder (MDD), but additional distinguishing features are found in PMDD that are generally not present in MDD. Table 49-2 depicts the similarities and differences between PMDD and MDD.

Daily Rating Scales

Daily prospective rating of symptoms is the only accepted method of confirming a diagnosis of PMS. Symptoms associated with PMS typically begin during the late luteal phase and resolve promptly with the onset of menstruation. Sometimes the onset is more gradual, beginning at ovulation, and the "offset" may involve a tapering over 2 to 3 days after the period begins. Symptoms that persist after menstruation suggest the presence of another diagnosis, since PMDD does not carry over into the follicular phase. A typical PMS rating scale is shown in Table 49-3.

Previous studies required a symptom increase of at least 30% between the late luteal phase as compared with the midfollicular phase in order to meet diagnostic criteria of PMS.[9] Studies suggest that an increase of 50% or more confirms the diagnosis.[9] Symptoms that increase by approximately 60 to 75% are indicative of women who meet PMDD criteria.[9]

Differential Diagnosis

Symptoms of PMS routinely present in a nonspecific manner. The clinician must approach a diagnosis by first excluding all other possible diagnoses and then evaluating a prospective record of the patient's daily rating of symptoms.

It is essential to differentiate PMS from other major mood and physical disorders because the nonspecific symptoms of PMS may overlap with psychiatric, endocrine, medical, or gynecologic disorders. A list of differential diagnoses should be carefully constructed, and each potential diagnosis should then be ruled out with the appropriate evaluations.

Mood Disorders

Both PMS and PMDD apply only to women who have luteal-phase symptoms and are symptom-free for at least 1 week after menses. Some women with mood disorders, such as major depressive disorder (MDD), may experience severe premenstrual worsening of their symptoms. These patterns are commonly referred to as perimenstrual exacerbation or perimenstrual magnification. Women with perimenstrual magnification will show premenstrual worsening of their symptoms during the late luteal phase, but will remain symptomatic throughout the menstrual cycle. Other noncyclic psychiatric conditions that can resemble PMS include anxiety disorders, personality

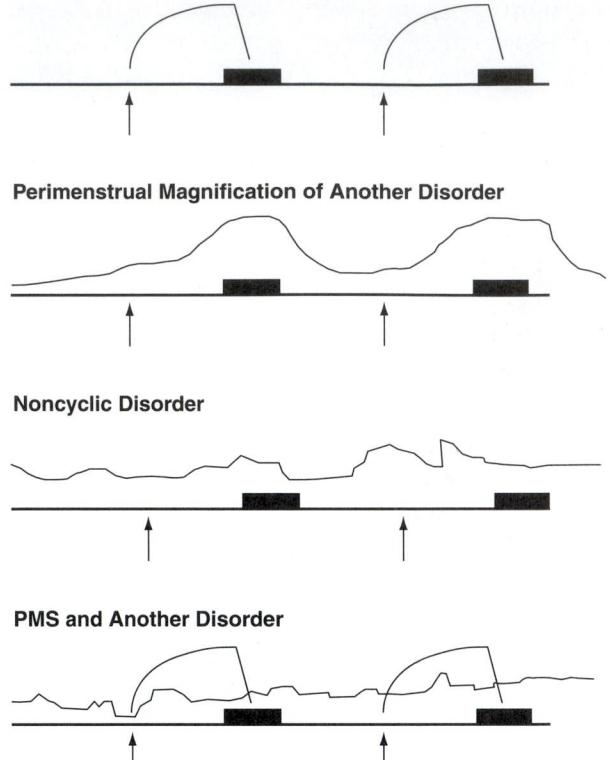

Figure 49-1 Pattern of symptoms associated with different menstrual cycle–affected conditions. Adapted with permission from Wallis LA, ed. Textbook of women's health. Philadelphia: Lippincott-Raven, 1998:693.

disorders, substance-abuse disorders, somatoform disorders, and eating disorders.[9] Finally, many women experience both a psychiatric disorder and PMS simultaneously. Dysthymia, a chronic minor depression, is the most common comorbid condition.[6] The diagnostic challenge is to sort out those with PMS only, another diagnosis only, or both diagnoses concurrently. Figure 49-1 illustrates the timing of symptoms in relation to ovulation and menses for the most common patterns.

Because of the similarity of PMS to other mood disorders, the diagnostic evaluation needs to include careful assessment of when these symptoms occur in the cycle. It is important to conduct mood assessments in the follicular phase, when the symptom levels are not confounded by PMS. High scores on mood measures in the follicular phase suggest that the problems extend beyond PMS. Prospective ratings can also help establish entrainment of mood disturbances to menstrual-cycle phase. If it appears that there are other mood disorders, but the severity is unclear, further psychiatric interview may be appropriate.

TABLE 49-3
DAILY SYMPTOM CHECKLIST

Month _____ Name _____

Date (day)	1	2	3	4	5	6	7	8	9	10	11	12	13	14	15	16	17	18	19	20	21	22	23	24	25	26	27	28	29	30	31
Check, if menstruating																															
Medication																															
Waking Temperature																															
Symptoms (Grade 0 to 4) 0 = not at all 1 = a little 2 = moderately 3 = quite a bit 4 = extremely																															
Mood swings																															
Irritability																															
Out of control																															
Nervous tension																															
Depression																															
Low interest level																															
Fatigue																															
Energetic																															
Confused																															
Crave sweets																															
Sleeplessness																															
Headaches																															
Breast tenderness																															
Feel bloated																															
General aches/pains																															
Other:																															

Medical Conditions

Medical conditions such as epilepsy, anemia, chronic fatigue syndrome, and autoimmune disorders, as well as endocrine diseases such as diabetes mellitus or hypothyroidism, can present with nonspecific symptoms, such as feelings of lethargy, weight gain, abdominal pain, bloating, and mood changes. Although classic examples of these disorders should not present any diagnostic dilemma, atypical presentations can be confused with symptoms of PMS. If suspicion is high for any of these disorders, appropriate evaluations should be undertaken.

Up to 72% of women with epilepsy have been reported to have catamenial seizures. Seizure exacerbation before and during menses has been documented in two-thirds of women with epilepsy, with nearly a doubling in frequency at the peak immediately premenstrually. No particular type of seizure is more prone to catamenial exacerbation than any other.[10]

There is a general impression that glucose tolerance is somewhat reduced during the luteal phase in nondiabetic women and that metabolic control is erratic during the late luteal phase in diabetic women. One study showed that three-fourths of hospital admissions for diabetic ketoacidosis (DKA) in the 14- to 42-year-old age group were female, and half of these were menstruating or just premenstrual at the time of admission.[10] However, currently, the nature of catamenial fluctuations in energy metabolism and their clinical significance for diabetes management remains inconclusive.

Gynecologic Conditions

Perhaps the most common misdiagnosis of PMS is that of dysmenorrhea. The reason for this misdiagnosis is usually not because of confusion of the symptoms, but because of confusion over definitions or inadequate history. Primary dysmenorrhea, by definition, is menstrual pain in the absence of pelvic pathology. The onset of dysmenorrhea is hours before menstruation and lasts up to 72 hours. Dysmenorrhea does not have prodromal affective symptoms. The pain of dysmenorrhea is characterized by intermittent crampy lower abdominal pain concentrated in the midline (suprapubic) region, and may be associated with diarrhea, nausea, or vomiting. The cause of primary dysmenorrhea is uterine prostaglandins causing painful uterine contractions. An initial conservative approach may include nonsteroidal antiinflammatory drugs or oral contraceptive agents.[11]

The hallmark of endometriosis is pain preceding the onset of menses. Endometriosis must therefore be clinically ruled out before a diagnosis of PMS is firmly established. A woman with fibroids may experience discomfort premenstrually due to increased engorgement of the intrauterine blood supply. As a result, fibroids, too, must be considered in a differential diagnosis of PMS.[11]

Both endometriosis and uterine fibroids cause menstrual pain because of an underlying pelvic pathology, and are considered secondary dysmenorrhea. If a patient presenting with symptoms of PMS has abnormal results on pelvic examination or has a suggestive history for gynecologic pathology, such as abnormal vaginal bleeding or severe dysmenorrhea, a more extensive work-up may be necessary.

If a woman reports breast tenderness and engorgement, the presence of breast masses or cysts must be excluded before a diagnosis of PMS is considered.[11] The differential diagnosis for such cyclic changes should include a condition of fibrocystic breast.

TREATMENT

Both nonpharmacologic and pharmacologic therapies are used to treat premenstrual symptoms. Management is based on a stepwise approach, accounting for type and severity of premenstrual symptoms. If presenting symptoms are mild, infrequent, or of short duration, use of nonpharmacologic approaches such as dietary changes, exercise, relaxation techniques, and behavior modification are warranted. If symptoms are more severe, frequent, or longer-lasting, drug therapy such as nonsteroidal antiinflammatory drugs (NSAIDs), hormonal agents, diuretics, and psychotropics should be considered. Figure 49-2 illustrates an algorithmic approach to the treatment of PMS.

Nonpharmacologic Treatment

Diet

Although there is no evidence that nutritional deficiencies cause PMS, poor dietary habits may exacerbate symptoms. A variety of nutritional factors have been evaluated in PMS, including appetite changes, glucose tolerance, carbohydrate intake, sodium and caffeine intake, and vitamin and mineral deficiencies.

Glucose abnormalities have been considered to contribute to PMS due to the presence of hypoglycemic-like symptoms such as food cravings, irritability,

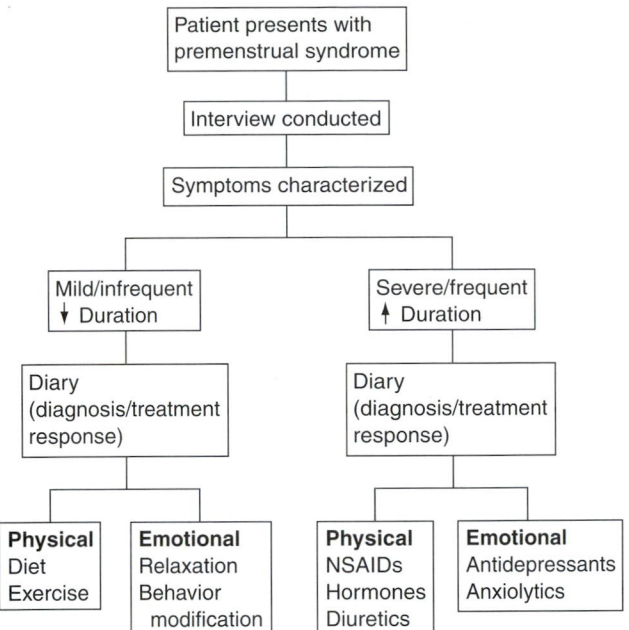

Figure 49-2 Approach to treatment of premenstrual syndrome. Adapted from DeMonico SO, Brown CS, Ling FW. Premenstrual syndrome. Curr Opin Obstet Gynecol 1994; 6:499.

nervousness, and fatigue. There has been no proven relationship, however, between premenstrual symptoms and changes in glucose concentrations in women with PMS. Consuming meals that are high in carbohydrate-rich foods and low in protein, particularly during the premenstruum, may improve symptoms such as depression, tension, anger, confusion, fatigue, and alterness.[12] "PMS escape," a dietary supplement that contains specially formulated carbohydrates to increase brain serotonin levels, has been marketed. Its efficacy may be based on the fact that deficiencies in serotonin-mediated brain neurotransmission may play a key role in the mood and appetite-related disturbances caused by PMS.[12]

SODIUM RESTRICTION Salt intake has been associated with premenstrual bloating and edema.[12] Although there is no evidence to support excess salt as the cause of PMS, increased salt intake can increase water retention and associated weight gain. Thus, it is reasonable to restrict salt intake to reduce sodium associated with water retention.

CAFFEINE RESTRICTION Caffeine has been associated with an increase in severity of premenstrual symptoms, particularly anxiety, tension, depression, and irritability.[12] Although caffeine intake is not related to

the cause of PMS, decreasing or avoiding caffeine intake may reduce symptoms. Care must be taken when stopping caffeine consumption, as abrupt cessation can be associated with withdrawal symptoms of irritability, nervousness, lethargy, and headache.

VITAMINS, MINERALS, AND NUTRITIONAL SUPPLEMENTS Use of vitamin E in the treatment of PMS originated from its use in fibrocystic breast disease. Although high-dose treatment with vitamin E (400 IU daily) has been associated with reduced mood symptoms and food cravings, no reduction has been noted in physical symptoms, including breast tenderness.[12] Low-dose vitamin E supplementation (150 to 300 IU) has not been shown to be effective in reducing PMS symptoms.[12] Although toxicity has not been noted with high-dose treatment with vitamin E, little evidence exists demonstrating its effectiveness as a treatment for PMS.

Vitamin B_6 supplementation has been advocated since the 1940s, even though there is no evidence of a deficiency in women with PMS. Open-label trials have supported the use of vitamin B_6 in PMS.[12] However, well-controlled studies have failed to demonstrate efficacy, due to use of suboptimal doses, inadequate samples, and noncomparable samples.[12] There is, moreover, a direct dose–response relationship for the development of reversible peripheral neuropathy in the use of vitamin B_6 at greater than 500 mg/day.[12] Therefore, the use of vitamin B_6 is limited by the absence of proven benefit and the risk of adverse events in high doses.

Use of evening primrose oil (which contains linoleic acid, γ-linoleic acid, and essential fatty acids) has been promoted as effective in PMS, even though a meta-analysis concluded no effect.[12] Vitamins, such as Optivite, which are high in magnesium, essential fatty acids, and vitamins E and B_6 have also been advocated in PMS, but efficacy has not been demonstrated in well-controlled studies.[12]

There are data from randomized, placebo-controlled trials demonstrating the efficacy of calcium supplementation. Administration of 1200 mg of calcium a day results in significant improvement in water retention, negative affect, cravings, and pain.[13]

Despite equivocal evidence for nutritional treatments, many clinicians recommend a nutritional approach in the initial treatment of PMS. Dietary changes that enhance nutritional status and promote good health are often recommended. This approach is relatively safe and has the added advantage that it is patient-controlled. Dietary approaches alleviate symptoms in some women; and maintaining a well-balanced diet promotes well-being. A PMS diet consists of 60% complex carbohydrates, 20% protein, and 20% fat.[12] If premenstrual food cravings are a predominant symptom, particular care should be taken to eat at more frequent intervals rather than to increase caloric intake. Caffeine and sodium intake should be minimized.

Exercise

The effect of exercise on PMS has not been fully elucidated. Increasing aerobic exercise reduced some of the physical symptoms and depressed mood in women with PMS in an open trial,[14] whereas another study reported that aerobic exercise was superior to strength training in reducing premenstrual symptoms in normal women.[14] Although further research is needed to confirm these observations, it is sensible to advocate exercise for most patients since it may improve bloating, self-esteem, and depression. A 20- to 30-minute moderate workout at least four times per week is recommended.

Psychotherapy and Relaxation Techniques

Preliminary controlled studies suggest efficacy for cognitive, behavioral, and relaxation techniques in the treatment of PMS.[14] Cognitive therapy focuses on changing distorted thought processes, such as negative thinking, which may lead to depressed feelings. Behavioral modification treatments, such as diet, exercise, and weight loss, help patients gain greater control over their lives and hence produce a positive impact. Relaxation techniques lead to a state of relaxed wakefulness and may lessen pain; they include deep breathing, mental imagery, progressive relaxation, meditation, and yoga. Although more well-controlled trials are needed to evaluate these treatments fully, it seems reasonable to conclude that they may be beneficial in helping women cope with their symptoms. In one trial of reflexology, patients were randomly assigned to reflexology or placebo reflexology. Patients receiving the true reflexology demonstrated significant improvement versus placebo.[15]

Pharmacologic Treatment

Nonsteroidal Antiinflammatory Drugs

PMS is associated with a number of symptoms (breast tenderness, abdominal cramps, general achiness, joint pain, headaches, backache) that may be prostaglandin (PG)-mediated. PG molecules are ubiquitous and present in nearly every human tissue. They participate in a variety of regulatory processes by interacting and/or modulating the activity of other hormones.

Many of the painful symptoms of PMS resemble symptoms of PG excess. There is ample evidence that PG inhibitors, or nonsteroidal antiinflammatory drugs (NSAIDs) effectively treat the pain component of PMS. NSAIDs administered 3 to 4 days premenstrually reduce breast tenderness.[16] Breast size may increase 30 to 40% premenstrually in affected women and be associated with mastalgia. PGE_1 and PGE_2 are found in human breast tissue and may mediate this breast swelling and tenderness; it is suspected that high local estrogen concentrations promote the biosynthesis of PG in the breast.[16]

A longer duration of nonsteroidal therapy is needed to treat other pain-related symptoms of PMS. Naproxen sodium (Naprosyn), 550 mg three times daily for 1 week premenstrually reduces symptoms of pain more effectively than placebo.[17] Mefenamic acid (Ponstel), 500 mg three times daily for 1 week premenstrually, reduces symptoms of pain more effectively than placebo.[17] Administered for 1 to 2 weeks, mefenamic acid effectively relieves lower abdominal/pelvic pain, backache, general aches and pains, and headache in 80 to 100% of women.[17]

A variety of NSAIDs are available for use, although only naproxen sodium and mefenamic acid have been evaluated for PMS therapy. The NSAIDs, as a group, have antiinflammatory, analgesic, antipyretic, and platelet-inhibitory properties.[17] The major mechanism of action of NSAIDs is the inhibition of cyclooxygenase activity and PG synthesis. Comparative trials of NSAIDs seldom demonstrate clinically important differences between agents, but variability between patients in efficacy and preference for different NSAIDs is commonly seen in clinical practice.[17]

The most frequent adverse reactions to NSAIDs are gastrointestinal, with dyspepsia being most common.[17] Gastric erosion, peptic ulcerations, and gastrointestinal hemorrhage are much less common, and are usually seen in patients with a history of peptic ulcer disease. Misoprostol (Cytotec) is the only drug approved to prevent NSAID-induced ulcers, and it effectively prevents both duodenal and gastric ulcers. However, the potential teratogenicity, incidence of diarrhea, and frequent dosing make misoprostol an unattractive option for many women. Sucralfate (Carafate) and H_2-antagonists usually do not prevent the more common gastric ulcers. In contrast, omeprazole (Prilosec), 20 mg taken once daily, is better tolerated than misoprostol and effectively treats both ulcer types in high-risk patients on NSAIDs.[18]

Renal toxicity is the second major category of side effect.[17] NSAIDs can cause reduced glomerular filtration, acute renal failure, interstitial nephritis, papillary necrosis, chronic renal failure, and hyperkalemia. Since therapy is generally given cyclically for 1 to 2 weeks per month in patients with PMS, the risk of significant gastrointestinal or renal toxicity is low. However, patients with preexisting renal impairment and hypovolemia are at greatest risk. Moreover, diuretics in combination with NSAIDs are associated with an increased risk of renal failure, and potassium-sparing diuretics in combination with NSAIDs increase the risk of potassium retention and hyperkalemia. Consequently, any patient with PMS receiving both medications should have serum electrolytes, blood nitrogen, and creatinine monitored.[17]

Sulindac (Clinoril) and nabumetone (Relafen) have been reported to cause less renal insufficiency because of the absence of active urinary nephrotoxic metabolites. In contrast, fenoprofen (Nalfon) has been implicated in 71% of NSAID-induced nephrotic syndrome cases.[17]

In addition to gastrointestinal and renal side effects, NSAIDs have caused undesirable nervous system and hepatic adverse effects. Table 49-4 compares the side-effect profiles of the NSAIDs.

An NSAID should be selected based on previous history of response, efficacy, tolerability, safety, and cost. Generically available NSAIDs include meclofenamate, ibuprofen, fenoprofen, ketoprofen, and naproxen. Patients who fail to benefit from one NSAID should be prescribed an agent from a different pharmacologic class. For instance, if the acetic acid etodolac (Lodine) does not adequately relieve pain, it would be useful to try a propionic acid, such as ketoprofen (Orudis) rather than another acetic acid, such as ketoralac (Toradol) (see Table 49-4).

Pain-related symptoms begin in the luteal phase and persist until menstruation. NSAID therapy should be initiated just prior to the onset of pain, and therapy should continue until menstruation begins. If dysmenorrhea is also a problem, NSAID therapy is continued until menstruation ceases. Once an NSAID has been selected, the doses should be increased until pain has been relieved or the maximum tolerable dose has been achieved. Some clinicians have used rather large doses with remarkable success.

Hormones

Hormonal treatments are based on the theory that the hypothalamic–pituitary–ovarian (HPO) axis plays a role in the generation of PMS symptoms. Therefore, changing the hormonal milieu may lessen symptoms and result in therapeutic benefit.

PROGESTERONE Though most well-controlled studies investigating natural progesterone (administered in suppository or micronized oral form) or the closely related progestins have demonstrated no benefit in treating premenstrual mood symptoms,[12,20] occasional reports have suggested efficacy. Moreover, many women as well as clinicians maintain strong advocacy for this treatment. Natural progesterone appears to be a benign treatment without major side effects.

ORAL CONTRACEPTIVES Oral contraceptives (OCs) may be beneficial to women with PMS because they inhibit ovulation by suppressing the release of the pituitary gonadotropins FSH and luteinizing hormone (LH).[21] OCs have been shown to be effective in treating some physical symptoms of PMS,[12] but their effect on emotional symptoms, particularly depression, is less clear. Evidence is also inconclusive as to whether monophasics (continuous estrogen–progestin dosing) or triphasics (continuous estrogen and titrated progestin dosing) are more beneficial in PMS.

In one study, no significant differences were found between the effects of placebo or OCs on women's sense of well-being over three treatment cycles.[12] A triphasic OC was found to significantly decrease breast pain and edema as compared with placebo in a 3-month, placebo-controlled, randomized trial in 59 women.[12] Women in the active treatment group who had premenstrual depression reported greater improvement in energy levels, less work impairment, and decreased hypersomnia. However, there was no significant difference between placebo and the triphasic OC in the relief of mood symptoms. In another study, triphasics caused more mood changes than monophasics.[12]

OC-related depression has been attributed to estrogen excess, progestin excess, estrogen deficiency, and pyridoxine (vitamin B_6) deficiency in approximately 5 to 6% of OC users.[22] Thus, either a low-dose monophasic or triphasic should be prescribed to minimize depressive symptoms that might be due to either estrogen or progestin excess. Figure 49-3 lists

TABLE 49-4
RELATIVE SIDE EFFECTS OF NONSTEROIDAL ANTIINFLAMMATORY DRUGS BY PHARMACOLOGIC CLASSIFICATION

Pharmacologic Class	Typical Dosage	Gastrointestinal	Central Nervous System	Hepatic	Renal
Salicylates					
Aspirin	325 mg four times a day	++++++	+	++	++
Diflunisal (Dolobid)	500 mg twice a day	++	+	+	+
Fenamates					
Meclofenamate (Meclomen)*	50 mg three times a day/ four times a day	++	+	+	++
Mefenamic acid (Ponstel)	250 mg four times a day	++	+	+	++
Acetic acids					
Etodolac (Lodine)	200–400 mg twice a day/ three times a day	++	+	+	++
Diclofenac (Voltaren, Cataflam)	50 mg twice a day/three times a day	++	+	+	++
Indomethacin (Indocin)	25–50 mg three times a day	++	+++	++	++
Ketoralac (Toradol)	10 mg three times a day/four times a day	++	+	+	+
Nabumetone (Relafen)	500–750 mg twice a day	++	++	+	+
Sulindac (Clinoril)	150–200 mg twice a day	++	++	+	+
Tolmetin (Tolectin)	200–600 mg three times a day	+	++	+	++
Propionic acids					
Ibuprofen (Motrin)*	200–800 mg four times a day	++	+	+	++
Fenoprofen (Nalfon)*	200–300 mg three times a day/ four times a day	++	++	+	++
Flurbiprofen (Ansaid)	100 mg twice a day/three times a day	++	++	+	+
Ketoprofen (Orudis, Actron)*	5–75 mg three times a day	++	+	+	++
Naproxen (Naprosyn)*	250–500 mg twice a day	++	+	+	++
Naproxen sodium (Anaprox)	275–550 mg twice a day	++	++	+	++
Oxaprozin (Daypro)	1200 mg a day	++	++	+	+
Oxicams					
Piroxicam (Feldene)	20 mg a day	+++	++	+	+

+ = minimum; ++ = mild; +++ = moderate.

*Available generically.

Adapted with permission from Dipiro JT, Talbert RL, Yee, GC, et al, eds. Pharmacotherapy: a pathophysiologic approach. 4th ed. Stamford, CT: Appleton & Lange, 1999:1018.

the relative hormonal potencies of the currently available OCs. Women who become depressed while taking OCs may be candidates to receive pyridoxine replacement therapy at 50 mg/day.[22]

Patients may be particularly sensitive to the estrogen, progestin, or androgenic effects of OCs. For example, a progestin-sensitive woman with PMS may have a history of depression and fatigue. This patient may benefit from a pill with very low progestational activity. An estrogen-sensitive woman with PMS may have a history of migraine, heavy menstrual cramps, and premenstrual nausea. This patient may benefit from an OC containing a very low dose of estrogen. However, she should be cautioned that spotting may occur, menses may be light or skipped, and missed pills could result in breakthrough ovulation. An androgenic-sensitive woman with PMS may report severe acne and would benefit from an OC with estrogenic activity and almost no androgenic activity. Table 49-5 lists the estrogenic, progestational, and androgenic side effects that may exacerbate specific premenstrual symptoms.

Clearly, more long-term prospective studies are required to critically test monophasic and triphasic OCs in the treatment of PMS. However, since OCs are such commonly prescribed medications, both patients and clinicians may feel more comfortable with their use as initial therapy and when physical rather than emotional symptoms predominate.

GONADOTROPIN-RELEASING HORMONE AGONISTS
More recently, attention has focused on the efficacy of gonadotropin-releasing hormone (GnRH) agonists in the treatment of PMS. GnRH agonists are synthetic analogs of naturally occurring GnRH, which suppress ovulation by inhibiting the release of pituitary

Progestin		Very Low	Intermediate	High
↑	**High**	*Loestrin 1/20** Mircette†	*Demulen 1/35†* Desogen† *Estrostep†§* *Loestrin 1.5/30** Ortho-Cept† *Zovia 1/35†*	Demulen 1/50† **Ogestrel*** **Ovral*** Zovia 1/35†
	Intermediate		Jenest†§ Levlen‡ Levora‡ Low-Ogestrel‡ LoOvral‡ Necon 1/35‡ Necon 10/11†§ Nelova 1/35‡ Nelova 10/11†§ Nordette‡ Norethin 1/35E‡ Norinyl 1/35‡ Ortho-Novum 1/35‡ Ortho-Novum 7/7/7†§ Ortho-Novum 10/11†§	Necon 1/50M‡ Nelova 1/50‡ Norethin 1/50‡ Norinyl 1/50‡ Norlestrin 1/50‡ Ortho-Novum 1/50‡ Ovcon 1/50‡
↓	**Low**	*Alesse†* *Levlite†* *Micronor†* *Nor-QD†* *Ovrette†*	*Brevicon†* *Modicon†* *Necon 0.5/35†* *Nelova 0.5/35†* Ortho-Cyclen†§ Ortho TriCyclen†§ Ovcon35† Tri-Levlen†§ *Tri-Norinyl†§* Triphasil†§ Tribora	
		Very Low	**Intermediate**	**High**
			← **Estrogen** →	

Figure 49-3 Relative estrogenic, progestational, androgenic, and endometrial activities of commonly prescribed oral contraceptives. *High androgenic activity. †Low androgenic activity. ‡Intermediate androgenic activity. §Multiphasic oral contraceptives. All others are monophasic oral contraceptives. *Italics* font shows low endometrial activity (increased spotting) Regular font shows intermediate endometrial activity **Bold** font shows high endometrial activity (decreased spotting) Adapted with permission from Dickey RP, ed. Managing contraceptive pill patients. 10th ed. Dallas, TX: EMIS Medical Publishers, 2000:98.

gonadotropins. They have been evaluated in nine studies, six of which were controlled.[12] Specific agents have included nafarelin (Synaref), goserelin (Zoladex), and leuprolide (Leupron) administered subcutaneously, intramuscularly, and nasally. All studies have found GnRH agonists to be effective in treating behavioral and physical symptoms of PMS, with the greatest response occurring with breast tenderness, bloating, irritability, and tension.

Three studies have shown that women with PMS and severe premenstrual dysphoria or premenstrual exacerbation of a mood disorder do not improve with GnRH agonists as compared with those without depressive symptoms.[12,23] These findings are consistent

TABLE 49-5
RELATIONSHIP OF HORMONE CONTENT TO EXACERBATION OF PREMENSTRUAL SYMPTOMS

Estrogen		Progestin	
Excess	**Deficiency**	**Excess**	**Deficiency**
Nausea, bloating	Early or midcycle breakthrough bleeding	Depression	Late cycle breakthrough bleeding
Breast tenderness		Tiredness, fatigue	
Edema	Hypomenorrhea	Increased appetite	Hypermenorrhea
Migraine headache	Increased spotting	Acne, oily scalp*	Dysmenorrhea
Weight gain (cyclic)	Nervousness	Weight gain (noncyclic)	
Hypermenorrhea	Vasomotor symptoms	Hypomenorrhea	

*Androgenic activity of progestin.

Adapted with permission from Dickey RP, ed. Managing contraceptive pill patients. 10th ed. Dallas, TX: EMIS Medical Publishers, 2000:102.

with some studies conducted with OCs,[11] and suggest that women should be evaluated for a mood disorder prior to initiation of both OCs and GnRH agonist therapy.

The main concern with long-term use of GnRH agonist therapy is osteoporosis and loss of cardioprotective effects of endogenous estrogen. The use of these agents alone is therefore recommended for no more than 6 consecutive months. Although adding back estrogen and progesterone can theoretically protect against the long-term consequences of ovarian steroid deficiency and prolong the use of these agents, studies[12] investigating "add-back" therapy found improvement was greatest for PMS subjects receiving GnRH agonists alone, followed by GnRH agonists and add-back therapy, and then placebo. Until more data are available, GnRH agonists should be reserved for patients with severe physical symptoms refractory to other treatments without a previous or current history of depression, and as a reversible medical trial when surgical oophorectomy is being considered. Leuprolide (Lupron) 3.75 mg intramuscularly monthly with low-dose estrogen/progestin add-back therapy is generally prescribed.

Diuretics

Abdominal bloating, edema, and weight gain are common premenstrual symptoms that should be initially treated by sodium restriction. Diuretics may be considered if dietary alterations are unsuccessful in reducing fluid retention.

Treatment of premenstrual symptoms have been evaluated in four controlled studies of spironolactone (100 mg/day)[12,24] and one controlled study of metolazone (2 to 5 mg/day).[12] Four of five studies found a reduction in abdominal bloating, one reported decreased weight gain, and one reported improved mood. The majority of women receiving metalozone 5 mg/day experienced excessive diuresis, with resulting weakness and electrolyte disturbances.[12]

Spironolactone is the agent of choice because of the larger number of controlled studies conducted and its improved tolerance. It is a mild potassium-sparing diuretic, acting as an aldosterone antagonist at the level of the distal renal tubules. Short-course, low-dose therapy (25 to 50 mg twice daily) during the luteal phase is recommended in women who experience severe bloating or fluid retention uncontrolled by diet.

By evaluating a patient's symptom calendar, it is possible to identify the day in the menstrual cycle on which water retention and weight gain begin. Diuretic therapy is best initiated at the time of onset of water retention and administered daily until the onset of menstruation, when spontaneous resolution of symptoms usually occurs. Diuretics effectively eliminate disturbing premenstrual weight gain and water retention when they are administered in this fashion.

Diuretics may cause intravascular depletion, electrolyte disturbance, and side effects such as fatigue, headache, irregular bleeding (in the case of spironolactone) and adverse drug interactions. Consequently, the clinician should use the lowest effective dosage in a cyclic manner, monitor electrolytes, blood urea nitrogen, and creatinine intermittently, and generally reserve diuretic use for patients with PMS who document premenstrual weight gain on their daily diary.

Antidepressants

Because the most troubling symptoms of PMS are usually mood-related, the antidepressants offer an important treatment option. Moreover, since alterations in neurotransmitters such as serotonin (5-HT) and norepinephrine (NE) may be associated with PMS, there is a theoretical basis for investigating the efficacy of antidepressants. Controlled trials have been conducted with antidepressants to determine whether they are more effective than placebo in the treatment of PMS.

TRICYCLIC ANTIDEPRESSANTS Noradrenergic (e.g., nortriptyline [Pamelor], desipramine [Norpramir]) and serotoninergic (e.g., clomipramine) tricyclic antidepressants (TCAs) have been evaluated in the treatment of PMS. An open-label trial evaluating the use of nortriptyline (50 to 125 mg/day), and controlled studies of continuous and luteal-phase dosing of clomipramine (Anafranil) (25 to 75 mg/day) have reported significantly improved symptoms in women with PMDD.[12]

Comparative trials have favored the efficacy and tolerability of serotoninergic over noradrenergic antidepressants in the treatment of PMS. An open-label comparison of 32 women with PMS receiving the serotoninergic antidepressant sertraline (Zoloft) (mean, 87 mg/day) showed decreased premenstrual symptoms more than the adrenergic antidepressant desipramine (mean, 110 mg/day), but not significantly, and was better tolerated.[12] In a larger double-blind, placebo-controlled trial of 81 patients with PMS, the serotoninergic antidepressant paroxetine (Paxil) was superior to the noradrenergic antidepressant

TABLE 49-6			
COST FOR 30 DAYS OF TREATMENT ACCORDING TO ANTIDEPRESSANT AND TYPICAL DOSAGE			

Medication	Typical Dosage	Cost for 30 Days of Treatment	Daily Dose Range
Generic nortiptyline	75 mg four times a day	$66.41	20–150 mg
Nortriptyline (Pamelor)	75 mg four times a day	$105.61	20–150 mg
Generic desipramine	150 mg four times a day	$65.70	75–300 mg
Desipramine (Norpramin)	150 mg four times a day	$98.86	75–300 mg
Fluoxetine (Prozac)*	20 mg four times a day	$79.22	20–80 mg
Sertraline (Zoloft)*	100 mg four times a day	$72.29	50–200 mg
Paroxetine (Paxil)*	20 mg four times a day	$69.86	20–50 mg
Fluvoxamine (Luvox)*	100 mg four times a day	$84.66	50–300 mg
Nefazodone (Serzone)*	200 mg twice a day	$74.11	100–600 mg
Venlafaxine (Effexor)*	100 mg twice a day	$88.43	75–375 mg

*Not available generically.

†Prices for drugs represent the average wholesale price of the drug, which reflects the average acquisition cost.

Adapted with permission from Cardinale V, ed. 2000 Drug topics red book. Montvale, NJ: Medical Economics, 2000.

maprotiline (Ludiomil) for some symptoms (e.g., irritability, food cravings, bloating, breast tenderness), but both antidepressants were superior to placebo in reducing premenstrual depression and anxiety.[12] Similarly, a study comparing fluoxetine (Prozac) with bupropion (Wellbutrin) and placebo found that fluoxetine led to greater improvement than either bupropion or placebo.[25] These preliminary data suggest that serotoninergic antidepressants may be more effective in treating the overall symptom distress of PMS, but both types of antidepressants are effective in improving mood. While serotoninergic antidepressants are generally more tolerable, generic noradrenergic antidepressants may be a choice when cost is a concern. Table 49-6 compares the cost of antidepressants at standard dosages. Additional controlled trials are needed to provide definitive information on the comparative efficacy of serotoninergic and noradrenergic compounds in the treatment of PMS.

SELECTIVE SEROTONIN REUPTAKE INHIBITORS
Newer studies have focused on serotoninergic antidepressants because of the underlying theory of serotonin involvement in PMS.

Fluoxetine was the first selective serotonin reuptake inhibitor (SSRI) to be investigated. Eight double-blind, placebo-controlled trials have demonstrated acute efficacy and one study has shown a sustained response.[12] Notable among the fluoxetine studies was a 6-month placebo-controlled multicenter study that investigated a 20 mg/day dose versus a 60 mg/day dose in 180 women with LLPDD.[26] Fluoxetine was superior to placebo at both doses, but subjects receiving the higher dose reported significantly more side effects. Although this was the first large multicenter study of fluoxetine, the focus was on three of the most common symptoms of PMDD, rather than on the spectrum of symptoms stipulated by the DSM-IV; also, functional impairment was not assessed. Recently, fluoxetene (Sarafem) was approved for the treatment of PMD by the Food and Drug Administration (FDA), and other SSRIs are currently being evaluated for a similar indication.

Yonkers and colleagues[27] conducted a 3-month multicenter study of sertaline in 200 women with PMDD. Sertraline (50 to 150 mg/day) was significantly better than placebo in reducing DSM-IV criteria symptoms as well as in improving relationships, social activities, and work production. Sertraline has also been used as luteal-phase treatment in 11 patients in a crossover study.[12] One open and one controlled study have shown paroxetine to be effective in decreasing premenstrual dysphoric symptoms in women with PMS.[12] Fluvoxamine (Luvox) (150 mg/day) was found to be no more effective than placebo in a 2-month controlled trial in 20 women with premenstrual symptoms, but in a more recent 2-month open study, 10 women with PMDD who received fluvoxamine (100 mg/day) showed significant improvement in premenstrual symptoms over base line.[12] The discrepancy in results may be related to differences in populations and dosages selected. Citalopram (Celexa) has also been reported for the treatment of premenstrual irritability or depressed

TABLE 49-7
SIDE-EFFECT PROFILES OF ANTIDEPRESSANTS USED TO TREAT PREMENSTRUAL DEPRESSION

Drug	Gastrointestinal Effects	Anticholinergic Effects	Sedation	Hypotension	Conduction Effects	Sexual Dysfunction	Weight Gain
Citalopram	0	+	+	0	0	++++	+
Desipramine	+	++	++	++	++	+++	+++
Nortriptyline	+	++	++	+	++	+++	+++
Fluoxetine	++	0	0	0	0	++++	0
Fluvoxamine	+++	0	0	0	0	++++	0
Paroxetine	++	+	+	0	0	++++	++
Sertraline	++	0	0	0	0	++++	+
Nefazodone	++	0	+++	+++	+	0	+
Venlafaxine	+++	+	+	0	+	++	+

0 = none; + = very low; ++ = low; +++ = moderate; ++++ = high.

Adapted with permission from Dipiro JT, Talbert RL, Yee GC, et al., eds. Pharmacotherapy: a pathophysiologic approach. 4th ed. Stamford, CT: Appleton & Lange, 1999:1148.

mood.[36] Intermittent luteal-phase dosing was more effective than placebo.

The primary benefits of the SSRIs over TCAs include tolerability, which is evidenced by substantially lower treatment termination rates due to side effects, and safety in overdose situations. As a class, the SSRIs lack significant sedative, anticholinergic, or cardiovascular effects, and are especially useful in women with coexisting medical illnesses. The adverse-effect profiles of the different SSRIs are similar, and include mild to moderate nausea, headache, dizziness, tremor, insomnia, and sexual dysfunction. Notable differences may be a higher incidence of anxiety and insomnia with fluoxetine, greater degrees of sedation, constipation, and dry mouth with paroxetine, and more diarrhea with sertraline.[28] Table 49-7 compares the side-effect profiles of the TCAs, SSRIs and the newer serotoninergic antidepressants.

Sexual dysfunction, including decreased libido, and anorgasmia, are associated with the SSRIs.[29] All of the drugs in this class seem equally likely to cause these problems. Management of sexual dysfunction includes allowing for tolerance to develop over time, or a reduction in dosage, as the degree of dysfunction is dose-related. If these measures are unsuccessful, then yohimbine (Yohimex, 5.4 mg), cyproheptadine (Periactin, 4 mg), bethanechol (Urecholine, 25 to 50 mg), or amantadine (Symmetrel, 100 to 300 mg) administered 1 hour prior to intercourse may be useful.[29] If the above methods are ineffective, switching to nefazodone (Serzone) or bupropion, which are not associated with sexual dysfunction, might be preferable.

While the side-effect profiles of the SSRIs are similar, there are important pharmacokinetic differ-

ences within this class. The primary difference is that fluoxetine has a longer elimination half-life of 1 to 3 days and also has an active metabolite, norfluoxetine, with an even longer half-life (7 to 10 days).[28] In contrast, sertraline, paroxetine, and fluvoxamine have elimination half-lives of about 1 day or less and are metabolized to clinically inactive compounds.[28]

The longer half-lives of fluoxetine and norfluoxetine may produce some clinical disadvantages. Since it takes several weeks to reach steady state with fluoxetine and response may not occur until after 3 weeks, allowance of adequate time for antidepressant response at lower doses (4 to 6 weeks) should occur before making dosage increases.[28] Moreover, a period of at least 5 weeks is required for elimination of fluoxetine from the body, whereas paroxetine, sertraline, and fluvoxamine are eliminated in 1 to 2 weeks. Finally, in the event of need for abrupt drug discontinuation due to pregnancy or an adverse reaction, fluoxetine's effects will persist.[28]

The SSRIs and other new antidepressants have varying effects on hepatic microsomal enzyme systems, and increasing knowledge about these effects provides useful information for predicting potential drug interactions. Fluoxetine and paroxetine are potent inhibitors of the CYP2D6 isoenzyme that is involved in the metabolism of TCAs, antipsychotics, and type 1C antiarrhythmics (e.g., propafenone, Rythmol).[30] Fluoxetine coadministration has been reported to increase serum TCA levels by two- to fourfold and can produce severe toxicity. Similar interactions have also occurred using TCAs shortly after fluoxetine discontinuation, due to its long elimination half-life. Sertraline and fluvoxamine are less potent inhibitors of the 2D6 isozyme in vitro and

TABLE 49-8
POTENTIAL CYTOCHROME P450 INTERACTIONS FOR SEROTONINERGIC ANTIDEPRESSANTS

CYPP450 Isoenzyme and Target Drugs	Inhibitory Effects of:					
	Fluoxetine	Fluvoxamine	Paroxetine	Sertraline	Nefazodone	Venlafaxine
CYP2D6						
Antiarrhythmics, antipsychotics, β-blockers, *opiates, TCAs*	+++	+	+++	+	+	+
CYP3A4						
Antiarrhythmics, TCAs, bupropion, *benzodiazepines,* calcium blockers, *nonsedating antihistamines*	++	++	−	+	+++	+
CYP2C9						
NSAIDs, TCAs, *warfarin*	−	−	−	+	−	−
CYP2C19						
TCAs, benzodiazepines, β-*blockers,* phenytoin, barbiturates, omeprazole	++	+++	?	+	−	−
CYP1A2						
Antipsychotics, β-blockers, TCAs, calcium blockers, *warfarin, theophylline,* tacrine	+	+++	+	+	−	−

− = none; + = minimal; ++ = mild; +++ = moderate; ? = no data.

Adapted with permission from Perry PJ, Alexander B, Liskow BI, eds. Psychotropic drug handbook. 7th ed. Washington, DC: American Psychiatric Press, Inc. 1997:453; and Preskorn SH. Cytochrome P450 enzymes: interpretation of their interactions with selective serotonin reuptake inhibitors, Part II. J Clin Psychopharmacol 1996;16:347.

*Drugs in italic type have moderately severe drug interactions. All others have mildly severe drug interactions.

may be less likely to produce significant drug interactions by this mechanism.

Other potential drug interactions with the SSRIs and drugs eliminated by the CYP3A4, CYP2C9, CYP2C19, CYP1A2 pathways are indicated in Table 49-8. The clinical effect of the drug interactions between SSRIs and other agents is dependent on the half-life of the particular SSRI and the target drug, the doses of both agents given, and the extent of inhibition by the SSRI. Using SSRIs in patients maintained on warfarin (Coumadin) should be accompanied by careful monitoring of the international normalized ratio (INR) and for excessive anticoagulation, since SSRIs inhibit the CYP2C9 and CYP1A2 pathways.[30]

One property of fluoxetine and paroxetine is that the usual starting dose of these agents, 20 mg/day, is often the effective antidepressant dose, thus avoiding the need for dose titration. The daily dose of paroxetine may be increased up to 50 mg, according to therapeutic effects and tolerability, but maximal response is seen in the range of 20 to 30 mg/day. Sertraline is usually initiated at 50 mg/day, and most patients require 100 mg/day for response. Patients with a significant anxiety component to their premenstrual symptoms should be started at lower doses, such as 10 mg/day of fluoxetine or paroxetine or 25 mg/day of sertraline, and titrated up to the standard dosage range over 8 to 12 weeks.

Because most SSRIs have been shown to be effective in treating premenstrual symptoms, what remains to be determined is the optimal timing of their administration. Studies of clomipramine[35], citalopram[36], and sertraline[37] suggest that half-cycle dosing may be effective and, if so, would certainly be more convenient and less costly for the patient. Future research should be designed to address this point.

NEWER SEROTONINERGIC ANTIDEPRESSANTS Initial studies with nefazodone (Serzone), an antidepressant structurally similar to trazodone, and venlafaxine (Effexor), an antidepressant pharmacologically similar to the TCAs, have been conducted in women with PMS. Daily treatment with nefazodone was evaluated in an 8-week open-label study in 23 women with PMS and 24 women with PMS and concurrent major depression or dysthymia.[12] Premenstrual symptoms significantly improved for both the PMS and premenstrual exacerbation groups, and nefazodone was well tolerated at doses of 100 to 600 mg/day.

One clinical disadvantage of nefazodone is that twice-daily dosing is required. However, it is not associated with sexual dysfunction and its cost may be lower than the SSRIs. Since nefaxodone's mechanism of action is distinct from other available antidepressants, it may also be a reasonable choice for women who do not respond to other therapies.

Venlafaxine also shows promise for the treatment of PMDD. A large multicenter trial employed rigorous standards, including DSM-IV criteria, subjective and objective measures, and measurement of both follicular and luteal phases. Women were found to have very few side effects when venlafaxine was started at a dose of 25 mg twice daily, then increased by 25 mg/day each cycle if needed. During treatment, daily ratings showed stabilization in symptoms of mood, irritability, and anger as well as in somatic symptoms.[31]

Venlafaxine has a similar pharmacologic profile to TCAs, but it has a more attractive side-effect and safety profile (see Table 49-7), and it does not significantly affect hepatic enzyme systems (see Table 49-8). Venlafaxine's adverse-effect profile is similar to that of the SSRIs (primarily nausea, sedation, and dizziness) with one notable exception—venlafaxine-treated patients have experienced mild increases in diastolic blood pressure, which is most common with doses greater than 200 mg/day. Venlafaxine therapy should be accompanied by blood pressure monitoring, especially at higher doses and in women with preexisting hypertension. Like nefazodone, venlafaxine requires divided daily dosing. Twice-daily dosing has been found to have effectiveness comparable to three-times-daily dosing, and is preferred to enhance compliance. Even though venlafaxine requires multiple dosing and is as expensive as the SSRIs, it may be helpful in patients with PMDD who have not responded to other treatments or in cases when the drug interaction profile of other antidepressants is problematic.

Anxiolytics

Treatment with the anxiolytic alprazolam (Xanax; 0.75 to 2.25 mg/day) in the luteal phase has met with some success, although not all studies showed effectiveness.[12] The initial side effect of drowsiness usually subsides in a short time.[12,32] Dependence, which is always a concern when treating with benzodiazepines, has not been demonstrated in patients carefully diagnosed with PMS when dosing is limited to the luteal phase.[12]

Effective treatment of PMS has also been noted with buspirone (Buspar), a nonbenzodiazepine 5-HT_{1A}

partial agonist anxiolytic, during luteal-phase dosing (30 mg/day).[33] Buspirone may be particularly helpful for anxious patients with PMS who are inappropriate candidates for benzodiazepines, such as women with a history of alcohol or substance abuse, chronic pain, or personality disorders, and for those in whom irritability is a major symptom. Results from a large trial are needed to confirm or refute these preliminary findings.

In women in whom premenstrual panic attacks develop, alprazolam, clonazepam (Klonopin), and lorazepam (Ativan) are the high-potency benzodiazepines most commonly prescribed; however, alprazolam is the only benzodiazepine labeled for use in treating panic disorder.[34] Benzodiazepines are better tolerated and ameliorate panic attacks and anticipatory anxiety more rapidly than TCAs.[34] Benzodiazepines are often administered during the first 8 to 12 weeks of antidepressant therapy to reduce drug-induced panic attacks.

Benzodiazepine doses must be gradually increased to avoid sedation and psychomotor impairment. Alprazolam can be initiated in doses of 0.25 mg to 0.5 mg four times/day, with gradual increases of 0/25 mg to 0.5 mg every 3 to 4 days until panic attacks abate.[34] Most patients respond to daily doses of 2 to 4 mg to maximally reduce premenstrual panic attacks. Breakthrough anxiety and panic attacks may occur at 3 to 5 hours after the last alprazolam concentrations. A higher dose, more frequent alprazolam dosage intervals, or a switch to clonazepam can alleviate this problem.[34] Clonazepam, because of its longer half-life, is associated with fewer interdose symptoms, and a less frequent dosage schedule of once or twice daily. For women with significant generalized anxiety, but without panic attacks, lower doses of benzodiazepines (1 to 2 mg/day of alprazolam in divided doses or its equivalent) may be titrated premenstrually.

The primary differences among the benzodiazepines are in their pharmacokinetic properties, and these often are among the main factors associated in drug selection. The benzodiazepines, which are metabolized by oxidation, are longer-acting and more likely to interact with other drugs as compared with those metabolized by conjugation. The lipophilicity (fat solubility) of the agent determines its onset of action and degree of abuse potential. Table 49-9 illustrates the currently available benzodiazepines according to equipotent dosage, onset and duration of action, and metabolic pathway.

TABLE 49-9
PHARMACOKINETIC COMPARISON OF BENZODIAZEPINES

Drug	Equipotent Dose	Rate of Onset	Duration of Action	Metabolic Pathway
Chlordiazepoxide (Librium)*	10	Intermediate	Long	Oxidation
Diazepam (Valium)*	5	Very fast	Long	Oxidation
Oxazepam (Serax)*	15	Slow	Short	Conjugation
Clorazepate (Tranxene)*	7.5	Fast	Long	Oxidation
Lorazepam (Ativan)*	1	Intermediate	Short	Conjugation
Alprazolam (Xanax)	0.5	Intermediate	Short	Conjugation
Clonazepam (Klonopin)	0.25	Fast	Intermediate	Oxidation

*Available generically.

Adapted with permission from Dipiro JT, Talbert RL, Yee GC, et al., eds. Pharmacotherapy: a pathophysiologic approach. 3rd ed. Stamford, CT: Appleton & Lange, 1997:1449.

Surgery

Ovariectomy has been reported to be successful in extreme recalcitrant cases of PMS.[12] Surgical therapy should be a last resort and should always be preceded by treatment with a GnRH agonist as a reversible medical oophorectomy.

REFERENCES

1. Smith S, Schiff I. Premenstrual syndrome: controversy and consensus. In: Smith S, Schiff I, eds. Modern management of premenstrual syndrome. New York: Norton, 1993:3.
2. Sondheimer SJ. Etiology of premenstrual syndrome. In: Smith S, Schiff I, eds. Modern management of premenstrual syndrome. New York: Norton, 1993:46.
3. World Health Organization. International statistical classification of diseases and related health problems. 10th rev. Geneva: World Health Organization, 1992.
4. American Psychiatric Association. Diagnostic and statistical manual of mental disorders. 3rd ed. Washington, DC: American Psychiatric Association, 1987.
5. American Psychiatric Association. Diagnostic and statistical manual of mental disorders. 4th ed. Washington, DC: American Psychiatric Association, 1994.
6. Yonkers KA. The association between premenstrual dysphoric disorder and other mood disorders. J Clin Psychiatry 1997;58(Suppl 15):19.
7. Chuong CJ, Burgos DM. Medical history in women with premenstrual syndrome. J Psychosom Obstet Gynecol 1995;16:21.
8. Schmidt P, Rubinow DR. Parallels between premenstrual syndrome and psychiatric illness. In: Smith S, Schiff I, eds. Modern management of premenstrual syndrome. New York: Norton, 1993:71.
9. Biddleman M, Seidman S. Premenstrual dysphoric disorder: assessment, diagnosis, and treatment options. Primary Psychiatry 1997;Oct:68.
10. Isaacson K, Balasubramanyam A. Relationship of medical illness to the menstrual cycle. In: Smith S, Schiff I, eds. Modern management of premenstrual syndrome. New York: Norton, 1993:82.
11. Severino SK, Moline ML. Diagnostic evaluation. In: Severino SK, Moline ML, eds. Premenstrual syndrome: a clinician's guide. New York: Guilford Press, 1989:142.
12. Brown CS, Freeman EW, Ling FW. An update on the treatment of premenstrual syndrome. Am J Man Care 1998;4:115.
13. Thys-Jacobs S, Starkey P, Bernstein D, et al. Calcium carbonate and the premenstrual syndrome: effects on premenstrual and menstrual symptoms. Am J Obstet Gynecol 1998;179:44.
14. Pearlstein T, Rivera-Tovar A, Frank E. Nonmedical management of late luteal phase dysphoric disorder. J Psychother Pract Res 1992;1:49.
15. Oleson T, Flocco W. Randomized controlled study of premenstrual symptoms treated with ear, hand, and foot reflexology. Obstet Gynecol 1993;82:906.
16. Budoff PW. Use of prostaglandin inhibitors in the treatment of PMS. Clin Obstet Gynecol 1987;30:453.
17. Brooks PM, Day RO. Nonsteroidal antiinflammatory drugs—differences and similarities. N Engl J Med 1991:324:1716.
18. Pharmacist's letter. Gastroenterology 1998;14(5):25.
19. Pharmacist's letter. Pain 1998;14(4):19.
20. Freeman E, Rickels K, Sondheimer SJ, Polanski M. Ineffectiveness of progesterone suppository treatment for premenstrual syndrome. JAMA 1990;264:349.
21. Barnhart KT, Freeman EW, Sondheimer SJ. A clinician's guide to the premenstrual syndrome. Office Gynecol 1995;79:1457.
22. Leeton J. Depression induced by oral contraception and the role of vitamin B_6 in its management. Aust NZ J Psychiatry 1974;8:85.
23. Brown CS, Ling FW, Andersen RN, et al. Efficacy of depot leuprolide in premenstrual syndrome: effect of symptom severity and type in a controlled trial. Obstet Gynecol 1994;84:779.
24. Smith S. Treatment for the physical symptoms of premenstrual syndrome. In: Smith S, Schiff I, eds. Modern management of premenstrual syndrome. New York: Norton, 1993:112.
25. Pearlstein TB, Stone AB, Lund SA, et al. Comparison of fluoxetine, bupropion, and placebo in the treatment of premenstrual dysphoric disorder. J Clin Psychopharmacol 1997;17:261.

26. Steiner M, Steinberg S, Stewart D, et al. Fluoxetine in the treatment of premenstrual dysphoria. N Engl J Med 1995; 332:1529.

27. Yonkers KA, Halbreich U, Freeman E, et al. Symptomatic improvement of premenstrual dysphoric disorder with sertraline treatment: a randomized controlled trial. JAMA 1997;278:983.

28. Grimsley SR. Mood disorders. In: Carter BL, Angaran DM, Lake KD, et al., eds. Pharmacotherapy self-assessment program. 2nd ed. Kansas City, MO: American College of Clinical Pharmacy; 1995:77.

29. Woodrum S, Brown CS. The management of SSRI-induced sexual dysfunction. Ann Pharmacother 1998; 32:1209.

30. Harvey AT, Preskorn SH. Cytochrome P450 enzymes: interpretation of their interaction with selective serotonin reuptake inhibitors. Part II. J Clin Psychopharmacol 1996;16:345.

31. Yonkers KA. Antidepressants in the treatment of premenstrual dysphoric disorder. J Clin Psychiatry 1997; 58(Suppl 14):4.

32. Freeman EW, Rickels K, Sondheimer SJ, et al. A double-blind trial of oral progesterone, alprazolam and placebo in treatment of severe premenstrual syndrome. JAMA 1995; 274:51.

33. Rickels K, Freeman E, Sondheimer S. Buspirone in treatment of premenstrual syndrome. Lancet 1989;1:777.

34. Kirkwood CK, Melton ST. Anxiety disorders. In: Carter BL, Angaran DM, Lake KD, et al., eds. Pharmacotherapy self-assessment program. 2nd ed. Kansas City, MO: American College of Clinical Pharmacy, 1995:111.

35. Sundblad C, Hedberg MA, Eriksson E. Clomipramine administered during the luteal phase reduces the symptoms of premenstrual syndrome: a placebo-controlled trial. Neuropsychopharmacol 1993;9:133.

36. Wikander I, Sundblad C, Andersch B, et al. Citaloprom in premenstrual dysphoria: is intermittent treatment during luteal phases more effective than continuous medication throughout the menstrual cycle? J Clinn Psychopharmacol 1998;18:390

37. Freeman EW, Rickels K, Arredondo F, et al. Full- or half-cycle treatment of severe premenstrual syndrome with a serotonergic antidepressant. J Clin Psychopharmacol 1999;19:3.

Chapter 50

Management of Menopause

Raymond W. Ke

Five Key Points

- Menopause is a physiologic state of oocyte depletion in mid-life women resulting in a relative estrogen deficiency.
- Estrogen deficiency results in numerous short- and long-term symptoms and disease.
- Treatment of the menopausal woman involves management of diet and lifestyle and promotion of preventive care.
- An integral component of preventive care for most menopausal women is estrogen replacement therapy.
- For certain women, there are risks and side effects associated with estrogen replacement, and treatment plans need to be individualized.

A mountain of articles and books written on various aspects of the menopausal period in women have recently appeared. The interest is not surprising since there are currently more than 30 million women past menopause in the United States, all of whom can reasonably expect to live over a third of their lifetimes in the postmenopausal period. This figure will increase to 37.9 million women by the year 2010 and 45.9 million by 2020.[1] Approximately 70% of women will experience at least one troublesome menopausal symptom, leading to an estimated 10 million visits to physicians annually. Since this encounter may be the first for many of these women in several years, it can serve as an opportunity for a timely reevaluation of health maintenance. A consideration of diet, exercise, smoking, alcohol consumption, and other lifestyle choices is important and should not be ignored. In addition, a logical decision to take or not to take estrogen-replacement therapy (ERT) or hormone-replacement therapy (HRT), based on an assessment of the risks and benefits, should form a part of this reevaluation. The management of menopause and the postmenopausal years should continue to be a major focus of health-care providers.

DEFINITIONS

To provide consistency and clarify any confusion surrounding the terminology associated with menopause, the following set of definitions, published in the WHO Technical Report, will be used[2]:

Natural menopause is defined as the permanent cessation of menstruation, resulting from the loss of ovarian follicular activity. Natural menopause occurs with the final menstrual period and is recognized with certainty only in retrospect, to have occurred after 12 months of amenorrhea for which there is no obvious pathologic or physiological cause. An adequate, independent biological marker for this event does not exist.

Perimenopause includes the period immediately prior to menopause (when the clinical features of approaching menopause commence) and the first year after menopause. In the past, this was referred to as the climacteric, a much less precise term that should be abandoned to avoid confusion.

Premenopause refers to the entire reproductive period prior to menopause.

Induced menopause is defined as the cessation of menstruation that follows either surgical removal of both ovaries, with or without hysterectomy, or iatrogenic ablation of ovarian function (e.g., by chemotherapy or radiation).

Postmenopause is defined as the period of time dating from the final menstrual period, regardless of whether the menopause was induced or spontaneous.

Premature menopause is defined as menopause that occurs at an age more than 2 SD below the mean age of menopause in the reference population. In practice, without reliable estimates of the distribution of age of natural menopause in developing countries, the age of 40 years is frequently used as an arbitrary cut-off point, below which menopause is said to be premature.

PATHOPHYSIOLOGY

The average age at menopause of 51 years has remained remarkably constant throughout the centuries, unaffected by improving nutrition and reduction of disease. However, certain chemotherapeutic agents, radiation, smoking, and even hysterectomy, can contribute to an earlier onset of menopause. Many younger women have had their ovaries surgically removed, and a smaller number who have had premature ovarian failure undergo menopause before the age of 40.

Assuming a natural course of events, beginning around age 40, as a woman's finite store of oocytes begins to deplete, ovarian follicles show a progressive increase in resistance to stimulation from pituitary gonadotropins as reflected in a compensatory rise in circulating follicle-stimulating hormone (FSH) and luteinizing hormone (LH). These changes are accompanied by diminished ovarian estradiol secretion and, ultimately, by sporadic ovarian activity. As a consequence, menstrual cycles are more likely to be anovulatory, with prolonged or erratic intermenstrual intervals and variable (at times excessive) menstrual flow. With the eventual loss of gametes, ovarian estradiol and progesterone production decreases to the point at which it cannot sustain endometrial development,

and amenorrhea ensues. High menopausal levels of FSH may rarely initiate follicular development of an isolated follicle or two in the menopausal years, while high LH levels continue to stimulate the interstitial cells of the ovary to secrete the weak androgen androstenedione. Androstenedione secreted from both the ovary and adrenal gland is converted in peripheral fat to biologically weak estrone, the predominant estrogen of the menopausal years.

Since estrogen receptors are present in many organs throughout the female body, a multisystem effect can be attributed to estrogen deficiency in menopause. Furthermore, the classic estrogen receptor model has been supplanted with the discovery of a second estrogen receptor. Traditional estrogenic effects on target tissues must now be understood through the differential expression of two or possibly more receptors and how different estrogen molecules interact with each receptor. Estrogen receptors have been detected within the urogenital tract, breasts, bones, skin and connective tissue, cardiovascular system, liver, and central nervous system. Long-term effects of estrogen deprivation, in which aging, genetic predisposition, and disease processes interact to produce a series of silent and potentially fatal changes, include osteoporosis, cardiovascular disease and, perhaps, Alzheimer's disease and colon cancer.

CONSEQUENCES OF ESTROGEN LOSS

The loss of estrogen associated with menopause is accompanied by many short- and long-term physical changes (Figure 50-1). Early changes associated with estrogen loss include vasomotor instability (hot flashes), mood changes, sleep disturbance, and vaginal irritation. While these symptoms can be disturbing and are commonly the reason women seek the advice of their physicians, the most significant concerns should be those associated with long-term estrogen deprivation, such as osteoporosis and cardiovascular disease, as these will ultimately have the greatest effect on life expectancy and quality.

Menopausal Hot Flashes

Significant advances have been achieved in the characterization of menopausal hot flashes (also known as vasomotor symptoms). Eighty-five percent of all postmenopausal women will experience vasomotor symptoms, typically described as an intense sensation of warmth, accompanied by perspiration, palpitations,

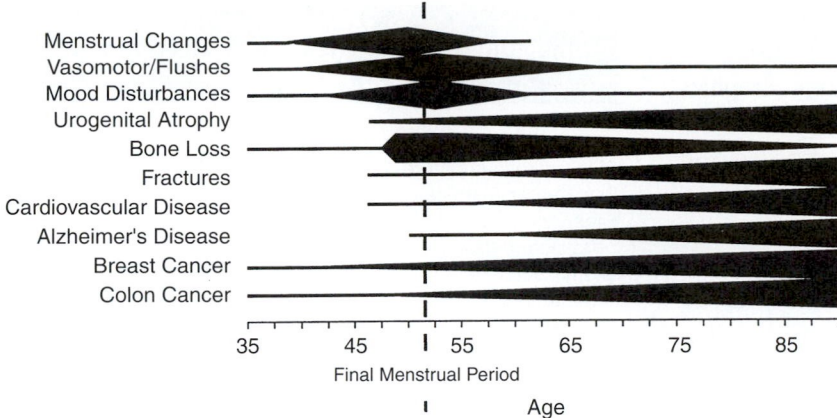

Figure 50-1 Symptoms and diseases associated with menopause and aging.

or sleep disturbance, and often followed by a cold chill. Although the symptom is generally self-limited and will spontaneously resolve within 1 to 5 years, the distress associated with this symptom is the primary motivation for most menopausal women seeking medical treatment. It is now believed that estrogen deficiency (not elevated gonadotropins) leads to acute intermittent changes in the set point for hypothalamic temperature regulation. Neuroendocrine discharges within the hypothalamus trigger peripheral vasodilation and perspiration, leading to an initial rise in skin temperature and decrease in skin conduction time. Simultaneously, a variety of acute endocrine changes have been noted, including a rise in LH, cortisol, androstenedione and dehydroepiandrosterone sulfate (DHEAS), together with sleep disruption if the episode occurs at night. The vasodilation and perspiration of the hot flash rapidly cools the body to satisfy the lower hypothalamic set point for temperature regulation, giving the secondary sensation of a cold chill.

It is hypothesized that hot flashes may result in irreversible loss of neurons, such that women who enter their 70s and 80s with a history of hot flashes have a decrease in neuronal reserve and are thus more likely to have Alzheimer's disease at an earlier age. Tests of verbal memory demonstrate a significant association with hot-flash severity.[3] These changes could not be explained by corresponding changes in symptoms of depression, anxiety, or insomnia.

Vaginal Bleeding

The definition of natural menopause includes loss of menses as a criterion, but menstrual periods rarely simply stop at a set point in time. Anovulation along with wide fluctuations in estradiol levels is a hallmark of the perimenopausal period and often leads to ab-

normal vaginal bleeding. Menses are often heavier than the patient is used to and the loss of a regular pattern is distressing. An assessment of the bleeding is indicated as pathology such as uterine leiomyomas and endometrial polyps are common and contribute to the high rate of hysterectomy in this age group.

Skin

Skin undergoes a natural aging process. The epidermis becomes thinner and dermal papillae less pronounced. These changes, together with loss of collagen in elastic tissue, frequently lead to the development of skin creases and breast atrophy after menopause. The vaginal skin is partially derived from müllerian origin and remains a target organ for estrogen. Loss of estrogen in the menopausal years leads to thinning of the vaginal epithelium and overall vaginal atrophy. Manifestations of this condition include vaginal irritation and itching, both of which respond promptly to estrogen replacement. Vaginal mucosal atrophy may present as loss of libido because of dyspareunia, reinforcing the admonition to obtain a careful history in order to elucidate the cause of sexual dysfunction in these women.

While ovarian androgen production in postmenopause does not increase, there is loss of ovarian estrogen secretion resulting in a relative hyperandrogenicity that, at times, may lead to postmenopausal hirsutism. It is not uncommon 5 to 10 years after menopause for women to present with concerns over slowly progressive growth of facial hair.

Urogenital Tract

Estrogen receptors have been detected in the female introitus, vagina, bladder, urethra, and pelvic-floor musculature, with all of these structures sharing their embryologic origins from the primitive urogenital sinus. After menopause, the urethral mucosa atrophies, resulting in a reduction in mean urethral closure pressure. Urethral collagen and elasticity also decrease, further compromising function and favoring the development of urethral sphincter incompetence (genuine stress incontinence). In the bladder, mucosal thinning with estrogen loss lowers the sensory threshold for detrusor contraction, resulting in irritative symptoms, including urinary frequency, nocturia, and urge incontinence. Thinned urogenital tissues are more susceptible to trauma or infection, with an increased incidence of lower-urinary-tract infection. Finally, estrogen deprivation may contribute to a loss of pelvic-floor tone and contractility.[4] Pelvic-organ prolapse can thus be considered a consequence of urogenital aging, though this is a multifactorial problem not solely related to hypoestrogenism.

Bone

Change in the bony skeleton is one of the most profound risks menopausal women face. Bone is not static. Rather, it is always in an active process of remodeling, which is a reflection of bone resorption by osteoclasts and formation by osteoblasts. Due to an increase in bone destruction relative to bone formation, bone mass normally declines with age. Peak bone density in women is actually achieved relatively early in reproductive life, around 24 to 28 years of age, and gradually decreases throughout life. The amount of bone present later in life is determined both by bone mass accumulated before the age of 28 years and the rate at which this store of bone declines. Estrogen deficiency following menopause is a major contributor to the pathogenesis of bone loss, with almost one-fifth of lifetime bone loss occurring in the first 5 to 7 years after menopause.[5]

Osteoporosis is characterized by low bone mass and microarchitectural deterioration, with a consequent increase in fragility and susceptibility to fracture, particularly in trabecular bone such as the neck of the femur (hip fracture), head of the radius (Colles fracture), and vertebrae (loss of height and kyphosis). While there is a reduction in the quantity of bone, there is no alteration in its chemical composition.

The medical and social consequences of these fractures make osteoporosis an important public health problem. In the United States, osteoporotic fractures,

TABLE 50-1
INDEPENDENT RISK FACTORS FOR OSTEOPOROSIS AND FRACTURES

Age
Slender body structure
Estrogen or testosterone deficiency
Lifestyle
  Calcium deficiency or low intake
  Smoking
  Sedentary lifestyle
Medications
  Corticosteroids
  Thyroid replacement
  Heparin
  GnRH analogs
Prolonged immobilization
Falls
  Alcohol
  Immobility
  Arrhythmias
  Poor vision
  Medications
  Hazards in home and workplace
Predisposing medical conditions
  Hyperparathyroididsm
  Malabsorption
  Hyperthyroidism
  Renal failure

including hip, Colles, vertebral, and humerus total 1.5 million annually. Most (90%) of the total annual cost of osteoporosis, estimated at $13.8 billion, is directly attributable to the treatment of women and does not include the cost of assisted-living facilities or home health care. Osteoporosis is preventable and treatable, but there are no clinical warning signs until a fracture occurs. Along with estrogen deficiency, age is a major contributor to risk, with 15% of women in their mid-60s suffering vertebral fracture, rising to 35% by the mid-80s. These figures are believed to be significantly underreported.[6]

For obstetricians and gynecologists, assessing a woman's risk for osteoporosis may be unfamiliar. Since it is a disease with no warning sign or symptoms and is particularly amenable to treatment at perimenopause, the importance of risk assessment and screening cannot be overemphasized. Table 50-1 lists the independent risk factors for osteoporosis and fractures. Factors that are associated with an increased risk of falls should be identified, especially in older women (Table 50-1). A physical examination should be performed, noting body habitus and any evidence of height loss or kyphosis. Unfortunately, clinical assessment of risk will identify only 30% of women with low bone mass at the time of menopause. Clearly, a quantitative assessment is needed, and currently, the best available tool to measure bone densitometry is dual-energy x-ray absorptiometry (DEXA). Standard bone x-ray films are highly insensitive, as more than 30% of the bone must be lost before an abnormal result is apparent. DEXA should be offered to women who are undecided about therapy and if the decision regarding treatment is dependent on the results. In addition, women with risk factors for osteoporosis and fractures should have bone densitometry determined as early as possible for base-line measurement. DEXA, however, has limited value in follow-up since it cannot detect subtle bone changes and should not be performed more frequently than every other year. To monitor therapy, biochemical markers of bone resorption and formation may prove to be useful and convenient as they are easily measured in urine. They provide information on whether short-term therapy has stopped the loss of bone but at present, do not give an accurate assessment of current bone density or fracture risk.

Cardiovascular

One in two women in the United States will eventually die from heart disease or stroke, as compared with 1 in 25 who will die from breast cancer.[7] While the incidence of symptomatic cardiovascular disease is low in premenopausal women, there is a dramatic change with menopause. Coronary artery disease becomes the most frequent cause of death in women age 50 years and older, followed by stroke, lung cancer, and breast cancer.[8] Since 1984, while the overall mortality rate for cardiovascular disease has declined in the United States, most of this decline has occurred in men, resulting in a increased mortality rate for women.

Two separate actions contribute to the apparent ability of estrogen to protect women from cardiovascular disease: lipid-dependent and lipid-independent mechanisms. In the lipid-dependent mechanism, estrogen prevents the adverse changes in lipid metabolism associated with menopause by raising high-density lipoprotein (HDL), lowering low-density lipoprotein (LDL), decreasing lipoprotein A, and decreasing LDL oxidation. Estrogen's lipid-independent effect involves direct modification of a function of the endothelium and vascular smooth muscle, such as increasing insulin sensitivity and vasodilatation,

while decreasing oxidative stress. Overall, studies have demonstrated that estrogen appears to have beneficial effects on retarding anatomic development of coronary atherosclerosis, improving lipid profiles and restoring normal vascular reactivity.[9]

Brain

Exposure to estrogen results in changes to brain structure and function. Subsequent withdrawal of estrogen after menopause may not only precipitate vasomotor symptoms, but may also have effects on serotoninergic, adrenergic, and cholinergic symptoms.[10] Estrogen deficiency may alter the threshold for clinical expression of various mood and cognitive disorders. Depression, irritability, loss of libido, and aggression have been commonly reported during the peri- and postmenopausal years. However, it has been difficult to establish a link between the psychological changes and the hormonal milieu of the menopause. Often, varied social factors occur at a time of physical change, emphasizing a biologic hurdle that is frequently, and unfortunately, perceived as the start of a downhill course. Just how psychosocial factors and hormonal changes interact to create the emotional changes that accompany menopause is unclear. Although the incidence of major depression does not change in association with menopause, other mood disorders are reported with increasing frequency during this transition. In addition, there is a second incidence peak for the development of schizophrenia in postmenopausal women, and women with premenopausal schizophrenia typically worsen after menopause.[10]

Estrogen appears to have a potent neuroprotective role, likely mediated by its antioxidant properties and its ability to enhance cerebral blood flow, improve cerebral glucose metabolism, reduce β-amyloid deposition, and decrease the resulting senile plaque formation.[11,12,13] Loss of this neuroprotective effect following menopause may contribute to the cognitive deterioration that occurs with normal aging and may partially explain the early expression of Alzheimer's disease among older women.

MANAGEMENT OF THE MENOPAUSAL WOMAN

It is important to realize that menopausal health care remains fragmented. This is, in part, because menopause is a normal transition and, in part, because the majority of women do not visit physicians specifically to discuss menopause, but usually for the control of short-term symptoms such as hot flashes. The perimenopausal period offers the obstetrician-gynecologist the opportunity to review each woman's health profile and to discuss, provide, direct, and encourage a program of preventive health care.

Needless to say, a complete history and physical examination should be performed. The guidelines for proper health maintenance and screening will be discussed elsewhere in this textbook. However, for perimenopausal women, the evaluation, including family history, should concentrate on a careful risk assessment for diseases such as coronary artery disease, stroke, Alzheimer's disease, cancer, and osteoporosis. It is important to inquire about social issues such as habits, mood, and sexual activity, as these will not usually be volunteered. This assessment should include a question regarding domestic abuse.

The physical examination is directed at cancer screening as well as an assessment of the chief symptom. Common physical findings may include thyroid enlargement, lymphadenopathy, breast lumps, hepatomegaly, and skin lesions. The pelvic and rectal examinations should be complete, including the evaluation of vulvar diseases and manifestations of urogenital aging. Screening for sexually transmitted diseases and testing for human immunodeficiency virus (HIV) should be offered in appropriate situations. Laboratory investigations, again, should concentrate on cancer screening. Routine testing for thyroid-stimulating hormone (TSH) and a full lipid profile is also indicated in this age group. If the patient reports abnormal vaginal bleeding, β human chorionic gonadotropin (βhCG), hematocrit (Hct), endometrial biopsy, transvaginal ultrasound, and/or hysteroscopy should be considered before initiation of hormone therapy.

In patients with an intact uterus, symptoms associated with menopause such as hot flashes can begin prior to the cessation of menstrual cycles. For many women, lifestyle adjustments are the initial response, but some symptoms will require the use of hormone therapy. Standard HRT may not be potent enough to suppress ovulation, and vaginal bleeding may still occur regularly or irregularly. In these patients, optimal control of symptoms and bleeding patterns may be achieved with the use of a low-dose (20 μg of ethinyl estradiol) combined oral contraceptive preparation. Healthy nonsmokers can be offered this treatment, provided they have no specific contraindications. It

provides effective cycle control, contraception, and relief from menopausal symptoms. Because the oral contraceptive (OC) suppresses the symptoms of menopause, the question of when to discontinue the OC, or to switch from OC to HRT inevitably arises. The traditional but insensitive method of diagnosing menopause in women taking OCs is the documentation of a serum FSH level greater than 30 mIU/ml on day 7 of the pill-free interval. Alternatively, the switch to HRT can arbitrarily be made at age 50, as the chance of spontaneous pregnancy by that point is remote.

Menopause itself does not require a diagnosis, and an adequate, independent biologic marker for this event does not exist. Most patients, however, are curious as to their menopausal status. If there has been at least 12 months of amenorrhea, in the absence of other possible causes, then natural menopause is diagnosed. The situation is more complicated in the patient with prior hysterectomy or who has significant menopausal symptoms and is still bleeding. Again, other possible causes accounting for the symptoms (e.g., pregnancy), need to be excluded. Perimenopause then becomes the diagnosis of exclusion, and therapy can be directed to the troublesome symptom or to the long-term prevention of disease without necessarily making a laboratory confirmation of menopause. Circulating FSH and estradiol levels fluctuate widely during perimenopause and should not be relied on. Rarely, FSH and estradiol levels may be used to check the adequacy of ERT/HRT, but tracking the patient's symptoms, particularly hot flashes, is easier and just as accurate.

Diet and Lifestyle Influence

Many of the leading causes of death are influenced by modifiable factors, including cigarette smoking, diet, exercise, and obesity. Counseling must include discussions about the importance of lifestyle changes, since it is around the time of menopause that the ill effects of a lifetime of unhealthy habits begin to surface and progress with age. This includes a discussion of not only how to best control the symptoms of menopause, but a discussion of a woman's existing conditions or her increased risk of such conditions, which may occur after menopause.

Cigarette smoking is a strong independent risk factor for cardiovascular disease, stroke, peripheral vascular disease, osteoporosis, and certain forms of cancer. Smoking cessation is the single most important change a woman can make to enhance her life expectancy. Similarly, the cardioprotective and anticarcinogenic effects of a diet low in saturated and trans-saturated fats and high in fiber cannot be overemphasized. Weight-bearing exercise enhances well-being, promotes balance and agility, and protects the heart and bone. Both regular aerobic exercise and periodic deep breathing exercises may result in a reduction in hot flashes. If a woman has hypertension, diabetes, or dyslipidemia, these should be brought under control and closely monitored.

Estrogen- and Hormone-Replacement Therapy (ERT/HRT)

Since the 1920s, a number of discoveries have led to the development of compounds for improving the health and quality of life of menopausal women. Unfortunately, no standard therapeutic regimen has been developed, but a variety of compounds, routes of administration, and dosages can be used to optimize individual therapy. Because of the symptoms and serious disease processes that are clearly associated with estrogen deficiency and the onset of menopause, therapy with exogenous estrogen to replace physiologic levels of circulating estrogen has been advocated, with the clear intention of preventing symptoms of the deficiency syndrome rather than treating them after they occur. However, several studies have demonstrated an increased risk of cancer of the endometrium in women receiving inappropriate estrogen treatment. Whether there is an increased risk of breast cancer, probably the most troubling aspect of ERT/HRT, has yet to be definitively determined. Nevertheless, the benefits do appear to outweigh the risks, and therapy does appear to lengthen and maintain quality of life, at least in a majority of selected patients. A woman who is experiencing early symptoms of menopause or who may have existing medical conditions or be at increased risk for certain diseases should be counseled specifically regarding ERT/HRT. Asymptomatic healthy women with no known risk factors for late-stage diseases should also be counseled, although the beneficial impact in this healthy group of women has yet to be elucidated.

Most physicians, especially obstetricians and gynecologists, are enthusiastic advocates for the use of ERT/HRT for the management of perimenopause and menopause. Unfortunately, we are not managing

TABLE 50-2 **APPROXIMATE EQUIVALENTS OF ORAL AND TRANSDERMAL ESTROGENS**	
	Dose Equivalent
Oral	
Conjugated equine estrogens	0.625 mg
Conjugated estrone sulfate	0.625 mg
Estropipate	0.625 mg
17β-estradiol	1.0 mg
Transdermal	
17β-estradiol	50-μg patch

to communicate that to our patients. Fewer than 20% of postmenopausal women in the United States have ever taken ERT/HRT and 50% of women who start will not complete 1 year of therapy.[14] Clearly, there are issues that concern patients that are not being addressed and we as physicians have to renew our efforts in effective counseling.

Estrogens

Estrone (E_1) and estradiol (E_2) are the only truly natural estrogens produced and secreted within a woman's body. To distinguish between different estrogens used in ERT, the terminology of natural versus synthetic is often confusing or misleading. The critical determinant of an estrogen preparation's usefulness is not its origin but its biologic effectiveness. The biologic equivalence of some standard estrogens currently available for ERT/HRT are listed in Table 50-2. These standard doses are approximately one-third to one-sixth the potency of the standard estrogen doses in low-dose oral contraceptive pills.

Estrogens are not readily absorbed by the gastrointestinal tract. To enhance oral bioavailability and prevent degradation, estrogens, either chemically produced or derived from plant or animal sources, can be conjugated and delivered as sodium sulfates or stabilized by adding piperazine or an ester group. Conjugated equine estrogen (CEE), extracted from pregnant mares, contains several sulfated estrogens in specific proportions and remains as the single most popular and most studied form of ERT.

Estradiol itself is available in oral, transdermal, parenteral, and vaginal delivery systems. To be absorbed orally, estradiol must be micronized in very small particles that result in an increase in surface area and rapid absorption. Once absorbed, all estrogens are converted in the liver to estrone. Because of the first-pass effect, orally ingested estrogens have a significant effect on the liver and produce a number of biologically active substances, which likely accounts for a major portion of bioactivity. It is associated with rapid increases in HDL cholesterol and triglycerides and may have an impact on coagulation factors. By contrast, transdermal estradiol application avoids hepatic first-pass metabolism, resulting in sustained concentrations of estradiol. While in theory transdermal estrogen should have less effect on lipoproteins, coagulation factors, and gallbladder disease, the clinical relevance of these findings has yet to be determined.

Progestins

The addition of a progestin to estrogen therapy has been shown to reduce, but not eliminate, the estrogen-attributed risk of endometrial hyperplasia/cancer in a dose- and duration-dependent fashion.[15,16] As this is the only current indication, only women with an intact uterus need to consider progestins. The effects are duration-dependent, and maximum protection is obtained with 14 days a month of exposure (Table 50-3).

Two different classes of progestins are commonly used in HRT: (1) Those related to progesterone or its metabolites, including medroxyprogesterone acetate (MPA), and (2) the 19-noretestosterone derivatives (norethindrone and norethindrone acetate). There are some notable differences between these agents. Oral micronized progesterone does not appear to antagonize the effects of estrogen on HDL cholesterol, whereas MPA attenuates the estrogen-induced lipid effects.[17] In addition, differences in bleeding patterns may occur. A full secretory transformation occurs with the use of MPA, while doses of less then 300 mg of micronized progesterone demonstrate antimitotic

effects only, which may result in less predictable, albeit lighter, withdrawal menses.[18] The 19-noretestosterone derivatives differ from the former compounds because of varying androgenic as well as progestagenic properties. Similar to MPA, full secretory transformation occurs with these agents.

Treatment Regimens

There are many regimens of ERT/HRT in use in clinical practice. Regimens that contain estrogen and progestin should always be offered unless a woman has had a hysterectomy, in which the endometrial protective effects of progestin will not be necessary.

CYCLIC Estrogen and progestin have been traditionally used in a cyclical manner (Figure 50-2). It typically consisted of estrogen taken from day 1 to 25 of the calendar month, with the addition of a progestin from days 10 to 25 each month, followed by a pill-free interval. A modified schedule uses uninterrupted estrogen dose without a pill-free interval. The physiologic rationale for the pill-free interval is unclear as withdrawal bleeding will occur in either case following progestin withdrawal. Many women report the return of distressing symptoms in the days when they are not taking hormones, and eliminating the pill-free interval may provide maximal symptomatic relief.

Current evidence suggests that 0.625 mg of CEE or its equivalent is the minimum fully effective dose for prophylaxis and treatment of osteoporosis.[19] Although lower doses of estrogen in combination with high doses of calcium may afford protection from osteoporosis, data are not sufficient to determine whether these doses will provide adequate cardioprotection. Cyclical progestin therapy generally involves 12 to 14 days of progestin use; typical doses are listed in Table 50-3. When doses larger than 0.625 mg CEE or its equivalent are used, larger doses of progestins are required.

CONTINUOUS COMBINED An alternative approach to cyclic ERT is continuous daily treatment with both an estrogen and progestin (see Figure 50-2). This method was developed in order to avoid the withdrawal bleeding associated with cyclic regimens. Women with progestin-related side effects also benefited from the corresponding decrease in dosage. Most of the available data are from studies that combined 0.625 mg of CEE with 2.5 to 5.0 mg of MPA per day.[20] Other progestins can be used, and their

---

**TABLE 50-3
DAILY PROGESTIN DOSAGE FOR
ENDOMETRIAL PROTECTION**

	Cyclic*	Continuous
Oral		
Medroxyprogesterone acetate	5–10 mg	2.5 mg
Megesterol	20 mg	
Micronized progesterone	200–400 mg	100 mg
Norethindrone	0.35–0.70 mg	0.35 mg
Norethindrone acetate	2.5 mg	
Transdermal		
Norethindrone acetate†	0.25 mg	

*At least 12 days of progestin per month.

†Currently only available in combination with a 17β-estradiol patch.

Cyclic

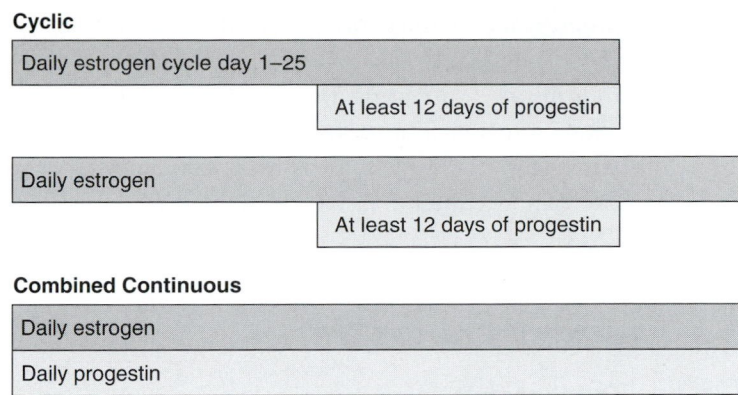

| Daily estrogen cycle day 1–25 | |
| At least 12 days of progestin | |

| Daily estrogen | |
| At least 12 days of progestin | |

Combined Continuous

| Daily estrogen |
| Daily progestin |

Figure 50-2 Hormone replacement monthly treatment regimens.

theoretical dose equivalents are listed in Table 50-3. Unfortunately, 40% of women receiving this therapy, far from avoiding vaginal bleeding, experience irregular, breakthrough bleeding during the first 3 to 6 months. Fortunately, the majority of patients who persist with this regimen become amenorrheic by 12 months and only 5% have breakthrough bleeding after 1 year of use.

ESTROGEN-ONLY Estrogen-only therapy is recommended only in women who do not have a uterus. This is the regimen of choice for women who have undergone hysterectomy. In these women, the addition of a progestin does not add any benefit and needlessly complicates ERT.

The role of unopposed estrogen in the development of endometrial neoplasia has been well documented and needs to be respected.[17] However, the development of estrogen-dependent endometrial carcinoma follows a well-defined course from preinvasive lesions that generally present early in its course and can be readily detected. Infrequently, despite the risk, a woman with a uterus may elect to take unopposed estrogen, usually because of previous bleeding problems or adverse progestin-related side effects. However, these women need close follow-up and the clinician needs to be confident of that patient's understanding and compliance. Endometrial assessment needs to be performed at least annually, and if there is evidence of premalignancy, immediate treatment sought.

ADVERSE REACTIONS The use of estrogens can result in unpleasant side effects in 5 to 10% of women using typical dosages of ERT/HRT. Common symptoms include breast tenderness, nausea, headache, and bloating. These side effects are often dose-related and

may resolve with continuous use or a decrease in dosage. Because the side effects vary among currently available estrogen preparations, if one product is not tolerated, another may be tried. Residual vasomotor symptoms or vaginal dryness may indicate the need for increasing the dose, whereas breast tenderness or leukorrhea may signal a need for dose reduction.

Adverse reactions to progestins are more frequent and unpredictable. Most commonly, women report breast tenderness, weight gain, bloating, and alterations in mood that can be debilitating. Cyclic-progestin-associated side effects may be reduced or eliminated by switching to a continuous combined regimen, likely because of a corresponding decrease in dosage. Like estrogens, each progestin preparation has a different side-effect profile. For example, micronized progesterone can cause sedation and therefore should be administered at bedtime. The clinician should not hesitate to try another progestin product if side effects become troublesome.

The most irritating symptom with HRT is vaginal bleeding, since the single, most eagerly awaited symptom of menopause is amenorrhea. Bleeding while on HRT tends to be light but sometimes unpredictable, particularly early in the continuous combined regimen. While the bleeding associated with the start of HRT is likely to be breakthrough in nature, there are instances when the endometrium should be evaluated. Further investigation is required in a perimenopausal woman if her bleeding is too heavy (particularly if associated with anemia), too long (lasting for more than 7 days), or too frequent (occurring at intervals of less than 21 days). In postmenopausal women, any bleeding after 6 months of amenorrhea warrants investigation. Similarly, if a patient is experiencing regular withdrawal menses from cyclic HRT, the appearance of unexpected, irregular bleeding should be evaluated. While transvaginal ultrasound measurement of endometrial thickness has proven useful in detecting endometrial pathology, the "safe" criteria for patients taking HRT are not well defined. Any postmenopausal woman, whether using HRT or not, with an endometrial thickness greater than 5 mm should have a biopsy performed for a histologic diagnosis.

ESTROGEN ANDROGEN THERAPY Following menopause, a woman's total estrogen production decreases by 80% and androgen production decreases by as much as 50%. Following bilateral oophorectomy, estrogen and testosterone concentrations drop precipitously. This deficiency in androgens, particularly in women who have surgically induced menopause, has been associated with decreased libido in some, but by no means all, women. Testosterone replacement appears to enhance libido in patients who have undergone surgically induced menopause, but its role in natural menopause is less clear.[21,22] It does appear to have a complementary, beneficial effect on relieving vasomotor symptoms when combined with ERT.

The most common preparation used is oral methyltestoterone, with a daily dosage of 2.5 mg. Adverse effects associated with the supraphysiologic dosages used for typical androgen supplementation in men does not occur with the much lower dose combined with estrogen and used in ERT/HRT for postmenopausal women. Such symptoms of androgen excess, including hirsutism, voice changes, and clitorimegaly, have an incidence of less than 3% with the low dosages currently available in commercial preparations indicated for hormone replacement. There are some concerns about the effects of androgens on plasma lipoproteins, and androgen-replacement therapy should not be given without concomitant estrogen therapy. Testosterone is partly metabolized to estrogen and should be opposed by progestin in a woman with a uterus. Hepatotoxicity is a theoretical concern with oral methyltestosterone, but has not been seen with the typical replacement dosages used in women.

Follow-up

Adherence to treatment is facilitated by involving the woman in the decision-making process, anticipating start-up problems, and arranging suitable follow up. An invitation for a return visit indicates the clinician's willingness to work through problems and monitor progress and reassures the patient that she will not be abandoned. This visit should occur no later than 3 months after initiating therapy. Regular follow-up allows a reevaluation of the treatment plan, especially when new evidence, such as from randomized clinical trials, becomes available.

BENEFITS OF ERT/HRT

Osteoporosis

Optimally, the prevention of osteoporosis should start during teenage years with adequate exercise and calcium intake in order to maximize peak bone mass once young adulthood is reached. A discussions of the dangers of smoking should include, among its other health implications, the risk to bone. As women age, their ability to absorb adequate calcium diminishes and intake requirements need to be increased. Perimenopausal women should ingest 1000 mg of calcium a day, increasing to 1500 mg a day by age 60. Women should also ingest 400 to 800 IU of vitamin D a day, especially if there is scant exposure to the sun. Unfortunately, calcium and vitamin D alone will not prevent the substantial bone loss seen immediately after menopause. However, the addition of ERT/HRT maintains and reverses the bone-mass depletion observed in these women, as it inhibits osteoclastic activity and tilts the balance between bone resorption and formation toward formation.

The beneficial effect of ERT/HRT on bone mineral density has been confirmed by the Postmenopausal Estrogen/Progestin Intervention (PEPI) trial,[23] which specifically examined the spine and hip in postmenopausal women, who on average were 52 years of age. After 3 years of continuous ERT with 0.625 mg of daily CEE, bone mineral density actually increased by 3.5% at the spine and by 2% at the hip, as compared with a decrease of 2 to 3% in placebo treated patients. Addition of continuous MPA further improved the bone-sparing effect at the spine over CEE alone or cyclic CEE/MPA.[23] While ERT/HRT appears to offer nearly equivalent bone-conserving benefit at any age, therapy should be initiated as soon as possible after symptoms of estrogen deficiency, because lost bone mass may never be recovered. Therapy initiated early in the postmenopausal period and continued until late life is associated with the highest bone mineral density.[24]

Because the highest incidence of radial and vertebral fractures occur mainly between 50 and 75 years of age, the effect of ERT/HRT on these fracture rates is easier to detect than that for hip fractures, which generally start in the late 70s. Although there are no randomized data, most observational studies confirm that ERT/HRT is useful in the prevention of both spine and hip fracture, with the overall reduction in relative risk ranging from 20 to 60%. Both oral and transdermal ERT/HRT decrease bone loss, reduce the incidence of fracture, and prevent loss of height.[25,26] However, there is evidence to state that several years of compliant ERT/HRT is required before the beneficial effects on fracture risk are noted. Furthermore, it appears that the beneficial effects of estrogen on bone dissipate once ERT is discontinued.

In addition to ameliorating osteoporosis, ERT/HRT may provide benefit for another condition that involves the skeletal system—tooth loss. Approximately 32% of U.S. women age 65 have no teeth. Although the prevention of periodontal disease is the most important factor of maintaining teeth, it has been hypothesized that some tooth loss may occur as a result of resorption of alveolar bone and, therefore, may reflect osteoporotic bone loss. The Nurses Health Study demonstrated over a 30% decrease in risk of tooth loss in current ERT users.[27]

Bisphosphonates

In addition to ERT/HRT, there are other agents and interventions that have proven to be useful alternatives for women at risk of osteoporosis and who cannot or choose not to take estrogen or those who choose not to take ERT/HRT. Bisphosphonates, a new class of drugs used in the prevention and treatment of established osteoporosis, are useful alternatives to ERT/HRT in the treatment of postmenopausal women. All bisphosphonates bind permanently to mineralized bone surfaces and, by inhibiting osteoclastic activity, reduce the amount of bone degraded during the remodeling cycle. In a randomized, 2-year trial, 5 mg of alendronate demonstrated a protective effect on spine and hip bone density over placebo, equivalent to the effect seen with ERT/HRT.[28] At a dose of 10 mg a day, alendronate is an effective treatment for osteoporosis, reducing the incidence of spine and hip fracture.[29] It is not yet known if there is a bone benefit to the addition of alendronate to existing ERT/HRT.

Selective Estrogen-Receptor Modulators (SERM)

The discovery of the second estrogen receptor has ignited a reevaluation of the way estrogen interacts with receptors in different tissues to produce a cellular effect. Considerable effort has been applied to the development of selective estrogen receptor modulators (SERMs), which could theoretically retain the cardioprotective and skeletal benefits of estrogen while avoiding the undesirable breast and endometrial effects. Tamoxifen, a first-generation SERM, has been used for many years as a selective antiestrogen in women with breast cancer. It can increase bone mineral density in postmenopausal women, but can also cause endometrial hyperplasia.[30] Overall, data are consistent with the hypothesis that tamoxifen exerts an agonist effect on bone, but the response is typically less than the maximal effect observed with estrogens or bisphosphonates.

By contrast, newer SERMs (e.g., raloxifene and droloxifene) have antiestrogenic activity in the uterus as well as in the breasts. While they appear to retain some of the favorable lipid and skeletal effects of estrogen, they do not provide any relief of vasomotor symptoms or urogenital atrophy. Results from a clinical trial in postmenopausal women indicate that raloxifene (60 mg a day) has modest bone-sparing effects without uterine stimulatory effects.[31] Raloxifene induces mild estrogen-like changes in the lipid profile and may reduce the risk of breast cancer in the short term without stimulating endometrium proliferation. It offers an alternative for preserving bone mass in some women who are at risk for osteoporosis and who are not candidates for ERT/HRT.

Coronary Heart Disease (CHD)

The fact that estrogen loss and aging are associated with a dramatic increase in cardiovascular disease among women has focused research on the cardioprotective effects of estrogen. Although ERT/HRT does not yet have an approved indication for the treatment of CHD, there is a preponderance of evidence to suggest that it should. Observational studies show a consistent reduction in relative risks for CHD, and a meta-analysis of these data indicates a dramatic risk reduction of 50%. Even if only partly true, the impact of this reduction, considering the high prevalence of cardiovascular disease in modern society, would catapult ERT/HRT to the status of a major medical advancement.

It has been known for some time that oral conjugated estrogens cause a favorable alteration of the lipid profile. The PEPI trial found that ERT produced an increase in HDL and lowered LDL and lipoprotein A levels. Therapy with synthetic progestins, but not progesterone, attenuated the increase in HDL, but most prospective studies show a similar protective effect with HRT as ERT.[17] Transdermal therapy also lowers LDL and lipoprotein A but has little effect on HDL. Oral, but not transdermal, ERT raises triglyceride levels but is clinically insignificant except to women with underlying hypertriglyceridemia.

Changes to the lipid profile with ERT/HRT cannot entirely explain the observed reduction in CHD incidence. Estrogen also has a direct vasodilatory effect on arterial and coronary vessels. Circulating estrogen promotes vasodilatation, likely by induction of nitric oxide production from the endothelium. Estrogen also exhibits antioxidant properties, reducing free radical damage to the endothelium and circulating LDL cholesterol, both risk factors for the development of atheromatous plaques. These receptor-mediated effects appear quickly after ERT is initiated and may, in part, explain how ERT augments coronary blood flow.[32,33] It is likely that postmenopausal women will require long-term exposure of ERT to first up-regulate the concentration of estrogen receptors, thus enhancing these vascular effects.

SERMs such as raloxifene appear to have some but not all of the cardioprotective effects of estrogen. In healthy postmenopausal women, raloxifene and tamoxifen both reduce plasma LDL levels. Raloxifene does not, however, exert any influence on HDL cholesterol.[31] There are no available data on whether SERMs have any beneficial impact on clinical cardiovascular outcomes.

Despite the observational evidence demonstrating a cardioprotective effect, there is still no clinical trial that proves that ERT/HRT can prevent cardiovascular events such as myocardial infarction in postmenopausal women. Observational data can be misleading because of the inevitable bias inherent in such studies. A sobering reminder of this fact is the result from the recently published Heart and Estrogen/Progestin Replacement Study (HERS) which was a large-scale, randomized, placebo-controlled, clinical trial.[34] It studied over 2700 older women with existing CHD and evaluated the efficacy of HRT in secondary prevention of cardiovascular events. Surprisingly, in this high-risk group, HRT did not reduce the overall risk

for myocardial infarction and cardiovascular death. By the fourth year of treatment, HRT treatment did result in fewer deaths, but unfortunately, this was counterbalanced by an increased mortality rate in the first year of the study. However, the study may have had too many study participants drop out and may not have been continued long enough to detect a significant difference. Furthermore, significantly more women in the placebo group were given lipid-lowering treatment, and the study group may have had inadequate medical treatment. These criticisms demonstrate how difficult it is to conduct large-scale clinical trials properly. Nevertheless, data from HERS is important and gives us caution when starting continuous combined HRT for women with existing CHD. Unfortunately, it does not clarify the issue on the use of ERT/HRT as primary prevention in healthy, postmenopausal women. Those data are currently being collected in the federally funded Women's Health Initiative, with results expected in 2005.

Alzheimer's Disease

Both in terms of prevalence and incidence, Alzheimer's disease is a major health issue for women. Women comprise 72% of the population over 85 years of age, and roughly half of this group has Alzheimer's disease. Not only do women constitute a greater proportion of the older population, but Alzheimer's disease is expressed earlier in women than in men. This is thought to be related to estrogen loss, since men typically have higher circulating estrogen than women by age 70.

Therapy with estrogen replacement appears to have a beneficial effect on memory in elderly women who may or may not have Alzheimer's disease. In a double-blind, placebo-controlled trial of 20 women who received 0.625 mg of CEE or placebo for 9 months and cycled every third month with MPA 5 mg for 13 days, 80% of those who were treated with estrogen showed an improvement in nine domains of behavior in cognitive function, especially verbal memory, as compared with none who had received placebo.[35] Furthermore, of those on placebo, half demonstrated no change in cognitive function and half became worse. There is substantial evidence that estrogens may reduce a woman's risk of Alzheimer's disease by delaying its expression and progression. Estrogen-treated women have a significant improvement in memory over base-line equivalents to about 1.5 years of Alzheimer's disease progression. The clinical significance was to delay disease progression by approximately 2 years.[36] Observational data, primarily in postmenopausal women who have used unopposed conjugated estrogens, consistently show a 40 to 60% reduction in the relative risk of Alzheimer's disease.[37] The minimum duration of ERT necessary to protect cognitive function is unknown. However, there is evidence to suggest that even as short a period as 4 months can delay onset of Alzheimer's disease.[38] Clinical data on the role of progestins in Alzheimer's disease risk and treatment are not yet available.

The mechanism for estrogen's neuroprotective effect is unknown. Estrogens may directly protect cognitive function in women by preventing oxidative damage in the brain and by protecting neurons from β-amyloid toxicity. In vitro, certain estrogenic compounds stimulate the production of critical neurotransmitters and have the ability to regenerate damaged neurons. Finally, ERT/HRT appears to improve cerebral glucose metabolism and augment regional blood flow in patients afflicted with Alzheimer's disease.

Other Benefits

Cancer of the colon remains the third leading cause of cancer deaths. Current use of ERT/HRT may impart a protective effect against the risk of colon cancer.[39] The precise mechanism of this action is not yet known. One hypothesis is that ERT/HRT affects bile acid metabolism and promotes tumor-suppressive activity through estrogen receptors. To assist in early detection of colon cancer, the American Cancer Society recommends that women aged 50 years and older received an annual digital rectal examination and fecal occult blood test, with flexible sigmoidoscopy every 5 years or colonoscopy every 10 years.

Early-stage age-related macular degeneration (AMD) is usually asymptomatic. However, it affects 17% of the population over the age of 43 and 35% of those age 75 years or older, with late-stage macular degeneration increasing after age 75 years. Late-stage disease is the leading cause of legal blindness in the United States, accounting for 25 to 60% of new cases. AMD may benefit from estrogen therapy. The 1988–1990 Beaver Dam Eye Study also suggests that ERT/HRT produces a small reduction in risk for early-stage and late-stage AMD.[40] Other aspects of ERT/HRT on eye function include a protective effect in postmenopausal women against cataract formation.[41]

RISKS AND CONCERN WITH ERT/HRT

Contraindications

The number of contraindications continue to decrease with increased knowledge and use of ERT/HRT. The Food and Drug Administration has established contraindications to ERT/HRT that advise against the use of this therapy in certain postmenopausal women (Table 50-4). If any of these conditions exist, an appropriate evaluation and treatment plan should be initiated, including lifestyle modifications that focus on the specific diagnosis. If HRT is contraindicated, other treatment options should also be considered that are specific for each women's disease risk, needs, and preferences.

Some of these contraindications may not be absolute. For example, ongoing research now suggests that the benefits of ERT/HRT for selected women with a history of treated breast or endometrial cancer may prove to outweigh potential risks. The woman must be fully informed that an increased risk for recurrence potentially still exists and must make the decision herself whether or not to take ERT/HRT if she has had breast or endometrial cancer. All relative contraindications must be discussed with each woman and weighed against the risk of not prescribing HRT.

Many women have concerns about HRT or may harbor misconceptions about the effects such therapy may have on their bodies. For example, women can be reassured that it does not restore fertility or produce weight gain. By far, a women's greatest fear, however, is that it will increase her risk of breast cancer. All of the issues listed in Table 50-4 should be discussed, even if a woman does not raise them.

TABLE 50-4
CONTRAINDICATIONS TO ERT/HRT

Known or suspected pregnancy
Known or suspected breast cancer
Estrogen-dependent neoplasia
Undiagnosed, abnormal genital bleeding
Active thrombophlebitis or thromboembolic disorders
Acute liver or gallbladder disease

Liver and Gallbladder Disease

The use of oral estrogen may carry a 1.5- to 2-fold increase in the risk of gallbladder disease. The risk of cholecystectomy appears to increase with dose and duration of use and to persist for 5 years or more after stopping treatment.[42] If a woman contemplating use of ERT/HRT has preexisting gallbladder disease, it may be advantageous to deliver estrogen by a nonoral route in order to avoid exacerbation of her condition.

Thromboembolic Disease

Two case–control studies of venous thromboembolism (VTE) have found a three- to four-fold increase in risk for current users of ERT.[43,44] While these studies show statistical significance, the clinical relevance is less impressive. The increase in putative risk corresponds to an additional two to three cases of VTE in 10,000 women per year, a small number for a condition that generally carries a low risk of mortality. A similar increase in risk has been observed with raloxifene. There is also an increase in relative risk in ERT/HRT users for pulmonary embolism, a dangerous form of VTE. The HERS study demonstrated a nearly threefold increase in relative risk of pulmonary embolism for HRT users over placebo, with two of them experiencing fatal pulmonary emboli.[34] Grodstein et al., from the Nurses Health Study, found that current users of ERT had a twofold risk of primary pulmonary embolism.[45] The absolute risk among women aged 50 to 59 years was found to be 5 additional cases per 100,000.

The low absolute risk of these conditions despite frightening increases in relative risk suggests that the majority of perimenopausal women who have no prior history may be reassured about the risk of thromboembolism. However, patients with risk factors such as antiphospholipid syndrome or factor V Leiden mutation have to be counseled carefully. While there may be a theoretical advantage to the use of transdermal estrogen preparations in women at risk, clinical data are not yet available. For women with existing thrombophilia who are appropriately anticoagulated, ERT/HRT is not contraindicated.

Cancer

Since several established risk factors for breast and endometrial cancer are associated with endogenous estrogen exposure, there exists a theoretical concern that ERT/HRT might increase the incidence of these cancers. Still, the hormonal regulation of these cellular events is not completely understood. Whereas estrogens are generally accepted as promoters of endometrial and breast epithelial-cell proliferation, its actions within the ovaries are less well known.

Breast Cancer

A 40-year-old woman in the United States has a 1 in 10 risk of developing breast cancer by the time she is 80. Since the 1940s, there has been an increase in the overall instance of breast cancer, but the mortality rate has remained relatively stable. The greatest increase has been seen in the incidence of carcinoma in situ, possibly as a result of improved screening and detection.

Many postmenopausal women may discontinue or not begin ERT/HRT because of fear of breast cancer. Based on a meta-analysis of over 90% of the epidemiological studies published on this subject, current users of HRT or those who ceased 1 to 4 years previously had a small increased relative risk of breast cancer, which was comparable to the effect of a delayed menopause.[46] The combined analysis reported an increased risk only for ERT/HRT use of more than 5 years, with the average relative risk of breast cancer increased by approximately 2% per year of use. Translated into real estimates, this reported relative risk for breast cancer with HRT would account for an excess of 2, 6, or 12 cases per 1000 ERT/HRT users after 5, 10, or 15 years of use, respectively. Within 5 years of discontinuation, the increased relative risk virtually disappeared. Furthermore, cancers diagnosed in women who had used ERT/HRT tended to be less advanced clinically than those who have never used it, possibly because ERT/HRT users had higher cancer screening rates. This supports the suspicion that the association between HRT and breast cancer may be the result of surveillance bias.[47] Others have found that despite an increase in breast cancer diagnosis, ERT/HRT use is associated with decreased breast cancer mortality.[48]

The magnitude of this putative risk can be appreciated better by comparing it to other known risk factors for breast cancer. There appears to be a greater risk of breast cancer due to excessive alcohol consumption or by failure to exercise regularly than that attributable to ERT/HRT. Indeed, data from the Nurses Health Study suggest that only women who consumed alcohol manifested increased risk of breast cancer with estrogen administration.[49] Estrogen plus progestin use does not result in a difference in risk as compared with estrogen alone.

Unfortunately, there is no reliable information guiding practitioners in the treatment for women at risk for breast cancer or who have been previously treated for breast cancer. Women with a family history of breast cancer in a first-degree relative carry a fourfold higher risk of its developing, with the risk increasing even more if two first-degree relatives are affected. There are some reassuring data that suggest that a positive family history, defined as a mother or sister with breast cancer, does not further influence the risk of developing cancer while on ERT/HRT.[50] More ominous is the detection of a specific genetic mutation (BRCA1 and BRCA2) in certain women, which would confer a 60 to 80% lifetime risk of breast cancer developing. The issue is even less clear for women who have previously been treated for breast cancer. While there is little information available to define the risks and benefits of ERT/HRT in breast cancer survivors, all cause mortality appears to be improved in estrogen users, likely from the cardioprotective action of estrogen. In 1996, the National Cancer Institute initiated a randomized prospective trial of HRT following the treatment of breast cancer in women with stage I and II disease to clarify this issue. All women in this category should receive expert individual counseling, which examines prognostic factors, quality of life issues, risk factors for osteoporosis, fractures and cardiovascular disease, and options for symptom control and disease prevention.

Breast cancer survivors frequently report symptoms such as hot flashes, vaginal dryness, and decreased libido, especially if the cancer occurred premenopausally or following chemotherapy. For patients who have decided against HRT, nonhormonal medications (clonidine, Bellergal-S) have been proven more effective than placebo in reducing hot flashes. Similarly, high-dose progestins are effective in alleviating vasomotor symptoms, although their safety has not been established in women previously treated for breast cancer. Certain forms of topical estrogen therapy, for example, sustained-release estradiol vaginal rings or low-dose vaginal cream can control vaginal symptoms with minimal systemic absorption. Other nonmedicated approaches may also be considered, including the use of lubricants or gels. For reduced libido, androgen therapy may be considered, although some androgens may be aromatized to estrogens. At present there is no evidence to support or refute the usefulness of adding androgens to an HRT regimen in breast cancer survivors.

Endometrial Cancer

Unopposed ERT in a woman with an intact uterus increases the risk of endometrial cancer by 5- to 10-fold depending on dose and duration. According to the PEPI trial, up to 30% of patients will have either simple and atypical endometrial hyperplasia when they take unopposed ERT.[17] Adding progestins to an ERT regimen markedly reduces, but does not eradicate, the risk of developing both endometrial hyperplasia and cancer in women with uteri. Whitehead et al. demonstrated the critical importance of duration of progestin therapy in stabilizing the endometrium.[16] They documented a 7% incidence of endometrial hyperplasia in patients taking unopposed ERT versus a 4%, 2%, and 0% incidence of hyperplasia in women taking MPA for 7, 10, and 12 days of each month, respectively. While the dose of progestin should be individualized, as a general rule, higher progestin doses should accompany higher-dose estrogen administration. Limited experience suggests that 14 days of higher-dose progestin therapy every 3 months may be sufficiently protective against the development of endometrial hyperplasia.

ERT/HRT has traditionally been withheld from women after treatment of endometrial cancer. The belief that it might increase the risk of recurrent disease, however, has never been substantiated. The American College of Obstetricians and Gynecologists has issued a committee opinion that HRT may be used in patients who have been treated for endometrial cancer and fall into a low-risk group: stage I disease, grade I or II histology, and less than 0.5 cm of myometrial invasion.[51] Although no data support this practice, estrogen administration tends to be started postoperatively, when the patient is ambulatory. The need to add a progestin to the regimen in these patients is unknown, and the use of androgens is controversial, because androgens may undergo aromatization to estrogen. The National Cancer Institute Gynecological Oncology Group is currently addressing these issues through a large randomized placebo controlled study in approximately 2000 women with stage I or II disease.

SPECIAL CONSIDERATIONS

Premature Ovarian Failure

Premature ovarian failure (POF) affects 1% of women under the age of 40. In the absence of a clear cause, there is a high incidence of biochemical, clinical, or familial autoimmune disorders, leading to the presumptive diagnosis of autoimmune POF. Due to the risks of premature osteoporosis and cardiovascular disease, long-term ERT/HRT should be offered to all women with POF. In these younger women, higher doses of estrogen may be needed for symptom relief than are usually required in older postmenopausal women. As women with POF would generally be exposed to a much longer duration of ERT/HRT but lower circulating estrogen levels than their peers, the long-term effects on such disorders as breast cancer are unclear. Until other data become available, it seems prudent to reevaluate the individual HRT risk–benefit profile when a woman with POF enters the usual menopausal age range.

Older Postmenopausal Women (60 and Older)

HRT may be of benefit for many women with such age-associated conditions as cardiovascular disease, osteoporosis and Alzheimer's disease. However, the incidence of breast cancer also increases with age and may be adversely affected by ERT/HRT. A careful risk–benefit assessment is necessary prior to ERT/HRT and should include a lipid profile and mammography. If there is existing CHD, the results from the HERS study cautions us about initiating ERT/HRT, although continuing established therapy is beneficial. Continuous combined therapy is the preferred regimen for the older woman with a uterus, as the return of cyclic menses is usually poorly tolerated. Breakthrough bleeding on this regimen is common in older hypoestrogenic women. To minimize mastalgia and other estrogen side effects, it is advisable to start therapy with the lowest possible estrogen dose, given daily or on alternate days, followed by slow increases to the minimum effective dose.

Migraines

In postmenopausal women who have a biologic predisposition to migraines, headaches may be precipitated by a fall in serum estradiol levels. A period of estrogen priming is a prerequisite. In other women, a rapid rise in serum estradiol may also provoke an attack. This implies that the constant hormone doses from the continuous combined regimen may be better tolerated than a cyclical regimen in headache-prone individuals planning HRT. There are few studies for guidance on whether ERT/HRT increases the risk of either provoking headaches or causing a permanent neurologic abnormality. If neurologic symptoms develop or worsen with use of ERT/HRT, it is advisable to withdraw treatment and seek a neurologic consultation for assessment of any abnormality.

Preoperative State

In the absence of reliable data, HRT with estrogen should be considered as constituting a risk for postoperative VTE. Women on ERT/HRT who undergo surgery without discontinuing treatment should be given specific prophylaxis, even if the excess risk is likely to be small. In most circumstances, women on ERT/HRT who undergo surgery will have additional risk factors (e.g., age, malignancy, reduced mobility) for VTE and will clearly need to receive prophylaxis.

Endometriosis

Combined estrogen and progesterone therapy in standard doses does not appear to cause regrowth of endometriosis in menopausal women or in women receiving estrogen–progestin add-back therapy following medical oophorectomy with GnRH agonists.[52] A small subgroup of women may experience recurrent pain and other symptoms during unopposed estrogen therapy, particularly if residual disease remains following definitive surgery. In the absence of evidence from randomized studies, this appears to be one of the few indications for progestin therapy following hysterectomy, either as part of a continuous combined regimen or as progestin-only therapy. There are no convincing data to support the prophylactic use of progestin-only therapy or the withholding of estrogen for 6 months following definitive surgery in order to allow regression of residual disease.

Fibroids

Uterine fibroids do not constitute a contraindication to HRT, but their presence should be documented in women considering therapy since uterine bleeding may be exacerbated. Although both estrogens and progestins can influence fibroid growth, doses in conventional HRT regimens are usually not sufficient to cause enlargement of fibroids. However, rapid growth or abnormal bleeding from a submucous fibroid requires investigation and possibly surgical intervention.

Diabetes Mellitus

HRT is not contraindicated in diabetes and should not be withheld from women with this condition. Estrogens alter glucose and insulin metabolism in different ways, depending on the compound used and the route of delivery. Both oral and transdermal 17β-estradiol reduce insulin resistance through improvement in insulin sensitivity and elimination. The PEPI trial noted that ERT had no effect on glucose tolerance but that addition of MPA to CEE elevated the 2-hour glucose value into the abnormal range.[17] The clinical significance of this finding is not known.

Alternative Approaches

In a 1997 survey conducted by North American Menopause Society, 80% of respondents reported the use of interventions other than prescription medication.[53] One out of every three Americans consulted an alternative-care provider in 1990, amounting to over 400 million visits and exceeding the number of visits to all U.S. primary care physicians. As mainstream medical journals begin to publish research about alternative therapies, health care providers face both the challenge and the opportunity to incorporate evidence-based alternative therapies into their practices.

There is a strong consumer-driven need for healthcare providers to be knowledgeable about complementary treatments for menopausal symptoms. While the risk–benefit ratio of conventional ERT/HRT is clear, adherence rates for such therapy are low, predominantly due to fear of cancer and dissatisfaction with menstrual bleeding. Women frequently combine ERT/HRT with herbal remedies, yet 70% of them fail to inform their physicians of this use.

Phytoestrogens

Phytoestrogens are plant compounds that have estrogen-like biologic activity and a chemical structure similar to that of estrogen. They have been marketed by some as a "natural SERM" and may exhibit mixed, albeit weak, agonist and antagonist actions on different target tissues. The three principal varieties are isoflavones (e.g., genistein and daidzein), coumestanes, and lignans. Phytoestrogens are present in the highest concentrations in soybean and flaxseed products. In addition to the commonly known soy foods (tofu, soya milk, and miso), newer products have been introduced that are more palatable in a Western diet. Fruits, vegetables, cereals, and seeds contain comparatively trivial amounts of phytoestrogens. Although there are no specific recommendations about dose and formulation, the epidemiologic evidence regarding phytoestrogens is derived from a typical Asian diet, which contains 20 to 150 mg of isoflavones or 20 to 50 g of soy protein per day.

Several clinical trials have demonstrated a mild, but significant, improvement in vasomotor symptoms and vaginal dryness in response to dietary phytoestrogen supplementation.[54] Although the results vary markedly, a high dietary intake of soy protein may offer some bone protection and is associated with variable, but significant, decreases in total cholesterol, LDL cholesterol, and triglycerides.[55] Phytoestrogens have been demonstrated to have a positive effect on bone density, although the doses used were much higher than those achieved through dietary intake.[54] There is almost no evidence to suggest that phytoestrogens may be protective against breast or endometrial cancer.

It should be noted that the benefits attributable to phytoestrogens may be derived, at least in part, from their incorporation into a low-fat, high-fiber Asian diet. Additional research is required to determine if increasing the phytoestrogen content in the relatively high-fat, processed, Western diet will have the same benefit or whether there is any benefit from over-the-counter phytoestrogen tablets. Gastrointestinal absorption of various phytoestrogens exhibits marked individual and sex-related differences, and it is not clear whether interaction with other foods or competition with exogenous or endogenous estrogens for the same receptors will alter their potential effect.

Vitamin Supplements

As noted earlier, calcium and vitamin D will reduce but not prevent postmenopausal bone loss. The strongest evidence for cardiovascular benefits involves the antioxidant potential of vitamin E. Supplementation with 100 to 800 IU daily of vitamin E have demonstrated a reduction in coronary heart disease and recurrent myocardial infarction.[56] However, the effects of dietary vitamin E of typically less than 100 IU/day appear to be ineffective. Vitamin E capsules are often used to relieve hot flashes and

	Indication	Dose	Comments
TABLE 50-5		
HERBAL PREPARATIONS COMMONLY USED BY POSTMENOPAUSAL WOMEN		
Black cohosh	Vasomotor symptoms	2 tablets daily	Can cause gastrointestinal upset or hypotension. May compete with ERT for receptors reducing efficacy of both.
St. John's wort	Depression	300 mg three times a day	Rare gastrointestinal upset or photosensitivity. Possible additive effect with other antidepressants esp. SSRI class.
Ginkgo biloba	Memory loss	120–160 mg daily	Can cause gastrointestinal upset, headaches, skin reactions. May potentiate anticoagulants.
Valerian	Sleep problems	400–900 mg at bedtime	Can cause headaches, excitability, cardiac arrythmia. May have additive effect with other hypnotics
Ginseng	Menopausal symptoms		Available data do not support use. Poor quality control.
Dong Quai	Menopausal symptoms		Available data do not support use.
Evening primrose oil	Vasomotor symptoms		Available data do not support use. No benefit over placebo.
Progesterone creams (nonprescription)			Available data do not support use.

vaginal dryness, but there is no evidence to support this use.

Herbal Medications

Herbal remedies are classified as food or dietary supplements and not as drugs. Consumers often consider them to be inherently safe, even though they may contain myriad biologically active compounds. Table 50-5 lists various herbal remedies that have been suggested for relief of menopausal symptoms. Although many of these remedies have provided short-term relief of symptoms, there are no data on long-term symptom relief or disease prevention. Herbal preparations notoriously exhibit little consistency or quality control, even in the same brand. Although they claim to treat menopausal symptoms, premenstrual syndrome, and osteoporosis, dosage, absorption, and bioavailability is highly variable.

CONCLUSION

Ultimately, our goal in the treatment of menopausal women is to improve the quality and quantity of postmenopausal life. While quality of life may be a subjective assessment, it has been demonstrated that women who use ERT/HRT for at least 5 years will live considerably longer than nonusers.[57] This reduction in mortality is largely due to the protective effect against coronary heart disease, with no significant difference in overall cancer mortality between estrogen users and nonusers. Therefore, the overall risk–

benefit assessment does appear to favor the use of ERT/HRT, as a small risk of breast cancer is more than overcome by the much lower risk of mortality from other causes. Each woman, after incorporation of a healthy lifestyle, should consider all the risk factors she may have for cancer, as well as for coronary heart disease, osteoporosis, and Alzheimer's disease; how much concern she attaches to these various conditions; and how much ERT/HRT would influence the quality of her life. Women who are considering only short-term ERT for the alleviation of menopausal symptoms may do so with the assurance that such use does not increase their risk of serious disease.

REFERENCES

1. U.S. Bureau of Census. Projection of the population of the United States: 1977–2050. Current Population Report Series P-25, 704.
2. WHO Scientific Group on Research on the Menopause in the 1990s. WHO Technical Report Series. Geneva: World Health Organization, 1996:866.
3. Phillips SN, Sherwin EB. Effects of estrogen on memory function in surgically menopausal women. Psychoneuroendocrinology 1992;17:485.
4. Cardozo LD. Role of estrogens in the treatment of female urinary incontinence. J Am Geriatr Soc 1990;38:326.
5. DiFasio J, Speroff L. Estrogen replacement therapy: current thinking and practice. Geriatrics 1985;40:32.
6. Cooper C, Atkinson EJ, O'Fallon WM, Melton LJ III. The incidence of clinically diagnosed vertebral fractures: a population based study in Rochester, Minnesota, 1985–89. J Bone Miner Res 1992;7(2):221.

7. Heart and Stroke Statistical Update. Dallas: American Heart Association, 1997.

8. National Center for Health Statistics. Vital Statistics of the United States, 1992. Vol. 2–Mortality, Part A. Washington, DC: Government Printing Office, 1993.

9. Rackley CE. Estrogen and coronary artery disease in postmenopausal women. Am J Med 1995;99:117.

10. Mortola JF. Estrogens and mood. J Soc Obstet Gynecol Can 1997;19:1.

11. Ohkura T, Teshima Y, Isse K, Matsuda H, et al. Estrogen increases cerebral and cerebellar blood flow in postmenopausal women. Menopause 1995;2:13.

12. Simpkins JW, Green PS, Gridley KE, Shi J. Estrogens and memory protection. J Soc Obstet Gynecol Can 1997; 19:14.

13. Henderson VW, Paganini-Hill A. Estrogen and Alzheimer's disease. J Soc Obstet Gynecol Can 1997;19:21.

14. Hammond CB. Women's concerns with hormone replacement therapy—compliance issues. Fertil Steril 1994; 62(Suppl 2):157S.

15. Beresford SA, Weiss NS, Voigt LF, McKnight B. Risk of endometrial cancer in relation to use of estrogen combined with cyclic progestin therapy in women. Lancet 1997;349:458.

16. Whitehead MI, Townsend PT, Pryse-Davies A, et al. Effects of various types and dosages of progesterones on the postmenopausal endometrium. J Reprod Med 1982; 27:539.

17. The Postmenopausal Estrogen/Progestin Interventions (PEPI) Trial Investigators. Effects of estrogen or estrogen/progestin regimens on heart disease risk factors in postmenopausal women: the postmenopausal estrogen/progestin interventions (PEPI) trial. JAMA 1995; 273:199.

18. Moyer DL, DeLingnieres B, Driguez P, Pez JP. Prevention of endometrial hyperplasia by progesterone during long term estradiol replacement: Influence of bleeding pattern and secretory changes. Fertil Steril 1993;59:992.

19. Lindsey R, Hart DM. The minimum effective dose of estrogen for prevention of postmenopausal bone loss. Obstet Gynecol 1984;63:759.

20. Weinstein L. Efficacy of a continuous estrogen/progestin regimen in the menopausal patient. Obstet Gynecol 1987; 69:1534.

21. Sherwin BB, Gelfand MM, Bender W. Androgen enhances sexual motivation in females: a prospective crossover study of sex steroid administration on surgical menopause. Psychosom Med 1985;47:339.

22. Casson PR, Carson SA. Androgen replacement therapy in women: myths and realities. Int J Fertil 1996;41:412.

23. The Postmenopausal Estrogen/Progestin Interventions (PEPI) Trial Investigators. Effects of hormone therapy on bone mineral density: results from the Postmenopausal Estrogen/Progestin Interventions (PEPI) trial. JAMA 1996;276:1389.

24. Barrett-Connor E. Risks and benefits of replacement estrogen. Annu Rev Med 1992;43:239.

25. Stevenson JC, Cust MP, Gangar KF, et al. Effects of transdermal versus oral hormone replacement therapy on bone density in spine and proximal femur in postmenopausal women. Lancet 1990;336:265.

26. Lufkin G, Wahner HW, O'Fallon WM, et al. Treatment of postmenopausal osteoporosis with transdermal estrogen. Ann Intern Med 1992;117:1.

27. Grodstein F, Colditz GA, Stampfer MJ. Postmenopausal hormone use and tooth loss: a prospective study. Am Dent Assoc 1996;127:370.

28. Hosking D, Chilvers CED, Christiansen C, et al. Prevention of bone loss with alendronate in postmenopausal women under 60 years of age. N Engl J Med 1998; 38:485.

29. Black DM, Cummings SR, Karpf DB, et al. Randomized trial of effect of alendronate on risk of fracture and with existing vertebral fractures: Fracture Intervention Trial Research Group. Lancet 1996;348:1535.

30. Fomander T, Rutqvist LE, Sjoberg AG, et al. Long term adjuvant tamoxifen in early breast cancer: effect on bone mineral density in postmenopausal women. J Clin Oncol 1990;8:1019.

31. Delmas PD, Djamson NH, Mitlak BH, et al. Effects of raloxifene on bone mineral density, serum cholesterol concentration, and uterine endometrium in postmenopausal women. N Engl J Med 1997;37:1641.

32. Luscher TF, Boulanger CM, Yang S, Noll G, Dohi Y. Interactions between endothelium derived relaxing and contracting factors in health and cardiovascular disease. Circulation 1993;87(Suppl V):V36.

33. Collins P, Rosano GMC, Sarrel PM, et al. 17 beta-estradiol attenuates acetyl choline induced arterial constriction in women but not men with coronary heart disease. Circulation 1995;92:24.

34. Hulley S, Grady D, Bush T, et al. Randomized trial of estrogen plus progestin for secondary prevention of coronary heart disease in postmenopausal women. JAMA 1998;280:605.

35. Birge SJ. The role of estrogen in the treatment of Alzheimer's disease. Neurology 1997;48(Suppl 7):S36.

36. Kantor HI, Michael CM, Shore H. Estrogen for older women. Am J Obstet Gynecol 1973;116:115.

37. Paganini-Hill A, Henderson VW. Estrogen replacement therapy and risk of Alzheimer's disease. Arch Intern Med 1996;156:2213.

38. Tang MX, Jacobs D, Stern Y, et al. Effect of estrogen during menopause on risk and age of onset of Alzheimer's disease. Lancet 1996;348:429.

39. Calle EE. Hormone replacement therapy and colorectal cancer: interpreting the evidence. Cancer Causes Control 1997;8:127.

40. Klein BE, Klein R, Jensen SC, Ritter LL. Are sex hormones associated with age-related maculopathy in women? Beaver Dam Eye Study. Trans Am Ophthal Soc 1994;92:289.

41. Coming RG, Mitchell P. Hormone replacement therapy, reproductive factors and cataracts: the Blue Mountain Eye Study. Am J Epidemiol 1997;145:242.

42. Grodstein F, Colditz GA, Stampfer MJ. Postmenopausal hormone use and cholecystectomy in a large prospective study. Obstet Gynecol 1994;83:5.

43. Daly E, Vessey MP, Hawkins MM, Carson JL, Gough P, Marsh S. Risk of venous thromboembolism in users of hormone replacement therapy. Lancet 1996; 348:977.

44. Jick H, Derby LE, Myers W, Vasilakis C, Newton KM. Risk of hospital admission for idiopathic venous thromboembolism among users of postmenopausal estrogens. Lancet 1996;348:981.

45. Grodstein F, Stampfer MJ, Goldhaber SZ, et al. A prospective study of exogenous hormones and risk of pulmonary embolism in women. Lancet 1996;348:983.

46. Collaborative Group on Hormone Factors and Breast Cancer. Breast cancer and hormone replacement therapy: collaborative analysis of data from 51 epidemiological studies of 52,705 women with breast cancer and 108,401 women without breast cancer. Lancet 1997;350:1047.

47. Bergkvist L, Adami H-O, Person I, Bergstrom R, Krusemo UB. Prognosis after breast cancer diagnosis in women exposed to estrogen and estrogen-progestin replacement therapy. Am J Epidemiol 1989;130:221.

48. Willis DB, Calle EE, Miracle-McMahill HL, Heath CW Jr. Estrogen replacement therapy and risk of fatal breast cancer in a prospective cohort of postmenopausal women in the United States. Cancer Causes Control 1996;7:449.

49. Colditz GA, Susan E, Hankinson S, Hunter D. The use of estrogens and progestin and the risk of cancer in postmenopausal women. N Engl J Med 1995;332:1589.

50. Sellers TA, Mink PJ, Cerhan JR, et al. The role of hormone replacement therapy in the risk for breast cancer and total mortality in women with a family history of breast cancer. Ann Intern Med 1997;127:973.

51. American College of Obstetricians and Gynecologists. ACOG Committee Opinion no. 126. Estrogen replacement therapy and endometrial cancer. August 1993.

52. Schlaff WD, Moghissi K, Lemay A, et al. Multi-center trial comparing 3.6 mg Zoladex therapy with or without hormone replacement therapy for the treatment of endometriosis. Fertil Steril 1995;64:S11.

53. Eisenberg DM, Kessler RC, Foster C, et al. Unconventional medicine in the United States: prevalence, costs, and patterns of use. N Engl J Med 1993;328(4):246.

54. Murkies AL, Wilcox G, Davis SR. Phytoestrogens. J Clin Endocrinol Metab 1998;83:297.

55. Anderson JW, Johnstone BM, Cook-Newell ME. Meta-analysis of the effects of soy protein intake on serum lipids. N Engl J Med 1995;333:276.

56. Rimm EB, Stampfer MJ. The role of antioxidants in preventive cardiology. Curr Opin Cardiol 1997;12:188.

57. Ettinger B, Friedman GD, Bush T, Quesenberry CP Jr. Reduced mortality associated with long-term postmenopausal estrogen therapy. Obstet Gynecol 1996;87:6.

Chapter 51

Recurrent Pregnancy Loss

William H. Kutteh

Five Key Points

- Recurrent pregnancy loss occurs in 2 to 5% of all couples of reproductive age.

- Increased maternal age is a significant risk factor in assessing abortion risks and a prior successful pregnancy gives a more favorable prognosis to couples with recurrent pregnancy loss.

- Causes that have been associated with pregnancy loss include genetic, endocrinologic, anatomic, immunologic, microbiologic, psychologic, and idiopathic. A complete evaluation after three losses will identify an associated cause in approximately two-thirds of cases.

- When the physician decides that an evaluation is warranted, a complete diagnostic evaluation should be initiated.

- Alcohol consumption (≥5 drinks per week) and tobacco use (≥10 cigarettes per day) increases the occurrence of pregnancy loss 1.5- to 2-fold over the age-adjusted risk.

DEFINITIONS

Recurrent pregnancy loss (RPL) has classically been defined as the occurrence of three or more consecutive spontaneous pregnancy losses. However, there is a continuing controversy about what constitutes a pregnancy loss, about what number of losses a couple should experience before an evaluation is initiated, and whether sporadic or only consecutive losses should be considered.[1] The spectrum of pregnancy loss ranges from preclinical losses (developmental failure, preimplantation loss) to clinical losses (embryonic loss, fetal loss, miscarriage, stillbirth) (Table 51-1). In this chapter, clinical losses will occupy the majority of the discussion.

Each pregnancy loss can be categorized as spontaneous, incomplete, or missed. A spontaneous pregnancy loss is the natural termination of pregnancy before the fetus is capable of external life, and is considered complete if the expulsion of the entire fetus and placenta from the uterus has occurred. An incomplete pregnancy loss is diagnosed in the presence of uterine bleeding with cervical dilation or ruptured membranes and products of conception that have partially passed through the cervix or remain in the vagina. Approximately 25% of pregnant women will have spotting in early pregnancy, but more than 50% of these pregnancies will progress to term.[2] An early ultrasound helps establish the prognosis. At the time of spotting, if the ultrasound reveals an embryo with

TABLE 51-1 **SPECTRUM OF PREGNANCY LOSS**

Preclinical loss
   Developmental failure—fertilized ova does not divide
   Preimplantation—blastocyst does not implant
   Preclinical—blastocyst lost with next menstruation
Clinical loss
   Embryonic—loss before 9 weeks of gestation
   Fetal—loss at or after 9 weeks of gestation
   Miscarriage (abortion)—loss before 20 weeks of
     gestation
   Stillbirth—loss after 20 weeks of gestation

TABLE 51-2
RELATION OF ABORTION FREQUENCY TO MATERNAL AND PATERNAL AGE AT CONCEPTION

Maternal Age (Years)	Percent Abortion	Paternal Age (Years)	Percent Abortion
<20	12.2	<20	12.0
20–24	14.3	20–24	11.8
25–29	13.7	25–29	15.7
30–34	15.5	30–34	13.1
35–39	18.7	35–39	15.8
40–44	33.8	40–44	19.5
>44	53.2	—	—

Data assembled from Warburton D and Fraser FC.[5]

a crown-to-rump length (CRL) of <5 mm and a heart rate of <80 bpm, it is almost universally associated with a subsequent embryonic death.[3] In embryos with a CRL of 5 to 9 mm, a heart rate of <100 bpm is indicative of a poor outcome, and for embryos with a CRL of 10 to 15 mm, a heart rate of <110 bpm is associated with a poor prognosis. A missed abortion occurs when the conceptus is retained in utero for more than 4 weeks after the death of a previously viable fetus as documented by sonography, Doppler ultrasound, or other means. More often than not, the nonviable fetus is retained for several weeks. In the absence of early ultrasound evaluation, these pregnancy losses may be considered to have occurred many weeks after the actual end of viability.[4] Thus, it is very important to obtain an accurate and detailed history of previous pregnancies in all couples with recurrent pregnancy loss.

OCCURRENCE AND RECURRENCE

The frequency of spontaneous pregnancy loss depends primarily on the method used to document pregnancy. It is well established that 10 to 15% of clinically recognized pregnancies will result in a fetal loss.[5] Originally, these losses were recognized after 8 weeks of gestation based on clinical observations such as bleeding, cervical dilation, passage of tissue, or pathologic determination of chorionic villi. More recently, the rate of pregnancy loss has been confirmed with the use of sensitive immunoassays specific for β-human chorionic gonadotropin (βHCG).[6-8]

In a study of 221 women followed for a total of 707 menstrual cycles, 198 pregnancies were detected (28%) based upon elevated urinary β-HCG.[6] There were 43 preclinical losses (22%), and in the remaining

155 clinical pregnancies there were 19 losses (12%), for an overall loss of 31%.

Maternal age has been shown to be a significant factor in assessing abortion risks.[5] The clinical pregnancy loss rate in women over 40 was more than double the rate in women younger than 20 (Table 51-2). Prior pregnancy history is also an important factor in assessing the risk of subsequent miscarriage based on the study of over 2000 couples with primary versus secondary pregnancy loss.[5] In couples with at least one live birth, the recurrence risk of pregnancy loss in a subsequent pregnancy increased from 12% to approximately 30% after three or four losses. However, in those couples who never had a live birth, the prognosis of recurrence was found to increase significantly with each additional loss (Table 51-3).[5,9] Importantly, these findings suggest that couples with a prior successful pregnancy and subsequent pregnancy loss have approximately a 70% chance of eventually producing a liveborn child. Those who have never delivered a liveborn offspring

TABLE 51-3
RECURRENCE RISK RELATIVE TO PRIOR GESTATIONAL EVENTS

Prior Outcome	Prior Losses	Recurrence (%)
Liveborn	0	12
	1	24
	2	26
	3	32
	4	26
Miscarriage	1	19
	2	35
	3	47
	4	54

Data collected from Poland BJ, Miller JR, Jones DC, Trimble BK[9] and Warburton D and Fraser FC.[5]

are faced with a lower overall success rate, about 50%.[10] Thus, both advancing maternal age and history of miscarriage are important factors in predicting future outcome and the possible effects of any treatment. The chance of a couple experiencing recurrent loss is between 1 and 2% per year.[11]

CAUSES OF RECURRENT LOSS

In general, the causes that have been associated with RPL have been categorized into genetic, endocrinologic, anatomic, immunologic, microbiologic, psychologic, and other factors.[12-16] Genetic abnormalities may occur in one or both of the parents in 1.8 to 4.6% of couples. Endocrinologic abnormalities have been reported in 5 to 29% of women with pregnancy loss. Immunologic factors have been associated with RPL in 15 to 50% of couples. Anatomic abnormalities, both of the congenital and acquired nature, have been reported in 5 to 28% of women with RPL. While microbiologic factors have not been shown to be a cause of multiple pregnancy loss, infectious agents are a factor in some cases of sporadic pregnancy loss. Recently, some authors have suggested that all women with RPL be evaluated for possible thrombophilia.[17] However, studies have not supported these recommendations.[18] Psychologic factors, which undoubtedly play a role in couples who have experienced the grief and suffering of even a single pregnancy loss, are more difficult to quantitate but often lend themselves to individual or group support sessions. After the basic evaluation for recurrent pregnancy loss is completed, as described later in this chapter, cause can be determined in over 65% of couples.[12,13]

GENETIC FACTORS

Losses attributed to genetic reasons can be divided into two large categories—parental and fetal. In recurrent pregnancy loss, a parental chromosomal anomaly (usually a balanced translocation) can be identified approximately 2 to 4% of the time.[19] The distribution of chromosomal abnormalities according to the sex of the carrier has been analyzed[20] (Table 51-4). Overall abnormalities were identified twice as frequently in the female partner in 16,661 couples studied. A karyotype of both partners should certainly be included in the workup for RPL.

Couples with normal karyotypes should be counseled that they may have a fetus with chromosomal abnormalities. In products of conception that have been karyotyped, the autosomal trisomies comprise the most frequent chromosomal complement in first-trimester spontaneous abortions. Of these, trisomy 16 occurs most frequently and is uniformly lethal. Trisomy 21 (Down syndrome) is usually the result of meiotic nondisjunction: the extra chromosome is maternal 80% of the time, which suggests a greater frequency of nondisjunction in oocytes than in spermatocytes. Monosomy X (45,X or Turner syndrome) is the most frequent individual karyotype found in the abortus of women with a single pregnancy loss. Triploidy (3n = 69) is the next most frequent group of chromosomal anomalies. The supernumerary haploid chromosome set originates from a paternal source in 80% of cases, suggesting that polyspermia is a possible mechanism. Tetraploidy (4n = 92), translocations, and mosaicisms occur less frequently. In addition, it has been shown that a correlation exists between the chromosomal complement of different spontaneous miscarriages in the same couple.[21-23] A

	TABLE 51-4		
	DISTRIBUTION OF CHROMOSOME ABNORMALITIES ACCORDING TO THE SEX OF THE CARRIER		
Abnormality	**Males** (n = 16,661)	**Females** (n = 16,661)	**Both** (n = 33,322)
Reciprocal translocations	150 (36.1)*	265 (63.9)	415
Robertsonian translocations	58 (30.4)	133 (69.6)	191
Inversions	25 (41.7)	35 (58.3)	60
Sex chromosome aneuploidy	7 (26.9)	19 (73.1)	26
Supernumerary chromosome	2 (18.2)	9 (81.8)	11
Total abnormalities	242 (34.4)	461 (65.6)	703

*Numbers in parentheses represent percentages of abnormalities listed that occurred in males as compared with females.

Data collected from DeBraekeleer M and Dao TN.[20]

pregnancy loss with a normal karyotype is most likely to result in a normal karyotype in the next pregnancy, whether it is a loss or a delivery. Furthermore, there is no increased risk of trisomy from a previous trisomic fetus. Finally, a nontrisomic but aneuploid loss results in an increased risk of nontrisomic aneuploidy in the next pregnancy.

ENDOCRINOLOGIC FACTORS

Widely divergent estimates of the significance of luteal-phase deficiency in RPL have been described ranging from 20 to 60%.[24,25] Two studies of RPL have noted a 15 to 20% incidence of a lag in endometrial maturation of 2 or more days in two consecutive cycles.[26,27] It is also of interest that evaluation of late-luteal-phase endometrial biopsies performed on regularly menstruating, fertile women with no history of pregnancy loss reveals a 26.7% incidence of at least a 2-day lag in sequential cycles.[28] These results bring into question the association of a luteal-phase defect with RPL as postulated by several authors.[24,25]

The optimal means of diagnosing a luteal-phase defect is also uncertain. The use of serum progesterone levels and of timed endometrial biopsies have been championed, and some clinicians use both.[29,30] In general, if a midluteal serum progesterone level is >10 ng/ml, an endometrial biopsy performed near the end of this cycle is unlikely to demonstrate a time lag greater than 2 days.[31] Biopsy studies appear to be more sensitive, but they are less specific. A diagnosis of luteal-phase defect is generally reserved for cases in which at least two consecutive biopsies have shown results consistent with a 2-day or greater lag in endometrial maturation.[32] Establishing ovulation more objectively via sonography or luteinizing hormone (LH) monitoring has been urged as a means to improve diagnostic testing and validity.[33]

Various treatments have been prescribed for luteal-phase deficiency,[25] including ovulation induction with either clomiphene citrate or human menopausal gonadotropins, HCG injection at the time of expected ovulation, and progesterone supplementation both during the luteal phase and up to 10 weeks of gestation. Bromocriptine therapy is recommended if the luteal-phase dysfunction is thought to be secondary to elevated prolactin levels.[34]

There is less information regarding other endocrinopathies and early pregnancy loss. Diabetes is more often associated with late pregnancy loss or stillbirth. Diabetic women with first-trimester elevations of blood glucose and glycosylated hemoglobin are at significantly greater risk of having a spontaneous abortion.[7] Insulin resistance, often associated with polycystic ovarian disease, is being investigated as a probable correlate to increased spontaneous pregnancy loss.[35] Significant thyroid and adrenal disorders usually result in infertility. However, both hypothyroidism and hyperthyroidism are associated with both early and late pregnancy loss, but data are insufficient to correlate thyroid disorders and recurrent early pregnancy loss.

ANATOMIC FACTORS

Women with a history of RPL have a significantly greater incidence of uterine abnormalities. This diagnostic group encompasses not only congenital uterine anomalies,[36] but also acquired abnormalities such as intrauterine synechiae, leiomyomatas, and the functional abnormality termed cervical incompetence. Müllerian anomalies have been diagnosed in 2 to 6% of women in populations with normal reproductive histories.[37-38] An even greater percentage of women evaluated for RPL have been found to have abnormalities of the upper genital tract.[37,39] Müllerian anomalies most likely originate from polygenetic or multifactorial causes, but some types of Müllerian malformations have been associated with in-utero diethylstilbestrol (DES) exposure.[40] All of these DES-exposed patients have increased rates of spontaneous abortion, preterm delivery, and ectopic pregnancy.[41] Unfortunately, data on the benefit of surgical therapy in patients with Müllerian anomalies are inconclusive because the majority of studies present the outcomes for groups of nonrandomized patients.[42-44] Patients with a history of DES exposure or the diagnosis of a unicornuate uterus are generally thought to have no improvement with metroplasty. Some investigators have advocated the liberal use of cerclage in patients with RPL,[45,46] particularly for individuals with a history of second-trimester losses. Women with RPL and a uterus didelphys or a bicornuate uterus can be considered for a cerclage or a Strassman unification procedure. A complete evaluation for other causes of RPL should be performed before recommending metroplasty. Operative hysteroscopy is the most popular therapy for a septate uterus when this anomaly is identified in a patient with RPL.[47,48]

These recommendations are based on favorable outcomes for patients carefully selected before surgery. Without data from a randomized prospective trial, the true benefit of these procedures for fertility and pregnancy maintenance remain uncertain.[49]

Acquired uterine abnormalities such as intrauterine synechiae are found in approximately 5% of women with RPL.[50] These adhesions and/or the accompanying uterine curettage may be causative of or secondary to pregnancy loss. The majority of cases of Asherman syndrome appear to result from uterine instrumentation. Good success rates have been reported following hysteroscopic removal of intrauterine adhesions.[51] The importance of leiomyomas as a cause of RPL is not well documented. Generally, submucous myomas or large intramural myomas that cause an endometrial impression are surgically removed.[52] The diagnosis and best treatment for cervical incompetence also remain areas of controversy rather than subjects of appropriately randomized clinical trials, although women with histories most clearly suggestive of cervical incompetence demonstrate excellent rates of term pregnancy achievement following an early gestation cervical cerclage procedure.[53,54]

IMMUNOLOGIC FACTORS

Two primary pathophysiologic models that support immunologic causes of RPL have evolved. The first is that some women's immune systems may produce phospholipid or other autoantibodies, which are thought to have a variety of deleterious effects on pregnancy. This is the autoimmune theory of RPL. The classical alloimmune theory is the model in which normal pregnancy maintenance requires that the immune system recognize an implanting embryo as foreign in order to protect the embryo from attack by the maternal system.[55] More recently, various alloimmune theories have been invoked to explain fetal loss, including T-helper embryotoxic cytokine factors, CD56-positive natural killer cells, and antipaternal cytotoxic antibodies.[56-59]

Autoimmune Association

An association between certain autoimmune conditions and RPL is now well established. During the past decade, the antiphospholipid syndrome (APS) has emerged as a heterogeneous autoimmune disorder associated with substantial risk for fetal loss.[60] The diagnosis of APS requires both clinical and serologic features, as outlined in Table 51-5.[61] The syndrome is designated as primary in patients with no apparent underlying disease and secondary when systemic lupus erythematosus (SLE) or a lupuslike disorder is also present. Women with antiphospholipid antibodies (APAs) but no clinical features, and those with fetal deaths and thromboembolic events but no laboratory abnormalities, are not currently classified. The most significant APAs have specificity against negatively charged phospholipids and are most commonly detected by determining lupus anticoagulant (LA) and anticardiolipin antibody (ACA) activity. Women with both previous early fetal loss and high levels of ACA may have a recurrent loss rate of 70%.[62] In referral populations of women with recurrent pregnancy loss, an approximate incidence of 15 to 20% positive APAs has been reported, while only 2 to 5% of low-risk

---

TABLE 51-5
SUGGESTED CLINICAL AND LABORATORY CRITERIA FOR THE ANTIPHOSPHOLIPID SYNDROME*

Clinical Features	Laboratory Features
Pregnancy morbidity	Lupus anticoagulant
≥1 unexplained death at ≥10 weeks or delivery at ≤34 weeks with severe PIH or three or more losses <10 weeks	
Thrombosis	IgG anticardiolipin antibodies (≥20 GPL)
Venous	
Arterial, including stroke	IgM anticardiolipin antibodies (≥20 MPL)

*Patients with antiphospholipid syndrome should have at least one clinical and one laboratory feature at some time during the course of their disease. Laboratory tests should be positive on at least two occasions more than 6 weeks apart. GPL = IgG phospholipid units; MPL = IgM phospholipid units; PIH = pregnancy-induced hypertension.

From Wilson WA et al.[63]

obstetrical patients with no history of recurrent loss will have LAs or ACAs.[11,63,64]

LA produces a paradoxical prolongation of phospholipid-dependent clotting assays which is not corrected on mixing with normal plasma. Tests commonly used to screen for LA are the activated partial thromboplastin time (APTT), dilute Russell viper venom time (dRVVT), and the kaolin clotting time (KCT).[65] The presence of LA must be confirmed by two additional tests when one identifies a prolonged phospholipid-dependent clotting assay.[66] Failure to correct the prolonged test with appropriate mixing studies and confirmation of phospholipid dependence are essential steps necessary to conclude that LA is present. In contrast, ACA is detected in an enzyme-linked immunosorbent assay (ELISA) using cardiolipin as antigen. For the results from a laboratory to be reliable, the ACA assay must be properly standardized.[67,68] Many APS patients have both LA and ACA, but they are not always concordant in a given patient. Therefore, both a coagulation assay for LA and an immunoassay for ACA should be performed if the presence of APAs is suspected. Low levels of IgG ACAs or IgM ACAs may represent nonspecific binding and are of questionable clinical significance.[69]

Some authors have suggested that autoantibodies other than LA or ACA contribute to the diagnosis or treatment of patients with recurrent autoimmune pregnancy loss.[70] β_2 glycoprotein is a cofactor for phospholipid binding, but its relevance to recurrent pregnancy loss is uncertain.[72] Women with recurrent pregnancy loss have a higher frequency of positive antinuclear antibody (ANA) titers, but their next pregnancy outcomes do not differ from women with negative ANAs.[73-79] The value of routine profiles for other phospholipids, nucleotides, histones, and their isotypes is still under investigation.[74-78] For example, as many as 10 to 15% of normal pregnant women have low ANA titers.[74] Autoantibodies to thyroglobulin and thyroid peroxidase or microsomal antigen are found in patients with Hashimoto thyroiditis, Graves disease, postpartum thyroiditis, and in some normal individuals. A correlation between the presence of thyroid antibodies and first-trimester pregnancy loss has been reported; however, antithyroid antibodies are present in 15 to 20% of normal pregnant women, which is comparable to women with a history of recurrent miscarriages.[79-82] Antithyroid antibodies may be a marker for other autoimmune diseases or may identify a subgroup of women who may not meet

the increased demand for thyroid hormones in early pregnancy, but the cause of thyroid-antibody–related pregnancy loss remains largely theoretical. More studies are needed to determine if effective treatment can be identified and to resolve whether these screening tests have any utility in the routine evaluation of patients with RPL.

Preconceptional counseling of patients with APS regarding the risk for serious medical problems is essential. Pregnancy complications include thromboembolic events, preeclampsia, fetal growth restriction, fetal distress, and a rare but serious postpartum cardiopulmonary syndrome.[65,83] Various treatment options are available for the patient with APS. Approximately 30% of patients have achieved live births without specific medical therapy. However, the prognosis is less favorable when previous pregnancies have been unsuccessful in the presence of LA or high levels of ACA. Comparison of studies is limited because of differences in study design, patient selection, and regimens used; however, data from controlled studies are summarized in Table 51-6.[83-90] Inclusion criteria used to select studies for this analysis were: (1) a study design that included a treated and a control group; (2) patients with at least two prior fetal losses; and (3) patients with serologic proof of LA or IgG ACA >20 IgG phospholipid units (GPL). All treatments appeared to improve the livebirth rate, but heparin and low-dose aspirin were superior to prednisone and low-dose aspirin when considering maternal and fetal complications.[83-90] Most clinicians use 10,000 to 20,000 units of heparin daily in two divided doses. Supplemental calcium, 1.5 g/day, may reduce the increased risk of osteopenia associated with higher doses. Concomitant use of prednisone and heparin is not recommended because this combination has not been shown to be better than either

---

TABLE 51-6
COMPARISON OF TREATMENTS OF WOMEN WITH ≥2 APA-ASSOCIATED PREGNANCY LOSSES*

Treatment	No. Treated	No. Liveborn (%)
None	166	33 (20)
Aspirin (80 mg/day)	81	39 (48)
Prednisone + aspirin	145	88 (61)
Heparin + Aspirin	151	113 (75)

*Data collected from controlled studies. Prednisone treatments included if at least 30 mg daily. Aspirin treatment was 60 to 100 mg daily. Heparin treatment was 10,000 to 20,000 units daily.

alone in achieving a live birth, and fracture risk may increase in women treated with the combination regimen. Some pregnant women with APS have been treated with intravenous immune globulin (IVIG).[91,92] Because this therapy appears less effective and is more expensive than heparin plus aspirin, IVIG for APS remains experimental at this time.

Alloimmune Association

Alloimmunity refers to immunologic differences between individuals of the same species. One example is the major-histocompatibility-antigen system. Because an embryo is the product of both maternal and paternal genomes, it is antigenically different from the mother. One rationale for an alloimmune cause for RPL is the assumption that unless the maternal immune system is suppressed, it would normally reject an implanting embryo. The process of blocking embryo rejection is believed to be maternally mediated. Alloimmune-mediated pregnancy rejection has been hypothesized to be due to the absence of dissimilarities between paternal and maternal antigens (i.e., HLA sharing). However, laboratory tests such as HLA typing or blocking antibodies are of no value in identifying patients with alloimmune-mediated pregnancy losses. More recently, several tests have been reported to be useful in identifying women with autoimmune abnormalities associated with RPL.[56-59] Tests that identify T-helper embryotoxic cytokine factors, such as interferon-γ and tumor necrosis factor-α, are being investigated.[57,58] Recent reports suggest that elevation of T-helper type 1 cytokines are associated with pregnancy loss (Table 51-7).[57,58] Immunophenotypes of endometrial cells from women with RPL as compared with normal fertile controls demonstrate alterations in large granular lymphocytes identified as natural killer cells.[93,94] One study suggested an association between elevated levels of peripheral blood natural killer cells (CD56+) and RPL, but the study was small and should be expanded and

confirmed.[59] Antipaternal cytotoxic antibody assays (leukocyte antibody detection) are also being evaluated as a possible marker for alloimmune-associated RPL.[60] However, to date, there are no specific tests to identify women with alloimmune RPL.

Even though definitive tests to diagnose patients with alloimmune-mediated RPL are lacking, two modes of alloimmunotherapy have been studied. These therapies are immunization with allogeneic blood mononuclear cells (an active immunization) and administration of IVIG (a passive immunization).

With leukocyte immunization, the patient with RPL is given either paternal or donor leukocytes before conception. Leukocytes have been administered intravenously, subcutaneously, intradermally, and as a combination of all three. Several randomized, controlled trials including a total of about 400 women have been published.[95-98] Perhaps all that can be concluded at this time is that roughly 60% of patients with RPL who have received paternal leukocyte immunization therapy have had successful pregnancies. From two independent analyses, the conclusion was reached that 11 patients have to be immunized to achieve one additional live birth.[99] The recent study by Ober et al.[100] investigated whether paternal mononuclear cell immunization improves the rate of successful pregnancies in women who had three or more spontaneous abortions. Women with other known causes of pregnancy loss were excluded in this double-blind, multicenter, randomized clinical trial. The successful pregnancy outcome in the group treated with paternal mononuclear cells was 31 out of 86 (36%), as compared with 41 out of 85 (48%) in the placebo group. This is the largest study performed to date and indicates that paternal mononuclear cell immunization therapy does not improve pregnancy outcome in women with recurrent miscarriage. The expense and potential morbidity associated with immunization therapy make full disclosure of relevant information and informed consent all the more important.[101,102]

The administration of IVIG has been evaluated as an alternative to allogeneic blood leukocyte therapy for the treatment of RPL. The mechanism by which IVIG modulates immune function is not known. The two most recent prospective, randomized, double-blind, placebo-controlled trials of the use of IVIG in the prevention of unexplained RPL demonstrated no differences in the subsequent pregnancy outcome when using IVIG versus placebo.[103,104] A total of six

TABLE 51-7 CD4+ T-HELPER CELLS AND EMBRYOTOXIC FACTORS		
	TH1	**TH2**
Response	Cellular	Humoral
Cytokines	TNF-α, IFNγ	IL-4, IL-5, IL-10
Function	Cytotoxicity	Protection
Associated	Pregnancy loss	Normal pregnancy

TABLE 51-8
INTRAVENOUS HUMAN IMMUNOGLOBULIN TREATMENT FOR RPL

Investigator	Entry* Criteria	IVIG (% Delivered)	Albumin (% Delivered)	P Value
Christiansen, 1992[106]	≥3 losses; normal HSG, P_4, TSH, chromosomes	9/17 (53%)	5/17 (29%)	0.16
GRSA/IVIG, 1994[107]	≥2 losses; normal uterus, chromosomes	20/33 (61%)	21/31 (68%)	0.17
Coulam, 1995[108]	≥2 losses; normal ANA, P_4, hysteroscopy, chromosomes	18/29 (62%)	12/32 (38%)	0.04
Perino, 1997[109]	≥3 losses; normal genetic, HSG, ANA, ACA cultures	16/22 (73%)	19/24 (79%)	0.73
Stephenson, 1997[104]	≥3 losses; normal gynecologic, genetic, HSG, and APA	11/19 (58%)	10/19 (53%)	0.50
Jablonowska, 1999[105]	≥3 losses; normal HSG, genetics, TSH, P_4, ANA, ACA	17/22 (77%)	15/19 (79%)	1.00
Total		91/142 (64%)	82/142 (58%)	0.33

*HSG = hysterosalpingogram; TSH = thyroid-stimulating hormone; ANA = antinuclear antibody; APA = antiphospholipid antibody.

randomized clinical trials evaluating the efficacy of IVIG for RPL have been published,[103-108] but results have not been in agreement (Table 51-8).[110,111] Enthusiasm over this treatment scheme should await the outcome of an appropriately designed, randomized, controlled trial for the use of IVIG for RPL.

MICROBIOLOGIC FACTORS

Maternal infections by a variety of organisms have been linked to pregnancy loss, including Mycoplasma (*M. hominis*),[111] Ureaplasma (*U. urealyticum*), group B β-hemolytic streptococci, Chlamydia,[112] *Treponema pallidum,* Toxoplasma, and viruses such as rubella, cytomegalovirus, herpes virus, and coxsackievirus. Most investigators interested in RPL have focused on *M. hominis* and *U. urealyticum* as possible causative agents. Two studies have reported a higher incidence of infection by these organisms in women with a history of multiple losses as compared with control women,[115,116] and two other nonrandomized studies have reported a higher proportion of good pregnancy outcomes following antibiotic therapy for infections of these organisms in women with RPL.[116,117] However, despite conclusive cause-and-effect relationships between *M. hominis* and *U. urealyticum* infection, antibiotic therapy, and RPL, many clinicians advise culture and treatment of these bacteria.

OTHER FACTORS

It has been postulated that RPL is caused by maternal exposure to a variety of environmental factors.[117,118] Few of the suggested agents have been conclusively demonstrated to cause abortion, however, except for ionizing radiation and several drugs such as antimetabolites (e.g., methotrexate), isotretinoin, and mifepristone.[117] Alcohol consumption (5 drinks per week) and cigarette smoking (10 cigarettes per day) have both been observed to increase the occurrence of pregnancy loss 1.5- to 2-fold.[119-121] Controversy continues over the association of caffeine use with spontaneous pregnancy loss.[122-125] Two reports indicate that the use of computer monitors and exposure to the accompanying electromagnetic fields do not put a woman at risk for spontaneous abortion.[126,127]

Increasing attention has been directed toward coagulation abnormalities in addition to APA as possible causes of RPL. Factor V Leiden (a point mutation [1691 → A] in the factor V gene), the prothrombin 20210 G → A mutation, and homozygosity for a common polymorphism in the methlyene tetrahydrofolate reductase (MTHFR) gene have been associated with arterial and venous thrombosis and arterial occlusive disease. MTHFR homozygosity is associated with increased homocysteine levels and pregnancy loss.[128] In view of the new recognition of the clinical importance of inherited disorders that predispose to venous thrombosis, women with recurrent miscarriages who have completed the standard workup (genetic, endocrinologic, anatomic, immunologic, microbiologic, iatrogenic) with no identified cause should consider hematologic screening.[129,130] This is definitely necessary in women with a previous episode or a close family history (parent or sibling) of thromboembolism.

Several investigators have presented results suggesting that psychological stress may be directly involved with RPL.[15,132] A selected subset of a group of patients with RPL who received supportive counseling demonstrated a better pregnancy outcome than patients not receiving this support. Interesting theoretical models linking stress to biologic changes detrimental to fetal development have been described.[133]

SUMMARY

Evaluation of a couple with RPL includes a directed history, physical examination, and laboratory evaluation. RPL, by definition, involves women who have had three or more losses, but factors such as advanced age or patient desire may often prompt evaluation of women with two losses. Both the evaluation and treatment must involve a sensitivity to psychological stresses that invariably accompany this problem. Appropriate counseling may lessen patient distress and marital dysfunction and may even improve the prognosis.[15,132]

When the decision to begin an evaluation is made, the complete evaluation should be recommended to all women (Table 51-9). Many have multiple factors contributing to RPL that can be identified only after a complete evaluation. Laboratory evaluations almost universally accepted include a karyotype of the woman and her partner, some assessment of luteal-phase adequacy and, when indicated, serum thyrotropin and prolactin levels. An assessment of uterine structure by hysterosalpingography, hysteroscopy, or sonohysterography is important.[134] Immunologic screening is complete only with appropriately performed assays for LA and ACA, such as the dRVVT and the ELISA. Cervical cultures for chlamydia and mycoplasma are often included and may be an occasional cause of miscarriage, but have not been associated with multiple losses.[135] Data from several well-designed studies argue against the use of expensive tests such as HLA typing (including HLA-DQα),[136] antipaternal antibody titers, or mixed lymphocyte blocking factor testing.[137,138] The role of tests for antithyroid antibodies, embryotoxic factors, and peripheral blood immunophenotypes remains unclear.

The use of alloimmunotherapy for unexplained RPL remains controversial.[60] At present, neither therapy can be recommended for routine clinical use for the treatment of recurrent spontaneous abortion.

TABLE 51-9
DIAGNOSIS AND MANAGEMENT OF RECURRENT PREGNANCY LOSS

Cause	Diagnostic Evaluation	Abnormal Result	Therapy
Genetic	Karyotype partners	3–5%	Genetic counseling
			Donor gametes
Anatomic	Hysterosalpingogram	15–20%	Septum transection
	Hysteroscopy		Cervical cerclage
	Sonohysterography		Myomectomy
Endocrinologic	Endometrial biopsy	5–8%	Progesterone
	Midluteal progesterone		Clomiphene citrate
	Thyroid-stimulating hormone		Levothyroxine
	Prolactin		Bromocriptine
	Fasting insulin/glucose		Glucophage
Immunologic	Lupus anticoagulant	15–25%	Aspirin
	Antiphospholipid antibodies		Heparin + aspirin
	(? Antithyroid antibodies)		Prednisone + aspirin
	(? Embryotoxicity assay)		(? IVIG)
	(? Immunophenotypes)		(? Leukocyte therapy)
Microbiologic	Cervical cultures	5–10%	Antibiotics
Thrombophilic (?)	Antithrombin III	(? 5%)	Aspirin
	Protein C, Protein S deficiency		Heparin + aspirin
	Factor V Leiden mutation		Low-molecular-weight heparin
	Dysfibrinogenemia		Folic acid
	Hyperhomocysteinemia		
Psychological	Interview	Varies	Support groups
	Questionnaire		Counseling
Iatrogenic	Tobacco, alcohol use	5%	Eliminate consumption
	Exposure to toxins, chemicals		Eliminate exposure

Thus, only patients who have had a complete evaluation that was negative and who have given informed consent should be considered for either leukocyte or IVIG therapy.

Clearly, a large number of couples with RPL experience profound grief, anger, and depression as a result of their reproductive failure. The ensuing sense of desperation may lessen their ability to cogently weigh pros and cons of various therapies. Couples with RPL who are having great difficulty dealing with their losses should be encouraged to undergo psychological counseling and join specific support groups such as SHARE.[140] Physicians are responsible for helping them resist the temptation of treatments that have not been scientifically validated. Finally, on an optimistic note, the couple should be reminded that 60 to 70% of women with a completely negative evaluation for RPL will ultimately deliver healthy offspring.[12]

REFERENCES

1. Plouffe L, Tho SPT, Hansen K. Basic workup of the couple with recurrent pregnancy loss. Infertil Reprod Med Clin N Am 1996;7:825.
2. Cunningham FG, MacDonald PC, Gant NF, et al. Abortion. In: Cunningham FG, McDonald PC, Gant NF, Leveno KJ, Gilstrap LC, eds. *Williams obstetrics,* 19th ed. Norwalk, CT: Appleton & Lange, 1993:661.
3. Doubilet PM, Benson CB. Embryonic heart rate in the first trimester: what rate is normal? J Ultrasound Med 1995;14:431.
4. Gilmore DH, McNay MB. Spontaneous fetal loss rate in early pregnancy. Lancet 1985;1:107.
5. Warburton D, Fraser FC. Spontaneous abortion risks in man: data from reproductive histories collected in a medical genetics unit. Am J Human Genet 1964;16:1.
6. Wilcox AJ, Weinberg CR, O'Connor JF, et al. Incidence of early pregnancy loss. N Engl J Med 1988;319:189.
7. Mills JL, Simpson JL, Driscoll SG, et al. Incidence of spontaneous abortion among normal women and insulin-dependent diabetic women whose pregnancies were identified within 21 days of conception. N Engl J Med 1988;319:1617.
8. Miller JF, Williamson E, Glue J, et al. Fetal loss after implantation: a prospective study. Lancet 1980;2:554.
9. Poland BJ, Miller JR, Jones DC, Trimble BK. Reproductive counseling in patients who have had a spontaneous abortion. Am J Obstet Gynecol 1977;127:685.
10. Stirrat GM. Recurrent miscarriage. I. Definition and epidemiology. Lancet 1990;336:673.
11. Kutteh WH. Recurrent pregnancy loss. In: Carr BR, Blackwell RE, eds. Textbook of reproductive medicine, 2nd ed. Stamford, CT: Appleton & Lange, 1998:679.
12. Harger JH, Archer DF, Marchese SG, et al. Etiology of recurrent pregnancy losses and outcome of subsequent pregnancies. Obstet Gynecol 1983;62:574.
13. Stephenson M. Frequency of factors associated with habitual abortion in 197 couples. Fertil Steril 1996;66:24.
14. Stirrat GM. Recurrent miscarriage. II. Clinical associations, causes, and management. Lancet 1990;336:728.
15. Stray-Pederson B, Stray-Pederson S. Etiologic factors and subsequent reproductive performance in 195 couples with a prior history of habitual abortion. Am J Obstet Gynecol 1984;148:140.
16. Tho PT, Byrd JR, McDonough PG. Etiologies and subsequent reproductive performance of 100 couples with recurrent abortion. Fertil Steril 1979;32:389.
17. Blumenfeld Z, Brenner B. Thrombophilia-associated pregnancy wastage. Fertil Steril 1999;72:765.
18. Kutteh WH, Park VM, Deitcher SR. Hypercoagulable state mutation analysis in white patients with early first-trimester recurrent pregnancy loss. Fertil Steril 1999; 71:1048.
19. Castle D, Bernstein R. Cytogenetic analysis of 688 couples experiencing multiple spontaneous abortions. Am J Med Genet 1988;39:549.
20. DeBraekeleer M, Dao TN. Cytogenetic studies in couples experiencing repeated pregnancy losses. Hum Reprod 1990;5:519.
21. Hassold TJ. A cytogenetic study of repeated spontaneous abortions. Am J Hum Genet 1980;32:723.
22. Warburton D, Kline J, Stein Z, et al. Does the karyotype of a spontaneous abortion predict the karyotype of a subsequent abortion? Evidence from 273 women with two karyotyped spontaneous abortions. Am J Hum Genet 41:465, 1987.
23. Geraedts JPM. Chromosomal anomalies and recurrent miscarriage. Infertil Reprod Med Clin N Am 1996; 7:677.
24. Karamardian LM, Grimes DA. Luteal phase deficiency: effect of treatment on pregnancy rates. Am J Obstet Gynecol 167:1391, 1992.
25. McNeely MS, Soules MR. The diagnosis of luteal phase deficiency: a critical review. Fertil Steril 1988;50:1.
26. Tulppala M, Björses U-M, Stenman U-H, et al. Luteal phase defect in habitual abortion: progesterone in saliva. Fertil Steril 1991;56:41.
27. Baird DD, Weinberg CR, Wilcox AJ, et al. Hormonal profiles in natural conception cycles ending in early, unrecognized pregnancy loss. J Clin Endocrinol Metab 1991;72:793.
28. Davis OK, Berkeley AS, Naus GJ, et al. The incidence of luteal phase defect in normal, fertile women, determined by serial endometrial biopsies. Fertil Steril 1989;51:582.
29. Rosenfeld DL, Garcia CR. A comparison of endometrial histology with simultaneous plasma progesterone determinations in infertile women. Fertil Steril 1976;27:1256.
30. Koninckx PR, Goddeeris PG, Lauweryns JM, et al. Accuracy of endometrial biopsy dating in relation to the midcycle luteinizing hormone peak. Fertil Steril 1977;28:443.
31. Heinsleigh PA, Fainstat T. Corpus luteum dysfunction: serum progesterone levels in diagnosis and assessment of therapy for recurrent and threatened abortion. Fertil Steril 1979;32:396.

32. Noyes RW. Uniformity of secretory endometrium. Obstet Gynecol 1956;7:221.

33. Peters AJ, Lloyd RP, Coulam CB. Prevalence of out-of-phase endometrial biopsy specimens. Am J Obstet Gynecol 1992;166:1738.

34. Pozo ED, Wyss H, Tolis G, et al. Prolactin and deficient luteal function. Obstet Gynecol 1979;53:282.

35. Kutteh WH. Treating PCOS-related infertility with insulin sensitizing agents. OBG Management 2000; 10:106.

36. Rock JA. Diagnosing and repairing uterine anomalies. Contemp Obstet Gynecol 1981;1:17.

37. Cooper JM, Houck RM, Rigberg HS. The incidence of intrauterine abnormalities found at hysteroscopy in patients undergoing elective hysteroscopic sterilization. J Reprod Med 1983;28:659.

38. Portuondo JA, Clmara MM, Echanojauregui AD, et al. Müllerian abnormalities in fertile women and recurrent aborters. J Reprod Med 1986;31:616.

39. Greiss FC, Mauzy CH. Genital anomalies in women: an evaluation of diagnosis, incidence and obstetrical performance. Am J Obstet Gynecol 1961;82:330.

40. American Fertility Society: The American Fertility Society classifications of adnexal adhesions, distal tubal occlusion, tubal occlusion secondary to tubal ligation, tubal pregnancies, Müllerian anomalies and intrauterine adhesions. Fertil Steril 1988;49:944.

41. Kaufman RH, Adam E, Binder GL, et al. Upper genital tract changes and pregnancy outcome in offspring exposed in utero to diethylstilbestrol. Am J Obstet Gynecol 1980;137:299.

42. Stillman RJ. In utero exposure to diethylstilbestrol: adverse effects on the reproductive tract and reproductive performance in male and female offspring. Am J Obstet Gynecol 1981;142:905.

43. Heinoven PK, Saarikoski S, Pystynen P. Reproductive performance of women with uterine anomalies. Acta Obstet Gynecol Scand 1982;61:157.

44. Rossi G, Diamond MP. Myomas, reproductive function, and pregnancy. Seminars Reprod Endocrinol 1992; 10:332.

45. Rock JA, Jones HW Jr. The clinical management of the double uterus. Fertil Steril 1977;28:798.

46. Ludmir J, Landon B, Gabbe SG, et al. Management of the diethylstilbestrol exposed pregnant patient: a prospective study. Am J Obstet Gynecol 1987;157:655.

47. Abromovici H, Faktor JH, Pascal B. Congenital uterine malformations as indications for cervical suture (cerclage) in habitual abortion and premature delivery. Int J Fertil 1983;28:161.

48. March CM, Israel R. Hysteroscopic management of recurrent abortion caused by septate uterus. Am J Obstet Gynecol 1987;156:834.

49. Perino A, Mencaglia C, Hamou J, et al. Hysteroscopy for metroplasty of uterine septa: report of 24 cases. Fertil Steril 1987;48:321.

50. Kirk EP, Chuong CJ, Coulam CB, et al. Pregnancy after metroplasty for uterine anomalies. Fertil Steril 1993; 59:1164.

51. Schenker JG, Margalioth EJ. Intrauterine adhesions: an updated appraisal. Fertil Steril 1982;37:593.

52. Lancet M, Kessler I. A review of Asherman's syndrome, and results of modern treatment. Int Fertil 1988;33:14.

53. Verkauf BS. Myomectomy for fertility enhancement and preservation. Fertil Steril 1992;58:1.

54. Golan A, Barnan R, Wexier S, et al. Incompetence of the uterine cervix. Obstet Gynecol Surv 1989;44:96.

55. Harger JH. Comparison of success and morbidity in cervical cerclage procedures. Obstet Gynecol 1980;56:543.

56. Coulam CB, Moore SB, O'Fallon WM. Association between major histocompatibility antigen and reproductive performance. Am J Reprod Immunol Microbiol 1987; 14:54.

57. Hill JA, Polgar K, Anderson DJ. T-helper 1-type immunity to trophoblast antigens in women with recurrent spontaneous abortion. JAMA 1995;273:1933.

58. Raghupathy R, Makhseed M, Azizieh F, Omu A, Gupta A, Farhat R. Cytokine production by maternal lymphocytes during normal human pregnancy and in unexplained recurrent spontaneous abortion. Hum Reprod 2000;15:713.

59. Beer AE, Kwak JYM, Ruiz JE. Immunophenotype profiles of peripheral blood lymphocytes in women with recurrent pregnancy loss and in infertile women with multiple failed in vitro fertilization cycles. Am J Reprod Med 1996;35:376.

60. Coulam CB. Immunotherapy for recurrent spontaneous abortion: early pregnancy. Biol Med 1995;1:13.

61. Lockshin MD. Antiphospholipid antibody syndrome. Rheum Dis Clin North Am 1994;20:45.

62. Wilson WA, Gharavi A, Koike T, et al. International consensus statement on preliminary classification criteria for definite antiphospholipid syndrome. Arthritis Rheum 1999;42:1309.

63. Dudley DJ, Branch W. Antiphospholipid syndrome: a model for autoimmune pregnancy loss. Infertil Reprod Med Clin North Am 1991;2:249.

64. Lockwood CJ, Romero R, Feinberg RF, et al. The prevalence and biological significance of lupus anticoagulant and cardiolipin antibodies in a general obstetric population. Am J Obstet Gynecol 1989;161:369.

65. Lockshin DW. Answers to the antiphospholipid antibody syndrome? N Engl J Med 1995;332:1025.

66. Martin BA, Branch DW, Rodgers GM. Sensitivity of the activated partial thromboplastin time, the dilute Russell's viper venom time and the Kaolin clotting time for the detection of the lupus anticoagulant: a direct comparison using plasma dilutions. Blood Coag Fibrinolysis 1996; 7:31.

67. Brandt JT, Triplett DA, Alving B, Scharrer I. Criteria for the diagnosis of lupus anticoagulants: an update. Thromb Haemost 1995;74:1185.

68. Peaceman AM, Silver RK, MacGregor SN et al. Interlaboratory variation in antiphospholipid antibody testing. Am J Obstet Gynecol 1992;166:1780.

69. Kutteh WH, Wester R, Kutteh CC. Multiples of the median: an alternative method for reporting antiphospholipid antibodies in women with recurrent pregnancy loss. Obstet Gynecol 1994;84:811.

70. Silver RM, Porter TF, Greenhill AE, et al. Anticardiolipin antibodies: clinical consequences of "low titers." Obstet Gynecol 1996;87:494.

71. Gleicher N, Pratt D, Dudkiewicz A. What do we really know about autoantibody abnormalities and reproductive failure? A critical review. Autoimmunity 1993;16:115.

72. Franklin RD, Hollier N, Kutter WH. β_2 glycoproteins as a marker of antiphospholipid antibody syndrome in women with recurrent pregnancy loss. Fertil Steril 2000; 73:531.

73. Osasawaram MM, Aoki K, Yagami Y. Are antinuclear antibodies predictive of recurrent miscarriage? Lancet 1996;347:1183.

74. Harger JH, Rabin BS, Marchese SG. The prognostic value of antinuclear antibodies in women with recurrent pregnancy losses: a prospective controlled study. Obstet Gynecol 1989;73:419.

75. Ober C, Karrison T, Harlow L, et al. Autoantibodies and pregnancy history in a healthy population. Am J Obstet Gynecol 1993;169:143.

76. Cowchock FS, Fort UG. Can tests for IgA, IgG or IgM antibodies to cardiolipin or phosphatidylserine substitute for lupus anticoagulant assays in screening for antiphospholipid antibodies? Autoimmunity 1994;17:119.

77. Yetman DL, Kutteh WH. Antiphospholipid antibody panels and recurrent pregnancy loss: prevalence of anti-cardiolipin antibodies compared to other phospholipid antibodies. Fertil Steril 1996;66:540.

78. Branch DW, Silver R, Pierangeli S, et al. Antiphospholipid antibodies other than lupus anticoagulant and anti-cardiolipin antibodies in women with recurrent pregnancy loss, fertile controls, and antiphospholipid syndrome. Obstet Gynecol 1997;89:549.

79. Stagnaro-Green A, Roman SH, Cobin RH et al. Detection of at-risk pregnancy by means of a highly sensitive assay for thyroid autoantibodies. JAMA 1990;264:1422.

80. Gilnoer D, Soto MF, Bourdoux P, et al. Pregnancy in patients with mild thyroid abnormalities: maternal and neonatal repercussions. J Clin Endocrinol Metab 1991; 73:421.

81. Singh A, Dantas ZN, Stone SC, et al. Presence of thyroid antibodies in early reproductive failure: biochemical versus clinical pregnancies. Fertil Steril 1995;63:277.

82. Pratt D, Novotny M, Kaberlein G, et al. Antithyroid antibodies and the association with non-organ-specific antibodies in recurrent pregnancy loss. Am J Obstet Gynecol 1993;168:837.

83. Branch DW, Silver RM, Blackwell JL, et al. Outcome of treated pregnancies in women with antiphospholipid syndrome: an update of the Utah experience. Obstet Gynecol 1992;80:614.

84. Kutteh WH. Antiphospholipid antibody-associated recurrent pregnancy loss: treatment with heparin and low-dose aspirin is superior to low-dose aspirin alone. Am J Obstet Gynecol 1996;174:1584.

85. Laskin C, Bombardier C, Mandel F, et al. Prednisone and ASA in women with autoantibodies and unexplained recurrent fetal loss. N Engl J Med 1997;337:148.

86. Hasegawa I, Takakuwa R, Goto S, et al. Effectiveness of prednisolone/aspirin therapy for recurrent aborters with antiphospholipid antibody. Hum Reprod 1992;7:203.

87. Kutteh WH, Ermel LD. A clinical trial for the treatment of antiphospholipid antibody associated recurrent pregnancy loss with lower dose heparin and aspirin. Am J Reprod Immunol 1996;35:402.

88. Passaleva A, Massai G, D'Elios MM, et al. Prevention of miscarriage in antiphospholipid syndrome. Autoimmunity 1992;14;121.

89. Rai R, Cohen H, Dave M, Regan L. Randomized, controlled trial of aspirin and aspirin plus heparin in pregnant women with recurrent miscarriage associated with phospholipid antibodies (or antiphospholipid antibodies). BMJ 1997;314:253.

90. Cowchock FS, Reece EA, Balaban D, et. al. Repeated fetal losses associated with antiphospholipid antibodies: a collaborative randomized trial comparing prednisone with low-dose heparin treatment. Am J Obstet Gynecol 1992;166:1318.

91. Spinnato JA, Clark AL, Pierangeli S, et al. Intravenous immunoglobulin for the antiphospholipid syndrome in pregnancy. Am J Obstet Gynecol 1995;172:690.

92. Valensise H, Vaquero E, de Carolis C, et al. Normal fetal growth in women with antiphospholipid syndrome treated with high-dose intravenous immunoglobulin (IVIG). Prenat Diagn 1995;15:509.

93. Clark DA, Vince G, Flanders KC, et al. CD56+ lymphoid cells in first trimester pregnancy decidua as a source of novel transforming growth factor-β2-related immunosuppressive factors. Hum Reprod 1994;9:2270.

94. Lachapell MH, Miron P, Hemmings R, Roy DC. Endometrial T, B, and NK cells in patients with recurrent spontaneous abortion. J Immunol 1996;156:4027.

95. Mowbray JF, Liddel H, Underwood JL, et al. Controlled trial of treatment of recurrent spontaneous abortion by immunization with paternal cells. Lancet 1985;1:941.

96. Ho H-N, Gill TJ, Hsieh HE, et al. Immunotherapy for recurrent spontaneous abortions in a Chinese population. Am J Reprod Immunol 1991;25:10.

97. Cauchi MN, Lim D, Young DE, et al. Treatment of recurrent aborters by immunization with paternal cells controlled trial. Am J Reprod Immunol 1991;25:16.

98. Gatenby PA, Cameron K, Simes RJ, et al. Treatment of recurrent spontaneous abortion by immunization with paternal lymphocytes: results of a controlled trial. Am J Reprod Immunol 1993;29:88.

99. Fraser EJ, Grimes DA, Schulz KF. Immunization as therapy for recurrent spontaneous abortion: a review and metaanalysis. Obstet Gynecol 1993;82:854.

100. The Recurrent Miscarriage Immunotherapy Trialists Group. Worldwide Collaborative Observational Study and Meta-Analysis on Allogenic Leukocyte Immunotherapy for Recurrent Spontaneous Abortion. Am J Reprod Immunol 1994;32:55.

101. Ober C, Karrison T, Odem RR, et al. Mononuclear-cell immunisation in prevention of recurrent miscarriages: a randomised trial. Lancet 1999;354:365.

102. Bux J, Westphal E, de Sousa F, et al. Alloimmune neonatal neutropenia is a potential side effect of immunization with leukocytes in women with recurrent spontaneous abortions. J Reprod Immunol 1992;22:299.

103. Katz I, Ovadia J, Fisch B, et al. Cutaneous graft-versus-host-like reaction after paternal lymphocyte immunization for prevention of recurrent abortion. Fertil Steril 1992;57:927.

104. Stephenson MD, Dreher K, Houlihan E, Wu V. Prevention of unexplained recurrent spontaneous abortion using intravenous immunoglobulin: a prospective,

randomized, double-blinded, placebo-controlled trial. Am J Reprod Immunol 1998;39:82.

105. Jablonowska B, Selbing A, Palfi M, Enerudh J, Kjellberg S, Lindton B. Prevention of recurrent spontaneous abortion by intravenous immunoglobulin: a double-blind placebo-controlled study. Hum Reprod 1999:14:838.

106. Christiansen OB, Mathiesen O, Husth M, et al. Placebo-controlled trial of treatment of unexplained recurrent spontaneous abortions and recurrent late spontaneous abortions with i.v. immunoglobulin. Hum Reprod 1995; 10:2690.

107. The German RSA/IVIG group. Intravenous immunoglobulin in the prevention of recurrent miscarriage. Br J Obstet Gynaecol 1994: 101:1072.

108. Coulam CB, Krysa L, Stern JJ, Busillo M. Intravenous immunoglobulin for treatment of recurrent pregnancy loss. Am J Reprod Immunol 1995:34:333.

109. Perino A, Vassiliadis A, Vucetich A, et al. Short-term therapy for recurrent abortion using intravenous immunoglobulins: results of a double-blind placebo-controlled Italian study. Hum Reprod 1977;12:2388.

110. Daya S, Gunby J, Clark A. Intravenous immunoglobulin therapy for recurrent spontaneous abortion: a meta-analysis. Am J Reprod Immunol 1998;39:69.

111. Kutteh WH. Recurrent pregnancy loss: an update. Current Opinion Obstet Gynecol 1999;11:435.

112. Riley LR, Tuomala RE. Infectious disease and recurrent pregnancy loss. Infertil Reprod Med Clin North Am 1991;2:165.

113. Witkin SS, Ledger WJ. Antibodies to chlamydia trachomatis in sera of women with recurrent spontaneous abortion. Am J Obstet Gynecol 1992;167:135.

114. Stray-Pederson B, Eng J, Reikvam T. Uterine T-mycoplasma colonization in reproductive failure. Am J Obstet Gynecol 1978;130:307.

115. Quinn PA, Shewchuk AB, Shuber J, et al. Serologic evidence of *Ureaplasma urealyticum* infection in women with spontaneous pregnancy loss. Am J Obstet Gynecol 1983; 145:245.

116. Quinn PA, Shewchuk AB, Shuber J, et al. Efficacy of antibiotic therapy in preventing spontaneous pregnancy loss among couples colonized with genital mycoplasmosis. Am J Obstet Gynecol 1983;145:239.

117. Toth A, Lessen ML, Brooks-Toth CW, et al. Outcome of subsequent pregnancies following antibiotic therapy after primary or multiple spontaneous abortions. Surg Gynecol Obstet 1986;163:243.

118. Polifka JE, Friedman JM. Environmental toxins and recurrent pregnancy loss. Infertil Reprod Med Clin N Am 1991;2:195.

119. Verp MS. Environmental causes of repetitive spontaneous abortion. Semin Reprod Endocrinol 1989;7:188.

120. Harlap S, Shiono PH. Alcohol, smoking, and incidence of spontaneous abortions in the first and second trimester. Lancet 1980;2:173.

121. Kline J, Shrout P, Stein Z, et al. Drinking during pregnancy and spontaneous abortion. Lancet 1980;2:176.

122. Kline J, Stein ZA, Susser M, et al. Smoking and the occurrence of congenital malformations and spontaneous abortions: multivariate analysis. Am J Obstet Gynecol 1983;145:61.

123. Mills JL, Holmes LB, Aarons JH, et al. Moderate caffeine use and the risk of spontaneous abortion and intrauterine growth retardation. JAMA 1993;269:593.

124. Kline J, Levin B, Silverman J, et al. Caffeine and spontaneous abortion of known karyotype. Epidemiology 1991;2:409.

125. Fenster L, Eskenazi B, Windham GC, et al. Caffeine consumption during pregnancy and spontaneous abortion. Epidemiology 1991;2:168.

126. Infante-Rivard C, Fernandez A, Gauthier R. et al. Fetal loss associated with caffeine intake before and during pregnancy. JAMA 1993;270:2940.

127. Roman E, Beral V, Pelerin M, et al. Spontaneous abortion and work with visual display units. Br J Indust Med 1992;49:507.

128. Schnorr TM, Grajewski BA, Hornung RW, et al. Video display terminals and the risk of spontaneous abortion. N Engl J Med 1991;324:727.

129. Nelen WLDM, Blom HJ, Thomas CMG, Steeger AP. Boers GHJ, Eskes TKAB. Methylenetetrahydrofolate reductase polymorphism affects the change in homocysteine and folate concentrations resulting from low dose folic acid supplementation in women with unexplained recurrent miscarriages. J Nutr 1998;128:1336.

130. Blumenfeld Z, Brenner B. Thrombophilia-associated pregnancy wastage. Fertil Steril 1999;72:765.

131. Kutteh WH, Park VM, Deitcher ST. Hypercoagulable state mutation analysis in white patients with early first-trimester recurrent pregnancy loss. Fertil Steril 1999; 71:1048.

132. Vlanderen W, Treffers PE. Prognosis of subsequent pregnancies after recurrent spontaneous abortion in first trimester. BMJ 1987;295:92.

133. Lapple M. Stress as an explanatory model for spontaneous abortions and recurrent spontaneous abortions. Zentralbl Gynakol 1988;110:325.

134. Keltz MD, Olive DL, Kim AH, Arici A. Sonohysterography for screening in recurrent pregnancy loss. Fertil Steril 1997;67:670.

135. Summers PR. Microbiology relevant to recurrent miscarriage. Clin Obset Gynecol 1994;37:722.

136. Townson DD, Nelson L, Scott JR, et al. Human leukocyte antigen DQ sharing is not increased in couples with recurrent miscarriage. Am J Reprod Immunol 1995; 34:209.

137. Coulam CB. Immunologic tests in the evaluation of reproductive disorders: a critical review. Am J Obstet Gynecol 1992;167:1844.

138. Cowchock FS, Smith JB. Predictors for live births after unexplained spontaneous abortions: correlations between immunologic test results, obstetric histories, and outcomes of next pregnancy without treatment. Am J Obstet Gynecol 1992;167:1208.

139. SHARE, Pregnancy and Infant Loss Support, Inc., St. Joseph Health Center, 300 First Capitol Drive, St. Charles, MO 63301-2893. 1-800-821-6819, www.nationalshareoffice.com.

Chapter 52

Endometriosis

Khaled Zeitoun
Debra Minjarez
Stephen Lincoln

Five Key Points

- **Endometriosis diagnosed at or shortly after puberty is frequently associated with the Müllerian disorders.**

- **Cases of endometriosis in the postmenopausal patient are rare, but when found are often associated with estrogen replacement therapy.**

- **Surgery remains the standard for diagnosis of endometriosis.**

- **Medical suppression of endometriosis for infertility patients seeking pregnancy has no proven beneficial effect.**

- **The endometriosis patients who suffer severe pelvic pain and undergo hysterectomy for control of symptoms experience a high recurrence rate of symptoms unless bilateral oophorectomy is performed.**

Endometriosis is a complex disorder characterized by the presence of endometrial glands and stroma outside their normal location within the endometrial cavity. Adenomyosis is the result of infiltration or invagination of the myometrium with endometrial glands and is considered a different entity from endometriosis.[1] Both conditions affect women throughout the world, resulting in infertility, pelvic pain, and decreased quality of life.

EPIDEMIOLOGY

It is estimated that 5 to 10% of women in the reproductive age period are afflicted with endometriosis.[2,3] However, the exact incidence or prevalence of endometriosis is really unknown. Diagnosis has been increasing with the use of laparoscopy and also with increased awareness of the disease and its various gross pathologic appearances. The prevalence of endometriosis in patients undergoing laparoscopy for chronic pelvic pain and infertility increases to 25 and 33%, respectively.[4-8]

Endometriosis is typically diagnosed at 25 to 29 years of age. The disease is generally considered to begin after puberty (with establishment of menses), to peak at 40 to 45 years of age, and to resolve with menopause. However, these rules do not always apply and approximately 5% of cases are diagnosed in postmenopausal women. Most, but not all, postmenopausal endometriosis cases are associated with estrogen replacement therapy.[9-14]

Moderate to severe endometriosis diagnosed at the time of puberty or shortly afterward is strongly associated with obstructive Müllerian anomalies, but there are reports of severe cases in adolescents with normal pelvic anatomy. Overall, about 10% of endometriosis cases are diagnosed in teenagers.[4,6,15-17]

The natural history of endometriosis, including time of establishment of lesions and clinical course, is not well understood and subject to speculation and debate. One reason may be the heterogenous nature of this disease with multiple factors affecting initiation and progression. Nonetheless, endometriosis remains one of the most common gynecologic disorders resulting in hospitalization and a leading cause of hysterectomy.[18]

CAUSE

Multiple theories have attempted to explain the cause of endometriosis. Unfortunately, no single theory can adequately explain the varied pathologic and clinical presentations. Endometriosis might actually present a spectrum of abnormalities where the exact line between normal and disease states is not completely defined.

One of the most widely accepted mechanisms explaining the development of endometriosis is the implantation of viable endometrium at an ectopic site.[19] Sampson's theory of retrograde menstruation hypothesizes that during menstruation endometrial tissue is deposited into the peritoneal cavity via the oviducts.[20] This theory is supported by animal studies wherein diversion of menstrual efflux into the peritoneal cavity led to the development of endometriotic lesions.[21,22] Human menstrual efflux contains viable endometrial cells that can grow in vitro and in immunologically compromised animals.[23-25] Sampson's theory is further supported by the findings of the frequent association of endometriosis with obstructive Müllerian anomalies and the most common location of endometriotic lesions in the dependent portions of the pelvis.[16,17,26] However, retrograde menstruation alone does not explain why only 5 to 10% of women develop pelvic endometriosis, while menstrual reflux is a universal phenomenon.[27-29]

Other forms of implantation are also possible. Iatrogenic implantation of endometrium in abdominal and episiotomy scars at the time of delivery resulting in endometriosis has been reported.[30-34] Also, lymphatic and hematogenous dissemination of endometrium explains some cases of endometriosis with implants in lymph nodes, or in distant sites like the lung or extremities.[35]

The occurrence of endometriosis when retrograde menstruation is not possible, such as in men treated with estrogens[36] or in patients with gonadal dysgenesis can only be accounted for by other theories.[37-39] Development of endometriosis from coelomic metaplasia or growth of lesions from embryonic rests, genetic predisposition, immune mediation, and toxin derivation have been other suggested hypotheses.

Coelomic metaplasia of the peritoneal lining or growth of lesions from embryonic rests were suggested to explain development of endometriosis when endometrial implantation is not possible.[40,41] The transformation of the coelomic epithelium lining the peritoneal cavity into endometrial-type tissue, as in the case of endometrioid tumors of the ovary, supports the latter theories. An initiating factor such as exposure to estrogen is needed, however.

The presence of immunologic abnormalities in patients with endometriosis has been suggested by studies demonstrating alterations in cell-mediated immunity and by demonstration of antibodies against the endometrium.[42-47] The absence of associated immune defects in cases with endometriosis, the complexity of the immune system, and the inconclusive nature of these studies cast doubts on theories implicating the immune system.

A genetic basis for endometriosis is suggested by the increased incidence in women with a positive family history of the disease. In these individuals endometriosis develops earlier in life and more severe degrees of the disease are observed. The inheritance pattern is probably polygenic or multifactorial.[48-51]

After demonstration of increased incidence of endometriosis in a colony of rhesus monkeys chronically exposed to the environmental toxin dioxin by Rier et al., in 1993, there has been a recent enthusiasm in the scientific community for clarifying the association between dioxin exposure and endometriosis in humans.[52] This was enhanced by the observation that elevated dioxin levels have been reported in a significantly higher number of patients with endometriosis compared with endometriosis-free controls in a population of women with infertility.[53] These and other studies were suggestive of an association between dioxin exposure and development of endometriosis.[54-56]

Rather than having one theory explaining the cause of endometriosis, a multitude of factors may be involved in the etiology of this enigmatic and complex disorder. Retrograde menstruation transports viable endometrium into the peritoneal cavity but may also act as an initiating factor for metaplasia of the coelamic epithelium into endometriotic lesions. At the same time defective clearance of shed endometrial fragments due to a local or general immunologic defect may further contribute to the development of endometriosis. An individual's genetic predisposition or environmental toxins may also impede clearance of the endometrial fragments from the peritoneal cavity or enhance implantation and then growth of lesions. These environmental factors may also enhance metaplasia of the coelomic endothelium into endometrial-like tissue. With further investigation, the future may provide more information as to the pathophysiologic origin of endometriosis.

PATHOLOGY

The diagnosis of endometriosis on microscopic examination usually requires the presence of a combination of endometrial glands and stroma.[1,57] Endometriomas are usually lined by a thin layer of endometrial epithelium with a surrounding layer of stroma.[31] Hemosidrin-laden macrophages are commonly seen in the stromal compartment of endometriosis lesions.[57]

The most common sites involved with endometriosis are the ovaries, peritoneum of the posterior and anterior cul-de-sac, and the uterosacral ligaments, but any pelvic or abdominal site may be involved. In fact, endometriosis can affect any organ or tissue, including remote sites like limbs or even the central nervous system.

Endometriotic foci involving the pelvic peritoneal surfaces are usually multiple. The classic appearance is usually that of a slightly raised spot with a red, blue, or brown discoloration.[58] The flame-red lesions are considered to be the most active. Adhesions are also very common and the lesions are usually surrounded by dense fibrosis. Atypical lesions are sometimes more difficult to recognize and vary in appearance.[59] These may appear as whitish spots or blisters on the peritoneal or serosal surfaces. Microscopic or hidden lesions are commonly present in peritoneal pockets.[60]

In more extensive cases massive adhesions may involve pelvic or abdominal organs leading to the formation of large amalgamated masses and nodules.[61] Endometriomas are usually within the ovary. These cystic structures have a fibrotic wall with a brown to yellow lining. Endometriomas (chocolate cysts) are usually small in size and rarely exceed 15 cm in diameter; they usually contain thick brownish fluid caused by altered blood in the cavity.[62]

MOLECULAR ABERRATIONS IN ENDOMETRIOSIS

Despite histological similarities, multiple molecular differences were reported between eutopic endometrium and endometrial-like tissue within endometriotic lesions. Alterations are also reported in eutopic endometrium and peritoneal fluid content of endometriosis patients compared to women without the disease.[42,63-65] Endometriotic lesions contain estrogen and progesterone receptors and are responsive to steroids, but studies indicate the presence of altered content throughout the menstrual cycle when compared with eutopic endometrium. Data from receptor studies, however, vary and conflicting results are reported.[66-68]

Several investigators have demonstrated aberrations in growth factors and cytokines such as interleukines and monocyte chemotactic protein-1.[69] Higher levels of expression of granulocyte-macrophage colony-stimulating factor (GM-CSF) and macrophage-CSF were demonstrated in endometriosis as well. These factors are chemoattractants and induce macrophage proliferation and angiogenesis.[70,71] Matrix metalloproteinases (MMPs) and their inhibitors are expressed in abnormal patterns and timing in endometriotic tissues compared to endometrium. These factors have important roles in growth, differentiation, and breakdown of normal endometrium. The altered balance between MMPs and tissue inhibitor of metalloproteinase-1 (TIMP-1) might favor progression and invasiveness of endometriosis through altered tissue remodeling.[72-74] Expression of cathepsin D, another enzyme involved in cell growth and invasion, is also increased in endometriosis.[75] Other alterations involve adhesion molecules (e.g., integrins) and complement component 3 (C3).[76,77]

With all the evidence indicating that endometriosis is an estrogen-dependent disorder, studying steroidogenic enzymes involved in estrogen biosynthesis was a natural step. Extremely high levels of aromatase P450 (P450arom) expression and activity in endometriotic stromal cells were demonstrated.[64] P450arom catalyzes the transformation of C_{19} steroids to estrogens. This enzyme is not expressed in normal endometrium and no local estrogen synthesis could be demonstrated in endometrial-derived cells.[64,78] In endometriotic lesions aromatase enzyme expression and activity is markedly stimulated by prostaglandin E_2 via a cyclic-AMP-dependent mechanism. The presence of P450arom allows local estrogen biosynthesis within endometriotic lesions; cytokines including prostaglandins in the peritoneal fluid of endometriosis patients are potential factors stimulating the local activity of this important steroidogenic enzyme.[63]

The transcription factor steroidogenic factor-1 (SF-1) is a mandatory factor for cyclic-AMP-dependent P450arom expression in the ovary.[79] Interestingly, abnormal SF-1 expression was recently demonstrated in endometriotic lesions. Again, this transcription factor is not present in significant levels in normal endometrium.[80]

17β-hydroxysteroid dehydrogenase type 2 (17βHSD-2) enzyme is another important steroidogenic enzyme involved in inactivation of the potent estrogen estradiol-17β in normal endometrium. This enzyme was found to be deficient in endometriotic lesions. The absence of 17βHSD-2 enzyme not only favors increased local concentrations of estradiol within the lesions but also might be a reflection of a partial progesterone resistance in endometriosis lesions. The imbalance created by increased local estrogen concentrations and progesterone resistance might have important etiological implications in this steroid responsive tissue.[81]

DIAGNOSTIC TESTS

The importance of an accurate noninvasive test for a common disorder like endometriosis cannot be overemphasized. Unfortunately available methods short of direct visualization of lesions during an invasive surgical procedure are still too insensitive or nonspecific.

CA-125 MEASUREMENT

CA-125 is a cell surface antigen and a useful marker in monitoring patients with epithelial ovarian cancer. This antigen is found in coelomic epithelial derived tissues, and thus is also expressed by the endometrium. Elevated CA-125 serum levels were demonstrated in patients with endometriosis, especially in advanced stages of the disease.[82-85] Unfortunately, the use of this assay as a screening test for diagnosis was disappointing because of low sensitivity (between 20% and 80%).[82,83,86] Its use in monitoring treatment and recurrences is also limited.[87] CA-125 elevations can also occur due to other concurrent conditions such

as nonendometriotic ovarian masses, pregnancy, menstruation, uterine leiomyomata, and pelvic inflammatory disease.[88] In conclusion, at the present time, there is no accurate marker for diagnosis of endometriosis.[89] However, several molecular aberrations in this abnormal tissue are currently being studied. The characterization of a marker that could predict the presence of the disease and be used to monitor therapy will be invaluable.

PELVIC IMAGING

Ultrasound would be a preferred imaging method for endometriosis. It is best performed using the vaginal probe because of better resolution. Ultrasound, however, is not very useful in detection of endometriotic implants and cannot differentiate these from other masses.[90] In contrast, endometriomas are diagnosed with excellent sensitivity and specificity.[91,92] The use of Doppler-flow studies to differentiate endometriosis from other ovarian masses, especially malignant tumors, has also been described.[93,94] A specific ultrasound description is reported with pericystic vessels, scanty blood supply, high resistance index, and an avascular cavity. The role of Doppler studies is not well defined.[93-95]

The utilization of magnetic resonance imaging (MRI) has been reported for diagnosis of endometriosis. MRI might be more useful in detection of endometriotic implants than ultrasound.[96] However, the sensitivity and specificity for detection of endometriomas is not improved.[91] At the present time, the use of MRI for diagnosis of endometriosis has a very limited role. Other imaging studies including computed tomography (CT) scans, barium enema, and chest radiographs may be needed in complicated and advanced cases involving extraabdominal sites or bowel.[97,98] These studies, however, are nonspecific and endometriotic lesions cannot be differentiated with certainty from other disease states.

Laparoscopy

Despite attempts to use imaging studies to diagnose endometriosis, surgical diagnosis remains the gold standard and a definitive diagnosis of endometriosis will need pelvic and abdominal exploration. Laparoscopy has assisted in the pathologic diagnosis of endometriosis while decreasing patient morbidity and has replaced laparotomy in all but very rare cases.

Tissue biopsy is recommended to obtain histological confirmation of endometriosis. However, with experienced examiners the presence of typical lesions is usually sufficient for diagnosis. The recent appreciation and description of different lesion types is probably one of the causes for the increase in frequency of diagnosis.[99] Atypical lesions such as clear papules might be difficult to detect and a thorough examination by a surgeon familiar with the disease is ideal.[59,100,101] Also, techniques like infusion of crystalloids into the cul-de-sac or painting of peritoneal surfaces with blood-tinged peritoneal fluid can be used to enhance detection of these subtle lesions.[102,103]

Deep infiltrating lesions are frequently extraperitoneal. They are difficult to visualize and can be missed by less-experienced surgeons.[104,105] Careful examination under anesthesia and palpation with a probe might aid in detecting these active and painful lesions.[106] Endometriomas are usually easily detected by laparoscopy, but sometimes aspiration of a suspicious cyst is helpful to confirm diagnosis before excision. Furthermore, inspection of the bowel is mandatory as a significant number of cases contain bowel lesions.[107]

CLASSIFICATION

Several classification systems have been suggested over the years to stage endometriosis according to severity of the disease. The goal was to divide the disease into stages that correlated with pregnancy rate or response to treatment, but this goal has never been completely realized. The staging systems were complex and not widely used, and studies did not show a good correlation between pregnancy rates and stage of the disease. The American Fertility Society (AFS) original and revised classifications were an effort to predict the probability of pregnancy following treatment of endometriosis, according to disease severity.[108,109] The revised AFS classification introduced in 1985 divided endometriosis into four stages (minimal, mild, moderate, and severe).[109] In this classification, higher scores were given to deep endometriosis, dense adhesions, and obliteration of the cul-de-sac. Numerous studies could not demonstrate a difference in pregnancy rates after treatment at different stages.[110,111] A new attempt at scoring the disease was made with the revised American Society for Reproductive Medicine (ASRM) classification of endometriosis in 1996.[112] The new classification encouraged recording of lesion

color and morphology. Like previous AFS classifications, it contained a standardized form to record findings. Again, data did not support any improvement in prediction of pregnancy after treatment in the ASRM classification.[113,114]

SYMPTOMS

Endometriosis is a leading cause of pelvic pain and is strongly associated with infertility. However, endometriosis has been implicated in a variety of other disorders including spontaneous abortions and abnormal uterine bleeding. In many instances associations cannot be confirmed by more recent studies.

Pain

Pain is a common symptom attributed to endometriosis.[115] More than half of patients presenting with pelvic pain and dysmenorrhea are diagnosed with endometriosis. The typical endometriosis-associated pain starts 1 to 2 days before onset of bleeding and lasts throughout menstruation, but it should be suspected in secondary or worsening primary dysmenorrhea. Dyspareunia also is a symptom of endometriosis and is usually associated with endometriosis of the uterosacral ligaments, deep pelvic implants, lesions of the rectovaginal septum, or a fixed retroverted uterus.[106] The presence of noncyclic pelvic pain, backache, and rectal pressure is also commonly described.[116,117] Endometriosis rarely presents by acute abdominal pain (3% of cases), but has been seen as a leaking or ruptured endometrioma.[118] Pain related to specific organ involvement such as urinary tract (dysuria and flank pain),[119,120] bowel (dyschezia),[121] lung (chest pain),[122] or nerves (sciatica),[123] is also described. Often endometriosis-related pain does not correlate with the severity of the lesion, and the actual pathophysiology of the pain in milder stages is not well understood, but may be related to prostaglandin production in the lesions.[117,124-127]

Infertility

Infertility is another symptom commonly attributed to endometriosis. Up to 30% of cases of infertility are associated with laparoscopially proven endometriosis and the disease has been detected in only a small percentage of fertile patients undergoing tubal ligation.[113,114,128] The exact incidence of endometriosis is, however, unknown and so the percentage of cases associated with infertility is difficult to assess. Furthermore, no correlation has been demonstrated between the different stages of endometriosis and pregnancy rates or response to therapy in infertile patients.[110,111,113] Another factor complicating the picture is that the exact mechanism causing infertility in milder forms of endometriosis is unknown, thus doubts still exist whether endometriosis is a direct cause of infertility.

Factors implicated in causing endometriosis-associated infertility include anatomic distortion and fibrosis of the fallopian tubes in severe cases, anovulation, luteal-phase defects, luteinized unruptured follicle (LUF) syndrome, autoimmune factors, spontaneous early abortions, altered peritoneal fluid environment by prostaglandins or inflammatory cells, and hyperprolactinaemia.[117]

Spontaneous Abortion

The older studies indicating an increased rate of spontaneous abortion in endometriosis could not be validated by newer controlled studies.[129,130]

Abnormal Uterine Bleeding

Many different patterns of abnormal bleeding are described with endometriosis including premenstrual spotting, hypermenorrhea, and oligomenorrhea. The incidence of annovulation and luteal-phase defects is, however, similar in endometriosis patients compared to women without the disease. Available data does not support an association between endometriosis and abnormal uterine bleeding.

Other Symptoms

Other uncommon symptoms related to specific organ involvement are sometimes seen, such as recurrent pneumothorax or hemoptysis in lung involvement;[122] rectal bleeding or hematuria in rectal or bladder involvement;[120,121] ureteric obstruction; and skin, perineal, or vaginal masses.[119]

CLINICAL EXAMINATION

Physical findings in endometriosis are not specific and in many instances do not correlate with disease severity confirmed at laparoscopy. In many cases minimal abnormalities are detected despite significant pelvic pathology and severe symptoms. Cul-de-sac tenderness is one of the most common findings. Nodularity along the uterosacral ligaments and in the cul-de-sac is also very suggestive. The lesions will be more prominent at the time of menstruation and tenderness will usually increase. Significant endometriomas will be appreciated as adnexal masses but other lesions, such as ovarian tumors, give a similar picture. Severe adhesions obliterating the cul-de-sac can cause the uterus to remain in a retroverted position, and movement of the uterus during examination will usually elicit tenderness. Deep lesions in the rectovaginal septum are better appreciated by a combined rectovaginal examination. This is important because they might be missed during laparoscopy.

TREATMENT

The inadequate number of prospective, randomized, controlled studies together with our lack of knowledge about the natural course of endometriosis makes assessment of treatment modalities a difficult task. Unfortunately, no ideal long-lasting treatment option is available to date and many of the current treatment options are temporary or associated with significant morbidity. Among other variables treatment will often depend on the presentation of the disease in an individual patient and the patient's desires and age.[117]

EXPECTANT MANAGEMENT AND PROPHYLACTIC TREATMENT

Until recently there was no evidence that medical or surgical therapy is superior to expectant management in infertile patients with milder forms of endometriosis. Expectant management has the advantage of being cheaper and avoiding side effects of therapy. On the other hand, surgical ablation of the lesions might prevent or slow progression of the disease, at least in some cases. In 1998 a Canadian prospective randomized study demonstrated that surgical ablation of lesions in minimal and mild cases of endometriosis enhanced fertility in this group of patients.[131] Although this is only one study, it nonetheless points in favor of ablation of even milder lesions discovered during laparoscopy. In younger patients not yet seeking pregnancy who have been diagnosed with endometriosis, the long-term use of oral contraceptives in an attempt to suppress the disease or slow its progression might be a reasonable option. Data demonstrating the long-term efficiency of such an approach, however, are not available.[117,132,133]

MEDICAL SUPPRESSION

The medical options available for treatment of endometriosis include oral contraceptives, Danazol, progestins, gonadotropin-releasing hormone (GnRH) agonists, and experimental modalities such as aromatase inhibitors. All medical modalities are of proven effectiveness in managing pelvic pain and in decreasing the size of the lesions. For treating infertility, these medical therapies have no proven beneficial effect. In fact, they may be a cause of delay in pregnancy due to their suppressive effect on ovulation. The effect of medical suppression is not permanent and recurrence rates after discontinuation of therapy are high. The different medications used are not expected to have any effect on adhesions or larger endometriomas.[134,135]

Danazol

Danazol is an isoxazol derivative of 17α-ethynyl-testosterone. Danazol is well absorbed and active when given orally. It has a central effect by which it attenuates the midcycle gonadotropin surge, and this is associated with anovulation and a reduction of estradiol levels.[134] Danazol's binding to the androgen receptor might have a local suppressive effect on the lesions but is the cause of some of its most disturbing side effects. The drug also inhibits steroidogenic enzymes within the ovary. Danazol is usually used in divided doses ranging from 400 to 800 mg per day for 6 to 9 months. The drug is very effective, relieving pelvic pain associated with endometriosis in about 90% of cases. Reports have also indicated its success in reducing the size of endometriotic lesions. The effectiveness of therapy is directly related to induction of amenorrhea. Side effects of Danazol are related both to its androgenic effect and to the resulting hypoestrogenic environment. Danazol is associated with weight gain, mood changes, depression, oily skin, muscle cramps, headaches, edema, altered appetite, acne, hirsutism, fatigue, decreased breast size, hot flashes, voice changes, and irregular bleeding. The drug has an adverse effect on the lipoprotein profile, resulting in a decrease of high-density lipoproteins (HDLs) and an increase of low-density lipoproteins

(LDLs) and may be associated with increased liver enzymes. Pregnancy has to be excluded because of the potential for virilization of a female fetus. The majority of patients taking the medication will experience side effects and at least 20% will discontinue the drug because of them. Recurrence rates are as high as 30% in 2 years after cessation of therapy. Danazol was once a very popular drug for use in the treatment of endometriosis but because of significant side effects, its use is now very limited and it is being replaced by GnRH agonists.[136-138]

Gestrinone

Gestrinone is a 19-nortestosterone derivative with progesterone agonist and antagonist effects. It has been studied extensively in Europe for treatment of endometriosis and it results in amenorrhea and endometrial atrophy. It has a long half-life and is given orally 1 to 3 times a week (2.5 to 7.5 mg). The potential side effects are similar to Danazol but are much milder and better tolerated. There is no adverse effect on lipoproteins or liver-function tests.[134,139-142]

Progestins

Progestins are believed to act by inducing decidualization and atrophy of the endometrial tissue within the endometriotic implants. Progestins also interfere with follicular growth probably via a central mechanism on the pituitary–hypothalamic unit but a local ovarian effect is also possible. These effects will result in decreased estrogen levels. Progestins can be given orally, e.g., medroxyprogesterone acetate (Provera) 20–30 mg orally per day or via the intramuscular (IM) route as in case of depomedroxyprogesterone acetate (Depo-Provera) in a dose of 150 mg IM every 1 to 3 months. The side effects of progestins include abnormal bleeding, mood changes, depression, headaches, weight gain, bloating, nausea, and a decrease of HDLs. Progestins are better tolerated than Danazol and few patients discontinue their medications due to side effects. Again, progestins do have a beneficial effect on pain and lead to regression of lesions, but the effect on pregnancy rate is no different from expectant management. Progestins are an effective and inexpensive alternative for patients who do not tolerate Danazol, GnRH agonists, or oral contraceptives.[133,138,143-145]

Oral Contraceptives

Oral contraceptive-induced amenorrhea was used to treat endometriosis, and this regimen was termed pseudopregnancy. Initially high-dose oral contraceptive pills were preferred, but the more recent low-dose estrogen pills seem to have similar effects on endometriosis. Oral contraceptives can be used in a continuous fashion, resulting in amenorrhea, or in a cyclic fashion. The therapeutic effect is probably due to the progestin in the pill causing decidualization and then atrophy of the endometriotic lesions. Side effects are similar to those of oral contraceptives and might be more severe in larger doses or continuous regimens. Oral contraceptives are a low-cost option for suppressive therapy and they seem to be effective in alleviating pelvic pain. The role of oral contraceptive therapy for decreasing recurrence is less clear but it seems to be a reasonable option in cases where pregnancy is not desired at the time of therapy.[146-148]

GnRH Agonists

GnRH agonists are modified GnRH peptides with a longer half-life and greater potency. Continuous administration of GnRH agonists downregulates the pituitary–hypothalamic unit, leading to decreased gonadotropin levels. The resultant hypoestrogenic environment due to ovarian inactivity seems to cause regression of endometriotic implants. GnRH agonists can be used as a nasal spray (Nafarelin in a dose of 200 to 400 mg twice daily) or in an injectable form (the depo form of leuprolide acetate in a dose of 3.75 mg every 4 weeks). Also available are a long-acting injectable form of leuprolide administered every 3 months and a subcutaneous implant (goserelin acetate).[149-151] GnRH agonists are used widely and have replaced Danazol for treatment of endometriosis. GnRH agonists do not have androgenic or progestogenic side effects, and no adverse effects on the lipid profile have been reported. The hypoestrogenic effect of GnRH agonists is, however, more profound and is the primary cause of the side effects from this agent. These include vaginal dryness, hot flashes, abnormal vaginal bleeding, insomnia, depression, libido changes, headache, fatigue, and skin changes. The most concerning side effect is the decrease of bone density with GnRH agonists. A decrease in trabecular bone density of up to 6% in 6 months

was reported. This effect is considered reversible after discontinuation of therapy but limits the time this agent can be used. Recent studies have also indicated the relative safety of a second 6-month course of GnRH agonist in cases with recurrence of symptoms. The long-term effect of multiple courses in these young women is not known, however, and there is a potential for delayed adverse effects on bone integrity. GnRH agonist treatment results in amelioration of pain in up to 90% of patients during therapy and this is comparable to the effect of Danazol. Reduction of lesion size is also reported. Side effects are more tolerable to patients than with Danazol. Again, similar to Danazol, there was no beneficial effect on pregnancy rates following discontinuation of GnRH agonist therapy.[152-155]

Add-back therapy combines GnRH agonists with other agents like estrogen and progestins or antiresorptive agents like biphosphonates. The goal is to decrease vasomotor symptoms and the detrimental effects on bone density with the possible use of GnRH agonists for prolonged periods of time. Medroxyprogesterone was not effective when used as add-back to GnRH agonists, and while norethindrone decreased side effects with no effect on therapeutic efficiency, it had an adverse effect on lipoproteins. The use of estrogen/progestin combination add-back therapy would be excellent for vasomotor symptoms and can help preserve bone density but it might decrease the efficiency of GnRH agonists in controlling endometriosis, and further studies are needed on the impact of this line of therapy. Preliminary studies using biphosphonates and norethindrone showed a beneficial effect in preserving bone mass. After discontinuation of these multidrug therapies, significant recurrence rates were reported as with other medical lines of management.[117,134]

Other Modalities

The antiprogesterone mefiprostone (RU 486) was reported to have a beneficial effect on endometriosis in small studies. The agent will disrupt the endometrium and inhibit ovulation. While this group of agents might prove to be of benefit, concerns about unopposed estrogenic effect on the endometrium need careful follow-up.[156]

Recently the aromatase inhibitor amastrozole was used in combination with alendronate and calcium to treat successfully a patient with severe recurrent endometriosis after total hysterectomy and salpingo-oophorectomy resistant to large doses of progestins. The agent caused a profound decrease of estrogen levels, and consequently resulted in the disappearance of a recurrent fungating endometriotic lesion in the vaginal vault. The successful alleviation of severe chronic pain in this patient was impressive.

Loss of bone, however, was significant (from 2.5% to 6.5% in 9 months), in spite of adding a biphosphonate. The effect of aromatase enzyme inhibitors merits further study in larger numbers of patients. It may have a role in treatment of resistant cases of endometriosis unresponsive to other medical modalities. It may also increase the pain-free interval after discontinuation of therapy.[157]

SURGICAL TREATMENT

Surgical therapy is the most common treatment modality used in endometriosis. Most cases affected with endometriosis are subjected to diagnostic laparoscopy, as this is still the only means of obtaining a definitive diagnosis. Since it is now possible to accomplish surgical resection and/or ablation in nearly all cases via laparoscopy, this route is preferred to laparotomy except in very special circumstances.

Surgical therapy for endometriosis is effective in relieving symptoms of pain and in debilitating lesions. Actually, large lesions like endometriomas and adhesions only can be treated surgically, as medical therapy is not effective.[158]

In contrast to medical treatment, surgical treatment of endometriosis has proven of value in improving pregnancy rates compared to medical modalities or no treatment. Surgical excision of endometriosis was considered beneficial in more severe cases of endometriosis, but the effect of surgery on milder stages of the disease was controversial.[159]

Recently, however, a prospective randomized study comparing surgical ablation of minimal and mild endometriosis with expectant management demonstrated a higher pregnancy rate in the surgically treated group. This study leads us to conclude that milder lesions should probably be treated when discovered at diagnostic laparoscopy.[131]

Recurrence after surgery will depend on the severity of the disease and the completeness of the procedure. Recurrence rates are approximately 20% over 5 years following complete surgical excision or

ablation.[158] The role of medical treatment modalities used with surgery is controversial. Preoperative medial suppression may be used in an attempt to decrease lesion size and vascularity before surgery. The disadvantage of this approach is potential changes in the appearance of lesions, making diagnosis and treatment more difficult. A delay in diagnosis will consequently also delay pregnancy.

Postoperative medical therapy may be used for patients with pain after incomplete excision, especially in severe disease. Postoperative medical therapy should never be used in patients seeking pregnancy, as this has not shown improved pregnancy rates and will delay pregnancy throughout the duration of therapy.[160-164] In conclusion, a beneficial effect of perioperative medical therapy is not supported by available data, and thus its use should be restricted to special circumstances. Patients with intractable pain who are awaiting surgery might benefit from such an approach.[160-164]

Principles of Surgery in Endometriosis

Surgery for endometriosis ranges from a simple ablation of small superficial lesions to complicated dissection and resection of massive adhesions involving nearby systems such as the bowel and the urinary tract.

- The goal during surgery is complete extrication of the disease whenever possible, so adequate definition of the extent of the lesions is important.
- Visualization should be adequate, and careful exploration of the pelvis is a must.
- In many cases anatomy is distorted and identification of vital organs (rectum, ureters, and bladder) is mandatory to prevent injury.
- Endometriotic lesions are in many instances deeper than they appear and the aim should be complete excision or ablation of the lesions.
- The surgeon has to be familiar with the use of electrocautery and laser as well as sharp dissection using laparoscopic scissors.
- It is important to recognize the need for help from a gastrointestinal surgeon or urologist in complicated cases.
- Adequate preoperative bowel preparation may be necessary in more advanced endometriosis.

In patients not desiring future fertility, removal of the uterus and the ovaries together with excision of the lesions constitutes definitive treatment.[111]

Recurrence rates after hysterectomy without bilateral salpingo-oophorectomy are significant, with 62% experiencing recurrent pain and 31% requiring further surgery. When the ovaries were excised recurrent pain occurred in only 10% of patients.[111,165]

THE ROLE OF ASSISTED REPRODUCTION

Controlled ovarian hyperstimulation (COH) with gonadotropins or clomiphene citrate followed by intrauterine insemination (IUI) unquestionably enhances monthly fecundity rates in endometriosis patients with patent fallopian tubes. The effect on cumulative pregnancy rates is controversial, however, with no demonstrated improvement over expectant management.[166] Ovarian stimulation with IUI seems to have better results than stimulation with timed intercourse. The use of COH/IUI is probably recommended for 3 to 4 cycles if pregnancy is delayed after surgical excision and earlier in older patients.[166-170]

Most patients with endometriosis have a least one patent fallopian tube, and in these patients, gamete intrafallopian transfer (GIFT), zygote intrafallopian transfer (ZIFT), or tubal embryo transfer (TET) are possible. Several groups reported excellent success rates with GIFT in patients who have endometriosis and who are seeking pregnancy. Presently with the decreasing frequency of GIFT secondary to the added cost of a laparoscopy procedure and increased information gained by in vitro fertilization, GIFT may have only a limited role.[171,172]

In vitro fertilization and embryo transfer (IVF/ET) is probably the preferred alternative when advanced assisted reproductive technology is needed. IVF/ET should be considered after 1 year of follow-up or after the failure of conventional therapy. The procedure should be used earlier in cases with extensive tubal damage, older patients, and in cases with associated factors leading to infertility.

The effect of endometriosis with more severe forms of the disease on pregnancy rates with IVF/ET is another debated issue. Endometriosis was implicated in decreased ovarian response, interference with monitoring, decreased fertilization and cleavage rates, decreased pregnancy rates, and increased early abortions.[173-178]

More recent studies, however, suggest no adverse effect of endometriosis on pregnancy rates with IVF/ET.[179] Downregulation of the ovary with a GnRH agonist for 6 months before IVF/ET was also suggested to improve outcome but presently there is no conclusive data to recommend this.[173-178]

In conclusion, COH/IUI seems to accelerate the occurrence of pregnancy but alone may not change the overall fertility. With improved techniques in IVF/ET, the pregnancy rates in endometriosis (even in severe cases) seem to be similar to tubal factor infertility. IVF/ET should be utilized after an adequate trial of less-invasive procedures.

REFERENCES

1. Clement PB. Diseases of the peritoneum (including endometriosis). In: Kurman RJ., ed. Blaustein's pathology of the female genital tract. 4th ed. New York: Springer-Verlag;1994:647.
2. Aral SO, Cates W Jr. The increasing concern with infertility: Why now? JAMA1983;250:2327.
3. Wheeler JM. Epidemiology of endometriosis-associated infertility. J Reprod Med 1989;34:41.
4. Goldstein DP, deCholnoky C, Emans SJ, Leventhal JM. Laparoscopy on the diagnosis and management of pelvic pain in adolescents. J Reprod Med 1980;24:251.
5. Hasson HM. Incidence of endometriosis in diagnostic laparoscopy. J Reprod Med 1976;16:135.
6. Eskenazi B, Warner ML. Epidemiology of endometriosis. Obstet Gynecol Clin North Am 1997;24:235.
7. Houston DE, Noller K, Melton LJ, Selwyn BJ. The epidemiology of pelvic endometriosis. Clin Obstet Gynecol 1988;31:787.
8. Kjerulff KH, Erickson BA, Langenberg PW. Chronic gynecological conditions reported by US women: Findings from the National Health Information Survey, 1984 to 1992. Am J Public Health 1996;86:195.
9. Vessey MP, Villard-Mackintosh L, Painter R. Epidemiology of endometriosis in women attending family planning clinics. Br Med J 1993;306:182.
10. Sangi-Haghpeykar H, Poindexter A. Epidemiology of endometriosis among parous women. Obstet Gynecol 1995;85:983.
11. Kempers RD, Dockerty MB, Hunt AB. Significant postmenopausal endometriosis. Surg Gynecol Obstet 1960; 111:348.
12. Punnonen R, Klemi P, Nikkanen V. Postmenopausal endometriosis. Eur J Obstet Gynaecol Reprod Biol 1980;11:195.
13. Djursing H, Peterson K, Weberg E. Symptomatic postmenopausal endometriosis. Acta Obstet Gynecol Scand 1981;60:529.
14. Punnonen R, Klemi PJ, Nikkanen V. Postmenopausal endometriosis. Eur J Obstet Gynecol Reprod Biol 1980; 11:195.
15. Chatman DL, Ward AB. Endometriosis in adolescents. J Reprod Med 1982;27:156.
16. Huffman JW. Endometriosis in young teen-age girls. Pediatr Ann. 1981;10:501.
17. Schifrin BS, Erez S, Moore JG. Teen-age endometriosis. Am J Obstet Gynecol 1973;116:973.

18. Velebil P, Wingo PA, Xia Z, Wilcox LS, Peterson HB. Rate of hospitalization for gynecologic disorders among reproductive-age women in the United States. Obstet Gynecol 1995;86:764.

19. Sampson JA. Perforating hemorrhagic (chocolate) cysts of the ovary. Arch Surg 1921;3:245.

20. Sampson JA. Peritoneal endometriosis due to the menstrual dissemination of endometrial tissue into the peritoneal cavity. Am J Obstet Gynecol 1927;14:422.

21. TeLinde RW, Scott RB. Experimental endometrium. Am J Obstet Gynecol 1950;60:1147.

22. Schenken RS. Effect of pregnancy in surgically induced endometriosis in cynomolgus monkeys. Am J Obstet Gynecol 1987;157:1392.

23. Geist SH. The viability of fragments of menstrual endometrium. Am J Obstet Gynecol 1933;25:751.

24. Keettell WC, Stein RJ. The viability of the cast-off menstrual endometrium. Am J Obstet Gynecol 1951;61:440.

25. Mungyer G, Willemsen WNP, Rolland R. Cells of the mucous membrane of the female genital tract in culture: A comparative study with regard to the histogenesis of endometriosis. In Vitro Cell Dev Biol 1987;23:111.

26. Olive DL, Henderson DY. 1987 Endometriosis and müllerian anomalies. Obstet Gynecol 69:412–415.

27. Blumenkrantz MJ, Gallagher N, Bashore RA, Tenckhoff H. Retrograde menstruation in women undergoing chronic peritoneal dialysis. Obstet Gynecol 1981;57:667.

28. Halme J, Hammond MG, Hulka JF, Raj SG, Talbert LM. Retrograde menstruation in healthy women and in patients with endometriosis. Obstet Gynecol 1984;64:151.

29. Liu DTY, Hitchcock A. Endometriosis: its association with retrograde menstruation, dysmenorrhea and tubal pathology. Br J Obstet Gynaecol 1986;93:859.

30. Scott RB, TeLinde RW, Wharton LR. Further studies on experimental endometriosis. Am J Obstet Gynecol 1953; 66:1082.

31. Gardner HL. Cervical and vaginal endometriosis. Clin Obstet Gynecol 1966;9:358.

32. Wolf GC, Singh KB. Cesarean scar endometriosis: a review. Obstet Gynecol 1989;44:89.

33. Chatterjee SK. Scar endometriosis: a clinicopathologic study of 17 cases. Obstet Gynecol 1980;56:81.

34. Paull T, Tedeschi LG. Perineal endometriosis at the site of episiotomy scar. Obstet Gynecol 1972;40:28.

35. Sampson JA. Metastasis of embolic endometriosis due to menstrual dissemination of endometrial tissue into the venous circulation. Am J Pathol 1927;3:93.

36. Melicow MM, Pachter MR. Endometrial carcinoma of the prostatic utricle (uterus masculinus). Cancer 1967; 20:1715.

37. Binns BA, Banerjee R. Endometriosis with Turner's syndrome treated with cyclic oestrogen/progesterone. Case report. Br J Obstet Gynaecol 1983;90:581.

38. El-Mahgoub S, Yassen S. A positive proof for the theory of coelomic metaplasia. Am J Obstet Gynecol 1980; 137:137.

39. Peress MR, Sosnowski JR, Mathur RS, Williamson HO. Pelvic endometriosis and Turner's syndrome. Am J Obstet Gynecol 1982;144:474.

40. Meyer R. Über den stand der frage der adenomyositis und adenomyome im allgemeinen und insbesondere über adenomyositis seroepithelialis und adenomyometritis sarcomatosa. Zentralbl Gynakol 1919;36:745.

41. Meyer R. Über endometrium in der tube, sowie über die hieraus entstenhenden wirklichen und vermeintlichen folgen. Zentralbl Gynakol 1927;51:1482.

42. Hill J, Anderson D. Lymphocyte activity in the presence of peritoneal fluid from fertile women and infertile women with and without endometriosis. Am J Obstet Gynecol 1989;161:861.

43. Hill JA. Immunology and endometriosis. Fertil Steril 1992;58:262.

44. Dmowski WP, Steele RW, Baker GF. Deficient cellular immunity in endometriosis. Am J Obstet Gynecol 1981;141:377.

45. Badawy SZ, Cuenca V, Stitzel A, Jacobs RD, Tomar RH. Autoimmune phenomena in infertile patients with endometriosis. Obstet Gynecol 1984;63:271.

46. Mathur S, Peress MR, Williamson HO. Autoimmunity to endometrium and ovary in endometriosis. Clin Exp Immunol 1982;50:259.

47. Wild RA, Hirisave V, Podczaski ES. Autoantibodies associated with endometriosis: Can their detection predict presence of the disease? Obstet Gynecol 1991;77:927.

48. Simpson JL, Elias S, Malinak LR, Buttram VC. Heritable aspects of endometriosis. I. Genetic studies. Am J Obstet Gynecol 1980;137:327.

49. Malinak LR, Buttram VC, Elias S, Simpson JL. Heritable aspects of endometriosis. II. Clinical characteristics of familial endometriosis. Am J Obstet Gynecol 1980; 137:332.

50. Lamb K, Hoffmann RG, Nichols RT. Family trait analysis: A case-control study of 43 women with endometriosis and their best friends. Am J Obstet Gynecol 1986; 154:596.

51. Ranney B. Endometriosis: IV. Hereditary tendency. Obstet Gynecol 1971;37:734.

52. Rier SE, Martin DC, Bowman RE, Dmowski WP, Becker JL. Endometriosis in Rhesus monkeys (Macaca mulatta) following chronic exposure to 2,3,7,8-tetrachlorodibenzo-p-dioxin. Fundam Appl Toxicol 1993;21:433.

53. Gerhard I, Runnebaum B. The limits of hormone substitution in pollutant exposure and fertility disorders. Zentralbl Gynakol 1992;114:593.

54. Cummings AM, Metcalf JL. Induction of endometriosis in mice: a new model sensitive to estrogen. Reprod Toxicol 1995;9:233.

55. Cummings AM, Metcalf JL. Methoxychlor regulates rat uterine estrogen-induced protein. Toxicol Appl Pharmacol 1995;130:154.

56. Cummings AM, Metcalf JL, Birnbaum L. Promotion of endometriosis by 2,3,7,8-tetrachlorodibenzo-p-dioxin in rats and mice: Time-dose dependence and species comparison. Toxicol Appl Pharmacol 1996;138:131.

57. Clement PB. Pathology of endometriosis. Pathol Annu 1990;25:245.

58. Dmowski WP. Pitfalls in clinical, laparoscopic and histologic diagnosis of endometriosis. Acta Obstet Gynecol Scand 1984;123:61.

59. Jansen RPS, Russell P. Nonpigmented endometriosis: Clinical, laparoscopic, and pathologic definition. Am J Obstet Gynecol 1986;155:1154.

60. Redwine DB. Peritoneal pockets and endometriosis. Confirmation of an important relationship, with further observations. J Reprod Med 1989;34:270.

61. Cantor JO, Fenoglio CM, Richart RM. A case of extensive abdominal endometriosis. Am J Obstet Gynecol 1997;134:846.

62. Egger H, Weigmann P. Clinical and surgical aspects of ovarian endometriotic cysts. Arch Gynecol 1982;233:37.

63. Noble LS, Takayama K, Putman JM, et al. Prostaglandin E_2 stimulates aromatase expression in endometriosis-derived stromal cells. J Clin Endocrinol Metab 1997; 82:600.

64. Noble LS, Simpson ER, Johns A, Bulun SE. Aromatase expression in endometriosis. J Clin Endocrinol Metab 1996;81:174.

65. Syrop CH, Halme J. Peritoneal fluid environment and infertility. Fertil Steril 1987;48:1.

66. Tamaya T, Motoyama T, Ohono Y, Ide N, Tsurusaki T, Okada H. Steroid receptor levels and histology of endometriosis and adenomyosis. Fertil Steril 1979;31:396.

67. Janne O, Kauppila A, Kokko E, Lantto T, Ronnberg L, Vihko R. Estrogen and progestin receptors in endometriosis lesions: comparison with endometrial tissue. Am J Obstet Gynecol 1981;141:562.

68. Lessey BA, Metzger DA, Haney AF, McCarty KS, Jr. Immunohistochemical analysis of estrogen and progesterone receptors in endometriosis: comparison with normal endometrium during the menstrual cycle and the effect of medical therapy. Fertil Steril 1989;51:409.

69. Tseng JF, Ryan IP, Milam TD, et al. Interleukin-6 secretion in vitro is up-regulated in ectopic and eutopic endometrial stromal cells from women with endometriosis. J Clin Endocrinol Metab 1996;81:1118.

70. Sharpe-Timms KL, Bruno PL, Penney LL. Immunohistochemical localization of granulocyte-macrophage colony stimulating factor (GM-CSF) in matched endometriosis and endometrial tissues. Am J Obstet Gynecol 1999;171:450.

71. Ueki M, Tsurunaga T, Ushiroyama T. Macrophage activation factors and cytokines in peritoneal fluid from patients with endometriosis. Asia-Oceania J Obstet Gynecol 1994;20:427.

72. Sharpe-Timms KL, Penney LL, Zimmer RL, Wright JA, Zhang Y, Surewicz K. Partial purification and amino acid sequence analysis of endometriosis protein-II (ENDO-II) reveals homology with tissue inhibitor of metalloproteinases-1 (TIMP-1). J Clin Endocrinol Metab 1995; 80:3784.

73. Sharpe KL, Vernon MW. Polypeptides synthesized and released by rat ectopic uterine implants differ from those of the uterus in culture. Biol Reprod 1993; 48:1334.

74. Sharpe KL, Zimmer RL, Griffin WT, Penney LL. Polypeptides synthesized and released by human endometriosis differ from those of the uterine endometrium in cell and tissue explant culture. Fertil Steril 1993; 60:839.

75. Bergqvist A, Fernö M, Mattson S. A comparison of cathepsin D levels in endometriotic tissue and in uterine endometrium. Fertil Steril 1996;65:1130.

76. Lessey BA, Castelbaum AJ, Sawin SW, et al. Aberrant integrin expression in the endometrium of women with endometriosis. J Clin Endocrinol Metab 1994;79:643.

77. Isaacson KB, Galman M, Coutifaris C, Lyttle CR. Endometrial synthesis and secretion of complement component-3 by patients with and without endometriosis. Fertil Steril 1990;53:836.

78. Bulun SE, Mahendroo MS, Simpson ER. Polymerase chain reaction amplification fails to detect aromatase cytochrome P450 transcripts in normal human endometrium or decidua. J Clin Endocrinol Metab 1993; 76:1458.

79. Michael MD, Kilgore MW, Morohashi K-I, Simpson ER. Ad4BP/SF-1 regulates cyclic AMP-induced transcription from the proximal promoter (PII) of the human aromatase P450 (CYP19) gene in the ovary. J Biol Chem 1995;270:13561.

80. Zeitoun K, Takayama K, Michael MD, Bulun SE. Stimulation of aromatase P450 promoter (II) activity in endometriosis and its inhibition in endometrium are regulated by competitive binding of SF-1 and COUP-TF to the same *cis*-acting element. Mol Endocrinol 1999;13:239.

81. Zeitoun K, Takayama K, Sasano H, et al. Deficient 17β-hydroxysteroid dehydrogenase type 2 expression in endometriosis: Failure to metabolize estradiol-17β. J Clin Endocrinol Metab 1998;83:4474.

82. Barbieri RL, Niloff JM, Bast RC Jr, Scaetzl E, Kistner RW, Knapp RC. Elevated serum concentration of CA-125 in patients with advanced endometriosis. Fertil Steril 1986;45:630.

83. Hornstein MD, Thomas PP, Gleason RE, Barbieri RL. Menstrual cyclicity of CA-125 in patients with endometriosis. Fertil Steril 1992;58:279.

84. O'Shaughnessy A, Check JH, Nowroozi K, Lurie D. CA-125 levels measured in different phases of the menstrual cycle in screening for endometriosis. Obstet Gynecol 1993;81:99.

85. Pittaway DE. The use of serial CA-125 concentrations to monitor endometriosis in infertile women. Am J Obstet Gynecol 1990;163:1032.

86. Hornstein MD, Harlow BL, Thomas PP, Check JH. Use of a new CA-125 assay in the diagnosis of endometriosis. Hum Reprod 1995;10:932.

87. Franssen AMHW, van der Heijden PFM, Thomas CMG, Doesburg WH, Willemsen WNP, Rolland R. On the origin and significance of serum CA-125 concentrations in 97 patients with endometriosis before, during, and after buserelin acetate, nafarelin, or Danazol. Fertil Steril 1992;57:974.

88. Pittaway DE, Fayez JA, Douglas JW. Serum-CA-125 in the evaluation of benign adnexal cysts. Am J Obstet Gynecol 1987;157:1426.

89. Mol BWJ, Bayram N, Lijmer JG, et al. The performance of CA-125 measurement in the detection of endometriosis: A meta-analysis. Fertil Steril 1998;70:1101.

90. Friedman H, Vogelzang RL, Mendelson EB, Neiman LH, Cohen M. Endometriosis detection by US with laparascopic correlation. Radiology 1985;157:217.

91. Guerriero S, Mais V, Ajossa S, et al. The role of endovaginal ultrasound in differentiating endometriomas from other ovarian cysts. Clin Exp Obstet Gynecol 1994; 22:20.

92. Volpi E, DeGrandis T, Zuccaro G, LaVista A, Sismondi P. Role of transvaginal sonography in the detection of endometriomata. J Clin Ultrasound 1995;23:163.

93. Kuriac A, Zulad I, Alfirevic Z. Elevation of adnexal masses with transvaginal colour. Ultrasound J Ultrasound Med 1991;10:295.

94. Kurjak A, Kupesic S. Scoring system for prediction of ovarian endometriosis based on transvaginal color and pulsed Doppler sonography. Fertil Steril 1994;62:81.

95. Aleem F, Pennisi J, Zeitoun K, Predanic M. The role of color Doppler in the diagnosis of endometriosis. Ultrasound Obstet Gynecol 1995;5:51.

96. Togashi K, Nishimura K, Kimura I, et al. Endometrial cysts: diagnosis with MR imaging. Radiology 1991; 180:73.

97. Elliot DL, Barker AF, Dixon LM. Catamenial hemoptysis: New methods of diagnosis and therapy. Chest 1985; 87:687.

98. Forsgren H, Lindhagen J, Melander S, Wargermark J. Colorectal endometriosis. Acta Chir Scand 1983; 149:431.

99. Redwine DB. Age-related evolution in color appearance of endometriosis. Fertil Steril 1987;48:1062.

100. Stripling MC, Martin DC, Chatman DL, Zwaag RV, Poston WM. Subtle appearance of pelvic endometriosis. Fertil Steril 1988;49:427.

101. Stripling MC, Martin DC, Poston WM. Does endometriosis have a typical appearance? J Reprod Med 1988;33:879.

102. Gleicher N, Karande V, Rabin D, Dudkiewicz A, Pratt D. The bubble test: a new tool to improve the diagnosis of endometriosis. Hum Reprod 1995;10:923.

103. Redwine DB. Peritoneal blood painting: an aid in the diagnosis of endometriosis. J Obstet Gynecol 1989; 161:865.

104. Koninckx PB, Martin DC. Deep endometriosis: A consequence of infiltration or retraction or possibly adenomyosis externa? Fertil Steril 1992;58:924.

105. Koninckx PR, Meuleman C, Demeyere S, Lesaffre E, Cornillie FJ. Suggestive evidence that pelvic endometriosis is a progressive disease, whereas deeply infiltrating endometriosis is associated with pelvic pain. Fertil Steril 1991;55:759.

106. Cornillie FJ, Oosterlynck D, Lauweryns JM, Koninckx PR. Deeply infiltrating pelvic endometriosis: histology and clinical significance. Fertil Steril 1990;53:978.

107. Prystowsky JB, Stryker SJ, Ujiki GT, Poticha SM. Gastrointestinal endometriosis: Incidence and indications for resection. Arch Surg 1988;123:855.

108. The American Fertility Society. Classification of endometriosis. Fertil Steril 1979;32:633.

109. The American Fertility Society. Revised American Fertility Society classification of endometriosis: 1985. Fertil Steril 1985;43:351.

110. Guzick DS, Bross DS, Rock JA. Assessing the efficacy of The American Fertility Society's classification of endometriosis: Application of a dose-response methodology. Fertil Steril 1982;38:171.

111. Adamson GD, Pasta DJ. Surgical treatment of endometriosis-associated infertility: meta-analysis compared with survival analysis. Am J Obstet Gynecol 1994; 171:1488.

112. Canis M, Donnez JG, Guzick DS, et al. Revised American Society for Reproductive Medicine classification of endometriosis: 1996. Fertil Steril 1997;67:817.

113. Guzick DS, Paul Silliman N, Adamson GD, et al. Prediction of pregnancy in infertile women based on the American Society for Reproductive Medicine's revised classification of endometriosis. Fertil Steril 1997;67:822.

114. Schenken RS, Guzick DS. Revised endometriosis classification: 1996. Fertil Steril 1997;67:815.

115. Muse K. Clinical manifestations and classification of endometriosis. Clin Obstet Gynecol 1988;31:813.

116. Vercellini P, Trespidi L, DeGiorgi O, Cortèsi I, Parazzini F, Crosignani PG. Endometriosis and pelvic pain. Relation to disease stage and localization. Fertil Steril 1996; 65:299.

117. Guarnaccia MM, Olive DL. Diagnosis and management of endometriosis. In: Carr BR, Blackwell RE, eds. Textbook of reproductive medicine. 2nd ed. Stamford, CT: Appleton & Lange, 1998:641.

118. Rossman F, D'Ablaing G, III, Marrs RP. Pregnancy complicated by ruptured endometrioma. Obstet Gynecol 1983;62:519.

119. Slutsky JN, Callahan D. Endometriosis of the ureter can present as renal failure: A case report and review of endometriosis affecting the ureters. J Urol 1983;130:336.

120. Stanley KE, Utz DC, Dockerty MB. Clinically significant endometriosis of the urinary tract. Surg Gynecol Obstet 1965;120:491.

121. Wynn TE. Endometriosis of the sigmoid colon. Massive intramural hematoma. Arch Pathol Lab Med 1971;92:24.

122. Wilhelm JL, Scommegna A. Catamenial pneumothorax. Bilateral occurrence while on suppressive therapy. Obstet Gynecol 1977;50:227.

123. Roth LM. Endometriosis with perineural involvement. Am J Clin Pathol 1973;59:807.

124. Moon YS, Leung PCS, Yuen BH, Gomel V. Prostaglandin F in human endometriotic tissue. Am J Obstet Gynecol 1981;141:344.

125. Vernon MS, Beard JS, Graves K, Wilson EA. Classification of endometriotic implants by morphologic appearance and capacity to synthesize prostaglandin F. Fertil Steril 1986;46:801.

126. Kauppila A, Puolakka J, Ylikorkala O. Prostaglandin biosynthesis inhibitors and endometriosis. Prostaglandins 1979;18:655.

127. Schenken RS, Asch RH, Williams RF, Hodgen GD. Etiology of infertility in monkeys with endometriosis. Measurement of peritoneal fluid prostaglandins. Am J Obstet Gynecol 1984;150:349.

128. Burns WN, Schenken RS. Pathophysiology. In: Schenken RS, ed. Endometriosis: contemporary concepts in clinical management. Philadelphia: Lippincott;1989;83.

129. Metzger DA, Olive DL, Stohs GF, Franklin RR. Association of endometriosis and spontenous abortion: Effect of control group selection. Fertil Steril 1986;45:18.

130. FitzSimmons J, Stahl R, Gocial B, Shapiro SS. Spontaneous abortion and endometriosis. Fertil Steril 1987; 47:696.

131. Marcoux S, Maheux R, Bêrubê S. The Canadian Collaborative Group on Endometriosis. Laparoscopic surgery in infertile women with minimal or mild endometriosis. N Engl J Med 1997;337:217.

132. Schenken RS, Malinak LR. Conservative surgery versus expectant management for the infertile patient with mild endometriosis. Fertil Steril 1982;37:183.

133. Hull ME, Moghissi KS, Magyar DF, Hayes MF. Comparison of different treatment modalities of endometriosis in infertile women. Fertil Steril 1987;47:40.

134. Kettel LM, Hummel WP. Modern medical management of endometriosis. Obstet Gynecol Clin North Am 1997;24:361.

135. Salat-Baroux J, Giacomini P, Antoine JM. Laparoscopic control of Danazol therapy on pelvic endometriosis. Hum Reprod 1988;3:197.

136. Seibel MM, Berger MJ, Weinstein FG, Taymor ML. The effectiveness of Danazol on subsequent fertility in minimal endometriosis. Fertil Steril 1982;38:534.

137. Bayer SR, Seibel MM, Saffan DS, Berger MJ, Taymor ML. The efficacy of Danazol treatment for minimal endometriosis in infertile women: A prospective randomized study. J Reprod Med 1988;33:179.

138. Olive DL. Medical treatment: Alternatives to Danazol. In: Schenken RS, ed. Endometriosis: Contemporary concepts in clinical management. Philadelphia: Lippincott; 1989:189.

139. Fedele L, Bianchi S, Viezzoli T, Arcaini L, Candiani GB. Gestrinone versus danazol in the treatment of endometriosis. Fertil Steril 1989;51:781.

140. Fedele L, Marchini M, Baglioni A, Antonio G, Motta T. Evaluation of histological and ultrastructural aspects of endometrium during treatment with gestrinone in women with amenorrhea or spotting. Acta Obstet Gynecol Scand 1990;69:143.

141. Hornstein MD, Gleason RE, Barbieri RL. A randomized double-blind prospective trial of two doses of gestrinone in the treatment of endometriosis. Fertil Steril 1990; 53:237.

142. Thomas EJ, Cooke ID. Impact of gestrinone on the course of asymptomatic endometriosis. Br Med J. 1987; 294:272.

143. Telimaa S, Puolakka J, Rönnberg L, Kauppila A. Placebo-controlled comparison of Danazol and high-dose medroxyprogesterone acetate in the treatment of endometriosis. Gynecol Endocrinol 1987;1:13.

144. Moghissi KS, Boyce CR. Management of endometriosis with oral medroxyprogesterone acetate. Obstet Gynecol 1976;47:265.

145. Johnston WIH. Dydrogesterone and endometriosis. Br J Obstet Gynaecol 1976;83:77.

146. Kistner RW. Management of endometriosis in the infertile patient. Fertil Steril 1975;26:1151.

147. Kistner RW. The treatment of endometriosis by inducing pseudopregnancy with ovarian hormones: a report of 58 cases. Fertil Steril 1959;10:539.

148. Moghissi KS. Treatment of endometriosis with estrogen-progestin combination and progestin alone. Clin Obstet Gynecol 1988;31:823.

149. Henzl MR, Corson SL, Moghissi K, Buttram VC, Berqvist C, Jacobson J. Administration of nasal nafarelin as compared with oral Danazol for endometriosis. N Engl J Med 1988;318:485.

150. Waller KG, Shaw RW. Gonadotropin-releasing hormone analogues for the treatment of endometriosis: Long-term follow-up. Fertil Steril 1993;59:511.

151. The American Fertility Society. Management of endometriosis in the presence of pelvic pain. Fertil Steril 1993;60:952.

152. Dmowski WP, Radwanska E, Binor Z, Tummon I, Pepping P. Ovarian suppression induced with buserelin or Danazol in the management of endometriosis: a randomized, comparative study. Fertil Steril 1989;51:395.

153. Fedele L, Bianchi S, Arcaini L, Vercellini P, Candiani GB. Buserelin versus Danazol in the treatment of endometriosis-associated infertility. Am J Obstet Gynecol 1989;161:871.

154. Barlow DH. Nafarelin in the treatment of infertility caused by endometriosis. Am J Obstet Gynecol 1990; 162:576.

155. Fraser IS, Shearman RPS, Jansen RPS, Sutherland PD. A comparative treatment trial of endometriosis using the gonadotrophin-releasing hormone agonist, nafarelin, and the synthetic steroid, Danazol. N Z J Obstet Gynaecol 1991;31:158.

156. Kettel LM, Murphy AA, Morales AJ, Ulmann A, Baulieu EE, Yen SS. Treatment of endometriosis with the antiprogesterone mifepristone (RU486). Fertil Steril 1996; 65:23.

157. Takayama K, Zeitoun K, Gunby RT, Sasano H, Carr BR, Bulun SE. Treatment of severe postmenopausal endometriosis with an aromatase inhibitor. Fertil Steril 1998;69:709.

158. Adamson GD, Nelson HP. Surgical treatment of endometriosis. Obstet Gynecol Clin North Am 1997; 24:375.

159. Olive DL, Lee KL. Analysis of sequential treatment protocols for endometriosis-associated infertility. Am J Obstet Gynecol 1986;154:613.

160. Buttram VC, Jr., Reiter RC, Ward S. Treatment of endometriosis with Danazol: report of a 6-year prospective study. Fertil Steril 1985;43:353.

161. Donnez J, Nisolle M, Clerckx F, Casanas F. Evaluation of preoperative use of Danazol, gestrinone, lynestrenol, buserelin spray, and buserelin implant, in the treatment of endometriosis asociated infertility. Prog Clin Biol Res 1990;323:427.

162. Rönnberg L, Järvinen PA. Pregnancy rates following various therapy modes for endometriosis in infertile patients. Acta Obstet Gynecol Scand 1984;123(Supp):69.

163. Chong AP, Keene ME, Thornton NL. Comparison of three modes of treatment for infertility patients with minimal pelvic endometriosis. Fertil Steril 1990;53:407.

164. Wheeler JM, Malinak LR. Postoperative Danazol therapy in infertility patients with severe endometriosis. Fertil Steril 1981;36:460.

165. Namnoum AB, Hickman TN, Goodman SB, Gehlbach DL, Rock JA. Incidence of symptom recurrence after hysterectomy for endometriosis. Fertil Steril 1995; 64:898.

166. Fedele L, Bianchi S, Marchini M, Villa L, Brioschi D, Parazzini F. Superovulation with human menopausal gonadotropins in the treatment of infertility associated with minimal or mild endometriosis: a controlled randomized study. Fertil Steril 1992;58:28.

167. Dodson WC, Haney AF. Controlled ovarian hyperstimulation and intrauterine insemination for treatment of infertility. Fertil Steril 1991;55:457.

168. Deaton AL, Gibson M, Blackmer KM, Nakajima ST, Badger GJ, Brumsted JR. A randomized, controlled trial of clomiphene citrate and intrauterine insemination in couples with unexplained infertility or surgically corrected endometriosis. Fertil Steril 1990;54:1083.

169. Chaffkin LM, Nulsen JC, Luciano AA, Metzger DA. A comparative analysis of the cycle fecundity rates associated with combined human menopausal gonadotropin (hMG) and intrauterine insemination (IUI) versus either hMG or IUI alone. Fertil Steril 1991;55:252.

170. Serta RT, Rufo S, Seibel MM. Minimal endometriosis and intrauterine insemination: Does controlled ovarian hyperstimulation improve pregnancy rates? Obstet Gynecol 1992;80:37.

171. Remorgida V, Anserini P, Croce S, Costa M, Ferraiolo A, Capitanio GL. Comparison of different ovarian stimulation protocols for gamete intrafallopian transfer in patients with minimal and mild endometriosis. Fertil Steril 1990;53:1060.

172. Schenken RS and Riehl RM. In vitro fertilization/embryo transfer and gamete intrafallopian transfer. In: Schenken RS, ed. Endometriosis: Contemporary concepts in clinical management. Philadelphia: Lippincott: 1989;293.

173. Matson PL, Yovich JL. The treatment of infertility associated with endometriosis by in vitro fertilization. Fertil Steril 1986;46:432.

174. Chillik CF, Acosta AA, Garcia JE, et al. The role of in vitro fertilization in infertile patients with endometriosis. Fertil Steril 1985;44:56.

175. Inoue M, Kobayashi Y, Honda I, Awaji H, Fujii A. The impact of endometriosis on the reproductive outcome of infertile patients. Am J Obstet Gynecol 1992;167:278.

176. Garcia JE, Tran T, Smith RD, Padilla SL. Relationship of endometriosis staging and in vitro fertilization outcome. Hum Reprod 6 1991;6(Suppl 1):74.

177. Gerday C, Jouan C, Demoulin A. IVF in patients with endometriosis: impact of severity of the disease. Hum Reprod 1991;6(Suppl 1):263.

178. Dicker D, Goldman JA, Levy T, Feldberg D, Ashkenazi J. The impact of long-term gonadotropin-releasing hormone analogue treatment on preclinical abortions in patients with severe endometriosis undergoing in vitro fertilization-embryo transfer. Fertil Steril 1992;57:597.

179. Olivennes F, Feldberg D, Liu HC, Cohen J, Moy F, Rosenwaks Z. Endometriosis: A stage by stage analysis—the role of in vitro fertilization. Fertil Steril 1995;64:392.

Chapter 53

Urogynecology: Urinary Incontinence and Sensory Disorders of the Female Lower Urinary Tract

Robert L. Summitt, Jr.

Five Key Points

- **Because symptoms of lower-urinary-tract dysfunction often overlap, particularly with regard to incontinence, a systematic stepwise evaluation utilizing specific tests is required.**

- **A urinalysis and culture should be one of the first tests obtained in patients presenting with complaints of urinary dysfunction. Infection must be ruled out before proceeding with further investigation.**

- **Stress incontinence is the most common cause of urinary incontinence in women, confirmed by direct observation of involuntary urine loss from the urethra with an increase in abdominal pressure in the absence of a detrusor contraction.**

- **Urge incontinence, the second most common cause of incontinence in women, is the involuntary loss of urine associated with a strong desire to void. In most cases it is associated with involuntary bladder contractions diagnosed by a cystometrogram.**

- **Bacterial cystitis occurs in up to 6 million women per year in the United States, with recurrent cystitis developing in up to 50% of those presenting for the first time.**

The field of urogynecology is relatively new with regard to its development as a subspecialty area in the care of women. It encompasses evaluation and treatment of lower-urinary-tract disorders ranging from urinary incontinence to irritative/sensory disorders such as urinary-tract infections, urethral syndrome, and interstitial cystitis. As obstetrician-gynecologists fulfill the role of primary care physician and specialist, they will have the constant opportunity of encountering women with lower-urinary-tract symptoms and therefore will be able to participate in or fully direct their evaluation and care.

Urinary incontinence affects over 13 million Americans, the majority being women. Among women aged 15 to 64 years of age, the incidence of urinary incontinence is 10 to 30%.[1] Urinary-tract infections will occur in 50% of women during their lifetimes, accounting for one of the most common reasons for visits to primary care physicians. Urethral syndrome and interstitial cystitis are less well known disease processes affecting women. However, their impact on quality of life and the need for proper diagnosis and treatment necessitate a greater understanding on the gynecologist's part.

conservative therapy. Avoidance techniques are common-sense measures used to change behaviors that result in urine loss. Examples include avoiding caffeine intake to reduce urine production, voiding prior to physical exertion, and avoiding heavy lifting. Bladder-training drills are a method of timed voiding, initially developed for overactive bladder problems, that have also been shown to be successful in reducing episodes of stress incontinence by over 50%.[11] Bladder drills will be discussed in more depth in the section on urge incontinence.

Pessaries and other mechanical devices treat stress incontinence by physically elevating the urethra and increasing urethral resistance, or simply by completely obstructing the urethra. Both standard pessaries (ring, Hodge, Smith) and specialized pessaries specific for treating stress incontinence have been shown to reduce urine loss by 60 to 80%. They elevate and stabilize the bladder, producing urodynamically confirmed changes that improve continence. In addition to pessaries, various other devices such as adhesive patches that fit over the external urethral meatus and urethral plugs that obstruct the lumen are available for patients. Their use must be carefully selected and tailored for a patient, depending on her needs and physical capabilities.

Medication use for the treatment of stress incontinence has been directed at increasing urethral tone. Although estrogen has been shown to improve urodynamic parameters in women with stress incontinence, more recent randomized, placebo-controlled trials have revealed that estrogen alone does not decrease the number and volume of incontinent episodes in women.[12,13] However, estrogen does provide benefits of improving coaptation of the urethral mucosal seal and increasing the density of α-adrenergic receptors in urethral smooth muscle. α-Adrenergic agonists stimulate urethral smooth muscle and increase tone. Medications such as phenylpropanolamine and phenylephrine, available in many over-the-counter drugs, can be used in cases of mild stress incontinence. Imipramine, a tricyclic antidepressant, has α-adrenergic agonist properties. Not only can it be used in the treatment of stress incontinence, but because it has anticholinergic properties, it can also be used when stress incontinence and urge incontinence coexist. Doses of 25 to 150 mg orally at bedtime are generally used.

Pelvic-muscle rehabilitation refers to strengthening of the supportive component of the pelvic diaphragm,

specifically the pubococcygeus muscle. The end result is augmentation of the closing muscles around the urethra and vaginal canal, leading to a greater ability to voluntarily and reflexively maintain continence with physical exertion. Kegel exercises have the patient voluntarily contract the pelvic muscles, typically for a specified time period and number of repetitions. Most advise that women contract the muscles for 10 seconds followed by a 10-second rest. The patient should start with 10 contractions, three to four times per day, gradually increasing repetitions weekly until she can perform sets of 25 to 30 contractions three to four times per day. This routine should be continued for at least 8 to 12 weeks, and in most cases indefinitely. With a well-followed pelvic-muscle exercise program, reductions in leakage of 50 to 60% can be expected.[14]

One drawback to Kegel exercises is that the patient may use the wrong set of muscles or may add accessory muscles such as the gluteals, upper leg adductors, or abdominals. In order to properly train and monitor exercise performance, biofeedback and vaginal cones have been used. Biofeedback usually uses either pressure or electromyographic recording of pelvic-muscle contractions to facilitate use of the correct muscles and to provide the patient with a goal for performance. Recording of either pressure or voltage increases over time demonstrates improvement in strength and generally correlates with improvement in incontinence. Patients return for regular biofeedback training sessions of a predefined number or until they are consistently performing exercises correctly. Weighted vaginal cones are another means for training the correct pelvic muscles. The patient receives a set of identically shaped cones of increasing weights, usually 20 to 100 g. The cones are inserted vaginally and retained in place by the pelvic muscles as part of a progressive resistance training program. Worn while ambulatory, the heaviest cone retainable is held 15 minutes twice a day. As increasing weight can be retained, pelvic-muscle strength increases and incontinence improves. In well-structured training programs using weighted cones, success rates in improvement of 60 to 80% have been demonstrated.[15]

Functional electrical stimulation is, in essence, another form of pelvic-muscle rehabilitation, but it uses electrical current to stimulate pelvic muscle contractions rather than having the patient perform them herself. Using a vaginally inserted electrode, current of a specific frequency and pulse duration is delivered, stimulating the pudendal nerve, which reflexively activates contraction of pelvic muscles. Treatment can be provided daily at home or on a less frequent basis at an office. Functional electrical stimulation is also useful in the treatment of urge incontinence. Success rates for treatment of stress incontinence using functional electrical stimulation range from 40 to 65%.

Surgical treatment of stress incontinence by far has the highest cure rates. When properly selected and performed, patients can expect surgical success rates of 82 to 90%. Over 150 surgical procedures for stress incontinence have been described. However, they all have basic goals in mind. The goals of surgery for stress incontinence due to urethral hypermobility should be to elevate the proximal urethra so that pressure transmission is restored, to stabilize and reduce urethral hypermobility, and to provide a stable platform for urethral compression. In addition, the surgical procedure must still allow proper voiding and emptying of the bladder.

It is not the goal of this section to describe surgical procedures for stress incontinence. Rather, proper selection of the surgical procedure will be described. Figure 53-6 provides an algorithm for selection of surgery based on several physical and urodynamic parameters.[16] Using urethral hypermobility and the presence or absence of intrinsic sphincter deficiency, patients can be roughly divided into several treatment categories. In the majority of cases, patients with stress incontinence will demonstrate urethral hypermobility with satisfactory urethral sphincter function. These women can best be treated with a standard

retropubic urethropexy such as a Burch procedure or a Marshall–Marchetti–Krantz procedure. Because failure rates with standard urethropexies are much higher when urethral hypermobility is accompanied by intrinsic sphincter deficiency, a suburethral sling procedure is recommended as success rates can approach 90% when used in this group of patients.[17] When urethral hypermobility is absent and intrinsic sphincter deficiency exists, supportive operative procedures have failure rates approaching 80%. In these cases, periurethral bulking procedures are recommended, using agents such as glutaraldehyde cross-linked collagen. Improvement rates of 70 to 80% are reported with repeat injections in these patients.

New surgical procedures for stress incontinence continue to be introduced, such as laparoscopic approaches and tension-free vaginal tape. Prudent selection of the correct operation, based on physical and urodynamic characteristics of the patient, will lead to good surgical outcomes.

Urge Incontinence

Urge incontinence is defined as the involuntary loss of urine associated with a strong desire to void.[1] In most cases, it is associated with urodynamic findings of involuntary detrusor contractions. The causes of urge incontinence are multiple. However, in the majority of cases, no recognizable pathology can be found (idiopathic). Other identifiable causes include bladder inflammation, neurologic disease, and bladder outlet obstruction. In the absence of neurologic disease,

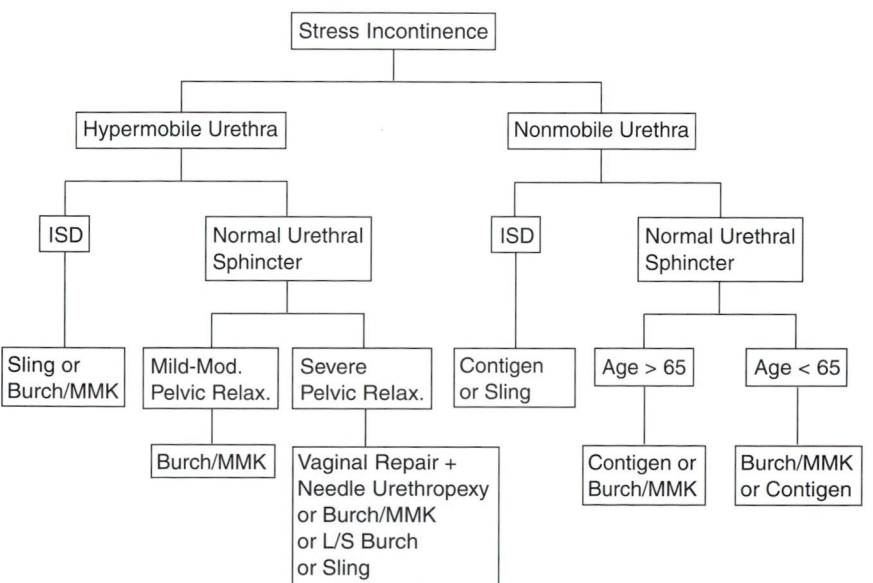

Figure 53-6 Algorithm for surgical management of stress incontinence.

the involuntary contractions associated with urge incontinence are called detrusor instability. When neurologic diseases exist, they are referred to as detrusor hyperreflexia. All patients with suspected urge incontinence should have a urine culture obtained and complete a voiding diary. However, the diagnosis is confirmed with a cystometrogram.

Treatments for urge incontinence are numerous, but in most cases bladder-retraining drills or pharmaceutical agents are used. Other therapies employed have included biofeedback, functional electrical stimulation, and surgery. More recently, surgical approaches have fallen out of favor and are reserved as a treatment of last resort.

Bladder-retraining drills, when properly performed and monitored, are associated with success rates of up to 80% in the treatment of urge incontinence.[11] They consist of a timed voiding schedule that is conducted during waking hours, asking the patient to attempt to avoid rising to void after going to sleep. Starting intervals of 30 to 90 minutes are used, selecting an interval slightly shorter than the average interval gleaned from the voiding diary. As the patient is successful in maintaining the interval with few or no leaking episodes, the voiding interval is gradually increased until reaching 3 to 4 hours. Patients keep written records of their voiding and incontinence episodes and maintain regular frequent office visits to review these records and receive positive feedback.

Medical therapy for urge incontinence uses a number of categories of drugs (Table 53-5). The most commonly used medications are anticholinergics or musculotropic drugs with significant anticholinergic properties. The musculotropic drugs (oxybutynin, tolterodine, flavoxate, dicyclomine) have direct smooth-muscle-relaxing properties, anticholinergic capabilities, and local anesthetic benefits. These two groups of drugs, in addition to the tricyclic antidepressant imipramine, have anticholinergic side effects of dry mouth, constipation, blurry vision, and

drowsiness. Calcium-channel blockers (nifedipine) have also been used for the treatment of urge incontinence. They may be particularly helpful in patients with narrow-angle glaucoma, for which anticholinergic agents may be contraindicated.

All medications must be carefully administered. Frequent regular visits are initially required in order to maximize the effective dose and minimize side effects. Patients should still be advised on maintaining a voiding schedule. Overall success rates with medical therapy approximate 60 to 70%.

Mixed Incontinence

Mixed incontinence refers to the presence of stress and urge incontinence existing simultaneously. When both conditions are diagnosed, treatment should be directed to the most significant symptom. Before contemplating surgery for the stress incontinence component, treatment should be maximized for urge incontinence. In many cases, the urge component may improve enough that no surgical therapy is desired. As noted earlier, medical therapy with imipramine may treat both components of mixed incontinence. When surgery is performed, some have noted that detrusor instability may improve in as many as 40% of cases. The reason for this is unclear, but it is postulated that surgery reduces vesical neck funneling, a stimulant to involuntary detrusor contractions.

Overflow Incontinence

Overflow incontinence is defined as the involuntary loss of urine associated with an overdistended bladder.[1] This results from either an underactive or acontractile bladder or bladder-outlet obstruction. An underactive bladder can result from peripheral neurologic disease such as diabetic neuropathy, or from nerve injury, as might result from radical pelvic surgery or trauma. Bladder-outlet obstruction in women

TABLE 53-5 MEDICAL THERAPY FOR URGE INCONTINENCE		
Category	**Drug Name**	**Dose**
Anticholinergic	Propantheline bromide	15 mg twice a day to 30 mg four times a day
Musculotropic	Oxybutynin chloride	2.5 mg twice a day to 20 mg three times a day
Musculotropic	Tolterodine	1–2 mg twice a day
Musculotropic	Flavoxate hydrochloride	100 mg twice a day to three times a day
Musculotropic	Dicyclomine hydrochloride	10 mg twice a day to 20 mg four times a day
Calcium-channel blocker	Nifedipine	10 mg twice a day to 120 mg a day
Tricyclic antidepressant	Imipramine hydrochloride	25–150 mg a day

is rare. However, it can result from severe anterior pelvic-organ prolapse that results in a kinking effect in the urethra. Patients with overflow incontinence generally have large postvoiding residual volumes and large capacities on cystometry.

Treatment for overflow incontinence is directed at the cause. When an underactive or acontractile bladder exists, medication is typically of little help. Instead, intermittent self-catheterization is the best means for maintaining an empty bladder and relieving incontinence. When outlet obstruction from prolapse exists, restoration of the prolapse surgically or with a pessary will often relieve the obstruction and overflow incontinence.

Functional Incontinence

Functional incontinence results from factors outside the lower urinary tract, such as chronic impairment of physical or cognitive functioning.[1] The diagnosis is often one of exclusion. Treatment addresses improvement in functioning. Examples of this include adjustment of medications in the elderly that affect cognition, or providing a patient who has debilitating arthritis with a free-standing commode.

Genitourinary Fistulas

Vesicovaginal and urethrovaginal fistulas are rare and are usually the result of surgery or trauma. In the United States, the most common cause of vesicovaginal fistula is complication from abdominal hysterectomy, the incidence being 0.1%.[18] Fistulas are commonly diagnosed by visual inspection after the patient presents with continuous urine loss from the vagina. They are confirmed by cystourethroscopy and/or radiologic contrast studies. In addition, they can be confirmed through instillation of a dilute dye solution in the bladder and noting passage of dye through the fistulous tract.

When initially diagnosed, catheter drainage of the bladder may allow spontaneous closure of small vesicovaginal fistulas. However, the majority will typically require surgical correction, as will all urethrovaginal fistulas. Repair should not be undertaken until 6 to 8 weeks after occurrence in order to allow resolution of inflammation. Most posthysterectomy vesicovaginal fistulas can be repaired transvaginally. However, complex fistulas or recurrent fistulas may require a transabdominal approach.

Ectopic Ureter

Ectopic ureter is an unusual condition. It is typically diagnosed in children, but can present in adulthood. It may be part of a single renal system or a duplicated system. The ureter typically implants into the urethra but can implant into the trigone. If it implants into the urethra, it can result in continuous incontinence.

Diagnosis is made with a combination of intravenous urography and cystourethroscopy. Management is surgical, ranging from ureteroureterostomy, ureteroneocystotomy, or partial nephrectomy.

SENSORY AND IRRITATIVE DISORDERS

Lower-Urinary-Tract Infections

Lower-urinary-tract infections can consist of cystitis (inflammation of the bladder) and urethritis (inflammation of the urethra). Bacterial cystitis occurs in up to 6 million women per year in the United States. Asymptomatic bacteriuria, defined as $>10^5$ bacterial colonies per milliliter, occurs in 3 to 8% of premenopausal women, the incidence rising significantly after menopause. Symptomatic bacteriuria (acute cystitis) can have as few as 10^2 to 10^3 bacterial colonies per milliliter. *Escherichia coli* is the most common cause of urinary-tract infections in women. *Staphylococcus saprophyticus* is the second most common cause of community-acquired urinary-tract infection. Other common bacteria causing urinary tract infections outside the hospital include Klebsiella, Proteus, and Enterobacter species.

In symptomatic patients, a number of tests, including microscopic urinalysis and rapid office detection kits, can be used. Unspun urine revealing one or more bacteria per high-power field correlates with $>10^4$ bacterial colonies per milliliter. For recurrent urinary-tract infections or with equivocal office testing, urine culture should be obtained.

As acute cystitis is an infection of the mucosal lining of the bladder, short-course therapy with antibiotics (3 days) is often quite effective. Trimethoprim–sulfamethoxazole is effective and inexpensive as a 3-day regimen. Newer, but expensive, quinolone derivatives are effective in 3-day courses, particularly for resistant strains. Nitrofurantoin has good activity versus *E. coli* but is best administered as a 7-day course.

Recurrent cystitis can occur in up to 50% of women who present for the first time. Recurrence of more than three infections per year deserves antibiotic suppression for 3 to 6 months using a single dose of nitrofurantoin or trimethoprim–sulfamethoxazole daily. If the bacteria is the same for all recurrences, structural urinary abnormalities or renal stones must be excluded.

Urethral Syndrome

Urethral syndrome is a complex of chronic irritative symptoms such as dysuria, urgency, frequency, suprapubic discomfort, and postvoiding fullness in the absence of a positive urine culture and any lower-urinary-tract abnormalities. Patients may also present with symptoms referable to pelvic pain and may experience dyspareunia.

The cause of urethral syndrome in unclear. Causes include inflammation of paraurethral glands due to infection, urethral spasm, hypoestrogenism, obstruction due to stenosis, and psychogenic and neurologic causes. The diagnosis is one of exclusion. Urine culture should be obtained to rule out urinary-tract infection. Pyuria may be present in the absence of a positive culture. Urethral cultures for Chlamydia are also helpful. Cystourethroscopy should be performed to rule out other causes of urethral and bladder pain such as diverticula and urinary-tract tumors. While no finding is diagnostic of urethral syndrome, mild urethral erythema with exudate and a white pseudomembrane are common findings.

Because the cause is poorly understood, numerous treatments for urethral syndrome have been proposed. Low-dose suppressive antibiotic therapy using a single tablet of nitrofurantoin 50 mg or trimethoprim–sulfamethoxazole daily for 3 to 6 months is useful, directing treatment at chronic paraurethral-gland infection. Others recommend 10 days of doxycycline therapy, suspecting Chlamydia as a source. Urethral dilations are recommended as treatment for urethral syndrome, adding urethral massage as an adjunct. This may be helpful in younger women when antibiotic therapy provides slow response. When hypoestrogenism is suspected, vaginal estrogen cream administered every other day for 2 to 3 months may provide relief.

Urethral Diverticula

A urethral diverticulum is an outpouching of the urethra that forms a sac-like structure. Typically forming on the inferior surface of the urethral lumen, diverticula result from obstruction, infection, and swelling of periurethral glands. The orifice eventually ruptures, leaving an opening from the urethral lumen into the sac. Diverticula can become reinfected, leading to recurrent pain, urinary-tract infections, and discharge. The historical triad of dysuria, dyspareunia, and postvoiding dribbling has been ascribed to urethral diverticula.

Diagnosis of a urethral diverticulum can be suspected from physical examination after finding a tender suburethral mass. Compression of the mass may result in expression of discharge from the urethra. Urethral diverticula can be confirmed by a combination of tests. A voiding cystourethrogram can demonstrate >80% of diverticula, revealing their number and contour. Urethroscopy can locate the diverticulum orifice, often demonstrating more than one. Urethral-pressure profilometry has been proposed as a method to locate the orifice in relation to the point of maximum urethral closure pressure, thus allowing planning of surgical correction. While a depression in pressure on the profile can be seen, it is very broad and is no more helpful in selecting the surgical approach than the combination of urethroscopy and voiding cystourethrography.[19]

Many diverticula are asymptomatic or have a wide orifice and require no treatment. However, when symptomatic, surgical therapy is usually used. When diverticula are distal and beyond the point of maximal urethral closure pressure, a marsupialization procedure (Spence procedure) can be used. For mid- or proximal urethral diverticula, a transvaginal excision with layer closure is recommended.

Interstitial Cystitis

Interstitial cystitis is a chronic inflammatory condition of the bladder wall for which no clear cause is known. It is manifested by severe suprapubic and bladder pain, frequency, urgency, nocturia, and dyspareunia. The pain is usually relieved for a short time after voiding. Generally, dysuria and incontinence do not exist.

Interstitial cystitis affects women in a ratio of 10:1 versus men, primarily occurring in middle age. While no clear cause is known, many have been proposed, including infection (bacterial or viral), allergic, neurogenic, and autoimmune. The most plausible cause is autoimmune, with the detection of certain serum markers in patients being documented. It is proposed that through an autoimmune reaction, damage to the glycosaminoglycan layer of the bladder epithelium occurs, creating a permeable lining that allows penetration of noxious agents into the interstitium of the bladder wall, leading to an inflammatory response. Typical inflammatory findings have been noted histologically, particularly documentation of mast cells in the detrusor muscularis.

The diagnosis of interstitial cystitis is based on the symptom complex and specific cystoscopic findings. Double-fill cystoscopy with hydrodistention, performed under general anesthesia, is required. On the second fill and distention, women with interstitial cystitis will demonstrate the typical findings of submucosal hemorrhages and petechiae, glomerulations, and in severe cases, Hunner ulcers and linear splits in the bladder mucosa. Bleeding may occur from the mucosa during filling, resulting in bloody effluent during the terminal drainage of the bladder. Although histologic findings of inflammation with mast cells have been documented, biopsy is not required for diagnosis. Biopsy is recommended to rule out preinvasive cancer of the bladder, which may resemble some of the findings of interstitial cystitis.

Treatment for interstitial cystitis is varied but generally is directed to relieving pain, reducing urinary frequency and nocturia, and improving overall well-being. In a few cases, hydrodistention of the bladder will provide relief. However, this is typically short-lived. Initial medical therapy using amitriptyline (25 to 100 mg nightly) may provide relief. It works through centrally acting pain pathways, while also serving sedative and antidepressant roles. Therapies developed specifically for interstitial cystitis have been used with moderate success. Dimethyl sulfoxide (DMSO) is a liquid used as a bladder instillation. A total of 50 ml is placed in the bladder for 15 to 20 minutes at 2-week intervals for approximately six treatments. DMSO has anti-inflammatory and analgesic properties, providing symptomatic relief in 60 to 70% of patients. Sodium pentosanpolysulfate (Elmiron) has been developed specifically for treating interstitial cystitis. It is a synthetic glycosaminoglycan given orally as a dose of 100 mg three times a day. Theoretically it replaces the defective layer lining the bladder. Success rates of up to 70% have been reported after a 3-month trial.

REFERENCES

1. Fantl JA, Newman DK, Colling J, et al. Urinary incontinence in adults: acute and chronic management. Clinical Practice Guidleline, No. 2, 1996 Update. Rockville MD: Department of Health and Human Services. Public Health Service, Agency for Health Care Policy and Research, March 1996. AHCPR Publication no. 96-0682.

2. Delancey JOL. Structural aspects of the extrinsic continence mechanism. Obstet Gynecol 1988;72:296.

3. Huffman JW. The detailed anatomy of the paraurethral ducts in the adult human female. Am J Obstet Gynecol 1948;55:86.

4. Delancey JOL. Structural support of the urethra as it relates to stress urinary incontinence: the hammock hypothesis. Am J Obstet Gynecol 1994;170:1713.

5. Summitt RL, Stovall TG, Bent AE, Ostergard DR. Urinary incontinence: correlation of history and brief office evaluation with multichannel urodynamic testing. Am J Obstet Gyecol 1992;166:1835.

6. Bergman A, Koonings PP, Ballard CA. Negative Q-tip test as a risk factor for failed incontinence surgery in women. J Reprod Med 1989;34:193.

7. McGuire EJ, Woodside JR, Borden TA, Weiss RM. Prognostic value of urodynamic testing in myelodysplastic patients. J Urol 1980;126:205.

8. Sand Pk, Bowen LW, Panganiban R, Ostergard DR. The low pressure urethra as a factor in failed retropubic urethropexy. Obstet Gynecol 1987;69:399.

9. McNicholas MMJ, Griffin JF, Cantwell DF. Ultrasound of the pelvis and renal tract combined with a plain film of abdomen in young women with urinary tract infection: can it replace intravenous urography? Br J Radiol 1991; 64:221.

10. Abrams P, Blaivis JG, Stanton SL, Anderson JT. The International Continence Society Committee on Standardisation of Terminology: the standardisation of terminology of lower urinary tract function. Scand J Urol Nephrol 1988;114(Suppl):5.

11. Fantl JA, Hurt WG, Dunn LJ. Detrusor instability syndrome: the use of bladder retraining drills with and without anticholinergics. Am J Obstet Gynecol 1981;140:885.

12. Hilton P, Stanton SL. The use of intravaginal oestrogen cream in genuine stress incontinence. Br J Obstet Gynecol 1983;90:940.

13. Fantl JA, Bump RC, Robinson D, et al. Efficacy of estrogen supplementation in the treatment of urinary incontinence. Obstet Gynecol 1996;88:745.

14. Ferguson K, McKey PL, Bishop KR, Kloen P, Verheul JB, Dougherty MC. Stress urinary incontinence: effect of pelvic muscle exercise. Obstet Gynaecol 1990;73:671.

15. Peattie AB, Plevnick S, Stanton SL. Vaginal cones: a conservative method of treating genuine stress incontinence. Br J Obstet Gyaecol 1988;95:1049.

16. Portera JC, Summitt RL. Common operations for stress incontinence: selecting the correct operation. Clin Obstet Gynecol 1998;41:712.

17. Summitt RL, Bent AE, Ostergard DR, Harris TA. Stress incontinence and low urethral closure pressure: correlation of preoperative urethral hypermboility with successful suburethral sling procedures. J Reprod Med 1990;35:877.

18. Thompson JD. Vesicovaginal and urethrovaginal fistulas. In: Rock JA, Thompson JD, ed. TeLinde's operative gynecology. Philadephia: Lippincott-Raven, 1997:1175.

19. Summitt RL, Stovall TG. Urethral diverticula: evaluation by urethral pressure profilometry, cystourethroscopy and the voiding cystourethrogram. Obstet Gynecol 1992; 80:695.

TABLE 54-4 NONSTEROIDAL ANTIINFLAMMATORY DRUGS FOR DYSMENORRHEA*		
Drug	**Initial Dose**	**Subsequent Dose**
Diclofenac (potassium)	50–100 mg	50 mg twice a day
Diclofenac (sodium)	75–150 mg	75 mg twice a day
Diflunisal	1000 mg	500 mg every 12 hr
Etodolac	400 mg	400 mg every 4 to 6 hr
Fenoprofen calcium	200 mg	200 mg every 4 to 6 hr
Flurbiprofen	50 mg	50 mg three times a day
Ibuprofen[†]	1200–1600 mg	800 mg every 4 hr
Indomethacin	25 mg	25 mg three times a day
Ketoprofen	75 mg	75 mg three times a day
Ketorolac	10 mg	10 mg every 4 to 6 hr
Meclofenamate[†]	100 mg	50–100 mg every 4 to 6 hr
Mefenamic acid[†]	500 mg	250 mg every 4 to 6 hr
Naproxen[†]	500 mg	250 mg every 4 to 6 hr
Naproxen sodium[†]	550 mg	275 mg every 6 to 8 hr
Sulindac	200 mg	200 mg twice a day
Suprofen	200 mg	200 mg every 4 hr
Tolmetin	400 mg	400 mg three times a day

* Consult full prescribing information before using any of these drugs.

[†] FDA approved for primary dysmenorrhea.

Reprinted with permission from Smith RP. Gynecology in primary care. Baltimore: Williams & Wilkins, 1996:399.

probability that a secondary cause is involved must also be heavily weighed.

In addition to NSAIDs, oral contraceptives are appropriate if contraception is desired. As with secondary dysmenorrhea, the thinner, more atrophic endometrium that results with these drugs will give a lighter, shorter, and more tolerable period. Some patients may consider the use of both oral contraceptives and NSAIDs to give even greater relief. Drugs such as calcium antagonists (nifedipine) or spasmolytic agents (isoxuprine, papaverine, ritodrine) may suppress uterine activity in the laboratory, but their side effects have limited their clinical usefulness.

Pelvic Pain Syndromes

The first and foremost treatment for any acute pain is the effective treatment of its cause. This may vary from emergency surgery to reassurance and simple support. Catastrophic events will require specialized, inpatient care. When the cause of pain is determined to be self-limited and does not threaten the long-term health or safety of the patient, primary, ambulatory care is suitable. For these patients, symptomatic therapy, or symptomatic therapy as an adjunct to pathology-directed therapy, is appropriate.

Patients with chronic pelvic pain offer a different therapeutic challenge. In these patients, in whom pain becomes the disease, care must be taken that the therapy offered does not potentiate the problem itself. Analgesics may be used, but sparingly, and every effort must be made to reduce the risk of both emotional and physical dependence. Suppression of ovulation may be useful as either a therapeutic method or to assist in evaluating ovarian or cyclic processes for causality. While analgesics, antispasmodics, birth control pills, and ovulation suppression may have some temporary benefit, only specific therapy aimed at correcting the cause will ultimately be successful. Since it may not be possible to relieve pain in all cases, it is sometimes necessary to settle for limited improvements, enhanced coping strategies, or behavioral modifications.

Analgesics are an obvious first step when nonspecific therapies are used. For mild pain, aspirin, acetaminophen, propoxyphene, or their compounds have found wide use. Unfortunately, the pain these patients experience is often of sufficient magnitude that these agents are less than fully effective. Potent analgesics are often required. Useful agents and their compounds are butalbital (Fiorinal, 1 or 2 every 4 hours), oxycodone (Percodan, 1 every 6 hours), pentazocine (Talwin, 1 every 3 to 4 hours), drocode (dihydrocodeine) bitartrate (Synalgos, 2 every 4 hours), codeine (30 to 60 mg every 4 hours), or meperidine (Demerol, 50 to 100 mg every 4 to 6 hours). While these agents, adjusted to the needs of the individual, may give good pain relief, their potential side effects may still render the patient unable to function normally. The use of these potent drugs should be limited and care exercised. Nonsteroidal agents may be used in place of these more potent agents, but because the main analgesic action of these drugs is via inhibition of prostaglandin synthesis, they will be of little value in pain processes that do not involve prostaglandin release.

When analgesics, especially stronger agents, are used care must be taken to avoid secondary gains that may contribute to, or worsen, the psychosocial aspects of the problem. Watch for direct positive reinforcement (such as special attention, care, or nurturing), indirect positive reinforcement (such as avoidance behaviors), and extinction or negative reinforcement of "well" behaviors. When analgesics are used, they should be given on a regular basis, not "as needed." The latter "requires" the patient to have pain and validates the patient's symptoms, often fueling the social aspects of pain behavior. Only enough medication should be given to get the patient to the next regular appointment. Neither the appointment nor the medication should be altered based on the pain. Both the patient and physician should understand the long-term nature of the illness and its treatment. It is important to directly involve the patient in the process of adaptation and rehabilitation. Having the patient take an active responsibility increases the success in establishing positive adaptive behaviors and decreases dependency and the "need to be ill."

Any agent that improves sleep, especially rapid-eye-movement (REM) sleep patterns, may improve chronic pain states. Some centers have reported success with medications such as amitriptyline (Elavil) in doses of 25 to 50 mg at bedtime. It is unknown if this success is due to a causal relationship between sleep disturbances and symptoms or pain, or merely reflects improved coping from more restful sleep.

Alternative treatment methods such as TENS, biofeedback, and nerve blocks may be useful in selected patients. Physical therapy and exercise programs may be of great help in patients with musculoskeletal components to their pain. Massage and tactile stimulation in the area of pain can suppress pain signals, and may possibly explain the pain relief obtained by liniments, rubbing, or acupuncture. The application of heat or cold, when not otherwise contraindicated, may provide relief for some patients. The use of TENS therapy can provide excellent pain relief for some patients without the side effects associated with pharmacologic agents. Nerve blocks and trigger-point injections may be of significant help in selected patients, while psychotherapy, biofeedback, relaxation therapy, acupuncture, or hypnosis may help others. Some patients respond well to antiinflammatory medications, muscle relaxants, mechanical support, active and passive exercise, stretch, diathermy, and other methods. Exercise programs directed toward enhancing strength or mobility may be therapeutic. Success with these methods will be influenced by patient motivation and the underlying physiology involved.

Surgical therapies are appropriate only when specific surgically treated pathologies are present and thought to be the cause of the patient's symptoms. Surgical therapy for chronic pelvic pain must be limited and carried out with the full knowledge by both doctor and patient that the pain may not be improved and may even be made worse by the surgical procedure. Only in the few patients in whom there is a specific, surgically correctable process that can be said with some probability to be the root of the patient's symptoms can there be a chance for successful surgical therapy. It should be noted that roughly 25% of patients referred for evaluation of chronic pelvic pain have previously undergone hysterectomy without resolution of their symptoms.

SELECTED READINGS

Dysmenorrhea

Akerlund M. Pathophysiology of dysmenorrhea. Acta Obstet Gynecol Scand 1979;87(Suppl):27.

Andersch B, Milson I. An epidemiologic study of young women with dysmenorrhea. Am J Obstet Gynecol 1982;144:655.

Anderson ABM, Hanes PJ, Fraser IS, Turnbull AC. Trial of prostaglandin-synthesis inhibitors in primary dysmenorrhoea. Lancet 1978;1:345.

Apgar BS. Dysmenorrhea and dysfunctional uterine bleeding. Primary Care Clin Office Pract 1997;24:161.

Bickers W. Uterine contractions in dysmenorrhea. Am J Obstet Gynecol 1941;42:1023.

Chan WY, Dawood MY, Fuchs F. Prostaglandins in primary dysmenorrhea: comparison of prophylactic and nonprophylactic treatment with ibuprofen and use of oral contraceptives. Am J Med 1981;70:535.

Chen FP, Chang SD, Chu KK, Soong YK. Comparison of laparoscopic presacral neurectomy and laparoscopic uterine nerve ablation for primary dysmenorrhea. J Reprod Med 1996;41:463.

Kresch .
  wo
  19:
Ling FV
  pai
Ling FV
  chr
  20:
Lipscon
  chr
  20:
Loeser J
  Ne
Longstro
  pai
Lundber
  tio
Magni (
  Pr
  syn
  56:
Malone
  me
Maruta
  foll
  in :
  199
Mathias
  Ste
  qua
  199
McDon:
  Gy
Milburn
  app
  N .
Nolan T
  tio
  pai
Ozaksit
  adc
  son
Peveler
  tor:
  wit
  son
Rachlin
  ma
Rapkin
  Ob
Rapkin
  His
  chr
Rapkin
  chr
Rapkin
  pel
Reiter F
  pel
Reiter F
  in
  Gy

ENDOCERVICAL CURETTAGE (ECC)

In the United States, colposcopy has traditionally included curettage of the endocervical canal. This was heavily influenced by early reports of patients in whom invasive cancer developed after cryotherapy for cervical dysplasia.[16,17] These studies concluded that failure to perform an ECC and take adequate numbers of biopsies were the most common colposcopic errors. However, subsequent studies have not fully supported these views.

Those advocating routine ECC generally cite the increasing incidence of adenocarcinoma and their precursors, the increasing incidence of squamous-cell cancer in young women, as well as the inexperience of many colposcopists. In one review, 122 of 1500 patients (8%) with abnormal cytology and adequate colposcopy had a positive ECC.[18] The majority of these (91%) had disease on conization (111 patients with CIN and one patient with microinvasion). However, this approach is not without drawbacks. Opponents of routine ECC note that the majority of positive results are false positives. Spiritos et al. found that all positive ECCs in a group of women with CIN and satisfactory colposcopy had disruption of a ectocervical lesion, indicating contamination during the curettage rather than endocervical disease.[19]

Most authorities agree that the ECC can be used by inexperienced colposcopists to avoid errors in colposcopic assessment and management. The use of ECC is also recommended by many authorities when no lesions are seen in patients with high-grade Pap smears. Endocervical curettage should not be performed on pregnant patients, as this increases the risk of rupture of the amniotic sac. The American Society of Colposcopy and Cervical Pathology (ASCCP) recommends that it is acceptable to routinely perform ECC on all patients or to selectively perform ECC based on risk factors for endocervical disease.[20] If ECC is not routinely performed on all patients, the ASCCP has the following recommendations for performing it:

1. Patients with low-grade lesions on Pap smears and unsatisfactory colposcopy should undergo ECC.
2. Conization or the loop electrosurgical excision procedure (LEEP) is recommended for unsatisfactory colposcopy and high-grade lesion on Pap smear.
3. ECC is not recommended for patients with satisfactory colposcopy showing a colposcopically negative endocervical canal.

ECC should sample the entire 360 degrees of the endocervical canal. After performing the curettage, the curette should be allowed to stay in place for approximately 1 minute. This allows the blood to coagulate around the curette and entrap the fragments of endocervical tissue. Rotating the curette during removal will further wrap this coagulum around the shaft and increase tissue recovery. The specimen may be placed either in a specialized container or on a brown paper towel before placing in fixative. Absorbent paper towels should not be used as they will disintegrate in the fixative solution.

Iodine Solution

Some authors have recommended the use of iodine staining during all colposcopic examinations. However, this procedure is not routinely performed by most colposcopists during cervical colposcopy. Iodine staining can be extremely useful when colposcopic findings are minimal or the colposcopist is inexperienced, or during the performance of vaginal colposcopy. It can also be used as part of a scoring system for differentiating low-grade from high-grade colposcopic lesions.[15]

Two different solutions are traditionally used during colposcopy. Schiller's solution is a mixture of 0.3% aqueous iodine and 0.6% potassium iodine in 300 ml of water, while Lugol's solution is 5% aqueous iodine and 10% potassium iodine in water. Lugol's solution is generally preferred for colposcopy because of its more pronounced effect. Lugol's solution stains normal glycogen-rich squamous epithelium a mahogany-brown, while glycogen-poor dysplastic epithelium and columnar epithelium are not stained. Unfortunately, Lugol's solution obscures vascular detail and should be applied only after these details have been noted.

CERVICAL BIOPSY

Biopsy of suspected areas of CIN are usually performed in this country prior to deciding on therapy. Treatment of lesions based on colposcopic findings without biopsy was once considered acceptable but can no longer be condoned. An exception is the removal of a colposcopically HGSIL with LEEP as part of a "see and treat" approach. This provides a histologic specimen to confirm disease and exclude more significant disease. Use of the colposcope to ensure that the intended biopsy site has actually been sampled is recommended. Although most patients do not require any analgesia for cervical biopsy or ECC, several options are available if needed. A nonsteroidal antiinflammatory agent 30 minutes prior to colposcopy, paracervical blocks, or topical 20% benzocaine spray can all be used to decrease the discomfort associated with ECC and cervical biopsy.

Biopsy specimens can be placed free in separate containers of formalin or more classically on brown paper towels and then placed in separate containers of formalin. If paper towels are used the specimen should be oriented on its side with the surface at right angles to the paper surface. It should be allowed to dry for a minute to ensure attachment and then placed specimen side down in fixative. This allows the pathologist to better orient the specimen and avoid tangential sectioning.

TREATMENT OPTIONS FOR CERVICAL DYSPLASIA

Cryosurgery

Cryosurgery came into widespread use in the 1970s and remains an excellent and relatively inexpensive option for treating cervical dysplasia. It is generally believed that temperatures of −20 to −40°C are needed to produce tissue necrosis.[21] These temperatures occur only within 2 mm of the leading edge of the ice ball. Therefore, it is necessary to produce an ice ball that goes well beyond the lesion to achieve adequate tissue destruction. The depth of freezing equates to the lateral spread of the ice ball. When cryosurgery was first introduced, Freon was the most common refrigerant, and it was common to freeze for 3 minutes and use time as an end point. Subsequently, cryosurgery units using carbon dioxide or nitrous oxide were developed and different protocols including a 5-minute freeze and double-freeze technique were introduced.

Currently, nitrous oxide is the most acceptable refrigerant, as it achieves very low temperatures and is bottled as a much cleaner gas than carbon dioxide, but there are no studies showing any differences in cure with different refrigerants. Although many studies have shown improved cure rates using a double-freeze technique, there is only one small randomized clinical trial comparing a single-freeze with a double-freeze technique.[22] This study showed an overall cure rate for CIN I and II to be 6.2% and 16.3% with

single- and double-freeze, respectively. One possible advantage of the double freeze is that the lesion can be reassessed and the second freeze used to ensure complete coverage of large or multifocal lesions. It is generally agreed that the appropriate end point is an ice ball that extends 5 mm past the edge of the lesion. Most modern units are designed so that the ice ball reaches near maximum size after 3 to 3.5 minutes. After this time, there is slow progression of the ice ball. As the ice ball expands, the amount of heat removed by the cryoprobe equalizes, with the heat replaced from warmer surrounding tissue. Maximum spread of the ice ball occurs after 5 to 7 minutes. Most authorities recommend reapplication if the ice ball has not reached the desired size by this time.

There are several techniques that may increase the success rate with cryosurgery. A thin layer of lubricating jelly applied to the probe tip will fill gaps between the probe and cervix, allowing better heat transfer to all surfaces. The tank pressure must remain adequate. If the needle on the pressure gauge falls below the green zone at any point during the freeze, the tank should be replaced and the freeze repeated. Probe tips vary in size. The tips most useful are the flat or slightly nippled probes. The long endocervical probes are not recommend except under very unusual circumstances, as these drive the squamocolumnar junction into the endocervical canal, making future evaluation of the endocervical canal extremely difficult.

General contraindications to cervical cryotherapy include known cervical cancer, unsatisfactory colposcopic examination, positive ECC, and pregnancy. Cryotherapy of the thin vaginal wall for vaginal dysplasia is contraindicated, as this may result in vesicovaginal or rectovaginal fistula formation. Cryotherapy in actively menstruating or premenstrual women may produce menstrual-flow obstruction from postoperative edema of the endocervical canal; cryotherapy is best avoided until later in the menstrual cycle. Relative contraindications include more than two-quadrant disease and lesions greater than 3 cm in size, as failure rates are increased in these patients.

Studies show excellent cure rate of cervical dysplasia with cryotherapy. A review of the literature in 1980 by Charles and Savage showed an overall cure of 89%.[23] If patients with failures who are retreated are included, the cure rate rises to 97%. It also must be realized that some of the series included in this review treated patients who probably would not be candidates today. Therefore, the overall cure rate of 89% in this review is probably conservative.

Some authorities now believe that cryosurgery should not be used with endocervical-gland involvement as the depths of the crypts may not be adequately treated.[24] However, there is no proof that this occurs. In fact, Anderson and Hartly have shown that in most cases CIN does not extend deeply into glands and that cryosurgery should be adequate in as many as 99% of patients.[25] However, maximum extension into glands could be as deep as 5.2 mm. As previously noted, adequate temperature for tissue necrosis with cryotherapy occurs only within 2 mm of the leading edge of the ice ball. If cervical neoplasia should extend 5 mm into a gland, an ice ball of 7 mm is required to achieve a successful freeze. Because of the difficulty in consistently achieving this size, many experts do not use cryosurgery to treat CIN with known gland involvement. In areas of widespread CIN, gland involvement may exist in an area where biopsy was not performed and remain undetected. This would further argue against treating widespread lesions with cryotherapy. The likelihood of gland involvement is also increased with increasing grades of dysplasia. Thus, many practitioners choose to limit cryotherapy to CIN II or focal CIN III.

Lesion size is also related to cure rate. Generally speaking, when more than two quadrants are involved with CIN, the cure rate is reduced to 50 to 60%.[26] Although lower cure rates with higher-grade lesions have been reported with some studies, Richart et al. did not find any differences in cure rates between the various grades of CIN after cryotherapy in a follow-up study of 40,000 woman-years.[27] Many believe that previous studies showing differential failure rates can be accounted for by lesion size as previously discussed.

All patients should be warned to expect profuse watery discharge that is occasionally blood-tinged and frequently malodorous. The cervix has, in effect, been frostbitten and undergoes the typical necrosis associated with frostbite. This appearance can be quite alarming to those unfamiliar with this effect if a speculum examination is performed during the resolution phase. Pap smear should not be repeated until 3 to 4 months after therapy, as the rapidly regenerating cells may be misinterpreted as malignancy on cytologic examination.

Conization

Cervical conization was first described by Lisfranc in 1834.[28] Conization may be performed with a scalpel or a laser. Each method has its advocates, but generally there seems to be little advantage in the use of laser for conization in a hospital setting. In the United States conization was initially used for diagnostic purposes only as earlier studies had shown a high incidence of residual disease in the uterus after conization. In contrast, Europeans used conization primarily for treatment. Despite early concerns about the efficacy of conization for CIN, Sze et al., in a comprehensive review of published studies, found the incidence of recurrent HGSIL to be under 3.5% in most studies and the incidence of subsequent invasive cancer generally less than 1%.[29] In patients treated with hysterectomy, recurrent HGSIL at the cuff was somewhat over 1%, but the incidence of invasive cancer was quite similar to and in some studies even higher than that following conization.[29] It has been suggested that the failure of many clinicians to perform Pap smears in patients who have had a hysterectomy may be one cause for the similar incidence of invasive cancer in both groups. However, the excellent follow-up of patients in several of the reviewed studies would seem to refute this explanation. As a result of the excellent cure rates achieved with conization with relatively little morbidity and mortality, most authorities no longer consider HGSIL alone to be an acceptable indication for hysterectomy.

Indications for a diagnostic conization are more limited than in the past. They include:

1. Endocervical curettage positive for dysplasia.
2. Two-step discrepancy between cytology and biopsy.
3. Inability to visualize the full extent of a lesion extending into endocervical canal.
4. Biopsy showing microinvasion or suggestive of invasive cancer.
5. Unsatisfactory colposcopy.
6. Extensive CIS of cervix.

Therapeutic indications include multifocal HGSIL, endocervical-gland involvement, and poor follow-up.

Complications of conization include hemorrhage, incompetent cervix, infertility, cervical stenosis, infection, and rarely, death. The most common of these complications is hemorrhage. This occurs in the first 24 hours in 0.2 to 17.5% of conizations.[29] Secondary hemorrhage occurs after the first postoperative day and has an incidence of 0.8 to 34%. This usually occurs within 12 to 15 days, but has been reported as late as 24 to 31 days.

Several techniques to decrease bleeding have been used with generally poor success. The most common technique is the use of lateral cervical sutures. Although lateral stay sutures aid in manipulation of the cervix, the published literature has not shown them to be helpful in reducing bleeding.[30-32] Likewise, Sturmdorf sutures have not been shown to reduce the incidence of postoperative bleeding.[29] Since the use of Sturmdorf sutures also often results in the new transformation zone being high in the endocervical canal, most authorities discourage their routine use. The volume of tissue removed has been considered a possible factor in subsequent hemorrhage, but there are conflicting reports in the literature about the importance of cone size and subsequent bleeding.[29]

The use of vasoactive agents has been the only method that has been shown in controlled studies to result in significantly less blood loss. An excellent review of these studies has been performed by Sze et al.[29] Generally, vasopressin 10 units in 20 to 30 cc of saline has been used, but solutions of neosynephrine and local anesthetic with 1% epinephrine have also been used. Fears of increased postoperative bleeding resulting from temporarily constricted vessels and rebleeding as the effect of these agents wear off has not been justified.

LEEP

Large-loop excision is essentially a modified conization performed with an electrosurgical loop. Cartier of France first proposed the use of loop excision for diagnosis and treatment of cervical dysplasia at the Fourth World Congress of Cervical Pathology and Colposcopy in London in 1981.[33] Pendiville et al. subsequently modified Cartier's loops and reported on a technique called large loop excision of the transformation zone (LLETZ) as an alternative to destructive therapy for cervical neoplasia.[34] This original acronym has now been replaced with loop electrosurgical excision procedure (LEEP).

As initially described, loop excision used small, thin (5 by 5 mm) wire loop electrodes to excise cervical tissue. Because of their small size, multiple passes were required. In addition to being time-consuming, these small loops produced marked thermocoagulation at the edges of the strips. Despite these drawbacks, the results of early studies were excellent, with cure rates approaching 95%. Complications were low and the squamocolumnar junction was colposcopically visible in 94% of patients after this type of loop excision.[33-35] LEEP has since been modified to make it easier to perform and interpret histologically. With the much larger loops used today, the entire transformation zone may be removed with one pass. The addition of modern electrosurgical generators allows the use of blended current that produces an excellent cutting effect as well as excellent hemostasis, with a minimum of thermal artifact.

The key advantage of LEEP is that it can be performed as an office procedure, but unlike other office procedures for dysplasia, it removes rather than destroys the affected tissue. Thus, tissue is available for histologic examination. The major disadvantages are that margins can be difficult to interpret, indications are more restricted and it cannot be tailored, as can traditional conization. If a procedure is to be done in an operating room under general anesthesia, conization is generally more appropriate than LEEP.

The indications for LEEP are controversial. Some authors have suggested that LEEP can be used for the same indications as traditional conization. However, the majority of authorities believe LEEP should not be used for cases of potential microinvasion or adenocarcinoma because of difficulty in assessing margins. The use of LEEP for patients with unsatisfactory colposcopy or a positive ECC is also unclear. Some suggest that LEEP be performed in patients with unsatisfactory colposcopy and a negative ECC. In addition, "top-hat" LEEP is used for patients with positive ECC in patients if colposcopy demonstrates a negative endocervical canal and ectocervical dysplasia, believing that a positive ECC in these patients is generally the result of contamination from an ectocervical lesion. It is thought that patients with a positive ECC and with incompletely visualized endocervical lesions, inadequate colposcopy, or an absence of visible dysplasia are generally better treated with conization.

LEEP is performed using standard electrosurgical techniques. This requires the use of an electrosurgical generator, return electrode or grounding pad, and electrosurgical handpiece. Specialized nonconductive speculums and sidewall retractors are also required. The use of a sidewall retractor is encouraged, as its use not only aids visualization but also provides some protection to the vaginal side walls. The standard plastic speculum used in many clinics should generally not be used because it has a tendency to close inadvertently, frequently during a procedure. A selection of loop electrodes of varying sizes should be available. A 2.0-by-0.8-cm loop is often the most practical for most excisions. The use of loops larger than 2.0-by-1.0 cm is not recommended because of the large amount of tissue removed with larger loops. A smoke evacuator is a requirement for LEEP in order to obtain adequate visualization during the procedure.

After the speculum is placed, the cervix is stained with Lugol's solution. Anesthesia is obtained with 1 to 2% lidocaine with 1:100,000 epinephrine. The use of a needle extender allows the use of standard 25-gauge needles for injection. Although paracervical blocks can be used, most operators find an intracervical block to provide equal anesthesia with less injection pain. Injections of 0.5 to 1 ml are made intracervically at 3, 6, 9, and 12 o'clock on the cervix. Part of the local anesthetic is injected to the depth of the proposed cone and a portion injected directly below the surface mucosa. The submucosal injection appears to provide the majority of anesthesia and is used without deeper injection by many clinicians, although the deeper injection may aid with hemostasis. Adequate anesthesia for LEEP is usually achieved within 3 minutes.

An idealized LEEP would remove the transformation and lesion in one pass (Figure 55-3). The use of multiple passes is acceptable, but result in increased difficulties for the pathologist in tissue orientation and thermal damages (Figure 55-4). The "top-hat" procedure may be used to remove a deep endocervical lesion (Figure 55-5). The LEEP may be performed in any direction that is most convenient. However the use of a top-to-bottom approach frequently allows the specimen to fall forward into the loop and is generally a less satisfactory technique than other approaches.

The power settings for LEEP will vary with the size of the loop used as well as the characteristics of the target tissue. Power requirements are decreased with decreasing loop size. Approximate starting-power settings for a given loop size are generally supplied by the manufacturer of the electrosurgical generator. A common mistake is to use too great a power setting to achieve easy loop passage through tissue. This excessive wattage will result in undesired thermal artifact. Tissue drag with appropriate power settings is generally the result of improper technique and speed rather than too little power. Power settings greater than 50 watts are not needed even for a 2.0-by-1.0-cm loop.

In general, a blended current using an off cycle of approximately 20% will produce the optimal combination of cutting and hemostasis for LEEP. For most generators this is the first blend setting (Blend 1). Electrosurgical generators produce blended current by altering the percentage of the time current is flowing. With pure "cut" or nonmodulated current, current is flowing 100% of the time. With pure "coag" or modulated current, the current is only on for approximately 5% percent of the cycle. Blend current is obtained by altering "cut" current. Thus, power settings for the various blend modes are set using the "cut" setting, not the "coag" setting. Blend current is not produced by "blending" the output from cut and coag current sources, as frequently believed.

Electrosurgical cutting is achieved by current vaporizing cells ahead of the electrode. The loop itself does not cut the tissue. Actual tissue contact with the electrode results in tissue desiccation not cutting. Thus, the power should be activated before touching tissue. The LEEP should be performed at a speed that allows the loop to float on its steam barrier through the tissue. Too rapid passage of the loop will overtake

Figure 55-3 Standard single-pass LEEP.

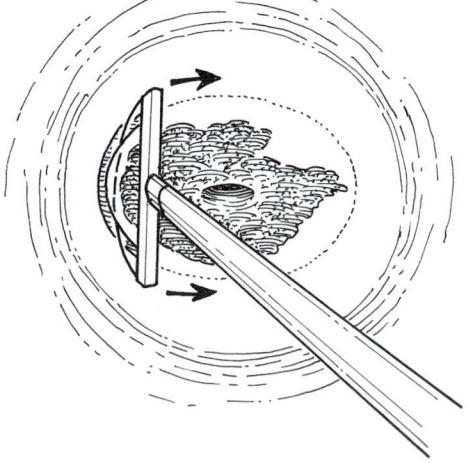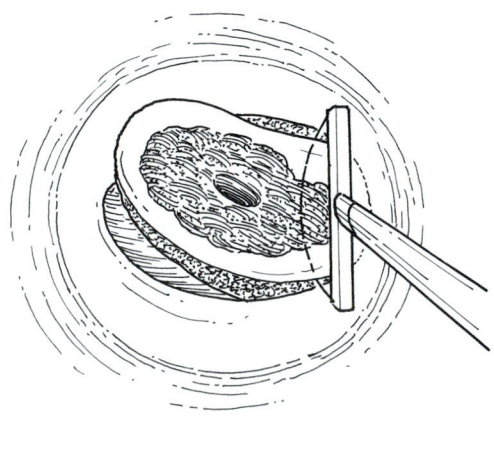

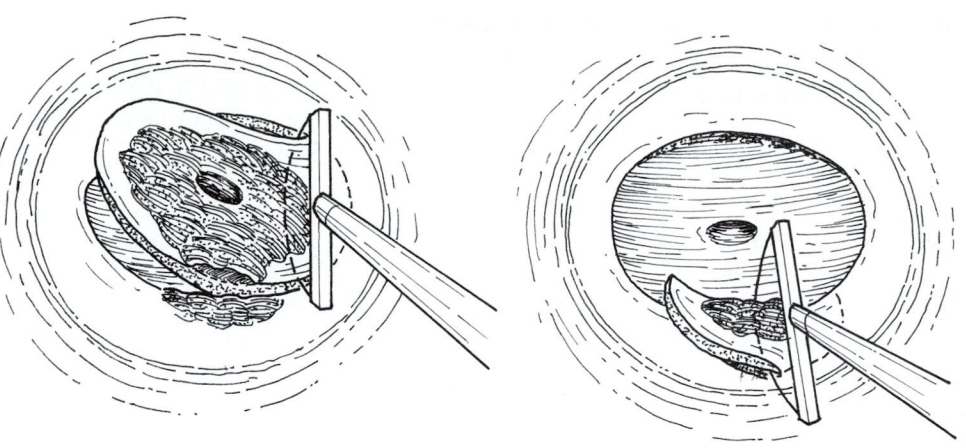

Figure 55-4 Multiple-pass LEEP.

the steam barrier and result in drag as the loop begins to desiccate the tissue. This effect will also occur if the power is inadvertently discontinued during the procedure. If this occurs, the loop should be removed and the procedure started from the opposite direction until the previous incision is joined.

The depth of excision for a LEEP is the same as needed for a laser ablation. This is generally 6 to 8 mm at the margins to a maximum depth of 8 mm at the endocervical canal. Studies have shown that the maximum depth of extension of dysplasia into the endo-

cervical gland is 5.2 mm.[25] The use of loops deeper than 1 cm removes excessive tissue and is discouraged.

Hemostasis after LEEP is obtained either with the use of a 5-mm ball electrode using pure modulated or "coag" current or alternatively with the use of a paste of Monsel's solution.

See-and-Treat LEEP

The use of LEEP to diagnose and treat cervical dysplasia in a single visit has been labeled see-and-treat

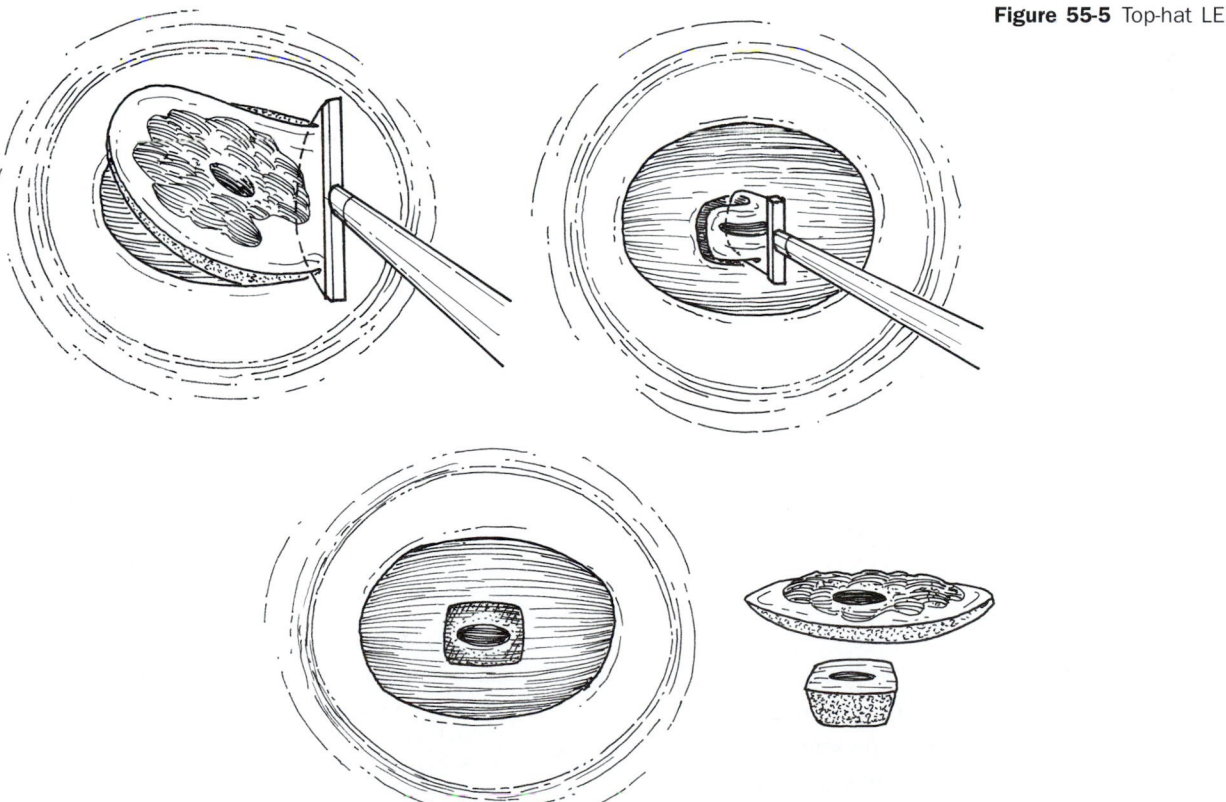

Figure 55-5 Top-hat LEEP.

LEEP. Patients with abnormal Pap smears undergo colposcopy and LEEP treatment during the first visit. Proponents argue that this approach is more cost effective than traditional options, reduces patient visits, and eliminates noncompliance with return visits for treatment. This approach has been used with some success in the United Kingdom. However, problems exist in the United States with incorporating this approach into the current system. In the United States, the term *HPV changes* on Pap smears is frequently used indiscriminately to describe cells with perinuclear halos without nuclear atypia. These changes are nonspecific and do not have the same significance or prognosis as true HPV changes (perinuclear halo and nuclear abnormalities). Under the Bethesda system, HPV changes are reported as LGSIL. In one large British series of see-and-treat LEEP, 25% were for HPV changes on Pap smear.[36] Many of these patients in the United States will have normal colposcopy and negative biopsy. Likewise, patients with LGSIL will also frequently have negative colposcopy. These patients generally represent either overdiagnosed or false-positive Pap smears. With increasing medicolegal concerns by pathologists over the missed diagnosis of abnormal Pap smears, many areas of the United States have seen a marked increase in the percentage of Pap smears reported as ASCUS and LGSIL. The use of see-and-treat LEEP under these conditions could result in overtreatment of large numbers of patients unless adequate precautions are taken.

For see-and-treat LEEP to be effective in the United States, patients with LGSIL should not be treated with LEEP without colposcopic evidence of dysplasia. One can also argue that patients with either HGSIL or LGSIL and lesions colposcopically consistent with only LGSIL should undergo biopsy and delayed treatment, as LGSIL can be effectively treated with less costly methods than LEEP or even followed conservatively without treatment. This is consistent with the position of the National Cancer Institute that routine excision or treatment of ASCUS or LGSIL Pap smears without histologic conformation is inappropriate.[9]

Immediate LEEP in patients with HGSIL with colposcopically high-grade disease is generally regarded as more practical. Likewise, see-and-treat LEEP in patients with HGSIL without colposcopic lesion also appears reasonable, as this represents a two-step discrepancy that would require subsequent conization or LEEP for further evaluation.

CONCLUSION

Using the principles outlined in this chapter, clinicians should be able to accurately interpret Pap smears reported as ASCUS or AGUS. They should also be able to understand the significance of these as well as other abnormal Pap smears and decide on appropriate diagnostic and treatment plans tailored to their patient's needs.

REFERENCES

1. Papanicolaou GN. New cancer diagnosis. In: Proceedings of the Third Race Betterment Conference. Battle Creek, MI: Race Betterment Foundation, 1928:528.
2. Babes A. Diagnostique du cancer uterin par les frottis. Presse Med 1928;36:451.
3. Koss LG. The Papanicolaou test for cervical cancer detection: a triumph and tragedy. JAMA 1989;261:737.
4. Ayres JE. Selective cytologic smear for diagnosis of cancer. Am J Obstet Gynecol 1946;53:609.
5. Richart RM, Barron BA. A follow-up study of patients with cervical dysplasia. Am J Obstet Gynecol 1969;105:386.
6. National Cancer Institute Workshop. The 1988 Bethesda System for reporting cervical/vaginal cytologic diagnosis. JAMA 1989;262:931.
7. Montz FJ, Monk BJ, Fowler JM, Nguyen L. Natural history of the minimally abnormal Papanicolaou smear. Obstet Gynecol 1992;80:385.
8. Taylor RP, Guerrieri JP, Nash JD, Henry MR, O'Connor. Atypical cervical cytology: colposcopic follow-up using the Bethesda system. J Reprod Med 1993;38:443.
9. Kurman RJ, Henson DE, Herbst AL, Noller K, Schiffman M. Interim guidelines for management of abnormal cervical cytology. JAMA 1994;271:1866.
10. Cox JT. ASCCP practice guidelines; management of glandular abnormalities in the cervical smear. J Lower Tract Dis 1997;1:41.
11. Kurman RJ, Malkasian GD, Sedlis A, Solomon D. From Papanicolaou to Bethesda: the rationale for a new cervical cytologic classification. Obstet Gynecol 1991;77:779.
12. Nasiell K, Roger V, Nashiell M. Behavior of mild cervical dysplasia during long-term follow-up. Obstet Gynecol 1986;67:6665.
13. Syrjanen K, Kataja V, Yliskoski M, Chang F, Syrjanen S, Saarikoski S. Natural history of cervical human papillomavirus lesions does not substantiate the biological relevance of the Bethesda system. Obstet Gynecol 1992; 79:675.
14. Nasiell K, Nasiell M, Vaclavinkova V. Behavior of moderate dysplasia during long-term follow-up. Obstet Gynecol 1983;61:609.
15. Reid R, Scalzi P. An improved colposcopic index for differentiation of benign papillomaviral infections from high-grade cervical intraepithelial neoplasia. Am J Obstet Gynecol 1985;153:611.
16. Towsend DE, Ostegard DR, Mischell DR, Hirose RM. Abnormal Papanicolaou smears. Am J Obstet Gynecol 1970;108:429.

17. Townsend DE, Richard RM, Marks E, Niesen J. Invasive cancer following outpatient evaluation and therapy for cervical disease. Obstet Gynecol 1981;57:145.

18. Soisson AP, Moloina CY, Benson WL. Endocervical curettage in the evaluation of cervical disease in patients with adequate colposcopy. Obstet Gynecol 1988;71:109.

19. Spiritos NM, Schlarerth JB, Ablang G, Morrow P. A critical evaluation of the endocervical curettage. Obstet Gynecol 1987;70:729.

20. Cox JT. ASCCP practice guidelines; endocervical curettage. J Lower Genital Tract Dis 1997;1:251.

21. Ferris DG. Cryotherapy of the cervix. J Lower Genital Tract Dis 1998;2:98.

22. Schantz A, Thormann L. Cryosurgery for dysplasia of the uterine ectocervix: a randomized study of the efficacy of the single- and double-freeze techniques. Acta Obstet Gynecol Scand 1984;63:417.

23. Charles EH, Savage EW. Cryosurgical treatment of cervical intraepithelial neoplasia. Obstet Gynecol Surv 1980; 35:539.

24. Burke L, Antonioli DA, Ducatman BS, eds. Colposcopy: text and atlas. Appleton & Lange, 1991.

25. Anderson MC, Hartly RB. Cervical crypt involvement by intraepithelial neoplasia. Obstet Gynecol 1980;55:546.

26. Townsend DE. Cryosurgery for CIN. Obstet Gynecol Surv 1979;34:828.

27. Richart RM, Townsend DE, Crisp WE, et al. An analysis of long-term follow-up results in patients with cervical intraepithelial neoplasia treated by cryotherapy. Am J Obstet Gynecol 1980;137:823.

28. Lisfranc MJ. Memoire Sur l'amputation der col de l'uterus. Gaz Med France 1834;2:385.

29. Sze EH, Rosenzweig BA, Bierenbaum DL, Silverman RK, Baggish MS. Excisional conization of the cervix uteri: a five part review. J Gynecol Surg 1989;5:235.

30. Chao S, McCaffrey RM, Todd WD, Moor JG. Conization in evaluation and management of cervical neoplasia. Am J Obstet Gynecol 1969;103:574.

31. Jones HW III. Cone biopsy in the management of cervical intraepithelial neoplasia. Clin Obstet Gynecol 1983; 26:968.

32. Claman AD, Lee N. Factors that relate to complications of cone biopsy. Am J Obstet Gynecol 1974;120:124.

33. Cartier R. Practical colposcopy. 2nd ed. Paris: Paris Laboratorie, 1984:139.

34. Pendiville W, Cullimore S, Norman S. Large loop excision of the transformation zone (LETZ): a new method of management for women with cervical intraepithelial neoplasia. Br J Obstet Gynaecol 1989;96:1054.

35. Mor-Yosef S, Lopes A, Pearson S, Monaghan JM. Loop diathermy cone biopsy. Obstet Gynecol 1990;72:884.

36. Luesley DM, Cullimore J, Redman CW, et al. Loop diathermy excision of the cervical transformation zone in patients with abnormal cervical smears. BMJ 1990;300:1690.

Chapter 56

Pediatric and Adolescent Gynecology

Joshua Sepesi
Claudette Jones Shephard

Five Key Points

- **The gynecologic evaluation of the pediatric or adolescent female requires a gentle touch and special instruments.**
- **Normal pubertal development occurs in a predictable sequential pattern.**
- **Vulvovaginitis is the most common gynecologic disorder among children.**
- **Irregular menstrual flow is fairly common in adolescents.**
- **Injuries limited to the genital area must be evaluated for possible sexual abuse.**

An awareness of the problems unique to pediatric and adolescent gynecology is essential for the appropriate treatment of the young female patient. The examination of the adolescent female should be approached with sensitivity, and the physician should be familiar with the structural and functional differences between the reproductive tract of children and that of the adult female. A basic understanding of normal pubertal development and its abnormalities is necessary for the evaluation of the adolescent. The physician should be able to provide these patients with educational information regarding female health issues, including sexuality and contraceptive counseling. In addition, the physician should have a working knowledge of common gynecologic disorders in the young female patient, including abnormalities of menstruation, vulvar disorders, and common genital tumors. Lastly, physicians should be comfortable in assessing the pediatric female with genital trauma or signs of sexual abuse,

while providing reassurance to the patient unaccustomed to or uncomfortable with examination of sexual areas. This chapter focuses on common gynecologic disorders in the pediatric and adolescent female and provides the physician with guidelines for the diagnosis and management of these problems.

GYNECOLOGIC EXAMINATION

Newborn

Maternal estrogens easily cross the placenta in utero, and because of this, it is not uncommon to find effects of estrogen stimulation during examination of the newborn female. Such findings may include breast budding or even marked breast enlargement. The labia are usually swollen, the clitoris may appear relatively large, and a vaginal discharge is frequently seen. The cervix-to-corpus ratio is about 3:1. These findings are normal and require no further investigation, as they usually will resolve within 6 weeks after birth.

Prepubertal

Because of limited estrogen stimulation during early childhood, the external genitalia of the prepubertal female are less prominent. The labia majora are flat, the labia minora and hymen are thin, the clitoris is small, and the vaginal mucosa is atrophic. The cervix is usually flush with the vaginal apex, and the uterus is small. By age 8 to 10, some signs of estrogenization have occurred and the cervix-to-corpus ratio decreases to about 1:1. When examining a patient in this age group, the physician must reassure her that the examination, although uncomfortable and embarrassing, will not be painful. Accompaniment by the mother or other guardian is often helpful, and examination of the young child (<5 years) while on the mother's lap may reduce anxiety. Older children should be asked to lie on the examination table in the frog-legged position with flexed knees and abducted hips. In addition, the mother can be next to the child throughout the examination. Stirrups are not necessary.

The examination should include the child's height and weight, general appearance, nutritional status, and the presence of any gross congenital abnormalities. The breasts should be inspected and palpated, and the Tanner stage noted. Abdominal examination should elicit the presence of any adnexal mass. Examination of the vulva and vestibule should be performed by applying light, lateral, downward pressure on either side of the perineum. Appropriate signs of hormonal stimulation for the patient's age should be noted, and patency of the hymenal orifice should be confirmed. The examiner should look for any abnormalities such as skin lesions or scars, vaginal discharge or odor, or signs of virilization. If a digital examination is necessary, rectoabdominal examination of the uterus and adnexae can be easily accomplished with little discomfort to the patient. However, for the apprehensive patient, a pediatric cocktail of meperidine (Demerol) 50 mg/ml, promethazine (Phenergan) 12.5 mg/0.5 ml, and chlorpromazine (Thorazine) 12.5 mg/0.5 ml can be administered at a dose of 1 ml per 20 lb (9 kg), with a maximum dose of 2 ml. If the child is being evaluated for an acute traumatic injury, or if she is extremely apprehensive, the aid of an anesthetist is advisable. Forceful examination should never be

performed, and general anesthesia is almost never necessary. If examination of the upper vagina is necessary, instruments such as vaginoscopes, anuscopes, otoscopes, or flexible urethroscopes can be used. The instrument as well as the patient's vaginal introitus should be lubricated with lidocaine jelly, and the patient should be allowed to see and touch the instrument prior to examination.[1,2]

Adolescent

For many females, the first gynecologic examination is during adolescence. Unfortunately, many patients are extremely fearful and anxiety-ridden because of horrible stories that they have heard from their friends or family about vaginal examinations. They often do not know why they need a pelvic examination or Pap smear, and are embarrassed to talk to a physician about their reproductive system and genitalia. This is an opportunity for the physician to adequately inform the patient regarding female health issues and to establish a good rapport with her. A patient's first gynecologic examination should never be rushed, and adequate office time should be allotted to complete the visit. If the patient does not feel in control of the gynecologic examination, she may make it her last.

A parent, usually the mother, may be present for the initial discussion and history taking, and a talk-through of the examination should be performed while the patient is still clothed. Explanations for why certain procedures are performed (e.g., Pap smears) should be incorporated into the discussion, and both the patient and parent should be reassured that her hymen will not be injured during the examination. At this time, the remainder of the visit should be without the parent. Questions about sexual behavior, sexually transmitted diseases, and contraception can then be discussed as appropriate, and the physician should inform the patient that all information between them is confidential. Under no circumstance should the physician undermine the patient's request for privacy unless legally bound to do so (e.g., in matters of sexual abuse).

The examination should then take place in the presence of a female assistant. Breast examination should be performed. This is an excellent time to provide instructions on breast self-examination. After inspection of the external genitalia, a long-bladed, narrow Huffman–Graves speculum should be inserted for visualization of the vagina and cervix. By this age, the vaginal mucosa is well estrogenized and the vaginal fornices can be visualized. The cervix-to-corpus ratio is now 1:2. Bimanual examination is performed by inserting a single finger into the vagina. Young girls who use tampons may tolerate this better. If the hymenal orifice is too small for digital examination, then a rectoabdominal examination should be performed. Explanations of what is being done are given throughout the examination, and the female assistant should give constant reassurance. After the examination, the patient should be allowed to get dressed, and then the physician can discuss any pertinent findings with her. If there are any findings that the physician believes are important to discuss with the parents, the patient should be so advised that, for her own benefit, this information should be released to the parents.[3]

NORMAL PUBERTY

Puberty is the period during which secondary sexual characteristics begin to develop, and the capability of sexual reproduction is attained. The cascade of physiologic changes that occurs during puberty is the result of complex neural and hormonal influences. In order for the physician to evaluate and treat abnormalities of puberty, a basic understanding of the physical and physiologic changes of puberty and their timing is necessary.[4]

Soon after birth, neonatal estradiol levels rise to near midfollicular phase levels, and associated waves of ovarian follicle maturation and atresia occur. This transient rise in estrogen is the result of the sudden withdrawal of maternal and placental estrogens and progesterones, resulting in release of newborn follicle-stimulating hormone (FSH) and luteinizing hormone

(LH). Approximately 24 months later, full negative feedback is obtained, and ovarian steroids and gonadotropin levels drop and remain low until about 8 to 10 years of age.[5,6] At this time, a cascade of neural and hormonal interactions occurs, which results in disinhibition of pulsatile gonadotropin-releasing hormone (GnRH) secretion and the initiation of puberty. The exact mechanism for the onset of puberty is still not clear, although it is recognized that a central nervous system (CNS) program in combination with a decrease in sensitivity to the negative feedback of estrogens likely plays a primary role. Some have postulated that an increase in adrenal androgens initiates the process.[7] In any event, the developmental changes that occur during puberty and their median age of onset proceed in the following manner:

1. Accelerated growth, 9.6 years
2. Breast budding (thelarche), 9.8 years
3. Pubic and axillary hair growth (adrenarche), 10.5 years (*Note:* pubarche specifically refers to the appearance of pubic hair.)
4. Peak height velocity, 11.4 years
5. Onset of menses (menarche), 12.8 years
6. Ovulatory cycles, 14.5 years

On average, this full sequence takes about 4.5 years to complete. Thelarche can normally occur between ages 8 to 13, and menarche should begin by age 16 in the presence of secondary sexual characteristics.

Any deviation from the aforementioned sequence or time frame of pubertal events should be considered abnormal. The Tanner classification (Table 56-1) is a useful system for following pubertal development in adolescents.[8] In addition to documentation of Tanner stages, the physician should note the child's height and weight at each visit to confirm normal growth patterns.

TABLE 56-1
TANNER STAGING OF BREAST AND PUBIC HAIR DEVELOPMENT

Breast Development
Stage 1: Preadolescent; elevation of papilla only
Stage 2: Breast bud stage; elevation of breast and papilla as small mound, enlargement of areolar diameter
Stage 3: Further enlargement and elevation of breast and areola with no separation of their contours
Stage 4: Projection of areola and papilla to form a secondary mound above the level of the breast

Stage 5: Mature stage; projection of papilla only caused by recession of the areola to the general contour of the breast

Pubic Hair
Stage 1: Preadolescent; no visible pubic hair
Stage 2: Sparse growth of long, slightly pigmented downy hair, straight or curled, primarily along labia
Stage 3: Considerably darker, coarser, and more curled; hair spreads sparsely over mons
Stage 4: Hair now adult-type, but area covered is still considerably smaller than in adult; no spread to medial surface of thighs
Stage 5: Adult appearance in quantity and type with classic female distribution and spread to medial aspect of thighs

ABNORMALITIES OF PUBERTY

Precocious Puberty

Sexual precocity is the appearance of secondary sexual maturation at an age greater than 2.5 SD below the mean, which correlates to age 8 for females in North America.[9] Precocious puberty is much more common in girls than in boys, with a ratio of 23:1.[10] Patients may present with increased growth, early breast development, premature pubic or axillary hair growth, or early onset of menses. They often have a combination of these findings, but may present with a single abnormality. Precocious puberty can be classified as either GnRH-dependent or GnRH-independent (Table 56-2). GnRH-dependent precocious puberty (also known as true precocious puberty) is the result of early activation of the hypothalamic–pituitary–ovarian (HPO) axis, usually from pulsatile secretion of GnRH from the hypothalamus. GnRH-independent precocious puberty (also known as precocious pseudopuberty) occurs when extrapituitary processes result in sex steroid production and/or secretion with subsequent early feminization.[11] In all forms of precocious puberty, it is important for the physician to be aware that the increased steroid secretion results in increases in height velocity, somatic development, and rate of skeletal maturation which ultimately can cause premature epiphyseal fusion and short adult height.[12]

GnRH-Dependent Precocious Puberty

By definition, signs of puberty will develop in 0.6% of normal females before age 8. This is known as idiopathic true precocious puberty and is the result of early, albeit normal, reactivation of the HPO axis and increased pulsatile GnRH secretion from the hypothalamus. Although this is the most common cause of precocious puberty, it is a diagnosis of exclusion, and other causes must first be ruled out.[13] Hypothalamic hamartomas are hyperplastic congenital malformations usually located in the floor of the third ventricle that secrete GnRH in a pulsatile fashion. Some CNS tumors can cause sexual precocity by impinging on the neural pathways between the hypothalamus and pituitary, resulting in feedback inhibition that may stimulate pulsatile GnRH secretion. Other CNS disorders such as head trauma, hydrocephalus, and encephalitis can stimulate precocious puberty through unknown mechanisms. There is usually a 1- to 2-month latent period from the time of injury to onset

---

TABLE 56-2
CLASSIFICATION OF PRECOCIOUS PUBERTY

GnRH-dependent precocious puberty
  Idiopathic true precocious puberty
  CNS disorders
    Hamartomas
    CNS tumors (craniopharyngioma, neuroblastoma, glioma, astrocytoma, ependymoma)
    Infectious processes (brain abcess, encephalitis, meningitis)
    Other CNS processes (head trauma, hydrocephalus, cerebral edema, cranial irradiation, cysts)
GnRH-independent precocious puberty
  Endogenous estrogen production
    Functional ovarian cysts
    Ovarian neoplasms
    Other hormone-producing neoplasms
  McCune–Albright syndrome
  Exogenous estrogens
    Medications
    Cosmetic and commercial products

---

of findings, and the precocity is usually reversible. In all cases of true precocious puberty, gonadotropin and estradiol levels will be elevated, and a regression of pubertal characteristics with GnRH therapy will be noted.[14, 15]

GnRH-Independent Precocious Puberty

Approximately 10% of females with precocious puberty will have an ovarian tumor. The tumor is usually an estrogen-secreting tumor such as a granulosa-cell or theca-cell tumor; however, teratomas, gonadoblastomas, and even ovarian cancers have been reported as causes of sexual precocity. Adrenal tumors can also cause early feminization, and although rare, they are usually associated with high levels of dihydroepiandrosterone sulfate (DHEAS). Functional ovarian cysts are also a common source of extrapituitary estrogen secretion, leading to precocious puberty, and a pelvic mass is palpable approximately 80% of the time. These patients often report irregular and heavy bleeding. Other sources of exogenous estrogen leading to precocious puberty include ingestion of oral contraceptives, hair and facial creams, anabolic steroids, and other estrogen-containing commercial products.[16]

McCune–Albright syndrome is described as a triad of polyostotic fibrous dysplasia, café-au-lait pigmentation, and precocious puberty. Other endocinopathies may be present as well, including hyperthyroidism, hyperparathyroidism, and Cushing syndrome. Sexual precocity in affected patients is the result of autonomous early production of estrogen by the ovary. Estradiol levels will be elevated; however, gonadotropin levels are low or normal. In addition, GnRH therapy fails to suppress hormone secretion or reverse the sexual precocity.[17,18]

Diagnosis and Treatment of Precocious Puberty

The cause of precocious puberty may be obvious by findings from the history and physical examination. Appropriate laboratory and radiologic tests may include serum FSH, LH, and human chorionic gonadotropin hormone (HCG), thyroid function studies (thyroid-stimulating hormone [TSH] and free thyroxine [T_4], serum DHEAS, total testosterone, estradiol, progesterone, and 17α-hydroxyprogesterone (17OHP), GnRH testing, bone age, head computed tomography (CT) or magnetic resonance imaging (MRI), and ultrasonography of the abdomen and pelvis. If all tests are normal, then idiopathic sexual precocity is the most likely diagnosis. Management and treatment of precocious puberty should be focused on the following:

1. Diagnosing and treating intracranial disease
2. Arresting of sexual maturation until normal pubertal range
3. Diminishing established precocious development when reversible
4. Maximizing eventual adult height
5. Reducing emotional and psychological stress and abuse

Treatment of true precocious puberty is with the initiation of a GnRH analog such as Lupron. Therapy is maintained until the epiphyses are fused or until appropriate pubertal and chronological age are matched. GnRH therapy is also effective in the treatment of GnRH-secreting hamartomas of the hypothalamus. For McCune–Albright syndrome, therapy is aimed at suppression of steroid production. This can be accomplished with either medroxyprogesterone acetate (Depo-Provera) or an aromatase inhibitor such as testolactone. If a specific cause for precocious pubertal development is identified, treatment is directed toward elimination of that cause. Some CNS tumors respond to radiation or chemotherapy, while others may warrant surgical excision. Ovarian and adrenal tumors also require surgical removal. Careful consideration should be given to possible psychosocial issues that arise in the child with precocious puberty. The patient should be reassured about her

health and sexuality, and additional counseling by a qualified professional may be beneficial to the child and the family.[19]

Isolated Precocious Development

Premature Thelarche

Premature thelarche is the isolated development of breast tissue, either unilateral or bilateral, before the age of 8. It is most common during the first few years of life, and is usually self-limited, requiring no therapy. On examination, growth patterns and bone age are normal, and estrogen levels are within the normal prepubertal range. Follow-up is required to identify patients in whom the premature breast development heralds the onset of true precocious puberty. The majority of patients have no further breast growth, and eventual pubertal development, menstrual pattern, and fertility are reported to be normal.[20,21]

Premature Menarche

Premature menarche implies the appearance of cyclic vaginal bleeding before the age of 10 in the absence of other signs of secondary sexual development.[22] Infection, the presence of a foreign body, abuse and trauma, and local neoplasm should first be considered, as isolated premature menarche is an exceedingly rare presentation of precocity. Normal growth, development, and fertility are not affected.[23]

Premature Adrenarche

Premature adrenarche is the isolated development of pubic or axillary hair before age 8 without other signs of precocious puberty, and it is the consequence of an early modest increase in adrenal androgen secretion. Sparse hair growth on the vulva does not constitute premature adrenarche. An enzyme deficiency (e.g., congenital adrenal hyperplasia) or tumor (e.g., Leydig-cell tumor) should be excluded with a thorough evaluation of both adrenal and gonadal function as well as assessment of androgen production. This can easily be accomplished by measuring levels of total testosterone, DHEAS, and 17OHP. In most cases however, premature adrenarche is idiopathic and of no clinical significance.[24] It does, however, appear to be more common among African-American and Hispanic girls.

Delayed Puberty

Delayed puberty is the lack of physical manifestations of sexual maturation at a chronologic age that is

TABLE 56-3
CLASSIFICATION OF DELAYED PUBERTY

Constitutional delay
Hypogonadotropic hypogonadism
  CNS disorders
    Tumors (e.g., craniopharyngiomas, germ-cell tumors)
    Congenital malformations
  Isolated gonadotropin deficiency
    Kallman syndrome
    Idiopathic hypopituitary dwarfism
  Miscellaneous disorders
    Prader–Willi syndrome
    Functional gonadotropin deficiency
      Nutritional deficiency
      Hypothyroidism
      Exercise- and stress-induced amenorrhea
      Cushing disease
      Diabetes
      Hyperprolactinemia
      Marijuana use
Hypergonadotropic hypogonadism
  Gonadal dysgenesis
    Turner syndrome
    Mosaicism
    True gonadal dysgenesis
  Primary ovarian failure
    Idiopathic
    Chemotherapy or radiation of ovaries
  Enzyme deficiencies

2.5 SD above the mean age of the onset of puberty. This correlates to age 13 for girls in the United States. Delayed puberty in girls is rare, and a genetic or hypothalamic–pituitary disorder must be suspected. Anatomic abnormalities of the reproductive and outflow tract must also be considered in the amenorrheic patient who otherwise has normal secondary sexual characteristics. Once anatomic causes have been eliminated, delayed puberty can be classified as either hypergonadotropic or hypogonadotropic hypogonadism. Constitutional growth delay is a diagnosis of exclusion. Table 56-3 lists the various causes of delayed pubertal development.

Hypergonadotropic Hypogonadism

Hypergonadotropic hypogonadism implies dysfunction of the end organ, in this case the ovary, resulting in elevated LH and FSH levels. The most common disorder of this type is gonadal dysgenesis, including Turner syndrome (45,X) as well as sex chromosome mosaicism (XO/XX or XO/XY). True gonadal dysgenesis (46,XX) can also occur. Primary ovarian failure can be the result of acquired damage to the ovaries such as torsion or radiation or chemotherapy, but often it is idiopathic. The most common enzyme deficiency associated with elevated gonadotropins and delayed puberty is 17α-hydroxylase deficiency, and this should be suspected in the adolescent female with sexual infantilism, hypertension, and elevated serum progesterone levels.

Hypogonadotropic Hypogonadism

Hypogonadotropic hypogonadism is caused by insufficient pulsatile secretion of GnRH. Tumors such as craniopharyngiomas can encroach on the pituitary stalk, resulting in decreased stimulation of the anterior pituitary. Kallmann syndrome is caused by agenesis or hypoplasia of the olfactory lobes, with resultant anosmia or hyposmia and GnRH deficiency. Nutritional deficiencies (anorexia, bulimia, malabsorption, chronic illness) and extreme exercise can also lead to low gonadotropin levels and delayed puberty. While physiologic growth delay accounts for 10% of all cases of delayed puberty, other causes of hypogonadotropic hypogonadism must first be ruled out.

Diagnosis and Treatment of Delayed Puberty

As with precocious puberty, the evaluation of the adolescent with delayed puberty begins with a thorough history and physical examination. Constitutional growth delay tends to be familial, and information regarding past general health, height and weight records, as well as relevant behavior such as extreme exercise or eating habits should be ascertained. Body measurements, Tanner staging, and the presence of any secondary sexual characteristics should be noted on physical examination. Laboratory and radiologic work-up should include LH and FSH levels, serum prolactin, progesterone, estradiol, testosterone, DHEAS, TSH and free T$_4$ levels, blood karyotype in patients with elevated gonadotropins, x-ray films for bone age, and CT or MRI of the head for individuals with low gonadotropin levels.

Treatment should be targeted at the removal or correction of the primary cause when possible. Timed gonadectomy should be performed in individuals with gonadal dysgenesis who are at risk for subsequent neoplasia. Hormonal therapy with 0.3 mg of conjugated estrogens daily should be initiated for hypogonadism. This will initiate and sustain maturation and function of secondary sexual characteristics and promote the achievement of full height potential. Adolescents in whom the diagnosis is constitutional delay require no therapy other than reassurance; however, early hormonal therapy may be worthwhile to minimize psychological stress.[25]

AMBIGUOUS GENITALIA

Ambiguous genitalia is a medical and psychological emergency that requires prompt evaluation of two major issues: the possibility of a life-threatening disease and the sex of rearing. Although most physicians will never see an infant with sexual ambiguity at birth, the need to assess the situation as quickly as possible makes this subject essential. It is vital for the physician not to make a gender assignment in the delivery room until all necessary data have been collected. It is equally important for the physician to reassure the parents that they have a healthy baby, but that the development of the external genitals is incomplete and tests are necessary to determine the sex. Furthermore, they should be informed that the cause of the problem will be identified and that a definite answer as to the sex of the baby should be available within a few days, or at most 1 to 2 weeks. Speculation as to the gender of the baby should be avoided and the infant should be referred to as "the baby" until a diagnosis has been made. In addition, the physician should educate the parents on common genital anlage for boys and girls.

Initial evaluation of the neonate with ambiguous genitalia includes history taking and physical examination, karyotype, appropriate serum hormone analyses, and radiographic studies. Parents should be asked about any family history of congenital adrenal hyperplasia (CAH), history of early neonatal death, consanguinity, metabolic disorders among family members,

---

TABLE 56-4
DIFFERENTIAL DIAGNOSIS OF AMBIGUOUS GENITALIA IN THE NEWBORN

Female pseudohermaphroditism
   Congenital adrenal hyperplasia
   Exogenous androgens
Male pseudohermaphroditism
   Testosterone biosynthetic defects
   Leydig-cell hyperplasia
   5α-reductase deficiency
   Androgen insensitivity syndrome
Gonadal disorders
   Gonadal dysgenesis
   True hermaphroditism
Malformation syndromes
   Chromosomal defects
   Single-gene defects
   Associations
Hypospadias
Cryptorchidism

---

maternal ingestion of steroid hormones during pregnancy, or maternal history of virilization. The infant should be examined for any signs of a malformation syndrome (e.g., dysmorphic features, abnormal body proportions, intrauterine growth restriction), hypertension, areolar hyperpigmentation, and evidence of dehydration. The number of gonads and their location should be well documented, characteristics of the labioscrotal folds should be noted, and measurements of the phallus should be precise. Identification of the urethra as well as vaginal and anal openings should also be made. Blood karyotype, 17OHP, DHEA, LH, FSH, total testosterone, and dihydrotestosterone (DHT) should be drawn. Pelvic/abdominal ultrasonography as well as either retrograde genitography or a voiding cystourethrography (VCUG) should be performed to better define internal structures. Table 56-4 lists the causes of ambiguous genitalia in the newborn.[26] Because the medical management and surgical correction of genital ambiguity are beyond the scope of the primary care provider, a multidisciplinary team approach is best suited for the comprehensive treatment of these patients.

COMMON DISORDERS IN PEDIATRIC AND ADOLESCENT GYNECOLOGY

Vulvovaginitis

Vulvovaginitis is the most common gynecologic disorder among children, as many factors predispose them toward its development.[27] Perineal hygiene is often overlooked among young girls, and contamination with stool and other debris is common. The vaginal mucosa is also more prone to infection due to the lack of estrogen stimulation.[28] Vulvovaginitis can be classified into three major groups:

1. Nonspecific vulvovaginitis: a disruption in the local microenvironment causes a polymicrobial infection with associated inflammation (e.g., foreign body, poor hygiene)
2. Secondary inoculation: a primary infection elsewhere (e.g., strep pharyngitis) is spread to the vagina by contamination (e.g., patient's hands) or bacteremia
3. Specific infections: refers to specific primary vaginal infections, usually sexually transmitted (e.g., gonorrhea)

The symptoms of vulvovaginitis can vary from mild discomfort to intense itching and burning or a foul-smelling discharge. Often it is the parents who first notice abnormal secretions. The irritating discharge often causes local inflammation and pruritus, and there may be scratch marks from the child, which can induce bleeding. This is especially true in the young unestrogenized child in whom the vulvar and vaginal epithelium is thin. Evaluation of secretions should include a Gram stain, appropriate bacterial cultures, and a wet preparation. Occasionally a urinalysis may also be helpful. The wet preparation should include a separate potassium hydroxide (KOH) preparation looking for mycotic organisms, and the presence of white and red cells, vaginal epithelial cells, trichomonads, and parasitic ova should be noted. Vaginoscopy can usually be reserved for patients with recurrent infections, those in whom initial treatment is refractory, or if the child has a foul-smelling and/or bloody discharge. In these situations, a thorough vaginal inspection is warranted to exclude the presence of foreign bodies or neoplasms.

Most instances of foreign bodies cause an intense inflammatory reaction with an associated bloody, foul-smelling discharge. The most commonly found objects are small pieces of toilet paper accidentally lodged in the vagina. The child usually does not recall the incident or does not admit to it. On examination, the object can easily be seen when the labia are separated and the perineum is stretched downward. They often appear as amorphous, grayish conglomerates along the posterior wall of the lower third of the vagina. They can usually be dislodged by irrigating with warm saline using a syringe, which produces little to no discomfort to the patient. Radiography is rarely warranted. Vaginoscopy is indicated for removal of large solid objects or to confirm that no other foreign body remains. Solid objects left in the vagina for prolonged periods can become embedded in the vaginal mucosa and can lead to vesicovaginal or rectovaginal fistulas, but this is a very rare occurrence.

Because most causes of vulvovaginitis in this age group are nonspecific, simple and practical measures usually alleviate the problem. Proper instructions should be given to the mother and child regarding vulvar hygiene. This should include the use of sitz baths and anal wiping from front to back. Keeping the perineum clean with warm water should suffice, as the additional use of creams, powders, and ointments will often exacerbate the problem. Occasionally mild bar soap may be used, but it should not contain any perfumes. The perineum should be patted dry with a soft terry cloth towel. Laundry detergents and fabric softeners should be free of perfumes, and the child may be advised to not wear undergarments to bed. Antibiotic treatment should be initiated only after a causative organism is identified. Rarely, empiric treatment is warranted (e.g., ampicillin 50 to 100 mg/kg/day) for intense inflammatory reactions while awaiting culture results, but a change in antibiotic regimen may be necessary if the isolated organism is resistant. A short course (twice a day for 5 to 7 days) of topical estrogen cream should restore any denuded vulvar and vaginal surfaces. For intense pruritus, a 1% hydrocortisone cream applied topically (twice a day for 5 to 7 days) to the affected area should alleviate any itching.[29]

Specific Infections

Vulvovaginitis can be the result of specific infections, either from direct contact or from secondary inoculation. Enteric and respiratory pathogens are the primary organisms responsible for secondary inoculation. Primary infections of the lower genital tract include sexually transmitted diseases (STDs), candida, toxic shock syndrome, pubic lice, and pinworms, among others. The diagnosis of STDs is fortunately rare in childhood, with an estimated incidence of 1 to 5%. It is important for the clinician to be aware of the various infectious causes of vulvovaginitis in the young female patient. The following section provides a brief overview of the clinical presentation, work-up, and treatment of various infectious causes of vulvovaginitis in this age group.

Sexually Transmitted Diseases

Gonorrhea

Neisseria gonorroheae is a fastidious gram-negative-diplococcus whose isolation requires proper culture techniques. Because prepubertal girls may harbor other Neisseria species that are not sexually transmitted, it is important that culture techniques are reliable so as to not falsely diagnose *N. gonorroheae*. This includes culture growth under high carbon dioxide tension, and culture swabs should always be plated directly onto the appropriate culture medium. DNA probes (e.g., GenProbe) are also acceptable means for isolating the organism, and they have the advantage of simultaneous testing for *Chlamydia trachomatis.*[30,31]

The prepubertal child with *N. gonorrhoeae* will usually present with a purulent vulvovaginitis rather than pain and cervicitis. Infection is usually caused by vulvar coitus or oral sex rather than vaginal penetration, so it is common to note an intact hymen on examination. The symptoms usually appear 2 to 7 days after the inoculation. The work-up in the young female patient should include the following:

1. Gram stain and culture of the discharge—if positive, then continue.
2. Interview of the child by either a social worker, psychologist, pediatrician, or other qualified health professional to elicit sexual abuse or misuse.
3. Culture all family members.
4. Perform rectal and pharyngeal cultures for *N. gonorrhoeae,* chlamydial cultures, and serology for syphilis; this should be done prior to treatment.
5. Treatment is with 125 mg of ceftriaxone intramuscularly.
6. Follow-up cultures of throat, rectum, and vagina 7 to 14 days after treatment; pedophiles are often repeat offenders.
7. All cases of gonorrhea must be reported to the mandated state agency.

Gonococcal infection in the sexually active adolescent should be diagnosed and treated in the same way as for an adult. Adjustments in antibiotic dosing may be necessary; consultation with a pharmacist may be indicated

Chlamydia

Chlamydia trachomatis is an intracellular organism that also requires special culture techniques for its isolation and proper identification. Cell culture with McCoy cells and fluorescent antibody stains remains the gold standard for identification of *C. trachomatis,* and this method should be used in the prepubertal patient for whom sexual abuse must be considered. Careful vaginal and urethral swabs should be obtained, and use of an adequate growth or transport medium should be utilized.[32] When the cultures grow *C. trachomatis,* freezing of the organism at −70°C is suggested for future confirmation by forensics. Other, less-sensitive techniques for diagnosis may be employed in the sexually active adolescent. The primary mode of transmission of chlamydia involves direct contact.[33] Neonates may be infected at birth through direct contact with colonized secretions of the vagina or rectum.[34] Vertical transmission at the time of cesarean section has also been reported.[35]

Children infected with *C. trachomatis* usually present with vaginitis, urethritis, or pyuria. Vulvar erythema, vaginal discharge or bleeding, and rectal pain can also occur, and concomitant infection with *N. gonorroheae* occurs in about 25% of cases. Erythromycin (30 to 50 mg/kg/day) is the treatment of choice in children 8 years and younger, and doxycycline (200 mg/day) should be used in older children. Prophylactic treatment is not recommended, and the practitioner should wait for the culture results before employing therapy.[36]

Syphilis

Syphilis in a child beyond the neonatal period is usually acquired through sexual contact. It is caused by the organism *Treponema pallidum,* and the gold standard for the diagnosis of primary syphilis is the identification of the spirochetes under darkfield microscopy obtained from the syphilitic chancre. Diagnosis of secondary and latent syphilis can be made using the VDRL and rapid plasma reagin (RPR) serum screening tests, followed by confirmation with either the fluorescent treponemal antibody-absorption (FTA-ABS) or the microhemagglutination–*Treponema pallidum* (MHA-TP) test.[37]

Primary syphilis in the pediatric patient has a similar presentation as in the adult, with the appearance of a painless genital chancre about 3 weeks after exposure. Primary lesions may also present in the oral cavity or in the perianal region.[38] Secondary syphilis often presents as a generalized skin rash (particularly palms and soles) approximately 4 to 12 weeks after initial exposure, but secondary syphilis is rare in the prepubarchal population. CSF samples should be obtained in children with evidence of neurologic involvement, or in whom congenital syphilis must be ruled out. As with other sexually transmitted diseases in the pediatric patient, sexual abuse must be considered, and all cases of confirmed syphilis must be reported to the proper authorities. After congenital syphilis and neurosyphilis have been ruled out, infected children should be treated with 50,000 units/kg of benzathine penicillin intramuscularly, not to exceed the adult dose of 2.4 million units. As with adults, serial RPR titers should be followed to confirm successful treatment.[39]

Genital Herpes

Herpes simplex virus (HSV) is transmitted via close contact with an individual who is shedding the virus, and although sexual transmission is the most common cause of genital herpes, autoinoculation from non-genital lesions has been documented in children. The virus (both HSV-1 and HSV-2) enters the mucosal surface through breaks in the epithelium and causes painful vesicular lesions to develop between 2 to 20 days after inoculation. Systemic symptoms such as fever, malaise, nausea, and headache, as well as inguinal lymphadenopathy, can also occur. Primary lesions are usually more severe, while recurrent genital lesions typically have less viral shedding and no systemic symptoms. The diagnosis in children is established by the isolation of the virus from suspicious lesions. Positive herpes cultures should be subjected to confirmatory testing because of possible false positive results from herpes zoster. False negative cultures can also occur if specimens are obtained from lesions in which there is little to no viral shedding. There are no treatment guidelines for genital herpes infection in children. Some clinicians use acyclovir since its safety has been demonstrated in the treatment of neonatal herpes simplex and childhood zoster, while others prefer to use symptomatic treatment such as sitz baths, topical anesthetics, and drying agents.[40-44]

Condyloma Acuminatum

There has been a dramatic increase in the incidence of condyloma in children. Transmission through casual and sexual contact as well as vertical transmission can occur, with the majority of perinatally transmitted human papillomavirus (HPV) occurring in children under the age of 2. Sexual transmission is more likely (up to 90% of cases) in children older than 2. The lesions can occur anywhere in the anogenital region, and they usually present as flesh-colored verrucous growths. The application of a compress dampened with 3% to 5% acetic acid will aid in the identification of lesions. The compress should be placed over the anogenital area for 10 to 15 minutes. The lesions will have a whitish appearance. Biopsy should be performed if the diagnosis is in question, especially if sexual abuse is a possibility. The use of the carbon dioxide (CO_2) laser for treatment of condyloma in children provides excellent results and allows for control over depth of tissue destruction. Topical agents such as podophyllin or imiquimod may also be employed, but may not be tolerated in this age group. Spontaneous regression may occur, but this is not recommended as a treatment of choice in children. Even with therapy, recurrence rates have been reported as high as 30%.[45-49]

Molluscum Contagiosum

Molluscum contagiosum is a benign skin disease caused by the poxvirus; it is spread by local contact. Unlike most STDs, molluscum is only mildly contagious and can be acquired from nonsexual contact. In adults it is usually asymptomatic and confined to the vulvar skin, but in children it can present over the entire body. The small 1- to 5-mm domed papules are usually pathognomonic, and the more mature nodules have umbilicated centers. Diagnosis can be confirmed by finding intracytoplasmic molluscum bodies on Wright or Giemsa stain from the expressed waxy material inside of a nodule. Because of the chance of autoinoculation, therapy should be aimed at removal of all lesions. Treatment of the nodules should include injection of a small subdermal wheal of 1% lidocaine followed by evacuation of the caseous material from each lesion. The nodule should then be excised with a dermal currette, and the base of the papule treated with ferric subsulfate (Monsel solution) or 85% trichloroacetic acid (TCA). For extensive disease, an alternative therapy may include cryosurgery or electrocautery.[50]

Pediculosis Pubis and Scabies

The crab louse (*Phthirus pubis*), or pedicularis pubis, is a parasitic infestation of the pubic hair; it is the most contagious of all sexually transmitted diseases, although it can be transmitted via towels or bedding. The predominant symptom of pubic lice is constant itching in the pubic area. The incubation period for pediculosis is about 30 days, but symptoms may develop after 5 days of exposure secondary to allergic sensitization. Examination of the vulva reveals tiny eggs and adult lice along with pepper-grain feces appearing next to the eggs. Definitive diagnosis can be made by placing the crust of a skin papule under oil immersion at 100× power. The louse looks like a six-legged miniature crab.

Scabies is a parasitic infection of the itch mite (*Sarcoptes scabiei*), and like the crab louse, is transmitted by close contact. Scabies infections are widespread, with no predilection for hairy areas. The female mite digs a burrow just beneath the skin and can travel up to 2.5 cm in a minute. The pathognomonic sign of scabies is the burrow, which has the appearance of a twisted line on the skin surface with a vesicle at one end. Patients have intermittent pruritus that is sometimes more intense at night, when the mites are more active. Hands, wrists, breasts, vulva, and buttocks are most often affected, and examination of these areas with the aid of a magnifying glass can be helpful in the diagnosis. Like the crab louse, scabies can be identified under the microscope by scraping the lesion and placing it on a slide with mineral oil. The mites lack claws on the side but do have two anterior triangular hairy buds.

The treatment of pediculosis pubis and scabies involves killing both the parasite and the eggs. The Centers for Disease Control and Prevention (CDC) recommends either permethrin (Nix Creme) or lindane (Kwell). They both come as a cream, but lindane is also available as a lotion or shampoo. Lindane is not recommended for children under the age of 2. Patients should be reexamined after 1 week of therapy and should continue treatment if necessary. Close household contacts should also be treated, and clothing and bedding should be decontaminated.[51]

Other Infections

Candida

Candidal vulvovaginitis can be common in adolescent females but is an uncommon finding in prepubertal girls. Predisposing factors in young females include a recent course of antibiotics, diabetes mellitus, and immunosuppression, among others. Diagnosis is made by the typical finding of a thick, white, cheesy, pruritic discharge with or without associated vulvar erythema and swelling. Wet preparation reveals budding yeast, and KOH preparation may accentuate the hyphae. Treatment should first include intravaginal or oral azole therapy (e.g., clotrimazole, miconazole), which has an 80 to 90% efficacy.

Recurrent vulvovaginal candidiasis (defined as four or more symptomatic episodes annually) warrants further investigation. The physician should first confirm the diagnosis of candida using appropriate cultures, and he/she should check for predisposing factors such as inappropriate or incomplete therapy, diabetes mellitus, or causes of immunosuppression such as human immunodeficiency virus (HIV).[52]

Toxic Shock Syndrome

Toxic shock syndrome (TSS) is a rare infection primarily affecting young menstruating women who use a single tampon for a prolonged period of time. Because it received such wide publicity in the 1980s, public awareness and changes in tampon products have significantly reduced the incidence of this dangerous infection. The disease is primarily caused by release of toxic shock syndrome toxin (TSST-1) and enterotoxin A (SEA) produced by *Staphylococcus aureus*. Not all cases of TSS are severe, and milder forms of the disease can occur in nonmenstruating females and during menses without tampon use. The CDC has set up the criteria for the diagnosis of the severe form of the disease, which requires four of five major criteria:

1. Fever of 38.9°C or higher
2. Rash: diffuse macular erythroderma (like a sunburn)
3. Desquamation, particularly of palms and soles, 1 to 2 weeks after the onset of the illness
4. Hypotension or orthostatic syncope/dizziness
5. Involvement of three or more of the following organ systems: gastrointestinal, muscular, mucous membranes, renal, hepatic, hematologic, CNS

In addition, cultures from CSF and blood must be negative. Management of TSS should include aggressive resuscitation with the administration of intravenous fluids and penicillinase-resistant antistaphylococcal antibiotics. Appropriate laboratory tests should be obtained, and the tampon should be promptly removed from the vagina. Some advocate irrigation of the vagina with saline, povidone–iodine solution, or antibiotic solution. For particularly severe cases, immunoglobulin therapy or steroids may be beneficial.[53]

Enterobiasis

Enterobiasis, or pinworms, is a common infection that affects all age groups but is most often symptomatic in children. It is caused by the organism *Enterobius vermicularis,* and infection begins by the ingestion of embryonated eggs, which are typically carried on fingernails, clothing, bedding, or house dust. The adult female worm deposits her eggs at night along the perianal region, which may cause symptoms of nocturnal anal pruritus and sleeplessness. Diagnosis is made by the finding of parasitic eggs, which can easily be detected by pressing adhesive tape to the perianal region early in the morning. Treatment should be given to all infected and symptomatic individuals and household members. This consists of a single 100-mg oral dose of mebendazole. There are no specific syndromes caused by *E. vermicularis.*[54]

Vulvar Skin Diseases

Lichen Sclerosus

Lichen sclerosus is a benign vulvar condition characterized by white, atrophic, parchmentlike skin with evidence of chronic ulceration, inflammation, and subepithelial hemorrhages. In more advanced cases, there can be loss of the demarcation of the labia, scarring of the clitoral hood, and thickening of the posterior fourchette. Involvement of the perianal area along with the labia often gives it an hourglass (or figure-of-eight) appearance. Patients often report itching, irritation, soreness, and sometimes bleeding. Although rare in the adolescent, this disease should be recognized and distinguished from vitiligo or other vulvar dystrophies. The diagnosis is usually made clinically, but a skin biopsy may be warranted. Histologic features on biopsy are quite typical, showing flattening of the rete pegs, hyalinization of the subdermal tissues, and keratinization.

Treatment is varied and somewhat controversial since the cause is unknown. Initial treatment should always include improved vulvar hygiene and elimination of local irritants and soaps containing perfume. An over-the-counter ointment (such as A and D ointment) can be helpful. For more severe cases, hydrocortisone cream (1% or 2.5%) can be used topically for 1 to 3 months. Clobetasol cream (Temovate) can also be applied twice a day for 2 weeks followed by once a day for 2 weeks. After a follow-up visit to document improvement, the cream can be applied every other day for an additional 2 weeks. Other treatments that have been suggested include topical progesterones and testosterones as well as other anti-inflammatory creams.[55]

Lichen Planus

Lichen planus is characterized by a unique eruption of tiny, flat, violaceous papules on flexor surfaces, mucous membranes, and the vulvar skin. Patients often have intense pain and/or pruritus, which may lead to linear scratch marks. The cause is thought to be autoimmune, and diagnosis is made by punch biopsy. This disease is rare in the adolescent but should be considered in the differential diagnosis of vulvar diseases. Treatment consists of topical steroid cream.[56]

Psoriasis

Psoriasis is a common skin disorder of unknown cause that affects the vulva in approximately 20% of cases. For most women psoriasis develops in the teenage years, with approximately 3% of adult women being affected. Vulvar psoriasis manifests as red to red-yellow papules along the intertriginous areas that tend to enlarge, eventually forming well-circumscribed dull-red plaques. The clinical presentation often resembles candida, but the classic silver scales and bleeding on gentle scraping help distinguish it from other vulvar skin disorders. Initial therapy should include application of topical 1% hyrocortisone cream. Refractory cases should be evaluated by a dermatologist.[57]

Contact Dermatitis

The vulvar skin is a frequent site of contact dermatitis, and the majority of chemicals that cause this condition are either cosmetic or therapeutic agents. Common examples include fabric dyes and softeners, soaps, bleaches, and local creams. More severe cases involve vulvar lesions after exposure to poison oak or poison ivy. Acute contact dermatitis is characterized by red, edematous skin that may become weeping and eczematoid. Patients often report vulvar tenderness, pruritus, and burning. Therapy is focused on removal of the offending agent followed by application of wet compresses of Burrow solution (diluted 1:20 with normal saline) for 30 minutes several times a day. The skin should be dried using cool air from a hair dryer, and application of lubricating jelly (e.g., petroleum jelly) will reduce the itching. For severe symptoms, low-dose hydrocortisone cream can be rubbed into the skin two to three times a day for a few days.[58]

Labial Adhesions

Labial adhesions (also known as adhesive vulvitis or labial agglutination) are thought to be the result of chronic vulvitis in which denuded epithelium of adjacent labia minora fuse together. Low estrogen levels likely play a role in their development as well. It is a benign self-limited condition that is relatively common in young girls between ages 2 and 6. It is not particularly serious, but can sometimes be misdiagnosed as congenital absence of the vagina. It is usually asymptomatic unless it is covering the urethral orifice, in which case there may be difficulty in voiding or associated urinary-tract infections. If scarring of the fourchette is noted in conjunction with labial agglutination, then sexual abuse must be considered. Diagnosis is made by the appearance of a translucent vertical line where the labia stick together. This thin avascular line is pathognomonic and may involve only part of the labia minora, usually the posterior aspect. Treatment is not necessary unless the child has problems urinating. Parents will often request active treatment even when it is not warranted. Topical estrogen cream applied twice daily will often result in spontaneous separation within 2 to 3 weeks. Forceful separation is unnecessarily traumatic and should not be done.[59] Recurrence of labial adhesions is common because the estrogen-deficient state exists until puberty. Proper perineal hygiene and removal of irritants may aid in the prevention of recurrence. The condition usually resolves after puberty.[60]

Urethral Prolapse

Urethral prolapse is a relatively common benign condition found in young girls. It is often mistaken as either a genital tumor, imperforate hymen, or sexual abuse by physicians not accustomed to seeing it, and because of this, it has been the source of much anxiety by concerned parents. Urethral prolapse occurs when the urethral mucosa protrudes through the meatus and forms a hemorrhagic, tender mass that can bleed quite easily. Some suggest that it is a result of redundant urethral mucosa while others postulate that there is some laxity of urethral support in the surrounding connective tissue. Despite these and other theories, the true cause remains unknown. The diagnosis is made by its typical appearance on examination, noting a doughnut-like mass superior to and separate from the vagina. Confirmation can be accomplished by passing a pediatric red rubber catheter through the center of the lesion followed by drainage of urine from the catheter. The tip of the catheter should first be coated with lidocaine gel prior to its insertion. The mainstay of treatment includes sitz baths three times a day along with a short course of topical estrogen cream (applied twice a day for 5 to 7 days). Resection of the prolapsed tissue should be considered for patients with urinary retention, large necrotic lesions, or in whom conservative therapy fails.[61-63]

Disorders of Menstruation

Dysmenorrhea

Pain with menses is common in young women, with some studies reporting up to 60% of adolescents experiencing significant dysmenorrhea. Most dysmenorrhea in adolescents is primary, but it may also be the result of pelvic pathology such as endometriosis or obstructing müllerian anomalies.

Typically, patients begin experiencing crampy lower abdominal pain with menses around age 14 or 15 (about 1 to 2 years after menarche). The pain may be accompanied by nausea, vomiting, diarrhea, low back pain, headache, or fatigue, and the pain usually begins a few hours before menstrual flow and lasts 24 to 48 hours. Dysmenorrhea can last up to 4 days or longer, with some girls even missing school because of their symptoms. Assessment of dysmenorrhea in the adolescent should include a thorough history and physical examination, with particular attention to the following questions:

1. Is she missing school, and if so, how many days?
2. Does she miss other activities or social events?
3. What other symptoms are associated with the cramps?
4. Is she sexually active?
5. What is the parent–daughter relationship?

Although most patients will simply have primary dysmenorrhea, the physician must recognize girls in whom the symptoms are disabling out of proportion to the cause. Such patients may have an aversion toward school, a history of physical or sexual abuse, or other significant psychosocial issues. It is important to obtain an accurate history regarding the use of nonsteroidal antiinflammatory drugs (NSAIDs) and degree of success, as many adolescents use subtherapeutic doses with little to no relief. Physical examination should include inspection of the genitalia and hymen, and a speculum examination should be performed for the sexually active adolescent. Rectoabdominal examination can be helpful in the virginal patient, and ultrasonography may be useful in defining suspected uterine and vaginal anomalies.

Once secondary causes have been eliminated, treatment should be aimed at symptomatic relief. The most common approach is the prescribing of NSAID compounds (ibuprofen, 800 mg; naproxen sodium, 220 or 275 mg; mefenemic acid, 250 mg) at appropriate intervals. The patient should be instructed to begin taking her medication as soon as her cramps begin, preferably before menstruation. In patients with severe symptoms, initiation of an oral contraceptive pill (OC) can be very helpful, as this will typically shorten her symptoms, and her menses will be more predictable. The OCs should initially be given for a short course (3 to 6 months). If severe symptoms recur with inadequate relief from NSAIDs alone, then long-term OC use may be necessary. Adolescents with primary dysmenorrhea should have regular follow-up visits (3 to 4 months) to monitor their symptoms and provide reassurance.[64]

Primary Amenorrhea

Primary amenorrhea is defined as the absence of menses by age 16 in the presence of normal secondary sexual characteristics or by age 14 when there is no visible secondary sexual characteristic development. Table 56-5 lists the causes of primary amenorrhea based on the presence or absence of secondary sexual characteristics. Work-up of the adolescent with primary amenorrhea should focus on a thorough history and physical examination as well as appropriate radiologic and laboratory studies. Pregnancy should always be considered in any patient of reproductive age. Referral to a specialist may be warranted in situations in which the cause is not easily identified.[65]

Abnormal Uterine Bleeding

Excessive or irregular menstrual bleeding in the adolescent is fairly common, and although most of these patients suffer from dysfunctional uterine bleeding (DUB), organic causes must first be excluded. The diagnosis of DUB is based on a thorough history and physical examination as well as appropriate laboratory tests. This includes a Pap smear, pregnancy test, urinalysis, complete blood count with peripheral smear, coagulation profile (prothrombin time [PT], partial thromboplastin time [PTT], and bleeding time), serum prolactin level, and thyroid-function tests. Endometrial biopsy is rarely indicated in the adolescent patient. The typical teenager with DUB has a history of prolonged, irregular periods since menarche that may last several days or even weeks. This is usually the result of anovulatory cycles and unopposed estrogen. The possibility of an underlying coagulopathy must be considered (18%), and specific questioning about episodes of easy bruising, gingival bleeding, epistaxis, or family history of coagulopathy is recommended. The most common bleeding disorders in the adolescent are von Willebrand disease and idiopathic thrombocytopenia purpura (ITP).

Once all organic causes of abnormal uterine bleeding have been eliminated, therapy should be initiated based on the severity of the anemia, if one exists. In patients whose hemoglobin is greater than 12 g/dl, reassurance and periodic evaluation is all that

TABLE 56-5
CAUSES OF PRIMARY AMENORRHEA

Amenorrhea associated with the presence of secondary sexual characteristics
　Müllerian abnormalities
　　Imperforate hymen
　　Transverse vaginal septum
　　Mayer–Rokitansky–Kuster–Hauser syndrome
　Androgen insensitivity
　True hermaphrodites
　Absent endometrium
　Ovarian failure
　　Chromosomal abnormality
　　Iatrogenic causes (radiation, chemotherapy, surgical damage to ovarian blood supply)
　　Galactosemia
　　Infections
　　Autoimmune disorders
　　Savage syndrome
　　Idiopathic
Amenorrhea associated with a lack of secondary sexual characteristics
　Hypogonadotropic hypogonadism
　　Physiologic delay
　　Kallmann syndrome
　　Central nervous system tumors
　　Hypothalamic and pituitary dysfunction
　Hypergonadotropic hypogonadism
　　Gonadal dysgenesis
　　Pure gonadal dysgenesis
　　Sex chromosome mosaicism
　　Partial deletion of X chromosome
　　Ovarian toxins (environmental and therapeutic)
　　17α-hydroxylase deficiency in XX individual
　　Other
Abnormal physical examination
　5α-reductase deficiency in XY individual
　　17-20 desmolase deficiency in XY individual
　　17α-hydroxylase deficiency in XY individual

is required. Iron supplementation may be helpful if the mean corpuscular volume is less than 80. The majority of these patients will revert to normal cycles within 1 to 2 years. Patients in whom the hemoglobin level is between 10 g/dl and 12 g/dl have a mild anemia that warrants some degree of medical therapy. This may include the use of cyclic progestin therapy such as medroxyprogesterone acetate (Provera), 10 mg daily for 7 days every 5 to 6 weeks. The initiation of OCs is an alternative therapy that has the additional benefit of contraception in the sexually active teenager. The addition of iron therapy is also warranted in this group. Patients whose hemoglobin levels are less than 10 g/dl require a thorough investigation for specific causes such as genital tract pathology, coagulopathies, and complications of pregnancy. Up to 20% of adolescents requiring hospitalization for abnormal uterine bleeding are found to have a coagulopathy. Once an organic cause for the bleeding has been ruled out, therapy such as OCs or cyclic progestins can be initiated. For patients with acute bleeding requiring intravenous (IV) fluid replacement and/or blood transfusion, the administration of conjugated estrogens (Premarin, 25 mg IV every 4 hours for 24 hours) is usually adequate for controlling the bleeding. Alternatively, patients may take a combination OC (e.g., OrthoNovum 1/35). The initial dose should begin as one tablet four times daily for 3 days, one tablet three times daily for 2 days, one tablet twice daily for 1 day, then one tablet daily for the remainder of the prescription. Vaginal bleeding that continues despite high-dose estrogen therapy is an indication for a diagnostic dilation and curettage.[66-69]

Genital Tumors

Ovarian

Ovarian masses in the pediatric and adolescent patient are the result of either functional cysts or neoplasms, both benign and malignant. Ovarian tumors are the most common genital neoplasm of childhood, and while the majority of these lesions are benign, ovarian torsion and malignant lesions need early diagnosis for optimal prognosis. Approximately 20 to 50% of ovarian tumors are actually functional cysts. They can be found in the fetus on routine obstetric ultrasound or on routine physical examination of the neonate, and they usually resolve on their own. Some authorities recommend elective cesarean section for fetuses with ovarian cysts >6 cm to reduce the risk of rupture during vaginal delivery, while others suggest antenatal cyst aspiration. The treatment for most ovarian cysts, however, is observation, with follow-up ultrasonography until resolution of the mass has been documented. If the cyst has not resolved by 4 months of age, the possibility of either neoplasia or torsion must be entertained, and surgery may be warranted.

Ovarian cysts in childhood and adolescence are usually the result of gonadotropin stimulation of the ovary, and these cysts may be hormonally active. Patients may present with vaginal bleeding, precocious pseudopuberty, or premature thelarche. Symptoms such as abdominal or pelvic pain, nausea, bloating, or increased abdominal girth may also be present. Simple cysts can be followed conservatively with a repeat physical examination and pelvic ultrasound about 6 to 8 weeks after the initial visit. If there are no inter-

TABLE 56-6
COMMON OVARIAN NEOPLASMS IN THE PEDIATRIC AND ADOLESCENT FEMALE

Benign neoplasms
  Functional cysts
    Follicular
    Corpus luteum
    Theca lutein
  Endometrioma
  Germ-cell tumors
    Gonadoblastoma
    Mature cystic teratoma
  Sex cord–stromal tumors (usually benign)
    Thecoma
    Granulosa cell
Malignant neoplasms
  Epithelial tumors
  Germ-cell tumors
    Dysgerminoma
    Mixed germ-cell tumor
    Endodermal sinus tumor
    Immature teratoma
    Embryonal tumor
    Choriocarcinoma
    Sertoli–Leydig-cell tumors

nal echoes on ultrasound and torsion is not suspected, this therapy can be continued safely. Laparoscopy or laparotomy is warranted in patients with severe pain, those in whom rupture or torsion is suspected, or for masses suspicious for neoplasia. OCs can be prescribed in the adolescent with a simple cyst in an attempt to prevent new cyst development.

Pediatric and adolescent patients who present with a solid adnexal mass, or in whom ultrasound suggests malignancy, should undergo exploratory laparotomy. Preoperative work-up should include appropriate tumor markers as well as the use of CT or MRI when indicated. Table 56-6 is a list of common benign and malignant ovarian tumors.[70]

Other

Most benign tumors of the vagina in children are unilocular cystic remnants of the mesonephric duct. Other benign vaginal neoplasms include teratomas, hemangiomas, simple cysts of the hymen, and paraurethral inclusion cysts. Gartner's duct (paraurethral) cysts are also relatively common. Large cysts that interfere with urination or vaginal drainage require surgical excision, but asymptomatic lesions can be left alone. Teratomas and cavernous hemangiomas also require surgical excision, whereas capillary hemangiomas usually disappear with time, requiring no surgical intervention.

Embryonal carcinoma of the vagina (sarcoma botryoides) is most often seen in children <3 years old. This tumor derives from undifferentiated mesenchyme and most often infiltrates the vaginal wall in the distal vagina. As the tumor spreads beneath the vaginal epithelium, the vaginal wall bulges into a series of polypoid growths containing edematous stroma and dilated blood vessels. This gives the lesion its characteristic soft, cluster-of-grapes appearance. Diagnosis of sarcoma botryoides (also known as childhood pelvic rhabdomyosarcoma) is confirmed by histologic examination and has a favorable prognosis with a combined treatment of chemotherapy with subsequent limited surgery or radiotherapy.[71]

GENITAL TRAUMA

Children at play are prone to injury. This may involve the genital region. Most injuries to the genitalia during childhood are accidental in nature; however, some may result from an abusive encounter. It is important to determine how the injury was sustained because abused children must be removed from an unsafe environment. Many genital injuries are of minor significance; few are life-threatening or require major surgical procedures. With severe trauma, or very young children, it may be necessary to perform the examination under general anesthesia.

Vulvar and Vaginal Injuries

Straddle injuries are fairly common in childhood. These are often the result of the active climber (monkey bars, cabinets, pools, etc.) sustaining a fall onto a very rigid object. Since the perineum and vulva are extremely vascular and the subcutaneous tissues are loosely arranged, an injury may cause blood vessels underneath the perineal skin to rupture. Blood accumulates under the skin and forms a hematoma, producing a rounded, tense, and tender swelling, the size of which depends on the amount of bleeding. A contusion of the vulva does not usually require treatment. A small vulvar hematoma can usually be controlled by pressure with an ice pack. A large hematoma, or one that continues to increase in size, should be incised, the clotted blood removed, and bleeding points ligated. If the source of the bleeding cannot be found, the cavity should be packed with gauze and a pressure dressing applied. The pack is removed in 24 hours. Prophylactic broad-spectrum antibiotics may be advisable. The vulva should be kept clean and dry. When the urethra is obstructed by the hematoma, it is necessary to insert a suprapubic catheter. Pelvic radiography may be necessary in some patients to rule out a fracture of the pelvis.

Since the vagina and hymen are recessed from the perineum and vulva, injuries to these structures are usually intentional. Most vaginal injuries occur when an object penetrates the vagina through the hymenal opening. Such penetration results in a laceration or a tear of the hymenal ring. Usually there is very little bleeding from a hymenal injury, but it indicates vaginal penetration, and thus the possibility of additional vaginal injuries. Therefore, a detailed examination is necessary to exclude injuries to the upper vagina. When a vaginal laceration extends to the vaginal vault, a laparotomy may be indicated to exclude extension of the tear into the broad ligament or the peritoneal cavity. Bladder and bowel integrity must also be confirmed.

Most vaginal wounds involve the lateral walls. Generally, there will be relatively little blood loss, and the child will not have much pain if the damage is only mucosal. The child will report intense pain when a lacerated blood vessel retracts underneath the vaginal mucosa and forms a hematoma. If the torn vessel is small, bleeding may stop spontaneously. Larger vessels may form large, tense hematomas that may distend the vagina, and require evacuation and ligation of the bleeding vessel.[72]

CHILD SEXUAL ABUSE

Child sexual abuse continues to plague our society in large numbers. It is a very serious problem that affects families, communities, and religious organizations among others. It transcends race, socioeconomic status, gender, and geographic location.[73] It is important to be aware of the possibility of sexual abuse when interacting with patients or being asked to assess a suspicious situation. Recognition of sexual molestation of a child is entirely dependent on the individual's inherent willingness to consider the diagnosis of suspected child abuse or molestation.[74] Because of the often-secretive nature of abuse, actual percentages are unknown. However, it is estimated to affect from 8 to 38% of all females younger than 18.

In order to standardize the definition of abuse, the National Center on Child Abuse and Neglect

(NCCAN) has adopted the following definition of child sexual abuse:

> Contact or interaction between a child and an adult, when the child is being used for the sexual stimulation of that adult or another person. Sexual abuse may also be committed by another minor, when that person is either significantly older than the victim, or when the abuser is in a position of power or control over that child.[75]

Although the legal definitions for crimes of sexual assault vary from state to state, most authorities agree that for rape to have taken place, the following must be present[72]:

1. A victim
2. Lack of consent or inability to consent (child, mental disability)
3. Threats or the actual use of force
4. Penetration

Not all sexual assaults are rapes.

The medical evaluation includes a thorough history and physical assessment. When the victim is a very young child, it may be difficult to exact a history. After rapport is established and a comfortable environment has been created, it is important to use age-appropriate language or interaction. Sometimes props such as anatomically detailed dolls are used for this purpose. The assistance of someone skilled in the use of these methods is very important.

The history is often given by a caretaker who has noted some behavioral changes (fear, anxiety, withdrawal, school problems, acting out behaviors, depression, increased sexual play, etc.) or physical changes (unexplained vaginal injuries or bleeding, bruises, recurrent vaginal infections, anogenital pain, recurrent atypical pain).[72] Disclosure may be readily given by the child in question, depending on the age and maturity.

During the physical examination, it is important not to focus solely on the genital area. A brief, general survey of the patient is helpful. Note should be made of any abnormalities of the skin (bruising, bite marks, lesions, etc.). The Tanner staging should be documented. Adequate visualization of the anogenital region is often realized with the patient in the frog-leg supine position. A systematic examination of the external genitalia, noting any abnormal markings, erythema, or discharge should be performed. Lateral or forward traction of the labia majora provides a good view of the vestibule, hymen, and lower vagina. The shape of the hymen (annular, crescentic, fimbriated, etc.) should be documented. Using the face of a clock as a base, any bumps, notches, or tears to the hymen are labeled. In the presence of discharge, a vaginal swab (calgi or regular) is obtained and a wet preparation done (Trichomonas vaginalis, bacterial vaginosis, candidias). Appropriate cultures (gonorrhea, chlamydia) should be obtained at this time.

In looking for specific patterns of injury, it is important to note that most injuries are to the vulva unless vaginal penetration occurs. Rubbing may result in erythema, skin bruising, or excoriations on the labia or vestibule. With time, healing occurs and may result in a relatively normal examination.[76]

Although many rely heavily on the physical evaluation of the child for evidence of abuse, it is often normal or nonspecific. Many patterns of abuse leave minimal, if any, marks. Fondling, oral sex, and caressing of the breasts are not likely to leave a trail. One classification of abnormal physical findings is as follows[72]:

Normal—No abnormalities detected

Nonspecific abnormalities—Redness, irritation, abrasions, friability of the posterior fourchette, labial adhesions, hymenal tags, hymenal bumps and clefts, nonspecific infections, bruising of the external genitalia

Specific findings—hymenal–vaginal tear, hymenal–perineal tear, sexually transmitted diseases, bite marks on the genitalia

Definitive abnormalities—presence of sperm, pregnancy (adolescent)

The absence of physical findings should not be construed to suggest a negative history for abuse. Perianal findings are often nonspecific; however, significant fissures and compromise of anal sphincter tone are red flags in the absence of specific gastrointestinal disease.

The health professional is obligated by law to report any suspicious findings (in the history or physical examination) to the appropriate local authorities. Collection of evidence should be left to those skilled in forensic evaluation and knowledgeable in the keeping the chain of evidence collection intact. Treatment of injuries and diseases should be carried out as medical protocol dictates.

ADOLESCENT PREGNANCY

Scope of the Problem

Children having children has been used to describe the problem of adolescent pregnancy. The United States remains at the forefront in this epidemic. Many are perplexed by the lower rates among several Scandinavian countries, where there is greater openness to sexual expression. The numbers are the same over the past three decades. Each year, approximately 1 million teenagers become pregnant.[77] Most of these pregnancies are unintentional. A little over half of these pregnancies result in deliveries. About 30% result in miscarriages and 20% in induced abortions.

Use of Contraception

Initial sexual intercourse is usually unplanned, although it is very important in the life of an adolescent. It may be the result of a coercive/abusive relationship, especially in the very young. As a result, effective contraception may not be involved. Six of ten 15- to 19-year-olds use birth control at first coitus.[78] In fact, the delay between first coital activity and seeking contraceptive advice is often 1 year, but 20% of first premarital pregnancies occur in the first month after the initiation of sexual intercourse and 50% within the first 6 months. Procrastination, not thinking that they could get pregnant, or being somewhat ambivalent about the whole subject, and worrying about confidentiality issues are the reasons given most often for the delay. When used, contraceptive practices may be inconsistent. As a result, teenagers are nearly twice as likely to experience contraceptive failure than women 30 years or older.[79]

Births to Adolescents

The birth rate for unmarried teens has doubled since the 1960s. Six of 10 babies born to adolescents are born to single mothers. Three of 10 adolescents who have their first child by 16 years or younger have their second child within 2 years. Only 4% of unmarried adolescent mothers put their babies up for adoption.

Adolescents and Abortions

Adolescents account for approximately 25% of the total number of abortions in the United States.[78] It is the outcome of about 44% of pregnancies among adolescents. There is a greater likelihood of delay in seeking an abortion until the second trimester, when the health risks of the procedure are increased.

Factors Associated with Adolescent Pregnancy

The psychosocial changes that are a natural part of adolescence play an important role in adolescent pregnancy. Unresolved dependency needs and insecure feminine identity lead to vulnerability and exposure to unplanned pregnancy. The impulsive nature of the adolescent does not often allow for advanced planning of such an encounter. "I didn't think it would happen to me" is a common response. In some settings, early childbearing may be common and regarded as the norm.

Consequences of Adolescent Pregnancy

Adolescence is the transition between childhood and adulthood. When pregnancy and parenting interrupt that transition, the development may be incomplete. Education is interrupted and may be incomplete as a result. The adolescent blessed with a very supportive family structure may overcome some obstacles to achieve career goals, but this is not common. A larger family at a younger age results from such pregnancies. Since parenting skills require some maturity, the infant of an adolescent mother may be at an increased risk for child abuse and neglect. Successive generations are at risk for repeating early pregnancy.

Complications of Adolescent Pregnancy

Health Risks to the Adolescent Mother

Pregnant teenagers are least likely to enter the health-care system early for prenatal care. Often the denial that exists or the desire to hide the pregnancy results in little or no prenatal assessment. Lack of familiarity with the symptoms of pregnancy may also play an important role in seeking prenatal care. Adolescent mothers are at an increased risk for first- and third-trimester bleeding. Poor nutrition with borderline iron stores result in anemia. Toxemia, low birth weight, and premature labor/delivery are often a problem. Maternal mortality and morbidity are increased. Social habits associated with high-risk behavior (use of tobacco, alcohol, or other drugs) increase the risk of having a baby with health problems. Sexually transmitted diseases are common in this population and may go undetected.[80] The small physical stature of the very young adolescent may necessitate delivery by Cesarean section.

The infants of an adolescent mother are at an increased risk for premature birth and its inherent complications (low birth weight, neonatal mortality, infant mortality). Unidentified/untreated sexually transmitted infections (gonorrhea, chlamydia, herpes, syphilis, HIV) or group B streptococcus can be detrimental to an infant's survival.

It is important for the health professional to take the opportunity of the prenatal encounter to educate the young pregnant patient and to assist in securing resources for the pregnancy, delivery, and beyond. It is also very important to be sensitive to the specific needs of this age group.

Sex Education and Contraceptive Counseling

Adolescent sexuality does not occur in a vacuum. It is the natural result of many of the psychosocial tasks of adolescence and sexual maturation. Early puberty and low socioeconomic status are associated with early sexual activity.[81] Adolescents who admit to sexual activity are more likely than their virginal peers to have low future and educational achievement orientation; they also are more likely to display attitudes of alienation, nontraditional attitudes toward sex, and other socially experimental behaviors.[82] Family characteristics (communication patterns, decision patterns, and moral judgments) have an impact on the decisions made by adolescents. The effect of influence exerted by peers (sex education, pressure) is significant, accounting in some studies for the major source of information.[83] The media (television, film, and magazines) are an important resource for information about some sexual behaviors. Models of sexual attractiveness, desirable behavior, and acceptance are portrayed at every opportunity.

It is important to establish a valid and informational education program for adolescents. This should start in preadolescence with acceptance of one's body. Knowledge of basic (age-appropriate) anatomy and physiology is an essential part of improved body image. Parents often fall short of providing this information, as they may feel uncomfortable or inadequate to provide it. Schools have taken up the task of educating our children in this area, but due to societal pressures the content of this instruction is far from adequate. Knowledge of sexually transmitted infections, acquired immunodeficiency syndrome (AIDS), the essentials about human reproduction, contracep-

tion, sexuality, and interpersonal relationships should be included in the curriculum.[84]

Contraceptive Counseling

An adolescent's decision to initiate or delay sexual activity is complex. The factors associated with early or later initiation of sexual intercourse include:[85]

Early Initiation	Later Initiation
Early onset of puberty	Emphasis on abstinence
Absence of a nurturing or supportive parent	Parental consistency and firmness in discipline
Sexual abuse	Goal orientation
Poor academic achievement	High academic achievement
Poverty	Regular attendance at a place of worship
Participation in other high-risk activities	

Availability of contraception is not causally related to sexual experimentation.[86,87]

Effective contraceptive use requires planning and preparation prior to having sexual intercourse. This task is often elusive for adolescents. Due to the impulsive, spontaneous, "just happened" nature of the initial coital encounter for adolescents, devising a good contraceptive plan is a challenge. As mentioned earlier, among adolescents the average delay in seeking contraceptive care is 1 year.

In counseling the adolescent, it is important to establish a "safe and comfortable" environment for discussion, one that would allow for the exchange of ideas on sexuality and dispelling myths concerning pregnancy prevention.

Factors to remember when choosing a contraceptive method for the adolescent:[88]

1. Acceptability: Is it a method the patient will continue to use consistently?
2. Effectiveness of method and frequency of intercourse: Does the method lend itself to the "unplanned" coital episode often seen in this age group?
3. Number of partners/concerns of sexually transmitted disease: Is the patient adequately protected?
4. Cost/access to medical care: Can the patient afford the method on a long-term basis?
5. Motivation/self-discipline of patient and male partner: Will reluctance to interrupt foreplay result in nonuse of the method?

6. Safety/risk: Will short-term convenience result in long-term drawbacks?
7. Personal and family religious and ethical philosophy: Will it influence usage?

Methods

ABSTINENCE. Abstinence is the only 100% effective method of contraception. It should include abstinence from anything that would place an exposed male penis near the female introitus. It is usually defined, however, as refraining from vaginal or anal insertive sex. Abstinence programs focus on the delay of initiating sexual activity until adulthood/marriage. To date, evidence regarding the efficacy of such interventions in the reduction of sexual behaviors remains controversial.[89] About 26% of adolescent couples trying to abstain from intercourse will become pregnant within 1 year. This method requires a lot of support from peers, society, and family. The clinician should be supportive in the patient's use of abstinence and teach negotiation and planning skills for its effective and safe use.[90] Periodic abstinence can be associated with a high failure rate among adolescent patients.

CONDOMS. Condoms are an effective barrier method of contraception for the responsible adolescent couple who uses them regularly and properly. They are essential in decreasing the transfer of sexually transmitted infections. Condoms require availability and willingness of the male partner to use at time of intercourse. They do not require a physical examination or prescription. They should be used with all forms of contraception in the sexually active female. Female condoms are relatively new to the scene and cost more.

SPERMICIDES. Spermicides have a relatively high contraceptive failure rate when used alone and must be applied with each act of intercourse to be effective. If used consistently with male condoms, the birth control effectiveness approaches that of OCs. Spermicides consist of two agents: nonoxynol 9 and octoxynol 9, applied intravaginally in a variety of forms (gel, foam suppository, and film). The combination of spermicide and condoms is a very effective means of contraception for adolescents because it provides effective prevention of pregnancy and STDs, is available without a prescription, and is inexpensive.[85] However, compliance is a concern.

TABLE 56-7
BENEFITS OF ORAL CONTRACEPTIVES

Protection against
  Ovarian and endometrial cancer
  Ectopic pregnancy
  Ovarian cysts
  Iron-deficiency anemia
  Benign breast disease
Possible decreased risks of bacterial STDs progressing to
    pelvic inflammatory disease
Therapy for dysmenorrhea
Other noncontraceptive uses
  Regulation of menses
  Treatment of dysfunctional uterine bleeding
  Decreased risk of osteoporosis
  Treatment of acne

ORAL CONTRACEPTIVES. OCs are reliable and effective for the prevention of pregnancy, are available by prescription, and are the most popular method of contraception among adolescents.[91] Currently, three forms of OCs are available: the fixed-dose combination (each tablet contains the same dose of estrogen and progestin), the phasic dose (the triphasic and biphasic packs containing varying doses of estrogen and progestin), and the minipill (progestin only). The newest generation of birth control pills have a low dose of estrogen (20 to 35 μg), and new forms of progestin. The standard 28-day pack of pills (21 days of hormone and 7 days of placebo) continues to be widely and successfully used by adolescents and should be encouraged over the 21-day pack for promoting daily compliance.[91] Benefits of the use of combination oral contraceptives are listed in Table 56-7.

Breakthrough bleeding is the most common side effect and, though usually limited to the initial 2 to 3 months, may be an annoyance to the adolescent. Weight gain, nausea, and headaches may also be a problem. The proper use of OCs is associated with a failure rate of <1%. However, the failure rate among adolescents may be as high as 15% because of inconsistent use.[92,93] One study suggests that adolescents miss an average of three pills per month.[94]

To minimize side effects such as hirsutism and acne, it is good to use an oral contraceptive agent with minimal androgenic potency. The following list gives the progestins commonly found in combination oral contraceptives in increasing androgenic progestin potency[88]: gestodene, desogestrel, norgestimate, norethindrone, norethindrone acetate, norgestrel, and levonorgestrel.

Adolescent compliance with OC use is of major concern. There is much room for patient education and anticipatory guidance. Ideally, adolescents should receive a complete gynecologic examination by the health care provider before taking OCs. In some circumstances (such as when a patient shows anxiety), the pelvic examination may be deferred and OCs prescribed if the patient is healthy, not pregnant, and has no contraindications to taking the pills. Therefore, OCs can be prescribed by the practitioner and the adolescent can be referred for an examination and Pap smear within the next 3 months.[85]

MEDROXYPROGESTERONE ACETATE (DEPO-PROVERA). Compliance issues are minimized with the use of a long-acting intramuscular dose of medroxyprogesterone acetate. Requiring administration every 12 weeks works well for the adolescent who cannot remember to take pills each day. However, many adolescent patients report irregular bleeding initially, weight gain, mood changes, and headaches. This contraceptive method may be safely recommended for adolescents who have chronic illnesses (e.g., seizures and sickle-cell disease), are developmentally disabled, are lactating, or are at risk for complications with estrogen.[85]

LEVONORGESTREL IMPLANTS (NORPLANT SYSTEM). Levonorgestrel implants are a highly effective long-acting progestin contraceptive that provides pregnancy prevention for up to 5 years. This contraception may be indicated in adolescents who desire long-term spacing between births, want an extended length of protection, have a history of problems with OCs, or are already mothers.[87,95] The high initial cost, potential side effects (breakthrough bleeding, headaches), and the need to have an experienced health-care professional remove the implant may present barriers for the otherwise interested adolescent.

INTRAUTERINE DEVICES (IUDs). The multiple-partner "serial monogamy" nature of adolescent sexual relationships makes the IUD an inappropriate method of birth control. They should be reserved for adolescent females who cannot use other contraceptive methods and whose sexual behavior does not put them at risk for STDs.

DIAPHRAGM/CERVICAL CAP. The diaphragm and cervical cap are effective barrier methods of contraception that require use of spermicides and condoms. These contraceptive methods have limited usefulness in adolescents, as they require a prescription, a visit with a health-care professional for a fitting, and a motivated adolescent who is comfortable and skilled with insertion. Consistent, correct use is critical.[85]

RHYTHM/WITHDRAWAL. Rhythm/withdrawal is not recommended in this group since it requires self-control and fairly predictable menstrual cycles. It also provides no protection from sexually transmitted infections.

EMERGENCY CONTRACEPTION. The "morning after" pill should be reserved for emergency situations such as rape. Teenagers, however, often have unplanned coital encounters, and access to this method is important. The failure rate is about 1 to 2%. It is important to initiate treatment within 72 hours of unprotected intercourse. This method consists of the use of two doses of oral contraceptives, 12 hours apart. It is associated with some degree of nausea, vomiting, headaches, and dizziness. Effective treatment regimens include:[79]

Ovral	2 tablets followed by 2 tablets 12 hours later
Alesse	5 tablets followed by 5 tablets 12 hours later
Lo Ovral, Nordette, Levlen, Triphasil, Tri-Levlen	4 tablets followed by 4 tablets 12 hours later

It is important to document compliance with the method chosen at interval visits. An adolescent who is content with her contraceptive choice has a higher decree of protection from pregnancy. Protection from STDs is also important.

REFERENCES

1. Muram D. Pediatric and adolescent gynecology. In: Ransom SB, McNeeley Jr SG, eds. Gynecology for the primary care provider. Philadelphia: Saunders, 1997:247.
2. Muram D. Vaginoscopy. In Stovall T, Ling F, eds. Atlas of benign gynecologic surgery. London, Mosby-Wolf, 1994: 191.
3. Muram D. Pediatric and adolescent gynecology. In: Ransom SB, McNeeley Jr SG, eds. Gynecology for the primary care provider. Philadelphia: Saunders, 1997:250.
4. Rebar R. Puberty. In: Berek JS, Adashi EY, Hillard PA, eds. Novak's gynecology. 12th ed. Baltimore: Williams & Wilkins, 1996:771.

5. Kaplan SL, Grumbach MM, Aubert ML. The ontogenesis of pituitary hormones and hypothalamic factors in the human fetus: maturation of central nervous system regulation of anterior pituitary function. Recent Prog Horm Res 32:161;1976.

6. Burger HG, Yfamada Y, Bangah ML, McCloud PI, Warne GL. Serum gonadotropin, sex steroid, and immunoreactive inhibin levels in the first two years of life. J Clin Endocrinol Metab 1991;72:682.

7. Grumbach MM, Kablan SL. The neuroendocrinology of human puberty: an ontogenetic perspective. In: Grumbach MM, Sizonenko PC, Aubert ML, eds. Control of the onset of puberty. Baltimore: Williams & Wilkins, 1990:1.

8. Muram D. Pediatric and adolescent gynecology. In: Ransom SB, McNeeley Jr SG, eds. Gynecology for the primary care provider. Philadelphia: Saunders, 1997:267.

9. Yen SSC, Jaffe RB. Reproductive endocrinology: physiology, pathophysiology and clinical management. 4th ed. Philadelphia: Saunders, 1997:361.

10. Bridges NA, Christopher JA, Hindmarsh PC, Brook CGD. Sexual precocity, sex incidence and aetiology. Arch Dis Child 1994;70:116.

11. Speroff L, Glass RH, Kase NG. Clinical gynecologic endocrinology and infertility. 5th ed. Baltimore: Williams & Wilkins, 1994:371.

12. Yen SSC, Jaffe RB. Reproductive endocrinology: physiology, pathophysiology and clinical management. 4th ed. Philadelphia: Saunders,1997:361.

13. Yen SSC, Jaffe RB. Reproductive endocrinology: physiology, pathophysiology and clinical management. 4th ed. Philadelphia: Saunders, 1997:362.

14. Maxwell M, Karacostas D, Ellenbogen RG, Brzezinski A, Zervas NT, Black PM. Precocious puberty following head injury. J Neurosurg 1990;73:123.

15. Attie KM, Ramierez NR, Conte FA, Kaplan SL, Grumbach MM. The pubertal growth spurt in eight patients with true precocious puberty and growth hormone deficiency: evidence for a direct role of sex steroids. J Clin Endocrinol Metab 1990;71:975.

16. Speroff L, Glass RH, Kase NG. Clinical gynecologic endocrinology and infertility. 5th ed. Baltimore: Williams & Wilkins, 1994:373.

17. Lee PA, Van Dop C, Migeon CJ. McCune–Albright syndrome: long-term follow-up, JAMA 1986;256:290.

18. Comite F, Shawker TH, Pescovitz OH, Loriaux DL, Cutler Jr GB. Cyclical ovarian function resistant to treatment with an analogue of luteinizing hormone releasing hormone in McCune–Albright syndrome. N Engl J Med 1984;311:1032.

19. Speroff L, Glass RH, Kase NG. Clinical gynecologic endocrinology and infertility. 5th ed. Baltimore: Williams & Wilkins, 1994:376.

20. Milles JL, Stolley PD, Davies J, et al. Premature thelarche: natural history and etiologic investigation. Am J Dis Child 1981;135:743.

21. Muram D, Dewhurst J, Grant DB. Premature menarche: a follow-up study. Arch Dis Child 1984;59:77.

22. Muram D. Pediatric and adolescent gynecology. In: Ransom SB, McNeeley Jr SG, eds. Gynecology for the primary care provider. Philadelphia: Saunders, 1997:274.

23. Muram D, Dewhurst J, Grant DB, Premature menarche: a follow-up study. Arch Dis Child 1983;58:142.

24. Muram D. Pediatric and adolescent gynecology. In: Ransom SB, McNeeley Jr SG, eds. Gynecology for the primary care provider. Philadelphia: Saunders, 1997:274.

25. Speroff L, Glass RH, Kase NG. Clinical gynecologic endocrinology and infertility. 5th ed. Baltimore: Williams & Wilkins, 1994:382.

26. Holm IA. Ambiguous genitalia in the newborn. In: Emans SJ, Laufer MR, Goldstein DP, eds. Pediatric and adolescent gynecology. 4th ed. Philadelphia: Lippincott-Raven, 1998: 49.

27. Grunberger W, Fisch LF: Pediatric gynecological outpatient department: a report on 600 patients. Wien Klin Wochenschr 1982;94:614.

28. Muram D. Pediatric and adolescent gynecology. In: Decherney A, Pernol M, eds. Current gynecologic and obstetric diagnosis and treatment. Norwalk, CT: Appleton & Lange, 1994;633.

29. Muram D. Pediatric and adolescent gynecology. In: Ransom SB, McNeeley Jr SG, eds. Gynecology for the primary care provider. Philadelphia: Saunders, 1997:251.

30. Whittington WL, Rice RJ, Biddle JW, et al. Incorrect identification of *Neisseria gonorrhoeae* from infants and children. Pediatr Infect Dis J 1988;7:3.

31. Hammerschlag M. Pitfalls in the diagnosis of sexually transmitted diseases in children. The Advisor, American Professional Society on the Abuse of Children (APSAC). 1989:4.

32. Emans SJ. Sexually transmitted diseases: gonorrhea, chlamydia trachomatis, pelvic inflammatory disease, and syphilis. In: Emans SJ, Laufer MR, Goldstein DP, eds. Pediatric and adolescent gynecology. 4th ed. Philadelphia: Lippincott-Raven, 1998:469.

33. Rettig PJ, Nelson JD. Genital tract infection with *Chlamydia trachomatis* in prepubertal children. J Pediatr 1981; 99:206.

34. Schachter J, Grossman M, Holt J. Infection with *Chlamydia trachomatis:* Involvement of multiple anatomic sites in neonates. J Infect Dis 1979;139:232.

35. Alexander ER. Maternal and infant sexually transmitted diseases. Urol Clin N Am 1984;11:131.

36. Muram D. Pediatric and adolescent gynecology. In: Ransom SB, McNeeley Jr SG, eds. Gynecology for the primary care provider. Philadelphia: Saunders, 1997:253.

37. Emans SJ. Sexually transmitted diseases: gonorrhea, chlamydia trachomatis, pelvic inflammatory disease, and syphilis. In: Emans SJ, Laufer MR, Goldstein DP, eds. Pediatric and adolescent gynecology. 4th ed. Philadelphia: Lippincott-Raven, 1998:490.

38. Dorfman DH, Glaser JH. Congenital syphilis presenting in infants after the newborn period. N Engl J Med 1990; 323:1299.

39. Centers for Disease Control. Sexually transmitted diseases treatment guidelines. MMWR 1993;42(RR-14):1.

40. Corey L. Genital herpes. In: Holmes KK, ed. Sexually transmitted diseases. New York: McGraw-Hill, 1990:391.

41. Gardner M, Jones J. Genital herpes acquired by sexual abuse of children. J Pediatr 1984;104:243.

42. Miller RG, Whittington WL, Coleman RM, et al. Acquisition of concomitant oral and genital infection with herpes simplex virus type 2. Sex Transm Dis 1987;14:41.

43. Sweet RL, Gibbs RS. Perinatal infections. In: Sweet RL, Gibbs RS, eds. Infectious diseases of the female genital tract. Baltimore: Williams & Wilkins, 1990:290.

44. Sweet RL, Gibbs RS. Perinatal infections. In: Sweet RL, Gibbs RS, eds. Infectious diseases of the female genital tract. Baltimore: Williams & Wilkins, 1990:144.

45. Bender ME. New concepts of condyloma acuminata in children. Arch Dermatol 1986;122:1121.

46. Hanson RM, Glasson M, McCrossin I, et al. Anogenital warts in childhood. Child Abuse Negl 1989;13:225.

47. DeJong AR, Weiss JC, Brent RL. Condyloma acuminata in children. Am J Dis Child 1982;136:704.

48. Herman-Giddens ME, Gutman LT, Berson NL. Association of coexisting vaginal infections and multiple abusers in female children with genital warts. Sex Transm Dis 1988;6:63.

49. Gale C, Muram D. The surgical treatment of condyloma acuminata in children. Adolesc Pediatr Gynecol 1990; 3;189.

50. Droegemueller W. Infections of the lower genital tract. In: Mishell DR, Stenchever MA, Droegemueller W, Herbst AL, eds. Comprehensive gynecology. 3rd ed. St. Louis: Mosby-Year Book, 1997:608.

51. Droegemueller W. Infections of the lower genital tract. In: Mishell DR, Stenchever MA, Droegemueller W, Herbst AL, eds. Comprehensive gynecology. 3rd ed. St. Louis: Mosby-Year Book, 1997:607.

52. Emans SJ. Vulvovaginal complaints in the adolescent. In: Emans SJ, Laufer MR, Goldstein DP, eds. Pediatric and adolescent gynecology. 4th ed. Philadelphia: Lippincott-Raven, 1998:431.

53. Emans SJ. Vulvovaginal complaints in the adolescent. In: Emans SJ, Laufer MR, Goldstein DP, eds. Pediatric and adolescent gynecology. 4th ed. Philadelphia: Lippincott-Raven, 1998:447.

54. Muram D. Pediatric and adolescent gynecology. In: Ransom SB, McNeeley Jr SG, eds. Gynecology for the primary care provider. Philadelphia: Saunders, 1997:252.

55. Emans SJ. Vulvovaginal problems in the prepubertal child. In: Emans SJ, Laufer MR, Goldstein DP, eds. Pediatric and adolescent gynecology. 4th ed. Philadelphia: Lippincott-Raven, 1998:90.

56. Droegemueller W. Benign gynecologic lesions. In: Mishell DR, Stenchever MA, Droegemueller W, Herbst AL, eds. Comprehensive gynecology. 3rd ed. St. Louis: Mosby-Year Book, 1997:476.

57. Droegemueller W. Benign gynecologic lesions. In: Mishell DR, Stenchever MA, Droegemueller W, Herbst AL, eds. Comprehensive gynecology. 3rd ed. St. Louis: Mosby-Year Book, 1997:475.

58. Droegemueller W. Benign gynecologic lesions. In: Mishell DR, Stenchever MA, Droegemueller W, Herbst AL, eds. Comprehensive gynecology. 3rd ed. St. Louis: Mosby-Year Book, 1997:475.

59. Droegemueller W. Pediatric gynecology. In: Mishell DR, Stenchever MA, Droegemueller W, Herbst AL, eds. Comprehensive gynecology. 3rd ed. St. Louis: Mosby-Year Book, 1997:268.

60. Muram D, Elias S. The treatment of labial adhesion in prepubertal girls. Surg Forum 1988;34:464.

61. Capraro VJ, Bayonet-Rivera NP, Magosas I. Vulvar tumor

62. Mercer LJ, Mueller CM, Hajj SN. Medical treatment of urethral prolapse. Adolesc Pediatr Gynecol 1988;1:182.

63. Muram D. Vaginal bleeding in children and adolescents. Obstet Gynecol Clin North Am 1990;17:389.

64. Laufer MR, Goldstein DP. Dysmenorrhea, pelvic pain, and the premenstrual syndrome. In: Emans SJ, Laufer MR, Goldstein DP, eds. Pediatric and adolescent gynecology. 4th ed. Philadelphia: Lippincott-Raven, 1998:373

65. Scherzer WJ, McClamrock H. Amenorrhea. In: Berek JS, Adashi EY, Hillard PA, eds. Novak's gynecology. 12th ed. Baltimore: Williams & Wilkins, 1996:809.

66. Claessens EA, Cowell CA. Acute adolescent menorrhagia. Am J Obstet Gynecol 1981;139:277.

67. Arvidsson B, Ekenved G, Rybo G, et al. Iron prophylaxis in menorrhagia. Acta Obstet Gynaecol Scand 1981; 60:157.

68. DeVore GR, Owens O, Kase N. Use of intravenous Premarin in the treatment of dysfunctional bleeding—a double-blind randomized control study. Obstet Gynecol 1982;59:285.

69. Southam AL, Richart RM. The prognosis for adolescents with menstrual abnormality. Am J Obstet Gynecol 1966;94:637.

70. Goldstein DP, Laufer MR. Benign and malignant ovarian masses. In: Emans SJ, Laufer MR, Goldstein DP, eds. Pediatric and adolescent gynecology. 4th ed. Philadelphia: Lippincott-Raven, 1998:553.

71. Muram D. Pediatric and adolescent gynecology. In: Ransom SB, McNeeley Jr SG, eds. Gynecology for the primary care provider. Philadelphia: Saunders, 1997:258.

72. Muram D. Child sexual abuse. In: Sanfilippo JS, Muram D, Lee RA, Dewhurst J, eds. Pediatric and adolescent gynecology. Philadelphia: Saunders, 1994:365.

73. Kemp C. Sexual abuse, another hidden pediatric problem. Pediatrics 1978;62:382.

74. Sgroi SM. Sexual molestation of children: the last frontier in child abuse. Child Today 1975;4:18.

75. National Center on Child Abuse and Neglect. Child sexual abuse: incest, assault and exploitation. Special report. Washington, DC: Department of Health, Education, and Welfare, Children's Bureau, August 1978.

76. Muram D. Child sexual abuse: relationships between sexual acts and genital findings. Child Abuse Negl 1989; 13:211.

77. Center for Population Options. Henshaw SK, van Vort J. Research note: teenage abortion, birth and pregnancy statistics: an update. Fam Plann Perspect 1989;March/April.

78. American College of Obstetricians and Gynecologists. Adolescent pregnancy, 2nd ed. The American College of Obstetricians and Gynecologists: Washington, DC, 1992.

79. Darney PD. Adolescent contraception in the new millennium. Alvin F. Goldfarb Lectureship: issues and answers in pediatric and adolescent gynecology, Atlanta, GA, April 2000.

80. March of Dimes Birth Defects Foundation Fact Sheet. White Plains, NY: March of Dimes Birth Defect Foundation, 1991.

81. Sanfilippo J. Adolescents and oral contraceptives. Int J Fertil 1991;36(Supp 2):65.

in children due to prolapse of urethral mucosa. Am J Obstet Gynecol 1970;108:572.

82. Chilman CS. Adolescent sexuality in a changing American society. 2nd ed. New York: Wiley, 1983.

83. Hayes CD, ed. Risking the future. Washington, DC: National Academy Press, 1987.

84. Risk and responsibility: teaching sex education in America's schools today. New York: The Alan Guttmacher Institute, 1989.

85. AAP Policy Statement—contraception and adolescents. Pediatrics 1999;104;1161.

86. Howard M, Mitchell M. Preventing teenage pregnancy. Pediatr Ann 1993;22:109.

87. Beach RK. Contraception for adolescents: part 1. Adolescent Health Update 1994;7:1

88. Slupik R. Contraception. In: Sanfilippo JS, Muram D, Lee PA, Dewhurst J, eds. Pediatric and adolescent gynecology. Philadelphia: Saunders, 1994:289.

89. Kirby D. No easy answers: research findings on programs to reduce teen pregnancy. Washington DC: The National Campaign to Prevent Teen Pregnancy, 1999.

90. Hatcher RA, Trussel J, Stewart F, et al. Contraceptive technology. 17th ed. New York: Ardent Media, 1998:299.

91. Piccinino L, Mosher W. Trends in contraception in the United States—1982-1985. Fam Plann Perspect 1998;30:46.

92. Trussell J, Hatcher RA, Cates Jr W, Stewart FH, Kost K. Contraceptive failure in the United States: an update. Stud Fam Plann 1990;21:51.

93. Jones EF, Forrest JD. Contraceptive failure rates based on the 1988 NSFG. Fam Plann Perspect 1992;24:12.

94. Blassone ML. Risk of contraceptive discontinuation among adolescents. J Adolesc Health Care 1989;10:527.

95. Grimes DA, ed. Contraception and adolescents: highlights from the NASPAG conference. Contraception Rep 1995;6:4.

Chapter 57

Ectopic Pregnancy

Gary H. Lipscomb

Five Key Points

- In pregnancies less than 41 days of gestation, a serum hCG rise of less than 50% every 48 hours is highly predictive of a non-viable gestation.

- The presence of a complex adnexal mass in a patient with hCG levels <2000 mIU/mL cannot be assumed to be an ectopic pregnancy.

- In single-dose methotrexate protocols, the serum hCG on days 4 and 7 are used to decide on repeat dosing.

- An initial serum hCG level at the time of methotrexate treatment >15,000 mIU/mL is associated with marked increase in failure rates.

- Patients treated with tubal-conserving surgical procedures should be followed with weekly hCG levels until persistent trophoblastic disease can be excluded.

In the United States, the incidence of ectopic pregnancies has increased dramatically during the past several decades. In 1948, the incidence of ectopic pregnancy was reported as 0.37 %.[1] Today the incidence of ectopic pregnancy as reported by the Centers For Disease Control and Prevention (CDC) is 1.9%.[2] There has been an almost fivefold increase in ectopic pregnancy since 1970, the first year accurate statistics were compiled by the CDC.[2] Fortunately, during the same time frame, deaths from ectopic pregnancy declined almost tenfold.

RISK FACTORS

Probably the most important factor responsible for the dramatic rise in ectopic pregnancy has been the increase in pelvic inflammatory disease (PID). However, numerous other risk factors for ectopic pregnancy, including previous tubal surgery, use of intrauterine contraceptive devices (IUDs), previous ectopic pregnancy, in vitro fertilization, use of progestin-containing contraceptives, smoking, previous abdominal surgery, and induced abortion have been identified. Several studies have attempted to better define the relative contribution of these risk factors in the development of ectopic pregnancy.

Using a population-based case–control study, Marchbanks et al. evaluated the association between ectopic pregnancy and 22 potential risk factors.[3] Nine variables associated with a significantly increased relative risk of ectopic pregnancy were initially identified. After conditional logistic regression, four variables remained as strong and independent risk factors:

1. Current IUD use
2. History of infertility
3. Prior PID
4. Prior tubal surgery (tubal sterilization, tuboplasty, or salpingectomy)

After simultaneously adjusting for the above factors, an increased risk for four other factors (previous abdominal/pelvic surgery, prior appendicitis, induced abortion, and in utero exposure to diethylstilbestrol [DES]) remained. However, the increased risk of these last four factors did not reach statistically significant levels.

In 1996, Ankum et al. reported a meta-analysis of all case–control and cohort studies published in the English literature between 1978 and 1994.[4] Previous ectopic pregnancy, previous tubal surgery, documented tubal pathology, and in utero exposure to DES were found to be strongly associated with the occurrence of ectopic pregnancy. Previous genital infection (PID, gonorrhea, and chlamydia infection), infertility, and lifetime number of sexual partners >1 were associated with a mildly increased risk.

Both of these studies confirm older previous studies showing that the risk for development of an ectopic pregnancy is increased by any agent that in some way slows or prevents the fertilized embryo from reaching the reaching the uterus. Patients with histories of such risk factors, particularly those strongly associated with ectopic pregnancy such as prior ectopic pregnancy or tubal surgery, should be screened early in pregnancy using the diagnostic methods described later in this chapter.

SIGNS AND SYMPTOMS

The classic triad of pain, vaginal bleeding, and amenorrhea still remains as the most common presenting symptoms seen with an ectopic pregnancy.[5] In the older literature, abdominal pain was reported to occur in 90 to 100% of ectopic pregnancies. Early in the course of tubal pregnancies this pain is probably due to tubal stretching, as it frequently begins many days in advance of actual tubal rupture. Other symptoms reported in association with ectopic pregnancy were dizziness, pregnancy symptoms, and vaginal passage of tissue.

The most common finding on physical examination remains adnexal tenderness. Classically this finding has been reported to occur in 75 to 90% of symptomatic patients.[5] An adnexal mass has also been described in approximately 50% of patients with an ectopic pregnancy. However, 20% of such masses are on the side opposite the ectopic pregnancy and probably represents a corpus luteum cyst. Other classic signs associated with ectopic pregnancy were abdominal tenderness, uterine enlargement, and orthostatic changes.

While these classical signs and symptoms still serve as useful indicators of possible ectopic pregnancy, it must be remembered that before the development of reliable and accurate techniques for evaluating patients with risk factors or minimal symptoms of ectopic pregnancy, most ectopic pregnancies were not diagnosed prior to tubal rupture. Thus, many of these signs and symptoms are associated with advanced or ruptured ectopic pregnancies that are frequently not amenable to conservative surgical or medical treatment. Ideally, pregnant patients with risk factors or minimal symptoms suggestive of possible ectopic pregnancy should be identified and screened for this diagnosis prior to development of overt indicators of tubal rupture.

DIAGNOSIS

The continued decrease in the death rate from ectopic pregnancy despite its rapidly increasing incidence appears to be the result of earlier detection and treatment rather than advances in operative management. Earlier detection has been made possible by more sensitive and specific radioimmunoassays for the β-subunit of human chorionic gonadotropin (hCG), and serum progesterone, as well as development of high-resolution transvaginal sonography and the widespread availability of laparoscopy.

Diagnostic algorithms using these tests have been developed to simplify the management of suspected ectopic pregnancies. As the sensitivity and specificity of the available diagnostic tests have increased, the need for laparoscopy to confirm the diagnosis has decreased. A nonlaparoscopic algorithm originally developed by Stovall et al has proven to be 100% accurate in a randomized clinical trial.[6] The updated version of this algorithm currently in use at the University of Tennessee, Memphis, is presented in Figure 57-1. The use of each of the diagnostic methods in this algorithm will be discussed in detail in the following section. Several other classic diagnostic tests not used in this algorithm along with the rationale for their exclusion will also be discussed.

At the University of Tennessee, patients presenting with mild pain or vaginal spotting are first screened with a quantitative hCG level and a serum progesterone. Patients with hCG levels ≥50,000 mIU/ml or a serum progesterone ≥25 ng/ml do not undergo further diagnostic evaluation unless they are at high risk for ectopic pregnancy. Common high-risk factors are previous ectopic pregnancy, previous tubal ligation or tubal surgery, or IUD currently in place.

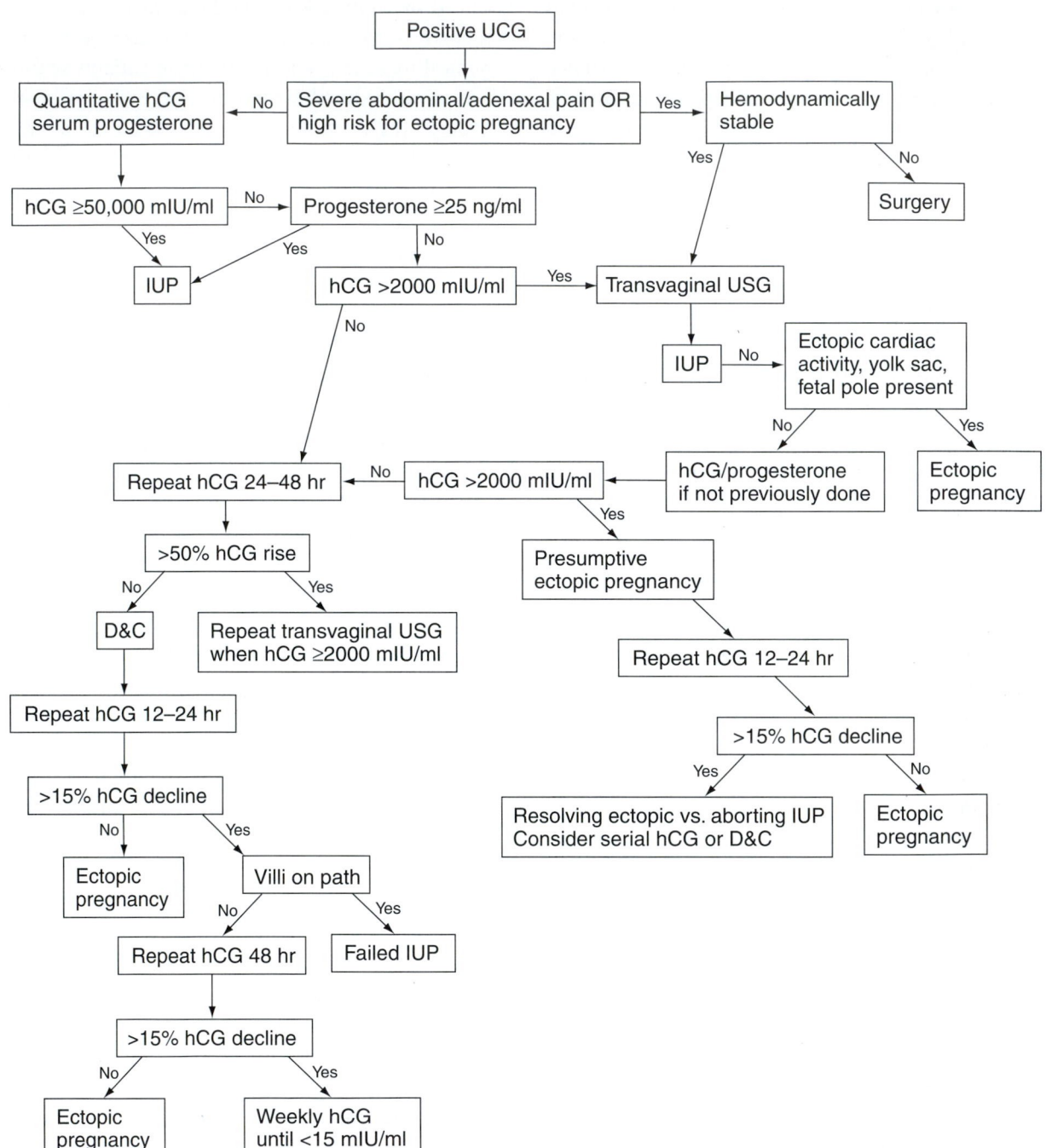

Figure 57-1 Diagnostic and treatment algorithm for ectopic pregnancy.

Human Chorionic Gonadotropin

In the past, the sensitivity of available pregnancy tests was such that only a positive test was useful. Biologic and immunologic tests were frequently not readily available in the mid-1970s and could require 24 hours or more to perform and could detect hCG only at levels of 1500 mIU/ml or greater. Using these tests, only 50% of ectopic pregnancies had a positive pregnancy test.[7]

The development of rapid, extremely sensitive enzyme-linked immunosorbent assay (ELISA) pregnancy tests has simplified the diagnosis of ectopic pregnancy. Currently available quantitative assays can be performed in minutes and will detect hCG at levels of 20 to 50 mIU/ml. Using these ELISA tests, hCG can be detected in first-voided maternal urine by day 21 of the menstrual cycle.[8] Prior to the development of ELISA pregnancy tests, the low sensitivity of available urine pregnancy tests made them unreliable with dilute urine specimens. However, the increased sensitivity of the ELISA urine pregnancy test should detect all but the earliest pregnancy without the need for a first-voided concentrated urine specimen. Likewise, these tests can be used as an initial screening test for pregnancy in patients presenting with symptoms consistent with ectopic pregnancy as all symptomatic ectopic pregnancies should have sufficiently high hCG levels to produce a positive urine test.

Quantitative hCG levels play a pivotal role in diagnosing the suspected ectopic pregnancy and allow for proper interpretation of the other diagnostic methods. Quantitative hCG levels are used not only to determine pregnancy viability but to confirm when an intrauterine pregnancy should be visible on transvaginal ultrasound. Unfortunately, in the past several different standards have been used to reference hCG. Currently, all modern laboratories report hCG levels standardized to the 1st International Reference Preparation (1st IRP). The 1st IRP was also previously referred to as the 3rd International Standard. Previous standards included the 1st and 2nd International Standard (IS). Clinicians should be aware that hCG levels referenced to different standards are not equivalent and that the reference standard is frequently not identified in much of the older literature. While the varying sensitivities to the α- and β-subunits make direct correlation between the different standards difficult, hCG levels referenced to the 1st IRP are approximately twice those of levels referenced to the 2nd IS. All hCG levels in this chapter are referenced to the 1st IRP unless otherwise stated.

Using radioimmunoassay methods, serum levels of hCG can be quantified down to 2 mIU/ml. The development of monoclonal antibodies to the entire hCG molecule has also reduced cross-reactivity to other hormones that share the same α-subunit (luteinizing hormone [LH], follicle-stimulating hormone [FSH], and thyroid-stimulating hormone [TSH]). Using these assays, hCG can be detected in maternal serum as early as 8 days after the LH surge. In intrauterine pregnancies, hCG levels rise in a curvilinear fashion until they plateau at approximately 100,000 mIU. However, the rise in hCG titers is essentially linear prior to 41 days of gestation.[9] Because of this linearity, the rate of hCG doubling can be used to assess viability of a pregnancy.

The mean doubling time for serum hCG in a normal intrauterine pregnancy (IUP) is 48 hours.[9-13] However, in patients with an ectopic pregnancy, the hCG will typically rise at a much slower rate. Based on studies of doubling times, serum level hCG will rise by at least 66% in 48 hours in 85% of normal pregnancies (1 SD from the mean).[10,12,13] Thus, 15% of normal IUPs will have rises less than this in 48 hours. A rise of less than 50% in 48 hours is more than 3 SD from the mean and would be associated with a nonviable pregnancy 99.9% of the time. However, this only indicates a nonviable pregnancy and is not indicative of whether the pregnancy is intrauterine or extrauterine. Since the interassay variability of hCG is 10 to 15%, a rise or fall of less than this is considered to be a plateau. Plateaued levels are the most predictive of ectopic pregnancy.

These doubling times apply only to early IUPs at less than 41 days of gestation. Although the rise in hCG remains linear with advancing age beyond 41 days, the doubling time increases progressively. While a normal 48-hour hCG rise for gestations less than 41 days is 103%, this rise falls to 33% for 41-to-57-day gestations and 5% for 57-to-65-day gestations.[9] Fortunately, all normal IUPs should reach the discriminatory zone for both transvaginal and transabdominal ultrasound prior to 41 days of gestation.

hCG levels $\geq$50,000 are rarely ($<$0.1%) associated with an ectopic pregnancy, thus the rationale for using this level as a cutoff for screening purposes. At hCG levels of $\geq$2000 mIU/ml, transvaginal ultrasound should visualize an intrauterine sac in all normal IUPs.[14] Patients with an abnormal rise in hCG (<50% in 48 hours) or plateaued levels (±15%) may undergo dilation and curettage (D&C) without fear of interrupting an ongoing viable intrauterine pregnancy. A plateaued or rising level after D&C indicates the presence of persistent trophoblastic tissue, usually an ectopic pregnancy.

Serum Progesterone

Historically, serum progesterone levels have been proposed as both a screening tool to identify patients with potential ectopic pregnancies, and to determine candidates for D&C to rule out ectopic pregnancy. Unfortunately, while preliminary studies suggested that all ectopic pregnancies were associated with serum progesterone levels below certain threshold levels, later studies have shown considerable overlap in progesterone values for viable IUPs, failed IUPs, and ectopic pregnancies. [15-18] While these data invalidated serum progesterone levels for the definitive diagnosis of an ectopic pregnancy, the authors of these studies suggested certain threshold levels for serum progesterone that could be used as part of a screening program for ectopic pregnancies.

Since only 1 to 2% of abnormal pregnancies (abortions or ectopic pregnancies) in the previously mentioned studies were associated with a progesterone level ≥25 ng/ml, this level has been used as the cutoff level in the current screening program. When ectopic pregnancies are associated with serum progesterone levels ≥25 ng/ml, it generally indicates a vigorous pregnancy that frequently exhibits cardiac activity on transvaginal ultrasound.

In earlier studies, a serum progesterone less than 6.5 ng/ml was always associated with a nonviable pregnancy, but did not indicate whether the failed pregnancy was intrauterine or ectopic. Since this progesterone level was considered diagnostic of a failed pregnancy, D&C to document the failed IUP could then be performed without fear of interrupting a viable pregnancy. This threshold level for pregnancy viability was subsequently lowered to 5 ng/ml and in 1996 two viable pregnancies with serum progesterones of 3.9 ng/ml were reported.[19] Thus, progesterone levels >5 ng/ml cannot be considered definitive proof of a failed pregnancy. However, progesterone levels <5 ng/ml are associated with a viable pregnancy in only 0.16% of cases.[19] Because of the extremely low probability of a viable pregnancy when

the serum progesterone is <5 ng/ml, D&C can be performed with minimal chance of interrupting a viable pregnancy. When coupled with abnormally rising hCG levels, the diagnosis of a failed pregnancy is essentially 100%.

Unfortunately, the turnaround time for serum progesterone levels in many laboratories may exceed several days. Unless results can be obtained within 24 hours, this test is of limited usefulness. In these circumstances, other screening and diagnostic tools, primarily hCG levels and ultrasound, must be used to diagnose the early unruptured ectopic pregnancy.

Transvaginal Ultrasound

Transvaginal ultrasound permits identification of an IUP at much lower hCG titers than is possible with transabdominal scanning. While an IUP will be apparent at hCG levels of 6000 to 6500 mIU/ml with transabdominal ultrasound scanning, an experienced transvaginal sonographer should always visualize a viable IUP at an hCG titer of 2000 mIU/ml.[14,20] However, the minimal hCG titer at which an intrauterine gestational sac should always be seen is not known, and thus each institution must develop its own lower limits for transvaginal detection of an IUP.

Identification of an intrauterine gestational sac by ultrasound essentially excludes an ectopic pregnancy, as the earliest sonographic finding of an IUP is a gestational sac. However, intrauterine fluid accumulations may produce a pseudosac, which may be falsely interpreted as a true gestational sac. Failing IUPs may also appear sonographically as a pseudosac. Prior to development of a yolk sac, the double decidual sac sign (two concentric echogenic rings separated by a hypoechoic space) is the best method to differentiate a true intrauterine sac from a pseudosac.

The addition of color Doppler to transvaginal sonography can help differentiate among a completed abortion, an incomplete abortion, and an early IUP before visualization of a gestational sac. Vaginal ultrasound can also accurately image oviducts and ovaries such that ectopic pregnancies and their dimensions can be defined.

The size of an identified ectopic pregnancy or the presence of ectopic cardiac activity is frequently used as a criterion for possible medical therapy. Typical size criteria for medical therapy range from 2 to 4 cm. In the protocol used at the University of Tennessee, ectopic pregnancies >4 cm in greatest dimension, or the presence of adnexal cardiac activity in ectopic pregnancies >3.5 cm, are both relative contraindications to methotrexate therapy. When determining candidates for methotrexate therapy in our protocol, only the gestational mass or sac size is considered, and not the overall size of the hematosalpinx or hematoma. If the gestational mass cannot be distinguished from the surrounding hematoma, then the size of the entire mass must be used. Since ectopic pregnancies are generally associated with lower hCG levels than IUPs of similar gestational age, they can often be visualized by transvaginal ultrasound at far lower hCG levels than an IUP. However, the finding of an adnexal mass in a patient with a presumed ectopic pregnancy and hCG levels <2000 mIU/ml should not automatically be assumed to be an ectopic pregnancy without the presence of a yolk sac, fetal pole or cardiac activity. Frequently such masses are, in reality, corpus luteum cysts associated with an early IUP.

In patients with hCG >2000 mIU/ml and no documented IUP by transvaginal ultrasound, a repeat hCG in 12 to 24 hours is recommended. This is particularly important in patients with a history of heavy vaginal bleeding, as a rapidly falling hCG may indicate a completed abortion. Such patients should be followed with serial hCG levels rather than using medical or surgical therapy. Because some of these patients may actually have resolving ectopic pregnancies, some clinicians may feel more comfortable treating these patients in a more aggressive manner rather than with observation. A more detailed description of observation as treatment for selected ectopic pregnancies is detailed later in this chapter.

Dilation and Curettage

With technical advances in ultrasound the differentiation between an ectopic and a failed intrauterine pregnancy at increasingly earlier gestations often eliminates the need for D&C. Nevertheless, D&C still plays an important role in the diagnosis of ectopic pregnancies with hCG levels below the ultrasound discriminatory zone. Except in the rare case of heterotopic pregnancy, the identification of chorionic villi in uterine contents obtained by curettage or from spontaneous passage essentially eliminates the diagnosis of ectopic pregnancy. The use of D&C also avoids giving methotrexate unnecessarily to a patient with a failed IUP.

The appropriate use of hCG doubling times and serum progesterone levels prior to D&C is necessary to avoid the possibility of interrupting a viable IUP. Patients with minimally falling hCG titers (<15% change) or a hCG rise of <50% in 48 hours should undergo D&C to differentiate between a failed IUP and an ectopic pregnancy. Since final histologic pathology may not be available for several days, hCG titers are followed postoperatively to avoid significant delays in diagnosis. As noted in the ectopic algorithm (Figure 57-1), a serum hCG drawn at the time of D&C is followed by a repeat measurement in 12 to 24 hours. Rising or inappropriately falling levels (<15% fall) after D&C are considered diagnostic of an ectopic pregnancy.

D&C, with its potential surgical morbidity and cost, can usually be avoided in patients with appropriately falling hCG titers. Most patients with falling hCG titers represent a resolving failed IUP, although a small number represent a spontaneously resolving ectopic pregnancy. Since the treatment protocol is essentially the same for spontaneously resolving ectopic pregnancies and as for resolving failed IUPs, D&C serves little purpose in these patients. However, since the actual success rate for expectant management is less certain than with other treatment options, many clinicians still prefer to perform a D&C to verify a failed IUP in these situations. Unfortunately, villi will be absent on final histology in up to 20% of these cases.[21] Since only the presence of villi is diagnostic, those without villi will still require serial HCG titers.

Laparoscopy

Laparoscopy remains the gold standard for the diagnosis of ectopic pregnancy. However, with the development of diagnostic algorithms that do not require the use of laparoscopy, laparoscopy may become a surgical method rather than a diagnostic tool. As one eliminates laparoscopy, the risks, costs, and morbidity associated with diagnosis and treatment of the ectopic pregnancy are decreased.

Culdocentesis

Culdocentesis has been widely used in the diagnosis of ectopic pregnancy. In the older literature, approximately 70 to 83% of all ectopic pregnancies had nonclotting blood (positive test) on culdocentesis.[22-24] Interestingly, 50 to 62% of these patients with positive culdocentesis were found to have an unruptured fallopian tube. Only serous fluid (negative culdocentesis) or no fluid/clotting blood (nondiagnostic culdocentesis) was found in 10 to 20% of ectopic pregnancies. False positive results were obtained in 2 to 3% of these culdocenteses. With modern diagnostic techniques, ectopic pregnancies are generally diagnosed far earlier than the ectopic pregnancies represented in these studies. Since these ectopic pregnancies were frequently ruptured or of advanced gestation at the time culdocentesis was performed, it is uncertain what proportion of ectopic pregnancies diagnosed today would have positive culdocentesis. Nor is it clear what percentage of these positive culdocenteses would have unruptured fallopian tubes.

Historically, culdocentesis was used to decide whether to perform a laparotomy for treatment of an ectopic pregnancy or other source of bleeding—i.e., blood was found—or to proceed with diagnostic laparoscopy to obtain a definitive diagnosis. With new instrumentation, laparoscopy is now a viable treatment option even in the presence of hematoperitoneum. As a result, culdocentesis offers little clinical utility when considering diagnostic and therapeutic options for ectopic pregnancy.

TREATMENT OPTIONS FOR ECTOPIC PREGNANCY

Prior to the development of surgical treatment options, mortality for presumed ectopic pregnancy was reported to be 67%.[25] In 1884, Tait reported a series of five patients treated with salpingectomy and subsequently reported a mortality of only 5%.[26] In 1887, the first case report of a tubal pregnancy removed by opening the tube, removing the trophoblastic tissue, and suturing the tubal incision was published by Martin in the German literature.[27] However, salpingectomy remained the treatment of choice for almost a century after this report. In fact, it was not until 1953 that a similar procedure was reported in the English literature by Strome.[28] Even today salpingectomy remains the most commonly performed procedure for ectopic pregnancies in many areas of the United States.

In the early 1970s laparoscopy became available for the diagnosis of ectopic pregnancy. Initially, the laparoscope was used only to diagnose a patient with an ectopic pregnancy before committing to a laparotomy, but in 1973, Shapiro and Adler reported the first laparoscopic salpingectomy for the treatment of an ectopic pregnancy.[29] In the 1980s, Bruhat and DeCherney along with their associates published their experiences with the performance of laparoscopic salpingostomies as treatment for ectopic pregnancy.[30,31]

Medical management with drugs such as methotrexate to avoid the need for surgical intervention are the most recent development in the treatment of ectopic pregnancy. Although initial protocols required prolonged hospitalization, and multiple doses of methotrexate were associated with significant side effects, current protocols are performed on an outpatient basis, frequently require only one dose of methotrexate, and are associated with minimal side effects.

Research also continues with agents such as potassium chloride, hyperosmolar glucose, dactinomycin, prostaglandins and RU 486 for the medical management of ectopic pregnancy. These agents may be given by direct injection into the ectopic sac, or in the case of dactinomycin, prostaglandins, and RU 486, given systemically by oral, intramuscular, or intravenous routes. However, due to the limited experience with these agents, their use cannot be recommended until further data are available.

The various surgical and medical treatment options for ectopic pregnancy are all effective, and the most appropriate option for any particular patient depends on the clinical circumstance, the experiences of the physician, and the wishes of the patient. Each of the treatment options will be discussed in detail below.

Surgical Therapy for Ectopic Pregnancy

Techniques for surgical treatment of tubal ectopic pregnancy include salpingectomy, partial salpingectomy, linear salpingostomy, linear salpingotomy, and fimbrial expression.

Salpingectomy

For patients who do not wish future fertility, removal of the entire fallopian tube (salpingectomy) with the ectopic pregnancy is generally the surgical treatment of choice. This procedure may also be appropriate in patients with a previous ectopic pregnancy in the same tube or with an extensively damaged tube.

Salpingectomy at the time of laparotomy is easily performed by placing clamps across the tubal mesosalpinx and removing the fallopian tube. In the past, removal of a portion of the interstitial segment of the tube (cornual resection) was also recommended. Some surgeons further advised suturing the round ligament to the posterior surface of the uterus (modified Coffey suspension) to cover the peritoneal defect produced by cornual resection. However, data to document the occurrence of a significant number of pregnancies in the tubal stump when cornual resection is not performed are lacking. Furthermore, deep resection of the cornu may predispose to uterine rupture with subsequent IUP. As a result, cornual resection is not routinely performed by most gynecologists.

Salpingectomy may also be performed with the use of a laparoscope. The proposed benefits of laparoscopic treatment over laparotomy include avoidance of laparotomy, decreased pain, shorter convalescence, and lower cost.[32] Laparoscopic salpingectomy may be

performed using electrosurgery, pre-tied sutures, mechanical stapling devices, or combinations thereof. One technique for laparoscopic salpingectomy is illustrated in Figure 57-2.

In the past, the performance of a "paradoxical" oophorectomy was recommended at the same time as a salpingectomy for the treatment of a tubal pregnancy.[33] In theory, ovulation would always occur on the side of the remaining tube rather than allow an ovary to function on a side where there was not a fallopian tube in close proximity, thus increasing the chance of conception. However, conception rates appear to be identical for patients treated with salpingectomy versus salpingo-oophorectomy.[34] Other arguments against this practice include the possibility of future loss of the one remaining ovary to other disease processes as well as the conservation of both ovaries to serve as sources of oocytes if in vitro fertilization techniques are required for future pregnancy. Thus, few authorities currently recommend

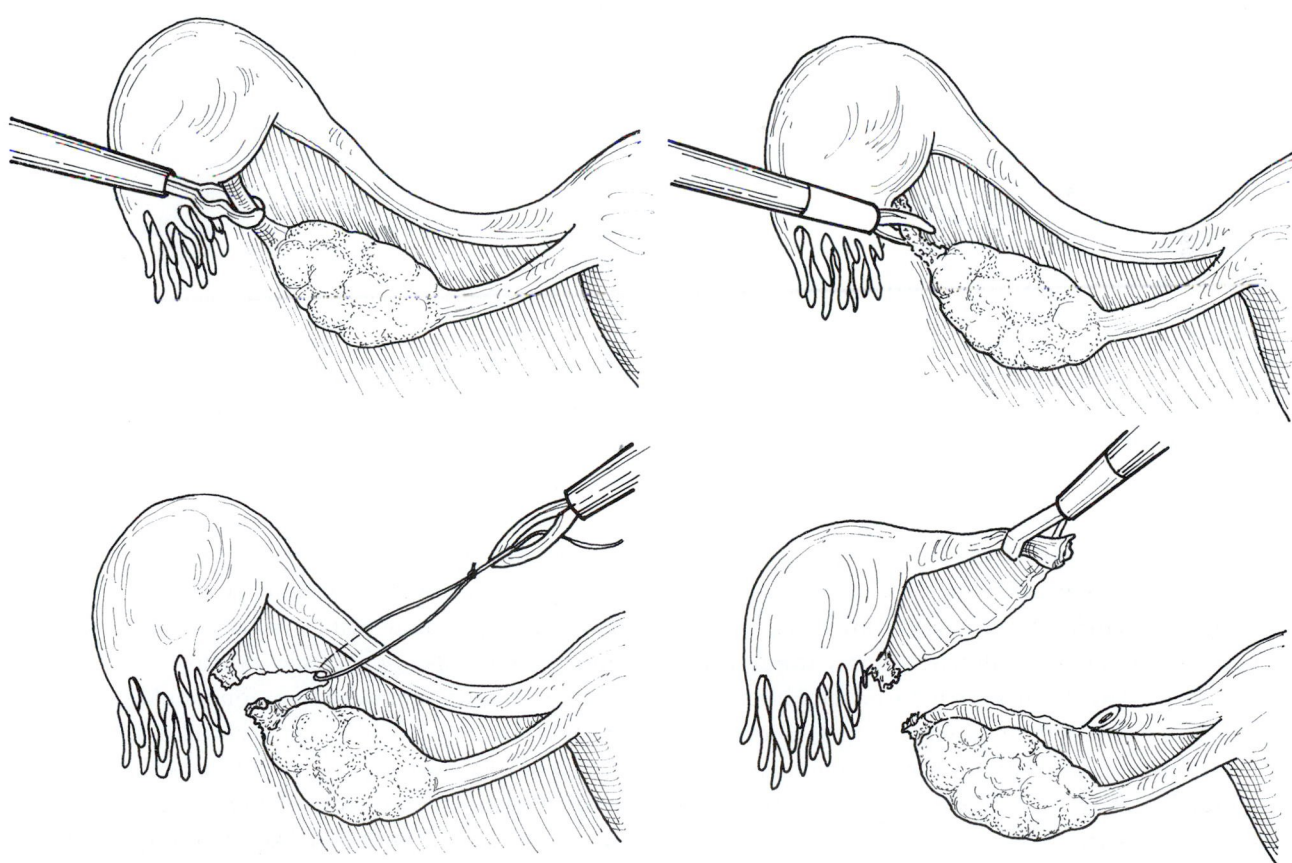

Figure 57-2 Technique of laparoscopic salpingectomy. The endoloop is placed around the tube and tightened. The fallopian tube and ovary are removed with scissors after additional loops are placed.

paradoxical oophorectomy at the time of salpingectomy for ectopic pregnancy.

Partial Salpingectomy

The removal of only the portion of the fallopian tube containing the ectopic pregnancy is termed partial salpingectomy. This procedure is generally performed when future fertility is desired and more conservative procedures are not possible due to extensive damage or continued bleeding after salpingostomy. A partial salpingectomy should not be performed unless reanastomosis is planned either immediately or as a second procedure at a later date, since repeat ectopic pregnancy in the blind distal tubal segment is possible unless the patient uses some form of contraception.[35,36] While minimal data exist to support either immediate or delayed repair, most surgeons prefer the delayed repair, believing repair is technically easier and more successful after resolution of the edema and inflammation accompanying an ectopic pregnancy.

Because of the low tubal patency rate following linear salpingostomy for isthmic ectopic pregnancies, partial salpingectomy has been advocated as the most appropriate procedure for this type of ectopic pregnancy.[37] However, other authors believe that the tubal patency rate following isthmic linear salpingostomy is acceptable.[38] Given the need for a second surgery for reanastomosis as well as the inability of many patients to afford a surgery that is generally not covered by health insurance in the United States, many surgeons are reluctant to perform a partial salpingectomy unless immediate reanastomosis is planned.

Salpingostomy

Opening the fallopian tube and removing the products of conception is the most common conservative surgical therapy for management of an ectopic pregnancy. The tubal incision may be closed with fine-caliber suture (salpingotomy), or allowed to heal by secondary intention (salpingostomy). Intrauterine pregnancies have been shown to occur earlier after salpingostomy than with salpingotomy.[39] In addition, the presence of sutures may also favor adhesion formation. Therefore, it is generally recommended that the tubal incision be left open.

Although the surgical technique is similar for both the laparoscopic and the open approach, laparoscopic salpingostomy requires a much greater degree of skill and dexterity than does the same procedure performed at laparotomy. The laparoscopic technique is illustrated in Figure 57-3.

The basics of linear salpingostomy involve the use of either a scalpel, needle-point electrode, or laser to incise the antimesenteric border of the fallopian tube over the ectopic pregnancy. The products of conception are then gently removed with laparoscopic graspers or thumb forceps. Vigorous removal is not recommended as this may lead to increased bleeding and damage to the tubal epithelium. The use of pressurized irrigation fluid has been suggested by some surgeons as a method of flushing additional trophoblastic tissue from the tube without increasing the risk of bleeding.

The injection of vasopressin (10 units in 20 to 50 ml of saline) prior to the linear salpingostomy can be used to markedly decrease bleeding. Injections are made in the antimesenteric portion of tube over the ectopic pregnancy, in the mesosalpinx beneath the ectopic and/or the region of the fimbica-ovarica, where branches of the ovarian blood vessels enter the mesosalpinx to supply the tube. These injections can be performed laparoscopically with special laparoscopic instruments or by using standard spinal needles passed transcutaneously. A 25-gauge spinal needle inserted using a shorter 18- or 20-gauge needle as an introducer will maintain optimal maneuverability, yet easily penetrate the tubal wall without the use of the excessive countertension on the tube frequently needed with larger needles.

Fimbrial Expression

The use of digital pressure to extrude a fimbrial ectopic pregnancy is probably the easiest of all the conservative surgical treatments to perform. However, some authors believe that in ampullary ectopic pregnancies the trophoblastic tissue rapidly erodes through the epithelium of the endosalpinx and develops between the tubal lumen and serosa.[40] If the growth of ampullary ectopic pregnancies is truly extraluminal, as some believe, fimbrial expression would potentially be more traumatic than a surgical incision. This factor could explain the high rate of both persistent trophoblastic disease and recurrent ectopic pregnancy associated with fimbrial expression.[41] If this technique is to be performed, it probably should be limited to fimbrial pregnancies already in the process of being spontaneously extruded from the tube.

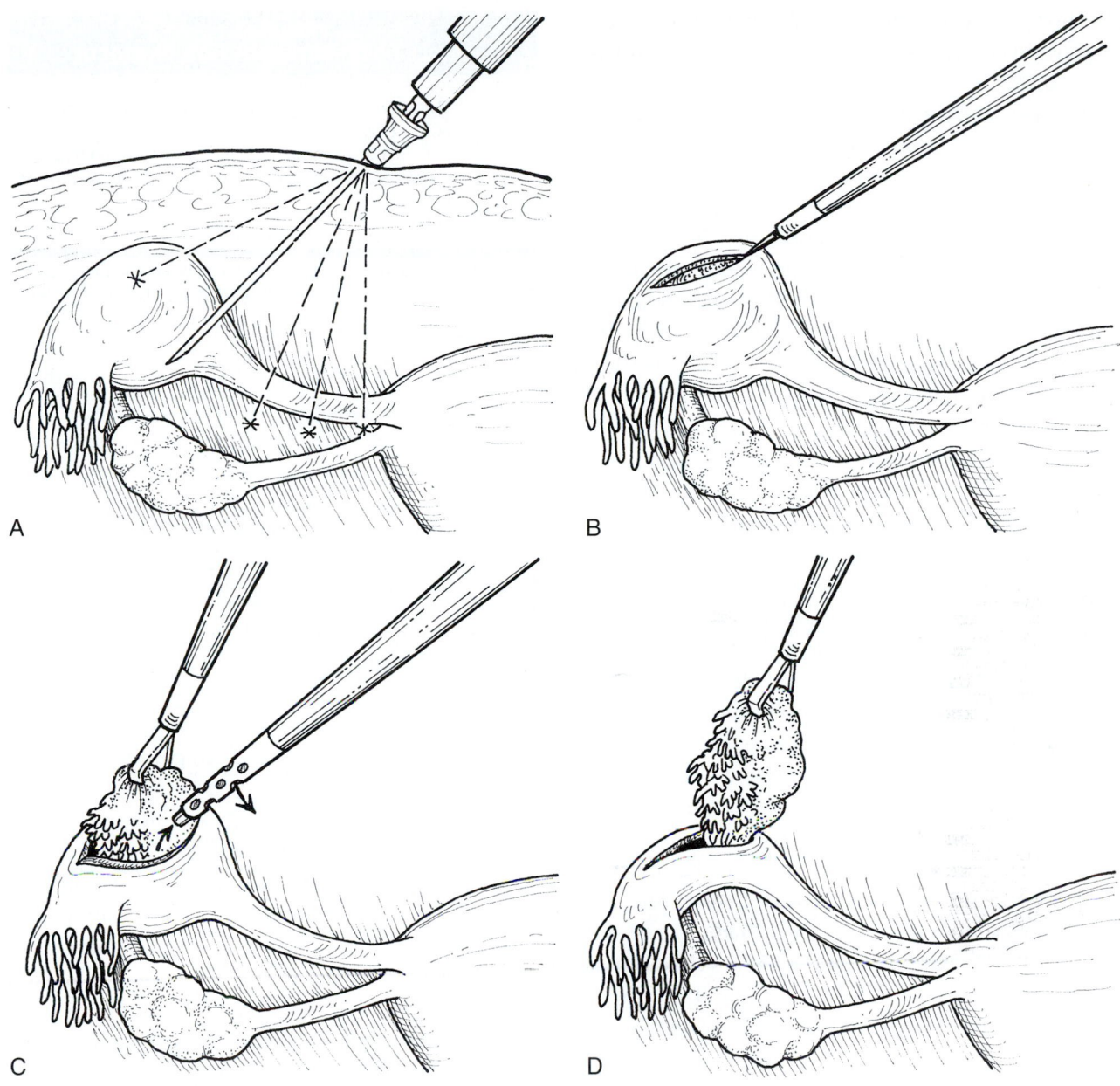

Figure 57-3 Technique of laparoscopic salpingostomy. A. Vasopressin injected. B. Tube open with unipolar needle. C. Products of conception removed. D. Completion of procedure.

METHOTREXATE

Methotrexate is a folic acid analog that has been used extensively in medicine for the treatment of certain neoplastic diseases, severe psoriasis, and adult rheumatoid arthritis. Methotrexate competitively binds to the enzyme dihydrofolic acid reductase, an enzyme that converts dihydofolate to tetrahydrofolate. This binding prevents the reduction of folate to its active form, tetrahydrofolate. Tetrahydofolate serves to transport one-carbon groups during the synthesis of purine nucleotides and thymidylate. Without tetrahydrofolate, DNA synthesis and repair, and cellular replication is impaired. Actively proliferating cells such as malignant cells, bone marrow cells, fetal cells, as well as mucosal cells of the mouth, intestine, and urinary bladder are generally the most sensitive to the effects of methotrexate. Methotrexate is rapidly cleared from the body by the kidneys, with 90% of an intravenous dose excreted unchanged within 24 hours of injection.[42]

Until recently, methotrexate was used in gynecology only for the treatment of gestational trophoblastic disease. In 1982, Tanaka et al. reported treatment of an interstitial ectopic pregnancy with a 15-day course of intramuscular methotrexate. This was the first report of methotrexate being used in the treatment of an ectopic pregnancy.[43] Subsequently, multiple reports describing the use of methotrexate for treatment of ectopic pregnancy have been published.

Initially, all methotrexate protocols for the medical treatment of ectopic pregnancy used multiple doses of methotrexate alternating with reduced folinic acid (citrovorum rescue factor). These protocols generally required prolonged hospital stays, lengthy courses of treatment, and higher-than-acceptable toxicity rates. Side effects encountered included changes in liver functions, bone marrow suppression, nausea, and stomatitis. Considering these side effects as well as patient costs, this form of treatment, although perhaps superior to surgical therapy, was not ideal.

In 1989, Stovall and co-workers at the University of Tennessee, Memphis, demonstrated that medical management of ectopic pregnancies could be performed safely on an outpatient basis.[44] In their protocol, intramuscular methotrexate, 1 mg/kg of actual body weight, was given on alternating days with citrovorum rescue factor 0.1 mg/kg. Methotrexate was continued only until there was a 15% decline in two consecutive daily hCG titers. A second course of methotrexate/citrovorum was given if previously falling levels changed ≤15% or rose between two consecutive hCG titers. Using this outpatient multidose regimen, a success rate of 96% with 100 patients was obtained. Five patients with ectopic cardiac activity were included in this series with four of five patient (80%). Of the 96 successfully treated patients, 17 patients (17.7%) required only one methotrexate injection, 38 (39.6%) required two doses, 22 (22.9%) required three doses, and 19 (19.8%) received four doses. No major side effects were reported. Minor side effects included three cases of transiently elevated liver functions and two cases of stomatitis.

Single-Dose Methotrexate Protocol

Since most patients treated with multidose methotrexate responded with falling levels before the peak

TABLE 57-1
SINGLE-DOSE METHOTREXATE PROTOCOL

Day	Therapy
0	hCG ±D&C
1	hCG, aspartate transaminase, blood urea nitrogen, complete blood count, creatinine, Rh, methotrexate
4	hCG
7	hCG

<15% decline between day 4 and 7 HCG, repeat methotrexate; >15% decline between day 4 and 7 HCG, follow weekly until HCG <15 mIU.

effect of the second and third injection, it was theorized that many patients could be successfully treated with only a single dose of methotrexate. Subsequently, a protocol using only single dose methotrexate without the use of citrovorum rescue factor was developed at the University of Tennessee, Memphis.[45] This protocol is detailed in Table 57-1. Because the majority of patients receive only one dose of methotrexate, this protocol is commonly referred to as "single-dose methotrexate." Compared to previous multidose methotrexate protocols, single-dose methotrexate is less expensive, has fewer side effects, requires less intensive patient monitoring, and has greater patient acceptance. Almost 400 patients to date have been treated with this protocol, with a success rate of approximately 93%. A summary of published results is included in Table 57-2. This success rate is similar to that obtained at our institution when a multidose protocol was followed. This success rate is particularly noteworthy since there was no upper limit placed on hCG levels and the limits on the size of an ectopic gestation that could be treated were liberalized several times. In addition, for purposes of our protocol size includes only the gestational mass if it can be delineated from surrounding hematoma. If a gestational

TABLE 57-2
SUCCESS RATES FOR ECTOPIC PREGNANCY BY SUBGROUP

	Overall Success	Method Success*
Total	287/315 (91.1%)	287/309 (92.9%)
Cardiac activity	35/44 (79.5%)	35/40 (87.5%)
Size >3.5 cm	9/10 (90.0%)	9/10 (90.0%)
Cornual	5/6 (83.3%)	5/6 (83.3%)
Cervical	2/2 (100%)	2/2 (100%)

*Success after elective withdrawals removed.

Based on data from Lipscomb GH, Bran D, McCord ML, Portera C, Ling FW. An analysis of 315 ectopic pregnancies treated with single-dose methotrexate. Am J Obstet Gynecol 1998;178:1354.

mass cannot be distinguished, the size of the entire mass is used. Currently, the upper limit of ectopic size for medical therapy at our institution is 4 cm if cardiac activity is not present and 3.5 cm with cardiac activity. The upper limit on ectopic size has been empiric, and some information suggests that ectopic size may not be a significant risk factor for failure.[46]

Before treatment with methotrexate, patients must be counseled extensively about the risk and benefits of treatment, the expected course and duration of treatment, and the importance of follow-up. Traditionally, all patients at our institution are screened with a base-line hCG, Rh factor, complete blood count (CBC), aspartate aminotransferase (AST), creatinine, and blood urea nitrogen (BUN). White-cell counts less than 1500, abnormal renal function, or elevation in the liver function values more than twice the upper limit of normal are contraindications to methotrexate. To date, no patient has not met these screening criteria, and it has been suggested by some that in the absence of a history of renal disease, previous hepatitis, liver dysfunction, or evidence of a depressed immune system, there is no need for a screening CBC, AST, creatinine, or BUN prior to initial methotrexate dosing. However, these tests should be performed prior to a second dose of methotrexate even if results are initially normal.

The presence of blood in the pelvis on ultrasound is considered by many to be a contraindication to medical therapy because of fears that this may indicate ongoing tubal rupture. As noted previously, 50% of unruptured ectopic pregnancies will have blood in the pelvis on culdocentesis and this alone is not considered in our protocol as a reason for surgical intervention. This blood may also produce mild peritoneal signs (i.e., rebound) on abdominal examination. Although there are no data to indicate the amount of blood in the pelvis above which it is unsafe to treat medically, we empirically consider blood in the upper abdomen a strong relative contraindication to medical therapy. Stable patients with smaller amount of bloods confined to the pelvis are routinely treated medically at our institution. If there is concern that this blood is the result of active bleeding, hospitalization with observation and serial hematocrits is indicated.

Methotrexate is given intramuscularly in a dose of 50 mg/m² based on actual body weight. For the average patient, this results in dosages of 75 to 100 mg, although obese patients frequently will require significantly more methotrexate. Methotrexate is generally

available in concentrations of 25 mg/cc. Using this concentration, a total volume of 3 to 4 cc is generally required to deliver the needed dose of methotrexate. Volumes greater than 3 cc are usually given with more than one injection, but can be administered in only one injection if necessary.

The day methotrexate is given is considered day 1 in our protocol. A repeat hCG is performed on days 4 and 7. If the hCG level declines <15% between days 4 and 7, a second dose of methotrexate is given and the protocol restarted at a new day 1. A repeat blood count and AST are obtained before redosing. We routinely obtain these laboratory tests with the hCG level on all day 7 patients to prevent delays if redosing is needed. If the hCG level declines ≥15%, hCG titers are then followed weekly until titers reach <15 mIU/ml. If the hCG level declines <15% in any week, repeat methotrexate dosing is performed and the protocol is again restarted at a new day 1. Although this protocol is referred to as single-dose methotrexate, approximately 20% of patients will require more than one treatment cycle.[47] The mean time to resolution in successfully treated patients is approximately 35 days.[47] However, resolution may take as long as 109 days. Tubal rupture also may be delayed, with the longest time from initial treatment to rupture in our database occurring at 31 days.

Ultrasound is generally not repeated for patients except to evaluate severe separation pain or for patients with positive ectopic cardiac activity. For patients with cardiac activity, ultrasound is repeated weekly until absence of cardiac activity is demonstrated. Patients with persistent cardiac activity on day 7 are redosed even if hCG titers are declining. No data exist on the number of doses of methotrexate that can be safely given. In patients with gestational trophoblastic disease, one common protocol uses a similar dose of methotrexate weekly until hCG levels are negative. Minimal side effects have been observed during this type of treatment. Nevertheless, our institution has traditionally restricted ectopic treatments to a maximum of three injections.

During treatment, patients are required to avoid alcohol and folate-containing vitamins. Sexual intercourse or pelvic examinations could potentially rupture the tubal hematoma commonly noted on ultrasound after methotrexate treatment and therefore should be avoided. Patients are also requested to avoid cabbage, onions, leeks, and other potential gas-producing foods to avoid the gastrointestinal distress from excess intestinal gas production that seems to be common following methotrexate treatment. Patients are instructed to use over-the-counter simethicone-containing anti-gas agents as needed for this problem.

Predictors of Success for Single-Dose Methotrexate

Since the development of methotrexate treatment for tubal ectopic pregnancies, many clinical variables have been suggested as prognostic of success with methotrexate therapy for ectopic pregnancy. The most commonly quoted predictors of success are hCG levels, progesterone levels, ectopic size, the presence of ectopic cardiac activity, and the presence of free peritoneal blood. Unfortunately, there is no consensus on which selection criteria are reliable. Because of the small numbers of treated patients previously available for analysis, it has been difficult to determine the true effect of these parameters on success rates. However, in one review the effect of ectopic size, mass volume, initial serum hCG levels, initial serum progesterone levels, and the presence or absence of ectopic fetal cardiac activity or free peritoneal blood were evaluated with respect to their effect on success with single-dose methotrexate treatment of 350 consecutive tubal ectopic pregnancies.[46] Preliminary univariate analysis showed only initial hCG level, initial progesterone, and the presence of ectopic cardiac activity to be statistically significant. Interestingly, ectopic size, hematoma volume, or the presence of free peritoneal blood confined to the pelvis were not significant risk factors for treatment failure. Logistic regression on these three statistically significant variables showed hCG to be the only significant contributing factor to the failure rate with a marked increase in the failure rate seen after 15,000 mIU/ml. This would seem to

indicate that many previous relative contraindications for medical therapy are invalid, with only hCG being predictive. Failure rates by hCG levels are presented in Table 57-3. The failure rates from this study can be used to counsel patients on their relative chance of success with single-dose methotrexate for ectopic pregnancy.

COMPLICATIONS OF METHOTREXATE THERAPY

Separation Pain

It is common for patients to experience an episode of increased abdominal pain during treatment.[48] Although the cause of this pain is unknown, it is likely that the pain results from either tubal abortion or tubal stretching due to hematoma formation. This pain is generally self-limiting and controlled with nonsteroidal antiinflammatory agents such as ibuprofen, 800 mg by mouth. Patients are also advised to rest after the ibuprofen and return for reevaluation if significant relief does not occur within 1 hour. Hemodynamically stable patients with severe pain are admitted and observed with serial hematocrits. An ultrasound can also be obtained to document the absence of blood outside the pelvis, indicating probable tubal rupture. As noted previously, the presence of presumed blood confined to the pelvis is not an indication for surgical intervention.

In an earlier review of our first 258 ectopic pregnancies treated with single-dose methotrexate, 34 patients required hospitalization for severe unrelieved pain and 22 other patients were evaluated as outpatients and released.[49] Twenty-seven of these 34 hospitalized patients (79%) did not require surgery during this hospitalization. Two hospitalized patients and one outpatient ultimately underwent surgery at a time remote from evaluation. Two of these surgeries were in patients who refused further medical therapy and requested surgery.

In many centers, patients with separation pain requiring evaluation undergo surgical therapy. Extrapolating from the above data, our success rate would have dropped to 82.5% if those patients hospitalized for separation pain underwent surgery and 74% if all patients with pain severe enough to require evaluation underwent surgery. We believe early surgical intervention in patients experiencing separation pain may be one reason for the lower success rate

---

TABLE 57-3
SINGLE-DOSE METHOTREXATE SUCCESS RATES BY HCG LEVELS

HCG Level (mIU/ml)	Success	Fail	% Success
<1000	118	2	98.3
1000–1999	40	3	93.0
2000–4999	90	8	91.8
5000–9999	39	6	86.7
10,000–14,999	18	4	81.8
>15,000	15	7	68.2

Based on data from Lipscomb GH, McCord ML, Huff G, Stovall TG, Ling FW. Predictors of success for systemic single-dose methotrexate for treatment of tubal ectopic pregnancy. Obstet Gynecol 1999;93:11S.

reported with single-dose methotrexate therapy by other institutions.

Hematoma Formation

Following treatment with methotrexate, 56% of ectopic masses will increase in size if followed by ultrasound.[50] We have observed hematomas 7 to 8 cm in size develop after treatment with methotrexate. Interestingly, most of these patients are asymptomatic. These masses will frequently persist for some time, with the longest documented time to resolution being 108 days.[50] Persistence after the disappearance of HCG is also common. These masses should not be interpreted as a treatment failure, as they probably represent resolving hematomas rather than trophoblastic tissue.

Side Effects

Potentially serious side effects, including marrow suppression, pulmonary fibrosis, nonspecific pneumonitis, liver cirrhosis, renal failure, and gastric ulceration, can occur with methotrexate. However, these are invariably seen when methotrexate is given in high doses with frequent dosing intervals—i.e., chemotherapeutic protocols for malignancy—but are rarely seen with the doses, dosing intervals, or treatment duration used for medical management of ectopic pregnancy. None of the approximately 400 patients treated at our institution have experienced serious side effects.

The most common side effect observed with the single-dose methotrexate protocol is excessive flatulence and bloating due to intestinal gas formation. This problem is usually self-limited and handled as previously described. Transient mild elevation of liver-function tests can occur but rarely exceed twice the upper limit of normal. These tests invariably return to normal within 2 weeks. Stomatitis may also be seen in patients receiving more than one methotrexate injection and is generally self-limited. If needed, viscous lidocaine can be used for symptomatic relief.

OBSERVATION WITHOUT INTERVENTION

The natural history of ectopic pregnancy is highly variable. At one extreme, there is acute pain, hemorrhage, shock, and even death. At the other, in an asymptomatic patient, the implantation may undergo resorption or tubal abortion. When hCG titers are falling and there is no evidence of tubal rupture, nonintervention offers freedom from chemotherapy toxicity and surgical morbidity. Success rates have been reported to be from 70 to 100%.[51] At our institution, all tubal ectopic pregnancies without cardiac activity have at least two hCG levels before treatment with methotrexate. Patients with falling levels are followed conservatively as long as hCG levels fall appropriately. However, since falling hCG levels are no guarantee against rupture, many physicians prefer to treat all diagnosed ectopic pregnancies with methotrexate regardless of the status of the hCG levels.

HETEROTOPIC PREGNANCY

The simultaneous occurrence of intrauterine and ectopic pregnancies is referred to as a heterotopic pregnancy. Classically, the incidence of naturally occurring heterotopic pregnancy has been reported as 1 in 30,000 pregnancies.[1] This figure, originally quoted in 1948, was arrived at by multiplying the ectopic rate (0.37% in 1948) by the dizygotic twinning rate of 0.8%. With the ectopic pregnancy rate now at 1.9%, the heterotopic rate for today would be 1 in 6579 pregnancies by the above formula. However, there is no evidence that these assumptions are valid.

Nevertheless, any increase in the ectopic rate or multiple pregnancy rate would be expected to similarly increase the heterotopic pregnancy rate. Patients treated with clomiphene citrate have been reported to have a heterotopic rate of 1 in 120 to 1 in 3000.[52] The use of menotropins for ovulation induction and in vitro fertilization techniques further increase the heterotopic rate with estimates as high as 1 in 100.[52] Because of the differing rates of HCG and progesterone produced by heterotopic pregnancies, the algorithms for the diagnosis of ectopic pregnancy described previously in this chapter cannot be reliably used in these situations.

PERSISTENT TROPHOBLASTIC DISEASE

Persistent trophoblastic disease is the continued growth of trophoblastic tissue in the fallopian tube of the abdominal cavity following surgical treatment for ectopic pregnancy. This condition is sometimes referred to as persistent ectopic pregnancy. This condition generally occurs after incomplete removal of an ectopic pregnancy during a conservative surgical procedure. Rarely, implantation of extruded trophoblastic tissue on peritoneal or visceral surfaces can also result in persistent trophoblastic disease. Untreated, persistent trophoblastic tissue may lead to tubal rupture and life-threatening intraabdominal hemorrhage.

The incidence of persistent trophoblastic disease after salpingostomy ranges from 3 to 20%.[53] Seifer et al. found that patients with amenorrhea less than 7 weeks or an ectopic size less than 2 cm were at increased risk for development of persistent trophoblastic disease.[54] hCG and progesterone levels prior to surgery can also be used to identify patients at increased risk. In one study, the risk of persistent trophoblastic disease was 23% for patients with a preoperative hCG >3000 mIU, but only 1.5% when the hCG was <3000 mIU.[55] Likewise, women with progesterone levels >35 ng/ml or with rising hCG levels (>100 mIU/ml in 24 hours) have been shown to be at increased risk for persistent trophoblastic disease.[56] The risk for persistent trophoblastic disease also appears to be slightly increased if the procedure is performed by laparoscopy rather than laparotomy. In a review of 157 salpingostomies for ampullary ectopic pregnancy, Seifer et al. reported persistent disease in 16 of 103 patients (16%) after laparoscopic salpingostomy, and in only one of 54 patients (2%) following salpingostomy by laparotomy.[54]

All patients treated for ectopic pregnancy with conservative surgical procedure should be followed with serial hCG levels to detect persistent trophoblastic disease. An initial hCG level should be obtained in the immediate postoperative period and repeated at least weekly until it is <15 mIU/ml. A decline of less than 15% on consecutive hCG titers indicates persistent trophoblastic activity. The percent fall of hCG on postoperative day 1 can also be used as a predictor of persistent trophoblastic disease. In one study, patients with a decline in hCG of <50% had a 3.51 relative risk to develop persistent disease, while no patient with a fall ≥77% developed persistent disease.[57]

Treatment for persistent ectopic pregnancy can be surgical or medical. Surgical therapy consists of repeat salpingostomy or, more commonly, salpingectomy. Methotrexate therapy may be preferable to surgical therapy for many hemodynamically stable patients. The fallopian tube is preserved and any trophoblastic tissue not confined to the tube is also treated. The same single-dose methotrexate protocol described previously is used for treatment of persistent trophoblastic disease.

At least one author has suggested the use of prophylactic methotrexate after salpingostomy to reduce the incidence of persistent trophoblastic disease.[58] Although prophylactic methotrexate reduced the incidence of persistent trophoblastic disease from 14.5 to 1.9%, one patient in each group still required repeat surgery. Such a treatment protocol would require treatment of 100 patients with methotrexate to prevent treating 12 patients. Furthermore, the time for the hCG levels to reach 15 mIU was only 2 days shorter (12 vs. 14) in the treated group. This difference was not statistically significant. Based on these data, prophylactic methotrexate cannot be advocated for routine use. However, the prophylactic use of methotrexate after conservative surgical surgery for ectopic pregnancy may be appropriate for patients unavailable for follow-up or at high risk for noncompliance.

SUMMARY

The incidence of ectopic pregnancy has reached epidemic proportions in the United States. Nevertheless, the mortality rate associated with this disease has steadily declined. This decline is primarily due to earlier diagnosis, which has allowed treatment prior to rupture. This earlier diagnosis is the result of improved assays for progesterone and hCG, transvaginal ultrasound, and the use of diagnostic algorithms that do not require the use of laparoscopy. Once diagnosed, numerous treatment options are now available, including the option of medical therapy. Future developments will hopefully provide for even earlier diagnosis as well as data on the optimal candidates for each form of treatment.

REFERENCES

1. DeVoe R, Pratt JH. Simultaneous intrauterine and extrauterine pregnancy. Am J Obstet Gynecol 1948;56:1119.
2. Centers for Disease Control. Ectopic pregnancy—United States, 1990–1992. MMWR 1995;44:46.
3. Marchbanks PA, Annegers JF, Coulam CB, Strathy JH, Kurland LT. Risk factors for ectopic pregnancy: a population-based study. JAMA 1988;259:1823.
4. Ankum WM, Mol BW, Van der Veen F, Bossuyt PM. Risk factors for ectopic pregnancy: a meta-analysis. Fertil Steril 1996;65:1093.
5. Weckstein LN. Current perspective on ectopic pregnancy. Obstet Gynecol Surv 1985;40:259.
6. Stovall TG, Ling FW, Carson SA, Buster JE. Nonsurgical diagnosis and treatment of tubal pregnancy. Fertil Steril 1990;54:537.

7. Hallatt JG. Repeat ectopic pregnancy: a study of 123 consecutive cases. Am J Obstet Gynecol 1975;122:520.

8. Lipscomb GH, Spellman JR, Ling FW. The effect of same-day pregnancy testing on the incidence of luteal phase pregnancy. Obstet Gynecol 1993;82:411.

9. Daya S. Human chorionic gonadotropin increase in normal early pregnancy. Am J Obstet Gynecol 1987;156:286.

10. Kadar N, DeCherney AH, Romero R. Receiver operating characteristic (ROC) curve analysis of the relative efficacy of single and serial chorionic gonadotropin determinations in the early diagnosis of ectopic pregnancy. Fertil Steril 1982;37:542.

11. Kadar N, Freedman M, Zacher M. Further observations on the doubling time of human chorionic gonadotropin in early asymptomatic pregnancies. Fertil Steril 1990; 54:783.

12. Kadar N, Caldwell BV, Romero R. A method of screening for ectopic pregnancy and its indications. Obstet Gynecol 1981;58:162.

13. Pittaway DE, Reish RL, Wentz AC. Doubling times of human chorionic gonadotropin increase in early viable intrauterine pregnancies. Am J Obstet Gynecol 1985; 152:299.

14. Bernaschek G, Rudelstorfer R, Csaicsich P. Vaginal sonography versus serum human chorionic gonadotropin in early detection of pregnancy. Am J Obstet Gynecol 1988; 158:608.

15. Marrs RP, Kletzky OA, Howard WF, Mishell DR Jr. Disappearance of human chorionic gonadotropin and resumption of ovulation following abortion. Am J Obstet Gynecol 1979;135:731.

16. Stovall TG, Kellerman AL, Ling FW, Buster JE. Emergency department diagnosis of ectopic pregnancy. Ann Emerg Med 1990;19:1098.

17. Stovall TG, Ling FW, Andersen RN, Buster JE. Improved sensitivity and specificity of a single measurement of serum progesterone over serial quantitative beta-human chorionic gonadotrophin in screening for ectopic pregnancy. Hum Reprod 1992;7:723.

18. Stovall TG, Ling FW, Cope BJ, Buster JE. Preventing ruptured ectopic pregnancy with a single serum progesterone. Am J Obstet Gynecol 1989;160:1425.

19. McCord ML, Muram D, Buster JE, Arheart KL, Stovall TG, Carson SA. Single serum progesterone as a screen for ectopic pregnancy: exchanging specificity and sensitivity to obtain optimal test performance. Fertil Steril 1996; 66:513.

20. Kadar N, DeVore G, Romero R. Discriminatory HCG zone: its use in the sonographic evaluation for ectopic pregnancy. Obstet Gynecol 1981;58:156.

21. Lindahl B, Ahlgren M. Identification of chorion villi in abortion specimens. Obstet Gynecol 1986;67:79.

22. Vermesh M, Graczykowski JW, Sauer MV. Reevaluation of the role of culdocentesis in the management of ectopic pregnancy. Am J Obstet Gynecol 1990;162:411.

23. Romero R, Copel JA, Kadar N, Jeanty P, Decherney A, Hobbins JC. Value of culdocentesis in the diagnosis of ectopic pregnancy. Obstet Gynecol 1985;65:519.

24. Cartwright PS, Vaughn B, Tuttle D. Culdocentesis and ectopic pregnancy. J Reprod Med 1984;29:88.

25. Parry JS. Extrauterine pregnancy: its causes, species, patho-logic anatomy, clinical history, diagnosis, prognosis, and treatment. Philadelphia: Lea & Febiger, 1876.

26. Tait RL. Five cases of extrauterine pregnancy operated upon at the time of rupture. BMJ 1884;1:1250.

27. Martin A. Zur Kenntniss der tubarschwangerschaft. Monatsschr Gerburtshilfer Gynakol 1887;5:244.

28. Strome WB. Salpingotomy for tubal pregnancy: report of a successful case. Obstet Gynecol 1953;117:472.

29. Shapiro HI, Adler DH. Excision of an ectopic pregnancy through the laparoscope. Am J Obstet Gynecol 1973; 117:290.

30. Bruhat MA, Manhes H, Mage G, Pouly JL. Treatment of ectopic pregnancy by means of laparoscopy. Fertil Steril 1980;33:411.

31. DeCherney AH, Romero R, Naftolin F. Surgical management of unruptured ectopic pregnancy. Fertil Steril 1981; 35:21.

32. Brumsted J, Kessler C, Gibson C, Nakajima S, Riddick DH, Gibson M. A comparison of laparoscopy and laparotomy for the treatment of ectopic pregnancy. Obstet Gynecol 1988;71:889.

33. Jeffcoate TNA. Salpingectomy or salpingo-ophorectomy? J Obstet Gynaecol Br Emp 1955;62:214.

34. Franklin EWd, Zeiderman AM. Tubal ectopic pregnancy: etiology and obstetric and gynecologic sequelae. Am J Obstet Gynecol 1973;117:220.

35. Cartwright PS, Entman SS. Repeat ipsilateral tubal pregnancy following partial salpingectomy: a case report. Fertil Steril 1984;42:647.

36. Diamond MP, DeCherney AH. Distal segment tubal pregnancy after segmental resection for an isthmic pregnancy: a case report. J Reprod Med 1988;33:236.

37. DeCherney AH, Boyers SP. Isthmic ectopic pregnancy: segmental resection as the treatment of choice. Fertil Steril 1985;44:307.

38. Smith HO, Toledo AA, Thompson JD. Conservative surgical management of isthmic ectopic pregnancies. Am J Obstet Gynecol 1987;157:604.

39. Tulandi T, Guralnick M. Treatment of tubal ectopic pregnancy by salpingotomy with or without tubal suturing and salpingectomy. Fertil Steril 1991;55:53.

40. Budowick M, Johnson TR Jr, Genadry R, Parmley TH, Woodruff JD. The histopathology of the developing tubal ectopic pregnancy. Fertil Steril 1980;34:169.

41. Kooi S, Kock HC. Surgical treatment for tubal pregnancies. Surg Gynecol Obstet 1993;176:519.

42. Bleyer WA. The clinical pharmacology of methotrexate: new applications of an old drug. Cancer 1978;41:36.

43. Tanaka T, Hayashi H, Kutsuzawa T, Fujimoto S, Ichinoe K. Treatment of interstitial ectopic pregnancy with methotrexate: report of a successful case. Fertil Steril 1982;37:851.

44. Stovall TG, Ling FW, Buster JE. Outpatient chemotherapy of unruptured ectopic pregnancy. Fertil Steril 1989; 51:435.

45. Stovall TG, Ling FW, Gray LA. Single-dose methotrexate for treatment of ectopic pregnancy. Obstet Gynecol 1991; 77:754.

46. Lipscomb GH, McCord ML, Stovall TS, Huff G, Portera SG, Ling FW. Predictors of sucess for systemic single-dose methotrexate for treatment of tubal ectopic pregancy. Obstet Gynecol 1999;93:11S.

47. Lipscomb GH, Bran D, McCord ML, Portera JC, Ling FW. Analysis of three hundred fifteen ectopic pregnancies treated with single-dose methotrexate. Am J Obstet Gynecol 1998;178:1354.

48. Stovall TG, Ling FW. Single-dose methotrexate: an expanded clinical trial. Am J Obstet Gynecol 1993; 168:1759.

49. Lipscomb GH, Puckett KJ, Bran D, Ling FW. Management of separation pain after single-dose methotrexate therapy for ectopic pregnancy. Obstet Gynecol 1999; 93:590.

50. Brown DL, Felker RE, Stovall TG, Emerson DS, Ling FW. Serial endovaginal sonography of ectopic pregnancies treated with methotrexate. Obstet Gynecol 1991;77:406.

51. Stovall TG, Ling FW. Expectant management of ectopic pregnancy. Obstet Gynecol Clin N Am 1991;18:135.

52. Tal J, Haddad S, Gordon N, Timor-Tritsch I. Heterotopic pregnancy after ovulation induction and assisted reproductive technologies: a literature review from 1971 to 1993. Fertil Steril 1996;66:1.

53. Seifer DB, Diamond MP, DeCherney AH. Persistent ectopic pregnancy. Obstet Gynecol Clin N Am 1991;18:153.

54. Seifer DB, Gutmann JN, Grant WD, Kamps CA, DeCherney AH. Comparison of persistent ectopic pregnancy after laparoscopic salpingostomy versus salpingostomy at laparotomy for ectopic pregnancy. Obstet Gynecol 1993; 81:378.

55. Lundorff P, Hahlin M, Sjoblom P, Lindblom B. Persistent trophoblast after conservative treatment of tubal pregnancy: prediction and detection. Obstet Gynecol 1991; 77:129.

56. Hagstrom HG, Hahlin M, Bennegard-Eden B, Sjoblom P, Thorburn J, Lindblom B. Prediction of persistent ectopic pregnancy after laparoscopic salpingostomy. Obstet Gynecol 1994;84:798.

57. Spandorfer SD, Sawin SW, Benjamin I, Barnhart KT. Postoperative day 1 serum human chorionic gonadotropin level as a predictor of persistent ectopic pregnancy after conservative surgical management. Fertil Steril 1997; 68:430.

58. Graczykowski JW, Mishell DR Jr. Methotrexate prophylaxis for persistent ectopic pregnancy after conservative treatment by salpingostomy. Obstet Gynecol 1997;89:118.

Chapter 58

Uterine Leiomyomas and Other Benign Pelvic Masses

Thomas E. Snyder
Thomas G. Stovall

Five Key Points

- Uterine myomas are smooth muscle, nonencapsulated, unicellular, hormone-dependent tumors of the female genitalia. These tumors demonstrate estrogen and progestin receptors.

- Uterine myomas decrease in size in response to GnRH agonists. Side effects of this therapy may include myoma degeneration and bleeding, bone loss, and delayed therapy of leiomyosarcomas. When antagonist therapy is discontinued, regrowth to approximately original size usually occurs within 6 months.

- Hysterectomy is the definitive therapy for symptomatic uterine leiomyomas in a woman who no longer desires the option of bearing children. GnRH therapy is useful in patients with uteri 14 to 18 weeks' size to enhance the possibility of vaginal hysterectomy or conversion from vertical to Pfannenstiel incision.

- Ovarian masses in children are malignant in a significant number of cases and require exploration. Clinical presentation is commonly abdominal pain, and germ-cell tumors predominate.

- The possibility of a sexually transmitted disease (STD) and pelvic inflammatory adnexal mass should be entertained in the adolescent female presenting with pelvic pain and/or mass. Most cases of pelvic inflammatory disease present without a mass. However, if multiple episodes or prolonged presence of disease is noted, the diagnosis of a tuboovarian abscess (TOA) must be entertained.

Evaluation of the pelvic or adnexal mass in the female represents one of the most common and challenging problems in gynecology. The diagnosis and subsequent therapy must be based on the characteristics of the mass, age at presentation, and the patient's desire for preservation of fertility. In addition, a pelvic mass must be differentiated as genital or extragenital in origin. While the potential for malignancy drives the need for accurate diagnosis and aggressive therapy, the majority of these masses, especially in the reproductive age group, are benign. However, the overlap in symptoms and presentation of benign and malignant lesions makes accurate diagnosis difficult. The usual textbook discussion of pelvic masses/benign ovarian conditions is a "laundry list" of possible pathologic entities, diagnostic methods, and therapies. In order to make the discussion more relevant to the practicing physician, this chapter will focus on a dynamic schema based on age at presentation, symptoms, and characteristics of the mass. Since uterine leiomyomas are the most common pelvic tumor in women of reproductive age, the pathophysiology, presentation, and management of these masses will be discussed in detail, followed by a review of common benign adnexal masses, both genital and extragenital in origin. Finally, a coherent management schema based on patient presentation and characteristics of the mass will be presented.

UTERINE LEIOMYOMAS

Uterine leiomyomas are the most common pelvic tumors in women of reproductive age, occurring in up to 50% of patients in autopsy series. They are more common in black women than white and are the most common indication for hysterectomy in the United States.[1] This results in 1 billion dollars in direct costs for inpatient care alone.[2] Leiomyomata account for approximately 30% of all hysterectomies, including 65.4% of hysterectomies in black women and 28.5% in white women (Figure 58-1).[3]

Prior to the 20th century, no therapy was available and these tumors occasionally grew to huge proportions and caused distortion of the abdominal wall, pain, bleeding, obstruction of vital organs, and death. Due to the surgical advances pioneered by H. A. Kelly and others, surgical manipulation of these tumors became possible. Thompson and Rock[4] quote the mortality rate at the Johns Hopkins Hospital between 1889 and 1906 as 5.75% before the development of surgery as compared with 1% between 1906 and 1909. Currently, approximately 175,000 hysterectomies are performed in the United States each year for leiomyomata or conditions arising from the presence of these tumors.

Often referred to as fibroids, myomas, fibromyomas, fibroleiomyomas, leiomyofibromas, or more correctly leiomyomas, these tumors may be found in any organ containing smooth muscle. They may be single or multiple and have been reported to weigh as much as 100 lbs.[5,6] Leiomyomas are categorized by location and may be subserosal, intramural (most common),

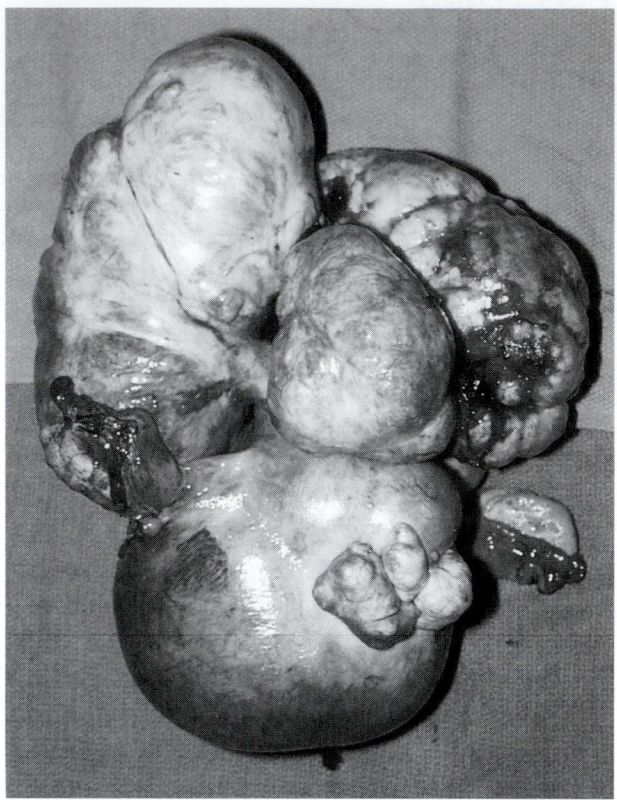

Figure 58-1. Uterine leiomyomas.

submucosal, pedunculated, or parasitic (Figure 58-2). In addition, submucosal leiomyomas may prolapse through the cervix and become infected or infarcted.

Infertility or recurrent pregnancy loss associated with leiomyomas may result from blockage of the tubal ostea or endometrial compression. These findings may lead to additional operations, adding even more morbidity or expense. Thompson and Rock point out that traditional management may change in the future because of (1) rising costs forcing review of less expensive methods of treatment, (2) surgical advances allowing minimally invasive therapy, (3) medical approaches with gonadotropin-releasing hormone (GnRH) agonists and perhaps antagonists in the future, and (4) changing social norms mandating a more conservative approach.[4]

Causes

Uterine leiomyomata are composed of smooth-muscle cells within a fibrous tissue matrix. Various terms have been applied; however, leiomyoma best describes the smooth-muscle origin and components of the tumors. The tumor is not encapsulated, but expansion of the

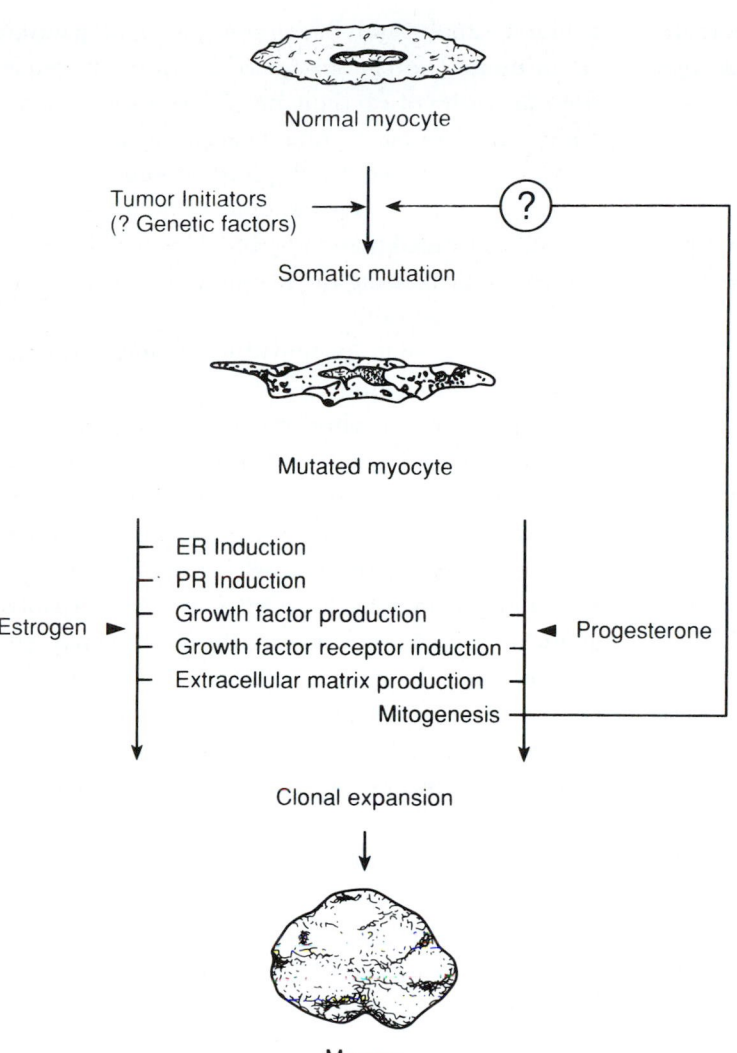

Normal myocyte

Tumor Initiators
(? Genetic factors)

Somatic mutation

Mutated myocyte

Estrogen ►

- ER Induction
- PR Induction
- Growth factor production
- Growth factor receptor induction ─── ◄ Progesterone
- Extracellular matrix production
- Mitogenesis ─

Clonal expansion

Myoma

Figure 58-2. Factors in leiomyoma growth. *Source: Rein MS, Barbieri RL, Friedman AS. Progesterone: a critical role in the pathogenesis of uterine myomas. Am J Obstet Gynecol 1995;172:14.*

borders gives rise to a pseudocapsule, which is often well delineated. Myomas are thought to be unicellular in origin, with all cells of a single glucose-6-phosphate dehydrogenase electrophoretic type.[7] Cytogenetic studies by Nilbert and Heim have suggested that certain translocations, especially on chromosome 12, may be important in their production.[8]

Steroid hormones, particularly estrogen, have long been recognized as promoting growth of myomas.[9] In addition, peptide growth factors are significant regulators of myoma growth.[1,10] Myomas are uncommon prior to menarche, regress after menopause, and increase in size during the reproductive years, apparently in response to estrogenic stimuli. Soules and McCarty[11] have demonstrated estrogen and progesterone receptors in myomas that vary with the menstrual cycle, and others have variably demonstrated increased receptors as compared with normal myometrium.[12-14] Pollow[15] et al. demonstrated decreased

conversion of estradiol to estrone in myomas possibly secondary to a deficiency of 17β-hydroxydehydrogenase. The subsequent relatively high estrogenic state within the myoma may explain growth of some myomas. The consistent response to GnRH agonists is perhaps the most convincing evidence of estrogen dependence.[16] Rein et al.[17] have shown that myoma growth may also be regulated by the mitogenic effect of progesterone. Their studies demonstrate that myoma proliferation is the result of clonal expansion and may involve the interaction of estrogen, progesterone, and local growth factors. Estrogen and progesterone may be equally important as promoters of myoma growth. The work of Anderson,[18] Brandon,[19] and Kastner and their colleagues[20] have further defined the role of progesterone and estrogen in regulating growth of myomas. While these factors have obvious importance in growth and development of these tumors, they may not totally explain the differences in speed with which the tumors grow. Other contributing factors may include differences in vascular supply, proximity to adjacent tumors, and degenerative changes (see Figure 58-2).

Histopathology

Leiomyomas may be single but are often multiple. They vary from less than 1 cm to large tumors weighing many pounds. The largest reported myoma was 65 kg by Hunt in 1888.[21] Myomas are originally located within the myometrium; however when noted clinically, they may be submucous, subserous, intraligamentous, pedunculated, or parasitic (Figure 58-3). The growth characteristics of the tumors influence the variety of locations noted at the time of surgery. Those tumors expanding toward the endometrial cavity become submucous, or if further growth occurs, they may expand on a pedicle and eventually protrude from the cervical os, becoming necrotic or infected (Figure 58-4). Growth toward the peritoneal cavity produces the typical irregular contours noted clinically. Protrusion into the broad ligament may cause confusion with adnexal masses. Pedunculated myomas grow on a pedicle into the peritoneal cavity. These may undergo torsion, with ischemia and loss of blood supply. The ischemic/partially necrotic mass may then be isolated by the omentum, reestablishing

a blood supply and becoming so-called parasitic leiomyomas. The cut surface of a myoma protrudes from the plane of excision and shows a smooth, glistening white to tan texture. There is no true capsule to myomas; however, the progressing borders produce compression of the surrounding tissue and production of a so-called pseudocapsule. This pseudocapsule is useful in delineating the margin of the tumors during surgical resection.

On microscopic examination myomas display a proliferation of mature smooth-muscle cells arranged in a trabeculated or whorled configuration. The muscle fibers are arranged in interlacing bundles. Fibrous connective tissue extends between the muscle bundles and is proportional to the amount of atrophy and degeneration (Figure 58-5). Many histologic variations of myomas have been described: cellular, atypical, epithelioid, myxoid, lipoleiomyomas, and leiomyoma with tubules.[22] Cellular leiomyomas are composed of small cells with scanty cytoplasm and may be confused with leiomyosarcomas. Atypical leiomyomas contain atypical cell clusters distributed throughout the tumor. These are called "bizarre" or "symplastic" and are also often confused with leiomyosarcomas. Epithelioid leiomyomas include leiomyoblastoma, clear-cell leiomyoma, and plexiform leiomyoma, as described by Kurman and Norris.[23]

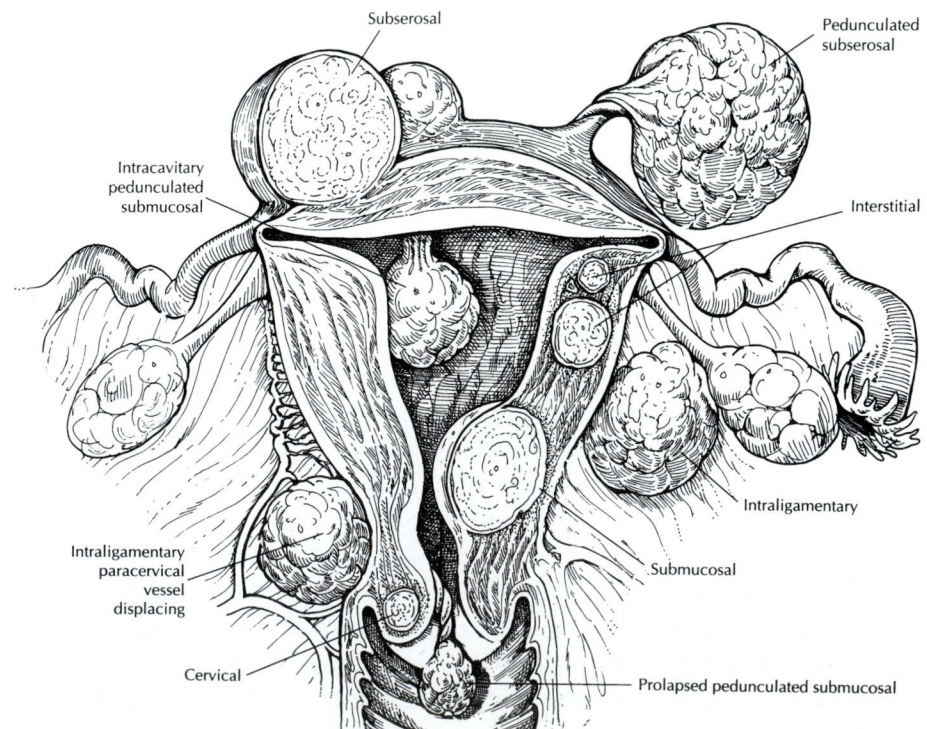

Figure 58-3 Location of uterine leiomyomas. *Source: Mann WJ, Stovall TG, eds. Myomectomy in gynecologic surgery, New York: Churchill Livingstone, 1996.*

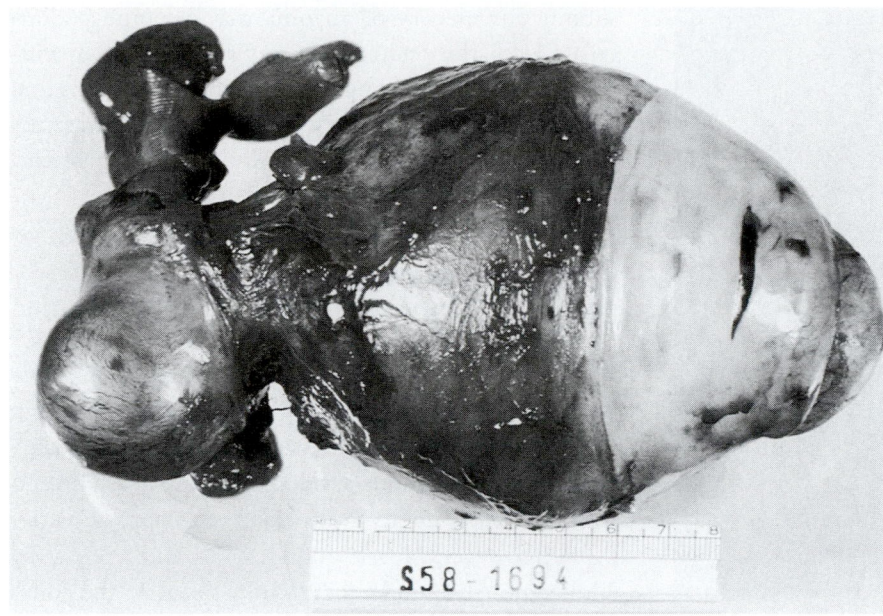

Figure 58-4 Uterine leiomyoma—cervical myoma. *Source: Breen SL, Jaffurs WJ. Gynecologic and obstetric pathology. Ortho Forum Educational Series.*

The clinical behavior of these tumors varies; however, small circumscribed tumors are benign. Myxoid leiomyomas have an amorphous myxoid substance that is circumscribed, and amitotic figures are absent. Lipoleiomyomas have large areas of fat and are diffuse or circumscribed. Leiomyomas with tubules have epithelium-lined tubules and are uncommon. Mesothelial differentiation also occurs.

Pathophysiology—"Degenerative" Changes

The long-term outcome of leiomyomas, like other tissues, depends on the maintenance of vascular supply.

Most leiomyomas have one to two arteries supplying the base of the tumor; therefore the amount of growth or degeneration depends on the maintenance of this blood supply: hyaline, myomatous, calcific, cystic, fatty, and red degeneration have been described. Hyaline degeneration is the most common and mildest form of degeneration, occurring in 60% of myomas. The smooth-muscle cells are replaced by fibrous connective tissue. The cut surface no longer demonstrates the original whorled appearance. Histologically, the cellular detail is lost as replacement by fibrous tissue continues. Cystic degeneration occurs when hyaline changes continue to affect the myoma. These tumors

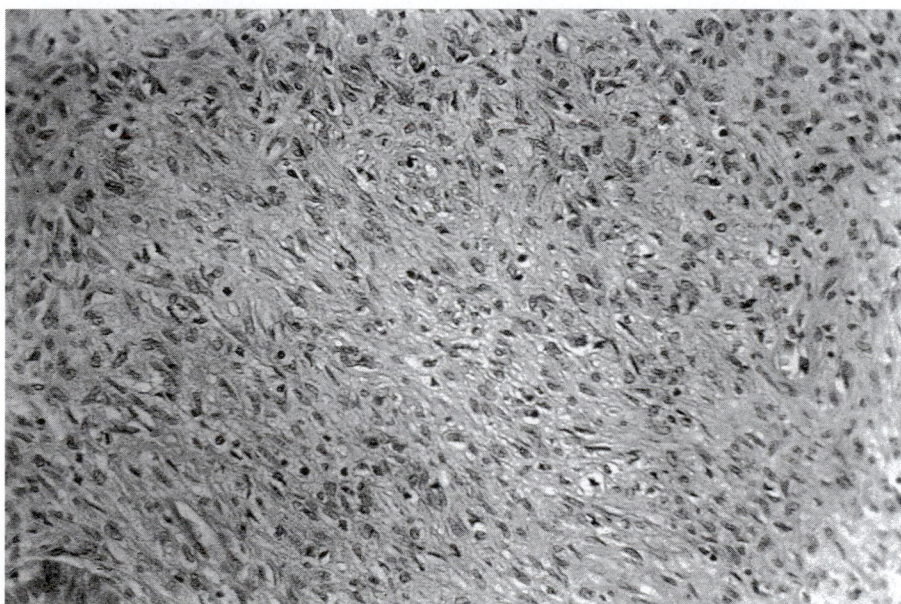

Figure 58-5 Uterine leiomyoma—microscopic. *Source: Breen SL, Jaffurs WJ. Gynecologic and obstetric pathology. Ortho Forum Educational Series.*

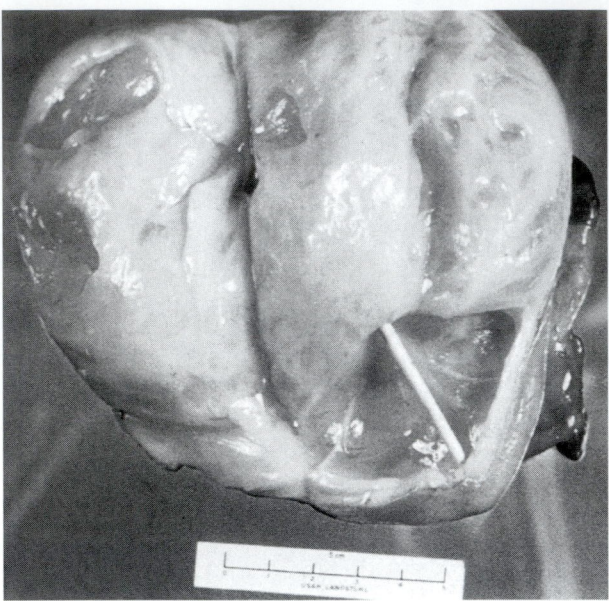

Figure 58-6. Uterine leiomyoma—cystic degeneration.
Source: Breen SL, Jaffurs WJ. Gynecologic and obstetric pathology. Ortho Forum Educational Series.

may become liquefied and form cavities filled with clear or gelatinous material. The change may be so severe that the myoma becomes a hollow cavity and develops the appearance of a cystic mass. Cystic change occurs in approximately 4% of myomas (Figure 58-6). Fatty degeneration is rare and results from severe hyaline degeneration. The presence of true fat in a myoma is uncommon; however, the degenerated myoma may develop a yellowish, fatty appearance. Calcific degeneration occurs in 4 to 10% of leiomyomas when calcium carbonate and phosphate are deposited in areas of necrosis. The calcification may be diffuse, solid, or circumferential. Thompson and Rock refer to these tumors as "wombstones" in their extensive treatise on the subject of leiomyomas.[4] These are seen on x-ray films and are more common in black than in white patients. Carneous or red degeneration occurs in rapidly growing myomas, e.g., during pregnancy. This may cause severe abdominal pain and the patient presents with symptoms of an acute abdomen. Red degeneration is essentially an ischemic, necrotic degeneration caused by loss of blood supply, e.g., torsion of a pedunculated myoma, and the "red" color is secondary to thrombosis and extravasation of blood into the myometrium.

Infections may occur in any myoma, but they occur more commonly in those with advanced degeneration or prolapse. Thompson and Rock quote one case of *Clostridium tetani* in a myoma.[4] More commonly, a submucous or cervical myoma may become pedunculated, fill the endometrial cavity, and become infected when protruding through the cervical os and exposed to vaginal flora. In severe cases of intramural necrosis and infection, frank peritonitis and sepsis may develop. However, these cases are rare.

LEIOMYOSARCOMAS AND UNUSUAL LEIOMYOMAS

According to current thought, leiomyosarcoma does not represent a degenerative change in preexisting myomas.[24] The exact incidence of degenerative change is difficult to determine although they are rare. Thompson and Rock quote the incidence as approximately 0.1%[4]; however, Novak quotes 0.7%, and a study by Montague et al. notes 0.29% in a series at the Johns Hopkins Hospital.[26] In fact, most leiomyosarcomas are noted incidentally on pathologic review following removal of the uterus for other reasons. While the malignancy may be suspected, especially in older women in whom rapid growth of an apparent uterine mass is noted, ovarian tumors are more often the true cause. Leibsohn et al.[27] noted no evidence of malignancy on endometrial sampling in his series of sarcomas, and none were suspected preoperatively (Figure 58-7).

The diagnosis of leiomyosarcoma is based on the finding of more than 10 mitotic figures per 10 consecutive high-power fields (HPFs) (Figure 58-8). Counts between 5 and 10 mitotic figures are called "cellular leiomyomas." Clinically, cellular leiomyomas exhibit benign behavior and if discovered at the time of myomectomy, it is not necessary to perform a hysterectomy. These tumors are also termed "smooth muscle tumors of uncertain malignant potential." The debate among pathologists regarding interpretation of the cellular patterns and nuclear appearance may make categorization of these tumors difficult.[28] Some authors believe histologic pattern is unreliable and that only metastatic tumors should be considered malignant.[29] Thompson and Rock believe mitotic count and histologic grade are important in tumors clinically confined to the uterus at surgery. They associate a poor prognosis with high mitotic counts and anaplastic cytologic features.[4] Others have found that mitotic index, degree of cytologic atypia, and presence of coagulative tumor-cell necrosis are important in prognosis.[30]

The term *malignant degeneration,* or *sarcomatous degeneration,* is often applied to leiomyosarcomas. However,

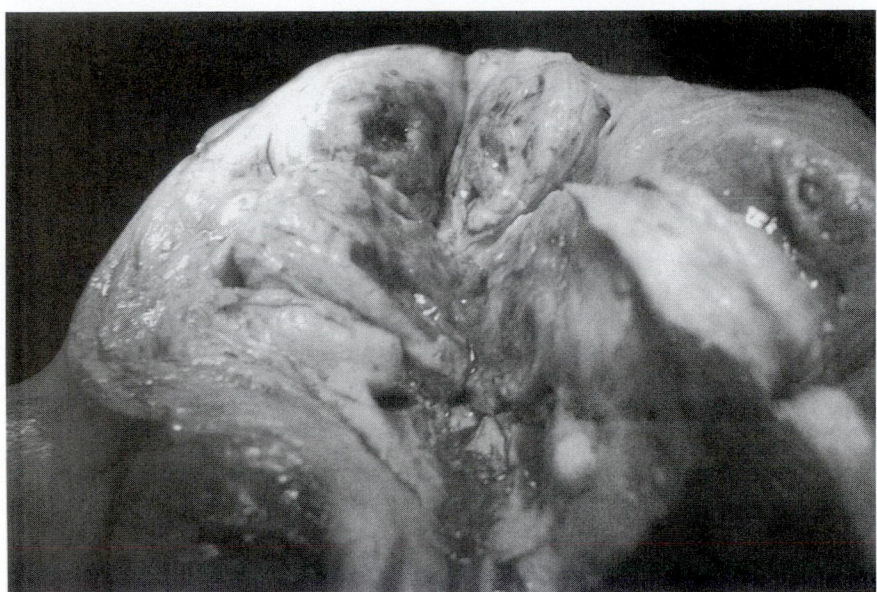

Figure 58-7 Uterine leiomyoma—leiomyosarcoma gross. *Source: Breen SL, Jaffurs WJ. Gynecologic and obstetric pathology. Ortho Forum Educational Series.*

it is uncertain whether these malignancies ever arise within an existing myoma or whether they represent a spontaneous smooth-muscle change. The incidence does increase with advancing age. A woman 60 years of age has 10 times the risk of a sarcoma as a 40-year-old. The data quoted above regarding higher incidence may reflect symptomatic older patients, while the lower incidences are associated with younger, more asymptomatic women. The patient usually experiences abnormal vaginal bleeding and on physical examination the uterus is noted to have increased significantly in size within a short period of time.[27] Hysterectomy may be curative in early tumors noted incidentally; however, tumors that exhibit blood-vessel invasion or external spread are usually lethal.

Unusual leiomyomas include epithelioid leiomyoma, which is an unusual smooth-muscle tumor consisting of rounded polygonal cells and multinucleate giant cells. These were first described in 1960 by Martin et al.[31] and are usually benign when confined to the uterus. Intravenous leiomyomatosis is a smooth-muscle tumor extending into the veins of the parametrium and broad ligaments. Approximately 100 cases have been described. The mitotic index is low (1 mitosis/15 HPF). The tumors usually exhibit a benign behavior after removal of the uterus. The tumor is thought to arise from vascular invasion from a leiomyoma or from the walls of veins in the myometrium. For further discussion the reader is referred to Thompson and Rock[4] and Edwards and Peacock.[32]

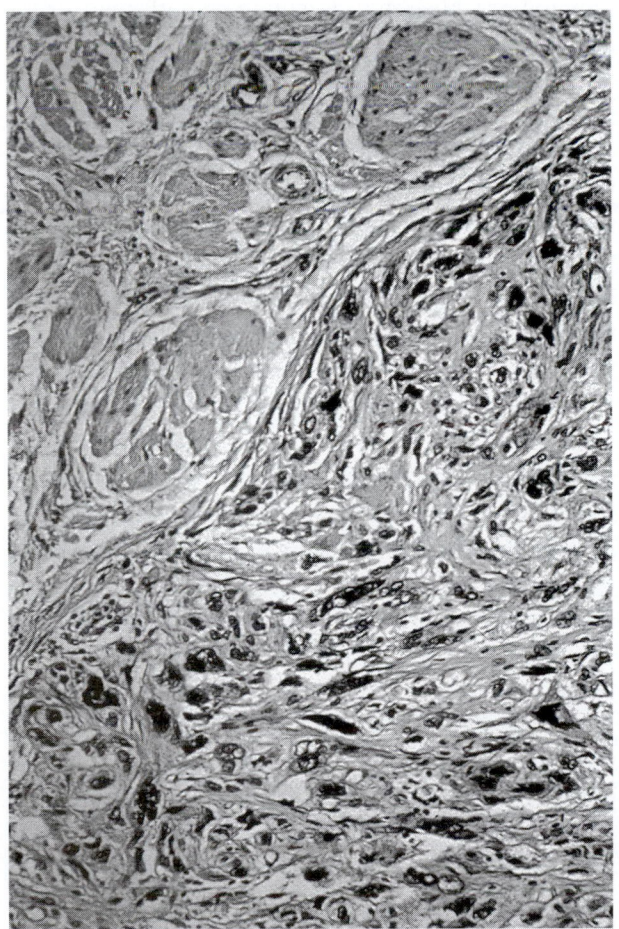

Figure 58-8 Uterine leiomyoma—microscopic leiomyosarcoma. *Source: Breen SL, Jaffurs WJ. Gynecologic and obstetric pathology. Ortho Forum Educational Series.*

Clinical Presentation

The estimates of symptoms caused by uterine leiomyomas range from 10 to 40%.[1] It is likely that the lower estimates more accurately reflect the incidence of symptoms due to the large number of known small asymptomatic myomas. Nevertheless, most leiomyomas remain asymptomatic. It is the consensus that smaller tumors (those <12-week gestational size) may be safely observed. If larger tumors are to be observed, it is mandatory that the diagnosis of myomatous uterus be made accurately. Physical examination, ultrasound, computed tomography (CT), or magnetic resonance imaging (MRI) may be useful to assure the clinician that the pelvic mass, especially in postmenopausal females, is uterine and not ovarian in origin. Confusion may easily arise if the tumor is located within the broad ligament or is pedunculated from the uterine fundus.

There are a number of misconceptions that relate to the diagnosis and management of leimyomas.

Size alone is classically quoted as an indication for hysterectomy in asymptomatic patients. "Twelve-week size" was usually the cutoff for allowing a uterus to remain in situ, even in an asymptomatic woman. Many women with a uterus of that size are likely to experience some of the symptoms noted below. However, there has been no evidence presented to indicate that such uteri should be managed surgically (see section on "Medical Management," below).

It was also commonly thought that the larger the uterus the more likely an increased blood loss at the time of hysterectomy. Reiter et al.[33] have established that blood loss was not significantly greater than those of lesser size, nor were operative complications greater.

Masking of ovarian pathology is often offered as a rationale for surgery. It is obvious that ovarian pathology must be ruled out, especially in the patient with a myoma that extends laterally or is pedunculated or in an older patient. However, advances in ultrasound and MRI have lessened their concerns. Studies by Zarvin et al.[34] suggest that MRI may be better than ultrasound in differentiating ovarian tumors from myomas; however ultrasound should be used as the initial screening tool.

Damage or obstruction of adjacent organs may be observed when the uterus enlarges above a 12-week size. Most clinicians are familiar with patients who have experienced frequency and urgency; more rarely, hydronephrosis may develop from obstruction of the ureters at the pelvic brim or urethral obstruction may

occur, causing urinary retention. Ureteral obstruction may be relatively asymptomatic; therefore, an intravenous pyelogram (IVP) or renal ultrasound may be useful as a screening tool if the patient is asymptomatic and has a uterus that extends above the pelvic brim.

Other rationales, including better potential for fertility and continued growth with hormone replacement, have been reviewed by Friedman and Haas,[35] without good support for intervention with the exception of the above findings.

SYMPTOMATIC LEIOMYOMA

The most common symptom associated with leiomyoma is abnormal uterine bleeding, most often menorrhagia defined as >80 cc blood loss over the course of a menstrual flow. Interestingly, >50% of women reporting excessive blood loss have measured blood loss that is within normal limits.[36] Indeed, many women with even large myomas may have regular menses of measurable duration and flow. Heavy bleeding does occur in approximately 30% of women with symptomatic bleeding presenting as both menorrhagia and metrorrhagia.[1]

Abnormal bleeding is commonly thought to be associated with submucous or pedunculated myomas on the basis of either ulceration or necrosis. However, ulceration is rarely observed in hysterectomy specimens or at hysterectomy. Indeed, a study by Rubin and Ford indicates that the incidence of submucous myomas (5%) is too low to explain the incidence of menorrhagia.[37] Sehgal and Haskins[38] indicate that the surface area of the endometrial cavity may increase greater than 10 times with large myomas. As noted previously, the areas involved with myomas may have increased estrogen receptors and be relatively hyperestrogenic, leading to overlying endometrial hyperplasia. Also, Farrer-Brown et al. have noted alterations in vasculature in the areas of leiomyomas that may alter normal hemostatic mechanisms.[39] Thompson and Rock[4] recommend endometrial sampling even for patients who have regular menstrual flow. Ultrasound, MRI, or more recently, sonohysterography may be useful in diagnosing submucous, pedunculated myomas, or other abnormalities that may influence bleeding patterns.

Pelvic pain is a common reason cited for either myomectomy or hysterectomy; however, myomas probably do not cause pain except in a few specific instances. Carneous degeneration or torsion, both of which may be caused by vascular ischemia, may cause pain or low-grade fever. Red degeneration and torsion are more common during pregnancy. Persand and Arjoon[40] found no correlation between the various degenerative processes and pelvic pain.

Pressure and Obstructive Symptoms

Pressure and obstructive symptoms may be reported in up to 30% of patients with uterine myomas. For example, uterine leiomyomas have purportedly caused urinary incontinence, and bulky myomas may cause frequency secondary to lack of adequate space for urinary bladder expansion. It is possible for an anterior myoma to impinge on the urinary bladder or a lower uterine segment or a cervical myoma to obstruct the urethra. Posterior myomas may press against the sigmoid, causing dyschezia and constipation. According to an ACOG Technical Bulletin, complete ureteral obstruction has not been reported, but we and others have observed significant hydronephrosis in the presence of massive leiomyomas placing pressure on the pelvic brim. Thompson and Rock[4] report that this hydronephrosis is generally reversible if no parenchymal damage has occurred. No studies appear to be available regarding degree of obstruction and alteration in renal function of patients with large, obstructing myomas or reversibility of the pathology if the obstruction is removed.

Reproductive (Spontaneous Abortion and Fertility Problems)

There are currently no specific data to document the anecdotal reports of association between uterine myomas and infertility. Buttram and Reiter[1] reported only 2.4% of myomectomies were performed for myomas in the absence of other factors for infertility. Infertility due to myomas per se is probably unusual.

On the other hand, the same authors reported a significant reduction in spontaneous abortions (41% vs. 19%) after myomectomy. The obvious possibility for causation of spontaneous, recurrent abortion may be present in the leiomyomatous uterus including endometrial obstruction, submucous myomas causing interference with implantation, placentation, and so forth. In addition, myomas have been associated with prematurity and stillbirth but no causal effects have been noted.

Uterine myomas may undergo torsion, infarction, and/or necrosis during pregnancy, causing the patient to present with acute abdominal pain. The outcome of these occurrences is usually favorable with conservative management. However, if surgical management is dictated by continued pain, infection, or other factors, several authors have reported satisfactory outcomes without excessive pregnancy loss.[41,42] Other pregnancy complications include placental entrapment, lower-uterine-segment or pelvic obstruction, or postpartum hemorrhage.

Evaluation

Physical examination may establish the diagnosis in >90% of cases.[43] The findings of an enlarged, firm, irregular mass contiguous with the cervix is almost always diagnostic. Uterine size should be estimated on the basis of gestational size. A uterus the size of a 12-weeks gestation weighs approximately 280 to 320 g.[33] The differential diagnosis includes pregnancy, adenomyosis, and especially in the late reproductive age and postmenopausal woman, ovarian neoplasm. If conservative management is elected, evaluation may include Pap smear, hemoglobin and hematocrit, and endometrial biopsy, especially if there is a history of irregular bleeding. Ultrasonography or MRI is useful in the assessment of uterine myomas. Advantages include objective measurement of size so that accurate follow-up of growth may occur. In addition, sonography will identify the ovaries as separate structures in the majority of patients. Andolf et al.,[44] however, have suggested that ultrasonography does not improve long-term outcome above clinical evaluation. Therefore, ACOG does not recommend routine ultrasonography for all patients with leiomyoma.

Treatment Options

Treatment options for uterine leiomyomas include expectant, medical, or medical/surgical management. Expectant/observational management is appropriate for the majority of leiomyomas, especially those that are asymptomatic regardless of size, within reason. Yearly physical examination and reassessment of bleeding patterns and associated symptoms is quite appropriate after an initial period of assessment to determine that rapid growth is not taking place. Nonsteroidal antiinflammatory drugs should be the first line of defense for menorrhagia and should be prescribed on a schedule for optimal results.

Medical Management

Medical therapy of myomas dates to 1946, when Goodman[45] reported the use of progesterone in six cases of uterine myomas. However, his results were disappointing. Poor results with progestational therapy were also reported by Goldzieher[46] and Segaloff[47] and their colleagues. The poor results may have been due to several factors: (1) pharmacologic progestins may act differently on endometrium and myometrium as demonstrated by Boulet and Fortier[48] in the rabbit model. In addition, studies of "add-back therapy" using progesterone have demonstrated regrowth of uterine myomas after an initial decrease in size, despite continued GnRH therapy.[49] (2) Estrogen and progesterone receptors appear to vary by location (myometrium vs. endometrium), area of the uterus sampled, and location of myomas (submucosal or subserosal).[50] Therefore, secondary to unpredictable and often undesirable response, progesterone is no longer advocated as a therapy for uterine myomas either preoperatively or long term.

GnRH AGONISTS

Clinical trials of GnRH agonists as medical or preoperative therapy date to 1985, when Maheux et al.[51] treated 10 women with subcutaneous buserelin. Following initial stimulation, the pituitary–ovarian axis was suppressed. After 3 weeks with estradiol levels in the postmenopausal range,[52,53] the treated myomas decreased in size by approximately 50%.[53] Since that initial trial, many studies have reported similar results.[54-56] All GnRH agonists have common effects on myomas, summarized in Table 58-1.[57] The most significant are: (1) consistent size reduction of approximately 40 to 60%; (2) maximum reduction by 8 to 12 weeks of therapy; (3) regrowth of myomas after discontinuance of therapy within 3 to 6 months; (4) relatively few side effects and complications.

Effects of GnRH Agonists on Uterine Myomas

Several studies have addressed the issue of physiologic effects of GnRH agonists on uterine myomas. Deligdisch et al.[58] reviewed the leiomyomatas removed

TABLE 58-1
GnRH EFFECTS ON UTERINE LEIOMYOMAS

Induction of hypoestrogenism occurs in all patients. The majority of side effects are related to estrogen deprivation.
45–60% reduction in myoma/uterine volume
Maximal rate of myoma reduction occurs in the first 8 wk
No significant size reduction occurs after 12 wk
Following discontinuation, there is regrowth of myomas to pretreatment size within 12 wk
Menorrhagia reported in approximately 1% of patients with light breakthrough bleeding occurring in 30–40%
Patients with severe anemia have correction of anemia within 8–12 wk
Preoperative use of agonists prior to hysterectomy increases the number of patients who are candidates for vaginal surgery
No consistent effect of agonists on the growth of leiomyosarcomas
Agonists coupled with estrogen replacement results in maintenance of a decreased uterine size and elimination of the hypoestrogenic side effects

Adapted from Stovall.[57]

from 30 control patients and 30 patients treated with leuprolide acetate. Nodular hyaline degeneration, hydropic degeneration, and obliteration of the interface between myoma and myometrium were found with greater frequency in treated patients than in controls. The findings were similar to those noted in involuting myomas from postmenopausal uteri. The authors concluded that a rapid decrease in size of treated myomas occurs secondary to hydropic degeneration and necrosis, perhaps because of a diminished vascular supply.

Similarly, Rutgers et al.[59] studied the sizes of arterial vessels in myomas from women treated with GnRH agonist and placebo for 3 months at the time of hysterectomy. Uterine volumes were noted to decrease by 30% and the diameter of the largest myomas by 27%. The diameter of intramyomatous arteries in the treated group were 24% smaller than arteries in myomas from the placebo group. In addition, arteriosclerotic changes, including intimal and medial fibrosis, were seen more often in GnRH-treated subjects. The authors concluded that estrogen deprivation may cause relative vasoconstriction of myomatous vessels. In contrast, Sreenan et al.[60] reviewed a series of 233 myomectomy specimens from 30 patients treated with leuprolide acetate versus 30 comparable controls. There was no significant difference noted in nuclear atypia, calcification, coagulation necrosis, hemorrhage, vascular change, myxoid change, hydropic degeneration, hyalinization, mitotic activity, or cellularity between treated patients and controls.

Therefore, the decreased volume of treated myomas may be related to GnRH-induced hypoestrogenism or decreased arterial blood supply to the myoma. However, resulting changes noted in myomas are not consistent in various study groups.

Effect of GnRH on Estrogen and Progestin Receptor Status in Leiomyomas

Leiomyomas clinically are estrogen-sensitive tumors. It is well known that these lesions develop during reproductive years and regress during menopause. In addition, premenopausal use of GnRH agonists results in a dramatic decrease in the size of myomas. However, following cessation of therapy with GnRH agonists, myomas rapidly regrow, almost reaching their original size within 6 months. Secondary to these findings, Regidor et al.[61] studied the estrogen and progesterone receptor content of myomas pretreated with GnRH agonist versus untreated premenopausal and postmenopausal controls. The GnRH-analog–treated myomas showed higher levels of estrogen and progesterone receptors than the untreated group. These data correlate with the estrogen and progestin receptor content of myomas from postmenopausal women. The authors hypothesized that this increased receptor content may be a partial explanation for the rapid regrowth of these tumors noted on withdrawal of GnRH agonist in premenopausal women.

Long-Term Therapy of Myomas with GnRH Agonists to Avoid Hysterectomy

The advantage of GnRH agonists appears to be limited to the short term secondary to development of osteoporosis and adverse lipid profiles with usage longer than 6 months. However, several articles have appeared analyzing the effect of estrogen, progestin, and estrogen/progestin "add-back" to delay surgery indefinitely or until a menopausal decrease in estrogen may favorably affect these tumors. Initially Bradham et al.[62] and Scailli and Jestila[63] reported the use of high-dose progestin (Depo Provera) and low-dose progestin (Provera, 5 mg per day) following treatment with GnRH agonists for 3 months. The authors reported a continued decrease in uterine size in the 6 months following cessation of GnRH agonist therapy. However, more than 50% of the patients dropped out of this study, mainly because of bleeding. Friedman et al.[49] reported a group of 51 premenopausal women with leiomyomas treated with the GnRH agonist leuprolide 3.75 mg every 4 weeks for 2 years. After 3 months of therapy, the patients were either given estropipate 0.75 mg daily plus norethindrone 0.7 mg daily for 14 days each month or norethindrone 10 mg daily. Uterine volume decreased by 40% in each group initially. However, mean uterine volume in the progestin-only add-back group increased to 80% of the pretreatment size by month 12 and 95% of pretreatment size by treatment month 24.[35] The estrogen/progestin (E/P) group did not demonstrate any subsequent change in uterine volume. The mean bone density decreased as expected during the initial 3 months of therapy but did not change in either group for the remainder of the study. Hematocrits increased in a parallel fashion as expected. Mean high-density lipoprotein (HDL) was unchanged in the E/P group but decreased by 36% in the progestin-only group. The authors concluded that the E/P group add-back regimen was clearly superior to progestin-only add-back in all parameters studied.

Finally, De Aloysio et al.[64] studied 34 perimenopausal women given leuprolide acetate each month for 6 months followed by a 5-month, drug-free interval and resumption of drug for an additional 6-month cycle. The premise of the study was that a normal perimenopausal decrease in estrogen would diminish the rapid regrowth of tumors noted in premenopausal women. As expected, there was a decrease in surgical intervention for symptomatic myomas, 8.8% as compared with 86.8% formerly. The results of this study obviously cannot apply to reproductive-age women with this problem.

Side Effects and Disadvantages

No medical therapy is without at least potential side effects and complications. Most side effects associated with preoperative treatment with GnRH agonists are minor, as are those associated with hypoestronism/menopause.[65] Essentially, all of these effects are self-limited and disappear 3 to 6 months after cessation of GnRH agonist therapy. More severe adverse effects are unusual and may be categorized as follows: (1) degeneration and bleeding; (2) bone loss; (3) possible relation to delayed therapy for leiomyosarcoma; and (4) others.

Hyaline degeneration and focal necrosis have been reported in 1 to 2% of cases treated with GnRH agonists. This finding is associated with pelvic pain and fever in patients with subserous tumors or intramural tumors and transcervical expulsion with submucous tumors. Friedman[66] reported good results with E/P contraceptive treatment in these cases. In addition, if myomectomy is to be performed, the degeneration may cause the plane normally made distinct by the pseudocapsule of the myoma to be obscured and necessitate piecemeal removal of the myoma.

Lee and Kazer[67] reported a case of massive ascites associated with pseudomeigs syndrome subsequent to a 3.75-mg injection of leuprolide acetate in a patient with a 20-week-size leiomyoma. Serra et al.[68] reported extrusion of four myomas through the cervix in a series of 110 patients treated with GnRH agonists. Five others required hysterectomy because of failure to relieve symptoms of bleeding or pressure. Hitti et al.[69] reported a case of massive necrosis within a uterine leiomyosarcoma during GnRH agonist therapy of a presumed benign leiomyoma in preparation for total abdominal hysterectomy. The issue of delayed diagnosis has been raised in these cases, but it probably is of relatively minor importance because of the scarcity of these tumors. McCoy[70] has reported a case of myocardial infarction following 2 months of leuprolide therapy in a patient with a strong family history of heart disease confirmed by electrocardiographic and enzymatic changes.

Prolonged use of GnRH agonists has been definitely associated with significant bone loss over several months. Therefore, the use of these agents for more than 6 months has not been recommended. Rivlin and others[65,71,72] have reported bone loss ranging from 3 to 11% with prolonged use of GnRH agonists, only part of which was reversible. Add-back therapy is partially successful at preventing further bone loss. However, progestin-only add-back has been variably associated with regrowth of myomas.

Medical/Surgical Therapy

Surgery alone or in combination with medical therapy has been the mainstay of therapy for uterine myomas for at least the past 7 to 10 years.[72]

Myomectomy versus Hysterectomy

Once the decision has been made to proceed with surgical management of leiomyoma, the next decision

point is for the patient to determine whether she desires to maintain the potential for future childbearing. If she does, and surgical intervention is required, myomectomy is the operative procedure of choice. The surgical approach to the patient undergoing myomectomy is somewhat dependent on the location of the myomas. Myomectomy can be performed by laparotomy, vaginally or laparoscopically or hysteroscopically as above.

Endoscopy/Laparoscopy

Hysteroscopic resection of myomas has been evaluated in several trials. Derman et al.[73] noted that approximately 20% of patients will require further therapy within 5 to 10 years of initial treatment. Laparoscopic resection of subserosal myomas has been reported, but long-term studies are lacking.[74]

Before performing a myomectomy, the physician should observe the precautions as outlined in Table 58-2. Most abdominal myomectomies are performed using a Pfannenstiel or other transverse incision. Surgical principles for myomectomy are similar to those used for other gynecologic surgical and infertility procedures. These techniques include meticulous hemostasis and avoidance of adhesiogenic materials. Hemostatic aids include myometrial injection of

---

TABLE 58-2
BEFORE PERFORMING A MYOMECTOMY

1. An absence of cervical malignancy should be documented by negative cervical cytology.
2. Anovlulation and other causes of abnormal bleeding should be eliminated.
3. When abnormal bleeding is present with ovulatory cycles, the possible presence of submucous fibroid should be assessed by dilation and curettage, hysteroscopy, or imaging techniques.
4. Surgical risk from anemia and need for treatement should be determined.
5. Advantages and disadvantages of myomectomy versus hysterectomy should be discussed with the patient and documented in the patient's record.

In addition, the physician should:

1. Evaluate other causes of male and female infertility or recurrent pregnancy loss.
2. Evaluate the endometrial cavity and fallopian tubes (e.g., by hysterosalpingography).
3. Document discussion that complexity of disease process may require a hysterectomy.

Note: In patients undergoing myomectomy because of infertility, there should not be a more likely explanation for failure to conceive or recurrent pregnancy loss.

Adapted from Stovall and Ling.[75]

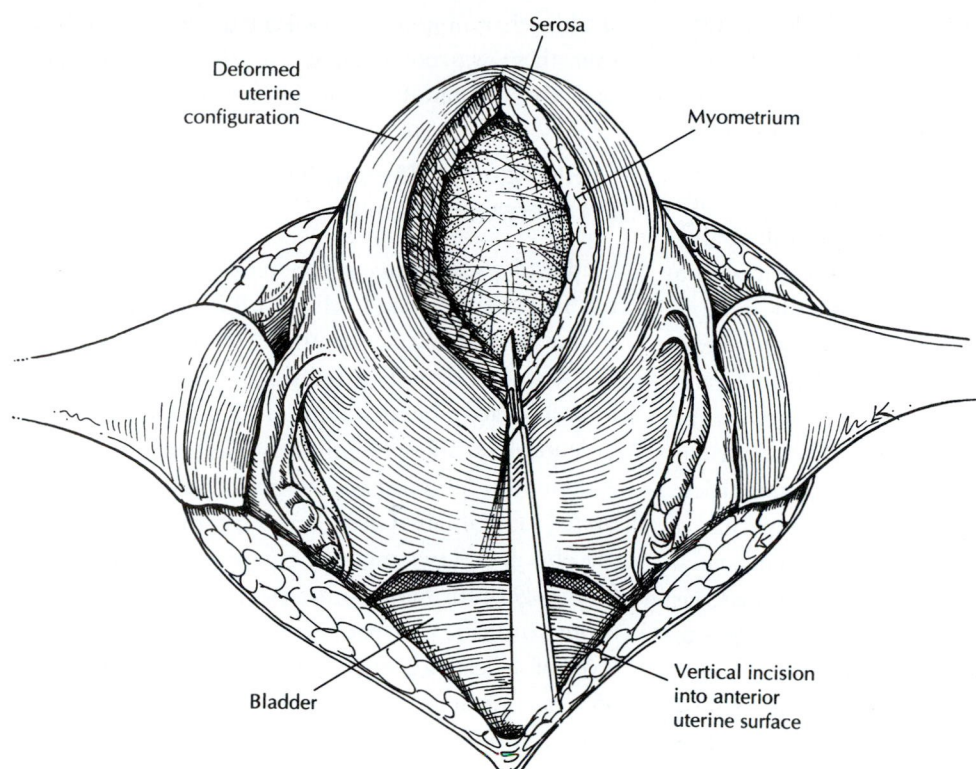

Serosa

Deformed
uterine
configuration

Myometrium

Bladder

Vertical incision
into anterior
uterine surface

Figure 58-9. Uterine
leiomyoma—myomectomy.
Source: Stovall and Ling.[75]

vasoconstrictors such as vasopressin (Pitressin). The incision is made to allow maximal removal of myomas in a vertical direction if possible, to avoid the more vascular areas of the uterus (Figure 58-9). For a detailed description the reader is referred to Stovall and Ling.[75]

Hysterectomy

Hysterectomy is the definitive therapy for symptomatic uterine leiomyomas in a woman who no longer desires to maintain her childbearing capacity. The reported risk of mortality as reviewed by several authors is approximately 1 in 1000 procedures.[76,77] Hysterectomy may be performed either with or without oophorectomy without apparent sequelae with reference to myomas. In general, asymptomatic uteri should be managed without surgery, as stated earlier. However, those that may be palpable abdominally and are a concern from the patient's point of view may be removed surgically. Patients with symptomatic uteri should be offered a trial of conservative management prior to hysterectomy. Symptoms of excessive uterine bleeding lasting longer than 8 days or bleeding either acutely or chronically to the point of anemia are considered adequate indications for surgery. In addition, acute or severe abdominal pain, chronic abdominal or

back pain, or pressure on contiguous organs to the point of discomfort is considered an adequate indication for operative intervention. The same procedures to rule out malignancy and evaluation of bleeding should be observed as prior to myomectomy. The procedure may be performed via a midline or Pfannenstiel incision, depending on the patient's body habitus, skeletal configuration, and the size and configuration of the uterine myomas. The same techniques as performed during hysterectomy for other reasons should be followed in the performance of hysterectomy for myomas.

The issue of GnRH agonists used preoperatively prior to hysterectomy has been investigated by several authors with relation to conversion from abdominal hysterectomy to vaginal hysterectomy, conversion from midline to Pfannenstiel incision, and therapy for preoperative anemia and operative complications.

Conversion from Abdominal to Vaginal Hysterectomy

Vaginal hysterectomy has been established as requring a shorter hospital stay, having decreased costs and lower overall morbidity, and requiring decreased convalescent time as compared with abdominal hysterectomy. Despite the reported safety of uterine morcellation at the time of vaginal hysterectomy, most gynecologic surgeons do not recommend vaginal hysterectomy for a "fixed" uterus or one greater than 10 to 14 weeks of gestational size. Conversion of abdominal hysterectomy to vaginal hysterectomy by reduction of uterine size would therefore be advantageous. To investigate this premise, Stovall et al.[78] studied a group of 90 premenopausal women with a uterine size of 14 to 18 weeks of gestation and another group of 60 premenopausal women with uterine size greater than 18 weeks. Patients were randomized to immediate surgery or 2 months of preoperative GnRH agonist therapy. All patients in the two groups with a pretreatment hemoglobin less than 11.0 g/dl randomized to agonist therapy had a significant ($\geq$1.5 g/dl) rise in hemoglobin. The criteria for performing vaginal hysterectomy required the uterus to be <14 weeks in size and mobile on examination. Patients in group 1 who received preoperative agonists were more likely to undergo vaginal hysterectomy (80 vs. 13%) than patients who did not receive preoperative agonist. Patients undergoing vaginal hysterectomy had a shorter hospital stay, decreased operative blood loss, and shorter convalescence than those undergoing abdominal hysterectomy. In the group with a uterine size of greater than 18 weeks despite a uterine volume reduction of 50%, intraoperative morbidity, operative blood loss, hospital stay, and postoperative convalescence did not differ between treatment arms similar to other studies.

Conversion of Midline Abdominal to Pfannenstiel Incision by GnRH Agonist Therapy

The issue of potential change in incision from midline to Pfannenstiel with GnRH therapy was addressed by Lumsden et al.[79] These authors studied 71 premenopausal patients undergoing abdominal hysterectomy for symptomatic myomas. Thirty-five patients received goserelin and 36 received placebo. Study parameters, including base-line uterine size and patients' demographics, were similar between the two groups. At the time of operation, uterine volumes were smaller, mean hemoglobin higher, and blood loss less in the treated group. Transverse incisions were elected more often in the treated group by surgeons who were blinded to treatment method. Surgery for 18% of those in the placebo arm was described as "dif-

ficult" versus none in the GnRH-treated group. However, there was no difference in operative time, postoperative complications, or duration of hospitalization.

GnRH Agonist Therapy and Preoperative Anemia

Studies demonstrating preoperative rise in hemoglobin in patients treated with GnRH agonists date to studies by Friedman and others[80,81] in the late 1980s. These studies demonstrated significant mean increases in preoperative hemoglobin and hematocrit with use of leuprolide. Subsequently, Stovall et al.[82] performed a double-blind, placebo-controlled trial of 265 patients to evaluate GnRH agonist plus iron versus placebo in the treatment of patients with anemia before surgery for leiomyomas. Seventy-four percent of agonist/iron-treated patients achieved a hemoglobin level of at least 12 mg/dl and hematocrit of at least 35% as compared with 46% of patients in the placebo iron group. The treatment group had a nearly twofold increase in autologous blood donation, which paralleled the increase in hemoglobin. The improved hematologic characteristics reduced the need for preoperative nonautologous blood transfusion. In addition, the authors proposed that the decreased uterine volume associated with agonist therapy may make surgery easier to perform.

However, among nonanemic patients with a pretreatment uterine size of 18 gestational weeks or more, preoperative treatment with a GnRH agonist did not appear to lower morbidity.

GnRH Agonist Therapy and Operative Complications

While GnRH agonist therapy reduces uterine size, the data regarding operative complications are contradictory. Lumsden et al.[83] used goserelin for 3 months prior to surgery in 13 symptomatic patients. They reported significantly reduced blood loss at abdominal hysterectomy (235 vs. 350 ml) and decreased febrile morbidity (15 vs. 43%). Later, the same authors reported on a series of 71 patients pretreated with goserelin.[83] As expected, uterine volume decreased and serum hemoglobin increased. Median blood loss at surgery was again significantly less in the treated group (187 vs. 301 ml).

Audebent et al.,[84] also in a randomized trial, found that operating time was marginally shorter (81 ± 18 vs. 98 ± 36) minutes in the treated group. However, they observed no differences in intraoperative blood loss or length of hospital stay. Vercelini et al.[85] performed a nonrandomized study of 133 premenopausal, anemic women treated with GnRH agonists prior to hysterectomy for leiomyomas. No treated patient required a blood transfusion, whereas 51% of the placebo-treated patients required transfusions, most on the basis of preoperative anemia. The authors noted no differences in operative blood loss or postoperative morbidity.

In comparison, Reiter et al.[33] in 1992 reported that patients with a uterine size greater than 12 weeks were no more likely to have perioperative complications than a uterus less than 12 weeks size. Perhaps Stovall et al.[78] refined this issue in a series of 60 patients with a preoperative uterine size >18 weeks, 30 of whom were treated and 30 of whom received placebo, as compared with a group of 90 patients with a preoperative uterine size of 14 to 18 gestational weeks. The authors found that the group with smaller uteri benefited from therapy with GnRH agonists. Both groups with larger uteri had very similar operative and postoperative morbidity.

The following conclusions may be reasonably drawn from the above and other similar studies. Patients with uteri 14 to 18 weeks in size treated preoperatively with GnRH agonist may have decreased operative time, shorter hospital stay, shorter convalescence, and decreased intraoperative blood loss, all because of increased use of vaginal hysterectomy. For those with larger uteri, the benefit derived from GnRH agonist pretreatment is marginal except for those who are anemic. This group of patients may benefit from the possibility of decreased preoperative morbidity secondary to menorrhagia and the ability to use autologous transfusions or perhaps avoid homologous blood transfusion at the time of surgery.

OTHER ADNEXAL MASSES (BENIGN DISORDERS OF THE OVARY)

While uterine leiomyomas are the most common benign tumors of the female genitalia, sources other than the uterus must be considered in the evaluation of benign pelvic masses. A discussion of those masses occurring in various age groups provides a convenient method of classifying possibilities to be included in the differential diagnosis. This section provides a systematic classification of these adnexal masses according to age group, their cause, and a rational management schema. Premenarchal masses will be considered first, then those encountered during reproductive years and postmenopausally, and finally those miscellaneous masses that may occur in various age groups.

Premenarchal Female

Malignancy in general and ovarian masses in particular are rare in childhood, accounting for approximately 1% of all cases. Conventional wisdom states that all pelvic/ovarian masses in young females are malignant until proven otherwise and require exploration. To some degree that is true, since older studies demonstrated approximately 80% of tumors in girls less than 9 years old, and 35% of all tumors in children and adolescents, are malignant.[86] Of these neoplasms, germ-cell tumors predominate (60%). However, more recent studies have shown that functional masses may occur in fetuses and young children. In one study of girls younger than age 10, only 60% of masses proved to be neoplasms, and two-thirds of those were benign.[87]

A pelvic mass in a premenarchal female may quickly become abdominal in location due to the small size of the pelvis. The child may then present with abdominal pain. Classic pelvic examination is difficult in this age group; therefore, abdominal examination and supplementary studies are the mainstay of diagnosis. Transabdominal ultrasonography is probably the most useful diagnostic tool in this age group. As in the postmenopausal female, simple unilocular cysts of small size are almost always benign and do not require surgical intervention. Observation over a period of 2 to 3 months is appropriate; however, these cysts tend to float in the abdominal cavity and may subsequently undergo torsion, giving rise to acute abdominal pain. New technologies with Doppler flow may aid in diagnosis, although this remains somewhat unclear. Tumor markers such as α-fetoprotein (AFP) or human chorionic gonadotropin (hCG) may also be used on occasion. However, any solid, multiloculated, persistent, or enlarging mass in this age group dictates surgical intervention.

Postmenarche/Adolescence

The postmenarchal/adolescent female in general is subject to the same variety of pelvic masses as the older woman of reproductive age, including uterine, adnexal, and extragenital masses. The possibility of functional adnexal masses increases and malignancy decreases as compared with the premenarchal female. The exception to this statement is the diagnosis of genital anomalies that may be recognized by the initial onset of menses and the appearance of a pelvic mass. This presentation includes a wide range of anomalies ranging from imperforate hymen to vaginal septae with noncommunicating upper Müllerian systems. The postmenarchal woman with vaginal septae, imperforate hymen, and obstructed unicornate uterus may present with abdominal/pelvic pain that may be acute or prolonged, depending on the degree of obstruction. Physical examination usually yields the diagnosis; however, again these young girls may be difficult to examine due to pain and lack of previous sexual activity or use of tampons. In these cases, examination under anesthesia and/or diagnostic laparoscopy will usually give the diagnosis.

Functional ovarian cysts occur frequently and may be found incidentally, present with acute abdominal pain secondary to torsion and ischemia, or rupture with peritoneal irritation. While endometriosis occurs less commonly than in older females, approximately 60% of patients of this age presenting with cyclic abdominal pain will be noted to have this problem.[88] In the absence of a mass, a trial of nonsteroidal analgesics is in order. If the patient presents with a pelvic mass, diagnosis is best accomplished by laparoscopy or laparotomy, depending on the size and characteristics of the mass. In most cases, endometriosis of the ovary may be repaired and the ovaries preserved. Following removal of visible disease, birth control pills will often give the triple advantage of pain relief, decreased incidence of recurrence, and pregnancy prevention.

The highest rate of pelvic inflammatory disease occurs in adolescents. Therefore, the possibility of a sexually transmitted disease (STD) and inflammatory adnexal mass should be entertained in the adolescent female presenting with pelvic pain and/or mass. The classic finding of cervical motion tenderness and uterine, adnexal, and lower abdominal pain, occasionally coupled with elevated temperature, suggests this diagnosis. Most cases of pelvic inflammatory disease present without a mass in these patients. However, if multiple episodes or prolonged presence of disease is noted, the diagnosis of a tubo-ovarian abscess (TOA) must be entertained (Figure 58-10). The diagnosis should be suspected when the patient presents with an adnexal mass on palpation or ultrasound or demonstrates a lack of response to standard antibiotic therapy. A TOA is a very serious condition, and while aggressive antibiotic therapy alone will cause resolution in the majority of cases, a ruptured TOA is a life-threatening complication that demands immediate surgical intervention. In the young age group, surgery may be conservative. Unilateral salpingectomy or oophorectomy or laparoscopic or CT-guided drainage have yielded good results. See Chapter 5 for further discussion of these entities.

Pregnancy in a postmenarchal female should be a primary consideration in any patient presenting with a pelvic mass. This group is also at risk for ectopic pregnancy, which may likewise present as a pelvic mass accompanied by pain. The diagnosis is suspected with a classic finding of amenorrhea, vaginal bleeding, and a positive pregnancy test. However, ectopic pregnancy is the great masquerader, mimicking appendicitis, pelvic inflammatory disease, or other disorders.

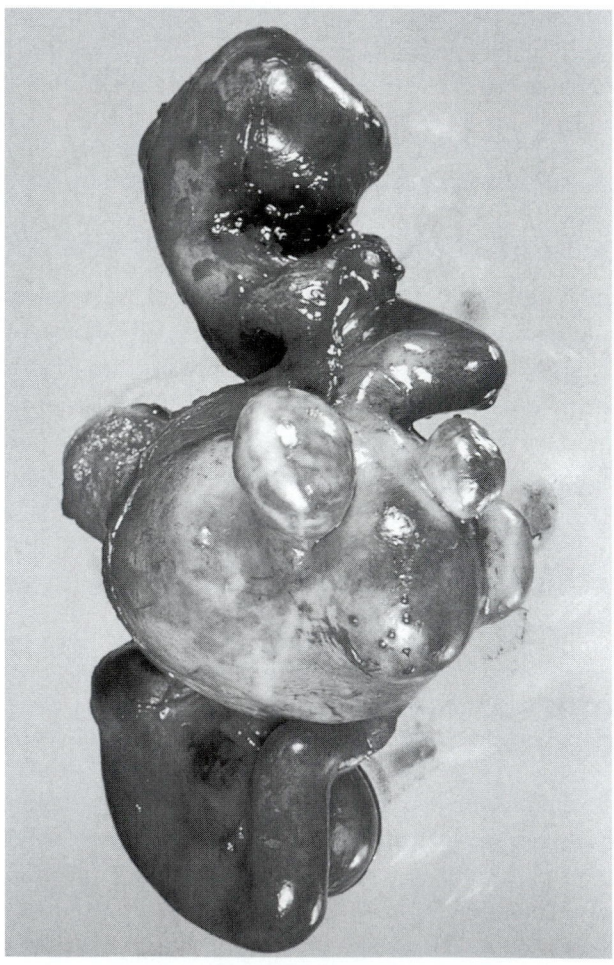

Figure 58-10 Tubo-ovarian abscess. *Source: Breen SL, Jaffurs WJ. Gynecologic and obstetric pathology. Ortho Forum Educational Series.*

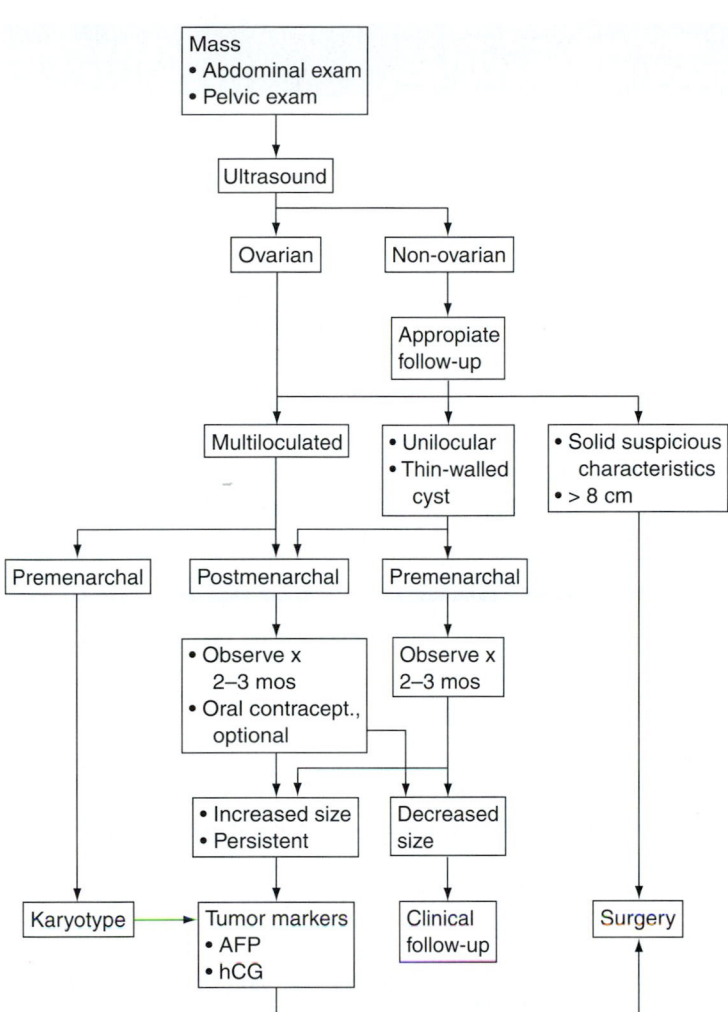

Figure 58-11 Management of pelvic mass in pre-menarchal and adolescent female. *Source: Hillard PA. Benign disease of the female reproductive tract: signs and symptoms. In: Berek JS, ed. Novak's gynecology. 12th ed. Baltimore: Williams & Wilkins, 1996.*

Like the premenarchal female, unilateral, unilocular cystic ovarian masses of small size may be managed conservatively because of the low incidence of malignancy. However, large, growing, solid, and/or multilocular masses require exploration. Surgical management should emphasize conservation of the ovary if at all possible. Even the presence of an apparent malignancy may be managed by unilateral oophorectomy in selected cases. A very coherent management schema for premenarchal and adolescent girls has been presented by Hillard (Figure 58-11).

Reproductive Age

Women of reproductive age are subject to the widest range of pelvic masses. In this age group, the frequency of pelvic masses is difficult to determine since many never present for surgery. Women of early reproductive age are at low risk for malignancy from pelvic masses, comprising only 10% of one group

studied at laparotomy. Most adnexal masses in this group less than 30 years old are functional cysts or dermoids and endometriomas, as compared with 33% and 25% of masses in women 31 to 49 years old (Table 58-3).[89]

While most ovarian tumors are asymptomatic, when symptoms are present they may include bloating or nonspecific pain that mimics gastrointestinal colic. The same generalizations that apply to masses in adolescents are true. Those that are less than 8 cm, unilocular, unilateral, and asymptomatic may be observed. Those that are solid, large, multilocular, or symptomatic require exploration. These masses may be conveniently divided into adnexal/ovarian, uterine, and extragenital (Table 58-4).[89]

Functional ovarian tumors comprise the largest group of adnexal/ovarian masses in women of reproductive age. They may be found accidentally or associated with acute abdominal pain secondary to torsion. Follicular cysts are usually thin-walled with clear

	TABLE 58-3	
	DIFFERENTIAL DIAGNOSIS OF ADNEXAL MASS	
Organ	**Cystic**	**Solid**
Ovary	Functional cyst	Neoplasm
	Neoplastic cyst	Benign
	Benign	Malignant
	Malignant	
	Endometriosis	
Fallopian tube	Tubo-ovarian abscess	Tubo-ovarian abscess
	Hydrosalpinx	Ectopic pregnancy
	Parovarian cyst	Neoplasm
Uterus	Intrauterine pregnancy in a bicornuate uterus	Pedunculated or interligamentous myoma
Bowel	Sigmoid or cecum distended with gas and/or feces	Diverticulitis
		Ileitis
		Appendicitis
		Colonic cancer
Miscellaneous	Distended bladder	Abdominal-wall hematoma or abscess
	Pelvic kidney	Retroperitoneal neoplasm
	Urachal cyst	

Adapted from DiSaia.[89]

fluid and a maximum diameter of 5 to 6 cm diameter and regress spontaneously within 1 to 3 months. Surgical intervention is necessary with persistence of a large cyst or a rupture that causes acute symptoms. Microscopically, these cysts are lined by a single layer of granulosa or theca cells.

Polycystic ovaries are the most common course of bilateral follicular cysts (Figure 58-12). This complex syndrome consists of a spectrum associated with increased secretion of luteinizing hormone and clinical androgen excess. These individuals commonly present with dysfunctional bleeding secondary to infrequency of ovulation and subsequent cyclic progesterone secretion. Grossly, the ovaries may exhibit a moderate size (usually less than 6 cm in diameter), bilaterality, and histologic evidence of infrequent ovulation.

TABLE 58-4
BENIGN OVARIAN TUMORS

I. Nonneoplastic tumors
  A. Germinal inclusion cyst
  B. Follicle cyst
  C. Corpus luteum cyst
  D. Pregnancy luteoma
  E. Theca lutein cysts
  F. Sclerocystic ovaries
  G. Endometrioma
II. Neoplastic tumors derived from coelomic epithelium
  A. Cystic tumors
    1. Serous cystoma
    2. Mucinous cystoma
    3. Mixed forms
  B. Tumors with stromal overgrowth
    1. Fibroma, adenofibroma
    2. Brenner tumor
III. Tumors derived from germ cells
  A. Dermoid (benign cystic teratoma)

Adapted from DiSaia.[89]

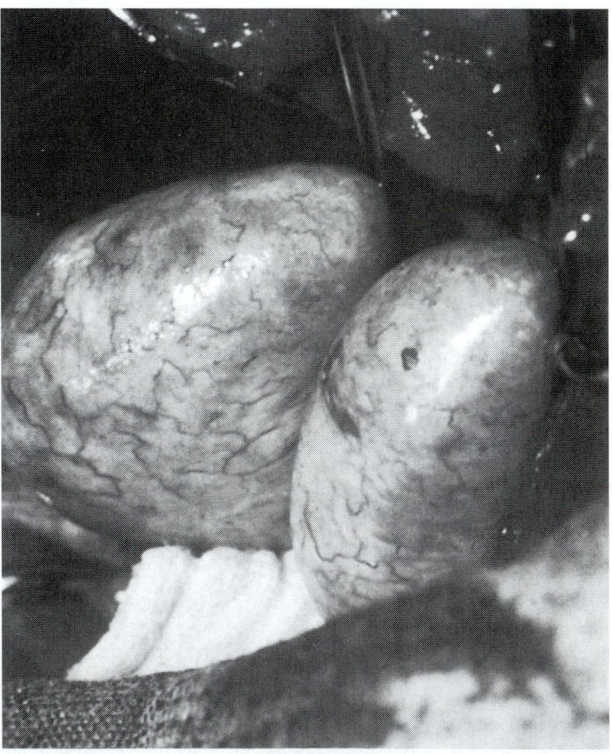

Figure 58-12. Polycystic ovaries. *Source: Breen SL, Jaffurs WJ. Gynecologic and obstetric pathology. Ortho Forum Educational Series.*

Corpus luteum cysts are less common but may give rise to more significant symptoms secondary to larger size and/or intraperitoneal bleeding. The cyst occurs as a consequence of normal ovulation and grossly contains characteristic yellow-orange material. Microscopic examination reveals luteinized theca and granulosa cells.

Theca lutein cysts are the least common of the functional cysts and are almost always bilateral and may attain large size (Figure 58-13). The histologic picture reflects their origin from hyperstimulation by hCG. Iatrogenic stimulation of the ovaries with any of the gonadotropin regimens for assisted reproduction may result in multiple follicular and/or theca lutein cysts. Conception may worsen the condition because of persistent hCG stimulation. Even with significant ovarian enlargement and development of ascites, surgical management is rarely indicated except in the event of torsion or rupture.

In the past, a trial of oral contraceptives has been suggested in order to suppress the ovaries while these functional cysts are observed for regression. More recent studies have questioned this philosophy, with no difference observed in time of cyst resolution between patients given oral contraceptives and those who are only observed.[90]

Uterine leiomyomas are the most common uterine masses and were reviewed extensively in the previous section.

Benign neoplastic adnexal masses in this age group are usually of three varieties. Dermoid cysts are the most common neoplasm in the reproductive years,

comprising 62% of ovarian neoplasms in one series of women under 40 years of age undergoing laparotomy for pelvic mass. Eighty percent of these cysts occur premenopausally. Malignant transformation is rare (<2%), and when it occurs it is squamous in origin.[91] Dermoids may present with acute abdominal pain more frequently than other ovarian masses because of their high fat content and tendency toward torsion. Diagnosis is facilitated by contained calcification, rendering these masses visible on abdominal x-rays and by a characteristic sonographic appearance. The surgeon should carefully inspect the opposite ovary and perform cystectomy only on the involved ovary if possible.

Epithelial tumors are the other major group of benign tumors in the reproductive age group. Serous cystadenomas are more common than mucinous tumors; they comprise 20% of all ovarian neoplasms and arise from invagination of the surface epithelium. They are also usually smaller than mucinous tumors and are unilocular with a cyst wall comprised of a single layer of cuboidal epithelium. Ten to twelve percent may be bilateral. Most are benign; only 20 to 25% are malignant in this age group. These tumors are often multilocular and contain a watery cystic fluid. Calcific psammoma bodies may be visible on x-ray.

Mucinous tumors are usually larger and less commonly bilateral as compared with serous tumors (10%). The cyst lining is usually smooth, although papillary projections may be seen. Cell types resembling endocervix and gastrointestinal epithelium may

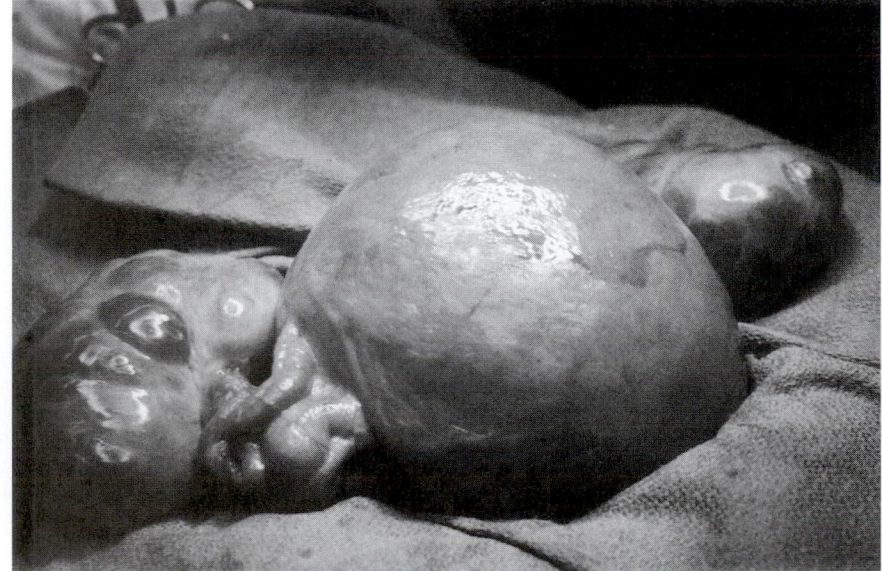

Figure 58-13. Theca lutein cysts. *Source: Breen SL, Jaffurs WJ. Gynecologic and obstetric pathology. Ortho Forum Educational Series.*

be observed microscopically. Pseudomyxoma peritonei is present in 2 to 5% of patients with mucinous tumors. Five to 10% of these tumors are malignant and may be difficult to distinguish from metastatic gastrointestinal malignancies.

Other benign ovarian masses presenting uncommonly include varieties of endometrioid tumors, mesonephroid tumors, Brenner tumors, and benign tumors of stroma origin.

Diagnosis of ovarian masses in this age group relies on standard physical examination coupled with ultrasound or occasionally CT scan. An endometrial sampling is indicated when both a pelvic mass and vaginal bleeding are present. The value of CA-125 is debatable in this age group because of the overlap with a wide range of other disease entities.

Surgical intervention for benign neoplasms should consider preservation of fertility and minimize the potential for postoperative adhesions. An elliptical incision is made over the most dependent area of the ovarian cyst. The cyst is then shelled out and the space closed in a layered fashion with fine suture. Ultrasound aspiration is discouraged because of the frequency of recurrence and the continuing debate about spilling a potentially malignant neoplasm.

POSTMENOPAUSAL ADNEXAL MASS

Proper identification and therapy of the adnexal mass in the postmenopausal female remains a challenge. The overall risk of malignancy in an ovarian cyst is 13% in a premenopausal and 45% in a postmenopausal woman. Dermoids are the most common premenopausal benign tumor. Serous cystadenoma is the most common postmenopausal mass and is the most common malignant tumor in both age groups.

With the development of sensitive ultrasound, the discovery of an incidental small ovarian mass may prove to be a diagnostic and therapeutic problem. Barber and Graker[92] proposed the concept that any ovary that is palpable in the postmenopausal female is abnormal and should be removed. Unfortunately, body habitus and other factors have demonstrated this dictum to be an unreliable predictor of malignancy. In addition, trends toward laparoscopic surgery and ancillary testing have raised new questions regarding the traditional management of adnexal masses in this age group.

Proper management of these patients hinges on the answers to several questions. (1) Can physical examination and ancillary techniques accurately differentiate malignant from nonmalignant masses on a preoperative or intraoperative basis? (2) What is the impact on survival, if any, of spill of a potentially malignant neoplasm? (3) Can a mass be accurately recognized as malignant at laparoscopic inspection? (4) What is the utility of ancillary laboratory studies in the definition of malignancy? (5) What is the significance of the asymptomatic small mass found incidentally on scanning of the pelvis in the postmenopausal female?

Clinical identification of pelvic masses is notoriously inaccurate, missing some 30% of ultrasonically detected masses <5 cm and 24% of masses >5 cm. Plain x-ray films and old contrast studies likewise have largely been replaced by ultrasound, and the technique of Doppler flow became the topic of interest in the 1990s.

Ultrasound parameters include size, number of loculations, presence of papillary excrescences, overall density, and Doppler pulsatility. Clinicians have known for many years that the larger the size, the more likely the mass is malignant. Larger cysts may give confusing ultrasound pictures. However, if a cyst is unilocular and without internal echoes, the likelihood of malignancy is small. Risk of malignancy is directly proportional to the number of internal echoes. Seventy percent of masses with multiloculations and solid components may be malignant. In addition, septations >3 mm in thickness and the presence of papillary excrescences and increased echo density may signal malignancy. However, one must remember the most echo-dense tumor is the dermoid. Doppler flow characteristics have shown good negative predictive value in several studies. However, the positive predictive value remains low. Therefore, if the mass appears benign by other characteristics and has no abnormal Doppler flow, the chance of malignancy is remote. Several authors have combined CA-125, ultrasound, and clinical examination, resulting in a relatively high sensitivity (86%) and specificity (97%) in the diagnosis of malignancy.[93]

Based on the above technology, invasive methods, such as ultrasound-guided aspiration of benign-appearing cysts, have been used to avoid open laparotomy. Unfortunately, the recurrence rate is high and examination of cyst fluid has a low sensitivity and negative predictive value. Therefore, this method may prove useful only in the limited cases in which operative intervention is not practical.

A second key question in the management of early ovarian cancer is the impact of tumor spill in otherwise early-stage ovarian malignancy. While this has been a relevant question because of the occasional spill at the time of laparotomy, it becomes even more important with the increasing use of laparoscopy in the diagnosis and attempted removal of ovarian masses. The relatively small number of cases of early disease makes determination of the significance of spill difficult. Early studies by Munnell[94] noted no difference in prognosis. However, most patients had either radiation or chemotherapy after surgery. A paper by Decker[95] implies that rupture may be detrimental; however, these lesions may have been more advanced. In a study by Dembo et al.,[96] histologic grade, dense adhesions, and ascites were the most significant predictive factors in Stage I disease with tumor spill. Intraoperative spill did not affect survival at a statistically significant level, even in patients followed without treatment postoperatively. Similar findings appear to apply to borderline epithelial tumors. Overall, current data suggest that tumor spill in well-differentiated tumors appears to have no significant impact, while Grade II and III lesions probably deserve postoperative therapy regardless of whether the lesion remains intact or ruptures at the time of surgery.

If laparoscopic management of an ovarian mass is undertaken, the clinician's ability to recognize malignant characteristics of a mass visually becomes important. Several series have reviewed this question in premenopausal and postmenopausal women. In premenopausal patients, 29% of masses subsequently found to be cancer in a series of 2526 adnexal masses had no visual characteristics of malignancy. A similar small number of malignancies were found in a series of postmenopausal females. Overall, these studies suggest that the probability of malignancy in a sonographically and visually benign mass is about 1%.[97]

When considering the role of laparoscopic removal of ovarian masses, one must consider whether tumor spill is more likely than with laparotomy. The usual procedure would be to place the excised mass within one of several bags designed for the purpose. The bulk of the cyst may then be removed by decompression and the sack extracted from the abdomen. It is more likely, however, that tumor spill would occur during dissection of masses adherent to adjacent structures, thus spilling those tumors more likely to be of higher grade. To date, no data are available to answer this question. Finally, one must question whether laparoscopic management leads to an increased number of oophorectomies rather than cystectomies.

What is the usefulness of laboratory studies such as CA-125 in the postmenopausal female? CA-125 is a monoclonal antibody raised as an immunogen to an ovarian cancer-cell line. CA-125 is expressed by normal tissues of müllerian origin in the premenopausal female, which limits its usefulness. The antibody is detectable in 80% of serous tumors and less in mucinous tumors. However, it is positive in only 50% of patients with Stage I disease, and therefore the positive predictive value of the test is low. Only 2% of females with an elevated CA-125 level as a screening test would theoretically have ovarian cancer. Usefulness may therefore be limited to follow-up of tumors found to have a positive marker and perhaps to screen some postmenopausal cases.[98]

Initial exploration with the laparoscope in masses with benign screening characteristics is appropriate. Intraoperatively, the mass should be carefully inspected for adhesions and surface excrescences. If no characteristics of malignancy are noted, selective drainage and removal may be performed. If findings suggestive of malignancy are noted, formal exploratory laparotomy, removal, and staging should be performed.[99]

Finally, with the increased use of imaging studies, the issue of the incidental, asymptomatic, small ovarian cyst arises. If CA-125 is elevated, the current data would suggest that the mass be removed. However, based on data now available, if the mass is cystic, unilateral, unilocular with no septae, no ascites, and <3 cm in diameter, follow-up without exploration appears acceptable. Follow-up should be frequent over the next year. If there is any progression in the mass over that period, exploration is indicated. One reasonable schema for management of the reproductive age and postmenopausal female with a pelvic mass is shown in Figure 58-14.[100]

Solid lesions, however, continue to deserve surgical removal. A reasonable approach to the late premenopausal or postmenopausal female would be preoperative ultrasound assessment, including Doppler flow studies and ancillary testing. If ultrasound suggests a benign lesion with findings of a small, unilateral,

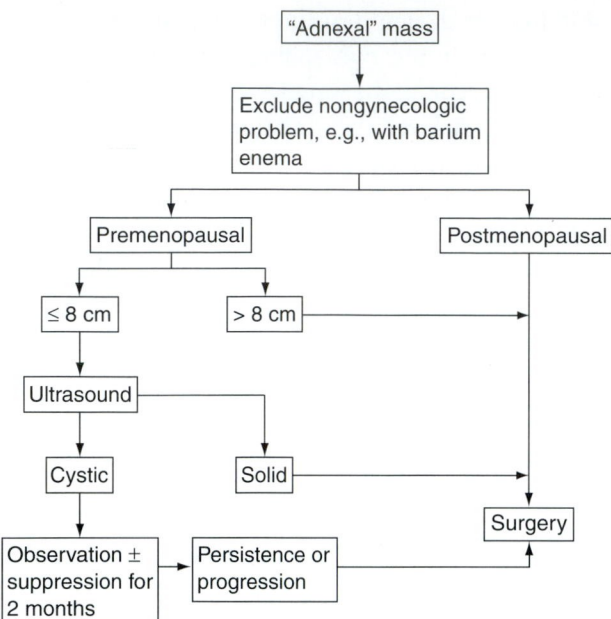

Figure 58-14 Management of adnexal mass in reproductive age and postmenopausal female. *Source:* Berek JS, Hacker NF. Practical gynecology oncology. 2nd ed. Baltimore: Williams & Wilkins, 1994.

unilocular, smooth mass without external or internal excrescence and the CA-125 is negative, it may be carefully observed.

SUMMARY

The proper diagnosis and management of uterine myomas and the adnexal mass in general continues to present a challenge to the practicing gynecologist. Uterine leiomyomas are the most common pelvic tumors in women of reproductive age. They may be small or large, single or multiple. These tumors may cause no symptoms at all, distort the uterus, cause irregular vaginal bleeding, increase the incidence of prematurity and other complications of pregnancy, and cause a multitude of other symptoms. They may cause confusion in the diagnosis of other pelvic masses, especially adnexal masses. Most myomas, especially those that are asymptomatic, should be managed conservatively. However, those causing symptoms or large enough to be of concern to the patient because of disfigurement should be removed. In the premenopausal woman, most adnexal masses are benign and may be managed conservatively either by observation or surgically with preservation of fertility. CA-125 is not an appropriate screening tool in either premenopausal or postmenopausal females but may

be used to follow the persistence or regression of existing disease. Transvaginal and Doppler ultrasound offer further definition of adnexal masses and may assist in management in the future after more experience is gained. Endoscopy is useful both for definition of questionable masses and removal in selected patients. Small, simple cysts are much more common than previously recognized in the asymptomatic, postmenopausal female and may be carefully followed if strict criteria are met.

REFERENCES

1. Buttram VC Jr, Reiter RC. Uterine leiomyomata: etiology, symptomatology and management. Fertil Steril 1981;36:433.
2. Graves, EJ. National Center for Health Statistics. National Hospital Discharge Survey: Annual Summary 1990. Vital and Health Statistics, Series 13 No. 112, Hyattsville, MD: Public Health Service, 1992.
3. Kjerulff KH, Guzinski GM, Langenberg PW, Stolley PD, Moye NE, Kazandjian VA. Hysterectomy and race. Obstet Gynecol 1993;82:757.
4. Thompson JD, Rock JA. Leiomyomata uteri and myomectomy. In: Rock JA, Thompson JD, eds. Te Linde's operative gynecology. 8th ed. Philadelphia: Lippincott-Raven, 1997:731.
5. Jonas HS, Masterson BJ. Giant uterine tumor: case report and review of the literature. Obstet Gynecol 1977;50:2S.
6. Singhabhandhu B, Akin JT Jr, Ridley JH, et al. Giant leiomyoma of the uterus: report of a case and review of the literature. Am J Surg 1973;39:391.
7. Townsend DE, Sparkes RS, Baluda MC, McClelland G. Unicellular histogenesis of uterine leiomyomas as determined by electrophoresis of glucose-6-phosphate dehydrogenase. Am J Obstet Gynecol 1970; 107:1168.
8. Nilbert M, Heim S. Uterine leiomyoma cytogenetics. Genes Chromosomes Cancer 1990;2:3.
9. Nelson WO. Endometrial and myometrial changes, including fibromyomatous nodules, induced in the uterus of the guinea pig by the prolonged administration of oestrogenic hormone. Anat Rec 1937;68:99.
10. Fayed YM, Tsibris JCM, Langenberg PW, Robertson AL Jr. Human uterine leiomyoma cells: binding and growth responses to epidermal growth factor, platelet-derived growth factor, and insulin. Lab Invest 1989;60:37.
11. Soules MR, McCarty KS Jr. Leiomyomas: steroid receptor content. Variation within normal menstrual cycles. Am J Obstet Gynecol 1982;143:6.
12. Lumsden MA, West CP, Hawkins RA, Bramley TA, Rumgay L, Baird DT. The binding of steroids to myometrium and leiomyomata (fibroids) in women treated with the gonadotropin-releasing hormone agonist Zoladex (ICI 118630). J Endocrinol 1989;121:389.
13. Tamaya T, Motoyama T, Ohono Y, Ide N, Tsurusaki T, Okada H. Estradiol-17-progesterone and 5-dihydrotestosterone receptors of uterine myometrium and myoma in the human subject. J Steroid Biochem 1979;10:615.

14. Wilson EA, Yang F, Rees ED. Estradiol and progesterone binding in uterine leiomyomata and in normal uterine tissues. Obstet Gynecol 1980;55:20.

15. Pollow K, Geilfub J, Boquoi E, et al. Estrogen and progesterone binding proteins in normal human myometrium. J Clin Chem Clin Biochem 1978;16:503.

16. Friedman AJ, Hoffman DI, Comite F, Browneller RW, Miller JD. Treatment of leiomyomata uteri with leuprolide acetate depot: a double-blind, placebo-controlled, multicenter study. Obstet Gynecol 1991;77:720.

17. Rein MS, Barbieri RL, Friedman AJ. Progesterone: a critical role in the pathogenesis of uterine myomas. Am J Obstet Gynecol 1995172:14.

18. Anderson J, Grine E, Eng CLY, et al. Expression of connexin-43 in human myometrium and leiomyoma. Am J Obstet Gynecol 1993;169:1266.

19. Brandon DD, Bethea CL, Strawn EY, et al. Progesterone receptor messenger ribonucleic acid and protein are overexpressed in human leiomyomas. Am J Obstet Gynecol 1993;169:78.

20. Kastner P, Krust A, Turcotte B, et al. Two distinct estrogen-regulated promotors generate transcripts encoding the two functionally different human progesterone receptor forms A and B. EMBO J 1990;9:1603.

21. Hunt SH. Fibroid weighing one hundred and forty pounds. Am J Obstet 1888;21:62.

22. Adelson MD, Adelson KL. Miscellaneous benign disorders of the upper genital tract. In: Copeland LS, ed. Textbook of gynecology. Philadelphia: Saunders, 1993:19.

23. Kurman RJ, Norris HJ. Mesenchymal tumors of the uterus. VI. Epithelioid smooth muscle tumors including leiomyoblastoma and clear-cell leiomyoma: a clinical and pathologic analysis of 26 cases. Cancer 1976;37:1853.

24. ACOG Technical Bulletin. Uterine leiomyomata. American College of Obstetricians and Gynecologists. no. 192. May 1994.

25. Novak ER. Benign and malignant changes in uterine myomas. Clin Obstet Gynecol 1958;1:421.

26. Montague A, Swartz DP, Woodruff JD. Sarcoma arising in leiomyoma of the uterus: factors influencing prognosis. Am J Obstet Gynecol 1980;138:16.

27. Leibsohn S, D'Ablaing G, Mischell DR, et al. Leiomyosarcoma in a series of hysterectomies performed for presumed uterine leiomyomas. Am J Obstet Gynecol 1990;162:968.

28. O'Connor DM, Norris HS. Mitotically active leiomyomas of the uterus. Hum Pathol 1990;21:223.

29. Corscaden JA, Smigh BP. Leiomyosarcoma of the uterus. Am J Obstet Gynecol 1958;75:149.

30. Bell SW, Kempson RL, Hendrickson MR. Problematic uterine smooth muscle neoplasm. Am J Surg Pathol 1994;18:535.

31. Martin JF, Bazin P, Feroldi J, et al. Tumeurs myoides intramuralei de l'estomac: considerations microscopiques aproposde 6 cai. Ann Anat Pathol 1960;5:484.

32. Edwards DR, Peacock JF. Intravenous leiomyomatosis of the uterus: report of 2 cases. Obstet Gynecol 1966;27:176.

33. Reiter RC, Wagner PL, Gambone JC. Routine hysterectomy for large asymptomatic uterine leiomyomata: a reappraisal. Obstet Gynecol 1992;79:481-485.

34. Zarvin M, McCarthy S, Scouth LM, et al. High field MRI and US evaluation of the pelvis in women with leiomyomas. Magn Reson Imaging 1990;8:372.

35. Friedman AJ, Haas ST. Should uterine size be an indication for surgical intervention in women with myomas? Am J Obstet Gynecol 1993;168:751.

36. Chimbira TH, Anderson ABM, Turnbull AC. Relation between measured menstrual blood loss and patient's subjective assessment of loss, duration of bleeding, number of sanitary pads used, uterine weight and endometrial surface area. Br J Obstet Gynaecol 1980;87:603.

37. Rubin A, Ford JA. Uterine fibromyomata in urban blacks: a preliminary survey of the relationship between symptomatology, blood pressure and haemoglobin levels. S Afr Med J 1974;48:2060.

38. Sehgal H, Haskins AL. The mechanism of uterine bleeding in the presence of fibromyomata. Am J Surg 1960;26:21.

39. Farrer-Brown G, Beilby JOW, Tarbit MH. Venous changes in the endometrium of the myomatous uteri. Obstet Gynecol 1971;38:743.

40. Persand V, Arjoon PD. Uterine leiomyoma: incidence of degenerative change and a correlation of associated symptoms. Obstet Gynecol 1970;35:432.

41. Burton CA, Grimes DA, March CM. Surgical management of leiomyomata during pregnancy. Obstet Gynecol 1989;74:707.

42. Hasan F, Arumwgan K, Sivanesaratrum V. Uterine leiomyomata in pregnancy. Int J Gynecol Obstet 1990;34:45.

43. Gambone JC, Reiter RC, Lench JB, Moore JG. The impact of a quality assurance process on the frequency and confirmation rate of hysterectomy. Am J Obstet Gynecol 1990;163:545.

44. Andolf E, Jørgensen C, Åstedt B. Ultrasound examination for detection of ovarian carcinoma in risk groups. Obstet Gynecol 1990;75:106.

45. Goodman AL. Progesterone therapy in uterine fibromyoma. J Clin Endocrinol Metab 1946;6:402.

46. Goldzieher JW, Maqueo M, Ricaud L, Aguilar JA, Canales E. Induction of degenerative changes in uterine myomas by high dose progestin therapy. Am J Obstet Gynecol 1966;96:1078.

47. Segaloff A, Wead JC, Sternberg WH, Parson W. The progesterone therapy of human uterine leiomyomas. J Clin Endocrinol 1949;9:1273.

48. Boulet AP, Fortier MA. Preparation and characterization of rabbit myometrial cells in primary culture: influence of oestradiol and progesterone treatment. In Vitro Cell Dev Biol 1987;23:93.

49. Friedman A, Daly M, Juneau-Norcross M, Gleason R, Rein M, LeBoff M. Long term medical therapy for leiomyoma uteri: a prospective, randomized study of leuprolide acetate depot plus either oestrogen-progestin or progestin "add-back" for 2 years. Hum Reprod 1994;9:1618.

50. Marugo M, Centonzi M, Bernasconi D, Fazzudi L, Bertha S, Geiodradarnuo G. Estrogen and progesterone reception in uterine leiomyomas. Acta Obstet Gynecol Scand 1989;68:731.

51. Maheux R, Giullotea UC, LeMay A, Bastide A, Fazekas

ATA. Luteinizing hormone-releasing hormone agonist in uterine leiomyoma: a pilot study. Am J Obstet Gynecol 1985;152:1034.

52. Friedman AJ. Use of gonadotropin releasing hormone agonists before myomectomy. Clin Obstet Gynecol 1993;36:650.

53. Friedman AJ. The biochemistry, physiology and pharmacology of gonadotropin releasing hormone (GnRH) and GnRH analogues. In: Barbieri RL, Friedman AJ, eds. Gonadotropin releasing hormone analogues: applications in Gynecology. New York: Elsevier,1991:10.

54. Adamson GD. Treatment of uterine fibroids: current findings with gonadotropin-releasing hormone agonist. Am J Obstet Gynecol 1992;166:746.

55. Watanabe Y, Nakamura G, Matsuguchi H, Nokaki M, Sano M, Nakano H. Efficacy of a low dose leuprolide acetate depot in the treatment of uterine leiomyomata in Japanese women. Fertil Steril 1992;58:66.

56. Vanleusden HA. Symptom-free interval after triptorelin treatment of uterine fibroids: long term results. Gynecol Endocrinol 1992;6:189.

57. Stovall TG. Gonadotropin-releasing hormone agonists utilization before hysterectomy. Clin Obstet Gynecol 1993;36:642.

58. Deligdisch L, Hirschmann S, Altchek A. Pathologic changes in gonadotropin releasing hormone agonist analogue treated uterine leiomyomata. Fertil Steril 1997; 67:837.

59. Rutgers JL, Spong CY, Sinow R, Heiner J. Leuprolide acetate treatment and myoma arterial size. Obstet Gynecol 1995;86:386

60. Sreenan JJ, Prayson RA, Biscotti CV, Thorton MH, Easley KA, Hart WR. Histologic findings in 107 uterine leiomyomata treated with leuprolide acetate compared to 126 controls. Am J Surg Pathol 1996;20:427.

61. Regidor PA, Schmidt M, Callies R, Kato K, Schindler AE. Estrogen and progesterone receptor content of GnRH analogue pretreated and untreated uterine leiomyomata. Eur J Obstet Gynecol Reprod Biol 1995; 63:69.

62. Bradham DD, Stovall TG, Thompson CD. Use of GnRH agonist before hysterectomy: a cost simulation. Obstet Gynecol 1995;85:401.

63. Scailli AR, Jestila JK. Sustained benefits of leuprolide acetate with or without subsequent nedroxymogesterone acetate in the nonsurgical management of leiomyomata uteri. Fertil Steril 1995;64:313.

64. De Aloysio D, Altieri P, Pretolani G, Romeo A, Paltrinieri F. The combined effect of a GnRH analogue at premenopause plus postmenopausal estrogen deficiency with the treatment of uterine leiomyomatas in perimenopausal women. Gynecol Obstet Invest 1995;39:115.

65. Friedman AJ, Juneau-Norcross M, Rein MS. Adverse effects of leuprolide acetate depot treatment. Fertil Steril 1993;59:448.

66. Friedman AJ. Combined oestrogen-progestin treatment of vaginal hemorrhage following gonadotropin releasing hormone agonist therapy of uterine myomas. Hum Reprod 1993;8:540.

67. Lee M-J, Kazer RR. Massive ascites after leuprolide acetate administration for treatment of leiomyomata uteri. Fertil Steril 1992;58:416.

68. Serra GB, Panetta V, Colosimo M, et al. Efficacy of leuprolide acetate depo in symptomatic fibromyomatous uteri. Ital Multicenter Study Clin Ther 1992; 14(Suppl A):57.

69. Hitti F, Glasberg SS, MacKenzie C, Meltzer BA. Uterine leiomyosarcoma with massive necrosis diagnosed during gonadotropin releasing hormone analogue therapy for presumed uterine fibroids. Fertil Steril 1991;56:778.

70. McCoy MJ. Angina and myocardial infarction with use of leuprolide acetate. Am J Obstet Gynecol 1994; 171:275.

71. Rivlin ME, Patel RB, Hess LW, Hess DB, Meeks GR. Leuprolide acetate depot for the treatment of uterine leiomyomas: changes in bone density, uterine volume and uterine vascular resistance index. Gen Reprod Med 1994;39:663.

72. Dawood MY, Lewis V, Ramos J. Cortical and trabecular bone mineral content in women with endometriosis: effect of gonadotropin releasing hormone agonist and danazol. Fertil Steril 1981;52:21.

73. Derman SG, Rehnstrom J, Neuwirth RS. The long-term effectiveness of hysteroscopic treatment of menorrhagia and leiomyomas. Obstet Gynecol 1991;77:591.

74. Dubuisson JB, Lecuru F, Foulot H, Mandelbrot L, Aubriot FX, Mouly M. Myomectomy by laparoscopy: a preliminary report of 43 cases. Fertil Steril 1991;56:827.

75. Stovall TG, Ling FW. Myomectomy. In: Mann WS, Stovall TG, eds. Gynecologic surgery. New York: Churchill Livingstone, 1986:445.

76. Dicker RC, Greenspan JR, Strauss, LT, et al. Complications of abdominal and vaginal hysterectomy among women of reproductive age in the United States. Am J Obstet Gynecol 1982;144:84.

77. Loft A, Anderson TF, Bronnum-Hansen H, Roepstouff C, Madsen M. Early postoperative mortality following hysterectomy: a Danish population based study 1977–1981. Br J Obstet Gynaecol 1991;98(2):147.

78. Stovall TG, Summit RL, Washburn SA, Ling FW. Gonadotropin releasing hormone agonist used before hysterectomy. Am J Obstet Gynecol 1994;170:1744.

79. Lumsden MA, West FW, Henry LC, et al. Treatment with the gonadotropin releasing agonist goserelin before hysterectomy for uterine fibroids. Br J Obstet Gynaecol 1994;101:438.

80. Friedman AJ, Harrison AD, Barbier L, et al. A randomized placebo controlled double blinded study evaluating the efficacy of leuprolide acetate depot in the treatment of uterine leiomyomata. Fertil Steril 1989;51:231.

81. Friedman AJ, Rein MS, Harrison-Atlas D, et al. A randomized placebo controlled, double blinded study evaluating a leuprolide acetate depot treatment before myomectomy. Fertil Steril 1989;52:728.

82. Stovall TG, Muneyyirci-delale O, Summit RJ Jr., Scialli AR. GnRH agonist and iron versus placebo and iron in the anemic patient before surgery for leiomyomas: a randomized controlled trial. Obstet Gynecol 1995;86:65.

83. Lumsden MA, West CP, Baird DT. Goserelin therapy before surgery for uterine fibroids. Lancet 1987;1:36.

84. Audebent AJM, Madenelat P, Querleu D, et al. Deferred versus immediate surgery for uterine fibroids: clinical trial results. Br J Obstet Gynaecol 1994;Suppl 10:29.

85. Vercelini P, Vendola N, Bocciolone L, et al. Gonadotropin releasing hormone agonist treatment before hysterectomy for menorrhagia associated with uterine myoma. Acta Obstet Gynecol Scand 1993;72:369.

86. Breen SL, Maxson WS. Ovarian tumors in children and adolescents. Clin Obstet Gynecol 1977;20:607.

87. Van Wintir JT, Simmons PS, Podratz KC. Surgically treated adnexal masses in infancy, childhood and adolescence. Am J Obstet Gynecol 1994;170:1780.

88. Hurd SJ, Adamson GD. Pelvic pain: endometriosis as a differential diagnosis in adolescents. Adolesc Pediatr Gynecol 1992;5:3.

89. DiSaia PJ. The adnexal mass and early ovarian cancer. In: DiSaia PJ, Creasman WT, eds. Clinical gynecologic oncology. 5th ed. St. Louis: Mosby Year Book, 1997:253.

90. Vessey M, Metcalfe A, Wells C, McPherson K, Westhoff C, Yeaks D. Ovarian neoplasms, functional ovarian cysts, and oral contraceptives. BMJ 1987;294:1518.

91. Horowitz IR, de al Cuesta RS. Benign and malignant tumors of the ovary. In: Carpenter SE, Rock JA, eds. Pediatric and adolescent gynecology. New York: Raven, 1992:397.

92. Barber HR, Graker EA. The PMPO syndrome (postmenopausal palpable ovary syndrome). Obstet Gynecol 1971;38:921.

93. Schuffer EM, Koneman P, Sohn C, et al. Diagnostic value of pelvic examination, ultrasound, and serum 125 in postmenopausal women with a pelvic mass: an international study. Cancer 1994;74:1398.

94. Munnell EW. Is conservative therapy ever justified in stage IA cancer of the ovary? Am J Obstet Gynecol 1969;103:641.

95. Decker DG, Webb MJ, Holbrook MA. Radiogold treatment of epithelial cancer of ovary: late results. Am J Obstet Gynecol 1973;115:751.

96. Dembo AJ, Davy M, Stenwig AE, Benle ES, Burk RS, Kjonstad R. Prognostic factors in patients with Stage I epithelial ovarian cancer. Obstet Gynecol 1990;75:263.

97. Masman M, Seltzer V, Boyce J. Laparoscopic excision of ovarian neoplasms subsequently found to be malignant. Obstet Gynecol 1991;77:563.

98. Einhorn N. Prospective evaluation of serum CA 125 levels for early detection of ovarian cancer. Obstet Gynecol 1992;80:14.

99. Steege J. Laparoscopic approach to the adnexal mass. Clin Obstet Gynecol 1994;37:392.

100. Berek JS, Hacker NF. Practical gynecologic oncology. 2nd ed. Baltimore: Williams & Wilkins, 1994:322.

Chapter 59

Pelvic-Organ Prolapse

Val Y. Vogt

Five Key Points

- Pelvic-organ prolapses are classified using the pelvic-organ prolapse quantification (POPQ) system.
- A variety of pelvic-floor defects can be addressed by using pessaries instead of surgery.
- Considerable controversy exists regarding which surgical procedures should be performed for the various types of pelvic-organ prolapse.
- Surgeons must have an armamentarium of procedures to accomplish surgical repairs and should not adhere to a single approach for all patients with symptomatic pelvic-organ prolapse.
- Colpoclesis is an alternative procedure that can be used for selected patients.

Pelvic-organ prolapse is a common condition, which leads to approximately 400,000 surgeries performed annually in the United States.[1] Women have a lifetime risk of 1 in 9 of requiring surgery for symptomatic pelvic organ prolapse and/or urinary incontinence. Not only are these conditions common but they are also challenging, as surgical management often provides less than optimal results. Surprisingly, failure rates have been estimated at 30%.[2] This demonstrates the inability to easily correct pelvic organ prolapse and/or urinary incontinence with surgery. Symptoms from prolapse can sometimes be relieved with a pessary, but if surgical correction is desired by the patient, a defect-oriented approach is recommended. Often, if all defects are not addressed at the initial surgery, recurrence, or in fact, increased degrees of the defects may develop postoperatively.[3] In addition, several types of procedures for pelvic-organ prolapse have been designed to correct these defects, but the best combination of procedures is debated. This chapter will describe techniques to fully evaluate pelvic-floor defects, review pessary management, and discuss various surgical options.

PREVALENCE

The exact prevalence of pelvic-organ prolapse is unknown. Current studies have determined the prevalence by examination in selected populations. Severe pelvic organ prolapse was present in 23% of 200 consecutive patients referred for a urogynecologic evaluation.[4] Another estimate is that 50% of parous women lose pelvic-floor support, resulting in prolapse: of these women, 10 to 20% seek medical care for their symptoms.[5]

DEFINITION

The definition of prolapse has varied in the current literature. Some reports describe prolapse in nondescriptive terms such as "small to large," or "mild to moderate" or compare the size to common fruit sizes such as the "size of a lemon." Using these terms makes

TABLE 59-1
BADEN AND WALKER CLASSIFICATION

Grade 0:	Normal position for each respective site
Grade 1:	Descent halfway to the hymen
Grade 2:	Descent to the hymen
Grade 3:	Descent halfway past the hymen
Grade 4:	Maximum possible descent for each site

Urethrocele, cystocele, uterine prolapse, culdocele, or rectocele: patient strains firmly. Grade descent of desired sites. Grade posterior urethral descent, lowest part at other sites.

the comparison of studies difficult. More objective classification systems that have been designed to address this issue have not been consistently used in the literature. From the late 1960s to the 1990s, Drs. Baden and Walker described a site-specific classification to identify all potential areas of loss of support.[6] The Baden and Walker classification was later modified to a halfway system (Table 59-1). Beecham described another classification with three grades of descent for "cystocele, uterine prolapse, apical prolapse, enterocele, and rectocele." The main differences between this system and the Baden and Walker system were the points of reference (introitus compared to the hymen) and the examination in the relaxed state compared to examination with straining.[7] The American College of Obstetricians and Gynecologists (ACOG) defines pelvic-organ prolapse as the protrusion of the pelvic organs into or out of the vaginal canal.[8] In the ACOG grading system the points of reference are the ischial spines and the hymen. A classification termed the POPQ (pelvic-organ prolapse quantification) was

designed to enable accurate quantitative description and comparison of pelvic support findings.[9]

PELVIC-ORGAN PROLAPSE QUANTITATION

The pelvic-organ prolapse quantitative standardization of terminology was adopted by the International Continence Society in 1995, by the American Urogynecologic Society in 1996, and by the Society of Gynecologic Surgeons in 1996. Prior to adoption by these societies, its clinical utility was evaluated as well as its interrater and intrarater reliability. Support by these societies encourages outcomes research to use this system to enhance comparison of studies. How to perform the POPQ will be described in detail, as this classification of prolapse will likely increase in use not only for outcomes research but also for clinical use. Initially, the POPQ may seem cumbersome to measure but with continued use it is easily performed. The POPQ is an adaptation of the Baden and Walker system, measuring eight sites to create a vaginal profile. The point of reference is the hymen, and the measurements in centimeters are determined with maximum strain. The hymen was chosen as the main reference point since it was considered more precise than the introitus. The measurements are in centimeters either into the vagina, which is described in negative values, or if the prolapse extends outside the hymenal ring, the centimeters are recorded in positive integers.

Two separate points are measured on the anterior, apical, and posterior aspects of the vagina as well as on the perineum (Figure 59-1 and Table 59-2). The

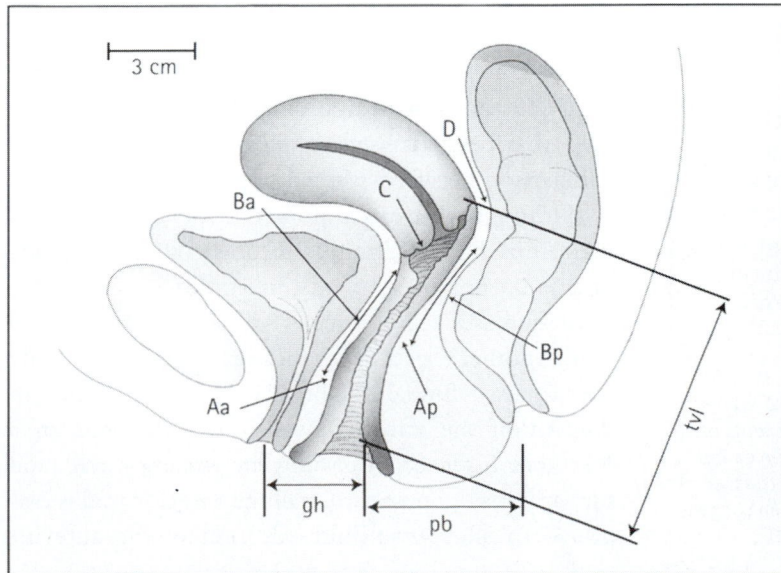

Figure 59-1 Diagram of the pelvic-organ prolapse quantitation (POPQ sites). This figure illustrates the anatomic positions of the POPQ sites. *From Benson JT. Urogynecology and reconstructive pelvic surgery. Vol 5. In: Stenchever MA, ed. Atlas of clinical gynecology. New York: McGraw-Hill, 2000.*

TABLE 59-2
SITES OF POPQ

The specific sites of the POPQ examination become more familiar with frequent use. These points are particularly helpful in recording the surgical outcomes in an objective manner. The conditions of the examination (patient position, use of strain, recording instrument) should be identical before and after surgery to obtain a meaningful comparison of any change.

Description	Range of Possible Values
Anterior wall	
Aa Single point 3 cm in from hymen	−3 to +3
Ab Using segment from 3 cm in (Aa) to apex, describes position of most distal point of anterior wall	−3 to + total vaginal length
Posterior Wall	
Pa Single point 3 cm in from hymen	−3 to +3
Pb Using segment from 3 cm in (Pa) to apex, describes position of most distal point of anterior wall	−3 to + total vaginal length
Apex	
C Position of apex when prolapse at maximum protrusion	
D If uterus present, position posterior fornix (helpful in determining extent of cervical elongation)	
Total vaginal length (to cuff or cervix)	

From Benson JT. Urogynecology and reconstructive pelvic surgery. Vol 5. In: Stenchever MA, ed. Atlas of clinical gynecology. New York: McGraw-Hill, 2000.

---

first point on the anterior vaginal wall (point Aa) is 3 cm proximal to the external urethral meatus and the second point (point Ba) is the point that represents the most dependent portion of the anterior wall. Likewise, on the posterior wall the first point (point Ap) is 3 cm proximal to the posterior hymen and the second point (point Bp) represents the most dependent portion of the posterior wall. Apically, the descent

Point Aa Anterior wall	Point Ba Anterior wall	Point C Cervix or cuff
Genital Hiatus	Perineal body	Total vaginal length
Point Ap posterior wall	Point Bp posterior wall	Point D posterior fornix

Figure 59-2 Recording the POPQ—numeric form. This figure shows a simple method of recording the POPQ values in an office chart. Although this method is convenient, each clinician may develop a method most suited to her or his situation. *From Benson JT. Urogynecology and reconstructive pelvic surgery. Vol 5. In: Stenchever MA, ed. Atlas of clinical gynecology. New York: McGraw-Hill, 2000.*

of the cervix (point C) and the posterior fornix (point D) are measured to the hymen. If a total hysterectomy has been performed, only descent of the vaginal cuff (point C) is measured. On the perineum, the midline distance between the external urinary meatus to the posterior hymen is measured, which is termed the genital hiatus (gh), and the midline distance between the posterior hymen to the midanal opening is measured which is termed the perineal body (pb). Also, total vaginal length (tvl) is measured with the prolapse reduced and is the only measurement taken in the relaxed state. These nine points can be recorded in a "tic-tac-toe" grid (Figure 59-2).

Once the vaginal profile with nine measured points has been determined, an ordinal staging system (Table 59-3) has been devised to allow useful analysis and comparison between studied populations.

Although the exact points to be measured are standardized, the technique to obtain these measurements has not been standardized. For example, one technique uses a ring forceps with centimeters etched on it. Another uses a paper measuring tape commonly used to assess fundal heights. To obtain the maximum descent of the anterior wall, one half blade of a speculum is placed displacing the posterior wall, and similarly, for the posterior wall the anterior wall is displaced to allow maximum descent of the anterior

TABLE 59-3
INTERNATIONAL CONTINENCE SOCIETY PELVIC ORGAN PROLAPSE ORDINAL STAGING SYSTEM

Stage 0	Points Aa, Ap, Ba, and Bp are all at −3 cm and either point C and D is at no more than −(X − 2) cm
Stage I	The criteria for Stage 0 are not met and the leading edge of prolapse is less than −1 cm
Stage II	Leading edge of prolapse is at least −1 cm but no more than +1 cm
Stage III	Leading edge of prolapse is greater than +1 cm but less than +(X − 2) cm
Stage IV	Leading edge of prolapse is at least +(X − 2) cm

X = total vaginal length in centimeters in Stages 0, III and IV. Stages I through IV can be subgrouped according to which portion of the lower reproductive tract is the leading edge of the prolapse, using the following qualifiers: a for anterior vaginal wall; p for posterior vaginal wall; C for vaginal cuff; Cx for cervix; and Aa, Bb, and D for the defined points of measurement (e.g., IV-Cx, II-a or III-Bp).

wall. Sometimes the leading edge of the prolapse can appear to be the anterior wall but truly is the posterior wall after placement of one half blade of the speculum or vice versa.

CAUSE

The cause of pelvic-organ prolapse is multifactorial. Vaginal delivery is considered the primary insult leading to prolapse. Vaginal delivery can lead to trauma of the supportive connective tissue and neuromuscular unit either by distinct breaks in the integrity or by traction injury. Damage to the levator ani complex and its innervation is common after vaginal childbirth.[10] Recovery from this damage can occur but may not be complete,[11] possibly increasing the risk for future stressors. Also, differences in the bony structure of the pelvis may predispose to pelvic-floor prolapse.[12] Other risk factors besides vaginal delivery that have been associated with prolapse include conditions that cause repetitive increased abdominal pressures to the pelvic floor, such as chronic cough or chronic obstructive lung disease, a long history of straining from constipation, repetitive heavy lifting, and obesity. These conditions are often implicated as contributing to prolapse but few data exist to substantiate this. One study describes an association of chronic straining from constipation prior to the onset of uterovaginal prolapse as compared with a control group.[13] Connective-tissue disorders and neuromuscular dysfunction other than that attributed to vaginal birth can also contribute to prolapse. Defec-

tive collagen and overall less collagen in pubocervical fascia has been seen in patients with prolapse as compared with controls.[14,15] Torpin reported that 28% of adult women with prolapse had spina bifida occulta as compared with 10% in a control population.[16] In addition, iatrogenic causes of prolapse can occur after surgery if the vaginal vault is not resuspended with the uterosacral–cardinal complex[17] or if the vaginal axis is altered. For example, after a Burch retropubic procedure, which elevates the anterior vaginal wall predisposing the posterior wall for prolapse, reoperation for prolapse was noted in 30% of patients.[3]

SYMPTOMS

Symptoms of pelvic-organ prolapse do not consistently correlate with the degree of prolapse. A patient can experience severe discomfort with minimal degrees of prolapse or absence of discomfort with complete vault prolapse. Prolapse can cause a variety of symptoms, which typically include pelvic pressure, pelvic heaviness, vaginal or perineal pain, sensation of tissue protrusion into or from the vagina, low back pain, observation or palpation of tissue from the vagina, and feelings of "sitting on something." Determining whether the prolapse contributes to all of the patient's symptoms can be difficult. Placement of a pessary can help determine if some of the symptoms are due to prolapse. If symptoms resolve or diminish after pessary placement, prolapse is a likely cause. Prolapse can obviously distort the anatomy but has varying ways of disrupting the physiology of the pelvic floor, leading to urinary, bowel, and sexual dysfunction. Specifically, urinary retention, urinary incontinence, dyspareunia, constipation, fecal incontinence, and feelings of incomplete emptying after urination and defecation are often associated with prolapse. Common symptoms of a rectocele are feelings of incomplete emptying after a bowel movement and requiring digital maneuvers for defecation. These symptoms need to be teased out of the common report of constipation. Current knowledge is lacking regarding the precise nature of symptoms that may be caused by the presence of a vaginal protrusion or bulge.

EXAMINATION

To address all pelvic-floor defects, patients should be examined to maximize the degree of prolapse and in

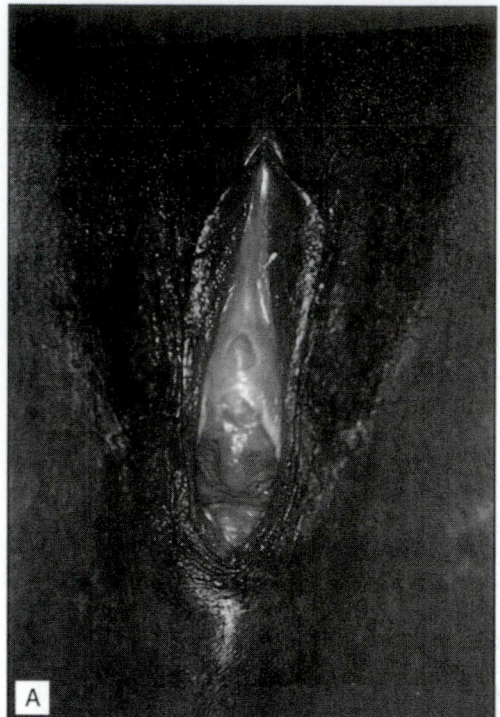
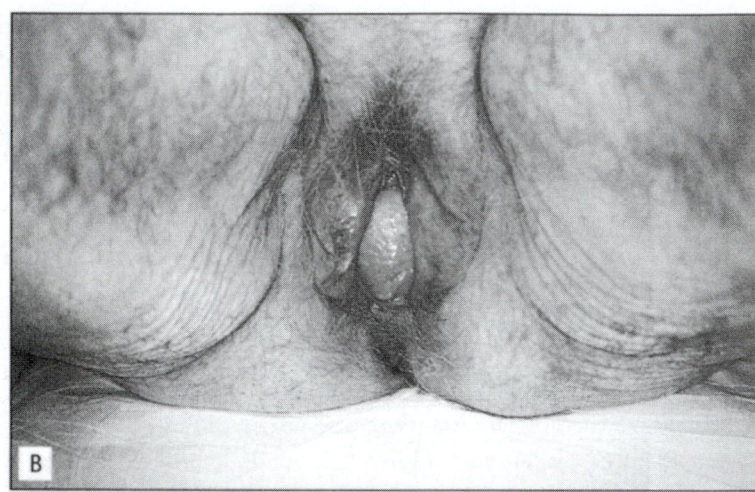

Figure 59-3 Parous. A. After vaginal delivery, the anterior vaginal wall commonly has altered topography. These changes can include loss of one or both lateral attachments, also called the paravaginal defect. This picture demonstrates the unilateral/bilateral loss of the lateral attachment. B. Other topographic changes may include loss of midline support. There may be less stability of the urethrovesical junction and external urethral meatus, although this is neither symptomatic nor clinically relevant in many women. Despite marked parity-induced alterations of the vaginal topography, the woman may remain asymptomatic. *From Benson JT. Urogynecology and reconstructive pelvic surgery. Vol 5. In: Stenchever MA, ed. Atlas of clinical gynecology. New York: McGraw-Hill, 2000.*

an organized fashion. To do this, the anterior, middle and posterior compartments should be evaluated separately. Most commonly a patient with prolapse has defects in all compartments, but occasionally only one compartment is affected (Figure 59-3). In addition, the patient should also be examined with a Valsalva maneuver, preferably in the standing position, to denote the degree of the prolapse. Evaluating a patient in the dorsal lithotomy position may be more comfortable for the patient as well as easier for the examiner but the severity of the prolapse may be minimized. Whether performed supine or standing, the examination can be awkward for the patient, and every effort should be made to put her at ease. Bearing down in front of an examiner may limit the amount of descent because of embarrassment and/or concerns about incontinence of urine, feces, or flatus. If the severity of the pelvic-floor defects does not seem consistent with the patient's symptoms, she should stand for the examination. and further evaluation with dynamic cystoproctography may be nec-

essary. This will be discussed later in the chapter. Ideally, the POPQ is measured and an ordinal stage is assigned.

Besides the degree of support, specific defects of anterior-wall prolapse can be delineated. As described by Richardson et al.,[18] defects of the anterior wall can be lateral, apical, distal, or midline (Figure 59-4). The lateral defect (also called paravaginal defect and traction defect) is considered detachment of the pubocervical fascia of the anterior wall from the fascia overlying the obturator internus at the arcus tendineus fascia pelvis. According to Richardson, 85% of anterior-vaginal-wall defects are paravaginal and bilateral defects are more common than unilateral. A midline defect (also termed a central defect) represents one or more disruptions in the pubocervical fascia beneath the bladder base. With a midline defect, the normal rugae of the anterior vaginal wall are absent. One way to determine if the anterior-wall defect is paravaginal or midline is to place an open ring forceps or two large swabs crossed at the introitus to support the

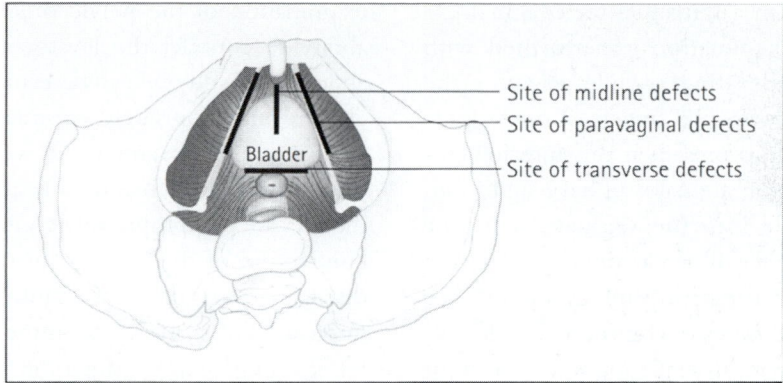

Figure 59-4 Sites of defects in the anterior vaginal wall. Defects in the anterior vaginal wall can result in cystocele, urethrocele, or anterior enterocele. Pictured are the most common sites for defects in the anterior vaginal wall. Paravaginal cystoceles are reported to be the most common, although no large epidemiologic study exists to confirm this. Other sites include the transverse and midline defects. Site-specific analysis examining the lateral sulci, apex, and midline is needed to identify these different defects. Because not all cystoceles have the same etiology, clinicians need different procedures to correct them. *From Richardson AC. Pelvic support defects in woman (urethrocele, cystocele, uterine prolapse, enterocele, and rectocele). In: Skandalakis J, et al. eds. Hernia: surgical anatomy and technique. New York: McGraw-Hill, 1989:238.*

lateral aspects of the anterior wall to the arcus tendineus fascia pelvis. If the prolapse is corrected with bearing down, the defect is paravaginal in nature. If the prolapse persists, the defect is most likely central, although a combination of defects can occur. An apical defect (also called a transverse defect) of the anterior wall occurs when the pubocervical fascia disrupts from its attachment to the pericervical ring to which the uterosacral–cardinal complex attaches posteriorly. The proximal apical defect of the anterior vaginal wall can occur despite a well-supported bladder neck. A rare distal defect occurs if the pubocervical fascia detaches from the urogenital diaphragm. The term "fascia" which has been used here and is commonly used in gynecologic literature, differs from the parietal fascia that overlies muscles such as the obturator internus and levator ani muscles. The term *adventitia* has been recommended when describing pubocervical "fascia."[19] Prolapse of the anterior wall has historically been called a cystocele since the bladder lies adjacent to this portion of the vaginal wall. Although uncommon, prolapse of the anterior vaginal wall, especially after a hysterectomy, can be an enterocele instead of a cystocele. Unless peristalsis is seen beneath the anterior wall, this is rarely diagnosed without dynamic cystoproctography, which determines which organ lies behind the prolapsed wall.

Apical prolapse is termed uterine prolapse or uterovaginal prolapse if the uterus is intact; if the uterus is absent, it is referred to as vault prolapse. Complete eversion of the vagina is simply termed vault eversion. Complete prolapse with a uterus intact can be termed procidentia. If significant anterior- and/or posterior-wall prolapse occurs, reducing these defects is necessary to accurately determine apical descent. One technique is pulling the intact speculum out of the vagina as the patient bears down. Using a speculum with both blades allows evaluation of the apex without distortion of anterior- or posterior-wall prolapse. Note the relationship of the cervix or cuff (point C) and the posterior fornix (point D) to the hymenal ring. The POPQ quantifies the percentage of descent of the apex. For example, if total vaginal length is 8 cm and maximum descent is 4 cm within the hymen, this can be termed 50% vault prolapse. The POPQ also evaluates cervical elongation if a significant difference occurs between the cervix (point C) and the posterior fornix (point D). Point D is meant to correspond to the uterosacral–cardinal complex, which may be useful when considering surgical correction.

Posterior prolapse can involve any or all of the following: rectocele, enterocele, and, rarely, sigmoidocele. Historically, rectoceles have been described by their size and location (low, mid, or high). With careful examination, further description of rectoceles can be delineated. A rectovaginal examination is required to evaluate posterior-vaginal-wall prolapse. One technique is to perform a bimanual rectovaginal examination. A rectal examination is performed with one's nondominant index finger while palpating the posterior vaginal wall with two fingers of one's dominant hand. A rectocele is present if the anterior rectal wall and the posterior vaginal wall have significant mobility and protrude into the vaginal canal. The normal rectovaginal space allows complete separation of vaginal and rectal function and independence from each other.[20] Although uncommon, a wide rectal lumen can occur with a well-supported posterior vaginal wall and is not considered a true rectocele. At present it is unclear if these patients should be treated differently from those with the more common finding of prolapse of both the anterior rectal wall and the posterior vaginal wall.

As with anterior-vaginal-wall prolapse, specific defects of the posterior wall have been described.[18] Most commonly, a distinct weakness is palpated transversely above the perineal body. This may represent a detachment of the rectovaginal septum (sometimes termed Denonvillier fascia) from the perineal body. Other less common defects are lateral, midline, and complex. Lateral defects are considered as separation from the pelvic sidewall and levator ani. Midline defects often extend to the vaginal apex and are associated with large rectoceles. Complex defects are L-shaped or U-shaped. Another type of defect of the posterior wall is a transverse apical defect that may represent detachment of the rectovaginal septum from the pericervical ring of support. An enterocele is abnormal descent of the peritoneum into the cul-de-sac.

The POPQ classification system does not distinguish whether posterior-wall defects include a rectocele, an enterocele, or a rare sigmoidocele. In a previously unoperated patient it is uncommon to have an isolated enterocele or rectocele pelvic-floor defect. Grading the severity of these defects separately is still helpful. Careful identification is necessary to determine which surgical procedures are required to repair these conditions.[21] On rectal examination, in addition to the above findings, note tone and the patient's ability to contract the external anal sphincter. If present, anal-sphincter defects can be palpated circumferentially by using a thumb perianally to map out the defects. With experience the internal and external anal sphincters can be palpated separately. Identifying anal-sphincter defects is mandatory when the patient reports fecal incontinence. After performing a bimanual examination of the pelvic organs, assess the patient's ability to contract the levator ani muscles. With the abdominal hand one can determine if abdominal muscles are inappropriately contracted with the attempt to contract the levator muscles. Also note if other assessory muscles such as the hip adductors or the gluteal muscles are inappropriately contracted with a "Kegel," contraction of the levator ani muscles.[22] Chapter 53 discusses other physical examination techniques for evaluation of urinary incontinence. For example, after the bimanual examination insertion of a cotton swab with sterile anesthetic gel and catheterization can determine postvoid residual. In addition, the catheterized urine can be cultured prior to more extensive urodynamic testing.

DEFECOGRAPHY

Defecography, also termed dynamic cystoproctography and evacuation proctography, is valuable in specifically identifying which structures are involved in prolapse. This radiologic examination is becoming increasingly available as other disciplines such as gastroenterology have noted its value, especially with defecatory disorders. Defecography in regards to prolapse is helpful primarily in two conditions: recurrence after pelvic reconstructive surgery, and when the symptoms and physical examination are incongruent. When considering surgical management after a recurrence, identification of all defects preoperatively is imperative. Recurrence after pelvic reconstructive surgery can result in rarer types of isolated defects or a combination of defects. For example, surgery may correct prolapse of the distal aspects of the anterior and/or posterior vaginal walls, but the more proximal components of the anterior and posterior vaginal walls are not addressed with surgery, or recurrence occurs. Another example is when the anterior- and posterior-vaginal-wall prolapse is corrected but the apical prolapse persists or recurs. Findings on defecography can aid in the diagnosis of the type of prolapse and, therefore, determine which surgical procedures offer the optimal results. In regards to a specific defect, an enterocele can easily be diagnosed on defecography but is easily missed on physical examination. In 74 consecutive patients with pelvic prolapse, Kelvin[23] noted 15 enteroceles on defecography when physical examination detected only 7.

Defecography is a technique in which contrast material in placed in the small bowel, colon, rectum,

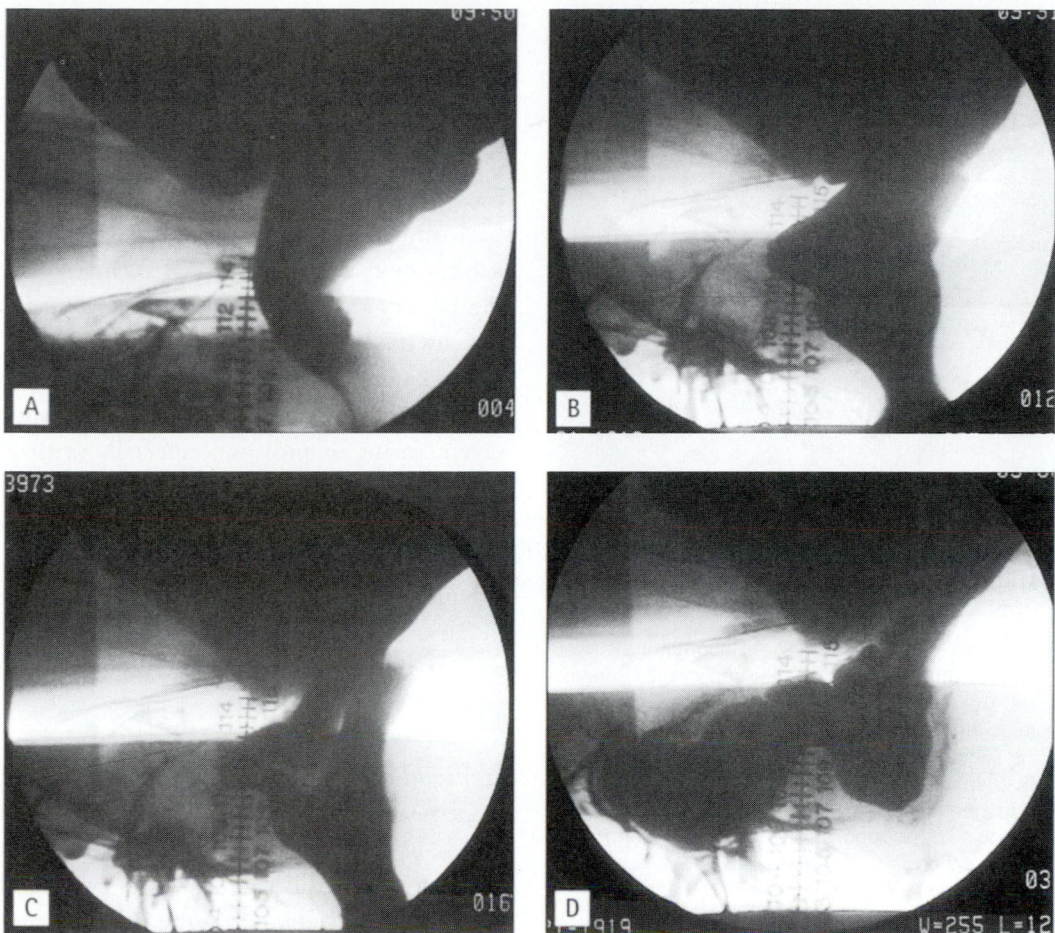

Figure 59-5 Enterocele with rectocele. These photographs demonstrate an apparently retaining rectocele that ultimately empties after maximal protrusion of the large enterocele. Although the patient may not report defecation difficulties, isolated enterocele repair may unmask rectocele symptoms. Thus, this possibility may warrant consideration if such symptoms have a new onset after reconstructive procedures. *From Benson JT. Urogynecology and reconstructive pelvic surgery. Vol 5. In: Stenchever MA, ed. Atlas of clinical gynecology. New York: McGraw-Hill, 2000.*

vagina, and bladder (Figure 59-5). Patients are radiographically evaluated while sitting on a special commode. Views are taken with the filled bladder at rest and after voiding. Also, views are taken before, during and after evacuation. While the physical examination evaluates the anatomic aspects of prolapse, defecography provides insight into the physiologic changes that occur with pelvic prolapse. A patient is more likely to perform an adequate Valsalva maneuver on a commode, especially if a contrast agent can stimulate evacuation. For example, one can assess how anterior-vaginal-wall prolapse affects the posterior-vaginal-wall prolapse and vice versa. A large cystocele may compress the posterior wall to prevent or augment bowel evacuation. Another type of defect, a sigmoidocele, which is abnormal descent of the sigmoid from its

sacral attachments, can be detected. If the patient has pelvic-prolapse symptoms and chronic constipation, repair of a sigmoidocele may be warranted, although this is controversial. At present, little is known about sigmoidoceles and the role they can play in patients with symptomatic pelvic prolapse. Defecography is not standardized and some centers do not evaluate the anterior compartment.

PESSARY

For symptomatic pelvic-organ prolapse, a pessary is a nonsurgical option. Pessaries were first described thousands of years ago.[24] The use of pessaries became more popular in the 1800s after Goodyear's discovery of rubber.[25] In the early 1900s prolapse was managed

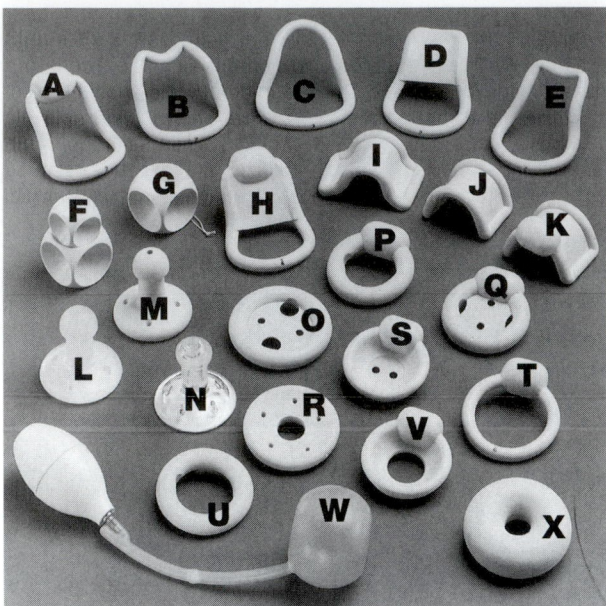

Figure 59-6 Available pessary models. A. Incontinence Hodge. B. Risser. C. Smith. D. Hodge with support. E. Hodge. F. Tandem cube. G. Cube. H. Incontinence Hodge with support. I. Gehrung with support. J. Gehrung with support. K. Incontinence Gehrung. L. Rigid gelhorn. M. Flexible gelhorn. N. Acrylic gelhorn. O. Ring with support. P. Incontinence ring. Q. Incontinence ring with support. R. Shaatz. S. Incontinence dish with support. T. Incontinence ring. U. Ring. V. Incontinence dish. W. Inflato Ball. X. Donut.

primarily surgically and pessaries were considered only for patients who were not surgical candidates. A resurgence of pessary use has occurred over the past few years in order to offer patients a nonsurgical option. Besides not being a surgical candidate, patients have several reasons for preferring pessary management. Reasons may be social, personal, or financial—for example, symptoms are not severe enough to require surgery or patients desire postponement of surgery for a specified period of time. In addition, patients with recurrence after surgical management may prefer a pessary to repeat surgery.

A variety of pelvic-floor defects can be addressed with a pessary to provide relief from symptoms. Several types and sizes of pessaries have been developed over the past 150 years to address these defects. The first modern-day pessary is the lever or Smith–Hodge type. Other types are ring, doughnut, gelhorn, Inflato Ball, Gehrung, and cube. Diaphragms are another and often less expensive option (Figure 59-6).

The ring pessary often provides the easiest insertion and removal by the patient. To place this pessary the ring is folded in half and placed within the vagina above the levator ani to allow the ring to sit parallel to the floor in the standing patient. The ideal fit is the largest size comfortable for the patient. As with most of the pessaries, insertion is often easiest for the patient lying down and removal is easiest standing while bearing down. Removal of the pessary is usually more difficult for the patient. A suture, coat thread, dental floss, or a washable shoestring can aid patients who have difficulty retrieving the pessary due to body habitus or manual dexterity. If such an "aid" is tied to the pessary the patient is encouraged to change it at her discretion.

A doughnut pessary is placed similarly to the ring but it cannot be folded. The doughnut works well for severe forms of prolapse, especially with a widened hiatus. Removal is more difficult than with the ring and a wide "aid" such as a shoestring can be helpful.

A gelhorn is placed to allow the knob to sit on the perineal body. The knob makes for easy removal. To insert, the flat part of the gelhorn is placed flat against the posterior vaginal wall and then rotated anteriorly once inside the vagina.

The inflatoball is an ideal pessary when insertion and removal is by a caretaker. Insertion of other types of pessaries can be uncomfortable for the patient; but this is usually not the case with the inflatoball. The deflated inflatoball is inserted and pumped to appropriate size, determined by the patient's comfort. The ball–valve mechanism that controls the inflation can be tucked inside the vagina if it is bothersome to the patient. The inflatoball is deflated for removal.

The Gehrung is unique in that it is malleable. Its convex design can be positioned to support primarily anterior or posterior prolapse. With an isolated anterior or posterior defect this pessary can be molded to the type and degree of the defect. This pessary can be placed in any position to provide the most comfort and reduction of the prolapse.

The cube pessary has its advantages and disadvantages. A cube will nearly always reduce the pelvic prolapse because it is dependent on suction for support and not on the support of the perineal body or levator ani muscles. The primary disadvantages include a malodorous discharge if not removed daily, and increased risk for vaginal-wall erosions or ulcerations. Before placing a cube pessary the patient must be willing to remove the pessary daily for cleaning or be willing to return frequently to assess vaginal integrity.

The primary contraindication for pessary management is a patient who refuses follow-up. Although rare, complications such as fistula formation have occurred from neglected care or poor follow-up.[26] Hormone-replacement therapy, if not contraindicated, is recommended for patients who desire pessary management. A small amount of estrogen cream can placed on the pessary with daily insertion. For those unable or unwilling to take hormone-replacement therapy, examinations for vaginal ulcers and erosions should be performed more frequently. Most patients remove their pessary before having intercourse, although some pessaries, such as the ring pessary, can remain in the vagina for intercourse. The patient may decide if keeping the pessary in the vagina for intercourse is more comfortable than with the pessary removed.

A pessary can also be a diagnostic tool. As stated earlier, symptoms from prolapse can be vague, and a well-fitted pessary can help determine if prolapse is contributing to the patient's symptoms. Pessaries have also been used to determine if urinary incontinence develops with the prolapse reduced. A large percentage of patients with moderate to severe prolapse have underlying urinary incontinence if the anterior vaginal wall is reduced. The urinary incontinence may be genuine stress incontinence, detrusor instability, mixed incontinence, or intrinsic sphincter deficiency. This is fully discussed in Chapter 53. Before surgical correction for symptomatic pelvic prolapse is undertaken, further evaluation of urinary incontinence or the potential for urinary incontinence is recommended. The surgical procedure preferred for correction of urinary incontinence may determine whether reconstruction of the prolapse is primarily abdominal or vaginal and also affect the combination of procedures for addressing all defects.

SURGICAL MANAGEMENT

Several factors need to be considered for surgical management—the patient's symptoms, including the presence of urinary and fecal incontinence, types and severity of prolapse defects on physical examination, previous surgical correction, general medical status, desire for future fertility, desire for retaining the uterus and/or cervix, and desire for retaining coital function. Considerable controversy exists regarding which procedures should be performed for the various types of pelvic prolapse. With the exception of at least one study, the vast majority of literature regarding the outcomes of surgical correction for prolapse is retrospective with short term follow-up; few comparative studies exist.[27] This limits the ability to determine

which types of procedures provide the best long-term success rates. As a variety of surgical operations exist, the most commonly performed procedures will be described. The surgical procedures will be described according to the specific defect they address. Laparoscopic techniques are becoming increasingly popular, but currently the literature regarding success rates and complications is insufficient for discussion of these techniques. Surgery needs to be carefully tailored to the specific defects and needs of the individual patient to provide her the optimal result. The surgeon must have an armamentarium of procedures to accomplish this and should not adhere to a single approach for all patients with symptomatic pelvic prolapse. The ultimate goal is to correct all defects while restoring normal anatomy and physiology of the pelvic floor.

ANTERIOR WALL PROLAPSE

The two most commonly performed procedures to correct a cystocele include anterior colporrhaphy for central, midline defects and paravaginal repair for lateral, paravaginal defects. The anterior colporrhaphy was first described by Kelly[28] in 1913 for treatment of stress incontinence (Figure 59-7). Several authors have described variations of this technique.[29] Although Kelly described this procedure for urinary incontinence, currently anterior colporrhaphy is performed solely for correction of a cystocele. Surgical correction of stress incontinence requires an additional procedure, such as a retropubic procedure or a suburethral sling procedure. Some authors advocate a suburethral fascial plication in addition to the anterior colporrhaphy for mild incontinence.[30]

A paravaginal repair can be performed abdominally or vaginally (Figure 59-8). It is considered one of the few true anatomical repairs for prolapse that does not depend on overcorrection or a compensatory mechanism for cure. The vaginal paravaginal repair was first described by White[31] in 1909. The pubocervicovaginal fascia is reattached to the arcus tendineus fascia pelvis overlying the obturator internus muscle. Distinct breaks in the fascia are commonly seen in the abdominal approach. Several interrupted permanent sutures are placed from the urethrovesical junction to the level of the ischial spines. Some authors advocate this procedure for stress incontinence in addition to correction of lateral defects. As with an anterior colporrhaphy, an additional procedure for stress incontinence is recommended

Figure 59-7 Technique of anterior colporrhaphy as described by Beck and colleagues. Placement of no. 1 chromic catgut, vertical mattress sutures (1, 2, and 3) plicating the fascia under the bladder base with long axis of the needle parallel to the fascial surface (bottom insert). Figure-of-eight no. 1 polyglycolic sutures (5 and 6) are inserted into the pubocervical fascia, scratching the back of the symphysis pubis with long axis of the needle held at right angles to the fascial surface (top insert). *From Benson JT. Urogynecology and reconstructive pelvic surgery. Vol 5. In: Stenchever MA, ed. Atlas of clinical gynecology. New York: McGraw-Hill, 2000.*

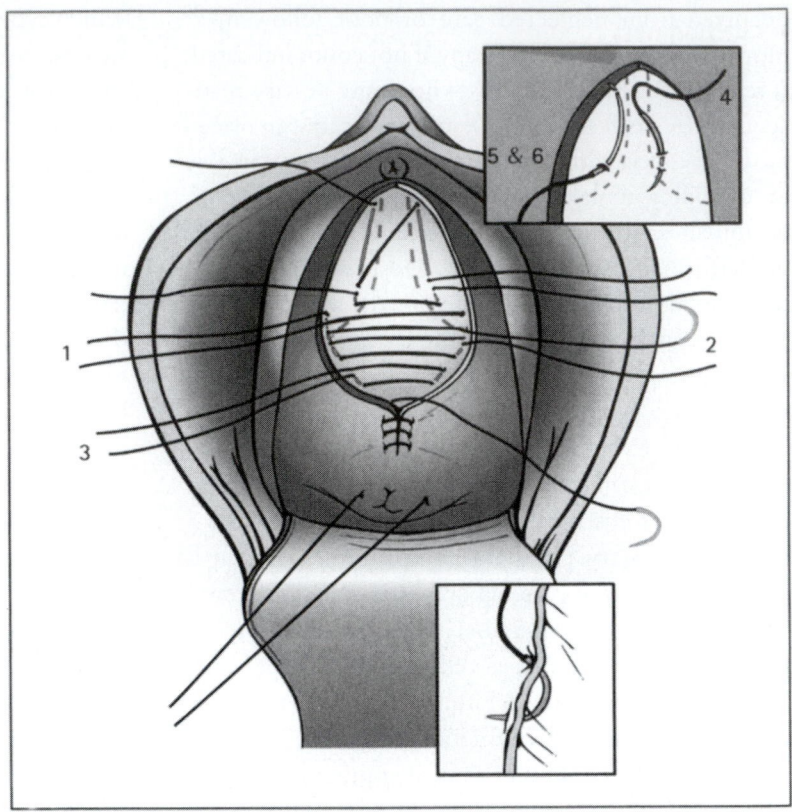

until further studies confirm adequate success rates for the paravaginal repair for stress incontinence.

The uncommon distal defect described by Richardson et al.[18] is rarely an isolated defect and is usually corrected when addressing the other types of cystocele defects. A specific repair for the distal defect has not been described. An apical defect often occurs, especially with recurrence of anterior-vaginal-wall prolapse. To correct an apical anterior-wall defect, reattachment of the anterior wall must be made to the pubocervical ring of support. A paravaginal repair reattaches the anterior wall to the arcus tendineus fascia pelvis from the level of the pubic symphysis to the ischial spines. Therefore, a paravaginal repair does not address the more proximal portion of the anterior wall. At present this is accomplished with correction of the vaginal apex, such as with a uterosacral vault suspension or abdominal sacrocolpopexy with the anterior leaf attached to the proximal anterior vaginal wall.

APICAL PROLAPSE

Vaginal procedures to correct apical prolapse include sacrospinous vault suspension, iliococcygeus suspen-

sion, and uterosacral vault suspension. Abdominal procedures include sacrocolpopexy and uterosacral vault suspension. Surgery for apical prolapse is to return the upper vagina to a horizontal axis in the standing position.[32] The sacrospinous vault procedure is performed unilaterally or bilaterally and suspends the vaginal apex to the sacrospinous ligament[33,34] (Figure 59-9). The iliococcygeus procedure is always performed bilaterally and suspends the vaginal vault from the fascia overlying the iliococcygeus muscle.[35] The uterosacral vault suspension can be performed abdominally or vaginally (Figure 59-10). The McCall culdoplasty reattaches the uterosacral ligaments to the posterior vaginal vault after a vaginal hysterectomy (Figure 59-11). The original McCall culdoplasty uses at least three interrupted permanent sutures, which are tied in the midline. Besides addressing vault support, this technique also obliterates the cul-de-sac, which corrects or prevents an enterocele.[36] Shortening of the uterosacral ligaments toward the sacrum is often required before reattachment to the vault if the ligaments are significantly attenuated. Another procedure, such as sacrospinous vault suspension, iliococcygeus suspension, or sacrocolpopexy, is recommended if adequate apical support cannot be obtained with a

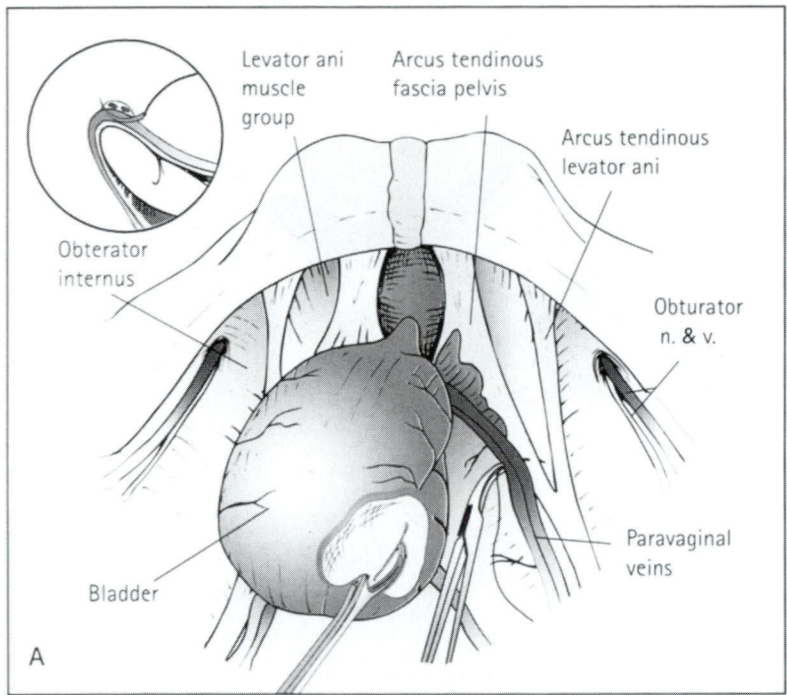

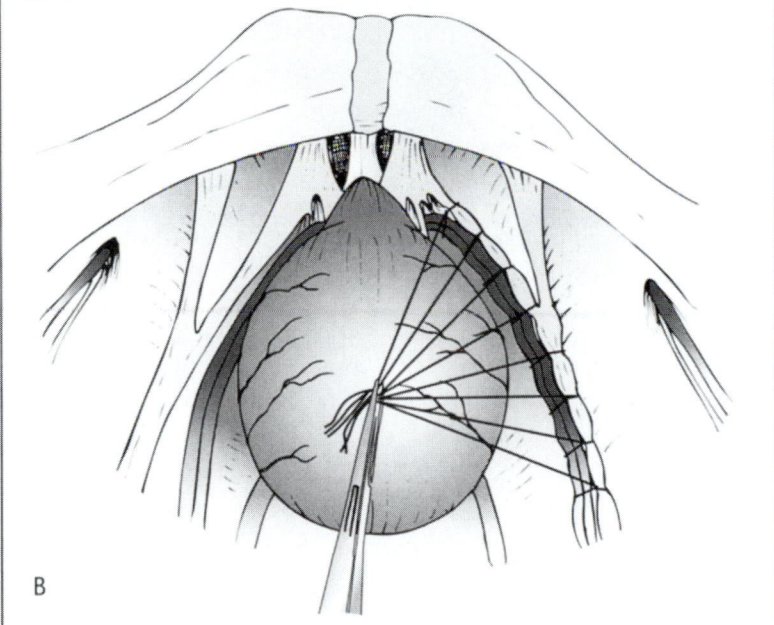

Figure 59-8 Correction of paravaginal cysto-cele. A. With the operator's nondominant hand intravaginally, the extent of the defect is palpated. The bladder is gently retracted medially over the vaginal hand, exposing the glistening white musculofascial tissue of the vagina. Before suture placement, pressure should be removed temporarily from the vaginal hand to ensure a vein is not being entered. B. Sutures are then placed close to the bladder medially; either encircling the paravaginal veins or placed just lateral to them. A full-thickness vaginal suture is used. The suture is completed by placement in the arcus tendineus fascia pelvis (ATFP) on the side wall or in the anatomic location of the ATFP if it has torn away. Successive sutures extending from the ischial spine to the ureth-rovesical junction are placed. When repairing a bilateral defect, the first side should be tied down before proceeding with the second side to prevent overcorrecting of the anterior vaginal wall. As the sutures are tied, the operator should feel the lateral vaginal sulci returning and correction of the cystocele oc-curring. *Panel A from Benson JT. Urogynecology and reconstructive pelvic surgery. Vol 5. In: Stenchever MA, ed. Atlas of clinical gynecology. New York: McGraw-Hill, 2000. Panel B from Richardson AC. Pelvic support defects in woman (urethrocele, cystocele, uterine prolapse, entero-cele, and rectocele). In: Skandalakis J, et al. eds. Hernia: surgical anatomy and technique. New York: McGraw-Hill, 1989:238.*

uterosacral vault suspension. There are several modifi-cations to the sacrocolpopexy. Modifications of the sacrocolpopexy are primarily extending the graft fur-ther down the vagina both anteriorly and posteriorly and not simply attaching the graft solely to the apex (Figure 59-12). The fascial or synthetic graft can con-sist of an anterior and/or posterior leaf, cone-shaped or Y-shaped depending on the type of defects that need to be addressed.[37,38] For example, a sacro-colpoperineopexy may be required if vault prolapse occurs with perineal descent. With this modification of the sacrocolpopexy, the posterior leaf of the graft is attached to the inferior edge of the fascial defect at the perineal body and suspended to the sacrum.[39] A vaginal stent facilitates attachment of the graft with interrupted, permanent sutures through the full

Figure 59-9 Pulley stitching. After securing the sutures to the ligament complex, a pulley stitch is placed at the site of the vaginal marking suture. *From Benson JT. Urogynecology and reconstructive pelvic surgery. Vol 5. In: Stenchever MA, ed. Atlas of clinical gynecology. New York: McGraw-Hill, 2000.*

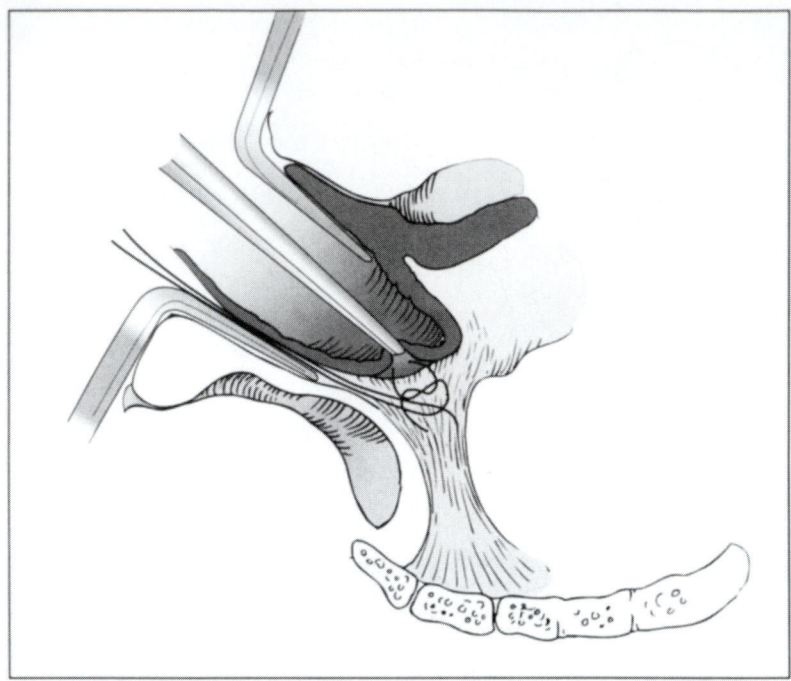

Figure 59-10 A vaginal stent rod placed intravaginally allows dissection of the vesicovaginal space anteriorly and the rectovaginal septum posteriorly. The uterosacral ligaments are freed distal to the previous tagged area. The most distal uterosacral segment is attached to the rectovaginal septum and the most proximal portion of the ligament is placed to the anterior vaginal wall just inferior to the cuff. Remaining sutures are placed along the posterior vaginal wall as needed. This technique will provide support to both the anterior apex and posterior apex. The laparoscopic approach is performed exactly as above, with the exception of a laparoscopic-assisted vaginal hysterectomy if indicated. The laparoscope is a means of access; its use should not change the way the basic procedure is performed. *From Benson JT. Urogynecology and reconstructive pelvic surgery. Vol 5. In: Stenchever MA, ed. Atlas of clinical gynecology. New York: McGraw-Hill, 2000.*

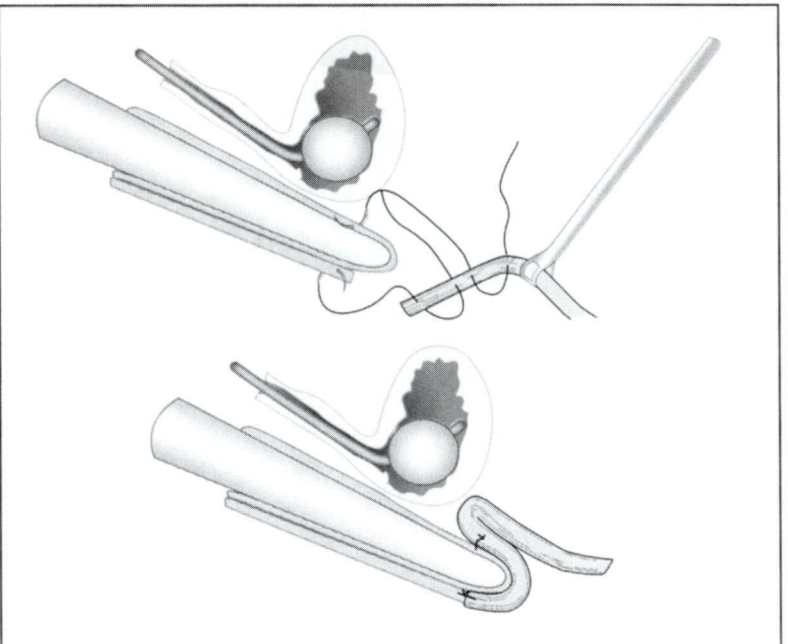

thickness of the vaginal walls. Typically, an enterocele repair is performed with a sacrocolpopexy and other defects are addressed as necessary.

POSTERIOR WALL PROLAPSE

Five of the most common procedures for treatment or prevention of enterocele include transvaginal en-terocele repair, McCall culdoplasty, and Torpin technique for vaginal procedures and Moschcowitz and Halban procedures for the abdominal approach. In the transvaginal enterocele repair the enterocele sac is identified, dissected from the rectum and vagina, and then excised. Several pursestring sutures close the cul-de-sac, and in addition, the uterosacral ligaments are shortened and reattached to the posterior vagina.

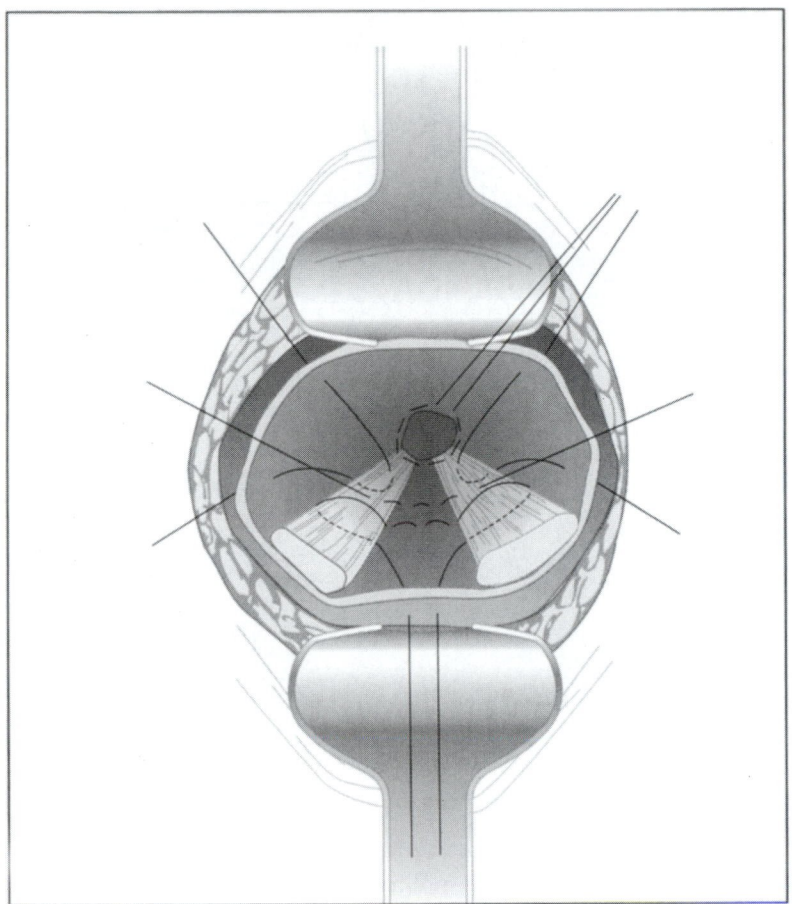

Figure 59-11 The anterior portion of the suture is placed through the anterior vaginal muscularis and held. The posterior suture is passed through the posterior peritoneum and posterior-vaginal-wall muscularis. The anterior and posterior muscularis sutrues are placed lateral to the midline approximately halfway to the vaginal angle. The cul-de-sac is closed with an internal McCall-type culdoplasty suture. The most distal segment of the uterosacral ligament is used for an external McCall suture. If strong cardinal ligaments were identified, they are placed through the vaginal angles and the cuff is closed last. *From Benson JT. Urogynecology and reconstructive pelvic surgery. Vol 5. In: Stenchever MA, ed. Atlas of clinical gynecology. New York: McGraw-Hill, 2000.*

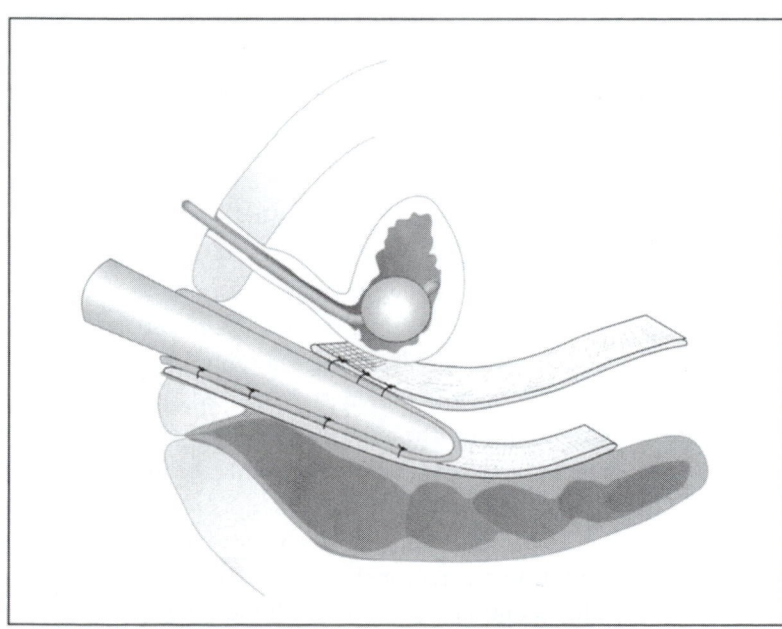

Figure 59-12 The anterior graft is secured by placing gentle retraction on the bladder, exposing the vesicovaginal space. With the vaginal stent serving as a guide, the graft is fixed to the anterior vaginal wall as laterally and as distally as possible. Typically, three to four rows of two sutures each are placed to secure this graft. *From Benson JT. Urogynecology and reconstructive pelvic surgery. Vol 5. In: Stenchever MA, ed. Atlas of clinical gynecology. New York: McGraw-Hill, 2000.*

Figure 59-13 The Moschowitz repair involves successive pursestring sutures placed around the cul-de-sac through the peritoneal and serosal surfaces only. The most superior suture should be 1 cm below the ureter to prevent kinking. Moschowitz sutures can be placed on either side of the sigmoid as shown or across the sigmoid as a single suture. The Halban and Moschowitz procedures possess little intrinsic strength themselves. Vaginal axis restoration over the levator plate is needed for these to be successful. *From Benson JT. Urogynecology and reconstructive pelvic surgery. Vol 5. In: Stenchever MA, ed. Atlas of clinical gynecology. New York: McGraw-Hill, 2000.*

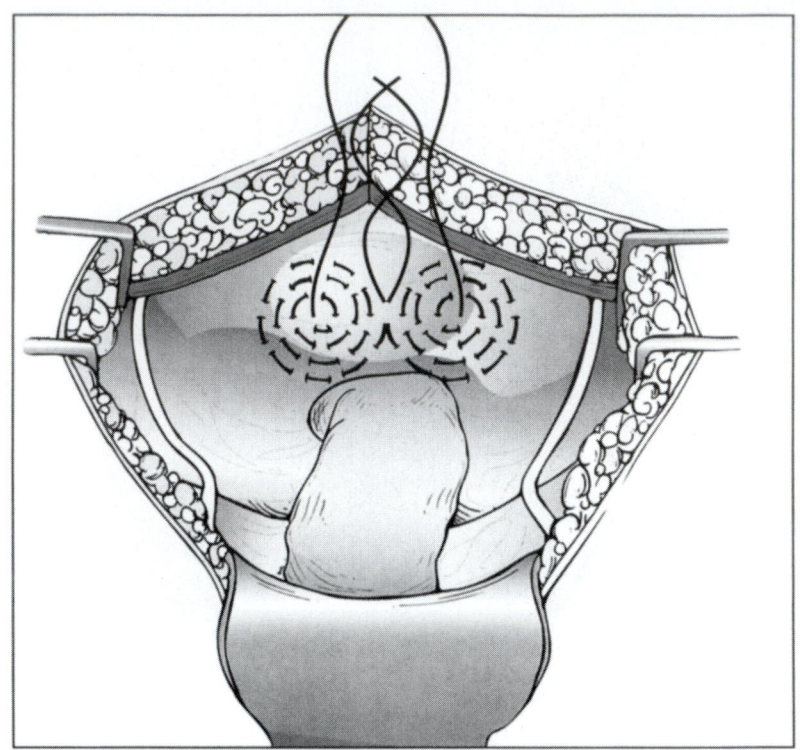

As described in the previous paragraph, the McCall culdoplasty closes the cul-de-sac by bringing the uterosacral ligaments together in the midline. The Torpin technique excises a triangular portion of "peritoneum, fascia and excessive vaginal vault wall"

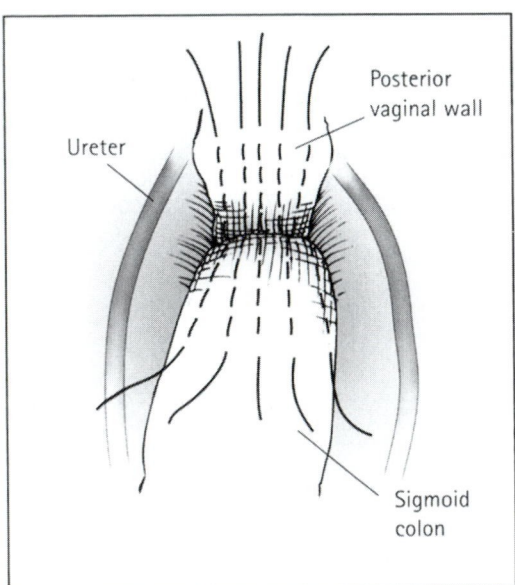

Figure 59-14 Appropriate apical support should be restored as needed and the Halban sutures tied down. *From Benson JT. Urogynecology and reconstructive pelvic surgery. Vol 5. In: Stenchever MA, ed. Atlas of clinical gynecology. New York: McGraw-Hill, 2000.*

through a posterior incision. The triangular incision is closed in the midline, providing vaginal length while narrowing the vaginal caliber.[40] In the abdominal procedure of Moschowitz, pursestring sutures are placed similarly to the transvaginal enterocele repair. In the original description the Moschcowitz procedure used several permanent concentric pursestring sutures to obliterate the cul-de-sac by approximating the peritoneum overlying the sigmoid to the posterior wall of the vagina[41] (Figure 59-13). The Halban enterocele repair similarly closes the cul-de-sac by suturing the peritoneum of the sigmoid to the posterior wall of the vagina. Instead of pursestring sutures, several rows of sutures are sagittally placed in a longitudinal fashion down the sigmoid, across the cul-de-sac, and up the posterior vaginal wall. Sutures are placed approximately 1 cm apart and medial to the ureters[42] (Figure 59-14).

The traditional posterior colporrhaphy for a symptomatic rectocele has had few modifications. This traditional procedure plicates the full length of the rectovaginal "fascia" in the midline.[43] (Figure 59-15). Differences in technique primarily revolve about whether or not to perform plication of the levator ani and to what degree of plication. New-onset dyspareunia after posterior colporrhaphy has been attributed to aggressive levator plication.[44] Also,

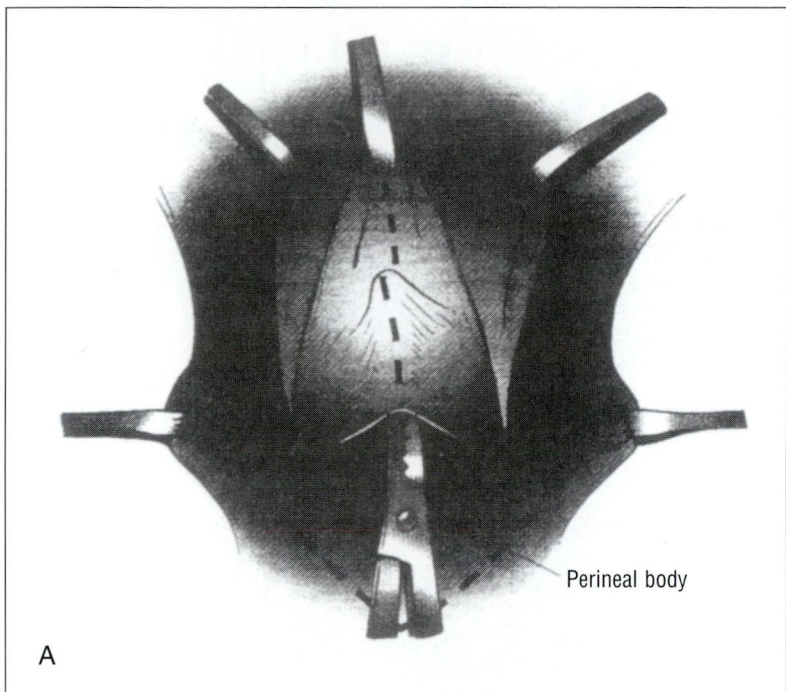

A

Perineal body

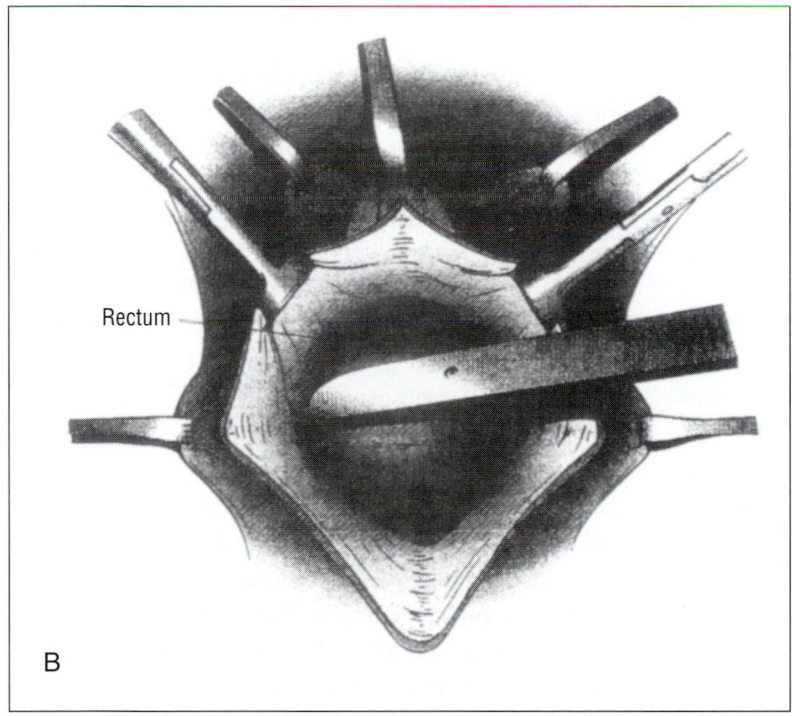

B

Rectum

Figure 59-15 Posterior colporrhaphy. A. The extent of the rectocele is ascertained and a posterior midline incision made through the vaginal epithelium only. B. Loss of rugation may indicate separation of the epithelium from the underlying musculofascial tissue and rectovaginal septum. The dissection is taken laterally to the crura of the levator muscles and superiorly as far as needed. *From Benson JT. Urogynecology and reconstructive pelvic surgery. Vol 5. In: Stenchever MA, ed. Atlas of clinical gynecology. New York: McGraw-Hill, 2000.*

(figure continues on following page)

Figure 59-15 Continued. C. A finger in the rectum delineates the deficient support tissue. The lateral musculofascial tissue and rectal vaginal septum are plicated in the midline, rebuilding this tissue. Epithelial trimming is done to remove redundant tissue only. The epithelium is closed and a perineorrhaphy completed as needed. Some surgeons recommend incorporating the levator muscles into this midline plication. This levator plication does not represent normal anatomy and should be avoided in the sexually active patient. A 30% rate of dyspareunia or apareunia follows a traditional posterior colporrhaphy.

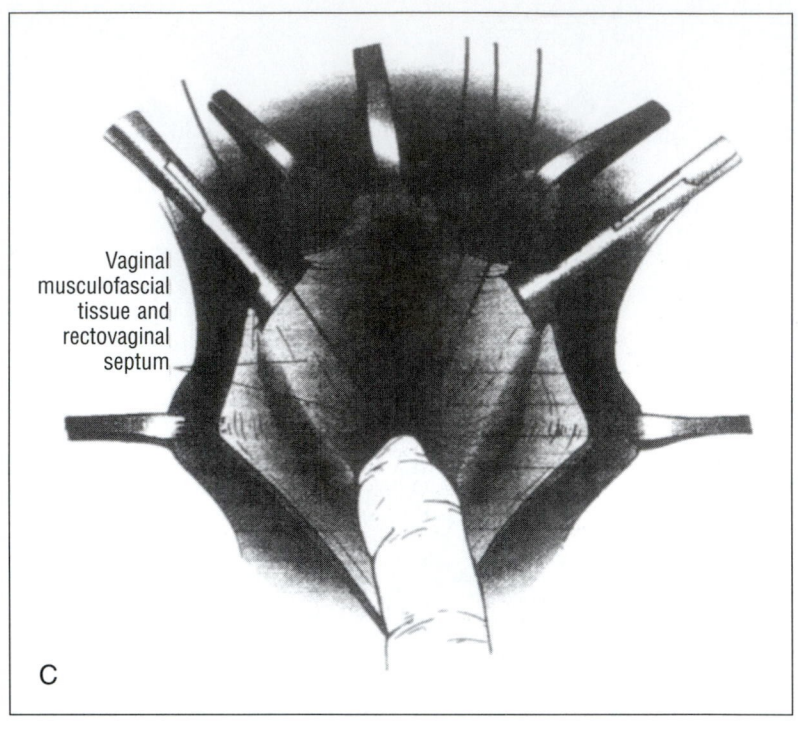

Vaginal musculofascial tissue and rectovaginal septum

C

perineorrhaphy is typically included in the posterior colporrhaphy if defects of the perineal body are encountered. Commonly the bulbocavernosus muscles require reattachment to the perineal body. Another type of rectocele repair is the site-specific repair[45,46] (Figure 59-16). In this technique the specific fascial defect is corrected. On bimanual rectal examination, commonly a "step-off" or a specific transverse defect of the rectovaginal septum can be palpated just cephalad to the perineal body. This defect is corrected with reattachment of the rectovaginal septum to the perineal body. Other fascial defects, if encountered with surgical dissection, are corrected with several interrupted sutures. Colorectal surgeons primarily repair rectoceles through a transanal approach. The transanal approach plicates the rectal muscularis and reattaches the muscularis to the levator ani.[47] The previously described sacrocolpoperineopexy reinforces the entire length of the posterior vaginal wall and can also be considered a type of rectocele repair.

ALTERNATIVE PROCEDURES

Colpocleisis is another alternative for a woman who has symptomatic pelvic-organ prolapse and does not desire the presence of a vagina (Figure 59-17). Careful selection of patients is required for this procedure. It cannot be assumed that a patient who does not

have vaginal intercourse or never expects to have vaginal intercourse is an appropriate candidate for colpocleisis; some patients simply desire to have a vagina separate from the issue of coital function. Colpocleisis can be performed for uterovaginal prolapse or vault eversion. The LeFort colpocleisis is closure of the anterior and posterior walls of the vagina without removing the uterus. Postmenopausal bleeding can be difficult to evaluate after a LeFort since the vaginal canal is obstructed. Therefore, dilatation and curettage is recommended prior to this procedure. A colpocleisis for vault eversion requires excision of the vaginal epithelium distal to the level of the levator ani. If an enterocele is present, it is addressed prior to aggressively plicating the levator ani and then performing a perineorrhaphy. Colpocleisis can be performed quickly and safely under regional or local anesthesia and is an option for patients who are not ideal surgical candidates. Support of the bladder neck is required because the alteration in the vaginal axis predisposes to stress incontinence. Preoperative evaluation of urinary incontinence, or the potential for it, determines which procedure provides the bladder-neck support.

When performing surgery for symptomatic pelvic-organ prolapse, all defects must be addressed in an organized fashion to obtain optimal anatomic and physiologic outcomes. Pelvic reconstruction is currently

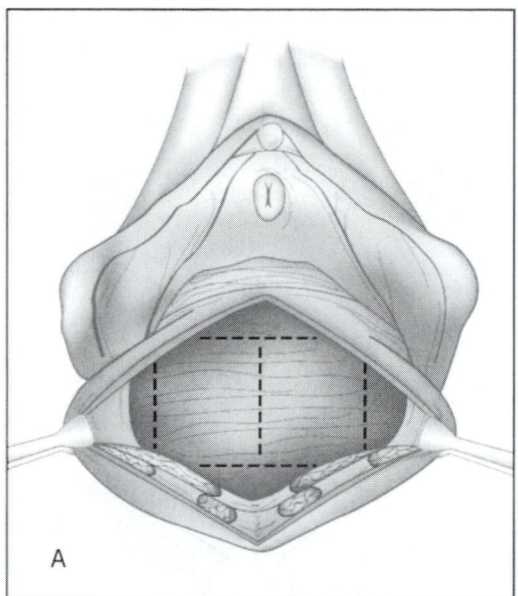

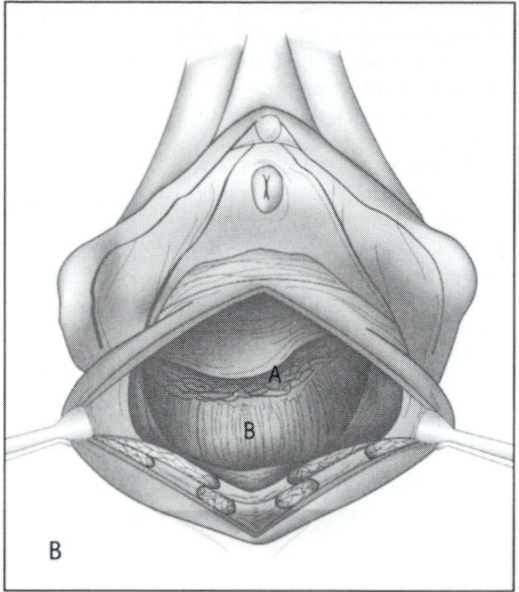

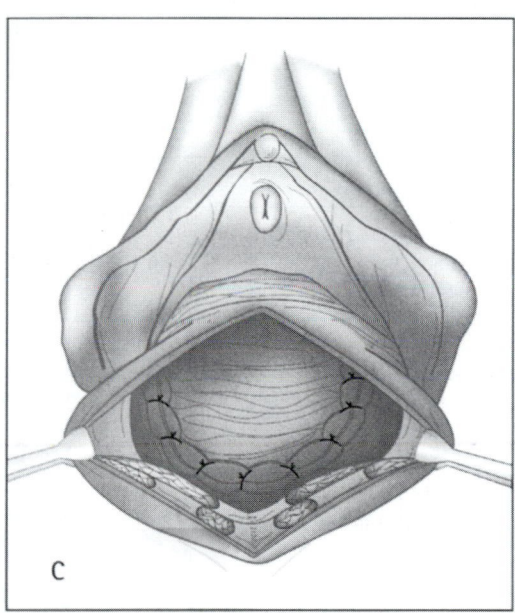

Figure 59-16 Sites and types of rectovaginal septal defects. Defects in the posterior vaginal wall may be enterocele, rectocele, or sigmoidocele. Ancillary imaging such a dynamic cystoproctogram may be helpful in differentiating these entities. Symptoms vary widely in patients with posterior-wall defects, a fact that underscores the importance of discussing patient's and physician's expectations for surgery. Successful correction of the bulging does not always equal relief of the patient's symptoms. Rectoceles have several methods described for their correction, although no one technique has proven superior. They include a defect repair, graft replacement, traditional posterior colporrhaphy, rectal-wall imbrication, and transanal repair. A. The defect approach to rectocele repair involves identifying the defect in the musculofascial tissue or the rectovaginal septum and correcting it. It avoids the mass closure technique of the posterior colporrhaphy. The support tissue may be torn at the perineal body, lateral side wall, or apex. The concept is the same as that for defects involved in the anterior wall. B. The dissection is begun in the posterior midline and carried out laterally. The dissection should be kept as thin as possible below the vaginal epithelium. A finger placed in the rectum will aid this dissection and help delineate the margins of the defect. *A* is the torn rectovaginal septum; *B* is the rectal muscularis. C. Once identified, the defect is repaired with interrupted sutures and the epithelium closed. *From Benson JT. Urogynecology and reconstructive pelvic surgery. Vol 5. In: Stenchever MA, ed. Atlas of clinical gynecology. New York: McGraw-Hill, 2000.*

Figure 59-17 Obliterative surgery is reserved for the patient who no longer desires sexual intercourse or in whom body self-image is not an issue. A LeFort colpocleisis may be used if the uterus is still present. An alternative approach uses a vaginal hysterectomy, if a uterus is still present, combined with a complete colpocleisis and levator plication. A. After performing a vaginal hysterectomy, the vaginal epithelium is undermined with a subepithelial solution of saline. Kocher clamps placed at the vaginal angles help maintain orientation as the dissection proceeds. Either a circumferential epithelial incision just inside the hymen can be made or a standard midline anterior and posterior incision is used. B. A wide perineorrhaphy is made by removing a large diamond-shaped area of perineum and distal vaginal epithelium.

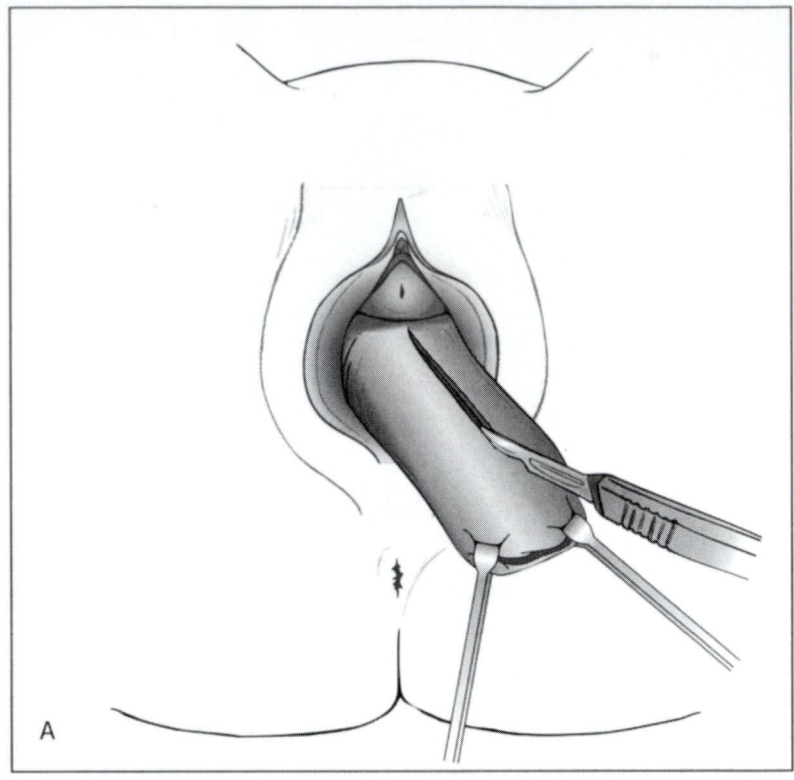

A

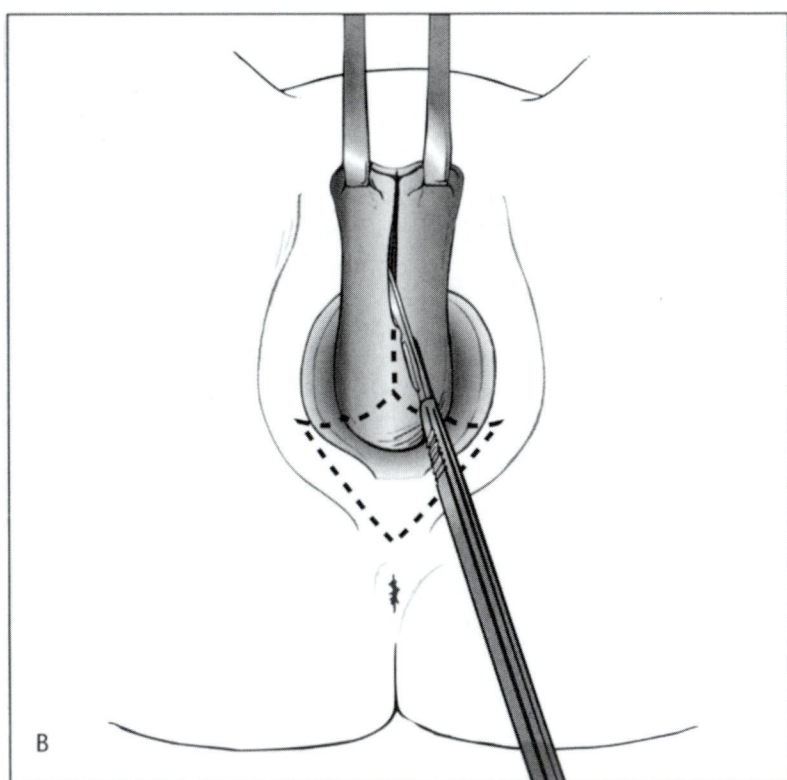

B

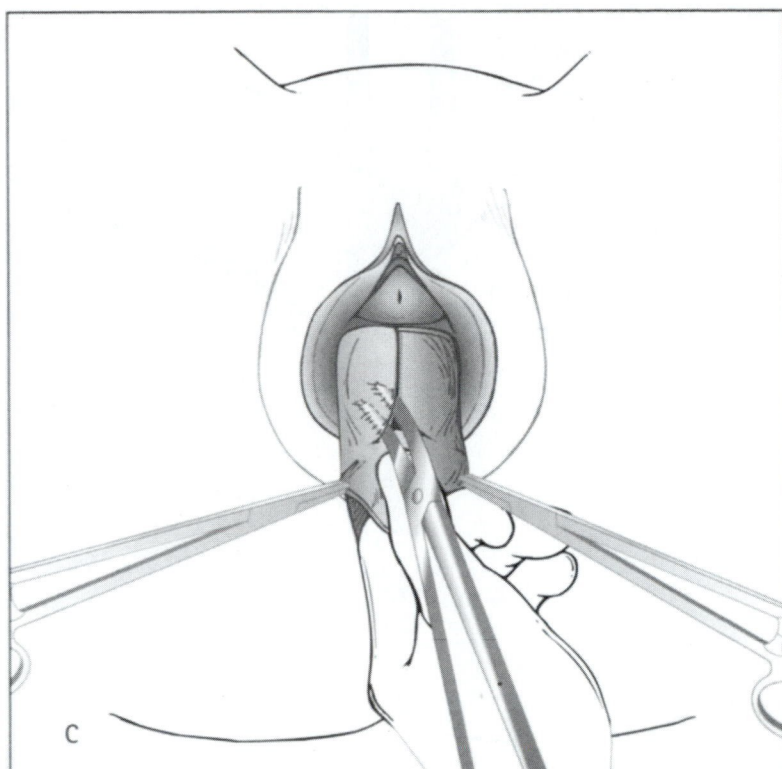

C

Figure 59-17 Continued. C–E. Using sharp and blunt dissection, the vaginal epithelium is dissected away from the underlying musculofascial tissue. The bladder, enterocele, and rectocele are all freed from the vaginal epithelium. The operator's nondominant hand is placed immediately on the vaginal epithelium and an assistant places countertraction on the prolapsing organs. Metzenbaum scissors are used to sharply divide the vaginal epithelium. The epithelium is removed leaving behind the prolapsing structures.

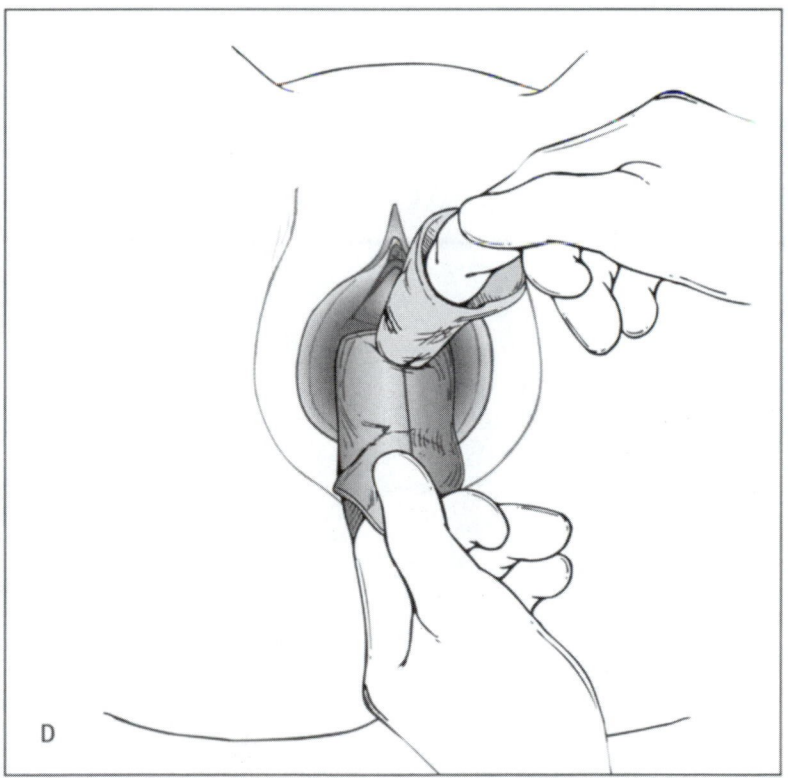

D

(figure continues on following page)

Figure 59-17 Continued. F. The leading edge of the prolapse is identified, and pursestring sutures are placed around it. As the suture is tied down and the tissue reduced, a hemostat is placed on the knot and the suture cut. The next pursestring suture is then placed with the tagged suture serving as the center. The hemostat helps reduce the tissue as the next suture is tied. This is carried on until the prolapsing tissue is above the level of the levator plate.

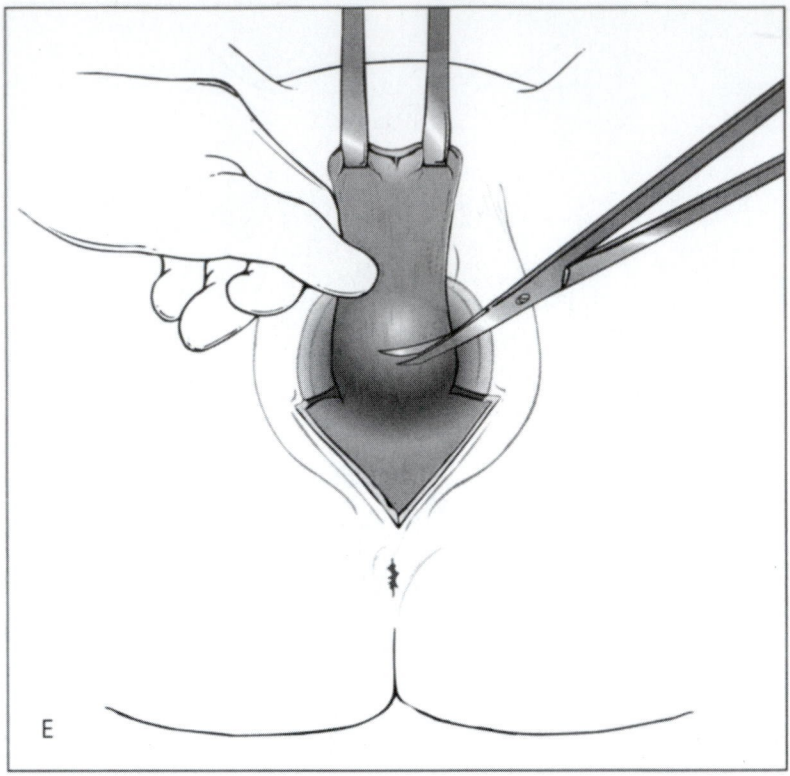

E

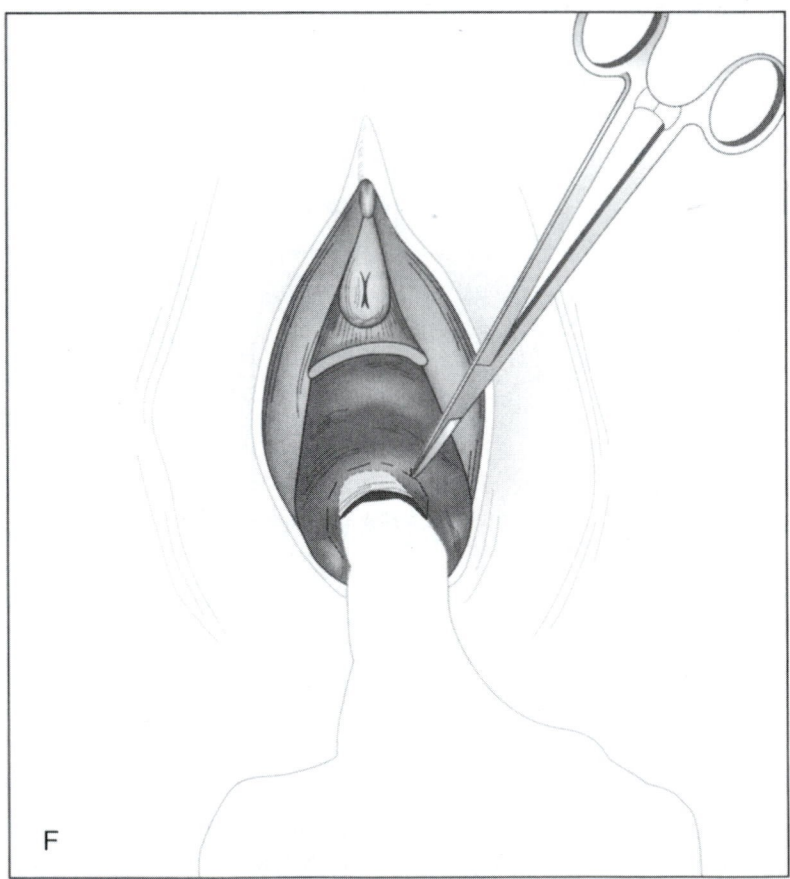

F

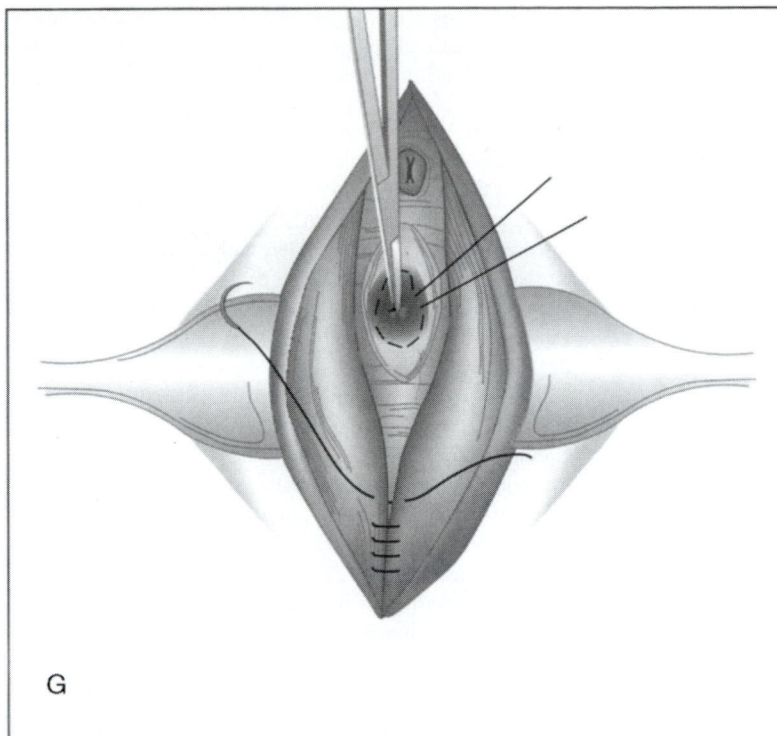

Figure 59-17 Continued. G. The levator muscles are palpated and approximated using a 0 or #1 permanent or delayed absorbable suture. They should be closed from above the rectum to the level of the urethrovesical junction (UVJ). The ureters must be clear of the levator muscles and the operator should place a finger rectally to help with suture placement. A Kelly-type plication at the UVJ helps prevent downward traction on the UVJ from the levator plication. A tight perineorrhaphy is performed so that at most one fingerbreadth can be placed below the urethra. At completion, the typical vaginal vault will be reduced to 3 cm in length and only one finger should fit below the urethra to the posterior fourchette. *From Benson JT. Urogynecology and reconstructive pelvic surgery. Vol 5. In: Stenchever MA, ed. Atlas of clinical gynecology. New York: McGraw-Hill, 2000.*

performed abdominally, vaginally, or with a combination of these routes. The literature regarding success rates and complications are at present insufficient for discussion of laparoscopic techniques for correction of prolapse. In the future and after further study, surgical management of pelvic-organ prolapse may include laparoscopic procedures solely or in conjunction with abdominal or vaginal reconstruction. Laparoscopic techniques will add to the current controversy regarding which procedures provide the highest success rates with the least morbidity. To reiterate, several factors must be considered before determining which procedures and which combination of procedures will provide the best overall outcome with the least morbidity for the individual patient.

REFERENCES

1. Pokras R, Hufnagel VG. Hysterectomies in the United States. Vital Health Statistics-13. 1987;92:1.
2. Olsen AL, Smith VJ, Bergstrom JO, Colling JC, Clark AL. Epidemiology of surgically mananged pelvic organ prolapse. Obstet Gynecol 1997;89:501.
3. Wiskind AK, Creighton SM, Stanton SL. The incidence of genital prolapse after the Burch colposuspension. Am J Obstet Gynecol 1992;167:399.
4. Bump RC. Racial comparisons and contrasts in urinary incontinence and pelvic organ prolapse. Obstet Gynecol 1993;81:421.
5. Beck RP. Pelvic relaxational prolapse. In: Kase NG, Weingold AB, eds. Principles and practice of clinical gynecology. New York: Wiley, 1983:677.
6. Baden W, Walker T. Surgical repair of vaginal defects. Philadelphia: Lippincott, 1992.
7. Beecham CT. Classification of vaginal relaxation. Am J Obstet Gynecol 1980;136:957.
8. American College of Obstetrics and Gynecologists. Pelvic organ prolapse. Technical Bulletin no. 214. October, 1995.
9. Bump RC, et al. The standardization of terminology of female pelvic organ prolapse and pelvic floor dysfunction. Am J Obstet Gynecol 1996;175:10.
10. Allen RE, Hosker GL, Smith ARB, Warrell DW. Pelvic floor damage and childbirth: a neurophysiologic study. Br J Obstet Gynecol 1990;97:770.
11. Snooks SJ, Swash M, Setchell M, Henry MM. Injury to the innervation of pelvic floor sphincter musculature in childbirth. Lancet 1984;8:546.
12. Sze EH, Kohli N, Miklos JR, Roat T, Karram MM. Computed tomography comparison of bony pelvis dimensions between women with and without genital prolapse. Obstet Gynecol 1999;93:223.
13. Spence-Jones C, Kamm MA, Henry MM, Hudson CN. Bowel dysfunction: a pathogenic factor in uterovaginal prolapse and urinary stress incontinence. Br J Obstet Gynecol 1994;101:147.
14. Jackson SR, Avery NC, Tarlton JF, Eckford SD, Abrams P, Bailey AJ. Changes in metabolism of collagen in genitourinary prolapse. Lancet 1996;347:1658.
15. Makinen J, Soderstrom KO, Kiilholman P, Hirvonen T. Histologic changes in the vaginal connective tissue of patients with and without uterine prolapse. Arch Gynecol 1986;239:17.

16. Torpin R. Prolapsed uteri associated with spina bifida and clubfeet in newborn infants. Am J Obstet Gynecol 1942; 43:892.

17. DeLancey JOL. Anatomic aspects of vaginal eversion after hysterectomy. Am J Obstet Gynecol 1992;166:1717.

18. Richardson AC, Lyons JB, Williams NL. A new look at pelvic relaxation. Am J Obstet Gynecol 1976;126:568.

19. Weber AM, Walters, MD. Anterior vaginal prolapse: review of anatomy and techniques of surgical repair. Obstet Gynecol 1997;89:311.

20. Benson JT. Rectocele, descending perineal syndrome, enterocele. Female pelvic floor disorders. Philadelphia: Norton, 1992:380.

22. Kegel AH. Progressive resistance exercise in the functional restoration of the perineal muscles. Am J Obstet Gynecol 1948;56:238.

23. Kelvin FM, Maglinte DD, Hornback JA, et al. Pelvic prolapse: assessment with evacuation procography. Radiology 1992;184:547.

24. Deger, RB, Menzin AW, Mikuta JJ. The vaginal pessary: past and present. Postgrad Obstet Gynecol 1993;13:12.

25. Miller DS. Contemporary use of the pessary. In: Sciarra J, ed. Clinical gynecology. Vol 1. New York: Harper & Row, 1991:1.

26. Goldstein I, Wise GJ, Tancer ML. A vesicovaginal and intravesical foreign body: a rare case of the neglected pessary. Am L Obstet Gynecol 1990;163:589.

27. Benson JT, Lucente V, McClellan E. Vaginal versus abdominal reconstructive surgery for the treatment of pelvic support defects: a prospective study with long term outcome evaluation. Am J Obstet Gynecol 1996;175:1418.

28. Kelly HA. Incontinence of urine in women. Urol Cutan Rev 1913;17:291.

29. Nichols DH. Gynecologic and obstetric surgery. St. Louis: Mosby-Year Book, 1993;334.

30. Schram M, Schram, D. Cystocele repair: a modified technique. Obstet Gynecol 1967;29:447.

31. White GR. Cystocele, a radical cure by suturing lateral sulci of vagina to white line of pelvic fascia. JAMA 1909; 53:1701.

32. Nichols DH, Milley PS, Randall CL. Significance of restoration of normal vaginal depth and axis. Obstet Gynecol 1970;36:251.

33. Nichols DH. Sacrospinous ligament fixation for massive eversion of the vagina. Am J Obstet Gynecol 1982; 142:901.

34. Morley GW, DeLancey JOL. Sacrospinous ligament fixation for eversion of the vagina. Am J Obstet Gynecol 1988;158:872.

35. Shull BL, Capen CV, Riggs MW, et al. Bilateral atachment of the vaginal cuff to the iliococcygeus fascia: An effective method of cuff suspension. Am J Obstet Gynecol 1993; 168:1669.

36. McCall ML. Posterior culdeplasty: surgical correction of enterocele during vaginal hysterectomy: a preliminary report. Obstet Gynecol 1957;10:696.

37. Timmons MC, Addison WA, Addison SB, et al. Abdominal sacral colpopexy in 163 women with posthysterectomy vaginal vault prolapse and enterocele: evolution of operative techniques. J Reprod Med 1992;37:323.

38. Timmons MC, Addison WA: Vaginal vault prolapse. In: Brubaker LT, Saclarides TJ, eds. The female pelvic floor: disorders of function and support. Philadelphia: Davis, 1996:263.

39. Cundiff GW, Harris RL, Coates K, Low VHS, Bump RC, Addison WA. Abdominal sacral colpoperineopexy: a new approach for correction of posterior compartment defects and perineal descent associated with vault prolapse. Am J Obstet Gynecol 1997;177:1345.

40. Torpin R. Excision of the cul-de-sac of Douglas for the surgical cure of hernias, through the female caudal wall, including prolapse of the uterus. J Int Coll Surg 1955; 24:322.

41. Moschcowitz AV. The pathogenesis, anatomy and cure of prolapse of the rectum. Surg Gynecol Obstet 1912;15:7.

42. Halban J. Gynakologische operationslehre. Berlin: Urban and Schwarzenberg, 1932.

43. Goff BH. A practical consideration of the damaged pelvic floor with a technique for its secondary reconstruction. Surg Obstet Gynecol 1968;46:866.

44. Kahn MA, Stanton SL. Posterior colporrhaphy: its effects on bowel and sexual function. Br J Obstet Gynecol 1997;104:882.

45. Richardson AC. The rectovaginal septum revisited: its relationship to rectocele and its importance in rectocele repair. Clin Obstet Gynecol 1993;36:976.

46. Cundiff GW, Weidner AC, Visco AG, Addison WA, Bump RC. An anatomic and functional assessment of the discrete defect rectocele repair. Am J Obstet Gynecol 1998; 179:1451.

47. Kahn MA, Stanton SL, Kumar DA. Randomized, prospective trial of posterior colporrhaphy versus transanal repair of rectocele: preliminary findings. In: Proceedings of the eighteenth annual meeting of the American Urogynecologic Society. International Urogynecology Journal and Pelvic Floor Dysfunction 1997;8:246.

Chapter 60
Vulvar Lesions

Roger P. Smith

Five Key Points

- When an obvious local cause of vulvar irritation is not present, the possibility of systemic disease must be considered.
- Estrogen or topical testosterone tend to thicken the epithelium of the vulva while topical steroids and estrogen deficit cause thinning.
- Biopsy of the vulvar skin or lesions is often the only reliable method of establishing the correct diagnosis.
- Viral infections account for the most common raised vulvar lesions (condyloma acuminata) and most common ulcers (herpes).
- The presence of an ulcerative lesion should suggest a sexually transmitted disease, though an advance malignancy must also be considered.

Vulvar irritations and vaginal infections are among the most common gynecologic ailments found in office practice. The tissues of the vulva and vagina represent a rich ecosystem, with many interactions between tissues, fluids, hormones, and microbes. This system is delicately balanced, and a disturbance in any element can result in discharge, irritation, odor, or discomfort. Lesions of the vulva are especially troublesome for both the patient and the provider; they represent a threat to a very private area and the very real possibility that they are the harbinger of significant disease.

The skin of the vulva is like that of other areas of the body with stratified squamous epithelium, hair follicles, and sebaceous, sweat, and apocrine glands. Just as in other areas of the body, the skin of the vulva is susceptible to inflammatory and dermatologic diseases. Intertrigo, hidradenitis suppurativa, psoriasis, seborrheic dermatitis, Fox–Fordyce disease, Forth disease, changes caused by Behçet or Crohn diseases, viral infections, and parasites may all affect the skin of the vulva. The skin of the vulva is also vulnerable to irritation from vaginal secretions, recurrent urinary loss, or contact with external irritants (such as soap residue, perfumes, fabric softeners, or infestation by pinworms). Changes may occur because of the effects of diabetes or hormonal alterations as well as dermatoses such as hypertrophic dystrophy, lichen sclerosis, psoriasis, and others. The possibility of premalignant or malignant change must always be considered as well.

IRRITATION AND ALLERGY

Contact Dermatitis

Diffuse reddening of the vulvar skin accompanied by itching or burning should suggest a secondary or allergic vulvitis. Contact dermatitis presents as a symmetric, red, edematous change in the tissues. Ulceration with weeping sores and secondary infection may occur, especially if itching has been severe. The list of possible irritants can be extensive, including feminine hygiene sprays, deodorants and deodorant soaps, tampons or pads (especially those with deodorants or perfumes), tight-fitting or synthetic undergarments, colored or scented toilet paper, and laundry soap or fabric softener residues. Spermicides, latex condoms, lubricants, sexual aids, or semen may be the source of irritation. Soiling of the tissues by urine or feces can also create significant symptoms for older patients. Severe dermatitis of the vulva due to contact with poison ivy or poison oak is occasionally encountered. Candida infection, which can mimic topical irritations, should be ruled out, especially in cases that do not respond, or in patients with risk factors such as immunosuppression or diabetes.

Contact dermatitis of the vulva is treated primarily by identification and removal of the offending substance. A careful history, combined with the withdrawal of the suspected cause, will usually both confirm the diagnosis and constitute the needed therapy. Wet compresses or soaks using Burow solution (three to four times daily for 30 to 60 minutes), followed by air drying or drying with a hair dryer (on the cool setting) will help relieve symptoms. Loose-fitting clothing and the sparing use of a nonmedicated baby powder may facilitate the drying process. Steroid creams, such as hydrocortisone (0.5 to 1%) or fluorinated corticosteroids (Valisone, 0.1%, Synalar, 0.01%) may be applied two to three times a day if needed. Antihistamines are of little benefit.

Infestations

In the absence of other obvious findings, vulvar itching may be caused by infestation with *Phthirus pubis* (the crab louse) or *Sarcoptes scabiei* (the itch mite). Suspicion should be increased when itching of the mons is one of the patient's symptoms. Pediculosis pubis is passed by close contact with a person already infected by the crab louse. Highly contagious, a single sexual encounter with an infected partner results in transmission in 90% of cases. Bedding or towels may also provide a less common source of infection. Infection generally occurs in hairy areas of the vulva and mons, though other hairy portions of the body may also be affected. The diagnosis is made by identifying small black specks (excreta) on the skin, or nits (eggs) at the base of hair shafts. The slow-moving louse itself may sometimes be directly observed.

Similar to the louse, the itch mite is transmitted by close contact. Unlike pediculosis, scabies is not

limited to hairy areas of the body, but may be found in any area. The more rapidly moving itch mite (up to an inch a minute) burrows beneath the skin, evoking an allergic response characterized by itching. Because allergic reaction is necessary for symptoms to develop, symptoms are rare before 5 to 7 days after the initial infection. This itching is cyclic and often worse at night, when the tissues are warmer and the lice are active. Inspection of the vulva will demonstrate eggs and adult lice. Confirmation of the diagnosis may be made by microscopic inspection of material scraped from inflamed papules.

Itching of the perineum and perianal areas should also suggest pinworms (*Enterobius vermicularis*), skin changes due to Crohn disease, anal fissures, or fistulae.

Pediculosis pubis and scabies require treatments aimed at both the adult parasites and the eggs. Treatment with 1% permethrin (Nix cream) with a second application 10 days after the first is generally effective. Local treatment of two applications over 2 days of a 1% gamma-benzene hexachloride (lindane) lotion, shampoo, or cream (Kwell) is also effective. Lindane must be left in contact with the eggs for at least 1 hour to be effective. Lindane is contraindicated in pregnant and breast-feeding women. Even with effective treatment, itching from scabies may continue for several days after therapy, and may require antihistamine treatment. Bedding, clothes, towels, and the home environment require careful cleaning and disinfection to avoid reinoculation.

Pruritus and Vulvodynia

Nonspecific pruritus and vulvodynia are perhaps the most frustrating vulvar symptoms encountered. The profound itching of vulvar pruritus leads to uncontrollable scratching, resulting in a repeating cycle of scratch, excoriation, healing, and itch that may lead to the development of what was called lichen simplex chronicus, or hyperplastic vulvar dystrophy, and now squamous-cell hyperplasia. Vulvodynia describes chronic and extreme burning, discomfort, and stinging, resulting in dyspareunia and general disability. Both pruritus and vulvodynia are nonspecific symptoms that often lack definite findings. Potential causes for these symptoms include local infections, sexually transmitted diseases, vulvar dystrophies, lichen sclerosis, and epithelial neoplasia, including cancer. Systemic disturbances such as diabetes, uremia, leukemia, and vitamin deficiencies must also be considered. Rarely, psychogenic processes may present in this manner.

Simple irritation of the vulva is common with most vulvar and vaginal pathologies. Treatment with cool sitz baths, moist soaks, or the application of soothing solutions such as Burow solution (Domeboro, aluminum acetate 5% aqueous solution, three to four times daily for 30 to 60 minutes) will be helpful. Patients should be advised to wear loose-fitting clothing and keep the area well ventilated and dry. To dry the perineum after bathing, a hair dryer set on cool will provide drying without the further irritation of towel drying. Systemic therapy with antihistamines is useful for some conditions, especially when night itching is intense and sedation better tolerated. Topical use of fluorinated steroids to combat irritation should be limited, as a steroid-induced dermatitis may result from prolonged use. Crotamiton (Eurax) may be applied topically, twice daily, to suppress itching. Occasionally, the use of a topical anesthetic, such as 2% lidocaine jelly, may be required.

Treatment is best driven by establishing an accurate diagnosis. When symptomatic therapy must be used, improved local hygiene, tepid soaks, and astringent agents (such as Burow solution) may all be effective in decreasing symptoms. Topical steroids, in small quantities and for a limited time only, may also be used.

Vulvar vestibulitis, also known as vestibular adenitis, presents with a history of progressively worsening vulvar tenderness and pain, leading to loss of function. Most often these women have been seen multiple times before the diagnosis is established. Typical histories include recurrent vaginal infections, recurrent urinary-tract infection, or new-onset entrance dyspareunia. These patients are unable to use tampons or have intercourse because of pain and tenderness localized to the posterior half of the vulva, the fourchette, and vestibule. Careful inspection (with magnification) may reveal small punctate erythematous patches located between the Bartholin glands, hymeneal ring, and middle portion of the perineum. Involvement of the periurethral (Skene) glands is also seen. Gentle palpation with a cotton-tipped applicator will reproducibly map the area of involvement. The cause of this process is currently unknown.

Vulvar vestibulitis undergoes spontaneous improvement in between one-third and one-half of patients over the course of 6 months. Some authors have suggested withdrawal of oral contraceptives, but strong evidence for either causation or significant improvement is lacking. Topical steroids may be tried, but success is generally poor. Local anesthetics

(2% lidocaine gel) may be used to improve symptoms or to allow intercourse, but the subsequent loss of pleasurable, as well as nociceptive, sensation is often unsatisfactory. Refractory cases may require surgical or laser excision, but there is a risk of scarring, resulting in continuing disability.

SKIN CHANGES AND DERMATOSES

Traditionally, vulvar disease has been classified by appearance using such terms as leukoplakia, kraurosis, and vulvar dystrophy. In 1987, the International Society for the Study of Vulvar Disease (ISSVD) established a three-tiered classification scheme that has gained wide acceptance (Table 60-1). This use of consistent terminology has helped to reduce some of the confusion surrounding the diagnosis and treatment of vulvar skin changes.

The skin of the vulva is susceptible to both dermatologic and systemic diseases. Psoriasis, seborrheic dermatitis and neurodermatitis, sebaceous or inclusion cysts, cutaneous candidiasis, and lichen planus may all affect the vulvar tissues. For many of these conditions, lesions elsewhere on the body may provide a clue to the diagnosis. The tissues of the vulva are also susceptible to acute cutaneous infections such as folliculitis, furunculitis, impetigo, and hidradenitis suppurativa.

In older patients, intense itching of the vulva may occur because of atrophic changes brought on by menopausal estrogen levels. Inspection of the vulva will reveal a symmetrically reddened, smooth, and somewhat shiny look to the skin of the vulva and perineum. A maturation index may be helpful, but is rarely required. Biopsy will reflect the hypoplastic nature of this disease and will help to differentiate this from lichen sclerosus (formerly lichen planus atrophicus), which has a similar gross appearance.

When atrophic change is the cause of irritation, treatment with estrogen replacement (locally, systemically, or both) is indicated. In patients with significant atrophic vulvar or vaginal changes, estrogen therapy

---

TABLE 60-1
ISSVD* CLASSIFICATION OF VULVAR DISEASE

I   Squamous-cell hyperplasia (formerly hyperplastic dystrophy)
II Lichen sclerosis
III Other dermatoses

*International Society for the Study of Vulvar Disease.

may take up to 6 months to give satisfactory results. In cases of lichen sclerosus, local application of testosterone propionate (2%) in petrolatum (applied two to three times daily, diminishing to once or twice weekly when satisfactory results are obtained) is generally effective. Hypertrophic dystrophy is best treated with fluocinolone acetonide (0.025% or 0.01%), triamcinolone acetonide (0.01%), or a similar corticosteroid applied two to three times daily. Fluorinated steroids should be used for short periods only, replacing them with hydrocortisone or nonsteroidal therapies as soon as possible.

Because estrogen therapy for atrophic vulvitis or vaginitis may take up to 6 months to give full relief, consideration should be given to adding vaginal moisturizers or lubricants. Newer products (such as Replens, Astroglide, or Lubrin suppositories) act to hold moisture in the vaginal tissues so that use may be as infrequent as three to four times a week.

A thinned, atrophic-appearing skin, with linear scratch marks or fissures, is found in lichen sclerosus. The skin is often described as having a cigarette-paper or parchment-like appearance. These changes frequently extend around the anus in a figure-eight configuration. Atrophic changes result in thinning, or even loss, of the labia minora and significant narrowing of the introitus. Fissures, scarring, and synechiae cause marked pain for some patients. Topical steroid therapy will generally make the condition worse. Topical application of testosterone (2% in petrolatum) is the preferred treatment.

Small, smooth nodules on the inner surfaces of the labia minora and majora suggest sebaceous or inclusion cysts of the labia, caused by inflammatory blockage of the sebaceous-gland ducts. The nodules contain cheesy, sebaceous material, confirming the diagnosis. Treatment consists of drainage and local hygiene to reduce the risk of recurrence.

Disorders of the apocrine glands of the labia may also be the source of vulvar symptoms. In hidradenitis suppurativa, chronic blockage leads to itching and burning that progresses to abscess formation and ulceration. These painful and tender lesions may coalesce, resulting in extensive scarring, chronic drainage, and sinus formation. Treatment consists of local therapy (sitz baths, incision and drainage, topical antibiotics) and systemic therapy with antibiotics or oral contraceptives. Local excision may be required in severe cases. When hidradenitis is suspected, a dermatologic consultation should be considered.

In Fox–Fordyce disease, the apocrine glands become blocked with plugs of keratin. Intense itching and tiny flesh-colored papules (without erythema) are the hallmarks of this disorder. The itching that the patient experiences is often inversely related to estrogen levels and, hence, is improved with pregnancy or estrogen-dominant oral contraceptives.

HYPERPLASIA, MALIGNANT, AND PREMALIGNANT CHANGES

Cancers of the vulva, vagina, Bartholin, or Skene glands are relatively rare. These cancers combined account for fewer than 5000 cases annually in the United States, with vulvar cancer far and away the most common. The best and only screening available for these lesions are genital self-examination and careful physical examination. Itching, irritation, cracking, or bleeding of the vulva may be present in vulvar cancer or premalignant lesions, and should increase clinical suspicion. Early skin changes may be overlooked if careful inspection is not made a part of the clinician's routine for pelvic examination.

Squamous-Cell Hyperplasia

Squamous-cell hyperplasia (formerly called hypertrophic vulvar dystrophy) causes a thickening of the vulvar skin over the labia majora, outer aspects of the labia minora, and clitoral areas. The tissues may have a dusky red to thickened white appearance, often with linear hyperplasia. Fissuring and excoriations are common because of intense itching. Constant vigilance is required to watch for possible premalignant or malignant changes that can often mimic these lesions and those of lichen sclerosis. Liberal use of 3- to 5-mm punch biopsy should be made any time there is uncertainty (Figure 60-1).

Once the diagnosis is established, treatment is directed to interrupting the itch–rash–itch cycle. This may be accomplished with antipruritic medications such as diphenhydramine hydrochloride (Benadryl) or hydroxyzine hydrochloride (Atrax) used at nighttime. Topical application of steroid creams (hydrocortisone (1 to 2%), triamcinolone acetonide (Kenalog, 0.1%), or β-methasone valerate (Valisone, 0.1%) may give relief. If significant improvement is not achieved in 3 months, biopsy is indicated.

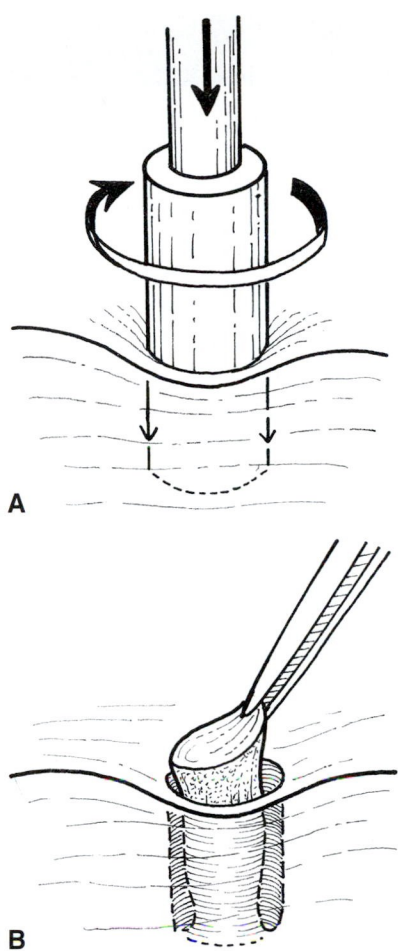

A

B

Figure 60-1 A. Punch biopsy is accomplished by pressing the instrument downward with a slight twisting motion until a loss of resistance is felt. B. The core of tissue created is elevated and excised at its base.

Vulvar Intraepithelial Neoplasia (VIN)

Vulvar intraepithelial neoplasia (VIN-I and VIN-II, mild and moderate atypia) are true neoplastic processes that carry a high risk of progression. The most common presenting symptoms are itching, chronic irritation, and the development of raised lesions. The lesions found in VIN are generally well localized and rough in texture. These lesions are most commonly found along the posterior vulva and perineal body, though they may be found in any location on the vulva. The diagnosis is established by biopsy.

Vulvar intraepithelial neoplasia, grade III (VIN-III) is diagnosed when there is full-thickness loss of maturation. The distinctions between this and carcinoma in situ are minimal and these conditions are often treated as the one and the same. Treatment of most VIN is by wide local excision, though for extensive lesions this may require simple vulvectomy.

The margins of intraepithelial change may often be suggested by the application of 3% acetic acid to the vulva, which produces acetowhite changes similar to those seen on the cervix.

Vulvar Cancer

Ninety percent of vulvar carcinomas are of squamous-cell origin. These tumors are most common between the ages of 65 and 70 years. The most common presenting symptom is itching, with red or white ulcerative or exophytic lesions found over the posterior two-thirds of the vulva. Because of the similarity of these symptoms and findings to the other vulvar dystrophies, biopsy must always be considered early in the diagnostic process. Aggressive surgical therapy, often performed by an experienced gynecologic oncologist, will be required.

Other Conditions

Paget disease is characterized by extensive intraepithelial disease, including the characteristic changes similar to those found in Paget disease in the breast. There is a high degree of association between Paget disease and carcinoma of the skin, colon, and breast. Wide local excision or simple vulvectomy are the usual treatments for Paget disease, but careful continuing follow-up for the possibility of recurrence must be maintained.

Melanoma of the vulva usually presents as a raised, irritated, pruritic, pigmented lesion. When melanoma is suspected, wide local excision is required for diagnosis and staging. If the melanoma is determined to be level I, this excision is considered adequate.

INFECTIONS

Whenever infection of the vulva is encountered, the possibility of a sexually transmissible infection must be considered. These infections may result in raised or ulcerated lesions, which may or may not be symptomatic. While the characteristics of the lesion facilitate the diagnosis, a general familiarity with the presentation of these infections is warranted (Table 60-2).

Swellings and Raised Lesions

Cystic, painful swelling of the labia in the area of the Bartholin gland suggests infection. Abscesses in the

TABLE 60-2
GENITAL LESIONS IN SEXUALLY TRANSMITTED DISEASES*

	Herpes	Genital Warts	Syphilis	Chancroid	Lymphogranuloma Venereum	Granuloma Inguinale
Organism	Herpes simplex virus	Human papillo-mavirus	*Treponema pallidum*	*Haemophilus ducreyi*	*Chlamydia trachomatis*	*Calymmatobacterium granulomatis*
Incubation	3–7 days	1–8 months	10–60 days	2–6 days	1–4 wk	8–12 wk
Primary lesion	Vesicle	Papule/polypoid	Papule	Papule/pustule	Papule/pustule/vesicle	Papule
Number	Multiple, coalesce	Variable	1	1–3	Single	Single or multiple
Pain	Yes	No	Rare	Often	No	Rare
Shape	Regular	Irregular	Regular	Irregular	Regular	Regular
Margins	Flat	Raised	Raised	Red, undermined	Flat	Rolled, elevated
Depth	Superficial	Raised	Superficial	Excavated	Superficial	Elevated
Base	Red, smooth	Normal, pink, white	Red, smooth	Yellow, gray	Variable	Red, rough
Induration	None	None	Firm	Rare, soft	None	Firm
Secretions	Serous	None	Serous	Purulent, hemorrhagic	Variable	Rare, hemorrhagic
Lymph nodes	Firm, tender	Normal	Firm, nontender	Tender, suppurative	Tender, suppurative	Pseudoadenopathy
Duration	5–10 days, recurrent	Months	Weeks	Weeks	Days	Weeks

*Boldfaced items are of particular help in making a differential diagnosis. Scabies, molluscum contagiosum, candida species, and other dermatologic conditions (e.g., hidradenitis suppurativa) may also cause genital lesions.

Modified from Sexually transmitted disease. In: Beckman CRB, Ling FW, Herbert WN, et al., eds. Obstetrics and gynecology. 3rd ed. Baltimore: Williams & Wilkins, 1998:348.

Bartholin gland develop rapidly over 2 to 4 days, producing extreme discomfort and disability, and may range to 8 cm or greater in size, usually requiring surgical drainage. Because these abscesses may be gonococcal in origin, further evaluation for other sexually transmitted diseases is prudent. Smaller, more chronic cysts, due to obstruction of the Bartholin duct, may be identified by gentle palpation at the base of the labia majora. These cysts are smooth, firm, and tender, with varying degrees of induration and erythema. The cysts may be clear, yellow, or bluish in color. Asymptomatic small Bartholin cysts require no therapy.

Mild infections of the Bartholin gland may respond to antibiotic or topical therapies. Over 80% of cultures of material from Bartholin's gland cysts are sterile. Most often, culture-positive cysts are secondarily infected by coliform organisms or are polymicrobial. Broad-spectrum antibiotic treatment will often successfully treat infections if abscess formation has not occurred. Warm to hot sitz baths will provide symptomatic relief and may promote pointing and drainage of small abscesses, with spontaneous drainage occuring in 1 to 4 days. When persistent, large, or particularly symptomatic abscesses occur, incision and drainage is indicated. Simple drainage of these abscesses is often associated with recurrence. Therefore, the placement of a Word catheter to form an epithe-

lialized tract, packing with iodoform gauze, or surgical marsupialization of the gland is preferred. Despite precautions, recurrences still happen to 5% to 10% of patients following marsupialization. Excision of the gland is often difficult and is associated with significant risk of morbidity, including intraoperative hemorrhage, hematoma formation, secondary infection, and scar formation with subsequent dyspareunia. As a result, excision is not generally recommended.

Mesonephric cysts of the vagina, lipomas, fibromas, hernias, hydroceles, and epithelial inclusion cysts may be confused with Bartholin gland cysts. Malignancy of the Bartholin gland is rare, but should be suspected in women over the age of 45, since benign cyst formation and infection is less common in this age group.

Like skin elsewhere in the body, fibromas, lipomas, papillomas, hemangiomas, inclusion or sebaceous cysts, and pigmented nevi may all be found in the tissues of the vulva and perineum. Though usually benign, pigmented lesions on the vulva or vagina are uncommon, and warrant biopsy to rule out malignancy (see above).

Vulvar hematomas will generally present with an obvious history of blunt trauma, such as a straddle injury or assault, but occasionally may result from sexual activities not volunteered in the initial history.

Hematomas are generally self-limited to the affected labia and respond to pressure and ice packs. Rarely, large or expanding hematomas may require surgical intervention.

The most common raised lesion of the vulva is condylomata acuminata, accounting for more than 500,000 cases a year, and earning it the distinction of most common sexually transmitted disease (other than pregnancy). Infection by human papillomavirus (HPV, most frequently serotypes 6 and 11) results in soft, fleshy, painless growths on the vulva, vagina, cervix, urethral meatus, perineum, and anus. Lesions that are symmetrical about the midline of the genital area are common. Condylomata may also be found on the tongue or within the oral cavity, the urethra, bladder, or rectum. The lesions may be single or multiple, and generally provide few symptoms by their presence; mild irritation or discharge may accompany secondary infections. The diagnosis of condylomata acuminata is made based on physical examination, but may be confirmed through biopsy.

Exuberant growth and frequent recurrences of condylomata are common in patients who are immunocompromised, who have diabetes, who are pregnant, or who are cigarette smokers. Condylomata may grow during pregnancy only to resolve when the pregnancy ends.

HPV is spread by skin-to-skin (generally sexual) contact and has an incubation period of from 3 weeks to 8 months, with an average of 3 months. It is thought that the presence of other vaginal infections such as candidiasis, trichomoniasis, or bacterial vaginosis increases the likelihood of infection by altering normal defense mechanisms, although coinfection is by no means required. Roughly 65% of patients will acquire the infection following intercourse with an infected partner. Condylomata are accompanied by Trichomonas or Gardnerella vaginal infections or other sexually transmitted disease in more than 10% of patients, making further screening of both the patient and her partner important to consider. Finding condylomata acuminata in a child should suggest the possibility of sexual abuse, but because close nonsexual contact can also result in infection, this is not sufficient evidence, by itself, to establish abuse.

Care must be taken to differentiate these from the smooth-topped condylomata lata of secondary syphilis, VIN, or dysplastic lesions. HPV infections (serotypes 16, 18, 31, 33, 35, 39, 45, 51, and 52) are also associated with cervical changes and an increased risk of cervical atypia and cancer, especially in smokers, requiring careful surveillance. Serotyping of HPV infections is currently of little clinical value since all patients, regardless of serotype, require careful follow-up and Pap smears.

Treatment of condylomata acuminata requires multiple visits and close follow-up. Treatment is directed toward reducing further spread, reduction of cancer risk, and cosmetic improvement. Complete eradication is unlikely and further spread remains a continuing possibility. Condylomata may be treated by the application of 20 to 25% podophyllin resin in tincture of benzoin, podophyllotoxin (0.5% solution, Condylox), or bichloroacetic and trichloroacetic acids (80 to 100% solution). Studies do not show definite superiority of one agent over another, though podophyllin is contraindicated for pregnant patients because of systemic absorption. This systemic absorption limits the size of lesions that should be treated with podophyllin to less than 2 cm, and restricts its use to lesions on the vulva, not the vagina. Podophyllin should be rinsed off the perineum in 30 minutes to 4 hours. With most topical therapy, sloughing of the treated lesions happens in 2 to 4 days. Scarring is rare. Reapplication of the topical agent is usually required, and should be carried out at a follow-up visit in 7 to 10 days. Topical therapy cure rates are good (50 to >75%), but recurrence generally exceeds 50% in 1 year. Injections with interferon alfa or interferon gel have been advocated, but success is limited, side effects are many, and the treatment is expensive and time-consuming, requiring multiple, frequent visits. Topical 5-fluorouracil (5-FU) may be applied two to three times a day by the patient, but significant chemical irritation often results. This is best reserved for severe cases. Severe cases, those with multiple recurrences, and pregnant patients with condylomata often require surgical, laser, or other specialized therapy.

Patients may self-apply podophyllotoxin to external lesions by applying the medication for 3 consecutive days each week for up to 3 weeks. Patients may also use imiquimod (Aldara) 5% cream, applied at night three times per week. The cream is left in contact with the lesions for 6 to 10 hours before it is washed away. Treatment continues until the lesions have cleared, but for no longer than 16 weeks. No matter what agent is used, if the lesions do not respond after several treatments, a reevaluation of the diagnosis should be made.

Small, raised, umbilicated lesions are typical of molluscum contagiosum. These asymptomatic lesions are caused by the poxvirus, a mildly contagious sexually transmitted disease. It takes several weeks to months for the lesions to develop after initial infections, and autoinfection is common. The lesions begin as domed papules and progress to mature lesions, 1 to 5 mm in diameter, with a umbilicated center filled with a caseous material. The papules may be found anywhere on the body except for mucous membranes. The diagnosis may be made clinically, or confirmed by expressing some of the waxy material from the lesion and examining it microscopically for intracytoplasmic molluscum bodies. Molluscum contagiosum is treated by curettage of the base of the papule, followed by cautery with either ferric subsulfate (Monsel solution) or 85% trichloroacetic acid. Cryosurgery or electrocautery may also be used but are more expensive and cumbersome. Follow-up should be in 1 month to look for new lesions.

Ulcers and Sores

The most commonly encountered ulcerative lesion of the vulva is that of herpes simplex infection. The vesicular lesions become ulcerated, may coalesce into running sores, and are extremely painful. These patients are often notable for their painful, "duck waddle" gait. Dysuria due to vulvar lesions or urethral or bladder involvement is common and may lead to acute urinary retention. Secondary infection of the ulcerated lesions is common. Additional symptoms of herpetic infections are reviewed in Chapter 59.

Viral cultures from suspected herpes vesicles, or the base of the ulcerated lesions, can recover the virus and confirm the clinical diagnosis, though care in the transport and storage of specimens is required. Culture success is inversely related to the duration of symptoms, with the best results obtained from cultures of the vesicles. Serologic typing of the virus is not necessary. Material scraped from the base of the lesions may also be smeared, fixed, and stained to show multinucleated giant cells and cells with intracellular inclusions. Antibody titers are of limited value because 30 to 100% of the sexually active groups studied have an elevated titer. Enzyme-linked immunoassay antigen detection test kits have been marketed, but a thorough evaluation of their sensitivity, specificity, and positive and negative predictive values is lacking. Preliminary studies indicate that false

negative rates of 30% are common. Other lesions that may be mistaken for herpes include primary chancres of syphilis, chancroid, lymphogranuloma venereum, granuloma inguinale, early condyloma, vaccinia, and Behçet syndrome (see Table 60-2).

Herpes infections in pregnancy deserve special mention. When herpes lesions are present near term or during labor, a significant risk of neonatal herpes infection exists. Roughly 50% of neonates delivered vaginally in the presence of herpes will develop infection. This infection carries a 80% mortality rate and significant risk of permanent ocular or central nervous system sequelae. To minimize this risk, cesarean delivery is often recommended for these patients.

General therapy for herpetic vulvitis is with analgesics and antipyretics, including topical applications of 2% lidocaine for pain relief, or an antimicrobial preparation to inhibit secondary infection. Approximately 10% of patients will need hospitalization for pain control or management of urinary complications. Direct therapy consists of acyclovir (Zovirax, 200 mg orally five times a day for 7 to 10 days) begun as soon as the diagnosis is made. Topical acyclovir ointment (5%) applied three to six times a day for 7 days, applied using gloves or a finger cot to prevent autoinoculation of other sites, may also be used, but is less effective than systemic management. Treatment with acyclovir will shorten the period of viral shedding and may improve symptoms if begun early enough in the course of the infection.

Suppressive therapy with acyclovir, 400 mg twice daily on a continuous basis for up to 12 months, may be used in patients with frequent (>6/year) recurrences. This prophylaxis significantly decreases both the frequency and severity of subsequent episodes by approximately 75%, but does not completely prevent them or prevent the patient from spreading the disease through viral shedding. Once prophylaxis is discontinued, the risk, frequency, and severity of recurrence may be unchanged.

Ulcerative lesions are a common presenting symptom for many veneral diseases ranging from the painless ulcers of primary syphilis to symptomatic lesions of chancroid or lymphogranuloma venereum. These must always be considered in the differential diagnosis. One such infection, chancroid, is more common than syphilis in some areas of Africa and Southeast Asia, but uncommon in the United States, with only about 1500 cases per year reported. *Haemophilus ducreyi*, the causative agent of chancroid, is not capable of infecting intact skin, thus the lesions of chancroid tend to be found in areas traumatized by sexual activity. *H. ducreyi* infection typically causes one to three painful "soft chancres" to appear 3 to 10 days after exposure. Though 10 times more common in men than in women, these vulvar chancres break down over about 2 weeks to form shallow, progressive ulcers with red, ragged, undermined edges, with little surrounding inflammation. Material from these ulcers is virulent and can infect other body sites.

In approximately 50% of patients, the unilateral adenopathy caused by chancroid will progress to massive enlargement and inflammation, called buboes. These may rupture and drain, causing extensive soft tissue and skin damage. The diagnosis is established on the basis of clinical findings, finding the gram-negative coccobacillus on smears from the primary lesion, or, rarely, on culture of aspirates of the bubo. Biopsy is also diagnostic, though not often performed. Treatment is with erythromycin, 500 mg four times a day, or trimethoprim–sulfamethoxazole 160 mg and 800 mg, twice a day. Both treatments must continue for no less than 10 days, or until the lesions heal. Fluctuant nodes may be drained by aspiration through adjacent normal tissue, but incision and drainage delay healing and should not be attempted.

Granuloma inguinale (also called donovanosis) is relatively common in the tropics, New Guinea, and Caribbean areas, but accounts for fewer than 100 cases per year in the United States. This infection is caused by the bipolar, gram-negative bacterium *Calymmatobacterium granulomatis*. With an incubation period of 1 to 12 weeks, this mildly contagious infection first presents with single or multiple subcutaneous papules. These evolve to form raised, red, granulomatous lesions that bleed on contact and undergo ulceration, necrosis, and extremely slow healing. These lesions are confined to the genitalia in 80% of cases. Unlike other ulcer-producing venereal diseases, granuloma inguinale does not produce marked adenopathy. The diagnosis is established clinically or through the identification of intracytoplasmic bacteria (Donovan bodies) in mononuclear cells. Treatment consists of tetracycline, 500 mg every 6 hours for 3 weeks. Secondary infection or significant scarring may occur in untreated cases. Because of relapse and late scarring, these patients should be followed carefully for several weeks.

Like other minor sexually transmitted diseases, lymphogranuloma venereum (LGV) is seen only sporadically in North America and Europe, but is prevalent in other parts of the world. Although it is 20 times more common in men than in women, LGV can still present both a diagnostic problem and a source of considerable morbidity for infected women. The primary lesion of LGV is an often-overlooked painless vesicle of 2 to 3 mm in size that appears 1 to 4 weeks after inoculation. A low-grade fever or malaise is often present, but mild. The lesions heal rapidly over the course of several days, leaving no scar. The secondary stage begins about 1 month later and is characterized by bubo formation, which is unilateral in two-thirds of cases. In 10 to 20% of patients, the accompanying edema and fibrosis may cause a linear depression parallel to the inguinal ligament, referred to as a groove sign. In one-third of patients, abscess, rupture, and fistula formation occur. Chronic progressive lymphangitis with chronic edema and sclerosing fibrosis may occur, causing extensive destruction of the vulva. Rectal stenosis may occur as well. Clinically, LGV may be mistaken for cancer.

LGV is caused by several serotypes of *Chlamydia trachomatis* and may be diagnosed by complement-fixation testing. Eighty percent of patients will have a titer of 1:16 or greater. Approximately 20% of patients with LGV will have false positive Venereal Disease Research Laboratory (VDRL) tests. Biopsy of the lesions is not diagnostic because of the nonspecific damage caused. Treatment should be begun even before confirmatory tests have returned. Treatment with tetracycline, 500 mg four times a day for 3 weeks, is recommended. Erythromycin or doxycycline may also be substituted.

One ulcerative condition that requires special mention is necrotizing fasciitis. While this process is not unique to the vulvar region, necrotizing fasciitis may begin in, or be mistaken for, secondary infections of other vulvar lesions or Bartholin gland abscesses. Any patient who is debilitated or is at increased risk (such as those with diabetes, alcoholism, or nutritional compromise) should be carefully monitored for the possibility of this life-threatening condition.

SELECTED READINGS

Aghajanian A, Bernstein L, Grimes DA. Bartholin's duct abscess and cyst: a case-control study. South Med J 1994; 87:26.

American College of Obstetricians and Gynecologists. Vulvar Dystrophies. ACOG Technical Bulletin no. 139. 1990.

Baker DA. Herpes and pregnancy: new management. Clin Obstet Gynecol 1990;33:253.

Bonnez W, Elswick RK Jr, Bailey-Farchione A, et al. Efficacy and safety of 0.5% podofilox solution in the treatment and suppression of anogenital warts. Am J Med 1994; 96:420.

Brennick J, Duncan L. Images in clinical medicine. Vulvar herpes simples infection. N Engl J Med 1993;90:38.

Bryson YJ, Dillon M, Bernsterin DI, Radolf J, et al. Risk of asquisition of genital herpes simplex virus type 2 in sex partners of persons with genital herpes: a prospective couple study. J Infect Dis 1993;167:942.

Bryson YJ, Dillon M, Lovett M, et al. Treatment of first episodes of genital herpes simplex virus infection with oral acyclovir: a randomized double-blind controlled trial in normal subjects. N Eng J Med 1983;308:916.

Cheetham DR. Bartholin's cyst: marsupialization or aspiration? Am J Obstet Gynecol 1985;152:569.

Cone RW, Swenson PD, Hobson AC, Remington M, Corey L. Herpes simplex virus detection from genital lesions: a comparative study using antigen detection (HerpChek) and culture. J Clin Microbiol 1993;31:1774.

Cunningham DS, Cutler GB Jr. Spontaneous vulvar necrotizing fasciitis in Cushing's syndrome. South Med J 1994; 87:837.

deRuiter A, Thin RN. Genital herpes: a guide to pharmacological therapy. Drugs 1994;47:297.

Farley DE, Katz VL, Dotters DJ. Toxic shock syndrome associated with vulvar necrotizing fasciitis. Obstet Gynecol 1993;82(Suppl):660.

Friedman-Kien AE, Eron LJ, Conant M, et al. Natural interferon alpha treatment of condylomata acuminata. JAMA 1988;259:533.

Friedrich EG Jr. Vulvar dystrophy. Clin Obstet Gynecol 1985; 28:178.

Goetsch MF. Vulvar vestibulitis: prevalence and histologic features in a general gynecologic practice population. Am J Obstet Gynecol 1991;164:1609.

Goldberg LH, Kaufman R, Kurtz TO, et al. Long-term suppression of recurrent genital herpes with acyclovir: a 5-year benchmark. Arch Dermatol 1993;129:582.

Gutman LT, St. Claire KK, Everett VD, et al. Cervical-vaginal and intraanal human papillomavirus infection of young girls with external genital warts. J Infect Dis 1994; 170:339.

Haddad J, Langer B, Astruc D, Messer J, Lokiec F. Oral acyclovir and recurrent genital herpes during late pregnancy. Obstet Gynecol 1993;82:102.

Horowitz BJ. Interferon therapy for condylomatous vulvitis. Obstet Gynecol 1989;73:446.

Johnson RE, Nahmias AJ, Magder LS, et al. A seroepidemiologic survey of the prevalence of herpes simples virus type 2 infection in the United States. N Engl J Med 1989;321:7.

Kawana T, Kawagol K, Takizawa K, Chen JT, Kawaguchi T, Sakamoto S. Clinical and virologic studies of female genital herpes. Obstet Gynecol 1982;60:456.

Mann MS, Kaufman RH. Erosive lichen planus of the vulva. Clin Obstet Gynecol 1991;34:605.

McKay M. Vulvodynia. J Reprod Med 1984;29:471.

Mertz GJ, Jones CC, Mills J, et al. Long-term acyclovir suppression of frequently recurring genital herpes simplex virus infection: a multicenter double-blind trial. JAMA 1988;260:201.

Nolan TE, King LA, Smith RP, Gallup DC. Necrotizing surgical infection and necrotizing fasciitis in obstetric and gynecologic patients. South Med J 1993;86:1363.

Randolph AG, Washington AE, Prober CG. Cesarean delivery for women presenting with genital herpes lesions: efficacy, risks, and costs. JAMA 1993;270:77.

Slater GE, Rumack BH, Peterson RG. Podophyllin poisoning: systemic toxicity following cutaneous application. Obstet Gynecol 1978;52:94.

Chapter 61
Preoperative Evaluation

Carol A. Glowacki
Thomas E. Nolan

Five Key Points

- A systematic approach to preoperative evaluation should be individualized to the needs of the gynecologic patient, based on the medical history of the patient and the procedure planned.

- Medical consultation is reserved for patients with severe systemic disease. Patients with a single, stable medical problem do not require medical consultation.

- Consideration should be given to antibiotic and DVT prophylaxis where appropriate.

- Preoperative informed consent should entail careful review and explanation of the planned procedure and the potential risks, allowing adequate time for patient questions.

- Careful preoperative care along with intraoperative skills and careful postoperative surveillance maximize the probability of successful surgical outcome.

The role of preoperative testing has changed substantially over the past 10 years, primarily to control costs. Admitting patients to the hospital the day prior to surgery to obtain laboratory work and medical clearance is no longer a luxury afforded patients and physicians. Preoperative laboratory use has been curtailed unless it has been proven to change patient treatment. Age criteria for certain tests and "cookbook" approaches to preoperative evaluation have also come under attack. The goal of this chapter is to reassess which studies are necessary and to outline a systematic approach to the preoperative gynecologic patient.

LABORATORY TESTING

Preoperative testing is valuable in assessment of a patient's operative risk and general health status. Many routine tests have been discontinued because of poor sensitivity and specificity in predicting less-than-optimal surgical outcomes or changing the surgical approach to the patient.[1] In addition, evaluation and treatment of borderline or false positive tests may impose further cost and risk to the patient.[2] Most normal diagnostic tests performed in the previous year do not warrant duplication if no clinical indication for reevaluation has occurred.[3] Imaging studies, such as preoperative assessment of masses by computerized topography (CT) or magnetic resonance imaging (MRI), are being used by gynecologists to assess the need for surgery, obtain tissue via fine-needle aspiration and biopsy for diagnosis, and improve planning of combined operative and adjunctive therapy. Despite more utilization of these technologies, there is no evidence that increased reliance on imaging has altered surgical outcome.[4] Age and underlying disease are useful in stratifying risk when ordering preoperative laboratory or imaging studies. However, many age-related examinations have been eliminated if patients have no risk factors or clinical evidence of disease.[5]

Urine pregnancy tests should be done on all women under 40 and all menstruating women who have not undergone a sterilization procedure. A urine or serum human chorionic gonadotropin (HCG) may be performed depending on availability and cost. Pregnancy tests should be performed no more than a week prior to surgery.

Clotting profiles, consisting of prothrombin time (PT), partial thromboplastin time (PTT), and fibrinogen, have not been shown to be cost effective in asymptomatic individuals. Clotting parameters should be ordered in patients currently taking anticoagulants known to affect the PT or PTT, in patients with a known clotting factor deficiency, or in patients with a history suspicious for bleeding disorders. The reliability of bleeding times as a predictor of perioperative bleeding complications has been questioned due to poor positive predictive value.[6]

Changes in the Health Care Financing Administration (HCFA) guidelines have resulted in changes for various electrolyte panels (i.e., renal and hepatic panels). Electrolytes such as the blood urea nitrogen (BUN), creatinine, and glucose (SMA7 or CHEM7) are good for 72 hours. BUN and creatinine should be ordered for patients with renal, cardiovascular, or hepatic disease and for patients over 60 years of age.

The value of preoperative chest radiography (CXR) in perioperative management is controversial. CXR is recommended for patients with pulmonary or cardiovascular disease and all patients over the age of 65. Cigarette smokers over the age of 50 or with a 20-pack-year or greater history should have a CXR.[2,7,8] Unless clinically indicated, a CXR performed in the past 6 months is adequate. Pulmonary-function tests have not been found to be of value in the perioperative setting. Incentive spirometry for postoperative atelectasis prevention should be taught to high-risk patients preoperatively.

Electrocardiography (ECG) is useful in females over age 50. Patients with risk factors for coronary artery disease (e.g., diabetes, hypertension, hyperlipidemia, and smoking) or a history of cardiovascular disease should also have an ECG.[2] ECGs within 6 months of the planned procedure are adequate in the clinically stable patient.

Evaluation for syphilis and human immunodeficiency virus (HIV) should be considered in select patients, primarily intravenous drug abusers, prostitutes, or individuals who have multiple sexual partners.

Patients with symptoms of a urinary-tract infection (UTI) or those undergoing operations with prosthetic material should have a preoperative urinalysis to avoid foreign-body infections secondary to an asymptomatic UTI. Intravenous pyelography (IVP) is valuable only when there is a suspicion of ureteral obstruction, ureteral entrapment from previous surgery, or an underlying disease process, such as malignancy, endometriosis, or pelvic inflammatory disease. Because the ureter is dynamic in position, the IVP is not useful in determining the location of the ureter preoperatively.[9]

CT scans and MRIs may be useful in defining disease spread and evaluating lymph nodes that may require biopsy. In suspected or known malignancies, imaging studies may alter management options toward radiotherapy or chemotherapy. Because of an increased focus for surgical staging in gynecologic malignancies, the usefulness of these studies may vary in the future.

Medical consultation is reserved for patients with severe systemic disease, particularly the unstable patient. Specific issues to consider perioperatively concern management of medications and potential fluid problems. Patients with a single, stable medical problem, such as those with well-controlled diabetes (blood sugar less than 200 mg/liter) or those with hypertension who are on monotherapy, do not require medical consultation. All patients with a history of cardiovascular disease (including myocardial infarction), unstable hypertension, history of pulmonary edema, steroid-dependent asthma, heavy smokers with suspected chronic obstructive pulmonary disease, or connective-tissue disease should receive preoperative medical clearance.[4]

BOWEL PREPARATION

In general, gynecologic surgery does not involve operative procedures on the bowel, but in some cases (malignancy, endometriosis, etc.) the risk of incidental bowel injury is high. Proper preoperative cleansing of the bowel reduces fecal mass, lessening the number of microorganisms within the lumen, and, in theory, decreasing the risk of infection and colostomy. During preoperative evaluation, assessment of the possibility of bowel surgery should be considered. If

---

TABLE 61-1
INDICATIONS FOR BOWEL PREPARATION

Potential for bowel resection is high (e.g., previous bowel surgery or ruptured appendix)

History of advanced benign pelvic disease such as endometriosis or pelvic inflammatory disease

"Frozen pelvis" on pelvic examination

Disease has obliterated the rectal vaginal septum

Suspected ovarian pathology or any suspicious adnexal mass, especially postmenopausally

Possible bowel involvement on preoperative imaging

History of diverticular disease

History of pelvic radiation

History of multiple pelvic surgeries or abdominal explorations

Possible gastrointestinal involvement or colonic carcinoma

Possibility of urologic pathology requiring conduit diversion

---

Reprinted with permission from Nolan TE. In: Mann WJ Jr, Stovall TG, eds. Gynecologic surgery. New York: Churchill Livingstone, 1990:7.

---

the potential exists, preparation of the gastrointestinal tract with mechanical cleansing and parenteral antibiotics is recommended. Some newer studies demonstrate no increased complications in colorectal surgery performed without preoperative bowel preparation, challenging traditional views (Table 61-1).[10,11]

There is no universally accepted regimen for bowel preparation. Effective bowel preparation should minimize patient discomfort and physiologic alterations, especially dehydration. When bowel preparation is performed, assessment of fluid status prior to surgery is important (see "Fluid Management," below). Fluid lost during bowel preparation is replaced by shifting fluid from the extracellular space into the intravascular space and then into the bowel lumen. The net result is a decreased intravascular volume, reflected by orthostasis or rising BUN. Hydration prior to induction of anesthesia compensates for the diminished intravascular volume.

Normal bowel flora contains over 20 species of aerobic bacteria and over 50 anaerobes. *Escherichia coli* is the major aerobic pathogen and *Bacteroides fragilis* the most common anaerobic pathogen contaminating septic wounds following colon surgery. In the absence of antibiotic prophylaxis, wound infection rates range from 32 to 58%, with infectious complications as high as 75%.[12]

There are few contraindications for bowel preparation. Exclusion criteria include patients unable to tolerate the mechanical aspects of the protocol, emergency surgery, and suspected bowel obstruction or ileus.[13] The use of osmotic high-volume bowel preparations in patients undergoing rectovaginal fisula

repair has been discontinued due to fecal leakage in the operative field. Simple enemas are given the night before surgery.

The ideal preparation for mechanical cleansing of the bowel alters the electrolytes and balance of body fluids minimally. There also should be no significant effect on nutritional and immunologic parameters. Basic preparations use enemas, cathartics, liquid diets, or whole-gut lavage with a variety of solutions such as Ringer's lactate, saline solutions, osmotics (e.g., mannitol), and nonosmotics (e.g., polyethylene glycol).

Extended preoperative clear liquid diets are associated with a negative nitrogen balance unless low-residue, nutritionally complete formulas are added. Any residue not absorbed by the small intestine creates a bacterial medium in the colon. Purgatives and enemas, frequently ineffective, may be time-consuming and stressful to the patient. They also result in a potentially hazardous loss of salt and water from the body.[14,15]

Whole-gut lavage, flushing 4 to 15 liters of electrolyte solution through the intestines, is an effective method of colonic cleansing. This technique may be associated with significant sodium and fluid retention, with up to 2 liters of free water absorbed. This creates a potential hazard in patients unable to readily excrete salt and water loads.[16] Symptoms ranging from nausea and vomiting to abdominal pain may be present in 28 to 48% of patients. Mannitol solutions create an overgrowth of *E. coli*, which can contribute to sepsis. Interestingly, mannitol is fermentable, and when metabolized by the colon, bacteria forms hydrogen, an explosive gas. Most importantly, it results in extracellular fluid shifts from the bowel wall to the bowel lumen, leading to systemic dehydration.[17] Currently there are better solutions than mannitol.

Polyethylene glycol solution combined with a balanced electrolyte solution is the preferred formula for mechanical bowel preparation. These solutions act as an isosmotic cathartic that is nonabsorbable in the gut and not fermentable. The sodium concentration is similar to that of plasma, and eliminates sodium diffusion. Sulfate substitution for chloride blocks absorption of sodium and chloride, eliminating the electrical and chemical gradient across the mucous membrane, preventing potassium exchange. As a result, there is minimal weight change, with minor alterations in water and electrolyte balance.[16] Caution must be exercised with elderly and frail patients, and instructions must be carefully worded to avoid either excessive or inadequate fluid intake at the time of bowel preparation.[18] Disadvantages to this preparation include a "salty taste" (which may be improved by chilling), nausea, a sensation of abdominal fullness, and bloating.

PROPHYLACTIC ANTIBIOTICS

Antibiotic prophylaxis is based on the principle that infection is prevented at the time of bacterial inoculation with subsequent inhibition of bacterial growth. The value of prophylactic antibiotics in clean-contaminated (operative fields containing or exposed to a normal bacterial flora) and clean operations where prosthetics are implanted has been established.[19,20] Routine use in clean surgical procedures has also been advocated.[21] Use of prophylactic antibiotics is common practice in obstetrics and gynecology, as many procedures involve the vagina, an area rich in microbes. Although a reduction in febrile morbidity from vaginal hysterectomy has occurred since the introduction of antibiotic prophylaxis, the benefit in abdominal hysterectomy remains controversial. Some studies report decreased postoperative infections, while others demonstrate no benefit.[22] The use of prophylactic antibiotics should be individualized based on the risks of each patient and the patient population.

Preoperative antibiotics are administered by mouth, enema, or parenterally. Controversy exists about whether oral or parenteral antibiotics are more effective in preventing postoperative wound infections. Neomycin, erythromycin, and metronidazole are the most common oral antibiotics used. All three have clinical efficacy in decreasing the colonic microflora. Erythromycin and metronidazole are well absorbed by the gut, attaining therapeutic serum levels. Erythromycin may produce significant gastrointestinal discomfort. Neomycin is not well absorbed, limiting its effectiveness in preventing sepsis. Due to questions of efficacy and side effects, many surgeons have abandoned oral antibiotics for parenteral antibiotics.[23]

Prophylactic antibiotics are given in the anesthesia staging area at the time the intravenous (IV) line is started to ensure adequate tissue levels. The current recommendation is 1 g of cefazolin. With a history of severe allergic reaction to penicillin (wheals, hives, respiratory distress), 900 mg of clindamycin is substituted. In the face of an infection, antibiotic choice is tailored to the specific organism involved. Prophylaxis should be individualized to the patient, patient population, and planned procedure.[24]

Before surgery, the anesthesiologist should be advised of any bowel preparation and the method to allow adequate perioperative fluid replacement. IV hydration and electrolyte replacement will help prevent intraoperative hypotension and oliguria, but often requires several hours of hospitalization. In most cases, 1 to 2 liters of balanced salt solutions prior to induction of anesthesia is adequate therapy.

PULMONARY COMPLICATIONS

The most common medical complications from surgery are pulmonary. Normal pulmonary function centers on the concept of work of breathing (WOB). WOB is the summation of the actions of the thorax, diaphragm, and intercostal, accessory, and expiratory muscles to perform oxygenation and ventilation. Elasticity and compliance of lung tissue require energy to enact effective respiration. Anesthesia, surgical incisions, and pain control (whether administered perioperatively or preoperatively) may alter the ability to ventilate and oxygenate. Lung capacity and transairway and transpulmonary pressures are also affected. Functional residual capacity (FRC) is decreased due to the effect of muscle relaxants on the respiratory muscles and cough reflex. In addition, mucous clearance is decreased and may lead to plugging of lower airways.[25]

Multiple risk factors for postoperative pulmonary complications have been identified. Patients older than 70 years of age have decreased lung compliance and elasticity.[26] Individuals with preexisting pulmonary disease (obstructive and restrictive), prior history of lung malignancy, and excessive sputum production, as in chronic obstructive pulmonary disease (COPD) are at higher risk for postoperative complications. Smokers, particularly those with a greater than 40-pack-year history, have a risk for postoperative hypoxemia and for pneumonia nearly twice that of nonsmokers.[27] Neuromuscular disease (myasthenia gravis or multiple sclerosis) may lead to restrictive lung disease and decreased respiratory drive. Obese patients ($>120\%$ of expected weight) are at higher risk. Surgical incisions extending into the upper abdomen inhibit the patient's ability to cough and to breathe deeply due to pain and diaphragmatic dysfunction of altered phrenic-nerve output.[28] These patients may benefit from preoperative pulmonary evaluation with CXR, spirometry, and arterial blood gas analysis.

Although the value of spirometric testing has been questioned,[29] it continues to be a mainstay of the preoperative pulmonary work-up. The two most important factors in spirometric evaluation are forced vital capacity (FVC) and forced expiratory volume at 1 second (FEV_1). The FVC measures the patient's ability to quickly expire as much air as possible without time limitations. The FEV_1 is a segment of FVC measured in the first second of expiration. A low FEV_1 (<2 liters) indicates obstructive airway disease, such as COPD, reversible bronchospasm (asthma), or poor patient effort. Spirometric standards vary with sex and age. Because of multiple variables in interpretation, abnormal results should be evaluated by a pulmonologist.

Arterial blood gases (ABGs) are a quick and easy means of measuring the ability of the patient to oxygenate and ventilate, with additional information concerning systemic acid–base balance. The ability to oxygenate decreases with age, thus ABG results are age-dependent. The normal partial pressure of oxygen (PaO_2) of a 60-year-old may be in the low 80s, while an 80-year-old may have a normal PaO_2 in the 60s (the rule of "60 = 80 and 80 = 60"). In general, a PaO_2 <70 mm Hg indicates a higher risk of pulmonary complications. Hypercapnia with a $PaCO_2$ >45 mm Hg is a serious risk factor in upper abdominal procedures, especially if not reversed with bronchodilators.[30,31] In lower abdominal surgery, no increased risk was found with a $PaCO_2$ >47 mm Hg.[30-32]

Pulmonary function tests (PFTs) assist in assessment of the need for prophylactic pulmonary measures perioperatively, and is valuable in select patients. Age alone, in the absence of pulmonary symptoms or history, is no longer an indicator for preoperative PFTs. The incidence of pulmonary conditions is increasing in women over the past 20 years, attributable to the rising number of smokers. Cigarette abusers with greater than 40-pack–years and individuals with a history of poorly controlled asthma should have PFTs. Clinical evidence of pulmonary disease (e.g., auscultated wheezes or dyspnea on exertion) warrants pulmonary-function testing.

Patients with evidence of restrictive lung disease, particularly those with a history of radiotherapy or sarcoidosis, should undergo pulmonary function testing. Certain central nervous system disorders, particularly neuromuscular diseases, may affect respiratory drive and should be evaluated. Knowledge of the extent of pulmonary dysfunction prior to surgery allows more careful monitoring in the perioperative period.

Smoking is an independent risk factor for pulmonary complications. Chronic phlegm production and air-flow obstruction contribute to a postoperative pneumonia rate twice that of nonsmokers. Goblet cells and ciliary cells may be damaged in smokers. Goblet cells secrete mucoid material that entraps infectious organisms and foreign material. In the normal patient, ciliary cells assist in moving the lower-respiratory-tract secretions into the upper respiratory tract. Anesthesia and endotracheal intubation may exacerbate the poor function of these cells, contributing to the development of pneumonia. More severe postoperative hypoxemia develops in smokers, and they have an increased incidence of atelectasis. These risks are unchanged for 8 weeks after cessation of smoking. Smoking is no longer an independent risk factor 6 months after cessation.[30]

Atelectasis is the failure of the lung to expand and is the most common postoperative pulmonary complication. Patients at high risk for postoperative atelectasis should be instructed preoperatively in the use of incentive spirometry. Early ambulation and incentive spirometry should be encouraged and narcotics used judiciously in the postoperative period. Parenteral nonsteroidal agents reduce the need for narcotics but should be used judiciously in the elderly or in individuals with compromised renal function. Elderly patients tend to have greater pain tolerance and may require only diphenhydramine hydrochloride and low doses of meperidine (10 to 25 mg intramuscularly) for pain relief. Patient controlled analgesia may also be used. Epidural analgesics are a useful alternative for pain control after major abdominal surgery, especially in individuals with compromised respiratory systems.

The primary function of the upper airway is to humidify and warm gases. In the immediate postoperative period, supplemental oxygen should be administered to prevent postanesthesia hypoxia. Humidification is important in avoiding lower-airway complications. Inadequate humidity in the upper airway may lead to lower-airway obstruction from dried, retained secretions. The natural ability of the mucociliary tree's ability to fight infections may be altered. Humidification in the spontaneously breathing patient is easily supplied by the bubbling diffusion technique (bubbling oxygen through water). In the intubated patient, the upper airway is bypassed and necessitates the use of warmed air and oxygen mixture.

The incision site is significant in the development of postoperative atelectasis and pneumonia. The incidence of pulmonary complications increases as the surgical field approaches the diaphragm. Therefore, upper abdominal procedures have a higher incidence of postoperative problems than lower abdominal procedures, and vertical higher than horizontal.[31] The patient's ability to cough and breathe deeply is compromised by postoperative pain and diaphragmatic dysfunction from altered phrenic nerve output.[28] These patients should use incentive spirometry for at least 48 to 72 hours postoperatively.

Asthma is a syndrome of recurrent airway obstruction, with an incidence of 1 to 5% in the adult population. Attacks of bronchospasm may resolve spontaneously or with bronchodilator therapy. Patients with evidence of bronchospasm on physical examination (wheezing or rales) should be considered for perioperative steroids.

Irritation of the airway by anesthetic agents may induce intraoperative bronchospasm. In the perioperative period, symptoms of dyspnea and difficulty breathing or speaking suggest acute bronchospasm. Physical examination usually reveals wheezing, rhonchi, and rales. The patient often appears anxious, perspires, and sits upright and occasionally uses the accessory muscles of the neck. Patients with asthma who have impending respiratory failure have cyanosis, with a decrease in audible wheezing on physical examination. Pulse oximetry has replaced ABGs in the evaluation of many patients. Oxygen saturation levels less than 90% should be considered for ABG evaluation. A respiratory rate greater than 30 breaths per minute, PCO_2 greater than 40 mm Hg, or hypoxia with PO_2 levels less than 60 mm Hg are indications for transfer to an intensive-care unit (ICU). If ICU admission is necessary, then an arterial line is recommended to allow repeat ABGs for continued monitoring.[4]

Treatment of acute asthma attacks involves sympathomimetic drugs such as metaproterenol (0.3 ml of a 5% solution in 2.5 ml of saline, every 4 hours as needed), or albuterol (0.5 ml of a 0.5% solution in 3 ml of saline, every 6 hours as needed). Methylprednisone, 1 to 2 mg/kg IV every 6 hours, should be initiated in patients with severe attacks that are unresponsive to sympathomimetic inhalation therapy after one to two doses. These patients should then be given oral prednisone.

Pneumonia diagnosed in the preoperative period should be treated prior to surgery if possible. Allow 2 to 3 weeks for resolution.[25] Nosocomial pneumonia is rare in the postoperative period and should be treated by an internist with knowledge of pathogen trends within the institution. Opportunistic infections are becoming more prevalent, with an increase in the number of resistant organisms, particularly in the ICU setting. The initial work-up includes posteroanterior and lateral view chest x-ray films. If evidence of pulmonary compromise exists, an ABG and bedside pulse oximetry should be obtained. Patients with sepsis, immunocompromise, or those who have received large volumes of blood products are prone to the development of adult respiratory distress syndrome (ARDS).

Respiratory failure is an uncommon complication in postoperative patients (Table 61-2). The most important cause of respiratory failure is unrecognized COPD followed by pulmonary embolus. Important preoperative predictors for postoperative mechanical

---

TABLE 61-2
CLINICAL CAUSES AND TYPES OF ACUTE RESPIRATORY FAILURE

Type	Mechanism	Causes	Clinical Conditions
Acute hypoxemia	Increased ventilation/perfusion shunt	Air-space congestion	ARDS Pneumonia Congestive heart failure Pulmonary edema
Hypoventilatory	Decreased respiratory drive	Decreased central nervous system drive	End-stage asthma Drug overdose Myasthenia gravis
Postoperative	Atelectasis Mucus plugging	Functional residual capacity	Obesity Anesthesia Smoking
Shock states	Hypoperfusion	Sepsis Myocardial damage Hemorrhagic shock	Pelvic abscess Cardiomyopathy Postoperative hemorrhage

Reprinted with permission from Nolan and Hankins.[33]

TABLE 61-3
EARLY CLINICAL MARKERS IN ARDS

Variable	Normal	Early ARDS	Respiratory Failure
Respiratory rate (breaths/min)	10–18	30–36	>30
PaO_2			
Room air (mm Hg)	>90	55–65	<55
Mask O_2 (mm Hg)	>150	80–100	<60
$PaCO_2$ (mm Hg)	36–42	32–45	>50
PaO_2/FiO_2	>350	200–350	<200
FEV_1 (m/kg)	50–60	10–20	<10

Reprinted with permission from Nolan and Hankins.[34]

ventilation are a FVC of less than 1 liter, or a PCO_2 greater than 45 mm Hg. Patients at high risk for pulmonary edema, particularly those with a history of congestive heart failure, should be monitored with bedside oximetry. Obese patients with evidence of sleep apnea (chronic snoring, inappropriate sleeping, and frequent headaches) should be evaluated prior to surgery. These patients may have sudden epiglottic occlusion and respiratory arrest postoperatively. All patients complaining of shortness of breath should have pulse oximetry (with an ABG if SaO_2 is <90%) and a CXR to assess for pulmonary edema and infiltrates. Pulmonary embolism should be considered, particularly in the patient with tachycardia and chest pain.

ARDS is a result of increased microvascular permeability at the alveolar level. Extravasation of intravascular fluid across the capillary bed into the alveoli results in poor oxygen exchange. Hypoxia ensues, characterized clinically as progressive dyspnea. Early physical findings include labored respiration, tachycardia, cyanosis, rales, and rhonchi. Early clinical markers are identified in Table 61-3. Diagnosis is confirmed in the presence of arterial hypoxemia, with a chest radiograph demonstrating diffuse infiltrates without cardiomegaly or pulmonary vascular redistribution. Early in the clinical course, the findings on chest x-ray films may initially be confused with pneumonia. A pulmonary artery wedge pressure of less than 18 mm Hg excludes congestive heart failure.

The most common predisposing factor to ARDS is sepsis, often secondary to aspiration or an abscess. Disseminated intravascular coagulation (DIC) is also a factor. Little is known about prevention, and it continues to be difficult to treat, with a mortality rate as high as 70%. ARDS is a diagnosis of exclusion, beginning with x-ray findings of hypoxia. Management continues to be primarily supportive by reacting to changing physiology with oxygen therapy, mechanical ventilation, and, if indicated, nutritional therapy (Table 61-4). The patient should be transferred to the ICU and a pulmonary consultation obtained. The provoking cause should be treated, if possible. If the patient survives, pulmonary function usually returns to normal.

Pulmonary thromboembolism remains a significant cause of morbidity and mortality. The majority of clinically significant pulmonary emboli in postoperative patients results from deep venous thrombosis (DVT) of the lower extremities. DVT is found in over 40% of surgical patients with radioactive fibrinogen scanning, however, 50% are asymptomatic.[35] The classic triad of DVT (calf pain or tenderness, edema, cord, and Homan sign) has been found unreliable. The diagnosis should be confirmed by Doppler flow studies or imaging studies (venography). Pulmonary emboli will present with anxiety, dyspnea, pleuritic chest pain, and cough. Acute pulmonary embolus may also present with hypotension or sudden death. Prevention with pharmacologic and/or nonpharmacologic measures continues to be the most effective treatment. A combination of these measures may be used in moderate- and high-risk patients.

TABLE 61-4
PHYSIOLOGIC CHANGES SEEN IN PATIENTS WITH ARDS

Rapid onset, 24 to 72 hours, following the inciting event
An increased ventilation rate at room air, with a decrease in PaO_2
Severe refractory hypoxia, despite supplemental oxygen
Chest radiography demonstrating diffuse pulmonary infiltrates
Capillary wedge pressure less than 18 mm Hg
Decrease in lung compliance
Increased pulmonary vascular resistance

Nonpharmacologic prevention of DVT includes graduated compression stockings (GCSs), intermittent pneumatic compression stockings (IPCs), and inferior vena cava interruption devices. GCSs use varying compression at different points in the stockings, reducing the incidence of DVT in low-risk patients by 50%.[36] These devices should be worn until the patient is walking well. When improperly worn, as in obese patients, the GCSs may function as a tourniquet. IPCs prevent venous stasis by intermittent inflation, and may stimulate the endogenous fibrinolytic system.[37] Often GCSs and IPCs are combined to minimize patient perspiration discomfort from IPCs alone.

Pharmacologic prophylaxis uses low-dose unfractionated heparin. A dose of 5000 U (7500 U in obese patients) is administered subcutaneously, beginning 2 hours prior to surgery and continuing postoperatively two to three times daily until the patient is fully ambulatory.

Low-molecular-weight heparins (LMWHs), although not yet approved by the Food and Drug Administration (FDA), are now available, and should simplify the treatment and prevention of thromboembolic disorders. These agents have several advantages over unfractionated heparin, and most clinical studies indicate the bleeding risk is equivalent to or less than heparin.[38] LMWHs are better absorbed after subcutaneous injection. Because of less protein binding, the bioavailability of LMWHs is greater than the unfractionated moieties. The longer half-life allows once or twice daily dosing.[39]

Three LMWHs are currently available in the United States: enoxaparin, dalteparin, and ardeparin. The recommendation for DVT prophylaxis with enoxaparin is 30 mg every 12 hours. The initial dose is begun 12 to 24 hours after surgery, although there is evidence it may be started prior to surgery without adverse bleeding sequelae. In established DVT, the recommended regimen is 1 mg/kg every 12 hours. Therapeutic international normalized ratio (INR) levels range from 2.0 to 3.0 for at least 48 hours.

On confirmation of the diagnosis of DVT, full-dose heparinization should be initiated. Activated partial thromboplastin time (PTT) should be maintained at 1.5 to 2.0 times normal to ensure full therapeutic effect. Once a therapeutic dose is reached on heparin, warfarin can be started. An INR of 2.0 to 3.0 should be maintained. Warfarin therapy should be maintained for 4 weeks if surgery is the only predisposing risk factor for DVT.[40]

STEROID THERAPY

Patients using steroids in the last year may be more susceptible to wound breakdown and adrenal insufficiency.[41] Patients receiving more than 20 mg of prednisone a day or 7.5 mg/day for more than 3 weeks in the previous year may require stress doses of steroids prior to surgery.[42] Minimally stressful surgery (most ambulatory cases) requires an additional 25 mg/day of hydrocortisone. Most major gynecology procedures fall into the moderate stress categories, requiring 50 to 75 mg/day of a hydrocortisone equivalent for 1 to 2 days, until the patient is tolerating oral intake. Severe stress (gynecologic oncology) procedures require 100 to 150 mg/day of a hydrocortisone equivalent for 2 to 3 days. Stress doses are added to maintenance doses (maximum of 240 mg/day) in those patients taking daily steroid doses, divided into intravenous doses every 8 hours until the stress is resolved. If indicated, patients should be restarted on oral maintenance doses in the postoperative period (Table 61-5).

Long-term steroid use increases the risk for wound infections and breakdown. This may be minimized by choosing procedures with a smaller risk of infection. Permanent sutures should be considered in closure.

CARDIOVASCULAR COMPLICATIONS

Cardiovascular disease affects 1 in 4 of all Americans and complications from cardiovascular disease continue to be a significant source of morbidity and death in the surgical setting. One-third to one-half of all perioperative deaths have a cardiac cause, although few studies actually include women.[43] Coronary

---

TABLE 61-5
STRESS DOSE REPLACEMENT OF STEROIDS

Indication
  Any patient who received more than 7.5 mg/kg day of prednisone for more than 5 days in the prior year
Preoperative regimen
  One hour before surgery—100 mg hydrocortisone intravenously
Postoperative regimen
  Day 1: 100 mg hydrocortisone intravenously every 8 hr
  Day 2: 100 mg hydrocortisone intravenously every 12 hr
  Day 3: 100 mg hydrocortisone intravenously once in morning
If patient begins oral feeding at any time: prednisone 20 mg the first day: decrease by 5 mg/day or until long-term dosage is reached.

Reprinted with permission from Nolan TE. Mann WJ Jr, Stovall TG, eds. Gynecologic surgery. New York: Churchill Livingstone, 1990:20.

artery disease (CAD) is responsible for nearly 50% of all female cardiovascular events and is more prevalent in the older population (>65 years). This group has a 55% higher rate of surgery than patients under 65 years, accounting for 75% of all surgical deaths.[44] Therefore, cardiovascular assessment is an integral part of the preoperative evaluation.

Myocardial Infarction

The incidence of perioperative myocardial ischemia and infarction is unknown. The majority of perioperative myocardial infarctions (MIs) follow sustained coronary ischemia. Most MIs occur up to 7 days postoperatively. Most myocardial events are silent, without typical chest pain, although some symptoms or changes in clinical status may occur. CAD significantly increases the risk of early MI after elective noncardiac surgery (from 0.1 to 0.2% in the general population to 4% with CAD).[45] Factors contributing to perioperative ischemia/infarction include vasospasm resulting from the release of stress-related humoral mediators and changes in coronary artery perfusion due to vascular tone, blood pressure, and cardiac contractility. In the presence of critical coronary artery stenosis, any decrease in flow may induce ischemia or infarction. The presence of CAD does not in itself predict a high risk for a perioperative cardiac event, and should be correlated with other factors. The American College of Cardiology/American Heart Association task force has stratified these factors into major, intermediate, and minor clinical predictors (Table 61-6).[46] The presence of major clinical predictors for a myocardial event warrants delay of surgery for medical management, risk-factor modification, and possibly coronary angiography. Postponement of surgery for intermediate and minor clinical predictors depends on the patient's functional capacity and the procedural risk. The functional capacity is the patient's ability to perform activities of daily living (e.g., climbing stairs). Most major gynecologic procedures are classified in the intermediate-risk category, while endoscopic procedures are considered low risk. Given the high mortality rate (between 36 and 83%), recognition of risk factors for coronary artery stenosis is extremely important in assessing perioperative risk and planning strategy.

Evidence of previous MI increases the risk for a perioperative MI, particularly if it occurred in the previous 6 months.[47] Advancing age is a significant

TABLE 61-6
CLINICAL PREDICTORS FOR A PERIOPERATIVE CARDIAC EVENT

Major clinical predictors
  Unstable coronary syndrome
  Decompensated congestive heart failure
  Significant arrhythmias
  Severe valvular disease
Intermediate clinical predictors
  Mild angina pectoris
  Prior myocardial infarction
  Compensated or prior congestive heart failure
  Diabetes mellitus
Minor clinical predictors
  Advanced age
  Abnormal electrocardiogram
  Rhythm other than sinus
  Low functional capacity*
  History of stroke
  Uncontrolled systemic hypertension

*Based on the patient's ability to perform the activities of daily living, e.g., climbing stairs.

risk factor because of decreased myocardial reserve and an overall increased risk for CAD. Several medical factors contributing to CAD are more prevalent after the age of 40, including important risk factors of diabetes mellitus and hypertension. Poorly controlled diabetes is associated with hyperlipidemia and accelerated atherosclerosis in peripheral and coronary arteries. Diabetic women have a greater post-MI mortality rate as compared with men.[43] Hypertension may cause myocardial thickening, decreased myocardial perfusion, and subsequent ischemia. Preoperative control of blood pressure may help reduce the potential for perioperative ischemia. Antihypertensive medications should be continued perioperatively.[46] Peripheral vascular disease and smoking are risk factors.

A thorough history is essential in the assessment of perioperative cardiac risk. Any history of chest pain, dyspnea, or syncope requires preoperative evaluation. Stable angina is chest pain that is predictable in onset, carrying no higher anesthetic or surgical risk than normal. Unstable angina is characterized by unpredictable chest pain, with changing patterns of frequency and intensity. It may predict an impending infarction. Modifiable risk factors for atherosclerotic disease should be noted, as well as associated diseases, such as cerebrovascular disease, diabetes, peripheral vascular disease, renal impairment, and pulmonary disease, particularly obstructive. Any history of angina, prior MI, CHF, or arrhythmias should be recorded. All medications, with dosages, should be carefully documented, and a thorough history taken with regard to smoking, alcohol, or illicit drug use.

An attempt should be made to determine the patient's functional cardiac capacity by assessing their ability to perform daily tasks. The capacity to perform activities of daily living, such as carrying a bag of groceries up one flight of stairs, correlates well with maximum oxygen uptake by treadmill testing.[46]

Physical examination should note general appearance, including cyanosis, dyspnea, nutritional status, and body habitus. Vital signs should be noted, and a thorough neck examination performed. Elevated jugular venous pressure, indicated by neck vein distention, is a reliable sign of hypervolemia or left ventricular dysfunction from venous overload. Carotid pulses and presence of bruits should be noted. Careful auscultation of the chest and precordial region is important. The posterior basilar region of the lungs is the most common site for pulmonary edema. Cardiac auscultation may reveal evidence of underlying cardiovascular disease. A third heart sound at the apical area suggests left ventricular failure. Murmurs should be closely assessed for evidence of valvular disease.

Laboratory studies in patients with cardiac abnormalities should include a complete blood count, ECG, and CXR. If the history or physical suggests hypoxia, ABGs may be helpful. Electrolyte counts may be indicated, depending on the patient's history and medications. A digoxin level should be drawn if indicated. Assessment of women for angina or cardiac insufficiency with ECGs or exercise stress testing is complicated by a relative lack of sensitivity and specificity, and, thus, are of poor prognostic value. A thallium scan may be more beneficial if the history or assessment of risk factors indicate a higher risk. Thallium, a potassium analog, is distributed throughout the myocardium, giving a dynamic representation of cardiac function. It provides highly sensitive and specific information on myocardial perfusion and viability. Motion abnormalities of the ventricular wall or decreased or absent myocardial flow suggest prior infarction, and cardiac catheterization should be considered. In the past, elderly patients unable to exercise have undergone a pharmacologic stress test with dipyridamole. More recent evidence suggests this test is a poor predictor of postoperative cardiac morbidity and mortality.[48,49]

A history of myocardial infarction warrants careful evaluation for myocardial dysfunction. The most widely used standards for assessment of cardiac risk are the Goldman criteria. These assess risk in 40-year-old men and have not yet been substantiated in women.[25] One study indicated that these criteria lacked sensitivity in the female population.[50] Many of the problems associated with testing of women stem from the overall low probability of heart disease in women, especially prior to age 65. Further investigation is necessary to differentiate risk factors in the female population, stratifying for things such as menopause and hormone-replacement therapy.

Valvular Disease and Cardiomyopathy

Careful cardiac auscultation may detect a heart murmur, suggesting possible valvular disease or a cardiomyopathy. New or worsening heart failure develops perioperatively in 20% of patients with valvular disease.[35] Echocardiography provides information on cardiac-wall dynamics, ejection fraction, and potential valvular disease. Aortic stenosis is the most common valvular lesion in the elderly, posing possible fluid management problems. The murmur of aortic stenosis is characterized by a grade II/VI to VI/VI systolic murmur in the right second intercostal space, radiating to the neck. Classic symptoms of severe aortic stenosis (angina, heart failure, or syncope) indicate a need to postpone surgery unless it is an emergency, so further evaluation and possible valve replacement may be performed.

Cardiac catheterization remains the gold standard for assessment of coronary artery stenosis, ventricular-wall function, ejection fraction, and valvular competence. Patients with mild, stable cardiac symptoms and ejection fractions greater than 40% (normal, 55 to 60%), generally are not at high surgical risk. With ejection fractions between 30 and 40%, a central venous access (subclavian or internal jugular) is recommended for surgery. Individuals with compromised ejection fractions can be extremely sensitive to salt solutions. A pulmonary artery catheter is recommended with an ejection fraction less than 30% because of higher surgical risk for cardiac events. Patients with an ejection fraction of less than 20% should only undergo emergency or life-saving procedures.

Prudent fluid management is vital in patients with cardiac abnormalities, particularly with demonstrable left ventricular dysfunction. If there is potential for difficult fluid management (procedures with high potential for blood loss or fluid shifts, such as ovarian cancer cases with ascites), central venous access and possibly pulmonary artery catheterization (PAC) is indicated. Central lines should be maintained in the postoperative period for higher-risk patients. Mobilization of third-space intraoperative fluids occurs 48 to 72 hours postoperatively. Careful monitoring for pulmonary edema should continue for this period. PACs are associated with certain complications, especially a higher risk of infection, and therefore should be removed when the patient is hemodynamically stable. Central access should remain until the third postoperative day, if feasible. Accurate calculation of estimated blood loss and fluid needs should be documented in the operating room and postoperative period.

A fluid management and medication plan should be developed prior to any operative procedure. The surgeon, anesthesiologist, and consultant internist or cardiologist should be involved and overall supervision decided prior to the case. Accurate calculation of estimated blood loss and fluid needs is vital during the procedure and the postoperative period. Preoperative fluid restriction, bowel preparation, and insensible intraoperative losses should be considered in these calculations, as well as any medication that alters intravascular volume (e.g., diuretics). Intake and urine output should be carefully monitored, particularly in the first 12 hours. *Fluid replacement should account for patient age, size, and stature. A frail, elderly patient does not require 125 ml/hr of fluid.* Patients over 60 years of age generally have decreased glomerular filtration rates (60 to 75 ml/minute or less). Fluid needs and drug metabolism should be addressed both intraoperatively and postoperatively. Consideration of postoperative monitoring in an ICU should be given to moderate-to high-risk patients.

Prophylactic Antibiotics and Subacute Bacterial Endocarditis

Subacute bacterial endocarditis (SBE) involves "seeding" of abnormal cardiac anatomy with microorganisms indigenous to the operative site, most commonly streptococci or staphylococci. Manipulation of the integumentary, intestinal, reproductive, or lower urinary tracts may release bacteria. The duration of bacteremia leading to SBE is brief, typically no longer than 15 to 20 minutes. Few cases occur in obstetric and gynecologic operative procedures. Reported cases often involve intrauterine devices, criminal abortion, and dilation and curettage. Only one reported case involved a hysterectomy.[51]

TABLE 61-7 **ANTIBIOTIC PROPHYLAXIS FOR ENDOCARDITIS:** **REGIMENS FOR GENITOURINARY PROCEDURES**	
Drug(s)	**Dosing Regimen**
Standard Regimen	
Ampicillin, gentamicin, and amoxicillin	Intravenous or intramuscular administration of ampicillin, 2.0 g, plus gentamicin, 1.5 mg/kg (not to exceed 80 mg), 30 min before procedure; followed by amoxicillin, 1.5 g, orally 6 hr after initial dose; alternatively, the parenteral regimen may be repeated once 8 hr after initial dose
Ampicillin/Amoxicillin/Penicillin—Allergic Patient Regimen	
Vancomycin and gentamicin	Intravenous administration of vancomycin, 1.0 g, over 1 hr plus intravenous or intramuscular administration of gentamicin, 1.5 mg/kg (not to exceed 80 mg), 1 hr before procedure; may be repeated once 8 hr after initial dose
Alternate Low-Risk Patient Regimen	
Amoxicillin	3.0 g orally 1 hr before procedure; then 1.5 g 6 hr after initial dose

Reprinted with permission from Dajani.[51]

Rheumatic heart disease, although decreasing in incidence in the United States, still accounts for 40 to 60% of infective endocarditis. Other lesions commonly associated with infection are tetralogy of Fallot, ventricular septal defect, patent ductus arteriosus, and valvular prosthesis. Mitral valve prolapse unless accompanied by mitral regurgitation is no longer a criteria for SBE prophylaxis. All IV drug abusers are at risk for acquired valvular lesions and may require prophylaxis. The recommendations of the American Heart Association for SBE prophylaxis are given in Table 61-7.

RENAL COMPLICATIONS

While postoperative renal insufficiency or failure is common in certain operative populations, preexisting renal disease in the gynecologic surgical population is unusual. Increased availability of hemodialysis and renal transplantation has led to more patients with renal diseases seeking elective surgery. A growing elderly population and more aggressive pelvic prolapse surgeries may lead to an increase in the number of gynecologic patients at risk for renal problems. Creatinine clearance declines approximately 1% per year with increasing age in the general population. Elderly patients are more susceptible to postoperative renal complications, particularly acute tubular necrosis

(ATN). Greater emphasis on preoperative imaging of pelvic masses involves increased use of IV contrast agents. Contrast-induced nephropathy may develop in patients with previously unrecognized renal insufficiency.

Patients with a BUN over 20 mg/liter or a creatinine (Cr) greater than 1.5 (1.0 in frail, elderly patients) require renal evaluation. The serum Cr must be adjusted for age and decreased lean body mass. It should also be considered in patients with chronic hypertension, particularly elderly patients with diabetes or those with documented CAD or left ventricular dysfunction. Other possible risk factors include malignancy, prior cardiac surgery, vascular disease, increased serum bilirubin, and decreased albumin.[22] A 24-hour urine collection may assist in evaluating early renal insufficiency. Estimated creatinine clearance (CrCl) is useful, and may be calculated by the following formula: $CrCl = (140 - age) \times$ weight (kg) divided by $(72 \times$ serum Cr). To correct for lower muscle mass this value should be multiplied by 0.85 in women.

Preoperative renal status is the best predictor of postoperative renal complications.[22] Renal insufficiency can be stratified into mild, moderate, and severe disease. Mild renal insufficiency is defined as a glomerular filtration rate (GFR) less than 80 ml/min but greater than 50, moderate between 25 and 50 ml/min, and severe or advanced renal insufficiency as a GFR between 10 and 25 ml/min. Surgical morbidity is directly related to the degree of preoperative renal insufficiency. Common problems encountered include infection, platelet dysfunction with subsequent bleeding tendency, anemia, nutritional problems, and poor wound healing. The fluid and electrolyte balance is affected when the GFR decreases to 25% below normal (moderate renal insufficiency). At this level, sodium retention begins and fluid and sodium restriction should be initiated. Hypertensive disorders are associated with renal insufficiency, possibly related to the kidneys' inability to remove sodium and volume. Antihypertensive agents, along with the underlying altered renin–angiotensin state, contribute to intravascular volume depletion.

Electrolyte abnormalities should be assessed in all patients with renal insufficiency, and preoperative dialysis performed, if indicated. Hyperkalemia (potassium ≥5.5 mEq/liter) may be treated with ion-exchange resins (e.g., Kayexalate). In emergency situations, IV glucose and insulin with bicarbonate will shift potassium intracellularly, but the effect is short,

and dialysis may be considered in the stable patient. ECG monitoring should be considered during these infusions. Postdialysis potassium levels will be artificially low, equilibrating over 24 hours. Potassium supplements should not be given.

Metabolic acidosis is common with severe renal failure. pH levels <7.25 should be corrected prior to surgery.[53] Rapid correction of the systemic pH may cause a drop in ionized calcium. It may be replaced with calcium-containing solutions.

Chronic renal failure is associated with anemia, frequently with hematocrits (Hcts) of 20 to 30%. Synthetic erythropoeitin is often instituted to reverse the level of anemia. An increased Hct (≥30 %) is associated with fewer bleeding problems, possibly secondary to increased viscosity.[54] Preoperative transfusion is indicated with Hcts of 20 to 25% and expected intraoperative blood loss of more than 500 to 1000 ml. Packed red blood cells should be given at preoperative dialysis to increase intravascular volume and minimize potassium toxicity. Bleeding problems may be attributable to uremia or platelet dysfunction (particularly with a serum creatinine greater than 6 mg/dl). A bleeding time is the most appropriate laboratory evaluation. Absolute platelet counts may be misleading due to platelet dysfunction. Cryoprecipitate is indicated if bleeding dysfunction persists despite frequent dialysis. DDAVP (desmopressin) can also be administered, which may potentiate von Willebrand factor. Heparin is given at dialysis; therefore, surgery should be delayed at least 2 hours postdialysis.

Nutritional status may be compromised in patients with renal disease secondary to malabsorption and anorexia. The patient's diet should be assessed and protein supplementation considered in preparation for the catabolic effect of surgery. Vitamin and iron supplements are important in patients on dialysis due to loss of water-soluble vitamins. Malnutrition is associated with immunocompromise and antibiotic prophylaxis is recommended.

Intraoperative hemostasis is extremely important. Shunt sites for dialysis should be well protected to avoid unnecessary pressure. Intravascular volume should be carefully monitored and maintained to avoid overhydration. Medications, including analgesics, should be carefully dosed and monitored, along with their metabolites. Early ambulation is encouraged. Dialysis should be performed within 48 hours of surgery. Skin closure devices should remain from 10 to 14 days because of delayed wound healing.

FLUID MANAGEMENT

Body fluids are divided arbitrarily into an intracellular compartment (45% of body weight) and extracellular compartment (20% of body weight). The extracellular compartment is subdivided into plasma and interstitial compartments. Fluid balance is maintained through the gastrointestinal (GI) tract, the skin, respiratory tract, and the renal system. The GI tract processes 6 to 9 liters per 24 hours, with fluid losses of 200 to 300 ml per 24 hours. Insensible losses through the skin and lungs are 600 to 800 ml per day. Absolute renal loss is approximately 600 ml per 24 hours. Compensation must be made for total daily insensible losses of 1000 to 1500 ml per 24 hours to calculate fluid balance and further insensible loss from fever or metabolic needs. The renal tract reflects the hydration status of the body, with urine output being an important indicator. Oliguria is urine output of less than 400 ml per 24 hours, while polyuria is greater than 3 liters per 24 hours.

Surgery affects the plasma space acutely, although fluid shifts, particularly free water, may take hours to equilibrate. Intravenous sodium equilibrates in as little as 30 minutes. Dehydration, in which fluid is removed from cells as a result of disease, exercise, or other causes, may not be reflected in total body losses. In addition, the thirst mechanism is blunted with age and vasopressin release is altered. Replacement of total body stores may require fluid boluses over 12 to 24 hours, despite initial increases in urinary output with 500- to 1000-ml fluid boluses.

Preoperative fluid status may profoundly affect intraoperative and postoperative fluid management. Same-day surgery admission may hamper preoperative hydration that in some cases should be done over days. Dehydration may result in hypotension at anesthesia induction. Fluid needs are magnified by the length of time the patient is without food or water, febrile illness, bowel preparation, and fistulas. Bowel preparation may result in an additional 1500 to 2000 ml of fluid loss. Patients living in warmer climates may be dehydrated in the summer. Medications such as diuretics or antihypertensives may affect fluid status. Patients on diuretics should have their electrolytes checked at least 1 week prior to surgery because total body potassium replacement may take several days. Potassium should be replaced with 40 mEq twice daily for 7 to 10 days in effervescent solutions, unless renal insufficiency is present. Antihypertensives may affect vascular tone, thereby modifying fluid requirements. Immediate perioperative fluid replacement should be the joint responsibility of anesthesia and preoperative caretakers. A minimum of 500 ml of fluid should be administered prior to anesthesia induction in the normal patient under 55 years of age, with additional fluid as indicated.

Intraoperative calculation of fluid balance should take into account estimated intraoperative and preoperative blood loss, patient size, and preoperative volume status. Urine output is an important variable in fluid status assessment, reflecting GFR and consequently, hydration. Extensive use of a retractor on the bladder may delay effective diuresis. Vital signs will reflect anesthetic agents (muscle blockers and halothane), the level of anesthesia (hypertension and tachycardia will develop in underanesthetized patients), and fluid status. Hemoglobin values measured on an ABG may be used in an emergency.

Isotonic saline solutions are used for fluid replacement in the intraoperative setting. Ringer's lactate solution, the most commonly given solution, consists of 130 mEq sodium, 4 mEq potassium chloride, 5 mEq calcium chloride, 109 mEq chloride, and 28 mEq lactate, which is converted to bicarbonate by the liver. Use of dextrose-containing solutions is important only in the patient with diabetes to provide glucose for ready metabolism. In the postoperative period, dextrose spares protein from gluconeogenesis. This may be important in the elderly patient with reduced muscle mass. Estimated intraoperative blood loss should be replaced with 3 ml of crystalloid solution for every 1 ml of blood.

Electrolyte balance should be monitored when replacing fluids, particularly in the elderly patients and those with significant medical problems. Sodium, potassium, and chloride are generally provided in balanced salt solutions. Fixed sodium losses of 100 to 200 mg/day through the skin and kidneys require replacement. Potassium losses equal approximately 1 mg/kg of body weight. Additional potassium may be administered through peripheral lines (40 mEq/liter) or central lines (80 mEq/liter).

Decreased urinary flow should be assessed systematically. Obstruction of the urinary catheter should be ruled out. The most important variable is unrecognized, ongoing blood loss. Crystalloid fluid bolus is administered only after evaluation of red-blood cell status with a hemogram or ABG hemoglobin. If vital signs are unstable, reexploration is performed immediately, and blood products given when indicated. A pulmonary artery catheter may be warranted, particularly in medically compromised or elderly patients. Furosemide may exacerbate hypovolemia and should be administered only in overt pulmonary edema.

Pulmonary artery catheter (PAC) placement is not warranted in patients with stable disease. Any patient with a reasonable chance for a PAC intraoperatively should have a central line access placed preoperatively. This may be converted to a PAC, over an introducer, with minimal delay.

DIABETES MELLITUS

Glucose control and adequate insulin levels are an important factor in surgical treatment for patients with diabetes. Insulin may be viewed as an anabolic hormone, and glucagon, cortisol, and growth hormone its counterregulatory hormones.[55] Patients with diabetes require approximately 0.75 to 1.0 U/hr of insulin to maintain euglycemia in a normal fed state. Surgical and metabolic stressors increase insulin resistance via increased circulating levels of adrenal glucocorticoids, catecholamines, and growth hormone, which may increase insulin requirements. The overall propensity in glucose balance is toward hyperglycemia. Fasting and operative stress can also lead to hypoglycemia with ketosis, protein loss, and poor wound healing. Diabetes also affects infection risks, acidemia, and electrolyte intravascular volume status. Renal and cardiovascular complications of diabetes further increase surgical risk.

Preoperative laboratory assessment of a patient with diabetes should include an ECG, serum chemistries, and urinalysis for protein and ketones. Diabetics with advanced renal disease may have a normal creatinine level, demonstrating only proteinuria.[56] Normalization of glucose levels (70 to 140 mg/dl) is important prior to surgery. Electrolytes should be carefully monitored in patients undergoing electrolyte bowel preparation.

Ideally, the surgery for a patient with diabetes should be the first one in the morning, to minimize fasting interval. One-half to two-thirds of the usual morning dose of intermediate- or long-acting insulin is given prior to surgery. Assuming normal renal function, intraoperative fluids should contain 5% dextrose solution with one-half normal saline and 20 mEq of potassium. Higher glucose levels (less than 250 mg/liter) are acceptable during surgery, due to an absence of reflexes to hypoglycemia under anesthesia. Intermittent intraoperative boluses of regular insulin are given in response to glucose levels. IV insulin infusion is the ideal method for intraoperative insulin control, but it is time-consuming and labor-intensive.

It is important to maintain good postoperative glucose control (70 to 140 mg/dl) to minimize infection risk and improve wound healing.[57] Once a liquid diet is well tolerated, the patient's usual insulin therapy and an American Diabetes Association (ADA) diet is started. Preoperative and postoperative metoclopramide may help prevent gastroparesis.

Insulin has multiple endocrinologic functions, including glucose transport into cells, gluconeogenesis, glycogenolysis, ketogenesis in the liver, and regulating lipid and fat metabolism with lipoprotein lipase activity. Insulin is necessary, even in the euglycemic state, or alternative metabolic pathways will be initiated. In the hypoglycemic state, glucose and insulin must be administered. Insulin is necessary to move glucose into cells and *should never be discontinued*.

The insulin infusion rate may be decreased to only 0.1 U/hr, but never stop administering insulin. Regular subcutaneous insulin should be given 2 hours prior to cessation of insulin drip. Patients with sepsis or infection have increased insulin requirements, and may respond erratically until the infection resolves. All postoperative patients with diabetes should be monitored for diabetic ketoacidosis (DKA) in the first 48 hours. Impending DKA may be heralded by increased respiratory rate or altered respiratory patterns. Respiratory rates greater than 24 to 28 per minute may represent respiratory alkalosis in response to metabolic acidosis. An ABG should be obtained to evaluate acid–base status.

Patients with Type 2 diabetes (previously called non-insulin-dependent diabetes, or NIDDM) generally require less perioperative glucose control. Thin type 2 patients have similar metabolic responses to type 1 (previously called IDDM) patients. The obese type 2 patient has high serum glucose levels secondary to insulin resistance and dietary indiscretion. These patients frequently become euglycemic within 24 to 36 hours of starting an ADA diet. Rarely, surgical or infectious stress will cause the type 2 patient to become ketotic and require insulin. If insulin is required, 10 U of regular insulin may be added to 1 liter of 5% dextrose solution, infused at 125 ml/hr. These patients often do not require postoperative insulin. Oral hypoglycemic agents should be restarted when tolerating a diet or at discharge.

Hyperosmolar coma differs from DKA, usually resulting from infection or stroke. It usually occurs in elderly type 2 patients who have become dehydrated. Total body water deficiency may be as high as 10 to 12 liters. These patients often present with serum glucose levels of 800 to 1000 mg/dl in the absence of ketosis. Fluid replacement should be initiated immediately, with a large normal saline bolus (2 to 3 liters) over the first 1 to 2 hours then decreased to 200 to 300 ml/hr to replace intravascular volume. Insulin infusion in low doses (1 to 2 U/hr) or subcutaneous insulin (5 to 10 U) will aid in lowering glucose. Electrolyte status should be monitored frequently. Once blood sugar is stabilized (200 mg/dl or less), 5% dextrose solution with 20 mEq potassium is started at 125 ml/hr. Diabetic diet and oral hypoglycemics are started once sensorium returns to normal.

Good perioperative glucose control is correlated with optimal wound healing and decreased infection. Patients with poorly controlled diabetes may be compromised at the cellular level, with poor phagocytosis, chemotaxis, opsonization, and bactericidal activities.[58] Prophylactic antibiotics are reasonable because of white-cell dysfunction. Patients with DKA may present with severe abdominal pain mimicking pelvic inflammatory disease with a ruptured tubo-ovarian abscess or appendicitis. Abdominal pain resolves with normalization of glucose.[58]

HYPERTENSION

Hypertension is among the most common chronic medical conditions. It is more prevalent in women than in men after 50 years of age. Severe, uncontrolled blood hypertension (systolic blood pressure [SBP] >170 mm Hg and diastolic [DBP] >110 mm Hg) increases the risk of intraoperative blood pressure lability and hypotension. Preoperative hypertension is associated with increased postoperative hypertensive episodes and myocardial ischemia.[59] Mild to moderate preoperative hypertension (SBP <170 mm Hg, DBP <110 mm Hg) is not associated with increased perioperative complications, although 25% of these patients will have a hypertensive or hypotensive episode perioperatively.

Preoperative evaluation should focus on identification of end-organ disease, such as myocardial ischemia, peripheral vascular disease, and renal insufficiency. Blood pressure medications should be taken the morning of surgery with a sip of water, to decrease blood-pressure lability. Problems in the patient with

hypertension may occur 48 hours to 1 week after surgery. Initial postoperative management should focus on avoiding hypoxia, fluid overload, and sympathetic stimulation from pain. Patients with LV dysfunction or renal insufficiency should be monitored carefully for pulmonary edema in the first 36 to 48 hours, when mobilization of third-space fluids may occur.

Although once the mainstay of hypertensive therapy, the usefulness of diuretics has been limited by their side effects. Thiazide and loop diuretics cause hypokalemia, unless combined with a potassium-sparing agent. Volume depletion may be a significant problem, as long-term diuretic use results in a "reset" of intravascular volume control. Assessment is done with a "tilt" test, measuring the blood pressure (BP) and heart rate (HR) in the supine position initially. The patient is then moved to a standing position, measuring the blood pressure and heart rate after a 5-minute interval. A positive tilt test notes a drop in DBP of 20 mm Hg, or an increase in heart rate of 20 beats/min. Volume replacement should be initiated prior to surgery, with a repeat tilt test to ensure adequate replacement.

Calcium-channel antagonists selectively inhibit slow inward calcium flux in vascular smooth muscle, causing direct arteriolar vasodilation. They are most useful in the African-American population and older patients resistant to β-blockers.[4] Caution should be exercised perioperatively, as these medications may result in acute drops in blood pressure when intravascular volume is low.

Angiotensin-converting–enzyme (ACE) inhibitors decrease peripheral vascular resistance by blocking the conversion of angiotensin I to the vasoconstrictor angiotensin II. When used in conjunction with diuretics, hypotension may result. As a result, diuretics are stopped 48 to 72 hours prior to the initiation of ACE inhibitors. The only ACE inhibitor in IV formulation is enalapril (1.25 mg every 6 hours with a 5.0 mg maximum), allowing improved perioperative control.

β-Blocker formulations are either lipid- or water-soluble. The water-soluble group (including atenolol and nadolol) have a long half-life, making them extremely useful in the perioperative setting. Propranolol is lipid-soluble, and comes in IV form (1 to 2 mg). β-Blocker withdrawal syndrome may occur in patients with CAD. Sudden withdrawal results in unstable angina and myocardial infarction.[60]

Central antihypertensive agents such as methyldopa and clonidine are rarely used as first-line therapy. Clonidine is occasionally useful in the perioperative setting, dispensed as a transdermal patch. The patch is active for 7 days and should be placed 48 to 72 hours before surgery to reach therapeutic levels.

Hydralazine is a direct arterial vasodilator with subsequent smooth-muscle relaxation. It may cause fluid retention. Common side effects of headache and tachycardia may be limited by the addition of a β-blocker. Given parenterally (0.5 to 1.0 mg every 15 minutes), it is extremely potent and may cause significant hypotension (in the patient with no preeclampsia). Because of the potential profound hypotensive effects, care must be taken to avoid confusion of drug-induced hypotension with hypovolemia. Minoxidil, another potent direct smooth-muscle relaxant, may cause beard growth.

α_1-Adrenergic blockers inhibit postganglionic norepinephrine-induced vasoconstriction in peripheral vascular smooth muscle. These agents decrease total cholesterol and low-density lipoproteins, while increasing high-density lipoproteins. They are often first-line treatment in antihypertensive therapy.

Anesthesia-induction agents may release catecholamines, exacerbating hypertension. Intravenous agents, such as nitroglycerin and nitroprusside, may be used in small boluses for short intervals. These are best managed by anesthetists and intensivists because of potency. The surgeon should be aware of their side effects, particularly tachycardia, in the postoperative period. To avoid confusion between hypotension due to medications and hypovolemia, close monitoring of urine output is warranted. More frequent measures of hematocrit may also be helpful, when indicated.

HEPATIC DISEASE

A thorough history should include questions regarding transfusions, bleeding history, and alcohol and drug abuse. Liver function studies (LFTs) should be ordered as appropriate. Alcohol abuse history may be difficult to elicit. Subtle elevations in LFTs may be the only indication of liver disease. Hepatitis should also be considered, with elevated LFTs and appropriate laboratory panels ordered. Patients receiving a blood transfusion prior to the late 1980s should be considered for hepatitis screening.

SUMMARY

A good history and physical examination is the foundation of sound perioperative care. Preoperative assessment should always be individualized and appropriate consultations obtained. The risk:benefit ratio must be assessed for each patient. The patient, based on clinical findings, may be adequately counseled about alternative management schemes and potential perioperative and postoperative complications. Careful preoperative care in combination with intraoperative skills and careful postoperative surveillance will maximize the probability of successful surgical outcome.

REFERENCES

1. Blery C, Charpak Y, Szatan M, et al. Evaluation of a protocol for selective ordering of preoperative tests. Lancet 1986;1:139.
2. Marcello PW, Roberts PL. "Routine" preoperative studies: which studies in which patients? Surg Clin N Am 1996; 76:11.
3. MacPherson DS, Snow R, Lofgren RP. Preoperative screening value of previous tests. Ann Intern Med 1990; 113:969.
4. Nolan TE. Optimization of the patient for surgery. In: Mann WJ Jr, Stovall TG, eds. Gynecologic surgery. New York: Churchill Livingstone, 1990:3.
5. Krenzien J, Roding H, Mummelthey R. Operative risk in octogenarians—a statistical prognostic index and its prospective validation. Theor Surg 1989;14:10.
6. Gewirtz AS, Miller ML, Keys TF. The clinical usefulness of the preoperative bleeding time. Arch Pathol Lab Med 1996;120:353.
7. Allison JG, Bromley HR. Unnecessary preoperative investigations: evaluation and cost analysis. Am Surgeon 1996; 62:686.
8. Velanovich V. Preoperative laboratory evaluation. J Am Coll Surg 1996;183:79.
9. Delancey JOL, Norton P, Wall LL. Practical urogynecology. Williams & Wilkins, Baltimore, MD, 1993.
10. Irving AD, Scrimglour D. Mechanical bowel preparation for colonic resection and anastamosis. Brit J Surg 1988; 75:1216.
11. Burke P, Mealy K, Gillen P, et al. Requirement for bowel preparation in colorectal surgery. Br J Surg 1994;81:907.
12. Condon RE, Nichols RL. Rational use of prophylactic antibiotics in gastrointestinal surgery. Surg Clin N Am 1975;55:1309.
13. Messing MJ, Nolan TE. Bowel preparations for gynecologic surgery. Female Patient 1993;18:15.
14. Levy AG, Benson JW, et al. Saline lavage: a rapid, effective and acceptable method for cleansing the gastrointestinal tract. Gastroenterology 1976;70:157.
15. Chung RS, Gurll NF, Berglund EM. A controlled clinical trial of whole-gut lavage as a method of bowel preparation for colonic operations. Am J Surg 1979;137:75.
16. Davis GR, Santa Ana C, et al. Development of a lavage solution associated with minimal water and electrolyte absorption or secretion. Gastroenterology 1980;78:991.
17. Jagelman DG, Fazio VW, et al. A prospective, randomized, double blind study of 10% mannitol mechanical bowel

preparation combined with oral neomycin and short-term, perioperative, intravenous Flagyl as prophylaxis in elective colorectal resections. Surgery 1985;98:861.

18. Lewis M, Rugg-Gunn F, Don C, Woods W. Bowel preparation at home in elderly people. BMJ 1997;314:74.

19. Condon RE, Wittman DH. The use of antibiotics in general surgery. Curr Probl Surg 1991;28:803.

20. Abramowisz M. Antimicrobial prophylaxis in surgery. Med Lett 1992;34:5.

21. Lewis RT, Weigand FM, et al. Should antibiotic prophylaxis be used routinely in clean surgical procedures: a tentative yes. Surgery 1995;118(4):742.

22. Thomas DR, Ritchie CS. Preoperative assessment of older adults. J Am Geriatr Soc 1995;43:811.

23. Panton ON, Atkinson KG, et al. Mechanical preparation of the large bowel for elective surgery: comparison of whole gut lavage with the conventional enema and purgative technique. Am J Surg 1985;149:615.

24. Hamsell DL. Prophylactic antibiotics in gynecologic and obstetric surgery. Rev Infect Dis 1991;13(Suppl 10):S821.

25. Monahan EG. Medical clearance for gynecologic surgery. Obstet Gynecol Surv 1998;53:117.

26. Nolan T. Surgery in the elderly. Postgrad Med 1992; 92:199.

27. Tait AR, Kyff JV, Crider B, et al. Changes in arterial oxygen saturation in cigarette smokers following general anesthesia. Can J Anaesth 1990;37:423.

28. Dureuil B, Viires N, et al. Diaphragmatic contractility after upper abdominal surgery. J Appl Physiol 1986;61:1775.

29. Lawrence VA, Dhanda R, et al. Risk of pulmonary complications after elective abdominal surgery. Chest 1996; 110:744.

30. Mohr D, Lavender RC. Preoperative pulmonary evaluation. Postgrad Med 1996;100:241.

31. Mohr D, Jett JR. Preoperative evaluation of pulmonary risk factors. J Gen Intern Med 1988;3:277.

32. Ravin MB. Comparison of spinal and general anesthesia for lower abdominal surgery in patients with chronic obstructive pulmonary disease. Anesthesiology 1971;35:319.

33. Nolan TE, Hankins GDV. Acute pulmonary dysfunction and distress: emergency care of the obstetric patient. Obstet Gynecol Clin N Am 1995;22:39.

34. Nolan TE, Hankins GDV. Adult respiratory distress. In: Pastorek JG, ed. Infectious disease in obstetric gynecology. Rockville, MD: Aspen, 1994:197.

35. Smith R, Osterweil D, Ouslander JG. Perioperative care in the elderly urologic patient. Urol Clin N Am 1996;23:27.

36. Merli GJ, Martinez J. Prophylaxis for deep vein thrombosis and pulmonary embolism in the surgical patient. Med Clin N Am 1990;71:380.

37. Knight MTN, Dawson R. Effect of intermittent compression of the arms on deep venous thrombosis in the legs. Lancet 1976;2:1265.

38. Hull RD, Pineo GF. Low molecular weight heparin treatment of venous thromboembolism. Prog Cardiovasc Dis 1994;37:71.

39. Hunt D. Low molecular weight heparins in clinical practice. South Med J 1998;91:2.

40. Research Committee of the British Thoracic Society.

Optimum duration of anticoagulation for deep-vein thrombosis and pulmonary embolism. Lancet 1992; 340:873.

41. Goforth P, Gudas CJ. Effects of steroids on wound healing—a review of the literature. J Foot Surg 1980; 19:22.

42. Salem M, Tainsh RE Jr, Bromberg J, et al. Perioperative glucocorticoid coverage: a reassessment 42 years after emergence of a problem. Ann Surg 1994;219:416.

43. Almany SL, Mileto L, Kahn JK. Preoperative cardiac evaluation: assessing risk before noncardiac surgery. Postgrad Med 1995;98:171.

44. Thomas DR, Ritchie CS. Preoperative assessment of older adults. J Am Geriatr Soc 1995;43:811.

45. Coley C, Eagle KA. Preoperative assessment and perioperative management of cardiac ischemic risk in noncardiac surgery. Curr Probl Cardiol 1996;21:296.

46. Eagle K, et al. ACC/AHA Task Force Report—guidelines for perioperative cardiovascular evaluation for noncardiac surgery. J Am Coll Cardiol 1996;27:910.

47. Svensson LG, Cruz H, et al. Timing of surgery after acute myocardial infarction. J Cardiovasc Surg 1996;37:467.

48. Baron JF, Mundler O, et al. Dipyridamole–thallium scintigraphy and gated radionuclide angiography to assess cardiac risk before abdominal aortic surgery. N Engl J Med 1994;330:663.

49. Mangano DT, London MJ, et al. Dipyridamole thallium-201 scintigraphy as a preoperative screening test. Circulation 1991;84:493.

50. Shackelford DP, Hoffman MK, et al. Evaluation of preoperative cardiac risk index values in patients undergoing vaginal surgery. Am J Obstet Gynecol 1995;173:80.

51. Seaworth BJ, Durack DT. Infective endocarditis in obstetric and gynecologic practice. Am J Obstet Gynecol 1986; 154:180.

52. Dajani AS, Bisno AL, Chung KJ, et al. Preventing bacterial endocarditis: recommendations by the American Heart Association. JAMA 1990;264:2919.

53. Burke JF Jr, Francos GC. Surgery in the patient with acute or chronic renal failure. Med Clin N Am 1987; 71:489.

54. Livio M, Mannucci PM, et al. Uraemic bleeding: role of anemia and beneficial effect of red cell transfusion. Lancet 1982;1:1013.

55. Schade DS. Management of diabetes in the surgical patient. Med Clin N Am 1988;72:1531.

56. Mogensen CE, Christen CK, Vittinghas E. The stages in diabetic renal disease: with emphasis on the stage of incipient nephropathy. Diabetes 1983;32(Suppl 2):64.

57. Rayfield EJ, Ault MJ, et al. Infection and diabetes: the case for glucose control. Am J Med 1982;72:439.

58. Campbell EW, Duncan LJP, et al. Abdominal pain in diabetic metabolic decompensations: clinical significance. JAMA 1975;233:166.

59. Goldman L, Caldera D. Risks of general anesthesia and elective operation in the hypertensive patient. Anesthesiology 1979;50:285.

60. Frishman WH. Beta-adrenergic blocker withdrawal. Am J Cardiol 1989;59:26F.

SECTION 3
Special Problems in Gynecologic Oncology

Chapter 62

Radiation Therapy and Chemotherapy

Douglas Horbelt
Jed Delmore

Five Key Points

- **Ionizing radiation disrupts DNA and renders cells incapable of clonogenic growth.**

- **Therapeutic radiation is described by the field exposed to radiation, the fraction (amount of radiation per administration), and the total dosage received.**

- **Long-term complications of radiation therapy include loss of organ parenchyma and replacement with fibrotic tissue based on hypoperfusion from radiation-induced endarteritis.**

- **Strategies for medical treatment of gynecologic malignances include the use of cytotoxic and hormonal agents.**

- **Combining chemotherapeutic agents attempts to use different cell-killing mechanisms to reduce cancer resistance to chemotherapy while trying not to produce additive complications.**

RADIATION THERAPY

Gynecologic malignancies are both sensitive to radiation and are surrounded by normal tissue that tolerates ionizing radiation well. A practicing gynecologist will be involved with the diagnosis and staging of these malignancies, and should have a functional knowledge of the indications and complications of radiation therapy. The success rate of radiation therapy is quite good,[1] and the gynecologist will be presented with problems that radiation has produced in normal tissue. Radiation-related symptoms and complications are infrequent and may happen after treatment or many decades later. It is in the patient's best interest that the gynecologist have a thorough knowledge of radiation therapy and its side effects.

Radiation has its effect on tissue when it is absorbed. Radiation causes ionization, which leads to oxygen free radical production.[2] It is this highly reactive free radical that adversely affects the DNA of the cells.[3] The structurally altered DNA is incapable of replication; hence the neoplastic cells are unable to continue clonogenic growth.[4]

The unit that describes the amount of radiation absorbed per unit mass of tissue is the gray. Formerly the unit was called a rad. One gray equals 100 rad and 1 rad is equivalent to 1 centigray (cGy). (The dose of radiation is expressed in these units.) Both the gray and centigray are in common usage. The total dose of external beam radiation to the pelvis may be written as 40 Gy (4000 cGy or 4000 rad). A single dose of radiation is termed a fraction.[5] It is the amount of radiation absorbed by the tissue during treatment. Usually it is once a day but it may be more than once a day (termed hyperfractionation). The centigray is usually used to describe the fractional dosage. The "standard" fraction size to the pelvis is 180 to 200 cGy. The radiation beam (also called a port or a field) is a stream of ionizing particles (high-energy x-rays, γ-rays, and electrons, etc.). The most common type of radiation beam used to treat pelvic malignancies consists of high-energy x-rays produced by a linear accelerator. In modern gynecologic oncology, beams are often combined in pairs such as anteroposterior–posteroanterior, right and left lateral, or four-field. The radiation emerges from the treatment unit as a diverging rectangle. Custom-made shielding is used to block portions of the beam that correspond to normal tissues that do not need to be treated. The blocked and shaped beam forms the actual radiation "port" that enters the patient. Anterior and posterior pelvic blocks often produce an octagon-shaped port.

Two- and four-field techniques are most commonly used for pelvic radiation of gynecologic malignancies. They are intended to treat the pelvic organs, ligaments (cardinal, uterosacral, and pubocervical) and the at-risk group of lymph nodes that drain the pelvic structures. The dose of radiation is prescribed with reference to the target organ (e.g., cervix). The skin surface dose varies depending on the diameter of the patient, the number of fields used, and the beam energy. As ionizing radiation passes through tissue it is absorbed in a predictable fashion. The further the photon beam passes through tissue the less intense it becomes.[6] The distribution of radiation dose within a treated volume is characterized by an isodose curve. Like a topographical map, it outlines the amount of radiation absorbed in tissue at various distances from the central field region. Each fraction of radiation is designed to deliver a quantity of radiation to the target organ. If it was given through only one port, the amount of radiation to the subcutaneous tissue and the preceding organs (e.g., bladder) would exceed the amount given to the cervix.[7] Therefore, each dose is usually administered through two or more fields. A portion of the dose is given anteriorly and a portion may be given posteriorly to the same pelvic field (anteroposterior–posterioanterior, AP-PA). The total dosage for that fraction may be 200 cGy, but if it is equally weighted then 100 cGy is given anteriorly and 100 cGy is given posteriorly. The resultant amount is still 200 cGy to the cervix, but because it is split,

less is given to the bladder and less is given to the colon than if it had been administered through one portal. The amount to the bladder and colon can be further reduced by increasing the number of fields. The four-field technique employs both the anteroposterior and the posteroanterior ports as well as two side ports.[8] The objective is to have the resultant amount of radiation absorbed by the cervix remain the same while sparing other pelvic organs. These side fields are approximately 15 cm by 9 cm. The 9-cm dimension is intended to minimize the amount given to the bladder and the rectocolon. There is also a rotational radiation administration technique that further increases the number of fields. Unfortunately, the greater the number of ports, the more are the technical difficulties encountered in daily setup. Therefore, when treating the full pelvis, it is customary to use either the two-field (AP-PA) or the four-field (AP-PA and two lateral) techniques.

The biologic effect of radiation on tissue is a function of the total amount administered, the daily fraction used, and the time over which it is administered. Therefore, the correct clinical description of radiation administered to a patient is the fractional dosage times the number of fractions in a certain time frame.[9] The complex interaction between the fractionation of radiation and its biologic effect on the tissue takes into consideration tissue repair, reoxygenation, repopulation, and redistribution.[10-12] These factors work on both the tumorous tissue and the normal organs that are treated. The daily dose (and total dose) must be great enough to irreparably damage abnormal tissue but not so great as to destroy normal organs. Therefore, 4000 cGy administered over 4000 fractions would have much less effect on the tissue than if 4000 cGy was administered in one fraction. The former would have minimal effect on the tumor and the latter would be fatal to the patient. The advantage in using fractionated radiation is based on exploiting differences in cell kinetics, inherent sensitivity, oxygenation, and molecular responses of tumor and healthy tissue.[3,13]

The curves in Figure 62-1 describe lethal damage to cells caused by administration of radiation. It requires multiple fractions before any biologic effect is seen.[14] There is a rapid upswing to a variable slope, which is linear until the few surviving cells are left. It then describes a flattening of the curve, requiring relatively more radiation to eradicate the residual surviving population. The curves are the same configuration for normal and neoplastic tissue. The distance

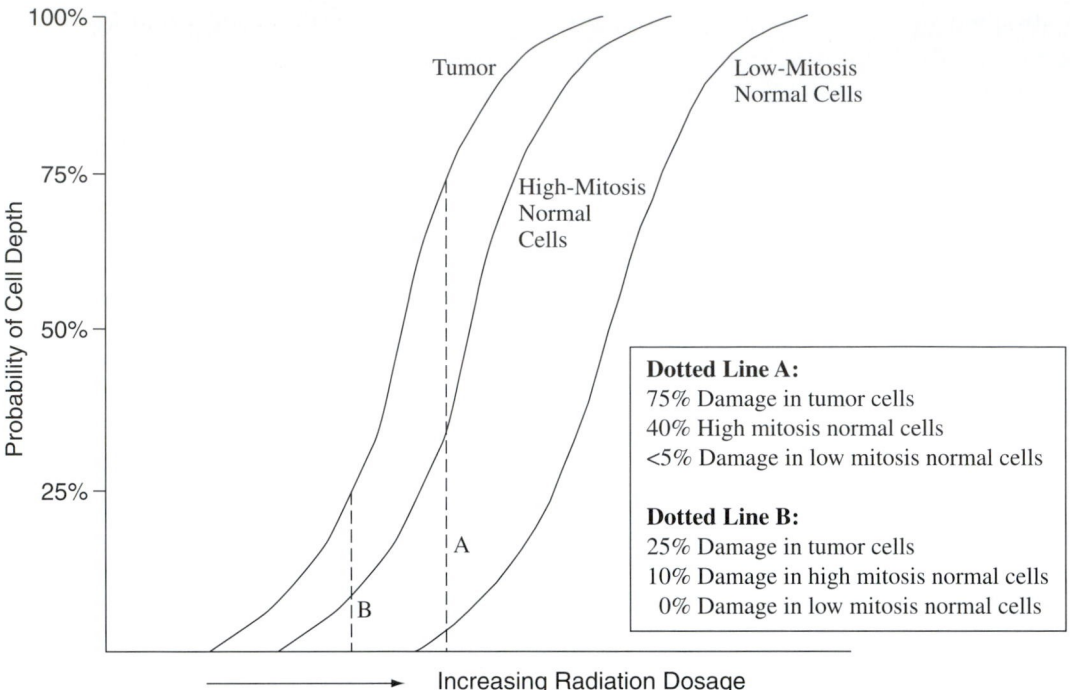

Figure 62-1 Tissue response to radiation dosages. Dashed line A = 75% damage in tumor cells; 40% high-mitosis normal cells; <5% damage in low-mitosis normal cells. Dashed line B = 25% damage in tumor cells; 10% damage in high-mitosis normal cells; 0% damage in low-mitosis normal cells.

between the curves (susceptibility to radiation damage) is a predictor of complications from radiation.[15,16] The more growth that is occurring in tissue, the greater the chance of tissue damage and the closer the normal curve is to the neoplastic one. Neurologic tissue, such as brain, has a low mitotic rate and therefore tolerates radiation well. Its curve is distant from the neoplastic curve. Small bowel has a high mitotic rate. It does not tolerate radiation as well. Its curve is close to the neoplastic one.

Fields are chosen in order to treat the primary tumor and the region at risk for spread. When a gynecologic tumor spreads lymphatically, treatment is directed at the first group of lymph nodes that is clinically unaffected and all the lymph nodes between that group and the primary tumor. In gynecology, there are four main lymph node groups. These are groin nodes, pelvic nodes, common iliac nodes, and paraaortic nodes. The groin nodes are defined by the femoral triangle both above and below the cribriform fascia. The femoral triangle is defined superiorly by the inguinal ligaments, medially by the adductor longus muscle, and laterally by the sartorius muscle. The pelvic nodes include external iliac, obturator, and parametrial nodes. This group is bounded by the bifurcation of the common iliac artery superiorly, the

circumflex iliac vein inferiorly, the superior vesical artery medially, and laterally by both the genital femoral nerve (anteriorly) and the obturator nerve (dorsally). The common iliac nodes begin at the bifurcation of the aorta superiorly and extend to the bifurcation of the common iliac artery. The nodes are around the artery and vein. The aortic bifurcation is at the level of the fourth lumbar vertebrae (L4) and a field that includes the common iliac nodes is sometimes referred to as an L4 field. The paraaortic nodes are defined by the renal arteries (12th thoracic vertebra) and the aortic bifurcation. The nodes are associated with the aorta and vena cava. This is called a paraaortic, or T12, field. Radiation is administered to the nodes and vessels so the upper fields become narrow to accommodate this lymphatic drainage pattern.

Adequate description of a teletherapy plan requires a number of factors. The total dose, fraction size, photon energy, field configuration, and the prescription point within the treated volume must be specified. For example, the description for a Stage I cervical cancer without clinical or radiologic evidence of spread to pelvic nodes might include a total dosage of 41.4 Gray (4140 cGy) in 23 fractions (180 cGy per fraction) in a pelvic four-field technique using high-energy photons. A computer is used to generate a dose distribution diagram (isodose distribution), which aids in specifying the prescription point. With these parameters, the biologic and therapeutic effects can be predicted and understood.

Brachytherapy is the implantation of a radioactive source either next to or into a tumor mass. The Fletcher–Suit[17] afterloading tandem and ovoids is an example of a device used to accomplish this for gynecologic malignancies. A hollow tube, called a tandem, is placed into the uterus through the cervix. The radioactive sources (usually cesium) are placed inside the tandem at a later time.[18] Ovoids are used in each lateral vaginal fornix. These also are afterloaded. Once loaded, the system of tandem and ovoids produce a dose distribution centered around the cervix and parametria.[19] Radiation from a source such as cesium is extremely intense next to the source but it dissipates quickly. This dissipation is described by the inverse square law.[20] The amount of radiation at 2 cm from a source is 1/4 ($1/2^2$) and at 3 cm is 1/9 ($1/3^2$) than at 1 cm. So the brachytherapy takes advantage of the high intensity in its immediate proximity to eradicate tumor cells and its rapid attenuation allows normal tissue such as bladder and colon to better tolerate its presence. Standard ovoids have the same shielding ventrally and dorsally in order to minimize the dosage to the bladder and colon. Brachytherapy is also divided into low-dose-rate (LDR) and high-dose-rate (HDR) strategies.[21] The HDR treatment is done on an outpatient basis, with less risk of operative complications and more convenience to the patient.[22] The LDR treatment produces fewer long-term side effects and is the time-tested gold standard. Both are effective methods of administering radiation to the central pelvis.[23,24]

Another technique uses steel needles, which are placed directly into the tumor mass, under anesthesia.[25,26] After placement, they are afterloaded with radioactive material such as iridium wires.[27] Divergent needles produce areas that do not have full radiation intensity (cold spots) and convergent needles have areas that have radiation effects that can exceed the tissue tolerance (hot spots). Placement and spacial alignment are critical to adequate therapy.[28,29] Pelvic templates such as the Syed template help maintain the proper spatial relationship between the radioactive (or iridium) sources.[30-33]

Radioactive phosphorus (^{32}P) is another isotope used to deliver radiation therapy.[34] It is a liquid form of radioisotope administered intraperitoneally and distributed throughout the peritoneal cavity.[35] The isotope decays quickly (half-life, 14.3 days) and the dose is delivered superficially along the tissue surfaces and within the peritoneal fluid. It is a method to address cytologic peritoneal malignant contamination.[36]

The effect of ionizing radiation on tissue is enhanced by the presence of oxygen.[7] Tissue that is well oxygenated has the ability to produce peroxide radicals that have a direct effect on cell DNA replication. Radiation can still affect relatively hypoxic tissue such as large tumor masses, but the amount required to achieve the same biologic effect is severalfold greater. Tumor masses may have hypoxic areas and therefore more radiation is needed to destroy those cells. The amount may be as high as threefold. This is known as the oxygen-enhancement ratio. Therefore, either smaller masses or well-oxygenated tissue have a more profound response to radiation than hypoxic tissue. The amount of radiation necessary for a hypoxic mass may exceed the tolerance of the normal tissue. Drugs can be used to enhance the effect of radiation on tumors.[37] Many drugs, including cisplatin, act as radiation enhancers.

Side effects from radiation therapy are considered as either short- or long-term. Short-term reactions occur in tissues that have a rapid cell turnover rate such as skin, intestinal mucosa, and bone marrow.[38] Radiation-related effects include erythema of the skin, diarrhea and radiation enteritis, fatigue, leukopenia, and thrombocytopenia. The side effects are transient and the patient usually recovers from these symptoms once radiation is stopped or the fractionation is modified. The degree of short-term reaction is not related to the degree of long-term effect.

Long-term effects develop after 6 months but may begin to manifest themselves as long as 20 to 30 years after administration. The effects are not usually severe but in some cases can be debilitating. Long-term complications deal with loss of tissue parenchyma (i.e., organ tissue such as kidney or liver). An endarteritis produces hypoperfusion of an area.[19,39] This area then loses parenchymal tissue and has it replaced with fibrotic tissue. This may produce some damage such as intermittent strictures of the bowel,[41] irradiation ulcers in the large bowel,[41-43] radiation-induced insufficiency fractures,[44] and osteomyelitis.[45] Radiation-induced cystitis[46] with bleeding and shrinkage of bladder capacity and bladder fistulas are other complications seen by the gynecologist.[47-49] Cellular recovery is usually not feasible and many times surgical intervention is necessary.[50] The cause of long-term radiation damage is multifactorial, but in general, damage increases with increasing dose per fraction, with increased total dose and with increased irradiated volume.[51]

CHEMOTHERAPY

The use of cytotoxic and/or hormonal therapies for the treatment of human malignancies is common and effective. A gynecologist may treat patients who have gynecologic as well as nongynecologic malignancies. It is important to have a working concept of the treatments in addition to the effects the regimens may have on other gynecologic or medical conditions. Strategies of prevention, such as tamoxifen for breast cancer, present special problems in hormonally responsive organs. Gynecology is one of the few specialties in which the treatment of its malignancies (surgery, chemotherapy, and radiation therapy) are closely and frequently interrelated. Physicians caring for women must have a functional understanding of these treatment methods.

Chemotherapy may be divided into cytotoxic and hormonal. Cytotoxic chemotherapy is intended to destroy or render the cancer cells incapable of reproduction. This usually is associated with disruption of the cell's reproductive process. Cytotoxic chemotherapy is further subdivided into cell-cycle-specific and cell-cycle-nonspecific drugs. When the therapy is active it influences the method and timing of administration.

The cell cycle is the reproductive process a cell goes through in order to replicate.[54,55] The cell-cycle stages are G1 phase, or growth after mitosis phase; S phase, or DNA synthesis phase; G2 phase, or growth after DNA synthesis phase; and M phase, or mitotic phase[56] (Figure 62-2). There is also an M0 phase that represents cells that are not actively dividing at the time. Cells may move in and out of the M0 phase.

Cell-cycle-specific chemotherapy affects the replication process during a distinct phase. An example is the vinca alkaloids such as vinblastine, which directly affect the spindle fibers during M phase. Cells that are not in M phase are therefore not damaged. Cell-cycle-nonspecific chemotherapy produces damage to the cell regardless of the phase of the active cycle (except M0). An example is the damage to DNA by intercalation that cisplatin produces.[58] It renders the cell nonclonogenic and not capable of correctly replicating its DNA.

Drugs that are cell-cycle-specific include vincristine[57] (Oncovin), vinblastine[57P] (Velban), 5-fluorouracil

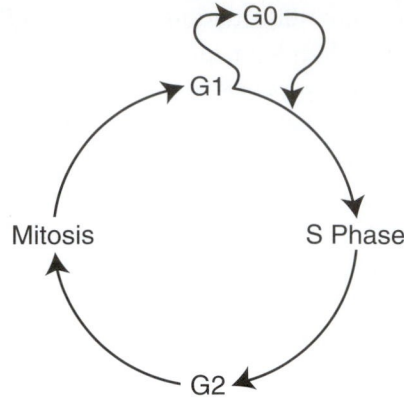

Figure 62-2 Cell cycle. G = growth after mitosis; S phase = DNA synthesis phase; G2 = growth after DNA synthesis; mitosis = cell division; G0 = cells not in the active division cycle.

(5-FU), methotrexate, and paclitaxel (Taxol).[57] Drugs that are cell-cycle-nonspecific include cisplatin, carboplatin, and doxorubicin (adriamycin).[57]

Cyclophosphamide

Chemotherapy can be administered as a single agent or in combination with other chemotherapeutic agents.[59] The concept behind combining agents has two main objectives. One is to combine drugs that do not use the same mechanism of cellular disruption.[60] Therefore, if a cell is resistant to one drug, it may be affected by the second or subsequent drugs. Using more than one drug also decreases the probability that the neoplastic cell will develop resistance to a drug.[61] The Golde–Coldman somatic mutation theory supports the concept of spontaneous somatic mutations that produce resistance to chemotherapy.[62,63] The strategy for combining drugs also takes into account the drug toxicities. Combinations try to avoid additive toxicities to specific organs or systems in order to allow the patient to tolerate the dosing schedule.

Gynecology has an array of malignancies with varying sensitivities to chemotherapy.[64] Gestational trophoblastic disease and germ-cell tumors of the ovary can be cured with chemotherapy.[65] Ovarian cancer and endometrial cancer do respond to chemotherapy and produce some prolongation of survival.[66] Cervical cancer has a similar response to chemotherapy but no demonstrable increase in survival.[67] Sometimes chemotherapy can be used in neoadjuvant settings. Neoadjuvant describes the use of chemotherapy prior to definitive surgery.[68,69] It is usually designed to be organ-sparing or at least to limit the degree of surgical extirpation required. Vulvar cancer is one example of neoadjuvant chemotherapy in gynecology.[70]

Chemotherapy may be used in a therapeutic or adjuvant fashion. Therapeutic administration is designed to address known disease—usually a mass or lesion that can be followed to assess response. Cytotoxic chemotherapy is believed to have a first-order kinetic kill pattern. That is, a certain proportion of cells are killed with each administration of chemotherapy. The larger the initial cell population, the more cycles of treatment are necessary to eradicate the tumor. Consider a tumor with a cell population of 10^9. This is approximately 1 cc of tumor. If there is a 90% kill ratio, then after one dose 10^8 cells still remain. Another dose would decrease the population to 10^7, and so forth. If a patient has 10^{12} cells (or 1 kg of tumor) it would require three more therapeutic cycles. This also assumes all cells are responsive to the chemotherapy and are not in the M0 or resting phase. Organisms can take only a limited number of doses of cytotoxic chemotherapy due to accumulative toxicities.

We also know from Gompertzian kinetics that after a certain tumor population has developed, tumor growth slows, and after 10^{12} cells are present, the host cannot sustain the tumor burden.[71] It is believed that tumor populations less than 10^5 can be controlled with immunologic mechanisms. More than 10^5 cells requires active therapy such as chemotherapy, surgery, or radiation therapy. It is at 10^9 cells, or 1 cc, that most conventional diagnostic methods can begin to make a diagnosis. Improvement in outcome will follow advances in technologies that allow diagnosis earlier and therefore require fewer cycles to control a more susceptible tumor population.

Adjuvant chemotherapy is proposed based on risk of recurrence and without a measurable lesion. It is based on the natural history of the tumor and its susceptibility to treatment. An example is a Stage I, Grade 3 epithelial ovarian malignancy that has been macroscopically completely excised. With no visual evidence of disease, the patient may be cured with surgery alone.[72] If chemotherapy is added adjuvantly, there is a greater probability of cure. Adjuvant therapy requires a tumor that is responsive to chemotherapy. Adjuvant chemotherapy is not used with mixed mesodermal sarcoma of the uterus in spite of its high

rate of recurrence because there is not a chemotherapeutic agent that has a good effect on the tumor.[73]

Treatment of cancer is a very individualized science. It requires the evaluation of the risk–benefit relationship.[74] It is also extremely important that the patient and her family have some realistic expectation for the treatment. The equation considers the patient's tumor type and tumor burden. It also considers any previous treatments and the patient's overall medical condition. Additional factors include availability of resources and the patient's emotional and social situation. A skilled practitioner must consider all these factors in weighing the benefits to be gained against the risks to be undertaken. Unrealistic expectations on the patient's and family's part only add to the anxiety of the clinical situation and further detract from the patient's quality of life. It is the physician's responsibility to educate and prognosticate in a clear and kind manner without removing hope or desire to survive.

Chemotherapeutic agents are cytotoxic and by their nature are toxic to both neoplastic and non-neoplastic cells[75] (Table 62-1). The therapeutic index

TABLE 62-1
ANTINEOPLASTIC AGENTS USED WITH GYNECOLOGIC MALIGNANCIES AND THEIR TOXICITIES

Agent	Toxicity
Dactinomycin (actinomycin D)	Myelosuppression, vesicant, mucosal ulceration
Bleomycin (Blenoxane)	Myelosuppression, pulmonary suppression, pulmonary fibrosis, fever
Carboplatin	Thrombocytopenia, neuropathy, nephropathy
Cisplatin	Nephrotoxicity, toxicity, peripheral neuropathy, nausea and vomiting
Cyclophosphamide (Cytoxan)	Myelosuppression, hemorrhagic cystitis, ovarian failure, alopecia
Dacarbazine (DTIC)	Myelosuppression, hepatotoxicity, nausea and vomiting
Doxorubicin (Adriamycin)	Myelosuppression, vesicant, cardiotoxicity, alopecia
Etoposide	Myelosuppression, alopecia, hypotension
5-Fluorouracil (5-FU)	Myelosuppression, mucosal ulcerations, alopecia
Hexamethylmelamine (Hexalen)	Myelosuppression, neurotoxicity
Ifosfamide (IFEX)	Myelosuppression, hemorrhagic cystitis, nephrotoxicity
Methotrexate	Myelosuppression, mucosal ulcerations, alopecia
Paclitaxel (Taxol)	Myelosuppression, peripheral neuropathy, alopecia, anaphylactic reactions

is the difference between the level that is toxic to cancer cells and that which is toxic to nonneoplastic cells. Since chemotherapeutic agents have their greatest effect on cells that are actively dividing, more active nonneoplastic cells have the greatest risk for complications. This is why the production of blood cells from the active marrow as well as hair follicles and mucous membranes are usually affected by chemotherapy treatments. Some agents have specific toxicities that are peculiar to that agent. Cisplatin is specifically neurotoxic and nephrotoxic while relatively sparing of the bone marrow.[76] Doxorubicin is toxic to the musculature of the heart, producing a type of heart failure usually refractory to cardiotropic medications.[77,78] Bleomycin, as well as the alkylating agents, may produce lung fibrosis.[79] Neurotoxicity, specifically peripheral neuropathy, is seen with cisplatin, paclitaxel, and hexamethylmelamine. Skin may show reactions to antineoplastic agents. The most common manifestation is alopecia, which occurs with many drugs. It is usually transient, with restoration of normal hair-follicle function within weeks of cessation of treatment. Some skin complications are greater in damage and recovery. Certain chemotherapies are known as vesicants.[80] These drugs can cause local necrosis if they extravasate from the vasculature. Vesicants used in gynecologic malignancies include doxorubicin, dactinomycin, and vinblastine. These drugs are usually administered into a large vessel with high flow, such as the superior vena cava. Central venous access for these drugs provides a degree of safety during their administration. Central venous catheters, especially the newer low-maintenance designs, provide the patient with a great degree of convenience with respect to administering other drugs and in drawing blood samples. Chemotherapy may also produce an allergic, hypersensitivity-type of skin reaction.[81] A special type of skin lesion occurs when doxorubicin is administered to a patient who has had external-beam radiation therapy. A red area develops in the skin that was radiated. It is known as radiation recall. It is not painful or uncomfortable, but the skin's appearance is altered. Doxorubicin may also produce hyperpigmentation in nail beds. Hypersensitivity skin reactions may also be attributed to the diluent of the chemotherapy. Paclitaxel, for example, is diluted in a substance that may produce a hypersensitivity reaction. Pretreatment with antihistamines and steroids usually ameliorates this manifestation.

Chemotherapeutic agents are mutagenic and may increase the chance of a second malignancy developing.[82] The use of alkylating agents, such as melphalan, for longer than 1 year can increase the risk of leukemia developing. Duration of treatment, the choice of chemotherapeutic agent, and the dosages used are significant determining factors. Intense combination therapies for trophoblastic disease or for germ-cell malignancies of the ovary that are short-term carry a lower risk of causing a second malignancy.

Chemotherapy may disturb gonadal function. Long-term use (longer than 6 months) of treatments that include cyclophosphamide or other alkylating agents may produce ovarian failure. As with mutagenesis, ovarian failure is associated with the prolongation and not the intensity of the treatment. This is especially true of the drug combination including alkylating agents. Usually patients become amenorrheic and follicle-stimulating hormone (FSH) levels are elevated. There is no treatment to correct ovarian failure.

Sometimes paraneoplastic syndromes develop in patients being treated with chemotherapy. A patient with lethargy, confusion, and altered mental status may be suffering from inappropriate antidiuretic hormone secretion (SIADH). Management consists of correcting the hyponatremia. Other metabolic abnormalities include hyperuricemia, hyperkalemia, and hypercalcemia. Correction of the metabolic abnormalities usually alleviates the symptoms.

Hematopoietic suppression and complications are many times the dose-limiting feature of a chemotherapy regimen.[83] When neutrophils are low, the patient is susceptible to infections that his/her body would otherwise easily control. Administration of pheresis packs of white cells is one option, but the development of growth factors that stimulate the bone marrow to produce the cells is the much safer and more effective option.[84] Hematopoietic growth factors include G-CSF (granulocyte colony-stimulating factor), GM-CSF (granulocyte–macrophage colony-stimulating factor), EPO (erythropoietin), and IL-3 (interleukin-3).[85]

G-CSF is clinically useful in increasing the production of neutrophils. It may also potentiate their function and survival. This allows a patient to maintain dosage levels of chemotherapy and decreases the incidence of fever associated with neutropenia. G-CSF also mobilizes progenitor cells and provokes maturation and production of these cells.

EPO and GM-CSF have limited use in the treatment of gynecologic malignancies.[84] Thrombocytopenia can also produce dose reductions or prolonged intervals of treatment. The availability of a megakaryocyte growth factor (thrombopoietin) will make it possible to maintain platelet levels as well as continue a dosage regimen. This factor should soon be available for clinical use.

Dose intensification has remained a goal in the management of tumors. Autologous stem-cell transplantation and hematopoietic growth factor support have accomplished the goal of augmenting a bone marrow that has been nearly eradicated by high-dose chemotherapy. Though still being explored as a potential dose-intensification strategy, stem-cell transplantation has not yet increased cure rates for the gynecologic malignancies.[86] Therefore, its use in ovarian and other gynecologic tumors should be confined to proscribed research protocols in order to develop the knowledge necessary to apply this technique in its most appropriate fashion.[87]

Adenocarcinomas of the female reproductive tract arise from tissue that is hormonally responsive. Endometrial and ovarian malignancies may express estrogen- and/or progesterone-receptor molecules.[88] With endometrial cancer, patients with progesterone receptors have a better prognosis. Tumors of hormonally responsive tissues may respond to hormonal signals. The administration of progesterone to patients with metastatic endometrial cancer is one example.[89] Normal endometrial tissue will convert from a proliferative to a nonproliferative secretory pattern under the influence of progestogens. When progestogens are administered to patients with metastatic endometrial cancer, a proportion will respond by having the tumor stop growing and then (over 12 to 16 weeks) begin to shrink as the tumor cells live their life and die.[90,91] They are not replaced because tumor replication is being suppressed by the progestin. The response to hormonal therapy in endometrial cancer is inversely proportional to the tumor's grade. Response rates for Grade 1 are 50%, Grade 2 35%, and Grade 3 12%. Progestogens have been reported to be active in ovarian malignancies as well. Progestogen therapy has few side effects and allows the hematopoietic system a respite from cytotoxic treatment for some previously treated patients.

Tamoxifen, a partial antiestrogen, is also effective in gynecologic adenocarcinomas. The gynecologist will see patients using this drug for treatment of hormone-receptor–positive breast cancer or for chemoprophylactic reasons.[92] While it has antiestrogenic effects in the breast, it has estrogenic properties on the endometrium. Some endometrial tissue responds with a hyperplastic pattern of growth, and a few develop endometrial cancers. The tendency to develop endometrial cancer seems to be dose-dependent. There is a higher rate of endometrial cancer when the dose is increased. Tamoxifen may be used to treat recurrent ovarian cancer.[63] Some adenocarcinomas of the müllerian tract have receptors for luteinizing hormone (LH). The administration of leuprolide, an LH agonist, has some therapeutic effect in a few patients. Other hormone strategies, such as androgens, have not demonstrated clinical usefulness for gynecologic malignancies.

Chemotherapy and drugs that either protect the organism from its effect or augment another treatment's efficacy are constantly being developed. The administration of hydroxyurea, cisplatin, or paclitaxel[61] during radiation augments the therapeutic effects of radiation therapy.[93-95] Protective strategies such as Mesna[61] bind with the active excretory products of ifosfamide and protect the bladder mucosa while allowing therapeutic levels of ifosfamide to be administered.[96,97] Advances in chemical treatments may come from antisense oligonucleotides. This class of drug is directed at the genetic lesion that produced the cancerous change. Direct gene therapies are also being developed, as well as drugs to turn on tumor-suppressor genes or turn off oncogene.[98] Tumors are known for active growth and increased vascularity. Indeed, the proliferating tumor cells are directly dependent on its vascular supply. Antiangiogenesis factors are designed to disrupt the vascular proliferation and therefore decrease cell growth.[64,95] Unique chemotherapy delivery systems and/or antibody-specific delivery systems are also being developed in order to have a greater effect on the tumor and a low index of side effects in the patient.

REFERENCES

Radiation Therapy

1. Eifel PJ. Intracavitary brachytherapy in the treatment of gynecologic neoplasms. J Surg Oncol 66;(2):141.
2. Churchill-Davidson I, Foster CA, Wiernik G, et al. The place of oxygen in radiotherapy. Br J Radiol 1966; 39:321.
3. Hall EJ. Radiobiology for the radiologist. 2nd ed. Philadelphia: Harper & Row, 1978.
4. Elking MM. DNA damage and cell killing: cause and effect. Cancer 1985;45:2123.
5. Hall EJ. Radiobiology for the radiologist. 4th ed. Philadelphia: Lippincott, 1988.

1236   Gynecology/Women's Health: Special Problems in Gynecologic Oncology

6. Fletcher GH, Shukovsky LJ. The interplay of radiocurability and tolerance in the irradiation of human cancers. J Radiol Electrol 1975;56:383.

7. Fletcher GH, ed. Textbook of radiotherapy. 3rd ed. Philadelphia: Lea & Febiger, 1980.

8. Fletcher GH. Keynote address: the scientific basis of the present and future practice of clinical radiotherapy. Int J Radiat Oncol Biol Phys 1983;9:1073.

9. Wong R, Thomas G, Cummings B, et al. In search of a dose–response relationship with radiotherapy in the management of recurrent rectal carcinoma in the pelvis: a systematic review. Int J Radiat Oncol Biol Phys 1998;40:437.

10. Kallman RF. The phenomenon of reoxygenation and its implications for fractionated radiotherapy. Radiology 1972;105:135.

11. Marples B, Lambin P, Skov KA, Joiner MC. Low dose hyper-radiosensitivity and increased radioresistance in mammalian cells. Int J Radiat Biol 1997;71:721.

12. Phillips RA, Tolmach LF. Repair of potentially lethal damage in x-irradiated HeLa cells. Radiat Res 1966; 29:413.

13. Fletcher GH. Clinical dose-response curves of human malignant epithelial tumors. Br J Radiol 1973;46:1.

14. Okunieff P, Morgan D, Niemierko A, Suit HD. Radiation dose-response of human tumors. Int J Radiat Oncol Biol Phys 1995;32:1227.

15. Fertil B, Malaise EP. Inherent cellular radiosensitivity as a basic concept for human tumor radiotherapy. Int J Radiat Oncol Biol Phys 1981;7:621.

16. Deacon J, Peckham MJ, Steel GG. The radioresponsiveness of human tumors and the initial slope of the cell survival curve. Radiother Oncol 1984;2:317.

17. Barillot I, Bone-Lepinoy MC, Horiot JC, et al. Organ preservation in cervix cancer. Rays 1997;22(3):410.

18. Decosse JJ, Rhodes RS, Wentz WB, et al. The natural history and management of radiation induced injury of the gastrointestinal tract. Ann Surg 1969;170:369.

19. Curtin JP, Shapiro F. Adjuvant therapy in gynecologic malignancies: ovarian, cervical and endometrial cancer. Surg Oncol Clin N Am 1997;6:813.

20. Joslin CA. Commentary: brachytherapy—clinical dosimetry and the integration of therapie gynaecological cancer. Br J Radiol 1996;69:689.

21. Stitt JA, Thomadsen BR. Innovations and advances in brachytherapy. Semin Oncol 1997;24:696.

22. Ogino I, Kitamura T, Okajima H, Matsubara S. High-dose-rate intracavitary brachytherapy in the management of cervical and vaginal intraepithelial neoplasia. Int J Radiat Oncol Biol Phys 1998;40:881.

23. Uno T, Itami J, Aruga M, et al. High dose rate brachytherapy for carcinoma of the cervix: risk factors for late rectal complications. Int J Radiat Oncol Biol Phys 1998;40:615.

24. Eifel PJ. Intracavitary brachytherapy in the treatment of gynecologic neoplasms. J Surg Oncol 1997;66:141.

25. Chyle V, Zagars GK, Wheeler JA, Wharton JT, Declos L. Definitive radiotherapy for carcinoma of the vagina: outcome and prognostic factors. Int J Radiat Oncol Biol Phys 1996;35:891.

26. Erickson B, Billit MT. Interstitial implantation of gynecologic malignancies. J Surg Oncol 1997;66:285.

27. Monk BJ, Tewari K, Burger RA, Johnson MT, Montz FJ, Berman ML. A comparison of intracavitary versus interstitial irradiation in the treatment of cervix cancer. Gynecol Oncol 1997;67:241.

28. Erickson B, Albano K, Gillin M. CT-guided interstitial implantation of gynecologic malignancies. Int J Radiat Oncol Biol Phys 1996;36:699.

29. Erickson B, Gillin MT. Interstitial implantation of gynecologic malignancies. J Surg Oncol 1997;66:285.

30. Chander S, Patel AK, Grover R, Rath GK. Evaluation of transperineal template implant technique in Indian cervical carcinoma patients. Indian J Med Sci 1997;51:231.

31. Corn BW, Lanciano RM, Rosenblum N, Schnall M, King S, Epperson R. Improved treatment planning for the Syed-Neblett template using endorectal-comagnetic resonance and intraoperative (laparotomy/laparoscopy) guidance: an integrated technique for hysterectomized women with vaginal tumors. Gynecol Oncol 1995;56:255.

32. Nath R, Wilson LD. Advances in brachytherapy. Cancer Treat Res 1998;93:191.

33. Brady LW, Micaily B, Miyamoto CT, Heilmann HP, Montemaggi P. Innovations in brachytherapy in gynecologic oncology. Cancer 1995;76(10 Suppl):2143.

34. Potter ME, Partridge EE, Shingleton HM, et al. Intraperitoneal chromic phosphate in ovarian cancer: risks and benefits. Gynecol Oncol 1989;32:314.

35. Fleay RF. Dosimetry in the use of collodial isotopes. Aust Radiol 1971;15:388.

36. Ott RJ, Flower MA, Jones A, McCready VR. The measurement of radiation doses from P^{32} chromic phosphate therapy of the peritoneum using SPECT. Eur J Nucl Med 1985;11:305.

37. Peters LJ, ed. Innovations in radiation oncology. New York: Springer-Verlag, 1987.

38. Wang CJ, Leung SW, Chen HC, et al. The correlation of acute toxicity and late rectal injury in radiotherapy for cervical carcinoma: evidence suggestive of consequential late effect (CQLE). Int J Radiat Oncol Biol Phys 1998; 40:85.

39. Rubin P, Casarett GW. Clinical radiation pathology. Philadelphia: Saunders, 1968.

40. Carratu R, Secondulfo M, deMagistris L, et al. Assessment of small intestinal damage in patients treated with pelvic radiotherapy.

41. Covens A, Thomas G, DePetrillo A, et al. The prognostic importance of site and type of radiation-induced bowel injury in patients requiring surgical management. Gynecol Oncol 1991;43:270.

42. Shiojima K, Mitsuhashi N, Yamakawa M, Sakurai H, Niibe H. Transrectal ultrasonography in evaluation of chronic rectal complications after radiation therapy for carcinoma of the uterine cervix. Invest Radiol 1998;33:74.

43. Babb RR. Radiation proctitis: a review. Am J Gastroenterol 1996;91:1309.

44. Libotte F, Autier P, Delmelle M, et al. Survival of patients with radiation enteritis of the small and the large intestine. Acta Chir Belg 1995;95(4 Suppl):190.

45. Blomlie V, Rofstad EK, Talle K, Sundfor K, Winderen M, Lien HH. Incidence of radiation-induced insufficiency fractures of the female pelvis: evaluation with MR imaging. AJR Am J Roentgenol 1996;167:1205.

46. Wignall TA, Carrington BM, Logue JP. Post-radiotherapy osteomyelitis of the symphysis pubis: computed tomographic features. Clin Radiol 1998;53:126.

47. Erbay N, Spencer RP. Late effects of postradiation cystitis noted on renal dynamic study. Clin Nucl Med 1998; 23:34.

48. McIntyre JF, Eifel PJ, Levenback C, Oswald MJ. Ureteral stricture as a late complication of radiotherapy for stage IB carcinoma uterine cervix. Cancer 1995;75:836.

49. Marks LB, Carroll PR, Dugan TC, Anscher MS. The response of the urinary bladder, urethra and ureter to radiation and chemotherapy. Int J Radiat Oncol Biol Phys 1995;31:1257.

50. Lentz SS, Homesley HD. Radiation-induced vesicosacral fistula: treatment with continent urinary diversion. Gynecol Oncol 1995;58:278.

51. Hamberger AD, Abdurrahman U, Jershenson DM, Fletcher GH. Analysis of the severe complications of irradiation of carcinoma of the cervix: whole pelvis irradiation and intracavitary radium. Int J Radiat Oncol Biol Phys 1982;9:367.

52. Withers HR, Peters LJ, Kogelnik HD. The pathobiology of late effects of irradiation. In: Meyn RE, Withers HR, eds. Radiation biology in cancer research. New York: Raven Press, 1980:439.

53. Deshpande DD, Shrivastava SK, Pradhan AS, Viswanathan PS, Dinshaw KA. Geometrical considerations in dose volume analysis in intracavitary treatment. Strahlenther Onkol 1996;172:326.

54. Johns HE, Cunningham JR. The physics of radiology. 4th ed. Springfield, IL: Charles C Thomas, 1983.

Chemotherapy

55. Baserga R. The relationship of the cell cycle to tumor growth and control of cell division: a review. Cancer Res 1965;25:581.

56. Young RC, DeVita VT. Cell cycle characteristics of human solid tumors in vivo. Cell Tissue Kinetics 1970; 3:285.

57. Tannock I. Cell kinetics and chemotherapy: a critical review. Cancer Treat Rep 1978;62:1117.

58. Rosenberg B. Cisplatin: its history and possible mechanisms of action. In: Prestayko A, Crooke S, Carter S, eds. Cisplatin: current status and new developments. New York: Academic Press, 1980:9.

59. DeVita VT, Young RC, Canellos GP. Combination versus single agent chemotherapy: a review of the basis for selection of drug treatment of cancer. Cancer 1985; 35:98.

60. Young RC. Drug resistance: the clinical problem. In: Ozols R, ed. Drug resistance in cancer therapy. Boston: Kluwer Academic, 1989;1.

61. Beck WT, Danks MK, Yalowich JC, et al. Different mechanisms of multiple drug resistance in two human leukemic cell lines. In: Wooley PV, Tew KD, eds. Mechanisms of drug resistance in neoplastic cells. San Diego: Academic Press, 1988:212.

62. Coldman A, Goldie J. Impact of dose-intense chemotherapy on the development of permanent drug resistance. Semin Oncol 1987;14:29.

63. Hatch KD, Beecham JB, Blessing JA, Creasman WT. Responsiveness of patients with advanced ovarian carcinoma to tamoxifen: a Gynecologic Oncology Group study of second-line therapy in 105 patients. Cancer 1991;68:269.

64. Krakoff IH. Systemic treatment of cancer. CA Cancer J Clin 1996;46:134.

65. Williams S, Blessing J, Slayton R, et al. Ovarian germ cell tumors: adjuvant trials of the Gynecologic Oncology Group (GOG). Proc Am Soc Oncol 1989;8:150.

66. Thigpen JT, Vance R, Balducci L, Blessing JA. Chemotherapy in the management of advanced or recurrent cervical and endometrial carcinoma. Cancer 1981;48:658.

67. Bonomi P, Blessing J, Ball H, et al. A phase II valuation of cisplatin and 5-fluororacil in patients with advanced squamous cell carcinoma of the cervix: a Gynecologic Oncology Group study. Gynecol Oncol 1989;34:357.

68. Frei A, Clark JR, Miller D. The concept of neoadjuvant chemotherapy. In: Salmon SE, ed. Adjuvant therapy of cancer. V. New York: Grune & Stratton, 1987:67.

69. Goldie JH. Scientific basis for adjuvant and primary (neoadjuvant) chemotherapy. Semin Oncol 1987;14:1.

70. Yordan E, Bonomi P, Wilbanks G. Chemotherapy of vulvar and vaginal neoplasms. In: Deppe G, ed. Chemotherapy of gynecologic cancer. New York: Alan R. Liss, 1984:85.

71. Fruchter RG, Maiman M, Sillman FH, et al. Characteristics of cervical intraepithelial neoplasia in women infected with the human immunodeficiency virus. Am J Obstet Gynecol 1994;171:531.

72. Cohen CJ. Surgical considerations in ovarian cancer. Semin Oncol 1985;12:53.

73. Gershenson DM, Kavanagh JJ, Copeland LJ, et al. High-dose doxorubicin infusion therapy for disseminated mixed mesodermal sarcoma of the uterus. Cancer 1987;59:1264.

74. Bonadonna G. Does chemotherapy fulfill its expectations in cancer treatment? Ann Oncol 1990;1:11.

75. Levin L, Hryuinuk W. Dose intensity analysis of chemotherapy regimens in ovarian cancer. J Clin Oncol 1987;5:756.

76. Kaplan RS, Wiernik PH. Neurotoxicity of antineoplastic drugs. Semin Oncol 1982;9:103.

77. Benjamin RS, Wiernik PH, Bachur NR. Adriamycin chemotherapy—efficacy, safety and pharmacologic basis of an intermittent single high-dosage schedule. Cancer 1974;33:19.

78. Allen A. The cardiotoxicity of chemotherapeutic drugs. In: Perry MC, ed. The chemotherapy source book. Baltimore: Williams & Wilkins, 1992:582.

79. McCarty KS, Jr, Barton TK, Fetter BF, et al. Correlation of estrogen and progesterone receptors with histologic differentiation in endometrial adenocarcinoma. Am J Pathol 1979;96:171.

80. Zweig J, Kabakow B. An apparently effective countermeasure for doxorubicin extravasation. JAMA 1978; 239:2116.

81. Dunagin WG. Dermatologic toxicity. Semin Oncol 1982; 9:14.

82. Kyle R. Second malignancies associated with chemotherapy. In: Perry M, Yarbro J, eds. Toxicity of chemotherapy. Orlando, FL: Grune and Stratton, 1984:479.

83. Hryniuk WM. The importance of dose intensity in the outcome of chemotherapy. In: Hellman S, DeVita V, Rosenbert S, eds. Important advances in oncology. Philadelphia: Lippincott, 1988:121.

84. Bociek RG, Armitage JO. Hematopoietic growth factors. CA Cancer J Clin 1996;46:165.

85. Demetri GD, Griddin JD. Hematopoietic growth factors and high-dose chemotherapy: will grams succeed where milligrams fail? J Clin Oncol 1990;8:761.

86. McGuire WP, Hoskins WJ, Brady MF, et al. Assessment of dose-intensive therapy in suboptimally debulked ovarian cancer: a Gynecologic Oncology Group study. J Clin Oncol 1995;13:1589.

87. Appelbaum FR. The use of bone marrow and peripheral blood stem cell transplantation in the treatment of cancer. CA Cancer J Clin 1996;46:142.

88. Ehrlich C, Young P, Cleary R. Cytoplasmic progesterone and estradiol receptors in normal, hyperplastic, and carcinomatous endometria: therapeutic implications. Am J Obstet Gynecol 1981;141:539.

89. Sall S, DiSaia P, Morrow CP, et al. A comparison of medroxyprogesterone serum concentrations by the oral or intramuscular route in patients with persistent or recurrent endometrial carcinoma. Am J Obstet Gynecol 1979;135:647.

90. Piotti P, Genitoni V, Comazzi R, et al. Relationship between pulmonary function tests and morphologic changes in the lung in bleomycin-treated patients. Tumori 1984;70:439.

91. Thigpen JT, Blessing J, DiSaia P, Ehrlich C. Oral medroxyprogesterone acetate in advanced or recurrent endometrial carcinoma: results of therapy and correlation with estrogen and progesterone receptor levels: the Gynecologic Oncology Group experience. In: Baulier E, Iacobelli S, McGuire W, eds. Endocrinology and malignancy. Park Ridge, NJ: Parthenon, 1986:446.

92. Bonadonna G, Valagussa P, Tancini G, et al. Estrogen-receptor status and response to chemotherapy in early and advanced breast cancer. Cancer Chemother Pharmacol 1980;4:37.

93. Stehman F, Bundy B, Keys H, et al. A randomized trial of hydroxyurea versus misonidazole adjunct to radiation therapy in carcinoma of the cervix. Am J Obstet Gynecol 1988;159:87.

94. Piver S. Hydroxyurea and radiation therapy in the treatment of carcinoma of the cervix. In: Surwit E, Alberts D, eds. Cervix cancer. Boston: Martinus Nijhoff, 1987:107.

95. Rosenthal DS. Cancer therapy—the 21st century. CA Cancer J Clin 1996;46:131.

96. Andriole GL, Sandlund JT, Miser JS, et al. The efficacy of MESNA as a uroprotectant in patients with hemorrhagic cystitis receiving further orazaphosphorine chemotherapy. J Clin Oncol 1987;5:799.

97. Antman RH, Ryan L, Elias A, et al. Response to ifosfamide and mesna: 124 previously treated patients with metastatic or unresectable sarcoma. J Clin Oncol 1989; 7:126.

98. Crystal RG. Transfer of genes to humans: early lessons and obstacles to success. Science 1995;270:404.

99. Rojansky N, Anteby SO. Gynecological neoplasias in the patient with HIV infection. Obstet Gynecol Surv 1996; 51:679.

100. Mandelblatt JS, Fahs M, Garibaldi K, et al. Association between HIV infection and cervical neoplasia: implications for clinical care of women at risk for both conditions. AIDS 1992;6:173.

101. Buckley SL, Molpus K, Carr MB, et al. Advanced ovarian carcinoma diagnosed during pregnancy in a patient with human immunodeficiency virus infection. Gynecol Oncol 1993;50:532.

102. Ojwang SB, Otieno MR, Khan KS. Human immunodeficiency virus states. In: DeVita VT, Hellman S, Rosenberg SA, eds. Cancer principles and practice of oncology, 3rd ed. Philadelphia: Lippincott, 1989:1953.

103. Shackney SE, McCormack GW, Cuchural GJ. Growth rate patterns of solid tumors and their relation to responsiveness to therapy. Ann Intern Med 1989;89:107.

104. Goldie J, Coldman A. A mathematical model for relating the drug sensitivity of tumors to the spontaneous mutation rate. Cancer Treat Rep 1979;63:1727.

Chapter 63
Vulvar and Vaginal Cancer

Jed Delmore
Douglas Horbelt

Five Key Points

- Symptoms of vulvar cancer include pruritus, bleeding, and the presence of a mass. Symptoms may be present for an extended period prior to evaluation and biopsy.

- Any suspicious lesion of the vulva should be evaluated by immediate biopsy.

- The therapy for vulvar cancer is determined on a case-by-case basis, and is becoming more conservative when it is safe to do so.

- Vaginal cancer is predominantly a disease of the elderly, with symptoms of vaginal discharge and bleeding.

- The success of therapy for vaginal cancer is limited by patient age, physical condition, and close proximity of other vital organs.

The objective of this chapter is to assist the practicing clinician in obtaining a solid, general knowledge of the natural history of carcinoma of the vulva and vagina. Diagnosis and evaluation of the patient with cancer of the vulva and vagina will be covered. Detailed descriptions of surgical techniques, radiation therapy, and chemotherapy have been avoided.

VULVAR CARCINOMA

Incidence of Vulvar Cancer

Cancer of the vulva is uncommon, and accounts for less than 0.5% of cancers in women. The American Cancer Society projects that 3400 new cases of vulvar cancer will be diagnosed in 2000. This contrasts with the prediction of 182,800 new cases of breast cancer and 36,100 new cases of uterine cancer.[1] The overall incidence of vulvar cancer is 1.5 in 100,000

women in the United States, and there has been no significant change in the incidence in the recent past.[2] Of importance to note is the progressive incidence with age.[3]

Epidemiology and Risk Factors

Early studies suggested an association between syphilis, lymphogranuloma venereum, granuloma inguinale, and epidermoid carcinoma of the vulva.[4,5] Those studies were based on Jamaican and African-American populations and appear not to account for most of the cases reported in the United States. Obesity, hypertension, and diabetes have also been associated with carcinoma of the vulva; however, studies have failed to confirm these as independent risk factors.[6] Currently agreed-on risk factors include other premalignant or malignant neoplasms of the genital tract, cigarette smoking, sexual activity, genital condyloma, and

	TABLE 63-1 **PROPOSED MODEL FOR VULVAR CARCINOMA**	
	Group I	Group II
Age	Relatively younger (35–65)	Older (55–85)
Previous condyloma	Common	Uncommon
Previous STD	Common	Uncommon
Preexisting lesion	VIN (carcinoma in situ)	Vulvar inflammation
		Lichen sclerosus
		Hyperplasia
Cofactors in development	Age	Vulvar "atypia"
	Immune status	Mutated host
	Viral integration	genes
Histopathology of tumor	Intraepithelial-like (basaloid) or	Keratinizing
	poorly differentiated	Well differentiated
Cervical neoplasia	High association	Low association
Smoking	High incidence	Low incidence
HPV nucleic acids	Frequent (>60%)	Seldom (<15%)

STD = sexually transmitted disease; VIN = vulvar intraepithelial neoplasia; HPV = human papillomavirus
Reprinted with permission from Crum.[13]

vulvar intraepithelial neoplasia (VIN).[6,7] The association between human papillomavirus (HPV) and vulvar cancer has been identified in as many as 60% of patients.[8] The association between HPV DNA and vulvar cancer is not as strong as the association between HPV and cervical cancer.[9] The risk of progression from carcinoma in situ to invasive carcinoma appears to be lower in younger women (3%) than in older women (19%).[10,11] Alani and Münger have summarized the basic biologic properties of HPV and the mechanisms of cellular transformation.[12] A review of the epidemiology and pathogenesis of vulvar cancer by Crum suggests at least two subsets of patients with vulvar cancer.[13] This model for vulvar carcinoma categorizes the groups by ages 35 to 65 versus 55 to 85 in addition to other factors (Table 63-1). A point should be made regarding chronic vulvar conditions and the risk of invasive carcinoma developing. Leukoplakia, lichen sclerosus, and vulvar dystrophy have been implicated as premalignant conditions for vulvar cancer. When atypical epithelial proliferation is excluded from this group and placed in the category of VIN, the risk of invasive cancer developing in the former group is very low.[14,15]

Presentation

The most common presenting symptom for patients with vulvar cancer is pruritus, followed by presence of a vulvar lesion, bleeding, and pain.[16] Whether because of the advanced age of the patients or the preceding vulvar dystrophy, a delay in diagnosis has been,

and still is, common. Symptoms have been reported to be present for a year or longer in 33 to 60% of patients.[4,16,17] The blame for the delay in diagnosis is evenly spread between patient and clinician.[18] After a delay by the patient in reporting symptoms, which may have resulted from a trial of home remedy, not uncommonly a protracted trial of topical therapy prescribed by the physician follows. The appearance of cancer of the vulva may vary from a large exophytic lesion, to a flat infiltrating lesion, to a necrotic ulcer. Size may vary from a few millimeters to a lesion large enough to replace the entire vulva. Most commonly, vulvar cancer originates on the labia majora, however, lesions of the labia minora, clitoris, or perineal body may develop. Over the past 15 years we have seen an increasing number of nursing home residents who were thought to have skin breakdown from incontinence and the regular use of diapers, when in fact, a vulvar carcinoma had developed.

Diagnosis and Evaluation

The diagnosis of carcinoma of the vulva is based entirely on biopsy or histologic evaluation. The type of biopsy performed is based on the size of the lesion. A lesion 1 cm or less is best approached with excisional biopsy in the office or as an outpatient. As lesions approach 2 cm, a full-thickness wedge biopsy or dermatome punch biopsy provides the best specimen. If an ulcerative lesion is present, the biopsy should be at the edge of the lesion and include the transition between normal skin and the lesion. Regardless of the type of instrument used for biopsy, full-thickness epidermis, dermis, and subcutaneous tissue should be included in the biopsy. As will be discussed later, the thickness of the lesion and depth of invasion must be evaluable in order to assess the risk of lymph-node spread. Biopsies with alligator or cervical biopsy forceps should be avoided because of the resulting crush injury of the tissue, which may hamper interpretation. If there is associated excoriation or skin disruption, several biopsies may be needed to allow the most accurate interpretation of the tissue. We prefer to use a number 15 scalpel blade for wedge biopsy or a disposable 4-mm Keyes punch for a core biopsy. If a wedge biopsy is performed, hemostasis is obtained with 3-0 or 4-0 synthetic absorbable suture. If a Keyes punch is used, the tip of a silver nitrate stick is placed in the biopsy site and pressure applied.

Histology

Squamous-cell carcinoma accounts for just over 90% of vulvar neoplasms. Malignant melanoma accounts for approximately 9% of primary vulvar malignancies.[19] A long list of rare histologic lesions of the vulva has been reported. Table 63-2 lists the malignant lesions of the vulva. As is true for all gynecologic malignancies, if questions exist pertaining to histologic interpretation, request consultation with a gynecologic pathologist. The pathology report for a vulvar biopsy, which describes carcinoma, should also include a statement regarding depth of invasion. Although not uniformly agreed on, depth of invasion is measured from the basement membrane of the adjacent, most superficial dermal papilla.[20] Depth of invasion becomes important when considering less radical treatment for superficial (early) invasive squamous-cell carcinoma, which will be addressed later.

Routes of Spread

Squamous-cell carcinoma of the vulva exhibits a predictable pattern of spread. Direct extension of the primary lesion to adjacent structures, mucosa, or skin is most common. Based on the location and size of the primary lesion, there may be spread to the vagina, urethra, or rectum. Extension of the primary lesion may also involve the mons pubis or adjacent thigh. In addition to direct extension, vulvar cancer may spread to regional lymph nodes, and late in the disease process

TABLE 63-2
HISTOLOGIC SUBTYPES OF VULVAR NEOPLASMS

Squamous-cell carcinoma
  Squamous-cell carcinoma (NOS)
  Basaloid carcinoma
  Warty (condylomatous) carcinoma
  Verrucous carcinoma
  Giant-cell carcinoma
  Spindle-cell carcinoma
  Acantholytic squamous-cell carcinoma (adenoid squamous carcinoma)
  Lymphoepithelioma-like carcinoma
  Basal-cell carcinoma
Adenocarcinoma
  Paget disease
  Bartholin gland tumor
  Breast carcinoma arising in ectopic mammary tissue
  Carcinoma of sweat gland origin
Malignant mesenchymal tumors
  Leiomyosarcoma
  Embryonal rhabdomyosarcoma (sarcoma botryoides)
  Dermatofibrosarcoma protuberans
  Malignant fibrous histiocytoma
  Epithelial sarcoma
  Malignant rhabdoid tumor
  Aggressive angiomyxoma
  Angiosarcoma and lymphangiosarcoma
  Hemangiopericytoma
  Kaposi sarcoma
  Alveolar soft-tissue sarcoma
  Malignant schwannoma
  Granular-cell tumor
  Liposarcoma
  Langerhans granulomatosis (histiocytosis X)
  Malignant melanoma
Other malignant tumors
  Yolk sac tumor (endodermal sinus tumor)
  Primary malignant lymphoma
  Merkel-cell tumor
Metastatic tumors
Tumors of the urethra

NOS = not otherwise specified.

may exhibit hematogenous spread. The lymphatic system of the vulva drains to the mons pubis and then laterally to the superficial inguinal nodes, deep femoral nodes, and then to the pelvic or iliac nodes.[21] Lymphatic drainage to the pelvic nodes from the perineum or clitoris has been demonstrated in cadavers but has occurred rarely in clinical practice.[17] Lesions that are clearly unilateral and do not involve the clitoris or perineum appear to have predictable spread patterns to the ipsilateral inguinal lymph nodes.[22-24] The pattern of spread from superficial inguinal to femoral to deep pelvic lymph nodes seems to be fairly predictable, with no cases of surgically documented pelvic-node metastases in the absence of inguinal–femoral node metastases.[17,23,25,26]

Staging and Prognostic Factors

Carcinoma of the vulva is staged according to the criteria proposed by the International Federation of Gynecology and Obstetrics (FIGO).[27] Previously staged clinically, vulvar cancer is now surgically staged. The older, clinical scheme relied on the size and extent of the primary lesion and palpation of the inguinal nodes. As a result of underestimation and over-estimation of nodal involvement, a more accurate surgical (pathologic) classification was proposed. Table 63-3 depicts the surgical/pathologic findings and the TNM classification. A combination of primary tumor characteristics, nodal involvement, and evidence of metastatic disease (TNM) constitutes the surgical/pathologic stage.

Accurate staging allows worldwide uniformity in reporting new cases. Ideally, staging should allow accurate prediction of treatment outcome and survival, and could be of benefit in the selection of specific treatments tailored to patient risk. Over the past 50 years great progress has been made in diagnosis, therapy, and outcome for carcinoma of the vulva. As accuracy and refinement of staging change so does the reporting of outcomes. For instance, many reports of the incidence of metastatic carcinoma to the inguinal

---

TABLE 63-3
FIGO STAGING OF VULVAR CANCER

FIGO Stage	TNM Classification	Clinical Characteristics
Stage 0	T_0	Carcinoma in situ
Stage I	$T_1N_0M_0$	Tumor confined to the vulva, perineum or both; 2 cm or less in greatest dimension. No nodal involvement.
Stage IA	$T_{1A}N_0M_0$	Stromal invasion no greater than 1.0 mm
Stage IB	$T_{1A}N_0M_0$	Stromal invasion greater than 1.0 mm
Stage II	$T_2N_0M_0$	Tumor confined to the vulva, perineum, or both; more than 2 cm in greatest dimension No nodal involvement.
Stage III	$T_3N_0M_0$	Tumor of any dimension with one or both of the following: (a) Adjacent spread to the lower urethra, vagina or anus; (b) Unilateral regional lymph node metastases
	$T_3N_1M_0$	
	$T_1N_1M_0$	
	$T_2N_1M_0$	
Stage IVA	$T_1N_2M_0$	Tumor of any dimension with one or more of the following: (a) Spread to upper urethra, bladder mucosa, rectal mucosa, or pelvic bone; (b) Bilateral regional node metastases
	$T_2N_2M_0$	
	$T_3N_2M_0$	
	T_4, any N, M_0	
Stage IVB	Any T, any N, M_1	Tumor of any size with distant metastases including pelvic lymph nodes

Tumor Characteristics

T_0 Carcinoma in situ
T_1 Tumor confined to the vulva, perineum or both; 2 cm or less in greatest dimension
T_{1A} Stromal invasion no greater than 1.0 mm
T_{1B} Stromal invasion greater than 1.0 mm
T_2 Tumor confined to the vulva, perineum, or both, more than 2 cm in greatest dimension
T_3 Tumor of any dimension with one or both of the following: Adjacent spread to the lower urethra, vagina, or anus
T_{4A} Tumor of any dimension with one or more of the following: Spread to upper urethra, bladder mucosa, rectal mucosa, or pelvic bone
T_{4B} Tumor of any size with distant metastases including pelvic lymph nodes

Regional Lymph-Node Status

N_x Regional lymph nodes cannot be assessed
N_0 Regional lymph nodes negative
N_1 Unilateral regional lymph node metastases
N_2 Bilateral regional lymph node metastases

Distant Metastases

M_x Presence of distant metastases cannot be assessed
M_0 No distant metastases
M_1 Distant metastases or positive pelvic lymph nodes

lymph nodes for clinical Stage I and II disease can no longer be applied to those stages. All patients currently found to have inguinal node metastases will by definition be described as having Stage III or IV disease. Therefore, the reader is cautioned to note which time frame and staging scheme is used when reviewing reports of recurrence or survival segregated by stage.

Factors proven to have prognostic significance, that is, predicting the risk of recurrence or death, have been extensively reported. These factors include lymph-node status, clinical stage, lesion size, depth of invasion, and presence of vascular space invasion.[16,28-32] The presence of metastatic carcinoma in the inguinal lymph nodes is the strongest indicator of risk of recurrent cancer, with a 90% survival in patients with negative inguinal lymph nodes, and a 37 to 57% survival in the face of positive nodes.[16,31,33] The number of involved lymph nodes seems to have an impact on the risk of recurrence and survival. In a summary from the Gynecolgic Oncology Group (GOG), patients with one or two microscopically involved inguinal lymph nodes were found to have a 75% survival, whereas patients with three or more lymph nodes involved had a 36% survival.[30] Primary lesions ≤ 2 cm in diameter have less than a 16% risk of inguinal-node metastases, whereas, lesions >2 cm in size have a 33 to 53% risk of positive inguinal nodes.[34] Table 63-4 depicts the percentage of patients by stage with positive and negative inguinal lymph nodes and survival. A striking similarity exists between the percentage of negative lymph nodes and percent survival. Survival data based on the most recent changes in FIGO staging have been retrospectively applied by the Gynecologic Oncology Group (GOG) and reported by Homesley and colleagues[37] and are depicted in Table 63-5.

The final point to be addressed pertaining to the risk of lymph-node metasases and prognosis is the lesion which has such limited depth of invasion that risk of lymph-node metastases is negligible. A distinction should be made between microinvasive carcinoma of the cervix and a comparable lesion of the vulva. Whereas invasion of ≤ 3 mm in the cervical stroma results in a minimal risk of pelvic-node metastases, the same criteria applied to the vulva results in a risk of inguinal node metastases of 5%.[20] As a result of this distinction, the International Society for the Study of Vulvar Disease (ISSVD) proposed the term early invasive cancer to include isolated lesions measuring ≤ 2 cm in diameter, with a depth of invasion of

≤ 1 mm.[38] In 1995, this definition was incorporated into the FIGO staging scheme as Stage IA. Using this definition, the risk of inguinal lymph node metastases is approximately 1%.[22,30,39-42] As will be discussed, this allows a less aggressive approach to treatment for the patient with the lowest risk of nodal metastases.

Therapy

The aggressive surgical management of carcinoma of the vulva, described in cadavers by Basset[43] and performed on patients by Taussig[44] and Way,[45] has resulted in increased survival in women suffering from the disease. This approach involves en bloc resection of the primary lesion and the vulva in association with the inguinal–femoral lymph nodes and in many cases a pelvic lymphadenectomy. Use of this technique from 1938 to 1971 resulted in a 48 to 71% 5-year survival, an operative mortality of 2.7 to 25.5%, and an average length of hospitalization of 23 to 90 days.[46] As knowledge of the disease has increased and surgical techniques have improved, survival, morbidity, and mortality have improved. As awareness of the disease increases, the number of women with earlier, less advanced disease has also increased. Over the past 15 years, reports have emphasized the possibility of individualized treatment.[47-49]

TABLE 63-4
SURVIVAL BY LYMPH NODE STATUS AND FIGO 1970 CLINICAL STAGE

Clinical Stage FIGO	Positive Nodes %	Negative Nodes %	5 Year Survival (%)
I	10	90	90
II	26	74	77
III	64	36	51
IV	88	12	18

Data from Green,[35] Iverson,[36] Hacker,[23] Rutledge,[4] Morley,[28] Benedet,[29] and Cavanagh.[33]

TABLE 63-5
1988 FIGO STAGING OF VULVAR CANCER AND SURVIVAL

Surgical Stage	Survival (%)
I	98
II	85
III	74
IV	31

Data from Homesley et al.[37]

Regardless of the technique chosen, therapy must address two points, removal of the primary lesion and treatment of the region at greatest risk for metastatic disease. Because vulvar cancers may vary from lesions less than 1 cm in size to lesions large enough to replace all recognizable parts of the vulva, one technique to remove the primary lesion should not be applied to all women. Recommendations for treatment made to individual patients must take into account lesion size, histology, knowledge of the lymphatic drainage of the site, and the overall condition of the patient. A more conservative surgical approach to the treatment of patients with vulvar cancer can result in decreased sexual dysfunction, decreased disruption of normal activity, decreased length of hospitalization, decreased risk of wound breakdown, and overall decrease in postoperative morbidity. However, a more conservative approach should not expose the patient to an increased risk of recurrence, as the mortality associated with recurrent disease to the groin is high.[23,50]

Management of the Primary Vulvar Lesion

This section will review the options of surgical management of the primary vulvar lesion. Following this section will be a description of the surgical options for management of the inguinal and pelvic lymph nodes. Application of the various options of therapy will then be described as applied to specific clinical situations. As mentioned previously, any treatment plan must address the primary lesion and the region at risk for metastatic disease. As is true for the surgical management of most malignancies treated with curative intent, a sufficient surgical margin is essential. Whereas the classical radical vulvectomy provides

Figure 63-1 A. Well lateralized vulvar carcinoma treated by wide local excision or radical hemivulvectomy. Ipsilateral lymphadenectomy through separate incision in invasion is >1 mm. B. Primary closure of both incisions. *Copyright © KUSM-Wichita Educational Technology, Wichita, KS.*

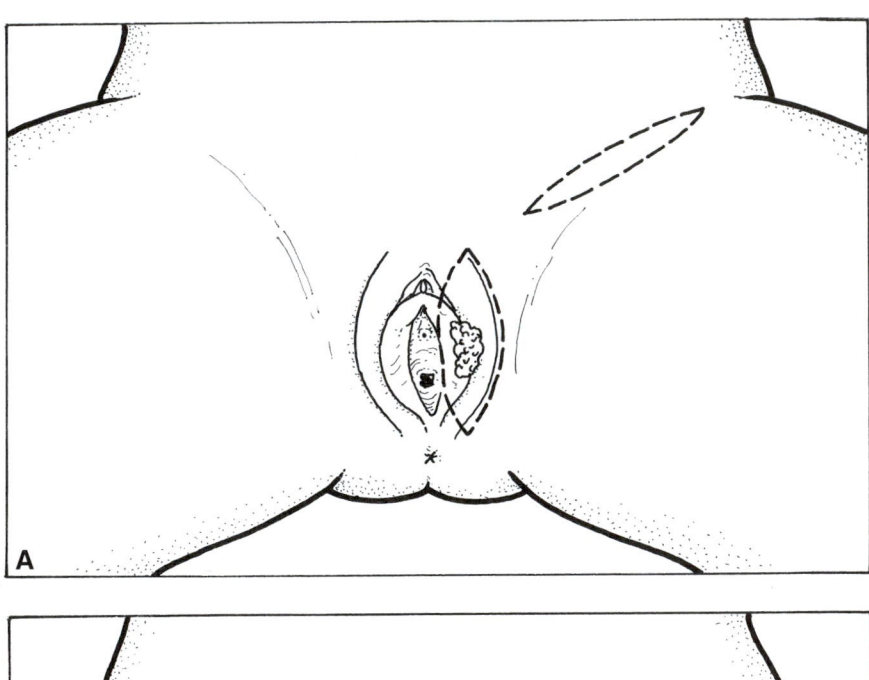

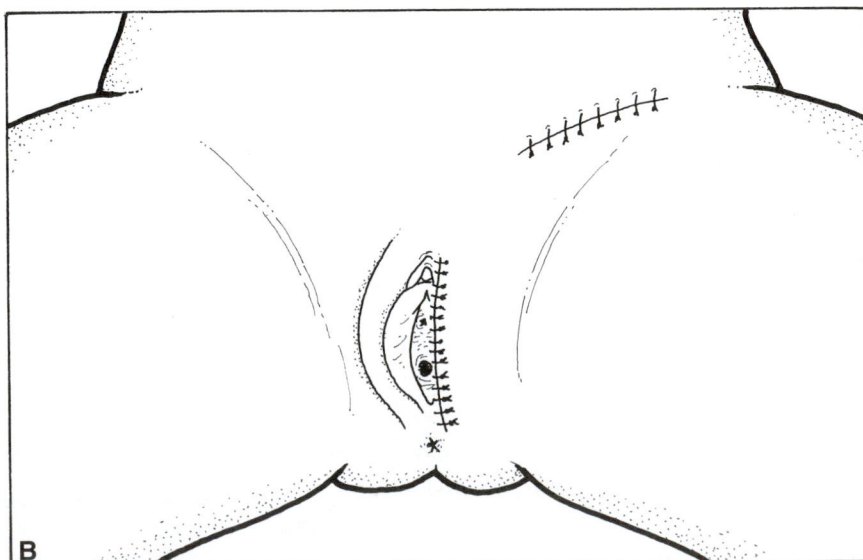

a wide lateral margin, the medial margin in most cases is not as wide. A surgical margin of 2 cm has been proposed as sufficient for clearance of T_1 and T_2 lesions.[51-53] Others have suggested that a margin of 1 cm is sufficient.[34,54] Regardless, the necessity of adequate, clear surgical margins is essential in that the presence of positive surgical margins is a significant predictor of failure to survive.[55] The options of surgical management of primary vulvar carcinoma are listed in increasing degrees of radical nature in Table 63-6. By most descriptions, wide local excision is defined as resection of a lesion with 2 cm lateral, medial, and deep margins. Radical local excision or radical hemivulvectomy implies 2-cm lateral and medial margins with deep dissection to the level of the inferior fascia of the urogenital diaphragm (Figure 63-1). In virtually all cases, primary, complete closure

of the skin defect is possible. Radical vulvectomy, originally described with en bloc dissection of the inguinal nodes, starts with a superior incision extending from the left anterior superior iliac spine (ASIS) to the mons pubis and on to the opposite anterior superior iliac spine (Figure 63-2). The inferior incision

TABLE 63-6
SURGICAL OPTIONS FOR TREATMENT OF PRIMARY VULVAR CARCINOMAS

1. Wide local excision
2. Radical hemivulvectomy, radical wide excision
3. Radical vulvectomy
4. Radical vulvectomy following preoperative chemotherapy or radiation therapy
5. Radical vulvectomy with (a) anovulvectomy, or (b) pelvic exenteration (anterior, posterior, or total)

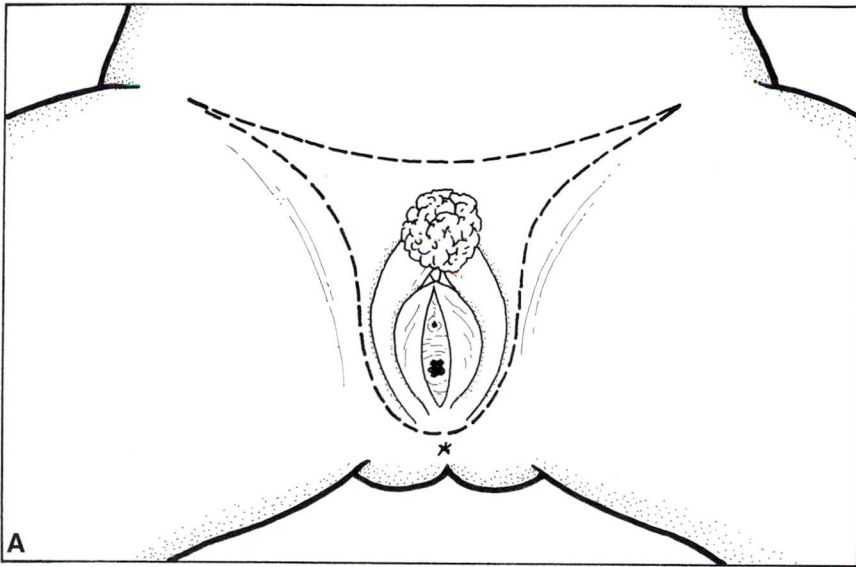

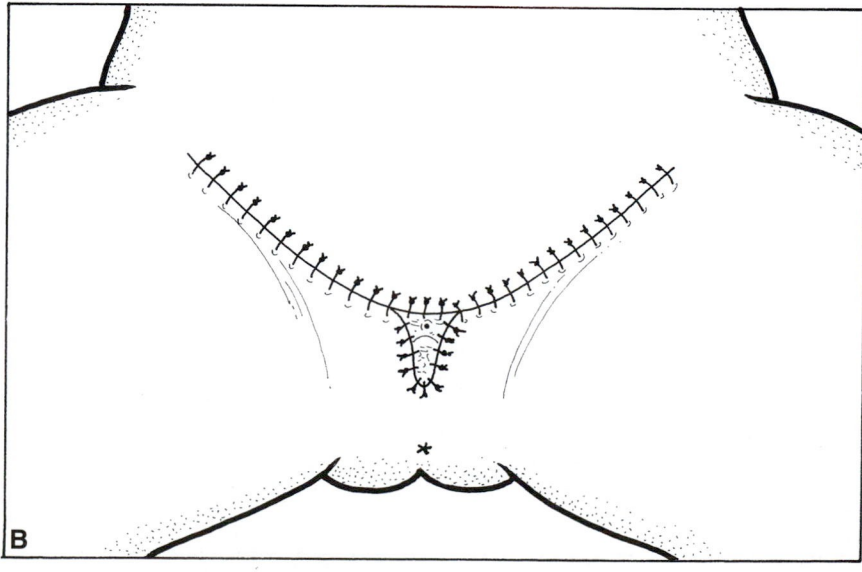

Figure 63-2 Large vulvar carcinoma, centrally located. Radical vulvectomy and bilateral inguinal lymphadenectomy (A) with primary closure (B). *Copyright © KUSM-Wichita Educational Technology, Wichita, KS.*

extends from the ASIS below and parallel to the inguinal canal across the adductor longus to the labial crural fold and inferiorly to the perineal body. The inner incision starts just superior to the urethral meatus and extends circumferentially around the vaginal mucosa. The specimen includes the entire vulvar skin and subcutaneous fat to the level of the urogenital diaphragm, the bulbocavernosus muscles, the clitoris, and may include the distal urethra if indicated. As would be expected, the complication rate associated with the traditional en bloc radical vulvectomy is quite high. The University of Michigan has published a comparison of en bloc resection of vulvar cancer and vulvectomy with separate groin incisions for the lymphadenectomy.[56] That report demonstrated a prolonged hospitalization, 64% wound breakdown rate,

20% wound infection rate, 21% incidence of cellulitis, and a 28% incidence of lymphocyst formation in women undergoing the classical en bloc radical vulvectomy (Figures 63-3 and 63-4). In addition, long-term treatment complications include lymphedema of the lower extremities, sexual dysfunction, and genital prolapse.[4,57-60]

Evaluation and Management of the Inguinal Lymph Nodes

Resection of the inguinal or inguinofemoral lymph nodes provides prognostic information and therapeutic benefit to the patient with carcinoma of the vulva. A brief description of inguinal anatomy may be of benefit, prior to a description of surgical techniques. The margins of the femoral triangle include

Figure 63-3 Large vulvar carcinoma, central, and superior location.
A. Radical vulvectomy and bilateral inguinal lymphadenectomy with preservation of perineal body.
B. Primary closure of three incisions.
Copyright © KUSM-Wichita Educational Technology, Wichita, KS.

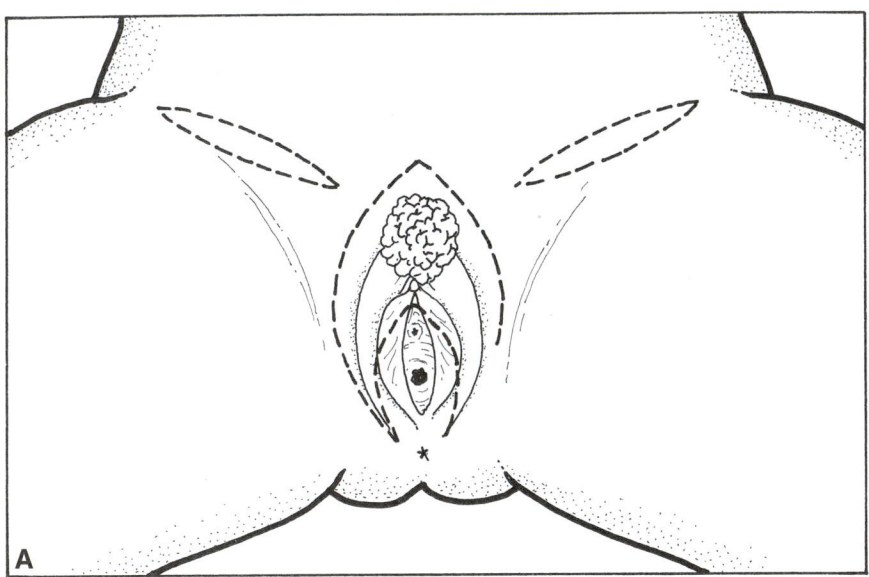

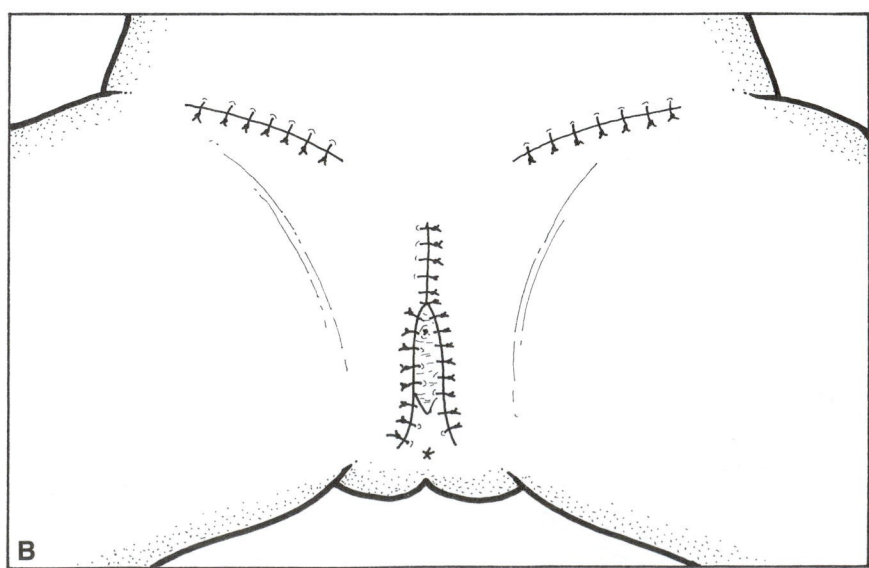

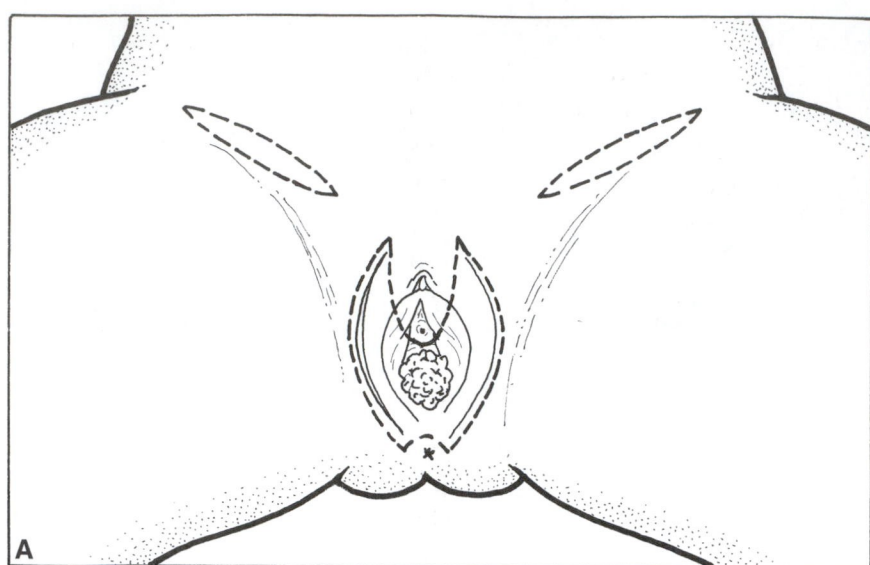

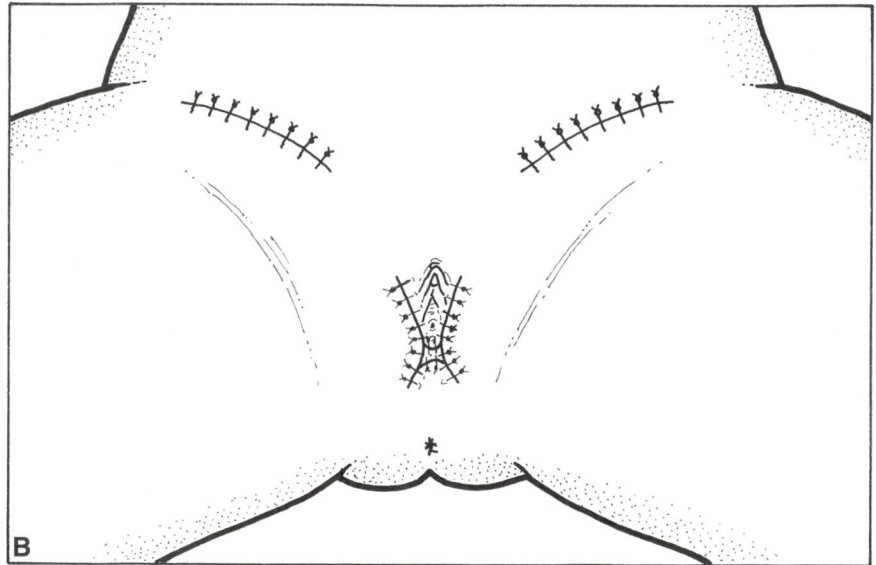

Figure 63-4 Large vulvar carcinoma, central, and inferior location. A. Radical vulvectomy and bilateral inguinal lymphadenectomy with preservation of the clitoris. B. Primary closure of three incisions. *Copyright © KUSM-Wichita Educational Technology, Wichita, KS.*

the inguinal ligament, extending from the anterior superior iliac spine to the pubic tubercle as the superior margin, the medial aspect of the sartorius muscle laterally, and the lateral aspect of the adductor longus muscle as the medial border. The floor of the inguinal triangle is composed of the pectineus, psoas, and iliacus muscles (Figure 63-5). The roof of the femoral triangle is composed of skin, subcutaneous fat, and superficial fascia, which is an extension of Scarpa's fascia of the abdominal wall. The contents of the inguinal triangle include two layers of lymph nodes. The superficial nodes are located between the cribiform fascia (an extension of the fascia lata from the sartorius muscle, which extends to the adductor longus muscle) and the superficial fascia. The superficial vessels of the groin pass through an opening in

the cribiform fascia, the fossa ovalis, to communica with the femoral artery and vein. Lymph nodes adj cent to the femoral vessels and below the cribifo fascia are called the deep inguinal or inguinofem nodes (Figures 63-6 and 63-7).

As originally described by Way, all patients d nosed with squamous carcinoma of the vulva treated with en bloc radical vulvectomy and bil inguinofemoral lymphadenectomy and pelvic phadenectomy.[61] Over time, the pelvic lymphad tomy has been performed much less frequen cause of information demonstrating absence o adenopathy unless multiple ipsilateral inguina are positive.[23-25] In addition, a GOG study strated a survival advantage and reduced gro rence in patients with positive groin nodes

Figure 63-5 Floor of the inguinal triangle. Borders include inguinal ligament, sartolius muscle, and adductor longus muscle. *Copyright © KUSM-Wichita Educational Technology, Wichita, KS.*

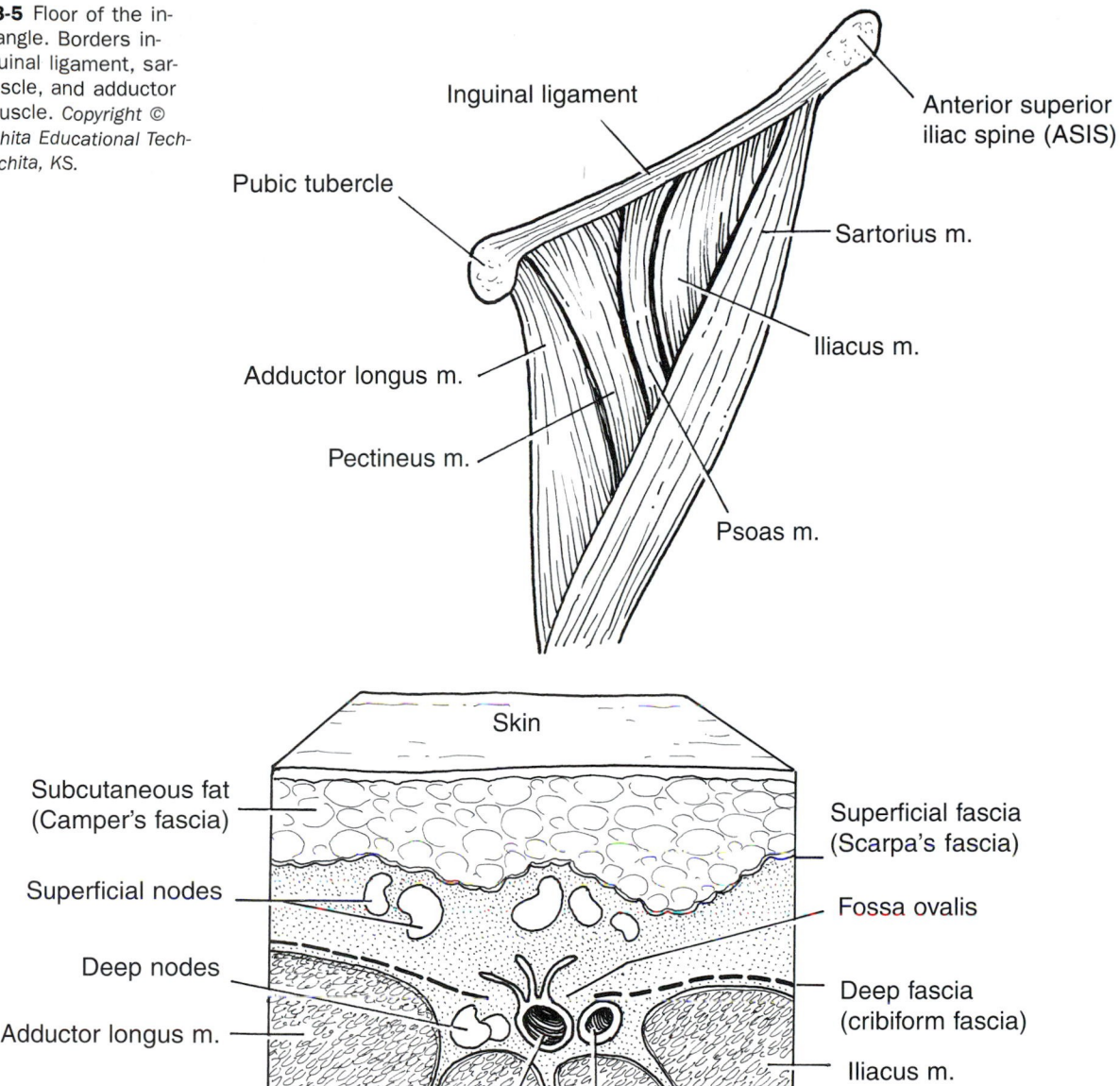

Figure 63-5 labels: Inguinal ligament · Anterior superior iliac spine (ASIS) · Pubic tubercle · Sartorius m. · Iliacus m. · Adductor longus m. · Pectineus m. · Psoas m.

Figure 63-6 labels: Skin · Subcutaneous fat (Camper's fascia) · Superficial fascia (Scarpa's fascia) · Superficial nodes · Fossa ovalis · Deep nodes · Deep fascia (cribiform fascia) · Adductor longus m. · Iliacus m. · Pectineus m. · Psoas m. · Femoral v. · Femoral a.

Figure 63-6 Roof of the femoral triangle includes skin, subcutaneous fat, and Scarpa's (superficial) fascia. Contents of the femoral triangle include vessels and nodes. Nodes below Scarpa's fascia and above the cribiform fascia are "superficial." Nodes below the cribiform fascia are considered "deep" nodes. *Copyright © KUSM-Wichita Educational Technology, Wichita, KS.*

pelvic and inguinal radiation as compared with those undergoing pelvic lymphadenectomy.[62] Primary radiation therapy of the groin has been proposed in place of groin dissection for patients without suspicious nodes. A GOG study designed to compare primary groin radiation with groin dissection in patients without suspicious nodes was closed early as a result of an unacceptable number of groin recurrences in the radiation group.[63] As will be discussed later, groin and

pelvic radiation have a role in preoperative and postoperative treatment of high-risk patients.

Three additional points must be addressed pertaining to the evaluation and treatment of inguinal lymph nodes. The first point is the use of separate groin incisions for the inguinal lymphadenectomy. As a result of high wound breakdown rates associated with en bloc, vulva, and groin dissection, several investigators have advocated the use of separate groin

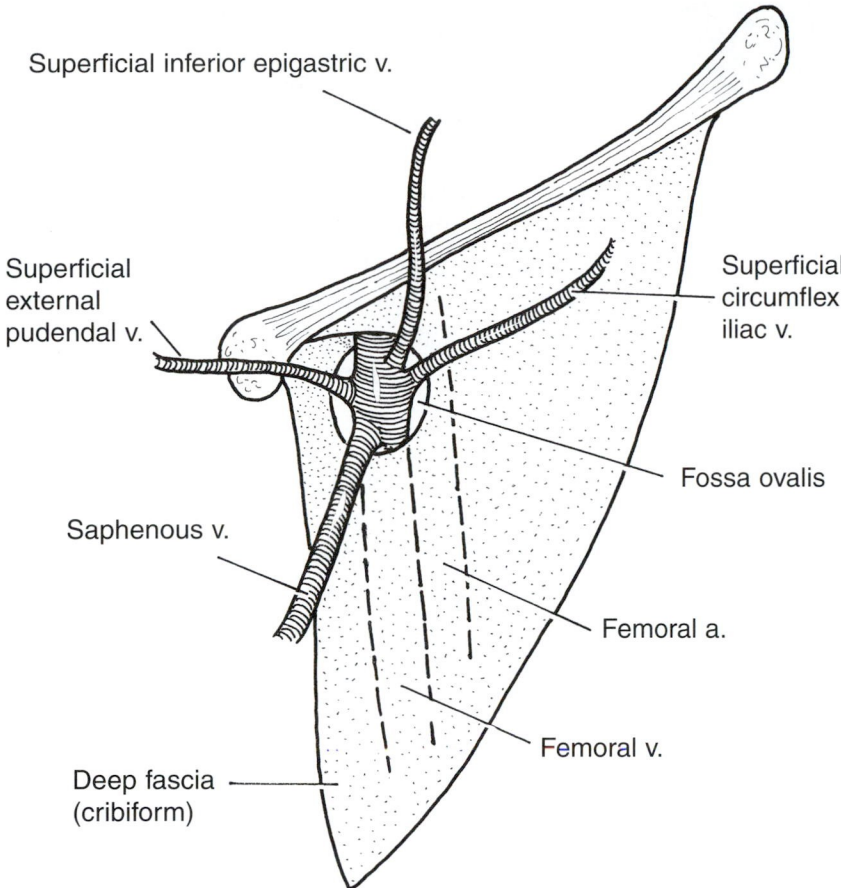

Superficial inferior epigastric v.

Superficial external pudendal v.

Saphenous v.

Deep fascia (cribiform)

Superficial circumflex iliac v.

Fossa ovalis

Femoral a.

Femoral v.

Figure 63-7 Cribiform or deep fascia with perforating vessels draining to the femoral vein, passing through the fossa ovalis. *Copyright © KUSM-Wichita Educational Technology, Wichita, KS.*

incisions for the inguinal lymphadenectomy[49,64-67] (see Figure 63-3). By leaving an intervening bridge of normal skin between the vulvectomy site and groin incision, the number of patients with groin incision breakdown has been greatly reduced.[66] The risk of recurrence within the skin bridge is low and is associated with clinically positive inguinal nodes.[57,66,68] The second point to address pertaining to inguinal lymphadenectomy for vulvar cancer relates to the need for unilateral versus bilateral node dissection. Cadaver dissection, in addition to historical surgical data, suggests a predictable lymphatic drainage from clearly lateralized lesions of the vulva to the ipsilateral groin nodes.[21-24] Spread to contralateral nodes appears to occur only after ipsilateral nodes are involved. This information has led to the use of unilateral inguinal lymphadenectomy for selected patients with laterally located vulvar lesions[47,52,57,69,70] (see Figure 63-1). Patients with midline lesions or lesions involving the labia minora are best treated with bilateral inguinal–node dissections.

The next point pertaining to inguinal-node assessment and therapy involves the question of superficial

inguinal lymphadenectomy versus complete, superficial, and deep inguinofemoral lymphadenectomy. As mentioned previously, the classical en bloc radical vulvectomy and bilateral inguinofemoral lymphadenectomy included removal of all superficial inguinal lymph nodes and removal of the cribiform fascia with full exposure and dissection of the femoral artery and vein, and transposition of the sartorius muscle over the femoral vessels. In addition to increasing the risk of lymphedema of the lower extremity, the risk of vascular injury is increased with this approach. DiSaia and colleagues described superficial inguinal lymphadenectomy as an alternate approach to early cancer of the vulva.[47] The basis for the use of superficial lymphadenectomy was the review of 79 patients undergoing radical vulvectomy and bilateral, full inguinal lymphadenectomy. No patient was found to have positive femoral nodes in the absence of negative superficial nodes. As a result of this pathology review, 18 patients with invasive lesions ≤1 cm in diameter, confined to the vulva or perineum, and invasion limited to ≤5 mm, were treated by wide local excision of the primary lesion and superficial lymphadenectomy.

1. No therapy
2. Ipsilateral superficial inguinal node dissection (separate incision)
3. Ipsilateral superficial inguinal and deep femoral node dissection (separate incision or en bloc dissection with vulvar lesion)
4. Bilateral superficial inguinal node dissection (separate incisions)
5. Bilateral superficial inguinal and deep femoral node dissection (separate incision or en bloc dissection with vulvar lesion)
6. Unilateral or bilateral superficial inguinal, deep femoral, and pelvic lymphadenectomy
7. Any of the above with postoperative radiation therapy

Subsequent to this report, deep femoral nodal metastases in the absence of superficial nodal involvement had been reported in a few patients.[23,71,72] In addition, 5% of patients reported by Burke et al.[52] and 6% of patients treated in a GOG study reported by Stehman et al.[42] with superficial lymphadenectomy developed recurrence in the dissected groins. Although it appears the risk of recurrence following superficial inguinal lymphadenectomy is low, a change in technique proposed by the group from the University of Turin may resolve the question of superficial versus superficial and deep lymphadenectomy.[73,74] In a study of 50 female cadavers, and 100 groin dissections, Borgno and colleagues found that all deep femoral nodes, ranging from one to four in number, were located within the opening of the fossa ovalis at the junction of the great saphenous and femoral veins.[73] Michelleti and colleagues demonstrated the same findings in 42 patients treated surgically for carcinoma of the vulva.[74] As mentioned previously, the adequacy of groin-node dissection in the management of vulvar carcinoma is extremely important given the dismal outcome associated with groin recurrences. Table 63-7 lists the options of inguinal-node management in increasing radicality.

The final point to address pertaining to the inguinal lymph nodes is the omission of the lymphadenectomy. As mentioned in the histology section, the lesion ≤2 cm in diameter with ≤1 mm of invasion carries a risk of metastasis to the inguinal lymph nodes of 1% or less.[22,36,48,75] This information would support omitting the groin-node dissection in those patients. In order to assess the possibility of groin radiation in lieu of groin dissection for patients with palpably negative groin nodes, the GOG compared the two methods in a randomized trial. Patients with T_1, T_2, or T_3 tumors with clinically negative nodes were randomized to node dissection versus radiation therapy. The trial was closed early as a result of an unacceptable number of recurrences in the radiation arm.[63] On occasion, very elderly patients with procedure-limiting medical problems or short life expectancy will undergo vulvectomy for hygiene purposes, with the groin dissection omitted.

Combination Therapy

As is true of carcinoma of the cervix, combination therapy with preoperative or postoperative radiation therapy, preoperative chemotherapy, or combination chemoradiation have been reported in the management of vulvar carcinoma. Almost by definition, combination therapy implies a patient at high risk for failure with conventional treatment, or who would otherwise require ultraradical surgical therapy such as exenteration or distal proctectomy. Boronow and colleagues reported the results of therapy and complications in 48 patients with advanced carcinoma of the vulva treated with preoperative radiation therapy.[76] Seventeen patients in that series were found to have no residual carcinoma in the final surgical specimen. Others have reported comparable results, with complication rates ranging from 4 to 23%.[22,77,78] These patients represent a highly selected group of women treated with a more limited resection following radiation therapy.

Patients with two or more microscopically positive inguinal lymph nodes appear to benefit from postoperative radiation to the groin and pelvis.[62] The GOG study reported by Homesley et al.[62] compared pelvic lymphadenectomy to inguinal and pelvic radiation therapy in patients with positive inguinal nodes. A survival advantage was demonstrated for the radiation group; however, the recurrence rate was primarily reduced in the inguinal area, not the pelvis. Patients with only one microscopically involved inguinal node appear to do well with surgical treatment alone.[23,62]

Combination chemotherapy and radiation therapy has been reported to provide excellent reduction in tumor size in large, locally advanced vulvar cancers that would otherwise have been inoperable or required exenterative surgery. Berek and colleagues reported good local control in 10 of 12 patients with Stage III and IV disease with the combination of cisplatin, 5-fluorouracil, and radiation therapy.[79] Eifel and colleagues from M.D. Anderson Cancer Center reported on 12 patients with advanced vulvar cancer treated with prolonged infusion of cisplatin and 5-fluorouracil, and concomitant radiation therapy. Four of eight patients who underwent vulvar resection at the completion of chemoradiation had no residual tumor.[80] The impact of combination therapy on long-term survival is still unclear.

Summary of Treatment Options

Although all possible clinical presentations cannot be addressed in this chapter, the following represent the most common presentation of patients with squamous-cell carcinoma of the vulva and reasonable approaches to therapy. For the purposes of the following summary, these definitions apply.

Limited lesion: Any lesion not involving the urethra or anal sphincter that is amenable to excision with a 1- to 2-cm margin in all directions.

Extensive lesion: Any lesion not amenable to excision without resection of portions of the urethra, anal sphincter, or anus. A lesion of such size that primary closure could not be accomplished after excision.

Lateral lesion: A lesion of any size that is amenable to excision with a 1- to 2-cm medial margin, while preserving the clitoris, urethra, and anus.

Nonsuspicious lymph nodes: Either nonpalpable, or smooth, small, mobile nodes. Does not imply absence of microscopic disease.

Abnormal lymph nodes: Enlarged, firm lymph nodes. Fixed, matted, or ulcerated lymph nodes.

SMALL LESION, ≤2 CM, WITH INVASION OF LESS THAN OR EQUAL TO 1 MM. Wide local excision or modified radical vulvectomy with 1- to 2-cm margins. Omit groin dissection.

LIMITED VULVAR LESION OF ANY SIZE WITH INVASION >1 MM, LATERALLY LOCATED, WITH NONSUSPICIOUS NODES, OR LYMPH NODES THAT ARE NOT ULCERATED OR FIXED. Wide local excision or modified or radical hemivulvectomy with 1- to 2-cm margins. Ipsilateral inguinal lymphadenectomy, including superficial inguinal lymphadenectomy, or superficial and deep inguinal lymphadenectomy, without removing the cribiform fascia (surgeon preference).

Primary lesion and inguinal nodes are removed with separate incisions. If any nodes are positive, a contralateral lymphadenectomy is performed. If two or more nodes are positive, postoperative radiation is given to both groins and the pelvic nodes.

LIMITED VULVAR LESION OF ANY SIZE WITH INVASION >1 MM, INVOLVING CLITORIS, MEDIAL LABIA MINORA, OR PERINEAL BODY, WITH NONSUSPICIOUS NODES. Radical wide excision, or modified radical vulvectomy with 1- to 2-cm margins. Bilateral, superficial, or superficial and deep inguinal lymphadenectomy without removing the cribiform fascia (surgeon preference). Primary lesion and inguinal nodes are removed through separate incisions. If two or more nodes are positive, postoperative radiation is given to both groins and pelvic nodes.

EXTENSIVE LESION WITH NONSUSPICIOUS NODES. Bilateral superficial and deep inguinal lymphadenectomy without removing the cribiform fascia. Radiation therapy or chemoradiation is proposed for reducing the size of the primary lesion. If two or more inguinal nodes are positive, include groins and pelvic nodes in radiation therapy port. Following radiation therapy or chemoradiation, resect any residual primary lesion. This approach may allow preservation of the urethra or anal sphincter if involved.

EXTENSIVE LESION WITH ABNORMAL NODES THAT ARE ULCERATED OR FIXED IN POSITION. Radiation therapy, or chemoradiation to vulva and both groins. Follow with bilateral inguinal lymphadenectomy and resection of any residual disease involving the vulva. This approach may allow preservation of the urethra and anal sphincter if involved.

Recurrent Vulvar Cancer

The factors most likely to predict survival for patients treated for invasive carcinoma of the vulva include lesion size, presence of positive nodes, and lymphatic vascular space involvement.[55] Sites of recurrent disease can be divided into local or vulvar, inguinal, or distant. Approximately 50% of patients experiencing an isolated vulvar recurrence will be cured with surgical therapy.[17,50] Few, if any, patients with groin, pelvic, or distant recurrence will be cured. Combinations of surgery, radiation therapy, and chemotherapy may be of benefit for palliative treatment of symptoms.

Paget Disease of the Vulva

Extramammary Paget disease of the vulva is a rare condition characterized histologically as intraepithelial proliferation of atypical gland-type cells. These cells seem to arise from multipotential cells derived from the stratum germinativum of the epidermis. Vulvar pruritus and burning are the most common presenting symptoms. The examination is characterized by thickened epithelium, hyperemia, excoriation, and in many cases a thin white exudate on the surface resembling "cake icing." The diagnosis is made by full-thickness punch biopsy. Although rare, invasive Paget disease with positive inguinal nodes has been reported.[81,82] Perhaps more common is the presence of an associated adenocarcinoma of sweat gland origin described in 14 to 19% of patients.[82,83] However, Bergen et al.[85] found no associated carcinomas in 14 patients, and Feuer et al.[82] identified one patient in 19 reported with extramammary Paget disease. An associated risk of metachronous carcinomas (breast, cervix, basal cell of skin, esophagus) at other sites has been reported to be present in 26 to 43% of patients.[82,84,86] The treatment of Paget disease of the vulva is surgical. Resections ranging from wide local excision to radical vulvectomy have been applied. All skin appendages and hair follicles must be included, which suggests a specimen depth of 4 to 5 mm. Paget disease of the vulva is not uncommonly associated with positive margins and increased risk of recurrence. In an effort to obtain clear margins at the time of surgery, extensive frozen-section evaluation or the use of fluorescein dye has been proposed.[85,87,88] In spite of these efforts and others, recurrent Paget disease is not uncommon. In a report of 14 patients with Paget disease of the vulva, Fishman and colleagues found 6 of 17 (35%) surgical specimens with clinically negative margins to be microscopically positive. In contrast, 3 of 8 (38%) specimens negative on frozen section were found to have positive margins on permanent section, suggesting a lack of benefit for frozen section evaluation.[89] The high recurrence rate may be explained by an elegant study reported by Gunn and Gallagher, histologically mapping surgical specimens with Paget disease.[90] Those investigators found irregular borders and multifocal lesions in all four specimens. Wide local excision with attempts to obtain negative margins would appear to be the best approach to the patient with extramammary Paget disease of the vulva. Any recurrences are likewise treated by wide excision.

Vulvar Melanoma

Malignant melanoma is the second most common invasive neoplasm of the vulva, accounting for 10% or less of vulvar neoplasms.[19] Data from the Surveillance, Epidemiology, and End Results (SEER) study, reported by Weinstock, suggest an incidence of vulvar melanoma in the United States of 0.108 in 100,000 women per year.[91] This accounts for 1.3% of all melanomas in women. Occurring more often in white women than in black women, the incidence increases with advancing age. The median age for vulvar melanoma was 66 years. Similar data and age incidence were reported by Ragnarsson-Olding et al. from Sweden.[92] The most common presenting symptoms include vulvar irritation, a vulvar mass, and bleeding. The diagnosis is made by excisional biopsy or full-thickness dermatome punch biopsy. Histologically, vulvar melanoma subtypes include superficial spreading melanoma, nodular melanoma, and acral lentiginous melanoma.

Historically, patients with vulvar melanoma have been treated by radical vulvectomy and inguinal lymphadenectomy. As the treatment of squamous-cell carcinoma of the vulva has tended to become less radical and more individualized, the treatment of vulvar melanoma has followed. Likewise as surgical treatment of cutaneous melanomas in other parts of the body have become more conservative, the treatment of vulvar melanomas has changed. Reports from the Royal Marsden Hospital, Roswell Park Memorial Institute, Memorial Sloan-Kettering Cancer Institute, the Netherlands Cancer Institute, and the Gynecologic Oncology Group have failed to identify a survival advantage of radical vulvectomy over wide local excision with a 2-cm margin.[93-97]

Multiple staging schemes have been applied to melanomas to aid in therapy decisions and to predict outcome. The FIGO/TNM staging system has been described earlier and was presented in Table 63-2. As tumor thickness and depth of invasion are better predictors of lymph node spread, microstaging systems have been proposed by Clark, Breslow, and Chung.[19,98,99] The Clark scheme depends on cutaneous, anatomic landmarks, whereas the Breslow system is based on depth of invasion. Because the subepithelial structures of the labia lack a well-defined papillary dermis, Chung et al.[19] proposed a modification of the Breslow system. Table 63-8 represents a comparison of the three microstaging systems. Trimble and colleagues reported on 80 patients,

TABLE 63-8
MICROSTAGING SYSTEMS OF MELANOMA OF THE VULVA

Clark System	Levels of Invasion	Breslow System	Depth of Invasion	Chung System	Levels of Invasion
I	In situ lesions; confined to the epithelium	I	≤0.75 mm	I	Confined to the epithelium
II	Lesion penetrates the basement membrane and extends into the papillary dermis	II	0.76–1.50 mm	II	Penetrates the basement membrane and extends into dermis or lamina propria to ≤1 mm from the granular layer or its estimated position
III	Lesion involves the papillary dermis and invades the reticular dermis	III	1.51–2.26 mm	III	Penetrates between 1 and 2 mm into subepithelial tissue
IV	Invades the deep reticular dermis	IV	2.27–3.0 mm	IV	Invasion beyond 2 mm, but not into underlying fat
V	Invades the subcutaneous adipose tissue	V	>3.0 mm	V	Invasion of subcutaneous adipose tissue

From Clark et al.,[98] Breslow,[99] and Chung et al.[19]

expanding on the original series by Chung, and found the Chung microstaging system more predictive of survival than the Breslow system.[95] Reporting a GOG study, Phillips found the AJCC (American Joint Committee on Cancer) staging system to be the only independent prognostic factor in 71 patients treated for vulvar melanoma.[97] The AJCC staging system is presented in Table 63-9. On the basis of available data, the AJCC staging system would seem to be the best system currently available for staging vulvar melanoma.

The role of lymphadenectomy in the management of vulvar melanoma is as much in question as it is with cutaneous melanomas found in other parts of the body. Depth of invasion is an accurate predictor of risk for nodal metastases. The presence of nodal metastases portends poorly for survival. Patients with cutaneous lesions <0.76 mm in depth have a very low risk of nodal metastases and would not be expected to benefit from lymphadenectomy. Likewise, patients with lesions >4.0 mm of invasion have a high risk of nodal disease and recurrence and are expected to benefit little from a lymphadenectomy. The patient with a primary lesion of 0.76 to 4.0 mm in depth may receive benefit from an elective regional-lymph-node dissection.[101] In the only prospective study to look at type of resection and lymphadenectomy, Phillips and colleagues could come to no conclusion pertaining to the advantage of lymphadenectomy when comparing lymphadenectomy with positive nodes to lymphadenectomy with negative nodes and no lymphadenectomy.[97]

Prospective trials of adjuvant therapy in women with vulvar melanoma at high risk for recurrence are not available. Relapse-free interval has been prolonged with the use of interferon alfa in high-risk patients with cutaneous melanoma.[102] Patients with high-risk vulvar melanoma should be encouraged to participate in clinical trials if available.

Posttreatment Surveillance of Vulvar Neoplasms

Posttreatment surveillance of patients with vulvar carcinoma is directed toward the early detection of local recurrences. A number of patients found to have small local recurrences involving the vulva may be saved with further surgery. Recurrent disease that is somewhat larger may be amenable to combination therapy with chemotherapy, radiation, and surgery. Frequent use of expensive radiologic tests such as computed tomography or magnetic resonance imaging in the asymptomatic patient has little use in the follow-up

TABLE 63-9
AMERICAN JOINT COMMITTEE ON CANCER STAGING FOR MELANOMA

Stage	Description
IA	Primary melanoma <0.75 mm thick and/or Clark level II (N0,M0)
IB	Primary melanoma 0.75–1.50 mm thick and/or Clark level III
IIA	Primary melanoma 1.51–4.0 mm thick and/or Clark level IV
IIB	Primary melanoma >4.0 mm thick and/or Clark level V
III	Regional lymph node and/or in-transit metastases (any T,N1–2,M0)
IV	Systemic metastases (any T, any N, M1)

of these patients. The identification of distant disease will result in symptomatic or palliative therapy. Because of the association between vulvar cancer and other premalignant and malignant lesions of the genital tract, cytologic screening of the cervix and vagina on a regular basis is suggested.

VAGINAL CANCER

Comprising 1.5 to 3.1% of all genital-tract malignancies, primary vaginal cancer is the least common gynecologic malignancy.[103-106] Malignancy involving the vagina is more common than the percentage stated above. As many as 90% of invasive malignancies involving the vagina are metastatic in nature, with spread from the cervix, uterus, vulva, or trophoblastic disease.[107] By convention, if an invasive carcinoma of the vagina involves the cervical portio it is classified as cervical cancer. Likewise, lesions involving the vagina and vulva are described as vulvar in origin. Primary carcinoma of the rectum, colon, bladder, or urethra may invade the vagina. If a patient has been treated for invasive carcinoma of the cervix within 5 years of the diagnosis of vaginal cancer, the lesion is considered to be recurrent cervical cancer rather than primary vaginal cancer.

Symptoms and Presentation

Primary vaginal cancer is predominantly a disease of postmenopausal women. The mean age at diagnosis is approximately 60 years.[104,106,108] However, 11 to 25% of patients are 50 years of age or younger.[106,108,109] Signs and symptoms at diagnosis include vaginal bleeding, vaginal discharge, and a palpable mass.[105,106,110] Eddy and Ball and their colleagues reported on 91 patients with primary vaginal cancer and found a mean duration of symptoms of 3 months.[104,106] As many as 25% of women diagnosed with primary carcinoma of the vagina have a history of previous therapy for cervical cancer, or a history of hysterectomy for carcinoma in situ of the cervix in the distant past.[105,106]

Causes

Because of the rarity of primary vaginal cancer, large-scale epidemiologic studies are unlikely. Multiple factors have been associated with the development of vaginal cancer, however, true cause and effect factors have not been identified. An excellent review of the role of infectious and environmental factors in the development of vaginal cancer was published by Marino in 1991.[111] A strong association between human papillomavirus (HPV), diethylstilbestrol (DES), immunosuppressive therapy, chronic vaginal irritation (i.e., pessary use), irradiation for cervical cancer, and the subsequent development of vaginal cancer is described. Similarities between squamous-cell carcinoma of the cervix and primary vaginal cancer help explain some or most of these associated factors. Embryologic development of the uterus, cervix, and upper two-thirds of the vagina from the same müllerian mesoderm would intuitively suggest a shared predisposition for malignant conversion. This accounts for the "field" theory of simultaneous malignant conversion of multiple locations in the genital tract. The role of HPV as a cocarcinogen in the development of cervical cancer has also been proposed for squamous lesions of the vagina.[112-114] A history of hysterectomy for any reason in women subsequently diagnosed with primary squamous-cell carcinoma of the vagina has been reported in 32 to 59% of patients.[103,106,115] Herman and colleagues found that when age and prior cervical disease are controlled for, there is no increased risk of vaginal cancer developing in women who have had a hysterectomy.[116] Patients previously treated for dysplasia of the genital tract do appear to have a greater risk for dysplasia or cancer of the vagina.[117-119]

Diagnosis

Punch biopsy of visible lesions or colposcopically directed biopsy of subclinical lesions is used to diagnose carcinoma of the vagina. Regardless of how convincing a Pap smear report is, a biopsy confirming the diagnosis histologically is required. The great majority of vaginal malignancies are squamous-cell carcinomas. As will be discussed later, clear-cell adenocarcinoma related to DES exposure is very rare. The frequency of various histology types is depicted in Table 63-10. The most common location of primary vaginal cancer at diagnosis is the upper third to half of the vagina.[106,109,120] The gross appearance of the primary lesion may range from exophytic to infiltrating to ulcerating. The patient referred for evaluation of a high-grade lesion on Pap test with the findings of a normal cervix on colposcopy should have thorough evaluation of the entire length of the vagina.

TABLE 63-10
PRIMARY VAGINAL CANCER HISTOLOGY

	Benedet[109]	Ball[104]	Rubin[108]	Eddy[106]	Al-Kurdi[110]
Squamous	86%	86%	80.8%	84%	84%
Adenocarcinoma	14%	14%	9.6%	13%	5%
(clear-cell)		(2%)			(2%)
Sarcoma			6.4%		9%
Melanoma			3.2%		2%
Other				3%	

The anterior or posterior blade of the vaginal speculum may hide an early vaginal cancer. Peters and colleagues defined microinvasive carcinoma of the vagina as <2.5 mm of invasion from the surface epithelium, no lymph–vascular space involvement, diagnosed by partial or total vaginectomy, and arising within a field of carcinoma in situ.[121] Six patients with superficially invasive carcinoma of the vagina meeting these criteria were treated surgically without evidence of recurrence. In a report of six patients treated similarly, with the same criteria, Eddy and colleagues reported one recurrence and cancer-related death.[122] Given the small number of cases reported, firm recommendations regarding the diagnosis and management of minimally invasive carcinoma of the vagina cannot be made at this time.

Staging

Cancer of the vagina is staged clinically in a manner similar to cervical cancer. The International Federation of Gynecology and Obstetrics (FIGO) staging system is applied to patients with primary carcinoma of the vagina. Examination under anesthesia, chest x-ray, cystoscopy, sigmoidoscopy, intravenous pyelogram, and barium enema may be included as components of the clinical staging. Table 63-11 describes the FIGO staging system. Figures 63-8 through 63-11 illustrate the four stages. A modification of the FIGO scheme has been proposed by Perez and colleagues to subdivide Stage II.[123] This modification would classify Stage IIA as carcinoma extending into the submucosal area of the vagina but not into the true paracolpium. Stage IIB would significantly involve the paracolpium but not extend to the pelvic wall. This subclassification is associated with worsened survival for patients with Stage IIB disease. Surgical staging, specifically extraperitoneal lymphadenectomy, may more accurately describe extent of disease and guide therapy, but improved survival as a result of that staging has not been proven. Clinical staging reflects the dominant pattern of spread, which is direct extension through mucosa into adjacent structures. Lymphatic and vascular spread also occur. Lesions arising in the upper two-thirds of the vagina are more likely to demonstrate spread to the pelvic lymph nodes, similar to cervical cancer. Lesions of the lower one-third of the vagina may metastasize to the inguinal lymph nodes, similar to vulvar cancer. Hematogenous spread accounts for distant metastases. Table 63-12 depicts the distribution of vaginal cancer by stage.

(Text continues on page 1258.)

TABLE 63-11
FIGO STAGING OF VAGINAL CANCER

Stage 0   Carcinoma in situ, intraepithelial carcinoma
Stage I   Carcinoma is limited to the vaginal wall
Stage II   Carcinoma has involved the subvaginal tissue but has not extended to the pelvic wall
Stage III   Carcinoma has extended onto the pelvic wall
Stage IV   Carcinoma has extended beyond the true pelvis or has involved the mucosa of the bladder or rectum; bullous edema or tumor bulge into the bladder or rectum is not acceptable evidence of invasion of these organs
Stage IVa   Spread of the carcinoma to adjacent organs and/or direct extension beyond the true pelvis
Stage IVb   Spread of carcinoma to distant organs

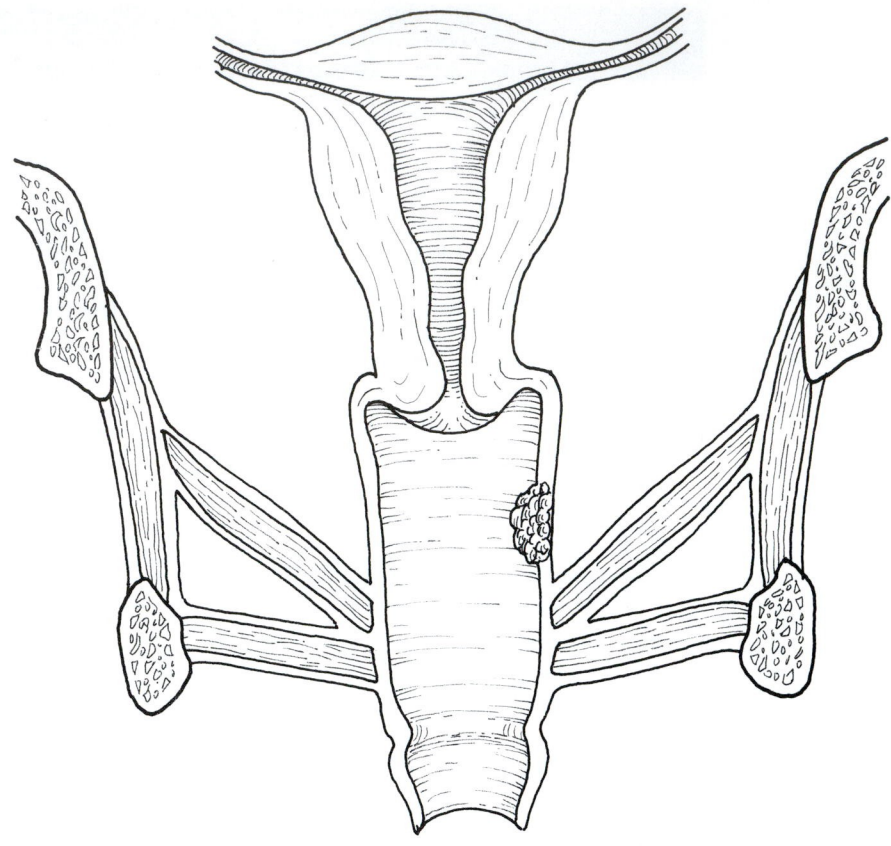

Figure 63-8 Stage I carcinoma of the vagina. Carcinoma limited to the vaginal wall. *Copyright © KUSM-Wichita Educational Technology, Wichita, KS.*

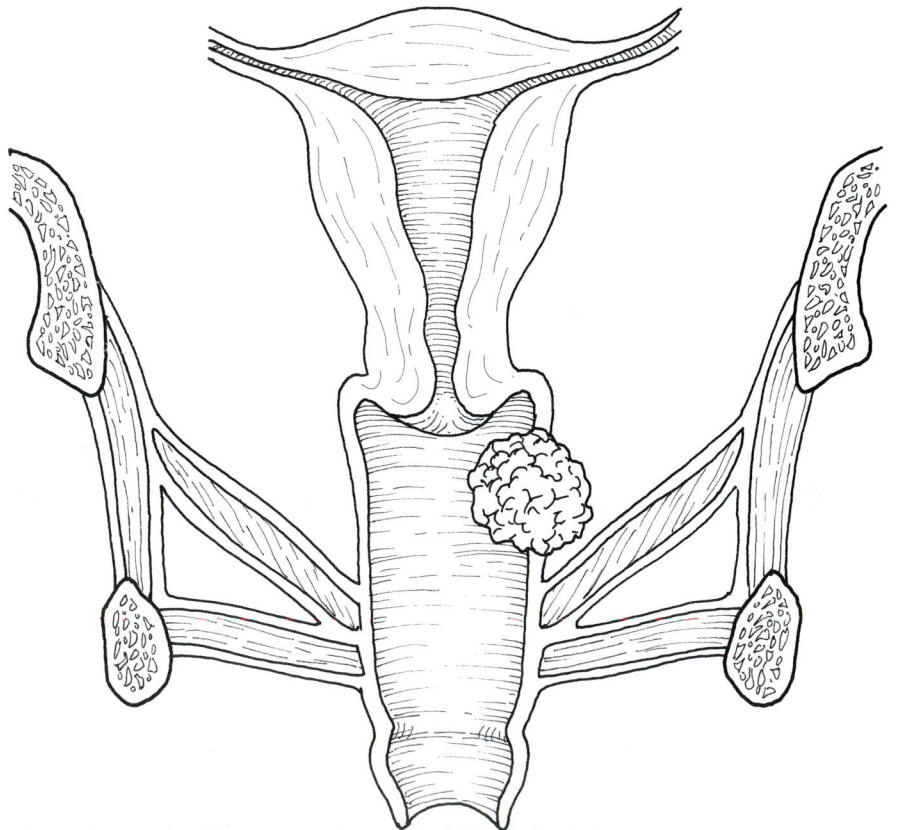

Figure 63-9 Stage II carcinoma of the vagina. Carcinoma has involved the subvaginal tissue but has not extended to the pelvic wall. *Copyright © KUSM-Wichita Educational Technology, Wichita, KS.*

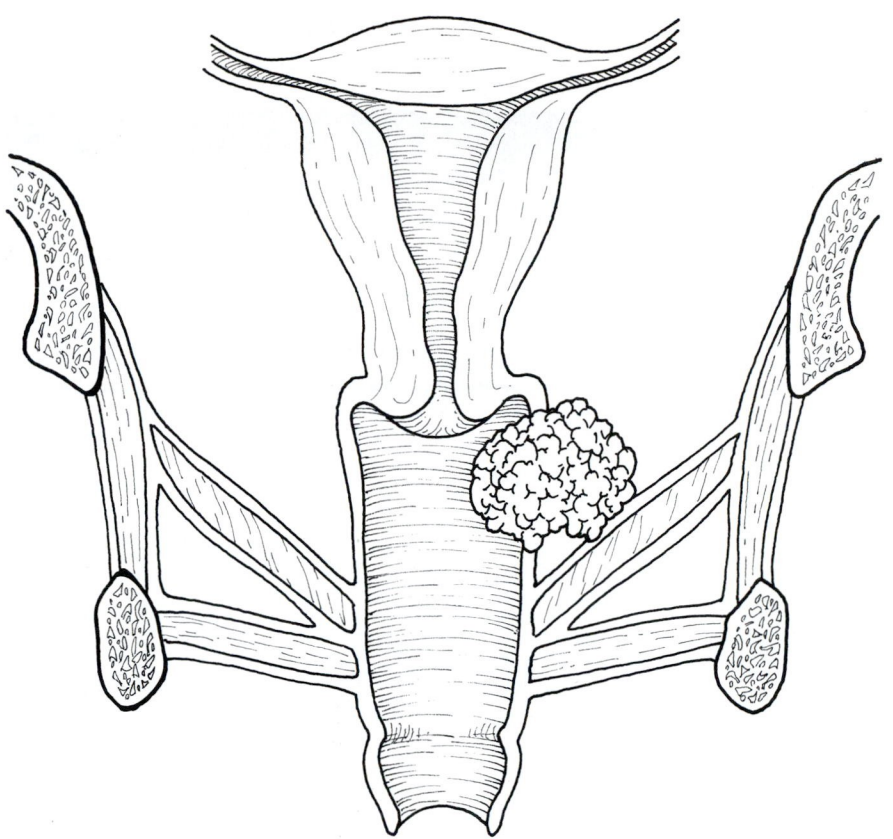

Figure 63-10 Stage III carcinoma of the vagina. Carcinoma has extended to the pelvic wall. *Copyright © KUSM-Wichita Educational Technology, Wichita, KS.*

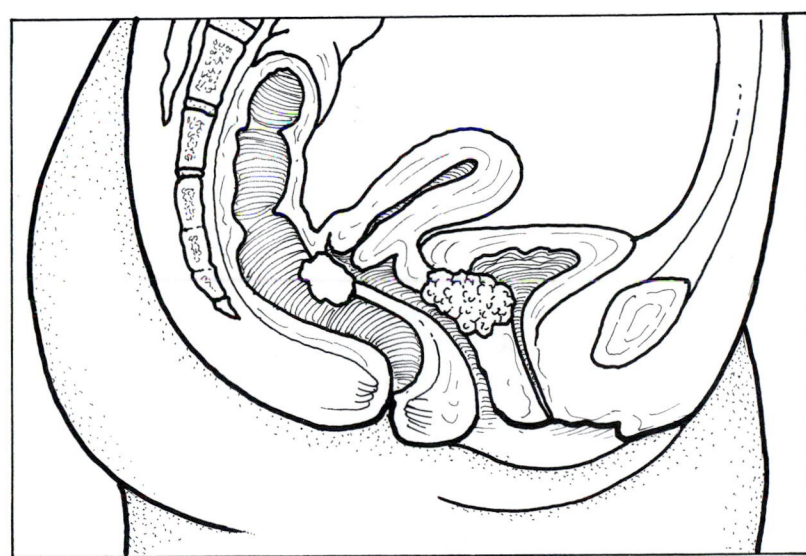

Figure 63-11 Stage IV carcinoma of the vagina. Carcinoma has spread to involve mucosa of bladder or rectum. *Copyright © KUSM-Wichita Educational Technology, Wichita, KS.*

	Stage I (no. of cases)	Stage II (no. of cases)	Stage III (no. of cases)	Stage IV (no. of cases)
TABLE 63-12 **VAGINAL CANCER: DISTRIBUTION BY FIGO STAGE**				
Eddy[106]	25	39	15	12
Manetta[124]	19	20	7	7
Rubin[108]	14	35	14	12
Benedet[109]	32	31	16	18
Urbanski[125]	33	37	40	15
Stock[126]	23	58	9	10
Kucera[127]	73	110	174	77
Total (%)	219 (22%)	330 (35%)	275 (28%)	151 (15%)

Evaluation and Therapy

Pretreatment evaluation of the patient diagnosed with primary vaginal cancer is directed toward the determination of extent and spread of disease. Tests acceptable for FIGO clinical staging purposes are listed in the previous section. Additional evaluation, although not allowed to alter the FIGO stage, will help direct treatment. Pretreatment computed tomography may be helpful in assessing the retroperitoneum for enlarged lymph nodes. In addition, CT scan may detect metastatic disease to the liver or the presence of ureteral obstruction. The extent of disease is most accurately determined by staging laparotomy or extraperitoneal lymphadenectomy. While surgical staging clearly establishes the extent of disease and may allow for changes in the radiation fields, a clear improvement in survival has not been demonstrated.

As compared with cervical cancer, surgical therapy plays a much smaller role in the therapy of primary vaginal cancer. Advanced patient age, large lesions, and the close proximity of the vagina to the bladder and rectum preventing wide surgical margins contribute to the reduced use of surgery and the greater use of radiation therapy. As demonstrated in Table 63-12, only 22% of patients present as Stage I. Small, Stage I lesions and the earliest Stage II lesions (IIa) at the vaginal apex may be treated by radical hysterectomy and upper vaginectomy with pelvic lymphadenectomy. The extent of dissection and denervation of the bladder may limit this operation in older or medically unstable patients. Radical surgery in young patients with vaginal cancer would allow preservation of the ovaries. Most patients will be treated with combination external-beam and intracavitary or interstitial radiation therapy.[126,128-131] Lesions of the upper vagina will be treated with external radiation ports similar to those applied to patients with cervical cancer—upper vagina and whole pelvis. Lesions of the lower vagina require treatment of the whole pelvis, entire vagina, and inguinal nodes. If the uterus is present and the primary lesion is located in the upper vagina, tandem and colpostats may be used to complete therapy. Because of the extent of vaginal involvement and the close proximity of bladder and rectum, many patients will require interstitial or needle implants, usually using iridium as the radioactive source. Complications from radiation therapy for vaginal cancer are higher than those reported for treatment of cervical cancer.[108,131] Advanced patient age, length of vagina treated, and close

TABLE 63-13 VAGINAL CANCER: 5-YEAR SURVIVAL BY FIGO STAGE			
Stage	Number of Patients	5-Year Survival	%
I	166	123	74
II	273	130	48
III	215	75	35
IV	126	19	15
Total	780	374	48

From Kucera,[127] Eddy,[106] Urbanski,[125] Stock,[126] and Rubins.[108]

proximity of bladder, rectum, and vulva contribute to the increased complication rate. For the most advanced lesions, a combination preoperative radiation therapy and pelvic exenteration may offer the patient the only chance for local control and cure.[106] Intuitively, combination chemotherapy and radiation therapy may be beneficial in the cases with large lesions. Although beneficial in the treatment of cervical cancer, large-scale studies demonstrating this benefit in vaginal cancer therapy are lacking.

Prognosis and Survival

Tumor size, tumor location, histologic grade, and stage are predictors of survival.[129,131-133] Clinical stage appears to be the greatest predictor of survival when multivariate analysis is performed.[132] As compared with cervical cancer stage for stage, cancer of the vagina is associated with worse survival. Overall survival for vaginal cancer is 48%. Table 63-13 lists survival of vaginal cancer patients by stage.

Diethylstilbestrol (DES) and Clear-Cell Carcinoma of the Vagina

From the late 1940s through approximately 1971, between 1 and 2 million women received diethylstilbestrol (DES) during pregnancy in an effort to prevent spontaneous miscarriage. In 1971 Herbst and colleagues reported an unusual number of clear-cell carcinomas of the vagina in young women and the apparent association between those cancers and in utero exposure to the nonsteroidal estrogen diethylstilbestrol.[134] Subsequent reports confirmed the association between in utero DES exposure and the development of clear-cell carcinoma of the vagina and cervix.[135-137] Numerous structural changes of the vagina, cervix, and uterus have now been associated with DES exposure. Exposure during the first trimester and total dose exposed appear to be the major predictors of anomalies. Fortunately, the epidemic of clear-cell carcinoma of the vagina did not develop. The frequency of DES-associated clear-cell carcinomas of the vagina peaked in 1975. Current estimates suggest a risk of clear-cell carcinoma of the vagina of 1 per 1000 women exposed to DES in utero. By now, it is assumed that most women exposed to DES in utero have passed their greatest risk. Several vaginal epithelial changes, including vaginal hood, cox comb cervix, and vaginal adenosis are more likely to be found than premalignant or malignant changes of the cervix or vagina. In the event of a history of in utero exposure to DES without previous evaluation, colposcopic examination of the cervix and entire vagina is recommended. Pap test of the cervix and vagina and staining of the vaginal mucosa with Lugol's solution looking for nonstaining areas is included with the first visit. Palpation of the entire length of the vagina is performed to avoid missing submucosal nodules, which may represent undisclosed adenosis. Nonstaining areas of the vagina and submucosal nodules are biopsied. If the initial evaluation is negative, repeat colposcopy is not required unless an abnormal Pap test is reported. The distinction between clear-cell carcinoma of the vagina and other cancers of the vagina pertains to the age of the patient. The DES-related clear-cell carcinomas of the vagina may be diagnosed at a much earlier age than other vaginal cancers. Limited resection with clear margins and postoperative radiation may allow preservation of reproductive function in selected patients. With that exception, radical surgery and pelvic lymphadenectomy or whole-pelvis radiation therapy and interstitial therapy is required.

Vaginal Melanoma

As noted in Table 63-10, vaginal melanomas account for 3% or less of all vaginal carcinomas. This represents 0.3% of all melanomas in women in the United States.[91] Reviewing data provided by the National Cancer Institute SEER program, Weinstock[91] reports a median age of 70 years for women diagnosed with vaginal melanoma. Whereas vulvar melanoma more commonly afflicts white women than black women, there is no racial difference for vaginal melanoma. The most common presenting signs and symptoms include vaginal bleeding, vaginal discharge, or a vaginal mass.[138-140] The diagnosis of primary vaginal melanoma is made by punch biopsy. Tumor width

rather than depth appears to provide the best estimate of prognosis. A significant difference in survival was reported for patients with vaginal lesions <3 cm in width as compared with those with widths ≥3 cm.[138,141]

Treatment of patients with vaginal melanoma remains controversial. In a report of 8 new cases of vaginal melanoma combined with 111 cases obtained from a literature review, Van Nostrand and colleagues found a survival advantage for patients treated with radical surgery.[142] Reid and colleagues presented a clinicopathologic analysis of 15 new cases of vaginal melanoma and a literature review of reports up to 1988 for a total of 130 patients without finding an advantage for radical surgical therapy.[138] Buchanan and associates presented a case of a long-term survivor of vaginal melanoma and a literature review from 1988 to 1997 for a total of 67 patients, and also found no survival advantage for radical surgical therapy.[141] If technically possible, wide local excision with a 2-cm lateral margin appears to provide comparable outcome to more radical surgical therapy or surgery combined with radiation therapy.[138,141,143] Unfortunately, survival for patients with vaginal melanoma is very poor regardless of the treatment undertaken. Of 197 patients reported in the literature and described by Reid[138] and Buchanan,[141] 18 (9%) are 5-year survivors. Local and distant recurrences continue to result in death for most patients with vaginal melanoma.

Summary

Vaginal cancers are uncommon and account for the smallest number of gynecologic malignancies. Regardless of histologic type, most vaginal cancers occur in women of advanced age at advanced stages. Large lesions, medically compromised patients, and close proximity of other vital organs, which are affected by aggressive radiation therapy or surgical treatment, compromise cure rates. Because of all the above factors, each patient is assessed for individualized therapy.

REFERENCES

1. Greenlee RT, Murray T, Bolden S, Wingo PA. Cancer statistics, 2000. CA Cancer J Clin 2000;50:7.
2. Sturgeon SR, Brinton LA, Devesa SS, Kurman RJ. In situ and invasive vulvar cancer incidence trends (1973 to 1987). Am J Obstet Gynecol 1992;166:1482.
3. Cramer DW. Epidemiology of the gynecologic cancers. Compr Ther 1978;4:9.

4. Rutledge F, Smith JP, Franklin EW. Carcinoma of the vulva. Am J Obstet Gynecol 1970;106:1117.

5. Hay DM, Cole FM. Primary invasive carcinoma of the vulva in Jamaica. J Obstet Gynecol Br Commonw 1969; 76:821.

6. Brinton LA, Nasca PC, Mallin K, et al. Case control study of cancer of the vulva. Obstet Gynecol 1990;75:859.

7. Mabuchi K, Bross DS, Kessler I. Epidemiology of cancer of the vulva. A case-control study. Cancer 1985;55:1843.

8. Rusk D, Sutton GP, Look KY, Roman A. Analysis of invasive squamous cell carcinoma of the vulva and vulvar intraepithelial neoplasia for the presence of human papillomavirus DNA. Obstet Gynecol 1991;77:918.

9. Franco EL. Epidemiology of anogenital warts and cancer. Obstet Gynecol Clin N Am 1996;23:597.

10. Fiorica JV, Cavanagh D, Roberts WS, et al. Carcinoma in-situ of the vulva: twenty-four years' experience. South Med J 1988;81:589.

11. Crum CP, Liskow A, Petras P, et al. Vulvar intraepithelial neoplasia (severe atypia and carcinoma in-situ): a clinico-pathologic analysis of 41 cases. Cancer 1984;54:1429.

12. Alani RM, Münger K. Human papillomavirus and associated malignancies. J Clin Oncol 1998;16:330.

13. Crum CP. Carcinoma of the vulva: epidemiolgy and pathogenesis. Obstet Gynecol 1992;79:448.

14. Kaufman RH, Gardner HL, Brown DJ, Beyth Y. Vulvar dystrophies: an evaluation. Am J Obstet Gynecol 1974; 120:363.

15. Hart WR, Norris HJ, Helwig EB. Relation of lichen sclerosus et atrophicus of the vulva to development of carcinoma. Obstet Gynecol 1975;45:369.

16. Podratz KC, Symmonds RE, Taylor WF. Carcinoma of the vulva: analysis of treatment and survival. Obstet Gynecol 1983;143:340.

17. Cavanagh D, Fiorica J, Hoffman MS, et al. Invasive carcinoma of the vulva: changing trends in surgical management. Am J Obstet Gynecol 1990;163:1007.

18. Boutselis JG. Radical vulvectomy for invasive squamous cell carcinoma of the vulva. Obstet Gynecol 1972; 39:827.

19. Chung AF, Woodruff JM, Lewis JL. Malignant melanoma of the vulva: a report of 44 cases. Obstet Gynecol 1975; 45:638.

20. Wilkinson EJ, Rico MJ, Pierson KK. Microinvasive carcinoma of the vulva. Int J Gynecol Pathol 1982;1:29.

21. Plentyl AA, Friedman EA. Lymphatic system of the female genitalia. Philadelphia: Saunders, 1971.

22. Hacker NF, Berek JS, Lagasse LD, et al. Individualization of treatment for stage I squamous cell vulvar carcinoma. Obstet Gynecol 1984;63:155.

23. Hacker NF, Nieberg RK, Berek JS, et al. Superficially invasive vulvar cancer with nodal metastases. Gynecol Oncol 1983;15:65.

24. Hoffman JS, Kumar NB, Morley GW. Prognostic significance of groin lymph node metastases in squamous carcinoma of the vulva. Obstet Gynecol 1985;66:402.

25. Curry SL, Wharton JT, Rutledge FN. Positive lymph nodes in vulvar squamous carcinoma. Gynecol Oncol 1980;9:63.

26. Hacker NF, Berek JS, Lagasse LD, et al. Management of regional lymph nodes and their prognostic influence in vulvar cancer. Obstet Gynecol 1983;61:408.

27. Creasman WT. New gynecologic cancer staging. Gynecol Oncol 1995;58:157.

28. Morley GW. Infiltrative carcinoma of the vulva: results of surgical treatment. Am J Obstet Gynecol 1976; 124:874.

29. Benedet JL, Turko M, Fairley RN, et al. Squamous carcinoma of the vulva: results of treatment, 1938-1976. Am J Obstet Gynecol 1979;134:201.

30. Sedlis A, Homesley H, Bundy B, et al. Positive groin lymph nodes in superficial squamous cell vulvar cancer: a gynecologic group study. Am J Obstet Gynecol 1987; 156:1159.

31. Homesley H, Bundy B, Sedlis A, et al. Prognostic factors for groin node metastases in squamous cell carcinoma of the vulva: a Gynecologic Oncology Group study. Gynecol Oncol 1993;49:279.

32. Hacker NF. Current treatment of small vulvar cancers. Oncology 1990;4:21.

33. Cavanagh D, Roberts WS, Bryson SCP, et al. Changing trends in the surgical treatment of invasive carcinoma of the vulva. Surg Gynecol Obstet 1986;162:164.

34. Hacker NF, Berek JS. Vulva. In: Haskell CM, ed. Cancer treatment. 3rd ed. Philadelphia: Saunders, 1990:351.

35. Green TH. Carcinoma of the vulva: a reassessment. Obstet Gynecol 1978;52:462.

36. Iversen T, Aalders JG, Christensen A, et al. Squamous cell carcinoma of the vulva: a review of 424 patients, 1956–1974. Gynecol Oncol 1980;9:271.

37. Homesley HD, Bundy BN, Sedlis A, et al. Assessment of current international federation of gynecology and obstetrics staging of vulvar carcinoma relative to prognostic factors for survival (a Gynecologic Oncology Group study). Am J Obstet Gynecol 1991;164:997.

38. Microinvasive cancer of the vulva: report of the ISSVD task force. J Reprod Med 1984;29:454.

39. Wilkinson EJ. Superficially invasive carcinoma of the vulva. Clin Obstet Gynecol 1985;28:188.

40. Magrina JF, Webb MJ, Gaffey TA, et al. Stage I squamous cell cancer of the vulva. Am J Obstet Gynecol 1979; 134:453.

41. Kelley JL III, Burke TW, Tornos C, et al. Minimally invasive vulvar carcinoma: an indication for conservative surgical therapy. Gynecol Oncol 1992;44:240.

42. Stehman FB, Bundy B, Dvoretsky PM, Creasman WT. Early stage I carcinoma of the vulva treated with ipsilateral superficial inguinal lymphadenectomy and modified radical hemivulvectomy: a prospective study of the gynecologic oncology group. Obstet Gynecol 1992;79:490.

43. Basset A. Traitemant chirurgicale operatoire de l'epithelioma primitif du clitoris: indications-technique-resultats. Rev Chir 1912;45:456.

44. Taussig FJ. Cancer of the vulva: an analysis of 155 cases (1911-1940). Am J Obstet Gynecol 1940;40:764.

45. Way S. The anatomy of the lymphatic drainage of the vulva and its influence on the radical operation for carcinoma. Ann R Coll Surg Engl 1948;3:187.

46. Way S. The surgery of vulvar carcinoma: an appraisal. Clin Obstet Gynecol 1978;5:623.

47. DiSaia PJ, Creasman WT, Rich WM. An alternate approach to early cancer of the vulva. Am J Obstet Gynecol 1979;133:825.

48. Berman ML, Soper JT, Creasman WT, et al. Conservative surgical management of superficially invasive stage I vulvar carcinoma. Gynecol Oncol 1989;35:352.

49. Burke TW Stringer CA, Gershenson DM, et al. Radical wide local excision and selective inguinal node dissection for squamous cell carcinoma of the vulva. Gynecol Oncol 1990;38:328.

50. Tilmans AS, Sutton GP, Look KY, et al. Recurrent squamous carcinoma of the vulva. Am J Obstet Gynecol 1992;167:1383.

51. Hoffman MS, Roberts WS, Finan MA, et al. A comparative study of radical vulvectomy and modified radical vulvectomy for the treatment of invasive squamous cell carcinoma of the vulva. Gynecol Oncol 1992;45:192.

52. Burke TW, Levenback C, Coleman, et al. Surgical therapy of T1 and T2 vulvar carcinoma: further experience with radical wide excision and selective inguinal lymphadenectomy. Gynecol Oncol 1995;57:215.

53. Practice guidelines: Vulvar cancer—Society of Gynecologic Oncologists clinical practice guidelines. Oncology 1998;12:275.

54. Heaps JM, Fu YS, Montz FJ, et al. Surgical–pathologic variables predictive of local recurrence in squamous cell carcinoma of the vulva. Gynecol Oncol 1990;38:309.

55. Rutledge FN, Folen Mitchell M, Munsell MF, et al. Prognostic indicators for invasive carcinoma of the vulva. Gynecol Oncol 1991;42:239.

56. Hopkins MP, Reid GC, Morley GW. Radical vulvectomy: the decision for the incision. Cancer 1993;72:799.

57. Hoffman MS, Greenberg H, Roberts WS, et al. Management of locally advanced squamous cell carcinoma of the vulva. J Gynecol Surg 1991;7:175.

58. Boyce CR, Mehram AH. Management of vulvar malignancies. Am J Obstet Gynecol 1974;119:48.

59. Morley GW. Cancer of the vulva: a review. Cancer 1981;48:597.

60. Anderson BL, Hacker NF. Psychosexual adjustment after vulvar surgery. Obstet Gynecol 1983;62:457.

61. Way S. Carcinoma of the vulva. Am J Obstet Gynecol 1960;79:692.

62. Homesley HD, Bundy BN, Sedlis A, Adcock L. Radiation therapy versus pelvic node resection for carcinoma of the vulva with positive groin nodes. Obstet Gynecol 1986;68:733.

63. Stehman FB, Bundy BN, Thomas G, et al. Groin dissection versus groin radiation in carcinoma of the vulva: a Gynecologic Group Study study. Int J Radiat Oncol Biol Phys 1992;24:389.

64. Byron RL, Mishell DR, Yonemoto RH. The surgical treatment of invasive carcinoma of the vulva. Surg Gynecol Obstet 1965;121:1243.

65. Ballon SC, Lamb EJ. Separate inguinal incisions in the treatment of carcinoma of the vulva. Surg Gynecol Obstet 1975;140:81.

66. Hacker NJ, Leuchter RS, Berek JS, et al. Radical vulvectomy and bilateral inguinal lymphadenectomy through separate groin incisions. Obstet Gynecol 1981;58:574.

67. Helm CW, Hatch K, Austin JM, et al. A matched comparison of single and triple incision techniques for the surgical treatment of carcinoma of the vulva. Gynecol Oncol 1992;46:150.

68. Christopherson W, Buchsbaum HJ, Voet R, et al. Radical vulvectomy and bilateral groin lymphadenectomy utilizing separate groin incisions: report of a case with recurrence in the intervening skin bridge. Gynecol Oncol 1985;21:247.

69. Iverson T, Abeler V, Aalders J. Individualized treatment of stage I carcinoma of the vulva. Obstet Gynecol 1981;57:85.

70. Farias-Eisner R, Cirisano FD, Grouse D, et al. Conservative and individualized surgery for early squamous carcinoma of the vulva: The treatment of choice for stage I and II ($T_{1-2}N_{0-1}M_0$) disease. Gynecol Oncol 1994;53:55.

71. Chu J, Tamimi HK, Figge DC. Femoral node metastases with negative superficial inguinal nodes in early vulvar cancer. Am J Obstet Gynecol 1981;140:337.

72. Podczaski E, Sexton M, Kaminski, et al. Recurrent carcinoma of the vulva after conservative treatment for "microinvasive" disease. Gynecol Oncol 1990;39:65.

73. Borgno G, Micheletti L, Barbero M, et al. Topographic distribution of groin lymph nodes: a study of 50 female cadavers. J Reprod Med 1990;35:1127.

74. Micheletti L, Borgno G, Barbero M, et al. Deep femoral lymphadenectomy with preservation of fascia lata: preliminary report on 42 invasive vulvar carcinomas. J Reprod Med 1990;35:1130.

75. Wilkinson EJ. Superficially invasive carcinoma of the vulva. Clin Obstet Gynecol 1991;34:651.

76. Boronow RC, Hickman BT, Reagan MT, et al. Combined therapy as an alternative to exenteration for locally advanced vulvovaginal cancer. Am J Clin Oncol 1987;10:171.

77. Fairey RN, Mackay PA, Benedet JL, et al. Radiation treatment of carcinoma of the vulva: 1950-1980. Am J Obstet Gynecol 1985;151:591.

78. Rotmensch J, Rubin SJ, Sutton HG, et al. Preoperative radiotherapy followed by radical vulvectomy with inguinal lymphadenectomy for advanced vulvar carcinomas. Gynecol Oncol 1990;36:181.

79. Berek JS, Heaps JM, Fu YS, et al. Concurrent cisplatin and 5FU chemotherapy and external radiation for primary treatment of advanced stage squamous carcinoma of the vulva. Gynecol Oncol 1991;40:171 abstract.

80. Eifel PJ, Morris M, Burke TW, et al. Prolonged continuous infusion cisplatin and 5-fluorouracil with radiation for locally advanced carcinoma of the vulva. Gynecol Oncol 1995;59:51.

81. Parmley T, Woodruff J, Julian C. Invasive vulvar Paget's disease. Obstet Gynecol 1975;46:341.

82. Feuer GA, Shevchuk M, Canalog A. Vulvar Paget's disease: the need to exclude an invasive lesion. Gynecol Oncol 1990;38:81.

83. Hart WR, Millman RB. Progression of intraepithelial Paget's disease of the vulva to invasive carcinoma. Cancer 1977;40:2333.

84. Curtin JP, Rubin SC, Jones WB, et al. Paget's disease of the vulva. Gynecol Oncol 1990;39:374.

85. Bergen S, DiSaia PJ, Liao SY, et al. Conservative management of extramammary Paget's disease of the vulva. Gynecol Oncol 1989;33:151.

86. Fenn ME, Morley GW, Abell MR. Paget's disease of the vulva. Obstet Gynecol 1971;38:660.

87. Mohs FE, Blanchard L. Microscopically controlled surgery for extramammary Paget's disease. Arch Dermatol 1979;115:706.

88. Misas JE, Cold CJ, Hall FW. Vulvar Paget's disease: fluorescein-aided visualization of margins. Obstet Gynecol 1991;77:156.

89. Fishman DA, Chambers SK, Schwartz PE, et al. Extra-mammary Paget's disease of the vulva. Gynecol Oncol 1995;56:266.

90. Gunn R, Gallagher H. Vulvar Paget's disease: a topographic study. Cancer 1980;46:590.

91. Weinstock MA. Malignant melanoma of the vulva and vagina in the United States: patterns of incidence and population-based estimates of survival. Am J Obstet Gynecol 1994;171:1225.

92. Ragnarsson-Olding B, Johansson H, Rutqvist L, et al. Malignant melanoma of the vulva and vagina. Cancer 1993;71:1893.

93. Davidson T, Kissin M, Westbury G. Vulvo-vaginal melanoma—should radical surgery be abandoned? Br J Obstet Gynaecol 1987;94:473.

94. Rose PG, Piver MS, Tsukada Y, et al. Conservative therapy for melanoma of the vulva. Am J Obstet Gynecol 1988;159:52.

95. Trimble EL, Lewis JL, Williams LL, et al. Management of vulvar melanoma. Gynecol Oncol 1992;45:254.

96. Tasseron EWK, van der Esch EP, Hart AAM, et al. A clinicopathologic study of 30 melanomas of the vulva. Gynecol Oncol 1992;46:170.

97. Phillips GL, Bundy BN, Okagaki T, et al. Malignant melanoma of the vulva treated by radical hemivulvectomy: a prospective study of the Gynecologic Oncology Group. Cancer 1994;73:2626.

98. Clark WH, From L, Bernadino EA, et al. The histogenesis and biologic behavior of primary human malignant melanoma of the skin. Cancer Res 1969;29:705.

99. Breslow A. Thickness, cross-sectional areas and depth of invasion in the prognosis of cutaneous melanoma. Ann Surg 1970;172:902.

100. Beahrs OH, Henson DE, Hutter RVP, et al., eds. Manual for staging of cancer. 4th ed. Staging for malignant melanoma of the skin. Chicago: American Joint Committee on Cancer, 1992.

101. Balch CM, Soong SJ, Milton GW, et al. A comparison of prognostic factors and surgical results in 1786 patients with localized (stage I) melanoma treated in Alabama, USA, and New South Wales, Australia. Ann Surg 1982; 196:677.

102. Kirkwood JM, Strawderman MH, Ernstoff MS et al. Interferon alfa-2b adjuvant therapy of high risk cutaneous melanoma: the Eastern Co-operative Oncology Group Trial EST 1684. J Clin Oncol 1996;14:7.

103. Allen DG, Planner RS. Primary vaginal cancer after hysterectomy. J Lower Genit Tract Dis 1997;1:203.

104. Ball HG, Berman ML. Management of primary vaginal carcinoma. Gynecol Oncol 1982;14:154.

105. Gallup DG, Talledo OE, Shah KJ, Hayes C. Invasive squamous cell carcinoma of the vagina: a 14-year study, Obstet Gynecol 1987;69:782.

106. Eddy GL, Marks RD, Miller MC, Underwood PB. Primary invasive vaginal carcinoma. Am J Obstet Gynecol 1991;165:292.

107. Hilborne LH, Fu YS. Intraepithelial, invasive and metastatic neoplasms of the vagina. In: Wilkinson EJ, ed.

Pathology of the vulva and vagina. New York: Churchill Livingstone, 1987:184.

108. Rubin SC, Young J, Mikuta JJ. Squamous carcinoma of the vagina: treatment, complications, and long term follow-up. Gynecol Oncol 1985;20:346.

109. Benedet JL, Murphy KJ, Fairey RN, Boyes DA. Primary invasive carcinoma of the vagina. Obstet Gynecol 1983; 62:715.

110. Al-Kurdi M, Monaghan JM. Thirty-two years experience in management of primary tumours of the vagina. Br J Obstet Gynaecol 1981;88:1145.

111. Marino MJ. Vaginal cancer: the role of infectious and environmental factors. Am J Obstet Gynecol 1991;165:1255.

112. Zur Hausen H. The role of papillomaviruses in anogenital cancer. Scand J Infect Dis 1990;69:107.

113. Crum CP, Roche JK. Papillomavirus-related genital neoplasia. Cancer Detect Prev 1990;14:465.

114. Weed JC, Lozier C, Daniel SJ. Human papillomavirus in multifocal, invasive female genital tract malignancy. Obstet Gynecol 1983;62:832.

115. Bell J, Sevin B-U, Averette H, Nadji M. Vaginal cancer after hysterectomy for benign disease; value of cytologic screening. Obstet Gynecol 1984;64:699.

116. Herman JM, Homesley HD, Dignan MB. Is hysterectomy a risk factor for vaginal cancer? JAMA 1986; 256:601.

117. Benedet JL, Saunders BH. Carcinoma in-situ of the vagina. Am J Obstet Gynecol 1984;148:695.

118. Hoffman MS, DeCesare SL, Roberts WS, et al. Upper vaginectomy for in-situ and occult superficially invasive carcinoma of the vagina. Am J Obstet Gynecol 1992; 166:30.

119. Lenehan PM, Meffe F, Lickrish GM. Vaginal intraepithelial neoplasia: biologic aspects and management. Obstet Gynecol 1986;68:333.

120. Houghton CRS, Iversen T. Squamous cell carcinoma of the vagina; a clinical study of the location of the tumor. Gynecol Oncol 1982;13:365.

121. Peters WA, Kumar NB, Morley GW. Microinvasive carcinoma of the vagina: a distinct clinical entity? Am J Obstet Gynecol 1985;153:505.

122. Eddy GL, Singh KP, Gansler TS. Superficially invasive carcinoma of the vagina following treatment for cervical cancer: a report of six cases. Gynecol Oncol 1990; 36:376.

123. Perez CA, Arneson AN, Dehner LP, Galakatos A. Radiation therapy in carcinoma of the vagina. Obstet Gynecol 1974;44:862.

124. Manetta A, Gutrecht EL, Berman ML, DiSaia PJ. Primary invasive carcinoma of the vagina. Obstet Gynecol 1990;76:639.

125. Urbanski K, Kois Z, Reinfuss M, Fabisiak W. Primary invasive vaginal carcinoma treated with radiotherapy: analysis of prognostic factors. Gynecol Oncol 1996; 60:16.

126. Stock RG, Chen AS, Seski J. A 30-year experience in the management of primary carcinoma of the vagina: analysis of prognostic factors and treatment modalities. Gynecol Oncol 1995;56:45.

127. Kucera H, Vavra N. Radiation management of primary carcinoma of the vagina: clinical and histopathological

variables associated with survival. Gynecol Oncol 1991;40:12.

128. Perez CA, Camel HM. Long-term follow-up in radiation therapy of carcinoma of the vagina. Cancer 1982;49:1308.

129. Ali MM, Huang DT, Gopelrud DR, et al. Radiation alone for carcinoma of the vagina: variations in response related to the location of the primary tumor. Cancer 1996;77:1934.

130. Davis KP, Stanhope CR, Garton GR, et al. Invasive vaginal carcinoma: analysis of early-stage disease. Gynecol Oncol 1991;42:131.

131. Chyle V, Zagars GK, Wheeler JA, et al. Definitive radiotherapy for carcinoma of the vagina: outcome and prognostic factors. Int J Radiat Oncol Biol Phys. 1996;35:891.

132. Peters WA, Kumar NB, Morley GW. Carcinoma of the vagina: factors influencing treatment outcome. Cancer 1985;55:897.

133. Chu AM, Beechinor R. Survival and recurrence patterns in the radiation treatment of carcinoma of the vagina. Gynecol Oncol 1984;19:298.

134. Herbst AL, Ulfelder H, Poskanzer DC. Adenocarcinoma of the vagina: association of maternal stilbestrol therapy with tumor appearance in young women. N Engl J Med 1971;284:878.

135. Ruffolo EH, Foxworthy D, Fletcher JC. Vaginal adenocarcinoma arising in vaginal adenosis. Am J Obstet Gynecol 1971;111:167.

136. Lanier AP, Noller KL, Decker DG, et al. A follow-up of 1,719 persons exposed to estrogens in utero and born 1943–1959. Mayo Clin Proc 1973;48:793.

137. Noller KL, Decker DG, Symmonds RE, et al. Clear-cell adenocarcinoma of the vagina and cervix: survival data. Am J Obstet Gynecol 1976;124:285.

138. Reid GC, Schmidt RW, Roberts JA, et al. Primary melanoma of the vagina: a clinicopathologic analysis. Obstet Gynecol 1989;74:190.

139. Heller DS, Moomjy M, Koulos J, Smith D. Vulvar and vaginal melanoma—a clinicopathologic study. J Reprod Med 1994;39:945.

140. Chung AF, Casey MJ, Flannery JT, et al. Malignant melanoma of the vagina—report of 19 cases. Obstet Gynecol 1980;55:720.

141. Buchanan DJ, Schlaerth J, Kurosaki T. Primary vaginal melanoma: thirteen-year disease-free survival after wide local excision and review of recent literature. Am J Obstet Gynecol 1998;178:1177.

142. Van Norstrand KM, Lucci JA, Schell M, et al. Primary vaginal melanoma: improved survival with radical pelvic surgery. Gynecol Oncol 1994;55:234.

143. Levitan Z, Gordon AN, Kaplan AL, Kaufman RH. Primary malignant melanoma of the vagina: report of four cases and review of the literature. Gynecol Oncol 1989;33:85.

TABLE 64-4
HISTOLOGIC CLASSIFICATION OF UTERINE CERVIX MALIGNANCIES

Squamous-cell carcinoma
  Large-cell keratinizing and nonkeratinizing carcinoma
  Verrucous carcinoma
Adenocarcinoma
  Typical (mucinous) endocervical adenocarcinoma
  Endometrioid adenocarcinoma
  Clear-cell adenocarcinoma
  Papillary adenocarcinoma
  Medullary adenocarcinoma
Variants of adenocarcinoma
  Adenoma malignum (minimal-deviation adenocarcinoma)
  Adenoid cystic adenocarcinoma
  Mesonephric carcinoma
Mixed-epithelial-cell carcinoma
  Adenosquamous-cell carcinoma
  Glassy-cell carcinoma
  Mucoepidermoid carcinoma
Neuroendocrine carcinoma
  Carcinoid
  Small-cell carcinoma

carcinoma precursors, resulting in a decrease in the number of squamous-cell carcinomas. Table 64-4 presents a list of cervical cancer histology.

The prognostic significance of specific histologic types of cervical cancer has been extensively studied. In general, if small-cell undifferentiated carcinomas (neuroendocrine differentiation) are excluded from the squamous histology group, there appears to be no difference in prognosis for Stage IB lesions when segregated by grade.[18] Small-cell undifferentiated carcinomas occur in younger women and exhibit a more aggressive behavior.[19] When stratified by histologic grade and lesion size, there appears to be no prognostic difference when comparing squamous-cell carcinoma and endocervical adenocarcinoma of the cervix.[20] Reports are conflicting as to whether adenosquamous carcinoma of the cervix is an independent prognostic factor.[21,22]

PRESENTATION: SIGNS AND SYMPTOMS

Signs and symptoms of cervical cancer will vary with the size and extent of the primary lesion or metastatic sites. The very smallest cancers will produce no symptoms and will only be detected by Pap test. As the primary lesion enlarges, patients may give a history of intermenstrual and postcoital vaginal bleeding. Additional symptoms will include foul-smelling vaginal discharge and heavier menses. Symptoms of

pelvic or leg pain suggest extension of the primary or metastatic sites into adjacent organs. Leg edema and sciatic-nerve pain suggest that tumor has invaded the pelvic side wall and may also be associated with ureteral obstruction.

PRETREATMENT EVALUATION AND STAGING

Carcinoma of the cervix is staged using the scheme proposed by International Federation of Obstetrics and Gynecology (FIGO)[23] (Table 64-5; Figures 64-1 to 64-4). Although ovarian, uterine, and vulvar cancers are staged surgically, carcinoma of the cervix continues to be staged clinically. Clinical staging allows

TABLE 64-5
FIGO STAGING FOR CARCINOMA OF THE CERVIX

Stage	Description
0	Carcinoma in situ (Cases of Stage 0 should not be included in any therapeutic statistics for invasive carcinoma.)
I	Carcinoma strictly confined to the cervix (extension to the corpus should be disregarded.)
IA	Invasive cancer identified only microscopically. All gross lesions even with superficial invasion are Stage IB cancers. Invasion is limited to measured stromal invasion with maximum depth of 5.0 mm and no wider than 7.0 mm.
IA1	Measured invasion of stroma no greater than 3.0 mm in depth and no wider than 7.0 mm.
IA2	Measured invasion of stroma greater than 3.0 mm and no greater than 5.0 mm and no wider than 7.0 mm.
IB	Clinical lesions confined to the cervix or preclinical lesions greater than Stage IA.
IB1	Clinical lesions no greater than 4.0 cm in size.
IB2	Clinical lesions greater than 4.0 cm in size.
II	Carcinoma extends beyond the cervix, but has not extended onto the pelvic wall. Carcinoma involves the vagina, but not as far as the lower third.
IIA	No obvious parametrial involvement
IIB	Obvious parametrial involvement
III	Carcinoma has extended onto the pelvic wall. On rectal examination there is no cancer-free space between the tumor and pelvic wall. Tumor involves the lower third of the vagina. All cases with hydronephrosis or nonfunctioning kidney should be included, unless they are due to other causes.
IIIA	No extension onto the pelvic wall, but involvement of the lower third of the vagina.
IIIB	Extension to the pelvic wall or hydronephrosis or nonfunctioning kidney
IV	Carcinoma has extended beyond the true pelvis or has clinically involved the mucosa of the bladder or rectum
IVA	Spread to adjacent organs
IVB	Spread to distant organs

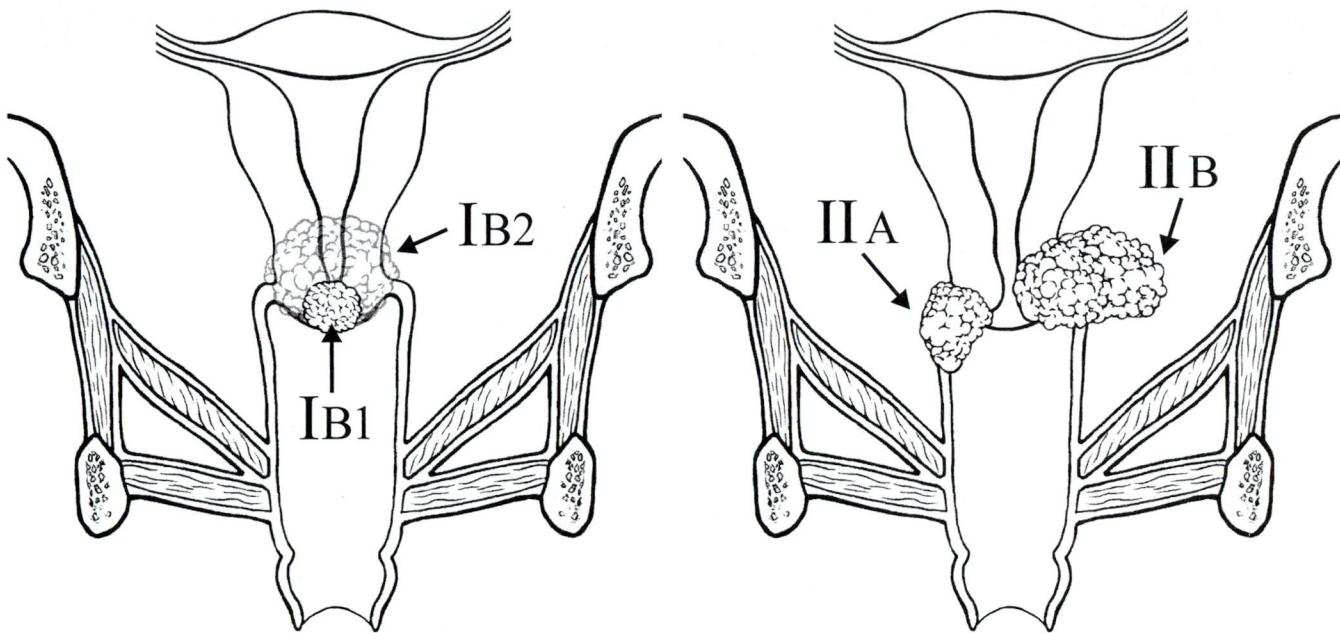

Figure 64-1 Stage IB carcinoma of the cervix. Stage IB1, Clinical lesion no greater than 4.0 cm in size. Stage IB2, Clinical lesion greater than 4.0 cm in size. *Copyright © KUSM-Wichita, Educational Technology, 1998, Wichita, KS.*

Figure 64-2 Stage II carcinoma of the cervix. Stage IIA, No obvious parametrial involvement. Involvement of upper two-thirds of vagina. Stage IIB, Obvious parametrial involvement. *Copyright © KUSM-Wichita, Educational Technology, 1998, Wichita, KS.*

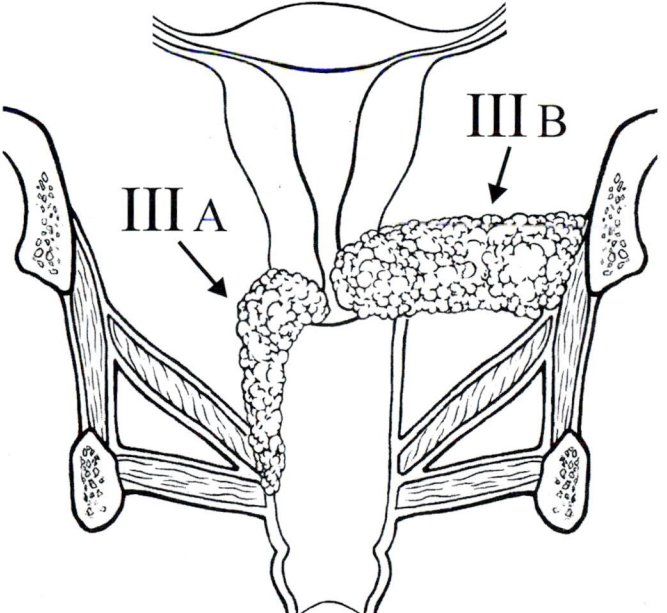

Figure 64-3 Stage III carcinoma of the cervix. Stage IIIA, No extension to the pelvic side wall, but involvement of the lower one-third of the vagina. Stage IIIB, Extension to the pelvic side wall, or hydronephrosis or nonfunctioning kidney. *Copyright © KUSM-Wichita, Educational Technology), 1998, Wichita, KS.*

radiographic tests that are available worldwide. These include chest radiography, barium enema, and intravenous pyelography. Other tests, such as computed tomography (CT) scan or magnetic resonance imaging (MRI) may be used in developing a treatment plan, but cannot be used to change the clinical stage. Routine use of barium enema or intravenous pyelography provides little benefit in the evaluation of

the asymptomatic patient with small Stage I or II disease. CT allows assessment of the pelvic and paraaortic nodes in addition to preliminary assessment of the kidneys and ureters in patients with large or advanced disease.[24] Cystoscopy and sigmoidoscopy may be helpful in establishing the diagnosis of Stage IV disease in the patient with a large cervical lesion.

Figure 64-4 Stage IV carcinoma of the cervix. Stage IVA, Spread to adjacent organs (bladder or rectum). Stage IVB, Spread to distant organs. *Copyright © KUSM-Wichita, Educational Technology), 1998, Wichita, KS.*

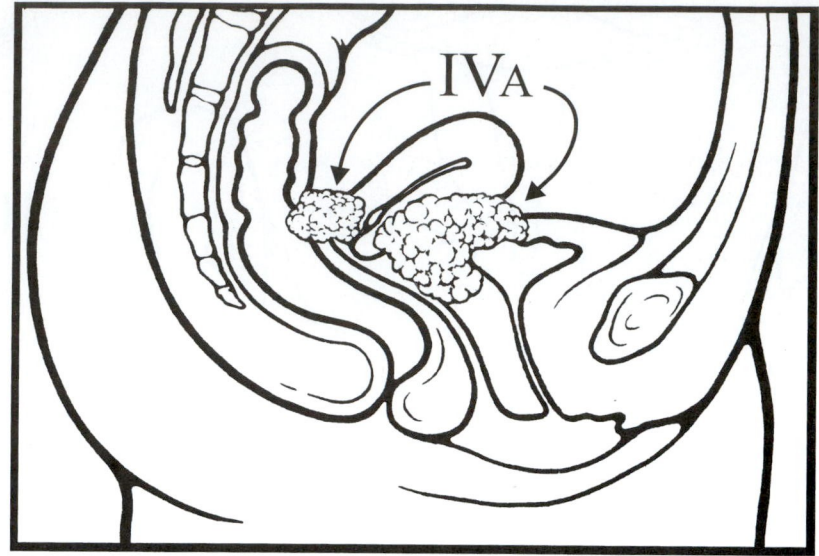

For patients with Stage IA and small Stage IB lesions who are considered good candidates for radical hysterectomy, the only pretreatment evaluation includes posteroanterior (PA) and lateral-view chest films, complete blood count (CBC), and chemistry profile. Surgical assessment of the abdomen and retroperitoneum are more accurate than radiographic evaluation. CT scan of abdomen and pelvis with intravenous, oral, and rectal contrast agents may best evaluate patients who are candidates for radiation therapy. MRI may provide better evaluation of tumor volume within the cervix, but does not provide the evaluation of renal function obtained with CT scan.[25] Lymphangiography is more accurate than CT scan or MRI in identifying aortic adenopathy but requires considerably more expertise by the radiologist interpreting the lymphgangiogram.[26] PA and lateral views of the chest, CBC, and chemistry profile are also beneficial prior to initiating radiation therapy.

Surgical staging of cervical cancer continues to be controversial. Surgical staging by extraperitoneal lymphadenectomy is required for some cooperative group clinical trials, and considered by some clinicians to be an essential part of the pretreatment evaluation of patients with cervical cancer. Extraperitoneal lymphadenectomy will identify evidence of metastatic carcinoma in some women with negative CT scan or MRI. However, most patients will have negative nodes or will be treated with the same external radiation portals as would have been proposed had the lymphadenectomy not been performed. This group will be exposed to the morbidity and expense without survival benefit.[27] A small group of patients found by staging lymphadenectomy to have microscopic foci of metastatic carcinoma in the aortic nodes will benefit from extended-field radiation therapy.[28] Cosin and colleagues reported on 266 patients undergoing staging lymphadenectomy prior to radiation therapy.[29] One hundred thirty-three of these patients were found to have surgically confirmed positive pelvic or paraaortic lymph nodes. Forty-four patients with positive lymph nodes survived for 5 years; these 44 patients accounted for 17% of the original 266 women undergoing surgical staging. Three of the 266 patients died from treatment-related causes, lymphedema developed in 18.4% of patients, and severe (Grade 4) complications developed in 10.5%. There was a survival advantage for the group of women with macroscopically positive nodes, which could be surgically debulked.

THERAPY OF CARCINOMA OF THE CERVIX

The management of cervical carcinoma requires treatment of the primary lesion and the region at primary risk for metastatic disease. The region at risk includes the parametria or paracervical tissues: the uterosacral, vesicouterine, and cardinal ligaments; and the pelvic lymph nodes. The region at risk may be excised by radical surgery or sterilized by radiation therapy. Although combinations of surgery and radiation therapy may be required in some circumstances, most patients are best served by treatment with a single method. The incidence of major complication for either method ranges from 3 to 11%, and is considered acceptable as compared with the risk of recurrent disease.[30] The combination of two radical therapies will result in a complication rate of 30% or greater.[31]

MICROINVASIVE CARCINOMA OF THE CERVIX

The concept of minimally invasive or microinvasive carcinoma of the cervix has been debated for decades. The definition must be sufficiently stringent to allow the identification of patients with cancer of the cervix who may be cured by nonradical means. Accepted as a component of the FIGO staging scheme and originally proposed by the Society of Gynecologic Oncologists (SGO) in 1973, the definition of microinvasion is that of neoplastic epithelium invading the cervical stroma to a depth of ≤3 mm or less[32]. Although absent from the FIGO scheme, the SGO definition excludes lesions of any depth with lymphatic or vascular space invasion from the microinvasive category. The importance of this definition rests in the ability to identify patients who have a negligible risk for pelvic lymph-node metastases (<0.5%), and a low risk for central recurrence (<1.0%).[33] Patients who meet this definition can be treated by conization alone, if continued fertility is desired, or by simple hysterectomy if fertility is not a concern. Lesions with depth of invasion >3 mm or vascular space invasion should be treated more aggressively as a result of increased risk of nodal metastases and central recurrence. Although there is increasing agreement about the natural history and therapy of minimally invasive or microinvasive squamous-cell carcinoma of the cervix, the same cannot be said for adenocarcinomas. There is no accepted definition of microinvasive adenocarcinoma of the cervix. Conservative treatment of the patient with minimally invasive adenocarcinoma of the cervix is decided on an individual basis after extensive pathologic review and discussion with the patient.

RADICAL HYSTERECTOMY AND PELVIC LYMPHADENECTOMY

Carcinoma of the cervix that is more extensive than microinvasion requires therapy that encompasses the central lesion and the region at risk. Patients with Stage IA2 or IB1, some Stage IB2, and small Stage IIA lesions may be candidates for radical hysterectomy and pelvic lymphadenectomy. Controversy exists

regarding the treatment of patients with large, barrel-shaped cervical carcinomas (Stage IB2).[34,35] The radical abdominal operation as described by Wertheim[35] and later modified by Meigs[36] forms the basis for the surgical approach to cervical cancer. Piver et al. described five classes of extended hysterectomy for cervical cancer.[38] The intent of the Class I hysterectomy is to ensure the removal of all cervical tissue. The ureters are not dissected from the ureteral tunnel. This procedure is used for those patients with large, barrel-shaped lesions of the cervix that have incompletely responded to radiation therapy. This is also referred to as an extrafascial hysterectomy.

The Class II extended hysterectomy is described as a moderately extended radical hysterectomy. More paracervical tissue is removed while preserving the blood supply to the distal ureters and bladder. Although the ureter is dissected out of the ureteral tunnel, the attachments to the pubovesical ligaments are left intact. The medial half of the uterosacral and cardinal ligaments is resected. A lymphadenectomy is elective, but it is performed by most clinicians. The procedure was described for use in the unusual circumstance of microinvasion when a question exists regarding depth of invasion following a conization of the cervix.

The Class III (Meigs) extended hysterectomy involves wide radical excision of the paravaginal and parametrial tissues, in addition to a complete pelvic lymphadenectomy. The uterine artery is ligated at the internal iliac artery. The ureter is completely dissected from the ureteral tunnel and the pubovesical ligament resected, with the exception of a small lateral portion between the distal ureter and superior vesical artery. This is done to reduce the risk of ureterovaginal fistula formation. The uterosacral ligament is resected at the sacrum and the cardinal ligament is transected at the pelvic side wall. The upper third of the vagina is removed. This is described as the optimal operation for the young patient with a small invasive lesion (Stage IB to IIA). Ovarian function may be preserved. The ovaries may be secured to the pelvic side wall or transposed to the paracolic gutter should postoperative radiation therapy be considered. Figure 64-5 depicts the extent of dissection for Class I to III extended hysterectomies.

The Class IV extended hysterectomy involves more extensive excision of paravaginal tissues, and, when indicated, excision of the internal iliac vessels along with that portion of the pelvic side wall. All

Figure 64-5 Extended hysterectomy. I = Class I, extrafascial. II = Class II, resection of the medial portion of the uterosacral and cardinal ligaments. III = Class III, resection of the uterosacral and cardinal ligaments at the pelvic side wall. B = bladder; C = cervix; and R = rectum. *Copyright © KUSM-Wichita, Educational Technology), 1998, Wichita, KS.*

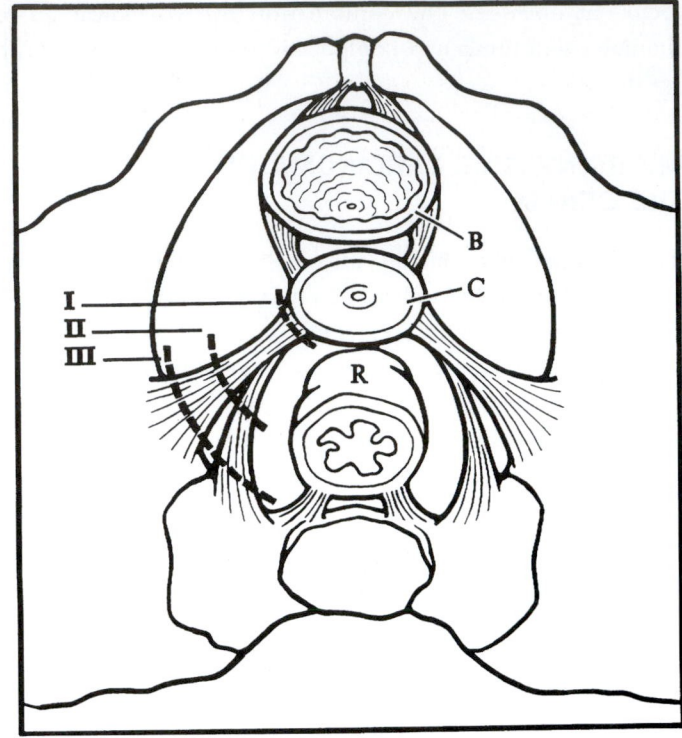

periureteral tissues are removed. In addition, the upper three-fourths of the vagina may be removed. This procedure was described for more anteriorly occurring central recurrences when preserving the bladder is possible. Removal of the hypogastric system, including the superior vesical artery, significantly increases the risk of postoperative fistula formation.

The Class V extended hysterectomy involves removal of central recurrent cancer involving portions of the distal ureter and bladder. The involved portions of the ureter, bladder, and hypogastric system are excised and the ureter is reimplanted into the bladder. In some cases, a ureteroileoneocystotomy was performed. Class IV and V extended hysterectomies are seldom used. Because of the significant risk of fistula formation, currently most clinicians would elect to perform an anterior pelvic exenteration with continent urinary diversion in patients with anteriorly

placed central recurrences in a previously radiated field.

Currently, most clinicians proposing surgical treatment for carcinoma of the cervix will perform a Class III (Meigs) radical hysterectomy for FIGO Stage IA2 or IB1, or small Stage IIA carcinoma of the cervix. As a result of the increased risk of metastatic disease associated with increasing size of the cervical lesion, there is less agreement on the use of radical hysterectomy in the treatment of patients with large (>4 cm) Stage IB2 cancers.[39,40]

The ideal candidate for radical hysterectomy is a healthy young patient with a small carcinoma of the cervix and a relatively low risk of nodal metastases. The advantages of radical hysterectomy are listed in Table 64-6.

RISKS AND COMPLICATIONS OF RADICAL HYSTERECTOMY

Following initial diagnosis and laboratory evaluation, the patient with cancer of the cervix is offered a treatment plan. Ideally, a multidisciplinary team including a gynecologic oncologist and radiation oncologist develops the plan. For patients with small or early cancer, choices of surgery or radiation therapy will be discussed. In order to make an informed choice regarding treatment, the patient must know

TABLE 64-6
ADVANTAGES OF RADICAL HYSTERECTOMY

Accurate assessment of the pelvis and abdomen for metastatic disease
Preservation of ovarian function if premenopausal
Decreased risk of distortion of the vagina and subsequent dyspareunia
Decreased risk of long-term bladder or rectal dysfunction

the advantages and disadvantages of all proposed treatments. Complications of radical hysterectomy include the potential for anesthetic complications or death; intraoperative bleeding, which may require transfusion; and intraoperative injury to the bladder, ureter, or rectum. Postoperative complications may include vesicovaginal or ureterovaginal fistula, pelvic abscess, deep venous thrombosis (DVT), or pulmonary embolus. The anticipated consequences of radical hysterectomy include some shortening of the vagina and temporary bladder dysfunction as a result of disruption of the autonomic nerve supply to the bladder. Prolonged suprapubic drainage of the bladder or intermittent self-catheterization will be required in almost all patients treated by Class III radical hysterectomy. For most patients, spontaneous bladder function will return within 4 to 6 weeks. The overall major complication rate following radical hysterectomy is 2 to 3%.[41]

The use of prophylactic antibiotics, autologous blood donation, improvements in surgical techniques, and DVT prophylaxis has greatly diminished the risk of major complications.

RADIATION THERAPY

The majority of patients diagnosed with carcinoma of the cervix will receive treatment with external-beam and intracavitary radiation therapy. External-beam radiation therapy, also referred to as teletherapy, is ionizing γ-radiation. Most external-beam radiation therapy is delivered by high-voltage linear accelerators, which results in 100% of the given dose accumulating 3 cm below the skin surface. This improved penetration of the photons results in a larger amount of radiation reaching the pelvis with less reaction on the skin surface. The portals for external-beam radiation therapy typically encompass the region at risk for spread of cervix cancer, which is from midvagina to the top of the L4 vertebral body. The lateral margin extends 1 cm lateral to the iliac vessels. The goal of external-beam radiation therapy is to sterilize the pelvic lymph nodes and paracervical tissues, in addition to reducing the size of the primary cervical lesion. In almost all cases, intracavitary cesium is used to complete therapy. Also referred to as brachytherapy, a radioactive isotope (usually cesium) delivers a high dose of radiation to the cervix and a small surrounding area. A uterine tandem and vaginal colpostats are positioned under general anesthetic and

---

TABLE 64-7
ADVANTAGES OF RADIATION THERAPY

May be used to treat almost any patient with cervical cancer
Better than surgery for treating large-volume cancer
No exposure to long surgery or anesthetic
Majority of the treatment is completed as an outpatient
Excellent cure rate

---

secured with gauze packing. After the position of the tandem and colpostats is confirmed by radiography, dosing simulation is computer generated for appropriate afterloading of the instruments. For safety purposes the instruments are loaded with cesium after the patient returns to her room. Some institutions use an interstitial needle template afterloaded with iridium (^{192}Ir) wire to complete the radiation therapy of the cervix and parametria. The advantages of radiation therapy are listed in Table 64-7.

RISKS AND COMPLICATIONS OF RADIATION THERAPY

Complications of radiation therapy can be divided into early or acute and late or chronic complications. Diarrhea occurs frequently during the course of external-beam radiation therapy. Diet changes and use of antidiarrheal medication control the symptoms in most patients. Skin reactions are much less common with the use of high-voltage therapy units. Moist desquamation may develop in intertriginous skin and skin folds in obese patients. Major complications include rectovaginal or vesicovaginal fistula, bowel obstruction, and necrosis of the vagina. Late effects of radiation may include fibrosis and agglutination of the vagina, proctitis, and cystitis. Approximately 6 to 14% of patients will experience major complications that may require surgical correction.[35,42,43] Complications may increase as the total dose of radiation and the area treated increase.

Every effort should be made to choose the single best method of therapy for each individual patient. Complication rates for radical surgery or radiation therapy are acceptable when viewed in the context of a fatal condition if left untreated. If possible, the combination of radical hysterectomy followed by radiation therapy is avoided. The risk of major complications is not the sum of the complication rates of the two treatments, but may be three times the rate of either treatment individually.[31]

UNEXPECTED INVASIVE CERVICAL CANCER FOUND AT THE TIME OF SIMPLE HYSTERECTOMY

Five groups of "cut-through" hysterectomy were described by Andras et al. in 1973.[44] The first two groups had clear surgical margins, and the remaining three had microscopic or gross tumor at the margins of resection. Reasons for the surprise finding of invasive cervical cancer in a simple hysterectomy specimen include a false negative preoperative Pap test, inadequate preoperative evaluation of an abnormal Pap test, failure to perform a Pap test preoperatively, and failure to perform a conization of the cervix to rule out invasive carcinoma. Other reasons include inadequate evaluation of the patient with abnormal vaginal bleeding prior to surgery and a preoperative diagnosis of endometrial carcinoma found to be cervical in origin on final pathology review.[45] In most circumstances, the situation can be avoided. Therapy for the patients found to have an unexpected diagnosis of cervical cancer in the postoperative period is most commonly radiation therapy. Radical parametrectomy, or resection of the vaginal apex, parametria and pelvic nodes, is also an option for patients who are thought to be good surgical candidates.[46,47] Although the cure rate appears not to be compromised in patients with no residual tumor in the simple hysterectomy specimen and who receive postoperative radiation therapy, the complication rates may be increased.

COMBINATION THERAPY

At times, preoperative or postoperative radiation therapy is required in order to provide the patient with the best chance for cure. Postoperative radiation therapy may follow a staging lymphadenectomy without hysterectomy. As mentioned previously, there is controversy about the extent of benefit for patients undergoing staging lymphadenectomy.[27,28] Regardless of the indication, the extraperitoneal approach to the paraaortic nodes has reduced the complication rate of radiation therapy following this operation.[29,47] We reserve the staging lymphadenectomy for selected patients and those in clinical trials. Postoperative radiation will also be proposed to patients explored for a radical hysterectomy but found to have multiple positive nodes or other evidence of high risk for recurrence. In those circumstances, the surgery is abandoned and the cervix and uterus left in place. Leaving the uterus may allow a better isodose distribution of the intracavitary cesium to the parametria. As mentioned previously, postoperative radiation may also be proposed to women who are found to have an unsuspected carcinoma of the cervix at the time of simple hysterectomy. Surgery may follow radiation therapy if there is incomplete or inadequate regression of a large barrel-shaped cervical carcinoma. This surgery may replace the final intracavitary cesium system. Although this approach may reduce the incidence of vaginal apex recurrences, the overall survival in this group of patients seems to be unchanged.[49] Other instances in which surgery and radiation are used in combination include the presence of a pelvic mass at the time of the original diagnosis, evidence of a pelvic abscess, a markedly enlarged uterus with leiomyomas, or uterine prolapse. It is important to reinforce the fact that the combination of surgery and radiation therapy in any sequence is associated with a higher complication rate than either therapy alone.

CERVICAL CANCER ASSOCIATED WITH PREGNANCY

It is hard to imagine a circumstance more emotional than the diagnosis of cancer associated with pregnancy. A Pap test is an essential part of the first prenatal visit. Colposcopy and cervical biopsy are performed to evaluate an abnormal Pap test during pregnancy. Endocervical curettage is usually not performed. A dysplastic process is followed with serial colposcopic examinations until the third trimester. Following delivery, full colposcopic examinations with endocervical curettage is performed and appropriate therapy proposed. If invasive cervical cancer during pregnancy cannot be excluded, conization of the cervix is performed. Because of the increased risk of miscarriage associated with conization and the inherent risk of miscarriage during the first trimester of pregnancy, we schedule the cervical conization at 13 to 14 weeks of gestational age. If invasive squamous-cell carcinoma is identified and satisfies the definition of microinvasion, conization alone is sufficient therapy, and the pregnancy continues to term. If invasive adenocarcinoma of any depth or squamous-cell carcinoma invading more than 3 mm is described, radical hysterectomy with pelvic lymphadenectomy is usually recommended. The decision regarding timing of the radical hysterectomy is based on the duration of gestation, patient desires, and usually involves

Chapt...

Uter...

Randall K. G...
Ward A. Kats...

14. Fink DJ. Change in American Cancer
    for detection of cervical cancer. CA C
    38:127.

15. Richart RM. Natural history of cervic
    neoplasia. Clin Obstet Gyecol 1968;1(

16. Lundberg G. The 1988 Bethesda syster
    vical/vaginal cytologic diagnoses. JAM

17. Broder S. Report of the 1991 Bethesd
    1992;267:1892.

18. Zaino RJ, Ward S, Delgado G, et al. H
    dictors of the behavior of surgically tr
    mous cell carcinoma of the uterine ce
    oncology group study. Cancer 1992;69

19. Abeler VM, Holm R, Nesland JM, Kjc
    cell carcinoma of the cervix: a clinicop
    26 patients. Cancer 1994;73:672.

20. Eifel PJ, Morris M, Oswald MJ, et al. /
    the uterine cervix: prognosis and patte
    376 cases. Cancer 1990;65:2507.

21. Averette HE, Nguyen HN, Donato D
    hysterectomy for invasive cervical canc
    prospective experience with the Mian
    Suppl 1993;71:1422

22. Harrison TA, Sevin BU, Koechli O, et
    carcinoma of the cervix: prognosis in
    treated by radical hysterectomy. Gynec
    50:310.

23. Creasman WT. New gynecologic stagi
    1995;58:157.

24. Moore DH, Dotters DJ, Fowler WC. (
    phy: does it really improve the treatmc
    noma? Am J Obstet Gynecol 1992;16'

25. Hofmann HMH, Ebner F, Haas J, et a
    nance imaging in clinical cervical canc
    tumor volumetry. Baillieres Clin Obste
    2:789.

26. Heller PB, Malfetano JH, Bundy BN,
    pathologic study of stages IIB, III, and
    the cervix: extended diagnostic evalua
    node metastases—a gynecologic oncol
    Gynecol Oncol 1990;38:425.

27. Barber HRK. Cervical cancer: pelvic
    lymph node sampling and its consequ
    Obstet Gynaecol 1988;2:768.

28. Heaps JM, Berek JS. Surgical staging (
    Clin Obstet Gynecol 1990;33:852.

29. Cosin JA, Fowler JM, Chen MD, et al
    cal staging of patients with cervical ca
    for lymph node debulking. Cancer 19

30. Lanciano RM, Martz K, Montana GS
    ence of age, prior abdominal surgery,
    dose on complications after radiation
    mous cancer of the uterine cervix: a p
    Cancer 1992;69:2124.

31. Barter JF, Soong SJ, Shingleton HM,
    of combined radical hysterectomy–po
    therapy in women with early stage ce
    necol Oncol 1989;32:292.

32. Seski JC, Murray RA, Morley G. Mic
    carcinoma of the cervix: definition, hi
    results of treatment. Obstet Gynecol 1

ENDOMETR...

Endometrial ...
malignancy er...
gynecologist. ...
common mali...
behind breast, ...
ican Cancer ...
33,000 new ...
about 1 in 100...
proximately 5...
this malignanc...
cer and more ...
of cervical car...
this cancer as ...
these women ...
prognosis with...
vival advantag...
ease of the pc...
cases are seen ...

consultation with a neonatologist to discuss neonatal outcome based on gestational age. For patients in the first and early second trimester, Porro radical hysterectomy with fetus in utero and pelvic lymphadenectomy is proposed. Toward the end of the second trimester and during the third trimester, cesarean radical hysterectomy is performed. We prefer to consult the maternal–fetal service to assess fetal viability prior to delivery. For patients with advanced-stage cancer (Stages II to IV), primary radiation therapy is used in the first trimester and early second trimester. For patients with larger or more advanced-cancers in the late second and third trimesters, cesarean delivery followed by radiation therapy is proposed. Emotional support to an extent much greater than usual is required for the pregnant patient with cervical cancer. In general, the prognosis for patients diagnosed with cervical cancer during pregnancy is similar to nonpregnant patients with comparable stage and tumor size.[50]

LARGE-VOLUME OR ADVANCED-STAGE CERVICAL CANCER

Initial tumor volume or size and extent or spread of disease predicts treatment failure. Patients with large Stage II to IV disease experience decreasing local or central control and increasing risk of distant or para-aortic nodal metastases.[39] Radiation therapy remains the mainstay of therapy for most women with advanced or large-volume cancer of the cervix. The practice of combining chemotherapy and radiation therapy continues to be investigated. Hydroxyurea or cisplatin given as radiation sensitizers to enhance the effects of radiation therapy in achieving local control has been reported.[51-53] Current clinical trials sponsored by the Gynecologic Oncology Group and the Radiation Therapy Oncology Group are addressing the clinical benefit of chemoradiation or radiation sensitizers. In this setting, chemotherapy is given during and following the radiation therapy. In contrast, neoadjuvant chemotherapy with cisplatin or a cisplatin-containing combination of drugs is given prior to radiation therapy to chemically reduce the tumor volume. Several studies have demonstrated an excellent response rate; however, the impact on overall survival was minimal.[54] Patients found to have large-volume or advanced disease at the time of initial diagnosis should be offered participation in clinical trials if available. Undue pessimism should be avoided;

even in patients with Stage IIIB cancer fixed to the pelvic side wall, the five-year survival rate will be approximately 30%. Extended-field radiation therapy will save a number of patients with documented para-aortic adenopathy.[55] Unfortunately, women found to have metastatic disease beyond the paraaortic nodes are seldom, if ever, cured. Protracted survival with a combination of chemotherapy and radiation therapy may be achieved in some patients.

UNIQUE PROBLEMS ASSOCIATED WITH THE DIAGNOSIS OF ADVANCED CERVICAL CANCER

Patients with advanced or large-volume cancer of the cervix may present with unilateral or bilateral ureteral obstruction, severe pain, or massive vaginal bleeding. Two of these problems—severe pain and massive vaginal bleeding—require immediate treatment. Ureteral obstruction is a unique problem, which may require more protracted discussion with the patient and her family. Women found to have ureteral obstruction secondary to cervical cancer, with disease confined to the pelvis or lower paraaortic region, are managed by placement of ureteral stents in a retrograde manner at the time of cystoscopy or antegrade by way of a percutaneous approach. If ureteral stents cannot be placed, temporary, percutaneous nephrostomy may be required. As radiation therapy reduces the tumor volume and ureteral obstruction, the stents are removed. On rare occasions, renal failure is the presenting problem of a patient with widely metastatic cervical cancer. Especially in a woman of advanced age with multiple medical problems and noncurable cancer, the patient and family must clearly understand the consequences and expected outcome prior to proceeding with a protracted, aggressive treatment and correction of the ureteral obstruction.

Eventually, most clinicians will be faced with the patient who presents to the office or emergency room with persistent, heavy, vaginal bleeding arising from a large, necrotic cervical cancer replacing the upper vagina. Fortunately, most of these patients can be treated by the judicious use of Monsel solution (ferrous subsulfate). If this fails, Monsel solution is applied to the bleeding tumor and a dry, 2-in. vaginal pack is used to apply pressure and fill the vagina. The pack is gently removed, usually as an outpatient, 24 hours later. Immediate consultation with a radiation oncologist is sought and may require initiation of therapy

Most clinicians will terminate t
performing the exenteration i
identified or if there is extensi
currence into the peritoneal ca

Historically, patients subject
procedure of any type were lef
urinary conduit stoma or both
low stapled anastomosis of the
the levator muscles have allowe
spared a permanent colostom
niques for continent urinary div
inated the need for a urostomy
ber of women.[68] Multiple te
described for vaginal reconstr
pelvic exenteration. Gracilis
myocutaneous flaps have provic
of tissue for vaginal reconstruc
for the elimination of ostomie:
of a neovagina, the physical anc
an exenterative procedure war
pretreatment selection and cou
patients. The late Dr. Felix Ru
all the gynecologic oncologists
a patient to undergo a pelvic
commitment to that patient fe

For patients undergoing p
risk of subsequent recurrent ca
62%.[67] Approximately 50% of i
tant disease and 50% recur in th
surveillance of patients under;
tion is directed toward identify
complications rather than exte
recurrent disease. Aggressive ra
in the asymptomatic patient m
recurrent disease; however, suc
recurrence is rare.

PALLIATIVE CARE

Patients with recurrent cervic
radiation therapy has failed, or
for radiation therapy, and whc
pelvic exenteration are offe
most cases this involves man
such as pain, bleeding, nausea,
of the ability to cure recurr
must be assured of the ability
toms of recurrent cancer. Opi
gesics and adjuvant drugs are
Rapid and aggressive contro

stages II
Int J Ra
52. Bonomi
trial of t
carcinor
study. J
53. Tseng (
concurr
vanced
1997;66
54. Souham
chemot
stage II
9:1991.
55. Podczas
radiatio
1990;66
56. Hoskins
tomy ar
of early
1976;4:
57. Perez (
alone ir
a 20 ye
58. Fletche
ture. Ar
111:22!
59. Perez (
therapy
ine cer
51:139.

their clinical behavior, diagnosis, and management as
well as therapy will also be presented.

Epidemiology

Endometrial adenocarcinoma affects women primarily in the postmenopausal and perimenopausal years
and is most frequently diagnosed between the ages of
50 and 65 years. As stated above, 75% of the women
are postmenopausal, while 25% are premenopausal,
and of this group 5% are diagnosed in women under
40 years of age. Rising sharply after 45 years of age,
the peak incidence of endometrial adenocarcinoma is
between 55 and 69 years of age, followed by a gradual decrease in its incidence thereafter. Two pathways
in the development of endometrial adenocarcinoma
have been postulated. The first and most common is
the recognized transition from atypical endometrial
hyperplasia to invasive adenocarcinoma that arises in
a background of unopposed estrogen. The second
pathway is the development of de novo adenocarcinoma without prior atypical hyperplasia or estrogen
use. These non–estrogen-related adenocarcinomas tend
to occur in the elderly, are associated with less favorable and aggressive histologic subtypes, are more
poorly differentiated, and carry an overall worse prognosis as compared with the initial subset.

Endometrial hyperplasias tend to develop earlier
than adenocarcinomas, with a peak incidence occurring between the ages of 40 and 60 years. In one
study 40% occurred between the ages of 40 and 50
years, 25% in the ages between 50 and 60 years, and
15% in patients less than 40 years of age.[1] These
findings support the basis of endometrial hyperplasias being precursors to adenocarcinoma of the
endometrium.

Many factors increase the likelihood of endometrial adenocarcinoma developing as well as endometrial hyperplasia; these factors are summarized in Table
65-1. Menopausal unopposed estrogen replacement
seems to be a primary factor, increasing a women's
risk for adenocarcinoma by 4 to 8 times. This risk is
higher with increasing doses of unopposed estrogen
as well as prolonged use. This risk is substantially reduced when progestins are used in combination with
estrogen. Similarly, combination oral contraceptives
also decrease the relative risk. Other forms of increased estrogenic stimulation also increase the risk.
Stein–Leventhal syndrome (polycystic ovary syndrome) or any state of chronic anovulation can also
lead to a hyperestrogenic state and hyperplasia and
subsequent adenocarcinoma. Estrogen-secreting tumors, such as granulosa-cell tumors, have also been
determined to increase the risk of developing adenocarcinoma. An association has been made between
prolonged tamoxifen use and the development of endometrial adenocarcinoma, with a risk that is 7.5
times higher than a nonuser of tamoxifen.[2] However,
when one weighs tamoxifen's role in reducing breast
cancer recurrence by 38%, the risk of developing a tamoxifen-induced endometrial adenocarcinoma is ac-
ceptably low.

MacMahon defined three of the most important
risk factors as obesity, nulliparity, and a late menopause,
occurring after 52 years of age.[3] Women who are 21
to 50 lb over ideal body weight have a 3-fold increased risk, whereas those more than 50 lb over ideal
body weight have a 10-fold higher risk for adenocarcinoma. This has been linked to the increased peripheral conversion of androstenedione to estrone in
morbidly obese women, as well as a potential link to
dietary fat intake. Nulliparous women carry a 2 times

TABLE 65-1
ENDOMETRIAL CARCINOMA RISK FACTORS

Increases the Risk	Diminishes the Risk
Unopposed estrogen stimulation	Ovulation
Unopposed menopausal estrogen-replacement therapy (4–8X)	Progestin therapy
Menopause after age 52 (2.4×)	Combination oral contraceptives
Obesity (21–50 lb., 3×) (over 50 lb., 10×)	Menopause prior to age 49
Nulliparity (2–3×)	Normal weight
Diabetes (2.8×)	Multiparity
Feminizing ovarian tumors	
Polycystic ovarian disease	
Tamoxifen	

increased risk for adenocarcinoma as compared with women who have had one child, and three times the risk as compared with women who have had five or more children. Age at menopause has also been identified as a risk, with women who undergo a "late" menopause (later than age 52) having a 2.5-fold increased risk.

Various other factors have been postulated. Diabetes mellitus carries a 2.8 times increased risk and is commonly associated with obesity. Idiopathic hypertension may also increase the relative risk 1.5 times, but its association with endometrial adenocarcinoma is not as strong. With regard to race, white women are twice as likely to have endometrial adenocarcinoma as their African-American counterparts.

Endometrial Hyperplasia

Endometrial hyperplasia occurs during long periods of unopposed estrogen such as chronic anovulation, especially around the perimenopause. Perimenopausal bleeding is usually marked by skips and delays in the woman's cycle. Any marked increase in the amount of flow or frequency of bleeding should warrant a thorough evaluation and biopsy. The current classification, which is accepted by the International Society of Gynecologic Pathologists, is based on the degree of cytologic atypia, since these are the only lesions that readily progress to endometrial adenocarcinoma. This classification system is presented in Table 65-2, and groups the hyperplasias into architectural as well as cytologic categories. Microscopically the architecture is described as simple (cystic) or complex, whereas cytologic atypia is either present or absent. If cytologic atypia is present, qualifications such as mild or severe may also be used. In general, hyperplasia is defined as a diffuse thickening of the endometrial lining with increased volume of tissue as well as an increase in the number and size of the endometrial glands.

Simple hyperplasia defines a thickened endometrium with large dilated glands in an abundant stroma. The outline of the glands has some invaginations and rare irregular outlines, giving this endometrial lining a "Swiss cheese" appearance. There is little or no progression to cancer.

Complex hyperplasia has increased thickness with crowded back-to-back glands and little intervening stroma. Most of the glands have an irregular outline, with some demonstrating papillary processes

TABLE 65-2
CLASSIFICATION OF ENDOMETRIAL HYPERPLASIAS

Types of Hyperplasia	Progressing to Cancer (%)
Simple (cystic) without atypia	1
Complex (adenomatous) without atypia	3
Simple with atypia	8
Complex with atypia	29

or bridges. This finding carries a low premalignant potential.

In atypical hyperplasias there is marked cytologic atypia of the nuclei within the glands. This is represented by marked nuclear enlargement, an increase in nuclear to cytoplasmic ratio, prominent nucleoli, and coarse abundant chromatin. This type of hyperplasia definitely identifies a significant premalignant state with frank progression to endometrial adenocarcinoma.

The percentage of hyperplasias progressing to endometrial adenocarcinoma are as follows: simple hyperplasia without atypia, 1%; complex hyperplasia without atypia, 3%; simple hyperplasia with atypia, 8%; and complex atypical hyperplasia, 29%.[4] Overall, most hyperplasias spontaneously regress; however, the ones with cytologic atypia have an increased risk of progressing to adenocarcinoma. This progression usually occurs over several years.

Management

The management of endometrial hyperplasia depends on the patient's age and whether future childbearing is desired, as well as the degree of cytologic atypia. Women 20 to 30 years of age who desire future childbearing can undergo conservative management after dilation and curettage reveals no cytologic atypia. Most of these hyperplasias can be managed expectantly with long-term follow-up since most of these will spontaneously regress. If abnormal bleeding recurs, endometrial sampling should be repeated; otherwise, these patients are sampled at 6-month intervals. Anovulatory or irregular menstrual bleeding can be managed with medroxyprogesterone acetate (Provera), 10 mg for 10 to 14 days, to induce withdrawal bleeding, or oral contraceptives can be used to cause a normal cycle. Younger patients with atypia require definitive treatment. Prior to beginning progestins, these patients should undergo a formal dilation and curettage to rule out an occult adenocarcinoma.

For mild atypia, medroxyprogesterone acetate, 10 mg for 10 to 14 days, will usually suffice. However, for severe atypia, higher doses of 40 to100 mg per day for 3 months may be necessary. Sampling should be repeated at 3 months to see if the atypia has persisted or resolved. Once the hyperplasia has resolved, ovulation induction can occur if childbearing is desired. If persistent atypical hyperplasia is identified after high-dose progestins, hysterectomy should be considered.

For older patients, the risk of endometrial adenocarcinoma and frank progression increases. Hyperplasias with moderate to severe atypia require hysterectomy. For mild atypia, progestins may be used to avoid surgical intervention, but if the atypia fails to respond or abnormal bleeding persists, hysterectomy should follow. If, for medical reasons, a hysterectomy is not advisable, long-term high-dose progestins and periodic sampling should be advised. Options include mesestrol acetate (Megace) 40 to 160 mg per day; medroxyprogesterone acetate (Provera), 40 to 100 mg per day; or intramuscular medroxyprogesterone acetate (Depo-Provera), 200 mg followed by 100 mg intramuscularly every month. Patients should remain amenorrheic with this regimen and any bleeding should raise suspicion for persistent disease or progression.

Symptoms and Signs

Symptoms of early endometrial adenocarcinoma are relatively few. The hallmark sign is postmenopausal bleeding, followed by abnormal perimenopausal bleeding, including increased frequency and amount of menses. Vaginal discharge is present in 90% of patients, and leukorrhea can be seen in 10%. Approximately 15% of all postmenopausal bleeding is due to endometrial carcinoma. There must be a high index of suspicion for patients under the age of 40 with chronic anovulation, as most of these cases are dismissed as "menstrual irregularities." Endometrial carcinoma should be considered in all females with postmenopausal bleeding, pyometra, perimenopausal patients with abnormal uterine bleeding and chronic anovulation, and the asymptomatic postmenopausal female with endometrial cells on a Pap smear. Incidentally, the routine Pap smear can detect endometrial carcinoma 50% of the time.

Signs of advanced disease include pelvic pressure or pain, increased urinary frequency, constipation, the presence of a palpable abdominal mass, or ascites.

Metastatic disease can be heralded by a chronic cough suggestive of pulmonary metastases to skeletal pain from bone involvement.

Diagnosis

The diagnosis of endometrial hyperplasia or adenocarcinoma is established by histologic examination of the sampled endometrium. This sample may be obtained from office endometrial biopsies or fractional dilation and curettage. Over 90% of endometrial carcinomas can be successfully detected with procedures that sample the endometrial cavity directly, making the office endometrial biopsy a safe and cost-effective tool for sampling the endometrium. Most patients tolerate the endometrial biopsy in the office without difficulty or analgesia. For patients in whom the procedure is difficult, a paracervical block or an oral antiprostaglandin 30 minutes prior to sampling may be used. If the endometrial biopsy is positive for endometrial carcinoma the diagnosis is definitive and a formal dilation and curettage is not necessary. Studies have confirmed that the endometrial biopsy correlates well with the fractional dilation and curettage.[5-7] However, if the patient continues to have symptoms despite a negative endometrial biopsy, a formal dilation and curettage is indicated since a 10% false negative rate exists for endometrial biopsies. A diagnosis of endometrial hyperplasia does not obviate the need for further work-up and evaluation if symptoms continue. All office procedures should be coupled with endocervical curettage to rule out a primary cervical cancer in questionable cases.

When an endometrial biopsy is impossible, such as with cervical stenosis, a formal fractional dilation and curettage is necessary. A fractional dilation and curettage is a systematic evaluation that involves an examination under anesthesia to look for other potential sites for vaginal bleeding, including the vulva, vagina, and cervix. Endocervical curettage is performed and the specimen is handed off separately so that histologic examination of the endocervix is not influenced by potential "drag down" from the uterine cavity. The uterus is then sounded, dilated, and a formal curettage is obtained from all four sides of the uterine cavity. The fractional dilation and curettage is considered the gold standard for determining the histologic nature of the endometrium.

In the general population and asymptomatic women, the cost of screening for adenocarcinoma and its precursors by endometrial biopsy is prohibitive.[8]

Women on hormone-replacement therapy do not need a biopsy prior to beginning therapy or during therapy unless abnormal bleeding occurs. Other methods for detecting endometrial abnormalities are transvaginal ultrasound and hysteroscopy. Transvaginal ultrasound may be useful in detecting endometrial abnormalities in patients with abnormal bleeding. Atrophic endometrium was associated with an endometrial stripe <3 mm, whereas women with postmenopausal bleeding and an endometrial stripe ≥10 mm had a high incidence of harboring an endometrial carcinoma.[9] Hysteroscopy is being used more frequently in conjunction with the fractional dilation and curettage. This procedure has several advantages, including the ability to directly biopsy focal lesions that might be missed by biopsy alone, and the ability to evaluate the endocervical canal directly.

Pathology

Endometrial carcinoma may start as a discrete focal lesion as in a polyp, or it may also be diffuse in several different areas. In some situations it may involve the entire lining of the endometrial surface. Almost all endometrial carcinomas are primarily adenocarcinomas. The various types of endometrial carcinoma are listed in Table 65-3. Histologic grading can be determined by the architectural growth pattern of the tumor or by the tumor's nuclear features. Both are equally accurate in defining the degree of differentiation of the tumor, and this is expressed as the grade.[10] Both the architectural and nuclear grade are used in the current FIGO staging (1988).[11]

Architecturally speaking, Grade 1 carcinomas comprise a 5% or less non-squamous solid growth pattern. Grade 2 carcinomas have between a 6 to 50%

TABLE 65-3
CLASSIFICATION OF ENDOMETRIAL CARCINOMAS

Endometriod adenocarcinoma
    Papillary villoglandular
    Secretory
    Adenocarcinoma with squamous differentiation
      (adenoacanthoma)
Mucinous carcinoma
Serous carcinoma
Clear-cell carcinoma
Squamous-cell carcinoma
Undifferentiated carcinoma
Mixed types (adenosquamous carcinoma)
Metastatic carcinoma

---

solid growth pattern, and Grade 3 carcinomas have greater than 50%. In nuclear Grade 1 carcinomas the nuclei are oval, uniform in appearance, and have evenly dispersed chromatin. Nuclear Grade 3 carcinomas have large pleomorphic, somewhat bizarre, nuclei, coarse chromatin clumps, and noticeable nucleoli. Nuclear Grade 2 carcinomas are intermediate to these two categories. Notable nuclear atypia inappropriate for the architectural grade, usually a two-grade discrepancy, will raise the grade of the carcinoma by one category. In serous, squamous-cell, and clear-cell carcinomas the nuclear grading takes precedence over the architectural grade. Higher-grade carcinomas are associated with increased depth of myometrial invasion, as well as increased chance of lymph-node metastases.[12]

Endometrioid adenocarcinomas are the most common carcinomas found in the endometrium, representing 75 to 80% of all carcinomas. These carcinomas most closely resemble the endometrial cells. One-third to one-half of these carcinomas will contain squamous differentiation or metaplasia, and most are well differentiated, conferring a good prognosis. Endometrioid adenocarcinomas with greater than a 10% mature squamous component have been labeled in the past as adenoacanthomas. These carcinomas were thought to behave in a less aggressive manner; however, the prognosis is similar to an adenocarcinoma if comparable myometrial invasion, stage, and presence of lymph-node metastases are accounted for. Adenosquamous carcinomas are truly a mixed type but are described as such because the squamous component is also malignant. These carcinomas tend to be less differentiated and to carry a worse prognosis as compared with the other types.

Papillary and secretory adenocarcinomas are variants of endometrioid adenocarcinomas. Papillary endometrioid adenocarcinoma is so named when the tumor takes on a papillary architectural form. This condition is not to be confused with a papillary serous adenocarcinoma. Secretory adenocarcinomas are rare, are usually found in postmenopausal women, and have a well-differentiated glandular pattern. These usually carry a good overall prognosis.

Clear-cell adenocarcinomas are rare, and account for approximately 4% of all carcinomas. These carcinomas resemble the clear-cell adenocarcinomas of the ovary, cervix, and vagina. These tend to develop in older postmenopausal females and also carry a poor prognosis. Survival rates of 39 to 55% are quoted, which is much less than the standard 65% for endometrioid adenocarcinomas.

Serous adenocarcinomas are also highly aggressive, but uncommon. These tumors demonstrate papillary growth patterns and closely resemble papillary serous adenocarcinomas of the ovary and fallopian tube, and psammoma bodies are frequently present on microscopic examination. They are usually found in advanced stages, with early myometrial and lymphatic invasion as well as intraperitoneal spread. Fortunately these carcinomas represent less than 10% of all carcinomas.

Mucinous adenocarcinomas typically have columnar or pseudostratified epithelium resembling the endocervix or ovary and comprise less than 5% of these cancers. This finding carries the same prognosis as an endometrioid adenocarcinoma, but a primary endocervical carcinoma must be ruled out.

Primary squamous-cell carcinomas of the endometrium are very rare and the prognosis is poor. This carcinoma is often found in elderly postmenopausal women and associated with pyometra, chronic inflammation, and cervical stenosis.

Metastatic disease from any extragenital site can give rise to an endometrial carcinoma, with the most common being breast, stomach, colon, pancreas, and kidney. The most common genital-tract metastasis is from an undiagnosed ovarian carcinoma.

Pretreatment and Staging Studies

After the diagnosis of endometrial adenocarcinoma is made, a thorough evaluation to define the extent of disease should be performed. A complete history and physical examination is needed to detect extrapelvic disease. At this time, evaluation of other medical problems that may affect surgery or therapy are brought under reasonable control. Routine preoperative tests include a complete blood count (CBC), basic metabolic profile, liver-function tests (LFTS), urinalysis, electrocardiogram, and posteroanterior and lateral chest radiography.

For locally advanced disease, nonroutine tests such as cystoscopy or proctoscopy, as well as examination under anesthesia, may be necessary to accurately locate and define the extent of disease. A barium enema or colonoscopy should also be performed if guaiac-positive stools are encountered. A computed tomographic (CT) scan of the abdomen and pelvis should be considered for abnormal LFTs, clinical evidence for hepatomegaly, suspicion of ascites, a palpable abdominal mass, or for suspected extrauterine disease.

At present, the only way to accurately assess and diagnose the extent and depth of myometrial invasion is by histologic examination of the gross uterine specimen. Both CT and magnetic resonance imaging (MRI) and to some extent ultrasound have been used preoperatively to assess the degree of myometrial invasion. Until more information is available these studies in this context should be considered experimental.

Serum levels of CA-125 have been measured in many patients and are usually elevated in patients with extrauterine spread or advanced disease.[13] The CA-125 becomes most useful in patients with suspected advanced disease, known Stage II, III, and IV disease, Grade 3 tumors, or tumors that have a serous or clear-cell histology.[14] In this patient population, serial measurements were elevated in 94% of the cases with recurrent disease, and the CA-125 level correlated well with the patients' response to therapy.

Staging

Once pretreatment studies have been completed the patient undergoes primary therapy consisting of either surgery or radiation therapy. Two classification systems exist to stage endometrial carcinoma, as outlined by the International Federation of Gynecologists and Obstetricians (FIGO). The old classification system is outlined in Table 65-4 and is entirely clinical. This staging system was in use between 1971 and 1988. This is the primary staging system used when patients are given radiotherapy as their initial treatment, and it should be designated as such. Of interest, most statistics quoted on endometrial carcinoma

TABLE 65-4
FIGO STAGING CLASSIFICATION OF ENDOMETRIAL CARCINOMA (1971–1988)[15]

Stage	Characteristic
I	Confined to the corpus
IA	Uterine cavity ≤8 cm
	G1: Well differentiated
	G2: Moderately differentiated
	G3: Poorly differentiated
IB	Uterine cavity >8 cm, any grade
II	Involvement of corpus and cervix
III	Extension outside the uterus but not outside the true pelvis, may involve bladder or parametrium but not mucosa of bladder or rectum
IV	Extends outside the true pelvis or involves the mucosa of the bladder or rectum

TABLE 65-5
FIGO STAGING CLASSIFICATION OF ENDOMETRIAL CARCINOMA (1988 TO PRESENT)

Stages	Characteristic
IA G123	Tumor limited to the endometrium
IB G123	Invasion < 1/2 the myometrium
IC G123	Invasion > 1/2 the myometrium
IIA G123	Endocervical gland involvement only
IIB G123	Cervical stromal invasion
IIIA G123	Tumor invades serosa and/or adnexa, and/or positive peritoneal cytology
IIIB G123	Vaginal metastases
IIIC G123	Metastases to pelvic and/or paraaortic lymph nodes
IVA G123	Tumor invasion of bladder and/or rectum
IVB G123	Distant metastases, including intraabdominal and/or inguinal lymph nodes

come from the old data generated with this clinical staging. The new staging criteria was adopted by FIGO in 1988 and is represented in Table 65-5. Endometrial carcinoma is now surgically staged, with particular emphasis being placed on Stage 1 disease with regard to depth of myometrial invasion.

Prognostic Factors

There are many variables that affect the clinical behavior of endometrial adenocarcinomas. These variables can be either clinical or pathologic. Clinical variables include age, race, and clinical stage of disease. Pathologic variables include grade, histology, depth of myometrial invasion, the presence of lymphovascular space involvement, spread to the uterine cervix, adnexa, or peritoneal cavity, positive peritoneal cytology, and the presence of pelvic or paraaortic lymph-node metastases. Steroid hormone content has also been found to affect prognosis and is also listed as a potential prognostic factor.

Clinical Factors

It has been shown in retrospective reports that younger women with endometrial adenocarcinoma have an improved prognosis as compared with their older counterparts.[16] The survival rate for women less than 50 years of age is 95%, while for those over 50 years of age it is 75%. This is because older patients usually have tumors of a higher grade and stage than younger patients with a well-differentiated and less-invasive carcinoma. Overall survival rates for whites are 64%,

and 27% for African-Americans, again reflecting a higher stage and grade of tumor as compared with white women. Tumor stage is well recognized as the single most important clinical factor as far as overall survival is concerned. Survival at 5 years is as follows: Stage I, 76%; Stage II, 60%; Stage III, 29%; and Stage IV, 10%. Fortunately most endometrial adenocarcinomas are Stage I, representing approximately 70% of all carcinomas.

Pathologic Factors

Histologic subtype plays an important role as a pathologic factor. The best prognosis is found with the typical adenocarcinomas, such as endometrioid adenocarcinoma, adenoacanthomas, and secretory carcinomas. Several histologic subtypes, regardless of grade, carry a very poor and unfavorable prognosis and include serous, adenosquamous, and clear-cell histologies. Although these carcinomas represent less than 10% of all carcinomas, their overall 5-year survival rate is less than 33%.[17] This finding is probably secondary to their increased recurrence rates and findings of systemic or advanced disease at initial laparotomy.

Grade is one of the major determinants of prognosis, with increasing grade carrying an overall worse prognosis. Grade is one of the most sensitive indicators because as the grade of the carcinoma increases there is a greater tendency for myometrial invasion, and subsequent lymph-node involvement.[18] Fifty percent of all Grade 3 tumors have greater than one-half myometrial invasion; pelvic lymph nodes are found positive in 30% of the cases, and positive paraaortic lymph nodes in 20%. On the other hand, only 10% of Grade 1 carcinomas have deep myometrial invasion. Only 7% of all Grade 3 carcinomas are limited to the endometrium.

Another pathologic factor equally as important as grade is depth of myometrial invasion. Deep myometrial invasion (>50%) is associated with a higher probability of recurrence, treatment failure, and extrauterine spread of disease. This association is largely related to grade as well.[19] Depth of myometrial invasion is a better determinant for lymph-node metastases than grade. Regardless of grade, only 1% of endometrial carcinomas with superficial involvement have pelvic lymph-node metastases as compared with approximately 27% for deep myometrial involvement. Of interest, carcinoma being present in adenomyosis is not considered to be deep myometrial invasion but rather an extension into these glands from the endometrial surface.[20]

Isthmus or cervical extension is another factor that warrants discussion. The location of the tumor is important, as in endocervical gland versus stromal involvement, but so is extent of involvement. The risk of positive pelvic lymph nodes double if the isthmus or cervix is involved. Also, as can be expected, the incidence of positive paraaortic lymph nodes also increases.

Lymphovascular space involvement exists in approximately 15% of all carcinomas and is an independent risk factor. The rate of positive pelvic and paraaortic lymph nodes increases by four and six times, to 27% and 19%, respectively. Increases in recurrence rate and deaths have been reported with lymphovascular space involvement. In Stage IB adenocarcinomas the recurrence rate is 27% with lymphovascular space involvement to 9% without.[21]

In Stage I and occult Stage II disease there is a 6% finding of spread to the adnexa. In patients with microscopic or macroscopic adnexal involvement, 32% have positive pelvic nodes and 20% have positive paraaortic nodes.

Intraperitoneal spread is an ominous finding, and if this finding occurs without gross adnexal involvement it correlates highly with positive pelvic and paraaortic lymph nodes. Overall, 51% of the pelvic lymph nodes will be positive under these circumstances.

Peritoneal cytology is positive in 15% of all endometrial adenocarcinomas, and its significance is controversial. Thirty-five percent of these patients will have gross extrauterine disease with either adnexal involvement, intraabdominal spread, or enlarged nodal disease. However, 4 to 6% will not demonstrate any of the above findings. If a patient has positive cytology with obvious extrauterine spread, there is concern for a poorer prognosis, whereas those without may do well.[22]

Both the pelvic and paraaortic lymph nodes are negative predictors if found to be positive. The greatest predictor of positive paraaortic lymph nodes is positive pelvic lymph nodes, approaching 32%. The frequency for both increases with adverse histology, higher grades, deep myometrial invasion, isthmus or cervical involvement, lymphovascular space involvement, and extrauterine metastases.

Hormone-Receptor Status

The hormone-receptor status is an independent prognostic factor for endometrial adenocarcinoma. In endometrial adenocarcinomas the steroid-receptor level is lower than in normal endometrium. The mean number of estrogen and progesterone receptors is inversely proportional to the histologic grade; Grade 1 carcinomas are more likely to be estrogen- and progesterone-receptor–positive. Patients with carcinomas found to be positive for both receptors have a longer survival than those with negative receptors.[23] The progesterone receptor is a stronger predictor of survival than the estrogen receptor. Cutoff values for positivity are >70 fmol/picograms for the estrogen receptor and >30 fmol/pgm for the progesterone receptor.[24] Some studies say that it is always advisable to obtain a receptor measurement on the initial hysterectomy specimen. The absolute values named above may influence future responses to progestational therapy.

Summary of Prognostic Factors

Two large Gynecologic Oncology Group (GOG) trials were conducted in a surgically prospective randomized fashion in 1984 and 1987.[18,19] These studies defined the prognostic factors mentioned above and have helped create the current treatment approach for patients with this disease. Cell type and grade can be determined before hysterectomy by biopsy. It should be noted, however, that a 31% inaccuracy rate exists on determining grade by dilation and curettage.[25] Recognition of all the other factors requires laparotomy, cytology sampling, hysterectomy, and careful pathologic examination and interpretation of all tissue removed. Because of this, in 1988 FIGO redefined endometrial adenocarcinoma as a surgically staged disease and incorporated many of these risk factors into the staging process.

Patterns of Spread

Endometrial carcinoma can spread by four routes: direct extension of tumor to adjacent sites, transtubal passage of exfoliated cells, lymphatic spread, and hematogenous spread. The mechanism of direct spreading is the most common, with resultant penetration through the myometrium and serosa. Endometrial adenocarcinoma can also involve the cervix via direct extension from contiguous spread. Adnexal metastases may also result in this fashion.

The presence of cancer cells in pelvic washings and the development of widespread intraabdominal carcinomatosis in the face of early disease supports the concept of transtubal spread. This is especially true in the serous and clear-cell histologic type, which in-

[text obscured]

with

[text obscured]

that
...oral
...odes
...ent,
...libu-
...e in-
...posi-
...itive
...oc-
...agi-

...nost
...sites
...ther
...trial

...rci-
...my
...the
...lia-
...the
...to-
...re-
...all

patients. Postoperative radiation therapy is reserved for patients with high risk factors after reviewing all of the pathologic material from the initial staging operation.

After the diagnosis of endometrial carcinoma is confirmed and the cell type and grade have been determined, the patient undergoes the appropriate studies to assess extent of disease and to determine the patient's suitability for an operative intervention. Operability rates for endometrial cancer approach 87% despite many patients' comorbid illnesses.[26]

The operation commences with an adequate abdominal incision, which allows for a thorough abdominal exploration as well as possible lymphadenectomy. This usually occurs through a midline incision; however, a Pfannenstiel incision with a Maylard or Chearney modification may be used as well. A pelvic washing is then obtained using saline, or if ascites is present, this is aspirated and sent for cytology. Any suspicious or obvious areas of extrauterine disease

are biopsied. The surgeon then proceeds with a extrafascial hysterectomy with bilateral salpingo-oophorectomy after the ends of the tubes are occluded to prevent tumor spill during manipulation. It is not necessary to remove any vagina with this operation. The excised uterus is then opened off of the field and the depth of myometrial invasion as well as the presence or absence of cervical involvement is determined by gross observation, which is accurate 91% of the time.[27] If any questions persist or other abnormalities are noted, a frozen-section diagnosis may be obtained. If there is no gross evidence of extrauterine disease, a pelvic and paraaortic lymph-node sampling is performed for any of the following: myometrial invasion greater than one-half the full thickness, Grade 3 carcinomas with any amount of myometrial invasion, cervical extension, extrauterine spread, serous, clear-cell, or undifferentiated histologies are present, or for any suspicious or enlarged lymph nodes. Some gray zones exist and differ from institution to institution. Inner one-half myometrial invasion, especially the middle third, that is Grade 2 or 3, carries a 5% chance of having positive pelvic lymph nodes. It would be reasonable under these circumstances to proceed with a sampling procedure. Any time there is a question about the degree and depth of myometrial invasion, a full sampling should also occur. The overall surgical complication rate is approximately 15%, with 6% having serious complications.[28]

Alternative methods of surgery are now available. Laparoscopy-assisted vaginal hysterectomy with laparoscopic lymphadenectomy is being studied in Stage I disease.[29] Laparoscopy provides for an alternative approach that involves a shorter hospital stay. It has not been determined and as yet is unproven whether laparoscopy is equivalent to standard laparotomy in the treatment of this disease. Currently the GOG is conducting a randomized trial to answer this very question. Vaginal hysterectomy alone in patients with marked obesity, or severe medical problems that place them at risk for an abdominal operation, can also be considered. This can usually be accomplished without difficulty and is preferable to radiation therapy alone in the treatment of this disease. This approach is applicable to most Grade I lesions.

Both surgery and irradiation have been used effectively in the treatment of Stage I disease. As mentioned above, the cornerstone of treatment is total abdominal hysterectomy and bilateral salpingo-oophorectomy and this operation should be performed whenever feasible. For patients who are not able to undergo or tolerate a surgical procedure, irradiation can be used. It should be noted, however, that radiation alone has a poorer overall survival rate as compared with surgery in Stage I disease: 69% at 5 years as compared with 87% in the operated group.[30] The extent of the operation is based on the relative risk of spread of disease outside the uterus.

Stage I Grade 1

In apparent Stage I Grade 1 adenocarcinoma, the risk of spread to the pelvic lymph nodes is extremely small. A standard hysterectomy with bilateral salpingo-oophorectomy is performed and the routine sampling of retroperitoneal nodes is not necessary, but any enlarged or clinically suspicious lymph nodes need to be removed. If deep myometrial invasion (>50) is present, the tumor size is >2 cm, or involves the lower uterine segment or the cervix, lymph nodes should be sampled. Most patients with deep myometrial invasion would receive postoperative whole-pelvis radiation therapy to 5000 cGy.

Stage I Grade 2 or 3

In these carcinomas there is a definite risk of pelvic and paraaortic lymph node spread, especially with Grade 3 tumors. As a rough guideline, for Grade 2 tumors with middle-third invasion and for any invasive Grade 3 tumors the operative approach includes sampling of the pelvic and paraaortic lymph nodes. Grade 3 carcinomas with no evidence of myometrial invasion probably do not need to undergo sampling, but this group represents a very small proportion of all Grade 3 tumors. The use of postoperative radiation therapy depends upon the pathologic findings. For Grade 2 tumors with negative nodes with up to one-half myometrial invasion, these patients can receive vaginal-vault irradiation. This may also apply to Grade 3 lesions confined to the endometrium. For deeply invasive Grade 2 tumors and any invasion of a Grade 3 tumor, whole-pelvis radiation is recommended. If positive pelvic nodes are found, external radiation is employed to cover the lymph-node-bearing areas. Patients treated in this fashion have a 5-year survival of 72%. For positive paraaortic lymph nodes, extended-field radiation is employed, using 4500 to 5000 cGy for a cure rate of 36%. Adnexal involvement is another indication for whole-pelvis radiation therapy. In some cases, whole-abdominal radiation is given since transperitoneal seeding is common.

Stage II

Three essential options exist for the treatment of Stage II disease; primarily operative with a radical hysterectomy and lymph-node sampling, primarily radiation therapy followed by extrafascial hysterectomy, or irradiation alone. Radical abdominal hysterectomy with bilateral salpingo-oophorectomy is an effective treatment option, with an approximate 5-year survival rate of 75%.[31] Radiation therapy is added if there are positive pelvic or paraaortic lymph nodes. Most patients are treated with radiation followed by surgery. This approach uses 4500 cGy external to the pelvis followed by a single brachytherapy implant. This is then followed by an extrafascial hysterectomy and paraaortic lymph node sampling 4 to 6 weeks later. This approach may be the best for gross cervical involvement, attaining 5-year survival rates of 70 to 85%. If for some reason the disease is inoperable, the external-beam radiation therapy is followed by two brachytherapy implants. This results in inferior treatment, with a 5-year survival rate of only 50%.

Radiation Therapy Considerations

Adjuvant radiation therapy has not been shown to improve survival for patients with endometrial adenocarcinoma in any prospective randomized trials.[32] Since most patients have early Stage I disease and do well, a large number of patients would need to be studied to demonstrate a significant benefit from adjuvant radiation therapy. Vaginal-vault irradiation to 5500 to 6000 cGy significantly reduces the incidence of vault recurrences from 14% in the untreated group to 2% in those receiving vault irradiation.[33] Morbidity from this therapy is low and the only complication is vaginal stenosis and dyspareunia if a dilator is not used. Indications for external pelvic irradiation to 4500 to 5000 cGy are decreasing. Pelvic irradiation significantly reduces the risk of pelvic recurrence, especially those with poor prognostic factors such as Grade 3 tumors, deep myometrial invasion, and cervical extension.[34] Significant morbidity is in the 5% range with this procedure. Logical reasoning would suggest that the appropriate use of adjuvant radiation therapy in selected high-risk patients should improve overall survival based on the facts above.

Stage III

Stage III disease accounts for 7% of all known endometrial carcinomas. These carcinomas do not involve the bladder or rectum but are confined to the pelvis with locally advanced disease past the uterus. There are two groups of patients in this category. The first group is the most common and represents patients with clinical evidence of Stage III disease. This can be diagnosed with either parametrial, pelvic side-wall, or adnexal involvement with a mass, as well as vaginal extension. The other group is surgical Stage III patients with subclinical evidence of spread to the adnexal structures discovered at the time of surgery. Treatment is highly individualized. For grossly enlarged adnexal masses, surgical removal is warranted. For parametrial or vaginal involvement, radiation therapy alone or in combination with hysterectomy if possible can be performed. The operative removal of as much tumor as possible was of prognostic significance, especially with gross adnexal involvement. The 5-year survival for the first group is 16%, and for the latter group 40%.[35] For patients with gross intraperitoneal disease with residual tumor less than 2 cm or positive cytology, whole-abdominal irradiation may be effective in addition to whole-pelvis irradiation. The 5-year survival for this group of patients is 63%.[36] For carcinomas that extend to the pelvic side wall, radiation therapy alone is used. In this advanced-stage disease systemic metastases are a problem, but adjuvant systemic chemotherapy is at present unproven. Because most of these tumors are poorly differentiated, a response to progestins is unlikely in the face of low receptor content.

Stage IV

Stage IV disease accounts for 3% of the patients and is defined by tumor metastases outside the pelvis. The lung is the most common site of extrauterine spread, accounting for 36% of the total. The management of Stage IV disease relies on a combination of surgery, radiation, and some form of systemic therapy: either progestins, chemotherapy, or both. Local control can be afforded by a hysterectomy followed by pelvic radiation therapy. Progestins and chemotherapy can also be used, and the treatment is highly individualized. Results of treatment are poor, with 10% of the patients being alive at 5 years. In special circumstances a pelvic exenteration may be considered for bladder or rectal involvement only.

Treatment after Incomplete Staging

In certain situations a patient may present who has not been appropriately staged for one reason or another. Any patient with intermediate- or high-risk

factors in the hysterectomy specimen should have at least postoperative vault irradiation and probably whole-pelvis radiation. Whether or not to use an extended field to cover the paraaortic lymph nodes needs to be individualized. An alternative is to perform a laparoscopic staging procedure to identify patients with microscopic disease who would benefit from extended-field irradiation. For Grade 1 or 2 carcinomas with inner third involvement the recommendation is to do nothing but closely observe.

Treatment of Recurrent Disease

Patients with recurrent disease must undergo a full evaluation to determine all sites of recurrence, since the form of treatment will depend heavily on this finding. Depending on the site of disease recurrence, the treatment may be curative or palliative. Treatment for recurrent disease consists of surgery, radiation therapy, endocrinologic therapy, and cytotoxic chemotherapy. Recurrences are rarely cured unless they are isolated to the vaginal cuff. Most occur within the first 3 years from diagnosis, and 90% by 5 years. Half of these recurrences are in the pelvis and vagina while the other half are distant. The most frequent nonpelvic recurrences are in the lung (17%), upper abdomen (10%), and bone (6%).[37]

Patients with recurrent disease in the pelvis without distant disease and no prior radiotherapy can be treated for their recurrence with radiation therapy. The 5-year survival rate for an isolated vaginal cuff recurrence after irradiation is 40%, while the rate for those recurring in the parametria is 20%. Recurrent disease in the pelvic lymph nodes is a poor prognosis, with few survivors despite radiation therapy.[38] It should be noted that if a recurrence occurs outside a previously irradiated field primary irradiation can be used when localized disease is found.

Surgery can be used for recurrent disease if resectable disease is found and when surgical intervention is deemed feasible and safe. Unfortunately, an isolated recurrence that meets the above criteria is rare. In some patients a pelvic exenteration can be performed for centrally recurrent nonmetastatic disease in patients who have already received radiation therapy. In these patients, in whom initial surgery and adjuvant radiation therapy have failed, this operation may remain the only potentially curative one available. Studies demonstrate a 20% chance for long-term survival.[39]

Endocrinologic therapy remains a valuable adjunct in patients with recurrent endometrial carcinoma.

The overall response rate using this approach is approximately 25%.[40,41] In using endocrinologic therapy the overall dose and route of administration does not seem to be correlated to response. Oral agents appear just as effective as intravenous or intramuscular preparations, so oral dosing is preferred. Because of their overall low toxicity profile, progestins should be used in all patients with documented recurrence. The overall survival for patients on progestins is 1 year, but approximately 15% of these patients achieve remission or stable disease and live 4 years or more.[40,42] There is an increased likelihood for response in patients with well-differentiated tumors and with tumors that exhibit both estrogen- and progesterone-receptor positivity. Agents that are most commonly employed are megestrol acetate, 160 to 320 mg/day, or medroxyprogesterone acetate, 200 mg/day to 1000 mg/week. Tamoxifen, 20 to 40 mg/day, has also been used as a form of salvage therapy. Tamoxifen is postulated to possibly increase the progesterone-receptor content, making combination therapy with a progestin more effective. Recently, gonadotropin-releasing analogues such as leuprolide or goserelin have also been used in salvage therapy following progestins.[43] Overall there is a 35% response rate noted with this regimen.

Cytotoxic chemotherapy has been used in the treatment of endometrial carcinoma but remains entirely palliative. As with progestins, responses are more likely to be seen in tumors that are well differentiated and at distant sites not previously treated with radiation. Most responses are short, usually 3 to 6 months in duration, and are usually partial responses. The median time of survival is 7 to 10 months. The most effective single agents against endometrial carcinoma are cisplatin, carboplatin, and doxorubicin. These agents demonstrate complete and partial responses in approximately 20% or so of the patients. Single-agent paclitaxel therapy has also been used in the treatment for this cancer, with a overall response rate of 36%.[44] Because of the low success rates with single-agent chemotherapy, combinations of the above have been utilized. The most common combination in use is cisplatin, doxorubicin, and cyclophosphamide. The response rate with this combination regimen is 31 to 81%. The majority of these responses are partial, with the duration of response between 4 and 8 months. Overall median survival is approximately 12 months. In most regimens the chemotherapy is combined with progestins in the treatment of metastatic disease, and the responses seen are not affected by prior progestational treatment. It becomes obvious when one looks at these results that newer chemotherapeutic agents or combinations are needed if we are to be successful in treating this condition.

Estrogen Replacement in Endometrial Cancer

Estrogen replacement in patients with endometrial carcinoma appears safe; however, the numbers of patients studied to date is small. Estrogen-replacement therapy is needed to prevent osteoporosis and heart disease, as well as for the treatment of menopausal symptoms. It appears from some studies that survival is not reduced by the postoperative use of estrogen in patients with early-stage disease (Stage I or II).[45] In a 5-year follow-up study, more patients died in the nonuser group (76 patients), as compared with only one in the estrogen-user group, suggesting a potential benefit in the group that was treated. The American College of Obstetrics and Gynecology has stated that estrogens can be used in patients with endometrial cancer as in any other woman except that the selection should be based on her prognostic indicators and the risk the patient is willing to assume.[46] Because of these concerns the GOG is currently evaluating a large prospective randomized trial comparing estrogen use to placebo in patients with early-stage endometrial carcinoma.

UTERINE SARCOMAS

Uterine sarcomas represent 3 to 5% of all uterine cancers and as such are extremely rare tumors. A classification system has been adopted by the International Society of Gynecologic Pathologists[47] to describe these tumors, since prior classification systems have become obsolete and updated. Essentially, two groups have been described, with the first representing pure nonepithelial uterine sarcomas and the second representing mixed epithelial and nonepithelial tumors. This classification system is outlined in Table 65-6. The order for most common to least common are the carcinosarcomas, leiomyosarcomas, endometrial stromal sarcomas, and adenosarcomas. Any discussion regarding these tumors is difficult because of the paucity of cases and the data surrounding them. Prior reports tended to place all uterine sarcomas into one group, whereas we now know that each behaves separately from the others. This section will attempt

---

TABLE 65-6
CLASSIFICATION OF UTERINE SARCOMAS

Endometrial stromal tumors
  Stromal nodule
  Low-grade stromal sarcoma
  High-grade stromal sarcoma
Leiomyosarcoma
Adenosarcoma
  Homologous
  Heterologous
Carcinosarcoma
  Homologous
  Heterologous

---

to present the current therapies involved in the management of these uncommon sarcomas.

Epidemiology

As stated above, these tumors are rare, with an annual incidence of 0.5 case in 100,000 women.[48] Carcinosarcomas are the most common entity in this group. The rate of uterine sarcoma is higher in the African-American population as compared with whites, and the reason for this disparity is not yet known. There are distinctive age-specific incidence curves for the two most common sarcomas. Carcinosarcomas present later in life, and are extremely rare in women under 40 years of age. After 40 years of age, the incidence of carcinosarcoma increases gradually. Leiomyosarcomas, on the other hand, occur earlier, with a plateau between the ages of 45 and 55, with a subsequent decline in incidence thereafter. There is strong evidence to suggest that prior radiation may lead to some sarcomas, with most occurring 2 to 20 years after the radiation. In a compilation of reports, approximately 9% of women with a uterine sarcoma had a prior history of pelvic irradiation. This relationship tends to favor the development of carcinosarcomas and adenosarcomas, not leiomyosarcomas.[49]

Symptoms and Signs

Abnormal uterine bleeding is documented in 77 to 95% of all the patients diagnosed with uterine sarcomas, and by far is the most common symptom.[50] This bleeding can range from postmenopausal to \perimenopausal to frank menorrhagia. Pelvic pain is seen as well in one-third of the patients and is usually associated with an enlarging abdominal mass, which is associated with a foul-smelling discharge. Occasionally, tissue may be seen prolapsing through the external cervical os, and this is almost entirely diagnostic for a carcinosarcoma.[51] An enlarging uterus is the usual chief symptom in patients diagnosed with a leiomyosarcoma; it is present in approximately 48% of the patients.[52] It should be noted, however, that the "classic" sign of a rapidly enlarging fibroid was only present in 3% of the cases with leiomyosarcoma.

Diagnosis

The general workup for uterine sarcomas follows an abnormal bleeding or postmenopausal bleeding outline. Dilation and curettage remains the gold standard for any diagnostic workup for abnormal uterine bleeding. The sensitivity of endometrial biopsy varies with the histology of the tumor involved. Most patients with a carcinosarcoma will have a correct diagnosis made on endometrial biopsy because of the mixed nature of the histologic components involved. Patients with leiomyosarcoma are only 25 to 50% successful in making the diagnosis by biopsy, probably relating to the fact that this tumor originates from the myometrium and superficial biopsy would be ineffective.[53] Most women who are diagnosed with leiomyosarcoma do not need a preoperative biopsy since abnormal bleeding is attributed to benign leiomyomata. After a thorough history and physical examination, the other recommended studies resemble the workup for an endometrial carcinoma. A CT scan can be obtained in uterine sarcomas to preoperatively determine if extrauterine disease is present, since the incidence of this is higher than for endometrial carcinoma.

Pathology

The histologic features of uterine sarcomas are very different and will be discussed individually. Carcinosarcomas are mixed tumors that contain malignant epithelial and stromal components. This term is synonymous with malignant mixed mesodermal tumor and malignant mixed Müllerian tumor. Of the mixed group of sarcomas, carcinosarcomas are the most common. This tumor generally occurs in postmenopausal women as large, solitary masses associated with abnormal bleeding. As mentioned previously, this tumor is associated with rapid growth and occasionally can prolapse through the cervix as a mass. On opening the specimen grossly, these tumors have large areas of hemorrhage and necrosis, and myometrial invasion is common. Microscopic examination usually reveals the epithelial component to be an adenocarcinoma. Endometrioid, serous, and clear-cell histologies predominate, and they are often poorly differentiated and associated with a squamous component as well.[54] The stromal component is a high-grade sarcoma that is either homologous, arising from a cell type already present in the uterus, or heterologous, from a foreign cell not encountered in the uterus normally. Once thought to be of importance, more recent studies have not confirmed any survival difference between these two types.[55] It is believed that carcinosarcomas arise from a single undifferentiated precursor cell that allows for the two types of cancer to develop. The frequency of metastases increases with a high-grade epithelial component, deep myometrial invasion, the presence of lymphovascular space involvement, and cervical extension.

Leiomyosarcomas represent 25% of all of the uterine sarcomas. These sarcomas rarely arise from a benign leiomyoma and are usually solitary. Grossly, they have fleshy, infiltrative borders with multiple foci of hemorrhage. This sarcoma is the only one that originates from the myometrium itself, whereas the others come from the endometrium. Microscopically, they have high cellularity, marked nuclear atypia, and numerous mitotic figures.[56] The emphasis for aggressive behavior is usually placed on the number of mitoses per 10 high-power fields. A diagnosis of leiomyosarcoma is made when >5 mitoses per 10 high-power fields are present with marked cytologic atypia, or if >15 mitoses per 10 high-power fields are present without any atypia. It is important to rule out other benign conditions such as intravenous leiomyomatosis and disseminated peritoneal leiomyomas. In intravenous leiomyomatosis, cords of benign leiomyoma extend into the vascular lumens of veins, whereas disseminated peritoneal leiomyomas are multiple fibroids throughout the peritoneal cavity that spontaneously regress after pregnancy or contraceptive use.

There are three categories to endometrial stromal sarcomas, and their distinction continues to be controversial.[57] The first is the stromal nodule, which is a well-circumscribed proliferation of uniform cells that resembles normal proliferative-phase endometrium. This is an entirely benign condition, with no known recurrences. Low-grade endometrial stromal sarcomas have identical cells to the stromal nodules except that the margin becomes infiltrative and destructive. There is also a strong predisposition to lymphovascular-space involvement, and these tumors usually are positive for the estrogen and progesterone receptors.[58] This tumor is malignant, but recurrences take years, and these are hormonally responsive to progestins and estrogen withdrawal. High-grade endometrial stromal sarcomas have marked cellular atypia and an increased mitotic count which is usually >10 mitoses per 10 high-power fields. These are extremely aggressive tumors with frequent relapses. Adenosarcomas are the other group of mixed tumors that contain a benign epithelial component and a malignant nonepithelial component. These tumors are usually diagnosed at a younger age than are carcinosarcomas; they are solitary and arise in the fundus of the uterus. Microscopically, the epithelial component is benign, cystically dilated glands, and the sarcomatous component is usually low grade. Overall, these tumors follow a benign course.

Staging

The current accepted staging system for uterine sarcomas is a modification of the endometrial staging system and is shown in Table 65-7.

Patterns of Spread

In general the uterine sarcomas demonstrate two patterns of activity, one of aggressive growth, with early lymphatic and hematogenous spread, or a slow growth with long disease-free intervals indicative of an indolent pattern. Carcinosarcomas, high-grade leiomyosarcomas, and high-grade endometrial stromal sarcomas are in the first group, while low-grade leiomyosarcomas, low-grade endometrial stromal sarcomas, and adenosarcomas comprise the last group. In the first group, overall survival is poor, with most deaths occurring within the first 1 to 2 years after diagnosis.

TABLE 65-6
CONVENTIONAL STAGING OF UTERINE SARCOMAS

Stage	Characteristic
I	Confined to the uterine corpus
II	Confined to the corpus and cervix
III	Confined to the pelvis
IV	Extrapelvic sarcoma

Lymphatic metastasis is an important factor in the natural history of carcinosarcoma and may even preclude hematogenous spread. Extraabdominal metastases are common, and patients who die from uterine sarcoma usually have widespread intraabdominal and pelvic disease. Leiomyosarcomas tend to have hematogenous spread early, with the lungs being the most common extraabdominal site of involvement. The recurrence rate for Stage I disease in carcinosarcomas is 53%, and in leiomyosarcomas it is 71%.[59]

Treatment

The standard treatment for uterine sarcomas is surgical removal by a total abdominal hysterectomy with bilateral salpingo-oophorectomy. At the time of surgery, the tumor should be analyzed for estrogen and progesterone receptors. Carcinosarcomas are frequently surgically upstaged (~40%) from Stage I disease at the time of initial laparotomy.[51] This is related to their pattern of spread, as it mimics a poorly differentiated adenocarcinoma. Surgical debulking at the time of laparotomy does not have an impact on or improve survival. Many patients with carcinosarcoma have positive lymph nodes.[59] The surgical procedure for leiomyosarcoma mirrors that for carcinosarcoma except in the case of a premenopausal female. In certain cases in which the patient is young, the ovaries may be left to prevent premature menopause and the need for estrogen-replacement therapy. A staging lymphadenectomy can be performed to gain important prognostic information, but the yield is usually low in this disease. For the endometrial stromal sarcomas, a full hysterectomy and bilateral oophorectomy is indicated as well. The ovaries need to be removed in this disease because these tumors are mostly estrogen-receptor positive, and recurrence is high if estrogenic stimulation persists. Total abdominal hysterectomy with bilateral salpingo-oophorectomy is curative in patients with an adenosarcoma, and no further staging is warranted.

Radiation therapy has traditionally been used in the adjuvant setting for uterine sarcomas. Its use parallels the same indications as for endometrial carcinoma. To date, no randomized controlled trials have addressed the effect of radiation therapy on survival. This is because of the heterogeneity of the group studied and the relatively small number of cases, which prohibits comparison. Because of this, local and regional tumor control is a more reliable measure of radiation's effectiveness. Adjuvant whole-pelvis radiation therapy significantly decreases the local failure rate in these diseases. Local failure rates for carcinosarcoma approach 26% for surgery alone, and are reduced to 16% with radiation. The same is also true for leiomyosarcoma, and the endometrial stromal sarcomas. Using radiation therapy as the primary and sole treatment for these conditions seems somewhat effective in the inoperable patient but does not approach the success of surgery combined with radiation.

Uterine sarcomas have two features that make systemic chemotherapy attractive: they have a significant recurrence rate of 50% in Stage I disease, and their propensity for early spread and recurrence at distant sites. To date, there is no proven role for adjuvant chemotherapy in the treatment of early-stage disease in which the disease has been completely excised. Chemotherapy is reserved for advanced or recurrent disease only. In carcinosarcomas, ifosfamide is the most active single agent to date, with an overall response rate of 32%.[60,61] Cisplatin is next, with an overall response rate of 19%. A current trial of the GOG is now looking at the combination of ifosfamide and cisplatin in the treatment of carcinosarcoma. Doxorubicin, an agent with activity in most other soft-tissue sarcomas, has no efficacy in carcinosarcoma. However, doxorubicin has demonstrated significant activity in leiomyosarcoma, with an overall response rate of 25%.[62] Ifosfamide has little or no activity in leiomyosarcoma. Because of the above limitations, new efforts are being made to identify additional active drugs as well as new combinations that may be helpful in the treatment of advanced or recurrent disease.

REFERENCES

1. Gusberg SB, Kaplan AL. Precursors of corpus cancer. IV. Adenomatous hyperplasia as stage 0 carcinoma of the endometrium. Am J Obstet Gynecol 1963;87:662.
2. Barakat RR. The effect of tamoxifen on the endometrium. Oncology 1995;9:129.
3. MacMahon B. Risk factors for endometrial cancer. Gynecol Oncol 1974;2:122.
4. Kurman RJ, Kaminski PF, Norris HJ. The behavior of endometrial hyperplasia: a long-term study of "untreated" hyperplasia in 170 patients. CA Cancer J Clin 1985;56:403.
5. Grimes DA. Diagnostic office curettage; heresy no longer. Contemp Obstet Gynecol 1986;27:96.
6. Mattingly RF, Thompson JD. Dilatation of the cervix and curettage of the uterus. In: Mattingly RF, Thompson JD, eds. Operative gynecology, 6th ed. Philadelphia: Lippincott, 1985;495.

7. Walters D, Robinson D, Park RC, Patow WE. Diagnostic outpatient aspiration curettage. Obstet Gynecol 1975; 46:160.

8. Koss LG, Schreiber K, Oberlander SG, et al. Detection of endometrial carcinoma and hyperplasia in asymptomatic women. Obstet Gynecol 1984;64:1.

9. Granberg S, Wikland M, Karlsson B, et al. Endometrial thickness as measured by endovaginal ulrasonography for identifying endometrial abnormality. Am J Obstet Gynecol 1991;164:47.

10. Zaino RJ, Kurman RJ. Squamous differentiation in carcinoma of the endometrium: a critical appraisal of adenoacanthoma and adenosquamous carcinoma. Semin Diagn Pathol 1988;5:154.

11. International Federation of Gynecology and Obstetrics. Annual report on the results of treatment in gynecologic cancer. Int J Gynecol Obstet 1989;28:189.

12. Creasman T, Boronow RC, Morrow CP, et al. Adenocarcinoma of the endometrium: its metastatic lymph node potential. Gynecol Oncol 1976;4:239.

13. Olt G, Berchuck A, Bast RC Jr. The role of tumor markers in gynecologic oncology. Obstet Gynecol Surv 1990; 45:570.

14. Rose PG, Sommers RM, Reale FR, Hunter RE, Fournier L, Nelson BE. Serial serum CA-125 measurements for evaluation of recurrence in patients with endometrial carcinoma. Obstet Gynecol 1994;84:12.

15. International Federation of Gynecology and Obstetrics. Classification and staging of malignant tumors in the female pelvis. Int J Gynecol Obstet 1971;9:172.

16. Christopherson WM, Connelly PJ, Alberhasky RC. Carcinoma of the endometrium. V. An analysis of prognosticators in patients with favorable subtypes and stage I disease. Cancer 1983;51:1705.

17. Wilson TO, Podratz KC, Gaffey TA, et al. Evaluation of unfavorable histologic subtypes in endometrial adenocarcinoma. Am J Obstet Gynecol 1990;162:418.

18. Creasman WT, Morrow CP, Bundy BN, et al. Surgical pathologic spread patterns of endometrial cancer (a Gynecologic Oncology Group study). Cancer 1987;60:2035.

19. Boronow RC, Morrow CP, Creasman WT, et al. Surgical staging in endometrial cancer: clinico-pathologic findings of a prospective study. Obstet Gynecol 1984;63:825.

20. Hall JB, Young RH, Nelson JH. The prognostic significance of adenomyosis in endometrial carcinoma. Gynecol Oncol 1984;17:32.

21. Aadlers J, Abeler V, Kolstad P, Onsrud M. Postoperative external irradiation and prognostic parameters in stage I endometrial carcinoma. Obstet Gynecol 1980;56:419.

22. Kadar N, Homesley HD, Malfetano JH. Positive peritoneal cytology is an adverse factor in endometrial carcinoma only if there is other evidence of extrauterine disease. Gynecol Oncol 1992;46:145.

23. Liao BS, Twiggs LB, Leung BS, et al. Cytoplasmic estrogen and progesterone receptors as prognostic parameters in primary endometrial carcinoma. Obstet Gynecol 1986; 67:463.

24. Palmer DC, Muir IM, Alexander AI, et al. The prognostic importance of steroid receptors in endometrial carcinoma. Obstet Gynecol 1988;72:388.

25. Saint Cassia LJ, Wepplemann B, Shingleton H, et al. Man-

26. agement of early endometrial carcinoma. Gynecol Oncol 1989;35:362.

26. Marziale P, Atlante G, Pozzi M. 426 cases of stage I endometrial carcinoma: a clinicopathological analysis. Gynecol Oncol 1989;32:278.

27. Doering DL, Barnhill DR, Weiser EB, et al. Intraoperative evaluation of depth of myometrial invasion in stage I endometrial adenocarcinoma. Obstet Gynecol 1989;74:930.

28. Morrow C, Bundy BN, Kumar RJ, et al. Relationship between surgical-pathological risk factors and outcome in clinical stage I and II carcinoma of the endometrium: a Gynecologic Oncology Group study. Gynecol Oncol 1991;40:55,.

29. Childers JM, Brzechffa PR, Hatch KD, Surwit EA. Laparoscopically assisted surgical staging (LASS) of endometrial cancer. Gynecol Oncol 1993;51:33.

30. Bickenbach W, Lochmuller H, Dirlich G, et al. Factor analysis of endometrial carcinoma in relation to treatment. Obstet Gynecol 1967;29:632.

31. Homesley HD, Boronow RC, Lewis JL. Stage II endometrial adenocarcinoma. Obstet Gynecol 1977;49:604.

32. Piver MS, Yazigi R, Blumenson L, Tsukada Y. A prospective trial comparing hysterectomy, hysterectomy plus vaginal radium, and uterine radium plus hysterectomy in stage I endometrial carcinoma. Obstet Gynecol 1979;54:85.

33. Lotocki RJ, Copeland LJ, DePetrillo AD, Muirhead W. Stage I endometrial adenocarcinoma: treatment results in 835 patients. Am J Obstet Gynecol 1983;146:141.

34. Salazar OM, Feldstein ML, DePapp EW, et al. Endometrial carcinoma: analysis of failures with special emphasis on the use of initial preoperative external pelvic radiation. Int J Radiat Oncol Biol Phys 1977;2:1101.

35. Aadlers JG, Abeler V, Kolstad P. Clinical (stage III) as compared to subclinical intrapelvic extrauterine tumor spread in endometrial carcinoma: a clinical and histopathological study of 175 patients. Gynecol Oncol 1984;17:64.

36. Greer BE, Hamburger AD. Treatment of intraperitoneal metastatic adenocarcinoma of the endometrium by the whole-abdomen moving strip technique and pelvic boost irradiation. Gynecol Oncol 1983;16:365.

37. Aadlers JG, Abelar V, Kolstad P. Recurrent adenocarcinoma of the endometrium: a clinical and histopathological study of 379 patients. Gynecol Oncol 1984;17:85.

38. Kuten A, Grigsby P, Perez C, Fineberg B, Garcia D, Simpson J. Results of radiotherapy in recurrent endometrial carcinoma: a retrospective analysis. Int J Radiat Biol Phys 1989;17:29.

39. Barakat RR, Patel DA, Curtin JP, Venkatraman ES, Hoskins WJ. Pelvic exenteration for recurrent endometrial adenocarcinoma. Gynecol Oncol 1966;250:163.

40. Thigpen JT, Blessing J, DiSaia P. Oral medroxyprogesterone acetate in advanced or recurrent endometrial carcinoma: results of therapy and correlation with estrogen and progesterone levels: the Gynecologic Oncology Group experience. In: Baulieu EE, Slacobelli S, McGuire WL, eds. Endocrinology of malignancy. Park Ridge, NJ: Parthenon, 1986:446.

41. Thigpen JT, Homesley HD. A randomized study of medroxyprogesterone acetate (MPA) 200 mg. versus 1000 mg. in the treatment of advanced, persistent or recurrent carcinoma of the endometrium. In: Gynecologic

Oncology Group statistical report—February 1990. Buffalo: Gynecologic Oncology Group, 1990;177.

42. Refenstein EC Jr. The treatment of advanced endometrial cancer with hydroxyprogesterone caproate. Gynecol Oncol 1974;2:377.

43. Gallagher CJ, Oliver RT, Oram DH, et al. A new treatment for endometrial cancer with gonadotropin releasing-hormone analogue. Br J Obstet Gynecol 1991;98:1037.

44. Ball H, Blessing JA, Lentz S, Mutch D. A phase II trial of Taxol in advanced and recurrent adenocarcinoma of the endometrium: a Gynecologic Oncology Group study. Proceedings of the Society of Gynecologic Oncologists Annual Meeting. 1995;102. abstract.

45. Creasman WT, Henderson D, Hinshaw W, Clarke-Pearson DL. Estrogen replacement therapy in the patient treated for endometrial cancer. Obstet Gynecol 1986;67:326.

46. American College of Obstetricians and Gynecologists. Estrogen replacement therapy and endometrial cancer. ACOG Committee Opinion. August 1993. no. 126.

47. Modified from Clement P, Scully RE. Pathology of uterine sarcomas. In: Coppleson M, ed. Gynecologic oncology. New York: Churchill Livingstone, 1981:591.

48. Harlow BL, Weiss NS, Lofton S. The epidemiology of sarcomas of the uterus. J Natl Cancer Inst 1986;76:399.

49. Clement PB, Scully RE. Mullerian adenosarcoma of the uterus: a clinicopathologic analysis of 100 cases with a review of the literature. Hum Pathol 1990;21:363.

50. Kahanpaa KV, Wahlstrom T, Grohn P, et al. Sarcomas of the uterus: a clinicopathologic study of 119 patients. Obstet Gynecol 1986;67:417.

51. Nielsen SC, Podratz KC, Scheithauer BW, O'Brien PC. Clinicopathologic analysis of uterine malignant mixed mullerian tumors. Gynecol Oncol 1989;34:372.

52. Hannigan EV, Gomez IG. Uterine leiomyosarcoma: a review of prognostic clinical and pathologic features. Am J Obstet Gynecol 1979;134:557.

53. Leibsohn S, d'Ablaing G, Mishell DR, Schlaerth JB. Leiomyosarcoma in a series of hysterectomies performed for presumed uterine leiomyomas. Am J Obstet Gynecol 1990;162:968.

54. Silverberg SG, Major FJ, Blessing JA, et al. Carcinosarcoma (malignant mixed mesodermal tumor) of the uterus: a Gynecologic Oncology Group pathologic study of 203 cases. Int J Gynecol Pathol 1990;9:1.

55. Podczaski ES, Woomert CA, Steven CH Jr., et al. Management of malignant, mixed mesodermal tumors of the uterus. Gynecol Oncol 1989;32:240.

56. Bell SW, Kempson RL, Hendrickson MR. Problematic uterine smooth muscle neoplasms: a clinicopathologic study of 213 cases. Am J Surg Pathol 1994;18:535.

57. Norris HJ, Taylor HB. Mesenchymal tumors of the uterus. I. A clinical and pathologic study of 31 carcinosarcomas. Cancer 1996;19:755.

58. Tosi P, Sforza V, Santopierto R. Estrogen receptor content, immunohistochemically determined by monoclonal antibodies, in endometrial stromal sarcoma. Obstet Gynecol 1989;73:75.

59. Major FJ, Blessing JA, Silverberg SG, et al. Prognostic factors in early-stage uterine sarcomas: a Gynecologic Oncology Group study. Cancer 1993;71:1702.

60. Sutton GP, Blessing JA, Rosenheim N, Photopoulos G, DiSaia PJ. Phase II trial of ifosfamide and mesna in mixed mesodermal tumors of the uterus (a Gynecologic Oncology Group study). Am J Obstet Gynecol 1989; 161:309.

61. Thigpen JT, Blessing JA, Beecham J, Homesley H, Yordan E. Phase II trial of cisplatin as first-line chemotherapy in patients with advanced or recurrent uterine sarcomas (a Gynecologic Oncology Group study). J Clin Oncol 1991;9:1962.

62. Omura GA, Major FJ, Blessing JA, et al. A randomized study of adriamycin in uterine sarcomas with and without dimethyl triazinoimidazole carboxamide in advanced uterine sarcomas. Cancer 1983;52:626.

Chapter 66

Ovarian Cancer

Brigitte E. Miller

Five Key Points

- The overall risk of ovarian cancer is about 1.7% in the general population; in 5% to 7% there is an inherited predisposition increasing the risk for other family members in some syndromes to as high as 50%.

- General screening for ovarian cancer is not cost effective and early symptoms are not characteristic; therefore it is important to always consider ovarian cancer in the differential diagnosis if a woman complains of ill-defined gastrointestinal problems not explained by adequate work-up, especially during the post-menopausal period.

- In early ovarian cancer, tumor removal and complete staging is important; in advanced ovarian cancer, adequate tumor reductive surgery significantly improves the outcome.

- Chemotherapy for epithelial ovarian cancer is administered intravenously or intraperitoneally and includes drugs such as a platin compound and paclitaxol as first-line therapy, and topotecan, gemcitabin, and to liposomal doxorubicin, among others, as second-line therapy.

- Cancer of the fallopian tube is very rare and treated like epithelial ovarian cancer.

Ovarian cancer is the most feared gynecological malignancy. Most patients are diagnosed in an advanced stage, when treatment is not very effective. The survival rates for early ovarian cancer are quite good and stage for stage not much different from endometrial cancer. But unfortunately there are no early symptoms, and therefore early diagnosis is rarely possible. In addition, there are no good screening tests for the general population, mainly due to the fact that the prevalence of ovarian cancer is low. The following chapter was written to explain the risk factors and epidemiology of ovarian cancer, discuss screening options, explain the pathology of ovarian tumors, and give recommendations for diagnosis and treatment.

EPIDEMIOLOGY

In 1999, about 25,200 women will be diagnosed with ovarian cancer and 14,500 will die.[1] This is due mainly to the fact that early diagnosis is not possible. Ovarian cancer is rare in the first four decades of life, after which the incidence rises significantly. The average age at diagnosis is 54 years. The United States has one of the highest incidences of ovarian cancer in the world—13 in 100,000 Caucasian women and 10 in 100,000 African–American women.

RISK FACTORS

Table 66-1 summarizes some of the risk factors for the development of ovarian cancer. These pertain to epithelial tumors, the most frequent diagnosis. Information regarding the other rare histological types is still very scant. Most factors are poorly defined. One model is called the "incessant ovulation theory," which postulates that persistent ovulation is involved in the development of ovarian cancer.[2] Every ovulation leads to injury to the ovarian epithelium, and during repair there is an increased risk of cellular injury leading to unregulated proliferation. This is supported by data showing that ovarian cancer is most frequent in countries with small family size and that prolonged periods of anovulation due to oral contraceptives or breast feeding reduce the risk of epithelial ovarian cancer.[3,4] After prolonged intake of oral contraceptives the risk decreases to as much as 50% in the general population and in women with a family history of ovarian cancer. More recently this effect has also been seen in patients at significantly increased risk for ovarian cancer due to mutations in the *BRCA1* gene.[5] On the other hand, there are some reports about an increased risk for ovarian cancer after infertility treatment, mainly after medication with clomiphene, a drug that induces ovulation for more than 1 year.[6] There is no definite answer to this question, as all studies are small and not always well controlled for confounding factors. Patients with infertility have an increased baseline risk, even if they do not receive any therapy. Another model, the "gonadotropin hypothesis," postulates that increased gonadotropin levels lead to higher estrogen levels, which then promote epithelial proliferation and thus increase the risk for malignant transformation. However, an increased risk for ovarian cancer has not been seen in women who delivered twins and on average have a higher gonadotropin level.[7] Medication with human choriogonadotropin has not been associated with an increased risk of ovarian cancer.[6] Among the environmental factors, excessive dietary intake of animal fat or red meat has the strongest inference and can also explain some of the geographical differences in the occurrence of ovarian cancer, which is most frequent in countries of the northern hemisphere, especially northern Europe, the United States, and Canada.

TABLE 66-1
RISK FACTORS FOR THE DEVELOPMENT OF OVARIAN NEOPLASMS
Family history
Long time periods with uninterrupted ovulations
High gonadotropin level
Nulliparity
Gonadal dysgenesis
Radiation
Talc exposure
Asbestos exposure
High coffee consumption
High fat intake
Low-fiber diet
Low-vitamin-A diet

Only about 5% to 7% of all ovarian cancers occur on a genetic background. The familial ovarian cancer syndrome has an autosomal dominant pattern of inheritance with variable penetrance; it is very rare, but leads to a 50% risk of ovarian cancer. The hereditary breast ovarian cancer syndrome is more frequent. It is related to a mutation in the *BRCA* genes, which are tumor-suppressor genes and affect transcription. The sequences of these genes are now known and the knowledge regarding their effect is increasing rapidly. Mutations in the *BRCA1* gene lead to a high susceptibility for carcinoma of the breast (lifetime risk up to 80%) and the ovary (lifetime risk up to 50%). Mutations in the *BRCA2* gene give rise to ovarian cancer in only 10% of the cases. The Lynch II syndrome (mutations in DNA repair genes) includes families with increased incidence of colorectal cancer, as well as adenocarcinomas of the endometrium and ovary.[8] All of these syndromes are quite rare. However, it is extremely important to obtain a careful family history as this could reveal a patient to be at increased risk for ovarian cancer. The lifetime probability for developing ovarian cancer is 1.6% in the general population, 9.4% in women with two affected first–degree relatives, and can be as high as 50% in the presence of inheritable syndromes.[9]

PREVENTION OF OVARIAN CANCER

Ovulation, specifically the number of ovulations, increases the risk of ovarian cancer. Oral contraceptives prevent ovulations and reduce the risk of ovarian cancer to about 50%.[10] As this effect is also seen in women with a family history of ovarian cancer, oral contraceptives may be used to reduce their risk. Although there are no prospective studies available, the retrospective reports are quite convincing. The individual risk profile regarding malignancy on the one hand and oral contraceptive-related complications on the other hand has to be assessed.[5]

SCREENING FOR OVARIAN CANCER

There is no good screening test for ovarian cancer. Most experience has been gathered using tumor markers such as CA-125 and transvaginal ultrasound.

Tumor Markers

CA-125 is a large glycoprotein found on serous surfaces with an antigenic determinant that is recognized by a monoclonal antibody. The upper limit of normal is usually defined at 35 U/ml, but is also dependent on the kit used for detection. It is the best marker for serous epithelial ovarian cancer; however, it is only elevated in 50% of the patients with Stage I disease. Furthermore, this marker is very unspecific. Table 66-2 shows other reasons for CA-125 elevations, which occur mainly in premenopausal women.[11] Therefore, CA-125 levels are more useful for screening in postmenopausal women. Since ovarian cancer is quite rare in the general population, a screening test has to be very specific (number of healthy patients with a negative test/all healthy patients). A large study from the Royal London Hospital involving 22,000

patients demonstrated a 98% specificity for CA-125 level. Still, 50 false positive values were seen for each diagnosed case of ovarian cancer.[12] Einhorn et al.[13] used sequential CA-125 determinations, achieving a sensitivity (number of patients with positive test/number of patients with cancer) of only 50%, but a specificity of 96% and a positive predictive value of 3.43% (patients with cancer and positive test/all patients with positive test). Using sequential values, a better test kit and regression analysis, Skates et al.[14] were able to increase the specificity in 5550 patients to 99.7%, leading to a positive predictive value of 16%. Using a combination of tumor markers may be another way to improve specificity. However, no other marker comes close to the effectiveness of CA-125 values.

In conclusion, the serum CA-125 level is not useful as a routine screening test for low-risk asymptomatic women. However, it should be used liberally in patients with symptoms suggestive of ovarian cancer and it may be worthwhile in patients with a positive family history of ovarian cancer. Asymptomatic premenopausal patients with negative physical examinations and normal transvaginal ultrasound, but moderately elevated CA-125 values (<100 U/ml) can be followed with repeat values in midcycle. Rising or high values in premenopausal patients and all elevated values in postmenopausal patients should be followed by transvaginal ultrasound and, if negative, mammography, barium enema, and even laparoscopy/laparotomy. On the other hand, a normal CA-125 value does not rule out ovarian cancer and should not delay further investigation or surgery in the presence of suspicious symptoms or findings on physical examination.

Ultrasound

Transvaginal ultrasound now is the most accurate diagnostic test for ovarian abnormalities. Over 6500 women have been screened in the University of Kentucky Ovarian Cancer Screening Project[15] and persistent abnormalities were seen in 1.4%. Surgical exploration demonstrated 37 benign tumors and 6 ovarian cancers, yielding a positive predictive value of only 6%. The CA-125 level was normal in all these patients. In over 17,000 screening years so far, no deaths from ovarian cancer have occurred. These results have been confirmed by other investigators. The average cost per screen can be reduced to $25.00 in a well-organized unit. The addition of color Doppler

---

TABLE 66-2
DIAGNOSES ASSOCIATED WITH ELEVATED SERUM CA-125

Gynecologic tumors	Nongynecologic tumors
Epithelial ovarian cancer	Pancreatic carcinoma
Dysgerminoma	Lung carcinoma
Sertoli–Leydig cell tumors	Breast carcinoma
Granulosa-cell tumors	Colon carcinoma
Fallopian-tube carcinoma	Nongynecologic conditions
Endometrial carcinoma	Pancreatitis
Endocervical carcinoma	Cirrhosis
Benign gynecologic conditions	Laparotomy
Cystadenoma	Peritonitis
Endometriosis	Peritoneal tuberculosis
Adenomyosis	Radiation
Leiomyomas	Intraperitoneal radio-
Normal pregnancy	colloid administration
Ectopic pregnancy	
Pelvic inflammatory disease	
Menses	

Reprinted with permission from Evans and Berchuck.[8]

flow imaging has not led to the expected increase in accuracy. Due to the low prevalence of ovarian cancer, the false positive rate is high. Karlan and Platt[16] calculated that 32 surgeries were necessary to detect one case of ovarian cancer in the general population. In women with a positive family history, however, only 17 surgeries were required for each case of cancer. Therefore, most screening programs now focus on women with a positive family history.

Screening studies have shown that simple ovarian cysts, 3 to 5 cm in diameter, are not infrequent in postmenopausal patients and can be followed with ultrasound evaluations provided the CA-125 level remains normal.[17] Cyst aspiration is an unreliable test to evaluate for malignancy and may increase the risk of dissemination; therefore, it should be avoided.

BRCA1 Testing

About 90% of inherited ovarian cancer is due to a mutation in the BRCA1 gene. In sporadic cancers, somatic mutations are seen in only 3%. The BRCA1 gene may be involved in the regulation of cell proliferation, functioning as a tumor-suppressor gene[1] regulating transcription. Unfortunately, the gene is very large, mutations can occur in many areas, and not all of these definitely lead to an abnormal protein. Complete sequencing of the gene is the most reliable and also the most labor-intensive way to detect a mutation. Other tests, such as single-stranded conformation analysis (screens segments of the gene for alterations) and the protein truncation test (evaluates the protein product for abnormalities), are not completely accurate. In view of these problems and other legal problems for patients in whom a mutation has been detected (health insurance, job qualification), the test should only be ordered after careful genetic evaluation and counseling, with discussion of all ramifications.[18]

SCREENING RECOMMENDATIONS

General Population

Screening is not recommended for the general population because efficacy and cost effectiveness have not been proven.

Positive Family History

Patients with one affected family member are at moderately increased risk (relative risk, 3.1). A careful family history should be obtained regarding all malignancies. Screening should be considered after age 35 using pelvic examinations, CA-125 levels, and transvaginal ultrasound examinations. Oral contraceptives may be advantageous unless pregnancy is desired. Prophylactic surgery is rarely indicated.

Strongly Positive Family History

Members of families with the ovarian cancer syndrome or the breast–ovarian cancer syndrome tend to develop their disease at a younger age. Patients considered at significantly increased risk are those with one or more first–degree relatives and in addition other second–degree relatives with ovarian or breast cancer. A careful family history regarding all malignancies should be obtained and indications for BRCA1 testing should be discussed. Beginning at age 25, annual CA-125 level determinations and vaginal ultrasound examinations should be performed. An increased incidence of benign changes should be expected in this premenopausal patient group. The patient should be placed on oral contraceptives unless she desires pregnancy. After she has completed her family, a prophylactic bilateral salpingo-oophorectomy should be considered, although this will not protect her completely against the risk of peritoneal adenocarcinoma, which occurs at a rate of 5% to 10%. Because many of these patients also are at increased risk for breast cancer, intense screening is important and again prophylactic surgery may become a consideration.[19]

SYMPTOMS

There are no early symptoms of ovarian cancer. The initial enlargement of the ovary does not uniformly cause discomfort. Occasionally, a tumor or nodularity in the cul-de-sac is felt during a routine examination. Sometimes the patient is the first to notice a mass. Once the tumor rises out of the pelvis, though, the patient may experience symptoms from pressure on the bladder or rectum. Most often, the diagnosis is made after abdominal dissemination has taken place, leading to impaired bowel function, decreased appetite, nausea, vomiting, changing bowel habits, and signs of peritoneal carcinomatosis,—i.e., weight loss, abdominal distention, and ascites.[20] Pain can also be caused by rapid enlargement of the ovarian tumor, as well as leakage of fluid into the peritoneal cavity and bleeding. This is more commonly seen in fast-growing tumors such as germ-cell malignancies. Often patients are initially referred for gastrointestinal evaluation, which is usually negative. Ultimately, ascites develops and the diagnosis of ovarian cancer is obvious. Decreased performance status and weakness are often present at this stage.

It is therefore very important to include ovarian cancer in the differential diagnosis, especially in postmenopausal patients with persistent, ill-defined gastrointestinal symptoms or persistent pelvic pain. Irregular vaginal bleeding or postmenopausal bleeding is rare.

PHYSICAL EXAMINATION

The pelvic examination is the most important means of evaluating an ovarian tumor. Perform a careful bimanual examination, as well as a rectovaginal examination. This is the best way to determine the size, position, fixation, and other characteristics of an ovarian lesion. Also, tumor implants or masses in the cul-de-sac can be sometimes felt as an early sign of disseminated disease. A Pap smear and a Hemoccult test should also be done. Follow this with a careful abdominal examination, evaluating for signs of ascites, an upper abdominal mass, an omental cake, or signs of bowel obstruction. Sometimes it may be difficult to distinguish an abdomen distended by ascites from an abdomen distended by a large cystic mass. In the presence of ascites, however, the flanks protrude and most of the dullness is percussed there, whereas the gas-filled loops of bowel float on top in the center of the abdomen. In contrast, a large cystic mass displaces the bowel loops to the flanks. In this scenario, bowel sounds are noted laterally and the dullness of the cystic mass is detected in the center of the abdomen. Other important features are a careful general physical examination with particular attention to the lymph-node survey, examination of the lungs to detect signs of pleural effusion, and a complete breast examination.

FURTHER WORK-UP

Tumor marker studies such as CA-125 levels are not clinically useful in young patients due to the many benign reasons for elevation. In postmenopausal patients with a pelvic mass, an elevated CA-125 level is a strong sign of malignancy.[21] On the other hand, a negative value never rules out ovarian cancer and should not discourage surgery if otherwise indicated. In the presence of gastrointestinal complaints, a carcinoembryonic antigen (CEA) value should be checked to rule out a large-bowel malignancy. However, this marker is also elevated in approximately 30% of ovarian malignancies. Tumor-marker studies are not helpful in guiding decisions regarding surgery in the presence of a pelvic mass. They may be helpful, however, to determine the overall risk and decide if a patient should be referred to an oncologist or if the lesion should be approached with the laparoscope. Adequate backup, however, should be available in any case so that appropriate therapy can be instituted if a malignancy is detected in the absence of tumor-marker elevations. Tumor markers are also important in a very young patient with a pelvic mass. In this age group, germ-cell tumors are frequent, so the α-fetoprotein (AFP), human chorionic gonadotropin (HCG), and lactate dehydrogenase (LDH) levels may be evaluated.

Routine preoperative evaluation should always include chest radiography to detect a pleural effusion, one of the most frequent presenting symptoms of Stage IV ovarian cancer. Evaluation of the gastrointestinal tract is not mandatory in all patients. However, if there are any gastrointestinal symptoms or a positive Hemoccult test, evaluation should not be delayed. In the presence of a large pelvic mass, a barium enema or sigmoidoscopy is helpful in determining the status of the sigmoid colon, which often is involved with advanced ovarian cancer. It is difficult even to evaluate at the time of surgery, because it is impossible to reach from below, and in the presence of advanced pelvic tumor, it may be difficult to evaluate from above. Patients should also be current regarding screening examinations, especially mammography.

Pelvic ultrasound, especially transvaginally, is the best way to evaluate ovaries. It demonstrates the presence and the size of a mass and also characterizes the inside of the mass. Findings suggestive of malignancy are solid areas, thick septations, and papillations. Scoring systems as suggested by Sassone et al.[22] evaluating inner wall structure, wall thickness, septation, and echogenicity are quite accurate in predicting ovarian malignancy. DePriest et al.[23] achieved a sensitivity of 89% and positive predictive value of 46% using a morphology index score consisting of the following parameters: ovarian volume, wall structure, and appearance of septations. In this respect, ultrasound is much more valuable than a CT scan. Although the

CT scan gives better information about the entire peritoneal cavity, this is rarely relevant to the decision to proceed with surgery. Doppler ultrasound evaluation of ovarian blood flow has not significantly improved the diagnostic accuracy. Using a malignancy index based on menopausal status, CA-125 value, and ultrasound, Tingulstad et al.[24] achieved a positive predictive value for ovarian cancer of 89% in a small group of patients. This information can be used to decide which patients should be referred to an oncologist.

LAPAROSCOPY

Laparoscopy is an invasive but accurate way to evaluate ovaries. Complete removal and frozen-section analysis of an ovarian tumor should be the goal, and all efforts should be made to avoid spillage of fluid. In cases of malignancy, appropriate surgery should be done as soon as possible. There is no definite evidence that laparoscopy has a negative effect on the outcome if an ovarian cancer is diagnosed, provided adequate therapy is instituted promptly.

PATHOLOGY OF OVARIAN CANCER

Sixty to 65% of all ovarian tumors are of epithelial origin. The relative frequency of epithelial tumors changes with age. During the first two decades of life, germ-cell tumors are more frequent. In older patients epithelial lesions increase in frequency. About 90% of all malignant ovarian tumors are of epithelial origin.[25] There are many different ovarian tumors, most of them quite rare (Table 66-3). Only the more important types will be discussed in the following paragraph.

Epithelial Tumors

The histologic classification of epithelial ovarian tumors corresponds to the epithelial differentiations found in the müllerian system: serous, mucinous, endometrioid, clear-cell, transitional-cell (Brenner tumor), mixed-epithelial-cell, undifferentiated carcinoma, and unclassified epithelial-cell tumors. These lesions can be benign, of low malignant potential (increased proliferation and atypia, but no invasion), or frankly malignant (increased proliferation, significant atypia, invasion).

TABLE 66-3
MODIFIED WORLD HEALTH ORGANIZATION COMPREHENSIVE CLASSIFICATION OF OVARIAN TUMORS

I. Epithelial Tumors
  Benign
  Borderline malignancy
  Invasive malignancy
    Serous
    Mucinous
    Endometrioid
    Clear-cell
    Brenner
    Mixed epithelial
  Undifferentiated
  Mixed mesodermal tumors
  Unclassified

II. Sex-cord stromal tumors
  Granulosa stromal cell
    Granulosa cell
    Thecoma-fibroma
  Androblastomas; Sertoli–Leydig
    Well-differentiated (Pick adenoma, Sertoli-cell tumor)
    Intermediate differentiation
    Poorly differentiated
    With heterologous elements
  Lipid-cell tumors
  Gynandroblastoma
  Unclassified

III. Germ-cell tumors
  Dysgerminoma
  Endodermal sinus tumor
  Embryonal carcinoma
  Polyembryoma
  Choriocarcinoma
  Teratomas
    Immature
    Mature (dermoid cyst)
    Monodermal (struma ovarii, carcinoid)
  Mixed forms
  Gonadoblastoma

IV. Soft-tissue tumors not specific to the ovary

V. Unclassified tumors

VI. Secondary (metastatic) tumors

VII. Tumor-like conditions (pregnancy, luteoma, etc.)

Regarding prognosis, tumor grading is very important. A well-differentiated tumor (Grade 1) consists primarily of papillary and glandular growth patterns. A Grade 3 tumor is composed of solid sheets of malignant cells, and the appearance of a Grade 2 tumor is somewhere in between. A variety of other pathologic characteristics has been evaluated; however, grade is the most important prognostic factor.

On gross inspection, it is often impossible to differentiate early-stage malignant tumors from benign lesions. However, in malignancy there is more frequent involvement of the ovarian capsule, solid areas, thick septations, and then disseminated peritoneal disease. Spread patterns are similar for all epithelial lesions. Initially the pelvic peritoneal surfaces are involved: tubes, uterus, pelvic side wall, and cul-de-sac. Transperitoneal tumor spread is most common, leading to disseminated small tumor nodules and, at a later stage, to coating of all peritoneal surfaces and an omental mass. The growth characteristics seem to be of some prognostic importance. A nodular growing tumor is easier to treat than a diffusely spreading tumor. Lymphatic spread is common. Figure 66-1 shows examples of early and advanced peritoneal tumor spread.

Serous Ovarian Tumors

These are the most frequent ovarian lesions, accounting for about 40% to 50% of the cases. Most patients are between 40 and 70 years old. Sixty percent of the malignant tumors are diagnosed in an advanced stage. A serous neoplasm is characterized by cystic structures, with papillations covered by ciliated cells. Under the microscope, significant nuclear atypia is noted, as well as signs of destructive stromal invasion with desmoplastic reaction. Psammoma bodies typical for serous tumors are formed by precipitation of calcium phosphate apatite crystals. They are seen in about 20% of the low-malignant-potential (LMP) tumors and in over 30% of the serous carcinomas.

LMP tumors reveal many complex papillations lined with two or more layers of atypical epithelial cells without evidence of invasion. Most of these tumors are Stage I at diagnosis. However, peritoneal implants may be seen and should be liberally biopsied. The peritoneal lesions can be either completely benign, such as endosalpingeosis, or they can be LMP without invasion, similar to the changes found in the ovary; rarely, invasive implants can be found leading to decreased survival. It is not absolutely certain if these peritoneal lesions are true metastatic implants or separate tumors developing due to a field effect.[26] Although LMP tumors can be diagnosed in all ages, the median age is 38 to 40.

Mucinous Neoplasms

About 20% of all ovarian tumors are mucinous. Of those, the vast majority (85%) are benign, 6% are of low malignant potential, and 9% are malignant. The benign mucinous cystadenoma is characterized by a tall columnar epithelium. LMP mucinous tumors show stratification of two or more atypical epithelial-cell layers; however, there is no evidence of invasion. The mucinous lining resembles either the endocervical or the intestinal epithelium. The endocervical type, composed of papillae covered by mucinous columnar cells, tends to occur in younger patients. For the intestinal-type mucinous borderline tumors, the mean age is 52 years. Here, tumors are often more complex and the intestinal-type mucin contained in goblet cells is seen. These tumors are associated with pseudomyxoma peritonei, leading to increased mortality of about 14% due mainly to recurrent intestinal obstruction caused by the tenacious mucin.[27] Mucinous ovarian carcinoma occurs in a wide age range, with a mean age of about 48 to about 54 years. Ten percent of localized tumors are bilateral. Fifty percent to 70% are diagnosed in Stage I. The diagnosis of malignancy is based either on stromal invasion with a desmoplastic reaction or the accumulation of more than three epithelial layers with significant atypia.

Endometrioid Tumors

Endometrioid tumors can arise from the ovarian epithelium; however, they can also arise in areas of endometriosis. Endometrioid tumors of low malignant potential are rarely diagnosed. Invasive endometrioid carcinoma is very similar in appearance to the typical uterine carcinoma. Most women are menopausal, with an average age of 55 years, although a broad age range is possible. Squamous metaplasia may be seen leading to benign or malignant components. In 35%, other epithelial differentiations are noted, such as clear-cell or mucinous or papillary serous patterns. In about 10% of the patients, a synchronous adenocarcinoma of the endometrium is also noted. In this case, it may be very difficult to distinguish if the ovarian tumor is a second primary or a metastatic lesion.

Sex-Cord Stromal Tumors

Most sex-cord stromal tumors are benign, while only a small percentage act malignant. These tumors arise from ovarian stromal cells such as granulosa cells, thecal cells, Sertoli cells, lipid cells, or fibroblasts.

Granulosa-Cell Tumors

The most frequent of these neoplasms is the granulosa-cell tumor. One subtype is the juvenile granulosa-cell

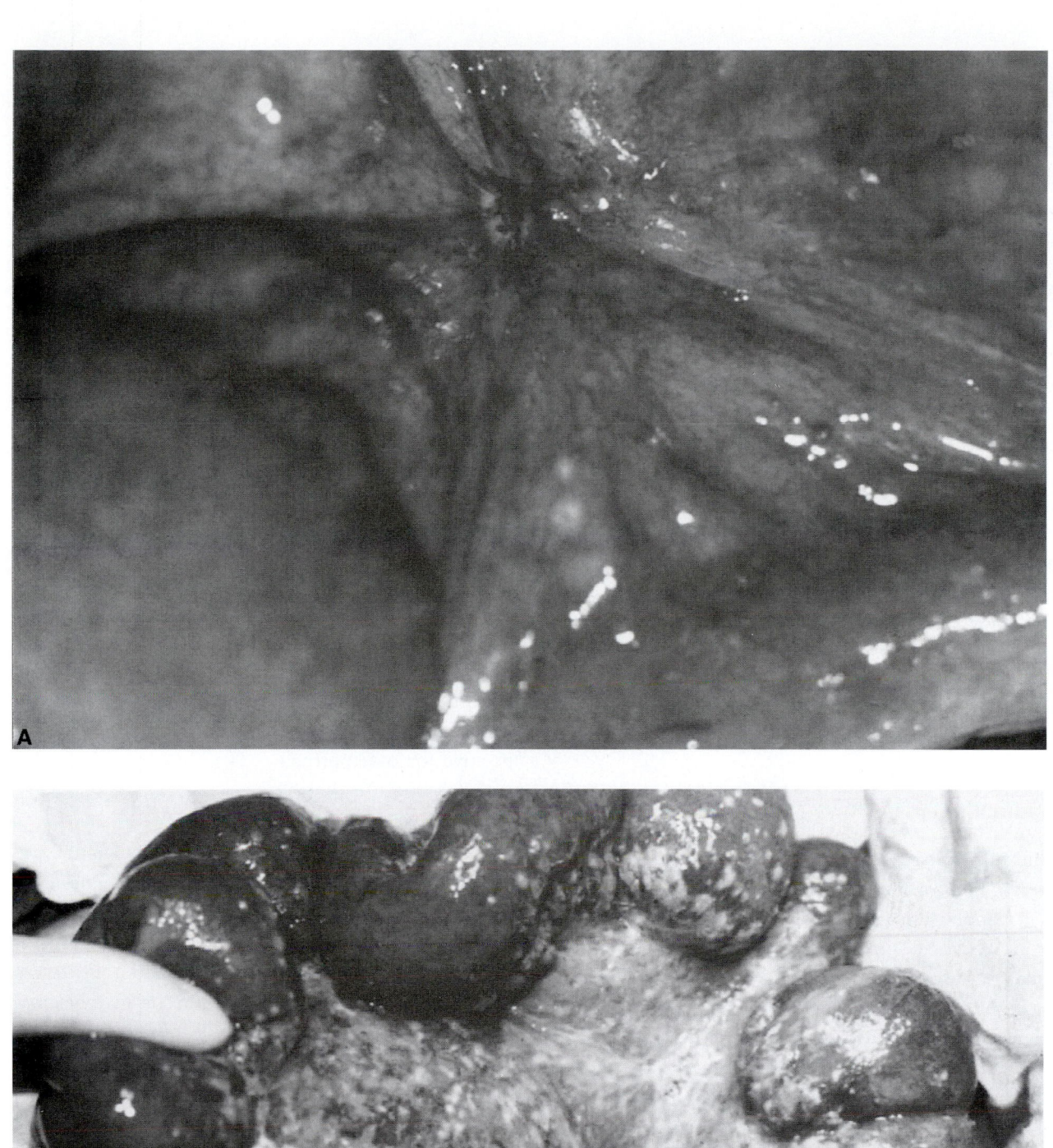

Figure 66-1 Examples of early (A) and advanced (B) peritoneal tumor spread.

tumor, which also can occur in patients over age 30 in up to 3% of the cases. These tumors are mostly solid with a diffuse tumor-cell pattern and often significant cytologic atypia and frequent mitosis. In spite of this appearance, the prognosis is good and only 5% will have a recurrence. Secondly, there are adult granulosa-cell tumors, which, however, can also occur in children. About 5% are also seen in premenarchal girls. These tumors are mostly unilateral, solid, smooth, and often quite hard. Large tumors have a worse prognosis. Under the microscope, a variety of different patterns can be seen. The characteristic Call–Exner bodies are small areas with nuclear debris surrounded by granulosa cells. Nuclear polymorphism and high mitotic rates are not frequent, but if present may lead to a worse prognosis. Recurrences are rare after resection of small lesions; however, in some reports, are noted in 25% or more of the cases, especially after prolonged follow-up. Recurrences can occur very late after initial treatment and have been reported even after 20 years. Tumor stage certainly is the most important prognostic factor, although this is rarely helpful, as most tumors present in Stage I. There is no proven benefit of adjuvant therapy for early lesions.

Androblastomas

Androblastomas are tumors derived from Sertoli or Leydig cells or a combination of both. Pure Sertoli-cell tumors (estrogen-producing) or Leydig-cell tumors (androgen-producing) are very rare. The combined variety of the Sertoli–Leydig-cell tumor is also quite rare and usually occurs in young women, mostly leading to a small ovarian lesion. The hormone effect is usually androgenic. Well-differentiated Sertoli–Leydig cell tumors are always benign, as well as most of those of intermediate differentiation. About 40% of the poorly differentiated tumors, mostly with high mitotic counts and heterologous elements, pursue an aggressive clinical course, and adjuvant chemotherapy should be considered.

Germ-Cell Tumors

Germ-cell tumors show evidence of differentiation into embryonic or extraembryonic tissue. Often, there is a mixture of different elements within a single tumor. Germ-cell tumors account for two-thirds of ovarian cancers in the first two decades of life. Overall, only 5% of germ-cell tumors are malignant. Most are benign dermoids.

Dysgerminoma

Most dysgerminomas arise in patients between 10 to 30 years old, some in patients with gonadal dysgenesis. They are bilateral in up to 50% of the cases. On macroscopic examination, the surfaces are smooth or slightly bosselated and the tumor is solid-appearing, gray on sectioning. Dysgerminomas can metastasize, leading to peritoneal implants, especially after rupture of the tumor, or to extensive lymphatic spread occurring early in the course of the disease. LDH often is elevated.

Endodermal-Sinus Tumors

Endodermal-sinus tumors (yolk-sac tumors) occur in young girls at an average age of 18 years. They usually form large, unilateral tumors with significant necrosis and often hemorrhage. The microscopic examination sometimes reveals the characteristic Schiller–Duvall bodies, which are small central capillaries surrounded by epithelial cells. The histological picture of yolk-sac tumors can vary considerably and frozen-section diagnosis is not easy. All tumors are positive for α-fetoprotein.

Teratomas

The prognosis of teratomas is not determined by the grade of differentiation but by the degree of the maturity of the tissue. The vast majority are mature, cystic teratomas, so-called dermoids. In about 1% to 2% of those lesions, malignancies can occur, mainly squamous-cell carcinoma, and rarely, adenocarcinomas. These patients are usually older, between 40 and 60 years old. Solid teratomas can contain a variety of tissue differentiations, but most solid teratomas are immature. The amount of immature neuroepithelium is an important prognostic factor, leading to an aggressive course.

TREATMENT OF OVARIAN CANCER

Preparation for surgery should include a complete discussion of all treatment options in case a benign, LMP, or invasive malignant tumor is found. All patients should undergo at least a mechanical bowel preparation; if bowel resection is anticipated, antibiotics should be added. If there is a suspicion that a malignancy may be present, a vertical abdominal incision should be used. This incision is the most versatile and can be enlarged as necessary. A transverse incision limits the evaluation of the upper abdomen. If a Pfannenstiel incision has been performed, it can be enlarged to a Cherney incision so that a large ovarian mass can be removed intact. One can also start with a Maylard incision. This incision then can also be extended laterally and even superiorly if necessary. In slim patients, adequate access to the lower paraaortic nodes and the omentum is achieved with this approach.

After the abdomen is entered, irrigation fluid should be taken from the pelvis and both gutters, as well as the subdiaphragmatic area, and sent for cytology unless there is gross peritoneal disease. Then a careful exploration of the entire pelvis and abdominal cavity should be performed, including evaluation of the large and small bowel, pelvic and paraaortic nodal areas, diaphragm, omentum, stomach, liver, gallbladder, and kidneys. This should be done in all patients with adnexal tumors.

Lesion Grossly Confined to Ovary

In this situation, initially a unilateral salpingo-oophorectomy should be performed in the postmenopausal patient. In young patients who still desire fertility, the tumor should be removed while trying to preserve as much of the ovary as possible. Even a small remnant of ovarian epithelium can be important for ovarian function. On the other hand, it is important to prevent rupture. As there are no definite gross features separating a benign tumor from a malignant tumor, all lesions should be treated as potentially malignant. If a cyst is very large, but otherwise not adherent, it can be drained by placing a pursestring suture, then inserting a gallbladder trocar into the tumor. Thus, spillage is minimized, but the tumor size is significantly reduced, making removal much easier.

Frozen-section analysis is paramount in planning the remainder of the procedure. If the result is benign, a conservative approach is indicated for the young patient. In postmenopausal patients, removal of the contralateral ovary should be recommended, and in patients over age 40 it should be considered. When a malignancy is diagnosed, a total abdominal hysterectormy and bilateral salpingo-oophorectomy (TAH/BSO) should be performed in most instances. Exceptions include the young patient with a LMP tumor or Stage IA Grade 1 epithelial ovarian adenocarcinoma or germ-cell tumor and who desires fer-

tility. Sometimes, the frozen-section diagnosis is inaccurate and is revised after the permanent sections are available. When in doubt, it is better to perform a conservative procedure in young patients. It is very important to discuss all possible outcomes with the patient whenever surgery for an adnexal mass is planned. The surgeon should know preoperatively the patient's plans for further children and if she is willing to accept a slightly increased risk for recurrence in order to preserve childbearing capacity.

The stage of an ovarian tumor is determined surgically. Especially if a malignant tumor appears localized to the ovary, a full staging procedure is of paramount importance, as it significantly determines the postoperative treatment and prognosis. Undertreatment should be avoided at all cost. All peritoneal surfaces should be carefully inspected. Suspicious areas or areas of adhesion should be biopsied. If no lesions are seen, random biopsies should be taken from the pelvis, the gutters, the diaphragm area (this can be substituted by cytology), and the large and small bowel. However, as these are random samples, they are frequently negative. About 30 to 40 samples should be taken; biopsies from the same area, pelvis versus upper abdomen, can be submitted together. This is followed by an infracolic omentectomy. Lastly, the lymph nodes of the pelvic and paraaortic area should be evaluated.[28] In clinical Stage I ovarian cancer, nodal metastases were noted in 4% to 12% of cases. The detection of nodal metastasis, however, upstages the tumor to Stage III and has a significant impact on postoperative treatment. Poorly differentiated lesions develop nodal metastases more frequently.[29] At this point, there is definite evidence that nodal evaluation is important for staging,[30] but it is less clear if it has any therapeutic benefit.[31]

Table 66-4 shows the staging system for ovarian cancer.

Bilateral Ovarian Tumors

Again, careful exploration of the entire abdomen should be done. The presence of bilateral tumors should always raise the suspicion of metastatic disease. It has been found in up to 25% of these cases. The most frequent primary tumors are endometrial, colon, breast, and gastric malignancies. The tumors should be removed and sent for frozen-section analysis. In case of a müllerian primary, removal of both ovaries and the uterus, followed by staging biopsies, are recommended. In case of a metastatic tumor of

TABLE 66-4
FIGO STAGING OF OVARIAN CARCINOMA (SURGICOPATHOLOGICAL)

Stage	Criteria
I	Growth limited to the ovaries
IA	Growth limited to one ovary; no ascites No tumor on the external surface; capsule intact
IB	Growth limited to both ovaries; no ascites No tumor on the external surfaces; capsules intact
IC	Tumor either Stage IA or IB, but with tumor on surface of one or both ovaries; or with capsule ruptured; or with ascites present containing malignant cells or with positive peritoneal washings
II	Growth involving one or both ovaries with pelvic extension
IIA	Extension and/or metastases to the uterus and/or tubes
IIB	Extension to other pelvic tissues
IIC	Tumor either Stage IIA or IIB, but with tumor on surface of one or both ovaries; or with capsule(s) ruptured, or with ascites present containing malignant cells or with positive peritoneal washings
III	Tumor involving one or both ovaries with peritoneal implants outside the pelvis and/or positive retroperitoneal or inguinal nodes. Superficial liver metastasis equals Stage III; tumor is limited to the true pelvis but with histologically proven malignant extension to small bowel or omentum
IIIA	Tumor grossly limited to the true pelvis with negative nodes but with histologically confirmed microscopic seeding of abdominal peritoneal surfaces
IIIB	Tumor involving one or both ovaries with histologically confirmed implants of abdominal peritoneal surfaces, none exceeding 2 cm in diameter. Nodes are negative.
IIIC	Abdominal implants greater than 2 cm in diameter and/or positive retroperitoneal or inguinal nodes
IV	Growth involving one or both ovaries with distant metastases. If pleural effusion is present, there must be positive cytology to allot a case to Stage IV. Parenchymal liver metastasis equals Stage IV.

gastrointestinal origin, a bilateral salpingo-oophorectomy should be done, followed by resection of the primary tumor if at all possible. In the presence of a peritoneal surface adenocarcinoma, again TAH/BSO and tumor-reductive surgery is recommended. If the ovarian metastasis is a sign of systemic disease, only the affected ovary should be removed in young patients with lymphoma or leukemia, and both ovaries should be removed in patients with breast cancer or postmenopausal patients.

In the case of an LMP tumor in a young patient who still desires fertility, a unilateral salpingo-oophorectomy or even just a tumor removal are necessary, although the risk of recurrence is slightly increased in this situation. Complete staging biopsies should also be done, but the risk of nodal metastasis is low.

Gross Evidence of Disseminated Malignancy

In this situation, tumor-reductive surgery is of major importance, whereas staging biopsies are less important. Initially, an ovary or a biopsy should be sent for frozen-section diagnosis to rule out the presence of metastatic disease. If a müllerian primary is diagnosed, the patient should be evaluated for tumor-reductive surgery. In a number of publications, tumor-reductive surgery has been shown to improve survival in patients with epithelial ovarian cancer.[32] Adequate tumor reduction or debulking means removal of all tumor down to a residual of 1 cm or less. These are the dimensions of the largest remaining tumor plaque.[33] Whether aggressive removal of all tumor plaques has an impact on survival remains controversial.[34] The impact of tumor biology and growth characteristics is difficult to specify in this situation. Patients with nodular tumor growth are better amenable to surgery and have a better prognosis than patients with diffuse, coating tumor spread.[35] The success of tumor-reductive surgery primarily depends on the extent of disease in the upper abdomen, where invasion of other organs such as extensive liver metastasis, large volume mesenteric disease, or upper aortic nodal metastasis may prevent adequate tumor reduction. However, large tumor masses in the pelvis can usually be adequately reduced, although resection of the rectosigmoid or loops of adherent small bowel may become necessary. A retroperitoneal approach is suggested by incising the peritoneum on the pelvic wall and identifying the ureter, pelvic vessels, and the infundibulopelvic ligament. The dissection then continues from lateral to medial and may include the rectosigmoid. Sigmoid resection is indicated in the face of obstruction or in cases in which this procedure will lead to optimal tumor reduction. Anteriorly, the peritoneum involved with tumor is dissected off the bladder, which is then freed from the cervix and upper vagina. Thus, the pelvic tumor, uterus, ovaries, and sigmoid can be removed in toto. Adequate tumor-reductive surgery is possible in 40% to 60% of patients.[36] Although morbidity can be significant with adequate postoperative care, mortality is only 1% to 2%.[37] If adequate tumor-reductive surgery is not possible, the least morbid procedure should be done because tumor removal to more than 2 cm of residual tissue does not improve survival.[38] Most patients will still derive symptomatic benefit from removal of a large omental cake or ovarian tumor, if this can be accomplished easily. In this situation bowel resection should only be done to relieve obstruction. Biopsies of the ovaries are important to confirm the diagnosis; an endometrial biopsy should also be considered if hysterectomy is not possible. These patients should then be treated with aggressive chemotherapy and may be evaluated for secondary tumor-reductive surgery if a good response is seen after two to three courses.[39] If there is no response to chemotherapy, surgery will not improve the outcome.

Young Patients Who Desire Reproductive Conservation

Conservative treatment can be recommended in young patients with borderline lesions, as well as early invasive lesions, Stage IA Grade 1 or 2. Complete staging biopsies should be done.[40] However, if the contralateral ovary looks normal, a biopsy is not recommended to avoid adhesion formation. Another option for patients with Stage I Grade 3 lesions has been suggested by DiSaia[41] and is to perform conservative surgery, but then add six cycles of combination chemotherapy. Especially in young patients, the ovaries recover quite well from chemotherapy. However, there are no randomized data proving the efficacy of this approach.

Low-Malignant-Potential Epithelial Tumors

If an LMP tumor is noted, removal of both ovaries and the uterus is indicated in most patients. However, in the young patient, it is sufficient to remove only the affected ovary or even dissect the tumor away from the ovary. With cystectomy, though, there is a slightly increased risk of recurrence.[42] Full staging is also recommended for patients with LMP tumors, although the clinical impact is limited.[43] The overall 5-year survival is around 95% for early-stage disease and as high as 75% for Stage III lesions.

Stromal Tumors

A bilateral salpingo-oophorectomy and hysterectomy is done for most patients. Again, unilateral removal is adequate in patients who desire further fertility. If the uterus is removed, it should be opened and at least inspected to rule out endometrial pathology. If the uterus is left in situ, then a dilation and curettage should be performed. If the tumor is large and signs of atypia or increased mitotic activity are noted, full staging procedures should be performed as recommended for epithelial ovarian cancer. In case of doubt, it is always better to be aggressive regarding the staging procedures.

Germ-Cell Tumors

Most tumors are confined to the ovary at the time of initial diagnosis. Minimally, a unilateral salpingo-oophorectomy should be done. This should be followed by complete staging procedures, including retroperitoneal nodal evaluation. If the contralateral ovary reveals any abnormalities such as masses or cysts, they should be removed, but an effort should be made to preserve the uterus and the contralateral ovary in these mostly young patients.

Patients with Significantly Reduced Performance Status

Sometimes patients with advanced disease present with a significantly reduced performance status, low albumin level, or significant medical problems. If the patient is unable to withstand aggressive tumor-reductive surgery, a diagnosis can often be made by evaluation of the ascites, if present, or by fine-needle aspiration biopsy. Chemotherapy should then be instituted using carboplatin as a single agent in the very frail patient to reduce the accumulation of ascites. In stronger patients, combination chemotherapy should be given. If the performance status improves and the tumor responds to chemotherapy, secondary tumor-reductive surgery should be considered.[44]

POSTOPERATIVE TREATMENT

Epithelial Tumors

After adequate surgery and staging, patients with Stage IA Grade 1 or 2 epithelial tumors do not need any further treatments.[45] If staging is incomplete, especially in Grade 2 lesions, the decision has to be made to either treat the patient prophylactically or to perform a staging procedure. In these early lesions, the importance of grade on survival is higher than that of substage.[46, 47] Patients with Grade III tumors or clear-cell carcinoma are at increased risk for recurrence and therefore adjuvant therapy is indicated. Treatment should also be discussed with patients after rupture of a malignant tumor and contamination of the peritoneal cavity with malignant cells. This can be given in mainly two ways. The most frequently used treatment is adjuvant chemotherapy using cisplatin or carboplatin as a single agent for six courses. There is no difference in effectiveness between these two drugs.[48] It is not known if combination treatment using a platin compound and paclitaxel is more effective or if three courses are equally as effective as six courses. Several large research studies to resolve these issues are ongoing. Usually, this treatment is well tolerated, especially medication with carboplatin, as it causes only mild nausea and no hair loss. Treatment with intraperitoneal radionuclides such as p32 is another option. This form of radiation therapy treats the peritoneal surfaces to a depth of only 2 to 3 mm. It does not deliver an adequate radiation dose to the retroperitoneal nodes. Several studies have shown that it is effective as adjuvant chemotherapy for Stage I ovarian cancer, especially when malignant cells are seen in peritoneal washings or if a malignant cyst ruptured at the time of removal.[49] However, the posttreatment course may be complicated by radiation bowel injury and dense adhesions, problems that are very difficult to treat. Therefore, most oncologists now use systemic chemotherapy.

In Stage II epithelial ovarian cancer, adequate staging is again of paramount importance. Postoperative treatment should consist of systemic chemotherapy using a combination of paclitaxel with carboplatin or cisplatin. This should be given for six courses. In patients without residual disease, a shorter regimen of three courses only may be adequate, but this is still under investigation.

Stage III epithelial tumors likewise are treated with adjuvant chemotherapy. The regimen most frequently used is systemic chemotherapy using cisplatin or carboplatin and paclitaxel. There is no difference in effectiveness between cisplatin and carboplatin in this combination, but the side-effect profile is better with carboplatin. This treatment is usually given for six courses. In patients with large-volume residual disease after surgery, the treatment may be extended to nine courses.[50] Initial response rates are around 80%; unfortunately, the recurrence rates are also high. If adequate tumor reduction has been achieved and there is minimal residual peritoneal residual disease, consid-

eration can be given to a combination of intraperitoneal chemotherapy with cisplatin, together with intravenous treatment with paclitaxel. While using the intraperitoneal route, a much higher concentration of the chemotherapeutic agent can be achieved. However, as it reaches the cancer cells by direct diffusion, it is only effective in small-volume disease. A large randomized study revealed a beneficial effect on tumor control and survival using the intraperitoneal route in these patients. Except for a few catheter-related complications, the overall side effects were reduced with intraperitoneal administration of cisplatin.[51] The benefit of high-dose chemotherapy with stem-cell support as the initial treatment for ovarian cancer so far has not been confirmed.

Stage IV disease is treated with aggressive combination chemotherapy.

In patients unable to undergo adequate tumor-reductive surgery, again combination chemotherapy is instituted. In patients who respond to treatment, consideration should be given to secondary tumor-reductive surgery after three courses. A large cooperative European study revealed increased tumor control and survival using this treatment approach.[52] A randomized American study is still in progress.

Low-Malignant-Potential Epithelial Tumors

Most of these tumors are Stage I and do not need further treatment. In the rare cases of Stage II or III lesions, the decision depends on the pathologic evaluation. Patients with invasive implants are at higher risk for recurrence and should be treated. Patients with noninvasive implants can be observed. Patients with bulky residual tumor after primary surgery benefit from treatment. A second-look laparoscopy after 1 year should be considered in patients with peritoneal implants. In the case of progressive disease, chemotherapy has to be instituted following the guidelines for invasive epithelial tumors.[53]

Stromal Tumors

Metastatic stromal tumors are treated with chemotherapy using combinations such as bleomycin and etoposide, bleomycin and vinblastine, or cisplatin with doxorubicin and cyclophosphamide. Unfortunately, the response is not as good as in epithelial ovarian cancer. Stage I granulosa-cell tumors or Sertoli–Leydig cell tumors[54] may not need any therapy unless they are large and contain other poor prognostic factors. Careful evaluation of the pathologic specimen should precede any treatment decision.

Germ-Cell Tumors

Malignant germ-cell tumors are always treated with adjuvant chemotherapy using drugs such as cisplatin, etoposide, and bleomycin for four to six courses. The response usually is excellent, and survival rates between 70% and 80% can be expected in early-stage lesions.

SECOND-LOOK LAPAROTOMY/LAPAROSCOPY

It is difficult to evaluate completely patients for residual ovarian cancer. General physical examination is not exact. On CT scan, only lesions more than 1 cm in diameter can be identified with certainty and the CA-125 level is not reliably elevated if the tumor volume is low. Therefore, the so-called second-look laparotomy was instituted. More recently, laparoscopy has been used with equal results.[55] It is a staging procedure that includes multiple peritoneal biopsies, as well as retroperitoneal node sampling if not done initially in patients who have completed their chemotherapy for ovarian cancer and have no evidence of residual malignancy on clinical examination and laboratory/radiologic evaluation. This procedure has been used less frequently during the past several years as it has not been shown to definitely improve the overall survival.[56] However, with the development of better second-line therapy, this assessment may change.[57] Second-look laparotomy is not indicated in patients with early-stage ovarian cancer after complete staging. In patients who did not have adequate staging procedures, specifically, peritoneal biopsies or retroperitoneal-node evaluation, a second-look surgery may be worthwhile. The most frequent indication now is a patient with an advanced Stage III ovarian cancer who is able and willing to accept further therapy or who is treated following a research protocol.[58] However, pros and cons of second-look laparotomy should be carefully discussed with the patient. In patients with advanced cancer, about 20% to 40% will have a negative second-look laparotomy. Another 20% will have only microscopic disease. Even if all biopsies are negative, patients with Stage III ovarian cancer still have a 40% to 50% chance for

developing recurrent disease.[59] After a negative second-look laparotomy, further treatment is under evaluation because of this high relapse rate. Options such as radiation therapy and intraperitoneal p32 application have been evaluated. Improved survival has been noted in some studies. In patients with advanced Stage III lesions, especially if there was a significant amount of residual disease, at least three more courses of chemotherapy should be given even if the second-look laparotomy is negative. In patients with very-low-volume tumor, intraperitoneal chemotherapy should be considered. Other options include further conventional-dose chemotherapy using drugs like topotecan, doxorubicin HCl liposome, gemcitabine, and others or high-dose treatments with stem-cell support.

The chance of discovering residual disease in patients with germ-cell tumors and negative tumor markers is very low. Therefore, a second-look laparotomy is not indicated.[60] Second-look laparotomy is not indicated for stromal tumors. Table 66-5 shows a summary of survival rates for patients treated for ovarian cancer.

FOLLOW-UP AFTER PRIMARY TREATMENT

The follow-up of an asymptomatic patient after therapy for epithelial ovarian cancer should include a complete interval history, physical examination, and rectovaginal pelvic examination and a CA-125 level if it was elevated at initial diagnosis. This is recommended every 2 to 3 months during the first year and at less frequent intervals thereafter. High-risk patients (Stage III lesions, Grade 3 histology) should be followed very closely for at least 2 years, than every 4 to 6 months until the 5-year limit is reached. A rising CA-125 level is a reliable predictor of relapse with a lead time of 3 to 4 months; however, a negative result does not exclude the presence of disease. Radiologic tests done on a routine basis are not cost effective. Their use should be individualized and guided by risk status and symptoms. Patients after treatment for early LMP tumors should be seen every 6 months. Late recurrences, even after 5 years, are possible. Patients with Stage III LMP tumors initially should be followed closely to determine the proliferation rate. CT scans after 6 and 12 months may be worthwhile. A laparoscopy after 1 year should be considered. Tumor markers are less effective for monitoring these lesions. Patients with residual large volume tumors

TABLE 66-5
FIVE-YEAR SURVIVAL RATES FOR SOME OVARIAN TUMORS

Epithelial tumors	
Low malignant potential, Stage I	91%
Low malignant potential Stage II	91%
Low malignant potential Stage III	75%
Invasive	
Stage IA	87%
Stage IB	71%
Stage IC	79%
Stage IIA	67%
Stage IIB	51%
Stage IIC	57%
Stage IIIA	41%
Stage IIIC optimal	35%
Stage IIIC suboptimal	13%
Stage IV	11%
Sex-cord stromal tumors	
Granulosa tumor	
Stage I	85%
Stage II-IV	33–53%
Fibroma thecoma	100%
Androblastomas	
Well differentiated	95%
Poorly differentiated	20%
Germ-cell tumors	
Dysgerminoma	
Early	100%
Advanced	95%
Other	
Completely resected	96%
Bulky residual	50–85%
Cancer of the Fallopian tube	
Stage I	83.6%
Stage II	51.6%
Stage III	35.9%
Stage IV	15%

after surgery should be treated similar to invasive carcinomas.

Patients with stromal tumors are followed as well, although due to the slower growth characteristics of most lesions, the examinations are scheduled less often, every 4 to 6 months. Patients with high-risk granulosa-cell tumors can also be followed with inhibin levels.

Patients with germ-cell tumors are followed very closely for at least 2 years, after which the risk of recurrence decreases significantly. Tumor markers such as α-fetoprotein and β-human chorionic gonadotropin are very reliable in these patients.

Management of Patients at Relapse

Therapy for patients with recurrent disease at this point is rarely curative. Secondary tumor-reductive surgery may be important for relief of symptoms such as the treatment of a bowel obstruction and may prolong survival in a small subset of patients.[61] However, overall survival is not improved.[62] Retreatment with platinum-containing regimens in patients who remain disease-free for more than 6 months after initial treatment is an option. Second-line chemotherapeutic regimens have a poor response rate, between 15% and 25%; however, stable disease and symptom control often can be achieved for a considerable length of time. Drugs such as topotecan, to liposomal doxorubicin, docetaxel, gemcitabine, altretamine, etoposide, and many experimental agents are used. In low-volume tumors that are still chemosensitive, high-dose chemotherapy with stem-cell support may be beneficial. Again, it is important to include as many patients as possible in research studies. At this time, quality of life becomes a major issue. In presenting treatment options, the physiologic status, not the chronologic age, should influence the physician's treatment recommendations. On one hand, the patient should not be given unrealistic expectations; on the other hand hope should not be destroyed. Some patients will place quality of life over aggressive treatments when the chance for cure is low, but for others treatment is very important even if the response rates are expected to be low. Decisions should be made on an individual basis.

ADENOCARCINOMA OF THE FALLOPIAN TUBE

Adenocarcinoma of the fallopian tube is diagnosed rarely, almost never prior to surgery. The clinical presentation is very similar to that of ovarian cancer. Vaginal bleeding is, however, more frequent and intermittent heavy discharge is a rare, but characteristic symptom. In advanced stages, it is impossible to distinguish from metastatic endometrial or ovarian cancer. Often patients present with a pelvic-abdominal mass and ascites.[63]

The staging is done surgically and the system is very similar to that devised for ovarian cancer. Most tumors are of papillary serous histology, but other müllerian differentiations are also possible.

Initial surgical therapy is similar to ovarian cancer. Staging biopsies are important in early lesions; in advanced disease tumor-reductive surgery is recommended.[64] The postoperative treatment again follows the guidelines for ovarian cancer using a platin compound and paclitaxel as the initial therapy. Hormonal therapy with progesterones or radiation therapy is also possible for palliation. Due to the rarity of the disease, comparative studies are not available. The overall survival rates are similar to ovarian cancer.[65]

REFERENCES

1. Cancer Statistics 1999. CA Can J Clini 1999;49(1).
2. Casagrande JT, Pike MC, Ross RK, et al. "Incessant ovulation" and ovarian cancer. Lancet 1979:170.
3. Whittemore AS, Harris R, Itnyre J, et al. Characteristics relating to ovarian cancer risk: collaborative analysis of 12 US case-control studies. Am J Epidemiol 1992;136:1184.
4. Banks E, Beral V, Reeves G. The epidemiology of epithelial ovarian cancer: a review. Int J Gynecol Cancer 1997; 7:425.
5. Narod SA, Risch H, Moslehi R, et al. Oral contraceptives and the risk of hereditary ovarian cancer. N Engl J Med 1998;339:424.
6. Rossing MA, Daling JR, Weiss NS. Ovarian tumors in a cohort of infertile women. N Engl J Med 1994;331:771.
7. Whiteman DC, Murphy MFG, Cook LS, et al. Multiple births and risk of epithelial ovarian cancer. J Natl Cancer Inst 2000; 92:1172.
8. Boyd J, Rubin SC. Hereditary ovarian cancer: molecular genetics and clinical implications. Gynecol Oncol 1997; 64:19.
9. Hartge P, Whittemore AS, Itnyre J, et al. Rates and risks of ovarian cancer in subgroups of white women in the United States. Obstet Gynecol 1994;84:760.
10. The Cancer and Steroid Hormone Study of the Centers for Disease Control and the National Institute of Child Health and Human Development. The reduction in risk of ovarian cancer associated with oral-contraceptive use. N Engl J Med 1987;316:650.
11. Evans AC, Berchuck A, Tumor markers. In: Hoskins WJ, Perez CA, Young RC, eds. Principles and practice of gynecologic oncology. 2nd ed. Philadelphia: Lippincott-Raven, 1997:177.
12. Jacobs I, Davies AP, Bridges J, et al. Prevalence screening for ovarian cancer in postmenopausal women by CA-125 measurement and ultrasonography. BMJ 1993;306:1030.
13. Einhorn N, Sjövall K, Knapp RC, et al. Prospective evaluation of serum CA-125 levels for early detection of ovarian cancer. Obstet Gynecol 1992;80:14.
14. Skates SJ, Xu FJ, Yu YH. Toward an optimal algorithm for ovarian cancer screening with longitudinal tumor markers. Cancer 1995;76:2004.
15. DePriest PD, Gallion HH, Pavlik EJ. Transvaginal sonography as a screening method for the detection of early ovarian cancer. Gynecol Oncol 1997;65:408.
16. Karlan BY, Platt LD. The current status of ultrasound and color Doppler imaging in screening for ovarian cancer. Gynecol Oncol 1994;55:S28.
17. Goldstein ST. Postmenopausal adnexal cysts: how clinical management has evolved. Am J Obstet Gynecol 1996; 175:1498.
18. American College of Obstetricians and Gynecologists. Breast–ovarian cancer screening. ACOG Committee Opinion no. 176, October 1996.
19. Lynch HT, Casey MJ. The role of prophylactic surgery for hereditary breast and ovarian cancer. Contemp Obstet Gynecol 1997:41.
20. Flam F, Einhorn N, Sjovall K. Symptomatology of ovarian cancer. Eur J Obstet Gynecol Reprod Biol 1988; 27:53.
21. Malkasian GD, Knapp RC, Lavin PT, et al. Preoperative evaluation of serum CA-125 levels in premenopausal and postmenopausal patients with pelvic masses: discrimination of benign from malignant disease. Am J Obstet Gynecol 1988;159:341.
22. Sassone AM, Timor-Tritsch IE, Artner A, et al. Transvaginal sonographic characterization of ovarian disease: evaluation of a new scoring system to predict ovarian malignancy. Obstet Gynecol 1991;78:70.
23. DePriest PD, Varner E, Powell J, et al. The efficacy of a sonographic morphology index in identifying ovarian cancer: multi-institutional investigation. Gynecol Oncol 1994;55:174.
24. Tingulstad S, Hagen Bjorn, Skjeldestad FE, et al. Evaluation of a risk of malignancy index based on serum CA-125, ultrasound findings and menopausal status in the preoperative diagnosis of pelvic masses. Br J Obstet Gynaecol 1996;103:826.
25. Fox H. Pathology of ovarian cancer. In: Kavanagh JJ, Singletary S, Einhorn N, et al., eds. Ovarian and fallopian tube cancer. Malden, MA: Blackwell Science, 1999:11.
26. Silva EG, Kurman RJ, Russell P, et al. Symposium: Ovarian tumors of borderline malignancy. Int J Gynecol Pathol 1996;15:281.
27. Fox H. Ovarian tumours of borderline malignancy: time for a reappraisal? Curr Diagn Pathol 1996;3:143.
28. Buchsbaum HJ, Brady MF, Delgado G, et al. GOG Protocol #41: Surgical staging of carcinoma of the ovaries. Surg Gynecol Obstet 1989;169:226.
29. Burghardt E, Girardi R, Lahousen M, et al. Patterns of pelvic and paraaortic lymph node involvement in ovarian cancer. Gynecol Oncol 1991;40:103.
30. Benedetti-Panici P, Greggi S, Maneschi F, et al. Anatomical and pathological study of retroperitoneal nodes in epithelial ovarian cancer. Gynecol Oncol 1993;51:150.
31. Spirtos NM, Gross GM, Freddo JL, et al. Cytoreductive surgery in advanced epithelial cancer of the ovary: the impact of aortic and pelvic lymphadenectomy. Gynecol Oncol 1995;56:345.
32. Allen DG, Heintz APM, Touw FWMM. A meta-analysis of residual disease and survival in stage III and IV carcinoma of the ovary. Eur J Gynaecol Oncol 1995;16:349.
33. Hoskins WJ, Bundy BN, Thigpen JT. The influence of cytoreductive surgery on recurrence-free interval and survival in small-volume stage III epithelial ovarian cancer: a Gynecologic Oncology Group study. Gynecol Oncol 1992;47:159.
34. Eisenkop SM, Halick RH, Wang HJ, et al. Peritoneal implant elimination during cytoreductive surgery for ovarian cancer: impact on survival. Gynecol Oncol 1993; 51:224.
35. van Geene P, Varma R, Dunn J, et al. The prognostic significance of intraperitoneal growth characteristics in epithelial ovarian carcinoma. Int J Gynecol Cancer 1996;6:219.

36. Hacker NF, Berek JS, Lagasse LD, et al. Primary cytoreductive surgery for epithelial ovarian cancer. Obstet Gynecol 1983;61:413.

37. Venesmaa P, Ylikorkala O. Morbidity and mortality associated with primary and repeat operations for ovarian cancer. Obstet Gynecol 1992;79:168.

38. Hoskins WJ, McGuire WP, Brady MF, et al. The effect of diameter of largest residual disease on survival after primary cytoreductive surgery in patients with suboptimal residual epithelial ovarian carcinoma. Am J Obstet Gynecol 1994;170:974.

39. Hoskins WJ. Surgical staging and cytoreductive surgery of epithelial ovarian cancer. Cancer 1993;71:1534.

40. Trimbos JB, Schueler JA, van der Burg M, et al. Watch and wait after careful surgical treatment and staging in well-differentiated early ovarian cancer. Cancer 1991; 67:597.

41. DiSaia PJ. Fertility-sparing treatment of patients with ovarian cancer. Cancer 1990;16:35.

42. Lim-Tan SK, Cajigas HE, Scully RE, et al. Ovarian cystectomy for serous borderline tumors: a follow-up study of 35 cases. Obstet Gynecol 1988;72:775.

43. Yazigi R, Sanstad J, Munoz AK. Primary staging in ovarian tumors of low malignant potential. Gynecol Oncol 1988;31:402.

44. van der Burg MEL, van Lent M, Buyse M, et al. The effect of debulking surgery after induction chemotherapy on the prognosis in advanced epithelial ovarian cancer. N Engl J Med 1995;332:629.

45. Young RC, Walton LA, Ellenberg SS, et al. Adjuvant therapy in stage I and stage II epithelial ovarian cancer; results of two prospective randomized trials. N Engl J Med 1990; 322:1021.

46. Sevelda P, Vavra N, Schemper M, et al. Prognostic factors for survival in stage I epithelial ovarian carcinoma. Cancer 1990;65:2349.

47. Ahmed FY, Wiltshaw E, A'Hern RP, et al. Natural history and prognosis of untreated stage I epithelial ovarian carcinoma. J Clin Oncol 1996;14:2968.

48. Taylor AE, Wiltshaw E, Gore ME, et al. Long-term follow-up of the first randomized study of cisplatin versus carboplatin for advanced epithelial ovarian cancer. J Clin Oncol 1994;12:2066.

49. Bolis G, Colombo N, Pecorelli, et al. Adjuvant treatment for early epithelial ovarian cancer: results of two randomised clinical trials comparing cisplatin to no further treatment or chromic phosphate (^{32}P). Ann Oncol 1995;6:887.

50. Gershenson DM, Mitchell MF, Atkinson N, et al. The effect of prolonged cisplatin-based chemotherapy on progression-free survival in patients with optimal epithelial ovarian cancer: maintenance therapy reconsidered. Gynecol Oncol 1992;47:7.

51. Alberts DS, Liu PY, Hannigan EV, et al. Intraperitoneal cisplatin plus intravenous cyclophosphamide versus intravenous cisplatin plus intravenous cyclophosphamide for stage III ovarian cancer. N Engl J Med 1996;335:1950.

52. van der Burg MEL, van Lent M, Buyse M, et al. The role of intervention debulking surgery in advanced epithelial ovarian cancer: an EORTC gynecological cancer cooperative group study. Int J Gynecol Cancer 1996; 6(Suppl 1):30.

53. Trimble CL, Trimble EL. Management of epithelial ovarian tumors of low malignant potential. Gynecol Oncol 1994;55:S52.

54. Zaloudek C, Norris HJ. Sertoli-Leydig tumors of the ovary: a clinicopathologic study of 64 intermediate and poorly differentiated neoplasms. Am J Surgical Pathol 1984;8:405.

55. Abu-Rustum NR, Barakat RR, Siegel PL, et al. Second-look operation for epithelial ovarian cancer: laparoscopy or laparotomy? Obstet Gynecol 1996;88:549.

56. Creasman WT, Gall S, Bundy BN, et al. Second-look laparotomy in the patient with minimal residual stage III ovarian cancer (a Gynecologic Oncology Group study). Gynecol Oncol 1989;35:378.

57. Friedman RL, Eisenkop SM, Wang HJ. Second-look laparotomy for ovarian cancer provides reliable prognostic information and improves survival. Gynecol Oncol 1997; 67:88.

58. Podratz KC, Kinney WK. Second-look operation in ovarian cancer. Cancer 1993;71:1551.

59. Rubin SC, Hoskins WJ, Saigo PE, et al. Prognostic factors for recurrence following negative second-look laparotomy in ovarian cancer patients treated with platinum-based chemotherapy. Gynecol Oncol 1991;42:137.

60. Gershenson DM, Copeland LJ, Junco GD, et al. Second-look laparotomy in the management of malignant germ cell tumors of the ovary. Obstet Gynecol 1986; 67:789.

61. Vaccarello L, Rubin SC, Vlamis V, et al. Cytoreductive surgery in ovarian carcinoma patients with a documented previously complete surgical response. Gynecol Oncol 1995;57:61.

62. Morris M, Gershenson DM, Wharton JT. Secondary cytoreductive surgery for recurrent epithelial ovarian cancer. Gynecol Oncol 1989;34:334.

63. Alvarado-Cabrero I, Young RH, Vamvakas EC, et al. Carcinoma of the fallopian tube: a clinicopathological study of 105 cases with observations on staging and prognostic factors. Gynecol Oncol 1999;72:367.

64. Eddy GL, Copeland LJ, Gershenson DM, et al. Fallopian tube carcinoma. Obstet Gynecol 1984;64:546.

65. Baekelandt M, Kockx M, Wesling F. Primary adenocarcinoma of the fallopian tube: review of the literature. 1993; 3:65.

66. Pecorelli S, Creasman WT, Pettersson F, et al., eds. FIGO Annual Report on the Results of Treatment in Gynaecological Cancer. 23rd Vol. J Epidemiol Biostat 1998:63.

SUGGESTED READINGS

1. DiSaia PJ, Creasman WT, eds. Clinical gynecologic oncology. 5th ed. New York: Mosby-Year Book, 1997.

2. Hoskins WJ, Perez CA, Young RC, eds. Principles and practice of gynecologic oncology. Philadelphia: Lippincott, 1997.

3. Morrow CP, Curtin JP, Townsend DE. Synopsis of gynecologic oncology. New York: Churchill Livingstone, 1993.

4. Rubin SC and Sutton GP, eds. Ovarian cancer. New York: McGraw-Hill, 1993.

Chapter 67

Gestational Trophoblastic Disease

Brigitte E. Miller

Five Key Points

- Gestational trophoblastic disease (GTD) includes several entities, such as complete mole, partial mole, transitional mole, invasive mole, choriocarcinoma, and placental site trophoblastic tumor.

- It is critical to follow β-human chorionic gonadotropin (β-HCG) values after a molar pregnancy, to determine β-HCG levels in patients with delayed postpartum hemorrhage, and in reproductive-age women presenting with widespread metastatic disease.

- In case of persistent or rising titers, work-up should include a laboratory survey, pelvic ultrasound, chest radiograph, and a computed tomographic (CT) scan of the abdomen and head to assess the category into which the GTD falls, i.e., nonmetastatic GTD, low-risk metastatic GTD, and high-risk metastatic GTD.

- Good response to single-agent chemotherapy with methotrexate or dactinomycin, as well as combination chemotherapy, can be expected.

- Close follow-up after completion of treatment with β-HCG values and examination is important. Effective contraception is mandatory.

The term gestational trophoblastic disease (GTD) includes several types of tumors ranging from benign to extremely malignant. In comparison with other gynecologic malignancies, GTD is characterized by several unique features. First, the exact pathologic diagnosis is not important for treatment decisions and follow-up in many instances. Second, a very accurate tumor marker is available by determining the β-HCG concentration. Third, on one hand, these tumors can be rapidly progressive; on the other hand, they are very curable with systemic chemotherapy even if advanced metastatic disease is present. Last, but not least, these tumors are derived from fetal tissue but mostly grow into maternal tissue. Many questions regarding the development of GTD are still unanswered. It is not known if GTD is related to deleterious recessive genes or to loss of tumor-suppressor genes.[1]

EPIDEMIOLOGY

Overall, gestational trophoblastic disease is rare in the United States. Reports vary from 1 in 923 to 1 in 1724 pregnancies or about 1.08 in 1000 pregnancies. The incidence of choriocarcinoma is 0.04 in 1000 pregnancies. Some of these differences may be related to methodologic problems. The figures in hospital-based studies are usually higher than in population-based studies. While the highest incidences are reported from Asian countries, such as Indonesia, Taiwan, China, or the Philippines, most of these reports are also hospital-based studies. In the United States, African-American women have been reported to have an increased, decreased, or similar risk of molar pregnancy as compared with Caucasian women. The risk of choriocarcioma, however, is about twice as high in African-Americans as in Caucasians. Native Alaskan women also seem to be at increased risk.[2]

A second risk factor is patient age. Complete molar pregnancies are more frequent at the extremes of the reproductive period. All reports state a higher incidence in women over age 40. In several studies an increased incidence has also been seen for women under age 20, but to a lesser extent.[3] Partial moles seem to occur with the same frequency throughout the reproductive period. The incidence may be underestimated, as many end as first-trimester miscarriages without the typical appearance of a mole so that the diagnosis is missed. The frequent occurrence of triploidy among early abortions may to some extent be due to partial molar pregnancies.[1] Some studies also found an increased risk of GTD if the paternal age was above 45.[4]

The strongest risk factor, however, is a previous molar pregnancy, which increases the risk of a second molar gestation to 1 to even 2.6%. After two molar pregnancies, there is about a 28% chance that a third pregnancy will likewise end as a mole.[5] In addition, the risk of molar pregnancy increases with a history of previous spontaneous abortions, some of which may have been very early molar pregnancies, and it decreases with a history of any term pregnancies. The protective effect increases with the number of normal pregnancies.

Other factors such as blood groups or dietary factors seem to be less important,[3] although a case control study by Berkowitz et al.[6] revealed vitamin A deficiency to be an important factor. Smoking, oral contraceptives, and other nutritional factors have been implicated in the development of GTD in some reports, but could not be confirmed in others.

TYPES OF GESTATIONAL TROPHOBLASTIC DISEASE

Molar pregnancies comprise three entities: complete mole, partial mole, and transitional mole. The complete mole is also called the classic mole. In most complete moles (95%), the tissue has a 46,XX composition. All chromosomes are of paternal origin. This occurs either by duplication of a single sperm within the ovum, leading to a 46,XX karyotype, or (in 25%) by two separate sperms entering an ovum, leading to the 46,XY or 46,XX karyotype. On examination, the uterus (in 33%) is often large for gestational dates and is filled with the typical vesicles if the diagnosis is made later in the course. If the diagnosis is made very early, the typical vesicles have not yet developed, and even some blood vessels may be seen.[7] There is no evidence of an embryo. On occasion, a normal twin pregnancy may develop in addition to a molar pregnancy. Using flow cytometry to determine ploidy and DNA analysis to compare polymorphisms, an accurate diagnosis can be made in most cases. On microscopic evaluation, there is significant hyperplasia of the cytotrophoblast as well as the syncytial trophoblast. The villi are swollen and do not contain vessels or fetal blood cells. Diagnosis is usually made early in the gestation, around 8 to 16 weeks. β-HCG values are often higher than in a normal pregnancy. The risk of malignant sequelae is reported to be between 15% to 25%.

The partial or incomplete mole usually develops with a triploid karyotype (80%). A fetus is usually present but often dies during the first trimester; rarely will it develop to term. The distortion of the villi is not as uniform, but more focal, with only mild hyperplasia. Fetal vessels and blood cells are seen. The diagnosis is usually made later in the pregnancy, between 10 and 20 weeks, and the β-HCG value is not as high as in complete moles. Because of the lower β-HCG values some of the typical complications such as severe hyperemesis and theca lutein cysts are rarely seen. Ultrasound findings also more frequently point toward a miscarriage than a GTD. The uterus is usually small or of adequate size for gestational age. The preoperative diagnosis is missed or noted as an incomplete abortion in the vast majority of the cases. The malignant potential seems to be

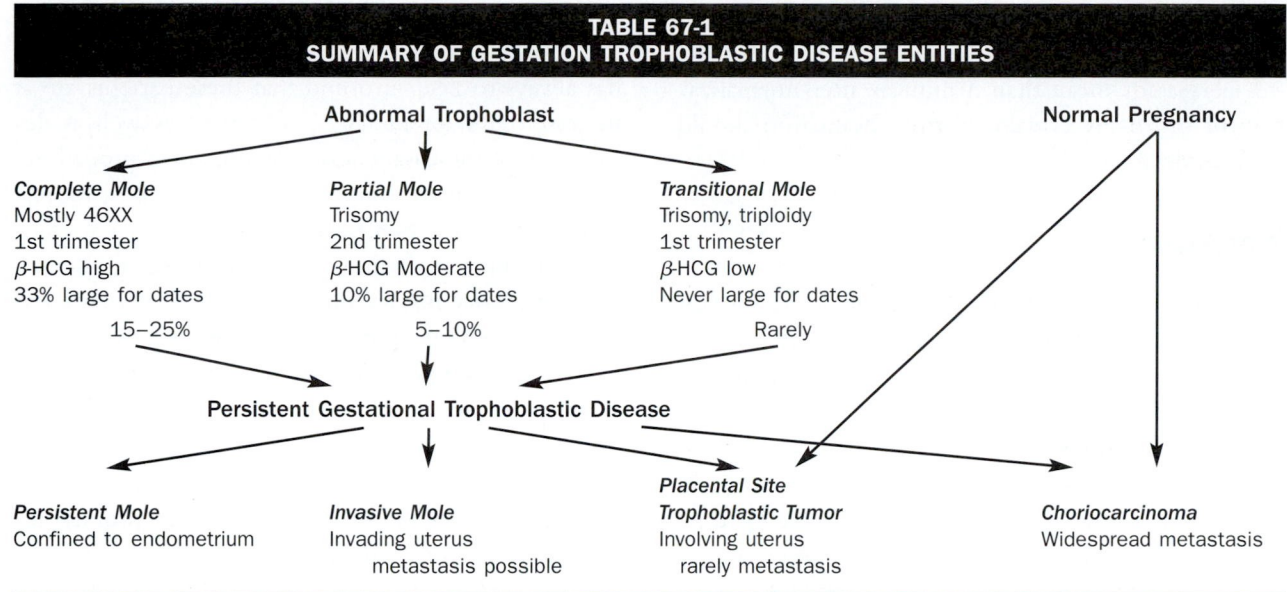

TABLE 67-1
SUMMARY OF GESTATION TROPHOBLASTIC DISEASE ENTITIES

lower, but reports vary significantly between 5% and 15%. The higher figure may be an overestimation, as many partial moles are probably diagnosed as abortions and not taken into account, thus significantly reducing the number of partial moles diagnosed.[1] In any case, all patients should be followed with serial β-HCG levels after the diagnosis of a partial mole.

The last component is the transitional mole or blighted ovum. Karyotyping often reveals a trisomic or triploid pattern. Hydropic villi are present; however, there is no evidence of hyperplasia. Remnants of embryonic development are often seen. The villi do contain capillaries. Diagnosis, again, is made early during the first trimester. The β-HCG value is usually low. The risk of subsequent malignancy is minimal.[8] A summary of the types of GTD is seen in Table 67-1.

SYMPTOMS

The early symptoms are similar to those of a threatened miscarriage, such as irregular uterine bleeding and cramping. Rarely, the typical vesicles are passed through the vagina. Due to the increased use of ultrasound, the diagnosis often is made early in the course of the pregnancy, before the typical symptoms occur. Complete moles mainly become symptomatic in the first and early second trimesters. In the presence of a partial mole, symptoms occur later in the second trimester. In contrast, a blighted ovum is also diagnosed early.

MEDICAL COMPLICATIONS

Due to the earlier diagnosis with ultrasound, most of the medical complications associated with molar pregnancy are seen less frequently. Vaginal spotting and bleeding may lead to anemia. The high β-HCG values can lead to severe hyperemesis, as well as toxemia, which otherwise is very unusual during the first part of the pregnancy. Thyroid dysfunction is another complication, due to the similarities between β-HCG and thyroid-stimulating hormone (TSH).[9] Clinical hyperthyroidism may occasionally develop. Treatment for all these problems consists of removing the molar pregnancy. These complications rarely develop in patients with partial moles.

If the molar pregnancy is advanced and diagnosed during the second trimester, there is an increased risk of high-output cardiac failure and pulmonary insufficiency. The incidence usually peaks about 4 hours after evacuation of the mole. It has been suggested that this event is due to massive embolization of fetal cells into the maternal circulation, but it may also be related to the anemia and to generous fluid administration.[10]

Due to the intense stimulation with β-HCG, both ovaries are often enlarged by multiple follicular cysts. This has been noted to complicate a complete molar pregnancy in 25 to 50% of cases. This is rarely seen with a partial mole. Occasionally, this enlargement can even further increase after evacuation of the mole and can lead to significant abdominal distention with ascites and dehydration. Usually these cysts regress spontaneously as the β-HCG level decreases, but sometimes regression can be delayed. If abnormalities persist for more than 3 months after normalization of the β-HCG value, further evaluation should be considered.[11]

DIAGNOSIS

It is impossible to establish a definite diagnosis on physical examination alone except when the miscarriage is in progress and the typical vesicles are expelled. In the presence of a complete mole, β-HCG values are very high, with an average of about 200,000 IU/ml. This is much higher than would be noted in a normal pregnancy. However, it is impossible to completely distinguish between a normal and a molar pregnancy on the basis of a β-HCG value. A variety of other measurements have been explored, such as estrogen, α-fetoprotein, HCG-α, and HCG-α and -β subunits. However, none of those provide a reliable diagnosis.

The best way to evaluate a possible molar pregnancy is to perform ultrasonography. Here, a characteristic picture is seen consisting of the absence of a gestational sac and a fetus, as well as a uterus filled with multiple, diffuse echoes. The examination is very reliable and also offers the ability to detect a fetus in the presence of a partial mole.

TREATMENT

As soon as the diagnosis is made, evacuation of the uterus should take place. Patients need to be prepared carefully as they are at increased risk for bleeding, injury of the uterus, and pulmonary complications. Chest radiography should be performed prior to the procedure. A β-HCG value should be determined, as well as a basic chemistry profile, including a thyroid-function test, although often the thyroid status has to be assessed on clinical findings only. Blood should be available for transfusion. If the pregnancy has reached the second trimester, intensive monitoring may be necessary and equipment should be available.

As most patients are young, a suction curettage with preservation of the uterus is the treatment of choice. An oxytocin drip should be started with the procedure. Dilatation should be done gently and the largest available suction curette should be used to remove the uterine contents. Blood loss is often overestimated due to dilution from the multiple vesicles.

At the end of the procedure, the uterine cavity should be carefully explored with a large sharp curette. One has always to keep in mind that these patients are at increased risk for uterine perforation, as well as destruction of the basal endometrium. These procedures have to be done cautiously, as there is a significant risk of complications. Schlaerth [12] reported a 67% complication rate, including infection, toxemia, anemia, and respiratory insufficiency among 277 patients. Especially when the procedure is done in the second trimester, this risk of respiratory insufficiency is increased. Oxygen monitoring in the recovery room is therefore recommended. The patients should also be watched carefully for signs of hyperthyroidism. As the placental tissue develops Rh antigens, Rh prophylaxis should be given to Rh-negative women, who do not have antibodies.

For older women who have completed their families and desire sterilization, hysterectomy certainly is an adequate treatment option. These patients still need to be followed with serial β-HCG levels. Although the risk of persistent trophoblastic disease is lower, it cannot be completely excluded.

Prophylactic administration of chemotherapeutic agents such as dactinomycin and methotrexate during evacuation of a hydatid mole has been shown to reduce the incidence of recurrent gestational trophoblastic disease. However, it is not completely effective. In some reports, a higher resistance to chemotherapy was noted in instances when GTD recurs. Therefore it cannot be recommended routinely.[13] It may be an alternative for patients in whom follow-up would be difficult.

SEQUELAE

Gestational trophoblastic disease can be divided into three entities—simple mole, invasive mole, choriocarcinoma, and placental trophoblastic tumor. The simple molar pregnancy is confined to the endometrium and is usually completely removed at the time of suction curettage. The characteristic feature of the invasive mole is that molar tissue invades the uterine muscle and blood vessels. Due to earlier diagnosis, this situation seems to be getting more rare. The diagnosis can only be made reliably at the time of hysterectomy. It seems that about 5 to 10% of molar pregnancies are invasive. In spite of the local invasion and the possible development of metastasis to the vagina and lung, the invasive mole is not a malignancy, as it is self-limited. The tumor regresses spontaneously.

About 3 to 7% of hydatid moles are followed by choriocarcinoma. This is a very fast-growing malignant tumor that tends to spread hematogenously. The lung is usually the first area of metastatic disease, as well as the lower genital tract. After that, it can spread to all areas of the body. The initial symptoms are often caused by organ damage due to the necrotic tumor with associated bleeding complications. It can, therefore, imitate a variety of other diseases such as brain tumor, liver tumor, or gastrointestinal ulcerations with chronic blood loss. The diagnosis should be considered every time a woman of reproductive age presents with a diffusely metastatic malignancy. Overall, 50% of choriocarcinomas develop after a molar pregnancy. The remainder of the cases follows a miscarriage or a normal pregnancy. The incidence is about 1000 times higher after a molar pregnancy than after a normal pregnancy. GTD that develops after a normal pregnancy is always a choriocarcinoma. Sometimes the initial symptom is delayed postpartum bleeding. It is, therefore, very important to check a β-HCG level in these patients.[14] However, in about 25%, the most recent pregnancy is not the causative pregnancy. These lesions can remain dormant for a prolonged period. Once proliferation has set in, this is one of the most rapidly growing tumors. Necrosis with bleeding is, therefore, not infrequent. Viable tumor is often seen only in the periphery of the lesion.

Very rarely is a choriocarcinoma in situ diagnosed. This is a focus of choriocarcinoma in an otherwise normal placenta. No treatment is necessary; however, baby and mother should be monitored with β-HCG level determinations.

The last type of gestational trophoblastic disease is the placental-site trophoblastic tumor, which usually occurs in women of reproductive age, but it also has been seen in postmenopausal women, although rarely. It may arise from a molar pregnancy or a normal pregnancy—sometimes even many years later. Although it usually follows a benign course by remaining localized, it rarely can lead to metastatic disease, which is quite difficult to treat, as the response to chemotherapy is not as good as with choriocarcinoma. Sometimes local invasion into the parametria is also seen. The uterus is usually enlarged and the β-HCG level slightly elevated, but never as high as in choriocarcinoma. Human placental lactogen (hPL) levels are frequently increased. The tumor does not

show a biphasic pattern and sometimes differential diagnosis from a poorly differentiated squamous carcinoma is difficult. Immunohistochemistry reveals moderate staining with β-HCG and intense staining with hPL. A high mitosis count and significant necrosis signifies a poor prognosis.[15] The initial treatment includes a hysterectomy. In the presence of metastatic disease, combination chemotherapy is necessary. Local metastases also respond to radiation therapy. [16,17]

FOLLOW-UP AFTER A MOLAR PREGNANCY

On physical examination, the patient needs to be evaluated for theca lutein cysts, involution of the uterus, as well as lower-genital-tract metastasis. If a lesion is seen (often as a dark purple nodule), biopsy should be avoided, as bleeding can be significant. A thorough pelvic examination should be done 1 week after and again in 1 month after evacuation of a molar pregnancy. The most accurate way, however, to follow these patients is to determine the β-HCG values (Table 67-2).

Like other stimulating hormones, the β-HCG molecule is a glycoprotein with two subunits, α and β. The β-subunit conveys the biologic activity. In the presence of gestational trophoblastic disease, there is also a variety of incomplete β-HCG molecules present to a much greater extent than during a normal pregnancy. Therefore, it is important to know exactly which test is used in the laboratory to determine the β-HCG values. Most new test kits use a molecular antibody technique in a sandwich assay;

TABLE 67-2
FOLLOW-UP FOR GESTATIONAL TROPHOBLASTIC DISEASE

During regression
  Weekly HCG
  Pelvic exam 1 wk after evacuation and every 2–4 wk until
    negative for HCG
After remission
  HCG weekly for 4 wk
  HCG monthly for 6–12 mo
  Contraception for 12 mo
  HCG if patient symptomatic
  HCG 6 wk after any subsequent pregnancy
Indication for treatment
  Rising HCG (3 weekly values)
  Plateau ($\pm$10% for 3 wk)
  Metastatis
  Biopsy with chorioca, PSTT

however, there is considerable variability regarding measurement of the incomplete forms. The preferred β-HCG test should measure not only the complete but also the incomplete β-HCG molecules. These are quite accurate and can detect the presence of 100,000 cells. The β-HCG values should be followed weekly until they return to normal, and then on a monthly basis for 6 to 12 months, depending on the time to regression. Usually, the initial drop is very rapid and then the slope flattens. Sometimes, regression is slower, but patients can be followed conservatively as long as the downward trend is continued. The average length of time to reach negative values is 73 days. Fifty percent of patients still have elevated values at 9 weeks.[18] About 60 days after molar evacuation, 70% of the patients will have normal β-HCG values and in 15% the values continue to drop slowly. In the remaining 15%, a plateau or rise occurs and treatment may become necessary. The following results were reported by Lurain et al.,[19] who evaluated 596 patients. Complete regression occurred in 22.6% at day 30, in 42.6% between days 41 to 69, and in 34.6% between days 61 and 170. Nineteen percent of these patients needed treatment. All patients who experienced spontaneous regression remained free of disease. On the other hand, Bagshawe[20] even followed patients with vaginal and pulmonary metastasis as long as the β-HCG levels declined, which led to treatment of only 5.7% of his patients. In the United States, earlier treatment is advocated to decrease the risk of significant complications related to advanced metastasis, especially when close follow-up is not guaranteed. Hatch[21] treated patients with persistent β-HCG elevation at 12 weeks—a total of 32%. Use of regression curves by other authors also increased the percentage of patients receiving chemotherapy up to 36%[22] and 27%.[23] Urine pregnancy tests are inadequate to follow GTD because they are not sufficiently selective.

The longer the HCG elevation, the more likely is metatstatic disease. Lurain et al.[19] noted chemotherapy to be necessary in 36% of patients with elevated β-HCG titers after 60 days. Patients at increased risk for gestational trophoblastic disease are women with delayed postpartum hemorrhage, large theca lutein cysts, postevacuation pulmonary insufficiency, a large uterine size, and a very high β-HCG value. This is also true for patients who are over the age of 40 or who are diagnosed with a molar pregnancy for the second time.[24]

It is very important to avoid another pregnancy during this follow-up period. Oral contraceptives are the recommended method and should be started immediately after suction dilation and curettage. There is no evidence that the estrogen component of oral contraceptives increases the risk of trophoblastic neoplasia.[25]

INDICATION FOR TREATMENT

Treatment should be instituted whenever there is a diagnosis of choriocarcinoma. Treatment is also indicated if there is an increase of the β-HCG values or a plateau for more than 3 weeks. Overall, around 20% of patients with molar pregnancy will have to receive chemotherapy.[19] The presence of metastatic disease is also an indication for treatment. The World Health Organization (WHO) criteria for treatment are as follows: (1) a serum HCG level greater than 20,000 IU/ml more than 4 weeks after evacuation; (2) progressively increasing β-HCG values; (3) evidence of choriocarcinoma or metastatic disease; (4) pulmonary metastasis greater than 2 cm in diameter or more than three in number.[26] In the United States, however, all patients with a rise in titer, the presence of metastatic disease, or choriocarcinoma are treated. There is difference of opinion how long a patient with a stable but not declining β-HCG should be followed. Most physicians treat if there is no decrease in 3 consecutive weekly titers. Kohorn recommended that patients who develop a plateau with low β-HCG values may even be followed longer provided complete follow-up is assured.[27] A repeat uterine curettage prior to treatment is not necessary. Rarely is there a significant amount of molar tissue inside the uterus. Repeat curettage rarely contributes significantly to treatment decisions and does not have a therapeutic effect.[28] Although pathologic evaluation of the curettage specimen can give some prognostic information, this is not accurate enough to base treatment on.

STAGING SYSTEMS

A variety of staging systems have been developed to define the prognosis of patients with persistent GTD. The International Federation of Gynecology and Obstetrics (FIGO)[29] staging system depends exclusively on the location of the metastasis (Table 67–3). It has a poor separation of categories, as about 75% of all cases fall into Stage III. It also is not useful for the

TABLE 67-3
INTERNATIONAL FEDERATION OF GYNECOLOGY AND OBSTETRICS (FIGO) STAGING FOR GESTATIONAL TROPHOBLASTIC DISEASE

Stage	Characteristics
I	Confined to uterine corpus
II	Extends outside the uterus, but limited to genital structures
III	Extends to the lungs, with or without genital-tract involvement
IV	All other metastatic sites

All stages are subdivided into:
  A—without risk factors
  B—one risk factor
  C—two risk factors

The risk factors are:
  1—β-HCG >100,000 mIU/ml
  2—>6 mo since pregnancy.

TABLE 67-4
CLINICAL CLASSIFICATION OF MALIGNANT GESTATIONAL TROPHOBLASTIC DISEASE

I. Nonmetastatic GTD: no evidence of disease outside the uterus, not assigned to any prognostic category
II. Metastatic GTD: any metastases
  A. Good-prognosis metastatic GTD
    Short duration (< 4 mo)
    Low HDC level (<40,000 mIU/ml serum β-HCG)
    No metastases to brain or liver
    No antecedent term pregnancy
    No prior chemotherapy
  B. Poor-prognosis metastatic GTD
    Long duration (>4 mo since last pregnancy)
    High pretreatment β-HCG level (>40,000 mIU/ml serum βHCG)
    Brain or liver metastases
    Antecedent term pregnancy
    Prior chemotherapy

decision if single-agent or multiagent chemotherapy should be given. Many other scoring systems have been developed; one of the best is the system developed by Bagshawe,[30] which was adapted by the WHO with some modifications (Table 67-4). The clinical classification system was originally used by Hammond and Soper and distinguishes between nonmetastatic and low- and high-risk metastatic disease.[31] High-risk factors identified in most studies include long duration, resistance to previous therapy, number of metastases, brain or liver involvement, and type of antecedent pregnancy.[31,32] The clinical staging system is quite accurate in identifiying prognostic categories. The WHO system adds some information to it and it

is semiquantitative and, therefore, a bit more complicated. It should not be used for patients without metatstatic disease, as a high score is possible in this situation; however, combination chemotherapy is not indicated. Not all prognostic factors are of equal importance. Patients who are at high risk mainly because of very high β-HCG levels can expect a good outcome.[33] The WHO scoring system is the best to determine the prognosis. It separates patients at high risk (score, 8 to 12) from patients at a very high risk (score >12) who are threatened by a death rate of 66%.[34] Recently modifications to the WHO staging system have been accepted by a group of experts such as (a) eliminating the ABO blood group as a risk

TABLE 67-5
WORLD HEALTH ORGANIZATION PROGNOSTIC INDEX SCORE FOR GESTATIONAL TROPHOBLASTIC DISEASE

Prognostic Factors	Score			
	0	1	2	4
Age (yr)	≤35	>39		
Antecedent pregnancy	Hydatidiform mole	Abortion	Term	
Interval (months)	<4	4–6	7–12	>12
β-HCG (IU/L)	<10	10^3–10^4	10^4–10^5	>10^5
ABO groups (female × male)	—	O × A	B	—
Largest tumor, including uterine tumor	3–5 cm	>5 cm	—	—
Site of metastases	Spleen, kidney	Gastrointestinal tract, liver	Brain	—
Number of metastases identified	1–4	4–8	>8	—
Prior chemotherapy	—	Single drug	Two or more	—

The total score for a patient is obtained by adding the individual scores for each prognostic factor. Total score 0–4 = low risk; 5–7 = intermediate risk; >7–8 = high risk.

factor; (b) increasing the factor for liver metastasis to 4; and (c) each lung metastasis to be included in the count must be ≥ 3 cm. There is also discussion about the definition of risk groups. Some experts felt that the intermediate risk group should be abandoned, that all patients with a score of 6 or less are low risk, and all patients with a score of 7 or more are high risk.[35]

WORK-UP FOR PERSISTENT GESTATIONAL TROPHOBLASTIC DISEASE

First, a careful history and physical examination are important. Pelvic examination should evaluate the patient for uterine or ovarian enlargement and lower genital metastasis. An ultrasonography should be performed to rule out an intrauterine pregnancy. Chest radiography should be done to check for metastasis. Certainly a CT scan identifies more patients with pulmonary metastasis;[36] however, this is not necessarily of clinical importance, especially as treatment is not different in patients with or without pulmonary metastasis. A higher incidence of resistance to methotrexate (MTX) has been reported in patients with small pulmonary metastasis seen only on CT scan by some authors[37]; however, this has not been confirmed by others.[36] Again, this finding does not change treatment decisions and therefore a routine CT scan is not necessary. In the absence of pulmonary metastasis, no further work-up may be necessary.[38] However, in case of a false negative pulmonary evaluation, other metastases could be missed.

A complete metastatic work-up should include a CT scan of the abdomen and brain to rule out poor prognostic metastasis.

Ultrasound evaluation is acceptable to check for liver metastasis. An MRI is the preferred method to diagnose brain metastasis, but it is not universally available and therefore not included in the FIGO staging recommendations. MRI is valuable to determine tumor volume within the uterus so that angiography is rarely necessary.[39] Exact documentation of intrauterine disease is rarely necessary unless surgery is contemplated in patients with recurrent or persistent disease. Blood chemistry determinations, including thyroid profile and liver-function tests, should also be done.

TREATMENT OF PERSISTENT GTD

Nonmetastatic GTD is highly curable. For a patient who also desires sterilization, a hysterectomy is the treatment of choice. β-HCG levels still need to be followed, but often regression continues without chemotherapy.

In those patients who would like to retain their uterus, single-agent chemotherapy with methotrexate and/or dactinomycin can be given (Table 67-6). The side-effect profile of the drugs is different. Methotrexate can cause moderate nausea and vomiting, as well as hematologic toxicity, and, rarely, severe acute and chronic liver injury, stomatitis, enteritis, interstitial pneumonitis, and renal and neurologic side effects, and should not be given if liver function is abnormal or if there is impaired renal function. Dactinomycin can cause severe tissue damage in cases of extravasation. In addition, patients may experience nausea, vomiting, stomatitis, bone marrow suppression, alopecia, acne, and liver damage. The most frequently used regimens are summarized in Figure 67-1. Remission rates between 85 and almost 99% can be expected. If the patient does not respond to one drug, she can be switched to the other drug and again a remission can be expected. One of the easiest regimens uses weekly methotrexate at a dosage of 30 mg/m^2 intramuscularly. Increasing the dose to 40 and 50 mg/m^2 does

TABLE 67-6		
SINGLE AGENT CHEMOTHERAPY FOR GTD		
Drug	**Dose**	**Response Rate**
Methotrexate (Soper)[60]	0.4 mg/kg daily × 5 every 2 wk	89%
Methotrexate (Homesley et al.)[40]	30 mg/m^2 IV every wk	81%
Methotrexate and	50 mg intramuscularly on days 1, 3, 5, 7	80%
Folinic acid (Berkowitz et al.)[41]	7.5 mg orally on days 2, 4, 6, and 8	
Dactinomycin (Pertrilli)[59]	1.25 mg/m^2 IV every other week	94%
Methotrexate alternating Dactinomycin	0.4 mg/kg daily × 5 alternating with 0.01 mg/kg daily	86%
(Freedman)[2]	× 5 every other week	

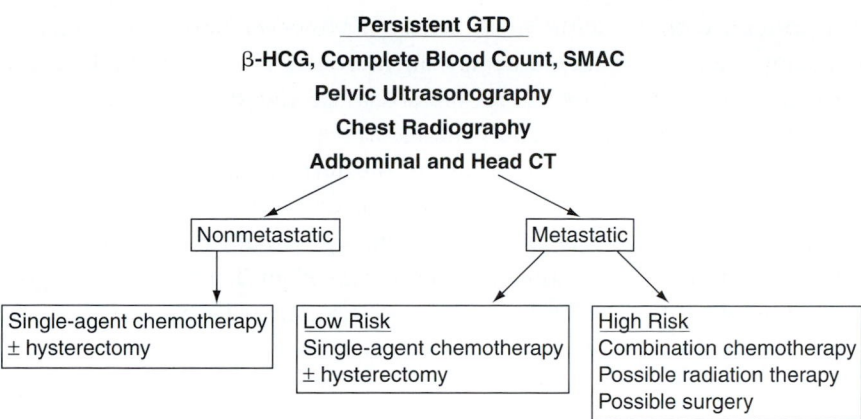

Figure 67-1 Work-up and treatment of persistent GTD.

not improve the response rate.[40] High-dose methotrexate with folinic acid rescue is more difficult to administer without improved outcome.[41] In addition, some reports state a higher rate of resistance with the combined therapy. Bagshawe et al.[42] noted resistance in 20% of the patients. The medication had to be changed due to toxicity in another 6%. At M.D. Anderson Cancer Center, an alternating treatment is used with methotrexate, 0.4 mg/kg for 5 days, followed by dactinomycin, 0.01 mg/kg day for 5 days two weeks later.[2] Other regimens include etoposide and 5-fluorouracil.[43] For patients who do not respond to single-agent treatment, combination chemotherapy is recommended.

Metastatic trophoblastic disease is clinically separated into low-risk or high-risk categories. The symptoms depend on the organ involvement. All women of reproductive age who present with an unexplained metastatic cancer should have their β-HCG level determined. Patients with low-risk metastatic disease, pulmonary metastasis only, and a WHO score below 8 can be treated with single-agent chemotherapy. Even in the presence of metastasis hysterectomy is an option for reducing the number of treatment courses necessary to achieve complete remission. In a patient with a higher score, metastatic disease to the brain and liver, or other tumors, combination chemotherapy should be instituted immediately.[44] This is an indication for emergency chemotherapy. Treatment delays should be avoided at all costs. The main threat to the patient does not come from the metastatic tumor, but from the associated bleeding, especially in the presence of brain or spinal cord metastasis. As these cases are quite rare, referral to a treatment center or a gynecologic oncologist is strongly recommended. Inadequate initial therapy may significantly decrease chances of survival.[45] Prognostic

factors are well summarized in the WHO system. Treatment regimens use combination chemotherapy such as MAC: methotrexate, dactinomycin, and cytoxan or chlorambucil[46] or the Bagshawe 7-drug regimen.[47] However, chemotherapy following the EMA-CO[48] regimen using dactinomycin, etoposide, methotrexate, vincristine, and cyclophosphamide is the preferred treatment most recently. Sometimes, especially in patients with refractory disease, etoposide and cisplatin are substituted for vincristine and cyclophosphamide (EMA-EP).[49] Even in this high-risk group, a complete response rate of 75% was seen. The treatment has to be given aggressively and delays are to be avoided.[44] Again, referral to a treatment center is strongly recommended. This regimen is also active against PSTT, but not as effective: only 4 out of 8 patients survived. Other combinations include cisplatin and etoposide or cisplatin, bleomycin, and vinblastine. Central nervous system disease should also be treated with radiation therapy. Although the blood–brain barrier is less effective in the presence of metastatic disease, systemic chemotherapy is not quite adequate to eradicate the central nervous system disease. Radiation[50] or intrathecal chemotherapy, therefore, should be strongly considered. If brain metastasis is diagnosed prior to chemotherapy and the distal disease can be controlled, a 5-year survival of 75% can be expected after radiation therapy and chemotherapy.[51] The prognosis for patients with recurrent disease and brain metastasis or patients in whom metastases develop during treatment is poor. Surgical decompression and sometimes resection is necessary. For liver metastasis, aggressive chemotherapy is the best option, and an overall survival rate of 27% can be expected. No significant differences were noted among the combination chemotherapy regimens.[52] A WHO score of >12 was a poor prognostic sign.

Occasionally surgery is an option in patients with recurrent or refractory GTD. A hysterectomy is effective for uterine disease. Rarely, a single metastasis to the lung or other areas can also be removed by surgery. A very thorough preoperative work-up is mandatory. Complete response rates up to 42% have been seen in these patients.[53] The response rate is better in patients who are a short time from diagnosis, have a small number of disease sites, have a lower WHO score, or have lesions other than choriocarcinoma.

FOLLOW-UP AFTER GESTATIONAL TROPHOBLASTIC DISEASE

Patients should avoid pregnancy at least for 1 year. If a pregnancy is planned after that time, an ultrasonography should be done as soon as possible to check for recurrence of a molar pregnancy. A good outcome can be expected in most cases.[54,55] If uterine instrumentation was aggressive, there is a slightly increased risk of placenta accreta. Following 445 patients after treatment for GTD, Rustin et al.[56] reported that 97% of those who desired more children conceived, and 86% had at least one live birth. Outcome was slightly worse after combination chemotherapy than after single-agent treatment. There is no definite evidence of an increased risk of fetal malformations in these patients.

Recurrent molar pregnancy is the most important risk after successful treatment. Reports in the literature vary significantly from a low estimate of 1%, still many times higher than the risk without previous GTD, to 4.4% and even as high as 9.6% in patients who were treated with chemotherapy.[57] As most of the patients are young, the risk of ovarian insufficiency due to chemotherapy is low. It may also be helpful that during this time most patients take oral contraceptives, which decrease the ovarian function and possibly ovarian injury. Alkylating agents as well as etoposide seem to have the strongest effect on ovarian function by destruction of resting oocytes. Even younger patients therefore are at increased risk for premature menopause and should be advised not to postpone childbearing until the late reproductive period. In older patients this can lead to menopause right away. The younger the patient, the better the recovery of ovarian function. Woolas et al.[58] followed patients after treatment with methotrexate and EMA-CO and reported subsequent pregnancies in 83%.

Secondary malignancies are another concern. No increased risk of malignancy was seen after therapy with methotrexate. However after combination chemotherapy, an increased risk of leukemia, colon cancer, and breast cancer was seen in patients who survived for more than 25 years.

In conclusion, the term gestational trophoblastic disease includes a variety of very different diseases ranging from completely benign to highly malignant. Treatment results are excellent. Therefore, the importance of close follow-up cannot be overstated, as it is the best assurance against a poor outcome.

REFERENCES

1. Newland ES, Paradinas FJ, Path FRC, Fisher RA. Recent advances in gestational trophoblastic disease. Curr Ther Issues Gynecol Cancer 1999;13:225.
2. Freedman RS, Tortolero-Luna G, Pandey DK, et al. Gestational trophoblastic disease. Obstet Gynecol Clin N Am 1996;23:545.
3. Grimes DA. Epidemiology of gestational trophoblastic disease. Am J Obstet Gynecol 1984;150:309.
4. Di Cinto E, Parazzini F, Rosa C, Chatenoud L, Benzi G. The epidemiology of gestational trophoblastic disease. Gen Diagn Pathol 1997;143:103.
5. Bracken MB. Incidence and aetiology of hydatidiform mole: an epidemiological review. Br J Obstet Gynaecol 1987;94:1123.
6. Berkowitz RS, Daniel W, Cramer MD, et al. Risk factors for complete molar pregnancy from a case control study. Am J Obstet Gynecol 1985;152:1016.
7. Paradinas FJ, Browne P, Risher RA, Foskett M, Bagshawe KD, Newlands E. A clinical, histopathological and flow cytometric study of 149 complete moles, 146 partial moles and 107 non-molar hydropic abortions. Histopathology 1996;28:101.
8. Morrow CP, Curtin JP. Tumors of the placental trophoblast. In: Morrow CP, Curtin JP, eds. Synopsis of gynecologic oncology, 5th ed. New York: Churchill Livingstone, 1998:315.
9. Curry SL, Hammond CB, Tyrey L, Creasman WT, Parker RT. Hydatidiform mole: diagnosis, management, and long-term follow-up of 347 patients. Obstet Gynecol 1975; 45:1.
10. Goldstein DP, Berkowitz RS. Current management of complete and partial molar pregnancy. J Reprod Med 1994;39:139.
11. Montz FJ, Schlaerth JB, Morrow CP. The natural history of theca-lutein cysts. Obstet Gynecol 1988;72:247.
12. Schlaerth JB, Morrow CP, Montz FJ, d'Ablaing G. Initial management of hydatidiform mole. Am J Obstet Gynecol 1988;158:1299.
13. Kim DS, Moon H, Kim KT, Moon YJ, Hwang YY. Effects of prophylactic chemotherapy for persistent trophoblastic disease in patients with complete hydatidiform mole. Obstet Gynecol 1986;67:690.
14. Tidy JA, Rustin GJS, Newlands ES, et al. Presentation and management of choriocarcinoma after nonmolar pregnancy. Br J Obstet Gynaecol 1995;102:715.

15. Dinh TA, Chiang S, Hannigan E, et al. Lower genital tract metastasis of placental site trophoblastic tumor: case report and review of the literature. J Lower Genital Tract Dis 2000;4:166.

16. How J, Scurry J, Grant P, et al. Placental site trophoblastic tumor: report of three cases and review of the literature. Int J Gynecol Cancer 1995;5:241.

17. Finkler NJ, Berkowitz RS, Driscoll SG, Goldstein DP, Bernstein MR. Clinical experience with placental site trophoblastic tumors at the New England Trophoblastic Disease Center. Obstet Gynecol 1988; 71:854.

18. Yuen BH, Cannon W. Molar pregnancy in British Columbia: estimated incidence and postevacuation regression patterns of the beta subunit of human chorionic gonadotropin. Am J Obstet Gynecol 1981;139:316.

19. Lurain JR, Brewer JI, Torok EE, Halpern B. Natural history of hydatidiform mole after primary evacuation. Am J Obstet Gynecol 1983;145:591.

20. Bagshaw KD, Dent J, Webb J. Hydatiform mole in England and Wales 1973-1983. Lancet 1986;ii:673.

21. Hatch KD, Shingleton HM, Austin JM, et al. Southern regional trophoblastic disease center. South Med J 1978; 71:1334.

22. Morrow CP, Kletzky OA, DiSaia PJ, et al. Clinical and laboratory correlates of molar pregnancy and trophoblastic disease. Am J Obstet Gynecol 1977;129:424.

23. Kohorn EI. Hydatiform mole and gestational trophoblastic disease in southern Connecticut. Obstet Gynecol 1982; 59:78.

24. Berkowitz RS, Cramer DW, Bernstein MR, Cassells S, Driscoll SG, Goldstein DP. Risk factors for complete molar pregnancy from a case-control study. Am J Obstet Gynecol 1985;152:1016.

25. Curry SL, Schlaerth JB, Kohorn EI, et al. Hormonal contraception and trophoblastic sequaelae after hydatidiform mole (A Gynecologic Oncology Group study). Am J Obstet Gynecol 1989;160:805.

26. World Health Organisation. Gestational trophoblastic disease. Technical report series 692. Geneva, WHO, 1983.

27. Kohorn EI. Evaluation of the criteria used to make the diagnosis of nonmetastatic gestational trophoblastic neoplasia. Gyn Oncol 1993;48:139.

28. Schlaerth JB, Morrow CP, Rodriguez M. Diagnostic and therapeutic curettage in gestational trophoblastic disease. Am J Obstet Gynecol 1990;162:1465.

29. Kohorn EI. The trophoblastic Tower of Babel: classification systems for metastatic gestational trophoblastic neoplasia. Gynecol Oncol 1995;56:280.

30. Bagshawe KD. Risk and prognostic factors in trophoblastic neoplasia. Cancer 1976;38:1373.

31. Soper JT, Evans AC, Conaway MR, Clarke-Pearson DL, Berchuck A, Hammond CB. Evaluation of prognostic factors and staging in gestational trophoblastic tumor. Obstet Gynecol 1994;84:969.

32. Lurain JR, Casanova LA, Miller DS, Rademaker AW. Prognostic factors in gestational trophoblastic tumors: a proposed new scoring system based on multivariate analysis. Am J Obstet Gynecol 1991;164:611.

33. Gordon AN, Gershenson DM, Copeland LJ, Stringer CA, Morris M, Wharton JT. High-risk metastatic gestational trophoblastic disease: further stratification into two clinical entities. Gynecol Oncol 1989;34:5.

34. Dubuc-Lissoir J, Sweizig S, Schlaerth JB, Morrow CP. Metastatic gestational trophoblastic disease: a comparison of prognostic classification systems. Gynecol Oncol 1991; 45:40.

35. Kohorn EI, Goldstein DP, Hancock BW, et al. Combining the staging system of the International Federation of Gynecology and Obstetrics with the scoring system of the World Health Organization of trophoblastic neoplasia. Intl J Gynecol Cancer 2000;10:84.

36. Ngan HYS, Chan FL, Au VWK, Cheng DKL, Ng TY, Wong LC. Clinical outcome of micrometastasis in the lung in stage IA persistent gestational trophoblastic disease. Gynecol Oncol 1998;70:192.

37. Mutch DG, Soper TJ, Baker ME. Role of computed axial tomography of the chest in staging patients with nonmetastatic trophoblastic disease. Obstet Gynecol 1986; 68:348.

38. Hunter V, Raymond E, Christensen C, Olt G, Soper J, Hammond C. Efficacy of the metastatic screening in the staging of gestational trophoblastic disease. Cancer 1991; 65:1647.

39. Preidler KW, Luschin G, Tamussino K, Szolar DM, Stiskal M, Ebner F. Magnetic resonance imaging in patients with gestational trophoblastic disease. Invest Radiol 1996;31:492.

40. Homesley HD, Blessing JA, Schlaerth J, Rettenmaier M, Major FJ. Rapid escalation of weekly intramuscular methotrexate for nonmetastatic gestational trophoblastic disease: a Gynecologic Oncology Group study. Gynecol Oncol 1990;39:305.

41. Berkowitz RS, Goldstein DP, Bernstein MR. Ten years' experience with methotrexate and folinic acid as primary therapy for gestational trophoblastic disease. Gynecol Oncol 1986;23:111.

42. Bagshawe KD, Dent J, Newlands ES, Begent RHJ, Rustin GJS. The role of low–dose methotrexate and folinic acid in gestational trophoblastic tumours (GTT). Br J Obstet Gynaecol 1989;96:795.

43. Kohorn EI. Single-agent chemotherapy for nonmetastatic gestational trophoblastic neoplasia: perspectives for the 21st century after three decades of use. J Reprod Med 1991;36:49.

44. Lurain JR. Management of high-risk gestational trophoblastic disease. J Reprod Med 1998;43:44.

45. Lurain JR, Brewer JI, Mazur MT, Torok EE. Fatal gestational trophoblastic disease, an analysis of treatment failure. Am J Obstet Gynecol 1982;144:391.

46. Gordon AN, Gershenson DM, Copeland LJ, et al. High risk metastatic gestational trophoblastic disease. Obstet Gynecol 1985;65:550.

47. Bagshawe KD. Treatment of high-risk choriocarcinoma. J Reprod Med 1984;29:813.

48. Schink JC, Singh DK, Rademaker AW, Miller DS, Lurain JR. Etoposide, methotrexate, actinomycin D, cyclophosphamide, and vincristine for the treatment of metastatic, high-risk gestational trophoblastic disease. Obstet Gynecol 1992;80:817.

49. Newlands ES, Mulholland PJ, Holden L, Seckl MJ, Rustin GJS. Etoposide and cisplatin/etoposide, methotrexate, and actinomycin D (EMA) chemotherapy for patients with high risk gestational trophoblastic tumors refractory to EMA/cyclophosphamide and vincristine

chemotherapy and patients presenting with metatstatic placental site trophoblastic tumors. J Clin Oncol 2000; 18:854.

50. Yordan, EL, Jr., Schlaerth J, Gaddis O, Morrow CP. Radiation therapy in the management of gestational choriocarcinoma metastatic to the central nervous system. Obstet Gynecol 1987;69:627.

51. Evans AC, Soper JT, Clarke-Pearson DL, Berchuck A, Rodriguez GC, Hammond CB. Gestational trophoblastic disease metastatic to the central nervous system. Gynecol Oncol 1995;59:226.

52. Crawford RAF, Newlands E, Rustin GJS, Holden L, Hern RA, Bagshawe KD. Gestational trophoblastic disease with liver metastases: the Charing Cross experience. Brit J Obstet Gynaecol 1997;104:105.

53. Lehman E, Gershenson DM, Burke TW, Levenback C, Silva EG, Morris M. Salvage surgery for chemoefractory gestational trophoblastic disease. J Clin Oncol 1994; 12:2737.

54. Song H, Wu P, Wu P, Wang Y, Yang X, Dong S. Pregnancy outcomes after successful chemotherapy for choriocarcinoma and invasive mole: long term follow up. Am J Obstet Gynecol 1988;158:538.

55. Berkowitz RS, Goldstein DP, Bernstein MR. Reproductive experience after complete and partial molar pregnancy and gestational trophoblastic tumors. J Reprod Med 1991;36:3.

56. Rustin GJS, Newlands ES, Lutz J-M, et al. Combination but no single-agent methotrexate chemotherapy for gestational trophoblastic tumors increases the incidence of second tumors. J Clin Oncol 1996;14:2769.

57. Kim JH, Park DC, Bae SN, et al. Subsequent reproductive experience after treatment for gestational trophoblastic disease. Gynecol Oncol 1998;71:108.

58. Woolas RP, Bower M, Newlands ES, Secki M, Short D, Holden L. Influence of chemotherapy for gestational trophoblastic disease on subsequent pregnancy outcome. Br J Obstet Gynaecol 1998;104:1032.

59. Petrilli E, Twiggs LB, Blessing JA, Teng NNH, Curry S. Single-dose Actinomycin-D treatment for nonmetastatic gestational trophoblastic disease. Cancer 1987;60:2173.

60. Soper JT, Clarke-Pearson DL, Berchuk A, et al. 5-day methotrexate for women with metastatic gestational trophoblastic disease. Gynecol Oncol 1994;54:76.

Chapter 68

Metastatic Tumor Spread to the Pelvis

Brigitte E. Miller

Five Key Points

- In the United States, endometrium, colon, breast, and stomach are the most frequent primary sites for ovarian metastasis.

- The ovary is the most frequent site of metastasis to the pelvis, followed by the vagina.

- If bilateral ovarian tumors are noted at the time of laparotomy, this is due to metastatic disease in about 20% of the cases.

- Preoperative evaluation should include a detailed medical history with close attention to symptoms regarding all organ systems, screening exams, and a complete general physical examination, including lymph node survey and breast exam, as well as a complete pelvic exam including Pap smear and hemoccult test.

- At the time of surgery, careful abdominal exploration should be done. In case of most gynecological primaries, peritoneal primaries, and colon primaries without liver metastasis, tumor reductive surgery should be done. Metastatic deposits from other primaries, as well as those with extensive peritoneal disease and liver metastasis should be treated palliatively only.

Metastatic tumor spread to the pelvis is not uncommon. Relative frequencies reported vary significantly depending on patient selection or the time of evaluation, such as presence at initial diagnosis versus autopsy studies, the type of lesions included (microscopic versus clinically apparent), and due to differing prevalence rates of various malignancies, the country where the report was generated. The most frequent pelvic metastatic sites are the ovaries (76%) followed by vaginal lesions (13%).[1] This is true for genital or extragenital primaries. Metastases to the pelvic lymphatic system can occur and may present as a separate lesion. Uterine or vulvar metastases are rare. Of all metastases to pelvic structures, 75% originate from extrapelvic tumors.[1] In addition, 60% of pelvic metastases are diagnosed during surgery for the primary lesion. The majority of the remaining cases are detected within 3 years of the initial diagnosis.[2]

Sometimes, however, the primary tumor is small and an ovarian metastasis is detected first.[3] The probability that a malignant ovarian tumor detected at the time of laparotomy is metastatic has been reported between 5 and 28%.[4,5] In the United States, the most frequent primary sites are the endometrium, colon, breast, and stomach. Overall, patients with ovarian metastases tend to be younger than patients with primary ovarian tumors[2] and also younger than patients with other metastatic tumors not involving the ovary.[6] The increased blood supply to the premenopausal ovary may account for this difference. In 75% of cases, the ovarian metastases are bilateral, and frequently metastatic deposits are found in other sites as well. Conversely, 15 to 20% of all malignant bilateral ovarian tumors are metastatic. Sometimes, metastatic involvement of the ovary causes stromal-cell luteinization, estrogen and progesterone production, and elevated testosterone levels due to peripheral conversion.[7] This can lead to menstrual irregularities, postmenopausal bleeding, or signs of virilization.

Metastatic deposits can reach the pelvis by several routes.[2] Direct extension or embolic metastasis can occur at the pelvic wall from genitourinary or colon tumors. Lymphatic spread from pelvic tumors is frequent, but blockage of the lymphatics and retrograde spread is also possible from extrapelvic malignancies such as breast cancer. Hematogenous metastasis is another route, usually as a sign of advanced disease and seen mainly in the ovary. Migration of tumor cells from the endometrium or endocervix through the fallopian tubes is another way of dissemination to the ovaries and peritoneum. Surface spread of malignant cells throughout the peritoneal cavity likewise can lead to metastatic implants on the pelvic peritoneum and pelvic organs.

In this chapter, an overview will be given about metastatic lesions to the pelvis, mainly the ovary. This will be followed by recommendations for workup and surgical therapy.

PRIMARY TUMORS LEADING TO PELVIC METASTASIS

Gynecological Tumors

Details regarding diagnosis and treatment of metastatic gynecologic tumors are to be found in the chapters dealing with the primary lesions. Lymph-node metastasis to the pelvic wall from vulvar, vaginal, or cervical primaries may present as a pelvic mass at the time of initial diagnosis or as the first sign of recurrent disease. Overall, the ovary is the organ most frequently involved with metastatic disease, mainly from endometrial adenocarcinoma. Adenocarcinomas of the endometrium account for approximately one-third of metastatic ovarian tumors.[8] However, it is sometimes difficult to distinguish ovarian involvement from a metastatic process or from a separate primary due to a so-called field effect. This has significant clinical implications. The prognosis for double primary tumors is much better than for metastatic disease.[9] Even in early disease, it may be difficult to make the distinction on clinical grounds.[10] Metastatic disease from the uterus is often multinodular, solid, and bilateral. In addition, there is no evidence of a premalignant lesion within the ovary and often other areas of metastasis are seen. Endometrioid tumors are seen, but more frequently the tumors giving rise to ovarian metastasis are undifferentiated lesions, adenosquamous, or papillary serous lesions. The tumor grade of the metastasis is not necessarily the same as that of the uterine primary. The uterine tumor usually is larger, deeply invasive, and involves the lymphovascular system. Flow cytometry and techniques of molecular biology may be used to establish clonality; however, the clinical value of these more complicated and expensive investigations has not been proven.[11] In the presence of advanced disease, the differential diagnosis is impossible to make and not clinically relevant.

Metastasis from a fallopian-tube carcinoma may also occur. Most often, it is impossible to establish the differential diagnosis from a primary ovarian tumor spreading to the tube; again, this distinction is not clinically relevant.

Metastasis to the ovary from cervical cancer is rare. A multicenter study by the Gynecologic Oncology Group, which evaluated almost 1000 patients with Stage IB cervical carcinomas treated with radical hysterectomy, showed the rate of ovarian spread to be 0.5% for squamous cell carcinoma and 1.7% for adenocarcinoma.[12] Tabata et al.[13] reported a 12% incidence of metastatic adenocarcinoma, but 56% of this study group consisted of patients with Stage II and III disease. Ovarian metastases occurred mostly in large-volume tumors exhibiting extensive lymphovascular space invasion or uterine fundal involvement, but were not related to nodal metastasis. Recurrent cervical cancer in the ovary is very rare and only case reports are available.

Historically, metastatic gestational trophoblastic disease involved the ovaries in 6 to 22% of cases. With improved technology and earlier diagnosis and treatment, ovarian metastases occur much less frequently.

Endometriotic lesions of the ovary undergo malignant transformation in less than 1% of cases. Endometrioid carcinomas predominate, but sarcomas and other rare cell types are also seen. Endometriomas larger than 10 cm or those growing rapidly and containing solid cystic or papillary areas should be submitted for intraoperative histologic analysis. Although the prognosis is quite good for lesions confined to the ovary (65% survival), it is poor for disseminated extragonadal lesions (10% survival).[14]

Gastrointestinal Tumors

Colon

Since the relative incidence of gastric carcinoma is decreasing, metastatic spread to the ovary from a colorectal carcinoma is now more common. In fact, colon cancer occasionally masquerades as a primary ovarian tumor because the metastasis often is much larger than the primary gastrointestinal (GI) tumor[15] (Figure 68-1).

Ovarian metastasis is seen in up to 7.4% of colon cancers at the time of initial laparotomy. Most ovarian metastases, however, are diagnosed during the first 3 years of posttreatment follow-up. About half of the patients have diffuse intraperitoneal spread at that time. Again, endocrine manifestations due to stromal luteinization may occur.

Most of the colorectal metastases, about 70%, are bilateral and quite large. The tumors are mostly lobulated, multinodular, or solid with minimal cystic areas. Often, there is also extensive necrosis.[16] In contrast, primary mucinous ovarian carcinomas are bilateral in only 20% of cases and metastases are mainly peritoneal. Cystic components are prominent, and necrosis is only mild to moderate. Histologically, metastatic colon cancer usually demonstrates a moderately differentiated adenocarcinoma with significant mucin production. Occasionally, the epithelium looks similar to an endometrioid or undifferentiated carcinoma. The stroma may show focal luteinization, edema, or even myxoid change. Extensive lymphatic involvement is seen at the ovarian hilus. Metastatic colon cancer stains negative for cytokeratin 7. A primary ovarian mucinous cancer, however, often has a fibrous capsule, is cytokeratin 7–positive, and demonstrates epithelial transitions. Stromal luteinization is uncommon. Carcinoembryonic antigen (CEA) is not a good marker to distinguish between the two. Although CEA is always positive in colonic carcinomas, it is also positive in approximately 37% of primary ovarian carcinomas.[17]

In women with a history of colon cancer who present with a pelvic mass, metastatic colon cancer is identified in 57% of cases, a benign ovarian tumor in 26%, and primary ovarian cancer in 17%. If a uterine malignancy is seen in these patients, a primary adenocarcinoma of the endometrium is seen in most cases (73%), but in 20%, metastatic colon cancer causes the intrauterine mass and gynecologic symptoms.[18]

Stomach

Krukenberg tumor is the best-described metastatic tumor to the ovary. It originates mainly from the stomach, although tumors of similar appearance can metastasize from the colon and rarely from the breast. As gastric carcinoma is more frequent in patients of Oriental origin, so are Kruckenberg tumors. On average, patients with Krukenberg tumor are quite young, about 45 years old. In up to 90%, the presentation is similar to patients with ovarian cancer, including abdominal pain, swelling, and ascites. Often, the ovarian masses are quite large. The primary carcinoma, mostly a diffuse-type gastric carcinoma, may be very small and difficult to detect, even at the time of laparotomy.[19] Peritoneal involvement is usually minimal. Krukenberg tumors are bilateral in over 80% of cases, with nodular, lobulated ovarian enlargement and an intact capsule. Cystic degeneration is common in larger lesions. Microscopic examination reveals the characteristic mixture of pleomorphic signet-ring cells and spindled stromal cells. The signet-ring cells are identical to those seen in gastric carcinomas. Immunohistochemical stains for epithelial markers are usually positive. Sometimes, the stroma can show significant collagenization, edema, or changes similar to a fibroma. As with many metastatic lesions, extensive lymphatic involvement of the hilus is frequent.

Carcinoid Tumors

These tumors account for only 2% of metastatic ovarian tumors, but may be difficult to distinguish from primary lesions. Most patients present with a pelvic or abdominal mass. The carcinoid syndrome is present in only about 40% of the cases. Frequently, the

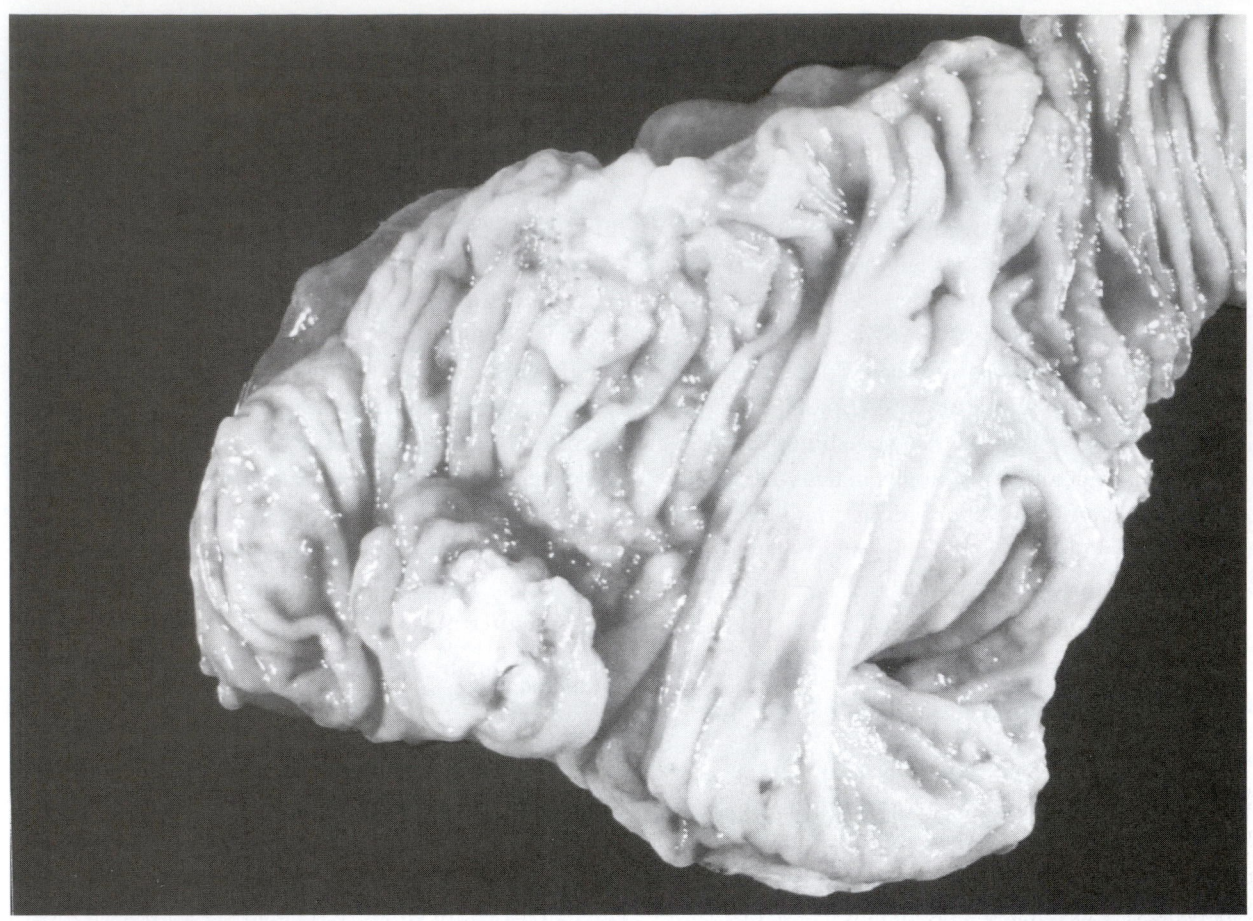

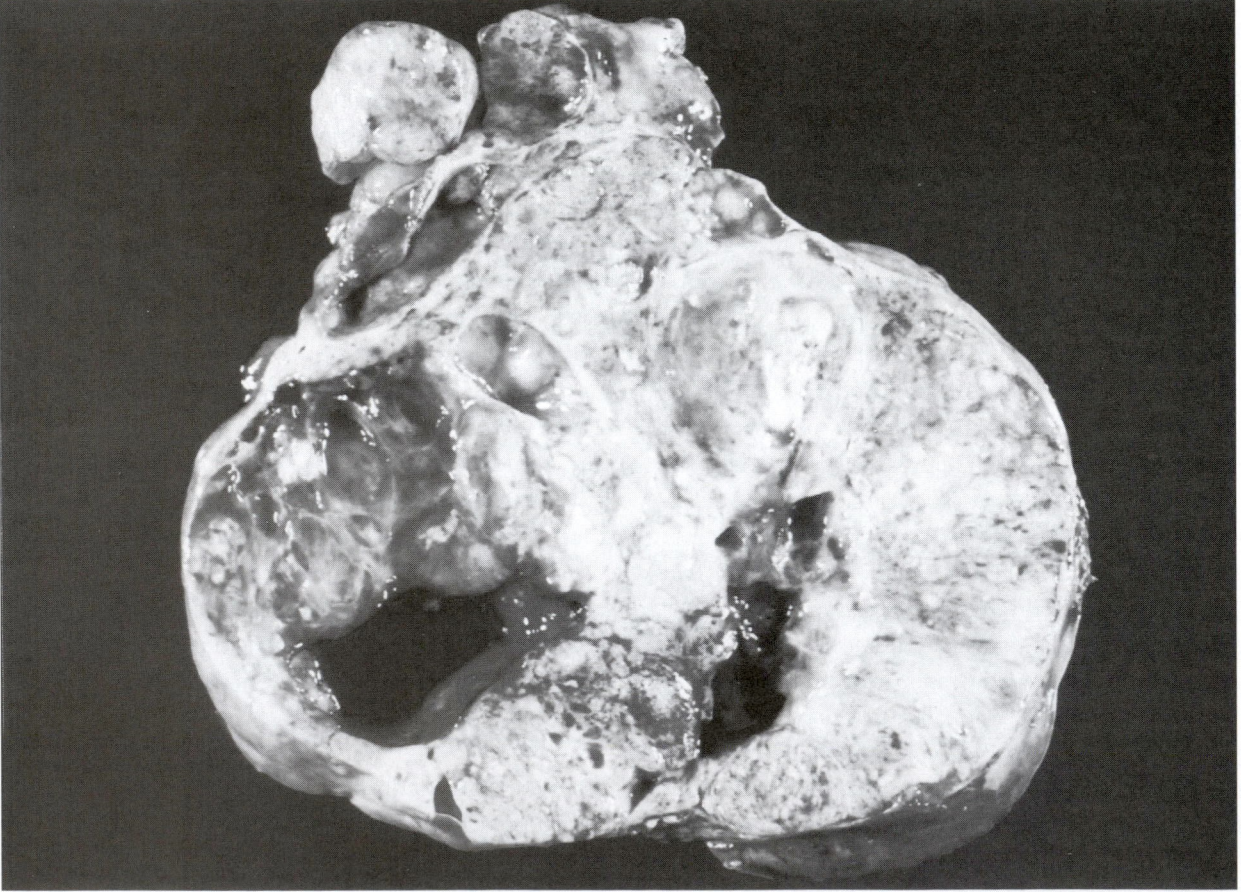

Figure 68-1 Large ovarian metastasis from a small adenocarcinoma in the cecum.

primary tumor is located in the ileum. However, it can be found in any other areas of the gastrointestinal tract.[16]

At the time of surgery, usually both ovaries are involved. Peritoneal and omental metastases are often present. The external surfaces of the metastatic ovarian tumors are smooth and lobulated. Histologically, all typical patterns of carcinoid tumors can be present, but the insular subtype is seen most frequently. On the other hand, primary ovarian carcinoids are almost always unilateral, lack extraovarian spread, and often demonstrate teratomatous elements on microscopic evaluation. The prognosis for patients with metastatic carcinoids is poor, with only one-third surviving for over 4 years.

Miscellaneous

All types of appendiceal tumors can cause pelvic metastases, mainly to the ovary. In patients with a low-grade mucinous adenocarcinoma of the appendix, there is a high incidence of pseudomyxoma peritonei, more frequent than after mucinous primary ovarian tumors.

Metastasis to the ovary from other organs of the GI tract such as the small bowel, pancreas, gallbladder, bile duct, and liver have been described in a few cases. Most often this occurs in the presence of widespread metastatic disease.

Peritoneal Tumors

Peritoneal carcinomatosis can lead to clinical symptoms very similar to ovarian cancer, as growth characteristics and tumor spread are similar. Commonly there is ascites, an omental mass, and often tumor deposits in the cul-de-sac. Initially tumor covers the outside of the ovary, but as the disease progresses, an ovarian mass may develop. These tumors may be due to widespread metastatic gastrointestinal malignancies or breast or lung cancer. Occasionally, a papillary serous carcinoma of the endometrium will present like this, without a history of uterine bleeding.

In addition, there is the serous surface papillary carcinoma or primary peritoneal serous carcinoma (PPSC), arising from müllerian remnants in the peritoneum. Clinical presentation and even histologic evaluation is very similar to serous ovarian tumors. The long-term survival, however, seems to be slightly higher in patients with PPSC.[20] Surgical findings include multiple small peritoneal tumor implants, which

in advanced disease can produce large masses. Initially, only the outside of the ovary is involved, while the omentum is usually diffusely infiltrated. Histologically, the tissue resembles papillary serous tumors of müllerian origin with psammoma bodies.

Malignant mesothelioma, another rare tumor, presents similarly. Asbestos exposure increases the risk significantly.[21] Histologically, these lesions are characterized by a biphasic pattern, with demonstration of both epithelial and sarcomatoid foci. Nonetheless, pathologic diagnosis may be difficult in these cases.

Tumors of the Urinary System

Metastases from a renal clear-cell adenocarcinoma to the ovaries are reported in less than 1% of autopsy cases. They may present many years after initial diagnosis and treatment. These lesions may be difficult to distinguish from a primary ovarian clear-cell adenocarcinoma. However, in most instances, metastatic lesions are bilateral and associated with other areas of metastatic spread. Microscopically, the typical hobnail cell of the ovarian clear-cell adenocarcinoma is often absent and the tumor reveals a striking sinusoidal vascular pattern instead.[22]

Very rarely, tumors from other areas of the urinary tract, such as transitional carcinomas of the renal pelvis, Wilms tumors, or bladder tumors can present with a pelvic mass due to extensive adenopathy. Over 90% are transitional cell tumors, and metastasis to the ovary has rarely been described.[23] However, nodal metastases to the pelvic wall are common.

Disseminated Systemic Disease

Breast Cancer

Breast cancer spreads to the ovaries, with adnexal involvement reported in up to 29% of patients with metastatic disease.[24] Up to 38% of all secondary ovarian tumors are from the breast.[25] Ovarian metastases rarely cause significant symptoms and are seldom diagnosed before the primary tumor. Recurrent breast cancer in the ovary has been reported as late as 16 years after initial diagnosis and treatment.[24] From reports describing therapeutic oophorectomy for metastatic breast cancer, tumor involvement was seen in 20 to 50%. When the ovaries are removed prophylactically, metastatic disease is noted less often (2 to 11%).[26] Metastatic breast cancer is seen bilaterally 75% of the time and is only microscopically apparent in two-thirds of the cases. Involved ovaries form solid tumors rarely larger than 5 cm with a white, nodular surface.[26] Microscopic examination shows that these multiple small nodules are often confluent. Although all growth patterns of breast cancer can be seen, the "Indian file" or the lobular pattern is most common. Typically, follicular structures are involved and there is extensive lymphovascular space invasion. Luteinization, however, is rarely seen.

Lymphoma

Ovarian involvement has been found in up to 25% of patients dying from widespread, metastatic lymphoma. In 0.3% of cases, an ovarian mass is the initial presentation of the lymphoma. At surgery, both ovaries are involved in 55% of patients and other metastases are seen in 64%.[27] Most of these patients are young, below age 40. There are also a few case reports of malignant lymphoma arising in the ovary as a primary extranodal lymphoma.

The clinical presentation is similar to other ovarian tumors, often leading to a large abdominal mass, ascites, and abdominal pain. The most frequent metastatic lymphoma is a non-Hodgkin lymphoma of B-cell type, mainly Burkitt lymphoma. Survival rates for patients with lymphoma presenting in the ovaries are around 40%.[28] However, rapid onset and systemic manifestations are poor prognostic factors.[29] The ovaries may be quite large, with a nodular surface and pale gray-white tissue. Edema and necrosis may be present. The microscopic picture is characterized by a diffuse monotonous infiltrate of neoplastic lymphoid cells with superimposed nodularity. The characteristic histologic pictures of the different lymphomas may be present. Often, a large number of macrophages are seen. The final diagnosis usually has to be confirmed with immunohistochemical stains.

Leukemia

Ovarian involvement with leukemia may be more frequent than with a lymphoma. Leukemic lesions are most often seen in children and have been noted in up to 66% of autopsy studies. Although these metastases are usually not clinically apparent, an ovarian tumor can rarely be the initial sign of relapse. Most often, these are cases of myeloid leukemia. Occasionally, granulocytic sarcomas can occur in the cervix, uterus, and ovary. These are extramedullary tumorlike masses of leukemic cells. Clinically, the initial hematologic evaluation may be negative, but signs of leukemia are sure to develop later. Immediate bone marrow aspiration often reveals leukemia. Sometimes the tumor tissue has a greenish tinge, which led to the original name "chloroma."[30] On microscopic examination, round multinodular leukemic infiltrates are seen in the cervix or may surround and invade the follicular structures of the ovary, usually without destroying them. Cordlike formation and diffuse masses similar to ovarian lymphoma are seen. Again, a variety of immunohistochemical stains may be necessary to confirm the diagnosis.

Melanoma

Ovarian metastases have been found in 16% of women dying of malignant melanoma. In Australia, where there is a high incidence of melanoma, it may constitute up to 10% of surgically resected ovarian metastases.[31] It may present up to 25 years after the primary lesion. Fifty percent of the patients have other signs of metastatic disease at that time. Macroscopically, the tumor is most often bilateral and multinodular and necrosis and cystic degeneration are present. Half of these tumors lack the characteristic melanin and because the microscopic features are variable, the differential diagnosis may be difficult. Again, immunohistochemical evaluation is helpful, especially positive staining for S-100 protein.[32] The rare primary ovarian melanomas arise in teratomas. The differential diagnosis between metastatic and primary ovarian melanoma may be difficult.

Miscellaneous

Small-cell carcinoma arising in the lung has been reported to spread to the ovary in less than 5% of the cases. A variety of other tumors can also spread to the ovary,[32] including thyroid carcinoma, neuroblastoma, and extragenital sarcomas.[33]

PREOPERATIVE EVALUATION

Medical History

A careful medical history is of paramount importance to avoid surprises. As stated above, metastatic melanoma for example can occur as long as 25 years after the primary lesion. Metastatic breast cancer can also occur after a prolonged interval. Most other metastases occur within a 5-year period from the original diagnosis. Sixty percent of recurrent colon cancers develop during the first 2 years. In addition, the patient's risk status for other malignancies should also be assessed. It is also important to know that the patient is current regarding screening examinations such as mammography and evaluation of the colon.

Recent History

All patients should be carefully questioned regarding general symptoms such as weight loss, weakness, and night sweats. Next, GI function should be carefully evaluated. The signs of a gastric carcinoma can be very subtle and difficult to distinguish from GI involvement of an ovarian carcinoma. In fact, many patients with ovarian cancer initially undergo a GI evaluation, with negative results. However, if symptoms are present, an upper endoscopy should be performed prior to surgery. Similarly, in cases of rectal bleeding or changing bowel habits, an evaluation of the colon is mandatory. The patient should be questioned regarding urinary symptoms such as pain, hematuria, or recurrent infections. Finally, a complete gynecologic history has to be obtained.

Physical Examination

A complete breast examination with palpation of the axilla should be done. Next, a careful lymph-node survey, including the supraclavicular and inguinal areas, is necessary. The skin should be checked for lesions and the lungs evaluated. This is followed by a complete abdominal examination to detect ascites, large masses, omental caking, hepatomegaly, or signs of bowel obstruction.

A complete pelvic examination, including recto-vaginal palpation, should be done. Is the mass separable from the uterus? Is ovarian enlargement felt? A cecal or sigmoid mass can feel very similar to an ovarian mass. Is there nodularity in the cul-de-sac? Is the mass originating from the pelvic wall? Is the mass mobile? During this examination a Pap smear should be done. A complete rectal examination with Hemoccult test should follow.

Laboratory and Radiologic Studies

Sometimes granulocytosis can also be seen with necrotic pelvic tumors; however, these values rarely are above 30,000. Very rarely, a leukemia is diagnosed this way. Significant anemia should alert the physician to the presence of a GI lesion. High platelet counts

TABLE 68-1
SUGGESTIONS FOR PREOPERATIVE EVALUATION TO IMPROVE DETECTION OF METASTATIC PELVIC TUMORS

Careful medical history and review of systems
Risk factor assessment for all malignancies
Careful physical examination, especially breast examination and lymph-node survey
Screening tests as indicated
Evaluation of the GI tract if even minor symptoms present

are usually related to a large tumor volume. Lactate dehydrogenase (LDH) and alkaline phosphatase may be elevated, and high values call for further evaluation to rule out metastatic disease. Results of tumor marker studies rarely influence the initial therapy if surgical evaluation is planned. Determination of CEA, CA-125, and to a lesser degree CA-15-3 and CA-19-9 may be useful if metastatic disease is suspected.

A preoperative chest x-ray film revealing nodular pulmonary lesions should also heighten suspicion for metastatic disease, as this is a very rare occurrence initially in gynecologic tumors. Pleural effusions, however, are frequently caused by metastatic ovarian carcinoma. Nodal metastases are often seen on computed tomographic (CT) scan in the presence of advanced gynecologic tumors. However, if the nodal enlargement is extensive, especially in the absence of a significant pelvic lesion, it could be due to a lymphoma. With a CT-directed biopsy, it is often possible to establish the diagnosis preoperatively. No specific finding on CT[34] or magnetic resonance imaging (MRI)[35] can be used to definitively distinguish between primary tumor and metastatic lesion. Although a barium enema is not routinely recommended for all patients with a pelvic mass, radiologic evaluation or endoscopy is necessary for patients with GI-tract-related symptoms or a positive Hemoccult test.

Suggestions for preoperative evaluation to improve detection of metastatic pelvic tumors are given in Table 68-1.

EVALUATION DURING SURGERY

Bilateral ovarian tumors should always raise the suspicion of metastatic disease. The same is true if the frozen-section analysis reveals a rare histologic pattern. Bilateral mucinous or endometrioid tumors are especially likely to be metastatic. On the other hand,